CARDIOLOGY
AN ILLUSTRATED TEXT/REFERENCE

CARDIOLOGY
AN ILLUSTRATED TEXT/REFERENCE

VOLUME 1

PHYSIOLOGY, PHARMACOLOGY, DIAGNOSIS

EDITORS

KANU CHATTERJEE, MB, FRCP
*Professor of Medicine
University of California,
San Francisco
Associate Chief of Cardiology
Moffitt/Long Hospital
San Francisco, California*

JOEL KARLINER, MD
*Professor of Medicine
University of California,
San Francisco
Chief of Cardiology
Ft. Miley Veterans
Administration Hospital
San Francisco, California*

ELLIOT RAPAPORT, MD
*Professor of Medicine
University of California,
San Francisco
Chief of Cardiology
San Francisco General Hospital
San Francisco, California*

MELVIN D. CHEITLIN, MD
*Professor of Medicine
University of California,
San Francisco
Associate Chief of Cardiology
San Francisco General Hospital
San Francisco, California*

WILLIAM W. PARMLEY, MD
*Professor of Medicine
University of California,
San Francisco
Chief of Cardiology
Moffitt/Long Hospital
San Francisco, California*

MELVIN SCHEINMAN, MD
*Professor of Medicine
University of California,
San Francisco
Chief of Electrophysiology
Moffitt/Long Hospital
San Francisco, California*

**FOREWORD BY
RICHARD GORLIN, MD**
*Mt. Sinai Medical Center
New York, New York*

J.B. LIPPINCOTT COMPANY
Philadelphia

GOWER MEDICAL PUBLISHING
New York ■ London

LIBRARY OF CONGRESS CATALOGING-IN-PUBLICATION DATA
Cardiology: an illustrated text/reference / editors, Kanu Chatterjee,
   William W. Parmley; foreword by Richard Gorlin.
      p.   cm.
      Includes bibliographical references.
      Includes index.
      Contents: v. 1. Physiology, pharmacology & diagnosis—v.
   2. Cardiovascular disease.
      ISBN 0-397-44611-X
      1. Cardiology.   2. Cardiovascular system—Diseases.
   I. Chatterjee, Kanu.   II. Parmley, William W. (William Watts), 1936-
   .
      [DNLM: 1. Heart Diseases.   WG 200 C26553]
   RC667.C383   1991
   616. 1'2—dc20
   DNLM/DLC   91-6641
   for Library of Congress   CIP

BRITISH LIBRARY CATALOGING IN PUBLICATION DATA
Cardiology.
   Rev. ed.
   1. Stet.
   I. Chatterjee, Kanu, 1934–   II. Parmley, William W. *1936*
   –
   616.12

   ISBN 0-397-44611-X

DRUG DOSAGE The authors and publisher have exerted every effort to ensure that drug selection and dosage set forth in this text are in accordance with current recommendations and practice at the time of publication. However, in view of ongoing research, changes in government regulations, and the constant flow of information relating to drug therapy and drug reactions, the reader is urged to check the package insert for each drug for any change in indications and dosage and for added warnings and precautions. This is particularly important when the recommended agent is a new or infrequently used drug.

© **COPYRIGHT 1991 BY GOWER MEDICAL PUBLISHING,** 101 Fifth Avenue, New York, NY 10003. All rights reserved. No part of this publication may be reproduced, stored in a retrieval system, or transmitted in any form or by any means electronic, mechanical, photocopying, recording, or otherwise without prior written permission of the publisher.

DISTRIBUTED IN USA AND CANADA BY:
J.B. Lippincott Company
East Washington Square
Philadelphia, PA 19105 USA

DISTRIBUTED ELSEWHERE (EXCEPT JAPAN) BY:
Wolters Kluwer Ltd.
Middlesex House
34-42 Cleveland Street
London W1P 5FB UK

DISTRIBUTED IN JAPAN BY:
Nankodo Co., Ltd.
42-6, Hongo 3-Chome
Bunkyo-Ku
Tokyo 113 Japan

EDITORS:
William B. Millard
Leah Kennedy

ART DIRECTOR:
Jill Feltham

DESIGNER:
Kathryn Greenslade

ILLUSTRATION DIRECTOR:
Laura Pardi Duprey

ILLUSTRATORS:
Susan Tilberry (schematics)
Patricia Gast
Vantage Art, Inc. (charts)

COMPOSITOR:
Tapsco, Inc.

10 9 8 7 6 5 4 3 2 1

**PRINTED IN SINGAPORE
BY IMAGO PRODUCTIONS (FE) PTE, LTD.**

DEDICATION

This book is dedicated to our wives Docey and Shanna. Their love, support, and understanding have been immeasurable in helping us put together this textbook of Cardiology.

KANU CHATTERJEE ▪ WILLIAM W. PARMLEY

FOREWORD

A textbook must meet a variety of criteria. Its contents must be authoritative without being dogmatic, comprehensive without being exhaustive, readable without losing scientific rigor, and, along with all of these characteristics, be able to incorporate significant changes in its field. These are daunting criteria for any text but even more so in the biomedical sciences and in the practice of clinical medicine, where articles are often outdated before publication. So how does one approach the problem for a text covering the field of cardiology? Kanu Chatterjee and William Parmley, renowned and respected cardiologists, have set out to do this. They bring to this book their different but complementary backgrounds in basic and clinical science, and bedside skill and judgment. These authors have edited a book in two volumes, achieving cohesiveness by employing six section editors, including themselves, each with special expertise, while at the same time drawing on a wide variety of recognized authorities in the field. They have imaginatively dealt with the issue of maintaining currency in changing times by making available to the reader a single conventionally bound book, or a looseleaf edition in which approximately 60 percent of the material is changed over a four-year period. Thus, they have bridged the important difference between a text accurate to a certain point in time, with the timeliness of a journal format.

The authors clearly have the practicing physician in mind; they have deliberately used color photographs, diagrams, and appropriate variation of print style to make the book readable and specific subsections identifiable. The authors have encouraged the individual contributors to express their personal opinions, and not necessarily to dwell exhaustively on all hypotheses concerning a controversial topic.

As a consequence, Chatterjee and Parmley have produced an innovative textbook of cardiology. They have combined their physiological and clinical perspectives to oversee and meld the contributions of over 150 authors, producing a text that should be of immense practical value to the cardiologist.

RICHARD GORLIN, MD
Mt. Sinai Medical Center
New York

PREFACE

When we received our cardiology training in the sixties, therapeutic options were relatively limited. The most exciting aspects of cardiology were in the realm of diagnosis through careful history, physical examination, and cardiac catheterization. Valvular heart disease taught us much about hemodynamics and valve function, and the potential for therapeutic benefit through cardiac surgery. Therapy for coronary artery disease was extremely limited during that time before the advent of bypass surgery. As one steps back and reflects on what has happened in the ensuing quarter-century, it is apparent that dramatic changes have occurred in our abilities to diagnose and treat all forms of heart disease. In a parallel fashion, extraordinary developments in molecular cardiology promise to revolutionize further our understanding of the pathophysiology of heart disease and to provide new avenues of treatment.

Of considerable importance has been the rapid pace of new developments in cardiology, especially in the last decade. This rapid explosion of knowledge and technology first prompted us to consider writing a looseleaf Textbook of Cardiology so that yearly revisions and additions could keep the textbook as current as possible. Cardiology was subsequently published in 1988 by J.B. Lippincott Company, and annual revisions of about 15% have helped to keep it up to date. In 1989, we were approached by Gower Medical Publishing who invited us to publish a hardbound edition of Cardiology and at the same time dramatically change illustrations by redoing them in color. This new project was so appealing that we immediately agreed and began the process of putting together this edition of the book.

Several factors encouraged us to move ahead with this project. First, although the looseleaf edition was doing well, it was clear that many readers still prefer a hardbound textbook. Second, the redoing of all illustrations, including producing them in color, offered an attractive option of giving the book a new look and more uniform illustrative material. Third, as chapters were revised and illustrations colored, they would feed back into the looseleaf edition and thus eventually upgrade the looseleaf version into an all-color illustrated book. Fourth, by taking a "snapshot" of the looseleaf text every few years, one could automatically provide updated hardbound copies and thus provide a current textbook in either published form.

We hope the reader will enjoy this hardbound copy of Cardiology: An Illustrated Text/Reference as much as we enjoyed putting it together. We are pleased with the new look of the book and with the expertise and dedication of the Gower staff in bringing this book to press in such a short time frame. We accept responsibility for any errors or shortcomings it may have and pledge to make each edition as readable, up to date, and informative as possible.

KANU CHATTERJEE ▪ WILLIAM W. PARMLEY

CONTRIBUTORS

Walter H. Abelmann, MD
Professor of Medicine,
 Harvard Medical School
Physician, Beth Israel Hospital
Boston, MA

**M. Thomas Abraham, MD,
 Doct Med (Cardiology), MRCP**
Consultant Cardiologist,
 Chest Diseases Hospital
Safat, Kuwait

Jonathan Abrams, MD
Professor of Medicine
University of New Mexico
 School of Medicine
Albuquerque, NM

Philip C. Adams, MRCP
Research Fellow, British Heart
 Foundation and American Heart
 Association
The Mount Sinai Medical Center
New York, NY

V. Paul Addonizio, Jr., MD
Assistant Professor of Surgery
University of Pennsylvania
 School of Medicine
Philadelphia, PA

Masood Akhtar, MD
Professor of Medicine
University of Wisconsin Medical School,
 Milwaukee Clinical Campus
Association Chief, Cardiovascular
 Disease Section
Director, Arrhythmia Service and
 Clinical Electrophysiology
Mount Sinai Medical Center
Milwaukee, WI

Edwin L. Alderman, MD
Professor of Medicine (Cardiology)
Director, Cardiac Catheterization
 Laboratory
Stanford University School
 of Medicine
Palo Alto, CA

Joseph S. Alpert, MD
Professor of Medicine and Director,
 Division of Cardiovascular Medicine
University of Massachusetts Medical
 School
Worcester, MA

Kelley P. Anderson, MD
Associate Professor of Medicine,
 Cardiology Division
University of Utah Medical Center
Salt Lake City, UT

Lina Badimon, PhD
Associate Professor of Medicine
Division of Cardiology
Mount Sinai School of Medicine of
 The City University of New York
New York, NY

John C. Bailey, MD
Professor of Medicine
Indiana University School of
 Medicine
Senior Research Associate
Krannert Institute of Cardiology
Indianapolis, IN

Neal L. Benowitz, MD
Professor of Medicine
Chief, Division of Clinical Pharmacology
 and Experimental Therapeutics
University of California, San Francisco
San Francisco, CA

Thomas P. Bersot, MD, PhD
Scientist, Gladstone Foundation
 Laboratories for Cardiovascular
 Disease
Cardiovascular Research Institute
Assistant Professor of Medicine in
 Residence
University of California, San Francisco
San Francisco, CA

Anil K. Bhandari, MD
Assistant Professor of Medicine
Director, Electrophysiology and
 Arrhythmia Service
University of Southern California
 Medical Center
Los Angeles, CA

**Margaret E. Billingham, MB, BS,
 FRCPath**
Professor of Pathology
Stanford University Medical School
Palo Alto, CA

C. Gunnar Blomqvist, MD
Professor of Internal Medicine and
 Physiology
Division of Cardiology
University of Texas Southwestern
 Medical Center at Dallas
Director, ECG and Noninvasive
 Cardiovascular Laboratories
Parkland Memorial Hospital
Dallas, TX

Elias H. Botvinick, MD
Professor of Medicine (Cardiology),
 Radiology (Nuclear Medicine)
Co-Director, Adult Cardiac Noninvasive
 Laboratory
Associate Director of Cardiac
 Rehabilitation
University of California, San Francisco,
 School of Medicine
San Francisco, CA

J. David Bristow, MD
Professor of Medicine and Director,
 Cardiovascular Research and Training
Oregon Health Sciences University
Portland, OR

Bruce H. Brundage, MD
Professor of Medicine
Chief, Section of Cardiology,
 University of Illinois
Chicago, IL

L. Maximilian Buja, MD
Professor and Chairman
Department of Pathology and
 Laboratory Medicine
University of Texas Medical School
Dallas, TX

Michael Callaham, MD
Professor of Medicine
Director, Division of Emergency
 Medicine
H. C. Moffitt/J. M. Long Hospitals
University of California, San Francisco
San Francisco, CA

Blase A. Carabello, MD
Professor of Medicine
Medical University of South Carolina
Charleston, SC

Shlomo Charlap, MD
Assistant Professor of Medicine
Downstate Medical Center
Physician in Charge, Coronary Care Unit
Long Island College Hospital
Brooklyn, NY

Kanu Chatterjee, MB, FRCP
Professor of Medicine
University of California, San Francisco
Associate Chief of Cardiology
Moffitt/Long Hospital
San Francisco, CA

Melvin D. Cheitlin, MD
Professor of Medicine
University of California, San Francisco
Associate Chief of Cardiology
San Francisco General Hospital
San Francisco, CA

**George Cherian, MD, Doct Med
 (Cardiology), FRCP, FAMS**
Professor of Medicine (Cardiology)
Faculty of Medicine, Kuwait University
Consultant Cardiologist, Chest Diseases
 Hospital
Safat, Kuwait

James H. Chesebro, MD
Professor of Medicine, Division of
 Cardiology
Mayo Clinic and Mayo Medical School
Rochester, MN

Alvin J. Chin, MD
Associate Professor of Pediatrics
University of Pennsylvania School of
 Medicine
Director, Non-Invasive Laboratories
Children's Hospital of Philadelphia
Co-Director, Adult Congenital Heart
 Disease Program
Philadelphia, PA

Arnold M. Chonko, MD, FACP
Professor of Medicine
Division of Nephrology and Hypertension
Director of Renal Dialysis, University of
 Kansas School of Medicine
Kansas City, KS

Kyung J. Chung, MD
Division of Pediatric Cardiology
University of California, San Diego,
 Medical Center
San Diego, CA

James L. Cox, MD
Evarts A. Graham Professor of Surgery
Chief, Division of Cardiothoracic
 Surgery
Washington University School of
 Medicine
Cardiothoracic Surgeon-in-Chief, Barnes
 Hospital
St. Louis, MO

Michael D. Cressman, DO
Department of Heart and Hypertension
Research Institute and Department of
 Hypertension and Nephrology
Division of Medicine, The Cleveland
 Clinic Foundation
Cleveland, OH

John Michael Criley, MD, FACC
Professor of Medicine and Radiological
 Sciences
University of California, Los Angeles,
 School of Medicine
Medical Director, St. John's Heart
 Institute
Santa Monica, CA

Michael Dae, MA
Associate Professor of Medicine
 (Cardiology) and Radiology (Nuclear
 Medicine)
Director of Cardiac Rehabilitation
Associate Director, Adult Cardiac Non-
 Invasive Laboratory
University of California, San Francisco,
 School of Medicine
San Francisco, CA

James E. Dalen, MD
Vice Provost for Medical Affairs
Dean, College of Medicine
Professor, Internal Medicine
University of Arizona
Tucson, AZ

Peter Danilo, MPhil, PhD
Department of Pharmacology
College of Physicians and Surgeons of
 Columbia University
New York, NY

Louis J. Dell'Italia, MD
Department of Medicine/Cardiology
University of Alabama at Birmingham
Birmingham, AL

J. Stephen Dummer, MD
Associate Professor of Medicine &
 Surgery
Division of Infectious Diseases
Vanderbilt University School of Medicine
Nashville, TN

L. Henry Edmunds, Jr., MD
Professor of Surgery and Chief, Division
 of Cardiothoracic Surgery
University of Pennsylvania School of
 Medicine
Philadelphia, PA

Neal Eigler, MD
Assistant Professor of Medicine
University of California, Los Angeles
Co-Director, Cardiac Catheterization
 Laboratory
Cedars-Sinai Medical Center
Los Angeles, CA

Robert S. Eliot, MD, FACC
Director, Stress Medicine Ltd.
Denver, CO

Myrvin H. Ellestad, MD, FACC
Clinical Professor of Medicine
University of California at Irvine,
 California College of Medicine
Chief, Division of Cardiology
Memorial Medical Center of Long Beach
Long Beach, CA

Avery K. Ellis, MD, PhD
Assistant Professor of Medicine
State University of New York at Buffalo
Medical Director, Memorial Heart
 Institute
Assistant Physician, Erie County
 Medical Center
Buffalo, NY

VII

Mary Allen Engle, MD, DSc
Stavros S. Niarchos Professor of Pediatric Cardiology
Professor of Pediatrics and Director of Pediatric Cardiology
The New York Hospital-Cornell University Medical Center
New York, NY

Gordon A. Ewy, MD
Professor of Medicine
Chief, Section of Cardiology and Associate Head, Department of Internal Medicine
University of Arizona College of Medicine
Director of Cardiology, University Medical Center
Tucson, AZ

T. Bruce Ferguson, Jr., MD
Assistant Professor of Surgery
Division of Cardiothoracic Surgery
Washington University School of Medicine
St. Louis, MO

Walter E. Finkbeiner, MD, PhD
Associate Professor, Department of Pathology
University of California, San Francisco
San Francisco, CA

Fabrice Fontaliran, MD
Staff Member, Pathologist
Hospital Jean Rostand
39 rue Jean Le Galleau
94200 Ivry - France

James S. Forrester, MD
Professor of Medicine, University of California, Los Angeles
George Burns and Gracie Allen Professor of Cardiovascular Research
Director, Division of Cardiology
Cedars-Sinai Medical Center
Los Angeles, CA

Fetnat M. Fouad-Tarazi, MD, FACC
Head of Cardiac Function Laboratory
Department of Heart and Hypertension, Research Institute
The Cleveland Clinic Foundation
Cleveland, OH

Guy Fontaine, MD, FACC
International Consultant
Director of Clinical Electrophysiology and Pacemaker Department
Hospital Jean Rostand
39 rue Jean Le Galleau
94200 Ivry - France

Robert Frank, MD
Associate Professor of Medicine
Hospital Jean Rostand
39 rue Jean Le Galleau
94200 Ivry - France

Michael Franz, MD
Assistant Professor of Cardiology
Stanford University Medical Center
Cardiology Division
Palo Alto, CA

Roger A. Freedman, MD
Assistant Professor of Medicine, Cardiology Division
University of Utah Medical Center,
Salt Lake City, UT

William F. Friedman, MD
J. H. Nicholson Professor of Pediatric Cardiology
Chairman, Department of Pediatrics
UCLA School of Medicine, UCLA Medical Center
Los Angeles, CA

William H. Frishman, MD
Director of Medicine
Hospital of the Albert Einstein College of Medicine
Montefiore Medical Center
Bronx, NY

Victor F. Froelicher, MD
Chief, Cardiology Section, Long Beach VA Medical Center
Professor of Medicine and Assistant Chief of Cardiology
University of California, Irvine
Irvine, CA

Edward D. Frohlich, MD
Vice President for Academic Affairs
Alton Ochsner Medical Foundation
Section of Hypertensive Diseases, Ochsner Clinic
New Orleans, LA

Valentin Fustler, MD
Arthur A. and Hilda M. Master Professor of Medicine
Chief, Division of Cardiology
Mount Sinai School of Medicine of the City University of New York
New York, NY

Hasan Garan, PhD
Associate Professor in Medicine, Harvard Medical School
Associate Physician, Massachusetts General Hospital
Boston, MA

Derek G. Gibson, MB, FRCP
Consultant Cardiologist, Brompton Hospital
Senior Lecturer, Cardiothoracic Institute, University of London
London, England

Ray W. Gifford, Jr., MD
Senior Vice Chairman, Division of Medicine
The Cleveland Clinic Foundation
Cleveland, OH

Emilio R. Giuliani, MD
Professor of Medicine
Mayo Medical School
Consultant in Cardiology, Mayo Clinic
Rochester, MN

Lee Goldman, MD
Professor of Medicine
Vice-Chairman of Department of Medicine
Harvard Medical School
Assistant Physician-in-Chief, Brigham and Women's Hospital
Boston, MA

Nora Goldschlager, MD
Professor of Clinical Medicine
University of California, San Francisco, School of Medicine
Director, Coronary Care Unit
San Francisco General Hospital
San Francisco, CA

J. Anthony Gomes, MD
Professor of Medicine
Director of Electrocardiography and Electrophysiology
Division of Cardiography, Department of Medicine
Mount Sinai School of Medicine of the City University of New York
New York, NY

Jared J. Grantham, MD, FACP
Professor of Medicine
Director, Division of Nephrology
University of Kansas School of Medicine
Kansas City, KS

Richard J. Gray, MD
Professor of Medicine (In Residence)
University of California, Los Angeles, School of Medicine
Los Angeles, CA

Frank J. Green, MD
Assistant Professor of Medicine
Krannert Institute of Cardiology
Indiana University School of Medicine
Indianapolis, IN

Gabriel Gregoratos, MD
Professor of Medicine
Director, Clinical Cardiology
University of California, Davis, School of Medicine
Davis, CA

Jerry C. Griffin, MD
Professor of Medicine in Residence
University of California, San Francisco, School of Medicine
San Francisco, CA

Bartley P. Griffith, MD
Associate Professor of Surgery
Division of Cardiothoracic Surgery
University of Pittsburgh School of Medicine
Pittsburgh, PA

Warren G. Guntheroth, MD
Professor of Pediatrics and Head, Division of Pediatric Cardiology
University of Washington School of Medicine
Seattle, WA

Jonathan L. Halperin, MD
Associate Professor of Medicine
Mount Sinai School of Medicine of the City University of New York
Attending Physician in Cardiology, Mount Sinai Hospital
Director of Clinical Services, Division of Cardiology
Mount Sinai Medical Center
New York, NY

Robert Hattner, MD
Associate Professor of Radiology (Nuclear Medicine)
Director, Section of Nuclear Medicine
University of California, San Francisco, School of Medicine
San Francisco, CA

John M. Herre, MD
Assistant Professor
Director, Eastern Virginia Medical School Cardiac Electrophysiology, Senbra Norfolk General Hospital
Norfolk, VA

Otto M. Hess, MD
Professor of Cardiology, Division of Cardiology
Medical Policlinic, University Hospital
Zurich, Switzerland

Charles B. Higgins, MD
Professor of Radiology
Chief, Section of Magnetic Resonance Imaging
University of California, San Francisco, School of Medicine
San Francisco, CA

Ronald Himelman, MD
Attending Physician
Desert and Eisenhower Hospitals
Palm Springs, CA

Norman K. Hollenberg, MD, PhD
Professor, Department of Radiology and Medicine
Harvard Medical School
Boston, MA

John H. Ip, MD
Division of Cardiology
Mount Sinai Medical Center
New York, NY

Joseph S. Janicki, PhD
Professor of Medicine
University of Missouri, Columbia School of Medicine
Division of Cardiology
Columbia, MO

Mark E. Josephson, MD
Robinette Foundation Professor of Medicine (Cardiovascular Diseases)
University of Pennsylvania School of Medicine
Philadelphia, PA

Martin A. Josephson, MD
Director of Cardiac Catheterization Laboratory
Wadsworth Veterans Administration Hospital
Assistant Professor of Medicine
University of California, Los Angeles, School of Medicine
Los Angeles, CA

John P. Kane, MD, PhD
Professor of Medicine, Biochemistry and Biophysics
Director, Lipid Clinic
University of California, San Francisco, School of Medicine
San Francisco, CA

Joel S. Karliner, MD
Professor of Medicine
University of California, San Francisco
Chief of Cardiology
Ft. Miley Veterans Administration Hospital
San Francisco, CA

Harold L. Kennedy, MD, MPH
Section of Cardiology
Professor of Medicine
Distinguished Cardiologist
Rush Medical School
Rush-Presbyterian-St. Luke's Medical Center
Chicago, IL

Thomas Killip, MD
Professor of Medicine, Mount Sinai School of Medicine
Executive Vice President for Medical Affairs
Beth Israel Medical Center
New York, NY

Francis J. Klocke, MD
Albert and Elizabeth Rekate Professor of Medicine and Cardiovascular Disease
Professor of Physiology and Chief, Division of Cardiology
State University of New York at Buffalo and Erie County Medical Center
Buffalo, NY

George T. Kondos, MD
Assistant Professor of Medicine
Associate Chief, Cardiology Section
Director, Cardiac Catheterization Laboratory
University of Illinois, College of Medicine
Chicago, IL

Richard J. Kovacs, MD
Department of Medical Research
Methodist Hospital of Indiana
Indianapolis, IN

Hans P. Krayenbuehl, MD
Professor and Chief of Cardiology
Medical Policlinic, University Hospital
Zurich, Switzerland

Jack Kron, MD
Associate Professor of Medicine, Division of Cardiology
Associate Director of Coronary Care Unit, Oregon Health Sciences University
Portland, OR

Gilles Lascault
Staff Member
Hospital Jean Rostand
39 rue Jean Le Galleau
94200 Ivry - France

Samuel Lévy, MD
Professor of Cardiology, University of Marseille
Chief, Cardiology Division
Hôspital Nord
Marseille, France

Wilbur Y.W. Lew, MD
Associate Professor of Medicine in Residence
University of California, San Diego
Veterans Administration Medical Center
San Diego, CA

Martin M. LeWinter, MD
Professor of Medicine, University of Vermont
Director, Cardiology Unit, Medical Center Hospital of Vermont
Burlington, VT

John H. McAnulty, MD
Professor of Medicine
Oregon Health Sciences University
Portland, OR

Dan G. McNamara, MD
Professor of Pediatrics, Baylor College of Medicine
Emeritus Chief of Pediatric Cardiology, Texas Children's Hospital
Houston, TX

Robert W. Mahley, MD, PhD
Director, Gladstone Foundation Laboratories for Cardiovascular Disease
Cardiovascular Research Institute
Professor of Pathology and Medicine
University of California, San Francisco
San Francisco, CA

Mary J. Malloy, MD
Clinical Professor of Medicine and Pediatrics
Director, Pediatric Lipid Clinic
University of California, San Francisco, School of Medicine
San Francisco, CA

Jay W. Mason, MD
Professor of Medicine
Chief, Cardiology Division, University of Utah Medical Center
Salt Lake City, UT

Jack M. Matloff, MD
Assistant Clinical Professor
University of California, Los Angeles, School of Medicine
Los Angeles, CA

Michael A. Matthay, MD
Associate Professor of Medicine and Anesthesia
Associate Director, Intensive Care Unit
Senior Scientific Staff, Cardiovascular Research Institute
University of California, San Francisco, School of Medicine
San Francisco, CA

James Metcalfe, MD
Professor, Department of Medicine
School of Medicine, Oregon Health Sciences University
Portland, OR

John M. Miller, MD
Assistant Professor of Medicine
University of Pennsylvania, School of Medicine
Philadelphia, PA

Fred Morady, MD
Professor of Internal Medicine
Director, Clinical Electrophysiology Laboratory
University of Michigan Medical Center
Ann Arbor, MI

Hugo Morales Ballejo, MD, FACC
Research Director
Institute of Stress Medicine, Inc
Denver, CO

Joel Morganroth, MD
Director, Cardiac Research and Developments
The Graduate Health System
Clinical Professor of Medicine
University of Pennsylvania, School of Medicine
Philadelphia, PA

Mary J. H. Morriss, MD
Associate, Pediatric Cardiology
Department of Pediatrics
The University of Iowa Hospitals and Clinics
Iowa City, IA

David W. Muller, MB, BS
Senior Fellow, Interventional Cardiology, Division of Cardiology
University of Michigan Medical Center
Ann Arbor, MI

Koolawee Nademanee, MD
Director of Clinical Electrophysiology
Wadsworth Veterans Administration Hospital
Associate Co-Director, UCLA-Wadsworth Arrhythmia Unit
Associate Professor of Medicine
University of California, Los Angeles, School of Medicine
Los Angeles, CA

Phuc Tito Nguyen, MD
Department of Medicine and Cardiovascular Research Institute
University of California, San Francisco, School of Medicine
San Francisco, CA

James T. Niemann, MD, FACEP
Associate Professor of Medicine
University of California, Los Angeles, School of Medicine, Los Angeles
Associate Chairman, Department of Emergency Medicine
Harbor-UCLA Medical Center
Torrance, CA

William O'Connell, BS
Computer Specialist
Director, Nuclear Medicine Computer Facility
University of California, San Francisco, School of Medicine
San Francisco, CA

Robert A. O'Rourke, MD
Division Chief of Cardiology
University of Texas Health Science Center Medical School at San Antonio
San Antonio, TX

Douglas Ortendahl, PhD
Assistant Professor of Physics, Radiology, and Radiology Imaging
Director, Nuclear Medicine Physics, University of California, San Francisco
San Francisco, CA

John A. Paraskos, MD
Professor, Department of Medicine, University of Massachusetts
School of Medicine
Worcester, MA

William W. Parmley, MD
Professor of Medicine
University of California, San Francisco
Chief of Cardiology
Moffitt/Long Hospital
San Francisco, CA

Carl J. Pepine, MD
Professor of Medicine and Associate Director of Cardiology
Department of Medicine, University of Florida
Chief, Cardiology Section, Veterans Administration Medical Center
Gainesville, FL

Robert W. Peters, MD
Associate Professor of Medicine, University of Maryland School of Medicine
Chief of Cardiology, Veterans Administration Medical Center
Baltimore, MD

Jeffrey M. Piehler, MD
Department of Cardiovascular Surgery
Mid American Heart Institute of St. Luke's Hospital
Kansas City, MO

Thomas A. Ports, MD
Professor in Medicine, Director Cardiac Catheterization Laboratory
Cardiovascular Research Institute, University of California, San Francisco
San Francisco, CA

Eric C. Rackow, MD
Chairman, Department of Medicine
St. Vincent's Hospital
New York, NY

Elliot Rapaport, MD
Professor of Medicine
University of California, San Francisco
Chief of Cardiology
San Francisco General Hospital
San Francisco, CA

Timothy J. Regan, MD
Professor of Medicine
Director, Division of Cardiovascular Diseases
Department of Medicine
University of Medicine and Dentistry of New Jersey
New Jersey Medical School
Newark, NJ

Leon Resnekov, MD, FRCP
Frederick H. Rawson Professor of Medicine (Cardiology)
University of Chicago
Chicago, IL

Dan M. Roden, MD
Professor of Medicine and Pharmacology
Vanderbilt University School of Medicine
Nashville, TN

Michael R. Rosen, MD
Departments of Pharmacology and of Pediatrics
College of Physicians and Surgeons of Columbia University
New York, NY

Jeremy N. Ruskin, MD
Associate Professor of Medicine, Harvard Medical School
Boston, MA

David J. Sahn, MD
Professor of Pediatrics and Chief of the Division of Pediatric Cardiology
University of California, San Diego
San Diego, CA

Melvin M. Scheinman, MD
Professor of Medicine
University of California, San Francisco
Chief of Electrophysiology
Moffitt/Long Hospital
San Francisco, CA

Nelson B. Schiller, MD
Professor of Medicine
University of California, San Francisco, School of Medicine
Director, Adult Echocardiography Laboratory, Moffitt/Long Hospital
San Francisco, CA

Robert C. Schlant, MD
Professor of Medicine (Cardiology)
Department of Medicine, Emory University of Medicine
Chief of Cardiology, Grady Memorial Hospital
Atlanta, GA

John Speer Schroeder, MD
Professor of Medicine, Stanford University School of Medicine
Palo Alto, CA

Ralph Shabetai, MD, FRCP (EDin)
Professor of Medicine and Associate Director of Cardiology
University of California, San Diego
Chief, Cardiology, Veterans Administration Medical Center
La Jolla, CA

Pravin M. Shah, MD
Professor of Medicine
Loma Linda University School of Medicine
Loma Linda, CA

Prediman K. Shah, MD, FACC, FCCP, FACP
Associate Professor of Medicine
University of California, Los Angeles, School of Medicine
Shappell and Webb Family Chair in Cardiology
Director of Inpatient Cardiology and Cardiac Care Units
Cedars-Sinai Medical Center
Los Angeles, CA

Jeffrey G. Shanes, MD
Assistant Professor of Medicine
Director, Cardiac Catheterization Laboratory
University of Illinois, Chicago, College of Medicine
Chicago, IL

John T. Shepherd, MD, DSc, FRCP
Professor of Physiology and Biophysics
Mayo Clinic and Mayo Foundation
Rochester, MN

Bramah N. Singh, MD DPhil (Oxon), FRACP, FRCP (London)
Director, Cardiovascular Research Laboratory
Wadsworth Veterans Administration Hospital
Director, UCLA-Wadsworth Arrhythmia Unit
Professor of Medicine
University of California, Los Angeles, School of Medicine
Los Angeles, CA

John A. Spittell, Jr., MD, FACP, FACC
Professor of Medicine, Mayo Medical School
Consultant, Cardiovascular Diseases
Mayo Clinic and Mayo Foundation
Rochester, MN

Peter C. Spittell, MD
Senior Clinical Fellow, Cardiovascular Disease
Mayo Graduate School of Medicine
Mayo Clinic
Rochester, MN

David H. Spodick, MD, DSc
Professor of Medicine, University of Massachusetts Medical School
Associate in Medicine, Tufts and Boston University Schools of Medicine
Director of Clinical and Cardiovascular Fellowship Program,
St. Vincent's Hospital
Worcester, MA

James P. Srebro, MD
Cardiology Consultants of Napa Valley
Assistant Professor of Clinical Medicine
Napa, CA

Jeremiah Stamler, MD
Dingman Professor of Cardiology
Department of Community Health and Preventive Medicine
Northwestern University Medical School
Chicago, IL

D. E. Strandness, Jr., MD
Professor of Surgery
University of Washington School of Medicine
Seattle, WA

Robert J. Stuart, MD
Director, Cardiac Rehabilitation, Memorial Medical Center of Long Beach
Clinical Instructor, University of California, Irvine, College of Medicine
Irvine, CA

Borys Surawicz, MD
Professor of Medicine, Indiana University School of Medicine
Senior Research Associate, Krannert Institute of Cardiology
Indianapolis, IN

H. J. C. Swan, MD, PhD, FACC
Professor of Medicine
University of California, Los Angeles, School of Medicine
Director, Division of Cardiology, Cedars-Sinai Medical Center
Los Angeles, CA

Robert Tarazi, MD
Department of Heart and Hypertension, Research Institute
The Cleveland Clinic Foundation
Cleveland, OH

Henry D. Tazelaar, MD
Fellow in Cardiac Pathology, Stanford University Medical School
Palo Alto, CA
Associate Professor of Pathology
Senior Associate Consultant
Mayo Clinic and Foundation
Rochester, MN

Nicholas A. Tepe, MD
Instructor in Surgery
University of Pennsylvania School of Medicine
Philadelphia, PA

Mark E. Thompson, MD
Division of Cardiology
University of Pittsburgh Presbyterian University Hospital
Pittsburgh, PA

Joelci Tonet, MD
Staff Member
Hospital Jean Rostand
39 rue Jean Le Galleau
94200 Ivry - France

Eric J. Topol, MD
Associate Professor, Internal Medicine
Director, Cardiac Catheterization Laboratories, Division of Cardiology
University of Michigan Medical Center
Ann Arbor, MI

Kent Ueland, MD
Professor Emeritus, Department of Gynecology and Obstetrics
Stanford University School of Medicine
Palo Alto, CA

Paul M. Vanhoutte, MD, PhD
Professor of Cardiology and Pharmacology
Mayo Medical School and Mayo Graduate School of Medicine
Rochester, MN

August M. Watanabe, MD
Professor, Department of Medicine and Pharmacology/Toxicology
Chairman, Department of Medicine, Krannert Institute of Cardiology
Indiana University School of Medicine
Indianapolis, IN

Karl T. Weber, MD
Professor of Medicine
Director, Division of Cardiology
School of Medicine
University of Missouri—Columbia
Columbia, MO

Max Harry Weil, MD, PhD
Distinguished Professor of Medicine, Physiology and Biophysics
Chairman of the Department of Medicine
Chief, Divisions of Cardiology and Critical Care Medicine
University of Health Sciences/The Chicago Medical School
North Chicago, IL

Nanette Kass Wenger, MD
Professor of Medicine (Cardiology)
Emory University School of Medicine
Director, Cardiac Clinics, Grady Memorial Hospital
Atlanta, GA

Pierre Wicker, MD
Associate Director
Pfizer Central Research
Pfizer, Inc.
Groton, CT

E. Douglas Wigle, MD, FRCP(C), FACP, FACC
Professor, Department of Medicine
Division of Cardiology, Toronto General Hospital
Toronto, Ontario, Canada

Joan Wikman-Coffelt, PhD
Professor, Department of Medicine
University of California, San Francisco, School of Medicine
San Francisco, CA

David J. Wilber, MD
Assistant Professor of Medicine, Loyola Stritch School of Medicine
Director, Electrophysiology Laboratory
Loyola University Medical Center
Maywood, IL

James T. Willerson, MD
Professor and Chairman, Department of Internal Medicine
University of Texas Medical School
Houston, TX

Gordon H. Williams, MD
Professor of Medicine, Harvard Medical School
Boston, MA

Patricia Wisler, MD
Assistant Scientist Department of Medicine
Indiana University School of Medicine
Krannert Institute of Cardiology
Indianapolis, IN

Raymond L. Woosley, MD, PhD
Professor and Chairman
Department of Pharmacology
Georgetown University Medical Center
Washington, DC

Paul G. Yock, MD
Assistant Professor of Medicine
Associate Director, Cardiac Catheterization Laboratory
University of California, San Francisco
San Francisco, CA

Douglas P. Zipes, MD
Professor of Medicine, Indiana University School of Medicine
Senior Research Associate, Krannert Institute of Cardiology
Indianapolis, IN

CONTENTS

VOLUME 1
PHYSIOLOGY, PHARMACOLOGY, DIAGNOSIS

Section 1
NORMAL AND ABNORMAL CARDIOVASCULAR PHYSIOLOGY
Section Editor: William W. Parmley

CHAPTER 1 *Cardiac Anatomy* 1.2
Melvin D. Cheitlin   Walter E. Finkbeiner

2 *Physiology of Cardiac Muscle Contraction* 1.19
William W. Parmley   Joan Wikman-Coffelt

3 *Cardiovascular Adrenergic and Muscarinic Cholinergic Receptors* 1.41
Patricia L. Wisler   Frank J. Green   August M. Watanabe

4 *Myocardial Hypertrophy, Failure, and Ischemia* 1.68
William W. Parmley   Joan Wikman-Coffelt

5 *Ventricular Function* 1.85
William W. Parmley

6 *Physiology of the Coronary Circulation* 1.101
Francis J. Klocke   Avery K. Ellis

7 *The Circulation in the Limbs: Normal Function and Effects of Disease* 1.114
John T. Shepherd   Paul M. Vanhoutte

8 *Physiology and Pathophysiology of Exercise* 1.129
C. Gunnar Blomqvist

9 *Pulmonary Edema* 1.144
Max Harry Weil   Eric C. Rackow   Carter E. Mecher

10 *Principles in the Management of Congestive Heart Failure* 1.154
William W. Parmley

11 *Orthostatic Hypotension* 1.163
C. Gunnar Blomqvist

Section 2
CARDIOVASCULAR PHARMACOLOGY
Section Editor: William W. Parmley

12 *Basic Principles of Clinical Pharmacology* 2.2
Raymond L. Woosley   Dan M. Roden

13 *Diuretics* 2.19
Arnold M. Chonko   Jared J. Grantham

14 *Digitalis, Catecholamines, and Other Positive Inotropic Agents* 2.34
Kanu Chatterjee

15 *Nitrates* 2.75
Jonathan Abrams

16 *The Alpha- and Beta-Adrenergic Blocking Drugs*   *2.91*
    WILLIAM H. FRISHMAN   SHLOMO CHARLAP

17 *Calcium Channel Blockers in Therapeutics*   *2.105*
    BRAMAH N. SINGH   MARTIN A. JOSEPHSON   KOONLAWEE N. NADEMANEE

18 *Vasodilator Drugs in the Treatment of Heart Failure*   *2.123*
    WILLIAM W. PARMLEY

19 *Hypolipidemic Agents*   *2.137*
    MARY J. MALLOY   JOHN P. KANE

20 *Antithrombotic Therapy in Cardiac Disease*   *2.143*
    JOHN H. IP   VALENTIN FUSTER   JAMES H. CHESEBRO   LINA BADIMON

21 *Cardiovascular Drug Interactions*   *2.172*
    NEAL L. BENOWITZ

Section 3
BEDSIDE EVALUATION OF THE PATIENT
SECTION EDITOR: KANU CHATTERJEE

22 *The History*   *3.2*
    KANU CHATTERJEE

23 *Bedside Evaluation of the Heart: The Physical Examination*   *3.11*
    KANU CHATTERJEE

24 *Examination of the Lungs*   *3.54*
    THOMAS KILLIP

25 *Bedside Diagnosis of Congenital Heart Disease*   *3.58*
    ALVIN J. CHIN   WILLIAM F. FRIEDMAN

Section 4
NONINVASIVE TESTS
SECTION EDITOR: KANU CHATTERJEE

26 *The Chest X-Ray Film and the Diagnosis of Heart Disease*   *4.2*
    MELVIN D. CHEITLIN

27 *Electrocardiogram*   *4.14*
    BORYS SURAWICZ

28 *Echocardiography and Doppler in Clinical Cardiology*   *4.33*
    NELSON B. SCHILLER   RONALD B. HIMELMAN

29 *The Scintigraphic Evaluation of the Cardiovascular System*   *4.107*
    ELIAS H. BOTVINICK   MICHAEL DAE   WILLIAM O'CONNELL   DOUGLAS ORTENDAHL   ROBERT HATTNER

30 *New Cardiac Imaging Modalities*   *4.163*
    CHARLES B. HIGGINS

31 *Exercise Stress Testing: Principles and Clinical Application*   *4.183*
    MYRVIN H. ELLESTAD   ROBERT J. STUART

32 *Exercise Evaluation of Cardiorespiratory Function*   *4.202*
    KARL T. WEBER   JOSEPH S. JANICKI

33 *Noninvasive Evaluation of Peripheral Vascular Disease*   *4.213*
    D. E. STRANDNESS, JR.

Section 5
INVASIVE TESTS
Section Editor: Kanu Chatterjee

34 *Cardiac Catheterization* 5.2
Blase A. Carabello

35 *Coronary Arteriography Including Quantitative Estimation of Coronary Artery Stenosis* 5.20
George T. Kondos Jeffrey G. Shanes Bruce H. Brundage

36 *Cardiac Digital Angiography* 5.43
Neal Eigler James S. Forrester

37 *Assessment of Ventricular Diastolic Function* 5.55
Derek G. Gibson

38 *Cardiac Biopsy* 5.67
Margaret E. Billingham Henry D. Tazelaar

39 *Bedside Hemodynamic Monitoring* 5.80
Kanu Chatterjee

Section 6
ELECTROPHYSIOLOGY
Section Editor: Melvin M. Scheinman

40 *Mechanisms of Cardiac Arrhythmias* 6.2
Richard J. Kovacs John C. Bailey Douglas P. Zipes

41 *Pharmacodynamics of Antiarrhythmic Drugs* 6.14
Peter Danilo, Jr. Michael R. Rosen

42 *Use of Antiarrhythmic Drugs: General Principles* 6.31
Kelley P. Anderson Roger A. Freedman Jay W. Mason

43 *Clinical Use of Newer Antiarrhythmic Drugs* 6.44
Samuel Levy

44 *Invasive Cardiac Electrophysiology Studies: An Introduction* 6.54
Masood Akhtar

45 *Measurements and Clinical Application of Monophasic Action Potentials* 6.68
Michael R. Franz

46 *Ambulatory Holter Electrocardiography: Technology, Clinical Applications, and Limitations* 6.87
Joel Morganroth Harold L. Kennedy

47 *The Sick Sinus Syndrome and Evaluation of the Patient with Sinus Node Disorders* 6.100
J. Anthony Gomes

48 *Bundle Branch Block and Atrioventricular Conduction Disorders* 6.111
Robert W. Peters Melvin M. Scheinman

49 *Supraventricular Tachycardia* 6.128
John M. Herre Melvin M. Scheinman

50 *Ventricular Arrhythmias* 6.142
John M. Miller Mark E. Josephson

51 *Right Ventricular Tachycardias* 6.156
    Guy Fontaine Robert Frank Fabrice Fontaliran Gilles Lascault Joelice Tonet

52 *Devices for the Management of Rhythm Disorders: Pacemakers and Defibrillators* 6.170
    Jerry C. Griffin

53 *Surgical Treatment of Cardiac Arrhythmias* 6.185
    T. Bruce Ferguson, Jr. James L. Cox

54 *Catheter Ablation for Cardiac Arrhythmias* 6.215
    Melvin M. Scheinman

55 *Syncope* 6.224
    Fred Morady

56 *Evaluation and Treatment of Patients with Aborted Sudden Death* 6.237
    David J. Wilber Hasan Garan Jeremy N. Ruskin

57 *Cardiopulmonary Resuscitation* 6.249
    James T. Niemann J. Michael Criley

58 *Congenital and Acquired Long QT Syndromes* 6.258
    Anil K. Bhandari Phuc Tito Nguyen Melvin M. Scheinman

VOLUME 2
CARDIOVASCULAR DISEASE

Section 7
CORONARY HEART DISEASE
Section Editor: Joel S. Karliner

59 *Epidemiology, Established Major Risk Factors, and the Primary Prevention of Coronary Heart Disease* 7.2
    Jeremiah Stamler

60 *Lipid Abnormalities: Mechanisms, Clinical Classifications, and Management* 7.36
    Robert W. Mahley Thomas P. Bersot

61 *Evaluation of the Patient with Signs and Symptoms of Ischemic Heart Disease* 7.48
    Louis J. Dell'Italia Robert A. O'Rourke

62 *Stable Anginal Pectoris* 7.62
    Joel S. Karliner

63 *Acute and Chronic Ischemic Heart Disease: Unstable Angina* 7.75
    Carl J. Pepine

64 *Silent Ischemia* 7.91
    William W. Parmley

65 *Variant Angina* 7.100
    John Speer Schroeder

66 *Acute Myocardial Infarction: Pathophysiology* 7.112
    Wilbur Y. W. Lew Martin M. LeWinter

67 *Measurement of Myocardial Infarction Size* 7.134
   L. Maximilian Buja James T. Willerson

68 *Management of Uncomplicated Acute Myocardial Infarction* 7.142
   Gabriel Gregoratos

69 *Reperfusion in Acute Myocardial Infarction* 7.163
   David W. Muller Eric J. Topol

70 *Complications of Acute Myocardial Infarction* 7.179
   Prediman K. Shah H. J. C. Swan

71 *Cardiac Rehabilitation* 7.204
   Victor F. Froelicher

72 *Management of the Postmyocardial Infarction Patient* 7.217
   Nora Goldschlager

73 *Transluminal Coronary Angioplasty and Newer Catheter-Based Interventions* 7.237
   Paul G. Yock

74 *Coronary Artery Bypass Surgery* 7.249
   Joel S. Karliner

75 *The Role of Cardiac Surgery in the Management of Acute Myocardial Infarction* 7.262
   Jack M. Matloff Richard J. Gray

Section 8
HYPERTENSION
Section Editor: William W. Parmley

76 *Pathophysiology of Essential Hypertension* 8.2
   Gordon H. Williams Norman K. Hollenberg

77 *Evaluation and Management of the Patient with Essential Hypertension* 8.16
   Edward D. Frohlich

78 *Evaluation of Secondary Forms of Hypertension* 8.28
   Michael D. Cressman Ray W. Gifford, Jr.

79 *Effects of Antihypertensive Treatment on Left Ventricular Hypertrophy and Coronary Blood Flow* 8.44
   Pierre Wicker Fetnat M. Fouad Robert C. Tarazi†

80 *Hypertension in the Elderly* 8.53
   Robert C. Tarazi†

†Deceased.

Section 9
VALVULAR HEART DISEASE
Section Editor: Elliot Rapaport

81 *The Use of Afterload-Reducing Agents in Acute Valvular Regurgitation* 9.2
   Jack Kron J. David Bristow

82 *Chronic Valvular Insufficiency* 9.11
   Hans P. Krayenbuehl Otto M. Hess

83 *Mitral Valve Prolapse Syndrome* 9.30
   Pravin M. Shah

84 *Valvular Heart Disease: Prosthetic Valve Replacement* 9.40
L. Henry Edmunds, Jr.   V. Paul Addonizio, Jr.   Nicholas A. Tepe

85 *Catheter Balloon Valvuloplasty* 9.54
James P. Srebro   Thomas A. Ports

86 *Infective Endocarditis* 9.73
Gabriel Gregoratos

87 *Tricuspid Valve Disease* 9.91
Gordon A. Ewy

88 *Aortic Stenosis* 9.106
Robert C. Schlant

89 *Mitral Stenosis* 9.116
Elliot Rapaport

Section 10
MYOCARDIAL, PERICARDIAL, AND ENDOCARDIAL DISEASES
Section Editor: Melvin D. Cheitlin

90 *Dilated Cardiomyopathy* 10.2
Ralph Shabetai

91 *Hypertrophic Cardiomyopathy* 10.18
E. Douglas Wigle

92 *Diseases of the Pericardium* 10.38
David H. Spodick

93 *Noninfective Endocardial Disease* 10.65
Edwin L. Alderman

94 *Pulmonary Heart Disease Including Pulmonary Embolism* 10.70
John A. Paraskos

95 *Myocarditis* 10.84
George Cherian   M. Thomas Abraham

96 *Rheumatic Fever* 10.98
M. Thomas Abraham   George Cherian

97 *Restrictive and Obliterative Cardiomyopathy* 10.107
Walter H. Abelmann

Section 11
CONGENITAL HEART DISEASE IN THE ADULT
Section Editor: Elliot Rapaport

98 *The Adult with Surgically Corrected Heart Disease: The Unnatural History* 11.2
Melvin D. Cheitlin

99 *Coronary Arterial Anomalies* 11.14
Melvin D. Cheitlin

100 *Cyanotic Congenital Heart Disease* 11.27
Mary Allen Engle

101 *Interatrial Septal Defect in the Adult* 11.43
Melvin D. Cheitlin   Elliot Rapaport

102 *Ductus Arteriosus and Ventricular Septal Defect in the Adult*   *11.51*
       Warren G. Guntheroth

103 *Congenital Valvular and Other Isolated Obstructive Lesions in the Adult*   *11.61*
       Mary J.H. Morriss   Dan G. McNamara

104 *Pulmonary Vascular Disease in Adults with Congenital Heart Disease*   *11.77*
       Joseph S. Alpert   James E. Dalen

105 *Echocardiography in Congenital Heart Disease*   *11.88*
       Kyung J. Chung   David J. Sahn

Section 12
OTHER DISORDERS OF THE CARDIOVASCULAR SYSTEM
Section Editor: Melvin D. Cheitlin

106 *Alcohol and the Heart*   *12.2*
       Timothy J. Regan

107 *Cardiovascular Injury as the Internist Sees It*   *12.13*
       Melvin D. Cheitlin

108 *Diseases of the Aorta and Peripheral Arteries*   *12.27*
       John A. Spittell, Jr.   Peter C. Spittell

109 *Cardiac Neoplasms*   *12.45*
       Emilio R. Giuliani   Jeffrey M. Piehler

Section 13
SECONDARY DISORDERS OF THE HEART
Section Editor: Melvin D. Cheitlin

110 *Collagen Diseases and the Heart*   *13.2*
       Jonathan L. Halperin

111 *Pregnancy in the Cardiac Patient*   *13.19*
       John H. McAnulty   James Metcalfe   Kent Ueland

112 *The Elderly Patient with Cardiovascular Disease*   *13.28*
       Nanette Kass Wenger

113 *Assessment and Management of the Cardiac Patient Before, During, and After Noncardiac Surgery*   *13.41*
       Lee Goldman

114 *Respiratory and Hemodynamic Management After Cardiac Surgery*   *13.52*
       Michael A. Matthay   Kanu Chatterjee

115 *The Relationship of Emotions and Cardiopathology*   *13.67*
       Robert S. Eliot   Hugo M. Morales-Ballejo

116 *Cardiac Complications of Substance Abuse*   *13.74*
       Michael L. Callaham   Kanu Chatterjee

117 *Endocrine Diseases and the Cardiovascular System*   *13.82*
       Leon Resnekov

118 *Cardiac and Cardiopulmonary Transplantation*   *13.92*
       Mark E. Thompson   J. Stephen Dummer   Bartley P. Griffith

**Section Editor
*William W. Parmley, MD***

NORMAL AND ABNORMAL CARDIOVASCULAR PHYSIOLOGY

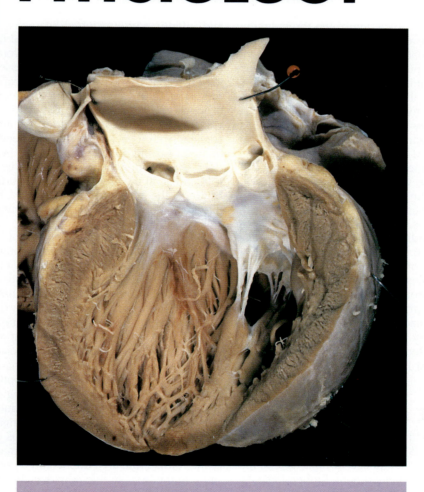

CARDIAC ANATOMY

Melvin D. Cheitlin • Walter E. Finkbeiner

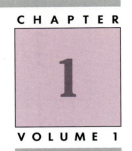

Although knowledge of the anatomy of the heart goes back to ancient times, the three-dimensional relationships of the various cardiac chambers have only recently interested clinical cardiologists. The early means of imaging the heart were projectional: chest radiography and, after cardiac catheterization began, angiocardiography. On the chest film the shadow of the cardiac silhouette was projected against a two-dimensional plane, and for the first time in the history of medicine it was important for the clinician to know the structures that formed the borders of the heart. With angiocardiography beginning in the middle of the 20th century, projection of the opacified chambers against the two-dimensional plane became possible and knowledge of the three-dimensional relationships of the cardiac structures became essential. Still, only those cardiologists and radiologists who performed these studies were really interested. It was not until echocardiography became a widely used clinical tool that knowledge of the three-dimensional anatomy of the heart became essential in understanding the coronal and cross-sectional planes that were exposed by these techniques. With the development of computed tomography and magnetic resonance imaging the ability to examine the heart in all planes became possible. To understand what these studies show requires an intimate knowledge of cardiac anatomy.

Knowledge of the interrelationships of the cardiac structures helps in understanding abnormalities that occur during pathologic derangement; for instance, the relationship of the conduction system to the valvular annuli explains why the patient with endocarditis that becomes extravalvular so often develops varying degrees of heart block. Because the His bundle perforates the right fibrous trigone it is also apparent why conduction system disease occurs so commonly with increasing age and increasing fibrosis and calcification of the valve rings. The relationship of the left bundle branches to the aortic valve ring explains the common occurrence of bundle branch block in calcific aortic stenosis. The relationship of the sinuses of Valsalva to the right and left cardiac chambers explains the sites of rupture of sinus of Valsalva aneurysms when they form aortic-cameral fistulas.

Detailed knowledge of the anatomy of the heart is obviously essential to the performance of the cardiac surgeon and the cardiologist. As the description of cardiac anatomy is available in great detail in a variety of anatomy books, this chapter will be devoted to details of cardiac anatomy that are of particular importance to the clinician—a type of "functional anatomy."

THE HEART AND THE MEDIASTINUM

The heart is a roughly conical structure composed of muscles surrounding two atria and two ventricles and anchored to the fibrous valvular annuli. The myocardial wall is composed of three layers: the endocardium, the myocardium, and the pericardium. Embryologically the heart invaginates the pericardial sac in such a way that it is surrounded by the pericardium, being suspended only by the reflections around the great vessels where the parietal pericardium is continuous with the myocardial visceral pericardium. These attachments consist of duplicated reflections of the pericardium, called the dorsal mesocardium; one set of the reflections is at the sinoatrial end around the venous inlets into the atria and the other set is at the great arteries as they leave the heart to form an arterial or conotruncal mesocardium. Within the mesocardium lie the cardiac nerves. The heart is otherwise free at all other surfaces within the pericardial cavity. The heart lying within the pericardial sac can move freely, lubricated with a small amount of pericardial fluid. With each beat the heart can change its volume in systole and diastole and twist as it ejects blood, all with minimal friction between it and the mediastinal contents and the lungs. The pericardium also serves to retain the heart within the mediastinum, especially during trauma, and forms an effective barrier to infection between the heart and the pleural cavities.

The visceral pericardium reflects off the great vessels in such a way that the proximal two thirds of the ascending aorta and the main pulmonary artery remain intrapericardial. About half of the superior vena cava is intrapericardial, but only 1 to 2 cm of the inferior vena cava lies within the pericardial sac. The inferior part of the pericardial sac is attached to the central tendon of the diaphragm. The anterior portion of the fibrous pericardial sac is attached to the sternum by the superior and inferior periretrosternal ligaments. The lateral pericardial sac is attached to the mediastinal portion of the right and left pleura.

Within the pericardial sac are several recesses of the pericardium caused by reflection off the great vessels (Fig. 1.1). The veins are all joined within the leaves of the pericardial reflection posteriorly in a ring, starting on the right from the inferior vena cava posteriorly and proceding in a semicircle to the inferior and superior right pulmonary vein and then to the left superior and inferior left pulmonary vein. This semicircle then encloses a space or recess within the posterior pericardium called the oblique sinus of the pericardial cavity. The other defined space within the pericardial cavity exists between the pericardial reflections off the great vessels: the aorta and pulmonary artery superiorly and the superior vena cava and two superior pulmonary veins inferiorly. This recess is called the transverse sinus of the pericardial cavity.

The importance of the position of these pericardial reflections is that the ascending aorta remains within the pericardial cavity. With dissection of the aorta or traumatic rupture of the ascending aorta, there is no tissue resistance to rupture and blood fills the pericardial sac, which is fibrous and relatively noncompliant, resulting in rapid cardiac tamponade. This explains why dissection involving the ascending aorta (type A dissection) is much more likely to be fatal than dissection that involves the descending aorta (type B dissection). The descending aorta is located in the posterior mediastinum and almost completely surrounded by the tough parietal pleura, which can support the aortic adventitia and contain a rupture.

The fibrous pericardium containing the heart is in the middle mediastinum, central in the chest, with about two thirds of its volume to the left of center and one third to the right. Between the right and left pleural cavities, right and left portions of the fibrous pericardium are completely covered, leaving only a small portion anteriorly on the left in the retrosternal area uncovered by pleura. Of importance is the position of the two phrenic nerves as they pass through the middle mediastinum. They lie to the left and right slightly posteriorly on the lateral surfaces of the pericardial sac. These nerves can be injured during open-heart surgery, resulting in paralysis of one or both leaves of the diaphragm, a serious problem complicating ventilation postoperatively. The posterior extent of pericardiectomy is usually limited by the position of the phrenic nerves and fear of injury to these structures. Posterior mediastinal structures include the esophagus, which is immediately posterior to the left atrium; the descending thoracic aorta, which is to the left of the esophagus; and the bifurcation of the trachea, located in the superior portion of the posterior mediastinum.

The blood supply of the pericardium consists of branches from the internal mammary artery, which are branches of the subclavian arteries and pass posteriorly to the anterior rib cage 0.5 cm laterally to the right and left edges of the sternum. These vessels pass to the diaphragm and divide into the musculophrenic and the superior epigastric branches. There are also contributions from the intercostal arteries, the subclavian arteries, and the posterior mediastinal arteries. At the root of the great vessels, around the pericardial reflections, are small interconnections between the epicardial coronary arteries and the internal mammary arteries.

The blood supply of the thoracic cage comes from the intercostal arteries that arise posteriorly from the aorta and anteriorly from the internal mammary arteries. The venous drainage of the chest wall follows the arterial distribution. The ten lower intercostal veins on the right enter the azygous vein posteriorly, which loops anteriorly and enters the superior vena cava in its posterior aspect. The upper two intercostal veins on the right enter the azygous or the innominate vein; the lower intercostal veins on the left enter the hemiazygous vein or accessory hemiazygous vein. The left hemiazygous vein crosses the midline posterior to the descending aorta at about the level of the eighth thoracic vertebra and enters the azygous vein on the right. With right-sided congestive heart failure, the dilated azygous vein as it joins the superior vena cava can be seen as a round structure on the chest film.

The great arteries and veins in the superior mediastinum have certain relationships that are clinically important. The innominate veins are formed by the joining of the subclavian veins, which pass over the first rib and inferiorly and posteriorly to the clavicle, and the internal jugular veins just behind the sternoclavicular joints. The right innominate vein enters the thoracic cavity and unites with the left innominate vein, which passes anteriorly to the aortic arch across the midline to form the superior vena cava. Posterior to these structures are the great arteries. The innominate artery arises as the first branch from the aorta. It divides into the subclavian artery, which lies posterior to the subclavian vein, and the common carotid artery, which again is posterior to the sternoclavicular joint. The second branch arising from the cap of the aortic arch is the left common carotid artery. The final major branch arising from the distal arch of the aorta is the left subclavian artery.

From this description it is apparent that the venous structures are anterior to the arterial structures and that both the left innominate vein and the arch of the aorta cross the midline. The left innominate vein is posterior to the sternum and could be injured during midsternal thoracotomy. The intimate relationship of the left innominate vein to the aortic arch explains the occasional aortic–left innominate vein fistula created by penetrating trauma.

EXTERNAL CONFIGURATION OF THE HEART

The external surface of the heart with the pericardium opened from the anterior approach reveals the right atrium at the right lateral border with a small portion of the inferior vena cava showing inferiorly and the superior vena cava forming the superior rightward border of the superior cardiac structures (Fig. 1.2). In the anterior mediastinum is the remnant of the thymus gland as the most anterior structure. Posterior to this is the ascending aorta. The root of the ascending aorta is hidden by the right auricular appendage, which extends as a medial superior structure from the right atrium. The inferior left border of the right atrium is along the atrioventricular groove in which runs the right coro-

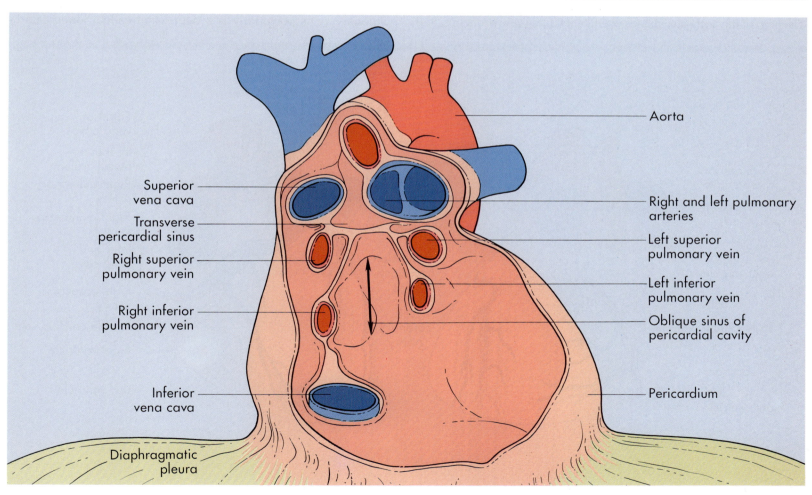

FIGURE 1.1 View of the dorsal wall of the pericardial cavity demonstrating the pericardial reflections. (Modified from Barry A, Patten BM: The structure of the human heart. In Gould SE [ed]: Pathology of the Heart. Springfield, IL, Charles C Thomas, 1968)

nary artery, usually buried in epicardial fat. The heart lies in the chest such that the right anterior atrioventricular sulcus runs almost vertically. The anterior and inferior portion of the heart is formed by the free wall of the right ventricle, which in the frontal plane forms a rough triangle with the apex, being the right ventricular outflow tract leading to the main pulmonary artery, which lies parallel to and just to the left of the ascending aorta. About 1 cm from the left cardiac border is the anterior interventricular sulcus, marked by epicardial fat, in which travels the left anterior descending coronary artery. The left border of the heart, including the apex that rests on the left diaphragm, is formed by the muscular, thick left ventricle. Between the left aspect of the main pulmonary artery and the left ventricle the tip of the left auricular appendage is just visible.

The parallel superior vascular structures from right to left, therefore, are the superior vena cava, the ascending aorta, and the main pulmonary artery. The main pulmonary artery is 4 to 5 cm in length and passes posteriorly across the ascending aorta, and at the upper margin of the transverse pericardial sinus directly superior to the roof of the left atrium it divides into right and left pulmonary arteries. The right pulmonary artery passes transversely directly posterior to the ascending aorta. Behind the right atrial–superior vena caval junction, the right pulmonary artery divides into a superior and an inferior branch at the right lung hilum. The left pulmonary artery passes in a direct line from the main pulmonary artery posteriorly and describes an arch posteriorly and leftward to reach the hilum of the left lung. The proximal left pulmonary artery is connected to the descending aorta by the ligamentum arteriosum. This causes the left pulmonary artery to rise superiorly and then after the ligamentum attachment to pass precipitously inferiorly.

The ascending aorta arises from the aortic fibrous ring, passes superiorly, anteriorly and rightward, and then turns leftward and posterior forming the aortic arch, giving off the great vessels mentioned. Directly posterior to the ascending aorta is the right pulmonary artery. The arch of the aorta also passes over the left mainstem bronchus, thus marking this aortic arch as "left-sided." If it passes over the right mainstem bronchus it is a "right-sided" aortic arch. After the left subclavian artery arises, the aorta assumes a left paravertebral position and passes down the posterior mediastinum to the left of the midline ridge as the descending aorta. The descending aorta gives rise to 12 paired intercostal arteries as well as a variably placed, anterior spinal artery and several bronchial arteries as the major branches in the thoracic cavity.

The cardiac silhouette in the frontal plane, therefore, proceeding clockwise from the right inferior border is formed by the inferior vena cava, the right atrium, the superior vena cava, the ascending aorta, the arch of the aorta, the main pulmonary artery, the left atrial appendage, and the left ventricle. The right ventricle is not a border-forming structure in this view.

From the right lateral aspect the right or anterior heart border is formed by the right ventricle, and the posterior border is formed by the right atrium inferiorly and the left atrium superiorly. The right ventricle gives rise to the right ventricular outflow tract and pulmonary artery. The superior portion of the cardiac structures is formed by the ascending aorta anteriorly. From the left lateral aspect the right ventricle is anterior, and the posterior aspect is formed by the left atrium superiorly and the left ventricle inferiorly (Fig. 1.2). In spatial orientation the right ventricle is anterior and right and the left ventricle posterior and left. The atria are posterior and superior to the ventricles, with the right atrium rightward and anterior to the left atrium.

Viewing the heart from the posterior aspect reveals the arch of the aorta rising superiorly to the pulmonary artery, which bifurcates into a left and a right branch above the left atrium (Fig. 1.2). The right pulmonary artery passes under the aortic arch behind the ascending aorta transversely to the right above the left atrium. The left atrium receives two right and two left pulmonary veins, a superior and an inferior vein on each side. Above the right pulmonary vein is the superior vena cava and below on the right the inferior vena cava. Just to the right of the pulmonary veins posteriorly is a depression called Sondergaard's

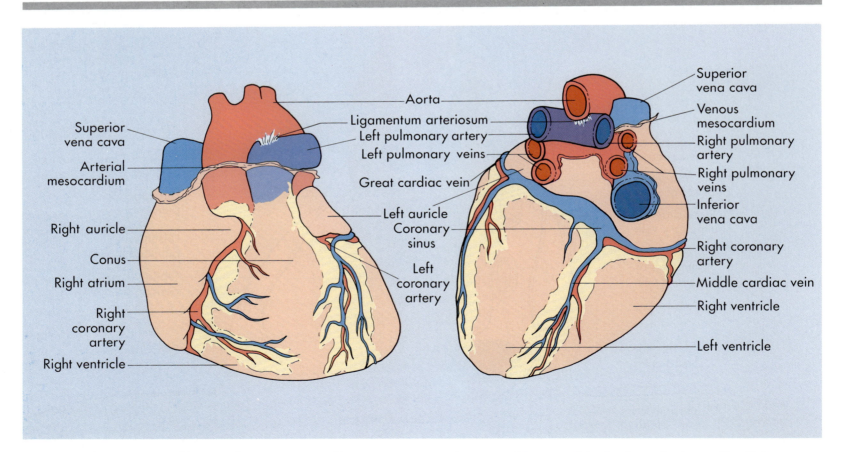

FIGURE 1.2 Left. Anterior view of heart. **Right.** Posterior view of heart. (Modified from Licata RH: Anatomy of the heart. In Liusada AA [ed]: Development and Structure of the Cardiovascular System. New York, McGraw-Hill, 1961)

groove, which is an external indentation marking the posterior interatrial septal attachment. An incision to the left of this groove brings the surgeon posteriorly into the left atrium and is one surgical approach to the mitral valve. To the right of Sondergaard's groove posteriorly is another groove, the sulcus terminalis, which corresponds to the crista terminalis on the lateral border of the smooth portion of the inner surface of the right atrium.

From this posterior view the proximity of the superior vena cava and right superior pulmonary vein can be appreciated, explaining the frequency of anomalous pulmonary venous drainage into the superior vena cava or into the right atrium. Inferior to the atria is the posterior atrioventricular groove. In the right side of this groove the right coronary artery passes posteriorly to the crux of the heart. At this point Sondergaard's groove, the left and right atrioventricular grooves, and the posterior interventricular groove all intersect. On the left side of the posterior atrioventricular groove is the coronary sinus as it passes rightward emptying into the posterior right atrium through the coronary sinus orifice.

INTERNAL STRUCTURE OF THE HEART
RIGHT ATRIUM

The interatrial septum separates the right and left atria, with the right atrium being anterior and rightward of the left atrium. During development, the interatrial septum is formed from partitioning embryonic walls, first the septum primum and later to the right the septum secundum. Neither of these embryonic septa are complete. In the embryo the septum primum fuses to the atrioventricular valve plane by contributions made from the endocardial cushions, thus closing the ostium primum orifice; as this occurs an opening appears in the septum primum that forms the foramen ovale. The septum secundum arises to the right of the septum primum and grows down as a crescent, starting superiorly and posteriorly to form a flap over the foramen ovale. Fusion of the flap to the septum primum usually occurs in the first postpartum year, but the foramen remains anatomically open in approximately 20% of adult hearts. The higher pressure in the left atrium compared with the right functionally keeps the flap pressed closed. Normally there is no left-to-right shunting of blood between the atria; however, a rise in right atrial pressure, even transiently, may open the flap creating a right-to-left shunt. This forms the basis for paradoxical emboli seen in patients who have normal hearts. If the foramen is patent, transient right-to-left shunting can be demonstrated by contrast echocardiography even in the normal heart during some phases of the cardiac cycle. This right-to-left shunting can be accentuated whenever the pressure of the right atrium is raised compared with the left atrium, for instance, after release of the Valsalva maneuver.

In the adult heart traces of these two embryonic septa can be seen. The foramen ovale is closed by the septum secundum, forming the fossa of the foramen ovale, which is about the size of a dime but occasionally the size of a quarter or even half-dollar. Because the fossa is formed mainly of fibrous tissue with some interspersed atrial muscle, it responds easily to changes in pressure on each side of the septum and can be seen by echocardiography to bulge into the atrium and form what has been called an aneurysm of the foramen ovale. With abnormally increased right atrial pressure, the fossa can be seen to bulge toward the left atrium.

Superior and posterior to the fossa is a ridge of atrial muscle, the limbus of the fossa ovale; this is an important landmark that is useful in the performance of trans-septal left-sided heart catheterization. In this procedure the Brockenbrough needle sheathed within the catheter is moved down from the superior vena cava into the right atrium. As the needle in the catheter is drawn into the right atrium, it presses against the atrial septum; and as it passes over the limbus it suddenly springs against the flexible fossa. This sudden movement of the catheter can be seen and felt, indicating to the operator that the catheter is in the proper place to accomplish atrial septal puncture.

The free wall of the right atrium can be seen to have fine muscular ridges, the pectinate muscles (Fig. 1.3). These are thin muscular col-

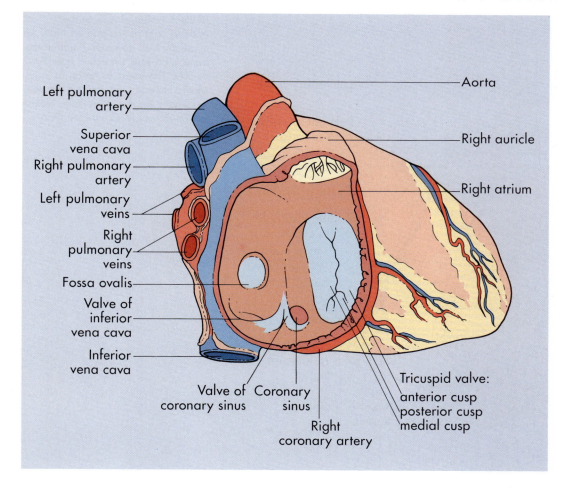

FIGURE 1.3 Right anterior oblique view of the opened right atrium. (Modified from Patten BM: The heart. In Anson BJ [ed]: Morris' Human Anatomy: A Complete Systematic Treatise. New York, Blakiston Division of McGraw-Hill, 1966)

umns, and between them the wall is only a millimeter or so thick; for this reason a catheter pressed against the wall of the right atrium looks as if it is right against the lung on fluoroscopy. If getting the catheter up against what appears to be lung is impossible, a thickened pericardium or pericardial effusion can be suspected. This thin atrial wall also explains the ease with which it can be perforated by stiff catheters.

The inferior vena cava enters the right atrium inferiorly. It is guarded by a thin, incompetent, valvular structure along its ventral aspect called the valve of the inferior vena cava or the eustachian valve. The orifice of the inferior vena cava is immediately rightward and inferior to the fossa ovalis, which embryonically was the foramen ovale (Fig. 1.4). In the fetus this arrangement allowed the oxygenated venous blood coming from the placenta to pass directly through the foramen ovale to the left atrium and left ventricle and thus out the aorta, bypassing the right side of the heart and lung. Its proximity to the fossa also explains the ease of catheter passage through secundum atrial septal defects when approached from the inferior vena cava. Immediately anterior to the inferior vena cava on the wall of the right atrium between the fossa ovalis and tricuspid annulus anteriorly is the ostium of the coronary sinus; it is guarded by another remnant valvular structure, the valve of the coronary sinus or thebesian valve.

Extending between the right side of the inferior and superior vena caval orifices is a muscle ridge, the crista terminalis, which fades inferiorly into the valve of the inferior vena cava. The wall of the right atrium between the crista terminalis laterally and the interatrial septum is smooth wall without pectinate muscles and is called the sinus venarum cavarum (Fig. 1.5). Embryologically this is derived from the right horn of the embryonic sinus venosus, whereas the trabeculated, pectinate-lined portion of the atrium is derived from the embryonic atrium.

The crista terminalis inferiorly gives rise to the thebesian and eusta-

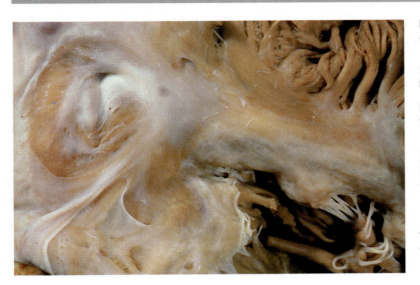
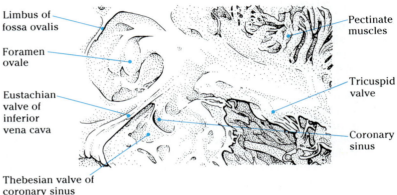

FIGURE 1.4 View of the inferior right atrium and a portion of the tricuspid valve orifice demonstrating various internal structures.

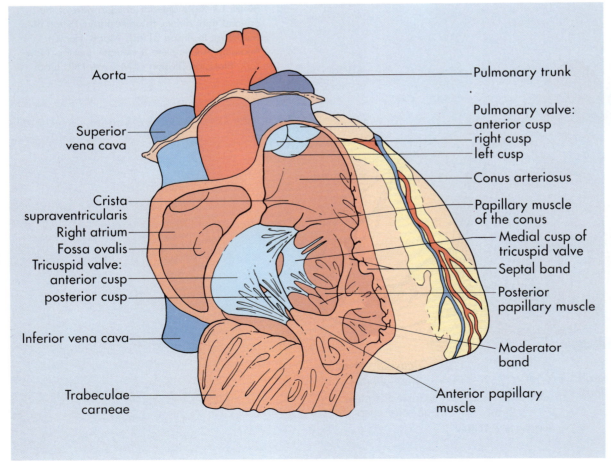

FIGURE 1.5 Ventral view of the opened right atrium and ventricle. An unusually well developed moderator band is present. (Modified from Patten BM: The heart. In Anson BJ [ed]: Morris' Human Anatomy: A Complete Systematic Treatise. New York, Blakiston Division of McGraw-Hill, 1966)

chian valves within the right atrial wall. From the place where the two valves come together a fibrous band called the tendon of Todara passes deep into the septal wall onto the pillar of the fossa ovalis and blends into the right fibrous trigone (see Fig. 1.4). Occasionally other strandlike structures can arise from this area, extending into the right atrial cavity. These fibrous structures, called the Chiari network, can be seen on two-dimensional echocardiography as structures moving in the cavity of the right atrium.

The superior vena cava enters the right atrium in the superior aspect and is unguarded by any valvular structure. It is in an almost direct line with the inferior vena cava but slightly anterior in its placement. Opening into the right atrium multiple small orifices of thebesian vessels can be seen, especially on the septal and lateral walls. The right atrioventricular orifice is situated in the floor of the right atrium, directed anteriorly, inferiorly, and leftward, and guarded by the tricuspid valve.

TRICUSPID VALVE

The tricuspid valve is attached to the right atrioventricular ring and hangs into the right ventricle. The leaflets have a continuous line of attachment running around the atrioventricular ring and crossing the middle of the membranous interventricular septum medially (Fig. 1.6). The free edges are notched, forming commissures that divide the valve roughly into three leaflets, the large anterior leaflet and smaller posterior and septal leaflets. The notchings of the edge of the leaflet are variable in depth. The leaflet is attached by fibrous chords called chordae tendineae to the papillary muscles. The chordae originate from the papillary muscles and branch once or twice before attaching to the leaflet (Fig. 1.7). Attachments are along the leaflet edge as well as on the ventricular surface of the leaflets for a variable distance from the free edge. The atrial surface of the valve is smooth and glistening; this is the surface that coapts during systole, closing the orifice by

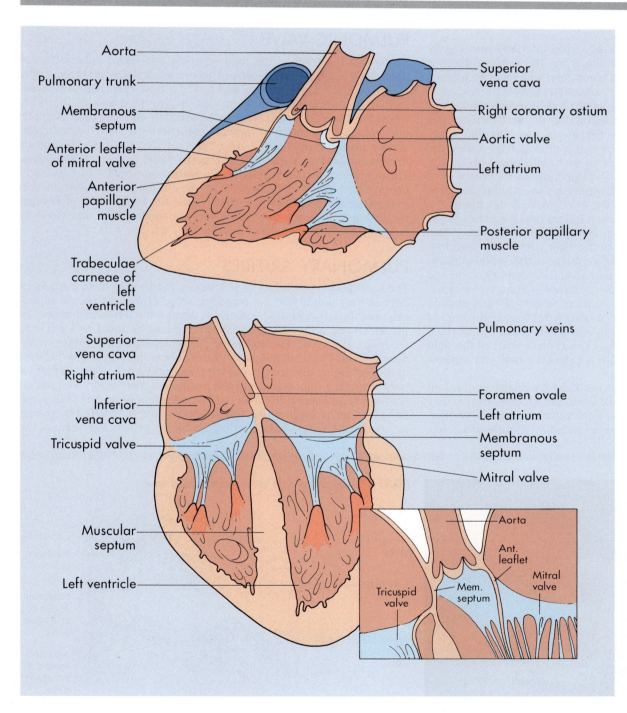

FIGURE 1.6 **A.** View of the opened left atrium and ventricle. **B.** Four-chamber view of the heart. (Modified from Licata RH: Anatomy of the heart. In Liusada AA [ed]: Development and Structure of the Cardiovascular System. New York, McGraw-Hill, 1961)

pressing the distal atrial surfaces of the leaflets together. The ventricular surface of the valve is roughened by the attachments of the chordae. The thinnest chordae are attached to the leaflet edge, and as the chordae are attached to the ventricular surface of the leaflet away from the free edge they become thicker. Each leaflet receives chordae from more than one papillary muscle, and each papillary muscle sends chordae to more than one valve leaflet (see Fig. 1.7).

The anterior leaflet arises from the sternocostal area of the tricuspid annulus and is reinforced by muscle inferiorly from the parietal band of the crista supraventricularis. The chordae to this leaflet arise primarily from the anterior papillary muscle. The septal cusp arises from an attachment related to the membranous septum. The chordae here are primarily from the papillary muscle to the septum. The posterior leaflet arises from the tricuspid annulus adjacent to the right atrial floor, and the chordae arise primarily from a number of small papillary muscles along the right ventricular floor. There can be supernumary leaflets at the intervalvular spaces.

RIGHT VENTRICLE

The right atrioventricular orifice leads anteriorly, inferiorly, and slightly leftward into the right ventricle (see Fig. 1.5). The right ventricle is roughly triangular with a thin wall that is enfolded with muscle columns called trabeculae carnae that make up about two thirds of the thickness of the wall with a narrow, compact layer of muscle externally. The inflow tract of the right ventricle is below the tricuspid orifice. The outflow tract forms the apex of the triangle at the pulmonic valve. Separating the inflow and outflow tracts is a muscle ridge called the crista supraventricularis, which forms an arch with one limb on the ventricular septum, the septal band, and one limb on the free wall of the right ventricle, the parietal band. It represents the inferior margin of the embryologic conus arteriosus. The third side of the triangle is formed by the ventricular septum, which bulges into the cavity of the right ventricle because the pressure on the left is so much higher than that on the right. The cross-section of the right ventricle is therefore crescentic. Characteristic of the right ventricle is the septal surface, deeply trabeculated with trabeculae carnae and columnar carnae and also a muscular trabecular column called the moderator band, which is present in many hearts and connects the distal portion of the septum to the free wall (see Fig. 1.5). This band usually terminates in the area of the anterior papillary muscle in the right ventricle and can be identified on two-dimensional echocardiography. The cephalic part of the right ventricle leading to the pulmonic valve is called the conus or outflow tract of the right ventricle.

The papillary muscles of the right ventricle are relatively constant but not as constant as those of the left ventricle. An anterior papillary muscle is on the anterior wall of the right ventricle near its junction with the septum; also, a constant, small papillary muscle arises just under the septal limb of the crista supraventricularis at the inferior border of the right ventricular outflow tract connecting to the septal leaflet of the tricuspid valve. Additionally, an inconstant group of posterior papillary muscles arises from the diaphragmatic wall of the right ventricle.

The right ventricle is thus characterized by several anatomical features: (1) the roughly triangular shape; (2) the separation of the right ventricular inflow from outflow tract by the crista supraventricularis; (3) the tricuspid valve, the septal leaflet of which embryologically is contributed by endocardial cushion tissue; (4) the discrete right bundle branch, which travels along the septum; (5) the papillary muscle of the conus; (6) the conus of the right ventricle or outflow tract; (7) the deep trabeculation of the right ventricular septal surface; and (8) the moderator band. Many of these features can be recognized by angiography, echocardiography, magnetic resonance imaging, or computed tomography. In patients with congenital heart disease, the ability to recognize the features of the right and left ventricles is key to understanding the anatomy of the congenital anomaly (see Fig. 1.5).

PULMONIC VALVE

Situated at the apex of the right ventricle and facing superiorly and posteriorly is the pulmonic valve. This semilunar valve has three cusps, a right and left anterior cusp and a single posterior cusp, which are named according to their orientation to the main axis of the body when the heart is in situ. The cusps are thin with fibrocartilaginous thickenings at the point of mutual coaptation, the noduli Arantii. Radiating from the nodule out over the fundus of the cusp are fibrous thickenings and along the edges crescentic thickenings called lunulae. The pulmonic cusps are similar to the aortic cusps but thinner, as might be expected owing to the lower diastolic closing pressure sustained in the pulmonary artery compared with that in the aorta. The leaflets open by flexing at the base into a rounded triangular orifice and close by coapting their distal ventricular surfaces (Figs. 1.8, 1.9).

PULMONARY ARTERIES

The main pulmonary artery or pulmonary trunk arises from the pulmonary fibrous ring above the pulmonic valve cusps and passes superiorly, slightly leftward, and posteriorly around the left medial aspect of the ascending aorta; it is about 3 cm in diameter and 4 to 5 cm long (see Figs. 1.2, 1.16). Just above the cusps are slight bulges, the pulmonary sinuses. The main pulmonary artery bifurcates just above the level of the left atrium into a right and left pulmonary artery. The left pulmonary artery is a continuation of the main pulmonary artery and passes posteriorly and superiorly over the left mainstem bronchus. This superior-posterior passage of the left pulmonary artery is aided by the attachment of a ligamentum arteriosus, which connects the origin of the

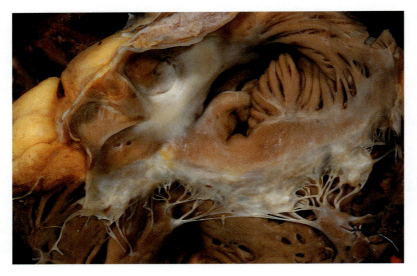

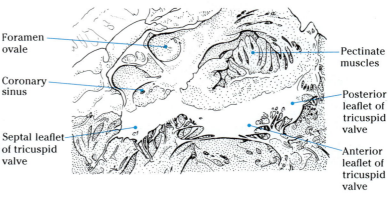

FIGURE 1.7 View of the right atrium and tricuspid valve.

left pulmonary artery with the initial portion of the descending aorta. The left pulmonary artery then continues sharply inferiorly. From the superior and anterior surface of the left pulmonary artery four branches to the upper lobe of the lung arise. The remainder of the left pulmonary vessels pass inferiorly to the lower lobe and lingula.

The right pulmonary artery passes rightward and slightly posteriorly behind the ascending aorta, lying on the superior surface of the left atrium, and enters the posterior mediastinum. The right pulmonary artery lies anterior to the right mainstem bronchus and posterior to the superior vena cava and the right superior pulmonary vein. The pulmonary artery at the hilum of the right lung divides into two major branches: the superior or ascending trunk, supplying the right upper lobe, and the descending or interlobular trunk, supplying the middle and lower lobes.

The pulmonary artery bifurcations generally follow the bronchial bifurcations and supply similar pulmonary segments. The relationship of the pulmonary arteries to the bronchi is important in that their positions can be seen on the chest x-ray film and they identify the "anatomical" right and left lungs. On the right the pulmonary artery passes anteriorly and inferiorly to the right bronchus and therefore the right bronchus is "eparterial." The left upper lobe bronchus is inferior to the left pulmonary artery, thus making this bronchus "hyparterial."

LEFT ATRIUM

The left atrium is to the left of and posterior to the right atrium; it is also inferior to the right pulmonary artery and lies posterior to the aortic root (see Figs. 1.8, 1.9). The left auricular appendage extends anteriorly to the left of the pulmonary trunk (see Fig. 1.2). The left atrial endocardium is more opaque than that of the right atrium. The pectinate muscles in the left atrium are confined to the tubular left atrial appendage. The rest of the left atrium is smooth. Four veins open into the left atrium posteriorly, two right and two left superior and inferior pulmonary veins. The right pulmonary veins drain into the left atrium near the atrial septum. The left pulmonary veins enter the left lateral wall of the left atrium. The atrial septum is smooth, although the limits of the fossa ovalis can usually be distinguished and represent the vestige of the original septum primum, which adhered to the developing septal wall of the septum secundum. Semilunar indentations can be seen, and occasionally these are not fixed to the wall, allowing probe patency of the interatrial septum. The left atrioventricular or mitral valve lies on the inferior anterior floor of the left atrium facing anteriorly, inferiorly, and to the left (Fig. 1.10).

MITRAL VALVE

The mitral valve, named fancifully for a bishop's mitre, guards the entrance to the left ventricle; it is attached to the mitral annulus and is composed of two leaflets, an aortic or anterior leaflet roughly oval in shape and a longer, narrower mural or posterior leaflet (see Fig. 1.9). The leaflets hang down into the cavity of the left ventricle in a curtain-like manner and are anchored to the left ventricle by chordae tendineae arising from papillary muscles and, in the case of the posterior leaflet, also directly from the left ventricular wall. The anterior leaflet actually hangs from a confluenced mitral ring and noncoronary and left coronary portions of the aortic ring (Fig. 1.11). The portion of the leaflet from its aortic ring attachment to the point of flexion of the anterior leaflet is known as the intervalvular membrane. The opening of the left ventricle, called the left ventricular os, is composed of nonmuscular fibrous structures and contains the mitral valve to the left and posterior and the aortic valve to the right and anterior. The left ventricle is separated by the aortic leaflet of the mitral valve into an inflow tract posteriorly and an outflow tract anteriorly (see Figs. 1.6, 1.11).

The mitral leaflet edges are scalloped, and "commissures," defined

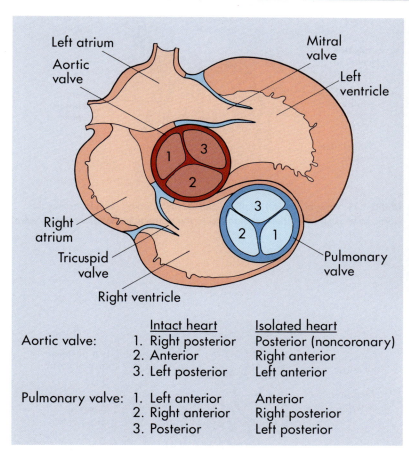

FIGURE 1.8 Diagram showing relationship of the cardiac valves. (Modified from Licata RH: Anatomy of the heart. In Liusada AA [ed]: Development and Structure of the Cardiovascular System. New York, McGraw-Hill, 1961)

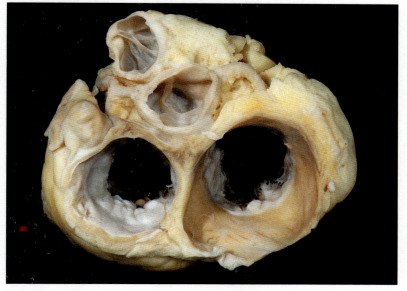

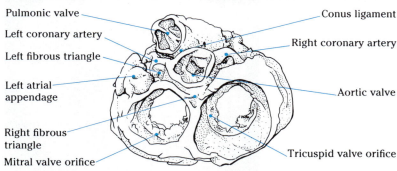

FIGURE 1.9 Superior view of the heart with the atria and epicardial fat removed.

as deepened clefts with fanlike chordae, can be identified. The two primary commissures separating the anterior and posterior leaflets are the anterolateral commissure and the posteromedial commissure (Fig. 1.10). The posterior leaflet may have two other minor commissural clefts dividing the posterior leaflet into three scallops: the anterolateral, the middle, and the posteromedial scallops. The importance of this relatively minor detail is that each of these scallops can prolapse into the left atrium individually and form a distinct angiographic picture.

The chordae tendineae attach to the leaflets along the free margins and also on the ventricular surface away from the free edge. This divides the valve into two parts: a rough, crescentic area adjacent to the edge that is the widest, about 1 cm at the center of the leaflet, narrowing as it approaches the commissures; and a smooth portion that extends medially and superiorly to become the intervalvular membrane, which attaches at the noncoronary and left coronary portions of the aortic annulus. The posterior leaflet hangs from the position of the mitral annulus situated adjacent to the coronary sinus.

The closure of the mitral valve in systole is accomplished by coapting or pressing the atrial surfaces of the mitral valve leaflets together. This overlap of coapted surfaces is important in the proper closing of the mitral valve. The valve is kept from inverting into the left atrium by the chordae. The chordae tendineae arise from the anterolateral and posteromedial papillary muscles and distribute to both leaflets (see Fig. 1.10). The chordae can be divided into three groups:

1. The first-order chordae originate as thickened fibroelastic chords at the tips of the papillary muscles and insert into the free edges of the valve. As they approach the leaflets they become thinner and divide once or twice.
2. The second-order chordae also arise as thickened, strong, tendinous chords at or near the papillary muscle tips and insert on the ventricular surface of the cusps. These are stronger chordae.
3. The third-order chordae originate from the left ventricular wall near the attachments of the cusps and attach to the ventricular surface of the posterior leaflet only.

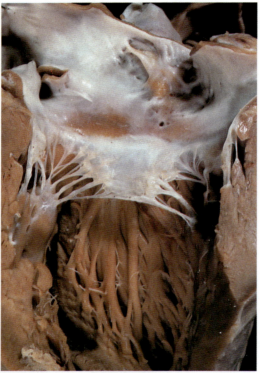

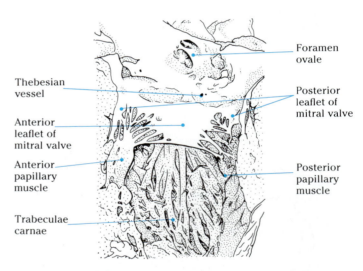

FIGURE 1.10 View of the left atrium and left ventricle. The cut bisects the posterior leaflet of the mitral valve.

FIGURE 1.11 View of the left ventricle and aortic opening demonstrating the aortic valve cusps and their relationship to the anterior leaflet of the mitral valve.

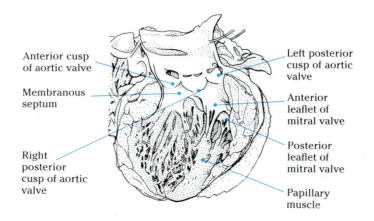

LEFT VENTRICLE

The left ventricle has a conal shape with an os or mouth filled by the aortic and mitral valves. The ventricle then tapers to the left ventricular apex (see Figs. 1.6, 1.11). The walls form the gently curving obtuse margin of the heart, about one half of the diaphragmatic wall, and the left-sided, narrow border of the anterior surface of the heart. The right anterior wall of the left ventricle is formed by the interventricular septum. The wall is about 1 cm thick and is divided into an outer two-thirds zone of compact muscle and an inner one-third trabeculated zone. The trabeculae carnae on the left are flattened because of the high pressure generated in the left ventricle. The septal surface of the ventricle has flattened trabeculae and, therefore, compared with the right ventricular surface of the interventricular septum, is smooth. The cavity of the left ventricle in diastole appears to be a football-like structure, an ellipsoid of revolution. Two papillary muscles, the anterolateral and posteromedial papillary muscles, project into the left ventricular cavity. The papillary muscles have a variable number of tips, usually two or three, with the posteromedial more variable than the anterolateral.

The left ventricle is admirably adapted to be a pressure-developing chamber. In cross-section it is circular; the interventricular septum, therefore, forms the right anterior wall of the left ventricle and is an integral part of the left ventricle and bulges into the right ventricular cavity. The outflow tract of the left ventricle is composed of the smooth, superior surface of the muscular septum, which at its apex becomes a membranous septum (see Figs. 1.6, 1.11). The other margin of the outflow tract is the anterior leaflet of the mitral valve, especially at its base. The membranous septum attaches to the right and noncoronary cusp portion of the aortic ring as well as to the tricuspid annulus and base of the atrial septum (see Figs. 1.6, 1.11).

Below the aortic valve is an area called the vestibule or subaortic sinus that is cylindrical and smooth walled. This vestibule lies relatively anterior to the rest of the left ventricle, and its borders are made of the ventricular muscle anterolaterally and by the posteromedial fibrous segments. This fibrous portion is made by the annular attachment of the anterior leaflet of the mitral valve and related membranous septum. The roof of the outlet of the subaortic sinus is the aortic valve cusps.

The ventricular septum is divided into a large, inferior muscular portion and a small, superior membranous portion. The membranous septum lies in the angle formed by the right and noncoronary cusps on the left side and attaches to the crest of the muscular septum (see Fig. 1.11). On the right side the septal leaflet and the anterior leaflet of the tricuspid valve attach to the middle of the membranous septum; therefore, part of the membranous septum on the right is above the tricuspid valve and is called the atrioventricular portion of the membranous septum and part is below the tricuspid valve (see Fig. 1.6). Defects in the membranous septum in these areas can produce either a left ventricular-to-right atrial tunnel or an interventricular septal defect.

The left ventricle is characterized by a number of "anatomical" features that distinguish it from the anatomical right ventricle: (1) the oval, football-like shape; (2) the smooth septal surface; (3) the lack of a conus or crista supraventricularis; (4) the fanlike left bundle branches; (5) the bicuspid atrioventricular valve; and (6) the intimate association of the aortic and mitral annuli, which cause the inflow and outflow tracts of the left ventricle to be separated only by the anterior leaflet of the mitral valve. Many of these features are identifiable on two-dimensional echocardiography, angiocardiography, and other imaging techniques.

Knowledge of the muscular architecture of the left ventricle is important in understanding the mechanisms of contraction of the left ventricle. The compact layer of the ventricular muscle is composed of syncytial layers of muscle cells. The muscular interventricular septum is the thickest muscle, composed of contributions from right ventricle and left ventricle, and therefore is trabeculated on both aspects.

The heart musculature is arranged in such a way that it appears to spiral inward from the superficial layers. The superficial layers run at right angles to the layers deeper in the wall. These layers are intimately interdigitated, preventing dissection into laminar structures. The origin or attachment of the muscular layers is from the fibrous skeleton at the base. These layers spiral around the ventricle and reinsert along different points of the same fibrous skeleton. One superficial layer, or aortospiral group, of muscles arises from the left half of the fibrous skeleton. The fibers arise from the aortic annulus and pass spirally around the obtuse margin of the heart and posteriorly over the diaphragmatic surface to end as muscle columns at the base of the posterior papillary muscle groups of both atrioventricular valves. A second superficial sinospiral layer arises around the orifice of the right atrioventricular valve and spirals over the anterior surface of the right ventricle. Both groups converge on the apex, forming a muscular vortex that results in anterior and posterior muscle columns in the ventricular wall and projects into the cavities as the papillary muscles.

The deeper muscle layers are less distinct. The middle layer, called the deep sinospiral muscle, originates from the mitral annulus and circles both ventricles at the base. Fibers from the deepest muscle layer posteriorly penetrate the interventricular septum along the posterior interventricular sulcus. The deepest muscle layer on the left is the deep bulbospiral muscle and originates from the septal portion of the left atrioventricular annulus. This muscle divides the left ventricular wall, forms a sphincteric band around the aortic outlet, and reattaches to the septal portion of the left atrioventricular annulus.

The fascicles of the deep bulbospiral and sinospiral muscles interdigitate in the muscular interventricular septum. The orientation of the major muscle bands results in shortening of the minor diameter on ventricular contraction. The spiral muscles on contraction pull the base of the ventricle, composed of the atrioventricular annuli, toward the apex.

AORTIC VALVE

The aortic valve guards the entrance into the aorta. It is a tricuspid, semilunar valve that is suspended from the aortic fibrous annulus. In the heart *in situ* the aortic cusps are named from their position relative to the main body axis, forming an anterior cusp and right and left posterior cusps. The coronary arteries arise just above these cusps, and the cusps also are named from the origin of the coronary arteries; thus, the anterior cusp is also known as the right coronary cusp, the left posterior as the left coronary cusp, and the right posterior as the noncoronary cusp (see Figs. 1.8, 1.11). Like the pulmonic cusps, the aortic cusps have noduli Arantii at the midportion of the free margins and crescentic lunulae.

The wall of the aorta adjacent to each cusp is dilated, forming the sinuses of Valsalva, which bulge well beyond the limits of the aortic annulus. The relation of the aortic sinuses to the rest of the heart is of interest. The anterior sinus bulges into the posterior portion of the right ventricular outflow tract. The left posterior sinus bulges over the interventricular septum anteriorly and faces the pericardial space posteriorly as well as the right pulmonary artery as it passes posteriorly to the aorta. The right posterior sinus is adjacent to the medial wall of the right atrium (see Fig. 1.8). Injury or aneurysmal formation in each of these sinuses can result in rupture and fistula formation into these respective chambers of the heart.

The three cusps close by coapting the ventricular surfaces near each free valve edge. The commissures extend to the aortic annulus. Commonly along the edges near the commissures the fibers of the cusp separate and form holes or fenestrations. These do not normally leak because they are occluded by the opposite leaflet on closure. Opening of the aortic cusps with systole results in a rounded triangular opening with flexion occurring at the base of the leaflet. Stenosis of the valve occurs if this flexion area becomes calcified.

The fibrous aortic annulus forms the junction of the connection between the aorta and the outflow (or subaortic sinus) of the left ventricle. This annulus marks the conotruncal junction, forming the transition from cardiac muscle of the left ventricle to smooth muscle of the aortic media. Not as well defined as the atrioventricular annuli, the aortic annulus consists of a wide, fibrous membrane around the base of the aorta extending inferiorly into the area of the membranous septum between the right and noncoronary cusps and into the mitral annular and anterior leaflet of the mitral valve between the left and noncoronary cusps.

CONDUCTION SYSTEM

Cardiac muscle has three fundamental properties: contractility, conductivity, and automaticity. The conduction system, both the nodes and the bundles, is composed of modified myocardial cells. The sinoatrial node and the atrioventricular node have cells where the property of spontaneous automaticity is highly developed and the His bundle and Purkinje system cells where the property of rapid conductivity is highly developed (Fig. 1.12).

The contraction of the heart is normally initiated in a mass of pacemaker nodal tissue lying subepicardially near the entrance of the superior vena cava, between the superior vena cava and the right atrial appendage on the roof of the right atrium in the superior portion of the sulcus terminalis. This mass of pacemaker cells is known as the sinoatrial (or SA node or node of Kent and Flack); it is a 3 × 7-mm structure and is derived from the myocardium of the right horn of the sinus venosus of the embryonic heart. The sinoatrial node receives its blood supply from the sinoatrial nodal artery, a branch of the artery to the orifice of the superior vena cava (Fig. 1.13). The impulse then spreads over the atrial muscle as a wave to the atrioventricular node (Fig. 1.14). At present it is believed that preferential pathways in the atrium, termed the anterior, middle, and posterior intra-atrial tracts, spread the innervation. Another pathway from the right atrium to the left atrium is called the bundle of Bachmann; however, these preferential pathways are controversial and difficult to demonstrate anatomically.

The impulse then enters the atrioventricular node (or node of Tawara), which is the slightly expanded, proximal end of the atrioventricular bundle located subendocardially in the floor of the right atrium in a fairly constant position in a triangle bounded by the orifice of the coronary sinus, the orifice of the inferior vena cava, and the small septal cusp of the right atrioventricular valve. The blood supply of the atrioventricular node is via the atrioventricular nodal artery, arising 90% of the time from the right coronary artery at the crux of the heart and 10% from the left circumflex coronary artery.

The impulse then is propagated from the atrioventricular node down the His bundle (Fig. 1.15). The His bundle runs anteriorly, perforates the right fibrous trigone, and enters the ventricular septum posteriorly and inferiorly to the membranous septum. The His bundle is 10 to 20 mm in length and 1 to 3 mm in diameter. In its central axis is found a constant artery arising from either the septal branches of the anterior descending coronary artery or from the posterior ventricular branches of either the right or the left coronary artery.

At its lower end the His bundle branches into two divisions, the right and left bundle branches (see Fig. 1.12). This bifurcation sits atop the crest of the muscular interventricular septum. The right bundle branch continues anteriorly and toward the apex for 10 to 20 mm. It is a thick branch, 1 to 3 mm in diameter, which is deeply buried in the muscle of the interventricular septum in the region of the crista supraventricularis. Near the junction of the interventricular septum and the anterior wall of the right ventricle the band becomes more compact and subendocardial and then can pass across the right ventricular cavity in the moderator band. More often the bundle runs through one of the columnae carneae to reach the right ventricular wall near the anterior papillary muscle of the right ventricle. From here it branches into a finely divided, subendocardial, anastomosing plexus. A small branch bends sharply back along the upper interventricular septum to the conus area. The blood supply to the right bundle branch is from the anterior descending coronary artery through the septal perforating vessels.

After its origin the left bundle branch crosses to the left side of the interventricular septum, spreads out as a subendocardial band of fibers, and emerges just below the membranous septum, below the commissure between the noncoronary and the right coronary cusp of the aortic valve. Functionally there are an anterior and a posterior group of branches and possibly an intermediate branch to the septum, but anatomically the divisions are not nearly so discrete. The anterior division runs anteriorly and toward the apex, forming a subendocardial plexus with branching at the area of the anterolateral papillary muscle. The posterior fascicles reach the area of the posteromedial papillary

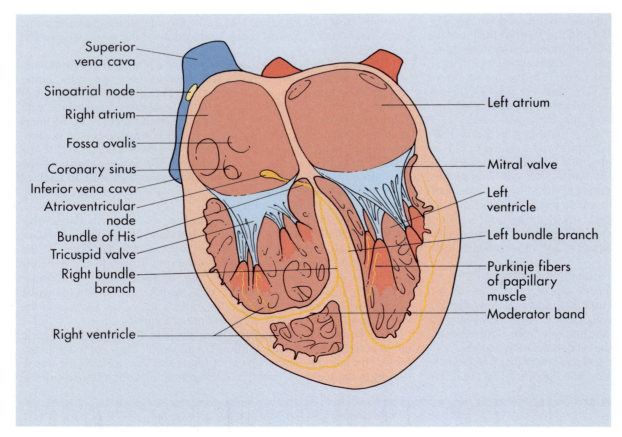

FIGURE 1.12 Diagram of the opened heart showing the location and relations of the conduction system. (Modified from Barry A, Patten BM: The structure of the human heart. In Gould SE [ed]: Pathology of the Heart. Springfield, IL, Charles C Thomas, 1968)

muscle. From there division occurs into the subendocardial plexus, spreading to the rest of the left ventricular muscle. The fibers distributing to the ventricular muscles are known as Purkinje fibers. These fibers are spread intramurally from subendocardium toward the epicardium.

Accessory atrioventricular bundles that connect atrium to ventricle in electrically low-resistance pathways that form the basis for Wolff-Parkinson-White syndrome or accelerated atrioventricular conduction have been described by Kent.[1] These so-called bundles of Kent can be situated anywhere along atrioventricular rings. Mahaim,[2] in 1931, also described "paraspecific" septal fibers leaving the left side of the bundle of His at the membranous septal area and reaching the upper left septum, and James[3] described fibers that bypass the atrioventricular node going into the His bundle. Each of these bypass tracts form the anatomical base for described electrocardiographic abnormalities.

CARDIAC VESSELS
CORONARY ARTERIES

The ostia of the coronary arteries are funnel-like depressions in the anterior and left posterior coronary sinus about the center of the sinus of Valsalva at the apex of the concavity of the sinus, usually at 1 to 2 mm above or below the level of the commissures (see Figs. 1.11, 1.16). There is usually one ostium for the left coronary artery in the left posterior coronary sinus and one ostium for the right coronary artery in the anterior sinus of Valsalva. Occasionally there will be two ostia from the right, one for the conus branch of the right coronary artery, and very occasionally two from the left, one for the anterior descending and one for the circumflex coronary artery.

The left coronary artery is a muscular artery arising from the lateral

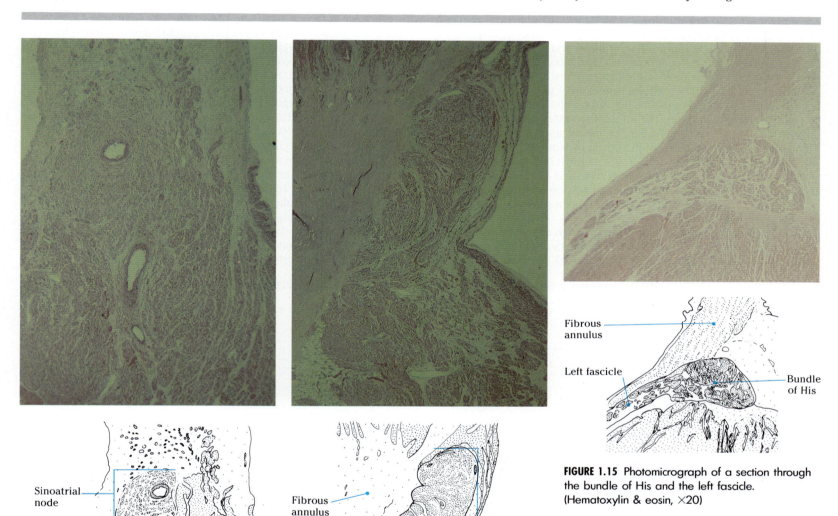

FIGURE 1.13 Photomicrograph of a section through the sinoatrial node. (Hematoxylin & eosin, ×25)

FIGURE 1.14 Photomicrograph of a section through the atrioventricular node. (Hematoxylin & eosin, ×31)

FIGURE 1.15 Photomicrograph of a section through the bundle of His and the left fascicle. (Hematoxylin & eosin, ×20)

wall of the left posterior sinus and passing behind the junction of the right ventricular outflow tract and pulmonary trunk to the left and anteriorly between the pulmonary artery anteriorly and the left atrium posteriorly (see Figs. 1.9, 1.16). The left main coronary artery can be 1 mm to over 1 cm long before it bifurcates, usually just under the left atrial appendage into the left anterior descending coronary artery and the left circumflex coronary artery. The coronary arteries lie in loose areolar connective tissue in epicardial fat. The anterior descending coronary artery passes to the anterior interventricular sulcus and down the anterior surface of the heart between the right and left ventricles to and frequently around the apex and onto the distal inferior surface of the heart (see Fig. 1.16). This vessel usually gives off a large septal perforator, which dives perpendicularly into the interventricular septum, and then a series of septal branches that supply the anterior two thirds of the muscular interventricular septum. On the surface of the right ventricle are small ventricular branches from the left anterior descending coronary artery. On the anterior surface of the left ventricle are one or more diagonal branches that can be a large and important source of blood supply for the anterior left ventricular wall.

As it travels in the left atrioventricular sulcus the left circumflex artery gives off one to three anterior branches, one lateral, and one posterior branch to the left atrium. Inferiorly it gives off varying numbers of obtuse marginal branches that supply the lateral and left posterior wall of the left ventricle. The circumflex artery continues in the left atrioventricular sulcus around the left lateral and posterior aspect of the heart and is buried beneath the coronary sinus as it passes posteriorly to the crux of the heart (Fig. 1.17). In most hearts it ends before it reaches the crux. Occasionally in the so-called left dominant circulation (about 15% of hearts) it continues across the crux and supplies the posterior descending coronary artery and even portions of the posterior right ventricle.

The superior vena cava ostial artery, which gives rise to the sinoatrial nodal artery arises from the left circumflex artery in about 25% of hearts and from the right coronary artery in 70%; in about 5% of hearts it arises from both circumflex and right coronary arteries. On occasion, instead of bifurcating the left main coronary artery trifurcates into an anterior descending, a circumflex, and a vessel between them termed the *intermedius artery*, which replaces a first obtuse marginal artery and supplies the anterolateral portion of the left ventricle.

The right coronary artery arises from its ostium in the anterior sinus of Valsalva and passes rightward and anteriorly behind the base of the pulmonary artery and its sinus and in front of and under the right auricular appendage. It passes into the right atrioventricular sulcus (see Fig. 1.16). The first branch, the branch to the right ventricular conus, passes anteriorly to the outflow tract of the right ventricle; in about 20% of hearts it arises as a separate orifice from the anterior sinus of Valsalva. It is important that this be known, as it forms a major source of collateralization to the left anterior descending coronary artery when this vessel is occluded and therefore should be visualized during coronary arteriography. An early branch of the right coronary artery is to the superior vena cava orifice. There are also branches to the right atrium. The right coronary artery gives one to three anterior ventricular branches to the free wall of the right ventricle, and at the acute margin of the heart a large vessel supplying the anterior wall of the right ventricle called the acute marginal coronary artery is given off. The right coronary artery continues in the anterior atrioventricular groove until it reaches the acute margin of the heart, where it turns posteriorly, passing under the arch of the inferior vena cava as it joins the right atrium. The right coronary artery continues to the crux of the heart, where it bends anterosuperiorly into the interatrial septum, giving off in 90% of hearts the artery to the atrioventricular node, which passes in the base of the interatrial septum superiorly and anteriorly to supply the atrioventricular node. The right coronary artery then turns inferiorly in the posterior interventricular sulcus, supplying the diaphragmatic wall of the left ventricle and right ventricle as the posterior descending coronary artery (see Fig. 1.17). This vessel gives off septal perforators shorter than those given off by the anterior descending coronary artery and supplying the posterior one third of the septum. The posterior

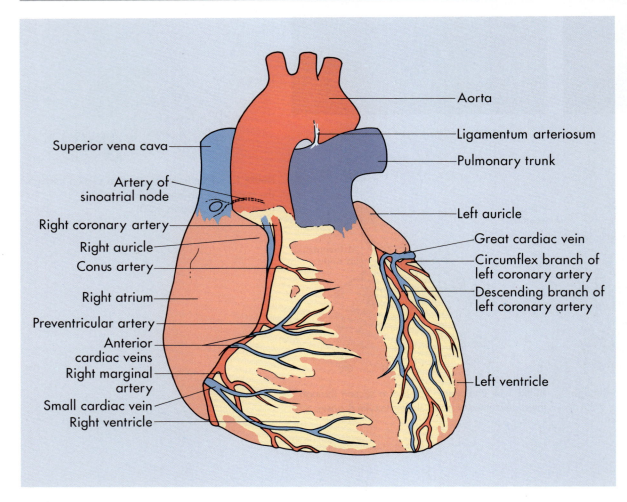

FIGURE 1.16 Coronary vessels of the ventral surface of the heart. (Modified from Barry A, Patten BM: The structure of the human heart. In Gould SE [ed]: Pathology of the Heart. Springfield, IL, Charles C Thomas, 1968)

descending coronary artery wraps around the apex and supplies the distal anterior wall of the left ventricle in a minority of hearts. In over 20% of the hearts the right coronary artery continues in the left atrioventricular groove, giving off one to three posterolateral branches supplying the posterior diaphragmatic wall of the left ventricle. The distribution of the terminal right coronary artery is reciprocally related to that of the left circumflex artery, and variations in coronary anatomy in the posterior aspect of the heart depend on whether the right coronary artery is dominant (75% of hearts) or the left coronary is dominant (10% of hearts). In about 5% of hearts both circumflex and right coronary arteries supply posterior descending branches to the diaphragmatic surface of the left ventricle. In about 5% of hearts the right coronary artery is very small congenitally, supplying only branches to the right ventricle, with the entire left ventricle supplied by the left coronary artery.

INTRAMURAL VESSELS

The superficial coronary arteries penetrate into the ventricular muscle at right angles. From these perforating vessels arise richly branching and anastomosing complexes of vessels in the walls of all four chambers, which eventually become the capillaries, forming a network of vessels around each muscle fiber. The exact nature of these branching vessels varies: some vessels perforate to the endocardium, where they branch in a treelike fashion; others are given off at right angles in comblike patterns at different levels of the ventricular wall (Fig. 1.18).

Ideas vary about whether there are anastomotic connections between perforating arteries in the subendocardial area or whether perforating arteries supply the muscle fibers in which they run and are thus end arteries. Probably both systems are present. The endocardium, especially in the papillary muscles and in the thick left ventricle are supplied either through the superficial epicardial coronary arteries, where they are at the extremity of the blood supply, or from the cavity of the ventricle through so-called luminal channels. There are also arterioluminal channels, described by Wearn and co-workers[4] in 1933, where arteriolar vessels empty directly through intertrabecular spaces into the ventricular cavity. Over the years various direct connections of coronary vessels to ventricular and atrial cavities have been described, the names depending on the histology of the small vessels involved. Other vessels found were thin walled, resembling capillaries, but with lumina variable in size and shape; these were called sinusoids, some of which empty directly into the cavity of the ventricle and some of which connect with venous structures, which then empty into the ventricular chamber. These have been called venoluminal channels. The lumina of these various vessels can be seen in the endocardium of the chambers. They are collectively known as thebesian veins but more appropriately should be called thebesian vessels, because they actually could be any of the four types of vessels. They are usually described as being more abundant on the right than on the left side and more abundant in the atria than in the ventricles.

From injection of hearts at autopsy with opaque material and postmortem x-rays and dissection, evidence is obtained that at the subarteriolar level there are collateral connections of approximately 100 μm and even over 200 μm between the various major arterial systems, most frequently about the apex and through the interventricular septum but also in the interatrial septum, at the crux of the heart, and also between the sinus node artery and other atrial arteries and over the anterior surface of the right ventricle. In the human there are few epicardial coronary artery collateral vessels in the heart with normal coronary circulation; these potential intramural collateral vessels, however, become large and important when coronary disease and obstruction

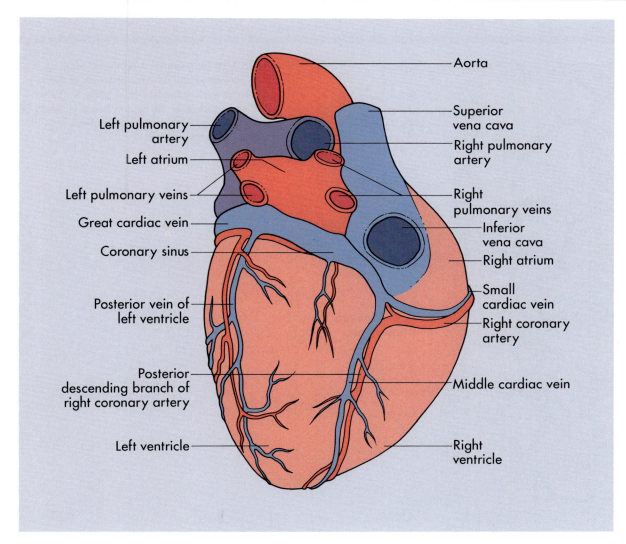

FIGURE 1.17 Coronary vessels of the dorsocaudal surface of the heart. (Modified from Patten BM: The heart. In Anson BJ [ed]: Morris' Human Anatomy: A Complete Systematic Treatise. New York, Blakiston Division of McGraw-Hill, 1966)

to the epicardial coronary vessels occurs. There are also extracoronary anastomotic connections between the coronary arteries and the systemic arteries, mostly at the base of the pulmonary artery and aorta and around the ostia of the pulmonary veins and the vena cavae; these structures connect branches of the pericardial vessels from the internal mammary and the intercostal arterial system and the coronary arteries, mostly at the pericardial reflections.

CORONARY VENOUS SYSTEM

The coronary veins in general follow distribution similar to the major coronary arteries and return blood from the myocardial capillaries to the right atrium, for the most part through the coronary sinus. The veins lie in the subepicardial fat, usually superficial to the coronary arteries (see Figs. 1.16, 1.17).

The *great cardiac vein* lies in the anterior interventricular sulcus and parallels the anterior descending coronary artery. It drains toward the base and then follows the circumflex artery posteriorly in the left atrioventricular groove and empties into the coronary sinus just beneath the left inferior pulmonary vein. This vein has valves at its entrance to the coronary sinus. Throughout its course it receives tributaries from the anterior interventricular septum, the walls of the left ventricle and right ventricle, and the left atrium, each guarded by valves at its entrance to the great cardiac vein. The posterior vein of the left ventricle drains into the coronary sinus at its distal end.

The *middle cardiac vein* runs in the posterior interventricular sulcus along with the posterior descending coronary artery. It receives tributaries from the posterior interventricular septum and ventricular walls and drains into the coronary sinus nearly at its ostium in the right atrium.

The *small cardiac vein* originates on the surface of the right ventricle, following the course of the acute marginal artery. It receives tributaries from the right ventricle and then parallels the right coronary artery in the right atrioventricular sulcus, receiving tributaries from the right atrium and the right ventricle and finally emptying into the coronary sinus near its entrance into the right atrium.

There are 3 to 12 *anterior cardiac veins* that lie on the anterior aspect of the right ventricle and drain through the wall of the right ventricle in the conal region, emptying into the small cardiac vein or directly into the right atrium through separate orifices.

The *coronary sinus* is formed as a continuation of the great cardiac vein and is 3 to 5 mm in diameter and 2 to 5 cm long. It runs in the posterior atrioventricular sulcus, receiving veins from the posterior left ventricle and the left atrium. A small vein draining down from the roof and posterior aspect of the left atrium between the right and left pulmonary veins, called the oblique vein of the left atrium or the vein of Marshall, is the remnant of the embryologic left common cardinal vein. In patients with a persistant left superior vena cava this vein persists as the communication to the coronary sinus.

CARDIAC LYMPHATICS

The lymphatic drainage of the heart is extensive. There is a subendocardial plexus of valved lymphatic vessels in the subendocardial connective tissue of all four chambers. This drains through the myocardial plexus of lymphatics, forming a weave of anastomotic lymphatic channels about the myocardial fibers. These drain in the interstitial connective tissue outward to the epicardium, where they form the epicardial plexus of lymphatic vessels. These join to form several constant large lymphatic channels that follow the coronary arteries and veins. Each of these major trunks drains into the atrioventricular sulcus and unite to form a single, large lymphatic trunk that courses over the top of the left main coronary artery under the arch of the main pulmonary artery and left pulmonary artery, passing leftward of the aortic valve and leaving the pericardium to join the left mediastinal plexus of vessels. These drain into the mediastinal lymph nodes and then into the thoracic duct.

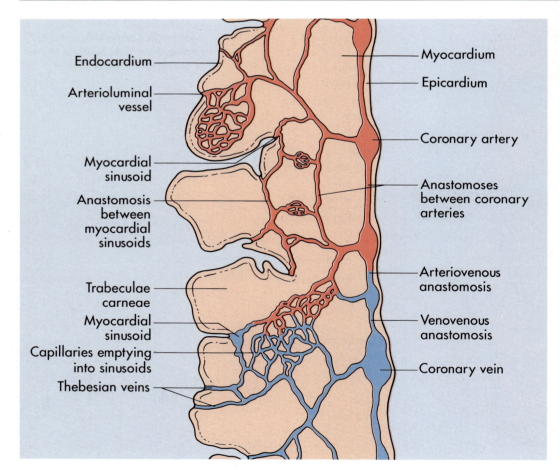

FIGURE 1.18 Diagram showing the relationship between intramural vascular channels of the ventricular wall. (Modified from Barry A, Patten BM: The structure of the human heart. In Gould SE [ed]: Pathology of the Heart. Springfield, IL, Charles C Thomas, 1968)

CARDIAC INNERVATION

The heart receives both parasympathetic and sympathetic afferent and efferent nerves. The preganglionic neurons of the sympathetic nervous system are located within the upper five or six thoracic levels of the spinal cord. These synapse with second-order neurons in the cervical sympathetic ganglia. The postganglionic sympathetic fibers terminate in the heart and great vessels. The preganglionic neurons of the parasympathetic system are located in the dorsal efferent nucleus of the medulla. These fibers pass as branches of the vagus nerve to the heart and great vessels, where they synapse with second-order neurons located in ganglia on the wall of the heart and great vessels (Fig. 1.19).

The autonomic nerves seen grossly for the most part carry both sympathetic and parasympathetic fibers entering the heart from the mediastinum by way of the dorsal mesocardia. The autonomic nerves are intimately interdigitated within two cardiac neuroplexuses, for convenience divided into a superficial cardiac plexus located on the anterior surface of the ascending aorta arch and over the pulmonary trunk and a deep cardiac plexus located to the right of the trachea above its bifurcation between the trachea and the right side of the aortic arch.

Because the left fourth and sixth embryonic aortic arches give rise to the arch of the aorta and ductus arteriosus, cardiac branches of the left vagus nerve and sympathetics from the left are distributed primarily to the aortic arch and pulmonary trunk to form the arterial or conotruncal plexus. In contrast to the arterial side, the venous side embryologically favors the right-sided structures. The right superior vena cava is retained, and the sinus venosus is shifted to the right from midline, entering the right atrium; therefore, the venous part of the heart is associated with the cardiac nerves from the right cardiac or sinoatrial plexus.

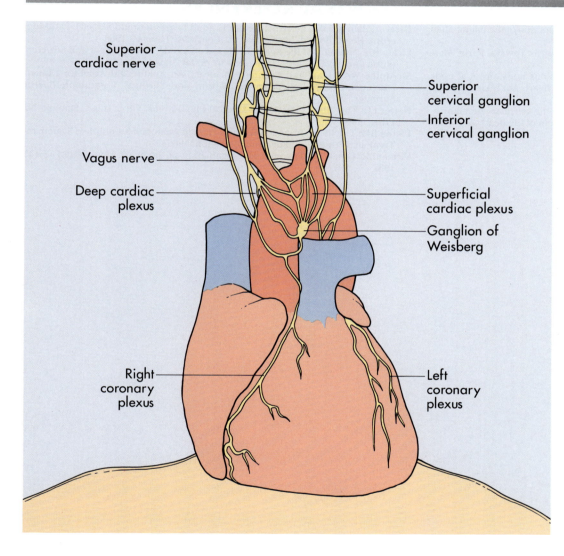

FIGURE 1.19 Nerve supply to the heart. (Modified from Tandler J. In Anson BJ [ed]: Lehrbuch der Systematischen Anatomie. Berlin, Springer-Verlag, 1926)

The sympathetic contributions arise from the superior and middle cervical ganglia, giving off, respectively, the superior and middle cardiac nerves. The inferior cardiac nerve arises from the fusion of the inferior cervical ganglion and the first thoracic ganglion, called the stellate ganglion. Each vagus nerve contributes to the cardiac plexuses by way of the superior and inferior cervical nerves and a thoracic cardiac branch from the recurrent laryngeal nerve. The superficial cardiac plexus derives its contributions from the inferior cervical cardiac branch of the left vagus nerve and the left superior cardiac nerves of the sympathetic nervous system. The ganglion of Wrisberg is associated with this plexus, lying between the aortic arch and the pulmonary trunk to the right of the ligamentum arteriosum.

The deep cervical plexus is formed by the three sympathetic cardiac nerves on the right and the three cardiac branches of the right vagus nerve; the superior, cervical, and thoracic cardiac branches of the left vagus nerve; the middle and inferior cardiac nerves of the sympathetic trunk; and direct branches from the five or six thoracic sympathetic ganglia.

From these plexuses the sympathetic and vagal nerves are distributed to the walls of the great vessels and atria, including the sinoatrial and atrioventricular nodes and the bundle of His. Sympathetic nerves and some parasympathetics are distributed to the ventricles in the atrioventricular sulcus and along the coronary arteries. In the same nerves and through the same pathways, afferent, sympathetic, and parasympathetic fibers pass back to the central nervous system.

REFERENCES

1. Kent AFS: Observations on the auriculoventricular junction of the mammalian heart. Q J Exp Physiol 7:193, 1913
2. Mahaim I: Les Maladies Organiques du Faisceau de His-Tawara. Paris, Masson, 1931
3. James TN: The connecting pathways between the sinus node and A.V. node and between the right and left atrium in the human heart. Am Heart J 66:498, 1963
4. Wearn JT, Mettier SR, Klump TG et al: The nature of the vascular communications between the coronary arteries and the chambers of the heart. Am Heart J 9:143, 1933

GENERAL REFERENCES

Barry A, Patten BM: The structure of the adult heart. In Gould SE (ed): Pathology of the Heart, 3rd ed. Springfield, IL, Charles C Thomas, 1968

Licata RH: Anatomy of the heart. In Liusada AA (ed): Development and Structure of the Cardiovascular System. New York, McGraw-Hill, 1961

McAlpine WA: Heart and Coronary Arteries: An Anatomical Atlas for Clinical Diagnosis, Radiological Investigation, and Surgical Treatment. Berlin, Springer, 1975

Netter FH: The Ciba Collection of Medical Illustrations, Vol 5, Heart. Summit, NJ, Ciba, 1969

Patten BM: The heart. In Anson BJ (ed): Human Anatomy: A Complete Systematic Treatise, 12th ed. Philadelphia, Blakiston, 1966

Virmani R, Ursell PC, Fenoglio JJ: Examination of the heart. Hum Pathol 18:432, 1987

Physiology of Cardiac Muscle Contraction

CHAPTER 2
VOLUME 1

William W. Parmley • Joan Wikman-Coffelt

A knowledge of cardiac muscle physiology is fundamental to an understanding of the performance of the heart. Furthermore, the function of the left ventricle represents one of the most important prognostic indices in patients with cardiac disease, a fact that emphasizes the necessity of understanding normal and abnormal cardiac muscle physiology. The purpose of this chapter is to emphasize principles of cardiac muscle performance, rather than to detail the vast number of physiologic studies that have been done over the years. In particular, those principles that have clinical relevance will be stressed more than observations of lesser clinical importance.

GENERAL PRINCIPLES

Before considering the techniques and indices used to describe muscle function, it is worthwhile to review three general principles (Table 2.1). First, all indices of performance are derived from two major contractile properties of heart muscle, namely its ability to shorten and to develop force. Second, cardiac muscle performance is altered by two principal mechanisms: (1) a change in initial muscle length (Frank-Starling mechanism) and (2) a change in contractile state. Lastly, there are four primary determinants of cardiac muscle performance that have relevance to the intact heart. The first is preload, which represents the initial load stretching the muscle to its diastolic length prior to contraction. The second, or afterload, represents the load facing the muscle as it develops force and attempts to shorten. Third, the contractile state represents the performance characteristics of heart muscle under a given set of loading conditions. The fourth factor is stimulation frequency, or heart rate. As we review these four determinants of cardiac muscle performance, it will be clear how the performance of the intact heart can also be described in terms of these same factors.

STRUCTURE–FUNCTION RELATIONSHIPS

Before discussing the details of cardiac muscle mechanics, it is worthwhile to review briefly the structure–function relationships of the intact heart. The right atrium forms the right border of the heart, whereas the left atrium forms the posterior-superior portion of the cardiac silhouette. The atria have three principal functions. During systole, the atria collect blood from their respective venous drainage. With the opening of the tricuspid and mitral valves during early diastole there is an initial rapid filling phase of the respective ventricles. During mid-diastole there is some continued filling, since each atrium serves as a conduit between venous drainage and its respective ventricle. Lastly, at the end of diastole, atrial contraction contributes a final amount of blood to the end-diastolic volume of each ventricle. An appropriately timed atrial contraction is extremely important for maintaining cardiac output and is progressively more important in patients with reduced compliance of the left ventricle, caused, for example, by coronary disease, or hypertrophy. In the setting of reduced ventricular compliance, an appropriately timed atrial contraction allows for the ventricle to reach a high end-diastolic pressure (preload), while maintaining a lower mean atrial pressure.

The right ventricle is the most anterior of the four cardiac chambers. Functionally, it has an inflow tract and an outflow tract. It is a thin-walled trabeculated ventricle that acts as a volume pump by delivering blood into the pulmonary artery at low pressures. The left ventricle is a conical ellipsoid structure, with the apex of the ventricle forming the apex of the heart. The interventricular septum is functionally more a part of the left ventricle than the right ventricle. With thicker walls than the right ventricle, the left ventricle is ideally suited as a pressure pump, since it works against the aortic pressure.

Fiber direction in the intact heart is relatively complex. In the left ventricle, fiber direction tends to run generally parallel to the long axis of the heart at the endocardial and epicardial surfaces, with a gradual 180° change in fiber direction as one moves from the inside to the outside of the heart. In the middle of the left ventricular wall, most of the fibers run circumferentially around the heart, perpendicular to the long axis. This accounts for the squeezing action of the ventricle, which is more important than shortening of the long axis in ejecting blood.

MYOCARDIAL CELLS
FIBERS

Myocardial cells or fibers are arranged in a syncytial fashion with intercalated disks at the ends of each cell. Myocardial cells have a centrally placed nucleus and are 40 μm to 100 μm in length and 10 μm to 20 μm in diameter (Fig. 2.1, A). Each fiber or cell is made up of numerous fibrils. Each fibril is a long chain of individual sarcomeres, which represent the fundamental contractile units. Because of the tremendous metabolic demands placed on the heart, and the need for a continuous supply of high-energy phosphates for contraction, there are numerous mitochondria, which are located between individual myofibrils (Fig. 2.1, B).

TABLE 2.1 GENERAL PRINCIPLES OF CARDIAC MUSCLE PHYSIOLOGY

Indices of performance are related to the ability of heart muscle to:
  Shorten
  Develop force
Cardiac muscle performance is altered by:
  Change in initial muscle length
  Change in contractile state
Determinants of cardiac muscle performance:
  Preload
  Afterload
  Contractile state
  Heart rate

SARCOMERES

Sarcomeres are composed of specific arrangements of two sets of overlapping myofilaments of contractile proteins: thick filaments of myosin molecules and thin filaments of actin molecules (Fig. 2.1, C). It is the biochemical and biophysical interaction occurring at precise sites between these strands of actin and myosin aggregates that produces contraction with generation of force and shortening of heart muscle. Within an individual myocardial cell, the neighboring sarcomeres are in register, so that the banded organization of contractile proteins inside the sarcomere imparts a cross-striated appearance to the muscle fiber.

The relative densities of the cross bands identifying the location of the contractile proteins within the sarcomere are shown in Figures 2.1, B and C. The myosin filaments are the broad, dark A band of constant length (1.5 μm in the center portion of the sarcomere); the stationary myosin units are held to each other by linkages at the midpoint of their filaments, shown by the dark M line. Surrounding the myosin units are the sliding actin filaments of constant length (1.0 μm) attached at either end of the sarcomere to the dark Z line, which also connects adjacent sarcomeres at this point. The Z bands and intercalated disks have an important generative function in the production of new sarcomeres. From the light I band of variable dimension, the actin filaments run centrally. Under physiologic conditions, overall sarcomere length (Z to Z distance) varies during the cardiac cycle between 2.2 μm and 1.5 μm, depending on the degree of end-diastolic fiber stretch and the extent of shortening during contraction. Immediately lateral on both sides of the M line is a thin light L line; this central area is the ML complex.

CONTRACTILE PROTEINS

The two primary contractile proteins of the sarcomere, actin and myosin, possess distinct structural and functional properties. The thin filament comprises two helical chains of globular actin molecules. As observed in cross-sections of the sarcomere, each thin filament is surrounded by three thick filaments and each thick filament is encompassed by six thin filaments. Although actin enhances the enzymatic action of myosin ATPase to more active actomyosin ATPase, there is no enzymatic participation of actin itself in the contractile mechanism. Instead, the physiologic role of actin is to combine reversibly at specific binding sites on the thin filament with the myosin crossbridges, one myosin head attaching to each active actin site. Thus, according to the sliding filament theory of contraction,[1] formation of crossbridges between active sites of actin and myosin causes inward movement of the thin filaments centrally along the fixed thick filament framework. In

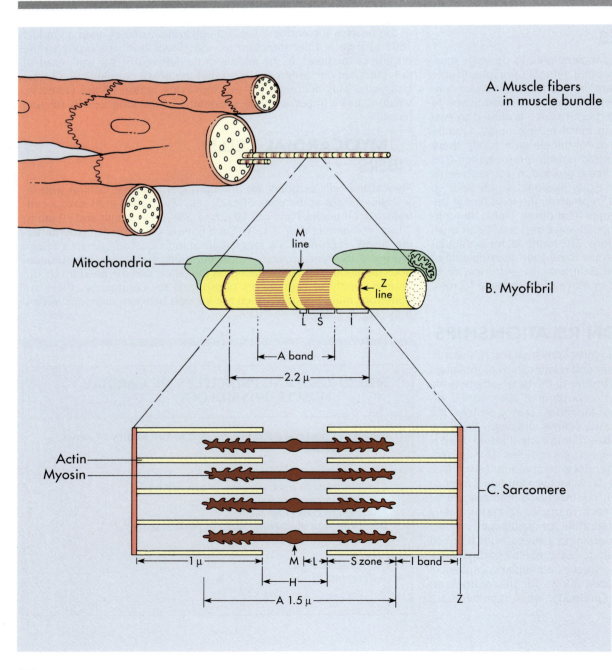

FIGURE 2.1 A. Myocardial structure viewed under light microscopy showing syncytium of cells or fibers. The intercalated disks demonstrate the cell boundaries. B. Ultrastructure of longitudinal section of an individual fiber schematized from electron microscope demonstrating parallel myofibrils composed of serially connected sarcomeres in register with sarcomeres of adjacent fibrils. Horizontal rows of mitochondria are situated throughout the cell. C. Diagrammatic representation of a sarcomere at L_{max} (resting length at which active tension becomes maximal) showing overlapping arrangement of thick (myosin) and thin (actin) filaments. (S, area of actin–myosin overlap; HMM, heavy meromyosin; LMM, light meromyosin) (Modified from Wikman-Coffelt J, Mason DT: Mechanisms of cardiac contraction. In Sodeman W (ed): Pathological Physiology, 7th ed. Philadelphia, WB Saunders, 1984)

this contractile process, the lengths of the filaments generally remain unchanged, although the thick filaments may display small conformational changes.

In addition to the two primary contractile proteins, actin and myosin, two regulatory proteins, tropomyosin and troponin, are located along the thin actin filament (Fig. 2.2). Tropomyosin and troponin are not contractile proteins as such. Instead, they serve a regulatory role in the contractile mechanism by inhibiting or activating the actin–myosin interaction. Tropomyosin molecules lie in elongated chains longitudinally along the paired actin strands of the thin filament. Troponin is attached at regular intervals to tropomyosin, coinciding with the grooves of the actin double helix. During relaxation of cardiac muscle, troponin, together with tropomyosin, prevents crossbridge reaction between actin and myosin. As demonstrated by Ebashi and coworkers,[2] troponin contains receptor subunits for the specific binding of calcium in the contractile system. Although calcium is considered as the activator of mechanical contraction, it actually functions as the specific inactivator of the troponin–tropomyosin complex's inhibition of actin–myosin linkage formation. Two further protein subunits complete the troponin structure (see Fig. 2.2), a tropomyosin-binding subunit and an actin–myosin interaction inhibitor. During polymerization, depolymerized globular actin is converted to the fibrous form, resulting in a double helix with seven actin molecules to a turn. Conversion of depolymerized actin occurs with the addition of adenosine triphosphate (ATP) and calcium. As also shown in Figure 2.2, A, tropomyosin is a long linear molecule composed of two subunits with a double helical conformation. Troponin is a globular molecule, affixed near the end of each tropomyosin molecule, consisting of three subunits termed *troponin I, C,* and *T.* As indicated in Figure 2.2, *B,* the reaction between actin and myosin is controlled by troponin and tropomyosin. During contraction, actin is turned on and reacts with myosin. During relaxation, actin is turned off, thus repulsing myosin, with the result that no interaction takes place; troponin I, like tropomyosin, has the ability to regulate the interaction between actin and myosin. Troponin T serves to bind the troponin complex to tropomyosin. Troponin C binds available Ca^{2+} for initiation of contraction and deactivates the inhibitory action of troponin I. Thus troponin $C-Ca^{2+}$ becomes a derepressor, exerting a conformational change that forces tropomyosin into the helical groove of actin, thereby exposing the actin sites for interaction with myosin. Evidence indicates that phosphorylation of troponin I plays an important role in the contraction process. This subunit is phosphorylated by myocardial cyclic adenosine monophosphate (AMP)–dependent protein kinase. Phosphorylation of troponin I, activated by catecholamines, decreases the calcium sensitivity of actomyosin by reducing the affinity of troponin C for calcium.

The thick filament is composed of staggered parallel clusters of a few hundred myosin molecules (Fig. 2.3), each characterized by an elongated rodlike core of interwoven paired helical coils (light meromyosin) with globular lateral endings or heads (heavy meromyosin). The globular projection contains the principal functional component of myosin: the crossbridge of the thick filament that interacts with actin of the thin filament to produce contraction. Furthermore, each globular crossbridge is paired with a light myosin subunit at its termination. These light subunits (light chains) of heavy meromyosin are thought to influence the level of regulated actomyosin ATPase activity in the remaining portion of the heavy meromysin (heavy chains).

The ultrastructure of interdigitating thick and thin filaments is illustrated in Figure 2.4 as they appear in longitudinal section. Three thick and four thin filaments are shown. Tropomyosin is in the groove of the double helix of actin molecules, and troponin is located at every seventh actin molecule. The thick filaments are composed of bundles of myosin molecules, each consisting of a central strand with lateral terminating heads that spiral outward from the core of the cylinder. These myosin molecules are grouped sequentially, so that the myosin heads spiral along both A band sections of the filament. Only the small middle zone of the filament is without myosin heads. With actin turned on during contraction, the myosin heads establish crossbridge contact with actin and enzymatic activity in the myosin heads takes place.

SUPERFICIAL MEMBRANE SYSTEM

In addition to the sarcomere contractile apparatus that occupies approximately one half of the myocardial fiber, there are other important specialized subcellular constituents. The individual myocardial fibers are covered by the sarcolemma membrane, of which the intercalated disks and transverse tubular system are derivatives of major significance. The intercalated disks are situated at intercellular junctions between the terminal sarcomeres of the cell, thereby locking fibers together at their ends. In ventricular myocardium, deep invaginations of the sarcolemma constitute the complex transtubular network or T system (Fig. 2.5). The intercalated disks and transverse tubular membranes provide pathways for rapid transmission of the depolarizing impulses. In addition to contributing a vehicle for excitation, the T system provides a comprehensive extension of the extracellular space throughout the cell, so that transmembrane cation transport of sodium, potassium, and calcium accompanying depolarization, repolarization, excitation–contraction coupling, and relaxation occurs quickly and synchronously. Furthermore, the T system furnishes a conduit for ready entry and egress of metabolites and other substances between the interstitial medium and the sarcoplasm.

MODULATORS OF MEMBRANE FUNCTION

An important biochemical factor in heart muscle that is involved in modulating the calcium sensitivity of the cardiac proteins is cyclic AMP, discovered by Sutherland and Rall.[3] Cyclic AMP is synthesized in the sarcoplasm from ATP by stimulation of the enzyme adenylate cyclase of the plasma sarcolemma and transtubular membranes. The activity of adenylate cyclase is enhanced by stimulation of β-adrenergic receptors, which are also in the sarcolemma. It has been suggested that the positive inotropic action of the catecholamines is mediated via cyclic AMP formation. The mechanism through which cyclic AMP increases myocardial glycogenolysis has been established (cyclic nucleotide stimulation of protein kinase causes phosphorylation of phosphorylase kinase from ATP, which, in turn, activates the phosphorylase enyzme, degrading glycogen).

Concerning the significance of cyclic AMP in the modulation of cardiac contraction, evidence suggests that myocardial cyclic AMP–dependent protein kinase phosphorylates protein components in the sarcoplasmic reticulum (phospholamban) and sarcolemma membrane (calciductin) governing calcium transport, and in troponin itself, thereby influencing the effects of calcium on the contraction reaction. Cyclic AMP is essential to contraction. It plays both a regulatory and a modulatory role in the cardiac cycle. Levels of free calcium appear to regulate cyclic AMP concentrations, and levels of cyclic AMP regulate calcium concentrations. Oscillations of cyclic AMP, along with calcium fluxes, occur with the cardiac cycle. Cyclic AMP increases with depolarization but is rapidly degraded; by the end of peak systole, the cyclic AMP values have returned to levels similar to those seen in the resting phase.[4]

Calmodulin is a small molecular weight protein with four high-affinity calcium binding sites. In the presence of calcium (5×10^{-7} M), it undergoes conformational changes, assuming a more helical, compact structure. In this calcium-bound state, it can activate several enzymes, including kinases and phosphatases involved in protein phosphorylation. By use of such regulators, the Ca^{2+} in the cytosol can accelerate its own removal by direct activation of enzymes, for which it is a substrate. Thus, contractility may be regulated in several ways, including covalent modification of membrane proteins, as well as regulatory and contractile components of the cell machinery.

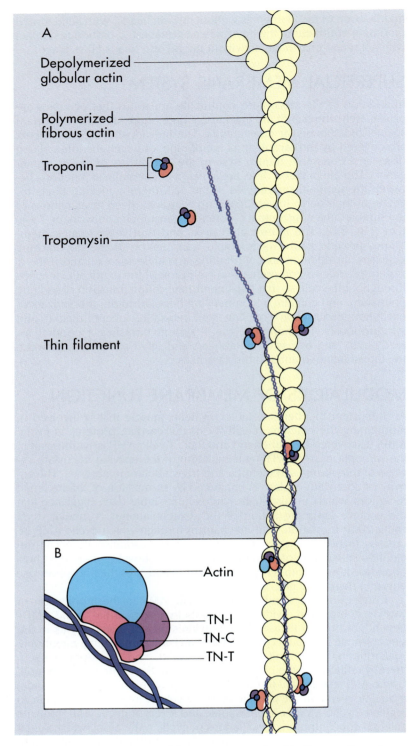

FIGURE 2.2 A. Representation of the components of a thin filament. From the top down are depolymerized globular actin, polymerized fibrous actin, tropomyosin, troponin, and the reconstituted thin filament. The latter is composed of fibrous actin with tropomyosin along side the actin grooves and troponin at each turn of the double helix of actin. **B.** Representation of the three subunits of troponin (*TN*) showing their relation to the other proteins of the thin filament. (*A* modified from Wikman-Coffelt J, Mason DT: Mechanisms of cardiac contraction. In Sodeman W (ed): Pathological Physiology, 7th ed. Philadelphia, WB Saunders, 1984; *B* modified from Wikman-Coffelt J et al: Myofibrillar proteins and the contractile mechanism in the normal failing heart. In Mason DT (ed): Congestive Heart Failure. New York, Yorke Medical Books, 1976)

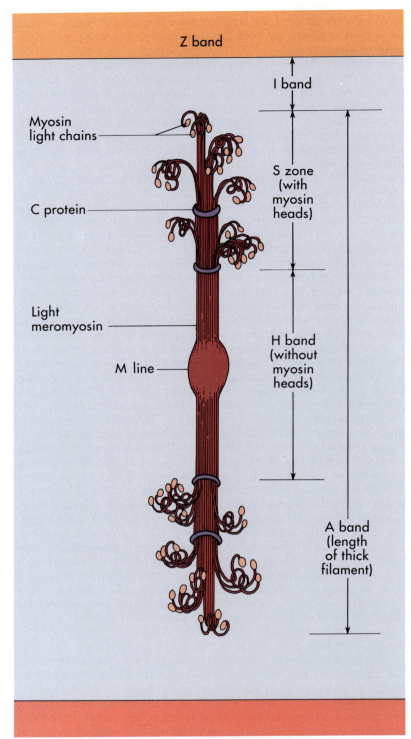

FIGURE 2.3 Three-dimensional view of a single thick filament containing myosin molecules. (Modified from Wikman-Coffelt J et al: Myofibrillar proteins and the contractile mechanism in the normal failing heart. In Mason DT (ed): Congestive Heart Failure. New York, Yorke Medical Books, 1976)

The action potential for cardiac cells is generated by the movement of ions across the cell membrane, which, in turn, is controlled by variations in membrane permeability and ion concentration gradient in a manner similar to that occurring in nerve cells. Studies with the aequorin technique in atrial and ventricular muscle have shown that changes in the rate of stimulation, in extracellular Ca^{2+}, and in catecholamines, all produce a greater increase in the flux of calcium. Catecholamines differ from other inotropic interventions in that they produce a smaller increase in tension production than would be expected from the increase in cytoplasmic Ca^{2+}. This decrease in sensitivity results from an increase in the degree of phosphorylation of troponin that is brought about by the cyclic AMP–induced activation of protein kinase.

There is evidence that the total force developed, the rate of tension development, and the rate of tension decline during relaxation can be related, respectively to the quantity of Ca^{2+} made available for binding to troponin, the rate of Ca^{2+} delivery to troponin, and the rate at which Ca^{2+} is removed from troponin. Many interventions that augment or depress the contractile state of heart muscle are associated with alterations in Ca^{2+} movement and concentrations in heart muscle.

Norepinephrine is a neurotransmitter directly linking cardiac sympathetic activity with β-receptor stimulation, resulting in elevated contractility and heart rate via cyclic AMP. The sympathetic nervous system normally exerts a major regulatory role in the augmentation of cardiovascular function in response to increased metabolic demands of the peripheral tissues, such as during physical exercise. The rich sympathetic innervation of heart muscle permits the heart to produce the majority of its own norepinephrine. In the terminals of the sympathetic nerves, norepinephrine is synthesized through a series of steps from tyrosine, in which tyrosine hydroxylase is the rate-limiting enzyme. The neurotransmitter is stored in the nerve ending in granules that protect it from enzymatic destruction by monoamine oxidase in the neuronal cytoplasm. In response to sympathetic impulses, norepinephrine is released to activate the synthesis of cyclic AMP and increase the myocardial influx of calcium. Catecholamines, by augmenting increases in cyclic AMP, do not appear to increase the size of the calcium channels or the rates at which the gates open but rather appear to recruit an additional number of active calcium channels that can open in response to depolarizing stimuli.

SARCOPLASMIC RETICULUM

An extensive intracellular tubular membrane system, the sarcoplasmic reticulum, complements the T system structurally and functionally in support of the process of excitation–contraction coupling and mechanical relaxation (see Fig. 2.5, *A*). The sarcoplasmic reticulum is entirely within the cell, and its general orientation is at right angles to the T system, so that the sarcotubular structure courses longitudinally along the rows of sarcomeres. The sarcotubular lateral sacs (terminal cisternae) store calcium; the intracellular transport of calcium from this area is important in linking membrane excitation with activation of the contractile apparatus. Also lateral sacs abut the intercalated disks and sarcolemma to provide each of the specialized membranes with a complete system for excitation–contraction coupling. An interesting exception is the Purkinje cell, which has no T system.

MITOCHONDRIA

The final myocardial substructure to be considered is the mitochondrion, which contains the aerobic biochemical systems of the fiber.

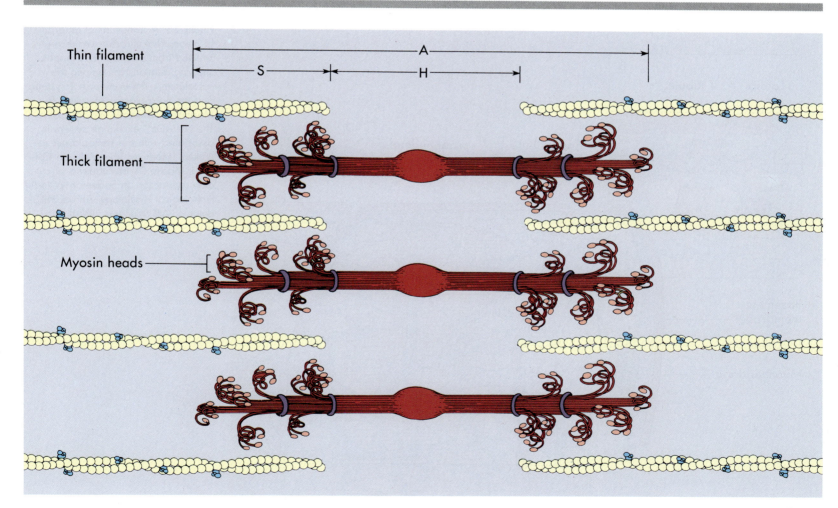

FIGURE 2.4 Diagrammatic representation of alternating myofilaments in longitudinal view in a portion of lateral section of thick filaments. (*H*, midzone ML band of the thick filaments) (Modified from Wikman-Coffelt J et al: Myofibrillar proteins and the contractile mechanism in the normal failing heart. In Mason DT (ed): Congestive Heart Failure. New York, Yorke Medical Books, 1976)

The mitochondria located between the myofibrils are abundant, in accordance with the heart's high requirement for oxygen, and they constitute nearly 30% of the myocardial cell. The mitochondria situated near the A bands (myosin) are the metabolic power plants in which oxygen and appropriate substrates are used to produce ATP, the final direct energy source of myocardial contraction and other biochemical reactions. The mitochondrial membranes also are capable of accumulating calcium, which might serve as an internal buffer against abnormal rises of sarcoplasmic calcium during the resting phase.

EXCITATION–CONTRACTION COUPLING AND THE CONTRACTILE PROCESS
ELECTRICAL EXCITATION

The electrical events constituting excitation of the myocardial fiber involve depolarization of the cell by rapid ingress of sodium into the sarcoplasm (phase 0 spike of the action potential), followed by an ingress of calcium through the slow calcium conductance channels (voltage-dependent) and an egress extracellularly of an equal amount of potassium (repolarization of the action potential). The change in charge distribution in the myofiber with depolarization and repolarization is shown in Figure 2.6.

The rapid Na^+ influx constituting complete phase 0 depolarization is a process that appears to be governed by activated Na^+ carriers (electrostatically controlled fast membrane channels or pores). The rate of rise of the spike action potential determines conduction velocity; relative to the surface electrocardiogram, phase 0 depolarization is denoted by the P wave in the atria and by the QRS complex in the ventricles.

The repolarization period is more complex (phases 2 and 3, Fig. 2.6). During systole, Ca^{2+} rises to between 10^{-6} M and 10^{-5} M, depending on the inotropic state of the heart and the cyclic AMP levels. The steepness of the calcium gradient across the membranes allows the use of Ca^{2+} as a fast trigger for a series of cytosolic events that open pores or channels in the sarcolemma and/or reticular membranes through which Ca^{2+} will flow down the gradient to increase 100-fold the cytosolic free calcium concentration. Sarcolemmal calcium is approximately 10^{-3} M and sarcoplasmic reticulum calcium approximately 10^{-2} M. The precise concentration of calcium during the resting phase is difficult to determine. Most of the light-sensitive reagents, such as aequorin, cannot detect levels less than 10^{-7} M. A resting calcium level of 10^{-7} M of cytosolic free calcium ions is high enough to inhibit the slow calcium channels (i.e., the I_{Ca}). The resting level of calcium is too low to activate most of the calcium-dependent enzymes. Thus, calcium-dependent enzymes are dependent on the calcium transients following depolarization for activation. The influx of calcium (phase 2) activates the K^+ conductance channels and promotes K^+ efflux, the rapid phase of repolarization (phase 3). The entire repolarization period constitutes the action potential duration that governs the refractory period of heart muscle and is represented on the surface electrocardiogram by the QT interval.

During diastole, following repolarization, the phase 4 recovery portion of the electrophysiologic cycle ensues, in which the depolarization Na^+ leaves the cell and the repolarization K^+ returns into the fiber. These cation exchanges during mechanical relaxation require the active energy-utilizing transport mechanism of the transtubular Na^+-K^+ ATPase pumps (Fig. 2.7). In addition, Ca^{2+} is removed from the fiber during the resting period by the sarcolemma Na^+-Ca^{2+} exchange transport system and Ca^{2+} ATPase.

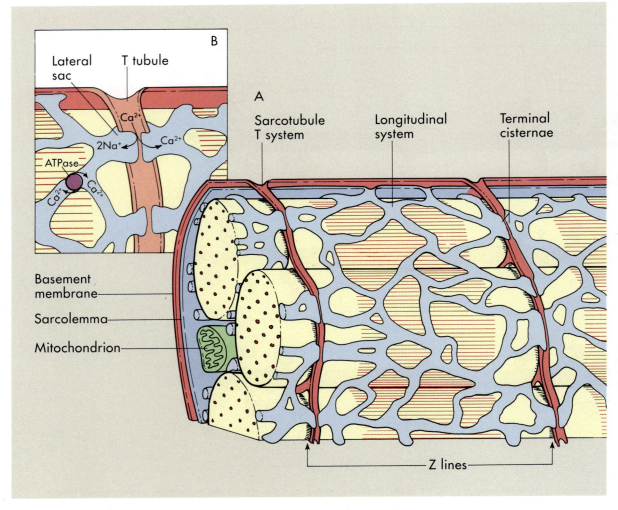

FIGURE 2.5 **A.** Longitudinal diagram of myocardial ultrastructure reconstructed from electron micrographs showing relationships among the sarcolemma, the transverse T system, and the sarcoplasmic reticulum. **B.** Magnified schematic view of above. The Na^+–Ca^{2+} exchange system is associated with the sarcoplasmic reticulum. (Modified from Wikman-Coffelt J, Mason DT: Mechanisms of cardiac contraction. In Sodeman W (ed): Pathological Physiology, 7th ed. Philadelphia, WB Saunders, 1984)

MECHANICAL ACTIVATION

When the stimulating impulse from the sinoatrial node arrives at the surface of a myocardial cell, an orderly sequence of events is initiated, in which calcium movement is the chief component linking electrical excitation of the fiber with mechanical activation of the contractile machinery in the sarcomere. Excitation of the individual cell proceeds as the depolarization wave spreads throughout the entire fiber along the sarcolemma and its interior transtubular membrane system. When the depolarizing current in the T system reaches the terminal cisternae, calcium depots of the sarcoplasmic reticulum, ionic calcium release is triggered from the lateral sacs into the sarcoplasm. Together with an apparently small but crucial quantity of ionic calcium influx across the sarcolemma-transtubular membrane occurring during phase 2 of the transmembrane action potential, this discharged calcium immediately diffuses to the sarcomeres, where it binds to the specific troponin C–Ca^{2+} receptor protein on the thin myofilaments in the overlap region (A band) between the thick and thin filaments.

Mechanical activation is then achieved by the binding of activator calcium to troponin C, which overcomes the troponin I–tropomyosin complex inhibition of actin and myosin interaction, with the result that actin–myosin electrostatic crossbridges are formed. Thus, Ca^{2+} binding to troponin C produces structural alteration of the troponin C protein, which is transmitted through troponin I to tropomyosin, so that tropomyosin moves deeper into the groove of the double helix of actin molecules. In this manner, these configurational changes of the troponin–tropomyosin complex free the actin binding sites to link directly with the myosin heads, thereby allowing actomyosin ATPase activity to occur with initiation of the contractile process. The temporal course of the entire excitation–contraction coupling process takes place rela-

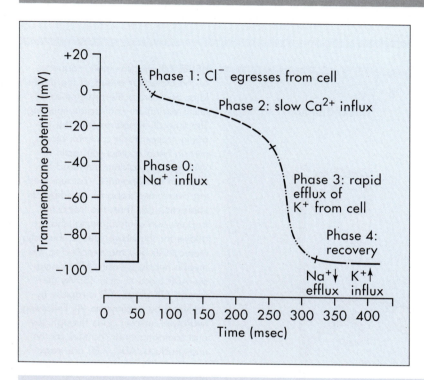

FIGURE 2.6 Intracellular action potential. See text for description of different phases. (Modified from Wikman-Coffelt J, Mason DT: Mechanism of cardiac contraction. In Sodeman W (ed): Pathological Physiology, 7th ed. Philadelphia, WB Saunders, 1984)

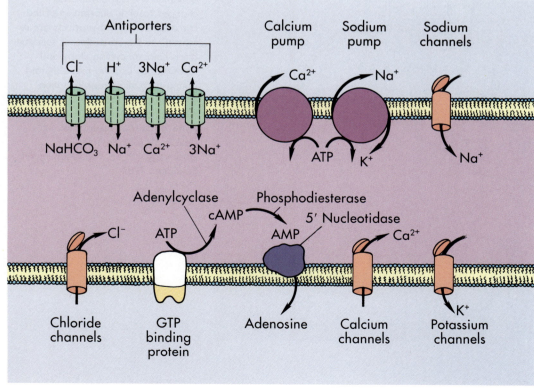

FIGURE 2.7 Transtubular cell membrane comprised of phospholipids interspersed with the Na^+–K^+ pump proteins. These operate during diastole to establish the Na^+ and K^+ gradients. (Modified from Wikman-Coffelt J, Mason DT: Mechanisms of cardiac contraction. In Sodeman W (ed): Pathological Physiology, 7th ed. Philadelphia, WB Saunders, 1984)

tively quickly, as indicated clinically by the average 0.06-second delay between the beginning of the QRS complex and the onset of isovolumic ventricular contraction.

CONTRACTILE MECHANISMS

The onset of contraction takes place with development of force and contractile element shortening by the cyclic interaction of actin–myosin linkage pulling the thin filaments along the immobile thick filaments toward the center of the sarcomeres. It is believed that the electrostatic links are next broken as myosin binds another ATP molecule. Thus, a repetitive sequence of making and breaking cross-linkages is established as the actin filament slides past the myosin filament during the entire course of ventricular contraction. For shortening of the sarcomere to occur, each actin–myosin crossbridge must perform sequentially. It is thus necessary for the myosin head to attach to actin, swivel, detach, and then reattach to the next actin binding site at a point farther laterally on the thin filament. The result is a rowing motion of the myosin heads, pulling the thin filaments together centrally and causing their overlap with decreasing distance between two lines, thereby producing sarcomere, myofilament, muscle fiber, and ultimately ventricular shortening.

RELAXATION

The phase of the excitation–contraction process in which calcium is delivered to the contractile apparatus does not require much ATP energy. The contractile reaction involving myosin ATP uses the great majority of total myocardial energy, which varies according to the muscle loading conditions and contractile state. Following development of the full active contractile state, the active process of relaxation ensues, with calcium rapidly binding to the sarcoplasmic reticulum. The cation is then pumped back into the lateral sacs by the sarcotubular calcium pump (relaxing factor), with the total energy needed for relaxation being relatively small. The biochemical process of contraction and relaxation is summarized in Figure 2.8.

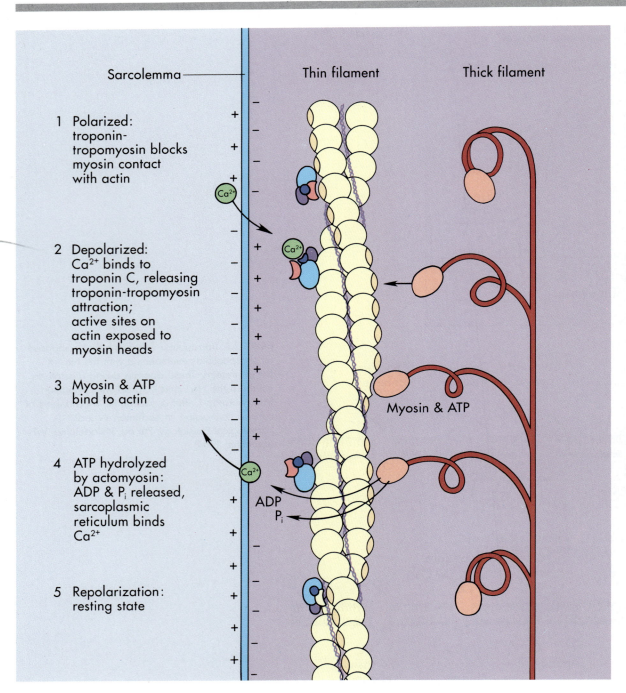

FIGURE 2.8 Diagrammatic sequence of the molecular events of the modulator and contractile proteins constituting excitation–contraction coupling. The time of depolarization: the troponin–tropomyosin complex blocks myosin head contact with actin (1). With greater calcium delivered to troponin C, troponin-C–calcium binding overcomes troponin–tropomyosin interaction (2). Thus, the troponin-tropomyosin conformational change allows for the active sites of the actin molecule to become exposed to the myosin heads. Myosin–ATP or myosin–ADP binds to actin (3). As the myosin-ATP binds, ATP is rapidly hydrolyzed by actomyosin (4). Following hydrolysis, myosin goes through several conformational changes as the end-products (ADP + Pi) are transferred to different positions in the oligomer. The conformational changes result in shortening of the sarcomere. The end-products are released. As the sarcoplasmic reticulum binds calcium, cycling stops and myosin goes into the relaxed state. During relaxation, repolarization takes place (5). (Modified from Wikman-Coffelt J, Mason DT: Mechanisms of cardiac contraction. In Sodeman W (ed): Pathological Physiology, 7th ed. Philadelphia, WB Saunders, 1984)

MECHANICS OF CONTRACTION

Most studies of the mechanics of heart muscle have been done with strips of cardiac muscle from different species of animals. A preferred preparation is the papillary muscle of either the right or the left ventricle. In this preparation, the muscle fibers all run in the same direction, a linear arrangement that allows for measurement of force and shortening at the ends of the muscle. Studies from isolated heart muscle will be used to illustrate the various principles of cardiac muscle contraction.

PASSIVE LENGTH–TENSION RELATION

The resting length–tension relationship of cardiac muscle is measured by attaching one end of the muscle to a fixed force transducer and gradually stretching out the other end of the muscle in a bath filled with an appropriate oxygenated nutrient solution. The shape of the passive length–tension relation is generally exponential (Fig. 2.9). At shorter lengths there is little rise in resting force as the muscle is stretched, whereas at progressively longer lengths there is an increasingly steep rise in resting force. Cardiac muscle, like other biologic tissue, however, is not perfectly elastic. If one keeps the muscle at a longer length, there is a slight reduction in force, which then stabilizes at a lower level (stress relaxation). As one returns the muscle to its initial length there will be a reduction in force below the original baseline, which will then tend to return to the control over time (creep). The implications of these passive properties of muscle are several. The ability to resist stretch at higher preloads is obviously important in preventing the ventricle from overdilating. This tends to keep the sarcomeres at a near optimal length, so that they can still function effectively with an acute volume overload. Stress relaxation occurs acutely during myocardial infarction, wherein the infarcted portion of the heart paradoxically bulges with each systole and ends up a longer length over a period of minutes to hours.

The passive length–tension relations of cardiac muscle remain relatively unchanged even with major changes in systolic function. With longstanding hypertrophy or heart failure, for example, there are only minimal changes in passive length–tension relations.[5] The slight increase in stiffness that does occur with longstanding hypertrophy may, in part, be due to the increase in collagen tissue that accompanies the hypertrophy. Even though the intrinsic passive properties of heart muscle may not change much with hypertrophy, there can be dramatic changes in passive pressure–volume relations of the left ventricle, with a decrease in compliance. For example, with the concentric hypertrophy that accompanies aortic stenosis there is a reduction in volume at a given diastolic pressure. The opposite effect occurs with volume overload, for example, in aortic regurgitation.

ACTIVE LENGTH–TENSION RELATIONS

The ability of heart muscle to generate force is dependent on the initial length of the muscle. A simple way to study this property of heart muscle is with isometric contractions. With each contraction muscle length is fixed (isometric), and there is force development but no shortening. In Figure 2.9, A, each isometric contraction at a given muscle length is represented by a vertical line. The series of contractions are obtained by successively increasing muscle length. At longer initial muscle lengths, the length of the developed force line becomes greater until one reaches an optimal muscle length (L_{max}), where the length of the developed force line is maximal. At longer muscle lengths there is a reduction in the developed force line, although the total force continues to rise owing to the more abrupt rise in resting force. This fundamental property of heart muscle, that is, the ability to increase force development at longer lengths (Frank-Starling mechanism), is, in part, responsible for the ability of the heart to respond to changes in the demand for cardiac output. It should be remembered, however, that the most important mechanism for increasing cardiac output is an increase in heart rate.

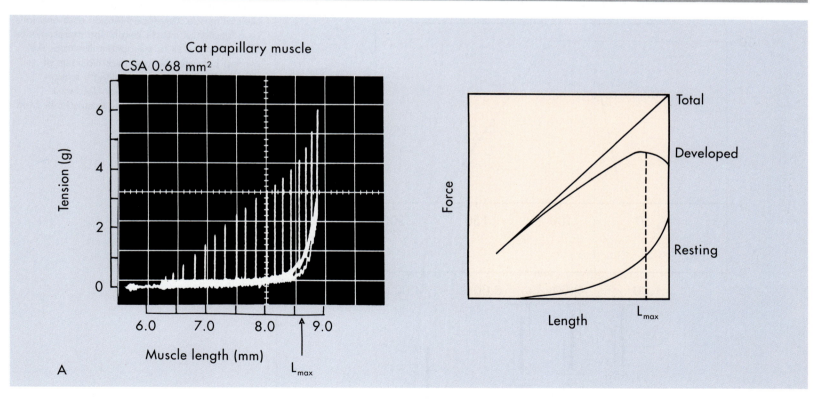

FIGURE 2.9 A. Polaroid photograph of superimposed passive and active length–tension relations of a representative cat papillary muscle. The bottom line represents the passive length–tension relation of the muscle as it is stretched. Each vertical line represents an isometric contraction at that given muscle length. L_{max} denotes that length at which the isometric contraction is maximal. **B.** Schematic representation of the data obtained in A. The developed force is obtained by subtracting the resting tension from the total tension. This defines L_{max} as that length at which developed tension is maximal.

ULTRASTRUCTURAL BASIS OF THE FRANK-STARLING MECHANISM

The relation between the length of the sarcomere and the force developed was defined in skeletal muscle by Huxley.[1] The general premise of this relationship is illustrated in Figure 2.10. The active length–tension relation of skeletal muscle has an ascending limb, a plateau, and a descending limb. As muscle length is increased *in vitro* it is possible to pull skeletal muscle out so that sarcomere length is greatly increased. Remember that skeletal muscle is attached to bony prominences *in vivo* so that its length is always near optimum. The descending limb of this ultrastructural relationship, therefore, represents a phenomenon seen only in the laboratory. An examination of the descending limb of force development shows that a reduction in force is related to a reduction in the overlap of the thin and thick filaments of the sarcomere. Force tends to approach zero as the overlap is eliminated. This fits well with the crossbridge theory of force development, that is, that force is related to the number of crossbridges that are formed. The plateau of the curve occurs at a sarcomere length of about 2.2 μm, wherein there is optimal overlap of actin and myosin filaments and, thus, the opportunity for maximal crossbridge formation. At the center of the myosin filament there are no active crossbridges, which accounts for the extension of the plateau beyond 2.0 μm. As one moves down the ascending limb of the active length–force relation, there is a reduction in force development. The crossbridge theory suggests that the thin actin filaments cross through the center of the sarcomere, interfere with the attachment of crossbridges at shorter muscle lengths, and thus reduce the developed force.

Other data suggest that additional mechanisms may be operative in determining force development along the ascending limb of the active length–tension relationship. For example, if one compares the active length–tension relations of skeletal muscle and cardiac muscle, they should be relatively the same, if the only determinant of developed force is the overlap of thin and thick filaments. As illustrated in Figure 2.11, however, the active length–tension relation for cardiac muscle falls inside that of the skeletal muscle.[6] This and other evidence suggest that there is length-dependent activation of cardiac muscle, so that the force that is generated tends to be proportionally greater at longer muscle lengths than that which would be dictated by the overlap of crossbridges alone. Recall that cardiac muscle tends to be incompletely activated during twitch contractions and cannot be tetanized as can skeletal muscle, another expression of its incomplete activation.

DIFFERENCES BETWEEN CARDIAC AND SKELETAL MUSCLE

At this point, it is worth reviewing some of the major differences between skeletal and cardiac muscle (Table 2.2). First, heart muscle has far more mitochondria than skeletal muscle, presumably reflecting its continual requirement for oxidative phosphorylation to supply the high-energy phosphates necessary for contraction. On the contrary, skeletal muscle can develop an oxygen debt, in that work performance can transiently exceed the oxygen requirements. Skeletal muscle has a much more richly developed sarcoplasmic reticulum than does cardiac muscle. This may reflect its greater dependence on internal stores of calcium for activation.

Skeletal muscle can tolerate large shifts in intracellular pH and even a complete loss of high-energy phosphates. When skeletal muscle is stressed, the phosphocreatine and ATP levels decrease, even falling to near zero with a concurrent increase in intracellular acidity. Garlick and associates have shown that the intracellular skeletal muscle pH when studied by ^{31}P nuclear magnetic resonance (NMR) falls as low as pH 6.0 during stressed working conditions.[7] It has long been known that in skeletal muscle lactic acid increases to high concentrations with an increase in work. The skeletal muscle then goes through a recovery

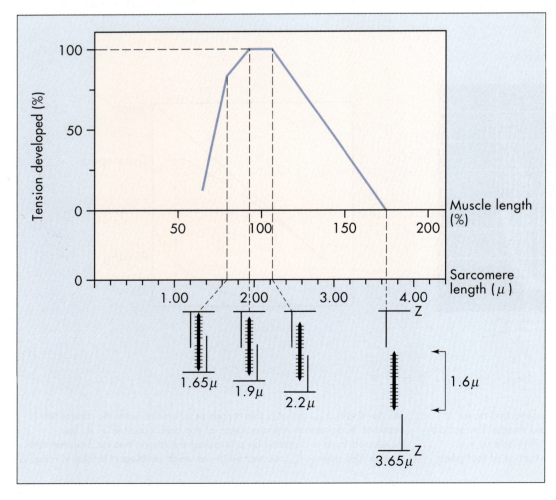

FIGURE 2.10 Active length–tension relation in skeletal muscle. Developed tension rises and falls as a function of muscle length. The representation of the sarcomeres at the bottom illustrates the overlap between thin and thick filaments at different points on the active length tension relation. (Modified from Hanson J, Lowy J: Molecular basis of contractility in muscle. Br Med Bull 21:264, 1965)

period in which the metabolites and pH again return to normal values. The heart, although a muscle, cannot tolerate the extreme conditions observed in skeletal muscle energetics, in part because it cannot remain quiescent, allowing recovery to take place.

As one stretches out skeletal or cardiac muscle, the resting force at L_{max} is relatively low in skeletal muscle, as compared with cardiac muscle. Since skeletal muscle is attached to two bony prominences that tend to fix its length, there is no need for a stiff, passive length–tension relation in skeletal muscle to prevent overdistention. The anatomical explanation for this stiffer length–tension relation in cardiac muscle is unclear, but it may relate to the greater content of collagen tissue and perhaps to the syncytial arrangement. Skeletal muscle *in vitro* can be stretched out to a length wherein sarcomeres are considerably extended. In cardiac muscle, as one stretches out sarcomeres, they tend not to go much beyond the optimum length of 2.2 μm, perhaps up to 2.4 μm.[8] In the patient who develops severe volume overload and heart failure with a marked increase in ventricular volume and mass, it is of interest that the sarcomeres remain at approximately the optimal length of 2.2 μm. This increase in volume and mass is accompanied by the addition of sarcomeres, both in series and in parallel, so that sarcomeres can remain at an optimum length.

Skeletal muscle can be tetanized. In addition, very fine movements are produced by intricate neural control of individual fibers. By contrast, cardiac muscle has an all or none twitch contraction and cannot be tetanized. Experimentally, one can use multiple stimuli and caffeine to approximate a tetanic contraction in cardiac muscle,[9] but this would never occur under physiologic circumstances.

Lastly, skeletal muscle fibers run the length of the muscle, so that individual cells are quite long. By contrast, cardiac muscle cells are bounded by intercalated disks. The multiple peripheral nuclei of skeletal muscle cells also distinguish them from the single, centrally placed nucleus of cardiac muscle cells.

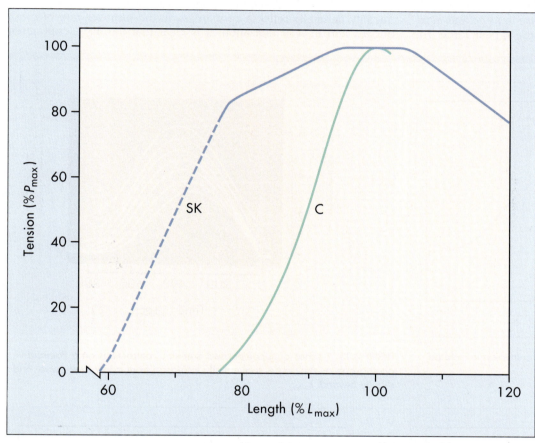

FIGURE 2.11 Relative active length–tension relations of skeletal (SK) and cardiac (C) muscle. Developed tension is expressed as a percent of maximum (100%), and relative length is expressed as a percent of L_{max} (100%). Note that the cardiac muscle curve falls considerably inside the skeletal muscle curve. (Modified from Allen DG, Jewell BR, Murray JW: The contribution of activation processes to the length–tension relation of cardiac muscle. Nature (Lond) 248:606, 1974)

TABLE 2.2 DIFFERENCES BETWEEN CARDIAC AND SKELETAL MUSCLE

Criteria	Skeletal	Cardiac
Mitochondria	+	++
Sarcoplasmic reticulum	++	+
Oxygen debt	+	0
Resting force at L_{max}	Low	High
Sarcomeres in overstretched muscle	>2.2 μm	2.2 μm
Tetanus	Yes	No
Contraction	Graded	All or none
Intercalated disks	No	Yes
Nuclei	Multiple, peripheral	Single, central

ISOMETRIC CONTRACTION

A standard way of studying isolated heart muscle in the laboratory is to fix the ends of the muscle so that when stimulated it can develop force but not shorten. This so-called isometric contraction is illustrated in Figure 2.12, where force is plotted as a function of time. Descriptors of the mechanics of this contraction, which are potentially useful, include the preload, the developed force (afterload), the time to peak force, the maximum rate of force development, and the time for force to decline 50% ($RT_{1/2}$). As one increases preload and moves up the Frank-Starling mechanism, sequential twitch contractions are produced, as illustrated by the superimposed contractions in Figure 2.13. Note that there is a slight prolongation of time to peak force and major increases in the maximum dF/dt and developed force.

If one increases contractility at a constant preload, the isometric contraction is altered as shown in Figure 2.14. With the use of catecholamines, there is a shortening of both the time to peak force and the overall contraction, accompanied by a dramatic increase in maximum dF/dt and peak force. If one increases contractility by increasing calcium in the perfusate, there is a similar increase in force and maximum dF/dt, although a lesser shortening of the time to peak force. The most dramatic difference between the two inotropic interventions is that the duration of contraction is not markedly shortened by a high calcium level and that relaxation time is prolonged.[10,11] This may relate to the direct effects of catecholamines in enhancing the uptake of calcium by the sarcoplasmic reticulum, so that relaxation is faster and the overall contraction is substantially shortened.

Because of the coupled relationship between maximum force, dF/dt, and the time to peak force, it is of interest to explore the question as to which of these indices is most useful as an index of contractile state. An ideal index of contractile state would be one that would change appropriately with a change in contractile state but be independent of loading conditions (*i.e.*, preload and afterload). Most positive inotropic interventions increase both maximum dF/dt and force, while shortening time to peak force. An example of an intervention that behaves differently is a change in temperature. The change in isometric contraction at a given preload when temperature is lowered from 30°C to 20°C is shown in Figure 2.15. Note that even though the maximum dF/dt is reduced at 20°C, the force is increased because of the marked prolongation of the duration of contraction. Since an increase in contractility generally reflects an increase in the turnover rate of crossbridges and in ATP utilization, it is clear that the 30°C contraction

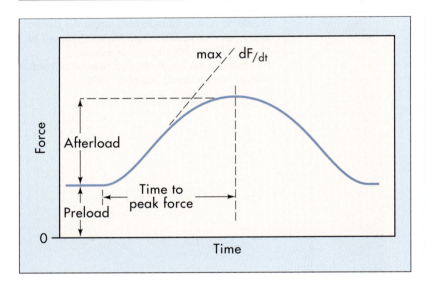

FIGURE 2.12 Schematic representation of an isometric contraction in isolated heart muscle plotting force versus time.

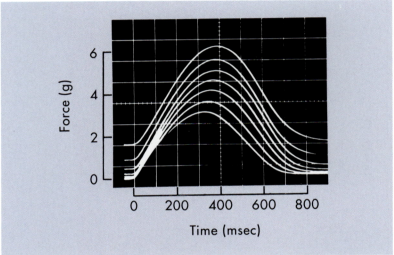

FIGURE 2.13 A series of superimposed isometric contractions on a Polaroid photograph as preload is sequentially increased from a low level up to, and slightly beyond, L_{max}.

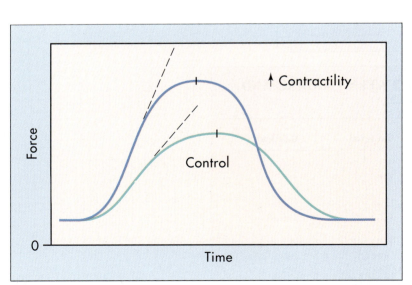

FIGURE 2.14 Schematic representation of the change in isometric contraction with an increase in contractile state. Usually, there is an increase in force development, a decrease in time to peak force, and an increase in maximum rate of force development (*dashed line*).

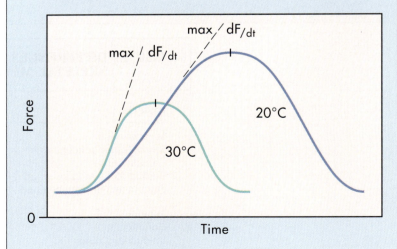

FIGURE 2.15 Relative change in isometric contraction with a change in temperature. Although the 20°C contraction develops more force, its maximum rate of force development is less than the contraction at 30°C owing to the prolonged time course of contraction.

would be considered to be at the higher inotropic state, even though developed force is less. Data of this kind led to the useful convention of using maximum dF/dt at a given preload as a good index of inotropic state when one is studying drugs in isolated heart muscle. Although such an index is useful under controlled loading conditions for evaluating the effect of inotropic agents, it is less useful in the intact heart, because of the dependence of maximum rate of pressure development (max dP/dt) on loading conditions and heart rate.

HEART RATE

In the heart muscle of most mammalian species an increase in stimulation frequency tends to produce an increase in contractility and force development, presumably by making more calcium available to the myocardium. Although dramatic changes in force development can be produced by altering stimulation frequencies at a low rate, changes in the physiologic range are of minor significance in altering contractility in patients. The major cardiovascular effect of increasing heart rate, for example, is to increase cardiac output during exercise. The change in contractile state of the myocardium is much less significant.

An illustration of the so-called positive force treppe with increasing frequency is shown in Figure 2.16. Another way of increasing contractile state is by paired electrical stimulation. If one adds a second stimulus immediately after the refractory period (during the declining phase of force development), there is a brief second mechanical response, as shown in Figure 2.17. The following contraction is markedly potentiated with a subsequent return to normal after a few beats. Presumably this increase in contractility is produced by enhancement of calcium entry with the paired stimulation. By using sustained paired stimulation in isolated heart muscle there is a fairly dramatic increase in contractile state, which can be sustained. Although such an intervention is quite potent in increasing contractile state, it has not been helpful in patients. Its major drawback appears to be the substantial increase in oxygen consumption that accompanies the increase in contractility, an effect that may lower high-energy phosphates and lead to subsequent deterioration of cardiac function.

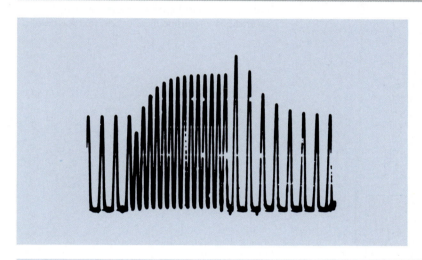

FIGURE 2.16 Slow-speed record of isometric contractions showing the positive force treppe with an increase in frequency of contraction. The descending staircase response is also seen as the stimulation frequency is returned to control. (Modified from Johnson EA: Force–interval relationship of cardiac muscle. In Berne RM (ed): Handbook of Physiology, Section 2, The Cardiovascular System, Vol I, The Heart. Bethesda, MD, American Physiological Society, 1979)

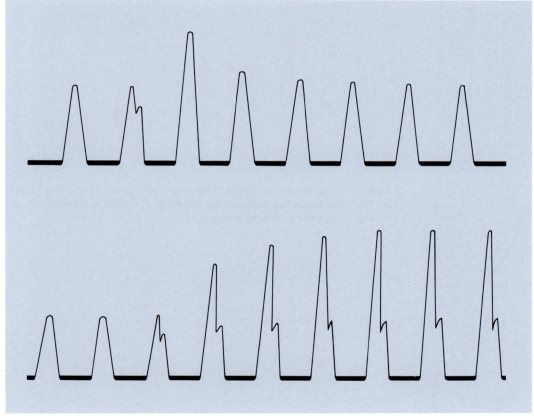

FIGURE 2.17 (Top). Isometric contractions with paired stimulation of the second contraction. The third contraction is augmented, with a return to control over a few beats. (Bottom) Isometric contractions with paired stimulation of each contraction beginning with the third one. This results in a sustained increase in contractile state. (Johnson EA: Force–interval relationship of cardiac muscle. In Berne RE (ed): Handbook of Physiology, Section 2, The Cardiovascular System, Vol I, The Heart. Bethesda, MD, American Physiological Society, 1979)

ISOTONIC CONTRACTION

Another contraction that is used in describing cardiac muscle mechanics is the isotonic contraction. A representative lever system that produces this contraction is illustrated in Figure 2.18. The lever rotates around a fulcrum with loads hanging from one end and the muscle attached to the other end. The lower end of the muscle is attached to a fixed force transducer, so that one can record force development by the muscle. Muscle shortening is recorded by a rotary length transducer at the fulcrum. By placing a preload on the other end of the lever system, the muscle will be stretched to an appropriate length along its passive length–tension relation. If a stop is then placed just above the muscle end of the lever system, any additional load (afterload) placed on the other end of the system will not be sensed by the muscle until it begins to contract. When the muscle is stimulated, it will develop force until it matches the load on the other end of the lever. At that point, it can shorten while lifting the load. The characteristic isotonic afterloaded contraction thus obtained is shown in Figure 2.19. The term *isotonic* comes from the fact that force remains essentially constant during the shortening phase of contraction. Several measurements can be used to describe this contraction, including the preload, the afterload, the distance the muscle shortens, and the velocity of shortening. It should be apparent that this kind of contraction is somewhat analogous to contraction in the intact heart, that is, the left ventricle develops isovolumic pressure until it opens the aortic valve and ejects blood while shortening. Of course, the isotonic force segment in isolated muscle is different from the rise and fall of aortic pressure and myocardial wall stress during ejection. Nevertheless, this kind of contraction in isolated heart muscle has been useful in developing certain principles that have application in the intact heart. A series of isotonic afterloaded contractions at a given preload is shown in Figure 2.20. As would be expected, the contractions with a higher afterload shorten

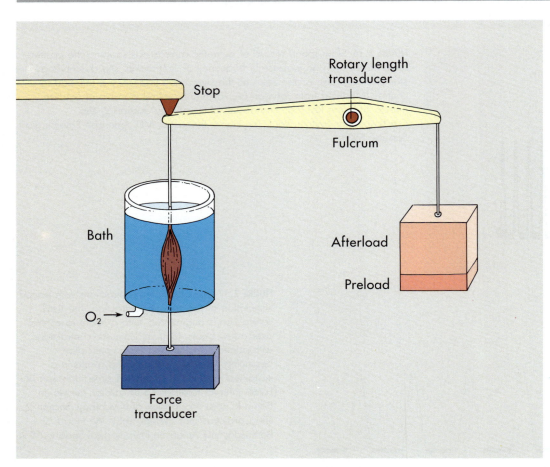

FIGURE 2.18 Schematic diagram of the isotonic lever system used to study isotonic afterloaded contractions in cardiac muscle. See text for details.

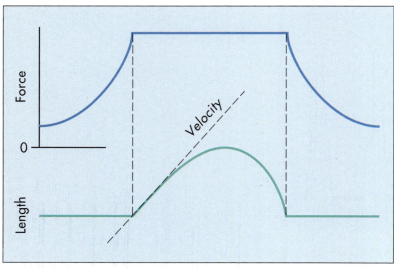

FIGURE 2.19 Representative isotonic afterloaded contraction. Shortening begins only after the muscle has matched the afterload. The initial velocity of shortening is shown as the dashed line.

less and have a lesser velocity of shortening. In some sense, this is a simple representation of the afterload principle: as the load is increased, shortening is reduced. Conversely, as load is reduced, the shortening is increased. The translation of this principle to the patient with heart failure illustrates the importance of vasodilator therapy in reducing the workload of the heart, which, in turn, will increase forward stroke volume. The relationship between shortening and load in a representative series of isotonic contractions is shown in Figure 2.21, to emphasize the importance of this principle.

When one takes the values for load and velocity of shortening at each afterload, one can plot a so-called force–velocity relation, as illustrated in Figure 2.22. There is a general inverse relationship between force and velocity, with the extension of the curve to zero load, representing theoretic maximal velocity of shortening, V_{max}. The force–velocity relation was emphasized by Hill in early studies in skeletal muscle,[12] because of the relationship between the constants of the hyperbolic equation and heat constants, representing energy flux during contraction. This relationship between energy and mechanics of contraction has led to the statement that the force–velocity relation is the most fundamental mechanical relation of contracting striated muscle.

In cardiac muscle, Sonnenblick noted characteristic changes in the

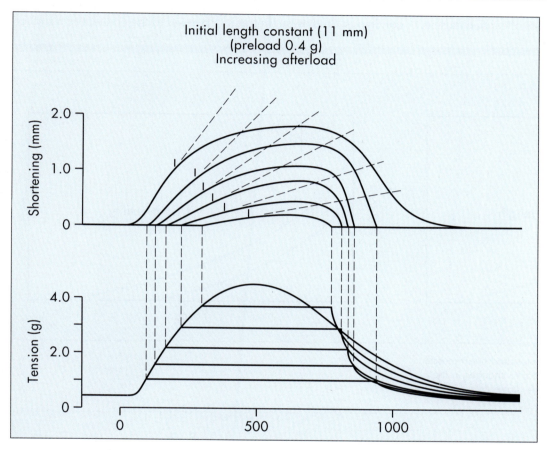

FIGURE 2.20 Superimposed series of isotonic afterloaded contractions with shortening shown at the top (dashed line represents initial velocity of shortening) and tension traces at the bottom. At higher afterloads, shortening and velocity of shortening are reduced. (Modified from Sonnenblick EH: Mechanics of myocardial contraction in the myocardial cell: Structure, function and modification. In Briller SA, Conn HL (eds): The Myocardial Cell: Structure, Function, and Modification. Philadelphia, University of Pennsylvania Press, 1966)

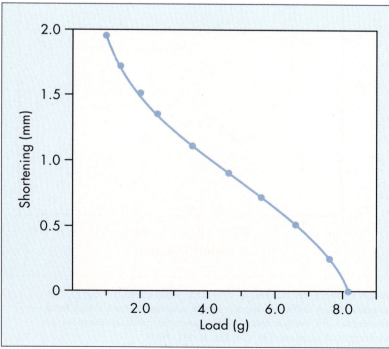

FIGURE 2.21 Relationship between load and the distance shortened in a representative series of isotonic afterloaded contractions in cardiac muscle.

force–velocity relation when comparing alterations in preload with alterations in contractility (see Fig. 2.22).[13] With alterations in preload, there was an increase in force development (Frank-Starling mechanism) with little change in V_{max} (maximum velocity of shortening). With alterations in contractile state, there was an increase in both V_{max} and in developed force. This led to the proposal that V_{max} be considered as an index of contractile state independent of loading conditions. A problem with using V_{max} as an index of contractile state relates to the fact that it is not totally independent of loading conditions.[14] Furthermore, there is great difficulty in calculating V_{max} in patients. More importantly, it has not proved to be any more useful than other indices of contractility, particularly those that describe the pump performance of the heart. For all of these reasons, V_{max} has not become useful in measuring contractility in patients, although it still remains a useful descriptor of the performance characteristics of cardiac muscle.

VELOCITY–LENGTH RELATIONS

Another property of cardiac muscle, which has been evaluated in some detail, is the relationship of instantaneous velocity and length during a series of isotonic contractions. A series of contractions during which the total load on the muscle remains the same but preload is decreased and afterload proportionally increased to maintain the same total load is shown in Figure 2.23. The instantaneous relationship between velocity and length is illustrated for each contraction. Note that after an initial rise much of the contractile course is along the same velocity–length relation during the balance of shortening. With an increase in contractility produced by norepinephrine (Fig. 2.23, *B*), the velocity–length relation is shifted upward. This suggests that this relationship could be used as an index of contractility, independent of loading conditions. Studies by Brutsaert[15] have led to the concept of a surface

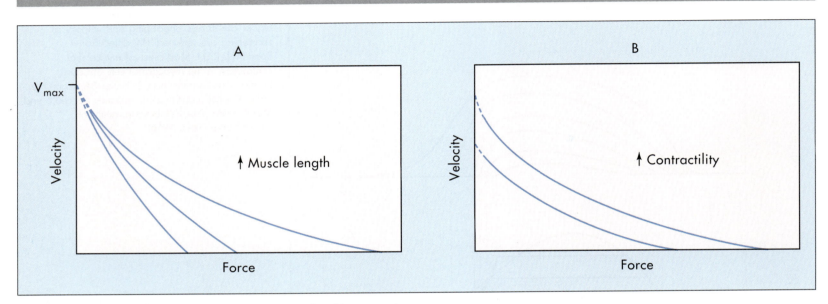

FIGURE 2.22 A. Representative force–velocity relations in isolated heart muscle obtained at three different muscle lengths. **B.** Representative changes in the force–velocity relation following an increase in contractile state.

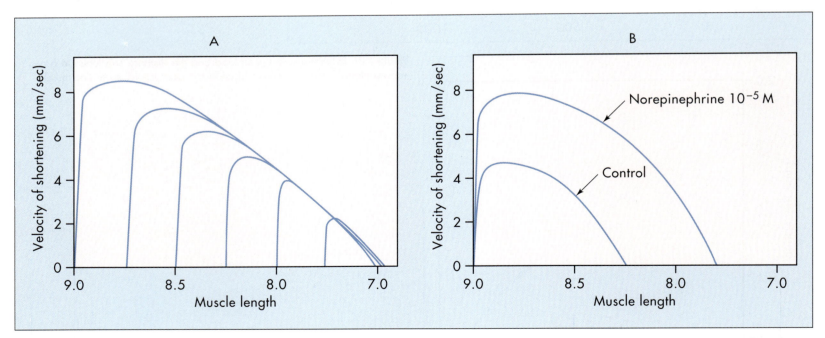

FIGURE 2.23 A. Superimposed velocity–length relations. Each contraction begins at a different muscle length, but contraction occurs with the same total load. Note that after an initial upstroke, the contractions proceed to the right and down along the same velocity–length line. **B.** When loading conditions remain constant, an increase in contractile state (produced by 10^{-5} M norepinephrine) shifts the velocity–length relation upward. (Modified from Sonnenblick EH: Instantaneous force–velocity length determinations in contraction of heart muscle. Circ Res 16:441, 1965)

of contractility that can be outlined on a three-dimensional grid, as seen in Figure 2.24. The relationship between force, velocity, and length is illustrated. The surface thus created would describe the contractility of cardiac muscle and its performance at any given point. Increases in contractility would shift this surface upward, while decreases in contractility would shift this surface downward. Although this is a useful descriptive scheme of the performance of cardiac muscle *in vitro*, it is almost impossible to apply clinically. Thus, like force-velocity relations, this method of describing cardiac muscle contractility has been restricted to the basic laboratory.

RELATIONSHIP BETWEEN ISOMETRIC AND ISOTONIC CONTRACTIONS

One of the more fundamental relationships of importance in cardiac muscle is illustrated in Figure 2.25. A series of isometric contractions define the active and passive length–tension relationship. Adding the two gives the total force line. A series of isotonic contractions are then obtained and plotted on the same graph. Note that with an individual contraction, force rises until it matches the afterload and then, with shortening, the line moves to the left and tends to end at the total force line. This is true irrespective of alterations in preload and afterload, at least within certain limits.[16] In other words, the endpoint of contraction falls on the total force line, regardless of the preload and afterload, and regardless of whether the muscle contracts isometrically or isotonically. A quantitative description of the total force line, therefore, would represent the contractile state of the heart, irrespective of the loading conditions.

With an increase in contractile state, this total force line is shifted up and to the left, as seen in Figure 2.26. It is shifted down and to the right with a decrease in contractile state. This relationship also holds in the intact heart when pressure–volume loops are plotted.

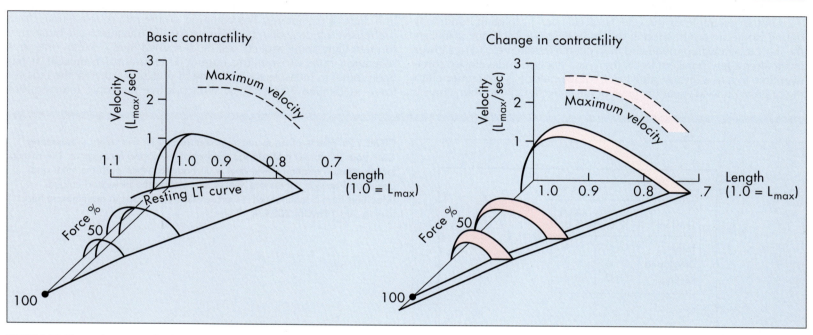

FIGURE 2.24 Three-dimensional relationship among force, velocity, and length. (*Left*) The velocity–length relationships are illustrated over a wide range. The velocity–length lines represent the contractile state of the muscle. (*Right*) With an increase in contractile state, there is a shift upward in velocity to a new surface, illustrated by the upper line in each shaded zone. Thus, contractility is represented by a given surface that shifts upward or downward in this three-dimensional relationship. (Modified from Brutsaert DL, Paulus WJ: Loading and performance of the heart as a muscle and pump. Cardiovasc Res 11:1, 1977)

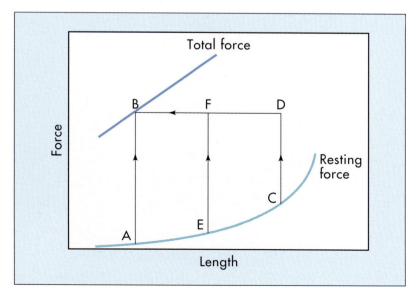

FIGURE 2.25 Schematic diagram of the relationship between force and length with isometric and isotonic contractions. The bottom line (resting force) represents the passive length–tension relation. The total force line is as defined in Figure 2.9. An isometric contraction, beginning at A, would develop force to B. An isotonic contraction beginning at point E, with an afterload equal to EF, would develop force to F and shorten to B. At a longer length (point C), an isotonic contraction, with an afterload equal to CD, would develop force to D and then shorten to B. Thus, all three of these contractions end at point B on the total force line. With differing preloads and afterloads than shown, both isometric and isotonic contractions would end on the total force line.

LENGTH AND LOAD-DEPENDENT CHANGES IN CONTRACTILE STATE

So far, the above description of cardiac muscle mechanics has paid little attention to the previous history of loading on its subsequent performance. In isolated heart muscle, however, a number of studies have shown that previous length and loading conditions can affect the subsequent performance. One of these phenomena is illustrated in Figure 2.27. If one changes the mode of contraction from isotonic to isometric between beats, the first isometric contraction develops more force than subsequent isometric contractions, which stabilize at a lower level.[17] After the muscle has stabilized, the mode of contraction is then switched back to isotonic. The shortening velocity of the first isotonic contraction is less than the subsequent shortening velocity, which stabilizes at a higher level. In other words, the muscle appears to be at a higher level of contractility during isotonic contraction, as compared with isometric contraction, as reflected by the increased shortening velocity of the stable isotonic beat and the increased force development of the first isometric beat.

Another example of the effects of changes in loading conditions during isometric contraction is shown in Figure 2.28. If one stabilizes the muscle at a high preload and then decreases the preload to a lower level, after a few transient beats there is a decline in developed force over time to a new steady-state level.[18] If the muscle is then returned to the original preload (near the peak of the active length–tension curve), there is a gradual rise in force to a new stable level. In other words, the muscle appears to be at a higher level of contractility at a longer muscle length and higher preload. Directionally, this would be helpful in improving muscle performance at higher preloads, which are generally used when there is a need to increase force development.

Although both of these phenomena (and other similar phenomena) have been described in isolated heart muscle, there is little evidence that they play an important role in the intact heart. Because one is unable to change the loading conditions as abruptly in the intact heart as one can in isolated heart muscle, these phenomena probably play no significant clinical role. Nevertheless, they emphasize the fact that cardiac muscle does have a memory for previous events such as loading and that these effects must be taken into account under certain experimental conditions.

RELAXATION

Considerable interest has been generated over the past decade on the diastolic properties of the ventricle and how they affect cardiac function. Part of this interest has centered on the rate of relaxation. Comprehensive studies of relaxation in cardiac muscle have been performed. Only some aspects will be described here.[11] When one plots relaxation rates of isometric contractions in cardiac muscle, it has been useful to measure the half-time of relaxation, that is, the time for force to decline 50% ($RT_{1/2}$). With positive inotropic interventions

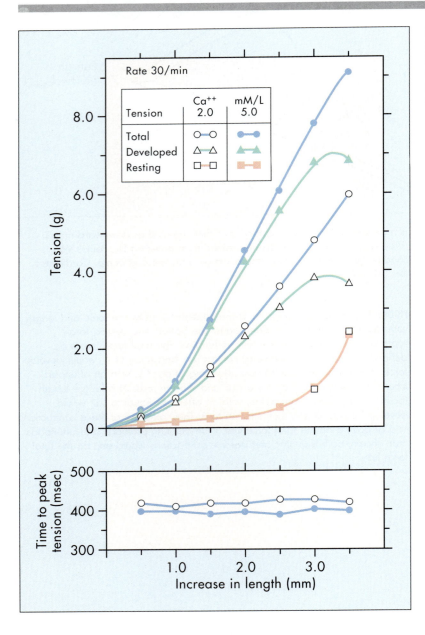

FIGURE 2.26 Effects of an increase in contractility (in this case by increasing Ca^{2+} from 2.0 to 5.0 mM) on the total and developed force curve. The resting length–tension relation (*lower line*) is unchanged, while both the total and developed tension curves are shifted upward by the increased calcium. (Modified from Sonnenblick EH: Force–velocity relations in mammalian heart muscle. Am J Physiol 202:931, 1962)

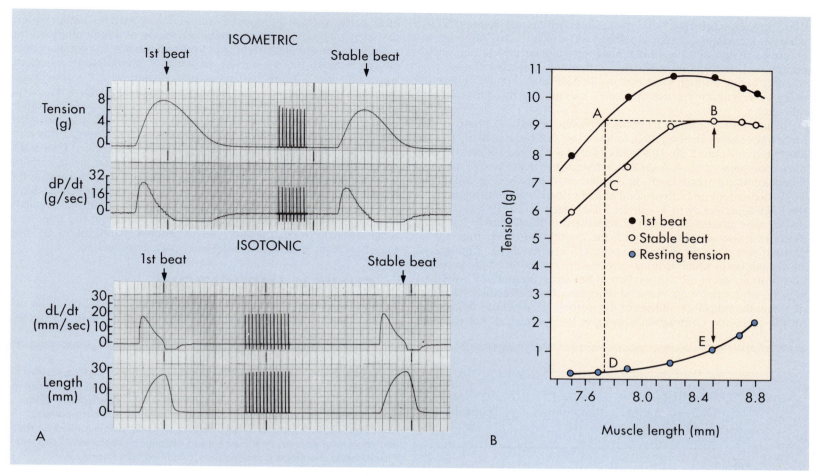

FIGURE 2.27 A. Sequential alteration of a series of contractions between isometric and isotonic. In the top panel, the first isometric contraction (first beat) was obtained after a series of isotonic contractions. The first beat and stable beat are shown at a rapid paper speed, while the intermediate beats are shown at a slow paper speed. Note the gradual reduction in force from the first beat to the stable beat, which is also accompanied by a reduction in maximum rate of force development (dP/dt). Subsequently, the contraction mode was switched from isometric to isotonic (lower panel). The first and stable isotonic beats are spread out at a rapid paper speed while the intermediate beats are recorded at a slower paper speed. Note that the stable isotonic beat has a greater shortening and velocity of shortening (dL/dt) than the first isotonic beat. Thus, there is an apparent alteration in contractility, which is reversible as one goes back and forth between series of isotonic and isometric contractions. **B.** This difference between the first and stable isometric contractions persists over the entire length–tension relation, as illustrated. The passive length–tension relation at the bottom is unchanged. The upper curve represents the first isometric contraction obtained after a series of isotonic beats, while the middle curve represents the stable isometric beats. Note for example, that the first isometric contraction, DA, develops more force than the stable beat EB at L_{max} (arrows). (Modified from Parmley WW, Brutsaert DL, Sonnenblick EH: The effects of altered loading on contractile events in isolated cat papillary muscle. Circ Res 23:521, 1969)

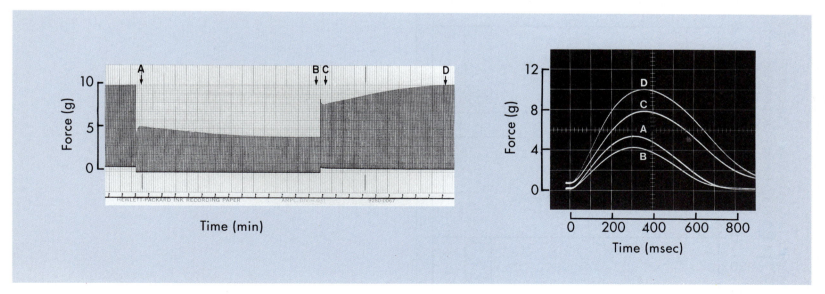

FIGURE 2.28 (Left) Slow speed record of a sequence of isometric contractions. Beginning at the left, contractions are obtained at L_{max}, the peak of the active length–tension relationship. Force is then reduced to a low level. After a transient phenomenon, isometric force is gradually reduced from A to B. Following an increase in the length of the muscle to L_{max} again, there is an increase in force from C to D back to control. (Right) The individual contractions, A, B, C and D, are spread out and superimposed on a Polaroid photograph. Thus, alterations in muscle length have a slow time-dependent effect on muscle contractility. (Modified from Parmley WW, Chuck L: Length-dependent changes in myocardial contractile state. Am J Physiol 224:1195, 1973)

there are characteristic changes. Catecholamines reduce $RT_{1/2}$, whereas increased calcium lengthens $RT_{1/2}$ (Fig. 2.29). Although increased calcium and catecholamines have similar effects on systolic contraction, they affect relaxation differently. Catecholamines, presumably acting through increased cyclic AMP, speed up the relaxation process by enhancing the uptake of calcium by the sarcoplasmic reticulum.

In isotonic afterloaded contractions, the relaxation phase of the force trace shows an abrupt fall, followed by an exponential decline, as illustrated in Figure 2.30. This lends itself to a $T_{1/2}$ measurement during the exponential decline. A similar technique has been used to measure relaxation in the intact heart. In isolated heart muscle (Fig. 2.31), this $T_{1/2}$ is dependent on both preload and afterload, which correlates with the load dependency of $T_{1/2}$ in the intact heart.

Another interesting aspect of relaxation in heart muscle has been the correlation of relaxation with the quantity of myocardial sarcoplasmic reticulum in different species.[19] For example, Figure 2.32 shows studies in which isotonic afterloaded contractions are superimposed on an isometric contraction at the same preload. In frog heart muscle, where there are reduced amounts of sarcoplasmic reticulum, note that the relaxation phases of the isotonic contractions tend to fall on the isometric contraction envelope. By contrast, in cat papillary muscle, the isotonic afterloaded contractions have a relaxation pattern that is initially outside the isometric envelope at a high afterload but rapidly falls inside this envelope at lower afterloads. Cat papillary muscle has a much more extensive network of sarcoplasmic reticulum, suggesting that a more avid uptake of calcium by the sarcoplasmic reticulum leads to a reduction in the duration of lightly loaded isotonic contractions. Rat muscle exhibits relaxation characteristics intermediate between those of cat muscle and frog muscle. It also has more sarcoplasmic reticulum than the frog but less than the cat. This phenomenon has been termed *load-dependent relaxation*. If one decreases the function of the sarcoplasmic reticulum by giving caffeine (which decreases uptake and increases release), and by making the muscle hypoxic (which also decreases sarcoplasmic reticulum function), one can change the load-dependent relaxation of cat papillary muscle to a load-independent state.[20] This points out the important relationship between the mechanical process of relaxation and the presence of an intact functioning sarcoplasmic reticulum.

CLINICAL IMPLICATIONS

An understanding of cardiac muscle mechanics is essential to an understanding of ventricular function in the cardiac patient. The princi-

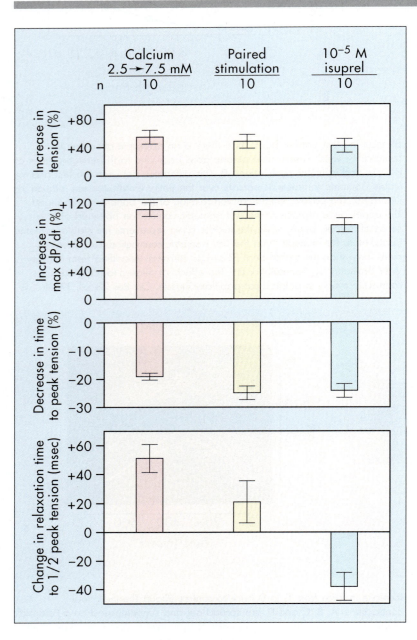

FIGURE 2.29 Effects of increased calcium, paired stimulation, and isoproterenol (Isuprel) on the isometric contraction. All interventions produced an increase in force (*top panel*), an increase in maximum rate of force development (dP/dt) (*second panel*), and a decrease in the time to peak tension (*third panel*). Note, however, that the interventions have a markedly differing effect on the relaxation time: whereas increased calcium prolongs it, isoproterenol shortens it, and paired stimulation is intermediate. (Modified from Parmley WW, Sonnenblick EH: Relation between mechanics of contraction and relaxation in mammalian cardiac muscle. Am J Physiol 216:1084, 1969)

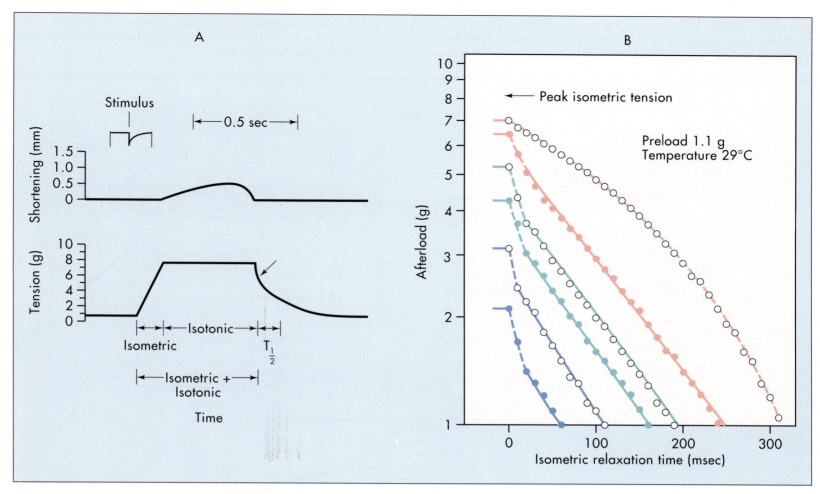

FIGURE 2.30 A. Representative afterloaded isotonic contraction in cat papillary muscle. During the decline of tension in the relaxation phase, there is an abrupt fall in tension (*arrow*) followed by an exponential decline. This is illustrated better in **B**, where the exponential decline in tension appears as a straight line on a log scale over a wide range of isotonic afterloaded contractions. This relationship no longer holds as one approaches peak isometric tension (*upper curve*). (Modified from Parmley WW, Sonnenblick EH: Relation between mechanics of contraction and relaxation in mammalian cardiac muscle. Am J Physiol 216:1084, 1969)

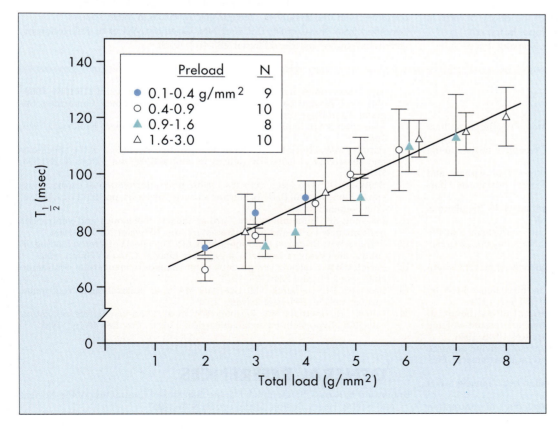

FIGURE 2.31 Load dependency of $T_{1/2}$ during relaxation obtained from isotonic afterloaded contractions (see Figure 2.30). At each preload, note that there is a relatively linear relationship between the $T_{1/2}$ of relaxation and the total load (preload plus afterload) over a wide range of preloads and afterload. (Modified from Parmley WW, Sonnenblick EH: Relationship between mechanics of contraction and relaxation in mammalian cardiac muscle. Am J Physiol 216:1084, 1969)

ples of this chapter have direct relevance to *in vivo* function and to the evaluation and management of patients with congestive heart failure, discussed in detail later in this volume. The four primary determinants of cardiac muscle performance (preload, afterload, contractility, and heart rate) form a useful framework with which to evaluate individual patients and to plan their therapy.

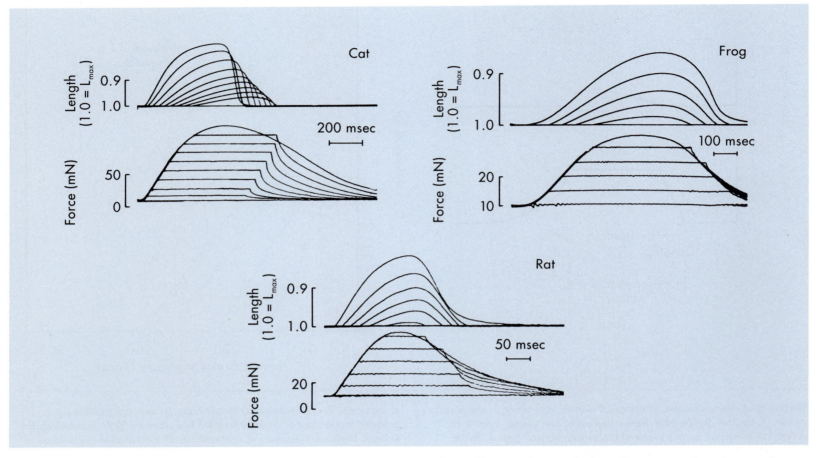

FIGURE 2.32 Series of superimposed isotonic afterloaded contractions in isolated ventricular muscle from cat, frog, and rat. In the force tracings (second panel of each set of two), note the relationship between the decay of force in isotonic contractions and the outer isometric force envelope. In the cat, relaxation of isotonic contractions occurs well inside the isometric force envelope; whereas in frog muscle, force decay occurs along the same line. Rat muscle is intermediate. The degree of "load-dependent relaxation" correlates with the amount of sarcoplasmic reticulum in these species. (Modified from Brutsaert DL, DeClerck NN, Goethals MM et al: Relaxation of ventricular cardiac muscle. J Physiol 283:469, 1978)

REFERENCES

1. Huxley AF: Muscle structure and theories of contraction. Prog Biophys Chem 7:255, 1957
2. Ebashi S, Ebashi F, Kodama A: Troponin as the Ca^{++}-receptive protein in the contractile system. J Biochem 62:137, 1967
3. Sutherland EW, Rall TW: The relation of adenosine-3'-5'-phosphate and phosphorylase to the action of catecholamines and other hormones. Pharmacol Rev 12:265, 1960
4. Wikman-Coffelt J, Sievers R, Coffelt RJ et al: The cardiac cycle: Regulations and energy oscillations. Am J Physiol 245:H354, 1983
5. Spann JF Jr, Covell JW, Eckberg DL et al: Contractile performance of the hypertrophied and chronically failing cat ventricle. Am J Physiol 223:1150, 1972
6. Jewell BR: Brief reviews: A re-examination of the influences of muscle length on myocardial performance. Circ Res 40:221, 1977
7. Garlick PB, Radda GK, Seeley PJ: Studies of acidosis in the ischemic heart by phosphorus nuclear magnetic resonance. Biochem J 184:547, 1979
8. Spotnitz HM, Sonnenblick EH, Spiro D: Relationship of ultrastructure to function in the intact heart: Sarcomere structure relative to pressure–volume curves in the intact left ventricles of dog and cat. Circ Res 18:49, 1966
9. Henderson AH, Brutsaert DL, Forman R et al: Influence of caffeine on force development and force frequency relations in cat and rat heart muscle. Cardiovasc Res 8:162, 1974
10. Sonnenblick EH: Force velocity relations in mammalian heart muscle. Am J Physiol 202:931, 1962
11. Parmley WW, Sonnenblick EH: Relation between mechanics of contraction and relaxation in mammalian cardiac muscle. Am J Physiol 216:1084, 1969
12. Hill AV: First and Last Experiments in Muscle Mechanics. Cambridge, England, Cambridge University Press, 1970
13. Sonnenblick EH: Implications of muscle mechanics in heart. Fed Proc 21:975, 1962
14. Parmley WW, Chuck L, Yeatman L: Comparative evaluation of the specificity and sensitivity of isometric indices of contractility. Am J Physiol 228:506, 1975
15. Brutsaert DL: The force–velocity–length–time interrelation of cardiac muscle. In Physiological Basis of Starling's Law of the Heart, pp 155–175. London, Ciba Foundation, 1974
16. Downing SE, Sonnenblick EH: Cardiac muscle mechanics and ventricular performance: Force and time parameters. Am J Physiol 207:705, 1964
17. Parmley WW, Brutsaert DL, Sonnenblick EH: The effects of altered loading on contractile events in isolated cat papillary muscle. Circ Res 23:521, 1969
18. Parmley WW, Chuck L: Length dependent changes in myocardial contractile state. Am J Physiol 224:1195, 1973
19. Brutsaert DL, DeClerck NM, Goethals MA et al: Relaxation of ventricular cardiac muscle. J Physiol 283:469, 1978
20. Chuck LH, Goethals MA, Parmley WW et al: Load-insensitive relaxation caused by hypoxia in mammalian cardiac muscle. Circ Res 48:797, 1981

GENERAL REFERENCES

Braunwald E, Ross J, Sonnenblick EH: Mechanisms of Contraction of the Normal and Failing Heart. Boston, Little, Brown & Co, 1967

Brutsaert DL, Paulus WJ: Loading and performance of the heart as a muscle and pump. Cardiovasc Res 11:1, 1977

Brutsaert DL, Sonnenblick EH: Cardiac muscle mechanics in the evaluation of myocardial contractility and pump function: Problems, concepts and directions. Prog Cardiovasc Dis 16:337, 1973

Chapman RA: Control of cardiac contractility at the cellular level. Am J Physiol 14:H535, 1983

Huxley AF: Muscular contraction. J Physiol 243:1, 1974

Opie Lionel H: Role of cyclic nucleotides in heart metabolism. Cardiovasc Res 16:483, 1982

Cardiovascular Adrenergic and Muscarinic Cholinergic Receptors

Patricia L. Wisler • Frank J. Green
August M. Watanabe

The major extrinsic regulation of the cardiovascular system occurs via the autonomic nervous system. The response of the heart and vasculature to autonomic influences is mediated by receptors located on the plasmalemma of myocytes in the heart and vessels. Our early understanding of these receptors was based on pharmacologic characterization of tissue responses to epinephrine and norepinephrine, which mediate the actions of the sympathetic nervous system, and to acetylcholine, which mediates the actions of the parasympathetic nervous system. Since the mid-1970s, the techniques associated with radioligand binding assays have made possible the direct study of receptors for the first time. Since the mid-1980s, recombinant DNA and immunological techniques have permitted subtyping and extensive characterization of the molecular structure of both adrenergic and muscarinic cholinergic receptors. These techniques for the direct study of receptors have enabled us to appreciate that they are physiologically regulated, and begin to understand how the binding of a neurotransmitter to its receptor is coupled biochemically to changes in cellular function. In this chapter we will confine our attention to the adrenergic and muscarinic cholinergic receptors. At the same time it must be noted that much work is currently being done on receptors for serotonin, dopamine, and angiotensin II, and that findings from these studies may affect the practice of cardiology in the future.

METHODOLOGY OF RECEPTOR BINDING ASSAYS

Radioligand binding assays are competitive protein binding assays similar in principle to radioimmunoassays (Fig. 3.1). The source of material for testing is an organ or tissue that, based on physiologic data, is thought to contain the receptor. The tissue is homogenized, and the receptor suspension produced by homogenization can then be used as is, or subjected to differential centrifugation to isolate partially purified cellular subfractions that contain the receptor. The receptor is detected by incubating the membrane suspension with a ligand that has extremely high affinity for the receptor and is radioactively labeled. Subsequently, radioligand bound to receptors is separated from the remainder, which remains free in the suspension. This is usually done by rapid vacuum filtration through glass fiber filter paper. The total radioactivity bound to the receptor protein can then be counted. The amount of radioactive ligand bound to nonreceptor material in the suspension must also be quantified. This determination of nonspecific binding is usually done in identical incubations that include a concentration of nonradioactive ligand sufficiently high to saturate the receptor. The remaining bound radioactivity is considered nonspecific binding of the radioligand. This is subtracted from the total bound radioactivity to yield the specifically bound radioactivity. The amount of receptors present can then be quantified. In general, radiolabeled receptor antagonists have proved easiest to study; for reasons that will become clear, the binding of radiolabeled agonists is more complex.

A number of criteria are used to verify that a particular ligand is indeed labeling the receptor of interest. Only organs and tissues that, based on pharmacologic and physiologic data, are presumed to possess the receptors being studied should bind the ligand specifically. Unlabeled drugs should be able to inhibit binding of the radioligand with the same rank order of potency that they display in eliciting a pharmacologic response. The biologically active stereoisomers should inhibit radioligand binding more potently than the inactive isomers. With increasing concentrations of the free radioligand, the amount of specifically bound radioligand should reach a plateau, *i.e.*, saturate. If these criteria of appropriate localization, pharmacologic specificity, stereospecificity and saturability can be met, then it is likely that the radioligand is binding to the receptor of interest. A number of technical considerations should also be met. The amount of radioligand bound should rise linearly with increases in the amount of tissue examined. There should be agreement between measurements of receptor affinity determined by different methods. There should be no metabolism of the radioligand by the tissue. Because radioligands bind to other material besides the receptor, this nonspecific binding should be determined appropriately. The specific binding should be rapid and reversible, appropriate to the rate of onset and reversibility of the pharmacologic effects of the unlabeled ligand.

The study of receptors rests on the assumption that the interaction of a receptor with a ligand follows the laws of mass action. A number of excellent reviews detail the mathematical features of the law of mass action, which provide a rationale for the kinds of experiments performed to study receptors.[1-3] The interaction of ligands with receptors can be studied under steady-state (equilibrium) conditions, during which the concentration of bound radioligand is constant and the reaction is allowed to proceed long enough to reach equilibrium. Receptor-ligand interactions can also be studied using kinetic experiments in which the rates of association and dissociation of the ligand with the receptor are directly measured.

Two types of equilibrium assay are used. The first is a saturation assay from which the affinity of the receptor for labeled ligands can be deduced, as well as the tissue concentration of receptors and the extent to which the interaction is a simple bimolecular reaction obeying the law of mass action. In a saturation assay, a fixed concentration of receptor is incubated with varying amounts of the radioligand (Fig. 3.2). As a function of increasing concentration of free radioligand (in this case the nonselective beta-adrenergic antagonist, [^{3}H]-carazolol),[4] specific binding rises and reaches a plateau, indicating saturation of the receptor. The equilibrium dissociation constant, K_D, of the receptor can be estimated from the concentration of free [^{3}H]-carazolol at which the concentration of receptor is half-maximal. Alternatively, as depicted in the inset, a Scatchard[5] analysis of the saturation data can be performed by plotting the ratio of bound to free radioligand versus the concentration of bound radioligand. This yields a line with a slope equal to $-1/K_D$ and an x intercept equal to the maximal receptor concentration, B_{max}. Thus, the K_D is expressed in a molar concentration, with lower K_D meaning higher affinity.

The second kind of equilibrium experiment used is a competition study, from which a number of parameters can be determined. They include:

1. The affinity of a receptor population for an unlabeled ligand
2. The concentration of receptors that bind the unlabeled ligand
3. The presence of receptor subtypes
4. The nature of the competition between the labeled and unlabeled ligands
5. Possible shifts in the affinity of the receptor population

An example of an equilibrium competition study is depicted in Figure 3.3. In this experiment, the specific binding of a fixed concentration of [^{3}H]-carazolol is examined in the absence and presence of ascending concentrations of unlabeled beta-adrenergic antagonists. Each of these antagonists is able to inhibit [^{3}H]-carazolol binding completely. One can measure the concentration of unlabeled antagonist at which [^{3}H]-carazolol binding is half-maximally inhibited, the IC_{50}. The competition data yielding the indicated sigmoid curves can be linearized using a logarithmic equation to yield a Hill plot.[6] If the slope of the line generated in a Hill plot is equal to one, then the unlabeled antagonist is likely to be a competitive inhibitor of [^{3}H]-carazolol. The K_D of the inhibitor, or K_i, can be calculated from the IC_{50}:[7]

$$K_i = \frac{IC_{50}}{1 + \frac{[L]}{K_D}}$$

where [L] and K_D are the concentration and K_D of [^{3}H]-carazolol. This is the case for both propranolol and carazolol in Figure 3.3. The slope factor for metoprolol, however, is significantly less than one. Using computer modeling techniques, it is possible to identify two classes of binding sites at which metoprolol and [^{3}H]-carazolol compete. One class of sites has a higher affinity for metoprolol, and presumably these are all beta-adrenergic receptors. The second class has a lower affinity for metoprolol, and these are presumably beta$_2$-adrenergic receptor sites.

One can also examine competition of unlabeled beta-agonists with labeled antagonists. In this case, however, even when the nonselective agonist isoproterenol is used, the curve generated may or may not be sigmoid. As illustrated in Figure 3.4, in membranes prepared in the absence of guanine nucleotides, competition of isoproterenol with [^{3}H]-carazolol yields a shallow sigmoid curve with a Hill plot slope less than 1. This is consistent with the presence of a small population of beta-adrenergic receptors with a high affinity for the agonist, and a larger population of beta receptors with a lower affinity for the agonist. In the presence of guanine nucleotides, all of the beta receptors exhibit the same low affinity for the beta-adrenergic agonist,[8] and the sigmoid curve described by the competition becomes steeper and shifted to the right, with a Hill plot slope of 1. Thus, the use of beta-adrenergic agonists, labeled or unlabeled, in binding studies is complicated by the necessity of identifying the presence or absence of guanine nucleo-

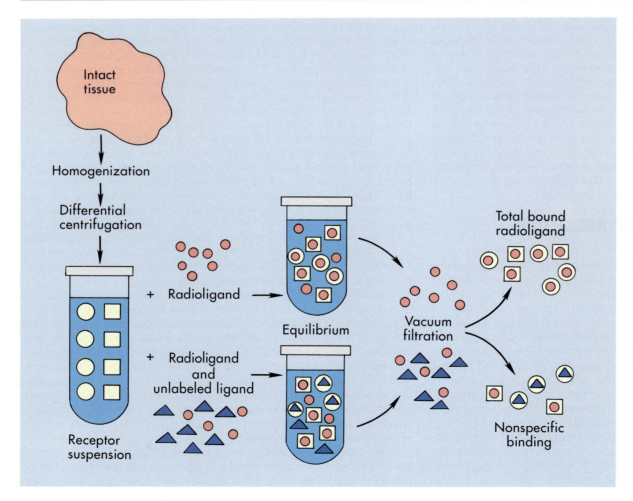

FIGURE 3.1 A source of receptors, in this case heart, is homogenized to yield a suspension of receptors. This suspension may be subjected to differential centrifugation or used as is. The suspension containing both receptors (open circles) and nonspecific binding sites (open squares) is then incubated with the radioligand (solid circles) in the absence or presence of a large concentration of unlabeled ligand (open triangles) until equilibrium is reached. The free ligands in solution are then separated from the bound ligand by vacuum filtration over glass fiber filters. In the presence of radiolabeled ligand alone, total binding of the radioligand by both receptor and nonreceptor sites can be determined. In the presence of a large concentration of unlabeled ligand, all receptor sites are occupied by the unlabeled ligand, and any binding of radiolabeled ligand is assumed to be due to nonspecific sites.

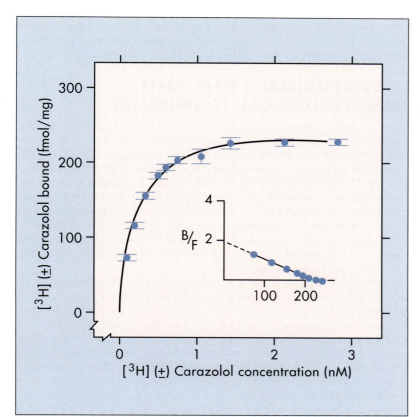

FIGURE 3.2 Saturation of specific [^{3}H]-carazolol binding, defined as that displaceable by 20 μM propranolol, is plotted as a function of increasing [^{3}H]-carazolol concentration. In the inset, a Scatchard analysis plots the ratio of bound to free [^{3}H]-carazolol (B/F) versus the concentration of bound [^{3}H]-carazolol (B). The slope of the Scatchard plot is equal to $-1/K_D$. The K_D is 135 pM, and B_{max}, 243 fmol/mg membrane protein. nM = 10^{-9} M, pM = 10^{-12} M and fmol = 10^{-15} moles. (Modified from Manalan AS, Besch HR Jr, Watanabe AM: Characteristics of [^{3}H](±)carazolol binding to beta-adrenergic receptor: application to study of beta-adrenergic receptor subtypes in canine ventricular myocardium and lung. Circ Res 49:326, 1981)

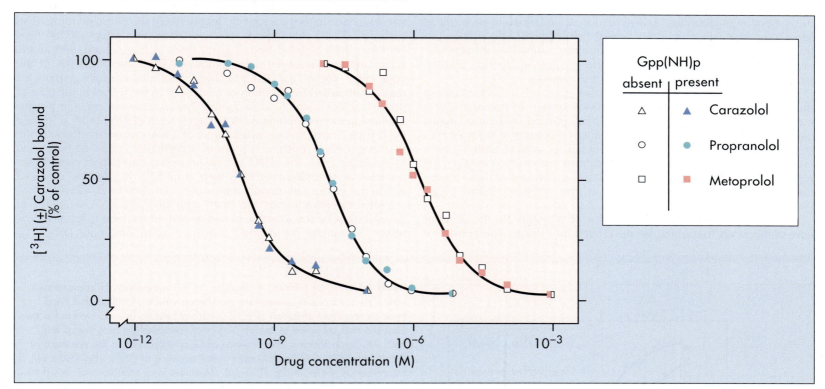

FIGURE 3.3 Competition of unlabeled beta-adrenergic antagonists with [^{3}H]-carazolol in canine ventricular myocardial membrane vesicles. Specific binding of a fixed concentration of [^{3}H]-carazolol in the presence of ascending concentrations of unlabeled antagonists is expressed as a fraction of that obtained in the absence of unlabeled antagonists. Unfilled and filled symbols represent the absence and presence of 5′ guanylylimidodiphosphate (Gpp(NH)p), 100 μM, which has no effect on antagonist competition. Slope factors: carazolol 0.96, propranolol 0.92, metoprolol 0.76. (Modified from Manalan AS, Besch HR Jr, Watanabe AM: Characteristics of [^{3}H](±)carazolol binding to beta-adrenergic receptor: Application to study of beta-adrenergic receptor subtypes in canine ventricular myocardium and lung. Circ Res 49:326, 1981)

tides in the preparation used. As will be described, this has enabled investigators to begin to understand how the binding of beta-adrenergic agonists to receptors is coupled to a sequence of biochemical events in the cell.

In addition to equilibrium studies, receptor-ligand interaction can also be studied using kinetic experiments. By measuring total and nonspecific binding of a radioligand to the receptor at various time points after the addition of the radioligand, one can calculate the rate of association of the ligand, or k_{+1}. When equilibrium is reached, a high concentration of unlabeled ligand can be added to the tube, and aliquots of protein removed for measurement of radioligand binding at various subsequent time points. From this experiment the rate of dissociation, k_{-1}, of the radioligand from its receptor can be calculated. The quotient k_{-1}/k_{+1} yields the K_D. It is important to determine K_D using both a kinetic and an equilibrium method, since discrepancies between the two may be clues that the reaction between the receptor and the radioligand is not a reversible molecular one. For example, many of the very high-affinity receptor antagonists exhibit a rapid phase of association and dissociation from the receptor as well as a second, more slowly reversible phase.

Thus, the direct study of receptors has enabled us to make a number of important discoveries. The existence of receptor subtypes has been confirmed using nonselective radiolabeled antagonists and unlabeled subtype-selective antagonists. Using unlabeled agonists in competition with labeled antagonists has enabled us to define a population of receptors that bind the agonists with high affinity in the absence of guanine nucleotides, and are shifted to a state of low affinity for agonists in the presence of guanine nucleotides. This observation, in turn, has led to the burgeoning study of membrane proteins regulated by these guanine nucleotides. As will be described below, these proteins seem to provide a mechanism by which the binding of a neurotransmitter by a receptor on the cell surface provides a signal for intracellular events. In providing such a signal these guanine nucleotide binding proteins also regulate receptor affinity for agonists.

Radioligand binding assays are also an approach to understanding the physiology of the autonomic nervous system in humans. Using currently available biopsy techniques, small portions of human organs can be made available for receptor studies. Circulating leukocytes possess beta-adrenergic receptors, and circulating platelets, alpha$_2$-adrenergic receptors.[9] These receptor populations are easily accessible for repeated study. Under certain circumstances, changes in these receptor populations may reflect changes in less easily accessible organ systems.

Radioligand binding assays also provide a system for the study of new compounds that could be developed into drugs. The activity of new compounds at receptor sites can be quickly and inexpensively assessed *in vitro* by these assays. This has been particularly useful in evaluating a variety of new inotropic and antihypertensive agents.

RECOMBINANT DNA AND IMMUNOLOGICAL TECHNIQUES

Until recently, receptors and other proteins were examined by biochemical and pharmacologic methods within the confines of extremely limited amounts of purified protein. Developments in recombinant DNA techniques have ushered in a new era of structure-function studies. Complementary DNA (cDNA) cloning provides material for hydridization to genomic DNA, enabling genes to be located on specific chromosomes and to be sequenced completely. cDNA clones can be altered by site-directed mutagenesis, so that functional domains of their expressed proteins may be identified. Protein cloning provides necessary amounts of pure protein for extensive structural, biochemical, and pharmacologic analyses.

Generally, receptors and regulatory proteins have now been characterized in molecular structural terms by a sequence of experiments. A typical sequence may begin with purification of the protein to electrophoretic homogeneity through the powerful techniques of affinity labeling and affinity chromatography. Partial sequencing of the purified protein provides amino acid arrangements from which codes for DNA can be derived. Using the deduced codes, matching DNA oligonucleotides can be chemically synthesized and radioactively labeled as probes. Such DNA probes are used to screen for matching DNA sequences in genomic and/or cDNA libraries. A genomic library is a collection of vector particles (lambda phage, plasmids, cosmids, or viruses), each harboring specific fragments of the entire genome of an organism. Using mechanical forces or restriction enzymes, the total genomic DNA isolated from a given tissue is fragmented, and all the fragments are packaged as recombinant DNA into the DNA of the appropriate vector, *e.g.*, lambda phage. The number of phage particles may be amplified by infection of a host cell (a bacterium in the case of phage vectors), which subsequently lyses, releasing multiple phages containing the recombinant DNA fragments. A cDNA library is formed by reverse transcriptase production of DNA complementary to the messenger RNA (mRNA) content of a particular tissue. As described for genomic DNA, the cDNA can be housed in carefully chosen vector particles as recombinant DNA, then amplified by infection of a cell where the vector can rapidly reproduce, and then be isolated.

After the DNA library has been amplified, the DNA sequence of interest must be found in the plated growth of bacteria that harbor the phage containing the desired sequence as recombinant DNA. The

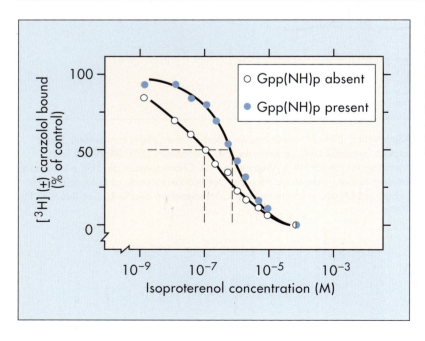

FIGURE 3.4 Effect of guanine nucleotides on the competition of isoproterenol with [^{3}H]-carazolol in canine lung membrane vesicles. Unfilled and filled symbols represent inhibition of [^{3}H]-carazolol binding by isoproterenol in the absence and presence of added 5'-guanylylimidodiphosphate (Gpp(NH)p), 100 μM. Slope factor in the absence of Gpp(NH)p, 0.42; in the presence of Gpp(NH)p, 0.74. K_i of isoproterenol in the absence of Gpp(NH)p, 0.026 μM; in the presence of Gpp(NH)p, 0.23 μM. (Modified from Manalan AS, Besch HR Jr, Watanabe AM: Characteristics of [^{3}H](±)carazolol binding to beta-adrenergic receptor: Application to study of beta-adrenergic receptor subtypes in canine ventricular myocardium and lung. Circ Res 49:326, 1981)

search is begun by blotting the plate, containing plaques that are sources of free phage particles, with a sheet of nitrocellulose. When the phage particles and DNA adhere to the nitrocellulose, a negative replica of the plate is formed. The phages are disrupted and phage DNA is denatured to single strands when the nitrocellulose sheet is exposed to high salt in basic solution. Then the phage recombinant DNA may be hybridized with a radioactively labeled DNA (or RNA) probe. Wherever binding of the labeled nucleic acid probe is detected by autoradiography of the nitrocellulose sheet, a corresponding plaque may be identified on the plate of bacterial growth. That plaque can be isolated and its phage reintroduced into bacteria to clone for increased purity and increased production of the desired phage. From the amplified phage growth, recombinant DNA can be isolated and analyzed for nucleotide sequence.

Alternatively, it is sometimes possible to detect the sought-after DNA sequence in the plate of bacterial growth by identifying some expression of its presence, such as a fusion protein formed by the protein of interest and a protein coded by the phage vector. In that case, an antibody probe to the targeted region of the expressed protein can locate the appropriate colony on the plate of bacteria, and the existence of DNA probes is not required. In any case, once the genomic DNA or cDNA corresponding to the protein has been sequenced, the entire amino acid sequence, or primary structure, of the protein can be deduced.

The protein itself can be cloned by transforming the appropriate vector containing recombinant DNA for the protein into a stable cell line which allows for transient or continuous expression of the protein. After the presence of the protein is detected by its particular binding, immunologic, or enzymatic properties, the cells which express it can be cloned. In this manner, sufficient pure protein becomes available, after further purification procedures, for analytic techniques such as electron diffraction that reveal secondary and tertiary protein structure.

A powerful new technique, the polymerase chain reaction (PCR), has begun to facilitate DNA sequencing by reducing cumbersome, time-consuming subcloning and biological amplification procedures.[10] PCR allows discrete fragments of DNA to be specifically amplified. Thus, DNA naturally present in amounts very difficult to detect can be amplified to become the most abundant fragment in a sample. The PCR method consists of denaturation of double-stranded DNA or cDNA made from mRNA, annealing of a pair of extension primers (synthetic oligonucleotides) to one end of the region to be amplified on each of the separated strands, and finally DNA polymerase-mediated extension of the two templates with primers attached. Cycling of this process provides an abundance of the DNA sequence targeted for study.

Immunological techniques are potent tools for locating and quantifying specific cellular proteins, as well as for differentiating protein subtypes that differ by as little as one amino acid. Antibodies are isolated from serum or other body fluids of animals immunized with the protein of interest as antigen. Antibody specific for the antigen can be purified by affinity chromatography from a polyclonal mixture of antibodies in serum. Alternatively, homogeneous monoclonal antibodies of the desired specificity can be formed by cloning a cell formed from fusion of the specific antibody-producing cell with a hybridoma cell. With antibody-based techniques, specific epitopes on a receptor molecule can be analyzed.

G PROTEINS

Adrenergic and muscarinic receptors constitute the initial step in a transduction system through which extracellular signals reach intracellular effectors that, in turn, produce particular cellular responses. Common to both receptor types are plasmalemmal guanine nucleotide regulatory proteins (G proteins) that couple agonist-bound receptors to effector enzymes or ion channels. The effectors are thus activated to initiate or modulate their special activities. G proteins may be more or less tailored for specificity in coupling receptors to particular effector proteins. Recently, several excellent publications have provided in-depth reviews of G protein research.[11-18]

The G proteins coupled to adrenergic and muscarinic receptors are members of a family of guanosine triphosphate (GTP)-regulated proteins. They commonly complex with one protein receptor to mediate reversible interaction with another macromolecular effector. Cell responses mediated by G proteins include adenylate cyclase activity, ion channel activation, cyclic guanosine monophosphate (cGMP) phosphodiesterase activity, protein synthesis, and microtubule aggregation-disaggregation. Members of the G protein family are heterotrimeric molecules composed of alpha, beta, and gamma subunits. The alpha subunits bind GTP and guanosine diphosphate (GDP) nucleotides, interact with effectors and receptors, and possess intrinsic GTPase activity. Alpha subunits endow trimeric G proteins with specificity, while the beta and gamma subunits are closely related, but not identical, among all the G proteins. G proteins identified to date are

TABLE 3.1 G PROTEINS IN CARDIOVASCULAR TISSUES

G Protein	Subunits	Molecular Weight kd	Receptors	ADP-Ribosylated By:*	Effector
G_s	$\alpha_s(4)$	44.5–46	β_1, β_2	Cholera toxin	Adenylate cyclase(+)
	$\beta(4)$	37.4			Ca^{2+} channel(+)
	$\lambda(3)$	8–10			Na^+ channel(−)
G_i	$\alpha_i(3)$	40.4–40.5	Muscarinic, α_2	Pertussis toxin	Adenylate cyclase(−)
	$\beta(4)$	37.4			Atrial K^+ channel(+)
	$\lambda(3)$	8–10			Phospholipase C(+)
G_o	$\alpha_o(1)$	39.9	Muscarinic	Pertussis toxin	?
	$\beta(4)$	37.4			
	$\lambda(3)$	8–10			
G_z	$\alpha_z(1)$	40	Muscarinic, α_1	Neither cholera toxin nor pertussis toxin	Phospholipase C(+)
	$\beta(4)$	37.4			
	$\lambda(3)$	8–10			

* Indicates the capacity of the G alpha subunit to be ADP-ribosylated by the listed bacterial toxin.

(Data from Robishaw JD, Foster KA: Role of G proteins in the regulation of the cardiovascular system. Annu Rev Physiol 51:229, 1989; Gilman AG: G proteins and regulation of adenylyl cyclase. JAMA 262:1819, 1989; Casey PJ, Fong HKW, Simon MI, Gilman AG: G_z, a guanine nucleotide-binding protein with unique biochemical properties. J Biol Chem 265:2383, 1990) listed in Table 3.1. Beta and gamma subunits form tightly cohesive complexes that interact with alpha subunits and with receptors. The beta-gamma complex is essential for the interaction of receptors with G protein. Beta-gamma complexes also function to inhibit interaction of alpha subunits with effectors by complexing with alphas. The beta-gamma subunits probably facilitate binding of G proteins to cell membranes, and perhaps interact directly with effector molecules.

The receptor proteins to which G proteins complex are themselves members of a family. This receptor family shares a number of protein structural features (Fig. 3.5). They include 1) an extracellular amino terminus, 2) an intracellular carboxy terminus, 3) seven domains that span the cell membrane, 4) three extracellular and three intracellular loops, 5) sites for glycosylation on asparagines at the amino terminus, and 6) sites for phosphorylation on threonine and serine residues on the third intracellular loop and the carboxy terminus. Experiments with cloned receptors expressed in mammalian cells suggest that the cytoplasmic segment of the protein between transmembrane segments V and VI is involved in selective coupling of receptor subtypes with distinct effector systems through specific G proteins.[19] In mammalian cells, all these structural traits are found in $alpha_1$- and $alpha_2$-, $beta_1$- and $beta_2$-adrenergic receptors, muscarinic cholinergic receptors, serotonin, substance K and angiotensin receptors, and rhodopsin. Recent studies with recombinant DNA indicate the existence of numerous other G protein-coupled receptors in diverse mammalian tissues.[20]

In cardiovascular tissue, G_s protein mediates stimulation of adenylate cyclase and production of second messenger cAMP via $beta_1$- and $beta_2$-adrenergic receptors. G_s also directly mediates beta-adrenergic modulation of voltage-dependent ion channels. G_i protein mediates inhibition of beta-adrenergic-stimulated adenylate cyclase activity by $alpha_1$ and muscarinic cholinergic receptor agonists. Probably G_i (or G_K) also directly couples muscarinic receptors to atrial and pacemaker cell K^+ channel activation. G_o is present in cardiovascular tissue, but its function is unclear. There is some evidence that it may regulate Ca^{2+} channels in the brain, where G_o is extremely abundant.

Recent and ongoing immunological and recombinant DNA studies of G proteins reveal unexpected diversity among all three subunits. To date, 12 species of alpha subunits, four beta subunits, and three gamma subunits have been distinguished in mammalian tissue. This heterogeneity becomes confusing in light of the fact that restrictions on subunit isotype interactions have not yet been shown. However, certain molecular characteristics are common to all forms of G protein subunits. The alpha subunits possess 1 or 2 sites for nicotinamide adenine dinucleotide-dependent adenosine diphosphate (ADP) ribosylation. This covalent modification of alpha subunits is catalyzed by bacterial toxins: by cholera toxin in the case of G_s alpha and G_t alpha, and by pertussis toxin in G_i alpha, G_o alpha, and G_t alpha. G_x alpha appears not to be ADP-ribosylated by either toxin. ADP-ribosylation of G_s alpha inhibits its GTPase activity, thus irreversibly activating the subunit to stimulate adenylate cyclase and ion channels. ADP-ribosylation of G_i alpha and G_o alpha disallows interaction between the subunits and receptors. These functional modifications make ADP-ribosylation a means for quantifying, localizing, and charting operational pathways for cellular G proteins. However, quantitation values from ADP-ribosylation alone are now recognized as insufficient data because of measurement variability and underestimation. Antibodies directed to interact with epitopes on G proteins are a more accurate quantitation tool, and should at least be used in combination with toxin-labeling methods.[21]

Other features common to G alpha subunits include homologous amino acid sequences that are the guanine nucleotide binding sites, domains that appear to bind receptors, beta-gamma subunits, and effectors, activation by AlF_4^-, and intrinsic GTPase activity. The structure-function relationships of G beta and G gamma subunits are currently being examined. Beta subunits seem to be highly homologous within and between tissue types, while gamma subunits appear more diverse.

The mechanism by which G proteins couple receptors to effectors is known in some detail for beta-adrenergic stimulation and $alpha_2$ and muscarinic cholinergic inhibition of adenylate cyclase (Fig. 3.6). Generally, when an agonist (hormone) binds to one of these receptors, a ternary complex is formed, composed of agonist, receptor, and trimeric G protein. Formation of this complex is associated with the rate-limiting dissociation from the G alpha of tightly bound GDP and its replacement by GTP. The association of GTP with the G alpha protein destabilizes the complex, so that the hormone and receptor dissociate

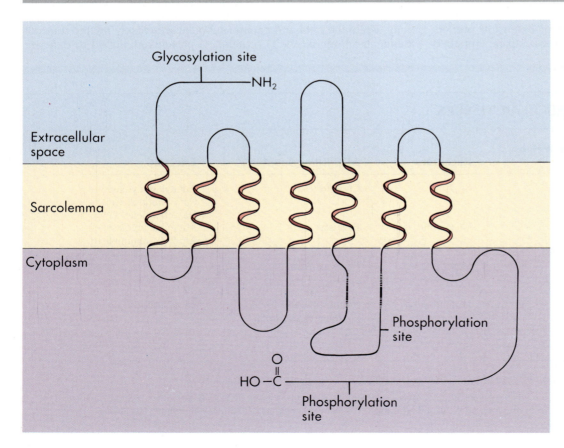

FIGURE 3.5 General schematic representation of the two-dimensional structure of the family of receptors that couple to G proteins. (Glyc) refers to possible sites for glycosylation and (P) denotes possible sites for phosphorylation. Amino acid sequences covered by shaded blocks are thought to be associated with coupling to G proteins. Secondary structure of receptor proteins appears to be alpha-helical in the seven membrane-spanning domains.

from the complex, with the receptor then reverting to its low-affinity form. The GTP-G alpha complex is then able to interact with its effector, leaving the beta-gamma subunits free for complexing with other unattached G alpha subunits.

The GTP-stimulated dissociation of the alpha from the beta and gamma subunits is the activation step for G proteins. This activation of the alpha subunits depends on the presence of Mg^{2+}. The subunit may be activated independently of receptor stimulation. This occurs in the presence of NaF and Mg^{2+}. Inactivation of the subunits is accomplished by hydrolysis of GTP to GDP. The GTPase activity is relatively slow, resides solely in the alpha subunit, and is stimulated by receptor agonists. GTPase-catalyzed hydrolysis is so slow that the freed receptor-hormone complex can activate 5 to 10 other G proteins during the time the first G protein is interacting with its effector. In this sense, the receptor-hormone catalyzes G protein activation. Slow GTPase activity also amplifies the effector enzyme reaction by allowing time for several molecules of product (cyclic AMP) to be generated before the G protein becomes inactive. GTP analogs that resist hydrolysis, such as 5'-guanylylimidodiphosphate (Gpp(NH)p) or GTP-gamma-S, irreversibly activate the alpha subunit. Similarly, cholera toxin is able to inhibit G_s GTPase activity, thus persistently activating the G_s alpha. On the other hand, pertussis toxin selectively prevents activation of G_i and G_o alpha subunits by blocking interaction of these G proteins with receptors.

Beyond the dissociation of GTP-bound alpha subunits from their complexes with beta-gamma subunits, the mechanisms of action for the various G proteins diverge. Activated G_s alpha subunits interact with adenylate cyclase to stimulate it and generate cyclic adenosine monophosphate (cyclic AMP) as second messenger in the generation of the cellular response (protein phosphorylation, ion channel opening, etc., and the ultimate physiologic response). Activated G_i and G_o alpha subunits are stimulatory or inhibitory regulators, depending on the receptors and effectors they connect. G_i alpha is believed to have a weak inhibitory influence on adenylate cyclase. The beta-gamma complex dissociated from activated G_i and G_o is thought to be the major adenylate cyclase inhibitory subunit. It presumably stimulates GTPase activity of G_s alpha by coupling to dissociated, activated G_s alpha. The coupling then results in an inactivated G_s alpha-beta-gamma-GDP complex.[22] G_i alpha also acts to produce other second messengers such as diacylglycerol (DAG) and inositol triphosphates (IP_3) that regulate protein phosphorylation and intracellular Ca^{2+} stores, respectively. G_i alpha may also modulate the second messenger cGMP.

The protein phosphorylation mentioned in connection with second messenger production is an important and principle mechanism by which extracellular signals control cell function.[23] Phosphorylation usually occurs on serine and threonine residues, and causes small conformational alterations that change biological properties of the protein. Thus, the functional status of many proteins depends on their state of phosphorylation which, in turn, depends on the balance of protein kinase and phosphatase activities. Both activities work through second messengers such as cyclic AMP and DAG.

G proteins are recognized as gates for cell membrane ion channels.[16] G protein gating can be indirect, acting in series by signal transmission from receptor stimulation, to G protein activation, to second messenger production, to membrane phosphorylation, to ion channel modulation. Indirect gating may employ such second messengers as cAMP, diacylglycerol, inositol triphosphate, and cGMP. Ca^{2+}, K^+, Na^+, and Cl^- channels in the heart have been associated with indirect gating. G protein gating can be direct, without interposition of a second messenger from the cytoplasm. Direct gating is faster and has been observed in Ca^{2+}, K^+, and Na^+ channels in cardiac membranes.

Several disease states exhibit changes in G protein function.[21] The severe diarrhea of cholera results from exaggerated water transport from serosa to lumen of the small intestine. The transport mechanism responds to persistent activation of G_s and overproduction of cAMP in the intestinal mucosa infected with *Vibrio cholera*. Whether the symptoms of whooping cough, caused by *Bordetella pertussis*, are secondary to inhibition of G_i is not known. There are suggestions of altered G protein function in heart failure from studies of animal models. The cardiomyopathic Syrian hamster is a genetic model of heart failure, the expression of a recessive autosomal genotype. Studies of cardiac membranes in the model revealed only half-normal G_s activity, but unexpectedly, no quantitative changes in G_s protein or in mRNA encoding G_s alpha.[24] However, in a canine model of heart failure, there were decreased activity and a decreased quantity of G_s.[25] In myocardium of mice with Chagas' disease, G_s protein was decreased by functional assessment. Genetically hypertensive rats displayed decreased function of G_s in their femoral arteries.[27]

In human hearts, studies have also suggested abnormalities of G proteins associated with cardiac disease. An increase in functional G_i in failing human hearts correlated with increased levels of mRNA encoding one of the G_i alpha subunits.[28] Additionally, indirect evidence of G_s reduction through assays of adenylate cyclase activity in cardiac membranes was observed in patients with the same disease.[29] Using mononuclear lymphocytes from patients suffering congestive heart failure as a surrogate tissue to reflect changes in myocardial tissue, an 80% reduction from normal values of G_s protein concentration was detected by cholera toxin-catalyzed ADP-ribosylation. Likewise, a 40% decrease in numbers of beta-adrenergic receptors was found.[30] But in another laboratory, G_s quantitation by ADP-ribosylation showed no difference between normal and failing hearts.[31] In a different cardiac disease, mitral valve prolapse with hyperresponsiveness to beta-adrenergic stimulation, G_s quantity was normal while its activity was increased above normal levels.[16]

ADRENERGIC RECEPTORS

In 1948 Ahlquist[32] first proposed the existence of subtypes of adrenergic receptors, alpha and beta, based on differential responsiveness of tissues to catecholamines. He designated alpha-adrenergic receptors as those mediating responses to catecholamines with the following

$$A + R\text{-}G_s\alpha\beta\gamma\text{-}GDP \rightleftharpoons A\text{-}R\text{-}G_s\alpha\beta\gamma\text{-}GTP + GDP \rightleftharpoons A\text{-}R + G_s\alpha\text{-}GTP + \beta\gamma$$

FIGURE 3.6 Formation of ternary complex between beta-adrenergic receptor (R), agonist (A), and G_s protein. Agonist binding to receptor and formation of the complex stimulates GDP dissociation and its replacement by GTP. Association of GTP with G_s alpha destabilizes the ternary complex so that the agonist and receptor dissociate from GTP-bound G_s protein, with the receptor reverting to a low-affinity form. Substitution of GTP for GDP also causes G_s beta-gamma subunits to dissociate from G_s alpha subunit. The activated G_s alpha-GTP is then able to interact with its effector, leaving the tightly associated beta-gamma subunits free for complexing with other unattached G alpha subunits.

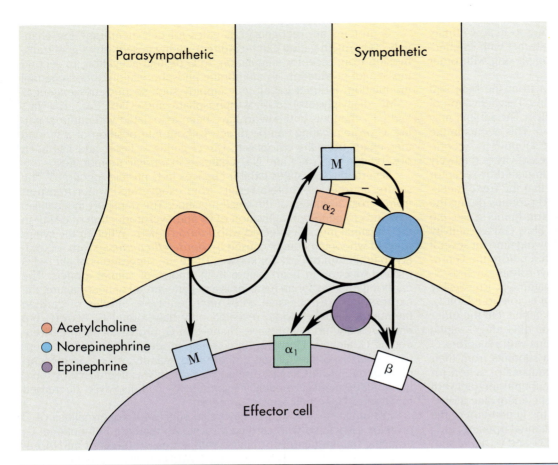

FIGURE 3.7 Interaction of sympathetic and parasympathetic nerve terminals and neurotransmitters. Sympathetic nerve terminal possesses muscarinic cholinergic (M) and alpha$_2$-adrenergic (alpha$_2$) receptors, which inhibit release of norepinephrine (NE) into synaptic cleft. Parasympathetic (vagal) nerve terminal contains acetylcholine (Ach). In addition to muscarinic cholinergic receptors, the myocardial cell possesses beta-adrenergic and alpha$_1$-adrenergic receptors. Epinephrine (E) from the circulation also has access to the alpha$_1$ and beta receptor. (Modified from Watanabe AM: Cholinergic Agonists and Antagonists, in Rosen MR, Hoffman BF (eds): Cardiac Therapy, p 95. Boston, Martinus Nijhoff, 1983)

TABLE 3.2 ADRENERGIC EFFECTS ON THE HEART AND VASCULATURE

Subtype	Mechanism	Location	Effect
Alpha$_1$	Increased phosphoinositide turnover	Ventricular myocardium	Positive inotropy
		Purkinje fibers	Negative inotropy
		Sinoatrial node	Negative inotropy
		Arterioles	Constriction
		Systemic veins	Constriction
Alpha$_2$	Inhibition of adenylate cyclase	Selected arterioles	Constriction
		Presynaptic adrenergic nerve terminals	Inhibition of norepinephrine release
	Increased phosphoinositide turnover	Platelets	Aggregation
		Inhibitory neurons, pontomedullary regions	Decreased peripheral sympathetic tone, enhanced vagal tone, vasodilation, negative chronotropy
Beta$_1$	Activation of adenylate cyclase	Sinoatrial node	Positive chronotropy
		Atrial myocardium	Positive inotropy
		Atrioventricular node	Positive chronotropy, dromotropy
		His-Purkinje system	Positive chronotropy, dromotropy
		Ventricular myocardium	Positive chronotropy, dromotropy; increased rate and extent of force development and relaxation
Beta$_2$	Activation of adenylate cyclase	Renal arterioles	Relaxation
		Sinoatrial node	Positive chronotropy
		Coronary, skeletal muscle, abdominal visceral, and pulmonary arterioles	Relaxation
		Systemic veins	Relaxation

(Data from Weiner N, Taylor P: Neurohumoral transmission: The autonomic and somatic motor nervous systems. In Gilman AG, Goodman LS, Rall TW, Murad F (eds): The Pharmacological Basis of Therapeutics, pp 69–99. New York, Macmillan, 1985; Rosen MR, Weiss RM, Danilo P Jr: Effect of alpha adrenergic agonists and blockers on Purkinje fiber transmembrane potentials and automaticity in the dog. J Pharmacol Exp Ther 231:566, 1984; Van Zwieten PA, Timmermans PBM WM: Cardiovascular alpha$_2$-receptors. J Mol Cel Cardiol 15:717, 1983; and Cotecchia S, Kobilka BK, Daniel KW et al: Multiple second messenger pathways of alpha-adrenergic receptor subtypes expressed in eukaryotic cells. J Biol Chem 265:63, 1990)

potency relationship: epinephrine > norepinephrine ≫ isoproterenol. The other subtype, which he termed beta-adrenergic receptors, had a different potency relationship: isoproterenol > epinephrine > norepinephrine. In 1967 Lands[33] proposed a further subtyping of the beta-adrenergic response: epinephrine and norepinephrine were equipotent in eliciting beta$_1$-adrenergic responses, while epinephrine was more potent than norepinephrine in eliciting beta$_2$-adrenergic responses. Beta$_1$ receptors were found in cardiac and adipose tissues, while beta$_2$ receptors were located in bronchial and vascular smooth muscle. Subsequently the alpha-adrenergic receptor has also been subdivided based on anatomic and pharmacologic criteria. Alpha$_1$ receptors were originally defined as post-junctional receptors that mediated smooth muscle contraction. Alpha$_2$ receptors were originally defined as pre-junctional receptors that were located on sympathetic nerve terminals and mediated feedback inhibition of norepinephrine release. Figure 3.7 illustrates these anatomic relationships, as well as the participation of the muscarinic cholinergic receptor, which will be described below. Subsequently it has been recognized that alpha$_2$ receptors can be found post-junctionally on tissues and on various circulating cellular elements. They have been identified on human platelets, adipose tissue, and hepatocytes. A post-junctional alpha$_2$-mediated pressor response has also been demonstrated. Consequently, alpha responses are now characterized on the basis of differential pharmacologic responses rather than on anatomy; prazosin exhibits up to a 10,000-fold more potent blockade of alpha$_1$ than alpha$_2$ responses, while yohimbine is a selective alpha$_2$ blocker. Table 3.2 details the location and responses mediated by adrenergic receptors, and Table 3.3 lists adrenergic agonists and antagonists.

THE BETA-ADRENERGIC RECEPTOR
RADIOLIGAND BINDING STUDIES

The beta-adrenergic receptors were the first cardiac autonomic receptors to be studied by radioligand binding techniques, with the earliest reports released in 1974. Subsequently, many useful ligands have been developed. [^{3}H]-CGP12177 is hydrophilic and is useful for detecting surface beta-adrenergic receptors, to the exclusion of intracellular ones. [^{125}I]-iodopindolol and [^{125}I]-iodocyanopindolol ([^{125}I]-ICYP) de-

TABLE 3.3 ADRENERGIC AGONISTS AND ANTAGONISTS

Subtype	Agonists	Antagonists
Alpha$_1$	Methoxamine Phenylephrine 6-F-norepinephrine Cirazoline	Doxazosin Prazocin (^{3}H) HEAT (^{125}I) WB 4101 (^{3}H) BE 2254 Oxymetazoline ARC 239
Alpha$_2$	Clonidine (^{3}H)	Yohimbine (^{3}H) Rauwolscine (^{3}H)
Alpha-nonselective	E ≥ NE ≫ PE > I	Phentolamine Dihydroergotamine (^{3}H) Phenoxybenzamine*
Beta-nonselective	Isoproterenol Dobutamine	Propranolol (^{3}H) Alprenolol Dihydroalprenolol (^{3}H) Pindolol (^{125}I)† Iodohydroxybenzyl pindolol (^{125}I)
Beta$_1$	I > E ≥ NE ≫ PE	Atenolol Metoprolol Betaxolol Bisoprolol Celiprolol
Beta$_2$	Salbutamol Terbutaline Procaterol Zinterol Dopexamine HCl Albuterol I > E ≫ NE ≫ PE	

* Irreversible

† Intrinsic sympathomimetic activity

(E, epinephrine; NE, norepinephrine; PE, phenylephrine; I, isoproterenol)

(Data from Stiles GL, Caron MG, Lefkowitz RJ: Beta-adrenergic receptors: Biochemical mechanisms of physiological regulation. Physiol Rev 64:661, 1984; Benfey BG: Function of myocardial alpha-adrenoceptors. Life Sci 31:101, 1982; Motulsky HJ, Insel PA: Adrenergic receptors in man: Direct identification, physiologic regulation, and clinical alterations. N Engl J Med 307:18, 1982; Corr PB, Heathers GP, Yamada KA: Mechanisms contributing to the arrhythmogenic influences of alpha-adrenergic stimulation in the ischemic heart, Am J Med 87 (suppl 24): 195, 1989; Brodde O–E: The functional importance of beta$_1$ and beta$_2$ adrenoceptors in the human heart. Am J Cardiol 62:24C, 1988; Feldman RD, Christy JP, Paul SL, Harrison DG: β-adrenergic receptors on canine coronary collateral vessels: characterization and function. Am J Physiol 257, H1634, 1989; and Frey MJ, Molinoff PB: Mechanisms of downregulation of beta-adrenergic receptors: Perspective on the role of beta-adrenergic receptors in congestive heart failure. J Cardiovasc Pharmacol 14 (suppl 5): S13, 1989)

tect both surface and internalized receptors, and possess high specific activity (2200 Ci/mmol). They can be used in assays of very small amounts of tissue. Most investigators have preferred to characterize the interaction of unlabeled agonists with the beta-adrenergic receptor by studying the competition of these agonists with labeled antagonists.

With the availability of sophisticated methods for separating membrane fractions of sarcolemma and sarcoplasmic reticulum, the beta receptors have been recognized as being located primarily on sarcolemma. A smaller population of beta receptors is located intracellularly in an extremely light density membrane fraction. These receptors are thought to be in dynamic equilibrium with those in the sarcolemma, and their translocation from cytoplasm to sarcolemma is probably dependent on the function of microfilaments.[34]

In general, the affinity of beta receptors for radiolabeled antagonists, expressed as K_D, is unaffected by most manipulations. Affinity of the receptors for agonists is subject to regulation by a number of conditions. In addition to guanine nucleotides, the presence of divalent cations including Mg^{2+}, Mn^{2+}, Ca^{2+}, and Sr^{2+} can affect beta receptor affinity for agonists.

As indicated in the discussion of receptor methodology, radioligand binding studies have provided direct confirmation of Land's classification of $beta_1$- and $beta_2$-adrenergic subtypes. In the majority of species studied, the $beta_1$ receptor predominates in myocardium, but the two subtypes may coexist. For example, pharmacologic studies done in human right atrial strips indicate that $beta_2$ agonists have a greater positive chronotropic effect, whereas $beta_1$ agonists have a greater inotropic effect.[35] This suggests that the coexistence of $beta_1$ and $beta_2$ receptors in human right atrium might subserve different physiological functions. In general, the relative proportion of $beta_2$ receptors is greatest in the right atrium. It is also clear that species differences exist, because rat and guinea pig right atrium possesses only $beta_1$ receptors. Table 3.4 summarizes a variety of experimental results in hearts from different species. Because most tissue preparations originate from organ homogenates, it is possible that the apparent coexistence of $beta_1$ and $beta_2$ receptors based on radioligand binding studies is due to the presence of a mixture of cell types. At least one study of cultured myocardial cells showed that $beta_1$-adrenergic receptors were located exclusively on muscle cells, while $beta_2$-adrenergic receptors resided exclusively on fibroblasts.[36] Cultured glioma cells, however, contain both $beta_1$ and $beta_2$ receptors.[37]

TABLE 3.4 DISTRIBUTION OF MYOCARDIAL BETA$_1$ AND BETA$_2$ RECEPTORS

Species	Chamber	Proportion (%) Beta$_1$/Beta$_2$
Frog	Left ventricle	20/80
Rat	Whole heart	83/17
	Ventricle	100/0
Guinea pig	Right atrium	77/23
	Left ventricle	100/0
Rabbit	Right atrium	72/28
	Right ventricle	92/8
	Left ventricle	93/7
	Left atrium	82/18
Cat	Right atrium	78/22
	Left ventricle	98/2
Dog	Left ventricle	85/15
Human	Right atrium	74/26
	Left ventricle	86/14

(Data from Stiles GL, Caron MG, Lefkowitz RJ: Beta adrenergic receptors: Biochemical mechanisms of physiological regulation. Physiol Rev 64:661, 1984)

BETA-ADRENERGIC RECEPTOR STRUCTURE

It is now possible to study the structure of the beta-adrenergic receptor, owing to the development of several biochemical techniques. First, beta receptors can be solubilized from membranes and purified by the technique of affinity chromatography. In this process the suspension of solubilized beta receptors is passed over a column to which a high-affinity beta-adrenergic antagonist such as alprenolol is bound. The beta receptors bind to the alprenolol and can then be eluted.[38] Using additional techniques such as high performance liquid chromatography, it is possible to obtain a population of biologically active beta receptors purified to near homogeneity. Specific protein components of the receptor to which the agonists and antagonists bind can be identified using photoaffinity labeling.[39] In this technique a radioligand is used that also contains a photoactive moiety such as an azide group ($-N_3$). It is apparent that both beta$_1$[40] and beta$_2$[41] receptors contain a ligand binding subunit protein with an apparent molecular weight of 62,000 to 67,000 daltons (62 to 67 kd). The intact beta receptors also display affinity for lectin affinity resins and are therefore thought to be glycoproteins.[42] Peptide mapping has revealed differences in the protein structure of beta$_1$- and beta$_2$-adrenergic receptors, suggesting that alterations in the primary protein sequence may ultimately be responsible for the different pharmacologic sensitivities of these receptors. It appears that purified 67-kd beta receptor protein can confer responsiveness to beta-adrenergic agonists when it is introduced into the cells of *Xenopus laevis*, the African clawed toad. These cells lack beta receptors, but contain the guanine nucleotide regulatory protein and catalytic component of the adenylate cyclase system to be described. Thus, the purified protein contains not only a radiolabeled ligand binding site, but also the site necessary to couple to adenylate cyclase.[43] This distinguishes the beta-adrenergic receptor from a variety of others, including the insulin, IgE, and nicotinic cholinergic receptors, which are composed of multiple subunits.[44]

Further understanding of receptor structure has been achieved by cloning the gene and cDNA for human beta$_2$ and beta$_1$ receptors.[45-49] The deduced amino acid sequence for beta$_2$ contains 413 residues, while beta$_1$ has 477 amino acids. The beta$_2$ receptor is 54% homologous with the beta$_1$ receptor. Both of them possess those characteristics listed above as representative of receptors that complex with G proteins. There are 7 membrane-spanning regions with accompanying cytoplasmic and extracellular loops, 2 sites for glycosylation, and 2 for phosphorylation. The gene for the beta$_2$ receptor is located on human chromosome 5. Along with the alpha$_2$ and muscarinic cholinergic receptor genes, the beta$_2$-receptor gene lacks introns (nontranslated DNA sequences) in its coding region. This feature is unusual in eukaryotic cells, and its significance is not known. Beta-adrenergic genes also contain sequences that bind glucocorticoids and cyclic AMP in their promoter regions. Glucocorticoid hormones and cyclic AMP may accelerate the rate of transcription of the DNA, thus increasing beta receptor levels in cell membranes.[46]

THE BETA-ADRENERGIC RECEPTOR–GUANINE NUCLEOTIDE REGULATORY PROTEIN–ADENYLATE CYCLASE COMPLEX

As previously indicated, the methodology of receptor binding studies has allowed us to consider the ways in which the binding of a hormone to its receptor leads to biochemical events within the cell and eventually to physiologic responses. This is generally referred to as receptor-effector coupling. Figure 3.8 summarizes several of these interactions. As indicated in Table 3.2, the mechanisms by which adrenergic receptors mediate their effects differ. Both beta$_1$ and beta$_2$ receptors cause stimulation of adenylate cyclase. There are data suggesting that in the human right atrium, norepinephrine, a beta$_1$-preferring but not totally selective agonist, stimulates adenylate cyclase predominantly with beta$_2$ receptors, even though the ratio of beta$_1$/beta$_2$ is about 65/35. This should be considered in the light of data showing that the positive inotropic and chronotropic responses to norepinephrine in both the right atrium and left ventricle normally occur through beta$_1$ receptors. But when larger amounts of catecholamines are circulating because of stressful conditions, beta$_2$ receptors also mediate increased contractile force and accelerate heart rate.[50] In contrast, alpha$_2$-adrenergic receptors and muscarinic cholinergic receptors inhibit adenylate cyclase activation. Adenylate cyclase is therefore dually regulated by inhibitory and stimulatory hormones. In addition, coupling of the beta receptor to adenylate cyclase is altered by exposure to catecholamines, a phenomenon described as *desensitization*.

A variety of experimental evidence provides support for the concept that the binding of beta-adrenergic agonists to their receptors leads to activation of adenylate cyclase, which in turn catalyzes the formation of cyclic AMP from ATP. Beta-adrenergic agonists affect cardiac tissue to cause increased force of contraction, increased heart rate, and increased rate of relaxation. All these effects appear dependent to some extent on increased cyclic AMP production. G$_s$ couples the beta receptor to the adenylate cyclase enzyme. This has been rigorously demonstrated by insertion of purified beta receptor, G$_s$ protein, and adenylate cyclase into artificial phospholipid vesicles, and observing the formation of a system for cyclic AMP synthesis responsive to hormonal stimulation.

Cyclic AMP causes dissociation of the regulatory subunit of protein kinase from its catalytic subunit, thereby activating the protein kinase. This kinase then activates a number of intracellular processes through phosphorylation of proteins, resulting in characteristic physiological responses to beta-adrenergic agonists. Alternatively, the beta agonist-activated G$_s$ protein may directly gate cell membrane ion channels, bypassing stimulation of cyclic AMP production.[16] Presumably, the molecular aspects of activated G$_s$ interaction with ion channels are similar to those of its interaction with adenylate cyclase enzyme. Pertinent to this presumption are preliminary data suggesting similarities of protein structure and topology of adenylate cyclase and ion channels.[18]

The catalytic subunit of adenylate cyclase has been purified and reconstituted with G$_s$ proteins and beta receptors in phospholipid membranes to form a beta agonist-stimulatable catalyst for conversion of ATP to cyclic AMP.[51] The catalytic subunit of bovine brain adenylate cyclase is a single glycopolypeptide with a molecular weight of 120 kd. It has been cloned and sequenced by recombinant DNA technology and shown to contain 1134 amino acid residues. It contains two sets of hydrophobic domains, each with six membrane spans which may be alpha helical. It also contains two large cytoplasmic hydrophilic domains, each with a possible catalytic region. In these structural aspects, the adenylate cyclase enzyme resembles several ion channels and a molecular exporter protein, P glycoprotein.[14,18,52]

As described above, formation of cyclic AMP leads to activation of cyclic AMP dependent protein kinase. This enzyme catalyzes the activation of a number of proteins through phosphorylation. Some proteins recognized to be phosphorylated by the action of beta-adrenergic agonists include the inhibitory subunit of troponin, the C protein of

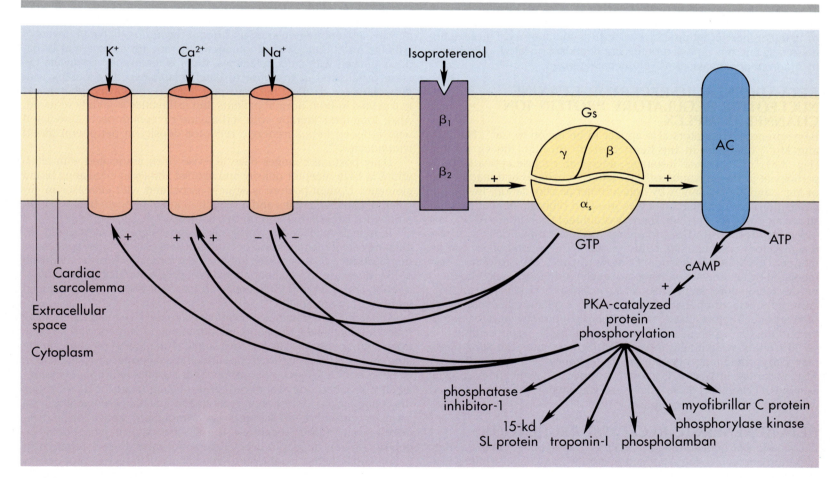

FIGURE 3.8 Beta-adrenergic receptor-effector coupling. Isoproterenol (iso) reacts with beta$_1$ and beta$_2$ adrenergic receptors. Both beta$_1$ and beta$_2$ receptors are coupled to G$_s$, which in the presence of GTP dissociates its G$_s$ alpha subunit to stimulate adenylate cyclase (AC). This results in formation of second messenger cyclic AMP (cAMP), which in turn stimulates protein kinase A (PKA) to phosphorylate various cellular proteins, including ion channels, involved in producing the positive inotropic, chronotropic, and dromotropic effects of beta-adrenergic stimulation. Activated G$_m$ alpha may also directly couple beta receptors to sarcolemmal Ca^{2+} channels for stimulation and sarcolemmal Na$^+$ channels for inactivation. (Data from Brown AM, Birnbaumer L: Ion channels and G proteins. Hosp Prac 24:189, 1939; Robishaw JD, Foster KA: Role of G proteins in the regulation of the cardiovascular system. Annu Rev Physiol 51:229, 1989; Gilman AG: G proteins and regulation of adenylyl cyclase. JAMA 262:1819, 1989; Schubert B, VanDongen AMP, Kirsch GE, Brown AM: β-adrenergic inhibition of cardiac sodium channels by dual G-protein pathways. Science 245:516, 1989; Yatani A, Brown AM: Rapid β-adrenergic modulation of calcium channel currents by a fast G protein pathway. Science 245:71, 1989)

myosin filaments, phospholamban, and a 15-kd sarcolemmal protein. Because increases in the slow inward calcium current occur in response to beta-adrenergic stimulation, it is thought that some components of the calcium channel are also phosphorylated. There is not a good temporal relationship of troponin I and C protein phosphorylation to the positive inotropic effects of beta-adrenergic agonists. Therefore, the role of phosphorylation of these proteins in contractile regulation is not clear. By contrast, after treatment of cardiac tissue with beta agonists, the onset of phosphorylation of phospholamban, a 22-kd membrane protein found in sarcoplasmic reticulum, is rapid and temporally associated with an increased rate of relaxation, and with an increase in the rate of calcium uptake attained by sarcoplasmic reticulum.[53] This effect on sarcoplasmic reticulum is thought to account in part for the characteristic shortening of the half-time of relaxation ($t_{1/2}$) of cardiac muscle under stimulation by beta agonists. The onset of phosphorylation of the 15-kd sarcolemmal protein is also quite rapid. It precedes the phosphorylation of phospholamban and shortening of $t_{1/2}$, and is temporally associated with increases in the maximal rate of force development under stimulation by beta-adrenergic agonists.[54]

Because increases in the slow inward calcium current occur in response to beta-adrenergic stimulation, it is thought that some components of calcium channels are also phosphorylated.[16] In addition, the sodium channel may be regulated by beta-adrenergic-stimulated phosphorylation. Isolated cardiac myocytes demonstrate that voltage-sensitive Ca^{2+} and Na^+ channels are linked to beta receptors in two ways: one through G_s and cyclic AMP, and the other through G_s alone. Therefore, beta agonists activate a sequence of enzymatic reactions, all coupled to the activation of adenylate cyclase via G_s. Upon withdrawal of beta-adrenergic agonists, cyclic AMP is metabolized by phosphodiesterase and the various proteins are dephosphorylated, presumably by different phosphatases as yet uncharacterized.

BETA-ADRENERGIC RECEPTOR–GUANINE NUCLEOTIDE REGULATORY PROTEIN–ION CHANNEL COMPLEX

Beta-adrenergic receptors also appear to be linked to Ca^{2+}, Na^+, K^+, and Mg^{2+} channels in the heart directly through the G_s protein (Fig. 3.8).[16,55,56] In these instances, adenylate cyclase appears not to participate in the activation of Ca^{2+} and K^+ channels and inactivation of Mg^{2+} and Na^+ channels by beta-adrenergic stimulation. Recent investigations with cardiac myocytes revealed biphasic beta-adrenergic stimulation of Ca^{2+} current. There was a direct (non-cyclic AMP), fast (10 msec) response to isoproterenol mediated by G_s. Diffusion was assumed to be rate-limiting in this reaction. The second phase was an indirect (cyclic AMP-dependent), slow (5 to 10 sec) response, also mediated by G_s. The accumulation of cyclic AMP in the cell seemed to be the rate-limiting step. This fast-slow biphasic modulation of Ca^{2+} current by beta-adrenergic stimulation may explain reflex stimulation of heart rate. The fast phase, where G_s protein directly links the receptor and the Ca^{2+} channel, has kinetics which fit the response time (1.5 sec) of reflex sympathetic modulation of heart rate. The slow phase may carry continuing beta-adrenergic enhancement of heart rate.[56] Also, in cardiac myocytes, G_s protein is implicated in the direct (as well as indirect) inhibition of Na^+ channels. The effect is more pronounced when membranes are depolarized.[55]

BETA-ADRENERGIC RECEPTOR REGULATION

Examination of beta-adrenergic receptor populations under a variety of perturbations has demonstrated that they are dynamic entities with respect to receptor number, subtype proportion, and receptor-effector coupling. Beta receptor regulation can be initiated at several different levels of metabolism.[46] Density and functional efficiency can be controlled by processes like desensitization that include down-regulation of receptor numbers, receptor internalization, and uncoupling from proteins essential in the chain of reactions leading to the physiological response. Beta receptors can also change as a result of alterations in their protein synthesis or degradation, or in their messenger RNA synthesis (gene regulation) and degradation. Furthermore, beta receptors can be modulated directly at the level of gene transcription.

DESENSITIZATION

The most extensively studied of these alterations is desensitization. When the beta-adrenergic receptor is exposed to catecholamines, a rapid increase in cyclic AMP accumulation is followed within five minutes by the progressive loss of responsiveness to further catecholamine exposure. *Homologous desensitization* is said to have occurred if the adenylate cyclase remains responsive to other classes of hormones whose responses are mediated by other receptors such as prostaglandin E_1 or histamine. Homologous desensitization is not mediated by cyclic AMP, and is generally thought to be due to a hormone-induced alteration in the receptor. *Heterologous desensitization* is defined as loss of responsiveness to all classes of hormones after exposure to one. It is thought to be due to alteration either in G_s or the catalytic subunit of adenylate cyclase, and is usually dependent on a prior increase in cyclic AMP. Desensitization can occur in response to exogenous administration of hormone, or to physiologic or pathologic conditions in which the receptor is exposed to increased concentrations of circulating hormone.

A number of human models of desensitization have been examined. These usually have evaluated beta receptors and adenylate cyclase responsiveness on circulating leukocytes rather than myocardial beta receptors. Changes in the circulating beta receptor population are presumed to reflect changes in myocardial receptors as well. In general, desensitization is associated with a decrease in beta receptor density, a phenomenon known as *down-regulation*. In lymphocytes of patients on chronic sympathomimetic therapy for asthma and of patients infused with catecholamines, there is diminished adenylate cyclase production in response to catecholamines. After therapy with terbutaline for six days, beta receptor number on polymorphonuclear leukocytes in both normal patients and asthmatics is greatly reduced. Also, long-term therapy with terbutaline or ephedrine is associated with reduced beta-adrenergic receptor density in peripheral blood lymphocytes.[44]

Daily postural changes have likewise been associated with alterations in beta receptor density and agonist affinity in circulating blood elements. Upright posture is acutely associated with increases in circulating catecholamines and a reduction in lymphocyte beta receptor affinity for isoproterenol in normal subjects.

In humans with severe congestive heart failure, an increase in circulating catecholamines also occurs. Left ventricular biopsy specimens demonstrate a 50% decrease in beta receptors. This is associated with a 45% decrease in maximal adenylate cyclase stimulation by isoproterenol, and a 54 to 73% decrease in maximal isoproterenol-induced increases in contractility.[57]

Other studies of humans in end-stage congestive heart failure have found a selective decrease in $beta_1$-adrenergic receptors, and no positive inotropic response to selective stimulation of $beta_1$ receptors in the atria and ventricles. However, nonselective isoproterenol stimulation of $beta_1$ and $beta_2$ receptors produced a positive inotropic response, albeit a reduced one. Therefore, in the failing heart, $beta_2$ receptors may compensate for lost $beta_1$ receptors to maintain contractility.[50] All forms of chronic heart failure show sympathetic activation and reduced levels of $beta_1$ receptors. The disease states in which $beta_2$ receptor numbers appear to fall include mitral valve disease, tetralogy of Fallot, and ischemic heart failure. No changes in $beta_2$ receptor density are observed in idiopathic heart failure and in aortic valve disease.[58]

When total tissue content of beta-adrenergic receptors is determined by quantitative light microscopic autoradiography of transmural slices of human heart, the failing heart clearly shows a reduction of these receptors. The down-regulation is more pronounced in subendocardial myocytes as compared with subepicardial myocytes and arterioles. This suggests that down-regulation cannot be solely attributed to increased levels of circulating catecholamines. Perhaps changes in patterns of sympathetic innervation and accompanying norepinephrine agonist availability are better explanations for the observed down-regulation.[59]

A variety of experimental designs has been used to elucidate the mechanism of catecholamine homologous desensitization. In mammalian cells the following sequence of events seems the most likely. As previously described, very soon after exposure to catecholamines, the beta-adrenergic receptor is converted to a form that is incapable of forming the high-affinity complex with G_s.[60] The receptor demonstrates a low affinity for agonist, and there is no effect on affinity when guanine nucleotides are added. Evidence suggests that these alterations are associated with phosphorylation of the receptors. A unique kinase, termed beta-adrenergic receptor kinase (βARK) phosphorylates only agonist-occupied beta receptors, probably on serine and threonine residues near the carboxy terminus. βARK is a ubiquitous cytosolic enzyme that translocates to the cell membrane when the beta receptor is stimulated by agonist occupation. It is likely that an additional protein is necessary for receptor phosphorylation to prevent receptor-G protein coupling efficiently. There are some suggestions that βARK phosphorylates other receptors coupled to adenylate cyclase.[45] After phosphorylation, the receptor is sequestered in an intracellular light buoyant density membrane fraction. While in the sequestering compartment, beta receptors remain fully functional, but in low-affinity, GTP-insensitive form. Dephosphorylation occurs in this compartment.[45] Sequestration is probably mediated by microfilaments, because it is inhibited by cytochalasin B in cultured chick myocytes.[35] The receptor may then be degraded, or, if the agonist is removed from the cell in time, the receptor may be recycled back to the cell surface. This recycling is not blocked by protein synthesis or glycosylation inhibitors, nor is it inhibited by colchicine, an inhibitor of microtubules. If agonist exposure is prolonged for 24 hours, for example, decreases in receptor number are blocked by colchicine. After agonist withdrawal following prolonged exposure, full recovery of receptor number takes a subsequent 72 hours, and this recovery can be blocked by protein synthesis inhibitors. Thus, there is an initial phosphorylation and uncoupling of the receptor, subsequent internalization presumably to the light buoyant density membrane vesicles, and either eventual recycling to the cell surface or degradation. These reactions are summarized in Figure 3.9. Species differences clearly exist. In avian erythrocytes, phosphorylation of the receptor occurs, but no internalization or down-regulation has been documented.[60-62] Receptor phosphorylation as well as internalization has been documented in S49 lymphoma cells and amphibian erythrocytes.[34]

The phenomenon of receptor internalization may have implications for experimental designs. If beta-adrenergic receptors are assayed in intact desensitized cells with lipophilic ligands that have access to internalized receptors, no change in total receptor number will be detected, even though some of them are uncoupled and internalized. Another potential pitfall is that if sarcolemmal preparations are assayed, internalized beta receptors on light vesicles will not be detected. Down-regulation, which refers to loss in total receptor number, must be clearly distinguished from receptor internalization.[16]

SUPERSENSITIVITY

The opposite perturbation, withdrawal of catecholamines, appears to increase beta receptor density, a phenomenon described as *up-regulation*. This mechanism may contribute to the phenomenon of *denervation supersensitivity*. This refers to the enhanced tissue responsiveness to catecholamines that occurs after surgical or chemical induction of sympathetic denervation. Use of such techniques experimentally has produced increases in beta receptor density in the denervated tissue.[63] In a human model of catecholamine suppression, subjects were fed a low or high salt diet to stimulate or suppress sympathetic nervous system outflow, as monitored by urinary and plasma catecholamines. The beta receptor density of leukocytes inversely correlated with circulating and 24-hour urinary catecholamine levels. This also correlated with

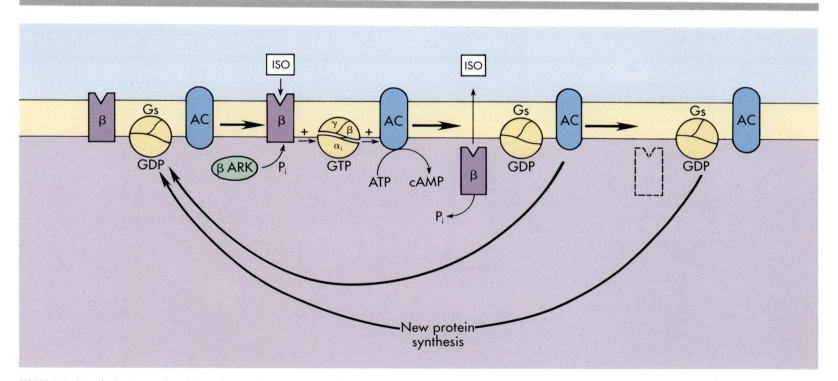

FIGURE 3.9 Catecholamine-induced homologous desensitization of the beta-adrenergic receptor. In mammalian cells, interaction of isoproterenol with the beta receptor is associated with activation of adenylate cyclase (AC) by G_s alpha-GTP. Agonist occupation is also associated with phosphorylation of the beta receptor by beta-adrenergic receptor kinase (βARK) which translocates to the sarcolemma from the cytoplasm when the beta receptor is stimulated by agonist occupation. The receptor is subsequently internalized in low-affinity form. It is dephosphorylated in the sequestering compartment and may return from there to the sarcolemma after removal of the desensitization stimulus. If the stimulus continues, the receptor may be degraded in the internal compartment, in which case new protein synthesis is required for resensitization at the cell surface. (Data from Lefkowitz RJ, Caron MG: Adrenergic receptors. Adv Sec Mess Phosphoprot Res 21:1, 1988)

an increase in their sensitivity to the positive chronotropic effect of isoproterenol.[64]

A related clinical phenomenon is the so-called "propranolol-withdrawal syndrome." Unstable angina and myocardial infarction have occurred in patients with ischemic heart disease after abrupt discontinuance of propranolol. Hypertensive patients who stopped their propranolol were demonstrated to have an increased inotropic and chronotropic response to isoproterenol. In another study, patients who stopped propranolol ingestion were noted to have an increased chronotropic response to isoproterenol as well as excessive sweating and palpitation two to 14 days after discontinuance. After treatment with propranolol, compensatory increases in beta receptors occurred in a variety of animal tissues and on circulating lymphocytes of human volunteers.[65] In the clinical studies, when propranolol was discontinued these subjects were noted to have increased heart rate, and heart rate-blood pressure product responses to standing. It must be pointed out that up-regulation of beta receptors is not uniformly found after propranolol treatment. In fact, the syndrome is probably uncommon. Also, it is not clear why it develops only in some patients. It may reflect individual differences in sympathetic tone prior to beta blockade. Before propranolol therapy, an individual with excessive sympathetic tone would be expected to have greater down-regulation of beta receptors secondary to the exposure to excessive catecholamines. With propranolol therapy the patient's beta receptors would up-regulate. After withdrawal of propranolol the patient's increased receptor density would be exposed to the usual circulating levels of catecholamines, and the patient would develop symptoms. A mechanism for receptor supersensitivity may simply be attenuation of a chronic, normal state of receptor down-regulation produced by continual exposure to catecholamine neurotransmitter. Receptors are also regulated at the level of gene expression. Several hormones that are not ligands for beta receptors modulate the beta-adrenergic system.[46] Glucocorticoids direct up-regulatory increases in beta receptor levels by direct interaction of the receptor for glucocorticoids with characteristic DNA sequences in the cloned gene for the $beta_2$-adrenergic receptor. The DNA sequences, called glucocorticoid response elements (GRE), seem to be positioned in the promoter region of the $beta_2$ receptor gene. Thus, a putative mechanism for the increase of $beta_2$ receptor numbers, messenger RNA for $beta_2$ receptor, and adenylate cyclase activity in the presence of glucocorticoids, is enhanced transcription of the $beta_2$ receptor.

RECEPTOR CHANGES IN PATHOLOGICAL CONDITIONS

Changes in either peripheral blood or myocardial beta-adrenergic receptors in association with a variety of medical conditions have been reported. In many instances the implications and mechanisms of these changes are not clear for a variety of reasons. First, beta receptor populations can change in response to changes in local or circulating catecholamines, the levels of which are not always determined. Second, it is important not only to define the beta receptor number and affinity with antagonists, but also the ability of isoproterenol to inhibit the antagonist binding and the maximal adenylate cyclase stimulation in response to agonists such as isoproterenol. These types of studies provide an indication of the proportion of receptors in the high-affinity state ($\%R_H$), and the efficiency of coupling of the beta receptor to adenylate cyclase. Third, the relationship between changes of beta receptor populations on peripheral blood lymphocytes and in other organs is not always clear. Thus, as our understanding of this receptor-effector complex has evolved, it has become clear that alterations can occur not only at the level of the beta receptor, but the G_s protein and adenylate cyclase as well. Therefore, the measurement of changes in beta receptor number and affinity alone provides an inadequate understanding of complex physiologic changes. Nevertheless, the fact that alterations in beta receptor number occur underscores their dynamic nature, and offers at least a clue to the mechanisms of physiologic changes produced. Some of the pathologic conditions which may alter beta receptors are summarized in Table 3.5 and amplified on in the subsequent text.

Myocardial ischemia is associated with changes in myocardial beta-adrenergic receptors.[66] In experimental myocardial infarction, increases in sarcolemmal beta receptors in the periinfarction tissue have been documented. Translocation of internalized beta receptors may be one mechanism for this up-regulation. As a function of increasing duration of reversible ischemia in guinea pigs, there is a progressive redistribution of beta receptors from intracellular light vesicles to the

TABLE 3.5 PATHOLOGIC STATES THAT REGULATE BETA-ADRENERGIC RECEPTORS

Condition	Tissue	Receptor Number	$\%R_H$*	Coupling Efficiency†
Hyperthyroidism	Myocardium	Increased	Increased	Increased
Hypothyroidism	Myocardium	Decreased	No change	No change
Corticosteroids	Myocardium	Increased		Increased
Adrenalectomy	Myocardium	No change or increased	Decreased	Decreased
Myocardial hypertrophy (pressure overload)	Myocardium	Increased		No change
Myocardial failure	Myocardium	Decreased		
	Peripheral lymphocytes	Decreased		
Hypertension, essential	Peripheral lymphocytes	No change	Decreased	Decreased
Myocardial ischemia	Myocardium	Increased		Increased
Myocardial infarction	Myocardium	Decreased		Decreased
Hypoxia	Myocardium	Decreased		Decreased
Aging	Peripheral lymphocytes	Decreased		Decreased

* Indicates the proportion of beta-adrenergic receptors that can form a high-affinity complex with isoproterenol.

† Indicates the efficacy of beta-adrenergic agonists in stimulating cyclic AMP accumulation.

(Data from Stiles GL, Caron MG, Lefkowitz RJ: Beta-adrenergic receptors: Biochemical mechanisms of physiological regulation. Physiol Rev 64:661, 1984; Horn EM, Corwin SJ, Steinberg SF, et al: Reduced lymphocyte stimulatory guanine nucleotide regulatory protein and β-adrenergic receptors in congestive heart failure and reversal with angiotensin converting enzyme inhibitor therapy. Circ 78:1373, 1988)

sarcolemma.[67] It is not clear whether this represents active cycling of receptors to the sarcolemma, or cessation of receptor internalization during myocardial ischemia. If the guinea pigs are pretreated with propranolol, a higher percentage of their beta receptors are located on the sarcolemma, and there is no further redistribution during ischemia. Increases in beta receptors have also been noted in isolated heart cells treated with inhibitors of cellular metabolism.[68]

Using cultured myocytes from neonatal rats, the coupling of beta-adrenergic receptors to transsarcolemmal Na^+ and Ca^{2+} channels through the G_s protein has been examined.[55] Results led to speculations that may explain the enhanced risk of arrhythmia with myocardial infarction. In ischemic heart disease, the decreased oxygen supply to tissue causes extracellular K^+ accumulation, which in turn causes membrane depolarization. There are also higher catecholamine levels. Thus, increased catecholamine stimulation of beta receptors that mediate increased Ca^{2+} current, and exaggerated inhibition of Na^+ current in depolarized cells, may both contribute to the risk of arrhythmia.

Changes in beta receptors in hyperthyroidism have been extensively studied. Clinically, hyperthyroidism is characterized by many symptoms suggestive of increased adrenergic tone, such as tachycardia, increased myocardial contractility, tremors, hyperthermia, and diaphoresis. In animal studies there is agreement that myocardial beta receptors increase and that there are also increases in the affinity of isoproterenol for these receptors, in the tendency of receptors to form the high affinity state, and in the extent of maximal stimulation of adenylate cyclase by isoproterenol.[44] A study in rats found no change in beta receptors on lymphocytes despite increases in myocardial beta receptors. In human peripheral lymphocytes, results have been conflicting, but at least in normal volunteers treated with triiodothyronine there was an increase in beta receptors, with each subject serving as his or her own control.[69] This suggests that biologic variability among human subjects may necessitate each individual serving as his own control. Other studies of heart tissue have revealed that circulating thyroid hormone levels correlated directly with numbers of $beta_1$ receptors, and that synthesis of new receptors was involved in the increases of $beta_2$ receptor density. In contrast, the correlation of thyroid hormone and beta receptors in liver was a negative one. Thyroid hormone-induced changes in hepatic beta receptors may be mediated through corticosteroids.[46] In studies of hypothyroid rats, decreases in myocardial beta receptor number have been documented. Although decreases in basal, isoproterenol- and NaF-stimulated adenylate cyclase activity in one study suggested alterations in multiple components of the adenylate cyclase system, another study of myocardial membranes prepared from hypothyroid rats noted no changes in agonist affinity or maximal adenylate cyclase stimulation. A reduced proportion of high-affinity binding sites and alteration of G_s has been noted in reticulocytes of hypothyroid rats, however.[44] From these various studies, it is clear that thyroid hormone affects multiple sites in pathways concerned with the function of the beta-adrenergic system. More research is necessary to unravel these relationships completely.

Although corticosteroid therapy is known to have a positive inotropic effect, the interaction between adrenal corticosteroids and the beta-adrenergic receptor system remains controversial. In rats, adrenalectomy has been observed either not to affect or to increase myocardial beta receptor number, and to increase the concentration of isoproterenol needed for half-maximal stimulation of adenylate cyclase. In human leukocytes there may be differential regulation of beta receptors, with receptor density increasing and decreasing by 40% in polymorphonuclear leukocytes and lymphocytes, respectively, in response to cortisone. Cortisone may also favor the formation of the high-affinity ternary complex.[44]

Myocardial hypertrophy is associated with beta-adrenergic receptor density changes. In pressure overload models in animals, myocardial hypertrophy was associated with depletion of tissue norepinephrine levels and an increase in beta receptor density. In one canine study in which animals were allowed to develop heart failure, this increase in beta receptor density persisted. The K_D of antagonist binding was also doubled, both in the absence and presence of left ventricular decompensation. There was a reduction in $\%R_H$, and levels of basal, isoproterenol-stimulated and fluoride-stimulated cyclic AMP generation were also reduced. Thus, although beta receptor density increased with the development of myocardial hypertrophy in this model, there was decreased ability of the receptor to interact with both agonists and antagonists, and impairment of coupling to adenylate cyclase as well.[70]

Alterations in the beta-adrenergic receptor-adenylate cyclase complex also occur in human hypertension. As compared with controls, leukocytes obtained from supine human subjects with essential hypertension showed no difference in beta receptor number, but they had a reduced agonist affinity, reduced $\%R_H$, and reduced maximal adenylate cyclase activation in response to isoproterenol. There was no change in the profile obtained from hypertensive patients with assumption of the upright posture, despite a twofold increase in plasma norepinephrine. This suggests that in essential hypertension there may be a failure of dynamic regulation of beta receptors.[71] Interestingly, there were no differences in levels of circulating catecholamines between normals and essential hypertensives. Studies in a variety of animal models of hypertension have given conflicting results, suggesting alterations of myocardial receptor density and coupling, sometimes in the absence of changes in beta receptors in other organs. While it seems clear that with the development of hypertension there is a decrease in the sensitivity of the myocardium to catecholamines and an attenuation of maximal adenylate cyclase activation by isoproterenol, these may be due to changes in one or more components of the beta-adrenergic receptor-adenylate cyclase complex.

Hypoxia has been studied in animal models, and observed to have effects on beta receptor number and coupling. Myocardium from hypoxic rats demonstrated a decrease in beta receptor number, diminished response to isoproterenol, and decreased basal, isoproterenol- and fluoride-stimulated adenylate cyclase activity. Hypoxia was associated with increased circulating norepinephrine, which suggests that there was homologous desensitization of the beta receptor. In addition, observed alterations in coupling suggested additional mechanisms. The beta receptor down-regulation was blocked by propranolol.[44]

Aging is associated with changes in beta receptors. It is known that heart rate and cardiac output tend to diminish with age. There is also a blunting of heart rate response to isoproterenol, in that higher doses are required to increase the rate of normal males by 25 beats per minute. In some studies, peripheral lymphocytes have been found to have lower beta receptor density as a function of age; other studies, however, have not detected any change. Animal studies also suggest age-related changes in beta receptors as well as in G_s and adenylate cyclase.[72] During fetal development of mice, acquisition of responsiveness to isoproterenol parallels an increase in beta receptor density. Senescent rats have a decreased rate of beta receptor synthesis.[73] Leukocyte adenylate cyclase activity in response to beta-adrenergic agonists is also reduced.[74]

CLINICAL IMPLICATIONS OF BETA-ADRENERGIC RECEPTOR STUDIES IN CARDIOVASCULAR DISEASE

The phenomenon of receptor regulation has implications in the management of patients with cardiovascular disease. One example of the clinical importance of beta-adrenergic receptor regulation is the propranolol withdrawal syndrome. The mechanism of withdrawal appears to be up-regulation of the beta receptor. It is less clear, however, why the incidence of this phenomenon is so small. Although this probably represents individual variations in sympathetic tone, there is at present no proof of this explanation. It appears prudent, however, to taper the dosage of beta-adrenergic blockers prior to their discontinuance.

A second prominent example of the clinical importance of beta receptor regulation is the striking reduction in morbidity and mortality of patients status post myocardial infarction with the early institution of beta-adrenergic blocking drugs.[75,76] The causes of this benefit are unclear. It is also unclear whether beta-adrenergic blocking drugs are reducing post infarction arrhythmia and sudden death. Experimental work indicates that during ischemia there is a translocation of beta receptors from internal light vesicles to the cell surface. If propranolol therapy is instituted prior to induction of ischemia, then the proportion of beta receptors located on the cell surface is greater, and no further translocation occurs during ischemia. It is uncertain whether propranolol therapy exerts a protective effect by blocking beta receptors, by preventing receptor translocation during ischemia, or both. Nevertheless, the beneficial effects of beta-adrenergic receptor blockade in this setting, combined with the observation that ischemia promotes externalization of beta receptors, suggest that regulation of these receptors is an important determinant of outcome after myocardial infarction.

A third example is still in the stage of clinical trial. This is the use of the $beta_1$-adrenergic blocker metoprolol in patients with severe heart failure. A number of such patients have been noted to improve over time on very low doses of metoprolol.[77,78] The conceivable explanations for this phenomenon are myriad. The mechanism probably depends on the actual beta receptor density in the myocardium of the patients in the study, but this is not definitely known. At least one possible explanation for the improvement, if indeed it does occur, is that these patients have $beta_1$-adrenergic receptor down-regulation due to prolonged exposure to elevated levels of circulating catecholamines. Treatment with metoprolol would tend to restore receptor density toward normal, and the heart would be more responsive to circulating catecholamines. Again, this interpretation is highly speculative.

Up-regulation appears to be beta receptor subtype-selective in the human heart.[50] Patients treated with the nonselective beta blockers sotalol, propranolol, and pindolol, and with $beta_1$ selective blockers metoprolol and atenolol, all exhibited increased atrial $beta_1$ receptor density. However, only sotolol and propranolol increased $beta_2$ receptor density. Pindolol, the other nonselective $beta_1$ and $beta_2$ antagonist, has sympathomimetic activity which probably caused the observed down-regulation of $beta_2$ receptors accompanying up-regulation of $beta_1$ receptors.

In the study mentioned earlier, where lymphocyte levels of G_s protein and beta receptors were depressed in patients with congestive heart failure,[30] angiotensin converting enzyme inhibitors (captopril and lisinopril) reversed the decreased status of both entities. The drugs promoted the expected clinical improvement in patients, but no association of enhanced receptor numbers or regulating proteins with changes in plasma catecholamine levels could be made.

It has become clear that in order to understand the mechanism of these phenomena, one must characterize not only circulating catecholamines, receptor density and affinity, but also myocardial catecholamine concentration, and levels and function of G_s, adenylate cyclase, and protein phosphorylation. A variety of biochemical events distal to stimulation of the beta-adrenergic receptor have profound influence on the physiologic response of the cell to catecholamines.

THE ALPHA-ADRENERGIC RECEPTOR
PHARMACOLOGY

Although alpha-adrenergic receptors are present in the myocardium, it is not clear whether they have any important physiologic effects under normal conditions. The density of myocardial alpha receptors varies substantially between species. Using light microscopic autoradiography of transmural slices of feline heart, the distribution of $alpha_1$ receptors (the predominant, if not the only, alpha subtype in myocardium) was examined.[79] They were found in highest density on myocytes, a three- to fourfold lower density on arterioles, and even lower density on coronary arteries. There appeared to be uniform myocytic $alpha_1$ receptor apportionment between subepicardial and subendocardial regions. The density of $alpha_1$ receptors measured in myocytes of cat left ventricle (9.1 fmol/mg protein) was about 20% of the density of beta receptors measured by the same method in human ventricle (52 fmol/mg protein). Positive inotropic effects of phenylephrine that are blocked by phentolamine have been reported in several different myocardial preparations from guinea pig, rat, rabbit, and dog.[80] In addition, increased functional refractory period, increased action potential duration, and decreased rate of phase 4 depolarization have been reported in response to treatment with phenylephrine, or epinephrine plus propranolol. Stimulation of alpha receptors in myocytes from rat heart leads to a reduction in cyclic AMP levels.[81] Recent studies have shown that this effect is mediated by $alpha_1$-adrenergic receptors, and that the mechanism for this effect is stimulation of phosphodiesterase activity.[82]

Alpha-adrenergic receptors may be important in a variety of pathologic conditions. In slowly beating preparations, alpha-adrenergic agonists exert a positive inotropic effect that is not detected at faster rates of stimulation. Unlike beta-adrenergic effects, there is no shortening of the duration of systole or increase in the rate of relaxation, no increase in myocardial cyclic AMP, and no increase in heart rate. This positive inotropic effect is probably mediated by an increase in calcium influx. Using low concentrations of catecholamines it is possible to demonstrate an alpha-adrenergic prolongation of the refractory period and action potential in myocardium, and a reduction of automaticity in isolated conducting tissue. At higher catecholamine concentrations these effects are overwhelmed by opposite beta-adrenergic effects. In partially depolarized ventricular myocardium, alpha-adrenergic stimulation has been reported either to depress or to restore electrical and mechanical activity.[83]

It is also important to remember the potential indirect effects on myocardial function from activation of alpha-adrenergic receptors located on other tissues, and from non-alpha-adrenergic effects of classic alpha-adrenergic agonists and antagonists. Stimulation of prejunctional $alpha_2$ receptors leads to inhibition of norepinephrine release from sympathetic nerve terminals. Therefore, alpha-adrenergic antagonists that block these prejunctional $alpha_2$ receptors can stimulate the heart by allowing greater norepinephrine release. Some examples of drugs that may do this include phenoxybenzamine, phentolamine, dibenamine, chlorpromazine, and tolazoline. Central $alpha_2$-adrenergic agonists stimulate central inhibitory neurons. This stimulation promotes a reduction in sympathetic tone and an enhancement of vagal tone, with a resulting fall in arterial blood pressure and heart rate. Therefore, clonidine can cause bradycardia due to its central effects; in addition, myocardial $alpha_2$ receptors may also have a role.[83] As previously described, these receptors, classically considered to be located in prejunctional nerve terminals, are now recognized not only to exist on extraneuronal sites as described in Table 3.2, but to mediate some forms of postjunctional vascular smooth muscle contraction as well.

A role of alpha-adrenergic receptors has been described in myocardial ischemia. The $alpha_1$ receptor density appeared to increase during myocardial ischemia, as well as in experimental congestive heart failure and hypothyroidism.[84] In cats it was evident that ventricular arrhythmia occurring during reperfusion after experimentally induced ischemia was associated with an increased responsiveness to alpha-adrenergic agonists.[85] Subsequent radioligand binding studies demonstrated a twofold increase in $alpha_1$ receptor density early after occlusion and a few minutes into reperfusion.[86] There was no change in beta receptor density in this model. However, it is known that arrhythmogenesis in the ischemic myocardium has ties to both alpha- and beta-adrenergic mechanisms. Elevated levels of intracellular Ca^{2+} have been measured in reperfused myocardium after a period of ischemia. The rise in intracellular Ca^{2+} could be prevented by alpha-adrenergic blockade.[84] In dogs, pretreatment with phentolamine or prazosin, an $alpha_1$-adrenergic antagonist, but not yohimbine, an $alpha_2$-adrenergic antagonist, prevented myonecrosis after embolization with 25-μM but not 50-μM microspheres. This was probably due to a nonuniform $alpha_1$-adrenergic influence on the coronary microcirculation.[87] $Alpha_1$ receptor stimulation also causes intramitochondrial Ca^{2+} concentration to rise. The increased Ca^{2+} is associated with impaired mitochondrial function, the extent and duration of which may be important in determining the reversibility of myocardial tissue damage after an ischemic episode.[84]

Based on trends in experimental findings, it may be surmised that alpha$_1$ receptors function as a backup inotropic system for conditions in which the beta-adrenergic response is compromised. The inotropic effects of alpha$_1$ receptor stimulation are ultimately Ca^{2+}-mediated. However, the relation of arrhythmogenesis to the increased intracellular Ca^{2+} is not documented.

RADIOLIGAND BINDING STUDIES

The study of alpha-adrenergic receptors in myocardium is less advanced than that of beta receptors, both because the alpha receptor has a more limited role and because of a slower development of useful radioligands. Currently the nonselective antagonists for alpha receptors include [^{3}H]-phentolamine, [^{3}H]-phenoxybenzamine, and [^{3}H]-dihydroergocryptine (DHE). DHE, however, also binds to dopaminergic and serotonergic receptors. The alpha$_1$-adrenergic subtype-selective antagonists include [^{3}H]-prazosin and [^{3}H]-WB4101. The alpha$_2$-selective adrenergic antagonists are [^{3}H]-yohimbine and [^{3}H]-rauwolscine. Less frequently used radiolabeled agonists include [^{3}H]-clonidine, which is alpha$_2$-adrenergic-selective, and [^{3}H]-norepinephrine, which is nonselective. A new alpha$_1$-adrenergic subtype-selective iodinated antagonist is [^{125}I]-IBE 2254 or [^{125}I]-HEAT.

These ligands have been used in saturation, time course, and competition studies to verify the existence of alpha receptors in a variety of tissues, as described in Table 3.2. In myocardium, alpha receptors are located in sarcolemma. With these studies the predominance of alpha$_1$ receptors in rat[88] and guinea pig[89] heart has been documented. The density of alpha$_1$ receptors in rat heart is greatest in membranes prepared from ventricles and interventricular septum, as compared with those from the atria. Populations of alpha$_1$ receptors in freshly isolated adult rat heart cells and neonatal cultured rat heart cells have recently been characterized using [^{3}H]-prazosin[90] and [^{125}I]-IBE 2254,[91] respectively. Alpha$_2$-adrenergic receptors in myocardium have not been extensively investigated. However, the limited studies that have been done suggest that alpha$_2$ receptors do not exist on myocytes. Arteries and veins possess both alpha$_1$ and alpha$_2$ receptors that mediate vasoconstriction. Alpha$_1$ receptors seem to be the preferentially innervated alpha receptors under normal circumstances. Alpha$_2$ receptors may be present on endothelial cells to control release of endothelium-derived relaxing factor.[92] Presently, at least four subtypes of alpha receptors have been recognized, using subtype selective drugs for their identification in binding assays. There are two alpha$_1$ subtypes, alpha$_{1A}$ and alpha$_{1B}$, and two alpha$_2$ subtypes, alpha$_{2A}$ and alpha$_{2B}$. These subtypes may be found alone or together in various tissues.[93]

ALPHA-ADRENERGIC RECEPTOR STRUCTURE

All alpha-adrenergic receptors are glycoproteins; subtypes may differ in the extent of glycosylation. Alpha$_1$ receptors are about 85 kd in molecular weight, and alpha$_2$ receptors about 70 kd. Cloning and sequencing cDNA and genes for alpha$_1$ and alpha$_2$ receptors have demonstrated their membership in the family of receptors that couple with G proteins. Thus, they share the family traits of seven membrane-spanning regions, an extracellular amino terminus and an intracellular carboxy terminus, three extracellular and intracellular loops each, and sites for phosphorylation and glycosylation. There are preliminary indications that screening cDNA libraries of various tissues will uncover more subtypes of alpha-adrenergic receptors. In humans, alpha$_{2A}$ has been mapped to chromosome 10 and alpha$_{2B}$ to chromosome 4.[93] Three subtypes have been cloned to date. The one alpha$_1$ receptor may correspond to the alpha$_{1B}$ subtype, while the two alpha$_2$ receptors probably correspond to the alpha$_{2A}$ and alpha$_{2B}$ receptors, as defined by ligand binding.[94]

THE ALPHA$_2$-ADRENERGIC RECEPTOR–G$_i$ PROTEIN–EFFECTOR COMPLEX

Schematic representations of alpha receptor-effector coupling are shown in Figure 3.10. Stimulation of alpha$_2$ receptors inhibits adenylate cyclase activation, and thus reduces the amount of cyclic AMP generated. GTP is also required. Agonist occupancy of the alpha$_2$ receptor seems to stabilize a ternary complex with an inhibitory guanine nucleotide regulatory protein, G$_i$.

As described previously, the activated G$_i$ protein can inhibit adenylate cyclase activity, which in turn can inhibit cellular responses to beta-adrenergic stimulation. There are data to indicate that the same alpha$_2$ receptor–G$_i$ protein complex can also stimulate phosphoinositol metabolism to produce the IP$_3$ and DAG second messengers (to be discussed below), albeit to a lesser extent than the complex inhibits adenylate cyclase.[94]

As is the case for beta receptors and G$_s$, alpha$_2$ receptor stimulation can act through the G$_i$ protein in another cyclic AMP-independent pathway. It is possible that alpha$_2$ receptors plus G$_i$ proteins inhibit voltage-sensitive Ca^{2+} and stimulate K^+ ion channels and a Na^+/H^+ exchange mechanism without mediation by cyclic AMP.[93] The concept beginning to emerge from these and similar studies is that cellular responses result from the receptor binding to one of the multiple G proteins that in turn couples to one of the multiple effector proteins. No longer tenable is the simple concept that one receptor interacts with a single type of regulatory protein that modulates one specific effector system.

THE ALPHA$_1$-ADRENERGIC RECEPTOR–G$_z$–EFFECTOR COMPLEX

The alpha$_1$-adrenergic receptor ligand binding site resides on a 78- to 85-kd protein.[96] This is coupled by a guanine nucleotide sensitive process[97,98] to the mobilization of intracellular calcium (Ca^{2+}) stores and to increased influx of extracellular Ca^{2+}. The G protein(s) that couple alpha$_1$-adrenergic receptors to their multiple effector systems are not well characterized. It is known that the G proteins that couple alpha$_1$ receptors to their major second messenger-producing phospholipase C pathway are pertussis toxin-insensitive. The stimulation of alpha$_1$ receptors in cardiac cells has been shown to result in a rapid fivefold increase in the production of [^{3}H]-inositol phosphate from [^{3}H]-inositol.[99] This has been interpreted as a mechanism for the mediation of alpha$_1$ receptor effects. The source of inositol phosphate is membrane phospholipid turnover. In the membrane there are several phospholipids, collectively called *phosphoinositides*. Phosphatidylinositol (PI) can be phosphorylated in the 4 and in the 5 position by specific kinases to form phosphatidylinositol 4-phosphate (PIP) and phosphatidylinositol 4,5-bisphosphate (PIP$_2$). In response to binding of the alpha$_1$ receptor agonist to its receptor, PIP$_2$ is hydrolyzed to form diacylglycerol (DAG) and inositol 1,4,5-trisphosphate (IP$_3$), as shown in Figure 3.10. These last two products are each second messengers for subsequent intracellular events. IP$_3$ acts by mobilizing intracellular Ca^{2+}, and DAG stimulates protein phosphorylation at seryl and threonine residues via activation of protein kinase C. Enhanced intracellular Ca^{2+} levels may also result from protein kinase C activation of Ca^{2+} channels in the cell membrane. In support of this hypothesis are the findings that a 15-kd sarcolemmal protein is phosphorylated in cardiac preparations on alpha$_1$ stimulation, and that increases in intracellular Ca^{2+} appear to follow that event.[100,101]

Additional data suggest that alpha$_1$-adrenergic receptor-G protein complexes are linked to other effector systems as well. They appear to activate, in addition to phospholipase C in IP$_3$-DAG second messenger production, phospholipase A$_2$, which produces arachidonic acid, the precursor of leukotrienes, thromboxanes, prostaglandins, and lipoxins. The alpha$_1$-adrenergic receptor-G proteins may also stimulate a phosphodiesterase for reduction of cellular cyclic AMP, activate a Ca^{2+} channel, and activate phospholipase D to produce phosphatidic acid for facilitation of inward Ca^{2+} transport.[93] Besides these effects, alpha$_1$

receptor stimulation increases cellular levels of cyclic AMP, putatively through either DAG-activated protein kinase C activating adenylate cyclase, or through increased intracellular Ca^{2+} stimulating Ca^{2+}-calmodulin adenylate cyclase.[94]

Thus, both alpha$_1$ and alpha$_2$ receptors are now recognized as being coupled to phosphoinositide metabolism for second messenger production. They are linked to the system by different G proteins (alpha$_1$ via pertussis toxin-insensitive, and alpha$_2$ via pertussis toxin-sensitive G protein). This coupling of alpha receptors to activation of phospholipase C is the dominant mechanism for alpha$_1$ receptor effects, and a secondary mechanism for alpha$_2$ effects.

Developmental changes in the response to alpha$_1$-adrenergic agonists have been linked to G proteins. Neonatal rat hearts respond to phenylephrine with an increase in heart rate. Adult rats, conversely, have a negative chronotropic response to phenylephrine. Each of these responses is blocked by the alpha$_1$-adrenergic antagonist prazosin. It is possible to assay for the presence of G protein, using pertussis toxin to label G with ^{32}P-labeled ADP. Data from cultured neonatal rat myocytes suggest that a negative chronotropic response to phenylephrine occurs when the cells are co-cultured with sympathetic neurons, that this response arises with the acquisition of functional pertussis toxin-sensitive G protein, and is blocked when tissue is treated with pertussis toxin.[102] Pertussis toxin-sensitive G protein seems to develop later than functional alpha$_1$ receptors. The negative chronotropic response to alpha$_1$-adrenergic agonists clearly appears to be dependent on the presence of functional pertussis toxin-sensitive G protein. In rat heart, the presence of a pertussis toxin-sensitive G protein that couples alpha$_1$ receptors to a negative chronotropic response depends on maturation of sympathetic innervation. In noninnervated neonatal rat hearts, where the alpha$_1$ response is positive chronotropy, the receptor appears to interact with another G protein, this one pertussis toxin-insensitive.[103]

ALPHA-ADRENERGIC RECEPTOR REGULATION

Two principal examples of alpha$_1$-adrenergic receptor regulation are known. A model of denervation up-regulation of alpha$_1$ receptors has been developed using 6-OH-dopamine, which depletes sympathetic nerve terminals of norepinephrine. Using this drug, a 40% increase in alpha$_1$ receptor density in rats has been demonstrated.[104]

The second example is an alteration by thyroid function in heart membranes. Unlike beta receptor, alpha receptor density decreases in hyperthyroidism, so that the ratio of beta to alpha increases. In hypothyroidism, both beta and alpha density decrease. The clinical implications of these findings are not clear.[105]

Platelet alpha$_2$-adrenergic receptors have also been shown to be regulated. In unstable angina there is a 26% decrease in alpha$_2$ receptor density, but an increase in the affinity of platelet alpha$_2$-adrenergic receptors for epinephrine, which correlates with an increased sensitivity to epinephrine.[106] During extracorporal circulation, platelet alpha$_2$-adrenergic receptors are down-regulated. This correlates with a reduced sensitivity to epinephrine and is prevented by therapy with prostaglandin.[107]

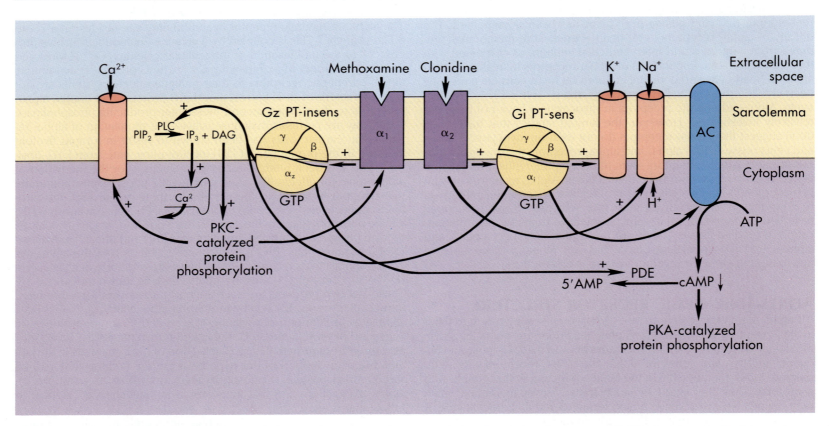

FIGURE 3.10 Alpha-adrenergic receptor-effector coupling. Methoxamine and clonidine react specifically with alpha$_1$ and alpha$_2$-adrenergic receptors, respectively. The alpha$_1$, receptor is coupled to G_z, which in the presence of GTP dissociates its G_z alpha subunit to stimulate phospholipase C (PLC). This results in the formation of second messengers inositol 1, 4, 5-trisphosphate (IP$_3$) and diacylglycerol (DAG), which increase intracellular Ca^{2+} levels, IP$_3$ by releasing Ca^{2+} from intracellular stores and DAG by stimulating protein kinase C (PKC) to phosphorylate sarcolemmal Ca^{2+} channels. PKC may also catalyze the phosphorylation of the alpha$_1$ receptor to inactivate it. In addition, activated G_z alpha may stimulate phosphodiesterase (PDE) to reduce intracellular cyclic AMP (cAMP) levels. The alpha$_2$-adrenergic receptor is coupled to G_i, which in the presence of GTP dissociates its G_i alpha and beta-gamma subunits to inhibit adenylate cyclase (AC) and the consequent protein kinase A (PKA) phosphorylation of cellular proteins. G_i alpha subunit also couples alpha$_2$ receptors directly to atrial K^+ channels for their stimulation. The alpha$_2$ receptor is also coupled via G_i alpha to stimulation of PLC. In addition, the alpha$_2$ receptor may directly activate a Na^+/H^+ exchange mechanism. (Data from Insel PA: Structure and function of alpha-adrenergic receptors. Am J Med 87:2A-12S, 1989; Cotecchia S, Kobilka BK, Daniel KW, et al: Multiple second messenger pathways of adrenergic receptor subtypes expressed in eukaryotic cells. J Biol Chem 265:63, 1990)

The mechanisms of alpha receptor regulation are less well detailed. However, data have recently implicated receptor phosphorylation in alpha$_1$ receptor down-regulation. Using the tumor-promoting substance phorbol ester myristate, which mimics diacylglycerol in activating protein kinase C, phosphorylation of alpha$_1$ receptor was demonstrated and associated with reduced sensitivity to norepinephrine and reduced alpha$_1$ receptor binding affinity for agonists.[108] The mechanisms of alpha receptor down-regulation have not yet been elucidated. However, there are recently proposed hypotheses concerning up-regulation that may help in understanding down-regulation as well.[84] A model system of hypoxic isolated canine myocytes was developed to refine a model of ischemic myocardium. The myocytes responded to hypoxia with a 200% reversible increase in alpha$_1$ receptors that exhibited no change in affinity for antagonist. The newly detected receptors did not originate from an intracellular compartment in a manner analogous to up-regulation of beta receptors. They appeared to have come from a location near the sarcolemma. Coincident with hypoxia and the appearance of additional alpha$_1$ receptors, a 70-fold increase in long-chain acyl carnitines was measured in sarcolemma. Acyl carnitines are known to perturb membranes and alter their fluidity. Therefore, it may be hypothesized that increased membrane fluidity allowed exposure of additional alpha$_1$ receptors on the cell membrane surface, resulting in up-regulation, increased cellular concentration of IP$_3$, increased intracellular Ca^{2+}, and increased risk of arrhythmogenesis.

CLINICAL IMPLICATIONS OF ALPHA-ADRENERGIC RECEPTOR STUDIES IN CARDIOVASCULAR DISEASE

The clinical implications of findings from alpha-adrenergic receptor studies are unclear at this time. Because alpha$_2$ receptor blockade would cause increased release of norepinephrine from synaptic sites, phentolamine has been judged deleterious in the therapy of acute myocardial infarction. Likewise, to the extent that alpha$_1$ blockers are less selective, they are less efficacious in antihypertensive therapy. Thus far, prazosin is the most selective and the most useful antihypertensive of the alpha$_1$-adrenergic antagonists. Preliminary reports also indicate that the alpha$_1$ antagonist doxazosin reduces the incidence of sudden death in patients with chronic heart failure.[84] Conversely, therapy with an alpha$_2$ blocker may prove helpful in hypotensive states.

The only clinical indication for therapy with a nonselective alpha antagonist is a pheochromocytoma with phentolamine or phenoxybenzamine.

THE MUSCARINIC CHOLINERGIC RECEPTOR
PHARMACOLOGY

The muscarinic cholinergic receptor mediates a variety of inhibitory inotropic and electrophysiologic effects in both the mammalian atrium and ventricle. These are detailed in Table 3.6, and muscarinic cholinergic agonists and antagonists are listed in Table 3.7. In general, the primary effects of muscarinic cholinergic receptor stimulation are to decrease heart rate and to decrease the force of contraction caused by beta-adrenergic agonists. Muscarinic receptors may act through one of several mechanisms. Muscarinic agonists may inhibit adenylate cyclase, or stimulate phosphoinositol hydrolysis, or act directly on certain ion channels in the myocardium. G proteins have been implicated as mediators in almost all of these mechanisms. The effect of muscarinic agonists is more pronounced in atrial than in ventricular tissue. In some cases the muscarinic effects are apparent in ventricular tissue only during concomitant beta-adrenergic receptor stimulation. The effects of acetylcholine clearly vary with cell type: there is an increase in the time-dependent potassium current, i$_{K1}$, in atrial, AV and SA nodal, and Purkinje fiber tissue, while it is unchanged in ventricular tissue.[109] The decrease in i$_{si}$ is not apparent in SA node but is in other cardiac tissue. Species differences also exist: in ovine Purkinje fiber i$_{K1}$ is decreased, but in canine Purkinje fiber it is increased.

The interaction of the muscarinic cholinergic responses with adrenergic responses has been the object of considerable interest. Choline esters have been demonstrated to antagonize beta-adrenergic effects on the heart. This is perhaps most evident in the response of the baroreceptor reflex to infusion of norepinephrine. Although the cells of the SA node are exposed to high levels of norepinephrine, the heart rate actually slows because of predominating vagal efferent activity elicited in response to elevated arterial blood pressure. Acetylcholine antagonizes the positive chronotropic and inotropic response to beta-

TABLE 3.6 RESPONSES MEDIATED BY THE MUSCARINIC CHOLINERGIC RECEPTOR

Location	Response	Mechanism
Sinoatrial node	Negative chronotropy	Hyperpolarization of resting membrane potential; reduction rate of diastolic depolarization; both the result of increase in i$_{K1}$, the time-dependent inward potassium current
Atrioventricular node	Negative dromotropy	Reduced rate of conduction, again due to increased i$_{K1}$, but also decrease in i$_{si}$, the slow inward calcium current
Atrial muscle	Negative inotropy	Increased i$_{K1}$, reduced i$_{si}$, associated with shortening of action potential duration, hyperpolarization of membrane, shortened refractory period
Purkinje fiber	Negative dromotropy	Same as for atrioventricular node; suppressed automaticity
Ventricular muscle	Altered ventricular repolarization, increased ventricular fibrillation threshold	Inhibition of i$_{si}$
Arterioles	Relaxation	Unknown; may require intact endothelium

(Data from Loffelholz K, Pappano AJ: The parasympathetic neuroeffector junction of the heart. Pharmacol Rev 37:1, 1985)

adrenergic agonists in both atrial and ventricular tissue. Acetylcholine also antagonizes the electrophysiologic effects of isoproterenol on atria and canine Purkinje fiber[110] and ventricular muscle. This antagonism is blocked by atropine. In continuously instrumented conscious dogs, blockade with atropine augments the positive inotropic effects of norepinephrine, epinephrine, isoproterenol, and dobutamine.[111] Muscarinic cholinergic agonists appear to have direct effects on atrial tissue, while in ventricular tissue muscarinic effects are indirect, manifested primarily in the presence of beta-adrenergic agonist stimulation.[112]

RADIOLIGAND BINDING STUDIES

The myocardial muscarinic cholinergic receptor has been characterized most commonly using [^{3}H]-quinuclidinyl benzilate (QNB), a nonselective muscarinic cholinergic antagonist. Another such antagonist used is [^{3}H]-N-methylscopolamine ([^{3}H]-NMS). A photoaffinity ligand, n-methyl-4-piperidyl-p-azidobenzilate, has been used to label membrane proteins prior to solubilization and electrophoresis. Another antagonist, pirenzepine, defines two QNB receptor populations in competition studies in the brain.[113] There is no conversion of pirenzepine sites in response to guanine nucleotides. The group with high affinity for pirenzipine has been designated subtype M_1, and the group with low affinity M_2. Rat cardiac tissue is presumed to contain predominantly M_2 because it has low affinity for pirenzepine; however, chick heart appears to contain M_1 receptors.[114] Another type of muscarinic receptor distinguished by pharmacologic and binding criteria is found in glandular tissue and may be designated M_3.

Studies with [^{3}H]-QNB have defined the regional distribution of cardiac muscarinic cholinergic receptors. In mammals the density of these receptors is greatest in the left atrium, followed in order by right atrium, interventricular septum, and right and left ventricles, which have about 12% as many receptors as the left atrium.[115] These numbers correspond with physiologic evidence for their distribution. In the frog there are 46% as many receptors in the ventricle as in the atrium, while in the embryonic and hatched chick there are 109% and 82%, respectively. The ventricles of these latter species also have a richer supply of parasympathetic innervation. Muscarinic receptors are located in the sarcolemma of myocardium, similar to beta- and alpha-adrenergic receptors. There is physiologic and histologic evidence that muscarinic receptors also exist on presynaptic sympathetic nerve terminals, and that muscarinic receptor stimulation can attenuate norepinephrine release, as shown in Figure 3.6. Indeed, sympathetic and vagus nerve terminals have been found to lie in close apposition to one another, and parasympathetic and sympathetic nerves are enclosed in the same Schwann cell.[112]

Studies of the muscarinic receptor using the agonist carbamylcholine (carbachol) to compete for [^{3}H]-QNB and [^{3}H]-NMS binding sites have revealed a super-high, a high, and a low affinity state of the receptor in chick atrium and in rat heart. Absence of the super-high affinity state has been noted in embryonic chick ventricle. In the presence of guanine nucleotide, the super-high affinity state is eliminated and the low affinity state predominates. The divalent cation Mg^{2+} also regulates binding; its addition increases the proportion of the receptors having super-high and high affinity states in chick heart, and also decreases the K_D of [^{3}H]-QNB, implying a higher affinity of the receptor for the antagonist. Monovalent cations decrease the receptor affinity for agonists. The addition of N-ethylmaleimide abolishes the effects of guanine nucleotide and Mg^{2+}, suggesting the participation of sulfhydryl groups in the interconversion of receptors between affinity states.[116] The association of the various affinity states with particular pharmacologic effects is unclear. Some reactions, such as a negative chronotropic response in embryonic chick atria, contraction of ileal smooth muscle, and inhibition of adenylate cyclase, appear to be associated with the low affinity form of the receptor. Other experiments, however, did not demonstrate muscarinic receptor responsiveness following 15 minutes of exposure to the muscarinic agonist carbachol, at which time there was a loss of high affinity binding of the receptor for agonist.[117] It seems most likely that desensitization of tissue to muscarinic agonists is associated with transition of the receptor from the high to the low affinity state. It is important to remember that agonist efficacy may not correspond to the affinity of the receptor for the agonist, due to multiple intervening steps between binding of the agonist by the receptor and the expected pharmacologic response. It is also possible that different affinity states of the muscarinic receptor are coupled to different pharmacologic responses, or represent a varying degree of coupling of receptor to effector response.

MUSCARINIC CHOLINERGIC RECEPTOR STRUCTURE

The muscarinic cholinergic receptor found in human myocardium is a glycoprotein with an apparent molecular weight of about 70 kd.[118] The polypeptide portion of the receptor contains 466 amino acid residues and has a molecular weight of about 52 kd.[119] Five subtypes of human muscarinic cholinergic receptors have been identified by molecular cloning techniques. They can be classified functionally into two groups. M_1, M_3, and M_5 generally stimulate phosphoinositol metabolism through pertussis toxin-insensitive and pertussis toxin-sensitive G proteins. These receptor subtypes also stimulate arachidonic acid release independently of effects on phosphoinositides. M_2 and M_4 generally decrease cyclic AMP in cells through G_i. A given receptor subtype can modulate more than one effector enzyme, but its predominant effect occurs via the enzyme it most efficiently regulates.[120,121]

The dominant structural characteristics common to receptors that complex with G proteins have been described in the discussion of G proteins. Muscarinic receptors belong to that group. Each of the subtypes is encoded by a unique gene. All of these genes lack introns in their protein-coding regions, an unusual feature also found in the genes for G protein-complexing beta$_2$-adrenergic and alpha$_2$-adrenergic receptors. A comparison of the primary, amino acid structure of the five subtypes reveals highly conserved amino acid sequences in the seven membrane-spanning regions and in the short connecting loops. This homology suggests that these may be regions involved with binding acetylcholine in the cleft made in the lipid bilayer membrane by insertion of such hydrophobic domains. The comparison also shows highly divergent primary structure in the large 5-6 loop in the cytoplasmic

---

TABLE 3.7 MUSCARINIC CHOLINERGIC AGONISTS AND ANTAGONISTS

Agonists	Antagonists
Acetylcholine (^{3}H)	Pirenzepine
Carbamylcholine	Atropine (^{3}H)
Oxotremorine	Scopolamine (^{3}H)
Muscarine	3-Quinuclidinyl benzilate (^{3}H)
Pilocarpine	N-methyl-4-piperidyl benzilate (^{3}H)
3-Acetoxy-quinuclidine	Propylbenzyloylcholine mustard (^{3}H)*
Cis-methyldioxolane (^{3}H)	N-methyl scopolamine (^{3}H)
	Benzhexol
	AF-DX 116
	Gallamine
	Methoctramine

* Irreversible

(Data from Sokolovsky M, Gurwitz D, Kloog J: Biochemical characterization of the muscarinic receptors. Adv Enzymol 55:137, 1983; Birdsall NJM, Chan S-C, Eveleigh P, Hulme EC, Miller KW: The modes of binding of ligands to cardiac muscarinic receptors. Trends Pharmacol Sci 10 (suppl Subtypes Muscarinic Recept IV):31, 1989)

domain and in the amino and carboxy termini. This lack of homology may relate to receptor interaction with different ion channels or effector systems. The subtypes appear to have some tissue specificity, as inferred from hybridization experiments with different tissues. It is believed that M_2 receptors predominate in heart muscle, while M_2 and M_3 are types found in smooth muscle.

That human M_2 cloned receptors are identical to the M_2 receptors identified by binding studies is suggested by the observation that the cloned M_2 receptor binds pirenzepine with affinity similar to that of M_2 isolated from rat and porcine atrium. Also, a receptor identical to human cloned M_2 is the only subtype found expressed in messenger RNA in rat heart.[119]

MUSCARINIC CHOLINERGIC RECEPTOR–G PROTEIN–EFFECTOR COMPLEXES

The muscarinic cholinergic receptor is coupled to adenylate cyclase via G_i, as previously described for the alpha$_2$-adrenergic receptor. Figure 3.11 schematically represents current understanding of muscarinic receptor-effector coupling. Reconstitution experiments of the muscarinic cholinergic receptor indicate that G_o likewise increases the affinity of the receptor for muscarinic cholinergic agonists.[122] It is not clear if G_o is also coupled to adenylate cyclase. The nature of the complex of muscarinic receptor with G_i and G_o proteins is such that interaction of receptor with regulatory protein is associated with high-affinity agonist binding to receptor, and with enhanced velocity of the GTPase activity intrinsic to the G protein. Release of GDP from the G protein appears to be the rate-limiting step accelerated by agonist-bound receptor complexing with G protein.[123] The muscarinic cholinergic receptor is also coupled to phosphoinositide turnover through a G protein, different from G_s, G_i, and G_o, and not yet isolated or fully characterized. The phosphoinositol metabolic pathway is the same as described for coupling with the alpha$_1$-adrenergic receptor. In chick embryo heart, phosphatidyl choline metabolism is also increased by muscarinic receptor stimulation. Putative second messengers produced by this pathway may increase intracellular Ca^{2+} levels.[124] Muscarinic receptors are also coupled directly to unique atrial K^+ channels by a pertussis toxin-sensitive G protein (G_i or G_k).[16] In addition, stimulation of myocardium by acetylcholine elevates cyclic 3'5' guanosine monophosphate (cyclic GMP).[125] There is a considerable body of evidence both for and against the hypothesis that cyclic GMP is a second messenger of muscarinic cholinergic agonists, and it may be that it is responsible

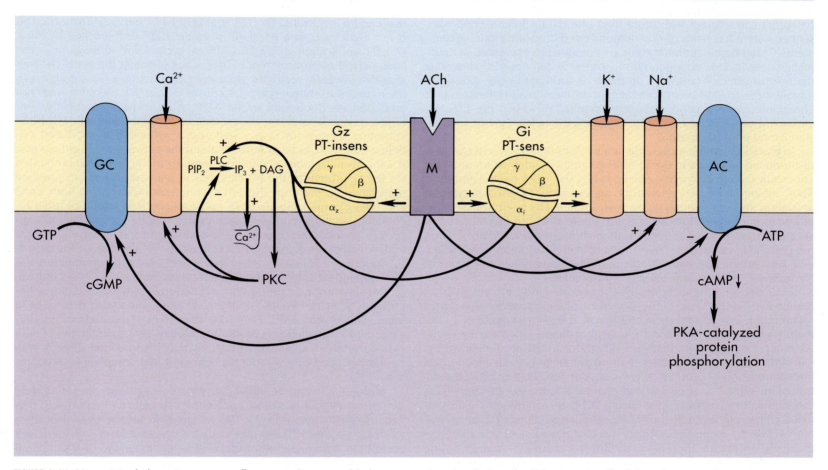

FIGURE 3.11 Muscarinic cholinergic receptor–effector coupling. Acetylcholine (ACh) reacts with a muscarinic receptor (M). The muscarinic receptor is coupled to G_z, which in the presence of GTP dissociates to G_z alpha to stimulate phospholipase C (PLC). This results in formation of second messengers inositol 1, 4, 5-trisphosphate (IP_3) and diacylglycerol (DAG) which enhance intracellular Ca^{2+} levels, IP_3 by releasing Ca^{2+} from the sarcoplasmic reticulum and DAG by stimulating protein kinase C (PKC) to phosphorylate sarcoplasmic Ca^{2+} channels. PKC may also phosphorylate PLC to inactivate it. Stimulation of the muscarinic receptor is associated with stimulation of guanylate cyclase (GC) to increase production of cyclic GMP (cGMP). The implications of this action are unclear. In addition, the muscarinic receptor is coupled to G_i, which in the presence of GTP dissociates its G_i alpha and beta-gamma subunits to inhibit adenylate cyclase (AC) and the consequent protein kinase A (PKA) phosphorylation of cellular proteins. G_i alpha subunit couples muscarinic receptors directly to atrial K^+ channels for their stimulation. The muscarinic receptor is also coupled via G_i alpha to stimulation of PLC. The muscarinic receptor may also directly activate Na^+ channels. (Data from Schimerlik MI: Structure and regulation of muscarinic receptors. Ann Rev Physiol 51:217, 1989; Bonner TI: New subtypes of muscarinic acetylcholine receptors. Trends Pharmacol Sci 11 (Suppl Subtypes Muscarinic Recep IV):11, 1989; Lechleiter J, Peralta E, Clapham D: Diverse functions of muscarinic acetylcholine receptor subtypes. Trends Pharmacol Sci (Suppl Subtypes Muscarinic Recep IV):34, 1989; Watanabe AM, Besch HR Jr: Interaction between cyclic adenosine monophosphate and cyclic guanosine monophosphate in guinea pig ventricular myocardium. Circ Res 37:309, 1975)

for some but not all muscarinic cholinergic responses. There are currently reports that phorbol esters, tumor-promoting substances that mimic the action of DAG in activating protein kinase C and blockade of arachidonic acid metabolism, have attenuated muscarinic-induced cyclic GMP increases.[118] Thus, muscarinic cholinergic receptors interact with multiple intracellular effector systems, including adenylate cyclase inhibition, phosphoinositide metabolism activation, direct ion channel activation or deactivation, and probably other intracellular entities that modulate the ultimate physiologic response to muscarinic receptor stimulation.

The coupling of muscarinic receptor to adenylate cyclase and to phosphoinositide turnover can be contrasted in several ways.[126] Although 2 muscarinic agonists, carbachol and oxotremorine, each inhibit adenylate cyclase, carbachol, but not oxotremorine, is able to increase phosphatidylinositol breakdown. Carbachol maximally inhibits cyclic AMP formation within several minutes, but inositol-1-phosphate production is detected only after 10 minutes of exposure to carbachol. Absence of extracellular calcium markedly attenuates phosphatidylinositol breakdown but not adenylate cyclase inhibition. Phosphatidylinositol breakdown is apparent even in the absence of beta-adrenergic agonists, whereas cyclic AMP inhibition is not. Finally, the half-maximal effect of carbachol on phosphatidylinositol breakdown is apparent only at a much larger concentration (20 μM) than that necessary to inhibit adenylate cyclase (0.2 μM). That muscarinic receptors can interact with more than one intracellular second messenger system has been clearly demonstrated in reconstitution experiments.[119] Recombinant muscarinic receptors were expressed in mammalian cells lacking endogenous muscarinic receptors, but possessing the normal effector pathways. In these reconstituted cells, carbachol inhibited cyclic AMP second messenger production and stimulated the phosphoinositide second messenger system. However, the ED_{50} for carbachol was 85 times lower for inhibiting adenylate cyclase than for stimulating phospholipase C.

In association with muscarinic attenuation of beta-adrenergic agonist-induced increases in cyclic AMP generation, attenuation of a variety of subsequent enzymatic reactions has also been demonstrated.[127] Thus, inhibition of beta-adrenergic agonist-induced phosphorylase a activation and glycogenolysis by acetylcholine has been noted. Phosphorylation of phospholamban is also attenuated, but this occurs to a greater extent than concomitant attenuation of cyclic AMP.[128] Thus, the possibility exists that muscarinic cholinergic agonists may antagonize beta-adrenergic agonist effects through additional mechanisms: for instance, through activation of phosphatases.

Four phosphatase enzymes have been identified in cytoplasm of mammalian cells. Type 1, the dominant phosphatase in myocardial membranes, is regulated by another protein known as inhibitor-1. The inhibitor protein is activated by phosphorylation catalyzed by cyclic AMP-dependent protein kinase.[23] When enhanced production of cyclic AMP acts as second messenger to stimulate cellular function via phosphorylation of proteins, the cyclic AMP also causes phosphorylation of inhibitor-1 to attenuate phosphatase activity, thereby amplifying the stimulatory response. See Figure 3.12. In experiments with perfused guinea pig ventricle, both beta-adrenergic stimulation of adenylate cyclase by isoproterenol and direct stimulation of adenylate cyclase by forskolin increased inhibitor-1 activity. Acetylcholine antagonized effects of both drugs on inhibitor-1. In parallel with these results, isoproterenol and forskolin decreased type 1 phosphatase activity in myocardial cell membranes, as expected if inhibitor-1 was activated. Acetylcholine not only antagonized the reduction of isoproterenol- and forskolin-induced phosphatase activity, but also increased basal phosphatase activity.[129] With these data, acetylcholine has been clearly implicated in regulation of protein phosphatase activity. Thus, muscarinic cholinergic receptors can reduce cellular protein phosphorylation by inhibiting cyclic AMP designated for cyclic AMP-dependent protein kinases. Additionally, muscarinic receptors can attenuate cellular protein phosphorylation by activating protein phosphatases. Because acetylcholine treatment raises cyclic GMP levels, its role in producing some of these effects has also been postulated. Recent data implicate decreased Ca^{2+} conductance in frog heart with decreased levels of cyclic AMP, which result from a cyclic GMP-dependent phosphodiesterase whose activity was increased by the enhanced generation of cyclic GMP clearly associated with muscarinic agonist action.[130]

A positive inotropic effect of acetylcholine occurs at concentrations equal to or greater than 10 μM. In this range, activation of phosphoinositide turnover has been reported. This response is not prevented by adrenergic blockade, nor does cyclic AMP increase. The response is blocked by atropine, suggesting that it is indeed receptor mediated. It is also associated with biochemical evidence of an increase in calcium flux.[117] Recent experiments now indicate that cyclic AMP levels can be increased by muscarinic receptor stimulation, but that this increase is secondary to muscarinic stimulation of phosphoinositol hydrolysis to form IP_3, which releases intracellular Ca^{2+} to stimulate Ca^{2+}-calmodulin-dependent adenylate cyclase.[120]

The interaction of the muscarinic receptor with inwardly rectifying potassium channels is different in different cell types. A potassium current with inward rectification occurs only in the presence of acetylcholine in sinoatrial and atrioventricular nodal cells, while in atrial muscle and Purkinje fiber cells this current is apparent in the absence, and increased in the presence, of acetylcholine. In atrial muscle cells this action of acetylcholine is clearly coupled to a GTP binding protein that can be inactivated by GTP analogs and by pertussis toxin.[131-133] It is not associated with elevation of cyclic GMP or mimicked by intracellular application of cyclic GMP or cyclic GMP analogs. It is not antagonized by isoproterenol. Thus, it appears that the acetylcholine-sensitive inwardly rectifying potassium channel ($i_{K(Ach)}$) is coupled to the muscarinic cholinergic receptor via G_i, but that the effects are not mediated via decreased cyclic AMP. A controversy presently continues, as one laboratory[134] has identified the alpha subunit of G_i as the activating species for $i_{K(Ach)}$, while other groups have produced evidence that the G_i beta-gamma subunit is the activator.[135] In either case, it is the M_2 muscarinic cholinergic receptor in the heart that is coupled via the G_i protein to the K^+ channels in pacemaker cells to produce diminished chronotropy. Recent experiments indicate that both alpha and beta-gamma subunits of G_i may independently activate atrial K^+ channels, each by a different mechanism.[121] Beta-gamma subunits appear to generate arachidonic acid through phospholipase A_2 stimulation. Arachidonic acid may then activate the K^+ channels. Blockade of this pathway eliminates activation by beta-gamma subunits but not GTP-dependent (alpha subunit) muscarinic activation.[136] In contrast, i_{si}, the slow inward current carried predominantly by calcium, is decreased by acetylcholine, primarily in association with decreases in intracellular cyclic AMP. Therefore, this effect of muscarinic cholinergic receptor stimulation is probably coupled via G_i to inhibition of adenylate cyclase. Cardiac Na^+ channels may also interact directly with muscarinic receptors without facilitation of their coupling by a G_i protein.[14,119]

Muscarinic receptor stimulation by some agonists, excluding oxotremorine, depolarizes atrial and ventricular cells pretreated with pertussis toxin to inactivate G_i. The stimulation also evokes a positive inotropic response. These effects are clearly associated with increased phosphoinositol metabolism and may reflect inhibition of a Na^+ pump or increased Na^+ influx.[137] Thus, interaction of cardiac Na^+ channels and muscarinic cholinergic receptors may represent a variation on the usual mechanism whereby G protein couples muscarinic receptor to ion channel. In this case, muscarinic agonists appear to open Na^+ channels without interposition of an activated G protein as coupler. However, persistent activation of a G protein with a nonhydrolyzable analog of GTP results in reversal of the agonist-induced increase in open Na^+ channels.[138]

The ontogenesis of two guanine nucleotide regulatory proteins has been illuminated in relation to the muscarinic cholinergic receptor. In embryonic chick heart cells, [^{3}H]-QNB receptor sites are demonstrable prior to the development of full responsiveness to acetylcholine.[139] It now appears that this responsiveness arises with development of two guanine nucleotide regulatory proteins, G_i and G_o, as assayed with pertussis toxin.[140] Whether each protein is coupled to the same or a different effector system is not clear.

MUSCARINIC CHOLINERGIC RECEPTOR REGULATION

Muscarinic receptor regulation has been extensively studied in neural tissue. Age-related decreases in muscarinic receptors have been documented. Denervation up-regulation has also been noted. Desensitization to carbachol has been demonstrated in embryonic chick heart. The concentration of carbachol producing half-maximal negative chronotropic effects increased 100-fold, while the number of [^{3}H]-QNB sites decreased 55%.[141] Subsequent studies have detected an early rapid (one to 15 minutes) loss of high affinity binding sites, followed after several hours of exposure by a loss of low affinity receptors. This second component could be inhibited by colchicine, suggesting involvement of microtubules.[117] The time course of these changes resembled that observed with the beta-adrenergic receptor. Muscarinic receptors were phosphorylated *in vivo* in the presence of agonists. Reconstitution experiments indicated that porcine atrial receptors depend on cyclic AMP-dependent protein kinase, while cerebral muscarinic receptors depend on protein kinase C for phosphorylation.[118] The role of phosphorylation of muscarinic receptors in down-regulation may not be closely analogous to that of beta-adrenergic receptors, although, in neuroblastoma cells, phosphorylation of muscarinic receptors appeared to mediate their rapid internalization and degradation.[142] Phosphorylation did not uncouple muscarinic receptors from G_i or change receptor affinity for ligand. Further experiments will be required to elucidate mechanisms of receptor loss.

Exaggerated myocardial sensitivity to the electrophysiologic effects of acetylcholine has also been documented in vagotomized cats.[143] In chronic canine preparations of cardiac sympathetic and parasympathetic denervation, an increase in beta-adrenergic receptor density and decrease in muscarinic cholinergic receptor density was reported.[63] More recent data show that chronic cardiac parasympathectomy in dogs converted ventricular myocardium from displaying only indirect

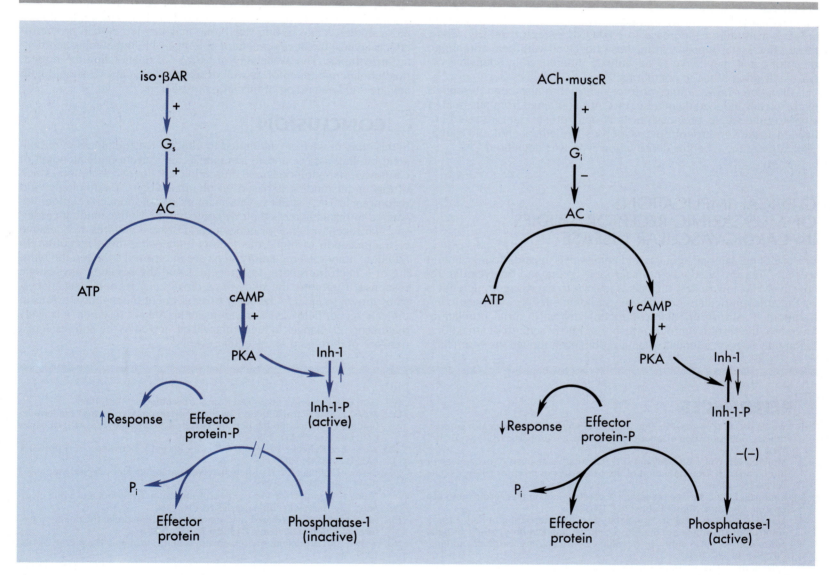

FIGURE 3.12 The role of phosphatase in modulating the effects of cardiovascular receptor stimulation. Isoproterenol (iso) stimulates the beta-adrenergic receptor (βAR) to stimulate adenylate cyclase (AC) for enhanced production of cyclic AMP (cAMP) through the stimulatory guanine nucleotide regulatory protein (G_s). Second messenger cAMP in turn stimulates protein kinase A (PKA), which catalyzes phosphorylation of various cellular proteins involved in the physiologic response. Among the proteins phosphorylated and activated is inhibitor-1 (Inh-1-P). Inh-1-P may then inactivate phosphatase-1 to prevent effector protein dephosphorylation (inactivation). This results in amplification of the cellular response. On the other hand, when acetylcholine (ACh) interacts with the muscarinic cholinergic receptor (ACh·muscR), the inhibitory guanine nucleotide regulatory protein (G_i) is activated to inhibit AC production of cAMP. Cyclic AMP-dependent PKA activity is thus attenuated, lifting inhibition of phosphatase-1 by Inh-1-P and allowing dephosphorylation of effector proteins. In this manner, the ultimate responses to PKA-mediated processes are curtailed. (Data from Cohen P: Protein phosphorylation and hormone action. Proc R Soc Lond 234:115, 1988)

responses to muscarinic stimulation (*i.e.*, acetylcholine-induced reduction of effects of beta-adrenergic stimulation) to displaying direct responses to acetylcholine. Thus, parasympathectomized hearts demonstrated shortening of the action potential duration on exposure to acetylcholine. In addition, selective parasympathectomy was associated with up-regulation of muscarinic receptors in the sarcolemma of canine ventricle, and with increased concentration of G_i and G_o proteins along with their intrinsic GTPase activities.[144] One implication of these studies is that there may be indirect influence on each limb of the autonomic nervous system. In view of this possibility, changes in both beta-adrenergic and muscarinic cholinergic receptor densities may need to be considered. It is also true that surgical vagotomy leaves the intrinsic cholinergic fibers in the heart intact, and these might influence muscarinic cholinergic receptor density in surgically decentralized preparations. When the effect of membrane depolarization on muscarinic receptor numbers was examined in cultured neuronal cells, membrane depolarization and resulting inactivation of voltage-sensitive Ca^{2+} channels appeared to increase muscarinic receptors by reducing the rate of their degradation.[145]

The effects of alteration in thyroid hormone status on muscarinic cholinergic receptors have also been described. After thyroidectomy, [^{3}H]-QNB receptor density increases. Therapy with triiodothyronine induces a moderate decrease in [^{3}H]-QNB receptor density. Thus, these effects are opposite from those observed with beta-adrenergic receptors, and may serve to accentuate differences in adenylate cyclase activation in those conditions.[117]

Alteration of muscarinic receptor density has also been described in chemically induced diabetes in rats. Atria obtained from rats treated eight to nine weeks previously with streptozotocin demonstrated enhanced negative chronotropic responses to bethanechol and carbachol. Muscarinic receptor density, however, was decreased.[146]

CLINICAL IMPLICATIONS OF MUSCARINIC RECEPTOR STUDIES IN CARDIOVASCULAR DISEASE

The use of cholinergic agonists and antagonists in cardiology is limited to acute therapy of supraventricular tachycardia and bradycardia, respectively. At low doses, digitalis is known to exert vagotonic effects on the atrioventricular node. These vagotonic effects contribute to impairment of atrioventricular conduction at rest in atrial fibrillation. Therefore the resting ventricular response rate in settings of atrial fibrillation may suggest adequate digitalization, even though the ventricular response rate is poorly controlled during exercise or after administration of atropine.

The antiarrhythmic drugs, disopyramide and quinidine, exert anticholinergic effects. In humans they may accelerate heart rate. This is particularly well demonstrated when quinidine is added to digitalis in the treatment of atrial fibrillation or flutter. If the patient is inadequately digitalized, atrioventricular conduction may be enhanced by the addition of quinidine. The ability of disopyramide and quinidine to compete with [^{3}H]-QNB has demonstrated that one mechanism for the anticholinergic effect of these agents is a direct action on the muscarinic receptor.[147]

There has been much speculation about the potential protective effects of vagal tone in humans. Loss of respiratory variation in heart rate has been associated with an increase in mortality.[148] There is experimental evidence that elimination of resting vagal tone in humans by the administration of atropine significantly shortens ventricular functional and effective refractory periods.[149] Case reports also document termination of ventricular tachycardia by enhancement of vagal tone.[150] In a canine model of reversible ischemia after anterior myocardial infarction, the blunting of an appropriate baroreceptor response is predictive of the development of ventricular fibrillation in association with exertional myocardial ischemia.[151] The implication of these studies is that resting vagal tone may provide certain protective effects against the development of potentially life-threatening ventricular arrhythmias. The availability of assays for quantitating the muscarinic cholinergic receptor as well as assays for G_i and G_o should help advance understanding of this area of research.

CONCLUSION

In this chapter we have attempted to indicate the usefulness of radioligand binding assays, and to summarize our current understanding of cardiovascular adrenergic and muscarinic cholinergic receptors. Much of this understanding is based on pharmacologic, immunologic, and recombinant DNA studies. The hallmark of autonomic receptors described in this chapter is their dynamic nature. Understanding cardiovascular receptor behavior in health and disease requires an adequate characterization of numerous factors influencing these receptors. In addition, numerous regulatory steps are interposed between the binding of a neurotransmitter to a receptor and the resulting physiologic response. Therefore, the study of cardiovascular receptors has necessarily grown to include the study of subsequent biochemical events in the cell. As our field of vision widens in this area of research, it is likely that observed changes in receptors will be viewed as the end result of a network of intra- and extracellular events.

REFERENCES

1. Weiland GA, Molinoff PB: Quantitative analysis of drug-receptor interactions: I. Determination of kinetic and equilibrium properties. Life Sci 29:313, 1981
2. Molinoff PB, Wolfe BB, Weiland GA: Quantitative analysis of drug-receptor interactions: II. Determination of the properties of receptor subtypes. Life Sci 29:427, 1981
3. Limbird LE: Cell surface receptors: A short course on theory and methods. Boston, Martinus Nijhoff Publishing, 1986
4. Manalan AS, Besch HR Jr, Watanabe AM: Characterization of [^{3}H]($\pm$)carazolol binding to beta-adrenergic receptors: application to study of beta-adrenergic receptor subtypes in canine ventricular myocardium and lung. Circ Res 49:326, 1981
5. Scatchard G: The attractions of proteins for small molecules and ions. Ann NY Acad Sci 51:660, 1949
6. Hill AW: The possible effects of the aggregation of the molecules of hemoglobin on its dissociation curves. J Physiol 40:iv–vii, 1910
7. Cheng YC, Prusoff WH: Relationship between the inhibition constant (K_i) and the concentration of inhibitor which causes 50 percent inhibition (I_{50}) of an enzymatic reaction. Biochem Pharmacol 22:3099, 1973
8. Maguire ME, VanArsdale PM, Gilman AG: An agonist-specific effect of guanine nucleotides on binding to the beta adrenergic receptor. Mol Pharmacol 12:335, 1976
9. Motulsky HJ, Insel PA: Adrenergic receptors in man: Direct identification, physiologic regulation, and clinical alterations. N Engl J Med 307:18, 1982
10. Oste C: Polymerase chain reaction. BioTechniques 6:162, 1988
11. Moss J: Signal transduction by receptor-responsive guanyl nucleotide-binding proteins: modulation by bacterial toxin-catalyzed ADP-ribosylation. Clin Res 35:451, 1987
12. Weiss ER, Kelleher DJ, Woon CW et al: Receptor activation of G proteins. FASEB J 2:2841, 1988
13. Casey PJ, Gilman AG: G protein involvement in receptor-effector coupling. J Biol Chem 263:2577, 1988
14. Numa S: A molecular view of neurotransmitter receptors and ionic channels. The Harvey Lectures, series 83:121, 1989
15. Allende JE: GTP-mediated macromolecular interactions: the common features of different systems. FASEB J 2:2356, 1988
16. Brown AM, Birnbaumer L: Ion channels and G proteins. Hosp Prac 24:189, 1989
17. Robishaw JD, Foster KA: Role of G proteins in the regulation of the cardiovascular system. Annu Rev Physiol 51:229, 1989
18. Gilman AG: G proteins and regulation of adenylyl cyclose. JAMA 262:1819, 1989
19. Fukuda K, Kubo T, Maeda A et al: Selective effector coupling of muscarinic acetylcholine receptor subtypes. Trends Pharmacol Sci, Dec suppl: 4, 1989
20. Libert F, Parmentier M, Lefort A et al: Selective amplification and cloning of four new members of the G protein-coupled receptor family. Science 244:569, 1989
21. Insel PA, Ransnäs LA: G proteins and cardiovascular disease. Circ 78:1511, 1988
22. Fleming JW, Strawbridge RA, Watanabe AM: Muscarinic receptor regulation

of cardiac adenylate cyclase activity. J Mol Cell Cardiol 19:47, 1987
23. Cohen P: Protein phosphorylation and hormone action. Proc R Soc Lond 234:115, 1988
24. Kessler PD, Cates AE, VanDop C, Feldman AM: Decreased bioactivity of the guanine nucleotide-binding protein that stimulates adenylate cyclase in hearts from cardiomyopathic Syrian hamsters. J Clin Invest 84:244, 1989
25. Longabaugh JP, Vatner DE, Vatner SF, Homcy CJ: Decreased stimulatory guanosine triphosphate binding protein in dogs with pressure-overload left ventricular failure. J Clin Invest 81:420, 1988
26. Morris SA, Tanowitz H, Factor FM, Bilezikian JP, Wittner M: Myocardial adenylate cyclase activity in acute murine Chagas' disease. Circ Res 62:800, 1988
27. Asano M, Masuzawa K, Matsuda T, Asano T: Reduced function of the stimulatory GTP-binding protein in β-adrenoceptor-adenylate cyclase system of femoral arteries isolated from spontaneously hypertensive rats. J Pharmacol Exp Ther 246:709, 1988
28. Feldman AM, Cates AE, Bristow MR, VanDop C: Altered expression of α-subunits of G proteins in failing human hearts. J Mol Cell Cardiol 21:359, 1989
29. Karliner JS, Scheinman M: Adenylate cyclase activity coupled to the stimulatory guanine nucleotide binding protein in patients having electrophysiologic studies and either structurally normal hearts or idiopathic myocardial disease. Am J Cardiol 62:1129, 1988
30. Horn EM, Corwin SJ, Steinberg SF et al: Reduced lymphocyte stimulatory guanine nucleotide regulatory protein and β-adrenergic receptors in congestive heart failure and reversal with angiotensin converting enzyme inhibitor therapy. Circ 78:1373, 1988
31. Feldman AM, Cates AE, Veazey WB et al: Increase of the 40,000 mol wt pertussis toxin substrate (G protein) in the failing human heart. J Clin Invest 82:189, 1988
32. Ahlquist RP: Study of adrenotropic receptors. Am J Physiol 153:586, 1948
33. Lands AM, Arnold A, McAuliff JP, Cuduena FP, Brown TG: Differentiation of receptor systems by sympathomimetic amines. Nature 214:597, 1967
34. Sibley DR, Lefkowitz RJ: Molecular mechanisms of receptor desensitization using the beta adrenergic receptor coupled adenylate cyclase system as a model. Nature 317:124, 1985
35. Marsh JD, Lachance D, Kim D: Mechanisms of beta-adrenergic receptor regulation in cultured chick heart cells: Role of cytoskeleton function and protein synthesis. Circ Res 57:171, 1985
36. Lau YH, Robinson RB, Rosen MR, Bilezikian JP: Subclassification of beta-adrenergic receptors in cultured rat cardiac myoblasts and fibroblasts. Circ Res 47:41, 1980
37. Ebersolt C, Perez M, Vassent G, Bockaert J: Characteristics of the beta$_1$ and beta$_2$ adrenergic sensitive adenylate cyclase in glial cell primary cultures and their comparisons with beta$_2$ adrenergic sensitive adenylate cyclase in meningeal cells. Brain Res 213:151, 1981
38. Shorr RGL, Lefkowitz RJ, Caron MG: Purification of the beta-adrenergic receptor: identification of the hormone binding subunit. J Biol Chem 256:5820, 1981
39. Lavin TN, Nambi P, Heald SL, Jeffs PW, Lefkowitz RJ, Caron MG: ^{125}I-labeled p-azidobenzylcarazolol, a photoaffinity label for the beta-adrenergic receptor: characterization of the ligand and photoaffinity labeling of beta$_1$ and beta$_2$ adrenergic receptors. J Biol Chem 257:12332, 1982
40. Shorr RGL, Strohsacker MW, Lavin TN, Lefkowitz RJ, Caron MG: The beta$_1$-adrenergic receptor of the turkey erythrocyte: molecular heterogeneity revealed by purification and photoaffinity labeling. J Biol Chem 257:12341, 1982
41. Benovic JL, Shorr RGL, Caron MG, Lefkowitz RJ: The mammalian beta$_2$-adrenergic receptor: purification and characterization. Biochem 23:4510, 1984
42. Stiles GL, Benovic JL, Caron MG, Lefkowitz RJ: Mammalian beta-adrenergic receptors: distinct glycoprotein populations containing high mannose or complex type carbohydrate chains. J Biol Chem 259:8655, 1984
43. Cerione RA, Strulovici B, Benovic JL, Lefkowitz RJ, Caron MG: Pure beta-adrenergic receptor: the single polypeptide confers catecholamine responsiveness to adenylate cyclase. Nature 306:562, 1983
44. Stiles GL, Caron MG, Lefkowitz RJ: Beta-adrenergic receptors: biochemical mechanisms of physiological regulation. Physiol Rev 64:661, 1984
45. Lefkowitz RJ, Caron MG: Adrenergic receptors. Adv Sec Mess Phosphoprot Res 21:1, 1988
46. Collins S, Bolanowski MA, Caron MG, Lefkowitz RJ: Genetic regulation of β-adrenergic receptors. Ann Rev Physiol 51:203, 1989
47. Frielle T, Collins S, Daniel KW, Caron MG, Lefkowitz RJ, Kobilka BK: Cloning of the cDNA for the human β_1-adrenergic receptor. Proc Natl Acad Sci USA 84:7920, 1987
48. Dixon RAF, Kobilka BK, Strader DJ et al: Cloning of the gene and cDNA for mammalian β-adrenergic receptor and homology with rhodapsin. Nature 321:75, 1986
49. Kobilka BK, Dixon RAF, Frielle T et al: cDNA for the human β_2-adrenergic receptor: A protein with multiple membrane-spanning domains and encoded by a gene whose chromosomal location is shared with that of the receptor for platelet-derived growth factor. Proc Natl Acad Sci USA 84:46, 1987
50. Brodde O-E: The functional importance of beta$_1$ and beta$_2$ adrenoceptors in the human heart. Am J Cardiol 62:24C, 1988
51. May DC, Ross EM, Gilman AG, Smigel MD: Reconstitution of catecholamine-stimulated adenylate cyclase activity using three purified proteins. J Biol Chem 260:15829, 1985
52. Krupinski J, Coussen F, Bakalyar HA et al: Adenylyl cyclase amino acid sequence: possible channel- or transporter-like structure. Science 244:1558, 1989
53. Lindemann JP, Jones LR, Hathaway DR, Henry BG, Watanabe AM: Beta-adrenergic stimulation of phospholamban phosphorylation and Ca^{2+}-ATPase activity in guinea pig ventricles. J Biol Chem 258:464, 1983
54. Presti CF, Jones LR, Lindemann JP: Isoproterenol-induced phosphorylation of a 15-kilodalton sarcolemmal protein in intact myocardium. J Biol Chem 260:3860, 1985
55. Schubert B, VanDongen AMP, Kirsch GE, Brown AM: β-adrenergic inhibition of cardiac sodium channels by dual G-protein pathways. Science 245:516, 1989
56. Yatani A, Brown AM: Rapid β-adrenergic modulation of calcium channel currents by a fast G protein pathway. Science 245:71, 1989
57. Bristow MR, Ginsburg R, Minobe W et al: Decreased catecholamine sensitivity and beta-adrenergic-receptor density in failing human hearts. N Engl J Med 307:205, 1982
58. Brodde O-E, Zerkowski H-R, Borst HG, Maier W, Michel MC: Drug- and disease-induced changes of human cardiac β_1 and β_2-adrenoceptors. Eur Heart J 10 (Suppl B):38, 1989
59. Murphree SS, Saffitz JE: Distribution of β-adrenergic receptors in failing human myocardium. Circ 79:1214, 1989
60. Mahan LC, Motulsky HJ, Insel PA: Do agonists promote rapid internalization of beta-adrenergic receptors? Proc Natl Acad Sci USA 82:6566, 1985
61. Sibley DR, Peters JR, Nambi P, Caron MG, Lefkowitz RJ: Desensitization of turkey erythrocyte adenylate cyclase: Beta-adrenergic receptor phosphorylation is correlated with attenuation of adenylate cyclase activity. J Biol Chem 259:9742, 1984
62. Strulovici B, Cerione RA, Kilpatrick BF, Caron MG, Lefkowitz RJ: Direct demonstration of impaired functionality of a purified desensitized beta-adrenergic receptor in a reconstituted system. Science 225:837, 1984
63. Vatner DE, Lavallee M, Amano J, Finizola A, Homcy CJ, Vatner SF: Mechanisms of supersensitivity to sympathomimic amines in the chronically denervated heart of the conscious dog. Circ Res 57:55, 1985
64. Fraser J, Nadeau J, Robertson D, Wood AJJ: Regulation of human leukocyte beta receptors by endogenous catecholamines: Relationship of leukocyte beta receptor density to the cardiac sensitivity to isoproterenol. J Clin Invest 67:1777, 1981
65. Aarons RD, Nies AS, Gal J, Hegstrand LR, Molinoff PB: Elevation of beta-adrenergic receptor density in human lymphocytes after propranolol administration. J Clin Invest 65:949, 1980
66. Mukerjee A, Wong TM, Buja LM, Lefkowitz RJ, Willerson JT: Beta-adrenergic and muscarinic cholinergic receptors in canine myocardium: effects of ischemia. J Clin Invest 64:1423, 1979
67. Maisel AS, Motulsky HJ, Insel PA: Externalization of beta-adrenergic receptors promoted by myocardial ischemia. Science 230:183, 1985
68. Buja LM, Muntz KH, Rosenbaum T et al: Characterization of a potentially reversible increase in beta-adrenergic receptors in isolated, neonatal rat cardiac myocytes with impaired energy metabolism. Circ Res 57:640, 1985
69. Ginsberg AM, Clutter WE, Shah SD, Cryer PE: Triiodothyronine-induced thyrotoxicosis increases mononuclear leukocyte beta-adrenergic receptor density in man. J Clin Invest 67:1785, 1981
70. Vatner DE, Vatner SF, Fujii AM, Homcy CJ: Loss of high affinity cardiac beta-adrenergic receptors in dogs with heart failure. J Clin Invest 76:2259, 1985
71. Feldman RD, Limbird LE, Nadeau J, Robertson D, Wood AJJ: Leukocyte beta-receptor alterations in hypertensive subjects. J Clin Invest 73:648, 1984
72. Scarpace PJ: Decreased beta-adrenergic responsiveness during senescence. Federation Proc 45:51, 1986
73. Pitha J, Hughes BA, Kusiak JW, Dax EM, Baker SP: Regeneration of beta-adrenergic receptors in senescent rats: a study using an irreversible binding antagonist. Proc Natl Acad Sci USA 79:4424, 1982
74. Feldman RD: Physiological and molecular correlates of age-related changes in the human beta-adrenergic receptor system. Federation Proc 45:48, 1986
75. Frishman WH, Furberg CD, Friedewald WT: Beta-adrenergic blockade for survivors of acute myocardial infarction. N Engl J Med 310:830, 1984
76. Friedman LM, Byington RP, Capone RJ, Furberg CD, Goldstein S, Lichstein E: Effect of propranolol in patients with myocardial infarction and ventricular arrhythmia. J Am Coll Cardiol 7:1, 1986
77. Engelmeier RS, O'Connell JB, Walsh R, Rad N, Scanlon P, Gunnar R: Metoprolol in dilated cardiomyopathy: improved exercise tolerance with chronic therapy. Circulation 70(II):II-117, 1984
78. Anderson JL, Lutz JR, Bartholomew MB: Low dose beta-blockade for dilated cardiomyopathy. A randomized study. Circulation 70(II):II-117, 1984
79. Saffitz JE: Distribution of α_1-adrenergic receptors in myocytic regions and vasculature of feline myocardium. Am J Physiol 257:H 162, 1989
80. Rosen MR, Weiss RM, Danilo P Jr: Effect of alpha adrenergic agonists and blockers on Purkinje fiber transmembrane potentials and automaticity in the dog. J Pharmacol Exp Ther 231:566, 1984
81. Watanabe AM, Hathaway DR, Besch HR Jr, Farmer BB, Harris RA: Alpha-adrenergic modulation of cyclic adenosine monophosphate concentrations

in rat myocardium. Circ Res 40:596, 1977
82. Buxton ILO, Brunton LL: Action of the cardiac alpha$_1$-adrenergic receptor: activation of cyclic AMP degradation. J Biol Chem 260:6733, 1985
83. Benfey BG: Function of myocardial alpha-adrenoceptors. Life Sci 31:101, 1982
84. Corr PB, Heathers GP, Yamada KA: Mechanisms contributing to the arrhythmogenic influences of alpha$_1$-adrenergic stimulation in the ischemic heart. Am J Med 87:2A-19S, 1989
85. Sheridan DJ, Penkoske PA, Sobel BE, Corr PB: Alpha adrenergic contributions to dysrhythmia during myocardial ischemia and reperfusion in cats. J Clin Invest 65:161, 1980
86. Corr PB, Shayman JA, Kramer JB, Kipnis RJ: Increased alpha-adrenergic receptors in ischemic cat myocardium: A potential mediator of electrophysiological derangements. J Clin Invest 67:1232, 1981
87. Eng C, Cho S, Factor SM, Sonnenblick EH, Kirk ES: Myocardial micronecrosis produced by microsphere embolization: Role of an alpha-adrenergic tonic influence on the coronary microcirculation. Circ Res 54:74, 1984
88. Williams RS, Dukes DF, Lefkowitz RJ: Subtype specificity of alpha-adrenergic receptors in rat heart. J Cardiovasc Pharmacol 3:522, 1981
89. Karliner JS, Barnes P, Hamilton CA, Dollery CT: Alpha$_1$-adrenergic receptors in guinea pig myocardium: Identification by binding of a new radioligand, (^{3}H)-prazosin. Biochem Biophys Res Commun 90:142, 1979
90. Skomedal T, Aass H, Osnes JB: Specific binding of [^{3}H]prazosin to myocardial cells isolated from adult rats. Biochem Pharmacol 33:1897, 1984
91. Kupfer LE, Robinson RB, Bilezikian JP: Identification of alpha$_1$-adrenergic receptors in cultured rat myocardial cells with a new iodinated alpha$_1$-adrenergic antagonist, [^{125}I]IBE 2254. Circ Res 51:260, 1982
92. Longer SZ, Schoemaker: Alpha-adrenoceptor subtypes in blood vessels: Physiology and pharmacology. Clin and Exper Theory and Practice A11:21, 1989
93. Insel PA: Structure and function of alpha-adrenergic receptors. Am J Med 87:2A-135, 1989
94. Cotecchia S, Kobilka BK, Daniel KW et al: Multiple second messenger pathways of α-adrenergic receptor subtypes expressed in eukaryotic cells. J Biol Chem 265:63, 1990
95. Regan JW, DeMarinis RM, Caron MG, Lefkowitz RJ: Identification of the subunit-binding site of alpha$_2$ adrenergic receptors using [^{3}H]phenoxybenzamine. J Biol Chem 259:7864, 1984
96. Leeb-Lundberg LMF, Dickinson KEJ, Heald SL et al: Photoaffinity labeling of mammalian alpha$_1$-adrenergic receptors: identification of the ligand binding subunit with a high affinity radioiodinated probe. J Biol Chem 259:2579, 1984
97. Blackmore PF, Bocckino SB, Waynick LE, Exton JH: Role of a guanine nucleotide-binding regulatory protein in the hydrolysis of hepatocyte phosphatidylinositol 4,5-bisphosphate by calcium-mobilizing hormones and the control of cell calcium: studies utilizing aluminum fluoride. J Biol Chem 260:14477, 1985
98. Goodhardt M, Ferry N, Geynet P, Hanoune J: Hepatic alpha$_1$-adrenergic receptors show agonist-specific regulation by guanine nucleotides: Loss of nucleotide effect after adrenalectomy. J Biol Chem 257:11577, 1982
99. Brown JH, Buxton IL, Brunton LL: Alpha$_1$-adrenergic and muscarinic cholinergic stimulation of phosphoinositide hydrolysis in adult rat cardiomyocytes. Circ Res 57:532, 1985
100. Lindemann JP: α-Adrenergic stimulation of sarcolemmal protein phosphorylation and slow responses in intact myocardium. J Biol Chem 261:4860, 1986
101. Presti CF, Scott BT, Jones LR: Identification of an endogenous protein kinase C activity and its intrinsic 15-kilodalton substrate in purified canine cardiac sarcolemmal vesicles. J Biol Chem 260:13879, 1985
102. Steinberg SF, Drugge ED, Bilezikian JP, Robinson RB: Acquisition by innervated cardiac myocytes of a pertussis toxin-specific regulatory protein linked to the alpha$_1$-receptor. Science 230:186, 1985
103. Han H-M, Robinson RB, Bilezikian JP, Steinberg S: Developmental changes in guanine nucleotide regulatory proteins in the rat myocardial α_1-adrenergic receptor complex. Circ Res 65:1763, 1989
104. Story DD, Briley MS, Langer SZ: The effects of chemical sympathectomy with 6-hydroxydopamine on alpha-adrenoceptor and muscarinic cholinoceptor binding in rat heart ventricle. Eur J Pharmacol 57:423, 1979
105. McConnaughey MM, Jones LR, Watanabe AM, Besch HR Jr, Williams LT, Lefkowitz RJ: Thyroxine and propylthiouracil effects on alpha- and beta-adrenergic receptor number, ATPase activities, and sialic acid content of cardiac membrane vesicles. J Cardiovasc Pharmacol 1:609, 1979
106. Mehta J, Mehta P, Ostrowski N: Increase in human platelet alpha$_2$-adrenergic receptor affinity for agonist in unstable angina. J Lab Clin Med 106:661, 1985
107. Wachtfogel YT, Musial J, Jenkin B, Niewiarowski S, Edmunds LH Jr, Colman RW: Loss of platelet alpha$_2$-adrenergic receptors during simulated extracorporeal circulation: prevention with prostaglandin E$_1$. J Lab Clin Med 105:601, 1985
108. Leeb-Lundberg LMF, Cotecchia S, Lomasney JW, DeBernardis JF, Lefkowitz RJ, Caron MG: Phorbol esters promote alpha$_1$-adrenergic receptor phosphorylation and receptor uncoupling from inositol phospholipid metabolism. Proc Natl Acad Sci USA 82:5651, 1985
109. Pappano AJ, Inoue D: Development of different electrophysiological mechanisms for muscarinic inhibition of atria and ventricles. Federation Proc 43:2607, 1984
110. Bailey JR, Watanabe AM, Besch HR Jr, Lathrop DR: Acetylcholine antagonism of the electrophysiological efforts of isoproterenol on canine cardiac Purkinje fibers. Circ Res 44:378, 1979
111. Vatner SF, Rutherford JD, Ochs HR: Baroreflex and vagal mechanisms modulating left ventricular contractile responses to sumpathomimetic amines in conscious dogs. Circ Res 44:195, 1979
112. Watanabe AM: Cholinergic agonists and antagonists. In Rosen MR, Hoffman BF (eds): Cardiac Therapy, p 95. Boston, Martinus Nijhoff, 1983
113. Birdsall NJM, Hulme EC: Muscarinic receptor subclasses. Trends in Pharm Sci 4:459, 1983
114. Brown JH, Goldstein D, Masters SB: The putative M$_1$ muscarinic receptor does not regulate phosphoinositide hydrolysis: studies with pirenzipine and McN-A343 in chick heart and astrocytoma cells. Mol Pharmacol 27:525, 1985
115. Fields JZ, Roeske WR, Morkin E, Yamamura HI: Cardiac muscarinic cholinergic receptors: biochemical identification and characterization. J Biol Chem 253:3251, 1978
116. Vickroy TW, Watson M, Yamamura HI, Roeske WR: Agonist binding to multiple muscarinic receptors. Federation Proc 43:2785, 1984
117. Loffelholz K, Pappano AJ: The parasympathetic neuroeffector junction of the heart. Pharmacol Rev 37:1, 1975
118. Schimerlik MI: Structure and regulation of muscarinic receptors. Ann Rev Physiol 51:217, 1989
119. Peralta EG, Winslow JW, Ashkenazi A, Smith DH, Ramachandran J, Capon DJ: Structural basis of muscarinic acetylcholine receptor subtype diversity. Trends Pharmacol Sci, Feb suppl:6, 1988
120. Bonner TI: New subtypes of muscarinic acetylcholine receptors. Trends Pharmacolog Sci, Dec suppl:11, 1989
121. Lechleiter J, Peralta E, Clapham D: Diverse functions of muscarinic acetylcholine receptor subtypes. Trends Pharmacol Sci 10 (Suppl Subtypes Muscarinic Recept IV):34, 1988
122. Florio VA, Sternweis PC: Reconstitution of resolved muscarinic cholinergic receptors with purified GTP-binding proteins. J Biol Chem 260:3477, 1985
123. Haga T, Haga K, Berstein G, Nishiyama T, Uchiyama H, Ichiyama A: Molecular properties of muscarinic receptors. Trends Pharmacol Sci, Feb suppl:12, 1988
124. Brown JH, Martinson EA, Jones LG: Muscarinic receptor stimulation increases phosphatidylcholine metabolism in embryonic chick heart cells. Trends Pharmacol Sci, Feb suppl:35, 1988
125. Watanabe AM, Besch HR Jr: Interaction between cyclic adenosine monophosphate and cyclic guanosine monophosphate in guinea pig ventricular myocardium. Circ Res 37:309, 1975
126. Brown JH, Masters SB: Muscarinic regulation of phosphatidylinositol turnover and cyclic nucleotide metabolism in the heart. Federation Proc 43:2613, 1984
127. Watanabe AM, Lindemann JP, Fleming JW: Mechanisms of muscarinic modulation of protein phosphorylation in intact ventricles. Federation Proc 43:2618, 1984
128. Lindemann JP, Watanabe AM: Muscarinic cholinergic inhibition of beta-adrenergic stimulation of phospholamban phosphorylation and Ca^{2+} transport in guinea pig ventricles. J Biol Chem 260:13122, 1985
129. Ahmad Z, Green FJ, Subuhe HS, Watanabe AM: Autonomic regulation of type 1 protein phosphatase in cardiac muscle. J Biol Chem 264:3859, 1989
130. Christie MJ, North RA: Control of ion conductances by muscarinic receptors. Trends Pharmacol Sci, Feb suppl:30, 1988
131. Breitwieser GE, Szabo G: Uncoupling of cardiac muscarinic and beta-adrenergic receptors from ion channels by a guanine nucleotide analogue. Nature 317:538, 1985
132. Pfaffinger PJ, Martin JM, Hunter DD, Nathanson NM, Hille B: GTP-binding proteins couple cardiac muscarinic receptors to a K channel. Nature 317:536, 1985
133. Sorota S, Tsuji Y, Tajima T, Pappano AJ: Pertussis toxin treatment blocks hyperpolarization by muscarinic agonists in chick atrium. Circ Res 57:748, 1985
134. Codina J, Yatani A, Grenet D, Brown AM, Birnbaumer L: The α subunit of the GTP binding protein G$_K$ opens atrial potassium channels. Science 236:442, 1987
135. Logothetis DE, Kurachi Y, Galper J, Neer EJ, Clapham DE: The $\beta\lambda$ subunits of GTP-binding proteins activate the muscarinic K$^+$ channel in heart. Nature 325:321, 1987
136. Kim D, Lewis D, Neer EJ, Graziadei L, Bar-Sagi D, Clapham DE: G-protein $\beta\lambda$-subunits activate the cardiac muscarinic K$^+$-channel via phospholipase A$_2$. Nature 337:557, 1989
137. Pappano AJ, Matsumoto K, Tajima T, Agnarsson U, Webb W: Pertussis toxin-insensitive mechanism for carbachol-induced depolarization and positive inotropic effect in heart muscle. Trends Pharmacol Sci, Feb suppl:35, 1988
138. Sokolovsky M, Cohen-Armon M: Cross talk between receptors: Muscarinic receptors, sodium channels, and guanine nucleotide-binding protein(s) in rat membrane preparations and synaptoneurosomes. Adv Sec Mess Phosphoprot Res 21:11, 1988
139. Galper JB, Klein W, Catterall WA: Muscarinic acetylcholine receptors in

140. Halvorsen SW, Nathanson NM: Ontogenesis of physiological responsiveness and guanine nucleotide sensitivity of cardiac muscarinic receptors during chick embryonic development. Biochemistry 23:5813, 1984
141. Galper JB, Smith TW: Properties of muscarinic acetylcholine receptors in heart cell cultures. Proc Natl Acad Sci USA 75:5831, 1978
142. Liles WC, Hunter DD, Meier KE, Nathanson NM: Activation of protein kinase C induces rapid internalization and subsequent degradation of muscarinic acetylcholine receptors in neuroblastoma cells. J Biol Chem 261:5307, 1986
143. Kovacs RJ, Bailey JC: Effects of acetylcholine on action potential characteristics of atrial and ventricular myocardium after bilateral cervical vagotomy in the cat. Circ Res 56:613, 1985
144. Hodges TD, Bailey JC, Fleming JW, Kovacs RJ: Selective parasympathectomy increases the quantity of inhibitory guanine nucleotide-binding proteins in canine cardiac ventricle. Mol Pharmacol 36:72, 1989
145. Subers EM, Liles WC, Luetje CW, Nathanson NM: Biochemical and immunological studies on the regulation of cardiac and neuronal muscarinic acetylcholine receptor number and function. Trends Pharmacol Sci, Feb suppl:25, 1988
146. Carrier GO, Edwards AD, Aronstam RS: Cholinergic supersensitivity and decreased number of muscarinic receptors in atria from short-term diabetic rats. J Mol Cell Cardiol 16:963, 1984
147. Mirro MM, Manalan AS, Bailey JR, Watanabe AM: Anticholinergic effects of disopyramide and quinidine on guinea pig myocardium: mediation by direct muscarinic receptor blockade. Circ Res 47:855, 1980
148. Eckberg DL: Parasympathetic cardiovascular control in human disease: a critical review of methods and results. Am J Physiol 239:H581, 1980
149. Prystowsky EN, Jackman WM, Rinkenberger RL, Heger JJ, Zipes DP: Effect of autonomic blockade on ventricular refractoriness and atrioventricular nodal conduction in humans: Evidence supporting a direct cholinergic action on ventricular muscle refractoriness. Circ Res 49:511, 1981
150. Waxman MB, Wald RW: Terminology of ventricular tachycardia by an increase in cardiac vagal drive. Circulation 56:385, 1977
151. Schwartz PJ, Billman GE, Stone HL: Autonomic mechanisms in ventricular fibrillation induced by myocardial ischemia during exercise in dogs with healed myocardial infarction: an experimental preparation for sudden cardiac death. Circulation 69:790, 1984

GENERAL REFERENCES

Berridge MJ: Inositol triphosphate and diacylglycerol as second messengers. Biochem J 220:345, 1984

Brodde O-E, Henderson AHH, Just H: Human cardiac β-adrenoceptor subtypes: Function, regulation and clinical significance. Eur Heart J 10 suppl B, 1989

Harden TK: Agonist-induced desensitization of the beta-adrenergic receptor-linked adenylate cyclase. Pharmacol Rev 35:5, 1983

Homcy CF, Graham RM: Molecular characterization of adrenergic receptors. Circ Res 56:635, 1985

Lefkowitz RJ, Caron MG, Stiles GL: Mechanisms of membrane-receptor regulation: Biochemical, physiological, and clinical insights derived from studies of the adrenergic receptors. N Engl J Med 310:1570, 1984

Limbird LE: Activation and attenuation of adenylate cyclase: the role of GTP-binding proteins as macromolecular messengers in receptor cyclase coupling. Biochem J 195:1, 1981

Watanabe AM: Cellular mechanisms of muscarinic regulation of cardiac function. In Randall W (ed): Nervous Control of Cardiovascular Function, pp. 130–164. Oxford University Press, New York, 1984

Watanabe AM, Jones LR, Manalan AS, Besch HR Jr: Cardiac autonomic receptors: recent concepts from radiolabeled ligand binding studies. Circ Res 50:161, 1982

MYOCARDIAL HYPERTROPHY, FAILURE, AND ISCHEMIA

William W. Parmley • Joan Wikman-Coffelt

Three of the most common pathophysiologic processes that affect the heart are hypertrophy, failure, and ischemia. One or more are encountered in a wide variety of cardiovascular disorders. Because these processes are fundamental to an understanding of cardiovascular pathology, they are discussed separately in this chapter as background for understanding their effects in specific clinical situations. Because myocardial calcium regulation is altered in these three states, both normal and abnormal calcium regulation will be discussed first.

ROLE OF CALCIUM IN REGULATION OF VENTRICULAR DEVELOPED PRESSURE

The chemical basis of cardiac mechanics is crossbridge interaction, associated with myofibrillar adenosine triphosphatase (ATPase) activity. Calcium, as a cofactor for myofibrillar ATPase, is in limiting concentration intracellularly and thus is the single most important regulator of ventricular developed pressure. There is a calcium gradient across the cell membrane: an approximate 10- to 20-fold gradient for total calcium ($40-80 \times 10^{-6}$ M), an approximate 1000-fold gradient for transients ($0.5-1.0 \times 10^{-6}$ M), and an approximate 3000-fold gradient for the resting level of calcium ($0.3-0.5 \times 10^{-6}$ M), assuming an interstitial calcium level of 1.0 mM.[1] The steepness of the gradient influences voltage of the cell and allows the calcium to act as a fast trigger for a series of cytosolic events using voltage-dependent channels in the sarcolemma and sarcoplasmic reticulum through which calcium flows into the cell down its ion gradient. The calcium concentration required for crossbridge interaction, that is, for regulating actomyosin ATPase activity, is between 0.5 and 1.0×10^{-6} M.[1]

REGULATION OF INTRACELLULAR CALCIUM

Ion gradients, voltage, cell volume, β-adrenergic activation, myofiber length, electrogenicity, the action potential, and hydrodynamics are important for regulation of intracellular calcium.[1] External calcium enters the cell through calcium channels and sodium–calcium exchange. Calcium is sequestered from the cytosol by sodium–calcium exchange and a calcium–ATPase pump.[1]

SARCOLEMMA CALCIUM CHANNELS

A family of diverse calcium channels is regulated by voltage and/or the calcium gradient across the membrane. In most species there are two voltage-dependent calcium channels in the sarcolemma of the ventricle: the fast channel (L) and the slow channel (N). Depolarization elicits a slow increase in intracellular calcium dependent on concentrations of both intracellular sodium and extracellular calcium and on membrane voltage.[2] The fast channel is activated by cyclic adenosine monophosphate (AMP). Nifedipine blocks the slow but not the fast calcium channel.[1] On the other hand, dihydropyridines increase the probability of fast channel opening. They prolong openings and shorten closings.[3,4] Thus the fast channels are referred to as the dihydropyridine sensitive channels. Verapamil blocks both the fast and slow channels. There are also low-threshold (T) channels in neural tissue. Amiloride at low concentrations selectively blocks the low-threshold channel and, at high concentrations, the fast channel.[3] Because all calcium channel blockers lower the influx of calcium and thus reduce developed pressure, they lower work and reduce oxygen consumption. In the absence of oxidative phosphorylation, work increases hydrogen ion production. Thus, by lowering work during ischemia or acidosis, calcium channel blockers protect the cell from severe acidosis.[5,6] Figure 4.1, for example, shows the protective effects of verapamil against acidosis in an isolated rat heart preparation.[6]

Calcium channel blockers can also be protective by augmenting coronary flow. Hypertrophy due to hypertension is related to a depressed coronary flow and flow reserve,[7,8] which, in turn, can result in acidosis. Calcium channel blockers can alleviate many of these deleterious effects.[7,8]

SARCOPLASMIC RETICULUM CALCIUM CHANNELS

Depolarization initiates calcium influx and release from the membrane, perhaps through the t-tubules, which contain calcium channels as shown in Figure 4.2.[9] The calcium channels in the sarcoplasmic reticulum are confined to the junctional cisternae,[10] which are 100 to 200 nm from the t-tubules.[11] Close proximity of the sarcolemma and sarcoplasmic reticulum is required as diffusion of calcium intracellularly is slow.[12] There is also nonuniform spatial distribution of intracellular calcium.[13] Mediation between the t-tubules and the sarcoplasmic reticulum may occur through breakdown of sarcolemmal membrane phosphotidylinositol 4,5-biphosphate (Ptd Ins [4,5] P_2), releasing insoluble inositol 1,4,5-triphosphate (Ins P_3), as shown in Figure 4.2. Intracellular receptors for Ins P_3 exist and when activated result in a release of cytosolic calcium.[14] This process is activated by depolarization. Inositol 1,4,5-triphosphate has been shown to couple excitation and contraction,[14] which may occur by opening calcium channels in the sarcoplasmic reticulum (see Fig. 4.2). The calcium channels of the sarcoplasmic reticulum are of a different nature from those of the sarcolemma as the former calcium channels are blocked with ryanodine but ryanodine does not react with sarcolemmal calcium channels.[15,16]

SODIUM–CALCIUM EXCHANGE

Sodium–calcium exchange has been shown to regulate the myocardial contractile state by augmenting cytosolic intracellular calcium following depolarization.[2] With depolarization the increase in intracellular calcium through sodium–calcium exchange depends on the intracellular sodium, extracellular calcium, and membrane potential.[2] Repolarization and intracellular calcium efflux depends on membrane current and voltage.[2] The influx of sodium during depolarization modifies the kinetics of sodium–calcium exchange in a manner that confers voltage dependence and electrogenicity on the enzyme.[17] Sodium–calcium exchange is regulated by the sodium and calcium gradients across the membrane and perhaps through a cyclic AMP–dependent phosphorylation of the sodium–calcium exchange enzyme.[18,19] Thus, factors such as hydrogen, depolarization, potassium, catecholamines, and so on that influence intracellular sodium also influence intracellular calcium.[1] Sodium–calcium exchange produces a membrane current that affects the membrane potential and indirectly influences all the potential dependent cellular processes. Inhibition of sodium–calcium exchange

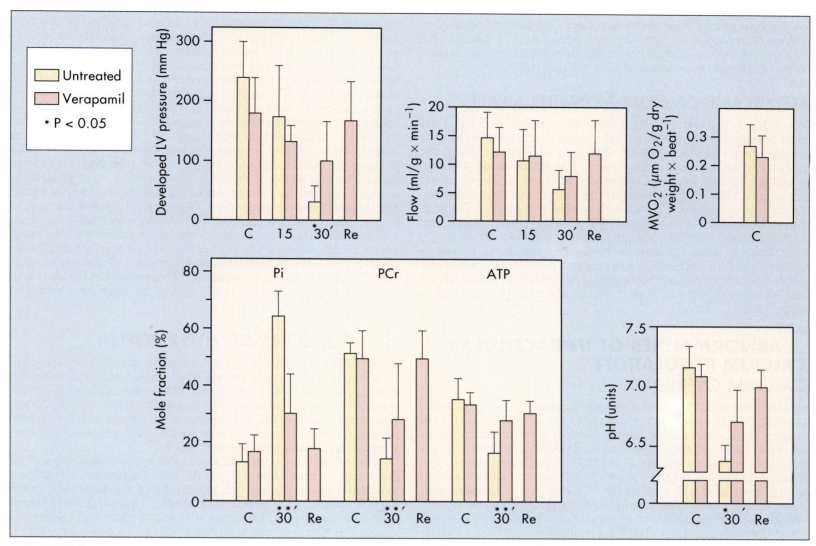

FIGURE 4.1 Effects of acidosis on isolated perfused rat hearts. After a 30-minute perfusion with an acidotic medium, hearts were reperfused with a normal medium. Rats pretreated with verapamil were compared with untreated rats (V—). **A.** Effects on left ventricular developed pressure and coronary flow. **B.** Effects on inorganic phosphate (Pi), phosphocreatine (PCr), adenosine triphosphate (ATP), and pH. (Modified from Markiewicz W, Wu ST, Parmley WW et al: Beneficial effects of verapamil during metabolic acidosis in isolated perfused rat hearts. Cardiovasc Drugs Ther 1:493, 1988)

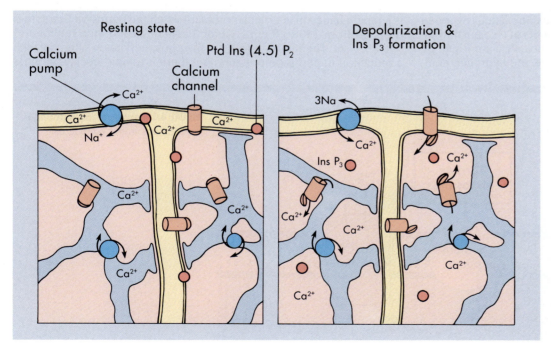

FIGURE 4.2 Effects of depolarization on calcium flux. See text for discussion.

causes cells to lose their electrical current. The sodium–calcium exchange is important for lowering the resting levels of calcium. The influence of sodium, and glycosides that increase sodium, on intracellular calcium concentrations is shown in Figure 4.3.

MEMBRANE CALCIUM-ACTIVATED ATPASE

Relaxation is initiated by sarcoplasmic reticular sequestering of calcium through an ATP-dependent calcium pump activated by catecholamine-induced phosphorylation.[20] This is an electrogenic pump, currents of which have been measured.[21] The sarcoplasmic reticulum contains a calcium-specific ATPase that constitutes 50% of membrane dry weight.[22] This enzyme transports the calcium ions into vesicles of the sarcoplasmic reticulum with high velocity and affinity.[1] The reaction proceeds with a stoichiometry of two calcium ions transported per ATP hydrolyzed.[1] Calcium-activated ATPase has a high affinity for calcium ions.[1] Calcium can also be transported out of the cytosol by sodium–calcium exchange.[2] A decrease in cytosolic cyclic AMP lowers the rate of calcium sequestering by calcium-activated ATPase and sodium–calcium exchange,[20] thus modulating the rate of relaxation.[1]

ABNORMALITIES OF INTRACELLULAR CALCIUM REGULATION
CALCIUM OVERLOAD

Calcium overload, that is, an excessive increase in total intracellular calcium, does not result in a positive inotropic effect because the calcium is sequestered and/or bound. Calcium overload has been observed in the cardiomyopathic hamster,[23] the calcium paradox,[24] and the ingestion of large amounts of alcohol.[25] An increase in free or total intracellular calcium does not augment cyclic AMP.[1] Calcium overload is often associated with an increase in acidity,[25] as in the cardiomyopathic hamster heart. The increase in hydrogen may be due to intracellular calcium displacement of intracellular hydrogen from protein sites.[26] Such competition will shift the concentration curve for calcium versus calcium-binding proteins toward higher calcium concentrations, so that a given concentration of calcium will have less effect; for example, less pressure will be generated for a given calcium release but more calcium will remain free during the resting phase. Calcium overload can also cause excessive calcium uptake by the mitochondria, resulting in inhibition of enzymes essential to the citric acid cycle, thus depressing mitochondrial function. In cases of calcium overload the free calcium may be normal while large amounts of calcium may be immobilized.[23] On the other hand, free intracellular calcium may be high but so may intracellular inorganic phosphate and hydrogen competing for the calcium-binding sites. Such competition occurs with membrane-bound ATPase sites that sequester calcium, as well as myosin and troponin.[27,28] Because different mechanisms may predominate in producing calcium overload, the effects of calcium channel blockers may differ in their protective effects. For example, treatment of the cardiomyopathic hamster with verapamil[29] but not diltiazem or nifedipine[30] results in improvement of cardiac performance and alleviation of the intracellular calcium overload.[30,31] Pretreatment of cardiomyopathic hamster hearts with verapamil helps protect the heart against cardiac depression associated with cardiomyopathy and helps preserve the high-energy phosphate levels *in vitro* (Fig. 4.4) and *in vivo*.[32] This may be due to the ability of verapamil but not diltiazem to augment intracellular calcium efflux via sodium–calcium exchange. The antimitotic agent doxorubicin (Adriamycin) has been shown to inhibit sodium–calcium exchange.[33] Pretreatment of rats with verapamil or a vasodilator helps protect the hearts against the depressive effects of doxorubicin.[34] In alcohol-induced cardiac dysfunction, ingestion of alcohol is associated with inhibition of sodium conductance[35] and intracellular dehydration.[36] Pretreatment of hamsters with verapamil helps protect the hearts against the depressive effects of alcohol.

HYPERTENSION AND HYPERTROPHY

Intracellular calcium levels may determine the presence or absence of hypertrophy. Hypertrophy occurs when protein synthesis is greater than degradation and/or metabolism supersedes catabolism. Physiologic calcium levels are known to regulate ribonucleic acid (RNA) and protein synthesis, as well as influence mitochondrial activity;[37] on the other hand, high concentrations of intracellular calcium activate proteolysis[38] and inhibit mitochondrial activity.[37]

The increase in calcium associated with hypertension may well be due to the hydrodynamics of a high perfusion pressure.[1] There is a rapid interchange of capillary fluid with that of interstitial fluid, resulting in a rapid increase in interstitial volume.[39] Interstitial and intracellular water are in rapid exchange, such that the half-life of water in a muscle cell is approximately 50 msec.[40] Sodium follows water movement because they may use the same channels.[41] Because sodium and calcium interchange are regulated by the gradients of each, sodium influences calcium concentrations. Thus, an increase in intracellular water may be associated with a positive inotropic effect owing to its indirect influence on intracellular calcium. With a decrease in perfusion pressure independent of any change in ventricular volume, there is a rapid change in ventricular pressure when the perfusion pressure is dropped from 140 to 0 cm H_2O for 10 seconds and then returned to 140 cm H_2O. There is no change in the phosphorylation potential with a reduction in perfusion pressure, but there is a rapid decline in intra-

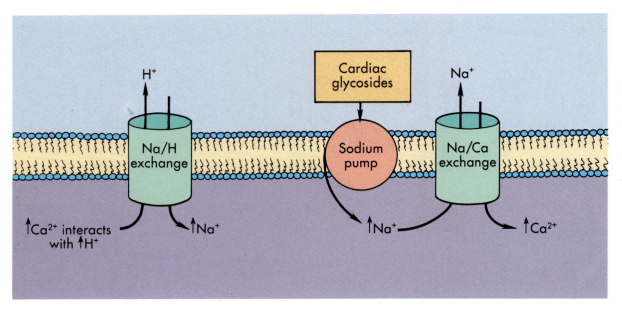

FIGURE 4.3 Important ion exchange mechanisms in the cardiac cell.

cellular water as determined by H-1 magnetic resonance imaging and a decrease in wall thickness as shown by two-dimensional echocardiography. The decrease in myocardial water content occurs both extracellularly and intracellularly. At the same time there is a decrease in the total amount of intracellular calcium.[42] Such an alteration may be an important mechanism eliciting hypertrophy, as total intracellular calcium levels increase with an increase in perfusion pressure.[42] Diltiazem prevents progression of hypertrophy in the spontaneous hypertensive rat,[7] and verapamil has been shown to decrease hypertrophy in the aortic constricted rat.[8] In both cases the calcium channel blockers prevented a decrease in coronary reserve normally associated with hypertension.

THE AGING PROCESS

The electrochemical gradient of calcium is maintained by the relative impermeability of the plasma membrane to calcium and by active extrusion. With aging the lipid composition of cell membranes change, resulting in higher quantities of docosahexanoic acid, a highly unsaturated fatty acid susceptible to peroxidation by free radicals.[43] A change in lipid composition and peroxidation of lipids comprising the cell membranes leads to alterations in membrane-bound proteins,[44] thus possibly influencing the permeability of the cell membrane to calcium and resulting in calcium overload with the aging process.[45] Among the many membrane changes occurring with aging there is also a decrease in intracellular cyclic AMP.[46] This decrease appears to be due to the uncoupling of the β-adrenergic site from the catalytic subunit.[46]

α-Adrenergic receptors do not involve cyclic nucleotides but are believed to involve stimulation of phospholipid metabolism and calcium mobilization.[47] α_1-Adrenergic receptor activation is important for glucose oxidation. With aging there is a decrease in α_1-adrenergic receptors and a decrease in glucose oxidation.[48] With a decrease in glucose oxidation there is a further decrease in delivery of pyruvate to the mitochondria, thus restricting developed pressure. Cardiac responsiveness to adrenergic agonists decreases with aging.[49] With a decrease in cyclic AMP there is a further decrease in glucose utilization and lipid oxidation.

ROLE OF GLUCOSE AND MITOCHONDRIAL ACTIVITY IN REGULATION OF DEVELOPED PRESSURE

With the heart working at maximum pressure and using high oxygen concentrations the energy metabolites ATP, inorganic phosphate, phosphocreatine, and glucose-6-phosphate are phased with the cardiac cycle.[50] This appears to be due to limited delivery of pyruvate to the mitochondria with glucose as the substrate.[50] With glucose as the substrate the redox state is lower than with pyruvate and is also phased with the cardiac cycle. However, with pyruvate as the substrate, reduced nicotinamide adenine dinucleotide is high and under maximum working conditions free adenosine diphosphate (ADP) becomes limiting for maximum mitochondrial activity.[1] The availability of free ADP sets limits to maximum work performance when oxygen and substrate are not limiting. On the other hand, with glucose as the substrate, delivery of pyruvate to the mitochondria becomes rate limiting. Phosphofructokinase is slow in the heart and thus limits the rate of glycolysis. This enzyme is further exacerbated by acidosis. The cardiomyopathic hamster heart shows intracellular acidosis and is depressed by glycolysis.[29] Likewise, when a normal heart is perfused with an acidotic medium, glycolysis is depressed.[5,51] In both models the developed pressure is 50% of the control. However, when the medium is switched to one containing pyruvate as the substrate, both the myopathic hamster heart and the acidotic healthy hamster heart express normal developed pressure when glycolysis is no longer limiting.[29] Even in the late heart failure stage this is important.[32] Similarly, when a heart is perfused with pyruvate versus glucose as the substrate, it recovers better following 30 minutes of coronary ligation. With pyruvate as the substrate there is little loss of the purine pool with reperfusion.[32] Figure 4.5 shows the use of pyruvate versus glucose as the substrate in the coronary ligated heart.[52]

Besides intracellular hydrogen regulation of phosphofructokinase and glycolysis, cyclic AMP and the purine nucleotides do the same. With a decrease in the high-energy phosphate ATP at steady-state level in the heart there is a similar decline in ADP and AMP owing to the

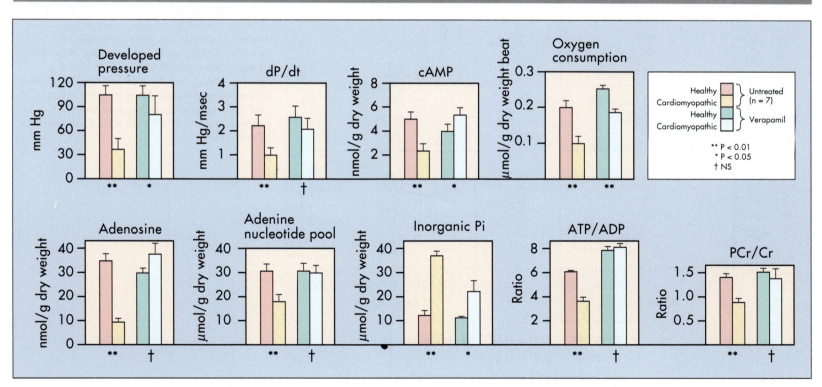

FIGURE 4.4 Physiologic and biochemical correlates in perfused hearts of healthy and cardiomyopathic Syrian hamsters treated and untreated with verapamil. Metabolic processes were terminated at diastole. Note the marked improvement both functionally and biochemically in the myopathic hearts treated with verapamil. (Modified from Wikman-Coffelt J, Sievers R, Parmley WW et al: Verapamil preserves adenine nucleotide pool in cardiomyopathic hamster. Am J Physiol 250:H22, 1986)

hydrolysis of AMP to adenosine and the efflux of adenosine and its products inosine and hypoxanthine from the cell. Loss of the purine nucleotide pool occurs in the cardiomyopathic hamster heart,[32] reperfusion of a normal heart following 30 minutes of coronary ligation,[52] reperfusion following 30 minutes of global ischemia,[53] or reperfusion of the normal heart following 30 minutes of perfusion in a medium of pH 6.8.[5] In most all of these cases pretreatment of the animal with verapamil prevents this loss of the purine nucleotide pool.[6,29,32] Also, use of pyruvate as the substrate helps alleviate the loss of the nucleotide pool.[29,32] With retention of the nucleotide pool, glycolysis proceeds at a better rate and developed pressure remains normal. Because high-energy phosphates are 50- to 100-fold in excess in the heart and the end products of ATP hydrolysis, namely inorganic phosphate and hydrogen, need to rise excessively high in order to inhibit developed pressure, energy does not normally limit cardiac function.

MYOCARDIAL HYPERTROPHY

Myocardial hypertrophy is increased growth of the heart due to an increase in cell size rather than cell division. As in other organs, this is due to augmented biosynthesis of proteins and RNA without a corresponding increase in degradation. The relative increase in size from a newborn cell to an adult cell and finally to a hypertrophied cell is shown in Figure 4.6. (Diameter size is taken from the reports of Zak[53] and Laks and co-workers[54] for the hypertrophied dog myocardium.) From these data, 125 times the contents of the newborn fiber can be placed in that of the hypertrophied fiber. Whereas the volume has increased tremendously, the surface area has only increased to one third of that of the volume; thus, exchange of gases, metabolites, and ions becomes more difficult.

The relative increase in cell surface area and cell volume during this enlargement process is shown in Figure 4.7. The greater flattening of the area curve at larger diameters illustrates the potential problem with exchange of metabolites and gases in hypertrophied cells, where surface area does not keep up with the increase in volume. Likewise, membrane-associated proteins such as adrenergic receptor sites, ion channels, and adenyl cyclase would all be reduced in relation to cell volume unless the density of these factors increased.

Normally, there is not an instantaneous diffusion of calcium across the membrane and throughout the cell. Due to protein binding, diffusion of calcium intracellularly is slower than the free diffusion coefficient. As a result, a variation in diffusion inside a cylindrically shaped cell occurs when submitted to a time-dependent flux at the sarcolemmal membrane. Calcium at the inner side of the membrane rises earlier and faster than calcium at the center of the cell, causing a gradient that increases with cell size. A variation in intracellular calcium concentration can alter the calcium-activated potassium channels, the inactivation of calcium channels, and the gradient of calcium at the membrane. Thus, as the cell hypertrophies there is a potential for cardiac performance to decrease simply due to a large cell volume in relation to cell surface and the inability of a large cell to function as rapidly and efficiently as a small cell.

EARLY STAGES

The sequence of events leading to increased protein synthesis in the stressed heart has been investigated both *in vivo* and *in vitro*, although an increase in the RNA ratio is used as an index of hypertrophy of all the cells constituting heart muscle and not simply myocytes. The heart

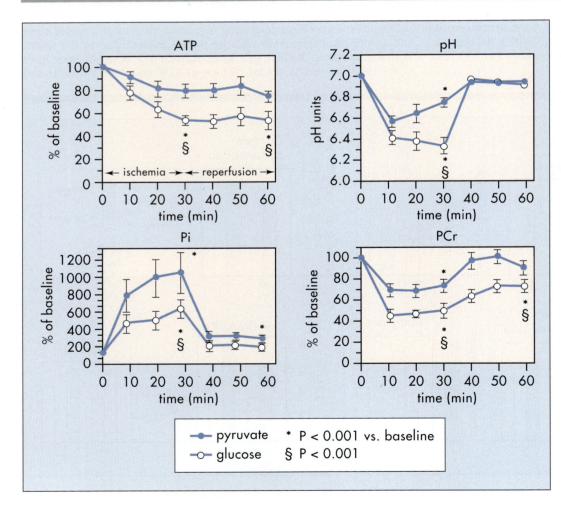

FIGURE 4.5 ATP, intracellular pH, inorganic phosphate (Pi), and phosphocreatine (PCr) values during 30 minutes of left coronary artery occlusion and 30 minutes of reperfusion. Values are means (SEM) for eight and nine hearts in the glucose- and pyruvate-perfused groups, respectively. *, $P < 0.001$ versus baseline values; §, $P < 0.001$ pyruvate- versus glucose-perfused groups. Statistical analysis was done for values at baseline, 30 minutes of ischemia, and 30 minutes of reperfusion. (Modified from Camacho SA, Parmley WW, James TL et al: Substrate regulation of the nucleotide pool during regional ischemia and reperfusion in an isolated rat heart preparation: A P-31 MRS analysis. Cardiovasc Res 22:193, 1988)

possesses a relatively high RNA to deoxyribonucleic acid (DNA) ratio, as compared with other organs. In addition, this ratio increases during hypertrophy. Present evidence suggests that within the first 30 minutes to 1 hour after the onset of an elevated workload, there is increased myocardial polyamine content and an increased adenyl cyclase activity associated with rises in RNA synthesis in the myocardium. This sequence of events is outlined in Figure 4.8. In response to increased ventricular wall stress and with the time required for transcribing messenger RNA, there is increased messenger RNA synthesis within 1 hour after an elevated workload. Within the time required for extranuclear transport of messenger RNA there follows (within 2 hours) an increase in specific messenger RNA types based on augmented synthesis of large-sized polysomes, presumably coding for large-molecular-weight proteins. There then follows an increase in myocardial protein biosynthesis. The nuclear events leading to regulation of RNA biosynthesis are shown in Figure 4.9.

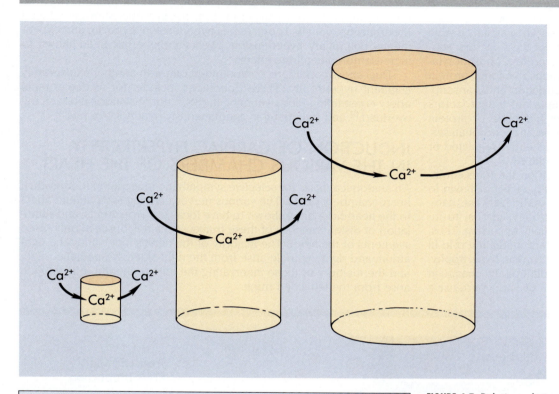

FIGURE 4.6 Diagrammatic representation of the volume of a muscle fiber at birth (6 μm diameter, *left cylinder*) of a dog, of an adult (18 μm diameter, *center cylinder*), and when hypertrophied (30 μm diameter, *right cylinder*). (Modified from Wikman-Coffelt J et al: Relation of myosin isozymes to the heart as a pump. Am Heart J 103:934, 1983)

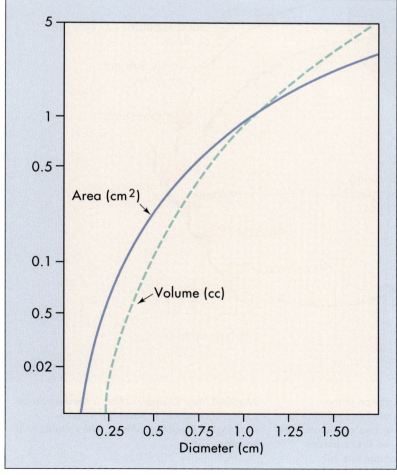

FIGURE 4.7 Relative relation of the augmentation of area to volume on the ordinate (semi-logarithmic scale) with increase in diameter on the abscissa for a spherical or cylindrical cell plotted according to mathematical calculations. (Modified from Wikman-Coffelt J et al: Chronological effects of mild pressure overload on myosin ATPase activity in the canine right ventricle. J Mol Cell Cardiol 7:219, 1975)

INDUCTION

Cardiac hypertrophy is known to result from those experimental and clinical conditions that put an increased load on the heart, such as increased pressure and/or volume. The response of the cardiac muscle cell has been studied extensively, but the nature of the intermediate link between the condition that evokes hypertrophy and the biochemical events that increase RNA (transcription) and protein biosynthesis (translation) in the muscle cell are still not completely understood. Most likely the factors that cause an increase of growth in the heart are similar to those observed for other organs. In other organs, important factors that increase RNA and protein synthesis are calcium, cyclic AMP, insulin, and modulators that increase one of these factors, subsequently leading to augmentation of cytosolic protein phosphorylation. Insulin, like calcium and cyclic AMP, augments ribosomal protein phosphorylation, leading to an elevation in translation and transcription. Calcium and cyclic AMP appear to be important trigger factors and not simply permissive factors required for induction of protein synthesis and hypertrophy. Most protein kinases and phosphatases, which modulate protein synthesis, are themselves either regulated or modulated by calcium via calmodulin and/or cyclic AMP.

Protein biosynthesis appears to be dependent on the transient influx of calcium with stimulation. Catecholamines have been shown to augment calcium fluxes as well as increase cyclic AMP. Likewise, catecholamines have been shown to induce hypertrophy, that is, to increase growth over and above that which is normally occurring. Thus, the sympathetic nervous system plays an important mediating role in the chain of events involved in the production of cardiac hypertrophy.

Catecholamines induce hypertrophy independent of any change in hemodynamics. For example, chronic infusion of subhypertensive doses of norepinephrine is a potent stimulus of hypertrophy in the dog heart.[55] Both α- and β-receptors have been implicated in this process.[56,57] Thus, excess norepinephrine secreted by the sympathetic nerve terminals can cause a greater influx of calcium, with depolarization leading over time to myocardial hypertrophy. As described in Chapter 2 there is a crosstalk between calcium and cyclic AMP, each modulating the other.[58]

There is increased cardiac sympathetic activity in many conditions that lead to compensatory cardiac hypertrophy. These include physical exercise, cold acclimatization, isoproterenol administration, constriction of the aorta, renal hypertension, deoxycorticosterone-induced hypertension, genetic spontaneous hypertension, hypoxia, and experimental pulmonary hypertension. Even thyroxine has been shown to increase norepinephrine effects.[59]

Dual stress conditions compounded one with another can severely augment hypertrophy. These conditions include, for example, renal artery constriction plus swimming in rats,[60] aortic stenosis plus volume overload,[61] and swimming in spontaneously hypertensive rats.[62]

INDUCTION OF CARDIAC HYPERTROPHY IN THE VARIOUS CHAMBERS OF THE HEART

An anatomical basis for selective sympathetic innervation to individual heart chambers exists. The various nerves carrying sympathetic fibers to the heart have been shown to have localized projections, and stimulation of distal branches of these trunks elicits responses in only those segments of the heart. The majority of the nerves innervating the right atrium and right ventricle arise from the right-sided sympathetic trunk, and the majority of those innervating the left atrium and left ventricle arise from the left-sided trunk.

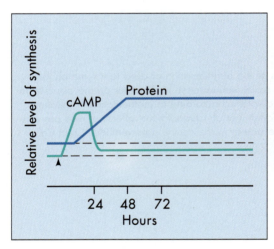

FIGURE 4.8 Diagrammatic representation of the increase in cyclic AMP and protein synthesis during the early stages of myocardial hypertrophy. Once the heart demonstrates an increased hypertrophied condition, cyclic AMP falls below normal and protein synthesis decreases. (Modified from Wikman-Coffelt J: Cardiac hypertrophy—biochemistry and experimental data. In Tarazi RC [ed]: Handbook of Hypertension. New York, Elsevier, 1985)

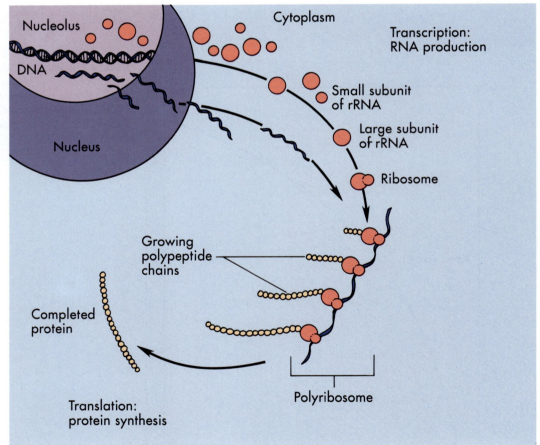

FIGURE 4.9 Diagram of transcription in the cytoplasm. The transcription of ribosomal RNA is restricted to the nucleolus. The two ribosomal RNA molecules are derived from the larger parent precursor molecules that separate into two. (Modified from Wikman-Coffelt J: Mechanism of cardiac contraction. In Sodeman W [ed]: Pathological Physiology, 7th ed. Philadelphia, WB Saunders, 1984)

Disproportionately greater hypertrophy appears to take place in the inner relative to the middle portion of the right ventricular wall in dogs after pulmonic stenosis. Spotnitz and co-workers[63] demonstrated a decreasing spectrum of sarcomere length from the inner to the outer wall of the normal left ventricle. The sarcomere length is consistent with the calculated and measured decrease in wall stress from the inner to the outer wall. Following 17 to 40 weeks of pulmonary artery banding in dogs, the sarcomere lengths in the midportion of the right ventricular wall were significantly greater than in the inner wall, suggesting decreased wall stress in the inner layers.

The degree of hypertrophy varies according to the region of the ventricle. The hypertrophy process begins at the base of the ventricle in right ventricular pressure overload and progresses apically.[64] The nonstressed left ventricle reflects the same response but to a lesser extent. Sarcomere lengths become the same at basal and apical sites in volume overload. Along with increases in wall thickness and cell lengths, there is also an increase in fiber width but not sarcomere length.

Meerson[65] observed that when hemodynamic overload is imposed on the left ventricle for prolonged periods, initially there is improvement in metabolic and mechanical function of the heart, but in later stages of hypertrophy the performance of the stressed ventricle gradually becomes impaired as the result of prolonged overload. Concomitantly, Meerson found that the hemodynamically nonstressed right ventricle eventually develops augmented function both biochemically and hemodynamically. This improved performance is sustained until the time of left ventricular dysfunction, when cardiac failure ensues.

Similar findings were noted in the hemodynamically stressed left ventricle and nonstressed right ventricle in experimental systemic hypertension.[66] In other studies of the nonstressed right ventricle in hearts with a pressure overloaded left ventricle, the inotropic state of right ventricular papillary muscles was elevated.[67] Moreover, investigations carried out on the pulmonary artery of aortic banded dogs demonstrated similar temporal alterations between the two ventricles.[68]

PROGRESSION

The mitochondrial cytochrome content per gram of tissue and the relative volume occupied by the mitochondria in cardiac fibers begin to decrease in relation to enhanced myofibrillar accumulation, depending on the animal model (e.g., 3 to 10 days after aortic banding in rats).[68] As a result, myofibrillar content increases substantially, so that the myofibrillar, mitochondrial ratio increases considerably. Thus, mitochondrial and myofibrillar masses respond to workload differentially. Collagen synthesis is augmented in animals that are undergoing cardiac hypertrophy and are subjected at the same time to hypoxic conditions. In other studies mild hypoxia was found by mass spectrometric tissue gas analysis 3 to 6 weeks after pulmonary artery banding in dogs. The lowered myocardial tissue Po_2 appears to result from an elevated myocardial respiratory rate, despite the coronary dilation evoked by decreased Po_2.

In the ensuing period (1 to 3 weeks, depending on the animal model) of the process of hypertrophy, the heart enlarges and other biochemical alterations appear. The cyclic AMP levels in the pressure-overloaded ventricle decrease if analyses are based on cardiac tissue weight. In addition, myocardial norepinephrine levels are diminished. Accompanying the decrease in cyclic AMP, there may be a concomitant reduction in RNA polymerase activity, which may result in return to a normal rate of protein synthesis, as reported by Everett and associates.[69] This eventually could cause a stabilization of ventricular weight at an increased load. Owing to the circumstances detailed below, partial or complete reversal of hypertrophy may occur, depending on the nature, degree, and duration of the initial stimulus as well as on the health and age of the animal and the species studied.

The maximum fiber size attained by myocardial hypertrophy is restricted partially by the ability of component organelles and other subcellular particles to increase in number proportionate to the demands of altered cellular dimensions. Although the heart's inherent use of the hypertrophic process serves the useful mechanical and hemodynamic process of maintaining circulatory integrity and alleviating the stress placed on single sarcomeres, the increase in contractile units so synthesized augments myocardial energetic requirements. Thus, the ability of mitochondria to increase in number proportionate to demands may determine, in part, the energy reserve of the heart.

Similar to the limited growth of mitochondrial mass in hypertrophy, there is restricted proliferative capillary development that does not keep pace with contractile protein synthesis during the hypertrophic process. There appears to be no proliferation of muscle fibers and only a limited proliferation of capillary networks during hypertrophy; therefore, the distance between capillaries increases due to muscle fiber hypertrophy. Under such circumstances, the degree of hypoxia may become considerable, particularly in the subendocardium.

RELATION OF ISOMYOSINS TO THE HEART AS A PUMP

The efficiency of the heart to function as a pump depends strongly on the composition of myosin. Myosin is the main protein comprising the thick filaments of a sarcomere. Each myosin in the thick filaments acts as a lever system to push the thin filament rods together and thereby shorten the muscle. Such mechanics are achieved by varying the tightness of the coils in the head region of myosin, a process requiring the splitting of ATP.

CARDIAC MYOSIN ISOZYMES

There are several types of myosins in the heart. When a specific enzyme has a slight modification in structure and rate of activity but the same general function the enzyme is referred to as an isozyme. The presence of myosin isozymes appears to be due to genetic regulation. For example, atrial myosin ATPase activity and velocity of shortening are about twice as great as corresponding values from the ventricular myocardium.[70] There are also disparities in both light and heavy chains of slow and fast skeletal muscle, as well as atrial and ventricular muscle. Studies have also shown that there are small differences in myosin ATPase activity of the left ventricle and right ventricle in the normal hearts of large dogs.

More recently, a new type of electrophoresis system was developed by Hoh and colleagues[71] in which atrial and ventricular myosin isozymes could be separated and identified. Differences in the ATPase activity among the three myocardial isozymes identified as V_1, V_2, and V_3 were shown to be due to two structurally different heavy chains, HCa and HCb. The latter can combine as a heterodimer or two different homodimers. The V_1 isozyme (homodimer of HCa) is common to the atria and is the dominant isozyme in the ventricles of rats at about 4 weeks of age. V_1 is the sole isozyme in adult rats treated with high doses of thyroxine. The homodimer of Hcb is the dominant isozyme heavy chain (V_3) in chronic hypophysectomized rats.

Later it was shown that HCa was the heavy chain of the atria and HCb was the main heavy chain of the ventricles in larger animals. With larger animals, differences in ventricular myosin heavy chains (V_3 designated HCb HCb and HCb' HCb') have been identified by structural studies as well as immunologically. Shifts in V_3 isomers can occur with hypertrophy in larger animals. However, shifts from atrial to ventricular and ventricular to atrial isozymes occur in the ventricles of rodents but seldom in larger animals.

INFLUENCE OF WORKLOAD ON SHIFTS IN ISOMYOSIN SYNTHESIS

The response of the heart to an increased workload depends not only on the ventricle, which is stressed, but also on the type of isomyosins present. This, in turn, varies with the age, species, and health of the animal. For example, if the stressed ventricle only contains a slow myosin, severe pressure overload causes no further decrease in myosin ATPase activity. Likewise, if the stressed ventricle contains only a myosin with high ATPase activity, then mild pressure overload causes no further increase in ATPase activity.

Thyroxine administration,[72] exercise,[73,74] and mild pressure overload[68] increase the workload on the heart and incite a shift in isomyosin synthesis toward a myosin with increased ATPase activity. On the other hand, severe pressure overload incites a shift in isomyosin synthesis toward a myosin with depressed ATPase activity.[68] Thus, some factor secondary to the increase in workload (i.e., secondary to the stretch in muscle fibers) is responsible for the induction of myosin isozyme synthesis. This is further demonstrated by the fact that ischemia without the corresponding development of hypertrophy does not appear to shift the synthesis of isomyosins.

PHYSIOLOGIC VERSUS PATHOLOGIC HYPERTROPHY

Enlargement of the heart is a natural consequence of the growth process, as mediated by hormonal and mechanical stimuli. During the middle years of life, heart size remains relatively stable. Physiologic hypertrophy can be produced during this time by a stimulus such as exercise training. A number of cardiovascular changes occur during this process. Depending on the type and duration of the training effort, considerable ventricular enlargement and hypertrophy can be produced. In this situation, the myocardium appears to retain a normal level of contractile state. This contrasts to the decrease in contractile state that accompanies severe long-term pressure or volume overload.[68] Even though the volume load on the left ventricle during maximum exercise in the athlete might be similar to the volume load imposed on the left ventricle with severe aortic regurgitation, the long-term result is different. The intermittent nature of the volume load in the athlete probably protects against the development of pathologic hypertrophy. Whether physiologic hypertrophy can ever become pathologic in the absence of a sustained load is unclear. If this phenomenon does occur, it must be quite uncommon. With removal of the excess loading conditions, regression of hypertrophy occurs almost uniformly in the individual with either physiologic or pathologic hypertrophy.

PATTERNS OF HYPERTROPHY

The best unifying hypothesis to explain patterns of ventricular hypertrophy is that the response of the ventricle is such as to maintain wall stress relatively constant.[75] A simplified form of the Laplace relation indicates that wall stress $(\sigma) = P \cdot R/2h$, where P is intraventricular pressure, R is the radius of curvature of that segment of the wall, and h is the wall thickness. This principle appears to account for the normal variations seen in wall thickness. For example, the apex of the left ventricle is thinner than the lateral free wall and also has a shorter radius of curvature. Thus, wall stress remains relatively constant in each location.

This principle appears to hold in general for the two main patterns of hypertrophy seen.[75] The first, which is represented by a lesion such as aortic regurgitation, is a diastolic volume overload that leads to both dilation and hypertrophy. If systolic pressure does not increase by much, then the increases in radius and wall thickness are relatively the same and wall stress is preserved. The second type of hypertrophy is pressure or systolic overload, as represented by aortic stenosis. Under these circumstances the increase in wall thickness and reduction in left ventricular radius with concentric hypertrophy counterbalance the rise in systolic pressure and tend to keep wall stress relatively constant.

Although the above description generally fits the facts, it is clearly too simple. For example, with diastolic overload and an increase in the size of the left ventricle, there will also be an increase in systolic wall stress during the isovolumic portion of the contraction. Thus, both increases in diastolic and systolic wall stress will play a role in the hypertrophy associated with volume overloading.

The increase in diastolic wall stress with volume loading leads to the laying down of new sarcomeres in series at the intercalated disks and Z lines. Even with extreme dilatation, the sarcomeres remain at approximately the optimum length of 2.2 μm, attesting to the dramatic increase in numbers of sarcomeres added in series. Systolic overload stimulates the laying down of sarcomeres in parallel in order to decrease wall stress by increasing wall thickness.

Two factors contribute primarily to the decreased function seen during the later stages of the hypertrophic process. If the hypertrophy is insufficient to reduce wall stress to normal in the face of a marked increase in wall stress, as for example with aortic stenosis, then the distance the muscle shortens will be reduced by the increased afterload (systolic wall stress). This reduction in ejection fraction reflects a mismatch between the afterload and the contractile reserve of the ventricle inherent in the Frank-Starling mechanism. The second mechanism by which ejection fraction is reduced is by reduction of the intrinsic contractility of the myocardium.

An example of these two different factors is seen in Figure 4.10. In patients with compensated left ventricular hypertrophy, the relationship between ejection fraction and wall stress falls on the same inverse relationship.[76] With decompensation due to a reduction in intrinsic contractility, this relationship is shifted down and to the left as the myocardium further loses its ability to shorten at a given wall stress.

Although the above discussion generally describes the patterns of hypertrophy and changes in function that occur with pressure or volume overload, it may not adequately account for the unusual patterns of hypertrophy seen in hypertrophic cardiomyopathy, which can affect principally the left ventricular septum or, in some cases, the ventricular apex.

Several factors might be playing a role under these circumstances. The left ventricle of the typical patient with hypertrophic cardiomyopathy is very hypercontractile, with a striking increase in ejection fraction. The possibility that increases in norepinephrine stimulation or calcium entry might directly contribute to both increased contractility and hypertrophy is a reasonable one. Regional variations in sympathetic stimulation could account for the predominance of hypertrophy in different locations. Alternatively, regional variations in wall stress due to geometrical considerations could also act as a potent stimulus for regional hypertrophy. Wall stress is inversely related to the radius of curvature in that area. Normally, the septum is concave to the left ventricle. If it becomes flat or convex (septal bulge), the calculated wall stress becomes enormous, owing to change in the radius of curvature. This could account, in part, for the predominant septal location of the hypertrophy.[77] With a flat septum, directional wall stress also becomes ill defined, which could account for the random direction of new fiber formation, or whorls.

Other factors, including genetic ones, may well play a more important role than the ones outlined previously. Nevertheless, the basic role played by catecholamines and wall stress undoubtedly influences the hypertrophic process under all circumstances.

HYPERTROPHY AND CORONARY FLOW

There is considerable evidence to suggest that the process of hypertrophy is accompanied by a relative reduction in coronary flow reserve. Clinically this would be manifest as exercise-induced angina in the absence of large-vessel coronary artery disease, a common phenomenon, for example, in the patient with severe aortic stenosis. A number of factors contribute to this. Studies of capillary density suggest that this index decreases with severe hypertrophy.[78] In a relative sense, the hypertrophied heart tends to outgrow its blood supply. Inadequate perfusion to the endocardium appears to be a particular problem in severe hypertrophy. The endocardium is always most vulnerable to a relative reduction in blood flow, as manifest, for example by ST-segment depression during exercise. Infarcts generally always involve the endocardium, while increasing degrees of transmural involvement reflect the severity of the ischemic insult. The penetrating arteries that traverse the myocardium from the large epicardial coronary arteries to the subendocardium are subject to greater systolic compression in hypertrophy. Calculated wall stress is highest near the endocardium, and high left ventricular diastolic pressures will also hinder endocardial flow. All of these factors contribute to the relative decrease in endocardial flow and the common occurrence of endocardial ischemia and fibrosis as a consequence of hypertrophy. In response to increased metabolic demand, both animal and human studies have documented this decrease in coronary flow reserve.[79,80] Whether this relative reduction in flow contributes directly to the reduced contractility seen in prolonged severe hypertrophy is unclear. It is probable that the major adverse effects are related primarily to the subendocardial ischemia and fibrosis just discussed.

REGRESSION OF HYPERTROPHY

As with all body tissues, there is continual turnover of muscle cells, with a steady state between formation and degradation. This is dramatically seen with skeletal muscle, where disuse leads to rapid atrophy, and conversely where isometric exercise can produce tremendous muscular enlargement. Obviously, the heart must work continuously, so that disuse atrophy is not possible. At least one clinical situation is analogous, however. In severe mitral stenosis, the left ventricle is volume underloaded and is characteristically small and hypofunctional. Sometimes, a very successful mitral commissurotomy can stress the left ventricle acutely, leading to decompensation. Over time, the ventricle dilates and thickens to restore compensation. Thus, mitral stenosis may be an example of mild "disuse atrophy."

In both animal and human studies, surgical correction of pressure or volume overload is accompanied by regression of hypertrophy. In spontaneous hypertensive rats with genetic hypertension there is an interesting difference in the effects of different blood-pressure lowering agents on regression of hypertrophy. For similar reductions in blood pressure, antihypertensive agents that interfere with the sympathetic nervous system have a much greater role in producing regression of hypertrophy than, for example, direct vasodilators.[81] Some human studies with antihypertensive drugs appear to support this conclusion. These data emphasize the role of the sympathetic nervous system in the hypertrophic process and may have important clinical implications for the selection of antihypertensive drugs.

In patients with longstanding pressure or volume overload with an associated reduction in contractility, surgical correction will often improve symptoms and produce some regression of hypertrophy, although contractility less often returns toward normal.[82,83] If prolonged volume overloading has produced a substantial laying down of collagen tissue, reduction in left ventricular volume may not occur with surgical correction of the overload. In animal models of hypertrophy and heart failure, relief of the pressure load may result in return of contractility,[84] although results are variable.[85] In the clinical setting, it may well be that the usual course of prolonged pressure or volume overload is so long that a return of intrinsic contractility is rarely possible and reductions in intrinsic contractility are mostly irreversible.

HEART FAILURE

In the process of the development of congestive heart failure there are a series of biochemical changes that occur in the failing myocardium. In many ways these changes are a progression of the changes that occur in severe left ventricular hypertrophy. They include a shift in myosin isozymes[68] with a decrease in actomyosin ATPase and associated velocity of contraction. Some data from experimental models of congestive heart failure suggest that calcium overload may be playing a pathophysiologic role.[32]

ISCHEMIA

Ischemia is the condition of oxygen deprivation produced by reduced blood supply. Ischemia is also accompanied by inadequate removal of metabolites consequent to reduced perfusion. Hypoxia is a state of reduced oxygen supply to tissues, despite adequate perfusion. Anoxia is the absence of oxygen supply, despite adequate perfusion.

For a given degree of reduced oxygen delivery, ischemia has more profound depressive effects on the myocardium than hypoxia. This presumably occurs because of reduced washout of metabolites with ischemia.[86]

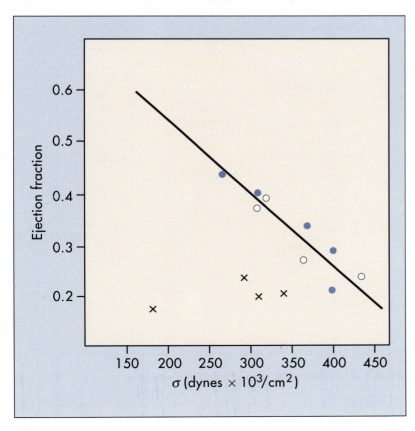

FIGURE 4.10 In patients with aortic stenosis, the preoperative ejection fraction is plotted relative to left ventricular wall stress. Patients with a satisfactory postoperative response (improvement in clinical class to class I or II) are illustrated by the circles. The crosses indicate postoperative deaths or class IV heart failure. (Modified from Carabello BA, Green LH, Grossman W et al: Hemodynamic determinants of prognosis of aortic valve replacement in critical aortic stenosis and advanced congestive heart failure. Circulation 62:42, 1980)

ENERGETICS

Normal heart muscle is uniquely dependent on aerobic metabolism for its energy supply. To satisfy this end, the myocardium requires the delivery of a continuous supply of large quantities of oxygen via the coronary circulation. The oxygen demand of the heart is considerably greater than for other organs, and, because myocardial oxygen extraction is near maximal at rest, increases in oxygen demand are primarily accomplished by elevations of coronary blood flow. Myocardial oxygen consumption of the ventricle[87] is principally determined by three hemodynamic related variables: (1) intramyocardial systolic tension or stress (primarily governed by systolic pressure and ventricular volume); (2) contractility; and (3) heart rate. Oxygen consumption may also vary with the type of isomyosin present. In addition to these three major determinants, external work or ventricular shortening (Fenn effect), energy of activation–relaxation, and basal diastolic energy requirements contribute to a relative minor degree to overall myocardial oxygen requirements.

OXIDATIVE PHOSPHORYLATION

Since ATP is the immediate energy source of the contractile apparatus and biochemical reactions elsewhere in the cell, myocardial energy metabolism is normally directed toward aerobic production of ATP in the mitochondria by substrate oxidation (dehydrogenation of citric acid intermediates requiring nicotinamide adenine dinucleotide), with discharge of carbon dioxide in the Krebs cycle (Fig. 4.11), consequent transport of hydrogen and its electron through the respiratory chain of flavoproteins and cytochromes (Fig. 4.12) (resulting in oxygen consumption and making of water), and oxidative phosphorylation, in which inorganic phosphate acquires a high-energy bond and combines with ADP to form ATP. In oxidative metabolism, almost 95% of the energy captured in ATP is derived from the transfer of electrons from carbohydrates or other substrates to oxygen.

The synthesis of ATP in the mitochondria is defined in Figure 4.13. Membranes provide a controlled internal milieu for the transfer of electrons and protons, resulting in the synthesis of high-energy ATP from ADP and inorganic phosphate.

Synthesis of ATP in the myocardium is by a rapid protonmotive force. The rate-limiting step in ATP synthesis is the movement of ATP out of the mitochondria and of ADP into the mitochondria. Muscle tissue must have the capability to synthesize ATP very rapidly and efficiently in the mitochondria and transport it to the muscle fibrils (site of utilization), where it is hydrolyzed to ADP and inorganic phosphate. ADP must return to the mitochondria for ATP resynthesis. The necessity for maintaining high values of ATP:ADP ratio in the muscle tissue results in very low concentrations of free ADP (less than 10^{-5} M). The concentration of ADP is too low to meet the required large diffusional fluxes to and from the mitochondria. Creatine, on the other hand, is a small molecule with a high diffusion rate and is present at free concentrations 100 times higher than that of ADP. Thus, the presence of creatine phosphokinase (an enzyme with a very high reaction rate)

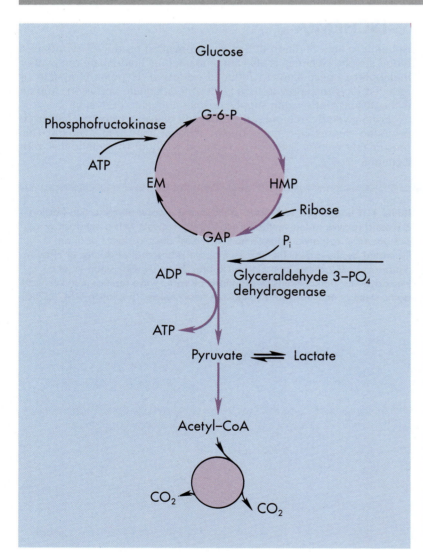

FIGURE 4.11 The pathway of glycolysis. (Modified from Wikman-Coffelt J: Cardiac hypertrophy—biochemical and experimental data. In Tarazi RC [ed]: Handbook of Hypertension. New York, Elsevier, 1985)

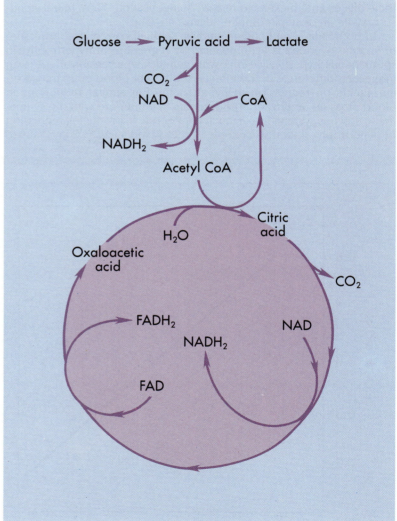

FIGURE 4.12 Diagrammatic representation of Krebs cycle.

throughout the cytoplasm enhances the rate of diffusion of the dephosphorylated forms of the high-energy phosphate compounds (ADP plus creatine) by approximately 100-fold in the heart. This ensures sufficiently rapid rates of ATP synthesis to sustain continuous muscular activity. Thus, in the mitochondria, the phosphocreatine:creatine ratio may be an important factor in regulating ATP synthesis.

The buffering action of phosphocreatine is depicted in Figure 4.14. Following the cleavage of ATP by myofibrillar ATPase to ADP and inorganic phosphate in the contraction reaction, and by additional myocardial ATPases in other biochemical processes requiring energy utilization, ADP is replenished with a high-energy phosphate from phosphocreatine or by oxidative phosphorylation to re-form ATP. The forward action of phosphocreatine to ATP uses a hydrogen ion. With the increase in intracellular acidity, the reaction increases in the forward direction. As a result, phosphocreatine is depleted before ATP in ischemia. In some types of heart failure, phosphocreatine also decreases more rapidly than ATP, whereas in the hereditary cardiomyopathy of hamsters, ATP is decreased to a greater extent than phosphocreatine.[88] The latter may be due to a deficiency in the nucleotide pool.

REGULATION OF MUSCLE ENERGY METABOLISM DURING THE CONTRACTION–RELAXATION CYCLE

Regulation of energy metabolism in a beating heart poses the question as to what extent the metabolic rate changes during each contraction–relaxation cycle. In the rat heart, each beat uses approximately 4.5% of the total ATP content of the heart during normal working conditions and 9% during stress conditions. If we assume that ATP hydrolysis occurs essentially instantaneously at a single point in the contraction–relaxation cycle, and that the measured value of ATP, ADP, and inorganic phosphate gives good approximations of their cytosolic concentrations, then hydrolysis of this much ATP increases ADP to 24% during normal working conditions and 48% during stress conditions. Consequently, the cytosolic (ATP)/(ADP)(Pi) would be expected to decrease by approximately 29% during normal working conditions. However, the heart contains a system that buffers changes in ATP and ADP. This consists of phosphocreatine, creatine, and the enzyme creatine phosphokinase, which catalyzes the near-equilibrium reaction. Because of the near-equilibrium relation between the adenine nucleotides and the creatine compounds, phosphocreatine serves to increase the available pool of ATP, whereas creatine fulfills the same function for ADP. Thus, during normal working conditions, there is only about a 2.1% decrease in the (ATP + phosphocreatine) pool, and this gives rise to a 4.6% increase in the (ADP + creatine) pool. Because the change in inorganic phosphate is the same as that calculated above 7.7%, the real decline in the ratio of (ATP)/(ADP)(Pi) during each contraction–relaxation cycle of the beating, perfused heart is only about 13% (Fig. 4.15).

MYOCARDIAL ENERGY SUBSTRATES

The predominant substrate for myocardial ATP synthesis consists of the circulating free fatty acids, consumption of which accounts for

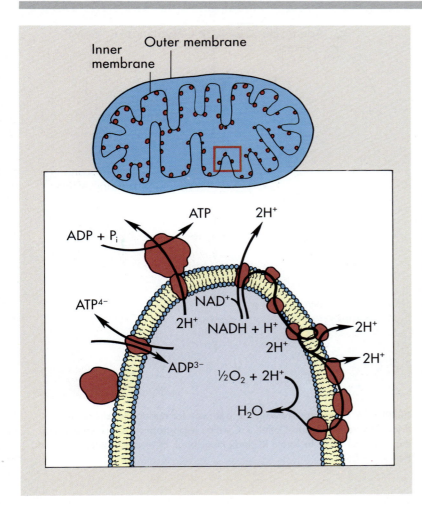

FIGURE 4.13 Diagrammatic representation of the mitochondrion (lower inset), showing the magnification of a portion of the membrane and a single crista depicting the transport of ATP and ADP, creatine kinase, the electron transport chain, and the cytochrome system. (Modified from Wikman-Coffelt J: Cardiac hypertrophy—biochemical and experimental data. In Tarazi RC [ed]: Handbook of Hypertension. New York, Elsevier, 1985)

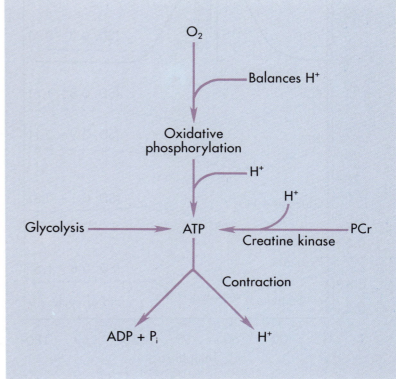

FIGURE 4.14 Diagrammatic representation of the balance of hydrogen ions via synthesis and utilization. (Modified from Wikman-Coffelt J: Cardiac hypertrophy—biochemical and experimental data. In Tarazi RC [ed]: Handbook of Hypertension. New York, Elsevier, 1985)

their large extraction by the heart. Fatty acids, however, cannot be used as the sole substrate due to the high acetate that accrues. Normally, blood glucose is used preferentially in the postprandial state. After transport across the sarcolemma-transtubular membranes, it is metabolized to glucose-6-phosphate. Under the influence of insulin, it may be stored as glycogen or undergo aerobic glycolysis to pyruvate in the sarcoplasm. In normal conditions, pyruvate is oxidized to acetyl-coenzyme A and undergoes aerobic metabolism in the citric acid cycle within the mitochrondria. Circulating lactate is also an important fuel, particularly when its concentration is elevated by prolonged skeletal muscle exercise. Blood pyruvate, like glucose, lactate, and free fatty acids, is readily taken up by the myocardium in proportion to its arterial blood concentration. Blood-borne ketone bodies and even amino acids may serve as substrates in certain abnormal conditions. Conversion of the substrate fuels into acetyl-coenzyme A is necessary for their entry into the citric acid cycle for aerobic ATP production.

NUCLEOTIDE POOL

In some pathophysiologic situations, such as experimental cardiomyopathy, recovery from lack of oxygen, cardiac hypertrophy, and stimulation with catecholamines, there is a decrease in the nucleotide pool. In such pathophysiologic situations, the degradation of ATP to ADP and AMP further proceeds to adenosine, inosine, and hypoxanthine, which are released and thus lost from the myocardial cell for restitution of adenine nucleotides through the "salvage pathways," as shown in

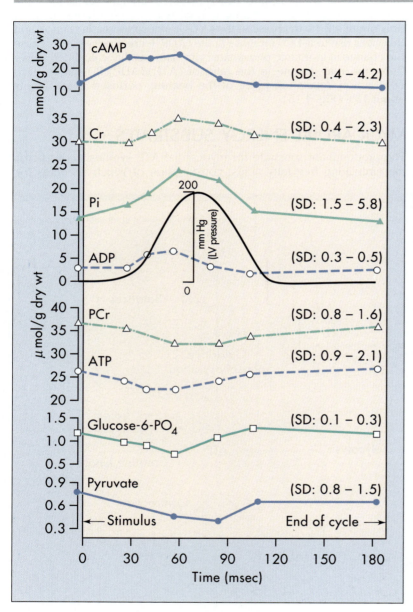

FIGURE 4.15 Pressure tracing curve of a single cardiac cycle in the rat heart. Stimulus is given at point zero, immediately after the point in late diastole is taken. Heart is freeze clamped at six points in the cardiac cycle and analyzed for cyclic AMP and various metabolites. Low-energy phosphates, inorganic phosphate (Pi), and ADP as well as creatine (Cr) and cyclic AMP are shown in the upper part. High-energy phosphates, creatine phosphate (PCr), and ATP as well as glucose-6-phosphate and pyruvate are shown in the lower part of the figure. (Modified from Wikman-Coffelt J et al: The cardiac cycle: Regulation and energy oscillations. Am J Physiol 14:H354, 1983)

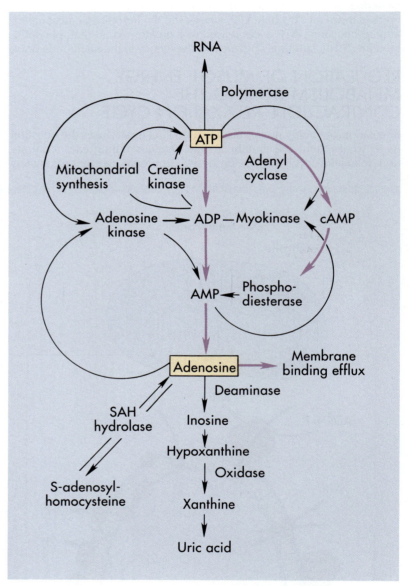

FIGURE 4.16 Flow chart showing the pathway for nucleotide utilization. (Modified from Wikman-Coffelt J: Cardiac hypertrophy—biochemical and experimental data. In Tarazi RC [ed]: Handbook of Hypertension. New York, Elsevier, 1985)

Figure 4.16. These pathways include the phosphorylation of adenosine to AMP through adenosine kinase and the conversion of hypoxanthine to inosine monophosphate, a reaction catalyzed by hypoxanthine guanine phosphoribosyltransferase.

EFFECTS OF ISCHEMIA ON MYOCARDIAL METABOLISM

During the first minutes of severe ischemia, the production of high-energy phosphates (the sum of ATP and phosphocreatine) declines and is greatly exceeded by the utilization; hence, tissue stores decline progressively, with phosphocreatine stores falling more rapidly than ATP stores. Phosphocreatine is depleted by transferring its high-energy phosphate to ADP in an attempt to maintain ATP stores. In the presence of normal aerobic mitochondrial function, ADP is converted to ATP, but in the absence of normal oxidative phosphorylation, AMP increases, which, in turn, is broken down into adenosine, inosine, and hypoxanthine with efflux from the cell. Such loss of nucleotides results in a depressed nucleotide pool. Such a depressed nucleotide pool can be alleviated experimentally by treatment with AICA-riboside, ribose, or precursors of nucleotides. In some instances, a return of the nucleotide pool to normal values is associated with a return of cardiac function to normal.

The technique of phosphorus-31 magnetic resonance imaging has provided important new information concerning high-energy phosphate stores and intracellular pH in ischemic myocardium. Multiple sequential measurements can be made on the same tissue and correlated with mechanical activity. This technique has demonstrated that the magnitude of intracellular acidosis and associated increase in inorganic phosphate correlate inversely with postischemic recovery of function. Phosphocreatine, but not ATP, content correlates with return of contractile function after reperfusion.

With ischemia and the reduction in oxygen delivery, a shift in metabolism occurs owing to the decrease in mitochondrial function. The production of reduced nicotinamide adenine dinucleotide during glycolysis is partially alleviated by production of lactic acid and alleviation of acetyl CoA by lipid synthesis. With a shift in metabolism during ischemia, adenosine increases[89] and depresses adenyl cyclase,[90] causing a decrease in myocardial cyclic AMP. This decrease in the inotropic state of the heart contributes to the decrease in contractile performance during ischemia.

Hypoxic myocardium produces more lactic acid than it consumes, with the result that coronary sinus blood will contain more lactic acid than systemic arterial blood. Normally, lactic acid concentration is greater in arterial blood than in the coronary venous effluent in the nonischemic heart, owing to myocardial lactic acid extraction for aerobic synthesis of ATP. In some patients with coronary artery disease and normal lactic acid extraction at rest, increased heart rate or stimulation of the heart with isoproterenol can cause lactic acid production by the heart.[91]

EFFECTS OF HYPOXIA ON THE MECHANICS OF CONTRACTION

Studies of isolated heart muscle have characterized the changes in contraction produced by hypoxia and subsequent reoxygenation (Fig. 4.17). Following the onset of hypoxia, there is a decline in developed force, in maximum dF/dt (maximum rate of force development), and in the time to peak force. With reoxygenation there is a striking prolongation of relaxation, as the contraction gradually returns to control levels.[92] This simple experimental model illustrates the profound effects of hypoxia on both contraction and relaxation. The prolonged relaxation may be due to depression of sarcoplasmic reticular function with decreased uptake of calcium.

EFFECT OF ISCHEMIA ON REGIONAL MYOCARDIAL FUNCTION

The dependence of various indices of regional function on blood supply is shown in Figure 4.18.[93] In this animal experiment, ultrasonic crystals were placed to measure a length segment and wall thickness. The coronary artery supplying this segment was then cannulated, and blood supply was sequentially reduced. Coronary supply to the rest of the heart remained normal. Note that a reduction in wall thickening was the most sensitive index of a decline in mechanical performance. Delayed relaxation is also an early mechanical sign of ischemia. It is of interest that local segment work (area of the stress-length loop) was directly related to the reduction in coronary flow. With sustained severe ischemia, regional contraction ceases rapidly and is replaced by paradoxical systolic expansion.

TIME COURSE OF NECROSIS

Following cessation of coronary flow by complete occlusion, the rate of necrosis of the affected myocardium is a time-dependent dynamic process. In the dog with coronary artery occlusion, myocardial necrosis begins within 15 to 20 minutes. The damage begins in the subendocardium and gradually progresses toward the epicardium (Fig. 4.19).[94] Collaterals play an important role in retarding this rate of progression in different species. For example, the rabbit and sheep have virtually no collaterals, whereas the dog and baboon may have well-developed collaterals. Without collaterals, as in the rabbit, myocardial

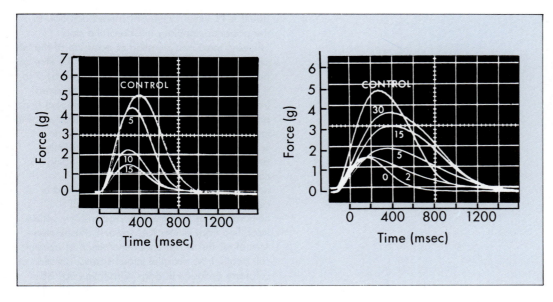

FIGURE 4.17 Time course of changes in the isometric contraction of an isolated cat papillary muscle during 15 minutes of hypoxia (*left*) and 30 minutes of reoxygenation (*right*). The numbers next to each curve indicate the time in minutes after the onset of hypoxia and after the onset of reoxygenation. (Tyberg JV, Yeatman LA, Parmley WW et al: Effects of hypoxia on mechanics of cardiac contraction. Am J Physiol 218:1780, 1970)

necrosis is virtually complete within 30 minutes. With collaterals, as in the dog, it may take up to 4 to 6 hours to complete necrosis (Fig. 4.20). The degree of collateralization in an individual patient with coronary artery disease will also greatly influence the rate of necrosis following coronary occlusion. This variability will certainly influence potential benefits of thrombolysis early after myocardial infarction.

EFFECTS OF REPERFUSION

Reperfusion following varying periods of complete occlusion is associated with a number of events.[95] Transient ventricular arrhythmias including ventricular fibrillation can occur. Reperfusion hemorrhage can occur in regions of advanced contraction band necrosis but is generally confined to necrotic myocardium only and generally does not interfere with myocardial healing or scar formation.[96] With reperfusion, there is a gradual return of function in the affected area, which may take up to days to complete. Reduced ATP levels in this area of "stunned myocardium" are also repleted only gradually.[89]

Reperfusion is followed by rapid return of electrocardiographic ST segment changes to normal and evolution of a Q wave infarct pattern. Washout of serum creatine kinase also occurs with reperfusion, with earlier and higher peaks.[97] All of the above may have considerable relevance to the patient receiving thrombolytic therapy following acute myocardial infarction.

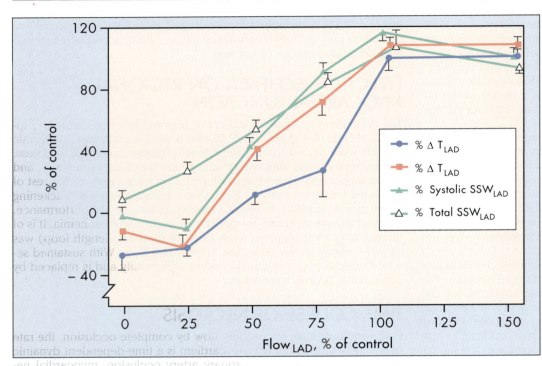

FIGURE 4.18 In the cannulated left anterior descending (LAD) coronary artery of the pig, graded reductions in flow were produced by decreasing LAD perfusion pressure. Reduction in wall thickening (ΔT_{LAD}) was the most sensitive indicator of reduced perfusion. Shortening of muscle ($-\Delta L_{LAD}$) and segmental systolic stroke work (systolic SSW_{LAD}) became negative (paradoxic systolic expansion) as LAD flow was reduced to 25% of control. Total segmental stroke work (total SSW_{LAD}) was linearly related to the reduction in LAD flow. (Modified from Stowe DF, Mathey DG, Moores WY et al: Segment stroke work and metabolism depend on coronary blood flow in the pig. Am J Physiol 234:H597, 1978)

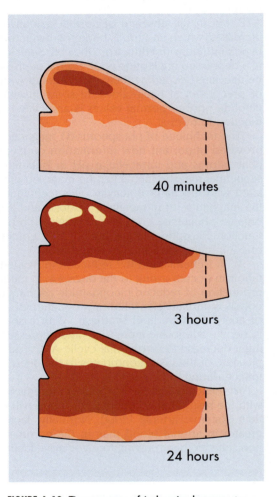

FIGURE 4.19 Time course of ischemic damage to the posterior papillary muscle of the dog following increased duration of occlusion of the left circumflex coronary artery of the dog. The time of occlusion is at the right and was followed by 2 to 4 days of reperfusion before sacrifice. Necrosis (red) is first seen in the subendocardium (top) and progresses toward the subepicardium (bottom) with increasing time of occlusion. The dashed line separates the perfusion zone of the circumflex artery (left) from the left anterior descending coronary artery (LAD) (right). Interstitial hemorrhage is represented by orange, and a central core of necrotic muscle devoid of hemorrhage or inflammatory response by yellow. (Modified from Reimer KA, Lowe JE, Rasmussen MM et al: The wavefront phenomenon of ischemic cell death. I. Myocardial infarct size vs. duration of coronary occlusion in dogs. Circulation 56:786, 1977)

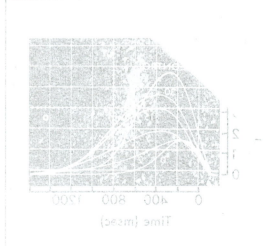

CLINICAL IMPLICATIONS

Hypertrophy, failure, and ischemia are commonly encountered in a wide variety of clinical conditions. A knowledge of the pathophysiology of these conditions is directly relevant to therapeutic decisions and to the interpretation of diagnostic tests. The current interest in producing regression of hypertrophy with sympatholytic agents is linked to an understanding of the trigger mechanisms for hypertrophy. Similarly, the role of calcium channel blockers in altering compliance of the left ventricle in hypertrophic cardiomyopathy is also related to the basic processes underlying the development of this syndrome. The rate at which ischemic myocardium becomes necrotic is also critical to the clinical intervention of thrombolysis in acute myocardial infarction. Furthermore, reperfusion may have important clinical effects. For all of the above reasons, a knowledge of basic research is helpful in these areas. It is probable that the next decade will see considerable further advances in our knowledge and ability to treat these conditions.

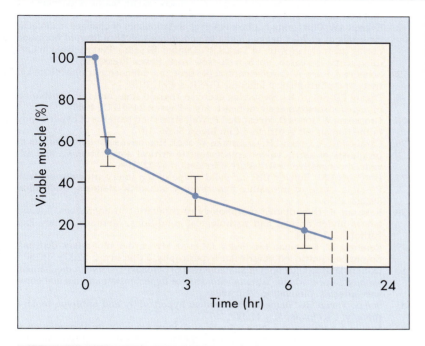

FIGURE 4.20 In the same study as Figure 4.19, the proportion of ischemic muscle that is viable is plotted as a function of time after coronary occlusions. (Modified from Reimer KA, Lowe JE, Rasmussen MM et al: The wavefront phenomenon of ischemic cell death. I. Myocardial infarct size vs. duration of coronary occlusion in dogs. Circulation 56:786, 1977)

REFERENCES

1. Wikman-Coffelt J, Wu ST, Watters T et al: Biochemical regulation of developed intraventricular systolic pressure. Am Heart J 115:876, 1988
2. Barcenas-Ruiz L, Beuckelmann DJ, Wier WG: Sodium-calcium exchange in heart: Membrane currents and changes in (Ca)i. Science 238:1720, 1987
3. Hirning LD, Fox AP, McCleskey EW et al: Dominant role of N-type Ca^{2+} channels in evoked release of norepinephrine from sympathetic neurons. Science 239:57, 1988
4. Chen J, Corbley MJ, Roberts TM et al: Voltage sensitive calcium channels: Normal and transformed fibroblasts. Science 239:1024, 1988
5. Watters TA, Wendland MF, Parmley WW et al: Factors influencing myocardial response to metabolic acidosis in isolated rat hearts. Am J Physiol 253:H1261, 1987
6. Markiewicz W, Wu ST, Parmley WW et al: Beneficial effects of verapamil during metabolic acidosis in isolated perfused rat hearts. Cardiovasc Drugs Ther 1:493, 1988
7. Tubau JF, Wikman-Coffelt J, Massie BM et al: Improved myocardial efficiency in the working perfused heart of the spontaneously hypertensive rat. Hypertension 10:396, 1987
8. Buser PT, Wagner S, Wu ST et al: Verapamil preserves myocardial performance and energy metabolism in left ventricular hypertrophy following ischemia and reperfusion. Circulation 80:1837, 1989
9. Schneider MF, Chandler WK: Voltage dependent charge movement in skeletal muscle: A possible step in excitation contraction coupling. Nature 242:244, 1973
10. McGrew SG, Boucek RJ, McIntryre JO et al: Target size of the ryanodine receptor from junction terminal cisternae of sarcoplasmic reticulum. Biochemistry 26:3183, 1987
11. Franzini-Armstrong C: Structure of the junction of frog twitch fibers. J Cell Biol 47:488, 1970
12. Fischmeister R, Horckova M: Variation of intracellular Ca^{2+} following Ca^{2+} currents in the heart. Biophys J 41:341, 1983
13. Harary HH, Brown JE: Spatially nonuniform change in intracellular calcium concentrations. Science 224:292, 1984
14. Vergara J, Tsien RG, Dely M: Inositol 1,4,5 triphosphate: A possible chemical link in excitation-contraction coupling in muscle. Proc Natl Acad Sci USA 82:6352, 1985
15. Wier WG, Yue DT, Marban E: Effects of ryanodine on intracellular Ca^{2+} transients in mammalian cardiac muscle. Fed Proc 44:2982, 1985
16. Blumlein SL, Sievers R, Wikman-Coffelt J et al: Effects of ryanodine on cat papillary muscle and isolated rat heart. Am Heart J 110:386, 1985
17. Reeves JP, Sutko JL: Sodium-calcium ion exchange in cardiac membrane vesicles. Proc Natl Acad Sci USA 76:590, 1979
18. Coroni P, Carfoli E: The regulation of the Na^+/Ca^{2+} exchange of heart sarcolemma. Eur J Biochem 132:451, 1982
19. Kostyuk PG, Krishtal OA: Effect of calcium and calcium chelating agents on the inward and outward current in the membrane of mollusc neurones. J Physiol 270:569, 1977
20. Katz AM: Role of phosphorylation of the sarcoplasmic reticulum in the cardiac response to catecholamines. Eur Heart J (Suppl)1:29, 1980
21. Hartung K, Grell E, Hasselbach W et al: Electrical pump currents generated by the Ca^{2+}-ATPase of sarcoplasmic reticulum vesicles absorbed on black lipid membranes. Biochem Biophys Acta 648:13, 1981
22. Murphy JG, Smith TW, Marsh JD: Calcium flux measurements during hypoxia in cultured heart cells. J Mol Cell Cardiol 19:271, 1987
23. Camacho SA, Wikman-Coffelt J, Wu ST et al: Improved myocardial performance and energetics in Syrian cardiomyopathic hamsters after isoproterenol treatment: A P-31 NMR study. Circulation 77:712, 1988
24. Nayler WG, Perry SE, Elz JS et al: Calcium, sodium and the calcium paradox. Circ Res 55:227, 1984
25. Wu ST, White R, Wikman-Coffelt J et al: The preventive effect of verapamil on ethanol-induced cardiac depression: Phosphorus-31 nuclear magnetic resonance and high pressure liquid chromatographic studies of hamsters. Circulation 75:1058, 1987
26. Mattiazzi AR, Cingolani HE, Spacapan de Castuman E: Relationship between calcium and hydrogen ions in heart muscle. Am J Physiol 237:H497, 1979
27. Srivastava S, Muhlrad A, Wikman-Coffelt J: Influence of myosin heavy chains on the Ca^{2+} binding properties of light chain LC2. Biochem J 193:925, 1981
28. Fuchs F, Reddy Y, Briggs FN: The interaction of cations with the calcium binding site of troponin. Biochem Biophys Acta 221:407, 1970
29. Markiewicz W, Wu ST, Parmley WW et al: Evaluation of hereditary Syrian hamster cardiomyopathy by 31P nuclear magnetic resonance spectroscopy: Improvement after acute verapamil therapy. Circ Res 59:597, 1987
30. Jasmin G, Proschek L: Comparative effects of Ca slow channel blockers on the hamster hereditary cardiomyopathy. In Sperelakis N, Caulfield J (eds):

Calcium Antagonists. New York, Martinus Nijhoff Publishing, 1983
31. Auffermann W, Wu ST, Parmley WW et al: Reversibility of acute alcohol cardiac depression: 31P NMR in hamsters. FASEB J 2:256, 1988
32. Wikman-Coffelt J, Sievers R, Parmley WW et al: Verapamil preserves adenine nucleotide pool in cardiomyopathic hamster. Am J Physiol 250:H22, 1986
33. Binah O, Cohen IS, Rosen MR: The effects of adriamycin on normal and ouabain-toxic canine Purkinje and ventricular muscle fibers. Circ Res 53:655, 1983
34. Wikman-Coffelt J, Rouleau JL, Parmley WW: Verapamil, propranolol, and hydralazine protect against the acute cardiac depression induced by adriamycin. Cardiovasc Res 17:43, 1983
35. Moore JW, Ulbricht W, Takata M: Effect of ethanol on the sodium and potassium conductances of the squid axon membrane. J Gen Physiol 48:279, 1964
36. Auffermann W, Wu ST, Parmley WW et al: Reversibility of acute alcohol cardiac depression: ^{31}P NMR in hamsters. FASEB J 2:256, 1988
37. Denton RM, McCormack JG: Calcium transport by mammalian mitochondria and its role in hormone action. Am J Physiol 249:E543, 1985
38. Reddy MK, Rabinowitz M, Zak R: Stringent requirement for calcium in the removal of Z-lines and alpha actinin from isolated myofibrils by calcium-activated neutral proteinase. Biochem J 209:635, 1983
39. Starling EH: On the absorption of fluids from the connective tissue spaces. J Physiol Lond 19:32, 1896
40. Mild KH, Lovtrup S: Movement and structure of water in animal cells. Ideas and experiments. Biochem Biophys Acta 822:155, 1984
41. Etchebest C, Pullman A: The gramacidin A channel energetics and structural characteristics of the progression of a sodium ion in the presence of water. J Biomolec Struct Dynam 3:805, 1986
42. Wikman-Coffelt J, Parmley WW: The role of calcium in myocardial hypertrophy. Heart and Vessels—An International Journal 4:128, 1988
43. Scarpace PJ: Decreased β-adrenergic responsiveness during senescence. Fed Proc 45:51, 1986
44. Feldman RD: Physiological and molecular correlates of age-related changes in the human β-adrenergic receptor system. Fed Proc 45:48, 1986
45. Hocman G: Biochemistry of aging. J Biochem 10:867, 1979
46. Nilius B, Nowycky MC: Mechanism of calcium channel modulation by β-adrenergic agents and dihydropyridine calcium agonists. J Mol Cell Cardiol 18:691, 1986
47. Butcher FR: Regulation of calcium efflux from isolated rat parotid cells. Biochem Biophys Acta 630:254, 1980
48. Roth GS: Effects of aging on mechanisms of alpha-adrenergic and dopaminergic action. Fed Proc 45:60, 1986
49. Scarpace PJ: Decreased β-adrenergic responsiveness during senescence. Fed Proc 45:51, 1986
50. Wikman-Coffelt J, Sievers R, Coffelt RJ et al: The cardiac cycle: Regulation and energy oscillations. Am J Physiol 245:H354, 1983
51. Wikman-Coffelt J, Parmley WW, Jasmin G: Cardiomyopathic and healthy acidotic hamster hearts: Mitochondrial activity may regulate cardiac performance. Cardiovasc Res 20:471, 1986
52. Camacho SA, Parmley WW, James TL et al: Substrate regulation of the nucleotide pool during regional ischemia and reperfusion in an isolated rat heart preparation: A P-31 MRS analysis. Cardiovasc Res 22:193, 1988
53. Zak R: Development and proliferative capacity of cardiac muscle cells. Circ Res (Suppl II)34/35:17, 1974
54. Laks MM, Morady W, Garner D et al: Temporal changes in canine right ventricular volume, mass, cell size, and sarcomere length after banding the pulmonary artery. Cardiovasc Res 8:106, 1975
55. Laks MM: Norepinephrine, the producer of myocardial cellular hypertrophy and/or necrosis and/or fibrosis. Am Heart J 94:394, 1977
56. Tarazi RC, Sen S, Saragoca M et al: The multifactorial role of catecholamines in hypertensive cardiac hypertrophy. Eur Heart J (Suppl A)3:103, 1982
57. Ostman-Smith I: Cardiac sympathetic nerves as the final common pathway in the induction of adaptive cardiac hypertrophy. Clin Sci 61:265, 1981
58. Le Peuch CJ, Ferraz C, Walsh MP et al: Calcium and cyclic nucleotide dependent regulatory mechanisms during development of chick embryo skeletal muscle. Biochemistry 18:5267, 1979
59. Ostman-Smith I: Prevention of exercise-induced cardiac hypertrophy in rats by chemical sympathectomy (guanethidine treatment). Neuroscience 1:497, 1976
60. Scheuer J, Malhotra A, Hirsch C et al: Physiologic cardiac hypertrophy corrects contractile protein abnormalities associated with pathologic hypertrophy in rats. J Clin Invest 70:1300, 1982
61. Mercadier JJ, Lompre A-M, Wisnewsky C et al: Myosin isoenzymic changes in several models of rat cardiac hypertrophy. Circ Res 49:525, 1981
62. Rupp H, Jacob R: Response of blood pressure and cardiac polymorphism to swimming training in the SHR. Can J Physiol Pharmacol 60:1098, 1982
63. Spotnitz HM, Sonnenblick EH, Spiro D: Relation of ultrastructure to function in the intact heart: Sarcomere structure relative to pressure-volume curves of intact left ventricle of dog and cat. Circ Res 18:49, 1966
64. Laks MM, Morady F, Swan HJC: Canine right and left ventricular cell and sarcomere lengths after banding the pulmonary artery. Circ Res 24:705, 1974
65. Meerson FZ: Contractile function of the heart in hyperfunction, hypertrophy and heart failure. Circ Res (Suppl II)24/25:9, 1969
66. Yamori Y, Tarazi RC, Ooshima A: Effect of β-receptor-blocking agents on cardiovascular structural changes in spontaneous and noradrenaline-induced hypertension in rats. Clin Sci 59:457S, 1980
67. Stewart D, Mason DT, Wikman-Coffelt J: Changes in cAMP concentrations during chronic cardiac hypertrophy. Basic Res Cardiol 73:648, 1978
68. Wikman-Coffelt J, Parmley WW, Mason DT: The cardiac hypertrophy process: Analyses of factors determining pathological vs. physiological development. Circ Res 45:697, 1979
69. Everett AW, Taylor RR, Sparrow WP: Protein synthesis during right ventricular hypertrophy after pulmonary artery stenosis in the dog. Biochem J 166:315, 1977
70. Wikman-Coffelt J, Refsum H, Hollosi G et al: Comparative force-velocity relations and analyses of myosin of dog atria and ventricles. Am J Physiol 12:H391, 1982
71. Hoh JFY, McGrath MA, Hale PT: Electrophoretic analysis of multiple forms of rat cardiac myosin: Effects of hypophysectomy and thyroxine replacement. J Mol Cell Cardiol 10:1053, 1977
72. Everett AW, Chizzonite A, Clark WA et al: Relationship of changes in molecular forms of myosin heavy chains to endogenous level of thyroid hormone during postnatal growth. In Tarazi RC, Dunbar JB (eds): Perspectives in Cardiovascular Research, Vol 8, p 83. New York, Raven Press, 1983
73. Scheuer J, Bhan A: Cardiac contractile proteins, adenosine triphosphate activity and physiological function. Circ Res 45:1, 1979
74. Pagani ED, Solaro RJ: Swimming exercise, thyroid state, and the distribution of myosin isoenzymes in rat heart. Am J Physiol 245:H713, 1983
75. Grossman W, Jones D, McLaurin LP: Wall stress and patterns of hypertrophy in the human left ventricle. J Clin Invest 56:56, 1975
76. Carabello BA, Green LH, Grossman W et al: Hemodynamic determinants of prognosis of aortic valve replacement in critical aortic stenosis and advanced congestive heart failure. Circulation 62:42, 1980
77. Hutchins GM, Bulkley BH: Catenoid shape of the interventricular septum: Possible cause of idiopathic hypertrophic subaortic stenosis. Circulation 58:392, 1978
78. Rakusan K: Quantitative morphology of capillaries in animal and human hearts under normal and pathological conditions. Methods Achiev Exp Pathol 5:272, 1971
79. Rembert JC, Kleinman LH, Fedor JM et al: Myocardial blood flow distribution in concentric left ventricular hypertrophy. J Clin Invest 62:379, 1978
80. Opherk D, Mall G, Zebe H et al: Reduction of coronary reserve: A mechanism for angina pectoris in patients with arterial hypertension and normal coronary arteries. Circulation 69:1, 1984
81. Sen S, Tarazi RC, Bumpus FM: Cardiac hypertrophy and antihypertensive therapy. Cardiovasc Res 11:427, 1977
82. Greves J, Rahimtoola S, McAnulty JH et al: Preoperative criteria predictive of late survival following valve replacement for severe aortic regurgitation. Am Heart J 101:300, 1981
83. Ross J Jr: Afterload mismatch in aortic and mitral valve disease: Implications for surgical therapy. J Am Coll Cardiol 5:811, 1985
84. Williams JF Jr, Mathew B, Hern DL et al: Myocardial hydroxyproline and mechanical response to prolonged pressure loading followed by unloading in the cat. J Clin Invest 72:1910, 1983
85. Coulson RL, Yazdanfar S, Rubid E et al: Recuperative potential of cardiac muscle following relief of pressure overload hypertrophy and right ventricular failure in the cat. Circ Res 40:41, 1977
86. DeBoer LMV, Ingwall JS, Kloner RA et al: Prolonged derangements of canine myocardial purine metabolism after a brief coronary artery occlusion not associated with anatomic evidence of necrosis. Proc Natl Acad Sci USA 77:5471, 1980
87. Parmley WW, Tyberg JV, Glantz S: Cardiac dynamics. In Knobil E (ed): Annual Review of Physiology, Chap 39, p 277. Palo Alto, CA, Annual Reviews, 1977
88. Sievers R, Parmley WW, James T et al: Energy levels at systole vs. diastole in normal hamster hearts vs. myopathic hamster hearts. Circ Res 53:759, 1983
89. Swain JL, Sabina RL, McHale A et al: Prolonged myocardial nucleotide depletion after brief ischemia in the open-chest dog. Am J Physiol 242:H818, 1982
90. Knab MT, Rubio R, Berne RM: Potential of slow action potential with theophylline or "micro" adenosine deaminase. Am J Physiol 244:H454, 1983
91. Gertz EW, Wisneski JA, Neese R et al: Myocardial lactate metabolism: Evidence of lactate release during net chemical extraction in man. Circulation 63:1273, 1981
92. Tyberg JV, Yeatman LA, Parmley WW et al: Effects of hypoxia on mechanics of cardiac contraction. Am J Physiol 218:1780, 1970
93. Stowe DF, Mathey DG, Moores WY et al: Segment stroke work and metabolism depend on coronary blood flow in the pig. Am J Physiol 234:H597, 1978
94. Reimer KA, Lowe JE, Rasmussen MM et al: The wavefront phenomenon of ischemic cell death. I. Myocardial infarct size vs. duration of coronary occlusion in dogs. Circulation 56:786, 1977
95. Murdock DK, Loeb JM, Euler DE et al: Electrophysiology of coronary reperfusion: A mechanism for reperfusion arrhythmias. Circulation 61:175, 1980
96. Fishbein MC, Y-Rit J, Lando V et al: The relationship of vascular injury and myocardial hemorrhage to necrosis after reperfusion. Circulation 62:1274, 1980
97. Roberts R, Ishikawa Y: Enzymatic estimation of infarct size during reperfusion. Circulation 68:I-83, 1983

VENTRICULAR FUNCTION

William W. Parmley

The biochemistry and physiology of individual muscle cells and strips of isolated heart muscle were described earlier. The basic principles of cardiovascular physiology have been determined in such preparations. In this chapter I will extend these findings to the intact heart, principally the left ventricle. Because the left ventricle delivers cardiac output to the body, and also plays the primary role in maintaining systemic blood pressure, most of the data on cardiac function in the literature refer to the left ventricle. Although it has received less attention, the right ventricle is also subject to the same principles. All of the concepts derived for the left ventricle can be applied to the right ventricle as well, although the quantitative description may be different. Since the prognosis of most patients with heart disease is primarily determined by the degree of left ventricular dysfunction, it is important to gain a detailed understanding of the performance of the left side of the heart and the various factors that can alter it.

Two traditional ways of describing left ventricular performance have emerged. The first is to take the principles derived from studies in isolated heart muscle and directly extrapolate them to the left ventricle. These indices have focused on wall stress, velocity of shortening, and rate of pressure development as indices analogous to those derived in isolated heart muscle. The second approach has been to concentrate on the hydraulic or pump performance of the left ventricle. This latter approach uses the measurements of pressure, volume, flow, and work as markers of the pump performance of the heart. Although both approaches are of interest, it appears that the clinical descriptors that have been most useful in patients with heart disease are those that describe the heart as a pump. Each of these approaches will be discussed in this chapter.

DETERMINANTS OF LEFT VENTRICULAR PERFORMANCE

The four mechanical determinants of cardiac muscle performance were detailed in Chapter 1. Their extension to the intact left ventricle requires some additional explanation.

PRELOAD

As defined in isolated heart muscle, the force used to stretch the muscle to an initial length represents the preload. In order to normalize for muscles of different thickness, the preload is divided by the cross-sectional area of the muscle to give force per cross-sectional area (stress). In isolated heart muscle, where all the fibers run in the same direction, this provides a reasonable estimate of the average force development per unit of muscle.

In the intact heart, however, it is clear that the situation is much different. Complex geometry and fiber direction make estimates of wall stress more difficult. Nevertheless, the data support the concept of calculating wall stress according to the various factors involved.[1] In translating force in a linear system to tension in the wall of the left ventricle, several factors must be considered. The first is fiber direction. Studies have shown that in general there is an approximate 180° shift in fiber direction as one moves from the endocardium to the epicardium in the free wall of the left ventricle.[2] Fibers tend to run parallel to the long axis in the endocardium and epicardium and perpendicular to the long axis in a circumferential fashion in the middle of the heart. The predominant mass of fibers run in a circumferential direction perpendicular to the long axis of the heart, thus accounting for the major squeezing action of the heart. In general, therefore, it has been common to calculate wall stress in a circumferential direction with the assumption that most fibers generally run in this direction.

Wall stress is then calculated as the force per cross-sectional area according to the Laplace relation. Without discussing more complex descriptions of this relation, a simplified form is shown below:

$$\text{Wall stress} = \frac{\text{left ventricular pressure} \times \text{radius of curvature}}{2 \times \text{wall thickness}}$$

It is clear from this relationship that wall stress can be increased by an increase in left ventricular pressure, dilation of the left ventricle, or thinning of the wall. For more complex formulas that relate wall stress to geometry, the reader is referred to other sources.[1]

The translation of preload to the intact heart, therefore, is to calculate end-diastolic wall stress. From the foregoing discussion, it is clear that this is not an easy or routine calculation. Other indices of the preload of the left ventricle have, therefore, been used. For example, left ventricular end-diastolic pressure and volume provide some information about the distensibility of the left ventricle. These two measurements determine a point on the passive left ventricular pressure–volume relation that is similar in shape to the passive length–tension relation in isolated muscle (Fig. 5.1). Because of the inherent difficulty in measuring end-diastolic wall stress, therefore, it is often more common to measure left ventricular end-diastolic pressure or volume as indices of preload. In critically ill patients with balloon-tipped catheters in the pulmonary artery, pulmonary capillary wedge pressure has been used as an indirect measure of left ventricular diastolic pressure and, thus, a clinically useful measurement of the preload of the left ventricle.[3] It should be restated, however, that a strict application of the principles of cardiac muscle mechanics to the intact heart dictates that end-diastolic wall stress be used as the preload of the left ventricle.

AFTERLOAD

Afterload was defined in isolated heart muscle as the additional load that the muscle faced as it developed force and attempted to shorten. By extension of the above discussion, wall stress encountered during systolic contraction represents the analogous measurement of afterload in the left ventricle. Because of the changing nature of left ventricular pressure, volume, and wall thickness during ejection, it is clear that wall stress during systole is a complex value to calculate and is not constant as is force in isotonic afterloaded contractions of isolated heart muscle.[4] Peak systolic wall stress is one important measure of afterload, although it appears that some more integrated measure of overall wall stress during systole is more appropriate.

Because of the difficulty in measuring instantaneous wall stress during systolic contraction, it has been more common to use other indices of afterload in the intact heart. One such index would be aortic pressure, which represents the load facing the left ventricle when it ejects blood. Hypertensive patients clearly have a greater load placed on the left ventricle. In patients with congestive heart failure in whom blood pressure may be low, however, aortic impedance[5] and systemic vascular resistance are increased and have been useful quantities in calculating the load faced by the heart. An increased peripheral resistance sets the stage for arteriolar vasodilators that can improve cardiac output by reducing peripheral vascular resistance.[6] In all cases, however, it should be appreciated that these latter indices only represent conceptually different ways of expressing afterload, but in fact they do not substitute for the precise definition of afterload, which is wall stress at any given instant during systolic contraction.

CONTRACTILE STATE

Contractile state refers to the ability of the heart to alter its performance at any given set of loading conditions. Heart muscle contractility is increased by a number of positive inotropic agents, such as catecholamines or digitalis. The quantitative measurement of the contractile state of the heart has always been difficult. A number of studies have attempted to identify various indices that accurately describe the contractile performance of the left ventricle independent of the loading conditions. These will be discussed in detail later. In general, it appears that the more clinically useful indices of left ventricular performance are those that deal with the pump performance of the heart and that indices extrapolated from isolated muscle mechanics have been less valuable in describing the performance of the left ventricle.

HEART RATE

Stimulation frequency in isolated heart muscle is directly translated to the intact heart as heart rate. In the intact left ventricle, the influence of heart rate is quite different from that in isolated heart muscle. Although changes in stimulation frequency over an appropriately low range are a potent way of altering contractile state in isolated heart muscle,[7] the usual range over which heart rate is altered in humans has little direct influence on cardiac contractility *per se*. Heart rate does remain the most important way of increasing cardiac output, particularly with exercise or in the face of a fixed stroke volume. Heart rate is also an important determinant of the myocardial oxygen supply–demand ratio. Increasing heart rate is a potent mechanism for increasing myocardial oxygen consumption.[8] In addition, since coronary blood flow occurs primarily during diastole, excessive heart rates may limit coronary blood flow by decreasing diastolic time. Intrinsic heart rate, that is, heart rate measured after both sympathetic and parasympathetic blockade,[9] appears to have some relationship to the state of left ventricular performance. It has not proved, however, to be an important measure of cardiac performance.

VENTRICULAR FUNCTION: INDICES OF MUSCLE PERFORMANCE
FORCE–VELOCITY RELATIONS

Initial studies in isolated heart muscle suggested that maximum velocity of shortening at zero load (V_{max}) was a useful index of cardiac muscle performance. Early studies suggested that this index of contractility was relatively independent of preload and changed in an appropriate fashion following interventions that changed the contractile state.[10] In the intact heart, one of the constant problems that the clinician faces is determining whether changes in ventricular performance are due to changes in intrinsic contractility or to an alteration of loading conditions. The potential application of force–velocity relations and V_{max}, therefore, to the intact heart led to several publications describing this particular application. In measuring velocity of shortening and V_{max} in isolated heart muscle, one needs to obtain shortening velocities at very low loads. Clearly, this was not possible in the intact heart, since aortic pressure remains within a fairly well-defined range and never approaches zero except in catastrophic circumstances. Since one could not directly measure velocity of shortening at low loads, calculation of contractile element velocity was done using mechanical models of left ventricular muscle performance with measurements made during the isovolumic phase of contraction.[11] During this time prior to the opening of the aortic valve, one can calculate the velocity of shortening of the contractile element by measuring the pressure development and instantaneous rate of pressure development (dP/dt). The formulas for such calculations are listed below.

A three-element mechanical model of muscle is used to describe velocity of contractile element shortening, even though the muscle does not change length (Fig. 5.2). In this model, the contractile element (CE) is assumed to be freely extensible at rest. Thus, the elastic properties of the parallel elastic (PE) define the exponential passive length–tension properties of the muscle. During isometric (isovolumic) contraction, the CE shortens and stretches the series elastic (SE). As measured in quick-release experiments in isolated heart muscle, the

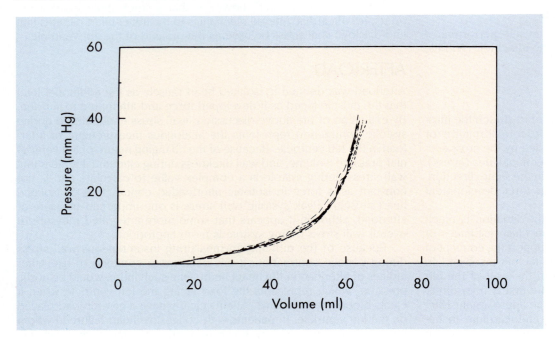

FIGURE 5.1 Repeated pressure–volume relations in a freshly excised left ventricle of a dog. Mitral and aortic orifices were closed. The generally exponential shape of the passive pressure–volume relation is illustrated.

SE also has an exponential length–tension relation.[12] By definition, therefore:

$$dF/dl(SE) = KF + C.$$

$dF/dl(SE)$ is the slope of the length-tension relation at any given force (F). K and C are constants. During isovolumic contraction,

$$dF/dt = dF/dl(SE) \times dl/dt(SE)$$

where $dl/dt(SE)$ = velocity of lengthening of the SE. If muscle length is not changing,

$$dl/dt(CE) = dl/dt(SE)$$

where $dl/dt(CE)$ is the velocity of shortening of the CE. Thus,

$$dl/dt(CE) = \frac{dF/dt}{dF/dl(SE)} = \frac{dF/dt}{K_1F + C}$$

C is generally small in relation to K_1F and has been dropped. During isovolumic contraction where radius of curvature and wall thickness are relatively constant, $F = K_2P$, where P is pressure and K_2 is a constant. Thus,

$$dl/dt(CE) = K_3 \frac{dP/dt}{P}$$

where K_3 is an overall constant. During isovolumic contraction, one could theoretically calculate the velocity of the contractile element (V_{CE}) from instantaneous measurements of P and dP/dt.[13]

An example of calculated V_{CE} obtained with this technique is shown in Figure 5.2. There are multiple problems with this calculation, however. It is not clear which mechanical model of muscle should be used in the calculation. Similarly, it is not clear that the elastic properties of the series elastic can be easily defined in the intact heart,[14] nor that they are necessarily constant in different hearts. These and other assumptions greatly affect the potential calculation of the force–velocity relation and its extrapolation to V_{max}. Because of these difficulties, different estimates of velocity have been obtained at different levels of developed pressure. It has been proposed that (dP/dt)/P at different levels of developed pressure be an index of cardiac contractility that is somewhat useful in the characterization of contractility of the intact heart.[15] It is apparent that such measurements require a high-fidelity pressure catheter within the left ventricle. A simple analog computer can then instantaneously calculate (dP/dt)/P as a function of pressure to provide an index of left ventricular function. The difficulties of assumptions, measurements, and calculations have made this approach less useful in describing left ventricular performance.

Two other factors have decreased the use of this approach. The first is that the normal range of such measurements is wide.[16] Second, in patients with heart disease, measurements did not appear to be clinically useful.[17] For example, in patients with acute myocardial infarction, calculations of V_{max} were often within the normal range, despite the presence of severe power failure and reduced ventricular function (Fig. 5.3). For all of these reasons, this approach appears to have little clinical usefulness in quantitatively describing left ventricular performance in patients. In addition, the development of other indices has overshadowed this approach.

VELOCITY OF CONTRACTILE FIBER SHORTENING

One other aspect of force–velocity relations has been used in measuring the contractile performance of the left ventricle. Measured velocity of fiber shortening at a given loading point would represent one point on a force–velocity relation.[18] It should be apparent that this velocity of shortening could be altered by preload, afterload, and contractile

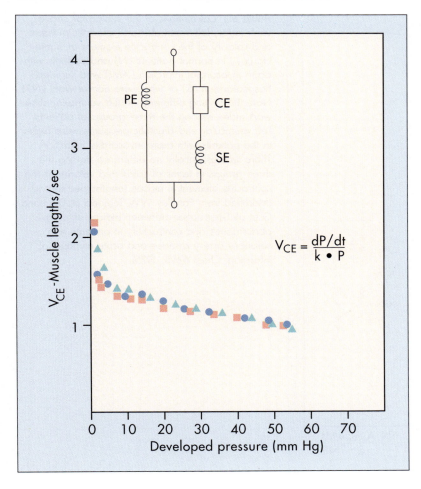

FIGURE 5.2 Calculation of velocity of the contractile element from instantaneous left ventricular pressure and dP/dt according to the three-element mechanical model shown. Calculations were made only during the isovolumic phase of contraction.

state. Theoretically, therefore, it might not be very useful in measuring left ventricular performance because of the confounding influence of all of these major hemodynamic determinants. Studies in patients with heart disease, however, have suggested that velocity of contractile fiber shortening (V_{CF}) is a reasonable index of left ventricular performance in the basal state.[18] Part of its appeal is that it can be measured noninvasively. For example, echocardiography and radionuclide ventriculography, in addition to ventriculography at the time of cardiac catheterization, can all be used to calculate the velocity of contractile fiber shortening. Despite its reasonable correlation with left ventricular performance, however, it also has been used less frequently. This reflects the utility of other indices of performance.

MAXIMUM RATE OF PRESSURE DEVELOPMENT

In isolated heart muscle, the maximum rate of force development (max dF/dt) is a useful index of cardiac muscle performance. If preload is held constant and the muscle contracts isometrically, a change in maximum dF/dt is always directionally related to a change in contractile state produced by a number of pharmacologic interventions. This fact makes it theoretically interesting to consider its counterpart in the left ventricle, namely maximum dP/dt, as an index of left ventricular performance.[19] First of all, it is clear that maximum dP/dt could only be an estimate of left ventricular performance. The direct analogue of maximum dF/dt in isolated heart muscle would be maximum rate of stress development in the left ventricle, which cannot be easily obtained. Furthermore, in order to measure maximum left ventricular dP/dt, one must have a high-fidelity catheter in the left ventricle. This invasive procedure is far less available than noninvasive indices of left ventricular performance.

More importantly, there are a number of factors that affect maximum dP/dt that have made it less useful as an index of contractile state. For example, an increase in left ventricular end-diastolic pressure increases maximum dP/dt, presumably through the Frank-Starling mechanism, in a manner similar to that seen in isolated heart muscle. In addition, the level of arterial pressure may influence maximum dP/dt. For example, maximum dP/dt occurs very close to the opening of the aortic valve, which represents the end of the isovolumic period of contraction. With a reduction in left ventricular pressure, the aortic valve may open and the isovolumic phase may terminate before maximum dP/dt is actually reached. This will artificially lower maximum dP/dt below the level that it would have attained if the arterial pressure had been slightly higher.[20] In addition, maximum dP/dt is markedly affected by an increase in heart rate. Thus, because of the dependence of maximum dP/dt on all four factors that determine left ventricular performance, it has been difficult to use it as an unambiguous measure of contractile state in the intact left ventricle.

Under certain circumstances, however, dP/dt could be used. For example, if heart rate does not change or goes down, and if left ventricular end-diastolic pressure is unchanged or goes down, and if aortic pressure is unchanged or goes down, then an increase in left ventricular maximum dP/dt represents a clear-cut increase in the contractile state of the left ventricle. This complexity of interpretation obviously limits the usefulness of this parameter.

Another difficulty surrounds the application of dP/dt when one attempts to compare one ventricle with another. For example, in the patient with severe aortic stenosis and left ventricular hypertrophy, there is a marked increase in systolic pressure and in maximum left ventricular dP/dt, as compared with a patient with normal blood pressure, even though these two hearts may be at the same level of contractile state. The maximum dP/dt is increased together with left ventricular systolic pressure, due to the hypertrophy. Thus, maximum dP/dt would have to be normalized in some way to account for hypertrophy or variations in aortic pressure in order to compare one heart with another. This is another way of stating that one must calculate wall stress if one is to directly compare one patient with another.[21] Thus, the most practical use of maximum left ventricular dP/dt has been in a given patient when one is administering therapeutic interventions. With

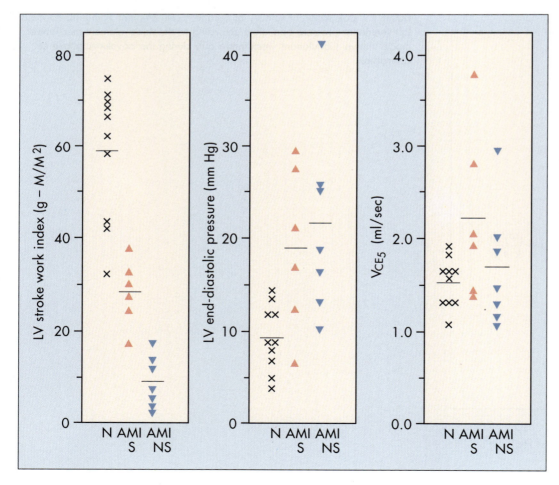

FIGURE 5.3 Calculations of left ventricular stroke work index, left ventricular end-diastolic pressure, and velocity of the contractile element at 5 mm Hg (V_{CE5}) in normal patients (N) and patients with acute myocardial infarction (AMI) who survived hospitalization (S) or who were nonsurvivors (NS). Note the striking difference in left ventricular stroke work index among the three groups of patients. Left ventricular end-diastolic pressures were higher in the patients with acute myocardial infarction. There was essentially no difference among the three groups in terms of calculated velocity of the contractile element in muscle lengths per second. (Modified from Parmley WW, Tomoda H, Diamond G et al: Dissociation between indices of pump performance and contractility in patients with coronary artery disease and acute myocardial infarction. Chest 67:141, 1975)

attention given to changes in heart rate and loading conditions as described above, it may be possible in some circumstances to use maximum dP/dt as an index of contractile state in the same patient.

AORTIC FLOW

Another measurement related to velocity of shortening is the instantaneous aortic flow in the ascending aorta. This can be measured in animal experiments by placing an electromagnetic flowmeter around the ascending aorta. The characteristic flow trace is shown in Figure 5.4. Integration of the area under this velocity time curve defines stroke volume. The maximum rate of increase of flow velocity (acceleration) is another measurement of left ventricular contractile state.[22] In patients in whom inotropic interventions increase contractile state there is frequently an increase in peak flow and in acceleration, even in circumstances in which there may be no change in stroke volume. Thus, peak velocity of blood flow or acceleration of flow are potentially useful indices of left ventricular inotropic state.[23] It should be apparent from the preceding discussions, however, that flow, like stroke volume and velocity of contractile fiber shortening, is very sensitive to preload, afterload, and heart rate. The influence of loading conditions, therefore, must be carefully considered when attempting to use such indices as measurements of contractile state. With new echo-Doppler technology, it is becoming increasingly easy to obtain noninvasive estimates of flow across various valves.[24] This has led to a resurgence of interest in this particular index of contractile state.

LEFT VENTRICULAR PERFORMANCE: INDICES OF PUMP PERFORMANCE
VENTRICULAR FUNCTION CURVE

One of the most clinically useful indices of left ventricular performance that can be measured in critical care units is the left ventricular function curve (Fig. 5.5). Some measure of left ventricular performance, such as stroke volume or stroke work, is plotted against some index of preload such as pulmonary capillary wedge pressure, obtained with a balloon-tipped catheter in the pulmonary artery. As illustrated in Figure 5.5, there is an increase in performance over the lower range of preloads until left ventricular performance reaches a plateau at a pulmonary capillary wedge pressure of 15 mm Hg to 20 mm Hg. This depiction of the Frank-Starling mechanism emphasizes the importance of volume loading or diuresis on left ventricular performance over a critical range of low left ventricular filling pressures. Alterations in left ventricular

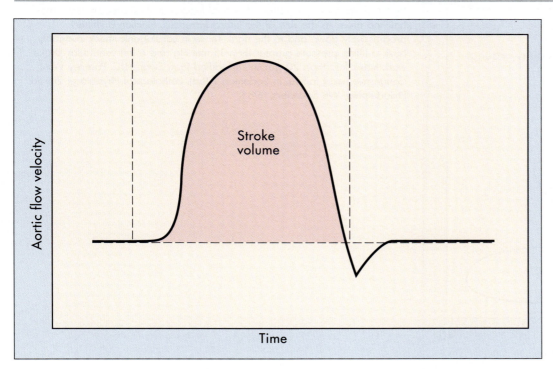

FIGURE 5.4 Representative aortic flow trace vs. time as obtained by an electromagnetic flowmeter. The area under the velocity–time curve represents the stroke volume.

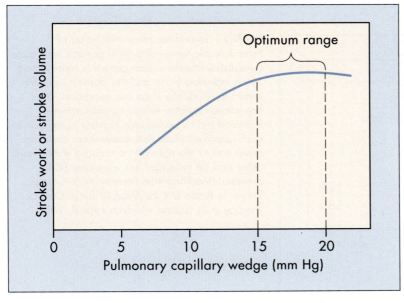

FIGURE 5.5 Representative left ventricular function curve as would be obtained, for example, in a patient with acute myocardial infarction. At a pulmonary capillary wedge pressure of 15 to 20 mm Hg, left ventricular performance (stroke work or stroke volume) is optimized. (Modified from Swan HJC, Parmley WW: Congestive heart failure. In Sodeman T (ed): Pathological Physiology, 7th ed. Philadelphia, WB Saunders, 1985)

performance as measured by this technique provide clinically useful information. Figure 5.6, for example, shows groupings of patients following acute myocardial infarction. Measurements of stroke work index and left ventricular filling pressure were used to place patients into different categories. The normal range is depicted as the crosshatched area.[25] Note that some patients with a small infarct may have function in the normal or hypernormal range. As the size of the infarct increases, however, function is shifted progressively down and to the right with a decrease in stroke work index and an increase in left ventricular filling pressure. Patients with severe power failure are invariably in the lower right hand quadrant of this graph. Thus, left ventricular performance is closely related to the size and clinical impact of myocardial infarction in individual patients.

The prognostic value of such measurements is indicated in Figure 5.7. In this group of patients with acute myocardial infarction, initial hemodynamics were correlated with the subsequent survival of the patients.[26] Note that those patients with the most severe hemodynamic derangements fall into the lower right-hand quadrant, with a stroke work index less than 20 g-m/m² and a pulmonary capillary wedge pressure greater than 15 mm Hg. This description of left ventricular performance is useful not only as a baseline for providing prognostic information but also in providing information about changes in response to therapeutic interventions. Figure 5.8, for example, shows the dramatic change that occurs in ventricular function in response to one of the new inotrope vasodilator drugs.[27] It appears, therefore, that the greatest clinical use of this method of describing left ventricular performance will be in patients who are hospitalized and can have measurements of cardiac output and pulmonary capillary wedge pressure. In critical care units this type of monitoring not only is routine but also has been extremely helpful in managing patients and selecting appropriate therapeutic interventions.

The relationship between right and left ventricular function deserves some discussion. In Figure 5.9, for example, both right and left ventricular functions are plotted on the same graph. This comparison is simplified if one uses stroke volume as the measure of left ventricular performance and the appropriate atrial pressure as the filling pressure of the respective ventricle. Since the right ventricle operates at a lower filling pressure (right atrial pressure) than does the left ventricle (left

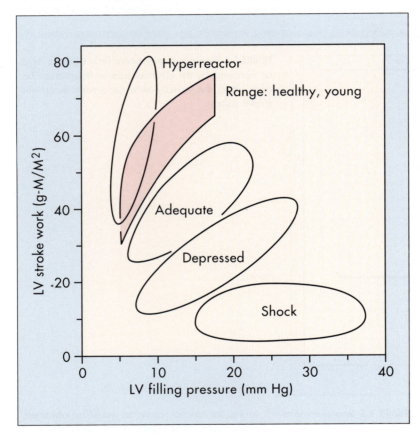

FIGURE 5.6 Groupings of patients following acute myocardial infarction in terms of their left ventricular function. Each area contains those patients designated by the description. The range of normal function is illustrated by the crosshatched area. As the size of the infarct increases, function is shifted progressively down and to the right. Those in cardiogenic shock invariably have a filling pressure greater than 15 mm Hg and a left ventricular stroke work index less than 20 g-m/m². (Modified from Swan HJC, Parmley WW: Congestive heart failure. In Sodeman T (ed): Pathological Physiology, 7th ed. Philadelphia, WB Saunders, 1985)

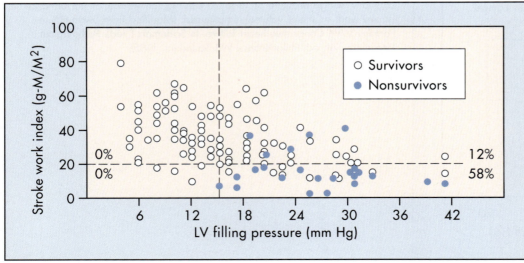

FIGURE 5.7 Immediate prognostic value of hemodynamic measurements in patients with acute myocardial infarction. Each patient is represented by an individual point and the dashed lines are drawn to divide the data into quadrants. The immediate mortality during hospitalization is indicated by the percentage number in the box in each quadrant. Note that nonsurvivors clustered down and to the right with a reduced stroke work index and an increased left ventricular filling pressure. (Modified from Parmley WW: Cardiac failure. In Rosen MR, Hoffman BF (eds): Cardiac Therapy, p 21. Boston, Martinus Nijhoff, 1981)

atrial pressure), the right ventricular function curve under normal circumstances is situated to the left of the left ventricular function curve. As averaged over any short period of time, the stroke volumes of the right and left ventricles are approximately the same, so that the two ventricles operate on the same horizontal line.

In this particular patient example, the patient suffered a myocardial infarction that affected primarily the left ventricle. Note that the left ventricular function curve was shifted down and to the right with a decrease in stroke volume and an increase in left ventricular filling pressure. Initially this did not affect the right ventricular function curve very much, so that there was even a slight decrease in the filling pressure of the right ventricle. If one then volume loaded the heart to try and take advantage of the Frank-Starling mechanism, one increased stroke volume somewhat, but because of the flat nature of the left ventricular function curve, one actually precipitated pulmonary edema by raising pulmonary capillary wedge pressure to high levels. Since the normal right ventricular function curve is a fairly steep curve, this volume-loading resulted in only a minimal increase in right atrial pressure. This representation of right and left ventricular performance emphasizes how useful this format can be in detecting individual changes in the function of the right or left ventricle. There are several clinical circumstances in which right ventricular performance can be reduced with little change in left ventricular performance. Examples of this would include right ventricular infarction or significant pulmonary embolus. Because of the rapidly changing nature of left ventricular performance in critical care units, this method of monitoring is ideally adapted to such an environment.

EJECTION FRACTION

One of the most useful single numbers of left ventricular performance is the ejection fraction. By definition, it is the stroke volume divided by the end-diastolic volume. In the normal left ventricle the ejection fraction is approximately two-thirds. In some studies, an ejection fraction

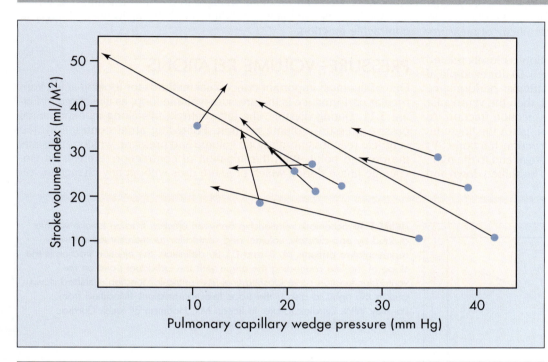

FIGURE 5.8 Representative effects of a potent oral inotrope-vasodilator (milrinone) in 10 patients with severe congestive heart failure. With an improvement in function, there is a shift upward and to the left in most patients, with an increase in stroke volume index and a reduction in pulmonary capillary wedge pressure.

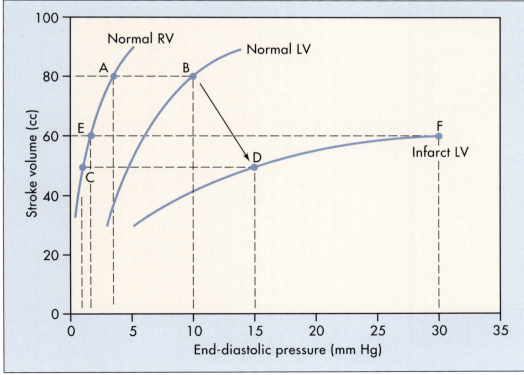

FIGURE 5.9 Right and left ventricular function in a patient before and after an infarct that affected the left ventricle. (See text for details.) The ordinate plots the end-diastolic pressure of the respective ventricle in millimeters of mercury. (Modified from Parmley WW: Hemodynamic monitoring in acute ischemic disease. In Fishman AP (ed): Heart Failure, p 105. Washington, DC, Hemisphere, 1977)

remains normal down to about 0.55 or slightly below. In the normal right ventricle, the ejection fraction is less than in the left side of the heart and is about 0.55.[28] As a measure of pump performance of the heart, the ejection fraction is relatively easy to measure by both noninvasive and invasive techniques that indicate relative left ventricular volumes. Its simplicity has made it a very useful index in categorizing patients. It should be clear, however, that because of the ejection nature of this index it is very sensitive to loading conditions. For example, increases in afterload can reduce ejection fraction without any intrinsic reduction in myocardial contractility.[29] An interpretation of ejection fraction, therefore, has to take into account any changes in loading condition. Problems in interpretation may arise, for instance, in patients with borderline normal left ventricular function who undergo exercise during the measurement of radionuclide wall motion studies. It is not uncommon in such patients to see a reduction in ejection fraction. This may be due, for example, to increased loading with poor ventricular reserve. Alternatively, the development of ischemia may also reduce ejection fraction by ischemic paralysis of a portion of the ventricle.[30] Thus, it is often not possible to state unequivocally what changes in ejection fraction mean in individual circumstances. Nevertheless, these tests are widely used because of simplicity of measurement and conceptual clarity.

It should be pointed out that the ejection fraction is closely related to a ventricular function curve. As shown in Figure 5.10, for example, if one plots stroke volume as the index of left ventricular performance and end-diastolic volume as the index of preload, then the ventricular function curve thus obtained is a measure of the ejection fraction. At any point on the ventricular function curve, the slope of the line connecting the origin to that point represents the ejection fraction (SV/EDV). As the ventricular function curve is shifted down and to the right, so the ejection fraction (slope of the line) will also be shifted down and to the right. This close relationship between ejection fraction and the ventricular function curve is important in relating the two in individual patients.

Despite the utility of the ejection fraction, however, it should be pointed out that there are many pitfalls to its interpretation. At very low preloads, the small end-diastolic volume of the ventricle leads to a reduction in the ejection fraction by the Frank-Starling mechanism. For example, in patients with reduced left ventricular end-diastolic volume, such as those with mitral stenosis, low normal ejection fractions may in part be due as much to a reduced preload as to reduced left ventricular function.[31] Similarly, as patients develop dilated ventricles, the influence of end-diastolic volume on ejection fraction can be considerable. For example, even at reduced ejection fractions, patients may have normal stroke volumes and thus may be able to maintain normal cardiac outputs, even in response to exercise. A body of data supports the concept that ejection fraction is not closely related to exercise tolerance.[32] The potential effect of afterloading on ejection fraction has also been discussed. Marked alterations in arterial pressure or systemic vascular resistance can produce changes in ejection fraction that represent the influence of loading conditions rather than intrinsic changes in contractile function.

PRESSURE–VOLUME RELATIONS

One of the most important conceptual methods for looking at left ventricular performance is the pressure–volume loop, as illustrated in Figure 5.11. During diastole, the left ventricle fills along its exponential passive pressure–volume relation. Following atrial contraction, the ventricle reaches end-diastolic volume and pressure, which represents the preload point. With the initiation of contraction, there is an isovolumic phase during which pressure rises without any change in vol-

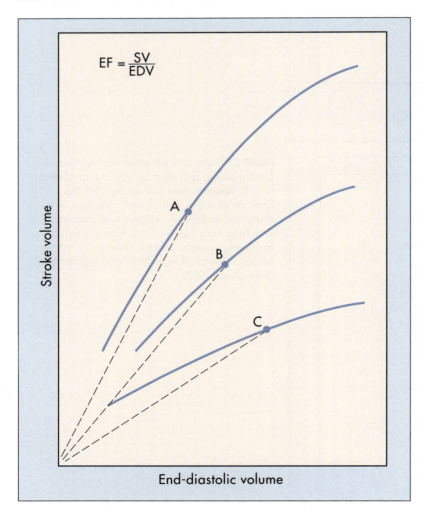

FIGURE 5.10 Schematic relationship between ejection fraction (stroke volume divided by end-diastolic volume) and ventricular function curves in three representative patients (A, B, and C). By definition, the ejection fraction is the slope of the line connecting the origin with the individual point on the ventricular function curve (*dashed line*). As ventricular function is shifted down and to the right, so also is the slope (ejection fraction). (Modified from Parmley WW: Cardiac failure. In Rosen MR, Hoffman BF (eds): Cardiac Therapy, p 21. Boston, Martinus Nijhoff, 1981)

ume. Following the opening of the aortic valve, there is an ejection phase with a rise and fall in pressure to aortic valve closing. Pressure then falls during relaxation until it matches left atrial pressure, following which the mitral valve opens and filling occurs again. This counterclockwise pressure–volume loop is a useful descriptor of the performance of the left ventricle. This same kind of diagram is used in physics to describe the performance cycle of an engine. By definition, the area inside a counterclockwise loop represents the external work done by the engine during that cycle. The area inside a clockwise loop would represent work done on the engine during such a cycle. By direct analogy, therefore, the area inside the counterclockwise pressure–volume loop of the left ventricle is the stroke work of the left ventricle (see Fig. 5.11, B). This is calculated by the formula shown below:

Stroke work = stroke volume × (mean left ventricular systolic ejection pressure − mean left ventricular diastolic pressure)

The width of the loop represents the difference between end-diastolic volume and end-systolic volume, or stroke volume. The height of the loop is the difference between mean left ventricular systolic ejection pressure and mean left ventricular diastolic pressure. Mean systolic pressure of the left ventricle is approximately one third the distance down from aortic systolic to diastolic pressure. Recall that mean arterial pressure is often estimated as one third of the distance up from aortic diastolic pressure to systolic pressure. Mean left ventricular diastolic pressure can often be estimated by mean pulmonary capillary wedge pressure. With very large systolic v waves seen with mitral regurgitation, however, the mean pulmonary capillary wedge pressure will be higher than the mean left ventricular diastolic pressure. Under most circumstances, however, this estimate can be used.

In order to normalize stroke work among patients of different sizes, it is customary to normalize for body surface area in square meters. Therefore, stroke work index is the calculated stroke work divided by body surface area. This index appears to be particularly sensitive in the evaluation of critically ill patients. One reason for its sensitivity is that each of the factors that affects left ventricular performance (heart rate, blood pressure, cardiac output, stroke volume, and pulmonary capillary wedge pressure) affects stroke work index in the appropriate direction. The cumulative influence of these various indices, therefore, is more sensitive than any single index alone in determining the state of left ventricular performance.

The other reason that the pressure–volume loop has gained recent favor as a descriptor of left ventricular performance is related to studies by Suga and Sagawa.[33,34] They performed a series of experiments in isolated hearts that are described below. By clamping the aorta so that the left ventricle could not eject blood, they obtained a series of isovolumic contractions, as illustrated in Figure 5.12. Note that the top of each of these isovolumic contractions, when connected, forms a fairly straight line, which is termed the isovolumic pressure line. Having thus determined this upper line, they next allowed the heart to contract normally, using different preloads and afterloads as illustrated in Figure 5.13. Note that with the alterations of preload and afterload, the endpoint of systolic contraction (end-systolic volume and dicrotic notch aortic pressure) tends to fall on the isovolumic pressure line regardless of the preload or afterload. This relationship, in fact, appears to be a more exact one in the intact heart than that obtained in isolated heart muscle. By quantitating the isovolumic pressure line, therefore, they described an index of the contractile state of the left ventricle, which was independent of the loading conditions. With an increase in contractile state,[33] the isovolumic pressure line was shifted up and to the left (Fig. 5.14); with a decrease in contractile state, the isovolumic pressure line was shifted down and to the right. The intercept with the volume axis (V_d) is little altered with these changes in contractile state. This relationship has spurred a considerable amount of research in recent years to use this technique as a measure of left ventricular performance.[35] There are several problems, however, that need to be emphasized. First of all, it is not precisely clear how one patient can be compared with another. For example, patients of different sizes will have different end-diastolic volumes. It is intuitive, therefore, that one would have to normalize in some way for left ventricular volume. Whether this is best done by expressing volume in terms of body surface area or other means is not clear at this time. Furthermore, with similar baseline contractile properties, left ventricles of different patients will develop different pressures. For example, the patient with hypertension or aortic stenosis will develop much higher left ventricular systolic pressures than the patient with normal arterial pressure. In

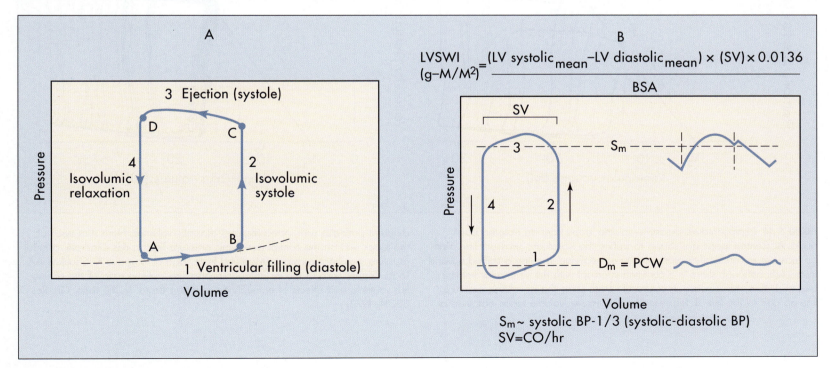

FIGURE 5.11 A. Representative pressure–volume loop of the left ventricle during a contraction cycle. Segment 1 represents ventricular filling during diastole. Segment 2 is isovolumic systole. Segment 3 is ejection and 4 is isovolumic relaxation. **B.** Calculation of left ventricular stroke work index (LVSWI) in g-m/m². Pressures are expressed in mm Hg and stroke volume in cc. (0.0136 converts mm Hg to the dyne-cm system.)

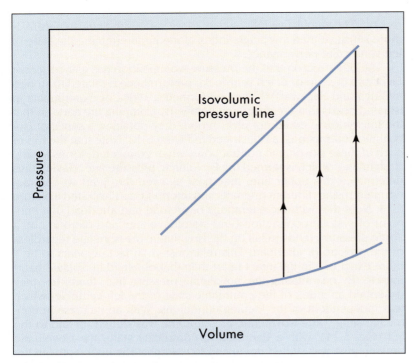

FIGURE 5.12 Representative isovolumic contractions obtained in an isolated dog heart with clamping of the aorta to prevent ejection. The heart contracts isovolumically up to a point and then relaxes along the same line, back to the passive pressure–volume relation. The peak of each contraction (three are shown) defines a line that has been termed the *isovolumic pressure line*.

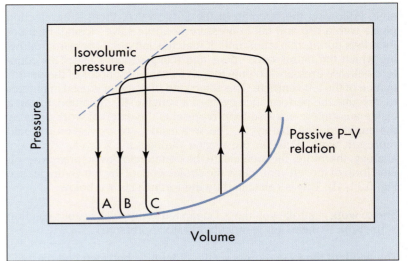

FIGURE 5.13 Three representative pressure–volume loops (A, B, and C) obtained at different preloads and afterloads. Note that the upper left hand corner of each loop ends on the isovolumic pressure line. This upper left hand point represents dicrotic notch aortic pressure and end-systolic volume.

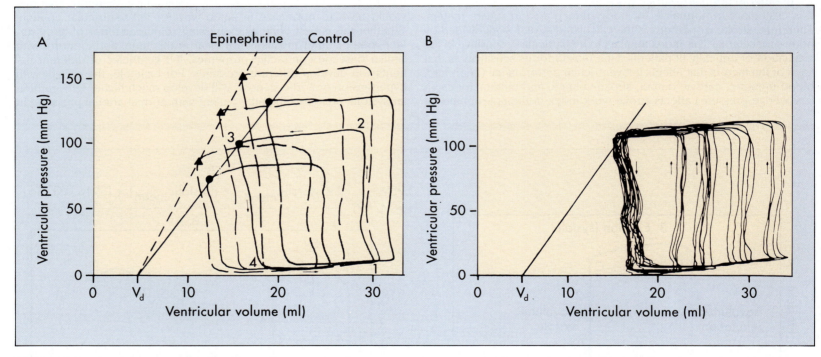

FIGURE 5.14 Representative pressure–volume loops from an isolated dog heart: **A.** Control loops are shown to define the isovolumic pressure line. With an increase in contractility produced by epinephrine, the line is shifted up and to the left, although there is a common intercept with the ventricular volume axis (V_d). Thus, an increase in contractile state shifts the isovolumic pressure line up and to the left. **B.** Representative pressure–volume loops obtained at different preloads with increasing end-diastolic volumes. Note that each of the loops end on the control isovolumic pressure line. In this example, arterial pressure was kept constant. (Modified from Suga H, Sagawa K, Shoukas AA: Load dependence of the instantaneous pressure–volume ratio of the canine left ventricle and effects of epinephrine and heart rate on the ratio. Circ Res 32:314, 1973)

the compensated state, where the intrinsic contractility of the left ventricle is the same, the isovolumic pressure line will be shifted upward in patients with higher left ventricular pressures (Fig. 5.15). It is intuitively apparent, therefore, that one must in some way normalize the pressure axis. Some attempts at normalization have used wall stress on the vertical axis: this may more nearly yield a measurement that can be used to compare different patients.

The influence of different types of valvular heart disease on the pressure–volume loop is illustrated in Figure 5.15. Shown together are pressure–volume loops from a normal patient, one with severe aortic stenosis, and one with aortic regurgitation. For the purposes of our discussion, let us assume that the patients with valvular disease are both in a compensated state. Therefore, the intrinsic contractility of the myocardium is the same in all three patients. Nevertheless, note the fairly dramatic changes in the pressure–volume loops. In the patient with aortic stenosis and concentric hypertrophy, there is a reduction in end-diastolic volume and a much greater pressure development. Thus, the isovolumic pressure line is shifted up and to the left. In the patient with volume overload due to aortic regurgitation, the end-diastolic volume is larger and, therefore, the passive pressure–volume relation is shifted to the right. These shifts, however, should not be interpreted to represent changes in contractile state but merely changes due to dilatation and hypertrophy in these two different states. Normalization of pressure as wall stress may help to obviate some of these differences,[21] although an appropriate normalization for volume is also required.

Despite some of these potential problems, the left ventricular pressure volume loop is an important technique for quantitating the performance of the left ventricle. In some studies, the data have been further approximated. Simplifications have included using peak systolic pressure rather than the endpoint of contraction on the pressure–volume loop, and drawing lines through the origin rather than through the intercept of the isovolumic pressure line on the volume axis.[36] Even these simplifications have appeared to provide useful information in comparing patient groups with different degrees of heart failure.

REGIONAL WALL MOTION

Virtually all of the above descriptors of left ventricular performance have assumed that there is a uniform contraction pattern of the left ventricle. This obviously is not true in patients with coronary artery disease or other disorders with segmental involvement of the left ventricle.[37] A complete description of left ventricular performance, therefore, must also include a description of the regional performance of the left ventricle. Numerous studies have quantitated this aspect of performance, using quantitative ventriculography at the time of cardiac catheterization, echocardiography, radionuclide ventriculography, gated CT scanning, or magnetic resonance imaging, just to name a few of the techniques employed. Some of the representative changes that can be seen in patients with coronary artery disease are illustrated in Figure 5.16. In general, a normal left ventricle has relatively uniform inward motion of all walls of the left ventricle. Shown in Figure 5.16 is a diagram of the left ventricle of a patient with a previous myocardial infarction where the anterolateral segment of the left ventricle is akinetic. Also seen in Figure 5.16 is a diagram of the left ventricle of a patient with acute myocardial infarction in which there is paradoxic systolic expansion of the acutely ischemic and infarcted zone. All variations of wall motion have been described in quantitative terms, since such information is extremely useful in locating the coronary arteries involved, and in detecting changes in wall motion caused by regional changes in the supply–demand relationships. For example, in patients with regional hypokinesis, normalization of wall motion may occur following paired electrical stimulation or unloading with nitroglycerin.[38] This suggests that some of these abnormalities are, in fact, related to regional ischemia, which can be influenced by transiently affecting oxygen supply or demand or contractility.

PASSIVE PRESSURE–VOLUME RELATIONS

Over the past few years there has been an intense study of the diastolic properties of the heart and so-called diastolic function. It is clear from these studies that in some cardiac disorders diastolic abnormalities may be the predominant problem. This occurs, for example, in patients with severe hypertrophy who have a marked decrease in diastolic compliance.[39] The stiffness of the left ventricle can lead to elevations of left ventricular filling pressures and the signs and symptoms of pulmonary congestion. As shown in Figure 5.17, the passive pressure–volume relation of the ventricle is generally an exponential curve. Shifts in this curve can occur both acutely and chronically. As seen in Figure 5.17, chronic shifts in the left ventricular pressure–volume relation occur, for example, in patients who undergo left ventricular dilatation or concentric hypertrophy. Only recently, however, have we appreciated acute shifts in the passive pressure–volume relations that can occur, particularly in response to changed loading conditions.[40] An example of such a shift in acute passive pressure–volume relations is seen in

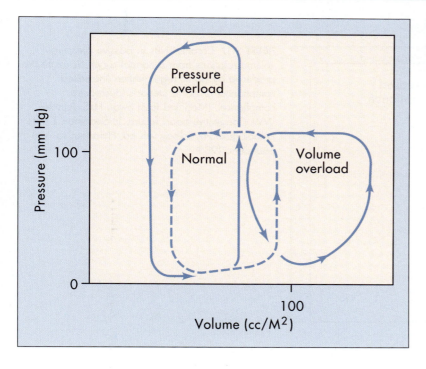

FIGURE 5.15 Representative changes over time in the left ventricular pressure–volume loop with severe pressure overload produced, for example, by aortic stenosis and severe volume overload produced, for example, by aortic regurgitation. (See text for details.)

Figure 5.18. In part, these changes appear to be related both to the influence of the pericardium and to the interaction of four chambers inside the pericardial sac. The influence of the pericardium on the left ventricular pressure–volume relation[41] is illustrated in Figure 5.19. In this particular dog experiment, the heart was volume loaded before and after pericardiectomy in order to determine the influence of the pericardium on the left ventricular passive pressure–volume relation. Note that following pericardiectomy, the passive pressure–volume relation of the normal left ventricle is shifted to the right. This suggests that as the ventricle is dilated, a stiff pericardium can restrict its filling and change the shape of the passive pressure–volume relation.

It should be remembered that the transmural filling pressure of the left ventricle is the left ventricular diastolic pressure minus the intrapericardial pressure. At larger volumes, when the stiff pericardium may be stretched, there is a rise in intrapericardial pressure that can effectively reduce the filling pressure of the left ventricle. Any influence that tends to reduce the volume of the heart, such as vasodilator drugs, can dramatically reduce the intrapericardial filling pressure and thus reduce left ventricular diastolic pressures without much change in left ventricular volume.[42] In addition, it appears that there is some interaction of the other heart chambers with the left ventricle inside the confines of the pericardial sac. That is, right ventricular distention can reduce left ventricular volume at a given left ventricular diastolic pressure.[43] One indirect estimate of intrapericardial pressure is right atrial pressure.

Acute changes in the passive pressure–volume relation of the left ventricle can also occur in response to ischemia, as indicated both in animal experiments[44] and in patients with coronary artery disease.[45] A

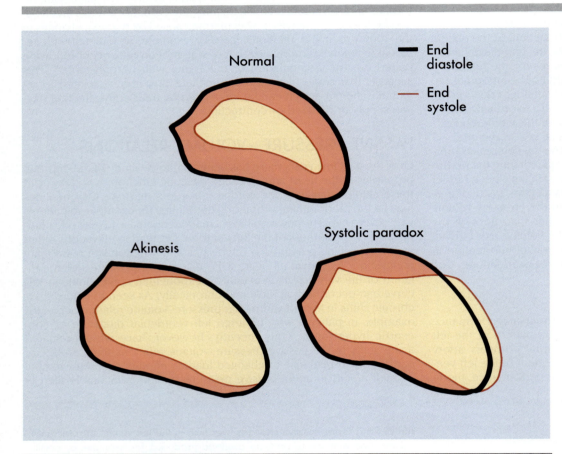

FIGURE 5.16 Representative alterations in left ventricular regional wall motion in patients with coronary artery disease. End-diastolic and end-systolic silhouettes of the left ventricle are shown in the right anterior oblique position. With acute myocardial infarction following coronary artery occlusion, there is systolic paradox of the anterior wall and apex (*lower right*). With healing of this myocardial infarction, this area would then become akinetic (*lower left*). (Modified from Swan HJC, Parmley WW: Congestive heart failure. In Sodeman T (ed): Pathological Physiology, 7th ed. Philadelphia, WB Saunders, 1985)

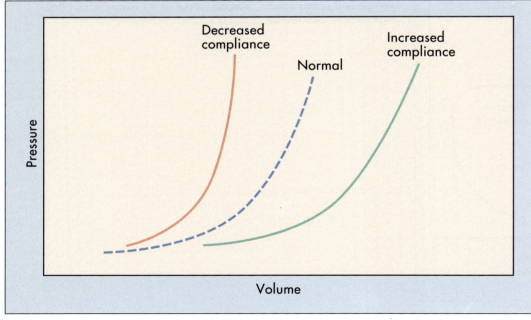

FIGURE 5.17 Chronic shifts in passive pressure–volume relations from a normal curve, as might be produced by aortic regurgitation (increased compliance) or aortic stenosis (decreased compliance). (Modified from Swan HJC, Parmley WW: Congestive heart failure. In Sodeman T (ed): Pathological Physiology, 7th ed. Philadelphia, WB Saunders, 1985)

number of other mechanisms have been postulated to affect the passive pressure–volume relations of the left ventricle.[46] They appear to be of lesser importance than ischemia, the influence of the pericardium, and interaction with the four chambers of the heart.

RELAXATION

The diastolic function of the heart is determined not only by the passive pressure–volume relations of the left ventricle but also by the rate of relaxation following contraction. A number of studies have been done to quantitate the rate of relaxation. As in isolated heart muscle, the terminal phase of left ventricular pressure during relaxation often follows an exponential curve. Thus, a $T_{1/2}$ can be derived as a measure of the rate of left ventricular relaxation.[47] Studies have shown that $T_{1/2}$ can be influenced by a number of variables that affect loading conditions and contractile state.[48,49] Delayed relaxation can certainly lead to higher diastolic pressures during the early filling phase of the left ventricular passive pressure–volume relation. However, this effect is dissipated by three half-lives. It is likely, therefore, that any change in relaxation rate may influence the first third, or at most, the first half of diastole, but probably has no effect on end-diastolic volume and pressure. At that time, relaxation effects have been dissipated and this data point can be used as a representative point on the passive pressure–volume relation of the left ventricle.

Measurements of flow rate into the left ventricle have been used widely as an index of left ventricular diastolic function. For example, in patients with coronary artery disease, it is frequent to have lower inflow rates during diastole.[50] As the ventricle becomes less compliant, in patients with coronary artery disease, it appears that atrial contraction and its contribution to end-diastolic volume become progressively more important. Similarly, in patients with hypertrophy,[51] or hypertrophic cardiomyopathy,[52] reduction of rapid filling rate during diastole is also reflective of the difficulty in filling a stiff ventricle. Acute ischemia can also reduce early filling rates. The measurement of filling rate during early diastole, therefore, may be a useful index not only of the relaxation rate of the ventricle but also of the stiffness or compliance of the ventricle and its ability to accept blood passively.

LEFT VENTRICULAR PERFORMANCE DURING STRESS

One of the most useful principles in the evaluation of left ventricular performance is the concept of obtaining measurements both at rest and after some form of stress.[53] I obtain such information from patients, for example, when I ask them if they develop dyspnea or fatigue with exercise. In a more quantitative way, this information is obtained following treadmill tests or during the imposition of other stresses, such as bicycle exercise, dye loading during ventriculography, and in-

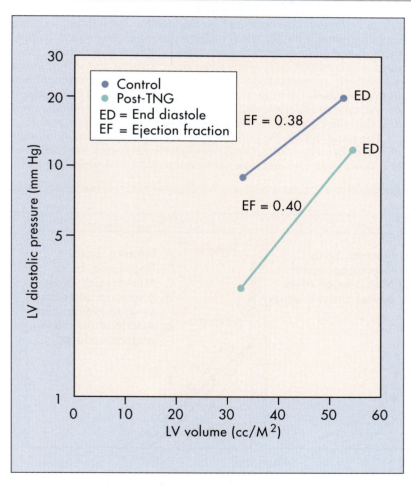

FIGURE 5.18 Acute shift in the passive pressure–volume relation produced by the vasodilator nitroglycerin (*TNG*) in a patient with heart failure. Left ventricular diastolic pressure is plotted on a log scale, so that the passive pressure–volume relation can be approximated by a straight line. The control passive pressure–volume relation is shown at the top with an ejection fraction of 0.38. Following sublingual nitroglycerin there is a dramatic reduction in left ventricular diastolic pressures with little change in volumes or ejection fraction. (Modified from Parmley WW, Chuck L, Chatterjee K et al: Acute changes in the diastolic pressure–volume relationship of the left ventricle. Eur J Cardiol 4(suppl):105, 1976)

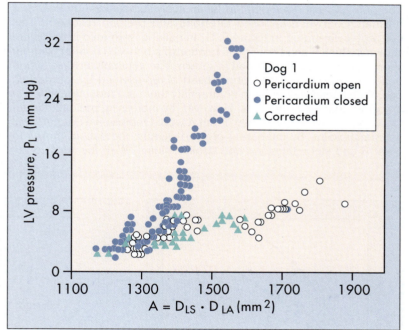

FIGURE 5.19 Changes in the diastolic pressure–volume relationship of an open-chest dog before and after pericardiectomy. Data were obtained following incremental volume loading. Note the stiffer left ventricular pressure–volume relationship with the pericardium closed (*closed circle*). With the pericardium open, the relationship is shifted to the right. By correcting for transmural left ventricular filling pressure (*triangles*), however, the passive pressure–volume relation is unchanged, even with the pericardium closed. (Modified from Tyberg JV, Misbach GA, Glantz SA et al: The mechanism for shifts in the diastolic, left ventricular, pressure–volume curve: The role of the pericardium. Eur J Cardiol 7(suppl): 1963, 1978)

creased afterload. The importance of this principle is illustrated from one study in Figure 5.20.[54] In this particular study an afterload stress was imposed on the left ventricle by having patients grip a hand grip dynamometer in order to increase arterial pressure through reflex mechanisms. This reflex produced by isometric exercise is presumably designed to maintain arterial pressure to perfuse exercising skeletal muscles.[55] The increase in arterial pressure also produces an afterload stress on the left ventricle. In order to overcome this afterload, the ventricle can use the Frank-Starling mechanism and an increased contractile state. A relatively normal integrated response to isometric exercise is shown in patient A on the ventricular function curve in Figure 5.20. Note that function shifts mostly upward, with an increase in stroke work index and little change in end-diastolic pressure. Patient B, however, has far less ventricular reserve; and with the onset of an afterload stress, function shifts markedly downward and to the right, with a decrease in left ventricular performance accompanying the increase in end-diastolic pressure. Without any reserve, in terms of the Frank-Starling mechanism or contractile state, the increased afterload decreases performance, and such patients readily develop symptoms during stress. The principle, therefore, of obtaining measurements before and during stress, is an extremely important one in attempting to describe left ventricular performance. Note, for example, that although the patients illustrated in Figure 5.20 had relatively similar resting function, they had a markedly different response to afterload stress.

AFTERLOAD MISMATCH AND PRELOAD RESERVE

The principle just discussed has been nicely summarized by Ross as a mismatch between imposed afterload and preload reserve.[56] This concept is illustrated in Figure 5.21. In patients with mild heart failure shown in the left hand panel, the relationship between contractile fiber shortening (V_{CF}) and afterload is shown. The generally inverse hyperbolic relationship for the normal heart is represented by the dashed line. With a mild reduction in contractility there is a reduction in V_{CF} at any given loading conditions. However, by increasing preload, the relationship is shifted to the right. Point A would represent a normal basal functional point. By increasing preload slightly, the patient moves to point B and still retains V_{CF} and stroke volume. With the stress of an increased afterload, the patient moves from B to C on a higher preload curve and can still maintain velocity of shortening at the higher afterload. With a severe increase in afterload, however, the patient has exhausted preload reserve and decreases function to point D. On the right hand panel, there is more severe depression of intrinsic function with a greater decrease in baseline V_{CF}. Point B represents the depressed basal function in this patient at maximum preload reserve. If there is any increase in afterload, function will be shifted down to point C. The use of vasodilators to reduce load might move the patient from point B to point D and better function. However, if one reduced preload and moved the patient to the farthest left hand curve (point E), there would be a marked decrease in function because of the lower preload.

This figure demonstrates the interaction between preload and afterload in determining left ventricular function. As ventricular reserve is decreased, patients become more sensitive to afterload with depression of function as afterload is increased. This occurs because of an exhaustion of preload reserve and no ability to further increase contractile state.

AUTONOMIC INFLUENCES ON CARDIAC PERFORMANCE

Neural regulation consists of the sometimes competing influences of the sympathetic and parasympathetic nervous systems.[9]

The sympathetic nervous system[57] has a right and left innervation of the heart. Via the right stellate ganglion, the sympathetic nerves supply primarily the sinoatrial node and the right atrium. The left cardiac nerve supplies primarily the posterolateral left atrium and left ventricle. Sympathetic nerve endings lie between muscle bundles in plexiform structures. Norepinephrine is synthesized from tyrosine and stored in the sympathetic nerve endings. Depolarization releases norepinephrine from granules that activate α- and β-receptors. The effect is terminated by reuptake of norepinephrine into sympathetic nerve endings, overflow into the circulation, or metabolism to vanillylmandelic acid.

The parasympathetic nervous system[58] is most important in terms of its effects on the sinoatrial and atrioventricular nodes. Vagal stimulation slows heart rate and slows atrioventricular nodal conduction. The

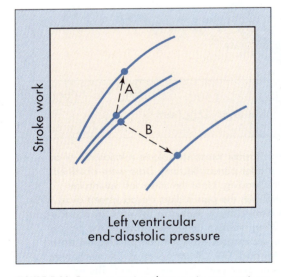

FIGURE 5.20 Representative changes in two patients who gripped a hand grip dynamometer to raise their arterial pressures. Although their resting measurements are virtually the same (two middle ventricular function curves), patient A has good ventricular reserve and shifts function upward in response to the increased arterial pressure produced by isometric exercise. On the other hand, patient B shifts down and to the right, indicative of poor ventricular reserve.

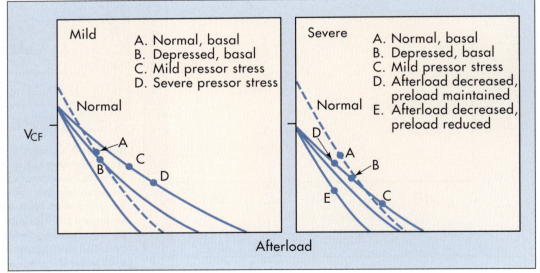

FIGURE 5.21 Concept of afterload mismatch and preload reserve in chronic myocardial failure. Velocity of contractile fiber shortening (V_{CF}) is plotted as a function of afterload. The normal inverse relationship is indicated by the dashed line. (See text for details of individual curves.) (Modified from Ross J Jr. Afterload mismatch and preload reserve: A conceptual framework for the analysis of ventricular function. Prog Cardiovasc Dis 18:255, 1976)

sometimes antagonistic effects of the sympathetic and parasympathetic nervous system have important effects on heart rate and the atrioventricular node. For example, resting heart rate is reduced by resting vagal tone, especially in those with exercise training effects. As one begins to exercise, the heart rate is initially increased by withdrawal of vagal tone.[59] At increasing levels of exercise, increased sympathetic tone then comes into play in producing further increase in heart rate.

Increased sympathetic tone and circulating catecholamines are important in maximizing cardiac performance, especially during maximal exercise or in the presence of both acute and chronic heart failure. The relation between catecholamine levels and left ventricular function, however, is a poor one.[60]

CLINICAL IMPLICATIONS

The four primary determinants of muscle performance (*i.e.*, preload, afterload, contractile state, and heart rate) can be extrapolated to describe the function of the intact left ventricle. It should be clear that an understanding of the effect of these four determinants is very useful in quantitating baseline performance and any change in response to therapeutic interventions. I have also detailed why indices of left ventricular performance based on indices of muscle performance have been less useful in describing left ventricular function in patients with clinical heart disease. Indices based on the hydraulic pump performance of the heart have been far more useful as descriptors of left ventricular performance. Of these, the ventricular function curve has proved to be the most useful in critically ill patients.

Overall, the ejection fraction is the single most useful number, although its sensitivity to loading conditions must be remembered. In addition, its dependence on end-diastolic volume must be taken into account in interpreting its numerical value. The pressure–volume loop appears to be the most important new way of evaluating left ventricular performance, although there are still considerable problems with normalization between patients. In patients with regional dysfunction, such as that associated with coronary artery disease, regional wall motion studies will always be critical in any kind of evaluation of left ventricular function.

It is also clear that evaluation of the passive pressure–volume relation of the ventricle and diastolic function are important in determining its clinical impact in any given patient. Diastolic abnormalities may be at least as prominent or in some cases more important in determining symptoms and signs in given patients. The pericardium has important restraining actions, particularly in the dilated ventricle, and the interaction with the pericardium can produce acute changes in the passive pressure–volume relation. An understanding of these principles and their application to patients will greatly help the clinician in evaluating and treating left ventricular dysfunction.

REFERENCES

1. Mirsky I: Elastic properties of the myocardium: A quantitative approach with physiological and clinical applications. In Berne RM (ed): Handbook of Physiology, Vol I, Section 2, The Cardiovascular System, p 497. Bethesda, MD, American Physiological Society, 1979
2. Streeter DD Jr, Spotnitz HM, Patel DJ et al: Fiber orientation in the canine left ventricle during diastole and systole. Circ Res 24:339, 1969
3. Swan HJC, Ganz W, Forrester J et al: Catheterization of the heart in man with use of flow-directed balloon-tip catheter. N Engl J Med 283:447, 1970
4. Rackley CE: Quantitative evaluation of left ventricular function by radiographic techniques. Circulation 54:862, 1976
5. Nichols WW, Conti CR, Walker WE et al: Input impedance of the systemic circulation in man. Circ Res 40:451, 1977
6. Chatterjee K, Parmley WW, Massie B et al: Oral hydralazine therapy for chronic refractory heart failure. Circulation 54:879, 1976
7. Johnson EA: Force interval relationship of cardiac muscle. In Berne RM (ed): Handbook of Physiology, Section 2, The Cardiovascular System, p 475. Bethesda, MD, American Physiological Society, 1979
8. Boerth RC, Covell JW, Pool PE et al: Increased myocardial oxygen consumption and contractile state associated with increased heart rate in dogs. Circ Res 24:725, 1969
9. Jose AD, Collison D: The normal range and determinants of the intrinsic heart rate in man. Cardiovasc Res 4:160, 1970
10. Sonnenblick EH: Force–velocity relations in mammalian heart muscle. Am J Physiol 202:931, 1962
11. Ross J Jr, Covell JW, Sonnenblick EH et al: Contractile state of heart characterized by force–velocity relations in variably afterloaded and isovolumic beats. Circ Res 18:149, 1966
12. Parmley WW, Sonnenblick EH: Series elasticity: Its relation to contractile element velocity and proposed muscle models. Circ Res 20:112, 1967
13. Mason DT, Braunwald E, Covell JW et al: Assessment of cardiac contractility: The relation between the rate of pressure rise and ventricular pressure during isovolumic systole. Circulation 44:47, 1971
14. Covell JW, Taylor RR, Ross J Jr: Series elasticity in the intact left ventricle by a quick release technique. Fed Proc 26:382, 1967
15. Mahler F, Covell JW, O'Rourke RA et al: Effects of acute changes in loading and inotropic state on left ventricular performance and contractility measures in the conscious dog. Am J Cardiol 35:626, 1975
16. Hugenholtz PG, Ellison RC, Urschel CW et al: Myocardial force–velocity relationships in clinical heart disease. Circulation 41:191, 1970
17. Parmley WW, Tomoda H, Diamond G et al: Dissociation between indices of pump performance and contractility in patients with coronary artery disease and acute myocardial infarction. Chest 67:141, 1975
18. Karliner JS, Gault JH, Eckberg DL et al: Mean velocity of fiber shortening: A simplified measure of left ventricular contractility. Circulation 44:323, 1971
19. Gleason WL, Braunwald E: Studies on the first derivative of the ventricular pressure pulse in man. J Clin Invest 41:80, 1962
20. Mason DT: Usefulness and limitations of the rate of rise of intraventricular pressure (dP/dt) in the evaluation of myocardial contractility in man. Am J Cardiol 23:516, 1969
21. Grossman W, Jones D, McLaurin LP: Wall stress and patterns of hypertrophy in the human left ventricle. J Clin Invest 56:56, 1975
22. Rushmer RF: Functional anatomy and control of the heart. In Cardiovascular Dynamics, 4th ed, p 76. Philadelphia, WB Saunders, 1976
23. Peterson KL, Uther JB, Shabetai R et al: Assessment of left ventricular performance in man: Instantaneous tension–velocity–length relations obtained with the aid of an electromagnetic velocity catheter in the ascending aorta. Circulation 47:924, 1973
24. Hattle L, Angelsen B: Doppler Ultrasound in Cardiology: Physical Principles and Clinical Applications, 2nd ed. Philadelphia, Lea & Febiger, 1985
25. Swan HJC, Parmley WW: Congestive heart failure. In Sodeman T (ed): Pathological Physiology, 7th ed, p 332. Philadelphia, WB Saunders, 1985
26. Chatterjee K, Swan HJC, Kaushik VS et al: Effects of vasodilator therapy for severe pump failure in acute myocardial infarction on short-term and late prognosis. Circulation 53:797, 1976
27. Kereiakes DJ, Viquerat C, Lanzer P et al: Mechanisms of improved left ventricular function following intravenous MDL 17043 in patients with severe chronic heart failure. Am Heart J 108:1278, 1984
28. Manyari DE, Kostuk WJ: Left and right ventricular function at rest and sitting positions in normal subjects and patients with coronary artery disease: Assessment by radionuclide ventriculography. Am J Cardiol 51:36, 1983
29. Osbakken MD, Boucher CA, Okade RD et al: Spectrum of global left ventricular responses to supine exercise: Limitation in the use of ejection fraction in identifying patients with coronary artery disease. Am J Cardiol 51:28, 1983
30. Campos CT, Chu HW, D'Agostino HJ Jr et al: Comparison of rest and exercise radionuclide angiocardiography and exercise treadmill testing for diagnosis of anatomically extensive coronary artery disease. Circulation 67:1204, 1983
31. Toutouzas P: Left ventricular function in mitral valve disease. Herz 9:297, 1984
32. Franciosa JA, Park M, Levine TB: Lack of correlation between exercise capacity and indexes of left ventricular performance in heart failure. Am J Cardiol 47:33, 1981
33. Suga H, Sagawa K, Shoukas AA: Load independence of the instantaneous pressure–volume ratio of the canine left ventricle and effects of epinephrine and heart rate on the ratio. Circ Res 32:314, 1973
34. Sagawa K: The end-systolic pressure–volume relation of the ventricle: Definitions, modifications, and clinical use. Circulation 63:1223, 1981
35. Grossman W, Braunwald E, Mann T et al: Contractile state of the left ventricle in man as evaluated from end-systolic pressure–volume relations. Circulation 56:845, 1977
36. Slutsky R, Karliner J, Gerber K et al: Peak systolic blood pressure/end-systolic volume ratio: Assessment at rest and during exercise in normal subjects and patients with coronary heart disease. Am J Cardiol 46:813, 1980
37. Gensini GC: Coronary arteriography: Role in myocardial revascularization. Postgrad Med 63:121, 1978
38. Klausner SC, Botvinick EH, Shames D et al: The application of radionuclide infarct imaging to diagnose perioperative myocardial infarction following

39. Benotti JR, Grossman W, Cohn PF: The clinical profile of restrictive cardiomyopathy. Circulation 61:1206, 1980
40. Alderman EL, Glantz SA: Acute hemodynamic interventions shift the diastolic pressure–volume curve in man. Circulation 54:662, 1976
41. Tyberg JV, Misbach GA, Glantz SA et al: The mechanism for shifts in the diastolic, left ventricular, pressure-volume curve: The role of the pericardium. Eur J Cardiol 7(suppl):1963, 1978
42. Parmley WW, Chuck L, Chatterjee K et al: Acute changes in the diastolic pressure–volume relationship of the left ventricle. Eur J Cardiol 4(suppl):105, 1976
43. Bemis CE, Serur JR, Borkenhagen D et al: Influence of right ventricular filling pressure on left ventricular pressure and dimension. Circ Res 34:498, 1974
44. Serizawa T, Carabello BA, Grossman W: Effect of pacing-induced ischemia on left ventricular diastolic pressure-volume relations in dogs with coronary stenoses. Circ Res 46:430, 1980
45. Mann T, Goldberg S, Mudge GH et al: Factors contributing to altered left ventricular diastolic properties during angina pectoris. Circulation 59:14, 1979
46. Glantz SA, Parmley WW: Factors which affect the diastolic pressure–volume curve. Circ Res 32:171, 1978
47. Weiss JL, Frederiksen JW, Weisfeldt ML: Hemodynamic determinants of the time course of fall in canine left ventricular pressure. J Clin Invest 58:751, 1976
48. Frederiksen JW, Weiss JL, Weisfeldt ML: Time constant of isovolumic pressure fall: Determinants in the working left ventricle. Am J Physiol 235:H701, 1978
49. Raff GL, Glantz SA: Volume loading slows left ventricular isovolumic relaxation rate: Evidence of load-dependent relaxation in the intact dog heart. Circ Res 48:813, 1981
50. Bonow RO, Bacharach SL, Green MV: Impaired left ventricular diastolic filling in patients with coronary artery disease: Assessment with radionuclide angiography. Circulation 64:315, 1981
51. Smith VE, Schulman D, Karimeddini MK et al: Rapid ventricular filling in left ventricular hypertrophy: II. Pathologic hypertrophy. J Am Coll Cardiol 5:869, 1985
52. Hanrath P, Mathey DG, Siegert R et al: Left ventricular relaxation and filling pattern in different forms of left ventricular hypertrophy. Am J Cardiol 45:15, 1980
53. Ross J Jr, Braunwald E: The study of left ventricular function in man by increasing resistance to ventricular ejection with angiotensin. Circulation 29:739, 1964
54. Kivowitz C, Parmley WW, Donoso R et al: Effects of isometric exercise on left cardiac performance: The grip test. Circulation 44:994, 1971
55. Donald KW, Lind A, McNicol GW et al: Cardiovascular responses to sustained (static) contractions. Circ Res 21(suppl 1):15, 1967
56. Ross J Jr: Afterload mismatch and preload reserve: A conceptual framework for the analysis of ventricular function. Prog Cardiovasc Dis 18:255, 1976
57. Randall WG: Sympathetic control of the heart. In Randall WC (ed): Neural Regulation of the Heart. New York, Oxford University Press, 1977
58. Levy MN, Martin PJ: Neural control of the heart. In Berne RM et al (eds): Handbook of Physiology, Section 2, The Cardiovascular System, p 581. Bethesda, MD, American Physiological Society, 1979
59. Robinson BF, Epstein SE, Beiser GD et al: Control of heart by autonomic nervous system: Studies in man on interrelation between baroreceptor mechanisms and exercise. Circ Res 19:400, 1966
60. Viquerat CE, Daly P, Swedberg K et al: Endogenous catecholamines in chronic heart failure: Relation to the severity of hemodynamic abnormalities. Am J Med 78:455, 1985

GENERAL REFERENCES

Braunwald E, Ross J Jr: Control of cardiac performance. In Berne RM (ed): Handbook of Physiology, Section 2, The Cardiovascular System, chap 15. Bethesda, MD, American Physiological Society, 1979

Cohn JN (ed): Drug Treatment of Heart Failure. New York, Yorke Medical Books, 1983

Parmley WW, Talbot L: Heart as a pump. In Berne RM (ed): Handbook of Physiology, Section 2, The Cardiovascular System, chap 11. Bethesda, MD, American Physiological Society, 1979

PHYSIOLOGY OF THE CORONARY CIRCULATION

Francis J. Klocke ▪ Avery K. Ellis

Since the primary function of coronary circulation is to supply the heart's metabolic needs, any discussion of the physiology of coronary circulation must begin by emphasizing the unusually close relationship between myocardial metabolism and perfusion. This is illustrated schematically in Figure 6.1. Because the heart has a limited and short-lived capacity for anaerobic metabolism, its steady-state metabolic needs can be considered solely in terms of oxidative metabolism. Myocardial oxygen uptake can be expressed as the product of coronary blood flow and the coronary arterial–venous oxygen difference. One of the unique features of coronary circulation is its high degree of oxygen extraction under basal conditions. The oxygen saturation of coronary sinus blood is typically only 20% to 30% (corresponding to a PO_2 of ~20 mm Hg), making it difficult for the heart to adjust to increasing metabolic needs by increasing oxygen extraction. Accordingly, changes in myocardial oxygen demand require changes in coronary flow, which are quantitatively similar. As will be discussed subsequently, coronary flow normally can increase four- to six-fold in response to increments in metabolic demand.

BALANCE BETWEEN MYOCARDIAL OXYGEN DEMAND AND SUPPLY
HEMODYNAMIC FACTORS GOVERNING DEMAND

Although the determinants of myocardial oxygen demand are complex, three factors predominate[1]:

1. *Afterload*. Afterload can be defined as the stress developed by myocardial fibers during shortening. Ventricular wall stress is expressed as force per unit area (g/cm^2) and is directly proportional to aortic systolic pressure and radius of curvature of the ventricle, and inversely proportional to ventricular wall thickness. Because of the ease with which it can be measured, systolic arterial pressure is a useful and frequently used index of ventricular wall stress. One must recognize, however, that changes in either radius of curvature or wall thickness affect wall stress independently of systolic pressure. Wall tension is less frequently substituted for wall stress. It is expressed as force per unit length (g/cm) and takes the chamber radius into account, but neglects the effects of wall thickness.
2. *Contractility (inotropic state)*. The difficulties involved in any quantitative assessment of myocardial contractility in the human are reflected by the numerous hemodynamic indices of this measurement that have been proposed. Substantial changes in myocardial oxygen uptake can result from changes in inotropic state caused by hemodynamic or metabolic interventions, for example, altered cardiac sympathetic neural activity or administration of calcium or another inotropic agent.
3. *Heart rate*. The effect of heart rate on myocardial oxygen demand is related primarily to the number of contractions per minute, although positive inotropic effects of increased rate also are involved.

Other factors affecting myocardial oxygen uptake are relatively minor. Under basal conditions, ~80% of the heart's total oxygen requirements can be related to the above three measurements. Although the heart's stroke volume can vary considerably with interventions, the independent effect of stroke volume on myocardial oxygen uptake is limited. Values of left ventricular oxygen consumption usually are expressed in terms of either the entire ventricle (cc of O_2 uptake per minute) or per unit weight of ventricle (cc/min/g).

RIGHT VERSUS LEFT VENTRICLE

The general features of the oxygen demand–supply relationship need to be considered for regions within the heart as well as for the entire organ. In keeping with the lower systolic pressure in the right ventricle, right ventricular oxygen demand normally is a small fraction of that in

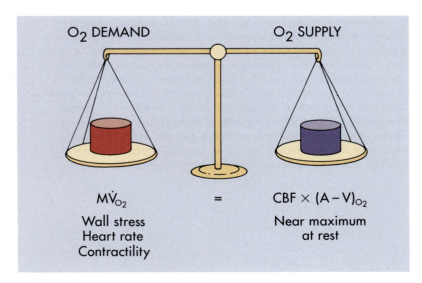

FIGURE 6.1 Schematic representation of the normal balance between myocardial oxygen demand and supply. ($M\dot{V}O_2$ = myocardial oxygen consumption; CBF = coronary blood flow; $(A-V)O_2$ = coronary arteriovenous oxygen difference)

the left ventricle. In most clinical circumstances, attention focuses on the left ventricle.

"DOUBLE PRODUCT" INDEX

USE IN EXERCISE TESTING. Because of the ease with which it can be measured, the "double product" of systemic arterial systolic pressure and heart rate is often used clinically as an index of total left ventricular oxygen consumption. The usefulness of the double product index in estimating increases in left ventricular oxygen demand during exercise testing is supported by experimental studies summarized elsewhere.[2] Rate-pressure products continue to correlate usefully with myocardial O_2 consumption in the presence of beta blockade, despite the reduction in contractility produced by this intervention.[3] An important feature of beta blockade is the altered relationship between left ventricular oxygen consumption and external workload during exercise. Any given level of workload is achieved at a lower value of double product and myocardial O_2 uptake. Conversely, any level of double product is associated with an increased external workload.

Among the other proposed indices of total left ventricular oxygen consumption are the "triple product" of systolic pressure, heart rate, and ejection time and the "systolic pressure–time index." The latter is obtained by integrating the area under the systolic portion of the left ventricular or central aortic pressure pulse (and multiplying by heart rate). As discussed elsewhere,[2] correlations between these indices and directly measured myocardial oxygen consumption do not appear better than the correlation between double product and oxygen consumption. As is the case with double product, these indices do not deal directly with effects of changes in contractility, ventricular volume or wall thickness.

It is of interest that myocardial O_2 requirements for a given level of exercise can be reduced by physical training. The reduction in oxygen demand is due mainly to the diminished heart rate during exercise in the conditioned individual.

TRANSMURAL, NONTRANSMURAL VARIATIONS WITHIN THE LEFT VENTRICLE

The oxygen demand/supply relationship is heterogenous within the left ventricle. A number of experimental observations indicate that oxygen consumption per gram of tissue normally is greater in the inner layers of the heart (subendocardium) than the outer (subepicardium). An inherently greater oxygen demand in the subendocardium seems consistent with models of transmural variations in developed stress[4] and with *in vivo* measurements of transmural variations in diastolic sarcomere length.[5] The greater oxygen consumption is accomplished by a transmural flow heterogeneity, that is, by a larger flow per gram in the subendocardium than the subepicardium[6] and by a larger subendocardial oxygen extraction.[7]

Over the years, attempts have been made to define hemodynamic indices that would predict an imbalance between subendocardial oxygen supply and demand.[6] Of particular interest has been the ratio of coronary diastolic to left ventricular systolic pressure-time per beat (DPTI:SPTI). Diastolic pressure time is taken as the area between the aortic and left ventricular pressure curves during diastole, and SPTI as the area under the left ventricular pressure curve during systole. The DPTI:SPTI ratio can be helpful in abnormalities that are not associated with coronary arterial obstruction (although potential limitations related to variations in hemoglobin concentration and other factors must be kept in mind). In the presence of coronary artery disease, diastolic pressure in the aorta exceeds diastolic pressure in the affected coronary arteries and DPTI cannot ordinarily be defined.

Myocardial perfusion also is heterogeneous in a nontransmural sense. Bassingthwaighte and colleagues[8] have reported a broad distribution of regional flow per gram in all layers of the left ventricle of the conscious baboon at rest and during stress. In dogs, regional flows vary similarly within transmural layers of the ventricle.[9] The laboratories of Klassen and Marcus suggested several years ago that flow within small areas of the left ventricle varies temporally as well as spatially.[10,11] An important consequence of normal flow variations is that any measured value for coronary flow represents an average of a distribution of flows within whatever area of myocardium is included in the measurement.

PHYSIOLOGIC FACTORS GOVERNING CORONARY FLOW

Physiologic factors governing coronary flow can be considered in terms of coronary driving pressure and impedance (Fig. 6.2). Traditional concepts of driving pressure and impedance have undergone significant revision during the past few years and continue to evolve.

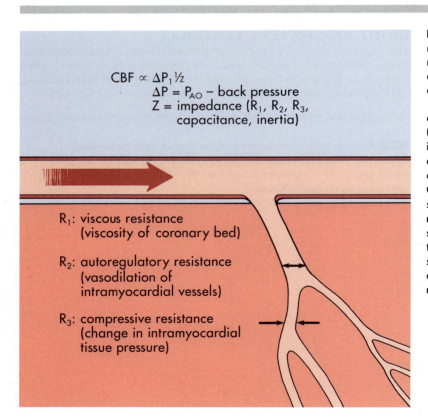

FIGURE 6.2 Schematic diagram of the coronary arterial circulation in the normal heart, illustrating the three functional components of coronary resistance. (Epi, subepicardium; Endo, subendocardium; $R_{1,2,3}$, viscous, autoregulatory, and compressive components of coronary resistance; ΔP, coronary driving pressure; P_{Ao}, aortic pressure; Z, coronary input impedance.)

As discussed in the text, coronary resistance may be viewed functionally as a time-dependent measurement resulting from the interaction of viscous (R_1), autoregulatory (R_2), and compressive (R_3) components. Viscous resistance is a relatively static factor on which more dynamic autoregulatory and compressive resistances are superimposed. Autoregulatory resistance can change greatly in magnitude but requires several cardiac cycles to do so. Compressive forces are especially important during systole and cause substantial variations in resistance during a single cardiac cycle. The magnitude of compressive resistance is greater in the subendocardium than subepicardium, but this is compensated for by a directionally opposite transmural adjustment in autoregulatory resistance and by a somewhat smaller subendocardial viscous resistance. Because of the transmural adjustment in autoregulatory resistance, coronary vasodilator reserve is normally less in the subendocardium than the subepicardium.

DRIVING PRESSURE

Driving pressure across the coronary bed has traditionally been taken as the difference between aortic and right atrial (*i.e.*, coronary venous) pressures, or as aortic pressure alone. Some workers have felt that the "back pressure" opposing coronary flow is influenced by tissue pressure within the myocardium and have suggested that left ventricular diastolic pressure is preferable to right atrial pressure as an index of back pressure. However, recent studies indicate that the minimum pressure required for forward flow in the coronary bed is at least a few millimeters higher than right atrial or left ventricular diastolic pressure, even during maximum vasodilation.[12] This back pressure is now commonly referred to as "zero-flow" pressure and abbreviated as $P_{f=0}$ or P_{ZF}. With arteriolar vasomotor tone operative, $P_{f=0}$ is substantially higher than during vasodilation (20 to 40 mm Hg) and probably plays a dynamic rather than static role in coronary flow regulation.[12] It, therefore, appears that intravascular pressure is regulated within the myocardium, perhaps at the level of the smaller arterioles, as might be advantageous for maintaining appropriate blood–tissue exchange of fluid and other substances.

IMPEDANCE

Although impedance to flow is often thought of only in terms of resistance it includes reactive as well as resistive components, that is, inertia, capacitance and resistance. Inertial effects have been studied infrequently in the coronary bed, but capacitive effects recently have received increasing attention. Capacitive effects relate to fluctuations of intravascular volume during a cardiac cycle, which result from changes in intra- and extravascular pressures including effects of systolic contraction. Differences in the phasic patterns of coronary inflow and outflow have long been appreciated. The preponderance of coronary inflow occurs during diastole (Fig. 6.3), whereas coronary outflow is accentuated by systolic contraction. Although capacitive effects cancel out over the entire cardiac cycle, they affect instantaneous patterns of flow throughout the cycle, particularly since the blood volume contained within the coronary vasculature constitutes as much as 6% to 15% of total heart weight.[13] The average value of myocardial blood volume during the cardiac cycle changes with interventions that involve vasodilation or vasoconstriction.

RESISTANCE

FUNCTIONAL COMPONENTS AND TEMPORAL VARIATIONS

The resistive component of coronary impedance remains the single most important factor controlling coronary flow. Coronary resistance can be modeled as the sum of three functional components (see Fig. 6.2).

1. *Basal viscous resistance,* designated R_1 in Figure 6.2, is defined as the minimum possible resistance of the entire coronary vascular bed and corresponds to the resistance during diastole with the coronary bed fully dilated. Since coronary vessels are distensible, R_1 varies with distending pressure.[14] In addition to depending on maximum vascular cross-sectional area, R_1 also varies with blood viscosity and any dynamic changes in the caliber of the epicardial (conductive) coronary arteries. In the absence of changes in hematocrit or other factors affecting blood viscosity or epicardial arterial caliber, R_1 can be considered to remain constant over relatively prolonged periods.

2. *Autoregulatory resistance,* designated R_2 in Figure 6.2, is the primary mechanism by which coronary flow adjusts to changing metabolic demand and is maintained constant in the face of changes in coronary arterial pressure at a constant level of demand.

   Autoregulatory resistance relates to arteriolar caliber and the number of open capillaries. Autoregulatory resistance is ordinarily 4 to 5 times larger than basal viscous resistance and can change over a few cardiac cycles in response to alterations in metabolic demand. Alterations in autoregulatory resistance are mediated primarily by arterioles or precapillary sphincters. As indicated by Poiseuille's law ($R = 8\eta l/\pi r^4$, where R = resistance, η = viscosity, l = vessel length and r = vessel radius), arteriolar resistance is inversely proportional to the fourth power of arteriolar radius. Thus, small changes in arteriolar luminal dimension can affect autoregulatory resistance profoundly.

   Under basal conditions autoregulatory tone is quite high. The ability of autoregulatory resistance to decrease in response to increased myocardial oxygen demand or decreased coronary arterial pressure is of pivotal importance in pathologic states and during stressful interventions. Because autoregulatory resistance is closely

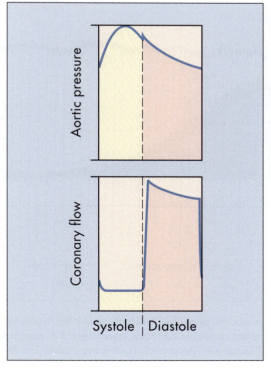

FIGURE 6.3 Variations of aortic pressure and instantaneous coronary artery flow during the cardiac cycle. Although aortic pressure is higher during systole than diastole, the compressive component of resistance increases markedly during systole, causing coronary inflow to be reduced to a small fraction of that occurring during diastole.

modulated by regional metabolic requirements, autoregulatory vasodilation can, at any one time, occur to different degrees in different areas within the ventricle. The magnitude of autoregulatory reserve is sufficient to allow coronary flow to increase by a factor of 4 to 6 at normal levels of arterial pressure.[15] Autoregulatory vasodilation also plays an important role in the occurrence of myocardial reactive hyperemia, *i.e.*, the increase in blood flow that follows a period of coronary arterial occlusion (Fig. 6.4).[16]

3. *Compressive resistance*, designated R_3 in Figure 6.2, represents the actions on coronary blood vessels of local forces within the ventricular wall. Compressive resistance varies during the cardiac cycle and is especially large during systole. When superimposed on basal viscous and autoregulatory resistance during systole, compressive resistance reduces instantaneous flow to a small fraction of that occurring during diastole (see Fig. 6.3). Although compressive resistance is smaller in magnitude in diastole, it becomes increasingly important when ventricular diastolic pressure (preload) or pericardial pressure is elevated.

TRANSMURAL VARIATION OF FUNCTIONAL COMPONENTS

All three functional components of coronary resistance vary transmurally as well as temporally (see Fig. 6.2). Basal viscous resistance (R_1) is normally less in the inner portion of the myocardial wall than in the outer, that is, there is an inherent transmural gradient of capillary density favoring the subendocardium.[17,18] Changes in compressive resistance (R_3) during the cardiac cycle involve important transmural variations. During systole there is a large pressure gradient across the myocardial wall. While the detailed pattern of this gradient is unsettled, intramyocardial pressure is near ventricular pressure in the subendocardium and decreases monotonically toward the epicardium.[6] An inner-to-outer diastolic gradient for compressive resistance also seems likely.[19,20]

Transmural variations in autoregulatory resistance (R_2) are illustrated schematically in Figure 6.2. As noted above, oxygen requirements are ordinarily greater in the inner layers of the heart than in the outer. In addition, flow to the inner layers of the heart is minimal during systole because of the "throttling" effect of systolic compressive resistance in the subendocardium. To compensate for these factors, flow to the inner layers of the heart during diastole must exceed that to the outer layers. Although some of the subendocardium's increased flow requirement is met by its inherently greater capillary density, the reduction in R_1 is not by itself adequate. Accordingly, some of the available R_2 reserve must be utilized. Autoregulatory vessels are, therefore, somewhat dilated even under basal conditions, for example, autoregulatory resistance normally is less in the subendocardium than in the subepicardium. This normal transmural difference in autoregulatory resistance implies that coronary vasodilator reserve is not uniform across the myocardial wall, and explains why the subendocardium is more vulnerable to circulatory-induced ischemia than the subepicardium. The degree to which subendocardial autoregulatory reserve is utilized under both normal and abnormal conditions varies considerably with heart rate.

STEADY-STATE RELATIONSHIPS BETWEEN CORONARY FLOW AND PRESSURE

Several of the hemodynamic factors just discussed are illustrated in Figure 6.5, which schematically represents steady-state relationships between mean coronary flow and mean coronary arterial pressure over a wide range of coronary pressures.

CALCULATION OF CORONARY RESISTANCE
LIMITATIONS OF ALL APPROACHES

Consideration also must be given to values of coronary resistance calculated from experimental measurements of pressure and flow. Calculations of resistance most often are performed in an effort to assess coronary vascular smooth muscle tone (R_2) and its response to interventions in normally autoregulating beds. Calculations also are made frequently under conditions of maximum vasodilation, usually to quantify autoregulatory vasodilatory reserve or to define changes in nonautoregulatory components of resistance in conditions, such as ventricular hypertrophy. Both mean and instantaneous values of pressure and flow have been used in these calculations, in at least 10 different approaches.[13]

The fundamental difficulty in all such calculations is that the relationship between coronary arterial pressure and flow depends not only on coronary vascular smooth muscle tone (R_2), but also on several

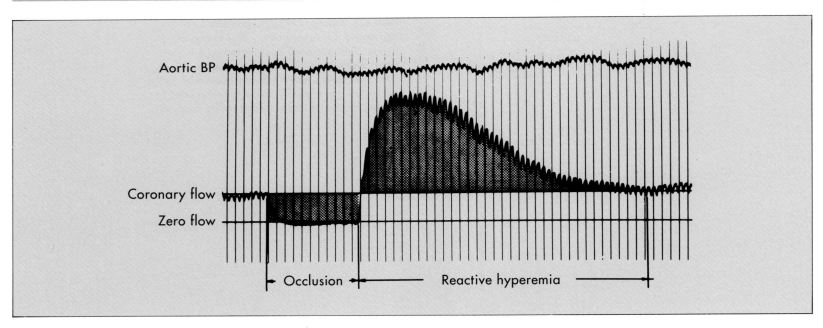

FIGURE 6.4 Coronary reactive hyperemia. Mean coronary artery pressure and flow are shown before, during, and after a brief period of coronary artery occlusion. During the postocclusion period, coronary flow rises severalfold above its preocclusion value. When the duration of occlusion is 20 seconds or more, the peak flow response during the hyperemic period is thought to reflect maximum coronary vasodilation (i.e., maximum coronary reserve). (Olsson RA: Myocardial reactive hyperemia. Circ Res 37:263, 1975. By the permission of the American Heart Association, Inc)

additional variables. Recently appreciated facts about the magnitude of coronary back pressure and its physiologic variation have been alluded to above, as have effects of nonresistive components of impedance. Effects of basal viscous or compressive resistance also are difficult to quantify. Since basal viscous resistance varies with distending pressure, R_1 is involved in changes in total resistance occurring in response to an intervention that alters arterial pressure. Changes in heart rate, myocardial contractility or ventricular preload produce alterations in compressive resistance (R_3) that are equally hard to quantify.

Because of these difficulties, modest changes in any calculated value of coronary resistance must be interpreted with great caution. This is especially true in man, in whom limitations of flow measurement techniques are, as discussed subsequently, greater than in experimental animals.

CONTROL OF AUTOREGULATORY RESISTANCE

The control of autoregulatory resistance is of primary importance in the regulation of coronary blood flow and has been the subject of intense investigation for decades. Mechanisms for adjusting autoregulatory tone can be classified under three headings.

METABOLIC FACTORS

Among the various factors potentially affecting autoregulatory resistance, metabolic factors continue to be thought to play the largest role. This conclusion is based on the close relationship between myocardial oxygen consumption and coronary flow observed in a myriad of investigations.

POSSIBLE REGULATORY FACTORS

Among the various substances or factors proposed at one time or another as *the* metabolic regulator of resistance are adenosine, oxygen tension, carbon dioxide tension, pH, lactic acid, potassium, and phosphate. Over the years, the largest body of evidence has been accumulated in favor of adenosine, particularly by Berne and coworkers.[21] It is possible that some vasoactive agents exert their influence indirectly by modulating local release of adrenergic transmitters.[22] In addition more than one agent is often active.[23]

ADENOSINE. Adenosine is a nucleoside composed of ribose and the purine base adenine. The concentration of adenosine in the interstitial space is presumed to relate directly to metabolic activity and to modulate the tone of resistance vessels. Adenosine is removed rapidly from

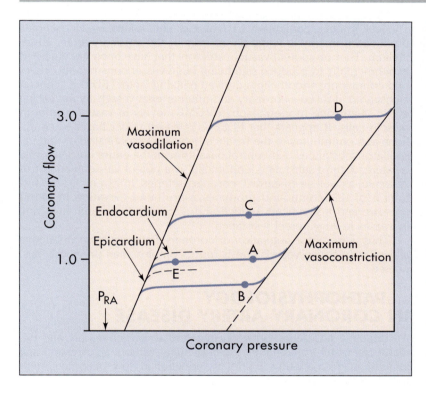

FIGURE 6.5 Steady-state relationships between coronary flow and coronary arterial pressure at varying levels of myocardial oxygen demand. The coronary bed can be considered to operate between the extremes of maximum vasodilation, on the left and above, and maximum vasoconstriction, on the right and below. Because the back-pressure to coronary flow exceeds coronary venous pressure, the minimum coronary arterial pressure required for forward flow exceeds right atrial pressure by at least a few millimeters of mercury.

The level of flow required to maintain an appropriate balance between myocardial oxygen demand and supply is determined by the level of cardiac metabolic activity. The heavy lines depict the average relationship between mean full-cycle flow and pressure for the entire myocardial wall at four levels of oxygen demand. The range of pressure over which flow remains relatively constant at any level of demand (i.e., the "autoregulatory" range) lies between the bounds of maximum vasodilation and vasoconstriction.

Point A may be considered to represent the normal basal condition, which is assigned a relative flow level of 1.0. *Point B* falls on a line corresponding to a lower metabolic demand and might represent the heart's operating point during the bradycardia of sleep. The reduced level of flow reflects autoregulatory vasoconstriction. *Point C* depicts a moderate increase in oxygen demand that might accompany pacing-induced tachycardia. There is relatively little change in arterial pressure, and the increase in flow primarily involves autoregulatory vasodilation. *Point D* represents a moderate level of muscular exercise. The increased myocardial metabolic demand causes coronary flow to increase to three times the resting value. The increased flow reflects a moderate increase in arterial pressure and a major decrease in autoregulatory resistance. Note that maximum vasodilation, which would correspond to at least a fourfold increment in flow at a normal level of coronary pressure, has not been reached.

Point E represents the situation in an area of left ventricle being perfused through a severely stenotic coronary artery. A pressure gradient across the stenotic lesion causes coronary pressure to be substantially less than simultaneous aortic pressure (which is at the level represented by *point A*). Flow in the area supplied by the stenotic artery is maintained at a normal (or near-normal) level by vasodilation, that is, autoregulatory reserve is used to a greater than usual degree under resting conditions to maintain the normal supply–demand relationship. Transmural differences in flow (corresponding to transmural differences in demand) are shown by the dotted lines above and below the line depicting average values for the entire myocardium. Should poststenotic pressure fall farther, or should metabolic demand increase, maximum vasodilation will be achieved earlier in the subendocardium.

the interstitial space, primarily by reentry into myocardial cells and local conversion to other substances. Although direct measurements of interstitial adenosine concentration have not been possible yet, a substantial body of indirect evidence suggests that interstitial adenosine concentrations vary with metabolic activity under both normal and abnormal conditions. The crucial question remains the causal implications of such a finding. In recent years it has been demonstrated that some autoregulatory responses are not altered substantially when the enzyme adenosine deaminase, which converts adenosine to inosine, is administered. This finding has caused some workers to conclude that adenosine is not essential in the regulation of coronary perfusion. Others are not convinced that adequate levels of adenosine deaminase have been achieved in the interstitial space to justify such a conclusion.

NEUROHUMORAL FACTORS

Arteriolar coronary vascular smooth muscle is subject to neurohumoral influences through direct autonomic innervation, as well as in response to vasoactive agents introduced via the coronary circulation. Neural adjustments in coronary vascular tone often are induced reflexly. Studies attempting to identify neural mechanisms for adjusting coronary resistance are technically difficult, in that direct neural effects need to be separated from secondary effects induced metabolically as a result of sympathetic stimulation or hemodynamic changes. In addition, neural effects during anesthesia can differ from those in the conscious state.

CONCLUSIONS FROM ANIMAL STUDIES

From studies in experimental animals, there is now agreement that direct adrenergic innervation of coronary resistance vessels involves both constrictor and dilator mechanisms. Evidence for α-adrenergic vasoconstriction is most persuasive. Reductions in coronary flow have been observed during intracoronary administration of α-agonists, during cardiac sympathetic nerve stimulation in the presence of β-blockade, and at the onset of sympathetic nerve stimulation in the absence of β-blockade.[23] Although α-receptors are fewer in the heart than in skeletal muscle, α-adrenergic vasoconstrictor activity appears able to compete with metabolically induced vasodilation even during interventions that substantially increase myocardial metabolic demand.[24,25]

β-Receptor- and cholinergic-mediated vasodilation have been demonstrated experimentally, but their functional role is not yet clear. The functional role of other vasoactive agents, for example, histamine, serotonin, prostaglandins, and leukotrienes, is also under continuing study.

HUMAN STUDIES

Although studies of neurohumoral influences are more difficult (and necessarily less conclusive) in man, studies contrasting normal subjects and cardiac allograft recipients suggest that α-adrenergic constrictor tone is present in the coronary bed under basal conditions.[26] Vasoconstrictor mechanisms at the arteriolar level have been suggested to be involved in the production of angina, in patients both with and without coronary artery disease.[27,28]

MYOGENIC FACTORS

According to the myogenic hypothesis, resistance vessels respond intrinsically to changes in transmural pressure, for example, distention of a vessel by an increase in intraluminal pressure stimulates contraction of vascular smooth muscle, whereas a decrease in transmural pressure results in vasodilation.[29] Although important myogenic influences have been demonstrated in other tissues, experimental studies that would enable influences of myogenic factors to be isolated from metabolic or neurohumoral factors have been difficult to formulate in the coronary bed. Some workers feel the myogenic response is especially important in maintaining flow constant during changes in coronary artery pressure, at a constant level of myocardial oxygen demand.

VASOMOTION OF THE CONDUCTIVE (EPICARDIAL) CORONARY ARTERIES

Although autoregulatory resistance (R_2) is of primary importance in the regulation of coronary vascular resistance, experimental work during the past few years has demonstrated that the caliber of epicardial (conductive) coronary arteries changes dynamically as a part of normal flow regulation. These large arteries have been known for some time to be subject to neural influences.[30] More recently, it has become apparent that their endothelium also contributes to the control of coronary flow through the synthesis of vasoactive compounds.[31]

One category of metabolites is the eicosanoids, metabolic products of arachidonic acid and the polyunsaturated fatty acids. These substances are precursors of thromboxane A_2, which is synthesized in activated platelets and induces platelet aggregation and vasoconstriction of the coronary vessels, and of prostacyclin (PGI_2), which is synthesized in endothelial cells, relaxes vascular smooth muscle, and inhibits platelet aggregation. It has been postulated that there exists a balance between the production of PGI_2 by endothelial cells and of thromboxane A_2 by platelets that is responsible for hemostasis and vascular integrity in the coronary, as well as in other vessels.

Other locally synthesized substances also affect large vessel tone. The leukotrienes, particularly LTC_4 and its metabolites, are eicosanoids produced primarily in white blood cells or the coronary artery endothelium. They are potent vasoconstrictors that have been documented experimentally to produce significant large vessel constriction. A second compound, endothelium-derived relaxing factor (EDRF), is not an eicosanoid; it relaxes coronary and other arterial vessels by increasing cyclic guanosine monophosphate (GMP) levels in vascular smooth muscle cells. It appears that EDRF is released under baseline conditions and contributes to the balance between vasoconstrictor and vasodilator substances that control basal tone in the entire coronary vasculature. A third substance, endothelin, is a potent vasoconstrictor of systemic, as well as epicardial, coronary arteries. Intravenous administration of this compound produces a profound elevation in blood pressure and a significant reduction in coronary flow, both involving increases in large vessel resistance.

Thus, vasomotor regulation of coronary flow involves conductive as well as resistive vessels and is more complex than previously suspected.

PATHOPHYSIOLOGY IN CORONARY ARTERY DISEASE

An ischemic imbalance between myocardial oxygen supply and demand can result from an increase in demand without a corresponding increase in coronary flow, a primary reduction in flow, or some combination of these processes.

AUTOREGULATORY COMPENSATION FOR PROXIMAL STENOTIC LESIONS

Adjustments in coronary circulation in response to occlusive lesions in the epicardial coronary arteries are illustrated schematically in Figure 6.6. The functional effect of an occlusive lesion may be modeled by adding a stenotic element upstream of the autoregulatory component of resistance. The increase in proximal coronary artery resistance produced by the stenosis is accompanied by a compensatory decrease in autoregulatory resistance, for example, the circulation calls on its normal vasodilator reserve to maintain total resistance at a normal level. Detailed information concerning compressive resistance in myocardium perfused by diseased vessels is limited; in this discussion, this component of resistance will be considered to remain unchanged.

Since modest increments in epicardial arterial resistance are readily compensated for by decreases in autoregulatory resistance, clinical manifestations of diminished perfusion are not evident in the initial phases of stenosis development. As the severity of a stenosis increases, autoregulatory reserve ultimately becomes exhausted during stress, at first with significant exertion, but subsequently with increasingly minor provocation and usually in the subendocardium before the subepicardium.

EFFECTS OF INDIVIDUAL STENOTIC LESIONS
FACTORS GOVERNING TRANSSTENOTIC ENERGY LOSSES

Important new insights into the static and dynamic factors governing the functional effects of a coronary stenosis have been developed during the past 10 to 15 years. In considering these factors, it is helpful to examine the stenotic lesion independently of the distal coronary vascular bed, focusing on factors affecting the pressure gradient across the stenosis itself.[32,33] Factors governing energy losses and, therefore, pressure drop across a stenosis are illustrated schematically in Figure 6.7. The transstenotic pressure drop varies with flow and is potentially influenced by viscous losses, separation losses and turbulence. Five points deserve mention. First, separation losses are proportional to flow raised to the second power and, therefore, become increasingly prominent as flow through a stenosis increases. Second, separation losses are also accentuated by increasing severity of stenosis in a nonlinear fashion. Third, for any given level of flow, the most important determinant of stenosis severity is the minimal cross-sectional area within the stenosis, which appears as a second-order term in the expression of both viscous and separation losses. Fourth, when evaluating an intervention that may change the resistance of a clinically important stenosis, emphasis ideally should be placed on the minimal cross-sectional area within the stenosis, expressed in absolute terms, for example, mm^2. (While the cross-sectional area in the poststenotic region does influence separation losses, it has limited importance when the degree of narrowing exceeds 50% of the vessel's internal diameter.) Fifth, since effects of length of stenosis are manifest through viscous rather than separation losses, stenosis length usually plays a less important role than minimal cross-sectional area in clinically important stenoses.

TRANSSTENOTIC PRESSURE DROP AS A FUNCTION OF FLOW
DEGREE OF STENOSIS VERSUS STENOSIS RESISTANCE: IMPORTANCE OF SMALL CHANGES IN CALIBER OF SEVERE STENOSES

Figure 6.8 illustrates the relationship between pressure drop across a stenosis and flow through the stenosis. Although the figure has been derived using fluid mechanics equations for steady flow of an incompressible fluid in rigid tubes with circular stenosis geometry, it applies in principle to the *in vivo* coronary circulation. The relationship between pressure drop and flow for any given stenosis is nonlinear; pressure drop increases more rapidly as flow rises. The relation between stenosis resistance and degree of stenosis is also nonlinear; resistance at any given flow increases progressively more rapidly as the degree of narrowing exceeds 50% of vessel diameter (see Fig. 6.8 inset). Because of this relationship between resistance and degree of stenosis, an important change in a patient's clinical status can result from a small increment in severity of an established stenosis, for example, from 80% to 90% diameter narrowing. Such an increment might represent a static progression of the underlying atherosclerotic process, but could also result dynamically from local vasomotion, a platelet aggregate, or a small thrombus or intramural hemorrhage. Conversely, small decreases in stenosis severity, either static or dynamic, can have potentially important therapeutic benefit. Because coronary lesions are frequently eccentric, with vascular smooth muscle retained in a portion of the arterial wall within the stenotic area, dynamic changes at the point of minimal cross-sectional area seem probable. Endothelial-dependent vasomotor responses may be blunted, or even reversed, directionally[34] in atherosclerotic coronary arteries.

FLOW-RELATED CHANGES IN FUNCTIONAL STENOSIS SEVERITY

When evaluating functional consequences of a stenotic lesion, flow-related changes in resistance that occur without any change in stenosis geometry also must be considered. Figure 6.9 makes two additional

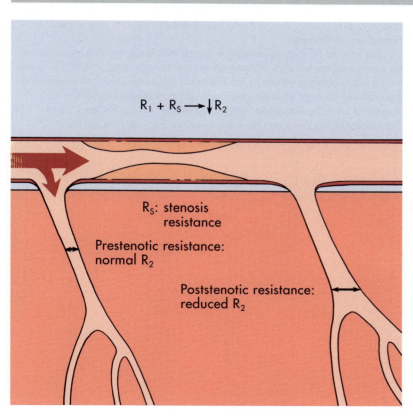

FIGURE 6.6 Schematic diagram of the coronary circulation with a portion of the ventricle supplied by a partially obstructed coronary artery. The three functional components of resistance show their usual patterns in myocardium perfused by the anatomically normal portion of the coronary artery (*left half of figure*). In myocardium located distal to the arterial obstruction (*right half*), autoregulatory resistance is reduced to compensate for the additional resistance offered by the stenosis. (*Epi* = subepicardium; *Endo* = subendocardium; $R_{1,2,3}$ = viscous, autoregulatory, and compressive components of coronary resistance; R_s = stenosis resistance)

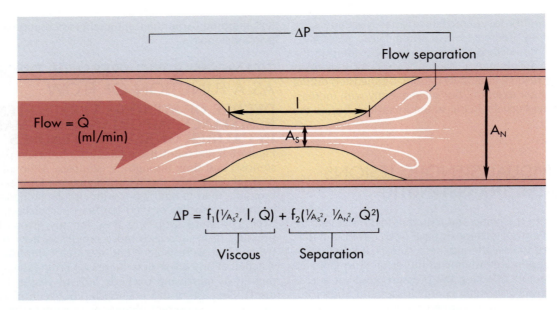

FIGURE 6.7 Factors governing energy losses across a stenosis. The figure illustrates a stenosed artery with a flow $\dot{Q}$, expressed as volume flow per unit time, that is, milliliters per minute. Minimal cross-sectional area within the stenosis is designated as A_s and stenosis length as l. The cross-sectional area of the normal portion of the artery beyond the stenosis is A_n. The fine lines indicate streamline laminar flow patterns before, within, and beyond the stenosis. Downstream of the stenosis, flow profiles show separation from the vessel wall, with resultant vortex formation.

The total pressure reduction across the stenosis, ΔP, is influenced by three factors: viscous losses, separation losses, and turbulence. Although the magnitudes of viscous and separation losses are both flow-dependent, separation losses are proportional to $\dot{Q}^2$ rather than $\dot{Q}$. The role of turbulence remains poorly defined. (Modified from Newsletter of the Council on Clinical Cardiology of the American Heart Association, Inc., vol 7, no. 3, 1982)

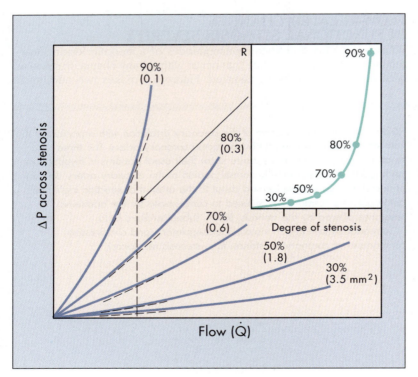

FIGURE 6.8 Relation between pressure drop across a stenosis (ΔP) and flow through the stenosis ($\dot{Q}$). Relations are shown for concentric stenoses of 30%, 50%, 70%, 80%, and 90% internal diameter. The numbers in parentheses below each percent diameter stenosis represent residual luminal cross-sectional area, calculated on the basis of a normal internal diameter of 3 mm and cross-sectional area of 7.1 mm². A potentially important advantage of absolute area measurements is the avoidance of underestimates of percent stenosis related to the inadvertent use of a narrowed segment adjacent to an arteriographic lesion when defining the severity of the lesion in relation to normal vessel diameter.

The level of flow corresponding to basal metabolic needs is represented by the vertical dotted line; stenosis resistances for this level of flow are shown as the dashed tangent lines to the individual pressure drop-flow relations. In the inset on the right, stenosis resistance (R_s) is plotted as a function of degree of stenosis. (Modified from Newsletter of the Council on Clinical Cardiology of the American Heart Association, Inc., vol 7, no. 3, 1982)

points: (1) Because of the nonlinear relationship between pressure gradient and flow, an intervention that produces an increase in flow results in an increase in stenosis resistance and, therefore, a reduction in coronary pressure distal to the stenosis. Potential effects of the reduced distal coronary pressure need to be considered in light of the information summarized in Figure 6.5. (2) Because of the phasic variations in flow occurring during each cardiac cycle, substantial changes in transstenotic pressure gradient occur during each cycle. These changes importantly limit the interpretation of measurements of mean gradient and flow for the entire cardiac cycle.

ARTERIOGRAPHIC ESTIMATES OF STENOSIS SEVERITY

Clinically, the arteriographic severity of a stenotic lesion is most often defined in terms of percent narrowing of luminal diameter in the arteriographic view showing the greatest degree of stenosis. Potential limitations of this approach are at least fourfold:

1. Even with technically excellent arteriograms, there remain important inter- and intraindividual variations in estimating degree of stenosis. These variations are most frequent with stenoses of moderate to marked severity, for example, 50% to 90% diameter narrowing. Few arteriographers would expect to distinguish regularly between 70% and 80% or 80% and 90% diameter narrowing. Yet, as shown in the inset of Figure 6.8, the functional severity of a stenosis approximately doubles between 70% and 80%, and doubles again between 80% and 90%.
2. The use of "percent" narrowing involves a comparison of the diameter of the stenotic lesion to the diameter of an adjacent area of coronary artery that is taken as a "normal reference," but which actually also is involved in the atherosclerotic process.
3. Most coronary stenoses are not concentric and, therefore, not optimally defined by any single diameter measurement.
4. As discussed earlier, many stenoses exhibit dynamic, as well as static, changes in functional severity. An arteriographic measurement reflects a single point, and is often made under the influence made from a vasodilating agent, such as sublingual nitroglycerin.

"Quantitative" arteriographic approaches have been developed in an effort to deal with limitations of usual clinical estimates of percent diameter narrowing and have been especially valuable in evaluating dynamic changes in individual stenoses.[35] As discussed elsewhere,[35,36] measurements of luminal cross-sectional area at the point of maximum narrowing are theoretically attractive in terms of dealing with noncentric lesion geometry. Absolute area measurements (mm^2) avoid the pitfalls of both a single diameter measurement and an expression of percent narrowing in relation to an adjacent area of coronary artery. However, the interpretation of an absolute value of minimum cross-sectional area is hampered by uncertainty concerning the area expected at the same point in the same artery in the absence of stenosis. In a normal coronary artery, luminal cross-sectional area decreases progressively with vessel size as one moves over the epicardial surface from base to apex. In addition, the cross-sectional area of even a single portion of a single vessel, such as the left anterior descending artery midway between the base and apex, varies with different patterns of coronary arterial arborization and probably also with sex, body size, ventricular hypertrophy, and other factors.

Because of this problem, quantitative arteriographic measurements are now sometimes reported in terms of percent reduction in luminal cross-sectional area rather than in absolute values. The measurement of percent reduction in area rather than diameter does minimize errors in the evaluation of nonconcentric lesions, but again uses an adjacent segment of a diseased artery as a "normal reference." The practical utility of either area or diameter estimates of percent narrowing may reflect the fact that atherosclerotic lesions often develop in an outward, as well as inward, direction, for example, when the lumen of a diseased area of artery adjacent to a lesion is used as the denominator in the calculation of percent stenosis, the error is less than would have occurred if arterial diameter had not increased.

Although these limitations of coronary arteriography need to be recognized, they should be considered in the context of the unique and continuing contributions of arteriography to both patient care and pathophysiology. The "test of time" is in many ways the ultimate one for a diagnostic or therapeutic technique. Coronary arteriography passed this test long ago and has become increasingly valuable as time

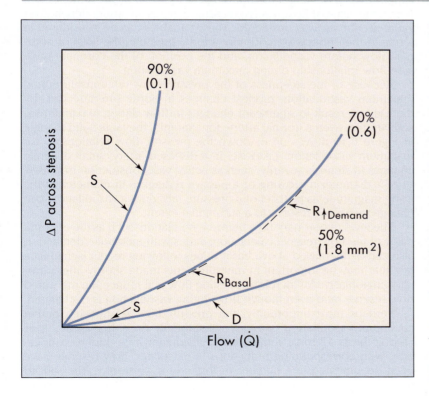

FIGURE 6.9 Relation between pressure drop across a stenosis (ΔP) and flow ($\dot{Q}$) through the stenosis. Because the magnitude of pressure drop varies with flow, important changes in pressure drop occur during each cardiac cycle. The letters S and D on the 50% stenosis line illustrate a situation in which diastolic flow is, as usual, three times greater than systolic flow and accompanied by a larger pressure gradient. Systolic (S) and diastolic (D) pressure gradients on the 90% stenosis line are much greater, and diastolic flow cannot increase in the usual amount because of the rapid increase in stenosis resistance with flow. In the *in vivo* situation, changes in pressure drop and flow during each cardiac cycle are modified further by instantaneous changes in downstream impedance related to ventricular contraction and intravascular capacitance. With the stenosis coupled to the downstream coronary bed, poststenotic systolic pressure is influenced by a "retrograde pumping effect" of ventricular contraction and by the stenosis itself. Systolic and diastolic flow patterns reflect associated capacitive effects, as well as the factors represented in the figure. The complexity of these various interrelations indicates important limitations of attempts to assess stenosis in terms of mean values of pressure gradient and flow for the entire cardiac cycle. Although phasic measurements of pressure gradient and flow are not yet feasible clinically, they should be included in experimental studies of stenosis behavior.

The figure also illustrates an increase in resistance related to increased flow for a 70% stenosis. Stenosis resistance, the tangent to the pressure-flow relation, is more than twice as great during augmented myocardial demand as under basal conditions, even though there is no change in stenosis geometry. Flow-related increases in stenosis resistance are probably an important feature of effort-related angina. One consequence of the pressure gradient-flow relationship is a reduction in coronary artery pressure beyond a stenosis during an intervention that increases flow across the stenosis without changing aortic pressure. (Modified from Newsletter of the Council on Clinical Cardiology of the American Heart Association, Inc., vol 7, no. 3, 1982)

has passed. Perhaps the most important reason for this is that arteriograms are rarely interpreted *in vacuo* but are instead synthesized into an overall clinical picture by an experienced physician. For example, in view of the information discussed earlier, it is appreciated that arteriographic progression cannot always be identified in a patient whose clinical status has worsened. Nor does one expect similar functional consequences from all lesions assigned a specific arteriographic severity. Thus, the physician has an essential cognitive role in combining arteriographic data with functional and other clinical information in the individual patient.

COLLATERAL CIRCULATION

Although the presence of coronary collaterals was considered as early as 1669, postmortem injection studies did not document their presence in animals until 1924 or in humans until 1964.[37] Preexisting collateral vessels are small and few in number, but can develop into a major vascular network, which can importantly modify the effects of coronary occlusive disease. Collateral vessels have been studied extensively in animals, but the extension of findings to humans is complicated by variations in the collateral circulation among different species and by limitations of animal models of human coronary artery disease.[38]

One important theoretic and practical aspect of coronary collaterals in man is their functional value in persons with coronary artery disease. There is agreement that collaterals develop only when a stenotic lesion is sufficiently severe to produce a substantial transstenotic pressure drop. In patients with an occluded native coronary vessel, the myocardial segment served by the occluded vessel has been reported to have better contractile function when collaterals are present than when they are absent.[39] It also is likely that preexistent collateral vessels decrease the rate or extent of myocardial necrosis at the time of acute coronary occlusion. This beneficial effect may be important when myocardial reperfusion is attempted after acute coronary occlusion and a significant time delay is involved.

Although coronary collateral vessels are able to preserve myocardial structure and function at rest, coronary flow per gram in collateral-dependent myocardium is reduced compared to normally perfused myocardium.[40] One reason for the reduced flow in collateral-dependent areas may be the pressure gradient across the collateral vessels. This gradient causes arterial pressure in the collateralized segment to be less than aortic pressure. Peripheral coronary pressure, such as the pressure measured in a distal coronary artery when the artery is occluded proximally, provides an index of the pressure available through collateral vessels and has been measured in man at surgery. In arteries with total or near total occlusive lesions, peripheral coronary pressures are only 25% to 50% of aortic pressure.[41-44] A low arterial perfusion pressure places a collateral-dependent segment of myocardium at or near the lower break point of the autoregulatory curve (see Fig. 6.5). Thus, it is not surprising that coronary reserve is limited, and that regional ischemia and dysfunction often occur in these segments during relatively moderate increases in cardiac workload.

CORONARY FLOW RESERVE

In recent years, there has been increasing interest in using measurements of coronary flow reserve to assess the functional significance of stenotic lesions. As noted earlier, the ultimate effect of a coronary stenosis depends on the degree to which the increased impedance to flow caused by the stenosis can be compensated for by autoregulatory processes. Coronary flow reserve is defined as the ratio of flow during maximum pharmacologic vasodilation to flow immediately before vasodilation. The quantitative magnitude of flow reserve varies inversely with severity of stenosis, that is, flow reserve decreases as stenosis severity increases and poststenotic coronary arterial pressure falls. Reserve becomes exhausted when coronary pressure reaches the point at which autoregulatory vasodilation is maximal.

Although the conceptual attractiveness of the evaluation of stenosis severity by quantitation of flow reserve has long been recognized, techniques potentially applicable to individual coronary arteries in man have only recently become available. Studies using an epicardial Doppler velocity probe in which vasodilation was produced with papaverine have established that coronary flow reserve is normally as great in man as in experimental animals, such as the dog, that is, as much as sixfold at usual levels of aortic pressure.[15] In retrospect, earlier human measurements reporting lower levels were probably compromised by the use of less-than-maximum vasodilator stimuli or flow measurement techniques that become inadequate at high levels of flow.

INTERPRETATION OF METHODOLOGICALLY SUITABLE MEASUREMENTS OF FLOW RESERVE

As measurements of flow reserve in man have been attempted more widely, important complexities of the flow reserve concept have been identified.[36] Several of these are illustrated schematically in Figure 6.10. Although some features of Figure 6.10 would differ if coronary flow were expressed in absolute rather than relative terms, the present formulation is more helpful for illustrating the points of greatest interest for measurement techniques currently used in man. As discussed earlier, the relationship between transstenotic pressure gradient and percent diameter narrowing is nonlinear, with progressively more rapid increases in gradient as the degree of stenosis exceeds 70%. Autoregulatory reserve is shown as being exhausted between 85% and 90% stenosis, with flow reduced slightly under basal conditions for a 90% diameter stenosis. The stenosis isopleths schematically represent the paths followed by individual stenoses when flow is increased by local vasodilation. Their intersections with the pressure-flow relationship for maximum vasodilation define the reciprocal variation of flow reserve with stenosis severity and demonstrate the attractiveness of the basic concept of using flow reserve measurements to define stenosis severity.

In specific clinical situations, it is more complex than often appreciated. Even assuming a methodologically perfect measurement technique, the value of flow reserve measured in a given artery depends on variables not always considered. These variables can be considered in terms of their effects on coronary arterial pressure, the level of coronary flow before vasodilation, and the position of the coronary pressure-flow relationship during maximum vasodilation.

Because of the steepness of the pressure-flow relationship during maximum vasodilation, modest changes in aortic pressure can, by themselves, result in significant changes in flow during maximum vasodilation in even a normal artery, for example, the large solid triangle in Figure 6.10 moves up or down the pressure-flow relationship for maximum vasodilation. Likewise, in a diseased artery, small dynamic changes in stenosis severity, such as active vasoconstriction from 80% to 85% diameter narrowing or a passive reduction in diameter of the same magnitude as poststenotic pressure falls during vasodilation, can change measured reserve to a substantial extent.

The level of coronary flow before vasodilation, such as the denominator of the flow reserve calculation, varies with metabolic demand. It also can be increased above basal values following recent ischemia, a fact that may be important in measurements made shortly after coronary angioplasty. An increase in resting flow will reduce the measured flow reserve ratio even though flow during vasodilation is unchanged.

Perhaps most importantly, the pressure-flow relationship during maximum vasodilation can vary substantially on either an acute or chronic basis. Chronic reductions in maximum flow during vasodilation, with corresponding reductions in calculated flow reserve, have been documented in a number of forms of hypertrophy. The shift to the right of the pressure-flow relationship in Figure 6.10 corresponds to a reduction in flow reserve from 5.0 to 3.0 at a normal coronary artery pressure. Reductions of this magnitude have been reported in patients with normal coronary arteries and a 30% increase in left ventricular mass due to essential hypertension; reductions of similar and even greater magnitude have been found in patients with hypertrophy related to valvular and congenital abnormalities.[13] In patients with coronary disease, variations in flow reserve for any given degree of stenosis might be expected solely on the basis of the frequent occurrence and variable degree of left ventricular hypertrophy. For example, in Figure 6.10, flow reserve would be essentially the same for an 80% stenosis supplying a normal ventricle and a 50% stenosis supplying a ventricle operating on the shifted pressure-flow relationship for maximum vasodilation.

In any given ventricle, the pressure-flow relationship during maximum vasodilation also can vary substantially with changes in hemodynamic factors such as heart rate, contractility, preload, and viscosity. Systematic measurements of coronary reserve during changes in these variables are not yet available in man.

Tachycardia affects flow reserve both by increasing myocardial metabolic demand, therefore increasing the prevasodilation flow level, and by reducing diastolic time per minute, therefore shifting the pressure-flow relationship during maximum vasodilation. Tachycardia also illustrates the potential importance of transmural variations in flow reserve, which are difficult to define with any technique presently used in man. Because the compressive effects of systolic contraction decrease progressively across the myocardial wall, tachycardia-induced shifts in the pressure-flow relationship for maximum vasodilation also vary transmurally, and are greatest in the subendocardium.[45]

Additional issues include effects of collateral flow and possible differences in the degree of vasodilation induced by ischemia and a pharmacologic agent. Measurements of flow in a single coronary artery fail to take into account collateral flow entering the arterial bed distal to the point of flow measurement. It seems likely that the proportional contribution of collateral flow to total myocardial flow would differ before and during pharmacologic vasodilation. With regard to pharmacologic versus ischemic vasodilation, a number of laboratories have now observed vasodilation in all ventricular layers in response to adenosine in the setting of reductions in flow sufficient to produce regional myocardial ischemia. Likewise, adrenergic constrictor influences seem able to limit flow increases during exercise as well as ischemia. Although the relevance of these observations for man remains to be clarified, they, too, potentially confound the interpretation of values of flow reserve measured using pharmacologic vasodilation.

The ultimate impact of these various complicating factors on the utility of flow reserve measurements for individual patient care decisions is difficult to anticipate, particularly since clinical experience is limited and short term. Experience with other indices of proven clinical value, such as ejection fraction, serves as a reminder that limitations of a measurement that initially seem major sometimes prove minor from a practical point of view as experience is accumulated. Flow-reserve measurements in groups of patients will clearly continue to play an important role in defining coronary pathophysiology.

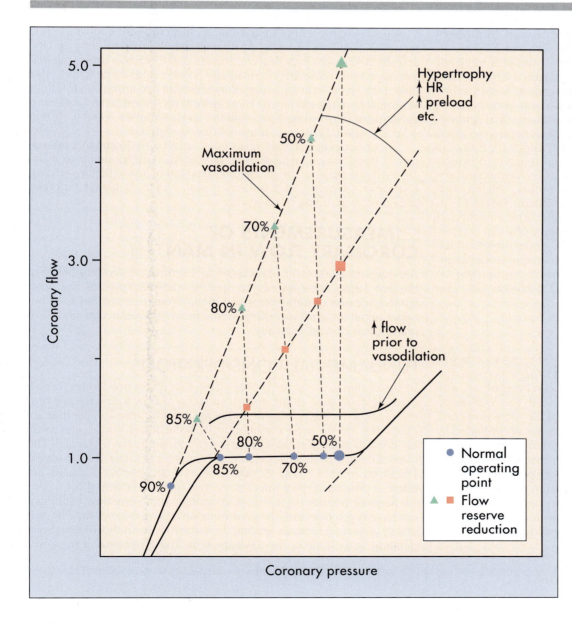

FIGURE 6.10 Complexities of the flow reserve concept. Effects of coronary stenoses under basal conditions are shown by the small circles. The horizontal distances between the normal operating point (*large circle*), and the individual stenosis points represent the transstenotic aortic-coronary pressure gradients for lesions of different severity, here expressed as percent diameter narrowing. The shift to the right of the pressure–flow relationship corresponds to a reduction in flow reserve from 5.0 (large triangle) to 3.0 (large square) at a normal coronary artery pressure. (Modified from Klocke F J: Measurements of coronary flow reserve: defining pathophysiology versus making decisions about patient care. Circulation 76:1183, 1987)

PATHOPHYSIOLOGY IN NONCORONARY ABNORMALITIES

TACHYCARDIA

In a normal person, tachycardia does not result in myocardial ischemia because increases in heart rate, with their associated increases in myocardial oxygen demand, cause autoregulatory coronary vasodilation (see Fig. 6.5). A healthy individual readily can perform sustained exercise at heart rates in excess of 150 beats per minute without developing ischemia. Extremely rapid tachycardias may be associated with ST depression on the electrocardiogram, suggesting subendocardial ischemia. In patients with abnormalities, such as aortic stenosis, coronary artery disease, or anemia, lesser degrees of tachycardia can result in significant subendocardial ischemia.[6] In addition to increasing myocardial oxygen demand, rapid heart rates limit the diastolic time available for subendocardial perfusion. Whereas diastole occupies approximately two thirds of the cardiac cycle at a heart rate of 60 beats per minute, diastolic time is only one quarter of the cardiac cycle at a heart rate of 180 beats per minute.

HYPERTROPHY

Cardiac hypertrophy, which usually results from a sustained pressure load on the left ventricle, for example, hypertension, aortic stenosis, can be associated with inadequate coronary perfusion. In conditions in which muscle mass is increased, oxygen consumption and coronary flow are increased under resting conditions for the entire ventricle, but remain relatively normal when considered on a per unit weight basis, for example, as cc O_2/min/g and ml flow/min/g. However, the proliferation of vascular channels may not keep pace with the increase in myocardial mass,[46] and the capillarity per gram of tissue is reduced, often by 20% to 30%. In the schema outlined in Figure 6.2, this reduction in vascularity may be considered as an increase in basal viscous resistance (R_1) if the latter is considered on a per unit mass basis. In order to compensate for the increased R_1, some of the normal autoregulatory reserve (R_2) is used to maintain a normal level of flow per gram under resting conditions. Similarly, in Figures 6.5 and 6.10, if flow is considered on a per gram basis, the slope of the maximum vasodilation line is decreased: that is, minimal resistance is higher. Maximum vasodilation therefore occurs at a higher-than-usual coronary arterial pressure. Thus, a patient with hypertrophy may be particularly vulnerable to myocardial ischemia during periods of hypotension. The limitation of coronary reserve associated with ventricular hypertrophy can be considerable, with ischemia developing at relatively modest levels of exercise or tachycardia.[47] The presence of subendocardial ischemia resulting from diminished coronary perfusion has been verified by pathologic studies in which diffuse subendocardial fibrosis has been noted in hypertrophied hearts.[48]

AORTIC STENOSIS

Myocardial oxygen demand is increased in aortic stenosis to a degree commensurate with the increased left ventricular systolic pressure (afterload). Concentric left ventricular hypertrophy can be extreme, with marked increases in systolic compressive forces (R_3) as well as an increased basal viscous resistance (R_1). Effects of the increased compressive forces on intramyocardial blood vessels are accentuated by the abnormal systolic gradient between left ventricular and coronary arterial pressures. It is not surprising, therefore, that subendocardial ischemia and angina occur frequently in the absence of coronary artery disease, and that subendocardial fibrosis is common in hearts at postmortem examination. A marked reduction in left ventricular coronary reserve has been documented in adult humans with normal coronary arteries and pressure-overload hypertrophy caused by aortic stenosis requiring valve replacement.[49]

AORTIC INSUFFICIENCY

Coronary reserve also has been reported to be diminished in the volume-overload hypertrophy associated with aortic insufficiency. An additional major consequence of aortic insufficiency is the reduced diastolic coronary arterial pressure. Diminished flow during diastole can put the subendocardium at particular risk. Because mean diastolic coronary pressure is in part related to heart rate (slow heart rates are associated with lower late-diastolic aortic pressures), mild degrees of tachycardia may be beneficial. In dogs, in which placement of an arterial–venous fistula simulated aortic insufficiency, mild tachycardia augmented mean diastolic aortic pressure and improved myocardial oxygen supply.[50]

ANEMIA AND POLYCYTHEMIA

Anemia in a euvolemic individual reduces the hemoglobin carrying capacity of the blood and limits myocardial oxygen delivery under conditions of basal coronary flow. Thus, the anemic patient requires a higher coronary flow to achieve normal oxygen delivery at any level of myocardial demand. As a result, there is coronary vasodilation at rest, and coronary blood flow, as well as oxygen extraction, increases substantially. In the schema of Figure 6.5, this would be manifest by an elevation in the horizontal autoregulatory portion of the flow-pressure relationship.[51] Studies in animals[52] have shown that there is an inverse relationship between coronary flow and hemoglobin level in awake dogs with anemia. In the presence of severe anemia, with hemoglobin < 5 g/dl, coronary reserve is so severely compromised that the reactive hyperemic response essentially is absent.

One favorable effect of anemia on the coronary circulation is a reduction in blood viscosity. As a result, basal viscous resistance (R_1) actually decreases. Experimental studies of the reactive hyperemia following a brief coronary occlusion in anemic dogs have found peak flow to be elevated in all layers of myocardium in comparison to values at normal hemoglobin levels. This can be represented by an increase in the slope of the maximum vasodilation line in Figures 6.5 and 6.10, that is, at any arterial pressure, maximal flow is higher.

Effects of polycythemia have been studied by Hoffman's laboratory.[53] Basal viscous resistance is increased, corresponding to a decrease in the slope of the maximum vasodilation line in Figures 6.5 and 6.10, and subendocardial underperfusion begins at higher coronary pressures than during normocythemia.

MEASUREMENTS OF CORONARY FLOW IN MAN

Although measurements of coronary blood flow in man were begun in the late 1950s, their impact on specific clinical problems has been limited because of conceptual and methodologic issues that have become apparent gradually. Measurements of left ventricular perfusion are of most interest clinically.

FUNDAMENTAL CONSIDERATIONS

In attempting to evaluate coronary flow, four issues need to be considered. First, because of the normal variation of flow within the left ventricle, any flow measurement technique must be able to take into account the rather wide distribution of local flows that is inevitably included in whatever single value is determined by the technique. The normal degree of flow variation is accentuated in many disease states. Localized areas of below average flow, as in an ischemic segment, are often of primary clinical importance, but easily overlooked.[54]

Second, because of the close coupling of coronary flow with myocardial oxygen demand, the interpretation of any value of flow as normal or abnormal requires relating the value to some index of metabolic demand at the time of the measurement. Third, because of the coronary circulation's large vasodilator reserve, coronary flow may be maintained at normal, or near-normal, levels under resting conditions or during moderate stress in disease states. Autoregulatory vasodilatory mechanisms are thought adequate to maintain resting flow in the subendocardium at diastolic coronary arterial pressures as low as 40 mm Hg.[55] And, fourth, because of the importance of regional reductions in flow within the left ventricle, transmural and nontransmural alike, clinically relevant flow measurements need to be regionalized to a much greater degree than originally anticipated. No currently available technique suitable for humans can identify a truly homogeneously perfused segment of myocardium. Important limitations also remain in approaches for isolating an area supplied by a given coronary artery. All currently available techniques for measuring coronary flow reserve have methodologic, as well as conceptual, limitations.[36]

CURRENT STATUS

At present, quantitative measurements of coronary flow in humans remain confined to centers that have a special interest in them and are able to implement appropriate methodology and to evaluate results in relation to metabolic demand, coronary reserve, and local flow heterogeneity. A detailed discussion of the strengths and limitations of individual flow measurement techniques is beyond the scope of the present chapter, but is available elsewhere.[13,32,54,56] More practical techniques for assessing regional flow in humans in a quantitatively reliable fashion continue to be investigated actively. Since flow abnormalities are most often of interest in relation to a supply–demand imbalance producing ischemia, improved techniques for assessing regional ischemia also deserve attention.

REFERENCES

1. Parmley WW, Tyberg JV: Determination of myocardial oxygen demand. Prog Cardiol 5:19, 1976
2. Klocke FJ, Ellis AK: Control of coronary blood flow. Annu Rev Med 31:489, 1980
3. Jorgensen CR, Wang K, Wang Y et al: Effect of propranolol on myocardial oxygen consumption and its hemodynamic correlates during upright exercise. Circulation 48:1173, 1973
4. Mirsky I: Left ventricular stresses in the intact human heart. Biophys J 9:189, 1969
5. Yoran C, Covell JW, Ross J Jr: Structural basis for the ascending limb of left ventricular function. Circ Res 32:297, 1973
6. Hoffman JIE, Buckberg GD: Transmural variations in myocardial perfusion. Prog Cardiol 5:37, 1976
7. Monroe RG, Gamble WJ, LaFarge CG et al: Transmural coronary venous O_2 saturations in normal and isolated hearts. Am J Physiol 228:318, 1975
8. King RB, Bassingthwaighte JB, Hales JRS, Rowell LB: Stability of heterogeneity of myocardial blood flow in normal awake baboons. Circ Res 57:285, 1985
9. Schänzenbacher P, Klocke FJ: Inert gas measurements of myocardial perfusion in the presence of heterogeneous flow documented by microspheres. Circulation 61:590, 1980
10. Sestier FJ, Mildenberger RR, Klassen GA: The role of autoregulation in spatial and temporal perfusion heterogeneity of the canine myocardium. Am J Physiol 235:H64, 1978
11. Falsetti HL, Carroll RJ, Marcus ML: Temporal heterogeneity of myocardial blood flow in anesthetized dogs. Circulation 52:848, 1975
12. Klocke FJ, Mates RE, Canty JM Jr, Ellis AK: Coronary pressure-flow relationships: controversial issues and probable implications. Circ Res 56:310, 1985
13. Marcus ML: The coronary circulation in health and disease. pp. 17, 117–109. New York, McGraw-Hill, 1983
14. Hanley FL, Messina LM, Grattan MT, Hoffman JIE: The effect of coronary inflow pressure on coronary vascular resistance in the isolated dog heart. Circ Res 54:760, 1984
15. Marcus M, Wright C, Doty D et al: Measurements of coronary velocity and reactive hyperemia in the coronary circulation of humans. Circ Res 49:877, 1981
16. Olsson RA: Myocardial reactive hyperemia. Circ Res 37:263, 1975
17. Wüsten B, Buss DD, Deist H, Schaper W: Dilatory capacity of the coronary circulation and its correlation to the arterial vasculature in the canine left ventricle. Basic Res Cardiol 72:636, 1977
18. Archie JP Jr: Minimum left ventricular coronary vascular resistance in dogs. J Surg Res 25:21, 1978
19. Rouleau J, Boerboom LE, Surjadhana A, Hoffman JIE: The role of autoregulation and tissue diastolic pressures in the transmural distribution of left ventricular blood flow in anesthetized dogs. Circ Res 45:804, 1979
20. Aversano T, Klocke FJ, Mates RE, Canty JM Jr: Preload-induced alterations in capacitance-free diastolic pressure-flow relationships. Am J Physiol 246:H410, 1984
21. Berne RM, Rubio R: Coronary circulation. In Berne RM (ed): Handbook of physiology. Section II: The cardiovascular system, p 873. Bethesda, MD, American Physiological Society, 1979
22. Shepherd JT: Alteration in activity of vascular smooth muscle by local modulation of adrenergic transmitter release. Fed Proc 37:179, 1978
23. Feigl EO: Coronary physiology. Physiol Rev 63:1, 1983
24. Mohrman DE, Feigl EO: Competition between sympathetic vasoconstriction and metabolic vasodilation in the canine coronary circulation. Circ Res 42:79, 1978
25. Murray PA, Vatner SF: Alpha-adrenoreceptor attenuation of the coronary vascular response to severe exercise in the conscious dog. Circ Res 45:654, 1979
26. Orlick AE, Ricci DR, Alderman EL et al: Effects of alpha adrenergic blockade upon coronary hemodynamics. J Clin Invest 62:459, 1978
27. Mudge GH, Grossman W, Mills RM Jr et al: Reflex increase in coronary vascular resistance in patients with ischemic heart disease. N Engl J Med 295:1333, 1976
28. Cannon RO III, Watson RM, Rosing DR, Epstein SE: Angina caused by reduced vasodilator reserve of the small coronary arteries. J Am Coll Cardiol 1:1359, 1983
29. Folkow B: Description of the myogenic hypothesis. Circ Res 15:1–279, 1964
30. Vatner SF, Pagani M, Manders T, Pasipoularides AD: Alpha adrenergic vasoconstriction and nitroglycerin vasodilation of large coronary arteries in the conscious dog. J Clin Invest 65:5, 1980
31. Cannon PJ: The role of the endothelium in coronary vasomotion: new insights. Primary Cardiol 15:15
32. Gould KL: Dynamic coronary stenosis. Am J Cardiol 45:286, 1980
33. Klocke FJ: Measurements of coronary blood flow and degree of stenosis: current clinical implications and continuing uncertainties. J Am Coll Cardiol 1:31, 1983
34. Ludmer PL, Selwyn AP, Shook TL et al: Paradoxical vasoconstriction induced by acetylcholine in atherosclerotic coronary arteries. N Engl J Med 315:1046, 1986
35. Brown BG, Balson E, Petersen RB et al: The mechanisms of nitroglycerin action: stenosis vasodilation as a major component of the drug response. Circulation 64:1089, 1981
36. Klocke FJ: Measurements of coronary flow reserve: defining pathophysiology versus making decisions about patient care. Circulation 76:1183, 1987
37. Fulton WFM: The Coronary Arteries. Springfield, IL, Charles C. Thomas, 1965
38. Gregg DE, Patterson RE: Functional importance of the coronary collaterals. N Engl J Med 303:1404, 1980
39. Schwarz F, Flameng W, Ensslen R et al: Effects of collaterals on left ventricular function at rest and during stress. Am Heart J 95:570, 1978
40. Arani DT, Greene DG, Bunnell IL et al: Reductions in coronary flow under resting conditions in collateral-dependent myocardium of patients with complete occlusion of the left anterior descending coronary artery. J Am Coll Card 3:668, 1984
41. Smith SC, Gorlin R, Herman MV et al: Myocardial blood flow in man: effects of coronary collateral circulation and coronary artery bypass surgery. J Clin Invest 51:2556, 1972
42. Goldstein RE, Stinson EB, Scherer JL et al: Intraoperative coronary collateral function in patients with coronary occlusive disease: nitroglycerin responsiveness and angiographic correlations. Circulation 49:298, 1974
43. Oldham HN Jr, Rembert JC, Greenfield JC Jr et al: Intraoperative relationships between aorta–coronary bypass graft flow, peripheral coronary artery pressure and reactive hyperemia. In Maseri A, Klassen GA, Lesch M (eds): Primary and Secondary Angina Pectoris. p. 363. New York, Grune and Statton, 1978
44. Flameng WF, Schwarz F, Hehrlein F, Boel A: Functional significance of coronary collaterals in man. Basic Res Cardiol 73:188, 1978
45. Bache RJ, Cobb FR: Effect of maximal coronary vasodilation on transmural myocardial perfusion during tachycardia in the awake dog. Circ Res 41:648, 1977
46. O'Keefe DD, Hoffman JIE, Cheitlin R et al: Coronary blood flow in experimental canine left ventricular hypertrophy. Circ Res 43:43, 1978
47. Hoffman JIE: Determinants and prediction of transmural myocardial perfusion. Circulation 58:381, 1978
48. Buchner F: Qualitative morphology of heart failure: light and electron microscopic characteristics of acute and chronic heart failure. Methods Achiev Exp Pathol 5:60, 1971
49. Marcus ML, Doty DB, Hiratzka LF et al: Decreased coronary reserve—a mechanism for angina pectoris in patients with aortic stenosis and normal coronary arteries. N Engl J Med 307:1362, 1982
50. Buckberg GD, Fixler DE, Archie JP, Hoffman JIE: Experimental subendocardial ischemia in dogs with normal coronary arteries. Circ Res 30:67, 1972

51. Hoffman JIE: Maximal coronary flow and the concept of coronary vascular reserve. Circulation 70:153, 1984
52. von Restorff W, Hö B, Holtz J, Bassenge E: Effect of increased blood fluidity through hemodilution on coronary circulation at rest and during exercise in dogs. Pflugers Arch 357:15, 1975
53. Surjadhana A, Rouleau J, Boerboom L, Hoffman JIE: Myocardial blood flow and its distribution in anesthetized polycythemic dogs. Circ Res 43:619, 1978
54. Klocke FJ: Coronary blood flow in man. Prog Cardiovasc Dis 19:117, 1976
55. Canty JM Jr: Coronary pressure-function and steady-state pressure-flow relations during autoregulation in the unanesthetized dog. Circ Res 63:821, 1988
56. Cannon PJ, Weiss MB, Sciacca RR: Myocardial blood flow in coronary artery disease: studies at rest and during stress with inert gas washout techniques. Prog Cardiovasc Dis 200:95, 1977

THE CIRCULATION IN THE LIMBS: NORMAL FUNCTION AND EFFECTS OF DISEASE

CHAPTER 7
VOLUME 1

John T. Shepherd ▪ Paul M. Vanhoutte

The blood flow to the limbs, as to any other organ or tissue, depends primarily on the systemic arterial blood pressure and the resistance to flow offered by the blood vessels, particularly the small arteries and arterioles (resistance blood vessels). The large systemic arteries act as a depulsator by storing part of the volume ejected from the left ventricle during systole, thus permitting it to drain to the periphery during diastole (Windkessel effect). The veins are the major determinants of vascular capacitance and hence of the cardiac filling pressure. The cardiovascular reflexes and direct control from brain centers regulate the sympathetic outflow, both qualitatively and quantitatively, to individual components of the cardiovascular system. As a consequence the arterial blood pressure is continuously adjusted to meet the varying stresses to the body. The complex interplay between local, humoral, and nervous events at the resistance blood vessels is the final determinant of their caliber and hence, together with the arterial blood pressure, of the tissue blood flow.[1,2] In addition, the endothelium can modulate the response of the underlying smooth muscle to various vasoactive substances.

In this chapter we will begin with a brief review of the principles governing the behavior of the limb circulation, followed by a description of the mechanisms involved in the regulation of vascular smooth muscle. Next, the regulation of the circulation to the skin, with its modest metabolic requirements and its prime role in temperature regulation, will be discussed and contrasted with that to the skeletal muscles, with their major metabolic requirements and their importance in the reflex control of arterial blood pressure. Finally, possible causes of vasospastic disorders will be mentioned and the hemodynamic consequences of atherosclerosis of the limb blood vessels summarized.

DYNAMICS OF THE LIMB CIRCULATION

The driving force for the flow of blood is the total energy imparted to it. This total fluid energy is determined by the sum of potential energy stored as pressure, kinetic energy, and potential energy from gravitational forces.

POISEUILLE'S LAW

The blood flow to the limb is controlled by the arterial blood pressure generated by contraction of the left ventricle and the resistance to flow imposed by the physical characteristics of the blood vessels and of the blood itself. Poiseuille's law states that, for a given cylindrical vessel, the resistance to flow is proportional to the viscosity of the fluid and inversely proportional to the fourth power of the radius of the vessel. Although this law applies strictly to the behavior of nonpulsatile laminar flow of a homogeneous fluid through a rigid tube of uniform caliber, it predicts that changes in resistance to blood flow through any vascular segment is most dependent on the radius of the small arteries and arterioles.[3]

PATTERNS OF BLOOD FLOW

As the blood flows through consecutive portions of the vascular tree it encounters a combination of inertial and frictional (viscous) forces. At low flow rates, viscous forces predominate and flow is streamlined and laminar. At high flow rates, the inertial forces predominate and flow may become turbulent. Turbulent flow is characterized by random fluctuations in the pressure and velocity of the fluid elements within the fluid stream. The energy transmitted to the vessel wall may be detected as a thrill and may be heard as a murmur.

LAPLACE'S LAW

Laplace's law states that the tension (T) in the wall of a spherical container is proportional to the product of the intraluminal pressure (P) and the radius (r) of the sphere. Hence the caliber of blood vessels is determined by the distending pressure and the wall tension. The latter can be altered actively by varying the degree of contraction of the smooth muscle in the blood vessel wall.

VISCOSITY

Viscosity of a Newtonian fluid is independent of the dimensions of the tube in which it flows and of the rate of flow, provided the latter is laminar and not turbulent. With a non-Newtonian fluid such as blood, which is a suspension of cells in a liquid, the viscosity and hence the resistance to blood flow varies depending on the rate of flow, the hematocrit, the caliber of the small vessels, the axial orientation of the red blood cells, and their deformability. The influence of vessel diameter on the apparent viscosity is due in part to changes in the orientation of the red cells in the plasma as the blood passes through the small vessels. Usually the cells occupy the center position of the vessel where the linear flow rate is highest, whereas the majority of the plasma flow is in the slower-moving outer layers. The red cells move with their long axis parallel to the direction of flow, provided turbulence does not occur, and the viscosity of the blood is inversely related to their deformability. This in turn depends on the Ca^{2+} concentration of the plasma. If excess Ca^{2+} enters the cell, as occurs when the blood contains less oxygen, the cell becomes stiffer and the viscosity of the blood increases.

The red blood cells are composed of a flexible lipoprotein membrane enclosing the hemoglobin-rich fluid. Red cell deformability is a complex function of the flexibility of the membrane and the viscosity of the internal fluid. The viscosity is directly affected by changes in the mean corpuscular hemoglobin concentration, by the type and physicochemical state of the hemoglobin, and by abnormal red cell inclusions.[3]

ENDOTHELIUM

The vascular endothelium is the monolayer of squamous cells in direct contact with the circulating blood. In addition to their role in the movement of fluids and solutes from the blood to the tissue cells, these cells are capable of many metabolic functions. The endothelial cells of the lungs extract norepinephrine and 5-hydroxytryptamine and degrade both monoamines, mainly through mitochondrial monoamine oxidase and/or catechol-O-methyltransferase. Endothelial cells also secrete the active products of the renin-angiotensin system and can inactivate bradykinin and encephalins. The endothelial cells also have a key role in coagulability.[4-6]

In addition to these roles, the endothelium can, in response to a large number of agents, form and release vasoactive substances that operate as autocrine and/or paracrine systems in the regulation of smooth muscle tone. The endothelial cells are a major site for the formation of prostacyclin by cyclooxygenase. This, by activating adenylate cyclase and augmenting the content of cyclic AMP in the underlying vascular smooth muscle, can cause its relaxation. By the same mechanism prostacyclin also inhibits platelet aggregation. Prostacyclin production can be stimulated by increases in blood flow as a consequence of the increase in shear stress and also by substances such as adenine nucleotides, bradykinin and thrombin.[7]

Similar physiologic stimuli, including platelet products (particularly adenosine and serotonin), thrombin, hormones (including catecholamines and vasopressin), and increases in shear stress can cause a nonprostanoid endothelium-dependent relaxation. Thus, relaxation is caused by the release of nitric oxide from its precursor L-arginine in the endothelial cells.[8-11] The nitric oxide causes relaxation of the underlying smooth muscle by activation of soluble guanylate cyclase in the vascular smooth muscle, leading to cyclic GMP-dependent protein phosphorylation, and inhibition of Ca^{2+} release from intracellular stores and of Ca^{2+} influx through receptor operated channels. There is also evidence for an endothelium-derived hyperpolarizing factor causing relaxation in some vessels. Endothelium-derived relaxing factor(s) is generally referred to as EDRF (Figs. 7.1, 7.2).[12,13]

Vasopressin in concentrations found during hemorrhage, by acting on V_1-vasopressinergic receptors on the endothelial cells of the cerebral vessels, causes relaxation of these vessels.[14] Oxytocin also has a similar action. By contrast, these hormones cause only constriction of the limb arteries and this is independent of whether the endothelium is present.

EDRF, like prostacyclin, can also inhibit platelet adhesion and aggregation, and together they act synergistically.[15,16] Thus, subthreshold concentrations of each inhibit platelet aggregation when given together. EDRF acts by activating soluble guanylate cyclase in the platelets, elevating the level of cyclic GMP and thus reducing cytosolic free Ca^{2+}. EDRF is a more potent relaxer of the smooth muscle than prostacyclin, and its release is the major contribution to the dilatation of the conduit arteries that accompanies the local metabolic relaxation of the resistance vessels in the active muscles during exercise. If platelets aggregate on normal endothelium, the products that they release, such as adenine nucleotides and serotonin, evoke endothelium-dependent relaxations.[17,18]

In addition to forming prostacyclin and EDRF, endothelial cells can produce contracting factors. Arachidonic acid and thrombin, for example, can cause endothelium-dependent relaxation of arteries, but endothelium-dependent contraction of veins. Thus, endothelial cells are characterized by the heterogeneity of their responses both within and between species. In cerebral coronary and peripheral arteries of

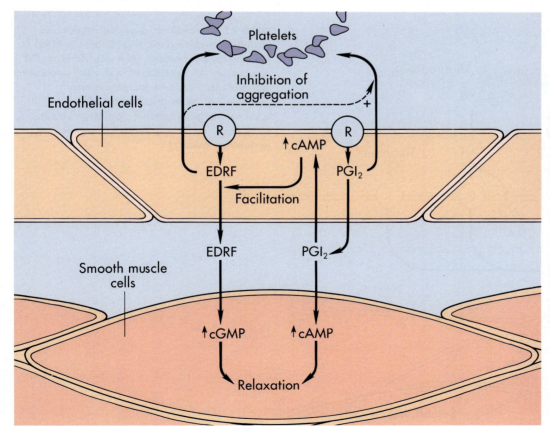

FIGURE 7.1 Endothelium-derived relaxing factor(s) (*EDRF*) and prostacyclin (*PGI₂*). EDRF and PGI₂ are formed in the endothelial cells in response to various agonists activating specific receptors (*R*) on the endothelial cell membrane. Distinct G proteins couple signals from activated membrane receptors to effector enzymes and ion channels. PGI₂ causes relaxation of the vascular smooth muscle by increasing the concentration of cyclic AMP, whereas EDRF operates by increasing the concentration of cyclic GMP. PGI₂ also facilitates the release of or protects the released EDRF. Both substances act synergistically to inhibit platelet aggregation.

the dog, anoxia and severe hypoxia can cause endothelium-dependent contraction. This cannot be explained by inhibition of the basal release of EDRF, since inhibition of endothelium-dependent relaxation by hemoglobin and methylene blue does not prevent it.[19]

Possible mediators of endothelium-dependent contractions include superoxide anions[20] and the potent vasoconstrictor peptide endothelin.[21]

REGULATION OF VASCULAR SMOOTH MUSCLE
AUTOREGULATION

The vascular transmural pressure dictates the length of the contractile components of the circular muscle of the blood vessels and thus the force the muscle generates in response to a given stimulus.[22,23] In certain blood vessels there is a basal activity of the smooth muscle (myogenic tone) that probably results from spontaneous depolarization of the cell membrane and the opening of Ca^{2+} channels; this myogenic activity may be either sustained or rhythmic. Elevating the transmural pressure causes the resistance vessels to contract to less than their initial diameter; they dilate when the transmural pressure decreases. These adjustments in vessel caliber serve to maintain a fairly constant flow and capillary hydrostatic pressure over a wide range of arterial blood pressure. This is the phenomenon of autoregulation of blood flow. Autoregulation may be explained by changes in the basal myogenic activity, possibly as a consequence of the changes in distending pressure altering ion fluxes across the membrane of the vascular smooth muscle cells. Thus an increase in pressure, and consequential increase in distention of the vessels, enhances the depolarization of the cell membrane and vice-versa. When the metabolic activity of the tissues surrounding resistance blood vessels increases, myogenic tone decreases owing to products of cellular activity; this decrease may be a consequence of hyperpolarization of the smooth muscle membrane and reduced entry of Ca^{2+}. Changes in the levels of such metabolites might account in part for autoregulation. Thus, with a rapid increase in pressure there is an initial transient increase in flow; this might "wash out" metabolites from the interstitial space with a resultant augmentation of the tone of the resistance vessels. Hence the question is whether blood flow or wall tension is being regulated. The myogenic mechanism may be important in the regulation of the precapillary vessels and thus in the maintenance of an appropriate capillary pressure and hence capillary nutritional exchanges. This implies a balance between the metabolic factors providing the appropriate flow to meet the metabolic needs by their action on the resistance vessels and the myogenic mechanism working in concert to prevent an excessive increase in capillary pressure.[24,25]

An increase in blood flow, and/or arterial diameter caused by an increase in pulsatile pressure, can cause an endothelium-dependent dilatation of large arteries as a consequence of the formation, by the endothelial cells, of a substance(s) that causes relaxation of the underlying smooth muscles.[26] This could provide an explanation for the increase in diameter of the larger arteries of the limb, during exercise of that limb, as the blood flow through them increases. In cerebral arteries, rapid stretch causes the endothelium to release a vasoconstrictor substance(s) that activates the underlying smooth muscle, suggesting a potential role of endothelial cells in autoregulation.

In humans, autoregulation of blood flow in the limb has been demonstrated by exposure of the forearm to subatmospheric pressures. Increasing the vascular transmural pressure by application of a negative pressure of 50 mm Hg to 100 mm Hg to the forearm is followed by a reduction of flow below the control level, whereas 100 mm Hg to 200 mm Hg is required to reduce calf blood flow. The latter may be because the arterial vessels of the calf are continuously exposed to much higher pressures during standing because of increased gravitational forces.[27]

CRITICAL CLOSURE

If the perfusion pressure is reduced below the autoregulatory range, the blood flow decreases. When this pressure falls below a critical value of 20 mm Hg to 40 mm Hg, the resistance vessels may close and flow ceases. The pressure at which this occurs is called the critical closing pressure. Critical closure may be explained by the resultant of the pressure difference across the wall (transmural pressure) and the wall tension, as defined by Laplace's law.

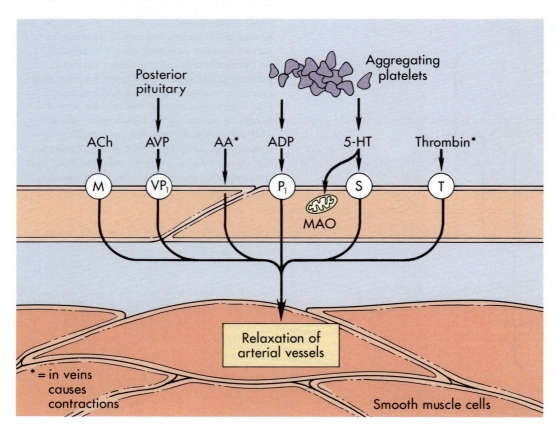

FIGURE 7.2 Formation of vasoactive substance(s) (endothelium-derived relaxing factor(s), or EDRF) by the vascular endothelium. (ACh, acetylcholine; AVP, vasopressin; AA, arachidonic acid; ADP, adenosine diphosphate; 5-HT, 5-hydroxytryptamine (serotonin); M, muscarinic receptor; VP_1, vasopressinergic receptor; P_1, purinergic receptor; S, serotonergic receptor; T, thrombin receptor; MAO, monoamine oxidase)

METABOLIC REGULATION

Changes in the composition of the extracellular fluid as a consequence of metabolic changes in the tissues decrease the activity of precapillary vascular smooth muscle both directly and probably indirectly by altering the output of norepinephrine from the sympathetic nerves. This permits the blood flow to be continuously adjusted to satisfy the metabolic requirements of the tissues. Local metabolic regulation of blood flow is of particular importance in the skeletal muscles because of rapid and large changes in their activity.[24] Hence current knowledge of the metabolic products responsible will be discussed in the section on the skeletal muscles.

ADRENERGIC NERVES

ADRENERGIC NEUROTRANSMISSION

RELEASE OF TRANSMITTER. When action potentials generated in ganglionic cell bodies reach adrenergic nerve endings in the blood vessel wall they activate the entry of extracellular Ca^{2+}. As a consequence, vesicles that contain stored transmitter migrate toward and fuse with the neuronal membrane. The site of fusion ruptures, and norepinephrine is released into the junctional cleft (exocytosis), diffuses to the smooth muscle cells, and activates adrenoceptors on the cell membrane. Although the exocytotic release of norepinephrine is dependent on the entry of Ca^{2+}, Ca^{2+} entry blockers, except at very high concentrations, does not seem to inhibit it, which implies that Ca^{2+} does not enter the neuronal membrane through slow Ca^{2+} channels (Fig. 7.3).

DISPOSITION OF RELEASED TRANSMITTER. Norepinephrine is removed from the junctional cleft by reuptake into adrenergic varicosities (neuronal uptake), overflow to the interstitial space, nonspecific binding to collagen, and uptake by smooth muscle cells. After neuronal uptake, part of the norepinephrine is destroyed by monoamine oxidase but most is returned to the vesicles. After uptake by the smooth muscle, norepinephrine is degraded by catechol-O-methyltransferase and monoamine oxidase (see Fig. 7.2).[1]

CIRCULATING NOREPINEPHRINE. The skeletal muscles form about 45% of the body mass, and the sympathetic nerves to their vessels provide the majority of the circulating norepinephrine. Most of the norepinephrine released from the nerves to the splanchnic vascular bed is metabolized by the liver and the pulmonary endothelium. Plasma levels of norepinephrine frequently are used as an index of sympathetic activity. Such levels are governed by the balance between release of norepinephrine from the sympathetic nerve endings, reuptake into the nerve endings, binding to nonneuronal sites, and extraneuronal catabolism of the amine. Only a small fraction of neuronal-released norepinephrine reaches the circulation so that local variations in sympathetic activity may occur without altering the plasma norepinephrine concentration.[28,29] However, although plasma norepinephrine levels and sympathetic activity to the skeletal muscles vary widely in humans, there is a significant positive correlation between a given subject's level of sympathetic activity and the plasma concentration of norepinephrine.[30] There is, however, no relationship between the mean level of sympathetic nerve activity and that of various blood pressure parameters in normotensive or hypertensive subjects.[31]

POSTJUNCTIONAL ADRENOCEPTORS

The α-adrenoceptors on smooth muscle cells can belong to at least two subtypes, classified as α_1 and α_2. In general, α_1-adrenoceptors predominate on arterial smooth muscle. Although both have been identified in venous smooth muscle the norepinephrine released from the sympathetic nerve endings acts predominantly on the α_2-adrenoceptors.[32-34] Measurements of transmembrane potentials from the smooth muscle cells of the canine saphenous vein suggest that α_1-adrenoceptor activation is a result of electromechanical coupling, whereas α_2-adrenoceptor activation depends on pharmacomechanical coupling.[35,36]

The smooth muscle cells of the resistance vessels of skeletal muscle contain adrenoceptors of the β_2-subtype, which are relatively sensitive to epinephrine and relatively insensitive to norepinephrine. On activation, these receptors cause relaxation of the smooth muscle that is attributable in part to activation, by hyperpolarization, of the enzyme adenylate cyclase located on the cell membrane; the adenyl cyclase

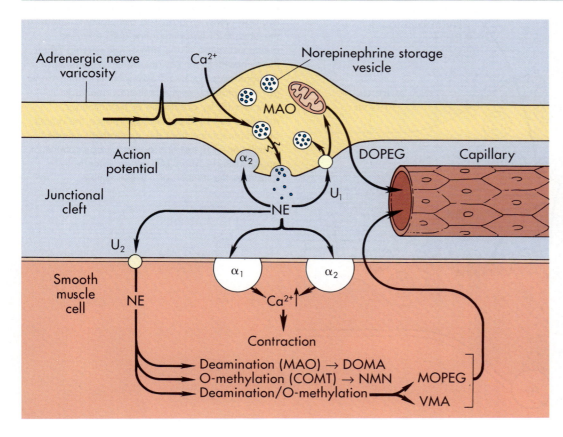

FIGURE 7.3 Release and disposal of the sympathetic neurotransmitter. The nerve impulse (action potential) activates the entry of Ca^{2+} ions into adrenergic nerve varicosities. This causes the norepinephrine-containing vesicles to migrate and fuse with the neuronal membrane, then to rupture and release norepinephrine into the junctional cleft. The norepinephrine (NE) activates α_1- and/or α_2-adrenoceptors on the smooth muscle cells. It may also activate α_2-adrenoceptors on the sympathetic endings and thereby reduce its own release. It is removed by (1) uptake into the nerve endings (U_1) where part of it is enzymatically degraded by the intraneuronal monoamine oxidase (MAO) to 3, 4-dihydroxyphenylglycol (DOPEG), but most is recycled to the storage vesicles; (2) uptake by the effector cells (U_2) and enzymatic degradation by the enzymes monoamine oxidase and catechol-O-methyltransferase (COMT) to 3, 4-dihydroxymandelic acid (DOMA), normetanephrine (NMN), 3-methoxy 4-dihydroxyphenylglycol (MOPEG), and 3-methoxy, 4-hydroxymandelic acid (VMA); and (3) diffusion to the capillaries. The metabolites of norepinephrine are inactive and diffuse to the extracellular fluid and the capillaries.

converts cytoplasmic adenosine triphosphate (ATP) to cyclic 3',5'-adenosine monophosphate (cyclic AMP). The increase in the intracellular cyclic AMP concentration facilitates removal of Ca^{2+}, and/or inhibition of Ca^{2+} influx, and this leads to disengagement of the contractile proteins. These receptors do not appear to be innervated and function primarily as hormone receptors for epinephrine released from the adrenal medulla. Their function in the regulation of muscle blood flow is unexplained. β-Adrenoceptor blockade of the vessels in the muscles does not interfere with the increase in blood flow to these muscles during exercise.[37,38] In fact, the additional blood supplied to the muscles by activation of these receptors with an infusion of epinephrine does not appear to be used for metabolic purposes during exercise.[39]

PREJUNCTIONAL ADRENOCEPTORS

In vitro studies have shown that norepinephrine released from the sympathetic endings can activate α-adrenoceptors of the $α_2$-subtype on prejunctional neuronal cell membranes, thus providing a mechanism for negative feedback on the further release of norepinephrine. $β_2$-Adrenoceptors are also present at this site, and when activated by epinephrine they enhance the exocytotic release of norepinephrine (Fig. 7.4).[40] In human saphenous veins, activation of prejunctional β-adrenoceptors augments the release of neurotransmitter more than in canine saphenous veins. As a consequence, in the human vein, β-adrenergic agonists augment, rather than depress, the contractile response to activation of the adrenergic nerve endings.[41,42]

OTHER PREJUNCTIONAL RECEPTORS

In addition to the $α_2$- and $β_2$-receptors on the sympathetic endings, other receptors have been identified (see Fig. 7.4). These include muscarinic receptors for acetylcholine, which when activated in isolated blood vessels reduce the output of norepinephrine during sympathetic nerve stimulation. Histamine and 5-hydroxytryptamine (serotonin) can also reduce the output of norepinephrine by activation of prejunctional H_2-histaminergic and S_1-serotonergic receptors, respectively.

Angiotensin II augments the vasoconstrictor responses to sympathetic nerve stimulation, in part because it facilitates the release of norepinephrine. The stimulation of adrenergic neurotransmission caused by the octapeptide, combined with the activation of central angiotensin receptor sites, and the facilitation of transmission at the sympathetic ganglia can augment the amount of norepinephrine present in the vicinity of the cardiac and vascular effector cells.

In living animals and humans, the importance of prejunctional regulation of norepinephrine release by any of these receptors, both in physiologic and pathologic conditions, has still to be determined.[40,43]

MODULATION OF NOREPINEPHRINE RELEASE BY METABOLITES

Metabolic acidosis and an increase in K^+ can reduce the output of norepinephrine from the sympathetic nerve endings in the face of a constant frequency of activation of the postganglionic sympathetic fibers, possibly by depressing Ca^{2+} entry into the nerve endings and a consequent inhibition of the exocytotic process. An increase in osmolality also reduces the release of norepinephrine during sympathetic nerve stimulation, as do adenosine and the adenine nucleotides (see Fig. 7.4). The effect of ATP is due to its rapid breakdown to adenosine; as the inhibition is antagonized by theophylline, the receptors mediating the inhibition of norepinephrine released by adenosine can be classified as P_1-purinergic receptors.[44,45]

LOCAL AXON REFLEX

Both in skin and muscle, a local sympathetic axon reflex can be triggered by venous congestion. The receptor site appears to be in small veins in skin, muscle, and subcutaneous adipose tissue and the effector sites in the arterioles supplying these tissues. This axon reflex may be

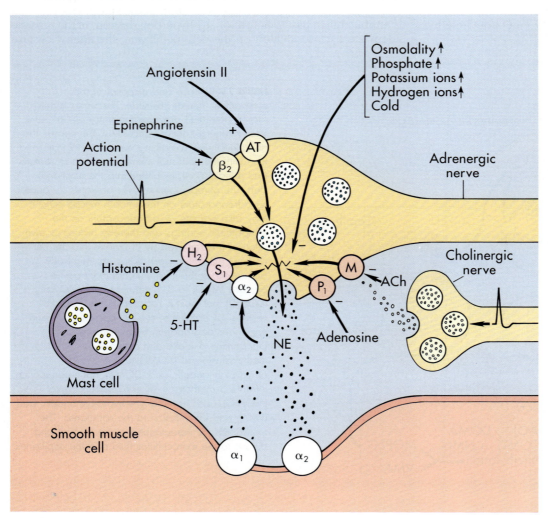

FIGURE 7.4 Alterations of transmitter release at the sympathetic nerve endings in vascular smooth muscle by local metabolic changes and by prejunctional receptors. An increased concentration in the interstitial fluid of adenosine, potassium ions, hydrogen ions, or increased osmolality can reduce the amount of norepinephrine (NE) released during activation of the adrenergic nerves. When the sympathetic nerves are active, stimulation of $α_2$-adrenoceptors by norepinephrine, of muscarinic (M) receptors by acetylcholine, of purinergic receptors (P_1) by adenosine or histaminergic receptors (H_2) by histamine can reduce the output of norepinephrine from the sympathetic nerves. Stimulation of $β_2$-adrenoceptors by epinephrine or angiotensin receptors (AT) by angiotensin II enhances the release of norepinephrine.

an important adjunct to the postural reflexes mediated through the central nervous system so that, on assuming the upright position, the resultant increase in hydrostatic pressure in the veins of the lower limbs causes a local constriction of the resistance vessels.[46,47]

SYMPATHETIC DENERVATION

Immediately following sympathetic neurectomy, the blood flow to normal limbs is increased due to dilatation of skin and muscle resistance vessels. The increased flow to the hand and forearm rapidly subsides to approach the preoperative level within about 2 weeks. In the vessels of the foot, however, the blood flow may remain at about twice the preoperative value. The mechanism by which vessel tone is regained remains obscure. Following preganglionic sympathectomy, nervous connection although absent after surgery is frequently reestablished. Since this takes some months, it is not likely to be the cause of the return of tone. Loss of neuronal uptake, which would increase the concentration of circulating catecholamines, and supersensitivity of the vessels to these amines may contribute. Since in humans tone returns to the vessels of the hands after sympathectomy, even to those that do not exhibit increased sensitivity to epinephrine and norepinephrine, the increase in tone cannot be attributed solely to supersensitivity to these amines.[26]

CHOLINERGIC NERVES

In several species, including the cat and the dog, stimulation of the sympathetic nerves after α-adrenergic blockade causes a transient vasodilatation in skeletal muscle. Since this is blocked by atropine and abolished by sympathectomy, it must be mediated by cholinergic nerves that accompany the sympathetic nerves to the muscle resistance vessels. The vasodilatation might be due to activation of prejunctional muscarinic receptors on the sympathetic nerve terminals, thereby reducing the norepinephrine output, and/or by a postjunctional action on muscarinic receptors on the vascular smooth muscle cells (see Fig. 7.4). The cholinergic nerves to skeletal muscle ordinarily are inactive but can be activated in animals by stimulation of specific hypothalamic areas to cause a defense reaction of fear or rage. Cholinergic vasodilatation has not been found in other species such as the rat or primate. However, in humans cholinergic fibers to the forearm muscles may be activated during emotional stress, fainting (vasovagal syncope), and the Valsalva maneuver and during application of ice to the forehead after α-adrenergic blockade.[26]

SKIN CIRCULATION
ANATOMY

The skin consists of the epidermis, composed of stratified squamous epithelium, and the dermis, composed of connective tissue and blood vessels, lymphatics, receptors, sensory nerves, sweat and sebaceous glands, and hair follicles. In addition to its role as a waterproof and protecting layer, the skin has a vital role in maintaining a normal body temperature. Thus, like the kidney, its blood flow usually far exceeds its small nutritional needs.

There are arteriovenous anastomoses in certain parts of the skin that are characterized by a thick muscular wall and rich sympathetic innervation. They are most numerous in the nail bed but are also present in the palmar surface of the hand and feet and in the ears. They have not been identified in the skin of the forearm or calf. These anastomoses provide a direct connection between the arterioles and the venules in the dermis. When they are open blood can bypass the high resistance arterioles and capillaries of the papillary plexus and be shunted directly to the capacious subpapillary venous plexus. The major fraction of the cutaneous blood volume is contained in the subpapillary venous plexus. During the very high skin blood flow associated with severe heat stress, the increased volume of this venous plexus may lead to a reduction of cardiac filling pressure.[48,49]

THERMOREGULATION
CENTRAL MECHANISMS

One of the principal control mechanisms in thermoregulation is the alteration of the circulation through the skin to govern the rate of heat flow from the body core to the environment (Fig. 7.5). Rapid, nervously mediated changes in skin blood flow provide fine tuning for the control of body temperature. Along with increased sweating this permits effective governance of the core temperature during heat stress. The thermoregulatory effector mechanisms are controlled by receptors in the skin, sensitive to cold and to heat, and by central thermal receptors in the hypothalamus, brain stem, and spinal cord. Some of the thermosensitive nerve endings in the skin travel with the sympathetic nerves to the spinal cord. Thus the body core and the skin are inputs to the thermoregulatory control system.[50] The skin resistance blood vessels and the cutaneous veins respond similarly, dilating with an increase in environmental temperature and constricting with a decrease. The cutaneous venoconstriction with body cooling not only decreases heat loss by decreasing the venous surface area but also directs venous flow through the venae comitantes where transfer of heat from the accompanying artery takes place. Such a countercurrent exchange creates a short-circuit that carries some of the arterial heat back to the body. With body warming the opposite occurs.[51,52]

Since in humans different skin areas have peculiarities in their control mechanisms during body heating, it is convenient to discuss them separately.

HAND AND FOOT. The cutaneous blood vessels in the hand and foot are supplied with sympathetic vasoconstrictor nerves. Interruption of the traffic in these nerves causes an increase in blood flow from control levels of 3 ml to 10 ml/dl of tissue per minute to 30 ml to 40 ml/dl of tissue per minute. There is no evidence for cholinergic nerves to hand blood vessels. In sensitive subjects when severe emotional sweating occurs, part of the vasodilatation in the hands or the feet may be secondary to the vasoactive products released by the activated sweat glands.[48]

FOREARM, UPPER ARM, CALF, AND THIGH. Under uncomfortably cool environmental conditions, interruption of the sympathetic nerve traffic to the skin vessels of the forearm results in a modest increase in skin blood flow. In a comfortably warm subject, this causes little if any change in flow, indicating that under these conditions the forearm skin resistance vessels are not subject to nervous influences. This is in contrast to the skin resistance vessels of the hands and feet, where the flow increases markedly when the sympathetic nervous activity to them is interrupted in comfortably warm subjects. With exposure to a generalized heat stress, the forearm blood flow increases well above the level reached when the cutaneous nerves are blocked with local anesthetic drugs. This increase is due to activation of vasodilator nerves. It is associated with the onset of sweating and can be delayed or reduced by injecting atropine into the brachial artery, indicating that it is due to a cholinergic mechanism. It appears that with sweating an enzyme is released into the tissue spaces from the sweat glands. This enzyme acts on proteins to produce a vasodilator peptide. One possibility is that a bradykinin-forming enzyme is released to form bradykinin and cause the vasodilatation.[26]

The pattern of vasomotor innervation of the skin of the upper arm, calf, and thigh appears similar to that of the forearm skin. Thus the linkage of dilatation to the regulation of sweating, which is induced by cholinergic nerves, and the change from the dominant to the limited control by sympathetic nerves occurs abruptly between the skin of the hands and feet and that of the rest of the limb.[48]

These conclusions from blood flow measurements have been confirmed by direct recordings of sympathetic nerve activity. Microelectrodes have been used to record from cutaneous sympathetic nerves to the hands and feet. The firing in these nerves occurs in bursts. With body cooling the interval between bursts decreases, whereas with body warming it increases. The outflow to both hands and feet is synchronized.[52] When sympathetic nerve activity is recorded simultaneously in human nerves to muscle and skin, there is no relationship in the timing or the amplitude of the bursts of activity. This indicates that the sympathetic ganglia contain at least two different neuronal populations with independent preganglionic inputs. Recordings of sympathetic activity to different skin areas in humans show that the reflex thermoregulatory functions in the distal glabrous skin areas are mediated mainly by the changes in activity of sympathetic vasoconstrictor fibers; sudomotor fibers only become active at relatively high temperatures. By contrast, sudomotor fibers predominate in the thermoregulatory control of the hairy skin on the dorsal side of the forearm and hand.[53,54]

LOCAL MECHANISMS

The responses to thermal stress are governed not only by changes in sympathetic outflow but also by the complex effects of temperature on the neuroeffector junction and vascular smooth muscle itself.[55]

COOLING. When isolated canine cutaneous veins are contracted by potassium ions, the contractions are depressed progressively as the local temperature is decreased. Since potassium causes contraction of vascular smooth muscle cells by depolarizing the cell membrane and increasing the influx of extracellular Ca^{2+}, this indicates that cooling depresses the complex sequence of events leading from depolarization of the cell membrane to activation of the contractile processes in vascular smooth muscle.[56] On the other hand, cooling from a control temperature of 37°C to 20°C to 15°C augments the contractile response to stimulation of the sympathetic nerves to the vein, despite the fact that cold depresses the release of norepinephrine. Earlier studies have suggested that the primary cause of the augmentation is an increased affinity of the postjunctional α-adrenoceptors for the neurotransmitter, with a minor contribution from inhibition of neuronal uptake and enzymatic degradation.[42] However, in calculating the affinity it was assumed that the smooth muscle of the cutaneous vein had a homogeneous population of α-adrenoceptors. The demonstration that this muscle has both α_1- and α_2-adrenoceptors prompted the examination as to whether or not they may be affected differently by cooling.[57] When the α_1-receptors are blocked by prazosin, cooling still augments the contractions to norepinephrine, but not following α_2-adrenoceptor blockade by rauwolscine. Also, cooling can augment the contractions caused by α_2-adrenoceptor agonists but depresses those caused by partial α_1-adrenoceptor agonists. Thus it seems that in the cutaneous veins cooling augments the responsiveness to activation of α_2-adrenoceptors and reduces that of α_1-adrenoceptors (see Fig. 7.5).

Studies of proximal and distal arteries of the human hand and foot, studied within 60 minutes of amputation, have shown that alpha$_2$-adrenoceptors are more prominent on distal arteries.[58] Also, the contractile responses to selective alpha$_2$-adrenoceptor agonists are increased by cooling, whereas those to alpha$_1$-adrenoceptor agonists are not. These studies, together with in vivo observations in healthy humans, support the conclusion that vasoconstriction with local cooling in the digits is mediated predominantly by alpha$_2$-adrenoceptors.[59]

WARMING. It has long been known that local warming of the hands, feet, or forearms causes an increase in blood flow due to relaxation of the resistance blood vessels and of the cutaneous veins.[26] Studies on isolated cutaneous veins have shown that warming directly enhances the contractility of the smooth muscle and does not affect the release of norepinephrine. Warming during stimulation of the sympathetic

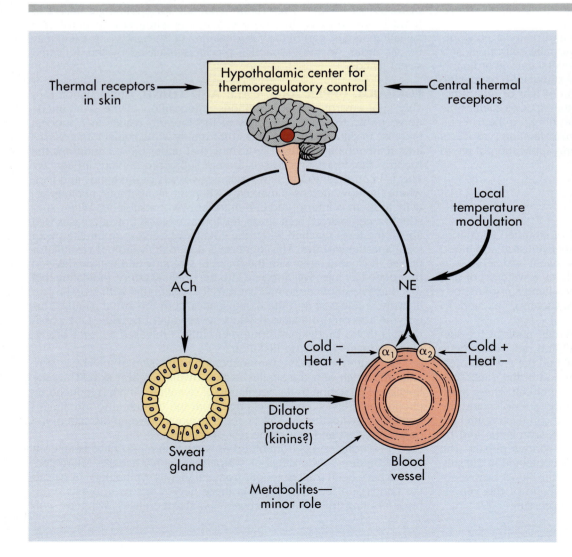

FIGURE 7.5 Resistance vessels in skin. Since the skin blood vessels require little flow to meet their metabolic needs, they are primarily governed by the thermoregulatory mechanisms. An increase in temperature of the thermosensitive cells of the hypothalamus reduces and a decrease augments the activity of the sympathetic nerves to the skin vessels. The norepinephrine (NE) that is released acts primarily on α_2-adrenoceptors on the smooth muscle cells and thus regulates their degree of contraction or relaxation. In a warm environment the release of acetylcholine (ACh) from the nerves to the sweat glands causes the formation of a dilator product(s). In addition, changes in local temperature cause complex changes at the neuroeffector junction and the vascular smooth muscle. Cooling, which decreases the output of norepinephrine, also augments the contractions caused by activation of α_2-adrenoceptors and depresses those caused by partial α_1-adrenoceptor agonists. Warming has little effect on the output of norepinephrine but causes relaxation of the smooth muscle by a specific inhibitory effect on the α_2-adrenoceptors on the smooth muscle.

nerves or administration of exogenous norepinephrine causes relaxation by a specific inhibitory effect on postjunctional α_2-adrenoceptors (see Fig. 7.5).[33]

COLD VASODILATATION

When the human extremities are immersed in water between 0°C and 10°C or 12°C there is a rapid constriction of the skin vessels. Provided the subject is comfortably warm, there is a rapid and marked dilatation of the skin resistance vessels after 5 to 10 minutes, and as exposure to cold continues, alternating periods of constriction and dilatation occur that are referred to as the hunting reaction.[26] This might be explained as follows. When the temperature of the tissue decreases with exposure to cold, the skin vessels constrict because of the increased responsiveness of postjunctional α-adrenoceptors for norepinephrine. As the blood flow decreases and cooling of the tissues continues, the vessels dilate owing to interruption of sympathetic transmission and hence of norepinephrine release and because of the direct inhibitory effect of cold on the smooth muscle cells. As the flow is reestablished the tissues are rewarmed. As soon as a certain temperature is reached, release of norepinephrine is resumed and acts on the sensitized α-adrenoceptors. As a consequence, the vessels constrict again and the cycle is repeated.[55,56]

The magnitude of the cold vasodilatation is inversely related to the sympathetic outflow to the skin vessels. If cold exposure is severe enough to cause the temperature of the body core to decrease, the resultant increased sympathetic activity dampens the cold vasodilatation due to the larger amount of neurotransmitter available to act on the α-adrenoceptors. This helps to preserve heat loss from the extremities but reduces the ability to use the hands for delicate tasks. However, if the core temperature is maintained, the large cold vasodilatation permits their normal function, especially in acclimatized subjects.[26]

REACTIVE HYPEREMIA

When the circulation to the skin is restored after a period of vascular occlusion, there is a rapid increase in blood flow followed by a gradual decline to the resting level. This increased flow is called reactive hyperemia. Current knowledge of the mechanisms involved is discussed in the section on the control of the muscle resistance vessels.

REFLEXES INVOLVING SKIN BLOOD VESSELS

In addition to the nervously induced changes in skin blood flow caused predominantly by thermoregulatory mechanisms, the skin vessels also respond by constricting with emotional stimuli and with respiratory maneuvers. The latter is due to a reflex resulting primarily from activation of receptors in the chest wall leading to a transient increase in sympathetic outflow to the skin resistance vessels and the veins. The skin blood vessels are usually unresponsive to alterations in the activity of the arterial and cardiopulmonary mechanoreceptors. Thus, with the change from the recumbant to the upright position, measurements of blood flow in the upper limbs show that there is no sustained mechanoreceptor-mediated reflex constriction of skin resistance vessels and cutaneous veins.[48] A local axon reflex caused by the increased venous distending pressure may help to maintain a constriction of the resistance vessels in the lower limbs. There is a sustained reflex constriction of the muscle resistance vessels, which together with the constriction of the splanchnic resistance and capacitance vessels acts to maintain the arterial pressure when standing upright.

Recordings from sympathetic nerves to skin and muscle blood vessels in humans reflect the changes observed in blood flow. Thus, in contrast to the sustained activity in sympathetic fibers of muscle nerves in the upright position, there is only a transient response in nerves to the skin.[52,60,61] Only in circumstances in which there is a marked decrease in the activity of the arterial and cardiopulmonary mechanoreceptors does a sustained constriction of cutaneous resistance vessels contribute to the increase in systemic resistance.[48]

INJURY (TRIPLE RESPONSE)

Light stroking of human skin with a blunt instrument can cause a white line to appear on the area stroked that is due to contraction of the vessels that contribute to the color of the skin. Heavy stroking leads to a red line at the site of the stroke due to dilatation of these vessels. This is followed by a flare appearing on either side of the red line that is attributed to local dilatation of the arterioles. Later a wheal appears along the red line, owing to transudation of fluid. This sequence of events, the flare, the red line, and the wheal, is named the triple response. The same phenomenon is seen with local injections of histamine, burns, ultraviolet radiation, cold injury, and antigen–antibody reactions affecting the skin. However, the nature of the chemical mediator(s) involved in the triple response remains to be established.[48]

SKELETAL MUSCLE
EXERCISE HYPEREMIA

Causal connections between the metabolic requirements of muscles and hyperemia during contraction is still not established. A single local metabolic factor that is a universal mediator of functional hyperemia in all the muscles of all species is unlikely. Indeed the evidence seems to support a multifactorial metabolic control system that may vary from one species to another and even in a single species, depending on the type of muscle and on the duration and severity and type of exercise. In addition, the factors that initiate the dilatation may not be those that maintain it. Most studies have been conducted under circumstances in which the flow is not permitted to increase normally during exercise. Thus the mechanism(s) involved may be different when there is an inadequate oxygen supply to the active muscles because of a restricted inflow, as compared with the normal circumstances in which the blood flow increases in proportion to the severity of the exercise. A very brief contraction of the forearm muscles is sufficient to elicit an increase in their blood supply, indicating the efficiency of the dilator mechanism. One possibility is that dilatation of the resistance vessels in the active muscles is the result of a decrease in the local oxygen content to a level insufficient to maintain the contractile process in the vascular smooth muscle cells. However, this has not been substantiated. Rather, the decrease in oxygen content causes the release of vasodilator substances from the active skeletal muscle cells. When the blood flow is not permitted to increase normally during the exercise, it seems that the initial dilatation is due probably to the release of potassium and to hyperosmolarity, with adenosine becoming increasingly important after 10 to 15 minutes (Fig. 7.6).[23,24]

REACTIVE HYPEREMIA

Although a myogenic mechanism contributes to reactive hyperemia in the limbs owing to the decrease in transmural pressure in the resistance vessels during the period of circulatory arrest, the accumulation of metabolites undoubtedly plays the key role. The longer the period of arrest of the circulation the greater is the subsequent hyperemia; the increase is mainly evident in the duration of the high flows, the peak flow being relatively stable. This implicates a vasodilator substance(s) whose concentration increases with time. The reactive hyperemia subsides exponentially in keeping with the washout or conversion of vasodilator metabolites. In addition to the substances described for exercise hyperemia, there is evidence suggesting that the local release of prostaglandins can contribute to the response although they are not the major cause. After prolonged arrest some of the hyperemia may be due to local release of histamine.[24]

The evidence to date suggests that there are both quantitative and qualitative differences in the factors involved in the hyperemia of the skeletal muscles during and after their contraction, and in the hyperemia that follows a period of circulatory arrest. Thus the myogenic response and endogenously formed prostaglandins have a more certain role in reactive hyperemia. However, adenosine and the adenine nucleotides may participate in both.[24]

MECHANICAL HINDRANCE TO BLOOD FLOW

During contraction the blood flow to skeletal muscles depends on the balance between the local metabolic changes causing relaxation of the resistance blood vessels, the architecture of the muscles, the degree of increase in intramuscular pressure causing hindrance to blood flow, and the perfusion pressure during the exercise. With intense exercise of the muscles, both dynamic and static, the metabolic consequences of the mechanical hindrance to flow presumably will cause additional metabolic changes similar to those that occur during arterial occlusion of the blood supply to the limb.

REFLEX CONTROL

At rest, the total flow to the muscles of the human body is about 1.2 liters/min. The blood flow to the resting forearm and calf muscle is 3 ml to 5 ml/dl of tissue/min, and with exercise it may be 10 to 15 times or more this about, owing to the action of local vasodilator metabolites. By contrast, blockade of the sympathetic nerves to the blood vessels of the resting limb muscles results in the twofold to threefold increase in blood flow; when the sympathetic nerves are activated maximally the resting blood flow is decreased to about 75% or more. Thus, as compared with the local mechanisms regulating muscle blood flow, the sympathetic nerves control a relatively small portion of flow capacity of the muscles. However, because of the large proportion of the body mass that is muscle, this permits reflex changes in vascular resistance in the muscles to make contributions to the reflex control of total systemic vascular resistance equivalent to that of the splanchnic and renal circulation.

CAROTID AND AORTIC BAROREFLEXES

Changes in activity of the arterial baroreceptors results in opposite changes in blood flow to the limb muscles. These changes are due to reflex alterations in the caliber of the small arteries and arterioles as a consequence of changes in the amount of norepinephrine released from the sympathetic nerves (see Fig. 7.6). The muscle veins react very weakly if at all. In animals the noradrenergic component of the baroreceptor reflex exerts a greater effect on the vascular bed of skeletal muscle than it does on the splanchnic or renal vessels.[24,62] In humans it seems that the arterial baroreceptors mainly exert a transient control over the muscle resistance vessels. Multi-unit recordings of the sympathetic impulses to the skeletal muscle vessels of the lower limbs show that these are grouped in pulse-synchronous bursts, which occur during a spontaneous reduction in arterial pressure and disappear during spontaneous elevations. The occurrence of bursts correlates with variations of diastolic but not systolic blood pressure; the changes of sympathetic activity per millimeter of mercury of blood pressure change are greater when the blood pressure is decreasing than when it is increasing. Thus acute decreases in arterial blood pressure are buffered more efficiently than acute increases, and variations of sympathetic activity to skeletal muscle are determined mainly by fluctuation in diastolic blood pressure. It appears that the carotid baroreceptors have a greater influence in modulating the vascular resistance in the skeletal muscles during dynamic than during static changes in arterial blood

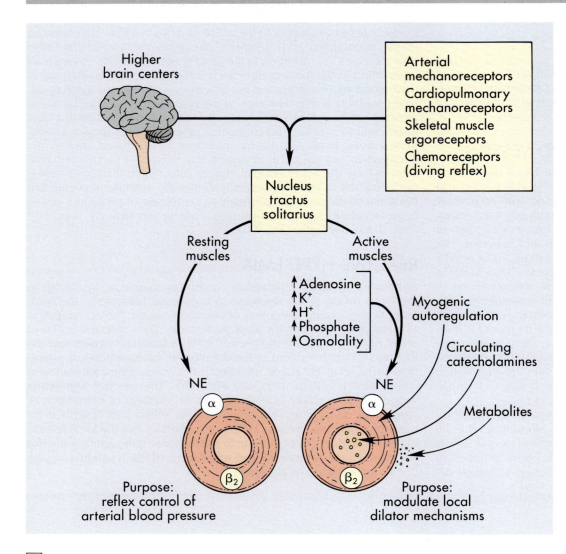

FIGURE 7.6 Regulation of resistance vessels in skeletal muscles. Metabolites play the major role in increasing the blood flow in accordance with metabolic needs during muscular exercise; this is due to their direct relaxing action on the vascular smooth muscle cells of the resistance vessels. They can also act on the sympathetic nerve endings where they decrease the amount of neurotransmitter released, which facilitates the vasodilation. Myogenic mechanisms at the precapillary microvessels help to balance the increase in blood flow and the capillary pressure to prevent edema of the tissues. During upright exercise, the muscle pump has a key role in reducing the venous pressure and hence the capillary pressure in the leg muscles. Because the muscles of the body constitute about 45% of the body mass they play an important role in the regulation of total systemic vascular resistance and hence the regulation of arterial blood pressure.

pressure. The absence of a correlation between static blood pressure levels and the sympathetic activity to skeletal muscle blood vessels implies that static control of arterial blood pressure depends more on the reflex control of other parts of the vascular system.[60] This contrasts to the major influence of receptors in the low-pressure side of the cardiovascular system on the resistance vessels in human skeletal muscles.

REFLEXES FROM HEART AND LUNGS

Procedures that increase intrathoracic blood volume in the human, such as raising the legs of a recumbent subject to the vertical position, negative-pressure breathing, and squatting, result in a reflex vasodilatation due to reduction in adrenergic nerve activity. Alternate positive and negative changes in intrathoracic pressure, which cause large changes in transmural pressure in the thoracic vascular structures without greatly altering mean transmural pressure, result in decreases in muscle vascular resistance. Conversely, procedures that decrease intrathoracic volume, such as tilting to the feet-down position, positive-pressure breathing, and the Valsalva maneuver, cause a reflex constriction of the muscle vessels. It is possible to demonstrate reflex changes in forearm blood flow with procedures such as lower body negative pressure or raising the legs of the recumbent subject before there is any change in arterial pulse pressure, rate of change of arterial pulse pressure, or change in heart rate. This indicates that the reflex changes in muscle blood flow are due primarily to alteration in the afferent traffic to the central nervous system from heart and lung mechanoreceptors and not to changes in carotid and aortic baroreceptor activity (see Fig. 7.6).[24,62]

CAROTID AND AORTIC CHEMOREFLEX

In animals, activation of the carotid and aortic chemoreceptors by decreases in Po_2 and/or increase in Pco_2 and pH leads to constriction of the skeletal muscle resistance vessels. There is no information on the role of the chemoreceptors in controlling the resistance blood vessels in human muscle. This is because it has not been possible to limit the effects of changes in Po_2, Pco_2, and pH solely to these receptors.

DIVING REFLEX

Mammals, including humans, and birds and reptiles can redistribute their circulation during diving. When the head is immersed in water the sensory endings of the trigeminal nerve are activated. This elicits a reflex cessation of breathing, vagally induced bradycardia, and adrenergically induced constriction of systemic resistance vessels in kidneys, skeletal muscles, and the splanchnic region (see Fig. 7.6). The apnea is followed by a decrease in Po_2 and an increase in Pco_2 in the arterial blood, which stimulates the arterial chemoreceptors. The continuous sensory input from the trigeminal nerve overrides the action of the chemoreceptors on the respiratory center. The circulatory effects of chemoreceptor stimulation augment those from the nose and face, leading to further cardiac slowing and constriction of the resistance vessels.[63]

MUSCULAR EXERCISE

During severe rhythmic exercise, particularly during isometric contractions the mean arterial pressure increases owing to a reflex increase in sympathetic outflow to the heart and systemic blood vessels. Thus, in spite of the marked vasodilatation in the exercising muscles the reflex constriction of other vascular beds permits the arterial pressure to increase. This is particularly helpful during isometric exercise where the increase in pressure may help to overcome the mechanical hindrance to blood flow to the active muscles. The rise in arterial pressure is reflexly mediated primarily by a central command from the cerebral cortex increasing the sympathetic outflow in proportion to the effort of the exercise, and by "ergoreceptors" in the exercising muscles, presumably owing to the action of metabolic products activating afferent fibers to the central nervous system that results in a reflex increase in sympathetic outflow (see Fig. 7.6). There follows an increase in resistance to flow in the vascular beds outside the active muscles, with the exception of the brain, and a constriction of the splanchnic capacitance vessels. The latter aids to maintain the filling pressure of the ventricles. The arterial baroreceptors are reset rapidly during exercise so that they continue to operate in the same manner but around a higher mean pressure.[64]

At the beginning of exercise the sympathetic control of the resistance vessels in the active muscles is lessened (functional sympatholysis). The mechanism by which this occurs is still debated. It is possible that the products of muscle metabolism that cause the dilatation of the resistance vessels in the active muscles also signal the afferent information that increases the sympathetic outflow and hence the blood pressure during exercise and at the same time reduces the output of norepinephrine from the sympathetic nerve terminals to the muscle resistance vessels by a prejunctional action (see Fig. 7.6). The other possibility is that these products of metabolism may alter the reaction between the norepinephrine released and the adrenoceptors on the vascular smooth muscle. After the initial period of sympatholysis, the sympathetic nerves operate again to adjust the blood flow to the active muscles in order to maintain the most economical ratio of blood flow to oxygen consumption.[65,66]

☐ LIMB VEINS
CUTANEOUS VEINS

Cutaneous veins are richly innervated by sympathetic noradrenergic nerves and have plenty of smooth muscle in their walls. The hypothalamic thermoregulatory centers dominate their neurogenic control and as the temperature of the body core is lowered the sympathetic outflow is increased selectively to these vessels and vice-versa. This neurogenic control is reinforced by the local effect of temperature. Local cooling augments and local warming depresses the cutaneous venomotor reactions to adrenergic nerve stimulation. These local responses are not due to alterations of neurotransmitter release but to actions of local temperature changes on the α-adrenoceptors on the smooth muscle cells.

A deep breath causes a transient reflex constriction of the cutaneous veins. This is a spinal reflex probably resulting from activation of receptors in the chest wall or diaphragm. Emotional stimuli also activate the noradrenergic nerves to the cutaneous veins. By contrast, the arterial baroreceptors and the cardiopulmonary receptors appear to exert little if any control of the cutaneous veins (Fig. 7.7).[51]

MUSCLE VEINS

The veins in the skeletal muscles have little or no sympathetic innervation, and the main factor contributing to the volume of blood in these veins is the muscle pump, especially in the leg veins in humans in the upright position (see Fig. 7.7). With each contraction of the leg muscles during rhythmic upright exercise, the mechanical compression and the resulting increase in intraluminal pressure in the deep veins causes them to empty. When the muscles relax, the intraluminal pressure in these veins decreases rapidly below that in the cutaneous veins so that blood flows to the latter. The emptying of the veins during and after the contraction restores the competence of the valves, so that the long hydrostatic column is broken into shorter segments and the pressure in the cutaneous veins is decreased. The decrease of the venous pressure increases the pressure differences between the arteries and veins and thus augments the blood flow through the lower limb. With a change from the supine to the standing position, the cardiac output and the volume of blood in the heart and lungs decreases by about 20% and the stroke volume is reduced. Exercise of the leg muscles restores the central blood volume and augments the filling pressure of the heart and hence the stroke volume.[51] When the valves of the leg veins are congenitally absent or damaged by thrombosis, there is an exaggerated pooling of blood in the upright position. During exercise the ability to displace blood from the legs is impaired so that the stroke volume and cardiac output do not increase normally.[67]

DISEASES AFFECTING LIMB BLOOD VESSELS
CONGESTIVE HEART FAILURE

In severe congestive heart failure, the circulating catecholamines and angiotensin II are increased due to increased sympathetic outflow to the renal and splanchnic vessels and the adrenal medulla. This helps to maintain the arterial blood pressure despite the reduced cardiac output. The primary cause of the increased neurohumoral excitation is the reduced ability of the arterial and cardiopulmonary mechanoreceptors to inhibit the vasomotor centers and hence the sympathetic outflow. During exercise, at the same workload as healthy subjects, the reflex constriction of the resistance vessels in these vascular beds and in the nonexercising muscles is exaggerated. Thus the limited increase in cardiac output is preferentially directed to the active muscles. The circulation to the brain and heart is relatively well preserved. The exaggerated reflex vasoconstriction may be due to a combination of the reduced inhibition of the vasomotor centers by the mechanoreceptors and a decreased ability of the resistance vessels in the active muscles to dilate. The latter would result in an increased activation of receptors in the muscle by the greater accumulation of metabolic products. These so-called ergoreceptors, when activated, cause a marked reflex increase in sympathetic outflow. In contrast to the dilatation of the skin vessels in normal subjects during prolonged exercise to permit loss of body heat, a constriction of these vessels often occurs in patients with heart failure, despite the needs for thermoregulation. The resulting failure to dissipate heat effectively is a further hazard to these patients.[68]

Abnormalities are also present in the local control of the circulation. This is most evident in the decreased ability of the resistance vessels in the skeletal muscles to dilate in response to the local metabolic stimulus of exercise or to a period of circulatory arrest. This results from an increased stiffness of the vessels as a consequence of their increased sodium content and of the interstitial edema. The edema also reduces the compliance of the limb veins.[68]

Studies on isolated systemic blood vessels have demonstrated that the cardenolides cause a release of norepinephrine from the sympathetic nerve endings.[69] This, rather than a direct effect on the vascular smooth muscle, is the primary cause of the contraction of the vascular smooth muscle. In normal humans digitalis causes an increase in arterial and venous tone, whereas in patients with heart failure the tone is decreased. It seems that, as a consequence of the improved cardiac performance by the drug, the enhanced sympathetic outflow is reduced and that this predominates over the local constrictor actions of the glycoside.[68] All the factors involved in causing the decreased sympathetic activity have still to be elucidated.

VASOSPASTIC DISORDERS

In susceptible subjects spasm of the digital arteries can be precipitated by cold exposure. Emotional disturbances are often contributory. However, the cause(s) is still undetermined. Patients without discernable other diseases that might contribute are referred to as having idiopathic or primary Raynaud's disease while those in whom it is a manifestation of several underlying disorders are said to have Raynaud's phenomenon. These secondary causes include connective tissue diseases, obstructive arterial diseases, neurologic disorders, and blood dyscrasias such as a high serum titer of cold agglutinins. Prolonged exposure to vibrating tools or certain drugs may also cause the phenomenon.[70]

While patients with idiopathic Raynaud's disease may have hand blood flows as large as normal subjects during local heating of the hands to 42°C, this does not imply that the distribution of flow within the digits is the same. Heating such patients in a 28°C environment increases arteriovenous shunt flow in the fingertip to normal values, but the capillary flow is lower than normal.[71]

Many suggestions have been made as to the cause of Raynaud's disease (Fig. 7.8). One factor is the intravascular pressure. For unknown reasons the digital blood pressure is lower than normal in patients with Raynaud's disease. This lower distending pressure would favor a greater decrease in vessel caliber even with a normal constrictor response to local cooling.[70] Any organic obstruction to the vessels, causing a lower pressure in the digital arteries, as occurs in certain types of Raynaud's phenomenon, could also contribute to the vasospastic attacks.

By contrast, in patients with serum cryoproteinemias or cold agglutinins, the aggregation of the red blood cells with digital cooling can result in mechanical obstruction to flow.[26]

In patients with Raynaud's disease, the β-adrenergic agonist isoproterenol decreases blood flow in the extremities. This could be due

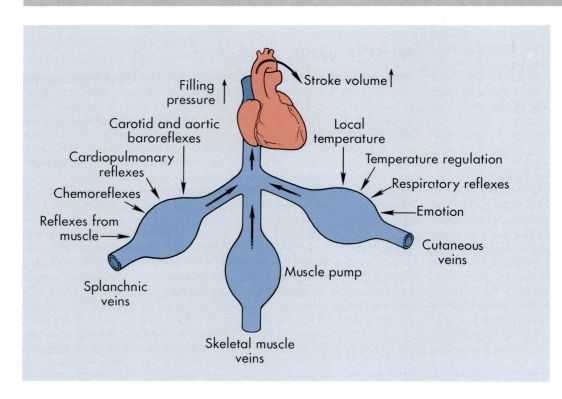

FIGURE 7.7 The regulation of the three major components of the systemic venous system: the splanchnic, skeletal muscle, and cutaneous veins. These components adjust the intrathoracic blood volume and hence the filling pressure of the heart by active expulsion of blood due to contraction of the venous smooth muscle and by passive expulsion due to a decrease in venous distending pressure resulting from constriction of the precapillary resistance vessels. The active expulsion of blood from the splanchnic venous bed is controlled primarily by the cardiovascular reflexes, while that from the cutaneous veins is governed mainly by local and central changes in temperature, by respiratory reflexes, and by emotion. The veins of the skeletal muscles have little or no sympathetic innervation, and are emptied passively by the pumping action of the skeletal muscles. (Modified from Shepherd JT: La Régulation de Système Veineux. Phlebologie 1:25, 1984)

to activation of presynaptic β-adrenoceptors and a resulting increase in the output of norepinephrine. Following an emotional stimulus, circulating epinephrine might activate these receptors and cause the digital vasoconstriction.[72] However, in patients with idiopathic Raynaud's disease stressful mental arithmetic causes a dilatation of fingertip resistance vessels.[73]

In patients with primary Raynaud's disease, but not in those with obstructive Raynaud's syndrome, the platelet α_2-adrenoceptor levels are elevated.[74] This suggests that there could be an increased number of these receptors on the digital arteries in Raynaud's disease, which would be consistent with Lewis's original postulation of a local cause.[27]

$5HT_2$-Serotonergic receptors also are present in the vasculature of the digits,[75] and patients with primary Raynaud's disease have increased circulating and platelet serotonin. In cutaneous arteries of the dog, cooling augments the contraction induced by autologous aggregating platelets, due to enhanced response to released 5-hydroxytryptamine. Thus, serotonin receptor activation may be another mechanism of vasoconstriction in raynaud's disease (Fig. 7.8).

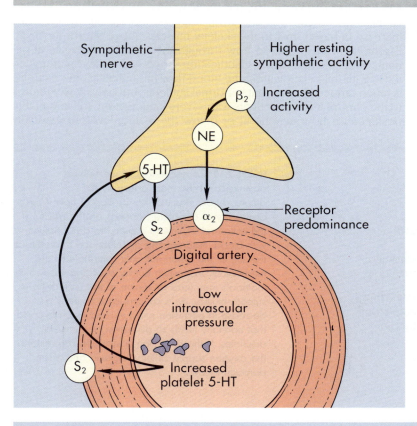

FIGURE 7.8 Possible mechanisms for digital vasospastic attacks in patients with idiopathic Raynaud's disease.

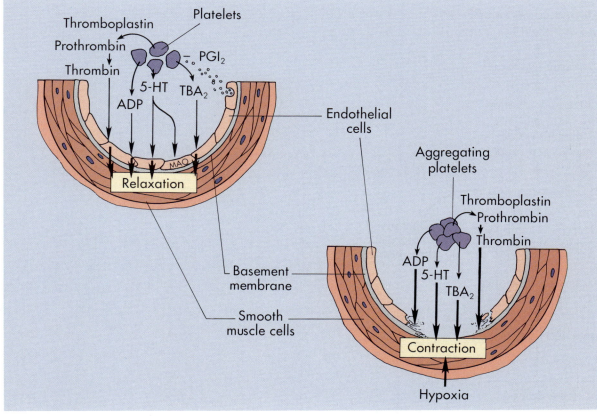

FIGURE 7.9 (*Top*) Role of the normal endothelium in causing relaxation of the underlying smooth muscle when exposed to substances released from aggregating platelets or formed in the coagulation process. (*Bottom*) When the endothelium is damaged these same substances cause vasoconstriction by their direct action on the vascular smooth muscle. (*ADP*, adenosine diphosphate; *5-HT*, 5-hydroxytryptamine; TBA_2, thromboxane A_2; PGI_2, prostacyclin; *MAO*, monoamine oxidase) (Modified from Shepherd JT, Vanhoutte PM: Spasm of the coronary arteries: Causes and consequences (the scientist's viewpoint). Mayo Clinic Proc 60:33, 1985)

Under resting conditions in a comfortable environment, the hand blood flow in healthy young females is lower than that of a control group of males. However, after total body warming, the hand blood flow in the women exceeded that in the men, indicating that the lower basal flow in women was due to increased sympathetic outflow to the extremities.[76]

Raynaud's disease is much more common in women. This would be consistent with the high resting sympathetic activity and the resultant greater wall tension in the digital arteries facilitating critical closure of these vessels. This would be consistent with Raynaud's postulate in 1812 that there is overactivity of the vasomotor nerves in these patients.[27]

Whether the endothelium in the digital vessels of patients with Raynaud's disease is capable of forming EDRF and prostacyclin has yet to be determined. Hyperfibrinogenemia may be present, even in primary Raynaud's phenomenon, and it is suggested that this might be secondary to endothelial injury.[77] It is possible that either as a consequence of an inherent defect, or because of repeated episodes of asphyxia, the endothelium might lose its ability to produce EDRF and prostacyclin, while retaining its ability to form vasoconstrictor autacoids. If it is damaged, and serotonin is released from aggregating platelets in the absence of the enzyme monoamine oxidase, this can not only cause constriction of the smooth muscle, but also be taken up by the sympathetic nerve endings and subsequently released along with norepinephrine to enhance the nervously induced vasoconstrictions.[78]

ATHEROSCLEROSIS OBLITERANS

Intermittent claudication is the early sign of atherosclerosis in limb vessels, since even a gentle stroll requires about a six to ten times increase in blood flow to the skeletal muscles above the resting level. Examination of the blood flow through the calf after exercise in patients with mild and severe claudication shows two distinct patterns. In those with mild claudication the blood flow immediately after exercise is much reduced below that in normal subjects and only slowly returns to the control level. In patients with severe claudication, the immediate postexercise flow may be at or below the resting level, to gradually

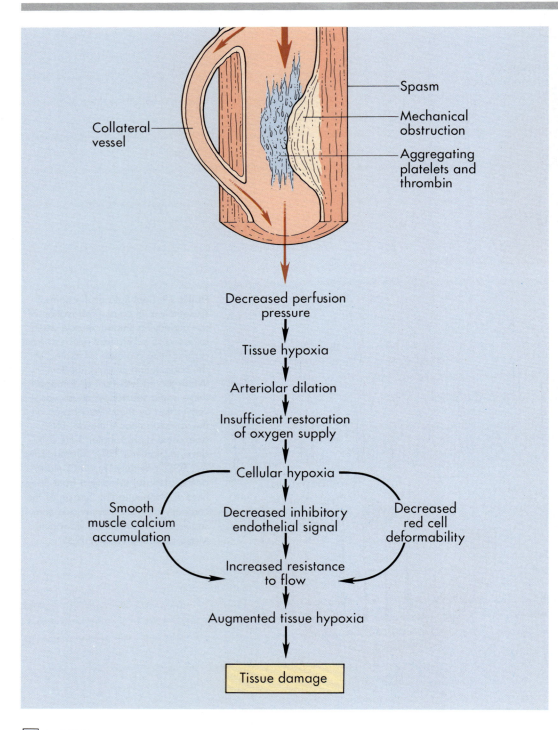

FIGURE 7.10 Consequences of mechanical obstruction of the main artery by the atherosclerotic process. Restoration of flow if the obstruction is complete depends on the ability of the collateral vessels to supply the distal tissues with blood. Aggregating platelets and thrombin at the site of the lesion not only contribute to the mechanical obstruction but by releasing vasoactive materials may lead to spasm of the underlying smooth muscle. As a consequence there is a decrease in perfusion pressure and tissue hypoxia that normally leads to dilatation of the distal arterioles. If this dilatation is insufficient to restore the oxygen supply, cellular hypoxia and tissue damage follows.

increase over the subsequent 10 or 15 minutes, peak at two or three times the resting level, and then very slowly subside. This illustrates the importance of the "steal phenomenon" in which the proximal part of the limb gets the limited amount of available blood before the more distal parts are satisfied. In patients with severe claudication the blood flow in the foot drops to zero immediately after exercise, to recover only when the metabolic requirements of the calf are satisfied. This accounts for the absence of pedal pulses after exercise. The steal of blood by the muscles helps to explain the frequent occurrence of necrotic lesions in more distal parts of the skin. A reduction of blood flow to the skin due to the mechanical obstruction is facilitated by the lower temperature of the limb with atherosclerosis, which tends to augment the constriction of the skin blood vessels.[26]

Many factors contribute to the deprivation of flow in limbs with obstructive vascular disease. The primary factor is the degree of mechanical occlusion caused by the atherosclerotic lesion, which determines the pressure drop across it. If this is large, the distending pressure in the resistance vessels distal to the lesion may decrease to the extent that critical closure occurs. Also, at the site of the lesion Bernouilli's principle is relevant. This states that transformation from potential energy (pressure) into kinetic energy (velocity) occurs when the cross-sectional area of the vascular system decreases. In arteries narrowed by atheroma, the velocity of flow through the stenotic area is increased and the radial pressure is reduced. Thus the stenosis is self-perpetuating. At the site of atheromatous plaques, the pressure at the edge of the plaque may be much greater than the pressure incident to its surface, thus predisposing to the shearing off of plaque material and the development of thromboembolism.[3]

At the site of the lesion, whether in systemic, coronary, or cerebral arteries, the damage to the endothelium may have an important role in determining the outcome (Fig. 7.9). The diminished secretion of prostacyclin at the site of damage favors platelet aggregation, with a resultant release of 5-hydroxytryptamine and thromboxane A_2. If any thrombin is formed, this, too, may enhance the constriction of the smooth muscle. The tissue hypoxia that follows the vasoconstriction may prevent any endothelium still intact from forming relaxing factor(s). Of interest is the fact that the endothelium of the veins may respond differently to that of the arteries to certain vasoactive substances. For example, thrombin causes an endothelium-dependent contraction of systemic veins.[79]

The sequence of events that may follow the mechanical obstruction of a major artery is shown in Figure 7.10. It emphasizes that the flow depends on the ability of the collateral vessels to bypass the obstruction and to deliver sufficient blood for the metabolism of the tissues. Unfortunately, because of their high resistance to flow, the ability to do so is limited. Spasm may cause a further decrease in blood flow and in perfusion pressure distal to the lesion. If the resultant metabolic dilatation of the distal resistance vessels is insufficient to compensate, the oxygen supply to the tissues will decrease and tissue hypoxia follows. This leads to a decrease in the ability of the endothelium to produce vasodilator substance(s); accumulation of Ca^{2+} of the vascular smooth muscle, leading to constriction of the blood vessels; and reduction in red blood cell deformability with the resultant increased viscosity.[80] These combine to augment peripheral resistance and further reduce blood flow, with a resultant increase in tissue hypoxia and tissue damage.

REFERENCES

1. Shepherd JT, Vanhoutte PM: The Human Cardiovascular System: Facts and Concepts. New York, Raven Press, 1979
2. Vanhoutte PM, Shepherd JT: Autonomic nerves to the systemic blood vessels. In Dyck PJ, Thomas PK, Lambert EH et al (eds): Peripheral Neuropathy, vol I, pp 301–326. Philadelphia, WB Saunders, 1984
3. McGrath MA: Dynamics of the peripheral circulation. Int Angiol 3:315, 1984
4. Tang S-S, Stevenson L, Dzau VJ: Endothelial renin-angiotensin pathway. Adrenergic regulation of angiotensin secretion. Circ Res 66:103, 1990
5. Chesterman CN: Vascular endothelium, hemostasis and thrombosis. Blood Reviews 2:88, 1988
6. Luskutoff DJ: The fibrinolytic system of cultured endothelial cells: Insights in the role of endothelium in thrombolysis. In Gimbrone M (ed): Vascular Endothelium in Hemostasis and Thrombosis, pp 129–141. Edinburgh, Churchill Livingstone, 1986
7. Gryglewski RJ, Botting RM, Vane JR: Mediators produced by the endothelial cell. Hypertension 12:530, 1988
8. Furchgott RF: Studies on relaxation of rabbit aorta by sodium nitrite: The basis for the proposal that the acid-activatable inhibitory factor from bovine retractor penis is inorganic nitrite and the endothelium-derived relaxing factor is nitric oxide. In Vanhoutte PM (ed): Vasodilatation, pp 4:401–14. New York, Raven Press, 1988
9. Ignarro LJ, Byrns RE, Wood KS: Biochemical and pharmacological properties of endothelium-derived relaxing factor and its similarity to nitric oxide radical. In Vanhoutte PM (ed): Vasodilatation: Vascular Smooth Muscle, Peptides, Autonomic Nerves, Endothelium, pp 427–436. New York, Raven Press, 1988
10. Palmer RMJ, Ferrige AG, Moncada S: Nitric oxide release accounts for the biological activity of endothelium-derived relaxing factor. Nature 327:524, 1987
11. Palmer RMJ, Ashton DS, Moncada S: Vascular endothelial cells synthesize nitric oxide from L-arginine. Nature 333:664, 1988
12. Feletou M, Vanhoutte PM: Endothelium-dependent hyperpolarization of canine coronary smooth muscle. Brit J Pharmacol 93:515–524, 1988
13. Taylor SG, Weston AH: Endothelium-derived hyperpolarizing factor: A new endogenous inhibitor from the vascular endothelium. Tr Pharm Sci 9:272, 1988
14. Katusic ZS, Shepherd JT, Vanhoutte PM: Vasopressin causes endothelium-dependent relaxation of the canine basilar artery. Circ Res 55:575, 1984
15. Radomski MW, Palmer RMJ, Moncada S: Endogenous nitric oxide inhibits human platelet adhesion to vascular endothelium. Lancet 2:1057, 1987
16. Sneddon JM, Vane JR: Endothelium-derived relaxing factor reduces platelet adhesion to bovine endothelial cells. Proc Natl Acad Sci USA 85:2800, 1988
17. Furchgott RF, Vanhoutte PM: Endothelium-derived relaxing and contracting factors. FASEB J 3:2007, 1989
18. Vanhoutte PM, Shimokawa H: Endothelium-derived relaxing factor and coronary vasospasm. Circulation 80:1, 1989
19. Rubanyi GM, Vanhoutte PM: Hypoxia releases a vasoconstrictor substance from the canine vascular endothelium. J Physiol (London) 364:45, 1985
20. Katusic ZS, Vanhoutte PM: Superoxide anion is an endothelium-derived contracting factor. Amer J Physiol (H Circ Physiol) 257:H33, 1989
21. Yanagisawa M, Inoue A, Ishikawa T et al: A novel potent vasoconstrictor peptide produced by vascular endothelial cells. Nature 332:411, 1988
22. Johnson PC: The myogenic response. In Bohr DF, Somlyo AP, Sparks HV Jr (eds): Handbook of Physiology, Section 2, The Cardiovascular System, Vol II, Vascular Smooth Muscle, pp 409–442. Bethesda, MD, American Physiologic Society, 1980
23. Dobrin PB: Vascular mechanics. In Shepherd JT, Abboud FM (eds): Handbook of Physiology, Section 2, The Cardiovascular System, Vol III, Peripheral Circulation and Organ Blood Flow, part I, pp 65–102. Bethesda, MD, American Physiologic Society, 1983
24. Sparks HV Jr: Effect of local metabolic factors on vascular smooth muscle. In Bohr DF, Somlyo AD, Sparks HV Jr (eds): Handbook of Physiology, Section 2, The Cardiovascular System, Vol II, Vascular Smooth Muscle, pp 475–513. Bethesda, MD, American Physiologic Society, 1980
25. Shepherd JT: Circulation to skeletal muscle. In Shepherd JT, Abboud FM (eds): Handbook of Physiology, Section 2, The Cardiovascular System, Vol III, Peripheral Circulation and Organ Blood Flow, part 1, pp 319–370. Bethesda, MD, American Physiologic Society, 1983
26. Busse R, Trogisch G, Bassenge E. The role of endothelium in control of vascular tone. Basic Res Cardiol 30:475, 1985
27. Shepherd JT: Physiology of the Circulation in Human Limbs in Health and Disease. Philadelphia, WB Saunders, 1963
28. Brown MJ, Jenner DA, Allison KJ et al: Variations in individual organ release of noradrenaline measured by an improved radioenzymatic technique: Limitations of peripheral venous measurements in the assessment of sympathetic nervous activity. Clin Sci 585, 1981
29. Fitzgerald GA: Peripheral presynaptic adrenoceptor regulation of norepinephrine release in humans. Fed Proc 43:1379, 1984
30. Wallin BG, Sundlöf G, Lindblad L-E: Baroreflex mechanisms controlling sympathetic outflow to the muscles in man. In Sleight P (ed): Arterial Baroreceptors and Hypertension, pp 101–107. Oxford, England, Oxford University Press, 1980
31. Wallin GB, Sundlöf G: A quantitative study on muscle nerve sympathetic activity in resting normotensive and hypertensive subjects. Hypertension 1:67, 1979
32. DeMey J, Vanhoutte PM: Uneven distribution of postjunctional alpha$_1$- and alpha$_2$-like adrenoreceptors in canine arterial and venous smooth muscle. Circ Res 48:875, 1981
33. Flavahan NA, Rimele TJ, Cooke JP et al: Characterization of postjunctional alpha$_1$- and alpha$_2$-adrenoceptors activated by exogenous or nerve-released

34. Cooke JP, Shepherd JT, Vanhoutte PM: The effect of warming on adrenergic neurotransmission in canine cutaneous vein. Circ Res 54:547, 1984
35. Matthews WD, Jim KF, Hieble JP et al: Post-synaptic alpha-adrenoceptors on vascular smooth muscle. Fed Proc 43:2923, 1984
36. Fowler PJ, Grous M, Price W et al: Pharmacological differentiation of post-synaptic alpha-adrenoceptors in the dog saphenous vein. J Pharmacol Exp Ther 229:712, 1984
37. Hartling OJ, Noer I, Svendsen TL et al: Selective and non-selective beta-adrenoceptor blockade in the human forearm. Clin Sci 58:279, 1980
38. Julin-Dannfelt A, Åström H: Influence of beta-adrenoceptor blockade on leg blood flow and lactate release in man. Scand J Clin Lab Invest 39:179, 1979
39. Marshall RJ, Shepherd JT: Effects of epinephrine on cardiovascular and metabolic responses to leg exercise in man. J Appl Physiol 18:1118, 1963
40. Shepherd JT, Vanhoutte PM: Local modulation of adrenergic neurotransmission. Circulation 64:655, 1981
41. Vanhoutte PM, Shepherd JT: Muscarinic and beta-adrenergic prejunctional modulation of adrenergic neurotransmission in the blood vessel wall. Gen Pharmacol 14:35, 1983
42. Verbeuren TJ, Lorenz RR, Aarhus LL et al: Prejunctional beta-adrenoceptors in human and canine saphenous veins. J Auton Nerv Syst 8:261, 1983
43. Vanhoutte PM, Verbeuren TJ, Webb RC: Local modulation of adrenergic neuroeffector interaction in the blood vessels wall. Physiol Rev 61:151, 1981
44. Verhaeghe RH, Lorenz RR, McGrath MA et al: Metabolic modulation of neurotransmitter release-adenosine, adenine nucleotides, potassium, hyperosmolarity, and hydrogen ion. Fed Proc 37:208, 1978
45. DeMey J, Burnstock G, Vanhoutte PM: Modulation of the evoked release of noradrenaline in canine saphenous vein via presynaptic receptors for adenosine but not ATP. Eur J Pharmacol 55:401, 1979
46. Henriksen O: Local sympathetic reflex mechanism in regulation of blood flow in human subcutaneous tissue. Acta Physiol Scand Suppl 450:100, 1977
47. Henriksen O, Sejrsen P: Local reflex in microcirculation in human skeletal muscle. Acta Physiol Scand 99:19, 1977
48. Roddie IC: Circulation to skin and adipose tissue. In Shepherd JT, Abboud FM (eds): Handbook of Physiology, Section 2, The Cardiovascular System, Vol III, Peripheral Circulation and Organ Blood Flow, part 1, pp 285–317. Bethesda, MD, American Physiologic Society, 1983
49. Rowell LB: Cardiovascular adjustments to thermal stress. In Shepherd JT, Abboud FM (eds): Handbook of Physiology, Section 2, The Cardiovascular System, Vol III, Peripheral Circulation and Organ Blood Flow, part 2, pp 967–1023. Bethesda, MD, American Physiologic Society, 1983
50. Hellon RF: Thermoreceptors. In Shepherd JT, Abboud FM, (eds): Handbook of Physiology, Section 2, The Cardiovascular System, Vol III, Peripheral Circulation and Organ Blood Flow, part 2, pp 659–673. Bethesda, MD, American Physiologic Society, 1983
51. Shepherd JT, Vanhoutte PM: Veins and Their Control. Philadelphia, WB Saunders, 1975
52. Hagbarth K-E, Hallin RG, Hongell A et al: General characteristics of sympathetic activity in human skin nerves. Acta Physiol Scand 84:164, 1972
53. Bini G, Hagbarth K-E, Hynninen P et al: Thermoregulatory and rhythm-generating mechanisms governing the sudomotor and vasoconstrictor outflow in human nerves. J Physiol (Lond) 306:537, 1980
54. Bini G, Hagbarth K-E, Hynninen P et al: Regional similarities and differences in thermoregulatory vaso- and sudomotor tone. J Physiol (Lond) 306:553, 1980
55. Shepherd JT, Rusch NJ, Vanhoutte PM: Effect of cold on the blood vessel wall. Gen Pharmacol 14:61, 1983
56. Rusch NJ, Shepherd JT, Vanhoutte PM: The effect of profound cooling on adrenergic neurotransmission in canine cutaneous veins. J Physiol (Lond) 311:57, 1981
57. Vanhoutte PM, Cooke JP, Lindblad L-E et al: Modulation of postjunctional α-adrenergic responsiveness by local changes in temperature. Clin Sci 68(suppl 10):121s, 1985
58. Flavahan NA, Cooke JP, Shepherd JT, Vanhoutte PM: Human postjunctional alpha$_1$ and alpha$_2$-adrenoceptors: Differential distribution in arteries of the limbs. J Pharmacol Exp Therap 241:361, 1987
59. Ekenvall L, Lindblad LE, Norbeck O, Etzell B-M: Alpha-adrenoceptors and cold-induced vasoconstriction in human finger skin. Amer J Physiol (H Circ Physiol) 24:H1000, 1988
60. Wallin GB, Sundlöf G, Delius W: The effect of carotid sinus nerve stimulation on muscle and skin nerve sympathetic activity in man. Pfluegers Arch 358:101, 1975
61. Burke D, Sandlöf G, Wallin BG: Postural effects on muscle nerve sympathetic activity in man. J Physiol (Lond) 272:399, 1977
62. Donald DE, Shepherd JT: Reflexes from the heart and lungs: Physiological curiosities or important regulatory mechanisms. Cardiovasc Res 12:449, 1978
63. Blix AS, Folkow B: Cardiovascular adjustments to diving in mammals and birds. In Shepherd JT, Abboud FM (eds): Handbook of Physiology, Section 2, The Cardiovascular System, Vol III, Peripheral Circulation and Organ Blood Flow, part 2, pp 917–945. Bethesda, MD, American Physiological Society, 1983
64. Walgenbach SC, Shepherd JT: Role of arterial and cardiopulmonary mechanoreceptors in the regulation of arterial pressure during rest and exercise in conscious dogs. Mayo Clinic Proc 59:467, 1984
65. Strandell T, Shepherd JT: The effect in humans of increased sympathetic activity on the blood flow to active muscles. Acta Medica Scandinavica Suppl 472:146, 1967
66. Joyner MJ, Lennon RL, Wedel DJ, Rose SH, Shepherd JT: Blood flow to contracting human muscles: Influence of increased sympathetic activity. J Applied Physiol 68:1453–1457, 1990
67. Bevegård BS, Lodin A: Postural circulatory changes at rest and during exercise in five patients with congenital absence of valves in the deep veins of the legs. Acta Med Scand 172:21, 1962
68. Zelis R, Longhurst J: The circulation in congestive heart failure. In Zelis R (ed): The Peripheral Circulations, pp 282–314. New York, Grune & Stratton, 1975
69. Aarhus LL, Shepherd JT, Tyce GM et al: Contractions of canine vascular smooth muscle cells caused by ouabain are due to release of norepinephrine from adrenergic nerve endings. Circ Res 52:502, 1983
70. Cohen RA, Coffman JD: Digital vasospasm: The pathophysiology of Raynaud's phenomenon. Int Angiol 3:47, 1984
71. Coffman JD, Cohen AS: Total and capillary fingertip blood flow in Raynaud's phenomenon. N Engl J Med 285:259, 1971
72. Giovanni B, Giuseppina CM, Susanna F et al: Altered regulator mechanisms of presynaptic nerve: A new physiopathological hypothesis in Raynaud's disease. Microvasc Res 27:191, 1984
73. Halperin JL, Cohen RA, Coffman JD: Digital vasodilatation during mental stress in patients with Raynaud's disease. Cardiovasc Res 17:671, 1983
74. Keenan EJ, Porter JM: α-Adrenergic receptors in platelets from patients with Raynaud's syndrome. Surgery 94:204, 1983
75. Coffman JD, Cohen RA: Serotonergic vasoconstriction in human fingers during reflex sympathetic response to cooling. Amer J Physiol 254 (Heart Circ Physiol) 23:H889, 1988
76. Cooke JP, Osmundson PJ, Shepherd JT: Sex differences in control of cutaneous blood flow. Circulation (in press, 1990)
77. Kallenberg CGM, Wouda AA, Haurethe T: Platelet activation, fibrinolytic activity and circulating immune complexes in Raynaud's phenomenon. J Rheumatol 9:878, 1982
78. Cohen RA: Platelet-induced neurogenic coronary contractions due to accumulation of the false neurotransmitter, 5-hydroxytryptamine. J Clin Invest 75:266, 1985
79. De Mey JG, Vanhoutte PM: Heterogeneous behavior of the canine arterial and venous wall. Circ Res 51:439, 1982
80. Reid HL, Dormandy JA, Barnes AJ et al: Impaired red cell deformability in peripheral vascular disease. Lancet 1:666, 1976

GENERAL REFERENCES

Roddie IC: Circulation to skin and adipose tissue. In Shepherd JT, Abboud FM (eds): Handbook of Physiology, Section 2, The Cardiovascular System, Vol III, Peripheral Circulation and Organ Blood Flow, part I, pp 285–317. Bethesda, MD, American Physiological Society, 1983

Rowell LB: Cardiovascular adjustments to thermal stress. In Shepherd JT, Abboud FM (eds): Handbook of Physiology, Section 2, The Cardiovascular System, Vol II, Peripheral Circulation and Organ Blood Flow, part 2, pp 967–1023. Bethesda, MD, American Physiological Society, 1983

Shepherd JT: Reflex control of arterial blood pressure. Cardiovasc Res 16:357, 1982

Shepherd JT: Circulation to skeletal muscle. In Shepherd JT, Abboud FM (eds): Handbook of Physiology, Section 2, The Cardiovascular System, Vol III, Peripheral Circulation and Organ Blood Flow, part I, pp 319–370. Bethesda, MD, American Physiological Society, 1983

Vanhoutte PM, Rimele T: Role of the endothelium in the control of vascular smooth muscle function. J Physiol (Paris) 78:681, 1982–1983

PHYSIOLOGY AND PATHOPHYSIOLOGY OF EXERCISE

C. Gunnar Blomqvist

Exercise physiology has become an important part of clinical cardiology. Concepts, methods, and procedures based on exercise appear at many levels in the diagnosis, treatment, and prevention of heart disease. This presence is appropriate and reflects basic physiology. The essence of normal cardiovascular function is the ability to transport oxygen, nutrients, and metabolites at rates sufficient to support optimal tissue function. The metabolic activity of skeletal muscle is a major determinant of systemic oxygen uptake and transport needs. Heavy dynamic or rhythmic exercise involving large muscle groups (e.g., running or climbing) presents a greater challenge to the cardiovascular system than any other physiologic stimulus and is most likely to precipitate symptoms in patients with heart disease.

DETERMINANTS OF PHYSICAL PERFORMANCE CAPACITY

The ability to perform any physical task is limited by the capacity of skeletal muscle to transform by aerobic and anaerobic mechanisms chemical energy to mechanical work, and the ability to activate and control these mechanisms. The oxygen transport capacity of the cardiovascular system is often the principal factor limiting the rate of energy transformation. The maximal rate is usually expressed as systemic maximal oxygen uptake, which is also a widely used measure of physical fitness. Maximal oxygen uptake is determined during treadmill or bicycle exercise and defined as the level at which an increase in work load no longer causes the expected increase in oxygen uptake. Increased energy demands must then be met by anaerobic metabolism. Muscular performance rapidly becomes limited by lactate formation and progressive intracellular acidosis.

Mean maximal oxygen uptake in healthy men reaches a peak of about 45 $ml \cdot kg^{-1} \cdot min^{-1}$ between ages 15 and 20. There is a gradual decline with increasing age to about 30 $ml \cdot kg^{-1} \cdot min^{-1}$ at age 60. The standard deviation is 10% to 15% of the mean. Mean values are similar in prepubertal boys and girls but maximal oxygen uptake in adult women is approximately 25% below corresponding age-specific male mean values. This sex difference is at least partially attributable to lower hemoglobin levels with lower oxygen-carrying capacity in women and higher body fat content measured as a percentage of total body weight.[1]

Groups of patients with various forms of acquired or congenital cardiovascular disease generally have a subnormal mean maximal oxygen uptake, but the proportion of the individuals with frankly abnormal values is variable. Fewer than 20% of patients with patent ductus arteriosus, but virtually 100% of patients with tetralogy of Fallot, have an abnormally low work capacity.[2] Patients with rheumatic heart disease have an average oxygen uptake about two thirds of normal.[3] Patients with angina pectoris or a recent myocardial infarction usually become symptomatic at a level corresponding to 50% to 60% of the normal age- and sex-specific maximal oxygen uptake.[4] The typical patient with healed myocardial infarction without angina has a higher work capacity and averages about 75% of normal values. The range of interindividual variation within this or any diagnostic category is very large (e.g., from 25% to 100% of expected maximal uptake in patients during the first 6 months following an acute myocardial infarction).[4]

Patients are often unable to satisfy the classical physiologic criteria for maximal oxygen uptake. A symptom-limited measurement is the functional equivalent of the more stringently defined maximum in normal subjects. In particular, many patients, for example, those with coronary or peripheral arterial disease, may be limited by defects in regional rather than systemic oxygen transport. However, angina pectoris, ventricular arrhythmias, or claudication effectively limits also the rate of systemic oxygen transport.

ENERGY SUPPLY

The immediate energy requirements for muscular work are covered by breakdown of adenosine triphosphate (ATP) to adenosine diphosphate (ADP) and inorganic phosphate. The total available ATP pool will only support a maximal running effort for a second but the ATP stores are normally replenished from muscle phosphocreatine. This source provides energy for a few more seconds. High-energy phosphate bonds must then be recreated. This can be done aerobically by mitochondrial oxidative phosphorylation using glycogen, glucose, or free fatty acids as fuels or anaerobically by glycogenolysis or glycolysis with lactate formation. Energy for work of a duration of more than a minute or two is provided mainly by oxidative phosphorylation. This requires cardiovascular transport of oxygen but provides much larger total amounts of energy than available from anaerobic sources. A 75-kg normal human subject stores some 5 kcal as high-energy phosphates, 1,100 kcal as glucose and glycogen, and at least 75,000 kcal as fat.[1]

Fats and carbohydrates supply equal amounts of energy at rest. Free fatty acids remain important during low-level steady-state exercise but the utilization of carbohydrates increases progressively with increasing levels of work. Maximal efforts are supported exclusively by carbohydrate metabolism. These changes in substrate utilization are reflected by a progressive increase in the respiratory quotient, that is, the ratio between carbon dioxide production and oxygen uptake (Fig. 8.1). The dependence on carbohydrates during heavy exercise limits endurance at work levels that approach but do not reach the capacity of the cardiovascular system to deliver oxygen. Under these circumstances, the main source of fuel is muscle glycogen and the onset of severe fatigue coincides with muscle glycogen depletion. Normal levels at rest are about 1.5 g/100 g skeletal muscle. A sequence of prolonged exercise to fatigue causing glycogen depletion, followed by rest and a carbohydrate-rich diet (carbohydrate loading) can establish a new higher glycogen level and improve endurance.[1]

Dynamic exercise involving large muscle groups (e.g., walking or running) does not significantly affect lactate levels in skeletal muscle or in blood until systemic oxygen uptake exceeds 50% to 60% of maximum in sedentary and 70% to 80% in well-trained individuals (Fig. 8.1). The onset of blood lactate accumulation has been taken as a sign of inadequate oxygen supply to active muscles and been referred to as the anaerobic threshold.[5,6] The rise in blood lactate usually coincides with a significant change in ventilatory pattern. There is an increase in the ventilatory equivalent for oxygen (the ratio ventilatory minute volume/oxygen uptake) without any change in the equivalent for carbon dioxide production.[7] The apparent anaerobic threshold as identified by respiratory gas analysis has been widely used to characterize systemic cardiovascular function both in normal subjects and in patients with heart disease.[7] The approach is potentially very useful since many patients with heart disease are unable to reach a true maximal oxygen uptake. However, the physiologic validity of the threshold concept is doubtful.[8] Skeletal muscle is most likely not hypoxic during submaximal exercise. Glycolysis with lactate production can occur even in the presence of adequate oxygen concentrations. Furthermore, blood levels reflect the balance between lactate production and removal rates rather than simply production. The ventilatory pattern associated with increasing blood lactate levels is nonspecific and present also in patients with McArdle's syndrome who lack skeletal muscle phosphorylase and are unable to produce lactate.[8] These considerations do not necessarily invalidate the use of the measurement as an empirical descriptor but it is prudent to refer to the onset or threshold of blood lactate accumulation rather than to an absolute anaerobic threshold.

Anaerobic states have often been regarded as abnormal and potentially dangerous but are part of the normal responses to exercise. Anaerobic mechanisms supply most of the energy during dynamic exercise of high intensity and a duration of less than 1 or 2 minutes, that is, less than the time normally required to reach an equilibrium between oxygen demand and transport. Heavy and sustained static exercise is also supported by anaerobic mechanisms. Intramuscular pressure generally exceeds the arterial pressure and the active muscle is ischemic.

SKELETAL MUSCLE CHARACTERISTICS

Striated muscle accounts for more than 40% of the total body weight in lean individuals.[9] Human skeletal muscle is a mosaic of fibers with different contractile and metabolic characteristics.[10] The contractile response is determined by the content of myosin ATPase. Slow-twitch or type I fibers have low levels of myosin ATPase but a high capacity for oxidative metabolism. The dominant fast-twitch fibers in untrained subjects, type IIb, have low oxidative but high glycolytic capacity. Type IIa, the common fast-twitch fiber in trained individuals, combines high potentials for anaerobic and aerobic metabolism. The average individual has equal numbers of type I and type II fibers but interindividual variations are large. The basic fiber type distribution is an inherited characteristic[11] but the metabolic properties, specifically the potential for oxidative metabolism, are greatly affected by the state of physical training. As would be expected, fiber type distribution is an important determinant of athletic performance. Sprinters tend to have a high proportion of type II and long-distance runners type I fibers.[10]

The metabolic range of skeletal muscle is very large. The quadriceps femoris muscle of a 75-kg normal individual weighs about 2.5 kg. Single leg dynamic knee-extension can be performed with little or no activity in other muscles. The systemic increase in oxygen uptake above resting levels may reach 1 liter $\cdot$ min^{-1} during fatiguing exercise, corresponding to a quadriceps uptake of 400 ml $\cdot$ kg^{-1} $\cdot$ min^{-1} with a blood flow of 2,500 ml $\cdot$ kg^{-1} $\cdot$ min^{-1}. The maximal perfusion rate represents a more than 60-fold increase above the normal resting blood flow level of about 40 ml $\cdot$ kg^{-1} $\cdot$ min^{-1}.[12]

Superior endurance athletes may have systemic maximal oxygen uptakes exceeding 6 liters $\cdot$ min^{-1} and cardiac output approaching 40 liters $\cdot$ min^{-1}. Extrapolation from the quadriceps data suggests that even this unusually high capacity for oxygen transport would have to be more than doubled to support prolonged maximal dynamic activity of all muscles of the body. Systemic oxygen transport is thus a rate-limiting function.[13,14]

SYSTEMIC OXYGEN TRANSPORT

The rate of oxygen transfer from ambient air to the tissue could theoretically be limited at any of several levels (*i.e.*, pulmonary, cardiovascular, or peripheral). Pulmonary transport includes ventilation, diffusion into blood, and chemical reaction with hemoglobin. Cardiovascular transport capacity is equal to the product of the maximal cardiac output and the arterial oxygen content. The peripheral links include distribution of cardiac output and diffusion to sites of tissue utilization.[15]

Table 8.1 details average pulmonary and cardiovascular functional capacities in groups of young college students and Olympic athletes. Measurements relating to pulmonary function were similar in both groups. The overall capacity for pulmonary oxygen transport also was similar, 5.6 liters $\cdot$ min^{-1} in the students after training and 6.2 liters $\cdot$ min^{-1} in the athletes. Most of the difference in maximal oxygen

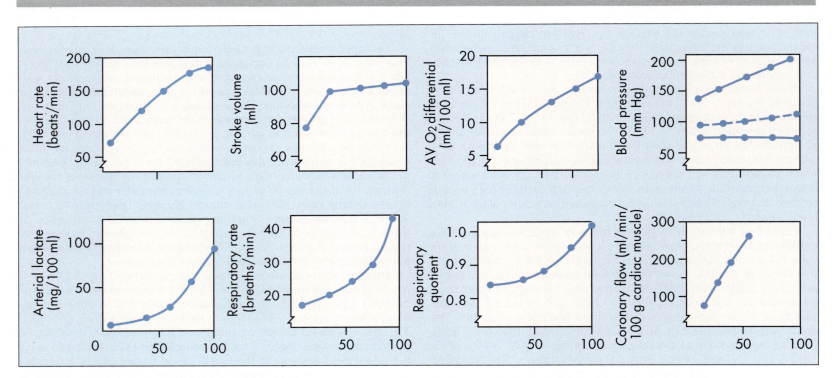

FIGURE 8.1 Characteristic features of normal cardiovascular, respiratory, and metabolic responses to dynamic exercise. Data points represent sitting rest, three levels of submaximal exercise, and maximal treadmill exercise. Values are plotted against relative load, that is, actual oxygen uptake percentage of maximal oxygen uptake. Blood pressure data include systolic, mean, and diastolic brachial artery pressures. (Modified from Blomqvist CG: Clinical exercise physiology. In Wenger NK, Hellerstein H (eds): Rehabilitation of the Coronary Patient, pp 179–196. New York, John Wiley & Sons, 1984)

uptake was accounted for by different capacities for cardiovascular oxygen transport with higher stroke volume and larger cardiac output in athletes. The data show that differences in physical activity and fitness have little effect on pulmonary function. However, cardiovascular and pulmonary oxygen transport capacities are closely matched in champion athletes whereas sedentary normal subjects utilize only about two thirds of their pulmonary capacity. Pulmonary rather than cardiovascular function is limiting performance at sea level in some individuals when maximal oxygen uptake exceeds 6 liters · min^{-1}. Athletes are also likely to have relatively larger declines in performance at altitude than average sedentary subjects.

ACUTE HEMODYNAMIC AND METABOLIC RESPONSES TO EXERCISE

Several major factors affect the normal responses to exercise, including the size of the active muscle mass, the mode of contraction (static and sustained versus dynamic and rhythmic), and the duration and intensity of the effort. Responses are modified by posture, environmental conditions (altitude, ambient temperature), and by individual characteristics (age, sex, state of health, and fitness).

DYNAMIC EXERCISE

Principal characteristics of the normal response to dynamic exercise (treadmill or two-leg bicycle exercise) are shown in Figure 8.1 and Table 8.2. The outstanding feature is a one-to-one match between the changes in peripheral oxygen demand and cardiovascular oxygen transport.

Cardiac output ($\dot{Q}$, liter · min^{-1}) during dynamic exercise is a linear function (Fig. 8.2) of oxygen uptake ($\dot{V}O_2$, liter · min^{-1}). Bruce studied healthy men during treadmill exercise and found $\dot{Q} = 4.1 + 5.6$ ($\dot{V}O_2$, liter · min^{-1}) (42 observations, linear correction coefficient [r] = 0.94, standard error of estimate [SEE] = 1.4 liter · min^{-1}).[16] Others have reported similar regression equations derived from measurements during bicycle exercise, including arm work and one-leg exercise.[17,18] This magnitude of change in cardiac output, corresponding to 5½ times the increase in oxygen uptake, provides for an effective increase in the rate of oxygen transport of 1 liter · min^{-1} for each 1 liter · min^{-1} increase in $\dot{V}O_2$. The arterial oxygen content is normally about 20 volumes % or 200 ml oxygen · liter^{-1} of blood and the maximal efficiency of oxygen extraction is significantly less than 100%. The slope (i.e., the ratio between change in cardiac output and change in oxygen uptake) is remarkably constant and largely unaffected by a variety of factors that alter the intercept or cardiac output at rest. Characteristics linked to variations in resting cardiac output include body size, age, sex, state of fitness, and posture.[16-19] A tight coupling between peripheral oxygen demand and cardiovascular transport is also evident at high altitude and in anemia.[20] In the absence of cardiovascular disease, decreases in arterial oxygen content are compensated by a proportional increase in cardiac output.

In the average healthy young man, transition from rest to maximal

TABLE 8.1 CARDIOVASCULAR AND PULMONARY FUNCTIONAL CAPACITIES DETERMINED DURING MAXIMAL EXERCISE IN COLLEGE STUDENTS AND OLYMPIC ATHLETES*

		Students		Olympic Athletes
	Control	After Bed Rest	After Training	
Maximal oxygen uptake (liters · min^{-1})	3.30	2.43	3.91	5.38†
Maximal voluntary ventilation (liters · min^{-1})	191	201	197	219
Transfer coefficient for O$_2$ (ml · min^{-1} · mm Hg^{-1})	96	83	86	95
Arterial O$_2$ capacity (vol%)	21.9	20.5	20.8	22.4
Maximal cardiac output (liters · min^{-1})	20.0	14.8	22.8	30.4†
Stroke volume (ml)	104	74	120	167†
Maximal heart rate (beats · min^{-1})	192	197	190	182
Systemic arteriovenous O$_2$ difference (vol%)	16.2	16.5	17.1	18.0

* Mean values, n = 5 and 6. Age, height, and weight similar. Adapted from Johnson[15] and Blomqvist and Saltin[74] by permission.

† Significantly different from college students, $P < 0.05$.

TABLE 8.2 CARDIOVASCULAR OXYGEN TRANSPORT AT REST (SITTING) AND DURING MAXIMAL EXERCISE (TREADMILL) IN NORMAL SEDENTARY YOUNG MEN

	Oxygen Uptake (l · min^{-1})	= Heart Rate (beats · min^{-1})	× Stroke Volume (ml)	× Arteriovenous O$_2$ Difference (ml · dl^{-1})
Rest	0.30	75	75	5.2
Maximal exercise	3.00	190	100	15.8
Ratio exercise/rest	10.0	2.5	1.3	3.0

treadmill or bicycle exercise causes a 10-fold increase in metabolic rate and systemic oxygen uptake. Oxygen transport and utilization are traditionally described in terms of the Fick equation: oxygen uptake = cardiac output × total arteriovenous oxygen difference, where cardiac output = heart rate × stroke volume. Typical normal data are illustrated in Table 8.2. Cardiac output increases by a factor of about 3.3, mainly due to an increase in heart rate. The magnitude of the increase in stroke volume varies with the body position in the resting control state and during exercise. Stroke volumes at supine rest and during mild upright exercise are similar and are within 20% of the maximal stroke volume. Venous pooling with decreased ventricular filling keeps stroke volumes at rest sitting and standing 20% to 40% below maximal levels.[19]

The relationship between oxygen uptake and heart rate is approximately linear in normal subjects during submaximal exercise (see Fig. 8.1). As previously discussed, cardiac output is also a linear function of oxygen uptake. It follows that heart rate during exercise at any given level of oxygen uptake varies inversely with stroke volume. The average maximal heart rate is 190 beats per minute in normal 25-year-olds. There is a gradual decrease with increasing age to an average of 160 beats · min^{-1} at age 65 years. The average decline approximates ¾ beat · min^{-1} per year but there are large interindividual variations.[1] These variations invalidate the use of a percentage of the estimated age-specific maximal heart rate as an end-point during exercise testing when the objective is to determine functional capacity.

The rate of oxygen transport normally greatly exceeds the demand at rest. Less than one third of the available oxygen is utilized (Table 8.2). These reserves are not maintained during exercise. The change in oxygen transport during exercise approximates the increased demand. Most of the increase in cardiac output is directed to working skeletal muscles, which operate with a high atrioventricular (A-V) difference already at submaximal loads.[13] The total blood flow to other tissues remains relatively unchanged but there is a major redistribution away from the splanchnic area and to the respiratory muscles and the myocardium. Cerebral flow changes very little. Cutaneous blood flow decreases steeply during exercise unless work is prolonged or performed in a hot environment.[21] The combined effect of increased systemic oxygen demand and redistribution of an increased cardiac output is an increase in the extraction to at least three fourths of the oxygen available in arterial blood.

Systemic resistance decreases progressively with increasing intensity of exercise. Metabolic vasodilation in working muscle more than offsets the vasoconstriction in inactive tissues. Mean arterial pressure increases only slightly, typically by less than 20 mm Hg, but there is a large increase in systolic pressure and pulse pressure. Systolic pressure during maximal work often exceeds 200 mm Hg in normal subjects (see Fig. 8.1).

Cardiac performance is normally significantly enhanced during exercise. The relative magnitude of contributions from increased preload (*i.e.*, the Starling mechanism) and from an increased contractile state is a matter of some controversy.[22] Both mechanisms are likely to be involved. End-diastolic volume and filling pressures increase on the transition from rest to exercise both in the upright and supine positions and there is a further increase with increasing work loads (Fig. 8.3). Left ventricular filling pressures may reach high levels, particularly in older subjects. Mean pulmonary artery wedge pressures of more than 20 mm Hg have been reported during supine exercise in healthy 60- to 80-year-old men.[23] End-systolic volume remains unchanged during supine exercise and decreases during upright exercise. These findings are consistent with an increased contractile state since systolic pressure may increase by as much as 100 mm Hg from rest to maximal exercise.[22]

At any submaximal workload or level of oxygen uptake, *arm exercise* produces a higher heart rate and arterial pressure than leg exercise but maximal oxygen uptake and maximal heart rate are lower.[24] Mechanical efficiency is also lower. Energy is expended gripping implements and stabilizing the torso. These efforts are largely static and do not translate into external work. Blomqvist and associates and Lewis and co-workers recently defined the general relationship between active muscle mass and cardiovascular response during dynamic exercise by examining two-leg, one-leg, and one-arm bicycle exercise and one-arm curl.[25,26] Cardiac output and systemic arteriovenous oxygen difference are strongly related to oxygen uptake irrespective of the mode of exercise. The slope of the relationship between heart rate and oxygen uptake is inversely proportional to active muscle mass, that is, the smaller the active muscle mass, the higher the heart rate at any absolute level of oxygen uptake. Arterial pressures (systolic, diastolic, and mean) are even more strongly affected by active muscle mass, with large increases in pressure at low levels of oxygen uptake during exercise involving a small muscle mass.

Schwade and associates compared arm and leg bicycle ergometry and included a group of patients with angina pectoris who often had chest pain during arm work but rarely during leg work.[27] This subpopulation had responses that were no different from patients who predominantly had their angina during leg work (*i.e.*, walking). The maximal workload that can be achieved during two-arm bicycle work varies

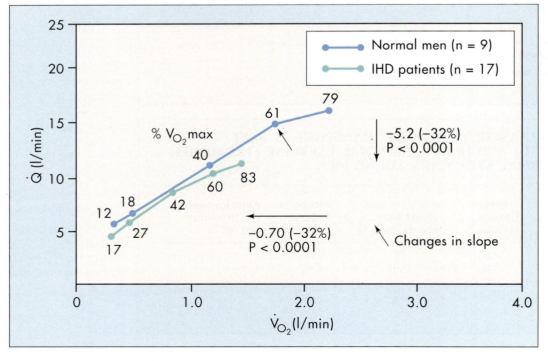

FIGURE 8.2 The relationship of cardiac output ($\dot{Q}$) to oxygen consumption ($\dot{V}O_2$) in normal men and in patients with ischemic heart disease (*IHD*). (Modified from Bruce RA, Petersen JL, Kusumi F: Hemodynamic response to exercise in the upright position in patients with ischemic heart disease. In Dhalla NS (ed): Myocardial Metabolism, pp 849–865. Baltimore, University Park Press, 1973)

from less than half to 70% of the load during two-leg work. Mechanical efficiency is highly variable but significantly lower during arm work, that is, oxygen uptake is higher at any given work load than during leg work. The lower mechanical efficiency combines with a steeper increase in heart rate and systolic blood pressure during arm work to cause a high myocardial oxygen demand relative to work load and systemic oxygen uptake. However, heart rate–blood pressure products at the onset of myocardial ischemia and the incidence of chest pain and ST segment abnormalities were similar during arm and leg work in the series studied by Schwade and co-workers. Others have reported a slightly higher rate–pressure product threshold for angina during arm work.[28] This is consistent with lower filling pressures[29] and, most likely, with lower ventricular volumes during arm work.

Thus, the cost of performing arm work is higher both in terms of myocardial work and systemic energy expenditure. There is little or no correlation between the peak work loads that can be achieved during arm and leg exercise. Arm work is therefore an effective alternate test method if the objective is to document myocardial ischemia, but large interindividual variations in mechanical efficiency and heart rate–blood pressure responses make it impossible to use arm work to derive a valid general estimate of systemic functional capacity.[28]

The normal one-to-one relationship between oxygen demand and oxygen transport is disrupted in severe chronic congestive heart failure (CHF). Patients with mild lesions are able to compensate for a depressed stroke volume by relative tachycardia. Cardiac output remains within normal limits at submaximal levels of exercise whereas maximal cardiac output and oxygen uptake are depressed in proportion to the decrease in stroke volume (see Fig. 8.2). In severe CHF, a more prominent reduction in stroke volume combines with regulatory abnormalities, including an attenuated heart rate response, to produce a subnormal cardiac output (Fig. 8.4).[30,31] However, patients with CHF retain a normal ability to extract the available oxygen.

The degree of functional impairment in CHF (determined from measurements of maximal oxygen uptake) cannot be predicted from data characterizing hemodynamics and ventricular function at *rest*.[32] There is also a striking lack of correlation between exercise capacity and measurements of ventricular performance *during exercise*.[32,33] The principal characteristic of patients with CHF is a lack of functional reserve. As previously discussed, normal subjects show a significant enhancement of contractile performance and a utilization of the Starling mechanism. An apparent lack of exercise-induced changes in ventricular function (perhaps at times overemphasized by the technical limitations inherent in radionuclide ventriculography of large hearts with severely depressed function) is characteristic of patients with severe CHF.[34] It is not surprising that under these circumstances the magnitude of the heart rate response becomes the principal determinant of exercise capacity.

A relative lack of diastolic reserve and attenuated cardiac responses to sympathetic stimulation are evident also in patients with lesser degrees of failure.[35] Univariate correlations between indices of ventricular function and exercise capacity are poor also in moderately severe CHF. However, exercise capacity is strongly related to cardiac output (*i.e.*, the product of stroke volume and heart rate). A patient with poor contractile performance may still achieve a relatively high cardiac output if (1) systemic resistance is relatively low, (2) the end-diastolic volume is large, and (3) the heart rate response is adequate.

STATIC OR ISOMETRIC EXERCISE

Sustained heavy static efforts produce large increases in systolic and diastolic arterial pressures with significant increases in heart rate and cardiac output. Peripheral resistance changes little in normal subjects, but vasoconstriction is the principal mechanism of the pressor response in patients with severe cardiac dysfunction. A pressor response mediated by vasoconstriction is also present in normal subjects after combined beta-adrenergic and parasympathetic blockade and in patients with transplanted, that is, denervated hearts.[36] The normal left ventricle is able to maintain stroke volume at resting levels with little or no increase in end-diastolic pressure despite the marked increase in systolic blood pressure and afterload. Stroke work increases markedly. These findings are consistent with enhanced myocardial contractility.

According to classical concepts, the magnitude of the pressor and heart rate responses is independent of muscle mass and absolute force development but closely linked to relative effort, that is, developed force expressed as a fraction of percentage of the force during a maximal voluntary contraction (MVC). Recent studies have demonstrated that the magnitude of the cardiovascular response (Fig. 8.5) is influenced not only by relative load but also by active muscle mass and absolute force development.[37] The relationship is nonlinear, with decreasing effects of increasing active muscle mass at high levels of force development.

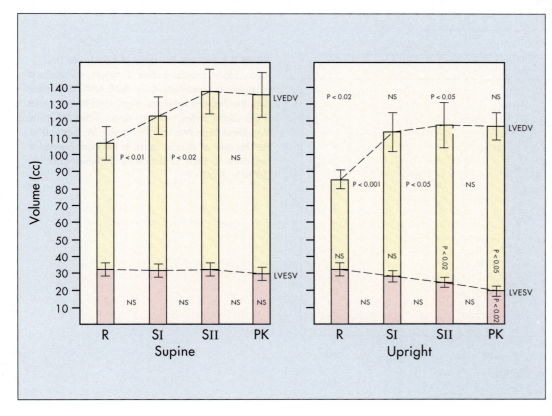

FIGURE 8.3 Left ventricular performance in normal subjects (n = 7). Absolute volume data derived by a nongeometric scintigraphic technique at rest (R), at two levels of submaximal exercise (SI and SII), and during peak effort (PK) in the supine and upright positions. The top of each bar represents left ventricular end-diastolic volume (LVEDV; mean ± SE); the pink portion, end-systolic volume (LVESV); and the yellow portion between LVESV and LVEDV, stroke volume. (Modified from Poliner LR, Dehmer GJ, Lewis SE et al: Left ventricular performance in normal subjects: A comparison of the responses to exercise in the upright and supine position. Circulation 62:528, 1980)

Hemodynamics during static exercise have often been characterized as a pressor response and contrasted to the volume or flow response during dynamic exercise. We have shown that this is an oversimplification and valid only for a comparison between dynamic exercise with large muscle groups (two-leg bicycle or treadmill exercise) and isometric exercise with small muscle mass (handgrip).[25,26] When dynamic exercise is performed with progressively smaller muscle groups, the hemodynamic response gradually assumes the characteristic "isometric" pattern. Heart rate and systolic blood pressure are virtually identical during static and dynamic exercise of identical small muscle groups at equivalent work loads (Table 8.3) and the similarities persist after combined beta-adrenergic and parasympathetic blockade.[26] This does not mean that all aspects of the cardiovascular responses are identical. The mode of contraction affects local hemodynamic conditions. There is vasodilation and a markedly increased blood flow to skeletal muscle during dynamic exercise, whereas static exercise causes mechanical obstruction of flow and local ischemia.

However, the different local conditions have little impact on systemic hemodynamics so long as the active muscle mass is small. The common denominator of the pressor responses to isometric and dynamic exercise of small muscle groups is a significant increase in cardiac output in the relative absence of metabolic vasodilation. Systemic vascular resistance remains near resting levels and any increase in cardiac output causes a proportional increase in blood pressure.

Heavy isometric efforts can be maintained only for short periods. The short duration of the hemodynamic response and the relatively small increase in heart rate explain why the pressor response to static exercise rarely causes angina pectoris. Heart rate and blood pressure responses to static exercise are also attenuated during the early phases of recovery from myocardial infarction.[4] Exercise-induced wall motion abnormalities may activate ventricular baroreceptors. Deformation of these receptors causes bradycardia and vasodilation, which oppose the normal reflex response to isometric exercise and protect against overload. An early study from our laboratory demonstrated more fre-

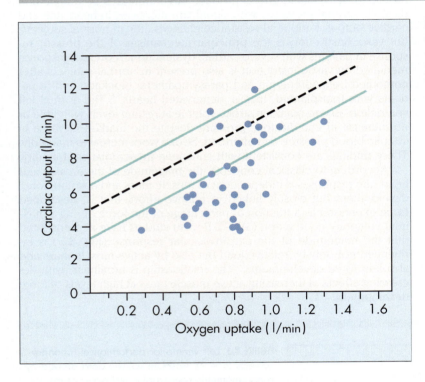

FIGURE 8.4 The relationship of cardiac output to oxygen uptake during bicycle exercise after myocardial infarction. (*Dashed line,* relationship in normal subjects; *outer lines,* two standard deviations; *solid circles,* data points from the patients) (Data from Wohl AJ, Lewis HR, Campbell W et al: Cardiovascular function during early recovery from acute myocardial infarction. Circulation 56:931, 1977)

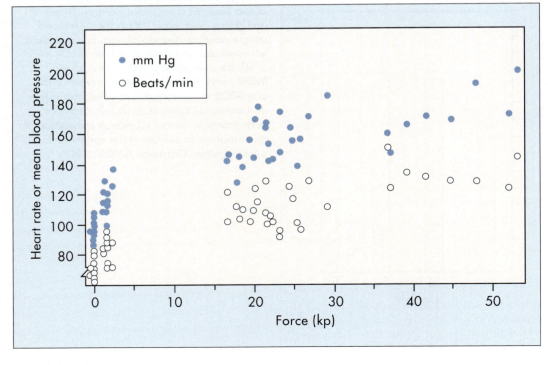

FIGURE 8.5 Individual values of heart rate and mean blood pressure after 1 minute, 45 seconds of sustained contractions at 40% MVC performed with the fingers, forearm, thigh, and forearm plus thigh. (*Solid circles,* mm Hg; *open circles,* beats/min) (Modified from Mitchell JH, Payne FA, Saltin B et al: The role of muscle mass in the cardiovascular response to static contractions. J Physiol (Lond) 309:45, 1980)

quent ventricular ectopic activity during handgrip at 30% MVC than during symptom-limited maximal bicycle exercise.[38] However, a majority of the patients in this series had severe left ventricular dysfunction. Subsequent studies have failed to support the concept that isometric exercise is arrhythmogenic and therefore dangerous.[4,39]

Static work and dynamic work are often combined in daily life, for example, when carrying a suitcase. The pressor response to isometric exercise is superimposed on the response to dynamic exercise at low work load levels[40,41] but the pressor effects gradually become less prominent as the intensity of dynamic exercise increases. Kerber and co-workers found no significant effect on the incidence of myocardial ischemia and suggested that the elevated diastolic pressure during combined exercise actually may improve myocardial perfusion.[41]

MYOCARDIAL PERFUSION

Exercise affects all major determinants of myocardial oxygen demand; left ventricular wall tension, contractile state, and heart rate all increase. The myocardium extracts a large fraction of the available oxygen at rest, that is, about two thirds as compared to less than one third in the systemic circulation. This means that increased myocardial oxygen demand during exercise must be met by an increase in coronary blood flow. In the normal heart, coronary blood flow closely parallels the increased *myocardial oxygen demand*.[42–45]

Coronary vascular resistance at the arteriolar level decreases markedly during exercise. Flow rates at rest are about 600 ml $\cdot$ kg^{-1} $\cdot$ min^{-1} of left ventricular myocardium per minute. Values exceeding 3000 ml $\cdot$ kg^{-1} $\cdot$ min^{-1} have been reported in normal young subjects during heavy upright exercise. The full capacity of the normal coronary bed is probably not reached even during maximal exercise.[46] Coronary artery atherosclerotic disease is associated with increased resistance to flow at the arterial level. Total coronary blood flow is usually normal in patients at rest, even if regional underperfusion is present. Flow rates at rest usually are not affected by large-vessel disease until the coronary arterial obstruction approaches the conventional arteriographic limit for significant obstruction of 50% of the vessel diameter, corresponding to a 75% reduction of cross-sectional area.[47] However, flow is a nonlinear function of lumen size and perfusion pressure. The length of the obstruction is also important. Conditions during exercise, with reduced myocardial arteriolar resistance, cause a relative increase in the flow limitations imposed by any obstruction of the large coronary vessels. Thus, even less severe lesions can cause measurable decreases in flow.[48]

Myocardial oxygen uptake in the normal heart is an excellent estimate of myocardial oxygen demand, since the myocardium is virtually unable to use anaerobic metabolic pathways. Oxygen uptake and coronary blood flow are closely correlated with the product of heart rate and systolic blood pressure. The *rate–pressure product* provides a measure of internal myocardial work but ignores the effects of changes in contractile state and ventricular volume. Nevertheless, the validity of the rate–pressure product has been well established by direct measurements of coronary blood flow and myocardial oxygen uptake in normal subjects under a variety of experimental conditions[42–45] and also by empiric studies in patients with angina pectoris.[49] Patients with typical effort angina have a well-defined threshold of myocardial ischemia, as measured by the rate–pressure product. Only interventions with marked effects on contractility and ventricular volume (*e.g.*, treatment with beta-adrenergic blocking agents) invalidate the rate–pressure product as an accurate estimation of myocardial oxygen demand.

Clinical studies during the late 1960s and early 1970s demonstrated that the onset of myocardial ischemia, precipitated by increased myocardial oxygen demand during dynamic exercise or by decreased oxygen supply in variant angina pectoris, is manifest by a well-defined set of pathophysiologic changes.[50–52] These include lactate production and potassium release as metabolic correlates of ST abnormalities and pain, and contractile dysfunction, apparent as regional and global depression of myocardial performance and an increase in left ventricular pressures.

REGULATORY MECHANISMS

The increased demand for oxygen transport during exercise is satisfied by a complex set of adjustments that affect both the central and peripheral components of the cardiovascular system.

REFLEX REGULATION

Neurogenic mechanisms have recently been reviewed by Shepherd and co-workers and Mitchell.[36,53] A summary is presented in Figure 8.6. Similar pathways are involved during static and dynamic exercise. With the onset of skeletal muscle contraction, signals are received by the cardiovascular centers from the motor areas of the brain where the voluntary contraction is initiated (central command), and from receptors that sense the degree of activity of the contracting muscles. The afferent impulses from skeletal muscle reach the spinal cord via slowly conducting small medullated (group III) and nonmedullated fibers (group IV or C-fibers) and ascend in the spinothalamic tract to the

TABLE 8.3 HEMODYNAMIC RESPONSES TO STATIC AND DYNAMIC HANDGRIP AND KNEE EXTENSION*

	Handgrip		Knee Extension	
	Static	Dynamic	Static	Dynamic
Heart rate (beats $\cdot$ min^{-1})	91 ± 4	99 ± 8	134 ± 11	128 ± 8
Arterial pressure (mm Hg)				
Systolic	150 ± 6	151 ± 4	193 ± 7	193 ± 10
Diastolic	94 ± 4	95 ± 3	114 ± 2	101 ± 2†
Cardiac output (liters $\cdot$ min^{-1})	6.8 ± 0.3	7.4 ± 0.4	10.1 ± 0.9	13.1 ± 1.0†

* Mean values and SE, n = 6

† Difference between static and dynamic difference significant at the 0.05 level

(Data from Lewis SF, Snell PG, Taylor WF et al: Role of muscle mass and mode of contraction in circulatory responses to exercise. J Appl Physiol 58:146, 1985)

cardiovascular centers in the brain. The receptors in the muscles are stimulated by the chemical changes produced by contractions. Experiments based on electrically induced rather than voluntary contractions and on exercise in subjects with sensory blockade suggest that the two mechanisms are capable of producing an appropriate cardiovascular response either working in conjunction or independently of each other. Both mechanisms appear to affect the same central and efferent neural circuits.

As a result of the impulse flow to the cardiovascular centers, the vagal activity to the heart decreases and the heart rate increases. The increased sympathetic noradrenergic outflow leads to increased cardiac contractility, increased tone of the splanchnic, renal, and other resistance vessels, constriction of the splanchnic capacitance vessels, and release of catecholamines, mainly epinephrine, from the adrenal medulla. Beta-adrenergic stimulation contributes to the heart rate response. As the arterial blood pressure begins to increase, the mechanoreceptors of the carotid sinus and aortic arch are activated, and presumably also the atrial and left ventricular deformation receptors. These baroreceptors may modify the increase in systolic arterial blood pressure, heart rate, and cardiac output.

VASOREGULATORY MECHANISMS

The activation of the sympathetic nervous system is manifest as elevated plasma catecholamines. The magnitude of the increase is related to relative intensity of work (actual oxygen uptake as a fraction of the individual's maximum) and to absolute oxygen uptake.[18] Most of the circulating norepinephrine is thought to constitute overflow from vascular receptors mediating vasoconstriction, particularly in resting skeletal muscle. Kinetics are complex and plasma levels do not necessarily provide an accurate measure of sympathetic nerve traffic. Exercise also activates local vasoregulatory mechanisms. There is a strong metabolic vasodilatory drive. In a young normal subject, the transition from rest to maximal exercise is typically associated with a threefold reduction

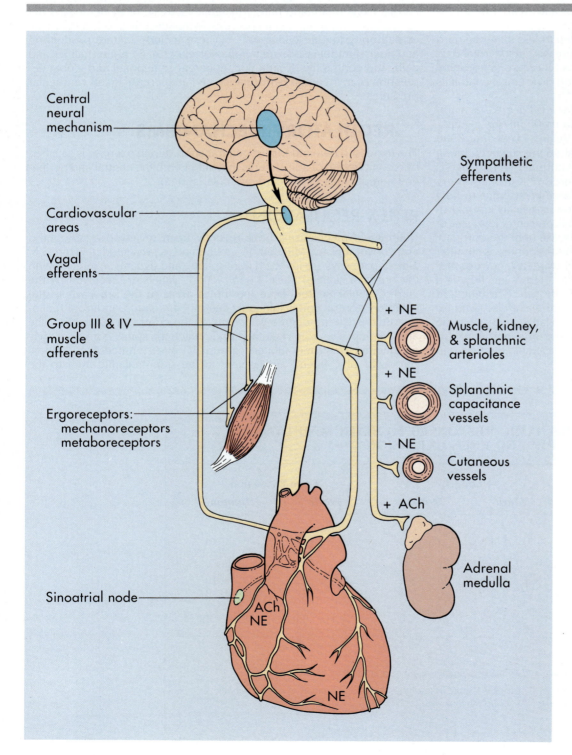

FIGURE 8.6 Cardiovascular control during exercise: central and reflex neural mechanisms. With onset of exercise, neural inputs are received by the cardiovascular areas from cerebral motor control areas ("Central Command") and from receptors in activated skeletal muscle. Receptors activated by exercise have been termed ergoreceptors. These receptors respond to metabolic and mechanical alterations and their afferent impulses are conducted by groups III and IV fibers to the spinal cord where they ascend to the cardiovascular areas. As a result of these two inputs to the cardiovascular areas, the parasympathetic activity to the heart decreases and the sympathetic activity to the heart, blood vessels, and adrenal medulla increases. (ACh, acetylcholine; NE, norepinephrine; SA, sinoatrial node) (Modified from Mitchell JH: Cardiovascular control during exercise. Am J Cardiol 54:34D, 1985)

in systemic resistance. Thus, at the systemic level the metabolic vasodilator activity overrides the neurogenic vasoconstrictor drive. Systemic resistance is actually minimal under conditions when the neurogenic constrictor drive is maximal (i.e., during maximal dynamic exercise involving both legs). Metabolic stimuli during submaximal exercise do not completely abolish the effects of the alpha-mediated vasoconstrictor drive in blood vessels supplying working muscle,[54] but there is no evidence for residual alpha-mediated constrictor activity during maximal one-leg quadriceps exercise.[55] It has previously been widely accepted that *maximal exercise* produces a metabolic vasodilatory activity that is of sufficient strength to override the alpha-mediated vasoconstriction. However, studies in normal subjects have clearly demonstrated that there is significant residual vasoconstrictor activity also during maximal exercise if it involves large muscle groups and requires rates of oxygen uptake and transport that equal or exceed maximal systemic capacity. Leg blood flow and conductance decrease when two-leg exercise is combined with arm exercise and when the maximally active muscle mass increases from one leg to two legs, that is, when a systemic flow that is inadequate relative to total metabolic demands is redistributed to provide optimal perfusion of all active tissues.[56-58]

Olsson has recently reviewed the regulation of blood flow in skeletal muscle.[59] In his generalized control system, the primary error signal producing vasodilatation is muscle activity rather than oxygen use and local P_{O_2}. Carbon dioxide and potassium fit the role as principal vasodilatory regulators better than other agents. They have release rates proportional to the contractile activity and the rate of energy transformation. The magnitude of exercise-induced concentration changes is consistent with a physiologically important role. Neither can explain all features of the exercise response, but these agents, combined with decreases in P_{O_2} and increases in osmolarity, markedly reinforce each other's vasodilatory effects. Adenosine is an important regulator of coronary flow but its role in skeletal muscle may be more limited and related primarily to conditions associated with ischemia and prolonged exercise. There is no current support for prostaglandins as major physiologic vasodilator agents during exercise.[59] The role of potassium as a principal metabolic vasodilator agent is intriguing. There is strong evidence that potassium release during exercise activates muscle afferents (groups III and IV) and mediates the reflex-induced increases in heart rate, cardiac output, contractile state, and arterial pressure.[60,61] The time course of the cardiovascular exercise response parallels potassium release.[62] Thus, the same agent may serve as a vasodilator (local effects) and a vasoconstrictor (reflex-induced alpha-adrenergic stimulation).

Autonomic dysfunction is an important feature in CHF. Dysfunction may be caused by changes affecting the basic functional characteristics of the autonomic nervous system or by abnormal patterns of activation of normal reflexes. Both mechanisms are present in CHF and they affect the responses mediated by both the sympathetic and parasympathetic systems.[63,64]

The failing heart has depleted stores of catecholamines.[65] Recent studies have revealed abnormal turnover rates of norepinephrine and its precursors.[66] At least in some forms of CHF, the end stage with depleted stores is preceded by increased turnover rates of norepinephrine (which serve as an indicator of overall sympathetic activity). Turnover rates may approach maximal rates of synthesis under basal conditions. This leaves little or no sympathetic reserve and may account for the apparent paradox of beneficial effects of long-term treatment with beta-adrenergic blocking agents in some patients with severe cardiomyopathy.[67]

Chronically increased levels of adrenergic activity at rest could be expected to cause down-regulation with decreased density of the adrenergic receptors. However, studies of responses to exogenous adrenergic agonists reveal no consistent pattern. Tilton and associates have recently reviewed receptor characteristics in CHF.[68] They concluded that end-stage CHF is associated with abnormal receptor density and responsiveness but it is uncertain whether similar dysfunction occurs also during the early stages of CHF.

Plasma catecholamines at rest are elevated and levels correlate with the degree of failure and ventricular dysfunction. An early paper by Chidsey and co-workers established the concept that in patients with CHF the response to exercise is hyperadrenergic.[69] Plasma norepinephrine levels in CHF are markedly elevated at intensities of exercise that produce little change in normal subjects. However, the rate of release of norepinephrine is determined by relative (percent of individual maximum) rather than absolute work load. Oxygen uptakes during exercise at 2 to 4 times resting levels correspond to loads well below 50% of maximal capacity in normal subjects but are maximal in patients with severe CHF.

Some patients with advanced CHF actually have subnormal catecholamine levels during maximal exercise. Markham and Firth found strong correlations between exercise capacity and the magnitude of the increase in norepinephrine and heart rate above resting levels.[70] Their data, presented in Table 8.4, suggest that patients with severe CHF have an attenuated rather than an excessive adrenergic response to exercise. The combination of high resting and low maximal levels of norepinephrine is consistent with the general concept of a diminished sympathetic reserve.[66]

EFFECT OF VARIATIONS IN THE LEVEL OF PHYSICAL ACTIVITY

Interindividual physiologic variations in physical performance capacity reflect a combination of genetic and environmental influences. Drastic changes in the habitual level of physical activity can, over a few weeks, decrease maximal oxygen uptake levels by one third (bed rest) or produce an increase of one third above control levels (strenuous physical training).[71] On the other hand, studies based on classical twin methodology[72,73] have demonstrated that inherited characteristics also have

TABLE 8.4 PLASMA CATECHOLAMINES AND HEART RATE AT REST, SITTING, AND DURING MAXIMAL UPRIGHT EXERCISE IN PATIENTS WITH SEVERE CONGESTIVE HEART FAILURE AND IN NORMAL SUBJECTS

	Epinephrine ($ng \cdot ml^{-1}$)	Norepinephrine ($ng \cdot ml^{-1}$)	Heart Rate ($beats \cdot min^{-1}$)
Rest			
CHF*	0.07	0.75	90
Normals†	0.04	0.38	80
Exercise			
CHF*	0.16	1.92	136
Normals†	0.46	3.67	194
Ratio Exercise/Rest			
CHF*	2.4	2.6	1.5
Normals†	11.5	9.7	2.4

* n = 16

† n = 6

(Data from Lewis SF, Taylor WF, Graham RM et al: Cardiovascular responses to exercise as functions of absolute and relative work loads. J Appl Physiol 54:1314, 1983; and Markham RW, Firth BG: *Personal communication*, 1983)

a major effect on maximal oxygen uptake (Fig. 8.7) and on the contractile and metabolic properties of skeletal muscle.[11]

PHYSICAL TRAINING

The principal features of the systemic cardiovascular responses to endurance training in normal subjects were well documented by the late 1960s and are illustrated in Table 8.1. The effects include an increase in maximal oxygen uptake, stroke volume, and cardiac output with no change or a small decrease in maximal heart rate. Systemic vascular conductance increases. There is also an increase in peripheral oxygen extraction and in the maximal systemic arteriovenous oxygen difference. Cardiac output at submaximal levels of work does not change significantly but the increase in stroke volume is associated with relative bradycardia at rest and at any given submaximal level of oxygen uptake. These cardiovascular changes are produced by a complex set of central and peripheral mechanisms operating at multiple levels (*i.e.*, structural, metabolic, and regulatory).[74]

EFFECTS ON SKELETAL MUSCLE

Endurance training produces large increases in the activities of the oxidative enzymes of skeletal muscle. The enzymes of the glycolytic pathway change very little. Saltin and Gollnick have reviewed the physiologic implications of these metabolic adaptations.[10] They noted that both longitudinal and cross-sectional studies on endurance training and detraining have demonstrated much larger and more rapid effects on the oxidative enzymes than on maximal oxygen uptake (Fig. 8.8). This implies that there is no direct causal link between enzymatic activity and systemic maximal oxygen uptake. However, the increased oxidative capacity following training is associated with an increased endurance capacity, defined as time to exhaustion at submaximal work load levels. The change in endurance is quantitatively related to an increased mitochondrial volume and increased capacity for oxidation in skeletal muscle. Levels may double after training whereas changes in maximal oxygen uptake rarely exceed 30%.[75]

Lack of substrate (glycogen) is a performance-limiting factor during prolonged exercise at high but still submaximal intensities. The training-induced cellular adaptations favor entry into the citric acid cycle of acetyl units derived from fatty acids.[76] The overall effects are an increased use of fats as substrate during exercise and a decrease in both aerobic and anaerobic utilization of carbohydrates, particularly muscle glycogen. These changes have no effect on maximal oxygen uptake, but the preferential use of fats improves endurance by postponing the development of performance limitations due to glycogen depletion or lactate accumulation, or both.

An increased systemic A-V O_2 difference after training has been a consistent finding in longitudinal studies of sedentary young men and patients with ischemic heart disease but not in women or older men.[74] A more efficient utilization of available oxygen may account for as much as one half of the improvement in maximal oxygen uptake produced by a short-term training program in young men (see Table 8.1). The widening of the systemic arteriovenous oxygen difference has been attributed to an increase in mitochondrial volume in skeletal muscle. However, it is unlikely that changes in mitochondrial volume are the primary cause. Immobilization causes a decrease of the aerobic capacity of skeletal muscle with no change or a decrease in mitochondrial volume, but the maximal A-V O_2 difference is maintained or increases slightly after bed rest (Table 8.1).[71,74]

The high systemic A-V O_2 difference after both training and deconditioning can be explained by *vascular adaptations*. A wide systemic A-V O_2 difference and efficient oxygen extraction after bed rest may reflect a relative prolongation of the mean transit time through skeletal muscle capillaries. Maximal cardiac output and, presumably, maximal skeletal muscle blood flow are significantly reduced after a bed rest period of less than a month whereas there is little or no short-term change in capillary density.[19,71] Increased usage of muscle causes a proliferation of the capillary bed with an increase in the number of capillaries and their dimensions, that is, an increase in capillary blood volume. A larger muscle blood flow following training can therefore be accommodated with little or no change in the capillary transit time. Furthermore, oxygen extraction is facilitated by the increased capillary density and the decreased diffusion distances.[13,74]

CARDIAC ADAPTATIONS

The improved utilization of the systemic capacity for oxygen transport only accounts for a small fraction of the large difference in maximal oxygen uptake between athletes and sedentary subjects. A superior systemic aerobic capacity clearly requires superior cardiac pump performance. The increased stroke volume that is a salient effect of training in normal subjects can be achieved simply by increasing cardiac dimensions or by improving the performance characteristics of the heart by (1) enhancing the intrinsic contractile properties of the myocardium and the responses to inotropic stimulation or (2) inducing extramyocardial adaptations that have secondary effects on performance (*e.g.*, by increasing ventricular filling or decreasing afterload and myocardial work).

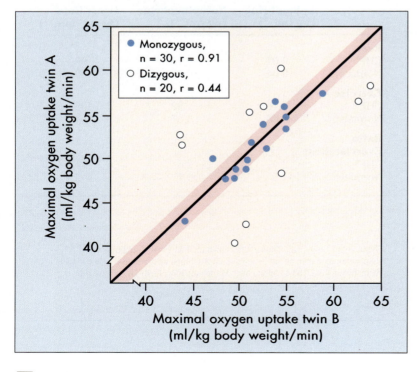

FIGURE 8.7 Intrapair differences in maximal oxygen uptake are much smaller in monozygous than in dizygous twins, suggesting that genetic factors strongly influence cardiovascular functional capacity. (Modified from Klissouras V: Heritability of adaptive variation. J Appl Physiol 31:338, 1971)

Cardiac adaptations and systemic adaptations with secondary cardiac effects have recently been reviewed by Blomqvist and Saltin and Schaible and Scheuer.[74,77] Cross-sectional results from early studies based on x-ray examinations and from more recent echocardiographic work have clearly demonstrated increased cardiac dimensions in athletes compared to sedentary controls. The cardiac adaptations vary with the specific demands imposed by the athletic activity. Endurance athletes have global cardiac enlargement. Left ventricular end-diastolic dimensions are increased with a proportional increase in ventricular wall thickness, suggesting that wall stress is being maintained at normal levels. Participants in sports that require isometric efforts tend to have normal end-diastolic volume but increased wall thickness, commensurate with the pressure load associated with heavy isometric efforts.

It is not known whether the marked cardiac enlargement that is seen in superior endurance athletes can be attributed solely to intense and prolonged training or if there is a genetic predisposition to cardiac hypertrophy. Former endurance athletes continue to have large hearts long after they turn sedentary. This is consistent with, but does not prove, predisposition. Most longitudinal training studies in human subjects have produced much smaller differences between active subjects and sedentary controls than cross-sectional studies.

Schaible and Scheuer recently reviewed five longitudinal echocardiographic studies of endurance training.[77] Only a single series documented significant increases in left ventricular diastolic wall thickness and myocardial mass. Left ventricular end-diastolic diameter increased in all five studies but the magnitude of change was very small (*i.e.*, +1% to +8% compared to changes in maximal oxygen uptake from +15% to +31%). Part of this apparent discrepancy can be attributed to the fact that left ventricular volume (and stroke volume) is a third power function of the linear cardiac dimension. The average increase in left ventricular diameter of 4% in the studies quoted by Schaible and Scheuer translates into volume change of 12.5%.

A large amount of data from animal studies is available but clear definitions of the cardiac effects of physical training have not emerged. Studies comparing wild and domesticated animal species have consistently shown larger heart weight relative to body weight in the wild species. This finding is consistent with hypertrophy induced by physical activity but not conclusive proof of a primary or causal relationship.[77] The results of experimental longitudinal studies vary with the species, the mode of exercise, and the sex of the experimental animal when hypertrophy is being defined as an increase in myocardial mass relative to lean body mass. However, under certain conditions both swimming and running are capable of producing hypertrophy and improved contractile performance. Recent experiments also suggest that physical training can restore to normal the depressed cardiac function in pathologic hypertrophy induced by renal hypertension in rats.[78] Enhanced contractility has been demonstrated in a variety of animal models, including isolated papillary muscles and isolated perfused hearts. Multiple myocardial subcellular and biochemical adaptations have been described. Adaptations affecting the contractile proteins or the systems regulating cellular calcium, or both, are particularly likely to be important.[77]

Conclusive detailed data are not available on ventricular performance before and after training during heavy exercise in normal human subjects. Hemodynamic data combined with radionuclide and echocardiographic exercise studies strongly suggest that physical training can increase cardiac pump capacity both in normal subjects and patients with ischemic heart disease.[79,80] However, it is not possible to discriminate clearly between changes in performance related to increases in myocardial mass and dimensions and changes caused by enhanced intrinsic contractile performance.

Several features differentiate physiologic and pathologic cardiac hypertrophy. Characteristically, the normal heart muscle grows to match the work load imposed on the ventricle, maintaining a constant relationship between systolic pressure and the ratio of wall thickness to ventricular radius, irrespective of ventricular size.[81] This means that wall tension is kept constant according to the law of Laplace. The weight lifter's increased mass-to-volume ratio is inappropriate relative to his blood pressure at rest, but the increased wall thickness is most likely appropriate to the hemodynamic conditions *during* isometric exercise and strength training, which induce a marked pressor response. By similar reasoning, an increase in ventricular volume with a secondary small increase in wall thickness is in line with the hemodynamic state during large-muscle dynamic exercise. The early stages of the myocardial responses to cardiac lesions that impose volume or pressure overloads are similar but pathologic hypertrophy has the po-

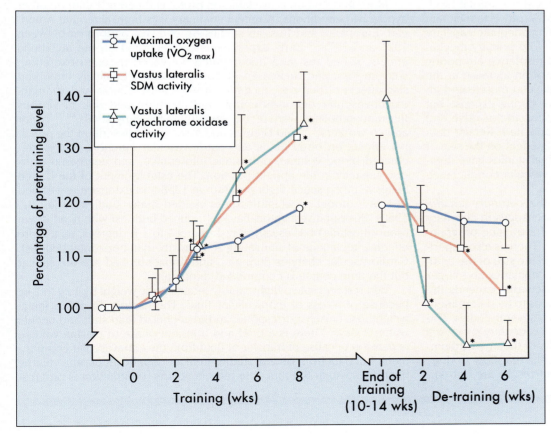

FIGURE 8.8 Time courses for changes in two mitochondrial enzymes and $\dot{V}O_{2max}$ during physical conditioning and deconditioning. Asterisks denote statistically significant changes in sequential measurements. Note that maximal oxygen uptake remains constant for at least six weeks during detraining. SDH and cytochromic activities decline. (Modified from Henriksson J, Reitman JS: Time course of changes in human skeletal muscle succinate dehydrogenase and cytochrome oxidase activities and maximal oxygen uptake with physical activity and inactivity. Acta Physiol Scand 99:91–97, 1977)

tential of causing a much larger increase in heart size. Weights higher than 500 g are rarely seen in athletes whereas valvular and myocardial disease may produce weights well above 1000 g.[82] The primary mechanism in both the abnormal and physiologic situation is hypertrophy of the individual muscle fiber. No convincing signs of hyperplasia have been described except in very young animals. The ratio of myocardium to interstitial tissue remains normal in physiologic hypertrophy but is decreased in failure.[83] The crucial difference between the stimuli producing physiologic and pathologic hypertrophy may be temporal, that is, intermittently increased load during physical activity versus a continuous increase in the presence of various congenital and acquired cardiac defects and in hypertension.

Adaptations in the *peripheral vasculature* are likely to have major effects on cardiac pump capacity. Ventricular filling or *preload* may be enhanced by physical training. The direct hemodynamic effects of skeletal muscle activity on cardiac filling and pump function are poorly understood, but increased skeletal muscle activity may be associated with enhanced extra-cardiac pump function. Increased levels of physical activity generally produce an expansion of total blood volume. A review of the combined results of several studies on the acute hemodynamic effects of blood volume expansion also suggests that high levels of physical fitness are associated with an increased ability to take advantage of the Starling mechanism and to improve stroke volume during exercise.[74]

Afterload reduction is a crucial component of the systemic cardiovascular responses to training. Based on data from both cross-sectional and longitudinal studies, Clausen has demonstrated a strong inverse and curvilinear relationship between maximal oxygen uptake and systemic peripheral resistance.[84,85] A marked reduction in peripheral resistance enables the athlete to generate a cardiac output of up to 40 liters per minute compared to 20 liters in the sedentary subject at similar arterial pressures during maximal exercise. Arterial pressures would be twice as high in the athlete if systemic resistance did not change and the same cardiac output were attained. However, analysis of the performance characteristics of the normal heart suggests that any potential gain in stroke volume that could be achieved by a training-induced increase in heart size would largely be negated by the increased afterload unless training also induced a decrease in systemic resistance.

The increase in the size of the capillary bed of skeletal muscle is a striking feature of the training response, but by far the largest portion of the resistance to systemic blood flow is exerted at the arteriolar level. The principal effect of an increase in the capillary density is to maintain optimal levels of oxygen extraction by maintaining adequate capillary transit times in the presence of high flow rates. The primary mechanisms responsible for the reduction in systemic resistance are poorly defined. It is likely that there is a combination of an increase in the anatomical capacity of the arteriolar bed and skeletal muscle and an enhancement of the metabolic vasodilator drive during exercise but the effects of training on alpha-adrenergic vasoconstrictor drive and beta-adrenergic vasodilation have not been quantitated. Recent data from our laboratory are consistent with a training effect on the size of the arteriolar bed. Cross-sectional and longitudinal studies have demonstrated a training-related increase in maximal vascular conductance of the leg as measured during reactive hyperemia.[80,86]

Physical training has significant effects on the *coronary circulation*.[74,77] Animal studies have demonstrated that changes in coronary flow patterns occur very early after the onset of a training program, which suggests significant regulatory adaptations. There is also experimental evidence for a training-induced increase in the size of the *coronary vascular bed* with changes involving both capillaries and larger vessels. The extent to which the increase in vascularity exceeds the increase in muscle mass in the normal heart remains to be determined. Neogenesis of coronary capillaries is suggested by several studies. The larger heart size in wild animals than in domestic sedentary species is also associated with an increased capillary density of the myocardium. Exercise training has been shown to promote collateral flow in dogs with experimental coronary artery narrowing but results are not uniform. Multiple studies in the dog and pig indicate that exercise produces no increase in collateralization in the absence of coronary lesions.[77]

Physical training clearly improves physical work capacity in most patients with angina pectoris or with healed myocardial infarction. However, human studies have failed to show any effect on stenotic lesions in major coronary vessels and much of the documented improvement has been attributed to a decrease in myocardial oxygen demand rather than to an increase in myocardial oxygen supply.

Physical training also induces significant changes in various *regulatory mechanisms* but our understanding of these effects is far from complete.

In Scheuer and Tipton's review,[87] ample evidence is presented that there is an increased parasympathetic activity at rest after training that causes bradycardia, but the results of various studies performed during exercise conflict.[74] Early experiments produced conflicting data on changes in adrenergic responses after training (*i.e.*, reduced, unchanged, and elevated plasma or myocardial epinephrine or norepinephrine levels). Recent studies have generated more uniform results. There are no significant changes in myocardial tissue concentrations or in the plasma levels of epinephrine or norepinephrine at rest. Plasma concentrations are lower at any absolute submaximal work load after training but there are no differences when comparisons are made on the basis of relative work intensity. Studies of cardiovascular responses to exogenous beta-adrenergic stimulation and of beta-adrenergic receptor numbers are inconclusive.[74]

PROLONGED BED REST AND RELATED CONDITIONS

The human responses to prolonged exposure to bed rest and to weightlessness during space flight have many important features in common. The hydrostatic intravascular and extravascular pressure gradients that are normally present in the upright position are abolished or minimized. This causes a central or cephalad fluid shift that initiates a complex series of adaptive changes in several organ systems. There is also a decrease in skeletal muscle activity. Reexposure to normal gravitational forces produces signs of orthostatic intolerance and there is a decreased capacity to perform exercise. The subject area has recently been reviewed in detail by Blomqvist and Stone.[19]

More information is available on prolonged bed rest than on other hypogravic conditions. A recent summary lists more than 500 American, European, and Russian studies on bed rest performed between 1921 and 1978.[88] Early experiments concentrated on the metabolic effects of bed rest and documented increased nitrogen excretion, calcium loss, and decreased glucose tolerance. Clinically important side-effects of bed rest, including loss of muscle mass and strength, cardiovascular deconditioning, and an increased risk of venous thromboembolism, were recognized during the early 1940s.[89,90] Taylor and co-workers[91,92] and Dietrick and associates[93] described the principal effects on body fluids and cardiovascular function, that is, decreased blood volume, orthostatic intolerance, and decreased exercise capacity in the upright position. The establishment of the United States manned space flight program in 1958 and extensive use of bed rest as a model of weightlessness yielded many studies during the 1960s. Russian investigators have introduced bed rest with head-down (antiorthostatic) tilt, usually at −4 degrees to −6 degrees, as a more effective technique of simulating zero gravity than horizontal bed rest. Cardiovascular changes during tilt and horizontal bed rest are similar but the time course is compressed during tilt.

Bed rest and space flight rapidly reduce body weight by 1 kg to 2 kg because of a loss of extracellular fluid. The magnitude of the initial weight loss closely corresponds to the cephalad fluid shift and occurs within 2 days. There is a brief and transient phase of plasma volume expansion because of transfer of fluid from the extravascular compartment, but data from several studies indicate significant plasma volume decreases within 6 hours. The plasma volume contraction is progressive during the first 3 days, but then a plateau is reached at an average loss level of 350 ml or about 12%. Similar losses also occur within 24 hours in space and during head-down tilt.[19]

There is no conclusive evidence that relatively short exposures to weightlessness (≤1 week) has any unique or specific effects on the cardiovascular system, that is, effects that cannot be reproduced at least in kind during earthbound simulation studies based on bed rest or head-down tilt. Similar considerations apply to the musculoskeletal system but the effects of zero gravity on the vestibular system are probably specific. A vestibular syndrome resembling motion sickness occurs in about 50% of all astronauts during the first few days of space flight. Weightlessness apparently alters the sensory inputs from the otoliths and from the musculoskeletal proprioceptors, which then conflict with the visual input on body position and motion.

Disuse atrophy of skeletal muscle, produced by bed rest or exposure to weightlessness, can cause secondary changes of cardiovascular function by affecting muscle tone, venous pooling, and the response to exercise. Disuse atrophy preferentially affects red fibers. The postural muscles, which contain a high proportion of red or slow-twitch fibers, are particularly vulnerable. The atrophy is reversible.[19] Loss of calcium is an important feature. Prolonged bed rest has produced losses at a rate of 0.5% of total body calcium per month. The process is progressive, and the rate tends to accelerate. The calcium loss appears to be more severe during weightlessness than during bed rest and there are as yet no effective countermeasures. Urolithiasis is a potential complication.

In normal young men, bed rest of 3 to 4 weeks' duration decreases maximal oxygen uptake as measured during exercise in the upright position by 13% to 28%.[19] Similar changes have recently been reported in 50-year-old men.[94] The effects on exercise performance in the supine position are smaller. Observations during submaximal exercise after space flight suggest reductions of the same order of magnitude as after bed rest. Recent studies in our laboratory have shown that a 24-hour period of head-down tilt produces similar changes in physical performance as bed rest of much longer duration.[95-97]

Studies based on radiographic and echocardiographic techniques indicate that bed rest and the related experimental conditions produce a significant decrease in heart size without change in contractile performance.[95,96,98,99] The combined data strongly suggest a reduction in filling pressures in the postadaptive state. Few direct pressure measurements have been made but significant decreases in central venous pressure after 24-hour head-down tilt have been recorded in our laboratory.[95-97] Systemic hemodynamic data are also generally consistent with decreased filling pressures after adaptation.

The principal effects on systemic hemodynamics of 3 weeks of bed rest in normal young men are illustrated in Figure 8.9. Similar results have been recorded after space flight and short-term head-down tilt. The most important change is a marked reduction in stroke volume at rest and during exercise, particularly in the upright position but also in the supine position. A relative tachycardia is present at rest and during submaximal exercise, but cardiac output is still significantly reduced. Maximal heart rate does not change. The systemic arteriovenous oxygen difference tends to be higher at rest and during submaximal exercise but unchanged during maximal work. The maximal oxygen uptake decreases in direct proportion to stroke volume. Mean arterial pressure remains unchanged at rest and during submaximal exercise but is significantly lower at the maximal level. Systemic peripheral resistance is generally higher, but the changes are small and nonsignificant.

Orthostatic intolerance is a universal finding after bed rest, head-down tilt, and space flight. The maximal heart rate difference between supine rest and head-up tilt typically increases from about +25 beats per minute before to +40 to +50 beats per minute. Arterial pressures during orthostatic stress are lower and the incidence of presyncope and syncope increases significantly.

Several lines of evidence argue against inactivity being the major cause of the decreased exercise performance and the orthostatic intolerance. Prolonged bed rest and short-term exposure to head-down tilt or weightlessness with a duration of as little as 24 hours produce similar changes in cardiovascular function. Myocardial and musculoskeletal adaptations to inactivity would require days to weeks to develop. Exercise in the supine position during bed rest generally fails to prevent the development of cardiovascular dysfunction.[19] In addition, if inactivity were a major factor, physical training should accelerate recovery, but this does not occur.[100] The primary cause of the cardiovascular dysfunction after bed rest, head-down tilt, and space flight is likely to be a response to an altered distribution of body fluids and intravascular pressures. The common denominator of these interventions is an initial cephalad fluid shift with a transient increase in central blood volume, cardiac filling pressures, ventricular volumes, and stroke volume. Apparently, the reference level or set-point for hemodynamic regulation in humans is the upright position. A successful adaptation to the supine position or to weightlessness includes decreased end-diastolic volume

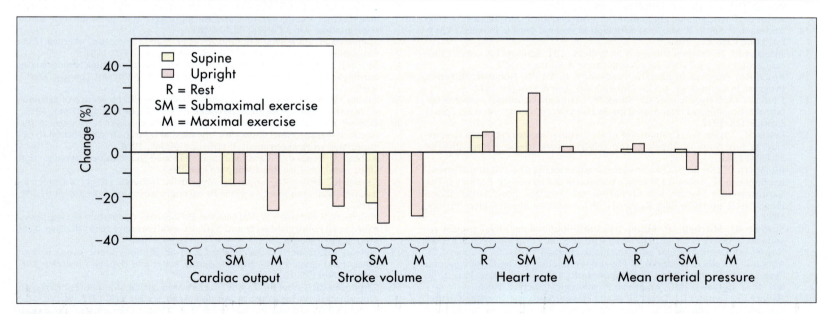

FIGURE 8.9 Hemodynamic effects of 3-week bed rest on cardiac output, stroke volume, heart rate, and mean arterial pressure supine and upright at rest during exercise in 5 normal young men. Control measurements before bed rest = 100%. (Modified from Blomqvist CG, Stone HL: Cardiovascular adjustments to gravitational stress. Handbook of Physiology, The Cardiovascular System, pp 1025–1063. Bethesda, MD, The American Physiological Society, 1983; data from Saltin B, Blomqvist G, Mitchell JH et al: Response to exercise after bed rest and after training. A longitudinal study of adaptive changes in oxygen transport and body composition. Circulation (Suppl) 7:1, 1968)

and filling pressures and decreased total blood volume. These losses and altered regulatory mechanisms make it impossible to cope effectively with a further decrease in central blood volume and filling pressures, when the upright position is resumed at normal gravity.[96]

Decreased intravascular volume is a significant factor. However, the response to an acute volume loss of 300 ml to 400 ml is much less severe than the orthostatic intolerance produced by bed rest and related conditions, strongly implying the involvement of other mechanisms. In addition, attempts to rehydrate subjects after bed rest or to prevent the blood volume loss have not fully corrected the deconditioning. Direct infusions of normal saline solution for administration of mineralocorticoid are only partially effective counter-measures.[19] Increased compliance of the leg veins with larger postural venous pooling could contribute, but several studies have failed to show any significant change. Alternatively, bed rest, head-down tilt, and space flight may cause relative impairment of the regulatory mechanisms that normally maintain arterial blood pressure and tissue perfusion in the upright position.[74]

These observations made in normal subjects are not directly transferable to the clinical situation. Patients with severe heart failure are generally resistant to orthostatic challenges. Nevertheless, the findings in various groups of normal subjects clearly document that bed rest has the potential to cause cardiovascular dysfunction, and they provide a rationale for reemphasis of a 40-year-old therapeutic approach. Levine and Lown in a classic study of chair rest for patients with acute myocardial infarction clearly demonstrated the importance of maintaining normal upright hydrostatic gradients in order to avoid adding the functional losses of cardiovascular deconditioning to the direct consequences of an acute myocardial infarction.[101]

REFERENCES

1. Åstrand PO, Rodahl K: Textbook of Work Physiology, 3rd ed. New York, McGraw-Hill, 1986
2. Goldberg SJ, Mendes F, Hurwitz R: Maximal exercise capacity in children as a function of specific cardiac defects. Am J Cardiol 23:249, 1969
3. Blomqvist CG: Exercise testing in rheumatic heart disease. Cardiovasc Clin 5(2):267–287, 1973
4. Wohl AJ, Lewis HR, Campbell W et al: Cardiovascular function during early recovery from acute myocardial infarction. Circulation 56:931, 1977
5. Hollmann W: Zur Frage der Dauerleistungsfahigkeit. Fortschr Med 74:439, 1961
6. Wasserman K, McIlroy MB: Detecting the threshold of anaerobic metabolism. Am J Cardiol 14:844, 1964
7. Davis JA: Anaerobic threshold: Review of the concept and directions for future research, Med Sci Sports Exerc 17:6, 1985
8. Brooks GA: Anaerobic threshold: Review of the concept and directions for future research. Med Sci Sports Exerc 17:22, 1985
9. Schutte JE, Longhurst JC, Gaffney FA et al: Total plasma creatinine—an accurate measure of total striated muscle mass. J Appl Physiol 51:762, 1981
10. Saltin B, Gollnick PD: Skeletal muscle adaptability: Significance for metabolism and performance. In Peachey LD, Adrian RH (eds): Handbook of Physiology. Section 10: Skeletal Muscle, pp 555–631. Bethesda, MD, American Physiological Society, 1983
11. Komi PV, Viitasalo JHT, Havu M et al: Skeletal muscle enzyme activation in monozygous and dizygous twins of both sexes. Acta Physiol Scand 100:385, 1977
12. Shepherd JT: Circulation to skeletal muscle. In Shepherd JT, Abboud FM (eds): Handbook of Physiology. Section 2: The Cardiovascular System, Vol III. Peripheral Circulation and Organ Blood Flow, Part 1, pp 319–370. Bethesda, MD, American Physiological Society, 1983
13. Saltin B: Hemodynamic adaptations to exercise. Am J Cardiol 55:42D, 1985
14. Andersen P, Saltin B: Maximal perfusion of skeletal muscle in man. J Physiol (Lond) 366:233, 1985
15. Johnson RL Jr: Oxygen transport. In Willerson JT, Sanders CA (eds): Clinical Cardiology, pp 74–84. New York, Grune & Stratton, 1977
16. Bruce RA: Progress in exercise cardiology. In Yu PN, Goodwin JR (eds): Progress in Cardiology, p 113. Philadelphia, Lea & Febiger, 1974
17. Faulkner JA, Heigenhauser GF, Shork MA: The cardiac output—oxygen uptake relationships of man during graded bicycle ergometry. Med Sci Sports Exerc 9:148, 1977
18. Lewis SF, Taylor WF, Graham RM et al: Cardiovascular responses to exercise as functions of absolute and relative work loads. J Appl Physiol 54:1314, 1983
19. Blomqvist CG, Stone HL: Cardiovascular adjustments to gravitational stress. In Shepherd JT, Abboud FM (eds): Handbook of Physiology. Section 2: The Cardiovascular System, Vol III. Peripheral Circulation and Organ Blood Flow, Part 2, pp 1025–1063. Bethesda, MD, American Physiological Society, 1983
20. Sproule BJ, Mitchell JH, Miller WF: Cardiopulmonary physiological responses to heavy exercise in patients with anemia. J Clin Invest 39:378, 1960
21. Rowell LB: Cardiovascular adjustments to thermal stress. In Shepherd JT, Abboud FM (eds): Handbook of Physiology. Section 2: The Cardiovascular System, Vol III. Peripheral Circulation and Organ Blood Flow, Part 2, pp 967–1023. Bethesda, MD, American Physiological Society, 1983
22. Poliner LR, Dehmer GJ, Lewis SE et al: Left ventricular performance in normal subjects: A comparison of the responses to exercise in the upright and supine positions. Circulation 62:528, 1980
23. Granath A, Jonsson B, Strandell T: Circulation in healthy old men, studied by right heart catheterization at rest and during exercise in supine and standing position. Acta Med Scand 176:425, 1964
24. Blomqvist CG: Upper extremity exercise testing and training. In Wenger N, Hellerstein H (eds): Exercise and the Heart, pp 179–196. New York, John Wiley & Sons, 1984
25. Blomqvist CG, Lewis SF, Taylor WF, Graham RM: Similarity of the hemodynamic responses to static and dynamic exercise of small muscle groups. Circ Res 48(Suppl I):87, 1981
26. Lewis SF, Taylor WF, Bastian BC et al: Hemodynamic responses to static and dynamic handgrip before and after autonomic blockade. Clin Sci 64:593, 1983
27. Schwade J, Blomqvist CG, Shapiro W: A comparison of the response to arm and leg work in patients with ischemic heart disease. Am Heart J 94:203, 1977
28. Blomqvist CG: Exercise testing and electrocardiographic interpretation. In Pollock ML, Schmidt DH (eds): Heart Disease and Rehabilitation, 2nd ed, pp 131–148. New York, John Wiley & Sons, 1986
29. Bevegård S, Freyschuss U, Strandell T: Circulatory adaptation to arm and leg exercise in supine and sitting positions. J Appl Physiol 21:37, 1966
30. Goldstein RE, Beiser GD, Stampfer M, Epstein SE: Impairment of autonomically mediated heart rate control in patients with cardiac dysfunction. Circ Res 36:571, 1975
31. Weber KT, Kinasewitz GT, Janicki JS, Fishman AP: Oxygen utilization and ventilation during exercise in patients with chronic cardiac failure. Circulation 65:1213, 1982
32. Ross J Jr: The failing heart and the circulation. Hosp Pract 18:151, 1983
33. Higginbotham MB, Morris KG, Conn EH et al: Determinants of variable exercise performance among patients with severe left ventricular dysfunction. Am J Cardiol 51:52, 1983
34. Firth BG, Dehmer GJ, Markham RV Jr et al: Assessment of vasodilatory therapy in patients with severe congestive heart failure: Limitations of measurements of left ventricular ejection fraction and volumes. Am J Cardiol 50:954, 1982
35. Dehmer GJ, Firth BG, Hillis LD et al: Alterations in left ventricular volumes and ejection fraction at rest and during exercise in patients with aortic regurgitation. Am J Cardiol 48:17, 1981
36. Shepherd JT, Blomqvist CG, Lind AR et al: Static (isometric) exercise. Retrospection and introspection. Circ Res 48(Suppl 1):179, 1981
37. Mitchell JH, Payne FC III, Saltin B, Schibye B: The role of muscle mass in the cardiovascular response to static contractions. J Physiol (Lond) 309:45, 1980
38. Atkins JM, Matthews OA, Blomqvist CG, Mullins CB: Incidence of arrhythmias induced by isometric and dynamic exercise. Br Heart J 37:465, 1976
39. DeBusk RF, Valdez R, Houston N et al: Cardiovascular responses to dynamic and static effort soon after myocardial infarction: Application to occupational work assessment. Circulation 58:368, 1978
40. Kilbom Å, Persson J: Cardiovascular response to combined dynamic and static exercise. Circ Res 48(Suppl I):93, 1981
41. Kerber RE, Miller RA, Najjar SM: Myocardial ischemic effects of isometric, dynamic and combined exercise in coronary artery disease. Chest 67:388, 1975
42. Holmberg S, Serzysko W, Varnauskas E: Coronary circulation during heavy exercise in control subjects and patients with coronary heart disease. Acta Med Scand 190:465, 1971
43. Nelson RR, Gobel FL, Jorgensen CR et al: Hemodynamic predictors of myocardial oxygen consumption during static and dynamic exercise. Circulation 59:1179, 1974
44. Jorgensen CR, Gobel FL, Taylor HL et al: Myocardial blood flow and oxygen consumption during exercise. Ann NY Acad Sci 301:213, 1977
45. Gobel FL, Nordstrom LA, Nelson RR et al: The rate pressure product as an index of myocardial oxygen consumption during exercise in patients with angina pectoris. Circulation 57:549, 1978
46. White FC, Sanders M, Bloor CM: Coronary reserve at maximal heart rate in the exercising swine. J Cardiac Rehab 1:31, 1981
47. Gould KL, Lipscomb K: Effects of coronary stenoses on coronary flow re-

48. serve and resistance. Am J Cardiol 34:48, 1974
48. White CW, Wright CB, Doty DB et al: Does visual interpretation of coronary angiograms predict the physiological importance of a coronary stenosis? N Engl J Med 310:819, 1984
49. Robinson BF: Relation of heart rate and systolic blood pressure to the onset of pain in angina pectoris. Circulation 35:1073, 1967
50. Parker JO, Chiong MA, West RO, Case RB: Sequential alterations in myocardial lactate metabolism, S-T segments, and left ventricular function during angina induced by atrial pacing. Circulation 40:113, 1969
51. Parker JO, West RO, Case RB, Chiong MA: Temporary relationships of myocardial lactate metabolism, left ventricular function, and S-T segment depression during angina precipitated by exercise. Circulation 40:97, 1969
52. Guazzi M, Polese A, Fiorentini C et al: Left ventricular performance and related haemodynamic changes in Prinzmetal's variant angina pectoris. Br Heart J 33:84, 1971
53. Mitchell JH: Cardiovascular control during exercise. Central and reflex neural mechanisms. Am J Cardiol 55:34D, 1985
54. Remensnyder JP, Mitchell JH, Sarnoff SJ: Functional sympathicolysis during muscular activity. Circ Res 11:370, 1962
55. Gaffney FA, Saltin B: Personal communication, 1985
56. Clausen JP, Klausen K, Rasmussen B, Trap-Jensen J: Central and peripheral changes after training of the arms and legs. Am J Physiol 225:675, 1973
57. Saltin B, Nazar K, Costill DL et al: The nature of the training response, peripheral and central adaptation to one-legged exercise. Acta Physiol Scand 96:289, 1976
58. Klausen K, Secher NH, Clausen JP et al: Central and regional circulatory adaptation to one-leg training. J Appl Physiol 52:976, 1982
59. Olsson RA: Local factors regulating cardiac and skeletal muscle blood flow. Annu Rev Physiol 43:385, 1981
60. Wildenthal K, Mierzwiak DS, Skinner NS Jr, Mitchell JH: Potassium-induced cardiovascular and ventilatory reflexes from the dog hindlimb. Am J Physiol 215:542, 1968
61. Tibes U: Reflex inputs to the cardiovascular and respiratory centers from dynamically working canine muscles: Some evidence for involvement of group III or IV nerve fibers. Circ Res 41:332, 1977
62. Saltin B, Sjøgaard G, Gaffney FA, Rowell LB: Potassium, lactate and water fluxes in human quadriceps muscle during static contractions. Circ Res 48(Suppl I):18, 1981
63. Eckberg DW, Drabinsky M, Braunwald E: Defective cardiac parasympathetic control in patients with heart disease. N Engl J Med 285:877, 1971
64. Abboud FM, Thames MD, Mark AL: Role of cardiac afferent nerves in regulation of circulation during coronary occlusion and heart failure. In Abboud FM, Fozzard HA, Gilmore JP, Reis DJ (eds): Disturbances in Neurogenic Control of the Circulation, pp 65–86. Bethesda, MD, American Physiological Society, 1981
65. Chidsey CA, Kaiser GA, Sonnenblick EH et al: Cardiac norepinephrine stores in experimental heart failure in dogs. J Clin Invest 43:2389, 1964
66. Sole MJ: Alterations in sympathetic and parasympathetic neurotransmitter activity. In Braunwald E, Mock MB, Watson JT (eds): Congestive Heart Failure: Current Research and Clinical Applications, pp 101–113. New York, Grune & Stratton, 1982
67. Swedberg K, Hjalmarson A, Waagstein F, Wallentin I: Beneficial effects of long-term beta-blockade in congestive cardiomyopathy. Br Heart J 44:117, 1980
68. Tilton GD, Bush L, Wathen M et al: What is wrong with the failing heart? Texas Med 79:35, 1983
69. Chidsey CA, Harrison DC, Braunwald E: Augmentation of plasma norepinephrine response to exercise in patients with congestive heart failure. N Engl J Med 267:650, 1962
70. Markham RV, Firth BG: Personal communication, 1983
71. Saltin B, Blomqvist CG, Mitchell JH et al: Response to exercise after bed rest and after training. Circulation 38(Suppl 7):1, 1968
72. Klissouras V: Heritability of adaptive variation. J Appl Physiol 31:338, 1971
73. Klissouras V, Pirnay F, Petit JM: Adaptation to maximal effort: Genetics and age. J Appl Physiol 35:288, 1973
74. Blomqvist CG, Saltin B: Cardiovascular adaptations to physical training. Annu Rev Physiol 45:169, 1983
75. Davies KJ, Packer L, Brooks GA: Biochemical adaptations of mitochondria, muscle, and whole-animal respiration to endurance training. Arch Biochem Biophys 209:539, 1981
76. Gollnick PD, Saltin B: Significance of skeletal muscle oxidative enzyme enhancement with endurance training. Clin Physiol 2:1, 1982
77. Schaible TF, Scheuer J: Cardiac adaptations to chronic exercise. Prog Cardiovasc Dis 27:297, 1985
78. Schaible TF, Ciambrone GJ, Capasso JM, Scheuer J: Cardiac conditioning ameliorates cardiac dysfunction associated with renal hypertension in rats. J Clin Invest 73:1086, 1984
79. Ehsani AA, Martin WH, Heath GW, Coyle EF: Cardiac effects of prolonged and intense exercise training in patients with coronary artery disease. Am J Cardiol 50:246, 1982
80. Martin WH, Montgomery J, Snell PG et al: Cardiovascular adaptations to intense swim training in sedentary middle-aged humans. Circulation 75:323, 1987
81. Ford LE: Heart size. Circ Res 39:297, 1976
82. Linzbach AJ: Heart failure from the point of view of quantitative anatomy. Am J Cardiol 5:370, 1960
83. Fuster V, Danielson MA, Robb RA et al: Quantitation of left ventricular myocardial fiber hypertrophy and interstitial tissue in human hearts with chronically increased volume and pressure overload. Circulation 55:504, 1977
84. Clausen JP: Circulatory adjustments to dynamic exercise and effect of physical training in normal subjects and in patients with coronary artery disease. Prog Cardiovasc Dis 18:459, 1976
85. Clausen JP: Effect of physical training on cardiovascular adjustments to exercise in man. Physiol Rev 57:779, 1977
86. Snell PG, Martin WH, Buckey JC, Blomqvist CG: Maximal vascular leg conductance in trained and untrained men. J Appl Physiol 62:606, 1987
87. Scheuer J, Tipton CM: Cardiovascular adaptations to physical training. Annu Rev Physiol 39:221, 1977
88. Nicogossian AE, Hoffler GW, Johnson RL, Gowen RJ: Determination of cardiac size from chest roentgenograms following Skylab missions. In Johnson RS, Dietlein LF (eds): Biomedical Results from Skylab, pp 400–405. Washington, DC, National Aeronautics and Space Administration, SP-377, 1977
89. Harrison TR: Abuse of rest as a therapeutic means for patients with cardiovascular disease. JAMA 125:1075, 1944
90. Dock W: The evil sequelae of complete bed rest. JAMA 125:1083, 1944
91. Taylor HL, Erickson L, Henschel A, Keys A: The effect of bed rest on the blood volume of normal young men. Am J Physiol 144:227, 1945
92. Taylor HL, Henschel A, Brozek J, Keys A: Effects of bed rest on cardiovascular function and work performance. J Appl Physiol 2:223, 1949
93. Dietrick JE, Whedon GD, Shorr E et al: Effects of immobilization on metabolic and physiologic function of normal men. Am J Med 4:3, 1948
94. Convertino VA, Sandler H, Webb P: The effect of an elastic reverse gradient garment on the cardiorespiratory deconditioning following 15 days bed rest, p 148. Preprints of the 1978 Annual Scientific Meeting, Aerospace Medical Association, New Orleans, LA, May 8–11, 1978
95. Nixon JV, Murray RG, Bryant C et al: Early cardiovascular adaptation to simulated zero gravity. J Appl Physiol 46:541, 1979
96. Blomqvist CG, Nixon JV, Johnson RL Jr, Mitchell JH: Early cardiovascular adaptation to zero gravity simulated by head-down tilt. Acta Astronautica 7:543, 1980
97. Gaffney FA, Nixon JV, Karlsson ES et al: Cardiovascular deconditioning produced by 20 hours of bedrest with head-down tilt ($-5°$) in middle-aged healthy men. Am J Cardiol 56:634, 1985
98. Henry WL, Epstein SE, Griffith JM et al: Effects of prolonged space flight on cardiac function and dimensions. In Johnston RS, Dietlein LF (eds): Biomedical Results from Skylab, pp 366–371. Washington, DC, National Aeronautics and Space Administration SP-377, 1977
99. Hung J, Goldwater D, Convertino V et al: Effects of bedrest deconditioning on exercise ventricular function in man (abstr). Am J Cardiol 47:477, 1981
100. DeBusk RF, Convertino VA, Hung J, Goldwater D: Exercise conditioning in middle-aged men after 10 days of bed rest. Circulation 68:245, 1983
101. Levine SA, Lown B: The "chair" treatment of acute coronary thrombosis. Trans Assoc Am Physicians 64:316, 1951

GENERAL REFERENCE

Mitchell JH, Blomqvist CG, Lind AR et al: Static (isometric) exercise: Cardiovascular responses and neural control mechanisms. Circ Res (Suppl) 48:II-I188, 1981

PULMONARY EDEMA

Max Harry Weil • Eric C. Rackow
Carter E. Mecher

With remarkable clarity, the English physiologist Ernest Starling[1] described the forces that govern the exchange of fluid between capillaries and their surrounding connective tissue spaces. Inherent in what has come to be known as the "Starling Law of the Capillary" are the six principal factors that determine the rate of fluid filtration across the capillary membrane. These are demonstrated, together with the Starling equation, in Figure 9.1 and include the hydrostatic pressure within the capillary and the hydrostatic pressure of the interstitium external to the capillary. It further includes the osmotic pressure generated by plasma proteins and predominately by albumin, namely the colloid osmotic or oncotic pressure of plasma within the capillary and the corresponding pressure in the interstitial fluid space external to the capillary. Finally, it describes the behavior of the membrane and more specifically the ease with which either water or plasma proteins may transit across the membrane. Two such transport coefficients are now recognized, namely a water transport coefficient and a protein transport coefficient.

PATHOPHYSIOLOGY

For practical purposes, the Starling equation provides a very good basis for understanding the primary defects that account for pulmonary edema. In the clinical setting, two primary mechanisms for fluid extravasation are recognized. The more frequent of these is hemodynamic pulmonary edema. This pulmonary edema state is most often due to increases in capillary hydrostatic pressure, which, in turn, is most often due to increases in pulmonary venous, left atrial, and left ventricular diastolic pressure during the course of left-sided heart failure. For this reason, it has often been referred to as cardiogenic pulmonary edema. Experimentally, hemodynamic pulmonary edema may be due to a reduction in the colloid osmotic pressure of plasma (*i.e.*, hypo-oncotic pulmonary edema).[2] However, for reasons that will be discussed in greater detail, even marked reductions in plasma colloid osmotic pressure may not be accompanied by pulmonary edema unless there is at least a moderate increase in capillary hydrostatic pressure.

Within the past 20 years, the importance of a second major cause of pulmonary edema due to increases in the permeability of the alveolar-capillary endothelial membranes to proteins has been identified. Appropriately referred to as "leaky capillaries," it is a defect due to increased protein flux from the capillaries into the interstitium. More specifically, the capillary endothelium is injured such that it can no longer function as a competent semi-permeable membrane by reflecting plasma proteins. In the Starling equation, it is identified as a reduction in the protein transport coefficient. Since permeability pulmonary edema develops in the absence of increased capillary hydrostatic pressures, it is also known as "noncardiogenic" or "low pressure" pulmonary edema. These major defects and their relationship to the Starling equation are shown in Figure 9.2.

CLINICAL DEFINITIONS

The clinical features of hemodynamic pulmonary edema may present as an acute event due to very rapid increases in pressures distal to the pulmonary capillaries that, with rare exceptions, reflect increases in left-sided heart filling pressures in the setting of cardiac crises. This follows extensive anterior myocardial infarction or acute myocardial ischemia superimposed on prior myocardial infarction in which left ventricular compliance is markedly reduced. The greater the clinical severity of heart failure, the larger is the increase in extravascular lung water.[3] This is in contrast to more protracted and persistent increases in pulmonary capillary hydrostatic pressures in patients with chronic pulmonary edema. Permeability pulmonary edema, on the other hand, is now commonly referred to as the adult respiratory distress syndrome

---

$$\dot{Q}_f = K_f[(P_c - P_i) - \sigma(P_{II_c} - P_{II_i})]$$

$\dot{Q}_f$ = Rate of fluid filtration

K_f = Water transport coefficient

P_c = Capillary hydrostatic pressure

P_i = Interstitial hydrostatic pressure

σ = Protein transport coefficient

P_{II} = Colloid osmotic (oncotic) pressure

FIGURE 9.1 Starling equation.

Pulmonary Edema ($\dot{Q}_f$)

Hemodynamic PE

    Hydrostatic ($\uparrow P_c$)

    Hypo-oncotic ($\downarrow P_{II_c}$)

Permeability PE

    Protein transport coefficient ($\sigma \downarrow$)

$$\dot{Q}_f = K_f[(P_c - P_i) - \sigma(P_{II_c} - P_{II_i})]$$

FIGURE 9.2 The two major causes of clinical pulmonary edema states and how they relate to the Starling equation.

(ARDS).[4] It is also known as primary pulmonary edema to call attention to the fact that the primary site of injury is within the lung.[5] This is in contrast to hemodynamic pulmonary edema in which the defect is almost always downstream and external to the lung.[6]

PULMONARY STRUCTURE AND FUNCTION

The predominant pulmonary alveolar epithelial cell is a so-called type I squamous pneumocyte that spreads over the blood–gas interface. A second cell, the type II pneumocyte, which is a granular, cuboidal epithelial cell, occurs in somewhat larger numbers and predominantly in the interstitial space more remote from the blood–gas interface. The interstitial space itself consists of loose interlobular, perivascular, and peribronchial connective tissue that communicates widely. It is also looked on as the thick alveolar capillary septum with an interstitial space separating the basement membrane of the capillary endothelium from the basement membrane of the alveolar epithelial cells. Richly supplied by lymphatic channels, which drain toward the hilum of the lung, it provides for storage of water and solute and its subsequent passage into the lymphatic channels. This contrasts to the thin septum in which there is close approximation between the basement membrane of the capillary endothelial cell and the basement membrane of the type I pneumocyte, thereby facilitating blood gas exchange.[7] Accordingly, there is a separation of the fluid storage and drainage function from that of gas exchange function.

Plasma water is stored in the interstitial spaces of the lung in gel state. This makes it possible to store a substantial amount of fluid with little increase in interstitial volume.[7] However, when the gel capacity is exceeded, interstitial pressure increases and free fluid accumulates. The lymphatic channels that course through perivascular and interlobular connective tissue then serve as drainage channels for this free fluid. Normally, interstitial pressure is believed to be negative. However, interstitial pressure is increased when free fluid accumulates in excess of the amounts that can be accommodated by the lymphatic channels. As the interstitial pressure rises, the so-called J receptors, which are stretch receptors in the interstitial space, are stimulated such that ventilation is increased.[8] This may be functionally useful because increased ventilation probably enhances lymphatic flow and therefore minimizes the risk of rapidly progressive interstitial edema and subsequent alveolar flooding.

The type II pneumocytes are believed to be the source of surfactant, a thin layer of phospholipid that lines the alveoli. It is the surfactant that reduces the surface forces at the air–tissue interface such as to maintain patency of alveoli. Surfactant therefore stabilizes alveolar units, prevents their collapse, and thereby reduces the risk of ventilation–perfusion mismatching with increased pulmonary venous-arterial shunting. It is also believed to have an antibacterial effect.[9]

COLLOID-HYDROSTATIC PRESSURE RELATIONSHIPS

Since the capillary endothelial membrane does not completely reflect plasma proteins, the interstitial colloid osmotic pressure normally ranges from one half to two thirds that of plasma and the protein transfer coefficient σ is approximately 0.7. Figure 9.3 diagrammatically illustrates the normal conditions of fluid flux across the capillary in which the interstitial colloid osmotic pressure is assumed to be at its highest, namely 19 mm Hg. The normal pulmonary capillary pressure is shown to be 7 mm Hg, and the normal colloid osmotic pressure of plasma is 25 mm Hg. Present evidence suggests that the interstitial

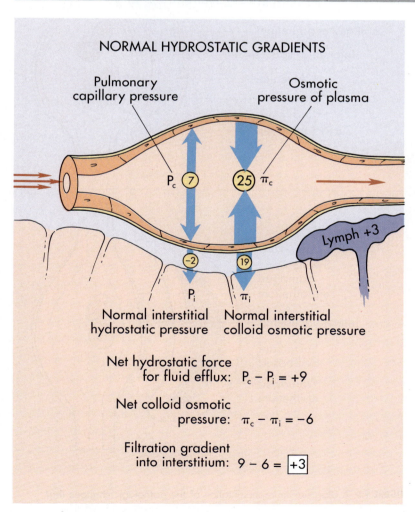

FIGURE 9.3 Normal pulmonary intracapillary and interstitial colloid–hydrostatic pressure relationships.

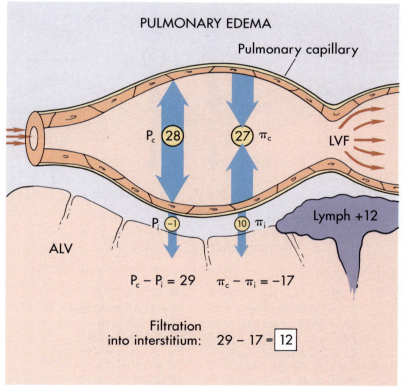

FIGURE 9.4 Pulmonary intracapillary and interstitial colloid–hydrostatic pressure changes during hemodynamic (hydrostatic) pulmonary edema.

hydrostatic pressure is normally negative and we assume it to be -2 mm Hg. Consequently, there is a net hydrostatic force for fluid efflux from the capillary of 9 mm and an opposing net colloid osmotic pressure of 6 mm. The net effect is a "normal" gradient of 3 mm Hg of pressure favoring fluid flow into the interstitium. This amount of fluid is well accommodated by the gel capacity of the interstitium. When the gel capacity is exceeded, it is effectively drained through the lymphatic channels.

This is in contrast to hydrostatic pulmonary edema (Fig. 9.4), in which the capillary hydrostatic pressure is increased to 28 mm. When the capillary hydrostatic pressure is increased to levels near or exceeding plasma colloid osmotic pressure, the resulting increase in fluid flux is believed to have two effects. Relatively larger amounts of protein are reflected, and therefore the interstitial colloid osmotic pressure is reduced. Consequently, the plasma colloid osmotic pressure within the capillary is progressively increased.[10] At the same time, there is less negative interstitial pressure probably due to the physical effects of augmented interstitial fluid. A capillary hydrostatic pressure of 28 mm Hg and an interstitial hydrostatic pressure of -1 mm Hg are illustrated. Accordingly, there is a net hydrostatic pressure of 29 mm. The capillary (plasma) colloid osmotic pressure is 27 mm, and the interstitial colloid osmotic pressure 10 mm Hg in the setting of left ventricular failure. Thus, there is a net filtration pressure of 12 mm. This gradient increases fluid flux such that both the gel capacity and the capability for lymphatic drainage is exceeded. With continued accumulation of interstitial fluid, there is overflow into alveoli and ultimately alveolar flooding. The surfactant concentration in fluid-filled alveoli is decreased; microatelectasis and both interstitial and alveolar fluid accumulations account for a marked reduction in pulmonary compliance.

The conditions that may prevail in the hypo-oncotic state are demonstrated in Figure 9.5. The data were obtained from a 75-year-old man who had nephrotic syndrome in consequence of amyloidosis. Plasma colloid osmotic pressure was markedly reduced in association with serum albumin concentrations of 1.5 g/dl. However, pulmonary artery occlusive pressure, measured with a Swan-Ganz catheter, was only 5 mm Hg. For the purpose of this and prior illustrations, the quantitative effects of pulmonary artery pressure on capillary hydrostatic pressure are not taken into account. However, since the capillary hydrostatic pressure was unusually low, the net effect was a normal filtration pressure of 3 mm Hg. Accordingly, the hemodynamic conditions did not favor pulmonary edema.

In the setting of ARDS, permeability pulmonary edema is attributed to alveolar-capillary injury (Fig. 9.6). Although the pathologic picture may vary from mild inflammatory change to those of hemorrhagic pneumonitis and hyaline membrane formation, the primary problem is believed to be due to damage of alveolar-capillary membranes at the

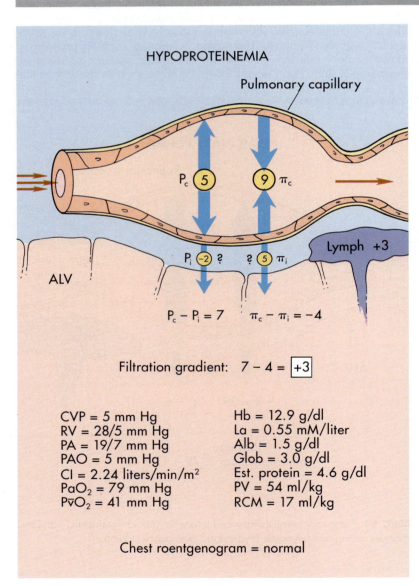

FIGURE 9.5 Pulmonary capillary colloid–hydrostatic pressure relationships in the pulmonary capillary for a patient with marked hypoproteinemia. (CVP, central venous pressure; PAO, pulmonary arterial occlusive pressure; La, blood lactate; PV, plasma volume; RCM, red cell mass)

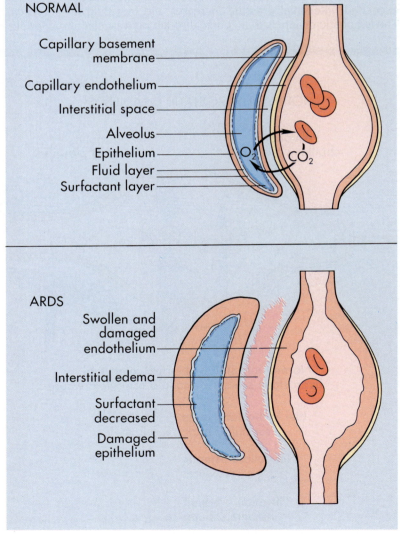

FIGURE 9.6 A diagramatic representation of the pathologic changes that account for permeability pulmonary edema in the setting of ARDS.

blood–gas interface. This accounts for interstitial and subsequent alveolar edema. There is usually no abnormality of either the capillary hydrostatic pressure or the colloid osmotic pressure of plasma. The colloid-hydrostatic pressure conditions during permeability pulmonary edema are diagrammatically illustrated in Figure 9.7. Permeability pulmonary edema therefore is, by definition, a consequence of the membrane injury and capillary leak of protein.

CLINICAL MEASUREMENTS

The capillary hydrostatic pressure of the lung can be estimated with current hemodynamic monitoring techniques using the flow-directed pulmonary artery catheter. Practical devices are also available for routine clinical measurement of colloid osmotic pressure and include the oncometer or colloid osmometer.[11] The so-called colloid-hydrostatic pressure gradient has been regarded by some workers, including us, as a helpful quantitator of the risk of pulmonary edema.[12-16] In normal subjects, the colloid-hydrostatic pressure gradient (*i.e.*, plasma oncotic pressure minus pulmonary artery occlusive pressure) exceeds 15 mm. When this gradient declines to less than 4 mm Hg in the setting of hemodynamic pulmonary edema, and especially if it persists at such levels for intervals exceeding 12 hours, the risks of pulmonary edema are believed to be greatly increased. The severity of hemodynamic pulmonary edema is progressively increased as the colloid osmotic minus pulmonary artery occlusive pressure gradient decreases to more negative levels. With decreasing colloid osmotic pressure in critically ill patients, there is also a progressive increase in mortality.[16,17] However, acute volume loading with non-colloid-containing fluids in both experimental animals and in patients, particularly in surgical settings, do not consistently support measurement of the colloid-hydrostatic pressure gradient as a reliable predictor of the risk of pulmonary edema.[18] The issue is not fully settled. It is likely, however, that in the setting of otherwise uncomplicated hemodynamic pulmonary edema in patients with decreased cardiac competence, the colloid-hydrostatic pressure gradient is a useful measurement. To the contrary, in settings in which there is a permeability defect, and this applies particularly to patients with traumatic injuries, following surgical operation, and/or sepsis, the colloid-hydrostatic pressure gradient may be invalidated because of a concurrent permeability defect.[19] As already cited, the hypo-oncotic state does not of itself provoke pulmonary edema unless there are concurrent increases in capillary hydrostatic pressures. The hydrostatic pressure exerts a larger effect than the colloid osmotic pressure, in part because reductions in plasma colloid osmotic pressure are associated with decreases in interstitial colloid osmotic pressure.[20]

HEMODYNAMIC (CARDIOGENIC) PULMONARY EDEMA
CLINICAL FEATURES

With increases in pulmonary venous pressure and consequently pulmonary capillary pressure, the onset of tachypnea followed by cough and wheezing signals the onset of pulmonary edema. Edema first appears in the perivascular connective tissue surrounding the small airways. Expiratory obstruction is accentuated by hyperventilation with high-velocity air flow. Initial hyperventilation accounts for mild respiratory alkalosis. Edema of the mucosa of the airways with bronchorrhea provokes cough and subsequently sputum production. With progressive alveolar flooding, restlessness and increasing respiratory distress with anxiety are observed. Crackles appear in the dependent portions of the lungs. The arterial blood *p*H declines with progressive alveolar flooding when respiratory alkalosis is gradually converted to respiratory acidosis and metabolic acidosis. The metabolic acidosis is primarily due to lactic acidosis. Even though cardiac output may be only moderately reduced, the increased work of breathing caused by progressive reductions in lung compliance together with anxiety and adrenergic stimulation increase the metabolic requirements for oxygen. With encroachment of fluid on the alveolar capillary exchange surfaces such that there is a critical reduction in functional alveoli, ventilatory gas exchange is curtailed. Accordingly, there is increased oxygen demand that cannot be met by the available oxygen supply. Hence anaerobic metabolism is in evidence with production of lactic acid. In more advanced stages of pulmonary edema, the patient appears pale with physical signs of both central and peripheral cyanosis accompanied by diaphoresis. With very severe pressure pulmonary edema, frothy and sometimes blood-tinged sputum indicates rapid transudation of fluid into the alveoli and the airways, with escape of red blood cells especially from congested mucosal blood vessels. In late stages of congestive heart failure, both cerebral blood flow and oxygen delivery are reduced and periodic breathing and especially Cheyne-Stokes respiration with intervening intervals of apnea and hyperventilation may appear. Highly variable blood gas results may be measured; during apnea there is a decline in arterial oxygen tension (Pa_{O_2}) and an increase in arterial carbon dioxide tension (Pa_{CO_2}). During hyperventilation, Pa_{O_2} is increased and Pa_{CO_2} is reduced.

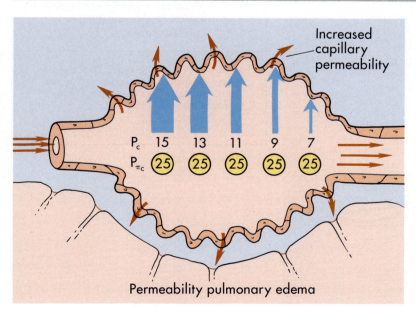

FIGURE 9.7 In capillary colloid-hydrostatic pressure conditions during permeability pulmonary edema no assumptions are made with respect to the interstitial capillary pressure. However, the interstitial colloid osmotic pressure approaches that of plasma.

PAROXYSMAL NOCTURNAL DYSPNEA

Contingent on the specific cause of left ventricular failure, a majority of instances of cardiogenic pulmonary edema are self-limiting. Typically, symptoms begin at night with cough, paroxysmal dyspnea, and orthopnea. This is largely explained by Starling mechanisms since there is nocturnal mobilization of edema fluid with expansion of the intravascular volume. In the upright posture, there is a large gravimetric effect on lower extremity venous pressure owing to the blood column that extends from the right atrium to the toes, even though it is in part moderated by venous valves. Normally, there is lower body extravasation of plasma water due to the higher venous pressure and, in turn, corresponding increases in systemic capillary pressures in the lower extremities. As shown in Figure 9.8, a difference of approximately 4 mm is observed between the colloid osmotic pressure in plasma of the human subject who has been upright for 4 hours in contrast to the colloid osmotic pressure in the supine posture. Corresponding increases in plasma protein occur in the upright posture and decreases in the supine position. Such "physiologic edema" fluid is reabsorbed when the patient resumes the supine posture. When this hypo-oncotic fluid reenters the intravascular compartment, the plasma protein concentration and colloid osmotic pressure is reduced.[21] As much as 20% of plasma water volume is augmented. The reabsorbed plasma water expands the intravascular volume and increases venous return and right- and left-sided heart preload. To the extent that there is impaired left ventricular function, the left-sided filling pressures and pulmonary capillary hydrostatic pressure is increased. The consequent pulmonary edema and the respiratory distress and sensation of suffocation that accompanies it arouses the patient from sleep. The patient typically sits up, then rushes to an open window with labored breathing and wheezing. In assuming the upright posture, preload and plasma volume are reduced and the symptoms of heart failure and, more specifically, those of hemodynamic pulmonary edema may be reversed.

CHRONIC HEART FAILURE

The majority of patients with paroxysmal nocturnal dyspnea and orthopnea are likely to have clinical signs of impaired cardiac competence with cardiac enlargement and a diastolic third heart sound that is accentuated during auscultation after mild exertion. In most instances there is concurrent right-sided failure with increases in jugular venous pressure, hepatojugular reflux, hepatomegaly, and peripheral edema. Cardiac output and the left ventricular ejection fraction are likely to be reduced at rest and fail to increase with exercise. Chronic fatigue is presumed to be due to decreases in blood flow to striated muscles, including respiratory muscles that have increased oxygen requirements. The increased work of breathing, stemming from reduced pulmonary compliance, adds to the muscular workload with increasing interstitial and alveolar pulmonary edema. The increased pulmonary water infringes on the exchangeable air volume. Therefore, there is substantial limitation in exercise capability not only because of reduction in cardiac output but also because of restraints in ventilation stemming from the restrictive defect caused by increases in lung water.

ROENTGENOGRAPHIC FEATURES

Routine roentgenographic examination of the chest typically demonstrates cardiac enlargement in patients with more chronic forms of

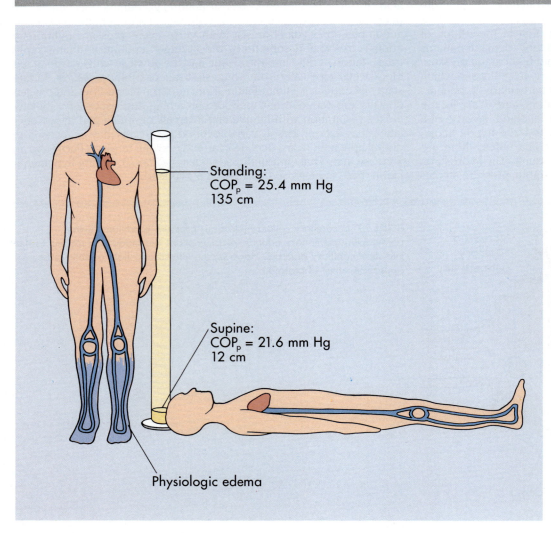

FIGURE 9.8 Differences in colloid osmotic pressure in the upright and supine postures and their relationship to the hydrostatic height of the venous fluid column in each of the postures.

TABLE 9.1 ROENTGENOGRAPHIC CRITERIA OF PULMONARY EDEMA

0	Normal
1+	Equal perfusion upper and lower lung fields
2+	Interstitial prominence; perivascular edema (vascular markings preserved)
3+	Septal lines (Kerley's B lines); diffuse reticular infiltrates (vascular markings obliterated)
4+	Bilateral confluent infiltrates; pleural effusion

(Turner AF, Lau FV, Jacobson G: A method for the estimation of pulmonary venous and arterial pressures from the routine chest roentgenogram. AJR 116:97, 1972)

congestive heart failure. In addition, there are changes that are characteristic of increases in pulmonary venous pressure and both interstitial and alveolar edema. These include increased venous perfusion of the upper lung fields (so-called cephalization), perivascular cuffing by edema fluid, prominence of interstitial lung markings, and the appearance of transverse, septal lines in the peripheral lung fields that are known as Kerley's B lines. With further progression in severity, diffuse reticular infiltration with obliteration of vascular markings, bilateral confluent infiltrates, and pleural effusion are observed. On the basis of these roentgenographic features, Turner and his associates[22] have developed useful criteria for the quantitation of severity of pulmonary edema and these are summarized in Table 9.1. The chest roentgenogram usually demonstrates bilateral opacification that typically fans out from the hilum to the bases. However, pulmonary edema may be asymmetrical and even unilateral in patients who habitually lie on only one side or who have concurrent lung disease.

Nevertheless, clinical and roentgenographic criteria for the differentiation of hemodynamic and permeability pulmonary edema are not consistently reliable. Permeability pulmonary edema is not likely to be accompanied by either cardiac enlargement or increases in pulmonary venous pressure. Fein and his associates[23] compared the differential diagnosis of hemodynamic and permeability pulmonary edema from clinical criteria alone with those that included hemodynamic measurements with measurements of pulmonary artery occlusive pressures. Only 62% of instances of hemodynamic edema were correctly diagnosed on the basis of the clinical criteria. However, this differentiation in critically ill patients may not be precise because it is likely that a significant number of patients have elements of both hemodynamic and permeability pulmonary edema. This is especially the case when congestive heart failure occurs in the setting of pneumonia or pulmonary embolization. Nevertheless, for patients who fail to respond to conventional therapy for acute pulmonary edema, current clinical practice would favor early hemodynamic study including the measurement and monitoring of pulmonary artery and pulmonary arterial occlusive (wedge) and systemic arterial pressure together with measurements of cardiac output and arterial blood gases. These measurements interpreted in conjunction with the clinical findings and especially the setting in which pulmonary edema develops usually allow for the differentiation between hemodynamic and permeability as primary causes of pulmonary edema.

ETIOLOGY

Hemodynamic pulmonary edema is almost always associated with either acute or chronic congestive heart failure. Heart failure, in turn, is due to ischemic, hypertensive, valvular, primary myocardial, or congenital heart disease. Congestive heart failure may also appear as a complication of extremes of cardiac rates and rhythms and especially tachycardia. The onset of atrial fibrillation with rapid ventricular rates may be the explanation of *de novo* onset of acute pulmonary edema. Between 10% and 20% of patients who have sustained acute myocardial infarction present with clinical signs of pulmonary edema.

Uncommonly, hemodynamic pulmonary edema is due to noncardiac causes. Increases in intracranial pressure following head injury or intracranial hemorrhage that provoke neurogenic pulmonary edema, excess α-adrenergic stimulation including that of pheochromocytoma associated with pulmonary edema, and high-altitude pulmonary edema are currently suspect as cases of pulmonary edema of hemodynamic cause. Current evidence implicates an initial episode in which arterial pressure is markedly increased and provokes acute left ventricular failure in these cases. However, there is likely to be a subsequent permeability defect in these unique types of pulmonary edema.[18,24-28] Very rarely, pulmonary edema may be due to an obstruction of pulmonary venous drainage due to congenital or acquired lesions and possibly due to the effects of endogenous and exogenous vasoactive constriction of pulmonary vessels distal to the capillaries. The common denominator is increased pulmonary venous pressure such that capillary hydrostatic pressure is raised to levels that typically exceed 25 mm Hg.

Although 25 mm Hg is regarded as the threshold value for development of hemodynamic pulmonary edema, substantially lower pressures may be observed in patients in whom colloid osmotic pressure is reduced. The opposite also applies. Not infrequently, pulmonary arterial occlusive or wedge pressure exceeding 30 mm Hg or even 40 mm Hg may be measured in the absence of pulmonary edema.[29] This is observed in patients with longstanding increases in pulmonary capillary pressures and patients with mitral valve disease and particularly mitral stenosis. However, it also applies to patients with either isolated aortic stenosis or aortic regurgitation in the absence of stenosis. It is uncommonly observed in patients with longstanding ischemic heart disease. It has been postulated that such high pressures are tolerated when cardiac output and therefore pulmonary blood flow are substantially reduced. However, in normal dog lungs, there is little change in capillary hydrostatic pressure over wide ranges of blood flow, although this may not apply under pathologic conditions. Other mechanisms have been suggested, such as increases in the efficiency of pulmonary lymphatic flow.[30]

CLINICAL MANAGEMENT

In patients with chronic congestive heart failure who have an acute exacerbation of pulmonary edema, there is high likelihood of prompt reversal following routine management with upright posture, increases in the inspired concentration of oxygen, and treatment with morphine and a potent diuretic such as furosemide. Indeed, such patients may be effectively managed in an appropriate emergency or outpatient setting over an interval of 4 to 8 hours. In view of the extreme respiratory distress with cough and wheezing, anxiety, pallor, cyanosis, and diaphoresis, the physician may be persuaded to undertake immediate aggressive invasive interventions, including endotracheal intubation, mechanical ventilation, and hemodynamic monitoring with flow-directed pulmonary artery and arterial catheters. This sets the patient on a course of more protracted inpatient care with initial admission to a cardiac or general intensive care unit. Unless the patient develops signs of circulatory shock or immediately life-threatening defects of cardiac rhythm, more conservative management is advised. If the patient fails to respond over the initial hour of management, more invasive interventions are justified.

When the patient is placed in an upright position, venous pressure and, therefore, preload is reduced. Both intrapulmonary and pleural fluid gravitate to the bases of the chest cavity such that the less-dependent lung is more effectively ventilated. In the sitting posture, compared with the supine posture, the work of breathing is lessened when the descent of the diaphragm is facilitated by gravity and unconstrained by the weight of congestive viscera.

Humidified oxygen is best administered by a face mask. Nasal prongs are not likely to be effective in the patient with marked respiratory distress or for one who breathes through the mouth. Reversal of hypoxemia is accompanied by decreases in pulmonary artery pressure and, therefore, pulmonary capillary hydrostatic pressure. Continuous positive airway pressure (CPAP) of 10 cm by face mask has been advised as an effective option for improving gas exchange.[31] A Venturi-type face mask may be used with inspired oxygen concentrations of 40%. Patients often struggle against the face mask and especially so when CPAP is added. Positive-pressure breathing with consequent increases in intrathoracic pressure also impedes venous return and therefore preload with theoretic benefit. However, this is at the risk of a disproportionate reduction in cardiac output. In extreme cases, the option of endotracheal intubation and mechanical ventilation may be used, together with positive end-expiratory pressure (PEEP). The ventilator, in conscious patients, should be on demand mode such that it assists rather than controls inspiration. PEEP is best maintained at levels not exceeding 15 cm H_2O or at a level that will not substantially compromise cardiac output.

Titrated doses of a narcotic are very effective. To 10 mg of morphine sulfate, one-half normal saline is added for a total volume of 20 ml. After an initial bolus of 4 ml (2 mg), between 1 ml and 2 ml is injected at intervals of 1 minute until anxiety is relieved. The patient then becomes more compliant and is much less likely to struggle against a face mask. Morphine also increases venous capacitance and thereby decreases preload. It depresses the pulmonary reflexes that account for dyspnea. The risk of increased bronchoconstriction stemming from histamine release by morphine and the risk of carbon dioxide narcosis has been greatly overstated. Since the patient is under close observation in an emergency facility, appropriate interventions can be promptly undertaken. If adverse effects do occur and especially apnea, naloxone in doses of 0.4 mg at 3-minute intervals serves as a specific antidote.

A loop diuretic such as furosemide in amounts of 40 mg to 80 mg is then injected intravenously. It has an immediate effect in that it also increases venous capacitance and decreases preload prior to inducing diuresis.

With the availability of vasodilator therapy, the clinician is provided with a very potent option for decreasing pulmonary capillary pressure and rapidly and effectively reversing cardiogenic pulmonary edema. The routine administration of sublingual nitroglycerin in amounts of 0.4 mg to 0.6 mg at 10-minute intervals is now recognized as effective and safe in the absence of hypotension. Its primary action is to increase venous capacitance and decrease preload. When pulmonary edema occurs as a complication of acute myocardial infarction and the patient is unresponsive to conventional management, intravenous infusion of nitroglycerin in amounts beginning with 10 μg/min and gradual increases to levels of 200 μg/min or more is an appropriate intervention. In the absence of acute myocardial infarction, and especially when the patient presents with hypertension, sodium nitroprusside administered at rates of 10 μg/min with increases of 5 μg/min at intervals of 5 minutes provides a secure option for arterial vasodilation and decreased afterload. When intravenous vasodilator drugs are administered under these conditions, hemodynamic monitoring is advised.

With the availability of vasodilator agents, rotating tourniquets and phlebotomy are now rarely used. Inotropic therapy with β-adrenergic agonists, digitalis glycosides, and nondigitalis inotropic agents such as amrinone are primarily used in the setting of more chronic states of congestive heart failure after acute pulmonary edema has been reversed. However, the mainstay of treatment of patients with chronic congestive heart failure with pulmonary edema now focuses on vasodilator therapy and especially angiotensin-converting enzyme inhibitors such as captopril or enalapril. When afterload and therefore pulmonary capillary pressure are reduced, the colloid-hydrostatic pressure conditions favor the rapid reversal of pulmonary edema. As plasma water, low in colloid content, is reabsorbed, the colloid osmotic pressure is decreased.[32] These features are demonstrated in Figure 9.9.

Conventional teaching held that intravascular volume is expanded during congestive heart failure and pulmonary edema. This, in fact, is not the case. The total body water is expanded, but intravascular volume may be substantially depleted when large amounts of protein-poor fluid are extravasated during the development of edema states.[33] When this fluid reenters into the intravascular space after reversal of pulmonary edema, plasma volume is expanded and colloid osmotic pressure is reduced. The effect of both vasodilator drugs and potent loop diuretics is an initial increase rather than a decrease in intravascular volume.[34]

During the development of acute pulmonary edema, the amount of fluid that is removed during edema formation may be so large as to produce hypovolemia with very marked reduction in cardiac output and clinical features of shock with near-normal pulmonary artery capillary pressures in spite of florid radiographic signs of pulmonary edema.[35] The reexpansion of intravascular volume promptly identifies such patients since there is a sharp rise in the pulmonary artery occlu-

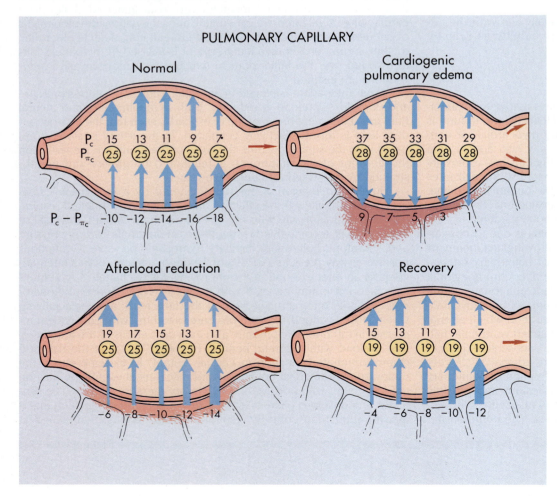

FIGURE 9.9 Diagrammatic demonstration of the capillary hydrostatic and colloid osmotic pressures in which normal conditions are compared with those of cardiogenic pulmonary edema and the effects of afterload reduction. During the development of pulmonary edema, the extravasation of fluids low in protein content accounts for increases in colloid osmotic pressure. Afterload reduction decreases capillary hydrostatic pressure and allows reabsorption of fluid low in colloid content, leading to reduction in colloid osmotic pressure.

sive pressure during fluid challenge. In this setting, a systemic fluid challenge with small volumes of colloid-containing fluids may be lifesaving and this is followed by more conventional management of congestive heart failure.

PERMEABILITY PULMONARY EDEMA
ETIOLOGY

Permeability pulmonary edema has a diversity of nonpulmonary as well as pulmonary causes. It occurs during the course of circulatory shock states and especially when these are associated with bacteremia, pancreatitis, and protracted hypovolemia following soft tissue injuries and major body burns. It appears as an adverse reaction to drugs and drug overdoses, including salicylates, heroin, methadone, propoxyphene, and colchicine. It is associated with acute increases in intracranial pressure due to intracranial injuries. Permeability pulmonary edema and ARDS follow near drowning and the ingestion of hydrocarbons and occur in the course of uremic renal failure. Primary pulmonary causes include viral and bacterial pneumonias and chemical and physical inhalants such as nitrous oxide, chlorine, ammonia, phosgene, cadmium, and smoke. It follows aspiration of gastric contents; contusion of the lungs; microembolization due to air, fat, or platelet-fibrin thrombi; and massive blood transfusion. Accordingly, pulmonary microvascular injuries result from a remarkable diversity of causes, all of which have in common an increase in pulmonary capillary permeability, low pressure pulmonary edema, impaired gas exchange, and a clinical course consistent with ARDS.[36,37]

MECHANISMS AND PATHOLOGY

The mechanisms of alveolar capillary injury are not well understood. Polymorphonuclear cells are sequestered at sites of vascular injury. Their activation with the production of superoxide, hydrogen peroxide, and hydroxy radicals have been viewed as major causes, although their role is still uncertain.[36,38] The granules of polymorphonuclear leukocytes also liberate elastase, collagenases, and myeloperoxidase. However, ARDS also appears in the setting of neutropenia, and this provides evidence that there are neutrophil-independent mechanisms of acute lung injury.[39]

A large number of blood-borne mediators have also been implicated. These include platelets and platelet activators, lymphocytes, complement, slow reacting substance of anaphylaxis, lysosomal (proteolytic) enzymes, histamine, bradykinin, and arachidonic acid metabolites including thromboxane, prostacyclin, prostaglandin E_2 and F_2, leukotrienes, and toxic oxygen radicals.

There is extensive destruction of type I pneumocytes. The alveoli are filled with proteinaceous edema fluid with large numbers of red cells. Sometimes a hyaline membrane is observed. White blood cells aggregate in small vessels. The lung is intensely congested and almost airless.

CLINICAL FEATURES

Within 6 to 24 hours after acute injury, the patient presents with respiratory distress characterized by dyspnea and tachypnea. The findings on physical examination are initially sparse, but widespread pulmonary rales subsequently appear. Roentgenographic examination of the lungs initially demonstrates subtle and diffuse interstitial infiltrates with evolution of patchy or confluent alveolar infiltrates that are equally prominent in the central and peripheral lung fields (Fig. 9.10). The clinical course is characterized by progressive hypoxemia with initial respiratory alkalosis followed by late respiratory and metabolic acidosis. There is a marked reduction in pulmonary compliance, and the course is fatal in approximately 50% of cases. It is characterized by terminal respiratory insufficiency and perfusion failure (shock). These features are summarized in Table 9.2.

In addition to the setting in which the manifestation presents, the initial differentiation between hemodynamic and permeability pulmonary edema is based on the measurement of pulmonary artery occlusive pressure. Permeability pulmonary edema is characterized by near-normal capillary pressures. Additional differentiation is made by analysis of endobronchial fluid aspirated from the airway. In patients with permeability pulmonary edema, the protein concentration and colloid osmotic pressure of the endobronchial fluid approximates that of simultaneously measured plasma. This is in contrast to hemodynamic pulmonary edema in which the endobronchial fluid is typically 50% or less of that simultaneously measured on plasma. These differences are demonstrated in Figure 9.11. The colloid osmotic pressure and protein content of endobronchial fluid in patients with permeability pulmonary edema is usually greater than 70% of that measured in plasma. It may even be greater than that of plasma because of evaporation of plasma water in the airways.[6,40–42] Isotopic methods have been used for detection of macromolecular leaks. These include the injection of radioactive macromolecules into the bloodstream such as albumin labeled with radioactive iodine and measurement of its clearance in the airway by the radioactivity of endobronchial fluid.[43] Clearance of radioactive small solutes administered by aerosol with surface monitoring of its dissipation over the anterior chest has also been used. Clearance was accelerated in patients with permeability pulmonary edema.[44] Extravascular lung water may be measured by double indicator dilution techniques, and instrumentation is commercially available, but it has not had wide clinical acceptance. The procedure is invasive and demanding, and the reliability of the measurement is limited. A cooled indocyanine green solution is injected into

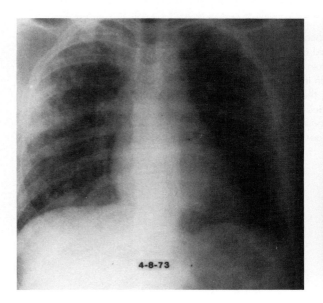
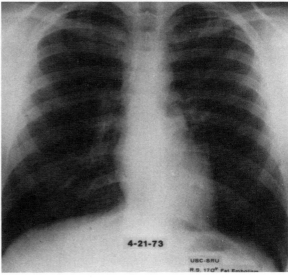

FIGURE 9.10 Roentgenographic changes characteristic of ARDS in a 17-year-old patient following a fracture of a long bone. The patient presented with post-traumatic respiratory distress. Radiographic resolution was demonstrated in a chest roentgenogram taken 15 days later.

the pulmonary artery, and the thermal and dye concentrations are detected in the aorta. Since the thermal tracer diffuses rapidly through lung water and the indocyanine tracer is only distributed through the vascular compartment on its first pass, the differences between these two measurements provide a measure of extravascular lung water.[45]

CLINICAL MANAGEMENT

No specific intervention for treatment of ARDS is currently available. The initial focus is on respiratory support and concurrent treatment of the underlying disease states. A marked reduction in pulmonary compliance greatly increases the work of breathing and early mechanical ventilation may be required. Because of the loss of functional alveolocapillary gas exchange units, the dead space/tidal volume ratio, which is normally 0.3, is more than doubled. To maintain adequate minute ventilation, a minimal tidal volume of 12 ml to 15 ml/kg is required. The additional risk of oxygen toxicity precludes increases in inspired oxygen concentrations of greater than 60%.

With the introduction of PEEP, the option for increasing the patency of the airways is such that a larger number of functional alveoli are recruited. Consequently, there is improved gas exchange and a reduction in ventilation–perfusion abnormalities. This is the option of choice for treatment of hypoxemia. However, increases in PEEP cause increases in intrathoracic pressure and thereby impede venous return to the heart and decreased cardiac output. There is now a consensus that more than 15 cm of PEEP, so-called super PEEP, may be counterproductive because of its cardiovascular effects and the risks of barotrauma. This is underscored by the fact that the ultimately lifesaving benefit of PEEP more generally is unproven.

Accordingly, the routine of ventilatory management includes endotracheal intubation and mechanical ventilation with a volume-cycled ventilator. Except for brief periods of resuscitation, the inspired concentrations of oxygen would best not exceed 60%. In instances in which the lesions are predominantly unilateral, the patient is best positioned such that the uninjured lung is below.

There is no evidence that prophylactic treatment with antibiotics, inotropic agents, or arterial vasodilator drugs improves outcome. The administration of pulmonary vasodilators may result in a deterioration of pulmonary gas exchange as a result of interference with hypoxic pulmonary vasoconstriction.[46–48] Glucocorticoids (more specifically, methylprednisolone), in pharmacologic doses of 30 mg/kg every six hours, have not been shown to alter outcome in patients with established ARDS.[49] Furthermore, early treatment with methylprednisolone in patients with sepsis neither prevents the development of ARDS nor improves survival.[50,51]

Prostaglandin E_1 (PGE_1), a vasodilator with anti-inflammatory properties, initially was shown to improve survival in surgical patients with ARDS.[52] However, this benefit of PGE_1 infusion could not be confirmed in subsequent studies.[53] In addition, when pulmonary hypertension is moderated by PGE_1, an increase in intrapulmonary shunt and a deterioration in pulmonary gas exchange has been observed.[54]

Fluid management is of importance. The issue of colloidal vs. crys-

TABLE 9.2 THE "NATURAL HISTORY" OF PERMEABILITY PULMONARY EDEMA (ARDS)

Time (hr)		
0		Catastrophic injury (usually with circulatory shock)
		Multisystemic trauma, hypovolemia, burn, disseminated systemic sepsis (bacteremia), pneumonia, intravascular coagulation
	Latent	Drug intoxication (heroin, methadone, propoxyphene, barbiturates, colchicine)
		Chemical and physical agents, inhalants NO_2, Cl_2, NH_3, phosgene, cadmium
		Pulmonary embolization (fat, thromboemboli)
		Pulmonary aspiration
		Oxygen toxicity
6–24		Tachypnea (>20/min); respiratory distress
		Total respiratory compliance < 50 ml/cm H_2O (i.e., tidal volume in ml/inspiratory plateau pressure in cm H_2O)
	Progressive	PaO_2 < 60 mm Hg at FIO_2 0.6
		Respiratory alkalosis (pH > 7.35, $PaCO_2$ < 40 mm Hg)
		Chest roentgenogram demonstrates diffuse interstitial and early alveolar infiltrate
		Increased dead space/tidal volume ratio
24–96		Loss of alertness
		Severely labored respiration
		Total respiratory compliance < 30 ml/cm H_2O
	Fatal	PaO_2 < 50 mm Hg at FIO_2 0.7
		Chest roentgenogram demonstrates progressive alveolar infiltrate, bilateral cannonball and/or ground-glass opacification
		Respiratory and metabolic acidosis: pH < 7.35, $PaCO_2$ > 40 mm Hg
		Lactic acidosis (arterial blood lactic acid > 2 mmol/liter)

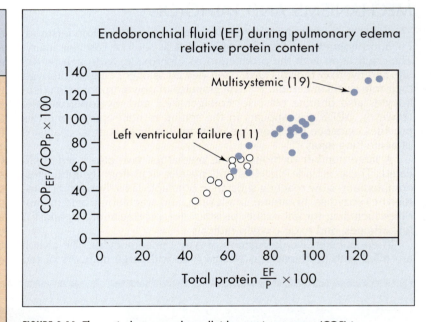

FIGURE 9.11 The ratio between the colloid osmotic pressure (COP) in endobronchial fluid and that of plasma is shown on the ordinate and the ratio of total protein concentration in endobronchial fluid and that of plasma on the abscissa. In instances of hemodynamic pulmonary edema, labeled left ventricular failure, the ratio was less than 0.7. In 16 of 19 patients with multisystemic injuries and clinical features of ARDS, the ratio exceeded 0.7. (Adapted from Carlson RW, Schaeffer RC Jr, Carpio M et al: Edema fluid and coagulation changes during fulminant pulmonary edema. Chest 79:43, 1981)

talloid fluids such that colloid osmotic pressure is kept within more optimal ranges is unsettled. There is excessive water retention owing to increased secretion of antidiuretic hormone. The vigorous use of potent diuretic agents, especially furosemide, may be of benefit, but the ultimate efficacy of these drugs is also unproven.

Fewer than half of patients with established ARDS survive.[55] However, selective types of permeability pulmonary edema have a more benign course. High-altitude and neurogenic permeability edema also have a much better prognosis. The same applies to pulmonary edema due to opiates, which are typically transient.[26] There is also a transient form of pulmonary edema after reexpansion of a pneumothorax that has been attributed to abrupt changes in alveolar pressure.[56-58]

CLINICAL IMPLICATIONS

The differential diagnosis of hemodynamic and permeability pulmonary edema is of practical importance since the mechanisms, management, and prognosis are dissimilar. In the case of hemodynamic pulmonary edema, measures that will reduce pulmonary capillary hydrostatic pressure and especially a reduction in left-sided filling pressures reverse pulmonary edema. In the instance of permeability pulmonary edema, no specific therapeutic options are currently available. The primary focus is on prevention and on management of the underlying cause.

REFERENCES

1. Starling EH: On the absorption of fluids from the connective tissue space. J Physiol (Lond) 19:312, 1896
2. Guyton AC, Lindsey AW: Effects of elevated left atrial pressure and decreased plasma protein on the development of pulmonary edema. Circ Res 7:649, 1959
3. Biddle TL, Khanna PK, Yu PN et al: Lung water in patients with acute myocardial infarction. Circulation 49:115, 1974
4. Ashbaugh DG, Bigelow DB, Petty TL et al: Acute respiratory distress in adults. Lancet 2:319, 1967
5. Tate RM, Petty TL: Primary pulmonary edema. In Stollerman GH (ed): Advances in Internal Medicine, pp 471–493. Chicago, Year Book Medical Publishers, 1984
6. Sprung CL, Rackow EC, Fein IA et al: The spectrum of pulmonary edema: Differentiation of cardiogenic, intermediate and noncardiogenic forms of pulmonary edema. Am Rev Respir Dis 124:718, 1981
7. Pietra GG: Biology of disease: New insights into mechanisms of pulmonary edema. Lab Invest 51:489, 1984
8. Paintal AS: The mechanism of excitation of type J receptors and the reflex. In Porter R (ed): Breathing: Hering-Breuer Centenary Symposium, Ciba Foundation Symposium, p 59. London, J & A Churchill, 1970
9. Nieman GF, Bredenberg CE, Clark WR et al: Alveolar function following surfactant deactivation. J Appl Physiol 51:895, 1981
10. Figueras J, Weil MH: Increases in plasma oncotic pressure during acute cardiogenic pulmonary edema. Circulation 55:195, 1977
11. Bisera J, Weil MH, Michaels S et al: An "oncometer" for clinical measurement of colloid osmotic pressure of plasma. Clin Chem 24:1586, 1978
12. Stein L, Beraud JJ, Cavanilles JM et al: Pulmonary edema during fluid infusion in the absence of heart failure. JAMA 229:65, 1974
13. DaLuz PL, Shubin H, Weil MH et al: Pulmonary edema related to changes in colloid osmotic and pulmonary artery wedge pressure in patients after myocardial infarction. Circulation 51:350, 1975
14. Stein L, Beraud JJ, Morissette M et al: Pulmonary edema during volume infusion. Circulation 52:483, 1975
15. Weil MH, Henning RJ, Morissette M et al: Relationship between colloid osmotic pressure and pulmonary artery wedge pressure in patients with acute cardiorespiratory failure. Am J Med 64:643, 1978
16. Rackow EC, Fein IA, Siegel J: The relationship of the colloid osmotic pulmonary artery wedge pressure gradient to pulmonary edema and mortality in critically ill patients. Chest 82:433, 1982
17. Morisette M, Weil MH, Shubin H: Reduction in colloid osmotic pressure associated with fatal progression of cardiopulmonary failure. Crit Care Med 3:115, 1975
18. Cheng CPK: Haemodynamic changes in adrenaline-induced acute massive lung oedema. Cardiovasc Res 9:105, 1975
19. Brigham KL, Snell JD Jr, Harris TR et al: Indicator dilution lung water and vascular permeability in humans. Circ Res 44:523, 1979
20. Vreim CE, Snashall PD, Staub NC: Protein composition of lung fluids in anesthetized dogs with acute cardiogenic edema. Am J Physiol 231:1466, 1976
21. Dixon M, Paterson CR: Posture and the composition of plasma. Clin Chem 24:824, 1978
22. Turner AF, Lau FV, Jacobson G: A method for the estimation of pulmonary venous and arterial pressures from the routine chest roentgenogram. AJR 116:97, 1972
23. Fein AM, Goldberg SK, Walkenstein MD et al: Is pulmonary artery catheterization necessary for the diagnosis of pulmonary edema? Am Rev Respir Dis 129:1006, 1984
24. Theodore J, Robin ED: Speculations on neurogenic pulmonary edema (NPE). Am Rev Respir Dis 113:405, 1976
25. Wray NP, Nicotra MB: Pathogenesis of neurogenic pulmonary edema. Am Rev Respir Dis 118:783, 1978
26. Naeije R, Yernault JC, Goldstein M et al: Acute pulmonary oedema in a patient with phaeochromocytoma. Intens Care Med 4:165, 1978
27. Fishman AP, Pietra GG: Stretched pores, blast injury and neurohemodynamic pulmonary edema. Physiologist 23:53, 1980
28. Minnear FL, Barrie PS, Malik AB: Effects of transient pulmonary hypertension on pulmonary vascular permeability. J Appl Physiol 55:983, 1983
29. Anderson FL, McDonnell MA, Tsagaris TJ et al: Absence of clinical pulmonary edema despite elevated wedge pressures. Arch Intern Med 141:1207, 1981
30. Sniderman A, Burdon T, Homan J et al: Pulmonary blood flow: A potential factor in the pathogenesis of pulmonary edema. J Thorac Cardiovasc Surg 87:130, 1984
31. Rasanen J, Heikkila J, Downs J et al: Continuous positive airway pressure by face mask in acute cardiogenic pulmonary edema. Am J Cardiol 55:296, 1985
32. Henning RJ, Weil MH: Effects of afterload reduction on plasma volume during acute heart failure. Am J Cardiol 42:823, 1978
33. Figueras J, Weil MH: Blood volume prior to and following treatment of acute cardiogenic pulmonary edema. Circulation 57:349, 1978
34. Schuster CJ, Weil MH: Blood volume following diuresis induced by furosemide. Am J Med 4:10, 1984
35. Figueras J, Weil MH: Hypovolemia and hypotension complicating management of acute cardiogenic pulmonary edema. Am J Cardiol 44:1349, 1979
36. Loyd JE, Newman JH, Brigham KL: Permeability pulmonary edema. Arch Intern Med 144:143, 1984
37. Tranbaugh RF, Lewis FR: Mechanisms and etiologic factors of pulmonary edema. Surg Gynecol Obstet 158:193, 1984
38. Glauser FL, Fairman RP: The uncertain role of the neutrophil in increased permeability pulmonary edema. Chest 88:601, 1985
39. Ognibene FP, Martin SE, Parker MM et al: Adult respiratory distress syndrome in patients with severe neutropenia. N Engl J Med 315:547, 1986
40. Gelb AF, Klein E: Hemodynamic and alveolar protein studies in noncardiac pulmonary edema. Am Rev Respir Dis 114:831, 1976
41. Fein A, Grossman RF, Jones JG et al: The value of edema fluid protein measurement in patients with pulmonary edema. Am J Med 67:32, 1979
42. Carlson RW, Schaeffer RC Jr, Carpio M et al: Edema fluid and coagulation changes during fulminant pulmonary edema. Chest 79:43, 1981
43. Anderson RR, Holliday RL, Driedger AA et al: Documentation of pulmonary capillary permeability in the adult respiratory distress syndrome accompanying human sepsis. Am Rev Respir Dis 119:869, 1979
44. Mason GR, Effros RM, Uszler JM et al: Small solute clearance from the lungs of patients with cardiogenic and noncardiogenic pulmonary edema. Chest 88:327, 1985
45. Lewis FR, Elings VB, Sturm JA: Bedside measurement of lung water. J Surg Res 27:250, 1979
46. Voelkel NF: Mechanisms of hypoxic pulmonary vasoconstriction. Am Rev Respir Dis 133:1186, 1986
47. Mélot C, Naeije R, Mols P, et al: Pulmonary vascular tone improves pulmonary gas exchange in the adult respiratory distress syndrome. Am Rev Respir Dis 136:1232, 1987
48. Radermacher P, Huet Y, Pluskma F: Comparison of ketanserin and sodium nitroprusside in patients with severe ARDS. Anesthesiology 68:152, 1988
49. Bernard GR, Luce JM, Sprung CL, et al: High dose corticosteroids in patients with the adult respiratory distress syndrome. N Engl J Med 317:1565, 1987
50. Bone RC, Fisher CJ, Clemmer TP, et al: Early methylprednisolone treatment for septic syndrome and the adult respiratory distress syndrome. Chest 92:1032, 1987
51. Luce JM, Montgomery AB, Marks JD, et al: Ineffectiveness of high-dose methylprednisolone in preventing parenchymal lung injury and improving mortality in patients with septic shock. Am Rev Respir Dis 138:62, 1988
52. Holcroft JW, Vassar MJ, Weber CJ: Prostaglandin E_1 and survival in patients with the adult respiratory distress syndrome. Ann Surg 203:371, 1986
53. Bone RC, Slotman G, Maunder R, et al: Randomized double blind, multicenter study of prostaglandin E_1 in patients with the adult respiratory distress syndrome. Chest 96:114, 1989
54. Mélot C, Lejeune P, Leeman M, et al: Prostaglandin E_1 in the adult respiratory distress syndrome: Benefit for pulmonary hypertension and cost for pulmo-

55. Fowler AA, Hammon RF, Good JT et al: Risk of the adult respiratory distress syndrome following common predispositions. Ann Intern Med 98:553, 1983
56. Mahajan VK, Simon M, Huber GL: Reexpansion pulmonary edema. Chest 75:192, 1979
57. Sprung CL, Loewenherz JW, Bauer H: Evidence of increased permeability in reexpansion pulmonary edema. Am J Med 71:497, 1981
58. Kernode DS, Di Raimondo CR, Fulkerson WJ: Reexpansion pulmonary edema after pneumothorax. South Med J 77:318, 1984

GENERAL REFERENCES

Boyd JE, Newman JH, Brigham KL: Permeability pulmonary edema. Arch Intern Med 144:143, 1984

Braunwald E: Heart failure: Pathophysiology and treatment. Am Heart J 102:486, 1982

Massie BM, Chatterjee K, Parmley WW: Vasodilator therapy for acute and chronic heart failure. Prog Cardiol 8:197, 1979

Staub N: Pulmonary edema. Physiol Rev 54:678, 1974

PRINCIPLES IN THE MANAGEMENT OF CONGESTIVE HEART FAILURE

William W. Parmley

CHAPTER 10 VOLUME 1

CLINICAL FEATURES

Congestive heart failure is a syndrome with multiple causes and manifestations. It is estimated currently that about 2 million Americans have congestive heart failure, with about 350,000 new cases appearing each year. Congestive heart failure is a syndrome with a high mortality. In the Framingham study, prospective data were gathered that showed that after the appearance of congestive heart failure, there was a 50% mortality in about 4 years.[1] Mortality is clearly related to the severity of left ventricular dysfunction.[2] In patients with New York Heart Association Class IV heart failure (symptoms at rest), the mortality is 50% in about 1 year.[3] Although most patients die because of worsening heart failure, a substantial number die suddenly.[4] Since serious ventricular arrhythmias are common in patients with heart failure, the potential role of antiarrhythmic agents deserves consideration. Some uncontrolled data suggest that such therapy might be helpful in selected patients.[5]

The relationship between the etiology of heart failure and survival has also not been clarified. Some data suggest that for the same degree of heart failure, those patients with cardiomyopathy may have a slightly more favorable course than those with coronary artery disease.[5] This difference appears to be minimal, however, if present at all.[6]

An often used definition of heart failure is the inability of the heart to deliver enough blood to peripheral tissues to meet metabolic demands. Certainly this definition describes the decrease in cardiac output that is characteristic of most forms of heart failure. In milder forms of heart failure, the decrease in cardiac output is manifested primarily during exercise as an attenuated rise in cardiac output during effort. As heart failure becomes more severe, there is an even greater attenuation of cardiac output during exercise and, finally, a reduction in cardiac output at rest.

The above description of congestive heart failure, however, does not take into account the congestive signs and symptoms caused by an elevation of right and left atrial pressures. During milder forms of heart failure, the left atrial pressure may be relatively normal, whereas there is an excessive rise during exercise. As heart failure becomes more severe, there is an increase in resting atrial pressures, together with an excessive rise with mild effort. In defining congestive heart failure, therefore, it is useful to consider both the inadequate cardiac output response and the excessive rise in atrial pressures as hallmarks of the syndrome.

CLINICAL FEATURES

The two major symptom complexes in patients with congestive heart failure are closely related to the two major hemodynamic abnormalities described previously. The most common limiting symptom in heart failure is dyspnea. In milder forms of heart failure, this is manifest primarily as dyspnea on exertion. As the heart failure becomes more severe, dyspnea is also manifest as orthopnea, paroxysmal nocturnal dyspnea, and dyspnea at rest.

Although the precise physiologic cause of dyspnea is uncertain, it is probably related to decreased compliance of the lungs, associated with a rise in left atrial pressure. The increased pulmonary pressures, interstitial fluid in the lung parenchyma, and increased airway resistance presumably contribute to the subjective sensation of an inability to take a breath without a greater inspiratory effort.[7] The fact that a transient increase in left atrial pressure and dyspnea are temporally associated emphasizes the close relationship between the two.

Certainly, dyspnea is not caused by hypoxia in the usual setting of congestive heart failure. Arterial oxygenation is often essentially normal. When abrupt reductions in left atrial pressure are produced, for example by venodilators, there may be a reduction in arterial oxygen saturation at the same time that dyspnea is disappearing.[8] This phenomenon is presumably due to a shift in lung perfusion to the lower lobes following a reduction in left atrial pressure. Reduction of ventilation to the lower lobes because of pulmonary congestion leads to a mismatch between ventilation and perfusion and a reduction in arterial oxygen content.

It should be noted that dyspnea is not a specific marker of congestive heart failure, although it represents one of its most important symptoms. Chronic pulmonary disease is a common cause of dyspnea, and it is often difficult to determine the relative importance of the heart and lungs in patients with combined disease. Obesity and poor physical conditioning are also common causes of dyspnea on exertion. Orthopnea is common to both cardiac and pulmonary disease. Assumption of the upright posture increases vital capacity as a common mechanism for symptomatic improvement in both conditions. Paroxysmal nocturnal dyspnea is more specific for heart failure and may relate additionally to decreased vital capacity and increased blood volume due to intravascular reabsorption of peripheral edema during recumbency.

The second major symptom complex in patients with heart failure is fatigue and decreased exercise tolerance. This is presumably related to an inadequate increase in cardiac output with exercise, with an inadequate increase in flow to skeletal muscle. Furthermore, there may be a relative reduction in flow to the kidneys, splanchnic circulation, and skin.

Other features associated with heart failure should be noted. An elevation in right atrial pressure leads to the signs and symptoms of systemic venous congestion. Hepatic congestion and enlargement may lead to right upper quadrant fullness or discomfort and tenderness to palpation. This is presumably related to stretching of the hepatic capsule. Peripheral edema may be accompanied by aching of the legs, discomfort with shoes, and concern over swollen ankles, particularly in women. Ascites is generally a late manifestation of heart failure, as manifested by abdominal swelling and discomfort and loss of appetite.

A myriad of other symptoms may accompany heart failure. Dizziness, lightheadedness, or presyncope may occur in some patients. Not only is blood pressure quite low in most patients with severe heart failure, but orthostatic changes may also exacerbate hypotensive symptoms. Transient arrhythmias or vasodilator therapy may contribute to dizzy episodes. Certainly, first dose effects with prazosin and angiotensin-converting enzyme inhibitors (captopril and enalapril) may cause abrupt falls in blood pressure in already hypotensive patients. Frequent ectopy and more serious arrhythmias are common in severe heart failure and may contribute to palpitations or dizziness. A careful analysis of all of the symptoms experienced by individual patients may provide important clues to the underlying hemodynamic and electrophysiologic abnormalities.

PATHOPHYSIOLOGY

The signs and symptoms of heart failure are caused by four syndromes that can appear alone or in combination. The syndromes include failure of the left ventricle as a pump, failure of the right ventricle as a pump, pulmonary venous hypertension, and systemic venous hypertension. The most common cause of right-sided heart failure is left-sided heart failure, through passive and reflex elevations of pulmonary artery pressure and vascular resistance. A number of processes can directly affect the right ventricle with minimal involvement of the left ventricle. These include chronic obstructive pulmonary disease, primary or secondary pulmonary hypertension, right ventricular infarction, pulmonary stenosis, and tricuspid regurgitation. The prototype example of the syndrome of elevated pulmonary venous pressure is mitral stenosis. Constrictive pericarditis is the prototype example of systemic venous hypertension.

The general factors that lead to these four syndromes are summarized in Table 10.1. Pressure overload is a relatively common cause of left ventricular hypertrophy and failure. Sustained hypertension and aortic stenosis are good examples of this phenomenon. With a sustained increase in left ventricular pressure there is compensatory hypertrophy, which can normalize wall stress. Compensatory hypertrophy with normal intrinsic muscle function can maintain left ventricular function at a near-normal level for years. With longstanding loading and excessive hypertrophy, however, there ensues an intrinsic decrease in cardiac muscle contractility that impairs left ventricular performance and leads to the syndrome of left-sided heart failure.

During this sequence, it is intuitively apparent that the best way to halt or potentially reverse this process is to reduce the load on the left ventricle. In animal models of pressure overload, it appears that the intrinsic decrease in contractility is frequently irreversible. Clinical experience tends to confirm this, which emphasizes the importance of unloading the ventricle before severe reductions in intrinsic contractility occur. In all circumstances, however, reducing the afterload on the left ventricle is effective in improving forward output. For example, in the patient with severe aortic stenosis, virtually no degree of left ventricular dysfunction should discourage one from replacing the aortic valve. The unloading effect will improve forward output no matter what the level of baseline left ventricular dysfunction.

Volume overload is produced by a number of common lesions. Among these are valvular regurgitation (*e.g.*, mitral or aortic), high output states (*e.g.*, anemia), or congenital lesions with shunts (*e.g.*, atrial septal defect, ventricular septal defect). Volume overload lesions generally result in combined dilatation and hypertrophy. Although wall thickness does not match that produced by pure pressure overload, overall chamber mass may be comparably increased. With prolonged severe volume overload, there ensues an intrinsic decrease in myocardial contractility, which is also mostly irreversible. In general, patients with volume overload do very well for many years. When intrinsic changes in contractility occur, however, they then pursue a more rapid downhill course. An appropriate management plan in patients with valvular regurgitation, therefore, is to replace the valve before a major intrinsic decrease in cardiac contractility has occurred. The specifics of these considerations will be covered in the chapters on valvular lesions.

It is worth mentioning, however, that different types of volume overloads must be considered separately. One example will suffice. Consider the difference between a patient with severe aortic regurgitation and one with mitral regurgitation. Valve replacement in severe aortic regurgitation reduces the loading conditions on the left ventricle. The decrease in end-diastolic volume that frequently occurs, together with a decrease in systolic pressure (due to a reduced stroke volume and pulse pressure), all help to unload the left ventricle and improve systolic function.[9] In the patient with mitral regurgitation, however, the situation is different. By unloading itself early in systole through ejection of blood backward into the left atrium, the left ventricle reduces wall stress and shortens further. Thus, mitral regurgitation enhances the ejection fraction if left ventricular contractility is preserved. When a prosthetic valve eliminates mitral regurgitation, left ventricular loading is increased and the ejection fraction is reduced.[10] This emphasizes the importance of replacing the mitral valve before a significant reduction of contractility has occurred.

Another pathophysiologic factor is loss of muscle, which is best exemplified by coronary artery disease with myocardial infarction. With acute infarction, the loss of 40% of left ventricular mass is sufficient to produce cardiogenic shock.[11] With smaller infarcts, the remaining normal muscle is subjected to increased wall stress and effectively experiences an increased volume overload. Additional ischemia may also contribute to a reduction in contractility.

The prototype example of decreased contractility is the patient with congestive cardiomyopathy. There are more than 20,000 new cases of congestive cardiomyopathy recognized annually in the United States. The overall incidence is about 1 in 10,000 of the population at large. There are multiple causes of cardiomyopathy: toxic causes include alcohol, cobalt, and doxorubicin; infectious or immunologic causes include viral or bacterial infections, rheumatic fever, and connective tissue disorders. A few cardiomyopathies are reversible, with some reversing spontaneously or with cessation of alcohol as a causative factor or with immunosuppressive therapy. Most severe cardiomyopathies tend to run a downhill course.

Mitral stenosis restricts filling of the left ventricle; constrictive pericarditis and pericardial tamponade restrict filling of the right ventricle. In addition to these examples, there are a number of situations in which ventricular filling is impeded. Endomyocardial fibrosis, severe hypertrophy, transient ischemia, and prior myocardial infarction all decrease the compliance of the left ventricle and impede diastolic filling. Infiltrative disorders and diabetes are additional examples of processes that can stiffen the left ventricle and impede filling. In almost all of these cases an appropriately timed atrial contraction assumes considerable importance in maintaining appropriate left ventricular filling. For example, when such patients go into atrial fibrillation there may be the onset of acute heart failure.

TABLE 10.1 PATHOPHYSIOLOGY OF CONGESTIVE HEART FAILURE: GENERAL FACTORS

Pressure overload	Decreased contractility
Volume overload	Restricted filling
Loss of muscle	

From the above discussion it is apparent that more than one factor may be playing a role in individual patients. For example, in patients with coronary artery disease, a number of factors contribute to the onset of heart failure, as outlined in Table 10.2. Not only does loss of muscle decrease ventricular function, but acute or chronic ischemia can also decrease regional function. The effect of an aneurysm depends not only on its size but also on the degree to which it can be paradoxically expanded during systole.[12] With acute occlusion of a coronary artery, there is rapid cessation of normal inward wall motion in the affected zone. This area is then paradoxically expanded, further reducing effective forward stroke volume. During the process of healing and the formation of a fibrous scar, the area becomes very stiff and noncompliant and paradoxic systolic expansion is virtually eliminated. Representative passive length–tension relations in human myocardium from an acutely infarcted zone, an aneurysm with muscle and fibrous tissue, and a fibrotic aneurysm are shown in Figure 10.1. The dramatic change in passive length–tension relations during the healing process is illustrated.

With larger infarcts, a process termed *infarct expansion* can also impose a mechanical disadvantage on the remaining normal myocardium by increasing left ventricular size and wall stress.[13] In a sense, this process mimics a "volume" overload on the remaining normal myocardium. If papillary muscles are affected, mitral regurgitation can ensue and produce a true volume load on the left ventricle. Both ischemic tissue and healed infarcts are stiffer than normal myocardium and, therefore, reduce ventricular compliance. In some cases, an elevation of pulmonary venous pressure can be due as much to decreased compliance as it can to systolic dysfunction.[14] The above discussion of coronary artery disease emphasizes how multiple factors may contribute to the pathogenesis of heart failure in a given patient. An evaluation of these factors is a useful exercise in each patient because of the differing therapeutic approaches that should be considered.

CAUSES OF CONGESTIVE HEART FAILURE

Any list of the common causes of heart failure will differ considerably, depending on the part of the world under consideration. The common causes of heart failure in the United States are listed in Table 10.3. At the institution where I am affiliated about two thirds of the patients referred for evaluation and treatment of severe heart failure have underlying coronary artery disease. Both hypertension and rheumatic valvular disease are declining as causes. This presumably reflects better recognition, treatment, and prevention of heart involvement in these patients. Myxomatous involvement of the mitral valve is currently

TABLE 10.2 PATHOPHYSIOLOGY OF CONGESTIVE HEART FAILURE IN CORONARY ARTERY DISEASE

Loss of muscle
Ischemia
Aneurysm (paradoxical expansion, increased wall stress)
Increased wall stress of remaining normal muscle
Mitral regurgitation
Decreased ventricular compliance

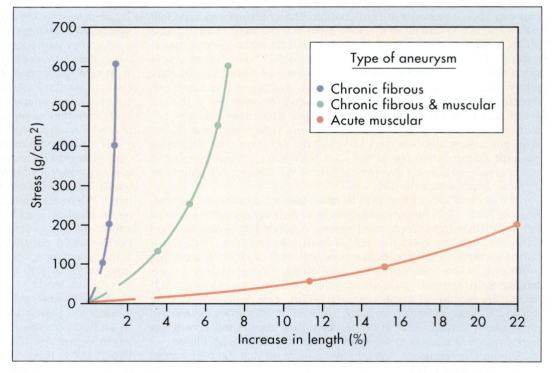

FIGURE 10.1 Representative length–tension relations of three different types of left ventricular aneurysms removed from patients.[6] The chronic fibrous aneurysm is the stiffest, while the acute infarction zone aneurysm is extremely compliant. The chronic aneurysm composed of fibrous and muscle tissue is intermediate. (Modified from Parmley WW, Chuck L, Kivowitz C et al: In vitro length–tension relations of human ventricular aneurysms: The relationship of stiffness to mechanical disadvantage. Am J Cardiol 32:887, 1973)

TABLE 10.3 COMMON CAUSES OF CONGESTIVE HEART FAILURE

Coronary artery disease	Cardiomyopathy
Hypertension	Cor pulmonale
Valvular heart disease	Congenital heart disease

TABLE 10.4 CAUSES OF HIGH CARDIAC OUTPUT

Hyperthyroidism	Atrioventricular fistula
Anemia	Dermatologic disorders
Paget's disease	Acute glomerulonephritis
Polyostotic fibrous dysplasia (Albright's disease)	Hepatic cirrhosis
	Beriberi
Hypernephroma with bone metastases	

the most common reason for surgically replacing the mitral valve. Calcific aortic stenosis, often on a bicuspid valve, remains a common cause of pressure overload of the left ventricle. Various forms of cardiomyopathy are also commonly seen as a cause of heart failure. Similarly, cor pulmonale due to chronic obstructive pulmonary disease or primary or secondary pulmonary hypertension is reasonably frequent. Congenital heart disease as a cause of heart failure is infrequently seen by the adult cardiologist. With better and more complete repair of complex congenital lesions, however, more of these patients will be seen in adult life in the future.

A number of less frequent disorders that cause an increase in cardiac output are listed in Table 10.4. Generally, these disorders are not the sole cause of heart failure but contribute to other causes by increasing the demands on the heart. General mechanisms include increased whole body oxygen consumption (e.g., hyperthyroidism), decreased oxygen delivery (e.g., anemia), arteriovenous shunting, or increased regional flow.

High-output cardiac states are relatively uncommon as causes of congestive heart failure. In patients with reduced ventricular reserve, however, any factor that increases cardiac output can manifest itself as a contributory cause to high-output failure. In general, the causes of high-output failure are those that lead to a marked reduction in peripheral vascular resistance. A normal, 70-kg man generally has a resting cardiac output of approximately 6.5 liters per minute. Since the total blood volume is approximately 5 liters, this indicates that the total blood volume circulates on average in slightly less than one minute. Of course, with exercise, the cardiac output can be increased dramatically in individuals with normal ventricular reserve. At rest, a normal adult consumes about 130 ml/m^2 of oxygen per minute. With normal oxygen saturation (95%), average cardiac output, and average hematocrit, there is approximately 20 ml oxygen per 100 ml of blood. Normally, the mixed venous oxygen content is about 75% saturated and has an oxygen content of approximately 15 ml per 100 ml blood. With a marked increase in tissue metabolism and/or a reduction in cardiac output, the body can, on occasion, extract up to 12 ml oxygen resulting in an approximate 35% oxygen saturation in the pulmonary venous blood. Generally, however, this kind of extraction occurs only with a marked increase in demand or a marked reduction in cardiac output.

A number of interventions can increase cardiac output. An increased body temperature may increase cardiac output more than 50%. This is due primarily to the increased skin blood flow required to dissipate heat. This increase in need for cardiac output may help explain the poor tolerance of patients with congestive heart failure to hot environmental conditions. Certainly with a limitation of the ability to increase cardiac output, there may also be a lesser ability to dissipate heat, which may add to discomfort in such patients.

Anemia is a common cause of an increase in cardiac output, because the decreased oxygen capacity of the hemoglobin must be compensated for by an increase in cardiac output. When the hematocrit falls below 25%, there is a consistent reduction in systemic vascular resistance accompanied by an increase in cardiac output. In patients with anemia who exercise, there is also an excessive increase in cardiac output in an attempt to maintain oxygen delivery to the exercising tissues. In patients with anemia that develops insidiously over time, very few symptoms may be found, although increased fatigue is the most common complaint. Other symptoms may develop if patients have underlying heart disease, such as angina in those with coronary disease. The evaluation of the anemia must be complete, particularly that due to chronic blood loss from the gastrointestinal tract. Treatment can often be specific, such as vitamin B_{12} for pernicious anemia.

Physical findings in patients with high-output failure are generally those expected with a high stroke volume and cardiac output. A slight tachycardia may be present, although the major factor associated with an increased cardiac output is an increased stroke volume associated with cardiomegaly. Bounding pulses with a wide pulse pressure and other peripheral signs similar to those in patients with aortic regurgitation may be present. Systolic flow murmurs and occasional mid-diastolic flow murmurs are present. Heart sounds are generally accentuated, and an S_3 may be heard at the apex. Cardiomegaly is the rule on chest radiograph.

In patients with hyperthyroidism there is a generalized increase in metabolic rate of all tissues in the body, mediated by thyroid hormone. This hormone also directly increases cardiac contractility and alters myocardial contractile proteins with a shift towards more rapidly contracting isomyosin V_1. Tachycardia and increased pulse pressure are characteristic of hyperthyroidism. There is some relationship to catecholamine stimulation, because administration of β-blockers tends to decrease these cardiovascular manifestations, although there is no change in the underlying thyroid state. This state may be due to a general up-regulation of β-receptors in patients with hyperthyroidism. Although β-blockers can decrease the tachycardia and cardiac output, therapy of the underlying thyroid disease is mandatory.

Arteriovenous fistulae of various kinds can also lead to an increase in cardiac output. The most common clinical manifestation of this form of decreased peripheral resistance is in patients with external arteriovenous shunts for hemodialysis. Various traumatic wounds, surgical interventions, or other causes can lead to acquired arterial venous fistulae. Uncommon causes include beriberi heart disease, which is appropriately treated with thiamine; Paget's disease of the bone, which is associated with a marked increase in vascularity of the bones; and fibrous dysplasia, which also leads to increased vascularity of bone. Cardiac output may also be increased in some individuals with cirrhosis or glomerulonephritis and in some patients with skin disorders such as psoriasis.

The so-called hyperkinetic heart syndrome has been described occasionally in young individuals with an increase in cardiac output who frequently complain of palpitations and atypical chest pain. β-blocker therapy may be helpful in this group of patients.

In managing patients with long-term heart failure, episodes of worsening heart failure are not uncommon. In evaluating such episodes, it is important to distinguish between a worsening of the underlying process and a precipitating cause that can be reversed. Some of the common precipitating causes of heart failure that should be considered in each patient episode are listed in Table 10.5. Reduction of therapy is probably the most common cause, since compliance with drug therapy is poor in many patients. Patients may run out of their prescribed pills or merely forget to take their medications. Once-a-day medications when possible, written instructions, and strong encouragement may be helpful in improving compliance.

Excessive salt intake is also a frequent cause of worsening heart failure. Obvious indiscretions such as eating pretzels, potato chips, dill pickles, or fast food "hamburgers and fries" are easily recognized. More often, however, careful questioning is required to discover the source of increased sodium.

Arrhythmias can be an important mechanism for precipitating left ventricular failure. A common example is the patient who develops atrial fibrillation with a rapid ventricular response. Such circumstances are particularly potent in producing heart failure in patients with mitral stenosis who depend on an appropriate diastolic time for blood to cross the stenotic mitral valve. Similarly, patients with hypertrophied ventricles, such as hypertrophic cardiomyopathy, may develop severe heart failure with the development of atrial fibrillation due to loss of the atrial kick. Less commonly, ventricular arrhythmias may precipitate heart failure. Ventricular tachycardia is a rhythm that frequently results in severe hypotension, reduced cardiac output, and elevated pulmonary capillary wedge pressure. Since it is rarely sustained for prolonged periods of time, it is generally manifested by transient symptoms of hypotension or heart failure.

Anything that increases the demands for cardiac output can also precipitate heart failure in a patient with poor ventricular reserve. This would include systemic infection and physical, environmental, or emotional stress. Either excess requirement for cardiac output or a marked increase in arterial pressure can greatly impair the heart with borderline compensation.

Pulmonary embolism appears to be more frequent than its recognized clinical expression. Inappropriate tachycardia with low cardiac output and evidence of right-sided heart failure may accompany multiple silent pulmonary emboli. This cause must be considered, for example, in the setting of a postoperative orthopedic patient or someone who has been in bed for a prolonged period of time. Myocarditis or bacterial endocarditis can also precipitate heart failure in susceptible patients and must be considered in patients in whom other causes do not appear to account for the change in symptoms. High-output states have been listed in Table 10.4 and need to be ruled out as causes for precipitating heart failure in patients with borderline compensation. Patients may also develop an unrelated illness as a cause of worsening heart failure. Perhaps most commonly, this may be a pulmonary or bronchial infection or the superimposition of influenza or other viral illnesses. Not infrequently, a patient may develop a second form of heart disease. For example, the development of coronary artery disease in a patient with preexisting valvular heart disease is a not uncommon sequence.

In summary, in approaching the patient with worsening heart failure, it is important to look carefully for precipitating causes, particularly those that can be treated or removed. If, in fact, there do not appear to be any causes that are apparent, then it becomes a more likely possibility that the underlying heart disease has intrinsically worsened.

THE MYOCARDIUM IN CONGESTIVE HEART FAILURE

A number of mechanical and biochemical factors are altered in cardiac muscle during the development of chronic congestive heart failure. A few of the more important ones are tabulated in Table 10.6 and briefly discussed below. In chronic congestive heart failure there is an intrinsic decrease in the contractility of individual myocardial fibers. This decrease in contractility is manifested as a decrease in velocity of shortening at a given load, a decrease in force development, and a decrease in maximum rate of force development. The elastic properties of cardiac muscle are little altered during the development of severe heart failure, although some data suggest that tissue from hypertrophied and failing hearts may be slightly stiffer than normal.

This intrinsic decrease in cardiac contractility is mostly irreversible. However, in the experimental setting, where one can produce hypertrophy and heart failure by pressure overloading, such as banding of the aorta or pulmonary artery, release of the bands at certain times can result in return of function toward normal.[15] In clinical circumstances, it is unclear that dramatic alterations in reversing depressed contractility can occur. This emphasizes the importance of considering relief of pressure or volume overload (e.g., with valve replacement) before irreversible changes in myocardial contractility have progressed.

A number of biochemical alterations have been noted in the failing heart. One of the more interesting ones includes a decrease in actomyosin ATPase activity. The enzymatic activity of the myosin crossbridge as it attaches to actin is responsible for breaking down high-energy ATP and generating the energy necessary for contraction at the crossbridge site. Over a wide range of species there is a general relationship between actomyosin ATPase activity and maximum velocity of muscle shortening.[16] This close relationship between mechanical performance and biochemistry is of interest, particularly when one considers what happens in chronic congestive heart failure. A decrease in actomyosin ATPase activity accompanies the decrease in velocity of shortening seen in chronic congestive heart failure.[17] This may be partially protective of the heart by reducing oxygen consumption for a given amount of external work. This change in actomyosin ATPase activity appears to be the result of synthesis of isoenzymes with a slower enzymatic activity.

A common accompaniment of hypertrophy and heart failure is increased collagen content of the myocardium. In part, this may contribute to the increased myocardial stiffness seen in patients with hypertrophy and heart failure. Certainly, increased collagen is common in the healing process that accompanies myocardial ischemic damage or myocardial infarction.

The autonomic nervous system is markedly affected with the development of heart failure. Because of a marked increase in sympathetic tone, there is a decrease in myocardial stores of norepinephrine. In part, this results because of the enhanced secretion of norepinephrine, although there is also evidence that decreased synthesis may occur. Tyrosine hydroxylase is a key enzyme in the synthetic pathway of norepinephrine and appears to be depressed, at least in experimental hypertrophy and heart failure.[18] A decrease in the function of the sarcoplasmic reticulum probably plays a major role in the genesis of some systolic dysfunction in congestive heart failure. The decreased ability to take up calcium, with lower calcium stores, may contribute directly to a decrease in contractility.

There has been some controversy about whether a decrease in high-energy phosphate stores may play a role in the genesis of congestive heart failure. Early studies in experimentally produced hypertrophy and heart failure suggested that ATP stores were not depleted and could not, therefore, account for the heart failure state.[19] Other studies in different models of heart failure have pointed out that there is a decrease in stores of high-energy phosphates, which may contribute to the heart failure state.[20]

TABLE 10.5 PRECIPITATING CAUSES OF HEART FAILURE

Reduction of therapy
High salt intake
Arrhythmias
Systemic infection
Physical, environmental, and emotional stress
Pulmonary embolism
Hypertension
Cardiac infection and inflammation
High output states
Development of an unrelated illness
Development of a second form of heart disease

TABLE 10.6 MYOCARDIUM IN CONGESTIVE HEART FAILURE

Mechanical Alterations	Biochemical Alterations
Decrease in velocity of shortening	Decreased actomyosin ATPase activity
Decrease in force development	Increased collagen
Decrease in maximum rate of force development	Decreased myocardial norepinephrine
Little or no change in passive length–tension relations	Decreased synthesis of norepinephrine
No change in series elastic	Decreased function of sarcoplasmic reticulum
	? Decreased high-energy phosphates
	? Excess myoplasmic calcium
	Decreased β_1-adrenergic receptors

One of the more intriguing hypotheses in recent years has been that excessive myocardial calcium plays a pathophysiologic role in the heart failure state. Excess myocardial calcium can be deleterious through several mechanisms. Excess calcium depresses mitochondrial function and also may activate proteases, which are deleterious to cellular integrity. One experimental model of heart failure is a hereditary congestive cardiomyopathy that develops in the Syrian hamster. In this animal model of heart failure, it has been demonstrated that excessive calcium may play a deleterious role. The use of calcium entry blockers in this model not only preserves histology but also preserves muscle function, emphasizing a negative effect of excessive calcium.[21] Whether excess calcium plays a role in other myopathies or other forms of heart disease is not clear at this time but deserves further investigation.

Important alterations have been noted in β-adrenergic receptors in patients with severe heart failure.[22] In the nonfailing human ventricle 77% of receptors were of the β_1 type, whereas 23% were of the β_2 type. In muscle removed from failing human ventricles, there was a 62% selective down-regulation of the β_1 receptors with little change in β_2 receptors. When studied in an isolated bath, β_2 stimulation became relatively more important in increasing contractility in failing human myocardium because of the relative increase in β_2 receptors.

COMPENSATORY MECHANISMS

A number of intrinsic compensatory mechanisms are available to the heart to counter the adverse physiology seen in the heart failure state. These are listed in Table 10.7. The increased preload that occurs with congestion of the right and left ventricles is initially beneficial by increasing stroke volume in accord with the Frank-Starling mechanism. The increase in sympathetic tone and circulating catecholamines may also be helpful in supporting the circulation through direct stimulation of contractility and through an augmentation of heart rate. Certainly, an increase in heart rate is one of the most important compensatory mechanisms for maintaining cardiac output in the face of a low fixed stroke volume. Under these circumstances, cardiac output and heart rate will be directly related. Thus tachycardia may not only be an important compensatory mechanism but is also a good marker of the severity of the underlying heart failure state. As patients improve spontaneously or with appropriate therapy, heart rate is often reduced. With a decrease in cardiac output, oxygen delivery to peripheral tissues can be maintained, in part, by increased extraction of oxygen from the blood. This results in an increased arteriovenous oxygen difference and decreased saturation of the mixed venous blood returning to the right side of the heart. This mechanism, however, is only a minor one and cannot compensate for a major reduction in cardiac output. A number of hormonal changes occur that might also be considered as compensatory, at least in their initial expression. In addition to increased circulating catecholamines there is activation of the renin-angiotensin-aldosterone system and increased levels of arginine vasopressin. The increase in angiotensin II might initially be helpful by maintaining blood pressure in the face of a decrease in cardiac output. Similarly, the production of increased amounts of aldosterone with retention of salt and water are helpful in terms of augmenting preload by the Frank-Starling mechanism. Increased arginine vasopressin might also be helpful as a vasoconstrictor in maintaining blood pressure when cardiac output falls.

The relative effects of these three hormonal systems have been studied in patients with congestive heart failure. Creager and co-workers[23] administered antagonists to each hormonal system in 10 patients with advanced congestive heart failure (Fig. 10.2). The arginine vasopressor antagonist did not produce major changes in hemodynamics, although its greatest effects were in patients whose plasma vasopressin was greater than 4 pg/ml. The renin-angiotensin antagonist, captopril, decreased systemic vascular resistance by 20%. Phentolamine, as an α-adrenergic antagonist, decreased systemic vascular resistance by 34%. This comparative study provides useful information about the relative importance of different hormonal vasoconstrictor mechanisms in patients with advanced heart failure. Their relative importance in increasing systemic vascular resistance appears to be that catecholamines are greater than angiotensin II, which is greater than vasopressin.

TABLE 10.7 COMPENSATORY CHANGES

Increased preload
Increased sympathetic tone
Increased heart rate
Increased arteriovenous oxygen difference
Increased circulating catecholamines
Increased renin-angiotensin-aldosterone
Increased arginine vasopressin

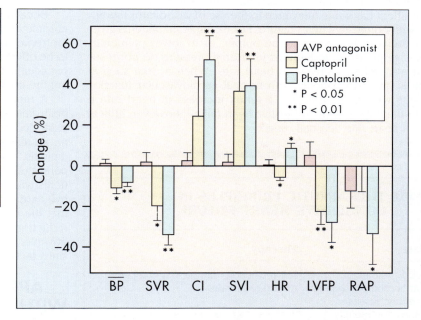

FIGURE 10.2 In ten patients the maximum hemodynamic response is illustrated (Mean ± SEM) for antagonists to arginine vasopressin (AVP antagonist), the renin angiotensin system (Captopril), and α-adrenergic constriction (phentolamine). ($\overline{BP}$ mean blood pressure: SVR, systemic vascular resistance; CI, cardiac index; HR, heart rate; LVFP, left ventricular filling pressure; RAP, right atrial pressure) (Modified from Creager MA, Faxon DP, Cutler SS et al: Contribution of vasopressin to vasoconstriction in patients with congestive heart failure: Comparison with the renin-angiotensin system and the sympathetic nervous system. J AM Coll Cardiol 7:758, 1986)

From the above description, however, it should be apparent that many of these compensatory mechanisms, while initially beneficial, may overshoot and produce adverse effects. A few brief examples will suffice. Although the initial increase in preload may be beneficial, excessive retention of salt and water produces the signs and symptoms of pulmonary and systemic congestion, which are deleterious to the patient with heart failure. Similarly, although catecholamines, angiotensin II, and arginine vasopressin may raise arterial pressure by vasoconstriction, in the face of a low cardiac output they become counterproductive by further reducing cardiac output due to the increased impedance placed on the circulation. This overshoot of systemic vascular resistance appears to be one of the most important factors that can be corrected by vasodilators in the patient with heart failure. Arteriolar vasodilator drugs have been extremely beneficial in lowering resistance and improving forward cardiac output. Similarly, venodilators, such as the nitrates, have been helpful in relieving venoconstriction and redistributing blood away from the chest, thus lowering right and left atrial filling pressures.

It is interesting to speculate whether or not excessive heart rates may be deleterious to the patient with heart failure. Under certain circumstances, β-blockers have been reported to be helpful to patients with congestive cardiomyopathy.[24] Although not a universal finding, this information does suggest that there may be circumstances in which excessive heart rate or catecholamines may be deleterious by increasing oxygen consumption or perhaps even affecting diastolic coronary blood flow.

The most important concept that should be emphasized in this section is that excessive overshoot of some compensatory mechanisms can be deleterious to the patient with heart failure and set the stage for many of the common therapeutic interventions that we use.

OTHER FACTORS

Congestive heart failure is associated with other effects on the cardiovascular system. Only a few will be discussed. Several studies have noted that there appears to be a decrease in baroreceptor and cardiac receptor responsiveness in patients with congestive heart failure. That is, alterations in blood pressure do not produce the same reflex effects on heart rate or contractility as in patients with more normal circulations.[25] This effect has some relevance to the use of vasodilator therapy in patients with congestive heart failure. For example, in patients given vasodilator drugs to improve cardiac output, or to lower pulmonary capillary wedge pressure, reductions in arterial pressure do not result in much, if any, reflex increase in heart rate. When a drug such as hydralazine is given to patients with normal cardiovascular function (*e.g.*, patients with hypertension), a reflex increase in heart rate is common. In the patient with congestive heart failure, however, little or no change in heart rate is usually seen.

There also appears to be a reduced ability to vasodilate peripheral blood vessels maximally, at least as measured in the forearm of patients with congestive heart failure.[26] Occluding the arm for a short period of time is a potent way of producing maximal vasodilation following release of the occlusion. In patients with congestive heart failure, this hyperemic response is considerably blunted. This may reflect increasing vasoconstrictor tone or, alternatively, may represent functional anatomical changes at the arteriolar level. For example, accumulation of salt and water at that level might make it more difficult for arterioles to vasodilate in response to the potent stimulus of short-term ischemia.

The blunted response of patients with congestive heart failure to a Valsalva maneuver is another expression of the reduced reflex response in patients with congestive heart failure. The lack of overshoot at various phases of the Valsalva maneuver presumably represents decreased reflex autonomic changes in these patients, in addition to the effects of congestion.[27]

The role of the kidney in congestive heart failure is a crucial one. Decreased renal perfusion leads to salt and water retention, a hallmark of congestive signs and symptoms. The role of the kidney in heart failure is discussed in detail elsewhere in this volume.

THERAPEUTIC PRINCIPLES

Some of the principles that we have been discussing in relation to therapy of congestive heart failure are outlined in Table 10.8. Four clinical expressions of the heart failure state are listed together with appropriate considerations for therapy. The increased preload that is responsible for the signs and symptoms of pulmonary and systemic congestion can be appropriately treated by salt restriction, diuretics, and venodilators. All of these will be effective in reducing excess salt and water retention, thereby reducing the excess volume load on the heart. Low cardiac output with its resultant symptoms of fatigue is, in part, related to the high systemic resistance, which is reflexly mediated by the vasoconstrictive mechanisms discussed. This high systemic resistance sets the stage for the use of arteriolar vasodilators, which can be effective in increasing forward cardiac output. In general, arteriolar vasodilators appear to be more effective (on a percentage basis) in patients with the highest systemic vascular resistance.

Because of the intrinsic decrease in contractility that occurs in chronic congestive heart failure, the stage is set for the use of positive inotropic agents. Digoxin is commonly used in this setting and appears to be effective in some patients. Both new intravenous and oral inotropic agents may also have a beneficial effect in heart failure by improving the contractile state of the left ventricle.

A rapid heart rate is frequently found in patients with congestive heart failure and is a common marker of the severity of the cardiovascular decompensation. In patients with atrial fibrillation, it is clear that an increase in atrioventricular block, with the use of drugs such as digitalis, can be extremely effective in improving left ventricular compensation. It is unclear whether a direct reduction of heart rate in patients with sinus tachycardia is also of benefit. In patients with congestive cardiomyopathy treated with β-blockers, there is some suggestion that the beneficial effects seen in some patients may be mediated by reduction of an excessive heart rate.[24] Further evidence is required, however, before we can confidently alter heart rate in patients with sinus tachycardia and produce beneficial effects.

APPROACH TO THE PATIENT WITH CONGESTIVE HEART FAILURE

The major elements that should be considered in the evaluation and management of the patient with congestive heart failure are listed in Table 10.9. First and foremost is the responsibility of the physician to determine the etiology of the heart failure. A knowledge of the cause of the heart failure determines, to a great extent, the subsequent ap-

TABLE 10.8 THERAPEUTIC PRINCIPLES IN CONGESTIVE HEART FAILURE

Problem	Therapy
Increased preload	Salt restriction, diuretics, venodilators
Low cardiac output, high systemic resistance	Arteriolar dilators
Decreased contractility	Positive inotropic agents
Rapid heart rate	
Atrial fibrillation	Increase atrioventricular block
Sinus tachycardia	Improve left ventricular performance (? β-blockade)

proach to therapy. Since many patients have precipitating causes that worsen their heart failure, it is also important to consider such causes each time a patient is seen with worsening of their heart failure. Correction of precipitating causes is always effective in helping patients to remain compensated.

Once the etiology of the heart failure is determined it is important to assess the severity of the disease and any associated problems that might affect the long-term course of the patient. In this respect, some determination of left ventricular function is a critical measurement. Since this can be obtained noninvasively by a variety of techniques, including echocardiography and radionuclide imaging, it should be quantitated as an important marker of the current stage and natural history of the disease in an individual patient. When patients are first seen, it is often difficult to be sure how rapidly their disease is progressing. Sometimes historical data can provide the information that is required. Alternatively, more objective data collected at two different times can provide quantitative information. The assessment of the time course of the disease in a given patient, especially when viewed against the background of the natural history of the disease, is helpful in assessing prognosis, response to therapy, and implications for surgery. In patients with valvular heart disease, or other correctable lesions, the timing of surgery becomes a key element in this ongoing assessment, as one attempts to intervene before major, irreversible changes have occurred in the intrinsic contractility of the myocardium.[28] Since cardiac transplant is a current, realistic goal in many patients, the potential availability and suitability of candidates should be considered, if the response to medical therapy is less than optimal.

In initiating medical therapy, a number of steps should be considered, as outlined in Table 10.9. Reduction of the workload of the heart has always been an appropriate way to improve left ventricular compensation. When this is accomplished by reduction in blood pressure, activity level, and weight or other restrictions, this practice has proven to be effective. A study by Abildgaard and co-workers[29] evaluated the effects of bed rest as an adjunct to increased diuretic therapy. The group with continuous bed rest for three days reduced their weight by 2.0 kg, while the group who was in bed only at night had a significantly smaller weight loss. Sodium restriction should also be employed. A common precipitating cause of heart failure is either a sodium load or inadequate diuretic therapy. Water restriction is rarely required. In some patients with New York Heart Association Class IV heart failure who are hyponatremic (despite excess fluid accumulation), water restriction may be required to bring the sodium up to more normal levels. These patients frequently have associated renal involvement with an inability to excrete a free water load.

Diuretics represent an effective form of therapy in patients with congestive heart failure. By and large it is prudent to start with the thiazide-type diuretics and then work up to more potent diuretics as required. In the patient with severe heart failure, a combination of diuretics may sometimes be helpful (e.g., metolazone plus furosemide). The role of digitalis in congestive heart failure will be discussed in more detail elsewhere in this volume. In patients with atrial fibrillation and a rapid ventricular response, digitalis is an effective drug in slowing the ventricular response and compensating the left ventricle. I believe that digitalis can be an effective form of therapy in some patients with congestive heart failure. Its inotropic effects are very modest, however. Those individuals in sinus rhythm who are most likely to respond have a dilated heart, congestive cardiomyopathy, and a third heart sound. Its once-a-day dosage is convenient and its potential benefit suggests that it be considered in the management of most patients with chronic congestive heart failure. Vasodilator drugs and inotropic agents will be discussed in other chapters in this volume.

Figure 10.3 illustrates the rationale for polypharmacy in congestive heart failure, using a combination of an inotropic agent (such as digoxin), a diuretic (such as furosemide), and a vasodilator (such as an angiotensin-converting enzyme inhibitor).

Another interesting form of therapy has been the use of β-blockers in congestive or dilated cardiomyopathy. Early studies in Sweden suggested that low-dose metoprolol might be of benefit in patients with excessive tachycardia.[24] Subsequent controlled studies have shown mixed results.[30,31] A multicenter trial was initiated in 1986 to answer this interesting question.

One of the major issues facing the clinician is how best to follow the patient who is treated for congestive heart failure. If a major clinical response occurs and is accompanied by a decrease in heart size on chest radiograph or echocardiogram, then there is no problem. Responses are often more subtle than this, however, and are complicated by the factors listed in Table 10.10.

Although ejection fraction is a good prognostic marker, it does not correlate with exercise tolerance. Similarly the acute hemodynamic effects of a given drug may not necessarily correlate with the chronic clinical response.[32] Although noninvasive techniques are an attractive way to follow patients treated with a new agent, they are very insensitive indices to change. Lastly, the patient's well-being can be adversely affected by drug side-effects, even though there may be important he-

TABLE 10.9 APPROACH TO THE PATIENT WITH CONGESTIVE HEART FAILURE

1. Determine etiology of heart failure.
2. Determine precipitating causes.
3. Assess the severity of heart failure and associated diseases.
4. Assess time course of the disease in light of its natural history.
5. Assess potential and timing of surgical therapy, if applicable.
6. Initiate medical therapy:
   a. Reduce workload of heart
   b. Reduce salt intake
   c. ? Water restriction
   d. Diuretics
   e. Digitalis
   f. Vasodilators
   g. New inotropic agents

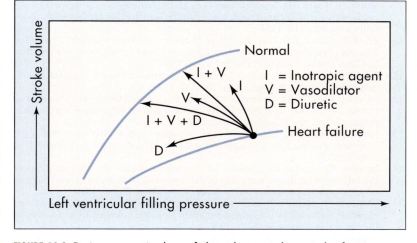

FIGURE 10.3 During congestive heart failure, the normal ventricular function curve is shifted down and to the right. Beginning at that point, the solid lines show the directional shifts (arrowhead) using single and combined therapy with each of the three classes of drugs. Note that the beneficial hemodynamic effects of each class are additive when combination therapy is administered. Thus, maximal beneficial hemodynamic effects are seen with triple therapy.

modynamic benefit. Amidst these difficulties, there are certain markers of clinical response. A careful history is important to detect how patients are doing. Serial weights are mandatory to judge the potential effects of diuretics in patients with fluid retention. Exercise tolerance on a treadmill is an important objective marker of improvement. One must use less severe graded exercise than tests such as the Bruce protocol, particularly in patients with considerable limitations. Measurement of total body oxygen consumption or anaerobic threshold may also be useful in judging efficacy.[33]

TABLE 10.10 PROBLEMS IN JUDGING EFFICACY OF THERAPEUTIC AGENTS

Ejection fraction does not correlate with exercise tolerance
Acute drug response may not predict chronic response
Noninvasive techniques may be insensitive indices
Drug side effects can mask hemodynamic benefit

CLINICAL IMPLICATIONS

The purpose of this chapter is to provide a pathophysiologic background underlying the development of congestive heart failure. An application of these principles is helpful in the appropriate evaluation and management of patients. It is especially recommended that the physician tailor his approach to the patient in an individual way. Interventions or drugs should be employed rationally to counteract or reverse the pathophysiologic changes of special importance to that patient. Combination therapy should likewise be synergistic and appropriate. One should avoid a "cookbook" approach to the patient and always attempt to individualize therapy so as to maximize benefit.

By evaluating alterations in preload, afterload, heart rate, and contractile state, one can select therapy designed to correct each of these specific abnormalities. Our major goals relate to attempts to improve symptoms and exercise tolerance. Of course, with surgically correctable disease, one should never prolong medical therapy at the expense of a continuing decline in intrinsic myocardial contractility. With the renewed interest in cardiac transplantation, this option has become more widely available for selected patients. The use of the artificial heart is clearly experimental at this time. Ultimately, prevention of heart failure will have the greatest beneficial impact in this syndrome.

REFERENCES

1. McKee PA, Castelli W, McNamara P et al: The natural history of congestive heart failure: The Framingham Study. N Engl J Med 85:1441, 1971
2. Massie B, Ports T, Chatterjee K et al: Long-term vasodilator therapy for heart failure: Clinical response and its relationship to hemodynamic measurements. Circulation 63:269, 1981
3. Franciosa JA, Willen M, Ziesche S et al: Survival in men with severe chronic left ventricular failure due to either coronary heart disease or idiopathic dilated cardiomyopathy. Am J Cardiol 51:831, 1983
4. Wilson JR, Schwartz JS, Sutton MSJ et al: Prognosis in severe heart failure: Relation to hemodynamic measurements and ventricular ectopic activity. J Am Col Cardiol 2:403, 1983
5. Simonton CA, Daly P, Kereiakes D et al: Survival in severe congestive heart failure treated with new nonglycosidic, nonsympathomimetic oral inotropic agents. Chest 92:118, 1987
6. Holmes J, Kubo SH, Cody RJ et al: Arrhythmias in ischemic and nonischemic dilated cardiomyopathy: Prediction of mortality by ambulatory electrocardiography. Am J Cardiol 55:151, 1985
7. Gold WM: Dyspnea. In Blacklow RS (ed): MacBryde's Signs and Symptoms, 6th ed, pp 335–348. Philadelphia, JB Lippincott, 1983
8. Pierpont G, Hale KA, Franciosa JA et al: Effects of vasodilators on pulmonary hemodynamics and gas exchange in left ventricular failure. Am Heart J 99:208, 1980
9. Stone PH, Clark RD, Goldschlager N et al: Determinants of prognosis of patients with aortic regurgitation who undergo aortic valve replacement. J Am Coll Cardiol 3:1118, 1984
10. Zile MR, Gaasch WH, Carroll JD et al: Chronic mitral regurgitation: Predictive value of preoperative echocardiographic indexes of left ventricular function and wall stress. J Am Coll Cardiol 3:235, 1984
11. Page DL, Caulfield JB, Kastor JA et al: Myocardial changes associated with cardiogenic shock. N Engl J Med 285:133, 1971
12. Parmley WW, Chuck L, Kivowitz C et al: *In vitro* length-tension relations of human ventricular aneurysms: The relationship of stiffness to mechanical disadvantage. Am J Cardiol 32:887, 1973
13. Eaton LW, Weiss JL, Bulkley BH et al: Regional cardiac dilatation after acute myocardial infarction: Recognition by 2-D echocardiography. N Engl J Med 300:57, 1979
14. Bristow JD, VanZee BG, Judkins MP: Systolic and diastolic abnormalities of the left ventricle in coronary artery disease: Studies in patients with little or no enlargement of ventricular volume. Circulation 42:219, 1970
15. Williams JF, Mathew B, Hern DL et al: Myocardial hydroxyproline and mechanical response to prolonged pressure loading, followed by unloading in the cat. J Clin Invest 72:1910, 1983
16. Barany M: ATPase activity of myosin correlated with speed of muscle shortening. J Gen Physiol 50:197, 1967
17. Alpert NR, Gordon MS: Myofibrillar adenosine triphosphatase activity in congestive failure. Am J Physiol 202:940, 1962
18. Pool PE, Covell JW, Levitt M et al: Reduction of tyrosine hydroxylase activity in experimental congestive heart failure. Circ Res 20:349, 1967
19. Pool PE, Spann JF Jr, Buccino RA et al: Myocardial high energy phosphate stores in cardiac hypertrophy and heart failure. Circ Res 21:365, 1967
20. Sievers R, Parmley WW, James T et al: Energy levers at systole vs. diastole in normal hamster hearts vs. myopathic hamster hearts. Circ Res 53:759, 1983
21. Rouleau J-L, Chuck LHS, Hollosi G et al: Verapamil and hydralazine preserve myocardial contractility in the hereditary cardiomyopathy of the Syrian hamster. Circ Res 50:405, 1982
22. Bristow MR, Ginsburg R, Umans V et al: B_1 and B_2 adrenergic receptor subpopulations in nonfailing and failing human ventricular myocardium: Coupling of both receptor subtypes to muscle contraction and selective B_1 receptor down-regulation in heart failure. Circ Res 59:297, 1986
23. Creager MA, Faxon DP, Cutler SS et al: Contribution of vasopressin to vasoconstriction in patients with congestive heart failure: Comparison with the renin-angiotensin system and the sympathetic nervous system. J Am Coll Cardiol 7:758, 1986
24. Swedberg K, Hjalmarson A, Waagstein F et al: Beneficial effects of long-term beta blockade in congestive cardiomyopathy. Br Heart J 44:117, 1980
25. Zucker IH, Earle AM, Gilmore JP: The mechanism of adaptation of left atrial stretch receptors in dogs with chronic congestive heart failure. J Clin Invest 60:323, 1977
26. Zelis R, Longhurst J: The circulation in congestive heart failure. In Zelis R (ed): The Peripheral Circulations, Clinical Cardiology Monographs, pp 282–314. New York, Grune & Stratton, 1975
27. Gorlin R, Knowles JH, Storey CF: The Valsalva maneuver as a test of cardiac function: Pathologic physiology and clinical significance. Am J Med 22:197, 1957
28. Ross J Jr: Afterload mismatch in aortic and mitral valve disease: Implications for surgical therapy. J Am Coll Cardiol 5:811, 1985
29. Abilgaard U, Aldershvile J, Ring-Larson H et al: Bed rest and increased diuretic treatment in chronic congestive heart failure. Eur Heart J 6:1040, 1985
30. Ikram H, Fitzpatrick P: Double-blind trial of chronic oral beta blockade in congestive cardiomyopathy. Lancet 2:490, 1981
31. Anderson JL, Lutz JR, Gilbert EM et al: A randomized trial of low dose beta-blockade therapy for idiopathic dilated cardiomyopathy. Am J Cardiol 55:471, 1985
32. Franciosa JA, Dunkman WB, Leddy CL: Hemodynamic effects of vasodilators and long-term response in heart failure. J Am Coll Cardiol 3:1521, 1984
33. Weber KT, Janicki JS: Cardiopulmonary exercise testing for evaluation of chronic cardiac failure. Am J Cardiol 55:22A, 1985

GENERAL REFERENCES

Cohn JN (ed): Drug Treatment of Heart Failure. New York, Yorke Medical Books, 1983
Fishman AP (ed): Heart Failure. Washington DC, Hemisphere, 1978

ORTHOSTATIC HYPOTENSION

C. Gunnar Blomqvist

CHAPTER 11

VOLUME 1

Orthostatic hypotension is a common and sometimes disabling condition. Likely causes include many different defects that singly or in combination affect major mechanisms controlling blood flow, vascular resistance, arterial pressure, and intravascular volume. The control systems are complex, and their interactions are poorly understood. As a consequence, obvious and straightforward therapeutic approaches sometimes prove ineffective but seemingly paradoxic measures are often helpful. These characteristics combine to make orthostatic hypotension a challenging topic.

■ CAUSES OF RECURRENT EPISODIC ARTERIAL HYPOTENSION

Syncope is a common manifestation of orthostatic hypotension. The principal mechanism of syncope, including the orthostatic variety, is a transient reduction in cerebral blood flow. Causes of recurrent episodes of arterial hypotension include cardiac *dysrhythmias*. Bradyarrhythmias, tachyarrhythmias, and intermittent atrioventricular conduction blocks can cause reductions in cardiac output of sufficient magnitude to impair cerebral perfusion, particularly in patients with coexisting cerebrovascular disease. *Mechanical obstruction* of systemic or pulmonary blood flow may produce global cerebral ischemia with syncope. Such conditions include valvular aortic or pulmonary stenosis, idiopathic hypertrophic subaortic stenosis, atrial myxoma, and pulmonary embolic or vascular disease with pulmonary hypertension.

A wide range of emotional and somatic afferent stimuli can precipitate *vasodepressor* or *vasovagal syncope*. Neither term is strictly accurate. The cardiovascular response usually includes both bradycardia and vasodilatation, and impulse flow is altered in both the parasympathetic and sympathetic portions of the autonomic nervous system. The typical psychological circumstances involve a perception of an actual or symbolic injury that the victim feels that he or she should be able to face without fear. Obligations to submit to painful or unfamiliar diagnostic or therapeutic procedures are prime examples.[1] Among the somatic mechanisms are carotid sinus hypersensitivity[2] and abnormal impact of afferent impulses from the ear, mouth, larynx, and pharynx (*e.g.*, in glossopharyngeal neuralgia).[3] Simple swallowing (deglutition syncope)[4] may precipitate vasodepressor syncope in some persons. The hemodynamic events have been well documented.[1,5-7] A typical sequence includes an initial phase with moderate tachycardia followed by a marked fall in heart rate and arterial pressure. The depressor phase of the response has many features in common with orthostatic hypotension that progresses to syncope and later will be discussed in some detail.

■ PATHOPHYSIOLOGY OF ORTHOSTATIC HYPOTENSION
PRINCIPAL FEATURES

Orthostatic or postural hypotension may be defined as the inability to maintain adequate arterial pressure and tissue perfusion in the upright position. The brain is almost always the organ most vulnerable to postural hemodynamic changes, but orthostatic angina pectoris has been described.[8] Syncope is the manifestation of grossly inadequate cerebral blood flow. Lesser degrees of hypoperfusion cause vague weakness and postural dizziness or faintness. Many different clinical conditions are associated with orthostatic intolerance. Some patients have severe and widespread structural neurologic and cardiovascular abnormalities. Others appear to have strictly functional disorders.

Two major mechanisms cause orthostatic intolerance: (1) relative central hypovolemia with postural decreases in cardiac filling and stroke volume to subnormal levels and (2) inadequate regulatory responses to the decrease in stroke volume and cardiac output.

The conventional terminology in this area is often inappropriate and confusing because it is based exclusively on the responses mediated by the sympathetic nervous system. It would be preferable to use dual descriptors referring to changes in intravascular volume and to regulatory responses. "Sympaticotonic orthostatic hypotension" may then be characterized as hypovolemic hyperreactive orthostatic hypotension. The "asympaticotonic" variety would be referred to as normovolemic hyporeactive orthostatic hypotension.

GRAVITY, CARDIOVASCULAR PRESSURE–VOLUME RELATIONSHIPS, AND STARLING'S LAW

All intravascular pressures have a gravity-dependent hydrostatic component (Fig. 11.1).[9,10] The interactions between the gravitational field, the position of the body, and the structural and functional characteristics of the blood vessels determine the distribution of intravascular volume. This, in turn, has major effects on cardiac filling and pump function.

Data on human blood volume, its distribution, and vascular pressure–volume relationships have been reviewed by Blomqvist and Stone.[10] Total blood volume in mammals is a linear function of body weight. Mean values in normal adult humans cluster around 75 ml/kg, corresponding to a total of 5 to 5.5 liters in a 70-kg person. High levels of physical activity and adaptation to a hot climate cause expansion of the blood volume with balanced increases in red blood cell mass and plasma volume.

Approximately 70% of the total blood volume is contained in the systemic veins; the heart and the lungs account for 15%, the systemic arteries for 10%, and the capillaries for 5%. Effective total vascular compliance represents the summed compliances of the various vascular compartments. It is dominated by the systemic veins. Measurements are derived by monitoring central venous pressure during acute changes in blood volume. Normal human compliance values are of the order of 2 to 3 ml/mm Hg/kg. Effective compliance is an empiric measurement, complicated by reflex hemodynamic adjustments with secondary redistribution of venous volume, by delayed compliance (viscoelastic creep of the vessel walls), and by adjustments in plasma volume by tissue filtration. Nevertheless, it provides a useful measure of the impact on right-sided cardiac filling pressures of acute hypovolemia and hypervolemia.

A simple Frank-Starling relationship (stroke volume as a function of end-diastolic volume or pressure) is a reasonably accurate descriptor of cardiac performance during postural changes in healthy persons at rest. There are normally no major changes in arterial blood pressure. Afterload, expressed as end-systolic wall stress, is usually slightly reduced in the upright position. The normal left ventricle ejects more than half of its end-diastolic volume, usually between two thirds and three fourths (Table 11.1).[11,12]

Stroke volume varies in direct proportion to changes in end-diastolic volume (Fig. 11.2).[13] Increases in ejection fraction with secondary increases in stroke volume, mediated by positive inotropism, are of only minor functional significance during acute interventions that primarily affect ventricular filling. Arterial pressure is maintained by adjustments in heart rate and systemic vascular resistance.

CEREBRAL PERFUSION

Cerebral blood flow is normally tightly controlled by autoregulation. It remains stable over a wide range of mean arterial pressure at normal levels of arterial carbon dioxide partial pressure. Cerebral blood flow usually starts to decrease significantly when driving pressure (mean arterial pressure at the eye level) falls below 50 mm Hg. Consciousness may be lost when blood flow falls below one fourth of normal, which usually occurs at a mean pressure of about 40 mm Hg.[14] The hydrostatic gradient between the levels of the heart and the brain in the upright position adds 30 mm Hg to the required pressure as measured at the heart level. A mean arterial threshold pressure of 70 mm Hg

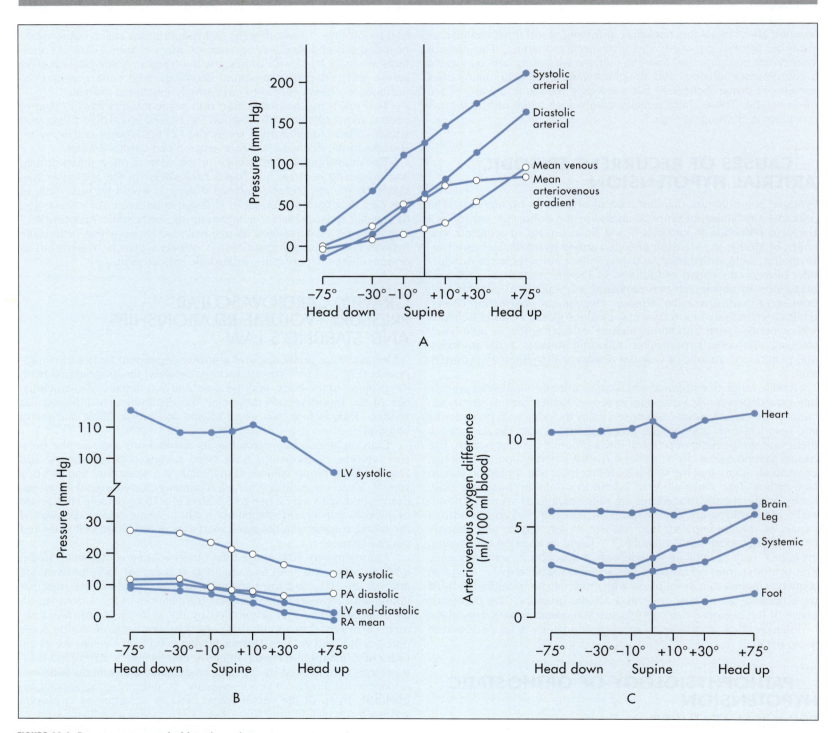

FIGURE 11.1 Responses to graded head-up tilt in ten young normal men. Intravascular pressures in foot (**A**) and in central circulation (**B**). (**C**) Arteriovenous oxygen difference. Angle of tilt (horizontal axis) plotted as sine function to provide linear scale for primary hydrostatic effects of body-position changes, based on data from Katkov and Chestukhin.[9] (LV, left ventricle; PA, pulmonary artery; RA, right atrium) (Modified from Blomqvist CG, Stone HL: Cardiovascular adjustments to gravitational stress. In Shepherd JT, Abboud FM (eds): Handbook of Physiology, Section 2, The Cardiovascular System. Volume III: Peripheral Circulation and Organ Blood Flow, Part 2, pp 1025–1063. Bethesda, MD, American Physiological Society, 1983)

corresponds to systolic and diastolic pressures of about 80/65 mm Hg. A significant shift of the autoregulatory range to the left is likely to occur in chronic autonomic dysfunction[15] with orthostatic hypotension, and a right-ward shift is a feature of systemic hypertension.

NORMAL RESPONSES TO ORTHOSTATIC STRESS

A change in body position from supine to standing or sitting initiates a well-defined sequence of events[10,16,17]:

1. Blood volume is redistributed away from the heart. About 500 ml is removed from the intrathoracic region to the legs. An additional volume of 200 to 300 ml is transferred to the veins in the buttocks and the pelvic area.
2. Cardiac filling pressures fall, and stroke volume decreases, usually by 20% to 30%.
3. An equally large acute decrease in arterial pressure is prevented by rapid baroreflex-induced increases in heart rate and systemic vascular resistance. Additional neurohumoral mechanisms are activated

TABLE 11.1 POSTURAL CARDIOVASCULAR ADJUSTMENTS IN NORMAL HUMAN SUBJECTS

Parameter	Supine	Sitting	p
Left ventricular volume (ml)*			
End-diastolic	107 ± 10	85 ± 6	<0.02
Endsystolic	34 ± 4	32 ± 5	
Stroke	76 ± 8	55 ± 5	<0.05
Ejection fraction (%)†	76 ± 2	72 ± 4	
Heart rate (beats per minute)	73 ± 4	84 ± 4	<0.001
Pressure (mm Hg)			
Brachial artery	96 ± 3	99 ± 4	
Systolic	130 ± 5	132 ± 5	
Diastolic	76 ± 3	82 ± 3	<0.05
Pulmonary artery	13 ± 1	13 ± 1	
Pulmonary capillary wedge	6 ± 1	4 ± 1	<0.001
Left ventricular end-diastolic	8 ± 1	4 ± 1	<0.001
Stroke index (ml/m²)	50 ± 5	35 ± 3	<0.001
Cardiac index (liters/min/m²)	3.5 ± 0.3	2.8 ± 0.2	<0.001

* Left ventricular scintigraphic data (mean ± standard error) from seven young normal subjects studied by Poliner and co-workers.[11]

† Hemodynamic measurements from ten sedentary men, aged 32 to 58 examined by Thadani and Parker.[12]

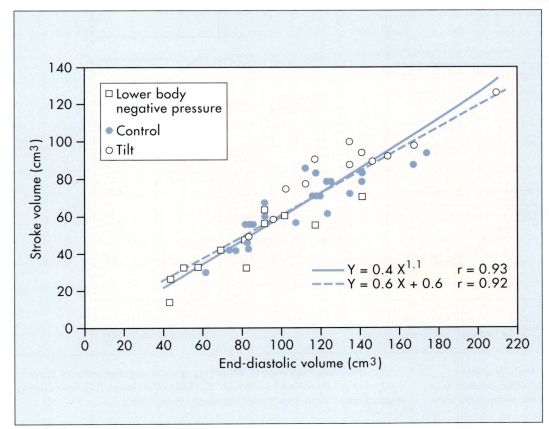

FIGURE 11.2 Relationship between left ventricular stroke volume and end-diastolic volume. Echocardiographic measurements in 12 normal young men. Large variations in preload were introduced by head-down tilt at 5° and lower body negative pressure at −40 mm Hg. (Modified from Nixon JV, Murray RG, Leonard PP et al: Effects of large variations in preload on left ventricular characteristics in normal subjects. Circulation 65:698–703, 1982)

within minutes to preserve adequate intravascular volume and to help maintain arterial pressure.

4. Cerebral perfusion pressure is kept within the autoregulatory range.

The principal features of the human cardiovascular response to orthostatic stress are shown in Figure 11.3. The data represented in the figure were collected during lower body negative pressure (LBNP). Application of LBNP produces a redistribution of intravascular volume similar to that which occurs during a transition from supine to sitting or standing. The use of LBNP facilitates many measurements. LBNP also gives the experimenter better control of the stimulus by minimizing skeletal muscle activity that has major effects on the blood volume distribution and on the dynamic cardiovascular response. Furthermore, in the microgravity environment of space, LBNP provides a means of studying the equivalent of gravitational postural shifts of intravascular volume.

Figure 11.3 shows a progressive decrease in right atrial pressure, left ventricular end-diastolic volume, stroke volume, and cardiac output. Aortic pressure during the early stages is maintained by vasoconstriction only. Initially this involves the skin and skeletal muscle (forearm), but later the splanchnic region is also involved. Further decreases in stroke volume are partially offset by increasing heart rate.

Plasma levels of norepinephrine increase, representing overflow from vascular receptors, and plasma renin activity levels are also elevated in response to large decreases in cardiac filling.[17-19]

TOTAL BLOOD VOLUME AND MECHANISMS CONTROLLING ITS DISTRIBUTION

Variations in total blood volume well within the physiological range may affect orthostatic tolerance.[20,21] The relative degree of peripheral pooling is also important. Patients with massive venous varicosities or a congenital absence of the venous valves have postural hypotension and decreased exercise capacity in the upright position.[22] Ambient temperature also affects the degree of peripheral pooling, probably mainly by altering skeletal muscle tone. Heat markedly reduces, and cold increases, orthostatic tolerance.[23] Relative rather than absolute magnitude determines the hemodynamic impact of peripheral redistribution of blood. Subsets of patients (e.g., those with mitral valve prolapse syndrome) with orthostatic hypotension and reduced total blood volume may pool no more or even less than normal controls in terms of absolute volume.[24] Other patients with intact autonomic function have a combination of increased absolute peripheral venous pooling and reduced total blood volume.[25]

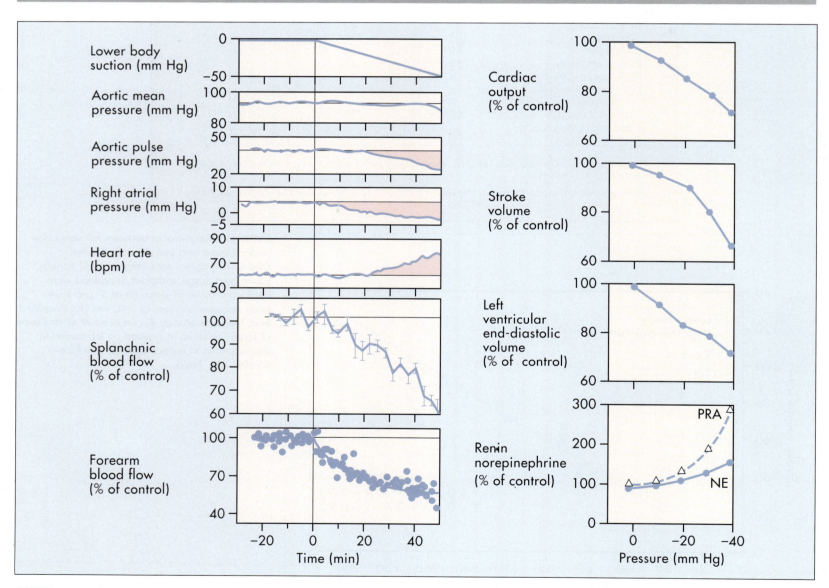

FIGURE 11.3 Cardiovascular responses to graded lower body negative pressure. Panels on the left show average responses to suction applied at a continuous rate of −1 mm Hg min^{-1} for 50 minutes.[18] Panels on the right show central circulatory responses to 10-mm Hg steps in negative pressure down to −40 mm Hg.[19] (Modified from Rowell LB: Human Circulation: Regulation During Physical Stress. New York, Oxford University Press, 1986)

Considerable controversy exists regarding the extent to which active reflex-mediated venomotor changes contribute to cardiovascular homeostasis during changes in posture.[17,26,27] In general, active venoconstriction may occur in the skin and in the splanchnic region. Veins supplying skeletal muscle are poorly innervated, and plasma concentrations of norepinephrine rarely reach levels that would produce venoconstriction. Furthermore, the deep veins in the leg have very thin walls. Venous compliance is largely determined by the characteristics of skeletal muscle. Mayerson and Burch measured intramuscular pressures in young persons who had had multiple episodes of orthostatic hypotension progressing to syncope.[28] Fainters had lower intramuscular pressures in the leg at rest and subnormal pressure increases during head-up tilt. Buckey and associates used a combination of magnetic resonance imaging (MRI) and occlusion plethysmography to examine the capacity of the deep leg veins.[29] At distending pressures equivalent to the hydrostatic venous pressures in the upright position, more than one half of the increase in leg volume was accommodated by the deep veins (Fig. 11.4). This finding implies that the properties of skeletal muscle are likely to affect significantly the distribution of venous volume and cardiac filling also at rest when the muscle pump is inactive.

Local reflex mechanisms may contribute to the vascular response to orthostatic stress. In experimental animals, activation of venous afferent fibers by distention produces reflex-induced leg muscle activity that may counteract postural pooling.[30,31] However, attempts to demonstrate a similar reflex in humans have been unsuccessful. Vasoconstriction with decreased limb blood flow in response to local venous distention mediated by a local (axonal) sympathetic reflex mechanism has been demonstrated by Henriksen and Sejrsen.[32,33]

CARDIAC PRESSURE–VOLUME CHARACTERISTICS

Cardiac pressure–volume characteristics during diastole (Fig. 11.5) are likely to modulate the systemic effects of any given decrease in intrathoracic blood volume. In the supine position in normal sedentary subjects, the left ventricle appears to be operating close to its maximal

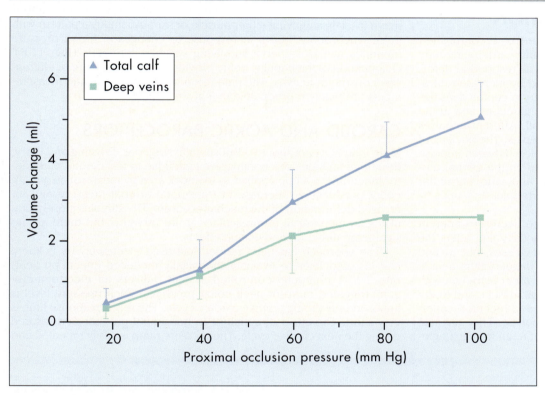

FIGURE 11.4 Changes in deep venous volume and total leg volume with increasing venous occlusion pressures. Measurements derived by quantitative analysis of cross-sectional magnetic resonance images of the lower leg. (Modified from Buckey JC, Peshock RM, Blomqvist CG: Deep venous contribution to hydrostatic blood volume change in the leg. Am J Cardiol 62:449–453, 1988)

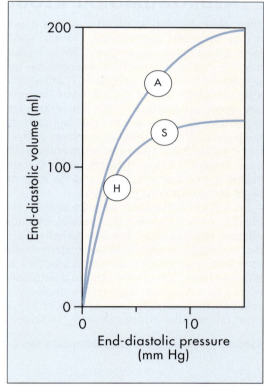

FIGURE 11.5 Potential mechanisms by which the diastolic pressure–volume characteristics of the normal left ventricle may affect orthostatic tolerance. In the supine position, sedentary subjects (S) operate at near-maximal volume, that is, on the relatively flat portion of the curve. Hypovolemia with a decrease in filling pressure (H) will cause a shift toward the steep portion and potentiates the effects on ventricular volume of further decreases in filling pressure. There is suggestive evidence that endurance athletes (who usually have large diastolic volumes) normally operate on the steep portion of the function curve (A). This provides a mechanism augmenting end-diastolic volume and stroke volume when filling pressures increase during exercise. However, there will also be a large orthostatic decrease in stroke volume that may help explain why high levels of aerobic fitness sometimes are associated with orthostatic hypotension. (Based on data in part from Chapter 5)

functional diastolic volume. Increases in filling pressure during exercise or intravenous fluid loading, or during the two interventions combined, produce only minor increases in end-diastolic volume and stroke volume.[10,34,35]

Hypovolemia decreases orthostatic tolerance for several different reasons. Large losses of intravascular volume lower supine filling pressure, end-diastolic volume, and stroke volume and magnify the orthostatic decreases in ventricular filling and stroke volume. Any absolute amount of postural venous pooling will represent a larger relative peripheral transfer in the hypovolemic subject. More importantly, hypovolemia alters the effective ventricular diastolic pressure–volume characteristics. The normal pressure–volume curve is nonlinear with a larger change in volume for any change in pressure at low filling pressures.[36] Hypovolemia causes a leftward displacement of the operating point away from the flat portion of the function curve (where moderate increases and decreases in filling pressure have little effect on end-diastolic volume and stroke volume) toward the steep portion of the curve where any further reduction in filling pressure will cause a large decrease in stroke volume.

NEUROHUMORAL REGULATION

Short-term regulation of arterial blood pressure is accomplished mainly by neural mechanisms. Carotid, aortic, and cardiopulmonary mechanoreceptors are involved. These receptors all respond to deformation, that is, to stretch or compression caused by increased intracavitary or transmural pressures. Cardiopulmonary receptor densities are particularly high at the left-sided atriovenous junctions and in the inferoposterior portion of the left ventricular wall. Afferent impulses travel with the vagus and the glossopharyngeal nerves. The nucleus of the tractus solitarius is the primary site of interaction between impulse traffic in the baroreceptor pathways and activity within the central nervous system.[37] Efferent fibers reach the sinus and atrioventricular nodes, the cardiac ventricles, and the systemic arterioles and veins by vagal and spinal cord pathways.

A fall in intravascular or intracardiac pressure decreases afferent impulse traffic. This releases central inhibitory activity and alters the efferent impulse flow. Parasympathetic drive decreases, but α- and β-adrenergic activities increase. Responses of the target organs include increased heart rate, increased contractility, and vasoconstriction with reduced blood flow to the skin, to inactive skeletal muscle, and to the renal and splanchnic regions. The majority of the β-receptors innervated by the sympathetic nerves are of the β_1 subtype. They regulate heart rate, cardiac contractile state, and release of renin from juxtaglomerular cells. The β_2-receptors of the resistance vessels in skeletal muscle have a vasodilator function but are not innervated.[38]

The existence of a triplicate system for neural control of blood pressure is well established,[39,40–42] but the interactions and degree of functional overlap between the three principal baroreflexes (carotid, aortic, and cardiopulmonary) are still poorly understood. Data from experiments in nonhuman species are not necessarily applicable to human physiology and medicine. Distributions of hydrostatic gradients and regional blood volume are markedly different in humans and quadrupeds, but interesting, minimally invasive and safe techniques have been developed for human use in the study of specific aspects of short-term reflex regulation of arterial pressure.

DIRECT MICRONEUROGRAPHIC STUDIES OF MUSCLE SYMPATHETIC NERVE ACTIVITY

A microneurographic technique for direct recording of human sympathetic nerve activity has been developed by Hagbarth and Vallbo[43] and has been applied extensively to the study of cardiovascular physiology by Wallin[44–46] and others.[47–51] The peroneal and median nerve are relatively easily accessible. A thin tungsten electrode is inserted into a nerve fascicle supplying either muscle or skin. An impulse pattern with pulse-synchronous bursts in response to changes in blood pressure identifies a muscle nerve supplying vascular terminals (Fig. 11.6). Quantitation of the impulse traffic provides a direct measure of efferent vasoconstrictor activity. The time resolution is excellent, and measurements are highly reproducible in a given subject.

CAROTID AND AORTIC BAROCEPTORS

More than 30 years ago, two British flight surgeons, Ernsting and Parry, described an ingenious noninvasive technique to test carotid baroceptor function.[52] Suction applied to the neck area by means of an airtight collar produces an increase in transmural arterial pressure and increased deformation of the mechanoceptors. The stimulus closely simulates an increase in intravascular carotid pressure, but there are no significant direct hemodynamic effects.

The approach has been refined and used extensively by Eckberg and his associates to evaluate the vagally mediated effects on heart rate.[53–57] A computer-controlled system delivers an electrocardiogram-triggered ramp of neck collar pressures. Each pressure level is imposed only during a single cardiac cycle. The reflex response time is very short. The effect of a change in transmural pressure is measured during the next cardiac cycle. The pressure ramp is easily repeated and

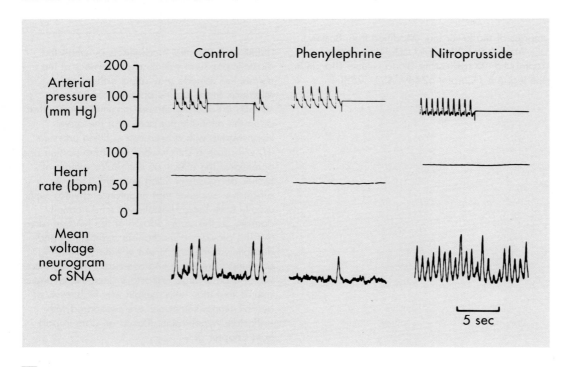

FIGURE 11.6 Arterial baroreceptor reflex responses: effect of elevating phasic and mean arterial pressure with phenylephrine and lowering pressure with nitroprusside on heart rate and efferent muscle sympathetic nerve activity (SNA) in a normal subject. SNA is pulse synchronous. An 8-mm Hg increase in arterial pressure (phenylephrine) caused marked reflex inhibition of SNA and a reflex fall in heart rate. A 15-mm Hg fall in arterial pressure (nitroprusside) caused an increase in SNA and heart rate. (Aksamit TR, Floras JS, Victor RG et al: Paroxysmal hypertension due to sinoaortic baroceptor denervation in humans. Hypertension 9:309–314, 1987)

stimulus–response curves (Fig. 11.7) can be based on multiple measurements. Characteristic abnormalities have been described in hypertension.[55] The operating point is reset in mild disease, and the sensitivity or slope is reduced in more advanced cases.

Major assets of this approach are the lack of effect on the native hemodynamic state and the relative ease by which complex quantitative data can be acquired. On the other hand, the procedure generates data only on the heart rate component of the reflex. Activation of the carotid baroceptors by increased transmural pressure of longer duration also affects the sympathetic nerve traffic to the resistance vessels in skeletal muscle.[51] At least theoretically, carotid baroreceptor function may be normal in the presence of attenuated heart rate responses if the vasomotor effects are enhanced.

The operating characteristics of the carotid and aortic baroreflexes appear to be different in different species. In dogs, the aortic reflex has a higher threshold and lower sensitivity than the carotid baroreflex. Ferguson and associates[58] and Sanders and co-workers[59] used a combination of the direct sympathetic nerve recording technique and the pressurized neck collar to examine the relationship between aortic and carotid reflexes in human subjects. Phenylephrine was infused with and without external pressure application to the neck to cancel the effects on transmural carotid sinus pressure. This approach left the aortic baroreceptors free to respond. The carotid baroreceptors were also activated separately by neck suction. The results confirm that both reflexes participate in the control of arterial pressure in human subjects and suggest that the aortic reflex is more powerful than the carotid. The greater sensitivity applies to the control of both heart rate and adrenergic vasoconstrictor activity.

LOSS OF ARTERIAL BARORECEPTOR FUNCTION

Aksamit and colleagues described a patient with loss of carotid and aortic baroreceptor function attributable to a combination of surgery and radiation therapy.[48] Large changes in arterial pressure, induced by infusions of phenylephrine and nitroprusside, failed to affect heart rate or directly measured adrenergic vasomotor nerve activity. The patient had retained cardiopulmonary reflex activity and responded to an LBNP-induced decrease in cardiac filling with a marked increase in sympathetic nerve activity. Arterial pressure was labile, but sustained hypertension was not present. Sinoaortic denervation in experimental animals produces a similar state. Thus, cardiopulmonary baroceptors may contribute to the control of arterial pressure but are by themselves unable to prevent rapid changes in arterial pressure. The patient was mildly orthostatic.

CARDIOPULMONARY RECEPTORS

The principal components of the cardiopulmonary receptor system are the left atrial and left ventricular receptors. Both sets respond to deformation. The atrial receptor population directly monitors atrial filling and indirectly monitors ventricular filling. The ventricular receptors discharge primarily during systole but are also influenced by diastolic events. Changes in ventricular wall stress, which is maximal during isovolumic systole, may be the common primary stimulus.

There are numerous and complex interactions between the mechanisms maintaining arterial pressure and body fluid homeostasis. Arterial pressure levels directly affect tissue filtration rates and renal excretion of sodium and water. The arterial and cardiopulmonary baroreflexes also control renal sympathetic activity (α-adrenergic vasoconstriction, β_1-mediated activation of the renin–angiotensin system). Vasopressin (antidiuretic hormone) is released from the neurohypophysis in response to increases in plasma osmolarity as detected by receptors in the hypothalamus. Vasopressin is also released when the atrial mechanoreceptors are unloaded by decreasing filling pressures, usually as a consequence of decreased central blood volume. Unloading of ventricular and arterial baroreceptors by decreases in transmural pressures also releases vasopressin. The relative importance of these receptor sites is not known in detail, but the atrial release mechanism may be less active in primates than in other species. Vasopressin may be physiologically important as a vasoactive substance, inducing vasoconstriction in skeletal muscle and the splanchnic area and vasodilatation in the coronary and cerebral circulations by a combination of endothelium-dependent (cyclo-oxygenase-me-

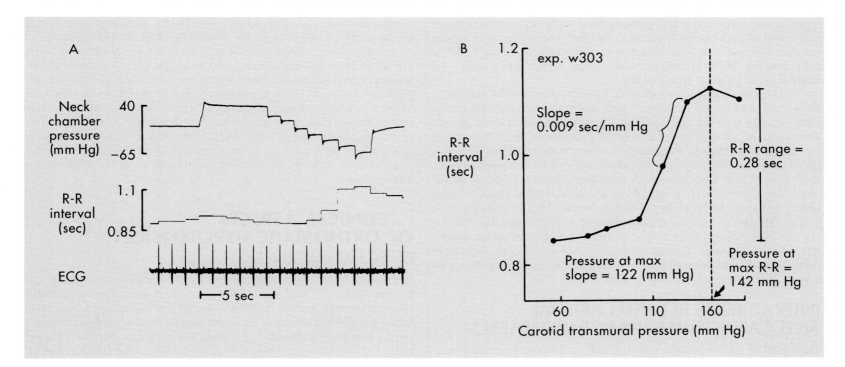

FIGURE 11.7 Experimental record (**A**) and average responses of one subject to seven applications of neck pressure sequence (**B**). **B** indicates method used to analyze baroreflex relations. Carotid transmural pressure was considered to be average systolic pressure minus neck chamber pressure. Pressure at maximum slope was taken as carotid transmural pressure halfway between pressures bracketing maximum slope. (Modified from Kasting GA, Eckberg DL, Fritsch JM et al: Continuous resetting of the human carotid baroreceptor–cardiac reflex. Am J Physiol 252 (Regulatory Comp Physiol 21:R732–R736, 1987)

diated, indomethacin-inhibited) and direct relaxation of smooth muscle.

Release of atrial natriuretic peptide (ANP) is caused by an increase in atrial transmural pressures. In addition to inducing natriuresis, ANP has multiple effects including vasodilatation and venodilatation, inhibition of renin and vasopressin release, and perhaps also a direct effect on capillary permeability.[17,38,60]

LBNP at nonhypotensive levels has been used as a means of unloading the low-pressure cardiopulmonary receptors without affecting the arterial sensors. LBNP in the range −5 to −10 or −15 mm Hg produces significant vasoconstriction, but there is no change in arterial systolic or diastolic pressures. Pulse pressure and aortic pulse contour also remain unchanged at moderate LBNP levels. These findings, combined with the absence of any heart rate change (see Fig. 11.3),[17] provide evidence for preferential involvement of the low-pressure receptor pathway and suggest that the principal response is vasoconstriction. However, cardiac filling pressures and stroke volume decrease. This is likely to cause a decrease in aortic and arterial pulse volume with a significant secondary change in carotid sinus and aortic wall stress. Some degree of activation of arterial baroreflexes cannot be ruled out, and the ventricular receptors may also respond.

LOSS OF CARDIOPULMONARY RECEPTOR FUNCTION

Current surgical technique in cardiac transplantation preserves the dorsal portion of the atria, including the neural pathways to and from the left atrial receptors. The efferent pathways to the right atrium and the sinus node are also intact, but the node is electrically isolated from the transplanted heart. The ventricular baroceptors are, of course, lost. Mohanty and associates reported marked attenuation of the normal reflex-induced increases in forearm vascular resistance and plasma norepinephrine levels during LBNP after cardiac transplantation.[61] The impaired responses were not caused by treatment with immunosuppressive agents. Renal transplant patients on similar regimens had enhanced vasoconstrictor responses. Furthermore, the vasomotor and norepinephrine responses to a cold pressor test were intact in the cardiac transplant patients. The combined data suggested to the authors that the impaired vasoconstrictor responses were caused by ventricular denervation. However, the patients in this series tended to be hypertensive; post-transplant patients tend to be hypertensive (as a side effect of cyclosporin treatment) and their mean forearm vascular resistance at rest was higher than in control subjects during LBNP at −40 mm Hg. Mean arterial pressure during LBNP was equally well maintained in patients and controls.

Victor and colleagues studied 12 patients after cardiac transplantation and six normal controls.[50] Left ventricular dimensions during LBNP at −14 mm Hg decreased to the same extent in both groups. There was no change in mean arterial pressure or heart rate in the control group. Muscle sympathetic nerve activity (MSNA) during LBNP, measured directly with the microelectrode technique, was twice as high as at rest. Compared with normal controls, the transplant patients had higher MSNA at rest but an identical relative change during LBNP. Sinus rate in the atrial remnant increased by 6 beats per minute in the patients, and mean arterial pressure fell by 3 mm Hg. The increases in MSNA and sinus node rate were abolished when mean arterial pressure was kept constant during LBNP by infusion of phenylephrine. These data indicate that arterial baroreflexes can compensate for loss of the ventricular receptor function.

INTERACTIONS BETWEEN ARTERIAL AND CARDIOPULMONARY BAROREFLEXES

Vasovagal or vasodepressor syncope and orthostatic syncope in subjects with intact autonomic nervous system have many common features.[1,5,6,39] There is an initial phase with moderate tachycardia and vasoconstriction, followed by a marked fall in heart rate and arterial pressure. There is little or no increase in plasma norepinephrine in response to the hypotension (Fig. 11.8). The cutaneous circulation is usually vasoconstricted but there is a large decrease in systemic resistance, caused by vasodilatation in skeletal muscle.[7] Paradoxic vasodilatation and bradycardia are also common features of hemorrhagic shock.[39,62] Data obtained by direct nerve recording techniques have documented a strong inhibition of impulse traffic in the α-adrenergic vasoconstrictor fibers supplying skeletal muscle during presyncope and syncope.[45,46]

The most likely cause of this sequence of events is conflicting inputs from arterial and cardiopulmonary baroreflexes. The left ventricular receptors are normally activated by increased intracavitary pressure and/or volume with increased wall stress. A progressive reduction in ventricular volume probably occurs during the presyncopal stage. Echocardiographic studies have demonstrated gradually decreasing left ventricular volumes with increasing degrees of peripheral venous pooling.[19] The left ventricular endocardial receptors will eventually be activated by direct compression. The salient stimulus is deformation, but the sensing system cannot differentiate between compression, which is associated with low volume and pressure, and distension, which is caused by high ventricular pressure and volume. The normal adjustments to reduced cardiac output and arterial pressure are negated, and bradycardia and vasodilatation are produced. An unstable autonomic state sometimes occurs during the presyncopal phase with large oscillations in heart rate and arterial pressure (Fig. 11.9).[63] This may reflect variations in the balance between opposing drives from ventricular and arterial receptors (*i.e.*, deformation of the ventricular receptors in an empty heart falsely signaling high left ventricular pressures at a time when the carotid and aortic receptors sense a low arterial pressure[16]) or represent an exaggeration of the intrinsic 0.1 Hz cyclical variations in adrenergic vasomotor activity.[64]

There is strong collateral support for an important role for the ventricular baroceptors. β-Adrenergic blockade increases left ventricular end-diastolic and endsystolic volumes and improves orthostatic tolerance after bed rest.[65] Activation of ventricular deformation receptors by high ventricular transmural pressure or direct contact is likely to be the principal cause of syncope in aortic stenosis and in idiopathic hypertrophic subaortic stenosis.[39] Bradycardia and arterial hypotension are also common features during the early stages of an acute inferior or inferoposterior myocardial infarction.[39] The activity of ventricular mechanoreceptors is likely to be enhanced by increased deformation of the ischemic segment of the ventricular wall. Reflex inhibition of renal sympathetic activity may, at least theoretically, limit the ability to conserve intravascular volume and to enhance vasoconstrictor responses (no renal vasoconstriction and no activation of the renin–angiotensin system). The hemodynamic effects at rest are usually transient, but relative bradycardia and hypotension are often present during the standard submaximal exercise test at discharge. The attenuated exercise responses are usually normalized within a few weeks when the healing process is completed (unpublished observations), and there is likely to be less deformation in or at the edge of the infarcted area.

CLINICAL ASPECTS OF ORTHOSTATIC HYPOTENSION
EFFECT OF AGING

Orthostatic hypotension from all causes becomes more prevalent with increasing age.[66] Caird and colleagues studied a large group of ambulatory men and women aged 65 and older.[67] Decreases in systolic blood pressure to 20+ mm Hg below supine resting levels after 1 minute of standing occurred in 24% and decreases of 30+ mm Hg occurred in 9% of the study population. A majority of the subjects had (1) two or more conditions likely to be associated either with hypovolemia or maldistribution of the blood volume (*e.g.*, anemia, chronic infection, or varicose veins) or with impaired cardiovascular control mecha-

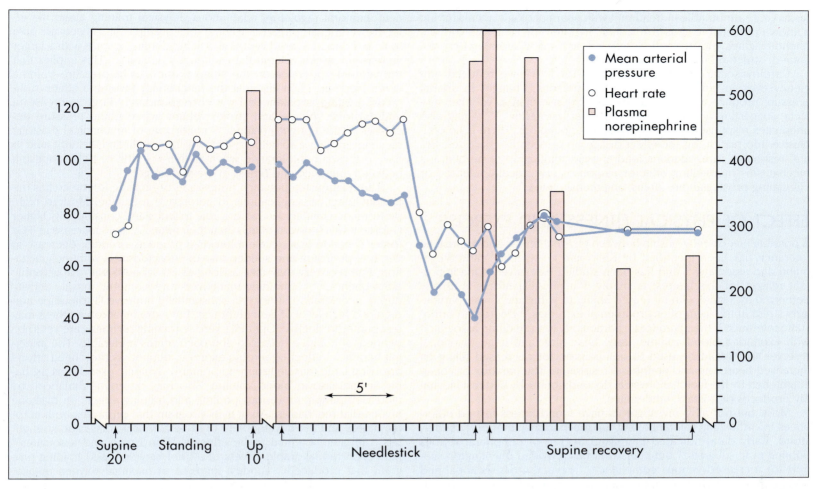

FIGURE 11.8 Mean arterial pressure (MAP), heart rate (HR), and plasma norepinephrine (NE) concentrations during syncope evoked by the emotional response to insertion of an intravenous needle in a 17-year-old female patient who suffered from recurrent syncopal episodes. Syncope was associated with severe hypotension and bradycardia. There was no norepinephrine response to hypotension during syncope, although the norepinephrine response to standing was intact. (Modified from Goldstein DS, Spanarkel M, Pitterman A et al: Circulatory control mechanisms in vasodepressor syncope. Am Heart J 104:1071–1075, 1982)

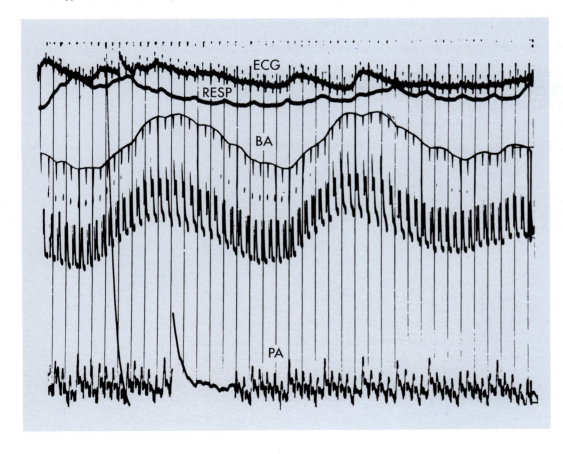

FIGURE 11.9 Vasomotor waves are present in the brachial artery pressure tracing (BA) but are not seen in the pulmonary artery pressure tracing (PA). Waves are unrelated to respiration (RESP) and are now believed to represent variations in α-adrenergic activity. The periodicity usually approximates 0.1 Hz. These waves were recorded during 70° head-up tilt after a 14-day bed rest period in a subject with reduced orthostatic tolerance. (Modified from Hyatt KH: Hemodynamic and body fluid alterations induced by bed rest. In Murray RM, McCally M (eds): Hypogravic and Hypodynamic Environments, pp 187–209. Washington, DC, National Aeronautics and Space Administration, 1971)

nisms (e.g., attributable to treatment with pharmacologic agents having a known potential to cause orthostatic hypotension such as levodopa, phenothiazines, tricyclic antidepressants, and vasodilators) or (2) presence of structural neurologic lesions.

Cardiovascular control mechanisms tend to have reduced efficiency even in generally healthy older persons. Changes in arterial pressure produce a smaller heart rate response than in younger subjects, suggesting a blunting of the arterial baroreflex.[68,69] Aging also attenuates responses mediated by β_1 adrenoceptors. There is no conclusive information on the effect of age on α-receptor characteristics and responses to exogenous α-adrenergic stimulation or on humoral mechanisms modulating effector responses (i.e., locally released or circulating prostaglandin, kinins, angiotensin, etc).[70]

EFFECT OF PHYSICAL FITNESS AND EXERCISE

A possible inverse relationship between physical fitness and orthostatic tolerance has been identified by Klein and co-workers[71] and Stegemann and associates[72] and has been studied extensively. One important reason for this interest is simply that physical fitness is usually perceived as a state with increased ability to withstand stress, particularly stress in the form of environmental extremes.[71] Decreased orthostatic tolerance is then paradoxic, particularly in a condition associated with expanded blood volume, large heart size, and large functional reserves that could be used to compensate for decreased filling by increased heart rate and peripheral resistance. The paradox has been heightened by the fact that physical deconditioning by bed rest inevitably produces orthostatic intolerance.

Most, but not all,[73] investigators have found fitness-related differences in orthostatic tolerance, but the mechanisms are poorly understood. Early data indicated increased degree of peripheral venous pooling in fit subjects,[74] but later work has provided only limited support for increased venous compliance.[75] Several cross-sectional and longitudinal studies have examined various aspects of baroceptor function. Fit persons have been shown to have attenuated heart rate[71,74,76-78] and vasoconstrictor responses to orthostatic stress.[77-79] Corresponding findings have been made in experimental animals.[80]

Significant group differences in orthostatic tolerance have also been reported in the absence of any major difference in baroreflex function.[81] It is possible that the decreased orthostatic tolerance to a significant extent is a consequence of cardiac mechanics rather than neurohumoral regulatory adaptations. Physical training alters the effective ventricular pressure–volume relationships. Fit subjects are able to respond to increased ventricular filling during exercise with a larger increase in stroke volume than sedentary persons.[35] This implies that the ventricle operates on the steep portion of its pressure–volume curve (see Fig. 11.5) and that the functionally favorable effect of increased filling is balanced by a correspondingly large decrease in end-diastolic volume and stroke volume when filling pressure decreases in the upright position. A major role of mechanical diastolic mechanisms may also help explain why the very fit and the unfit tend to have orthostatic intolerance whereas there is little or no relationship between tolerance and fitness in the mid range.

The relationship between fitness and orthostatic tolerance has important practical implications in aerospace medicine. Modern high-performance military aircraft are able to withstand considerably higher G-force levels (upward of 9G) than their pilots. A rapid increase in +Gz forces (head-to-foot acceleration) can produce a sudden decrease in cerebral perfusion and sudden loss of consciousness with incapacitation. Full recovery may take as long as 30 seconds with catastrophic consequences.[82,83] Straining maneuvers and isometric muscle activity during acceleration stress can substantially improve G tolerance and require a high level of general fitness, but extreme aerobic fitness may be counterproductive. Optimal exercise training regimens are yet to be defined, although a balanced approach seems preferable. The principal beneficial effect of aerobic exercise, defined as prolonged efforts involving large muscle groups in primarily dynamic exercise, is probably an increase in blood volume. This may be counterbalanced by increased peripheral venous pooling and training effects on diastolic myocardial mechanics. An activity program that promotes both aerobic fitness and the development of skeletal muscle mass and strength has a greater potential to be effective. Convertino and associates[84] have reported favorable effects of a brief bicycle-based training program that produced a modest increase in maximal oxygen uptake, whereas Pawelczyk and co-workers[75] found decreased tolerance after a running program.

Heavy exercise also has acute effects on orthostatic tolerance by producing a combination of transiently increased body temperature, metabolic acidosis, and hypovolemia with reduced central venous pressure and mean arterial pressure (Table 11.2).[85] This phase is followed[85] by increased orthostatic tolerance, probably due to an expansion of the plasma volume).[86]

TABLE 11.2 POSTEXERCISE HEMODYNAMIC DATA IN SIX NORMAL SUBJECTS

Variable	Preexercise Control Value	Postexercise Measurements			
		5 Minutes	25 Minutes	50 Minutes	110 Minutes
Heart rate (beats per minute)	60	105*	89*	79*	74*
Mean arterial pressure (mm Hg)	94	90*	88*	87*	93
Central venous pressure (mm Hg)	6	4*	3*	4*	4*
Bicarbonate (mmol/liter)	24	15*	20*	23	24
Plasma volume (%)	100	84*	89*	98	100

* $P < 0.05$, compared with control values. All measurements were taken with the subject in the supine position.
(Data from Bjurstedt H, Rosenhamer G, Balldin U et al: Orthostatic reactions during recovery from exhaustive exercise of short duration. Acta Physiol Scand 119:25-31, 1983)

HYPERREACTIVE HYPOVOLEMIC ORTHOSTATIC HYPOTENSION
ORTHOSTATIC INTOLERANCE CAUSED BY PROLONGED BED REST AND RELATED CONDITIONS

Prolonged bed rest is a common cause of orthostatic intolerance and decreased exercise performance.[10,87-89] The hemodynamic syndrome is of the hypovolemic hyperreactive variety. There is generally only a modest loss of blood volume (300 to 500 ml), and the degree of hemodynamic abnormality is greater than predicted from the magnitude of the hypovolemia. The development of cardiovascular dysfunction during bed rest has generally been attributed to the prolonged physical inactivity, but there is now strong support for the concept that a rapid response to the redistribution of body fluids is the primary mechanism.[90-92] Head-down tilt at moderate degrees was first introduced in the Soviet Union as a means of simulating the redistribution of fluids that occurs at zero gravity.[93] A 20- to 24-hour period of tilt at $-4°$ to $-6°$ produces a marked central shift of intravascular and interstitial fluid. Central venous pressure, left ventricular end-diastolic volume, and stroke volume all increase transiently, but the increased central volume promptly activates various compensatory mechanisms. There is also a significant humoral response with inhibition of vasopressin, renin, and aldosterone.[90]

A negative fluid balance is established within hours during head-down tilt. Filling pressures, stroke volume, and cardiac dimensions decrease to a level below the supine baseline within 24 hours.[90-92] In fact, at that time the hemodynamic state in the supine position is similar to that normally prevailing in the upright position. When the system is challenged with an intravenous volume load, the disposition of the infused volume is similar before and after head-down tilt with an equally rapid return to preinfusion intravascular volume in both states despite the significant tilt-induced hypovolemia.[94] This implies that adaptation produces a new operating point for the mechanisms controlling intravascular and interstitial volume. These observations are consistent with Gauer's view (see Blomqvist and Stone[10]) that the upright position defines the normal operating point for the human cardiovascular system. Once adaptation has occurred and supine hemodynamics approach the normal upright pattern, the subject will have lost the capacity to deal with the fluid shift that occurs during the transition from supine to upright position. Orthostatic intolerance becomes manifest. The degree of cardiovascular dysfunction is similar after a 3-week bed rest period and after 20 hours at head-down tilt.[92] A similar sequence of events is likely to occur during adaptation to the microgravity during space flight. Post-flight orthostatic intolerance is to some extent present in virtually all returning astronauts. The degree of orthostatic intolerance and the loss of exercise capacity following space flight is also significantly greater than would be predicted from the total blood volume loss. It has been shown that blood volume loss during bed rest can be prevented by the administration of 9α-fluorohydrocortisone or corrected by intravenous fluid administration. Neither intervention completely restores normal hemodynamics.[10] Exercise in the supine position during bed rest does not prevent the development of orthostatic intolerance, whereas a few hours per day spent in the standing or sitting position is an effective countermeasure.[10] Relative short daily periods of LBNP at moderate levels of negative pressure have been shown to be effective in preventing orthostatic intolerance induced by prolonged (120 days) periods of head-down tilt[95] and have also been used routinely by Soviet cosmonauts during long space flights.[96]

The exact regulatory adaptations that are responsible for the disproportionately large effect of the hypovolemia are still to be defined. On the other hand, there is little doubt that the fluid shift is the primary stimulus to the cardiovascular changes that develop during bed rest. This has clinical relevance and provides a rationale for reemphasis of the arm chair approach to the treatment of acute cardiovascular disorders as described by Levine and Lown.[97]

MITRAL VALVE PROLAPSE AND RELATED CONDITIONS

Much attention has been paid to a fairly large, but poorly defined, group of patients with functionally important circulatory abnormalities in the absence of any structural neurologic or major cardiovascular lesions. Symptoms suggesting orthostatic intolerance are common. Other complaints include atypical chest pain, palpitations, fatigue, and poor exercise tolerance. In the absence of any physical or echocardiographic findings of mitral valve prolapse (MVP), these patients are often given diagnosis of dysautonomia, vasoregulatory asthenia,[98] or hyperkinetic heart syndrome[99] or are considered to have cardiovascular symptoms related to anxiety neurosis. Starr[100] suggested that the primary defect in neurocirculatory asthenia is a "clumsiness of the circulation," analogous to the ordinary clumsiness of muscular movements. Clumsiness in a sense of lack of precise control is a prominent feature of the mitral valve prolapse syndrome (MVPS, the combination of prolapse and symptomatic autonomic dysfunction) and related disorders. Some patients with MVPS have either markedly attenuated or grossly enhanced vagally mediated cardiovascular responses to common stimuli, such as to the Valsalva maneuver or the diving reflex.[24,101]

Many aspects of MVPS have been examined in great detail by Boudoulas and Wooley.[102] A series of studies by Gaffney, Schutte, and associates have dealt with the nature of the autonomic dysfunction in MVP, including its links to the degree of valvular abnormality and its relation to similar functional abnormalities in patients without valvular defects.[24,103-106] The combined experience of these investigators has been reviewed.[107]

There is a tenuous relationship between the degree of anatomical abnormality and the severity of any symptoms. The characteristic click–murmur complex is only a marker that reflects an abnormal relationship between valvular and ventricular anatomy. Prolapse can be the consequence of a redundant valve or of reduced left ventricular size. At one extreme is a group of patients with a large valve and associated skeletal defects, including pectus excavatum and scoliosis. Schutte and co-workers described a distinctive habitus in women with MVP.[104] A discriminant function that used only height, arm span, and anteroposterior chest diameter produced correct classification of 75% to 85% of patients with MVP and controls. The combination of prolapse and these anthropomorphic features is inherited as a dominant trait. On the opposite side of the spectrum are patients who may be symptomatic with chest pain, palpitations, fatigue, exercise intolerance, and marked orthostatic hypotension and who have prolapse with normal valvular anatomy but a small left ventricle. Furthermore, MVP can be produced in perfectly normal asymptomatic persons by interventions that decrease the size of the left ventricle. Beattie and co-workers performed two-dimensional echocardiograms in 20 normal subjects during LBNP that induced a progressive reduction in left ventricular volume.[108] Almost one third of the subjects developed posterior bowing of the mitral leaflets and fulfilled classic echocardiographic criteria for MVP.

It has been suggested that many patients with prolapse have a primary hyperadrenergic state,[102,109,110] expressed primarily as increased β-adrenergic activity that produces a hyperkinetic circulatory state. However, most of our patients with MVP have had normal levels of plasma catecholamines and normal hemodynamic state during supine rest. The heart rate response to exogenous β-adrenergic stimulation by infusion of isoproterenol is also within normal limits. Some patients show large postural increases in plasma norepinephrine levels, but these persons tend to have large postural decreases in ventricular end-diastolic volume and stroke volume. Massive sympathetic activation with tachycardia and vasoconstriction is necessary to maintain normal blood pressure and cerebral perfusion in the upright position. However, some patients have an exaggerated vasoconstriction and produce blood pressures above control values even in the presence of an abnormally low cardiac output, suggesting true α-adrenergic hyperreactivity. Maintaining a normal activity pattern and spending the day in the upright position, sitting, standing, and walking then produces a chronic hyperadrenergic state.

Hypovolemia is a common feature of the prolapse syndrome. The combination of increased α-adrenergic activity and hypovolemia in MVPS is reminiscent of the findings in patients with pheochromocytoma, in whom excessive catecholamines cause a volume-contracted state. Other studies in normotensive and hypertensive subjects have also documented a strong, general, inverse relationship between blood volume and the levels of sympathetic stimulation. Increased vascular tone in both arterial and venous systems reliably produces a rapid and marked decrease in total blood volume. The hypovolemia will become chronic if the increase in sympathetic drive persists. Mechanisms by which chronic vasoconstriction, hypovolemia, and MVP and MVPS might interact are presented in Figure 11.10.

The hypovolemia and MVP combine to magnify the reduction in forward stroke volume that normally occurs during orthostatic stress. A vicious cycle is established when marked vasoconstriction is required to maintain arterial blood pressure and cerebral perfusion in the upright position. Substantial mitral regurgitation is not prerequisite for an exaggerated postural stroke volume reduction. The increasing volume contained by the ballooning mitral leaflets with decreasing ventricular size may produce, for any given reduction in left ventricular filling pressure, an exaggerated decrease in diastolic sarcomere length, fiber shortening, and forward stroke volume. These effects are likely to be further amplified by effects of hypovolemia on effective ventricular pressure–volume relationships (see Fig. 11.5). Measurements based on radionuclide ventriculography have shown marked reduction in left ventricular end-diastolic volume in patients with MVP during upright rest and exercise. This supports the concept that decreased ventricular filling and forward stroke volume in the upright position are critical features in the pathophysiology of this syndrome.[24,107]

This relationship between MVP, reduced blood volume, and chronic vasoconstriction may well provide an explanation for the complex overlap of features in MVP and in a variety of functional and psychiatric syndromes.[108] Excessive vasoconstriction caused by chronic anxiety with elevated catecholamines, high resting heart rates, and diminished plasma and ventricular volumes may produce functional MVP defined as abnormal motion of a structurally normal mitral valve. Similarly, autonomic dysfunction with orthostatic intolerance in patients with myxomatous MVP could be expected to increase the frequency of symptoms such as palpitations, easy fatigability, near-syncope, and resting tachycardia that often are interpreted as signs of psychoneurosis. Although studies specifically linking anxiety, vasoconstriction, and diminished blood volume are not available, a number of psychophysiologic studies document a strong relationship between acute and chronic stress, anxiety, and vasoconstriction. This relationship forms the rationale for the use of skin temperature as an indicator of the levels of stress and anxiety when training subjects in relaxation techniques and biofeedback. There is also evidence that hypovolemia can be found in patients with severe, chronic stress and anxiety directly related to serious somatic disease. The "missing blood syndrome"[111] refers to a profound hypovolemia in wounded Vietnam war casualties undergoing long-term reconstructive treatment. This "anemia" is actually a severe hypovolemia, characterized by a near-normal or even slightly elevated hematocrit. It is resistant to transfusion and iron therapy and is associated with significant hypotension during surgery. It eventually disappears spontaneously when the patient's underlying condition has improved to a point when he otherwise is ready for discharge home.

Fouad and associates[112] have described a previously unknown variety of hypovolemia by studying a group of 11 patients with orthostatic intolerance and a marked reduction (average −27%) in blood volume. Extensive diagnostic studies excluded pheochromocytoma and hypoaldosteronism. The hemodynamic pattern at rest supine was characterized by subnormal cardiac output and high peripheral resistance. The blood pressure tended to be labile, but catecholamine responses to head-up tilt and cardiovascular responses to the Valsalva maneuver, to the cold pressor test, and to exogenous β-adrenergic stimulation were all appropriate. The hemodynamic state at rest was temporarily normalized by blood volume expansion by intravenous human albumin. The syndrome was termed *idiopathic hypovolemia* in the absence of any identifiable cause of the abnormal cardiovascular state.

NORMOVOLEMIC HYPOREACTIVE ORTHOSTATIC HYPOTENSION

There is a wide spectrum of neurogenic causes of orthostatic hypotension. Bannister's[113] classification (Table 11.3) of autonomic failure includes (1) *primary defects*, in which the disease process is well defined and involves only a limited number of structural elements, (2) *secondary defects*, in which the involvement of the autonomic nervous system is part of a more general process, and, (3) *drug-induced autonomic failure*.

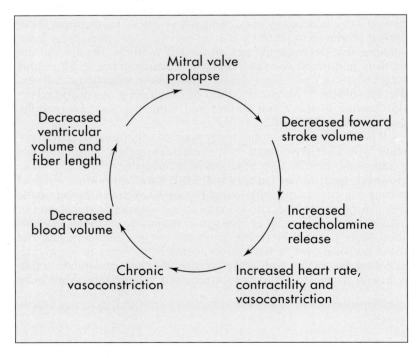

FIGURE 11.10 A proposed set of pathophysiologic mechanisms linking mitral valve prolapse and autonomic nervous system dysfunction in a vicious cycle. A hemodynamically significant prolapse is not a requirement. (Modified from Gaffney FA, Blomqvist CG: Mitral valve prolapse and autonomic nervous system dysfunction. A pathophysiological link. In Boudoulas H, Wooley CF (eds): Mitral Valve Prolapse and the Mitral Valve Prolapse Syndrome, pp 427–443. Mount Kisco, NY, Futura Publishing Co, 1988)

Orthostatic hypotension is often the first symptom of autonomic failure. Bannister suggested that the need for precise postural adjustments of the circulation arose during a late evolutionary stage and that the mechanisms preventing orthostatic cerebral ischemia therefore are less robust than other more basic control systems. However, many patients with autonomic failure present with apparent Parkinson's disease or with bladder symptoms and impotence. Most of the different conditions listed in Table 3 are discussed in great detail in a monograph by Schatz[114] and in Bannister's textbook.[115]

Schatz classified the neurogenic causes with respect to the anatomical site of the principal defect.[114] Involvement of afferent pathways is relatively rare but occurs in diabetes mellitus, alcoholic neuropathy, and the Holmes-Adie syndrome. Central lesions cause the autonomic failure in familial dysautonomia (Riley-Day syndrome). Multiple cerebral infarcts and Wernicke's encephalopathy may induce autonomic dysfunction with orthostatic hypotension. Mild orthostatic hypotension is also often present in idiopathic parkinsonism.

The majority of the causes of neurogenic orthostatic hypotension primarily involve the efferent pathways of the autonomic nervous system. Pure autonomic failure (formerly idiopathic orthostatic hypotension) is characterized by denervation-type hypersensitivity to direct-acting catecholamines but decreased response to tyramine and by low peripheral catecholamine stores but increased α-adrenergic receptor density, all of which are features consistent with a postsynaptic lesion. Multiple system atrophy (Shy-Drager syndrome) is a more diffuse degenerative process. Abnormalities have been documented in several areas, including the solitary nucleus and preganglionic vagal neurons. Norepinephrine levels at rest are normal, and the peripheral sympathetic system is probably intact. Spinal cord trauma may affect the function of the intermediolateral column and produce orthostatic hypotension.

Autonomic failure is often generalized in diabetes, and orthostatic hypotension may be a relatively late manifestation. Its emergence is usually caused by sympathetic vasoconstrictor nerve damage. Diabetic neuropathy may also involve afferent pathways. Any peripheral neuropathy may damage the adrenergic vasoconstrictor nerves. Chronic alcoholism may affect both the afferent and efferent limbs of the autonomic nervous system, but orthostatic hypotension usually occurs late.

TREATMENT OF CHRONIC ORTHOSTATIC HYPOTENSION
THERAPY FOR HYPOVOLEMIC HYPERREACTIVE ORTHOSTATIC HYPOTENSION

The following sequence of care is intended primarily for patients with hypovolemic hyperreactive orthostatic hypertension, such as patients with MVPS[107] and related conditions.

1. Information and reassurance. Many patients with orthostatic hypotension are anxious and should be given a liberal amount of attention with detailed explanations and reassurance.
2. Physical training and increased salt intake. A progressive physical fitness program is often helpful. Physical training causes a balanced increase in plasma volume and red blood cell mass. Adrenergic activity at rest and during submaximal exercise is reduced.[35] However, occasionally patients may have markedly impaired cardiac filling also during exercise.[103] They often have very low exercise capacity and derive little benefit from physical training when it is used as the initial intervention. These patients may respond favorably if exercise is reintroduced at a later stage of treatment. Swimming has been recommended as an ideal form of exercise. The external hydrostatic pressure effectively prevents any activity-induced orthostatic symptoms, but upright water immersion must be avoided since it is a powerful diuretic agent and rapidly induces acute hypovolemia.[10] With these precautions, swimming is appropriate as an initial step but should progress to a balanced exercise program, designed to improve both aerobic fitness and skeletal muscle mass and strength.

   Many persons have been impressed with the potential dangers of excess sodium chloride. Patients with MVPS, who have symptoms of chest pain and palpitations, may be particularly prone to self-imposed salt restriction, which certainly is not needed in the presence of hypovolemia and low blood pressure. On the other hand, increased salt and fluid intake is rarely effective unless combined with other measures.
3. Low-dose clonidine treatment. Clonidine is an α_2-adrenergic ago-

---

TABLE 11.3 GENERAL CLASSIFICATION OF AUTONOMIC FAILURE

I. Primary
  A. Pure autonomic failure (Bradbury-Eggleston syndrome, formerly idiopathic orthostatic hypotension)
  B. Autonomic failure with multiple system atrophy (Shy-Drager syndrome)
  C. Autonomic failure with Parkinson's disease

II. Secondary
  A. General medical disorders (diabetes, amyloid, carcinoma, alcoholism)
  B. Autoimmune diseases (acute and subacute dysautonomia, Guillain-Barré syndrome, connective tissue diseases)
  C. Metabolic diseases (porphyria, vitamin B_{12} deficiency, Tangier disease, Fabry's disease)
  D. Hereditary disorders (dominant or recessive sensory neuropathies, familial dysautonomia, familial hyperbradykinism)
  E. Central nervous system infections (syphilis, Chagas' disease, herpes zoster, human immunodeficiency virus)
  F. Central nervous system lesions (vascular lesions or tumors involving hypothalamus or midbrain, multiple sclerosis, Wernicke's encephalopathy, Adie's syndrome)
  G. Neurotransmitter defects (Dopamine β-hydroxylase deficiency)
  H. Aging

III. Drugs
  A. Tranquilizers (phenothiazines, barbiturates)
  B. Antidepressants (tricyclics, monoamine oxidase inhibitors)
  C. Vasodilators (nitrates, hydralazine, calcium antagonists)
  D. Adrenergic blocking agents (central or peripheral action)
  E. Angiotensin-converting enzyme inhibitors

(Modified from Bannister R, Mathias C: Management of postural hypotension. In Bannister R (ed): Autonomic Failure: A Textbook of Clinical Disorders of the Autonomic Nervous System, 2nd ed, pp 569–595. Oxford, Oxford University Press, 1988)

nist. It also has central effects that usually produce adrenergic inhibition. The onset of the action is gentle, and side-effects are mostly limited to sedation and dryness of the mouth. The α-antagonistic effects usually dominate in subjects with a grossly intact autonomic nervous system, and clonidine has the capacity to break the vicious circle of vasoconstriction, hypovolemia, and orthostatic intolerance in patients with MVPS or chronic anxiety.

Clonidine treatment for at least a month resulted in reduced postural catecholamine responses and relative vasodilatation in the upright position but markedly improved orthostatic tolerance in a series of 8 patients (Fig. 11.11) studied by Gaffney and associates.[105] The treatment also caused a 12% expansion of the plasma volume. Significant improvement was evident measured both by symptoms and by quantitative analysis of the postural hemodynamic responses. Clonidine treatment progressed at 2-day intervals from 0.05 mg orally at bed time to 0.4 mg/day, or to side effects. Coghlan has successfully used a similar regimen at the University of Alabama, Birmingham (personal communication to Dr. Gaffney). The patients with idiopathic hypovolemia studied by Fouad and associates[112] received clonidine in low doses (0.1 to 0.2 mg/day) as an effective adjunct to plasma expansion therapy with hydrofluorocortisone (0.1 mg twice daily) and a diet high in sodium.

Thus, the central adrenergic inhibitory action of clonidine that makes it effective in essential arterial hypertension produces equally beneficial effects in hypovolemic hyperreactive orthostatic hypotension. Clonidine has also proved to be a useful agent in patients with severe idiopathic hypotension and complete loss of peripheral neural sympathetic and parasympathetic control. In these patients, the α_2-agonist properties totally dominate and produce vasoconstriction and venoconstriction with a substantial increase in blood pressure.[115]

4. Progression to the treatment usually reserved for patients with normovolemic hyporeactive orthostatic hypotension is indicated if measures 1 through 3 prove ineffective.

THERAPY FOR NORMOVOLEMIC HYPOREACTIVE ORTHOSTATIC HYPOTENSION

The approach to therapy is generally more complex in the hyporeactive group. It is often very difficult to determine the exact nature, localization, and extent of the underlying disease process. As a consequence, the therapy will often have an empiric component.

Bannister and Mathias[15] have reviewed general principles for management and made several important points. Patients with chronic hyporeactive orthostatic hypotension tend to adjust their autoregulatory range for adequate cerebral blood flow. They are often able to maintain adequate cerebral perfusion at subnormal arterial pressures, such as at systolic levels of about 60 mm Hg compared with 80 mm Hg in most normal subjects. Therapy should therefore be guided by symptoms and signs of cerebral ischemia rather than by the blood pressure. Furthermore, consistently normal pressures in the upright position can often only be maintained at the cost of inducing hypertension in the supine position. Comprehensive approaches to treatment have been formulated by Schatz[114] and by Bannister and Mathias.[15]

GENERAL CONSIDERATIONS AND RECOMMENDATIONS

Trivial stresses can produce symptomatic hypotension in patients lacking essential elements of the blood pressure control system and include straining during micturition or defecation, exposure to a warm environment, and having an ordinary meal. Carbohydrates are more

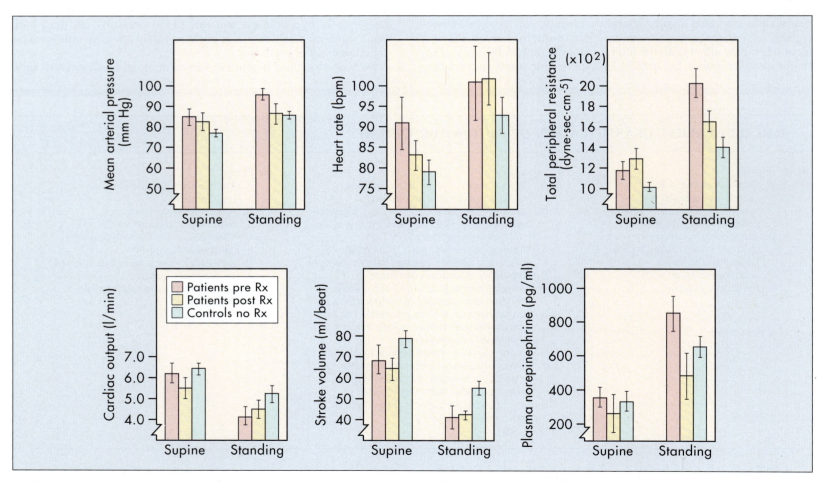

FIGURE 11.11 Hemodynamic and neuroendocrine measurements in controls and in patients before and after long-term oral administration of clonidine (values are means ± SE). (Modified from Gaffney FA, Lane LB, Pettinger W et al: Effects of long-term clonidine administration on the hemodynamic and neuroendocrine postural responses of patients with dysautonomia. Chest 83S:436S–438S, 1983)

likely to induce hypotension than fats or proteins, perhaps via release of insulin and gastrointestinal hormones with vasodilator properties. Alcohol is prone to cause further vasodilatation. On the other hand, caffeine has been found to minimize postprandial hypotension in a placebo-controlled study.[116] Vasoactive drugs should be avoided. The response to vasodilators is amplified for defense mechanisms and the effects of vasoconstrictors and venoconstrictors may be greatly magnified by denervation hypersensitivity.

Most patients with chronic orthostatic hypotension have a definite circadian rhythm with minimal pressures during the morning hours. Head-up tilt during sleep, first proposed by Maclean and Allen,[117] minimizes the redistribution of body fluids that otherwise occurs at night. Normally, the central fluid shift during supine bed rest increases cardiac filling and causes a diuresis with a loss of intravascular and interstitial fluid. These losses, which tend to be abnormally large in patients with autonomic failure, are contained by the use of the head-up tilt. There is often a significant improvement of the blood pressure levels during the day and nocturnal hypertension is avoided. External support, in the form of a custom-fitted counterpressure garment, is quite effective in many patients. The garment is constructed of an elastic mesh of graded firmness to match the postural hydrostatic gradients. The disadvantages of the approach become obvious in a hot climate.

PHARMACOLOGIC APPROACHES

A summary of current pharmacologic approaches is given in Table 11.4.[15] By the nature of these diseases, most agents have been used only in very small groups of patients, and it is difficult to provide adequate evaluation of any single specific approach. The use of clonidine has been discussed in an earlier section. Dihydroergotamine is a direct-acting α-adrenergic agonist that may preferentially cause venoconstriction. The principal disadvantage is its poor bioavailability. Indomethacin has been used to negate the vasodilator effects of prostaglandin but may be effective primarily by increasing smooth muscle sensitivity to norepinephrine. Fluorohydrocortisone (fludrocortisone) is the most widely used of all pharmacologic agents for the treatment of orthostatic hypotension. Its multiple actions include plasma volume expansion and sensitization of vascular receptors to pressor amines, perhaps by increasing the number of adrenergic receptors. The initial dose in autonomic failure is 0.1 mg daily.

TABLE 11.4 DRUGS USED IN THE TREATMENT OF POSTURAL HYPOTENSION

Site of Action	Drugs	Predominant Action
Vessels: vasoconstriction		
Adrenoceptor-mediated:		
Resistance vessels	Ephedrine	Indirectly acting sympathomimetic
	Midodrine, phenylephrine, methylphenidate	Directly acting sympathomimetics
	Tyramine	Release of norepinephrine
	Clonidine	Postsynaptic α-adrenoceptor agonist
	Yohimbine	Presynaptic α_2-adrenoceptor antagonist
Capacitance vessels	Dihydroergotamine	Direct action on α-adrenoceptors
Vessels: prevention of vasodilatation	Propranolol	Blockade of β_2-receptors
	Indomethacin	Blockade of prostaglandins
	Metoclopramide	Blockade of dopamine
Vessels: prevention of postprandial hypotension	Caffeine	Blockade of adenosine receptors
	SMS 201-995	Blockade of vasodilator peptides
Heart: stimulation	Pindolol	Intrinsic sympathetic action
	Xamoterol	
Plasma volume expansion	Fludrocortisone	Mineralocorticoid effects
		Increased plasma volume
		Sensitization of α-receptors to norepinephrine
Kidney: reducing diuresis	Desmopressin	Action: V_2-receptors of renal tubules

(Modified from Bannister R, Mathias C: Management of postural hypotension. In Bannister R (ed): Autonomic Failure: A Textbook of Clinical Disorders of the Autonomic Nervous System, 2nd ed, pp 569–595. Oxford, Oxford University Press, 1988)

REFERENCES

1. Engel GL: Psychologic stress, vasodepressor (vasovagal) syncope, and sudden death. Ann Intern Med 89:403–412, 1978
2. Trout HH III, Brown LL, Thompson JE: Carotid sinus syndrome: Treatment by carotid sinus denervation. Ann Surg 189:575, 1979
3. Khero BA, Mullins CB: Cardiac syncope due to glossopharyngeal neuralgia. Arch Intern Med 128:806, 1971
4. Wik B, Hillestad L: Deglutition syncope. Br Med J 3:747, 1975
5. Weissler AM, Warren JV: Vasodepressor syncope. Am Heart J 57:786–794, 1959
6. Epstein SE, Stampfer M, Beiser GD: Role of the capacitance and resistance

vessels in vasovagal syncope. Circulation 37:524–533, 1968
7. Goldstein DS, Spanarkel M, Pitterman A et al: Circulatory control mechanisms in vasodepressor syncope. Am Heart J 104:1071–1075, 1982
8. Hines S, Houston M, Robertson D: The clinical spectrum of autonomic dysfunction. Am J Med 70:1091–1096, 1981
9. Katkov VE, Chestukhin VV: Blood pressures and oxygenation in different cardiovascular compartments of a normal man during postural exposures. Aviat Space Environ Med 51:1234–1242, 1980
10. Blomqvist CG, Stone HL: Cardiovascular adjustments to gravitational stress. In Shepherd JT, Abboud FM (eds): Handbook of Physiology, Section 2, The Cardiovascular System. Volume III: Peripheral Circulation and Organ Blood Flow, Part 2, pp 1025–1063. Bethesda, MD, American Physiological Society, 1983
11. Poliner LR, Dehmer GJ, Lewis SE et al: Left ventricular performance in normal subjects: A comparison of the response to exercise in the upright and supine positions. Circulation 62:528–534, 1980
12. Thadani U, Parker JO: Hemodynamics at rest and during supine and sitting bicycle exercise in normal subjects. Am J Cardiol 41:52–59, 1978
13. Nixon JV, Murray RG, Leonard PP et al: Effects of large variations in preload on left ventricular characteristics in normal subjects. Circulation 65:698–703, 1982
14. Hainsworth R: Fainting. In Bannister R (ed): Autonomic Failure: A Textbook of Clinical Disorders of the Autonomic Nervous System, pp 142–158. New York, Oxford University Press, 1988
15. Bannister R, Mathias C: Management of postural hypotension. In Bannister R (ed): Autonomic Failure: A Textbook of Clinical Disorders of the Autonomic Nervous System, 2nd ed, pp 569–595. Oxford, Oxford University Press, 1988
16. Ziegler MG: Postural hypotension. Annu Rev Med 31:239–245, 1980
17. Rowell LB: Human Circulation: Regulation During Physical Stress. New York, Oxford University Press, 1986
18. Johnson JM, Rowell LB, Niederberger M et al: Human splanchnic and forearm vasoconstrictor responses to reductions of right atrial and aortic pressure. Circ Res 34:515–524, 1974
19. Ahmad M, Blomqvist CG, Mullins CB et al: Left ventricular function during lower body negative pressure. Aviat Space Environ Med 48:512–515, 1977
20. Murray RH, Krog J, Carlson LD et al: Cumulative effects of venesection and lower body negative pressure. Aerosp Med 38:243–247, 1967
21. Bergenwald L, Freyschuss U, Sjöstrand T: The mechanism of orthostatic and haemorrhagic fainting. Scand J Clin Lab Invest 37:209–216, 1977
22. Bevegård S, Lodin A: Postural circulatory changes at rest and during exercise in five patients with congenital absence of valves in the deep veins of the legs. Acta Med Scand 172:21–29, 1962
23. Raven PB, Pape G, Taylor WF et al: Hemodynamic changes during whole body surface cooling and lower body negative pressure. Aviat Space Environ Med 52:387–391, 1981
24. Gaffney FA, Karlsson ES, Campbell W et al: Autonomic dysfunction in women with mitral valve prolapse syndrome. Circulation 59:894–901, 1979
25. Streeten DPH, Anderson GH Jr, Richardson R et al: Abnormal orthostatic changes in blood pressure and heart rate in subjects with intact sympathetic nervous function: Evidence for excessive venous pooling. J Lab Clin Med 111:326–335, 1988
26. Shepherd JT, Vanhoutte PM: Veins and Their Control. pp 175–238. Philadelphia, WB Saunders, 1975
27. Rothe CF: Venous system: Physiology of the capacitance vessels. In Shepherd JT, Abboud FM (eds): Handbook of Physiology, Section 2, The Cardiovascular System. Volume III: Peripheral Circulation and Organ Blood Flow, Part 1, pp 397–452. Bethesda, MD, American Physiological Society
28. Mayerson HS, Burch CE: Relationship of tissue (subcutaneous and intravascular) and venous pressure to syncope induced in man by gravity. Am J Physiol 128:258–269, 1940
29. Buckey JC, Peshock RM, Blomqvist CG: Deep venous contribution to hydrostatic blood volume change in the leg. Am J Cardiol 62:449–453, 1988
30. Thompson FJ, Barnes CD, Wald JR: Interactions between femoral venous afferents and lumbar spinal reflex pathways. J Auton Nerv Syst 6:113–126, 1982
31. Thompson FJ, Yates BJ: Venous afferent elicited skeletal muscle pumping: A new orthostatic venopressor mechanism. Physiologist 26(suppl):S74–S75, 1983
32. Henriksen O: Local sympathetic reflex medium in regulation of blood flow in human subcutaneous adipose tissue. Acta Physiol Scand 450(suppl):7–48, 1977
33. Henriksen O, Sejrsen P: Local reflex in neurocirculation in human skeletal muscle. Acta Physiol Scand 99:19–26, 1977
34. Parker JO, Case RB: Normal left ventricular function. Circulation 60:4–12, 1979
35. Blomqvist CG, Saltin B: Cardiovascular adaptation to physical training. Annu Rev Physiol 45:169–189, 1983
36. Parmley WW: Ventricular function. In Parmley WW, Chatterjee K (eds): Cardiology, vol 1, chap 5. Philadelphia, JB Lippincott, 1988
37. Speyer KM: Central nervous system control of the cardiovascular system. In Bannister R (ed): Autonomic Failure: A Textbook of Clinical Disorders of the Autonomic Nervous System, pp 56–79. Oxford, Oxford University Press, 1988
38. Shepherd RFJ, Shepherd JT: Control of blood pressure and the circulation in man. In Bannister R (ed): Autonomic Failure: A Textbook of Clinical Disorders of the Autonomic Nervous System, pp 70–96. Oxford, Oxford University Press, 1988
39. Mark AL: The Bezold-Jarisch reflex revisited: Clinical implications of inhibitory reflexes originating in the heart. J Am Coll Cardiol 1:90–102, 1983
40. Mark AL, Mancia G: Cardiopulmonary baroreflexes in humans. In Shepherd JT, Abboud FM (eds): Handbook of Physiology, Section 2, The Cardiovascular System. Volume III: Peripheral Circulation and Organ Blood Flow, Part 2, pp 795–814. Bethesda, MD, American Physiological Society, 1983
41. Mancia G, Mark AL: Arterial baroreflexes in humans. In Shepherd JT, Abboud FM, (eds): Handbook of Physiology, Section 2, The Cardiovascular System. Volume III: Peripheral Circulation and Organ Blood Flow, Part 2, pp 755–794. Bethesda, MD, American Physiological Society, 1983
42. Bishop VS, Malliani A, Thorén P: Cardiac mechanoreceptors. In Shepherd JT, Abboud FM (eds): Handbook of Physiology, Section 2, The Cardiovascular System. Volume III: Peripheral Circulation and Organ Blood Flow, Part 2, pp 497–556. Bethesda, MD, American Physiological Society, 1983
43. Hagbarth KE, Vallbo AB: Pulse and respiratory grouping of sympathetic impulses in human muscle nerves. Acta Physiol Scand 74:96–108, 1968
44. Wallin BG, Delius W, Hagbarth KE: Comparison of sympathetic nerve activity in normotensive and hypertensive subjects. Circ Res 33:9–21, 1973
45. Wallin G: Sympathetic nerve activity underlying electrodermal and cardiovascular reactions in man. Psychophysiology 18:470–476, 1981
46. Wallin BG: Intramural recordings of normal and abnormal sympathetic activity in man. In Bannister R (ed): Autonomic Failure: A Textbook of Clinical Disorders of the Autonomic Nervous System, pp 177–195. Oxford, Oxford University Press, 1988
47. Mark AL, Victor RG, Nerhed C et al: Microneurographic studies in the mechanisms of sympathetic nerve responses to static exercise in humans. Circ Res 57:461–469, 1985
48. Aksamit TR, Floras JS, Victor RG et al: Paroxysmal hypertension due to sinoaortic baroceptor denervation in humans. Hypertension 9:309–314, 1987
49. Victor RG, Leimbach WN: Effects of lower body negative pressure on sympathetic discharge to leg muscles in humans. J Appl Physiol 63:2558–2562, 1987
50. Victor RG, Scherrer U, Vissing S et al: Orthostatic stress activates sympathetic outflow in patients with heart transplants (abstr). Circulation 78:II-365, 1988
51. Rea RF, Eckberg DL: Carotid baroreceptor-muscle sympathetic relation in humans. Am J Physiol 253:R929–R934, 1987
52. Ernsting J, Parry DJ: Some observations on the effect of stimulating the carotid arterial stretch receptors in the carotid artery of man (abstr). J Physiol (London) 137:45, 1957
53. Eckberg DK, Cavanaugh MS, Mark AL et al: A simplified neck suction device for activation of carotid baroreceptors. J Lab Clin Med 85:167–173, 1975
54. Eckberg DL, Eckberg MJ: Human sinus node responses to repetitive, ramped carotid baroreceptor stimuli. Am J Physiol 242:H638–H644, 1982
55. Eckberg DL: Carotid baroreflex function in young men with borderline blood pressure elevation. Circulation 59:632–636, 1979
56. Sprenkle JM, Eckberg DL, Goble RL et al: Device for rapid quantification of human carotid baroreceptor-cardiac reflex responses. J Appl Physiol 60:727–732, 1986
57. Kasting GA, Eckberg DL, Fritsch JM et al: Continuous resetting of the human carotid baroreceptor-cardiac reflex. Am J Physiol 252 (Regulatory Integrative Comp Physiol 21):R732–R736, 1987
58. Ferguson DW, Abboud FM, Mark AL: Relative contribution of aortic and carotid baroreflexes to heart rate control in man during steady state and dynamic increases in arterial pressure. J Clin Invest 76:2265–2274, 1985
59. Sanders JS, Ferguson DW, Mark AL: Arterial baroreflex control of sympathetic nerve activity during elevation of blood pressure in normal man: Dominance of aortic baroreflexes. Circulation 77:279–288, 1988
60. Hall JE (ed): Symposium: Arterial pressure and body fluid homeostasis. Fed Proc 45:2862–2903, 1986
61. Mohanty PK, Thames MD, Arrowood JA et al: Impairment of cardiopulmonary baroreflex after cardiac transplantation in humans. Circulation 75:914–921, 1987
62. Secher NH, Bie P: Bradycardia during reversible shock—a forgotten observation? Clin Physiol 5:315–323, 1985
63. Hyatt KH: Hemodynamic and body fluid alterations induced by bed rest. In Murray RM, McCally M (eds): Hypogravic and Hypodynamic Environments, pp 187–209. Washington, DC, National Aeronautics and Space Administration, 1971
64. Cohen M, Gootman PM: Periodicities in efferent discharge of splanchnic nerve of the cat. Am J Physiol 218:1092–1101, 1970
65. Sandler H, Goldwater DJ, Popp RL et al: Beta-blockade in the compensation for bed-rest: Cardiovascular deconditioning: Physiologic and pharmacologic observations. Am J Cardiol 55:114D–119D, 1985
66. Cunha UV: Management of orthostatic hypotension in the elderly. Geriatrics 42:61–68, 1987
67. Caird FI, Andrews GR, Kennedy RD: Effect of posture on blood pressure in the elderly. Br Heart J 35:527–530, 1973
68. Gribbin B, Pickering TG, Sleight P et al: The effect of age and high blood

pressure on baroreflex sensitivity in man. Circ Res 29:424–431, 1971
69. Shimada K, Kitazumi T, Ogura H et al: Differences in age dependent effects of blood pressure on baroreflex sensitivity between normal and hypertensive subjects. Clin Sci 70:489–494, 1984
70. Davies B, Sever PS: Adrenoceptor function. In Bannister R (ed): Autonomic Failure: A Textbook of Clinical Disorders of the Autonomic Nervous System. pp 348–366. Oxford, Oxford University Press, 1988
71. Klein KE, Wegmann HM, Bruner H et al: Physical fitness and tolerances to environmental extremes. Aerosp Med 40:998–1001, 1969
72. Stegemann J, Meier U, Skipka W et al: Effects of multi-hour immersion with intermittent exercise on urinary excretion and tilt-table tolerance in athletes or non-athletes. Aviat Space Environ Med 46:26–29, 1975
73. Convertino VA: Aerobic fitness, endurance training, and orthostatic tolerance. Exerc Sport Sci Rev 15:223–259, 1987
74. Luft UC, Myrhe LG, Leoppky JA et al: A study of factors affecting tolerance of gravitational stress stimulated by lower body negative pressure. Albuquerque, NM, Lovelace Foundation, 1976 (Contract NA59-14472, 2-60)
75. Pawelczyk JA, Kenney WL, Kenney P: Cardiovascular responses to head-up tilt after an endurance exercise program. Aviat Space Environ Med 59:107–112, 1988
76. Mangseth GR, Bernauer EM: Cardiovascular response to tilt in endurance trained subjects exhibiting syncopal reactions (abstr). Med Sci Sports Exerc 12:140, 1980
77. Raven PB, Rohm-Young D, Blomqvist CG: Physical fitness and cardiovascular response to lower body negative pressure. J Appl Physiol 56:138–144, 1984
78. Smith ML, Raven PB: Cardiovascular responses to lower body negative pressure in endurance and static exercise-trained men. Med Sci Sports Exerc 18:545–550, 1986
79. Mack GW, Xiangrong S, Hiroshi N et al: Diminished baroreflex control of forearm vascular resistance in physically fit humans. J Appl Physiol 63:105–110, 1987
80. Bedford TG, Tipton CM: Exercise training and the arterial baroreflex. J Appl Physiol 63:1926–1932, 1987
81. Levine BD, Buckey JC, Fritsch JM et al: Physical fitness and orthostatic tolerance: The role of the carotid baroreflex (abstr). Clin Res 36:295A, 1988
82. Burton RR: G-induced loss of consciousness: Definition, history, current status. Aviat Space Environ Med 59:2–5, 1988
83. Whinnery JE: Converging research on +Gz-induced loss of consciousness. Aviat Space Environ Med 59:9–11, 1988
84. Convertino VA, Montgomery LD, Greenleaf JE: Cardiovascular responses during orthostasis: Effects of an increase on VO_2 max. Aviat Space Environ Med 55:702–708, 1984
85. Bjurstedt H, Rosenhamer G, Balldin U et al: Orthostatic reactions during recovery from exhaustive exercise of short duration. Acta Physiol Scand 119:25–31, 1983
86. Convertino VA: Potential benefits of maximal exercise just prior to return from weightlessness. Aviat Space Environ Med 58:568–562, 1987
87. Taylor HL, Henschel A, Brozek J et al: Effects of bed rest on cardiovascular function and work performance. J Appl Physiol 2:223–239, 1949
88. Saltin B, Blomqvist CG, Mitchell JH et al: Response to exercise after bed rest and after training. Circulation 37(suppl VII):1–78, 1968
89. Chobanian AV, Lille RD, Tercyak A et al: The metabolic and hemodynamic effects of prolonged bed rest in normal subjects. Circulation 49:551–559, 1974
90. Nixon JV, Murray RG, Bryant C et al: Early cardiovascular adaptation to simulated zero gravity. J Appl Physiol 46:541–548, 1979
91. Blomqvist CG, Nixon JV, Johnson RL Jr et al: Early cardiovascular adaptation to zero gravity simulated by head-down tilt. Acta Astronautica 7:543–553, 1980
92. Gaffney FA, Nixon JV, Karlsson ES et al: Cardiovascular deconditioning produced by 20-hour bedrest with head-down tilt (−5°) in middle-aged men. Am J Cardiol 56:634–638, 1985
93. Kakurin LI, Lobachlk VI, Mikhallov VM et al: Antiorthostatic hypokinesia as a method of weightlessness simulation. Aviat Space Environ Med 46:1083–1086, 1976
94. Gaffney FA, Buckey JC, Hillebrecht A et al: The Effects of a 10-Day Period of Head-down Tilt on the Cardiovascular Responses to Intravenous Fluid Loading, p 45. Lyon, International Union of Physiological Sciences, Commission of Gravitational Physiology, 11th Annual Meeting, Preprints, 1989
95. Guell A, Gharib C, Pavy A et al: Cardiovascular Deconditioning Syndrome During Weightlessness Simulation and the Use of LBNP as a Countermeasure, p 5. Lyon, International Union of Physiological Sciences, Commission of Gravitational Physiology, 11th Annual Meeting, Preprints, 1989
96. Gazenko OG, Genin AM, Yegerov AD: Major medical results of the Salyut-6-Soyuz 185-day space flight. Rome, Preprints of the XXXII Congress of the International Astronautical Federation, 1981
97. Levine SA, Lown B: The "chair" treatment of acute coronary thrombosis. Trans Assoc Am Physicians 64:316–327, 1951
98. Holmgren A, Jonsson B, Levander M et al: Low physical working capacity in suspected heart cases due to inadequate adjustment of peripheral blood flow (vasoregulatory asthenia). Acta Med Scand 158:413–446, 1957
99. Gorlin R: The hyperkinetic heart syndrome. JAMA 182:823–829, 1962
100. Starr I: Ballistocardiographic studies of draftees rejected for neurocirculatory asthenia. War Med (Chicago) 5:155, 1944
101. Coghlan HC, Phares P, Cowely M et al: Dysautonomia in mitral valve prolapse. Am J Med 67:236–244, 1979
102. Boudoulas H, Reynolds JC, Mazzaferri et al: Metabolic studies in mitral valve prolapse syndrome: A neuroendocrine-cardiovascular process. Circulation 61:1200–1205, 1980
103. Gaffney FA, Huxley RL, Nicod P et al: Abnormal cardiovascular regulation in mitral valve prolapse (MVPS) during exercise (abstr). Circulation 64(suppl IV):248, 1981
104. Schutte JE, Gaffney FA, Blend LB et al: Distinctive anthropometric characteristics of women with mitral valve prolapse. Am J Med 71:533–538, 1981
105. Gaffney FA, Lane LB, Pettinger W et al: Effects of long-term clonidine administration on the hemodynamic and neuroendocrine postural responses of patients with dysautonomia. Chest 83S:436S–438S, 1983
106. Gaffney FA, Bastian BC, Lane LB et al: Abnormal cardiovascular regulation in the mitral valve prolapse syndrome. Am J Med 52:316–320, 1983
107. Gaffney FA, Blomqvist CG: Mitral valve prolapse and autonomic nervous system dysfunction: A pathophysiological link. In Boudoulas H, Wooley CF (eds): Mitral Valve Prolapse and the Mitral Valve Prolapse Syndrome, pp 427–443. Mount Kisco, NY, Futura Publishing Co, 1988
108. Beattie JM, Blomqvist CG, Gaffney FA: Mitral valve prolapse in normal subjects during orthostatic stress (abstr). J Am Coll Cardiol 5:404, 1985
109. Boudoulas H, Wooley CF (eds): Mitral Valve Prolapse and the Mitral Valve Prolapse Syndrome. Mount Kisco, NY, Futura Publishing Co, 1988
110. Pasternac A, Tubau JV, Puddu PE et al: Increased plasma catecholamine levels in patients with symptomatic mitral valve prolapse. Am J Med 73:783–790, 1982
111. Valeri DR, Altschule MD: Hypovolemic Anemia of Trauma: The Missing Blood Syndrome. Boca Raton, FL, CRC Press, 1981
112. Fouad FM, Tadena-Thome L, Bravo EL et al: Idiopathic hypovolemia. Ann Intern Med 104:298–303, 1986
113. Bannister R: Introduction and Classification. In Bannister R (ed): Autonomic Failure: A Textbook of Clinical Disorders of the Autonomic Nervous System, 2nd ed, pp 1–20. Oxford, Oxford University Press, 1988
114. Schatz IJ: Orthostatic Hypotension. Philadelphia, FA Davis, 1986
115. Robertson D, Goldberg MR, Hollister AS et al: Clonidine raises blood pressure in severe idiopathic orthostatic hypotension. Am J Med 74:193–200, 1983
116. Onrot J, Goldberg MR, Biaggioni I et al: Hemodynamic and humoral effects of caffeine in autonomic failure: Therapeutic implications for postprandial hypotension. N Engl J Med 313:549–554, 1985
117. Maclean AR, Allen EV: Orthostatic hypotension and orthostatic tachycardia: Treatment with the "head-up" bed. JAMA 115:2162–2167, 1940

GENERAL REFERENCES

Bannister R: Autonomic Failure. A Textbook of Clinical Disorders of the Autonomic Nervous System, 2nd ed. Oxford, Oxford University Press, 1988

Rowell LB: Human Circulation: Regulation During Physical Stress. New York, Oxford University Press, 1986

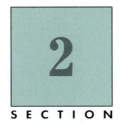

SECTION 2

Section Editor
William W. Parmley, MD

Cardiovascular Pharmacology

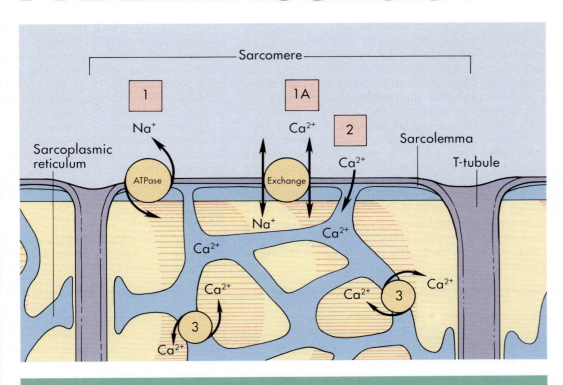

Basic Principles of Clinical Pharmacology

Raymond L. Woosley ▪ Dan M. Roden

Fundamental to the rational use of any drug is an understanding of the basic principles of pharmacology. The steps involved between drug administration and its effect can be broken down to several components amenable to modelling and measurement (Fig. 12.1). Pharmacokinetic parameters allow description and prediction of drug concentration in the body. Pharmacodynamic variables such as potency and efficacy describe drug action and are clinically most useful when related to drug concentration at the effector site. More often than not this cannot be sampled directly, but estimates can be made using pharmacokinetic variables. Thus, while admittedly complex, an integrated pharmacokinetic–pharmacodynamic approach to dose–response relationships is beginning to receive wider attention. In theory, pharmacokinetic–pharmacodynamic applications are powerful, allowing prediction of drug concentration, of onset and offset of drug effect, of the magnitude of the response, and of the dose necessary to achieve the desired effect. While these goals may be realized occasionally, the great interpatient variability in drug response requires that measurement and modelling be considered as additional information and used to support decisions based upon clinical judgment. Nonetheless, knowledge of the factors that influence a drug's disposition in the body (pharmacokinetics) and drug action (pharmacodynamics) can simplify the approach to therapeutics and help provide an optimum benefit-to-risk ratio for the patient.

DOSE–RESPONSE RELATIONSHIPS

The response to increasing doses of drug is usually graded, and reaches a maximum. For most drugs, the dose-response curve is described by a hyperbola, although in some cases a sigmoid relationship is apparent (Fig. 12.2). The classical approach has been to use a log dose–response curve that transforms a hyperbolic relationship to one that is sigmoid with a linear portion in the range of approximately 20% to 80% maximum effect, providing a convenient means of comparing drug potencies (Fig. 12.3). However, the application of nonlinear regression analysis to untransformed dose–response curves may be a more fruitful approach to exploring concentration-effect relationships.

In cases where the response is "all-or-none" (presence or absence of effect) or in which dose–response curves are flat, the relationship between dose and response is best described by probability statistics (*e.g.*, the cumulative frequency of patients responding at a given dose or concentration).

RECEPTORS

It was inferred at the turn of the century that the response to a drug is mediated by interaction of the drug with specific cellular binding sites —receptors. However, technological advances, notably affinity chro-

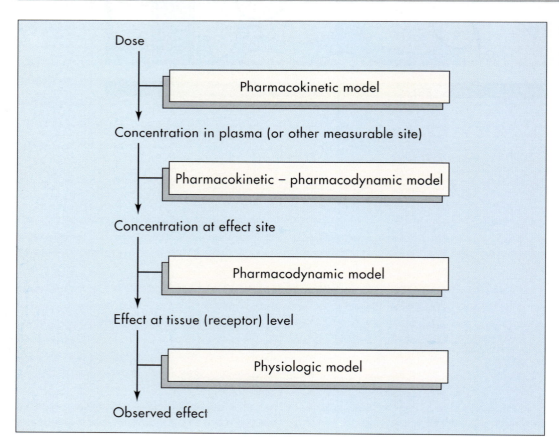

FIGURE 12.1 Sequence of steps involved in drug dose resulting in effect, illustrating the levels at which mathematical modelling can be used to describe and predict concentration and effect.

matography and photoaffinity labelling, have only recently allowed preliminary characterization of the receptor macromolecules themselves and the steps involved from initial recognition between a ligand–receptor (drug or endogenous substance) to the expression of effect. Ligand-binding studies have also aided our current understanding of receptor localization, specificity and structure–activity relationships, and receptor dynamics.

Receptors are heterogeneous, ranging from enzymes (digitalis glycosides bind to Na^+-K^+-adenosine triphosphate [ATP]) to nucleic acids (with which many antineoplastic agents interact). But ligand–receptor interactions generally result in either changes in ion permeability, or changes in some biochemical function such as activation of a cyclic nucleotide-dependent protein kinase, or both. To date, the best-studied receptor system is that of the adenyl cyclase-coupled β-adrenergic receptor. The current concept of this receptor system comprises three components: (1) the hormone receptor, (2) a "coupling" protein regulated by guanine nucleotides (e.g., guanosine triphosphate [GTP], guanosine diphosphate [GDP]) that couples ligand–receptor binding to activation of (3) adenyl cyclase (converts adenosine triphosphate [ATP] to cyclic adenosine monophosphate [AMP]) (Fig. 12.4).

The ligand–receptor activation process can be modelled to various degrees of sophistication, the simplest model being that of an equilibrium between two receptor states: resting/closed and activated/open. One theory proposes that the relative affinity of a ligand for these two receptor states will determine its biologic activity. For example, agonists (agents that elicit a response) shift the equilibrium in favor of the activated state (i.e., they promote the interaction of the receptor with the coupling protein), while antagonists (agents that prevent a response to agonist) show equal affinity for both receptor states and do not alter their equilibrium. A partial agonist (for example, a β-blocker with intrinsic sympathomimetic activity) may be thought of as having an only somewhat greater affinity for the activated state. Thus, it will cause only a slight shift of the equilibrium in favor of the activated state.

An important concept is that the receptor population is not fixed, and the number of receptors self-regulates in response to the degree of their stimulation. Thus, phenomena related to an attenuated or augmented response (tolerance, tachyphylaxis, desensitization, or increased sensitivity to the drug) can be due wholly or in part to changes in receptor density. For example, β-adrenergic receptor density increases ("up-regulation") during chronic treatment with propranolol. The effect appears to persist as long as propranolol is administered, and for some time after discontinuation, providing a possible explana-

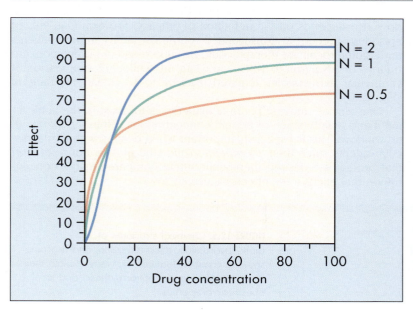

FIGURE 12.2 Typical dose–response curves, where N is a number influencing the slope of the curve. As N increases, the curve becomes progressively steeper and more sigmoidal. In some cases, but certainly not all, N may be related to processes at receptor level (e.g., the cooperative behavior of oxygen association with hemoglobin can be described by a curve where N = 4, reflecting the number of oxygen binding sites).

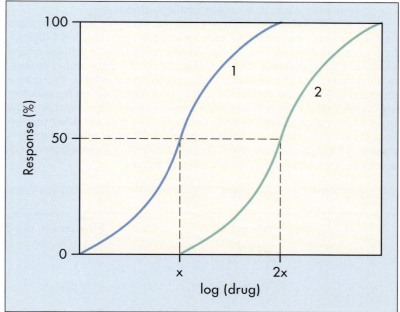

FIGURE 12.3 Log dose–response curves for two agonist drugs acting at the same receptor site. Agonist 1 is twice as potent as agonist 2. The two curves could apply equally well to a plot of agonist alone (1) and in the presence of a competitive antagonist (2).

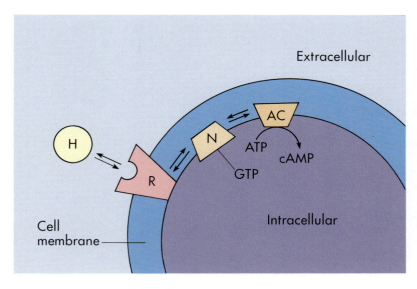

FIGURE 12.4 Schematic diagram of the components of hormone-responsive adenyl cyclase system. Association of H with R forms HR, which interacts with N, resulting in the exchange of GDP for GTP. R and N-GTP dissociate, allowing N-GTP to activate AC. The activation process results in hydrolysis of N-GTP to N-GDP. (R, beta adrenergic; N, guanine nucleotide regulatory protein; AC, adenylate cyclase; H, hormone or agonist) (Modified from Lefkowitz RJ, Michel T: Plasma membrane receptors. J Clin Invest 72:1185, 1983)

tion for the delayed supersensitivity to β-adrenergic stimulation seen after stopping propranolol therapy.[1] Clinically, this may be manifest as worsened angina, arrhythmias, and so forth. Chronic receptor stimulation, for example, the use of sympathomimetics in the treatment of asthma, may lead to a reduction ("down regulation") in receptor density, and therefore to a loss of efficacy. Treatment with antagonists possessing partial agonist activity also leads to receptor down-regulation, and may contribute to their efficacy.

Another mechanism of receptor sensitivity control may be modification of receptor coupling to a regulatory protein, so that ligand–receptor binding is divorced from the sequence of events leading to effect. Such a mechanism may be important in instances of acute desensitization to agonist.

STRUCTURE–ACTIVITY RELATIONSHIPS

The therapeutic usefulness of most drugs depends on their specificity, which in turn implies interaction with a receptor. The ability of a drug to interact with a receptor depends on its having the correct physical, chemical, and spatial configuration. Minor modifications in structure can yield compounds with widely differing potencies or loss of efficacy. The screening of a series of chemical compounds related in structure to a known active compound can not only produce information on chemical relationships crucial to pharmacologic activity but can also provide clues to receptor configuration.

The specificity of a drug for a particular receptor also determines biologic activity. For example, chlorpromazine, procaine, and diphenhydramine all have a large cyclic hydrocarbon and a tertiary amino group in their molecular structure (Fig. 12.5). All three drugs possess antihistaminic, local anesthetic, and antiarrhythmic effects. The extent to which these agents interact with the receptors involved in transducing these effects determines their relative potencies. Additionally, other chemical groupings provide the molecules with still other properties. Thus, of the three, diphenhydramine is the most effective antihistamine, procaine the best local anesthetic, and chlorpromazine possesses antiemetic and major tranquilizing activity.

In many cases, specificity extends to steric requirements. Thus, only the l-optical isomer of norepinephrine, and not the d-isomer, elevates blood pressure; the l-enantiomer of verapamil has more potent hypotensive and chronotropic effects than d-verapamil.[2]

However, not all drugs interact with specific receptors. For example, by generation of a nitric oxide free radical, nitrate vasodilators may initiate vascular smooth muscle relaxation mediated by increases in cyclic guanosine monophosphate (GMP).[3] Osmotic diuretics depend on their physical properties for therapeutic benefit.

THERAPEUTIC WINDOW

The therapeutic window for a drug encompasses the range of doses or plasma concentrations (when there is a reliable correlation with pharmacologic effect) that elicit a therapeutic effect in most patients with adverse effects in only a few. At some appropriately chosen low dose, most patients will not respond at all. Increasing doses will result in more and more patients showing a desired, therapeutic response, and this will be paralleled by an increasing number of patients who develop unwanted, adverse effects. The wider the margin between the concentrations that produce efficacy and those associated with side effects, the more leeway there is in dosing, and the wider the therapeutic window. Conversely, a narrow therapeutic window requires careful dose adjustment in order to avoid toxic effects. The therapeutic window also depends on the definition of efficacy. For example, 90% of episodes of recurrent nonsustained ventricular tachycardia in patients undergoing tocainide therapy could be suppressed at plasma concentrations of 2.8 µg/ml to 10 (mean 6) µg/ml, while 90% suppression of ventricular extrasystoles required 9 µg/ml to 13 (mean 11) mcg/ml (Fig. 12.6).[4]

One aim of studying pharmacokinetics is to assist in the achievement and maintenance of plasma concentrations within the therapeutic window. This is especially important when dealing with cardiovascular agents since their *therapeutic ratio* (the plasma concentration that produces a desired therapeutic effect compared to the concentration that elicits toxic effects) is usually low.

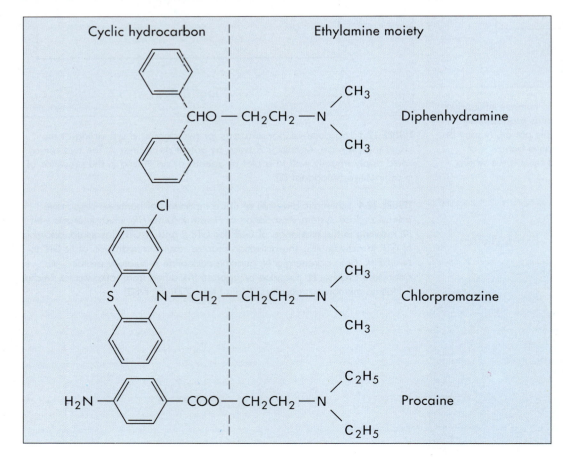

FIGURE 12.5 Chemical structures of diphenhydramine, chlorpromazine, and procaine showing common features that may explain their shared antihistaminic, antiarrhythmic, and local anesthetic properties.

ABSORPTION

FACTORS INFLUENCING ABSORPTION

Following administration (aside from intravenous injection), a drug must first be absorbed either from the gut, oral mucosa, muscle, and so forth, and must enter the systemic circulation before it can reach its site of action. Several factors influence the rate and extent of absorption from these sites, including the physicochemical properties of the drug, the surface area available for absorption, and regional blood flow. In general, lipid soluble drugs penetrate cell membranes more readily than hydrophilic agents; a nonionized drug permeates more readily than an ionized drug. Since many drugs are either weak acids or weak bases, differences in the pH of the gastrointestinal tract (strongly acid stomach, nearly neutral small intestine) will determine the extent of ionization and thus the rate of absorption following oral administration. For practical purposes, however, the greatest amount of absorption occurs in the small intestine by virtue of the large surface area available.

Gastrointestinal pathology can influence the amount of drug absorbed. Diarrhea or extensive small bowel resection, both of which reduce intestinal transit time, can result in markedly diminished absorption, especially of sustained-release preparations that are designed to allow prolonged absorption.

The same principles apply to other routes of administration. For example, following intramuscular injection, absorption is more rapid from deltoid rather than gluteal muscle since the former has a higher blood flow. Drugs that are insoluble at tissue pH, or those in an oily vehicle or microcrystalline suspension, will form a depot, releasing the drug slowly, which may allow less frequent injections.

BIOAVAILABILITY

Bioavailability is the proportion of an administered dose reaching the systemic circulation. By definition, following intravenous injection, a drug is 100% bioavailable. Thus bioavailability after, for instance, oral administration is determined by comparison of the area under the plasma concentration time curves following oral and intravenous dosing. Bioavailability can be lowered by incomplete absorption due to problems in the drug's formulation or to the presence/absence of food, or by concomitant administration of agents that alter gastric pH (e.g., antacids) or motility (e.g., narcotic analgesics and atropinelike drugs which slow gastric emptying or metoclopramide, which speeds it). Efficient presystemic extraction by the gut wall or, more usually the liver (first-pass effect), will also lower systemic availability.

The time course of absorption may also be important in instances where rapid attainment of a therapeutic plasma concentration is desirable following the initial (or single) dose. Although either rapid absorption or slow absorption can result in the same amount of drug becoming available systemically (equal area under the concentration-time curve), therapeutic concentrations are achieved sooner if absorption is rapid (Fig. 12.7). For some drugs (e.g., tocainide or mexiletine), avoiding rapid absorption and the resulting high peak plasma concentrations by giving drugs with food can reduce the incidence of dose-related side-effects but have efficacy unaltered since the extent of absorption is unchanged.

DISTRIBUTION

Having entered the systemic circulation, the drug distributes throughout the body, carried by the extracellular (vascular and interstitial) water in which it is dissolved. As in the case of absorption from the site of administration, the drug's passage into various body tissues depends on the lipid solubility of the drug, its degree of ionization, the vascularity of the tissue, and the size of the drug molecule, or drug-protein complex when the drug is bound to plasma protein. Lipid-soluble drugs readily diffuse across capillaries and all biological membranes (including the blood-brain and blood-cerebrospinal fluid barriers), while hydrophilic drugs depend on the permeability characteristics of the capillaries to allow access to extravascular sites. The capillaries in the liver and kidney are particularly permeable to all but protein-bound drugs, while those of the brain are virtually impermeable to water-soluble molecules of any size. Since quantification of the amount of drug in the various body spaces is not feasible, the plasma concentration usually serves as a guide to the drug's disposition.

VOLUME OF DISTRIBUTION

At any time following administration, the drug concentration in plasma will be defined by the amount of drug in the body and the volume in which it is distributed. Intracellular protein binding or tissue sequestration will result in only a small amount of drug left in the extracellular water. Thus, the plasma concentration will be low. On the other hand, the calculated variable—the (apparent) volume of distribution—will be large, since estimation of the volume of distribution is by comparison of the amount of drug in the body to the plasma concentration. Obviously, the larger the calculated volume of distribution, the smaller the fraction in plasma. Thus, the apparent volume of distribution should not be ascribed to actual anatomical volumes. For instance, the volume of distribution of mexiletine is about 600 liters to 700 liters,[5] far in excess of total body water. The usual reason for such a large value is extensive tissue binding, leaving little drug in the plasma.

There are substances, however, that are confined to certain physiological volumes and may be used as reference materials in pharmacokinetic studies. For example, certain dyes remain confined to plasma, inulin distributes throughout the extracellular water, and antipyrine

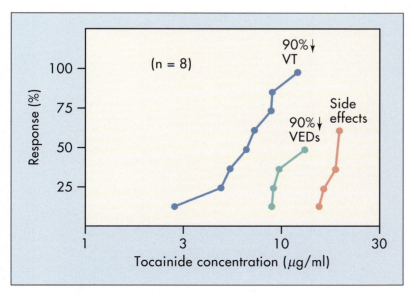

FIGURE 12.6 Relationship between drug plasma concentration, and therapeutic or adverse effects in treatment of ventricular ectopic depolarizations (VEDs) and ventricular tachycardia (VT) with tocainide. (Modified from Roden DM, Reele SB, Higgins SB et al: Tocainide therapy for refractory ventricular arrhythmias. Am Heart J 100:15, 1980)

occupies total body water. The corresponding volumes of distribution for a 70-kg individual are 3 liters, 13 liters to 16 liters, and 40 liters to 46 liters, respectively. In general, however, the volume of distribution relates to the extent of tissue localization of a drug rather than to any actual physiological volume.

METABOLISM AND ELIMINATION

As soon as a drug enters the circulation it is available for elimination. This usually occurs either by metabolic modification of the drug or by excretion via the kidneys (Table 12.1). The rate of removal of a drug is termed clearance, and is expressed as the volume of plasma from which a drug is completely removed per unit time (e.g., ml/min). Total body clearance is the sum of clearance at all sites of elimination.

HEPATIC CLEARANCE

The liver is the most important site of drug metabolizing activity in the body. Hepatic extraction may include biotransformation (metabolism), biliary excretion, and drug binding to intracellular proteins. Hepatic clearance is influenced by two independent variables: the activity of drug metabolizing enzymes, and liver blood flow. The relative importance of these two factors depends on the particular drug. For a drug with a low hepatic extraction ratio, increases in enzyme activity result in important changes in pharmacokinetic variables (increases in clearance and a shortened elimination half-life). On the other hand, for a drug with a high extraction ratio, increased metabolizing activity has little effect. Conversely, changes in hepatic blood flow affect high extraction drugs, but not low extraction drugs. Thus, changes in liver blood flow do not alter the disposition of phenytoin (a low extraction drug), while enzyme induction does not have a large effect on the disposition of lidocaine (a high extraction drug).

Some drugs are so extensively cleared by the liver after absorption by the gut and prior to entering the general circulation (the first-pass effect) that oral use is not feasible. One example is lidocaine, which is well absorbed but only about 35% is systemically bioavailable after oral administration. Increasing the oral dose to attain therapeutic plasma levels results in a corresponding increase in the levels of lidocaine's metabolites. These levels, unfortunately, result in unacceptable central nervous system side-effects, precluding the use of large oral doses of lidocaine.

ENZYME INDUCTION/INHIBITION

Certain agents (enzyme inducers) can promote synthesis of microsomal enzymes, resulting in increased drug metabolizing activity. In some cases, the increased activity results in more rapid destruction of the drug itself, and tolerance to the drug develops as a consequence. However, some drugs are able to induce enzymes for which they themselves are not substrates. Concomitantly administered agents, which happen to be substrates for the induced enzyme, may then be subject to increased hepatic metabolism. Enzyme induction is most likely to have important consequences for the disposition of drugs with a normally low hepatic extraction ratio.

A number of agents can inhibit drug metabolizing enzymes, increasing the systemic availability of drugs normally highly extracted by the liver. For instance, cimetidine increases the availability and prolongs the half-life of lidocaine[6] and propranolol.[7] Propranolol, both by reducing hepatic blood flow and by inhibiting microsomal enzymes, decreases the clearance of lidocaine.[8]

Obviously, careful patient observation is necessary whenever multiple medications are prescribed, but especially when stopping or starting a drug that alters the metabolism of other agents. Some drugs with known or proposed enzyme induction or inhibition effects in man are listed below.

HEPATIC ENZYME INDUCERS
  Phenytoin
  Phenobarbital
  Rifampin
  Ethanol
  Carbamazepine
  Glutethimide
  Griseofulvin

HEPATIC ENZYME INHIBITORS
  Cimetidine
  Allopurinol
  Disulfiram
  Anabolic steroids
  Chloramphenicol
  Metronidazole
  Quinacrine

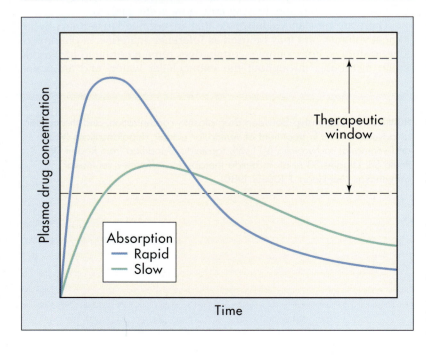

FIGURE 12.7 Plasma concentration with time following rapid and slow absorption of drug. Bioavailability in both cases is 100% because the area under each of the two curves equals that under the intravenous dose curve. However, therapeutic effect in the two situations may differ greatly.

Isoniazid
Estrogens/Oral contraceptives
Amiodarone

Unexpected toxicity or loss of therapeutic effect is likely, and may not be immediately apparent. For example, amiodarone, the concentration of which in the liver is about 1000 times that in the plasma, inhibits the hepatic clearance of many other drugs.[9] Since the elimination half-life of amiodarone ranges from 2 weeks to 15 weeks, it may take months before normal hepatic clearance of other drugs is restored after stopping amiodarone.

RENAL CLEARANCE

Metabolic products are usually more polar, and thus more water-soluble than the parent compound, facilitating excretion via the kidneys by either passive glomerular filtration or active tubular secretion.

The kidneys are by far the most important route of excretion of unchanged drug or drug metabolites. In some cases, excretion by the kidneys is the major route of elimination, and the means of terminating a drug's effect. In other cases, the kidneys simply excrete a drug's inactive metabolites.

Elimination by glomerular filtration is a passive process, dependent on the extent of plasma protein binding. Since only free drug can pass the glomerular membrane, a highly protein-bound drug that is not actively secreted into the urine will be eliminated slowly. If this is the main route of elimination and the volume of distribution is large (*i.e.*, little drug in plasma), a prolonged half-life can result. For example, diazoxide is 90% bound to albumin and eliminated by glomerular filtration with a half-life of about 30 hours. Changes in protein binding that result in an increase in free drug concentration will also increase renal elimination and shorten the elimination half-life.

While glomerular filtration always occurs, tubular secretion is an active process and may or may not occur, depending on the particular drug. When renal clearance exceeds clearance by filtration, tubular secretion can be inferred. As free drug is carried across into the tubular lumen, more free drug dissociates from the protein–drug complex to replace the "lost" drug. Protein-binding, therefore, does not limit tubular secretion as it does glomerular filtration.

Tubular reabsorption can also be important in reducing the renal clearance of drug. Since the nonionized form of a weak acid or base can diffuse readily from the tubular urine back across the tubule cells into plasma, an alkaline urine will promote excretion and prevent reabsorption of a weak acid, while an acid urine will diminish excretion and favor reabsorption. The opposite relationship is true for weak bases. For example, the half-life of mexiletine, a weak base, is approximately 9 hours when the urine is alkaline, and 3 hours when acidic.[10]

PROTEIN BINDING

In plasma, most drugs are reversibly bound to plasma proteins, including albumin, alpha-1-acid glycoprotein (AAG), lipoproteins, and

TABLE 12.1 DISPOSITION OF CARDIOVASCULAR DRUGS

Drug	Inactivation or Major Route of Elimination (%)	Oral Bioavailability (%)	Active Metabolites	Protein Binding (%)
Quinidine	Liver (50–90) Kidney (10–30)	70	Probable	50–95
Procainamide	Kidney (30–60) Liver (40–70)	75*	Yes	15
Disopyramide	Kidney (36–77) Liver (11–37)	80	Yes	20–60†
Lidocaine	Liver	35	Yes	40–70†
Phenytoin	Liver	70–100*,†	No	90
Mexiletine	Liver	90	No	70
Tocainide	Liver Kidney	100	No	50
Flecainide	Liver	95	No	40
Encainide	Liver	26‡; 89*,§	Yes‡	
Lorcainide	Liver	80–100	Yes	85
Propafenone	Liver	10–50*,†	Yes	90
Bretylium	Kidney	20	No	?(low)
Amiodarone	Liver	20–50	Yes	?(high)
Verapamil	Liver	20	Yes	90
Nifedipine	Liver	45–60*	No	90
Diltiazem	Liver	38–90†	Yes	80
Propranolol	Liver	30–40*	Yes	95
Metoprolol	Liver	50*	No	12
Timolol	Liver	75*	No	10
Nadolol	Kidney	20	No	30
Pindolol	Liver (60) Kidney (40)	90	No	57
Digoxin	Kidney	60–75	No	20
Digitoxin	Liver	?(100)	No	95

* Inherited differences in metabolism
† Dose- or concentration-dependent
‡ In "extensive metabolizers"
§ In "poor metabolizers"

gamma globulins. Although the most abundant protein, albumin, avidly binds acidic drugs, many cardiovascular agents are basic and bind peferentially to AAG.[11] AAG is an acute phase protein whose concentration increases dramatically in response to stress such as myocardial infarction and surgery. Increased levels have also been reported in chronic inflammatory diseases such as rheumatoid arthritis, inflammatory renal disease, and Crohn's disease.

The degree of protein binding has implications for both drug disposition and drug effect. Only the unbound, free drug is able to cross cell membranes or bind to receptor sites, thereby eliciting a pharmacological effect. A decrease in protein binding, as a result of disease or displacement by another drug, will increase the free fraction, which in turn increases the amount of drug available for equilibration with extravascular sites. This will increase the volume of distribution and may alter clearance as described below.

Changes in protein binding are most likely to be clinically important for those drugs that are highly protein bound. For example, for a drug which is 98% bound to plasma protein, a decrease in binding to 96% will double the free fraction from 2% to 4%. For a drug that is 60% bound, a similar decrease in binding will result in only an increase of one-twentieth (from 40% to 42%) in the free fraction. In the latter case, clinically important consequences of the change in protein binding are unlikely. In the former case, the clinical significance will depend on the total amount of drug present in the plasma and whether the increase in free fraction results in a corresponding increase in free drug concentration. This, in turn, depends on whether the increase in free fraction is accompanied by an increase in clearance.

Some drugs are cleared slowly and drug-protein dissociation during a single pass through a metabolizing or eliminating organ is small. For example, phenytoin is such a "low-extraction" drug that is extensively protein-bound. A decrease in phenytoin binding to albumin, as occurs in the presence of uremia or displacement by salicylate, results in an increase in the free fraction and, transiently, the free concentration. Since the clearance of low-extraction drugs is related directly to the free fraction, an increase in phenytoin free fraction results in an increased clearance. As more free drug is cleared, the free concentration returns to its original level, and the total plasma phenytoin concentration falls. Thus, while the same amount of free drug is available to exert pharmacological activity as before, reliance on total plasma concentration could be misleading. Both efficacy and toxicity may appear at lower than usual total plasma concentrations.

If the same decrease in protein binding occurs in the case of a highly extracted drug, such as lidocaine or propranolol, the net result may be different. Since both free and protein-bound drug are cleared, changes in binding do not affect clearance. Since clearance remains constant, the total concentration at steady state will remain the same. However, since the free fraction has increased, and less drug is protein-bound, the free concentration will also be increased. In such a case, exaggerated pharmacological activity, possibly resulting in unexpected toxicity, may occur at total plasma concentrations within the usual therapeutic range.

Plasma protein binding can therefore serve as a drug storage site, "protecting" drug from passive elimination processes in the liver and kidneys, or it can act as a delivery system for drugs that are highly cleared by the liver or kidneys as a result of active transfer processes.

CONCENTRATION-DEPENDENT BINDING

For most drugs, the fraction of drug bound to protein, at least for doses in the therapeutic range and well beyond, remains constant. However, some drugs (e.g., disopyramide) show nonlinear, saturable protein binding in the range of concentrations attained during routine clinical use (Fig. 12.8). Thus, as the total plasma concentration increases, so does the free fraction. For example, doubling the total disopyramide concentration from 2 µg/ml to 4 µg/ml may increase the free disopyramide concentration by as much as sixfold.[12]

PHARMACOKINETICS

Pharmacokinetics describes the relationship of the processes of absorption, distribution, and elimination of a drug with time. The fate of a drug in the body can be approximated by mathematical models which in turn allow prediction of dosing schedules.

CONCEPT OF COMPARTMENTS

The various spaces into which the drug distributes are viewed as "compartments" or discrete volumes containing a certain mass of drug, with rate constants for entry and exit of drug from each of these compartments. Entry and exit of drug occurs from a central compartment, which in practical terms may be thought of as the plasma (and perhaps highly perfused tissues such as brain, lung, heart, and kidneys, depending on the rapidity of distribution to these tissues relative to others). The drug may distribute more slowly into various tissues, which can then be regarded as peripheral compartments, with rate constants of entry to and exit from the central compartment (Fig. 12.9). Although the postulated compartments may correspond to drug distribution and elimination from discrete tissue groups, such physiological processes cannot be inferred from the model. It is important to recognize that the purpose of partitioning a drug into compartments is simply to allow convenient mathematical description of the time course of drug disposition.

The simplest case is that of rapid, intravenous injection of a drug that is not distributed to other compartments. In this case, a semiloga-

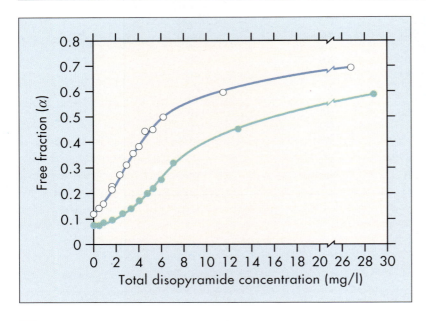

FIGURE 12.8 Saturable protein binding of disopyramide: As the total disopyramide concentration increases, so does the free fraction (unbound/bound drug). These are the extremes of values obtained in a population of 12 subjects. (Modified from Meffin PJ, Robert EW, Winkle RA et al: Role of concentration-dependent plasma protein binding in disopyramide disposition. J Pharmacokinet Biopharm 7:29, 1979)

rithmic plot of plasma concentration against time yields a straight line (Fig. 12.10).

Such a linear relationship describes a first-order process; the amount of drug cleared from the plasma depends, at any instant, on the amount remaining in the plasma. Thus, plasma concentration decreases by a constant fraction with each unit of time. The most useful unit of time is that required for the plasma concentration to decrease by half, and is termed the "elimination half-life."

Following intravenous administration of a drug, a plot of log plasma concentration against time (semilog plot) often shows an initial curvature. This departure from linearity represents the initial dilution of drug within the plasma and its distribution to other tissues. Once distribution is complete, drug in both the central and peripheral compartments is in equilibrium. The curve can be dissected into two, rather than one, straight lines; the first represents the distribution half-life, and the second already is familiar as describing terminal elimination (Fig. 12.11).

This concept of mass-action compartments wherein drug is distributed can be extended to multicompartment models. The semilog plot of plasma concentration with time following a single intravenous dose will then be described by a polyexponential equation, with rate constants for entry to and exit from each compartment. However, even with the aid of computers to fit the data to an equation, most drugs can

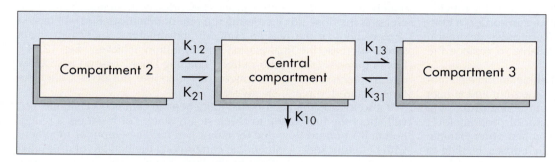

FIGURE 12.9 Schematic diagram of a multicompartment open model, in this case three compartments. Rate constants for drug transfer between compartments are the K values. Note that drug input and output occurs only via the central compartment.

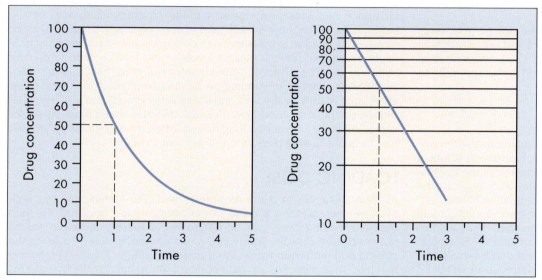

FIGURE 12.10 Drug concentration with time during first-order elimination for a single compartment plotted on an arithmetic scale (*left*) and on a semilog scale (*right*).

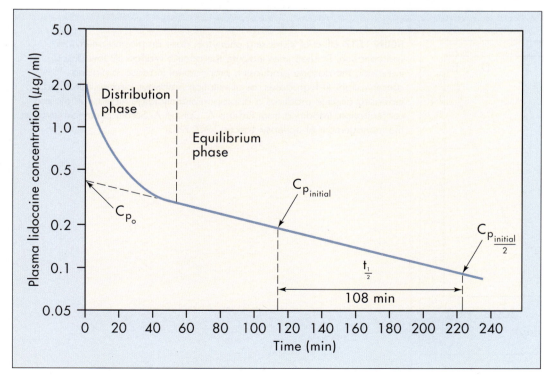

FIGURE 12.11 Semilogarithmic plot of drug concentration against time, two compartment model. The initial rapid fall in plasma concentration primarily reflects distribution.

VOLUME 1 ■ CARDIOVASCULAR PHARMACOLOGY

be modelled to one or two compartments. It is rare that more complex considerations are required.

If the drug is administered by some route other than intravenously, it first will have to be absorbed into the circulation. A semilog plot of plasma concentration against time shows an initial increase in concentration as drug is absorbed, followed by equilibration of drug between central and peripheral compartments, and a linear elimination phase with a slope identical to the slope that would have been evidenced had the drug been administered intravenously. Absorption, like elimination, is usually a first-order process; a constant fraction of the total drug present is absorbed per unit time. As the amount of drug remaining to be absorbed diminishes, so does the rate of absorption. However, sustained-release preparations, in which drug slowly dissolves out of a wax or polymer matrix, are designed to be roughly analogous to a constant-rate infusion. This may be zero-order: a constant amount of drug is absorbed per unit time. Zero-order absorption is the case whenever a reservoir of drug is available to replace the amount absorbed.

It should also be mentioned that pathways of elimination (*e.g.*, biotransformation, renal tubular secretion) may become saturated at high doses of drug, and elimination may change from a first-order to a zero-order process. This is the case for elimination of propranolol,[13] phenytoin,[14] and possibly diltiazem,[15] which exhibit first-order elimination at low doses and zero-order elimination at high doses, leading to disproportionately large increases in plasma concentration with increasing dose (Fig. 12.12).

The mathematical relationships describing the above processes provide the basis for constructing dosing schedules and are of practical utility in understanding and interpreting plasma drug concentration information.[16,17] These relationships are considered in the appendix to this chapter.

MULTIPLE DOSES

Most drugs are given as multiple doses in order to maintain an effective plasma concentration. In practice, there will be fluctuation about a mean plasma concentration between doses. The degree of the fluctuation will depend on the length of the dosing interval relative to the elimination half-life. If the dosing interval is short relative to the half-life, the fluctuation will be small, but the degree of accumulation will be large. Conversely, a long dosing interval combined with a short half-life will result in wide fluctuation, but little accumulation. By definition, the plasma concentration of a drug administered at intervals corresponding to its half-life will show a twofold fluctuation between minimum and maximum plasma concentration. The acceptability of a dosage regimen will depend in large part on the width of the therapeutic window (Fig. 12.13).[18]

STEADY STATE

By definition, following multiple dosing or continuous infusion a drug will reach "steady state" when the rate of entry into the body equals the rate of elimination. An important concept is that the time taken to reach steady state or to eliminate the drug completely is dependent only on the elimination half-life of the drug or active metabolites, if these accumulate. Table 12.2 illustrates the relationship between half-life and drug accumulation/elimination. It is evident that after approximately five half-lives, either process is virtually complete. Neither increasing the dose nor increasing the rate of administration will hasten achievement of the plasma concentration plateau; such maneuvers simply increase the final plasma concentration achieved (Fig. 12.14). Loading doses (see section titled "Loading Dose" below) may allow one to reach an effective concentration sooner but do not alter the time required to reach steady state.

It also follows that factors that influence the elimination half-life also will affect the time taken to reach steady state. For instance, a reduction in liver blood flow due to diminished cardiac output or treatment with beta-blockers or cimetidine can prolong the half-life of drugs that are extensively metabolized in the liver. Renal dysfunction can slow clearance and thus prolong the half-life of drugs eliminated by the kidneys. In either case it will take correspondingly longer to reach steady state, so that premature dose escalation based on the usual time taken to achieve plateau plasma levels would lead to excessive accumulation of drug. Chronic administration of drug can also be associated with changes in elimination kinetics, especially for those drugs eliminated mainly by the liver and those with hemodynamic effects that reduce splanchnic blood flow. For example, the elimination half-life of verapamil is about twice as long during longterm oral therapy,[19] so that less frequent dosing is required to prevent toxicity.

LOADING DOSE

In many instances, it is not feasible to wait four half-lives to five half-lives before effective plasma concentrations are attained. In such cases, a loading dose can be employed to initially increase plasma concentration rapidly, followed by maintenance doses to keep the plasma concentration within the therapeutic range. It will still take five half-lives to achieve steady state concentration, but an effective plasma

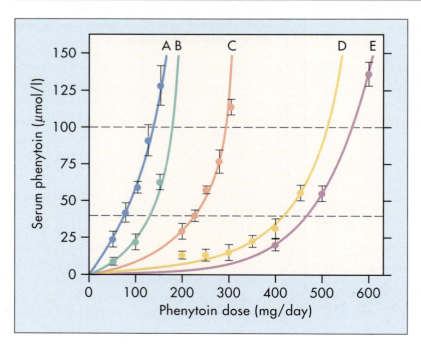

FIGURE 12.12 Effect of increasing phenytoin dose on plasma phenytoin concentration. Dashed lines indicate therapeutic window. At low doses, increasing the dosage produces a proportional increase in plasma concentration. At high doses, as elimination pathways become saturated, increased dosage produces a disproportionately large increase in plasma concentration. (Modified from Richens A, Dunlop A: Serum phenytoin levels in the management of epilepsy. Lancet 2:247, 1975)

concentration will be attained sooner. The price paid is an increased risk of attaining toxic plasma levels after an initial large dose. In addition, should the maintenance dose be too high or too low, side effects or loss of efficacy, respectively, will develop after an apparently beneficial effect due to the loading dose. Recognition that these changes in drug response are due to such simple pharmacokinetic phenomena is often delayed, or the connection is never made. If drug is given intravenously, greater control of plasma drug concentration can be achieved by combining bolus injection(s) with rapid or maintenance infusions (Fig. 12.15).

ACTIVE METABOLITES

Although in most cases drugs are metabolized to compounds with little, or clinically inconsequential pharmacological activity, in some instances metabolites can contribute significantly to the efficacy or toxicity observed after administration of parent drug. For instance, the monoethylglycine xylidide metabolite (MEGX) of lidocaine possesses some antiarrhythmic activity and the glycine xylidide metabolite potentiates the convulsant properties of both lidocaine and MEGX.[20] Certain metabolites of quinidine may be antiarrhythmic and may contrib-

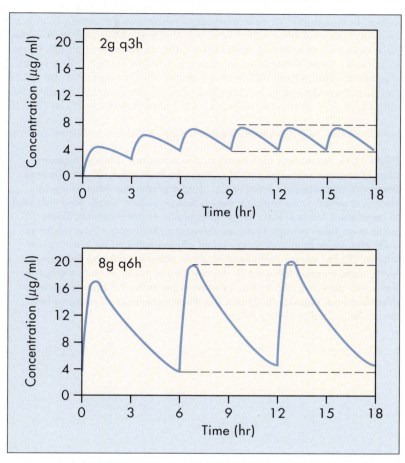

FIGURE 12.13 Relationship among the elimination half-life, the width of the therapeutic window and the frequency of dosing for a rapidly absorbed and eliminated drug (in this case, procainamide). These computer simulations of plasma concentrations show that frequent dosing is required when the therapeutic window is narrow (4 μg/ml to 8 μg/ml; top panel) to avoid excessively high or low values. If the therapeutic window were wider (e.g., 4 μg/ml to 20 μg/ml; bottom panel), larger doses could be given less frequently. Since elimination half-life (139 minutes) is not changed, the time to reach steady state conditions is the same. (Modified from Roden DM, Woosley RL: Application of pharmacologic principles in the evaluation of new antiarrhythmic agents. In Morganroth J, Moore EN (eds): Sudden Cardiac Death and Congestive Heart Failure: Diagnosis and Treatment, pp 13–30. Dordrecht, Holland, Martinus Nijhoff, 1983)

TABLE 12.2 RELATIONSHIP BETWEEN HALF-LIFE AND EXTENT OF COMPLETION OF A FIRST-ORDER PROCESS

Number of half-lives elapsed	Amount of Drug Excreted (%)*
1	50
2	75
3	87.5
4	93.8
5	96.9
6	98.4
7	99.2

* Or accumulated to steady state.

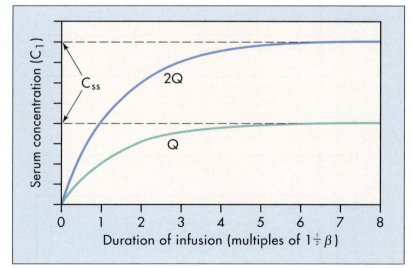

FIGURE 12.14 Plasma concentration against time for constant infusion of a drug at rates Q and 2Q. Note that plateau concentration is reached at the same time, independent of Q, but that the plateau concentration achieved depends on Q.

ute to QT prolongation seen during therapy.[21] N-acetylprocainamide (NAPA), the major metabolite of procainamide, can be antiarrhythmic in its own right with electrophysiological and clinical effects distinct from procainamide. Investigation of this metabolite has provided insight into the apparent great variability in response to procainamide. In a comparison of intravenous procainamide (before NAPA could be produced) with oral NAPA, about half the patients responded to procainamide but not NAPA, while some responded to both, and some to neither.[22] Therefore, NAPA may or may not contribute to the antiarrhythmic actions of procainamide. However, high concentrations of NAPA can certainly contribute to toxicity, including *torsades de pointes*, a syndrome of polymorphic ventricular tachycardia occurring in a setting of marked prolongation of QT interval. Acetylator phenotype, which markedly influences the response to procainamide and other drugs, including hydralazine and isoniazid, which serve as substrates for N-acetyltransferase, is genetically determined and bimodally distributed. In white and black populations, the distribution between slow and fast acetylators is approximately equal while oriental populations are virtually all (90%) rapid acetylators. Procainamide-induced lupus occurs more frequently and earlier, in slow acetylators. Unfortunately, there is no simple way of predicting acetylator phenotype, so that it may be wise to monitor both parent drug and metabolite levels on at least one sample in patients receiving these drugs. A NAPA/procainamide ratio greater than 1:1 when dosing is at steady state (and renal failure is absent) indicates a rapid acetylator phenotype. The clinician should be aware that the patient may be responding to parent drug and/or metabolite.

Bimodal distribution of enzymes involved in oxidative metabolism has been described for debrisoquine,[23] propranolol,[24] encainide[25] and propafenone.[26] It appears that 6% to 9% of the population lack the major enzyme responsible for biotransformation of these drugs. The clinical implications in these poor metabolizers will depend on the relative potencies and pharmacokinetics of the parent drug and metabolites. For example, in extensive metabolizers (approximately 93% of patients) the oral bioavailability of encainide is about 25% to 35% due to extensive presystemic metabolism; the elimination half-life of encainide in these individuals is about 2.5 hours (range 0.5–8 hours). Apparent elimination half-lives of active metabolites, on the other hand, are considerably longer (8–20 hours). In contrast, in poor metabolizers (7% of the population), oral bioavailability is about 80% to

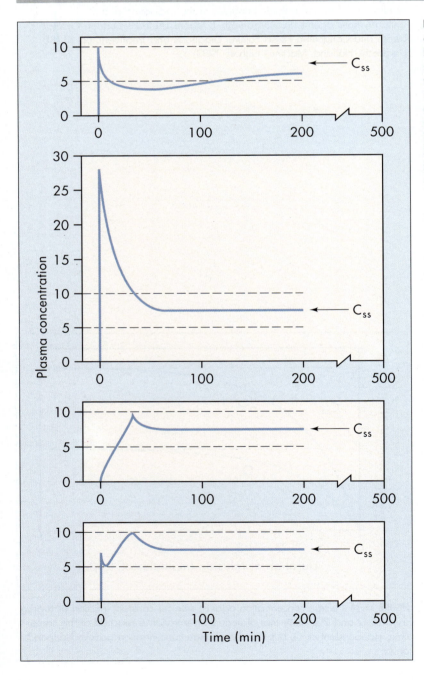

FIGURE 12.15 Alternatives for loading and maintenance (infusion) regimens after intravenous administration of a drug with half-life of 100 min. Dashed lines indicate therapeutic window; C_{ss}, drug concentration when a steady state is achieved. Dose regimens (*top to bottom panels*): single dose, adjusted to avoid peak levels in toxic range, later results in subtherapeutic levels; single dose large enough to ensure therapeutic levels throughout results in early plasma levels in toxic range; rapid infusion followed by maintenance infusion (double infusion technique) results in delay in achieving therapeutic levels; rapid injection followed by double infusion results in early therapeutic levels with plasma concentration maintained within the therapeutic window. (Modified from Woosley RL, Shand DG: Pharmacokinetics of antiarrhythmic drugs. Am J Cardiol 41:986, 1978)

90%, with an encainide elimination half-life of 8 to 20 hours. These differences result in a distinct plasma drug concentration profile (Fig. 12.16) and pharmacodynamic consequences (Fig. 12.17). This is caused by the fact that certain metabolites of encainide have antiarrhythmic activity equal to or greater than encainide itself. Although parent drug and metabolites, respectively, are the predominant active species in poor and extensive metabolizers, antiarrhythmic activity is seen in both populations at similar doses of encainide.

EFFECT OF DISEASE ON DRUG DISPOSITION

Drug disposition is usually determined at a fairly early stage in the development of a drug, usually using healthy, young men as study volunteers. Unfortunately, the disposition of a drug in the patients for whom it is intended is often markedly different (Table 12.3), and other disease processes and concomitant drug therapy can further complicate matters.

Although the choice of initial dosage regimens in individual patients with hepatic or renal disease is often empiric, some knowledge of the impact of various disease states on drug disposition can be a valuable adjunct to patient observation.

LIVER DISEASE

Chronic liver disease has the most impact on drugs that are normally highly cleared by the liver. Both drug metabolizing activity and hepatic blood flow may be reduced, with portosystemic shunting diverting portal blood (and unchanged drug) directly to the systemic circulation. These changes reduce hepatic clearance, and thus raise plasma concentrations of unchanged drug. For most drugs, reduction in dosage or dosage interval is necessary to avoid toxicity. For a drug with active metabolites, the net effect would depend on the pharmacokinetics and pharmacodynamics of the metabolites compared to the parent drug. In cases where therapeutic benefit is largely derived from active metabolites, another agent, not subject to hepatic metabolism, might be considered. Aside from changes in drug disposition, there is some evidence of pharmacodynamic change for certain drugs in patients with hepatic disease. For example, the central nervous system effects of chlorpromazine are exaggerated in such patients, particularly in the presence of hepatic encephalopathy.[27]

CARDIAC FAILURE

The decreased cardiac output and increased sympathetic tone in patients with congestive heart failure results both in diminished blood supply to the gut, to the liver and the kidneys, and in poor peripheral perfusion. These changes have implications for drug absorption, distribution, and elimination.

Delayed and incomplete absorption of drugs in patients with cardiac failure can be expected. For instance, cardiac patients may absorb approximately one-half as much quinidine as normal subjects, and take twice as long to reach peak plasma concentration.[28] However, because of the reduced volume of distribution, plasma concentrations attained by cardiac patients may be higher than those in control subjects (Fig. 12.18).

A decreased volume of distribution in cardiac failure has also been described for disopyramide[29] and lidocaine.[30] Cardiac failure may also result in significant changes in drug clearance, both for drugs whose clearance depends mainly on organ blood flow and those whose clearance is determined by drug metabolizing enzyme activity. Perfusion of the liver and kidneys is decreased, and a decrease in drug metabolizing enzyme activity has been found in liver biopsy specimens from patients with congestive cardiomyopathy. A direct relationship between plasma

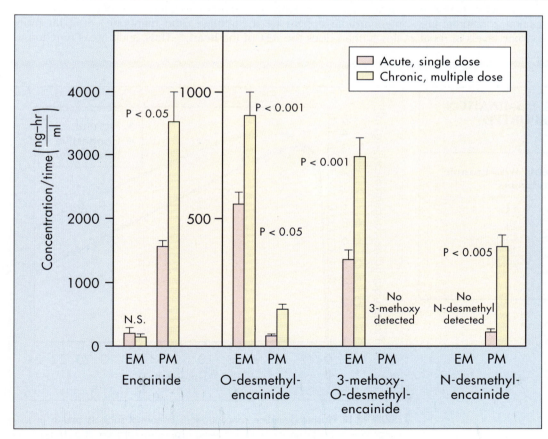

FIGURE 12.16 Areas (0 hr to 8 hr) under the plasma concentration/time curves for encainide and its metabolites after single and multiple oral doses (mean ± SEM [standard error of the mean]) in extensive (*EM*) and poor (*PM*) metabolizers. (Modified from Wang T, Roden DM, Wolfenden HT et al: Influence of genetic polymorphism on the metabolism and disposition of encainide in man. J Pharmacol Exp Ther 228:605, 1984)

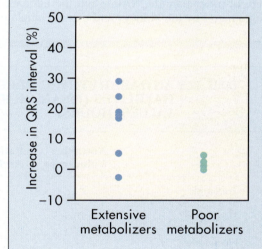

FIGURE 12.17 Percentage increase in QRS interval during an 8-hr dosing period after multiple oral doses of encainide in extensive and poor metabolizers. Prolongation of the QRS interval has been shown to correlate with plasma concentration of O-desmethylencainide. (Modified from Wang T, Roden DM, Wolfenden HT et al: Influence of genetic polymorphism on the metabolism and disposition of encainide in man. J Pharmacol Exp Ther 228:605, 1984)

clearance of lidocaine and cardiac output has been described, with a 39% decrease in lidocaine clearance among heart failure patients compared to normal subjects.[30]

Depending on the relative magnitude of changes in clearance and volume of distribution, the elimination half-life may be unaffected or prolonged. Despite changes in clearance, the mean elimination half-life of lidocaine,[30] procainamide,[31] and quinidine[28] appear similar in patients with and without heart failure, while those of disopyramide,[29] and mexiletine,[32] appear to be prolonged, with a proportionately longer time to reach steady state.

It is clear that drug therapy in patients with cardiac failure mandates the use of initial low doses with escalation under careful supervision. Prolongation of elimination half-life may also warrant less frequent dosing and less frequent changes of dose since the length of time to steady state plasma concentration is increased.

RENAL DISEASE

Obviously, renal disease will have the most impact on those drugs eliminated mainly by the kidneys (see Table 12.1). However, renal disease can also affect protein binding[33] (hypoalbuminemia; presence of binding inhibitors or altered affinity of protein for drug), drug metabolism (diminished activity of some enzyme systems including N-acetyltransferase), and urinary pH (alkalinization can alter tubular reabsorption of drugs and the degree of ionization of weak bases, resulting in diminished excretion).

It is difficult to predict the interplay and relative contribution of these various effects to changes in drug disposition. However, for drugs that are mainly eliminated by renal excretion, one can expect decreased clearance and prolongation of elimination half-life, often in direct proportion to the decrease in creatinine clearance. For example, the half-life of digitoxin, elimination of which involves mainly extrarenal pathways, does not change in renal failure, while the half-life of digoxin, which is largely eliminated by the kidneys, increases with severe renal failure from 36 hours to about four days. The active metabolite of procainamide, NAPA, and the lidocaine analog, tocainide, are eliminated by the kidneys and can accumulate to toxic levels in renal failure.[34,35] Obviously, if accumulation to toxic levels is to be avoided, less drug must be administered, by either increasing the dosing interval or decreasing the dose administered.

ACUTE MYOCARDIAL INFARCTION

The patient with acute myocardial infarction (MI) presents a special challenge with respect to drug therapy. Altered hemodynamics and increased levels of AAG can markedly affect the disposition of any drug administered following myocardial infarction.

Lidocaine is one of the most frequently administered and probably the most extensively studied drug in the setting of acute MI. Administration of lidocaine to patients suspected of having sustained an infarction results in a broad range of plasma levels with accumulation of lidocaine in plasma during a constant infusion in those patients with confirmed infarction (Table 12.4). These changes can be largely explained by an increase in plasma protein binding as a result of increased levels of AAG.[36] Although the total plasma concentration rises parallel to AAG concentration, the free fraction declines, and free lidocaine concentration remains fairly constant. Therefore, higher than usual plasma concentrations may be well tolerated in acute myocardial infarction (concentrations > 6 μg/ml, normally considered toxic, have been reported to be well tolerated several days after myocardial infarction) and indeed may be necessary to maintain adequate free lidocaine levels for antiarrhythmic effect. Similar high plasma concentrations of drug when administered to patients with myocardial infarction have been reported for quinidine[37] and disopyramide.[38] In addition to increased total plasma concentration of drugs binding to AAG, the changes in drug disposition described for lowered cardiac output and renal impairment may also apply following myocardial infarction.

A further consideration in drug therapy following myocardial infarction is that the usual temporal relationship between drug administration and effect may be altered. The heart is normally a highly perfused organ so that most drugs in plasma rapidly equilibrate with myocardial tissue. However, in infarction, the areas of poorly perfused myocardium appear to accumulate (and eliminate) drug far more slowly than does the rest of the heart.[39] Thus, such areas function as

TABLE 12.3 ANTIARRHYTHMIC DRUG ELIMINATION HALF-LIVES (MEAN OF REPORTED VALUES, HOURS)

	Normal Volunteers	Patients With Chronic Arrhythmias
Tocainide	11	14
N-acetylprocainamide	6.5	10
Mexiletine	10.5	12.5
Aprindine	22	48
Flecainide	14	20.3

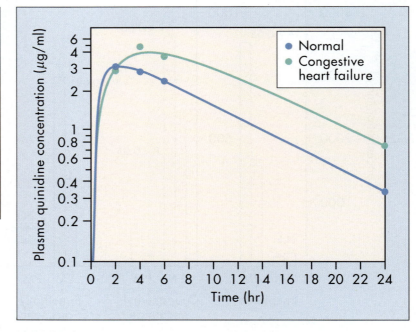

FIGURE 12.18 Plasma quinidine concentrations in normal subjects and in congestive heart failure patients following oral administration of 600 mg quinidine sulfate. The data points are the mean levels in ten subjects. (Modified from Crouthamel WG: The effect of congestive heart failure on quinidine pharmacokinetics. Am Heart J 90:335, 1975)

peripheral, rather than central, pharmacokinetic compartments and, depending on the drug's effector site, there may be a corresponding delay between drug administration and pharmacological effect.

AGE

Drug disposition in both the elderly and the very young can vary widely from that in the young adult population in which it is usually defined. Deterioration of renal and hepatic function, or immaturity of these processes, can result in significant changes in the pharmacokinetic variables. For example, the half-life of inulin (eliminated by glomerular filtration) in an infant is approximately three times that in an adult. In addition, the extremes of age may be associated with changes in sensitivity to drugs. For example, elderly patients have a reduced response to β-receptor agonists and antagonists. The likely explanation in this case is a reduction in the number of β-receptors with age.[40] On the other hand, an increased sensitivity to benzodiazepines[41] and coumarin anticoagulants[42] has been noted in elderly patients. Unfortunately, few drugs have been systematically evaluated in either the very young or elderly and information has often been gained through anecdotes or adverse clinical experiences, sometimes at considerable human expense (e.g., chloramphenicol and the "gray-baby" syndrome).

THERAPEUTIC DRUG MONITORING

The usefulness of drug plasma concentrations as a means of guiding therapy presupposes a correlation between pharmacological effect and plasma concentration of a drug. While this is generally true, there are instances when plasma concentration can be misleading. For example, a pharmacological effect may persist even after drug has been eliminated from plasma. Often, this may be accounted for by the presence of an active metabolite (e.g., encainide), or some irreversible action of the drug that requires physiological regeneration for termination of effect (e.g., depletion of catecholamine stores by reserpine). In some cases there may be a temporal delay between plasma concentration and effect which may be the result of the drug's receptor site residing in a poorly perfused tissue, or a tissue into which drug only diffuses slowly (e.g., digoxin diffuses slowly into myocardial tissue so that its cardiac effects are apparent an hour or more after intravenous administration)[43] (Fig. 12.19).

Further complications are poorly defined therapeutic ranges (the usually quoted therapeutic range for quinidine is derived using a nonspecific assay and is based mainly on 30-year-old data on conversion of atrial fibrillation[44]) and great interpatient variability in response. Part of this variability is explained by the fact that the free, unbound drug is considered pharmacologically active, while most therapeutic ranges are based on total plasma concentration of the drug (free drug plus that quantity bound to plasma protein). The extent of binding to plasma protein varies considerably. A range of 51% to 87% among normal subjects has been quoted for quinidine[45]; it is likely that variability among patients is greater. The situation could be improved by monitoring free drug rather than total plasma drug concentration, since this should correlate better with pharmacological effect. For example, acute ECG changes due to intravenous quinidine[46] and disopyramide[47] correlated well with free, but not total, drug levels. Unfortunately, free levels of drug are rarely measured, partly because they are often too low for accurate measurement by conventional methods. It also should be mentioned that drug concentrations in whole blood or serum are not equivalent to plasma concentration. The ratio of blood to plasma concentration is related to the hematocrit, the affinity of the drug for blood cells, and the protein binding. Determination in serum carries the potential of loss of drug adsorbed to clots.

The specificity of the drug assay also should be taken into consideration when interpreting drug level data. Is the assay specific for unchanged drug, or does it also include metabolites that may themselves possess pharmacological activity and distinct pharmacokinetics? Newer, more specific assays, measuring parent drug alone, may not correlate well with a therapeutic range based on older, nonspecific assays.

Drug level data can only be useful if accompanied by some knowledge of the dosing history, when the sample was obtained relative to the dosing interval, concomitant medication, and other disease processes. Only then can the measured concentration be evaluated in a meaningful way. Finally, drug levels are no substitute for clinical judgement. Some patients respond (or even develop side effects) at low concentrations, while others may require high concentrations and tolerate them without side effects.

TABLE 12.4 EFFECTS OF TIME ON TOTAL AND FREE PLASMA LIDOCAINE CONCENTRATIONS, AAG, AND PERCENT FREE LIDOCAINE IN EIGHT PATIENTS WITH MYOCARDIAL INFARCTION ON A CONSTANT 2 mg/min INFUSION (MEAN AND RANGE)

	Time (hr)			
	12	24	36	48
Total lidocaine (μg/ml)	3.15	3.38	3.61	4.23*
	(1.9–4.1)	(1.7–4.5)	(1.6–4.7)	(2.7–6)
Free lidocaine (μg/ml)	0.99	0.99	1.02	1.11
	(0.67–1.25)	(0.58–1.48)	(0.54–1.28)	(0.84–1.43)
AAG (mg/dl)	95	101	108	120*†
	(57–127)	(61–137)	(78–136)	(91–152)
Free lidocaine (%)	0.31	0.30	0.29	0.27†
	(0.25–0.39)	(0.22–0.34)	(0.22–0.39)	(0.21–0.32)

* $P < 0.03$ at 12, 24, and 36 hr

† $P < 0.03$ at 12 and 24 hr

(From Routledge PA, Shand DG, Barchowsky A et al: Relationship between alpha-1-acid glycoprotein and lidocaine disposition in myocardial infarction. Clin Pharmacol Ther 30:154, 1981)

CONCLUSION

Currently available cardiovascular agents are limited by side effects and the potential for exacerbating the condition being treated. In addition, altered disposition of drug as a result of changes in protein binding or concomitant disease processes, active metabolites, drug interactions, and poorly defined therapeutic ranges with great interpatient variability are some of the factors that complicate therapy. The considerations presented here can serve only as a first approximation in determining a suitable drug regimen. Clinical observation then allows at least some appreciation of how a particular patient handles a drug. With an understanding of basic pharmacological principles, the patient's response to and disposition of drug at other doses can then be predicted. A grasp of such principles is invaluable in both the choice of drug and the establishment of an optimum benefit-to-risk ratio for the patient.

APPENDIX
MATHEMATICAL CONSIDERATIONS

A number of simple mathematical relationships describe the fate of drug in the body. Following intravenous administration, the plasma concentration of a drug (Cp) declines with time (t) from its initial concentration (Co) at a rate proportional to Cp:

$$\frac{dCp}{dt} = -k_e Cp \qquad \text{(Eq. 1)}$$

where k_e is the proportionality or rate constant of elimination.

Integrating equation (1)

$$Cp = Co\, e^{-k_e t} \qquad \text{(Eq. 2)}$$

and taking logarithms

$$\log Cp = \log Co - \frac{k_e t}{2.303}$$

Thus, a semilogarithmic plot of Cp against t yields a straight line with y-intercept log Co and slope $-k_e/2.303$. Since the elimination half-life ($t_{1/2}$) is, by definition, the time taken for Cp to be reduced to Cp/2, substituting into equation (2) yields

$$\frac{Cp}{2} = Cp\, e^{-k_e t_{1/2}}$$

from which it can be shown that

$$t_{1/2} = \frac{0.693}{k_e} \qquad \text{(Eq. 3)}$$

(Note that these considerations should apply equally well to absorption kinetics, when absorption is a first-order process. Then the k is absorption rate constant, and $t_{1/2}$ the absorption half-life.) The semilogarithmic plot also allows calculation of volume of a distribution (Vd), since

$$Vd = \frac{D}{Co}$$

where D is the administered dose.

Since total clearance (Cl) is the volume of plasma from which drug is completely removed in unit time

$$Cl = k_e Vd \qquad \text{(Eq. 4)}$$

Combining equations (3) and (4):

$$t_{1/2} = \frac{Vd \times 0.693}{Cl}$$

Thus, elimination half-life depends on both the volume of distribution and the clearance.

In multicompartment models similar considerations apply. For intravenous injection with distribution and elimination phases

$$Cp = Ae^{-\alpha t} + Be^{-\beta t}$$

where the first term may be viewed as corresponding to the distribution process, while the second term describes elimination. Both terms

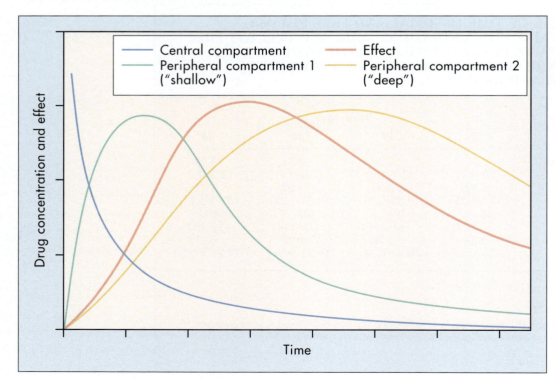

FIGURE 12.19 The relationship between changes in response and changes in concentration of drug throughout various body compartments of a 3-compartment pharmacokinetic model. Note that the effect curve is not in phase with drug concentration in any kinetic compartment and is least well represented by that in the central (plasma) compartment. Such a relationship is illustrative of data obtained after intravenous digoxin where the effect curve could reflect shortening of the QS2 interval or reduction in the left ventricular ejection time. (Modified from Whiting B, Kelman AW: The modelling of drug response. Clin Sci 59:311, 1980)

contribute to the calculation of Co and k_e, while several volumes of distribution can be defined. Equilibrium volume of distribution (often designated Vd_{ss}) will be the sum of all the compartment volumes in which the drug is distributed. Both the volume of the central compartment, (sometimes referred to as the "initial" or "central" volume of distribution) and Vd_{ss} are important in determining intravenous dose requirements.

CONSTANT INFUSION

If a drug is administered by constant infusion at rate Q into a simple one-compartment model then, assuming first-order elimination, Cp changes with time:

$$\frac{dCp}{dt} = \text{rate of infusion} - \text{rate of elimination}$$

$$\frac{dCp}{dt} = \frac{Q}{Vd} - k_e Cp$$

Integrating

$$Cp = \frac{Q}{k_e Vd}(1 - e^{-k_e t})$$

As t approaches infinity, $(1 - e)$ approaches 1, and

$$Cp = \frac{Q}{k_e Vd} = C_{ss} \qquad \text{(Eq. 5)}$$

where C_{ss} is the plasma concentration at steady state.

Stated another way, at steady state, drug input equals drug output:

$$\frac{Q}{Vd} = k_e C_{ss}$$

Since

$$k_e = \frac{Cl}{Vd}$$

Substitution into equation (5) yields

$$C_{ss} = \frac{Q}{Cl} \qquad \text{(Eq. 6)}$$

MULTIPLE DOSES

Multiple doses, whether intravenous, oral, or intramuscular, generally can be thought of as extensions of the case above. Thus, following oral administration, and assuming constant-rate absorption over the dosing interval (as an approximation to the more usual first-order kinetics of absorption):

$$Q = \frac{\text{amount of drug absorbed}}{\text{dose interval}}$$

$$= \frac{\text{Dose (D)} \times \text{fraction bioavailable (f)}}{\text{dose interval }(\tau)}$$

Substituting in equation (6) for Q

$$C_{ss} = \frac{f \times D}{Cl \times \tau}$$

Recall that if a drug is completely bioavailable, $f = 1$.

Although the arguments presented here adequately describe the kinetics of many drugs, they do, of course, represent a very simplified approach to complex physiological processes, more detailed analyses of which are always possible.

REFERENCES

1. Raftery EF: Cardiovascular drug withdrawal syndromes. A potential problem with calcium antagonists? Drugs 28:371, 1984
2. Giacomini JC, Nelson WL, Theodore L et al: The pharmacokinetics and pharmacodynamics of d- and dl-verapamil in rabbits. J Cardiovasc Pharmacol 7:469, 1985
3. Murad F, Rapoport RM, Fiscus R: Role of cyclic-GMP in relaxations of vascular smooth muscle. J Cardiovasc Pharmacol (Suppl 3)7:5111, 1985
4. Roden DM, Reele SB, Higgins SB et al: Tocainide therapy for refractory ventricular arrhythmias. Am Heart J 100:15, 1980
5. Prescott LF, Clements JA, Pottage A: Absorption, distribution and elimination of mexiletine. Postgrad Med J (Suppl 1)53:50, 1977
6. Bauer LA, Edwards WAD, Randolph FP, Blouin RA: Cimetidine-induced decrease in lidocaine metabolism. Am Heart J 108:413, 1984
7. Feely J, Wilkinson GR, Wood AJJ: Reduction of liver blood flow and propranolol metabolism by cimetidine. N Engl J Med 304:692, 1981
8. Bax NDS, Tucker GT, Lennard MS, Woods HF: The impairment of lignocaine clearance by propranolol-major contribution from enzyme inhibition. Br J Clin Pharmacol 19:597, 1985
9. Marcus SI: Drug interactions with amiodarone. Am Heart J 106:924, 1983
10. Kaye CM, Kiddie MA, Turner P: Variable pharmacokinetics of mexiletine. Postgrad Med J (Suppl 1)53:56, 1977
11. Piafsky KM: Disease-induced changes in the plasma binding of basic drugs. Clin Pharmacokinetics 5:246, 1980
12. Meffin PJ, Robert EW, Winkle RA et al: Role of concentration-dependent plasma protein binding in disopyramide disposition. J Pharmacokinet Biopharm 7:29, 1979
13. Wood AJJ, Carr RK, Vestal RE et al: Direct measurement of propranolol bioavailability during accumulation to steady state. Br J Clin Pharmacol 6:345, 1978
14. Richens A, Dunlop A: Serum phenytoin levels in the management of epilepsy. Lancet 2:247, 1975
15. McAllister RG, Hamann SR, Blouin RA: Pharmacokinetics of calcium-entry blockers. Am J Cardiol 55:30B, 1985
16. Greenblatt DJ, Koch–Weser J: Clinical pharmacokinetics, Part II. New Engl J Med 293:964, 1975
17. Woosley RL, Shand DG: Pharmacokinetics of antiarrhythmic drugs. Am J Cardiol 41:986, 1978
18. Roden DM, Woosley RL: Application of pharmacologic principles in the evaluation of new antiarrhythmic agents. In Morganroth J, Moore EN (eds): Sudden Cardiac Death and Congestive Heart Failure: Diagnosis and Treatment, pp 13–30. Dordrecht, Holland, Martinius Nijhoff, 1983
19. Schwartz JB, Keefe DL, Kirsten E et al: Prolongation of verapamil elimination kinetics during chronic oral administration. Am Heart J 104:198, 1982
20. Narang PK, Crouthamel WG, Carliner NH, Fisher ML: Lidocaine and its active metabolites. Clin Pharmacol Ther 25:654, 1978
21. Holford NHG, Coates PE, Guentert TW, Riegelman S, Sheiner LB: The effect of quinidine and its metabolites on the electrocardiogram and systolic time intervals: concentration-effect relationships. Br J Clin Pharmacol 11:187, 1981
22. Roden DM, Reele SB, Higgins SB et al: Antiarrhythmic efficacy, pharmacokinetics and safety of N-acetylprocainamide in human subjects: Comparison with procainamide. Am J Cardiol 46:463, 1980
23. Mahgoub A, Idle JR, Dring LG, Lancaster R, Smith RL: Polymorphic hydroxylation of debrisoquine in man. Lancet 2:584, 1977
24. Alvan G, von Bahr C, Seidman P, Sjoquist F: High plasma concentrations of β-receptor blocking drugs and deficient debrisoquine hydroxylation. Lancet 1:333, 1982
25. Wang T, Roden DM, Wolfenden HT et al: Influence of genetic polymorphism on the metabolism and disposition of encainide in man. J Pharmacol Exp Ther 228:605, 1984
26. Siddoway LA, McAllister CB, Wang T et al: Polymorphic oxidative metabolism of propafenone in man. Circulation (suppl III) 68:III-64, 1983
27. Maxwell JD, Carrella M, Parkes JD et al: Plasma disappearance and cerebral effects of chlorpromazine in cirrhosis. Clin Sci 43:143, 1972
28. Crouthamel WG: The effect of congestive heart failure on quinidine pharmacokinetics. Am Heart J 90:335, 1975
29. Landmark K, Bredesen JE, Thaulow E et al: Pharmacokinetics of disopyramide in patients with imminent to moderate cardiac failure. Eur J Clin Pharmacol 19:187, 1981
30. Thomson PD, Melmon KL, Richardson JA et al: Lidocaine pharmacokinetics in advanced heart failure, liver disease, and renal failure in humans. Ann Intern Med 78:499, 1973

31. Kessler KM, Kayden DS, Estes D et al: Procainamide pharmacokinetics/pharmacodynamics in acute myocardial infarction or congestive heart failure. Circulation (suppl II) 70:II-446, 1984
32. Leahey EB Jr, Giardina EGV, Bigger JT Jr: Effect of ventricular failure on steady state kinetics of mexiletine. Clin Res 26:239A, 1980
33. Reidenberg MM, Drayer DE: Alteration of drug–protein binding in renal disease: Clin Pharmacokinet (suppl) 9 1:18, 1984
34. Drayer DE, Lowenthal DT, Woosley RL et al: Cumulation of N-acetylprocainamide, an active metabolite of procainamide, in patients with impaired renal function. Clin Pharmacol Ther 22:63, 1977
35. Weigers U, Hanrath P, Kuck KH et al: Pharmacokinetics of tocainide in patients with renal dysfunction and during haemodialysis. Eur J Clin Pharmacol 24:503, 1983
36. Routledge PA, Shand DG, Barchowsky A et al: Relationship between alpha-1-acid glycoprotein and lidocaine disposition in myocardial infarction. Clin Pharmacol Ther 30:154, 1981
37. David BM, Whitford EG, Ilett KF: Disopyramide binding to alpha-1-acid glycoprotein: Sequential effects following acute myocardial infarction. Clin Exp Pharmacol Physiol 9:478, 1982
38. Kessler KM, Kissane B, Cassidy J et al: Dynamic variability of binding of antiarrhythmic drugs during the evolution of acute myocardial infarction. Circulation 70:472, 1984
39. Wenger TL, Browning DJ, Masterton CE et al: Procainamide delivery to ischemic canine myocardium following rapid intravenous administration. Circ Res 46:789, 1980
40. Vestal RE, Wood AJJ, Shand DG: Reduced β-adrenoreceptor sensitivity in the elderly. Clin Pharmacol Ther 26:181, 1979
41. Reidenberg MM, Levy M, Warner H et al: Relationship between diazepam dose, plasma level, age, and central nervous system depression. Clin Pharmacol Ther 23:371, 1978
42. Husted S, Andreasen F: The influence of age on the response to anticoagulants. Br J Clin Pharmacol 4:559, 1977
43. Whiting B, Kelman AW: The modelling of drug response. Clin Sci 59:311, 1980
44. Sokolow M, Ball RE: Factors influencing conversion of chronic atrial fibrillation with special reference to serum quinidine concentration. Circulation 14:568, 1956
45. Kates RE, Sokoloski TD, Comstock TJ: Binding of quinidine to plasma proteins in normal subjects and in patients with hyperlipoproteinemias. Clin Pharmacol Ther 23:30, 1978
46. Woo E, Greenblatt DJ: Pharmacokinetic and clinical implications of quinidine-protein binding. J Pharmaceut Sci 68:466, 1979
47. North FC, Mitchell LB, Wyse DG, Duff HJ: Electrophysiologic responses to free and total disopyramide concentrations in patients with inducible sustained ventricular tachycardia. Circulation 70:II-442, 1984

GENERAL REFERENCES

Benet LZ, Massoud N, Gambertoglio JG (eds): Pharmacokinetic Basis for Drug Treatment. New York, Raven Press, 1984

Holford NHG, Sheiner LB: Understanding the dose-effect relationship: Clinical application of pharmacokinetic–pharmacodynamic models. Clin Pharmacokinet 6:429, 1981

Kupersmith J: Monitoring of antiarrhythmic drug levels: Values and pitfalls. Ann NY Acad Sci 432:138, 1984

Lefkowitz RJ, Michel T: Plasma membrane receptors. J Clin Invest 72:1185, 1983

Molinoff PB: α- and β-Adrenergic receptor subtypes. Properties, distribution and regulation. Drugs 28(suppl 2):1, 1984

Sweeney GD: Variability in the human drug response. Thromb Res (suppl) IV 30:3, 1983

Williams RL: Drug administration in hepatic disease. N Engl J Med 309:1616, 1983

Woosley RL, Roden DM: Importance of metabolites in antiarrhythmic therapy. Am J Cardiol 52:8C, 1983

Diuretics

Arnold M. Chonko ▪ Jared J. Grantham

Many cardiovascular diseases interfere with the normal renal excretion of sodium, chloride, and water, leading to their retention in an expanded extracellular fluid compartment. Diuretic drugs promote the renal loss of solutes and water and by these actions are extremely useful in the treatment of edematous states.

The principal mechanisms and clinical utility of diuretics are best understood in the context of the perturbed physiology of renal salt and water handling that occurs in various cardiovascular abnormalities. But first a brief review of normal renal salt and water handling is in order.

▢ REVIEW OF RENAL PHYSIOLOGY: SALT AND WATER HANDLING

Figure 13.1 is a schematic diagram of the mammalian nephron and the various transport processes that occur along its course. Each kidney is composed of about 1 million nephrons. Renal plasma flow averages about one tenth of the cardiac output under usual circumstances (500 ml/min).[1]

Renal blood flow is critically dependent on cardiac output and

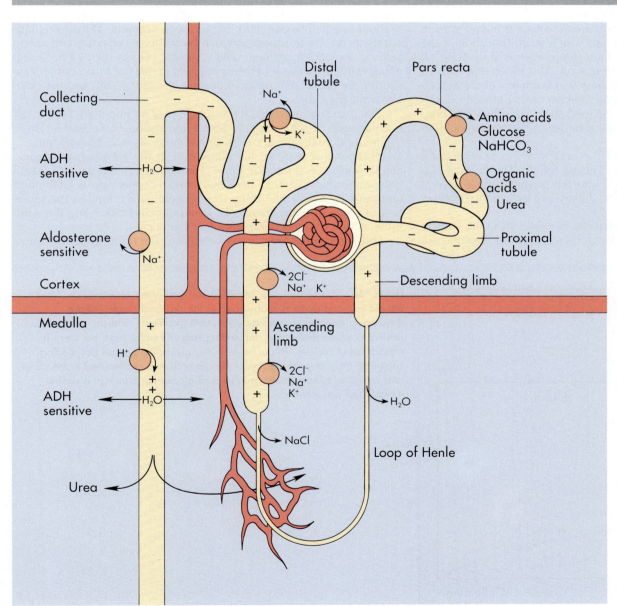

FIGURE 13.1 Sites of tubule salt and water absorption. Sodium is reabsorbed with inorganic anions, amino acids, and glucose in the proximal tubule against an electrical gradient that is lumen negative. In the late part of the proximal tubule (pars recta), sodium and water are reabsorbed to a lesser extent and organic acids (hippurate, urate) and urea are secreted into the urine. The electrical potential is lumen positive in the pars recta. Water, but not salt, is removed from tubule fluid in the thin descending limb of Henle's loop, but in the ascending portion salt is reabsorbed without water, rendering the tubule fluid hyposmotic with respect to the interstitium. Sodium, chloride, and potassium are reabsorbed by the medullary and cortical portions of the ascending limb; the lumen potential is positive. Sodium is reabsorbed and potassium and hydrogen ions are secreted in the distal tubule and collecting ducts. Water absorption in these segments is regulated by antidiuretic hormone (ADH). The electrical potential is lumen negative in the cortical sections and positive in the medullary segments. Urea is concentrated in the interstitium of the medulla and assists in the generation of maximally concentrated urine.

systemic arterial blood pressure. In the range of mean arterial pressures from 80 to nearly 200 mm Hg the normal kidney keeps renal blood flow and glomerular filtration rate (GFR) nearly constant. Below these limits both renal blood flow and GFR appear to vary directly with mean arterial blood pressure. Glomerular filtration ceases at a pressure of about 40 mm Hg in normal subjects. In diseased kidneys, however, renal blood flow and GFR may not be regulated to constant levels at pressures above 80 mm Hg owing to the loss of vasomotor control. Normally, one fifth of the plasma entering the glomeruli is filtered.[2-5] The volume of ultrafiltrate depends on the net driving force across the glomerular capillary, which normally averages 10 to 15 mm Hg. This small gradient is enough to filter 100 to 125 ml/min (150 to 180 liters/day) on the average.

The kidney expends most of its energy to reclaim 99% of the glomerular filtrate under normal circumstances, allowing only about 1% of the filtrate to be excreted eventually as urine. Obviously, failure of the heart to pump effectively will reduce the GFR and urine output.

In the proximal segments large amounts of filtered salt and water are reabsorbed without developing major differences between urine and blood in the concentrations of solutes. By contrast, the distal nephron, which arbitrarily begins at the bend of Henle's loop, absorbs salt and water at a slower rate than the proximal nephron but generates great transtubule differences in concentration. The proximal tubule is composed of at least three distinct portions: the convoluted segment (S_1 segment), a terminal straight (pars recta) portion (S_3), and an intermediate section (S_2). Salt and water are absorbed at higher rates in S_1 than in S_2 or S_3. Henle's loop begins with a sharp transition of the epithelium into a thin descending limb that curves sharply back on itself and becomes the thin ascending limb. The ascending limb of Henle's loop has papillary and medullary thin segments and a medullary and cortical segment that is clearly thicker and composed of different types of epithelial cells than the medullary part. The distal convoluted tubule is a transitional segment between the ascending limb and the cortical collecting tubule.

The collecting system begins in the cortex where several distal tubules unite to form the cortical collecting tubule. The cortical collecting tubule descends unbranched into the medulla where several collecting tubules unite to form the medullary and thence the papillary collecting ducts.

There are also two distinct populations of nephrons in the kidney: superficial and juxtamedullary. Although these nephrons have the potential to affect renal salt and water excretion in different ways, studies have not clearly resolved these differences, and for this discussion both nephron populations are considered to be identical.

Figure 13.2 shows the fraction of water and sodium remaining at various sites along the renal tubule. The proximal tubule is the principal site of salt and water reabsorption since approximately 60% of the filtered fluid and sodium is reabsorbed in this segment under normal circumstances. The structure of the epithelial cells of the S_1 proximal segment reflects the high volume flux from lumen to blood that occurs across this segment. There is a prominent luminal brush border, numerous deep invaginations of the basal cell membrane, large numbers of mitochondria, and relatively "leaky" intercellular junctions. High concentrations of carbonic anhydrase are located within these cells and their luminal membranes. This enzyme has a prominent role in bicarbonate reabsorption.

Fluid reabsorption in the proximal tubule is closely linked to the volume of the plasma or extracellular fluid compartment. Thus, with contraction of the extracellular fluid volume, proximal tubule reabsorption is enhanced, whereas with expansion of the extracellular fluid, proximal tubule reabsorption is diminished. The controls for this system remain uncertain but may be linked to natriuretic hormones such as atrial natriuretic factor or effects of the concentration of the peritubular plasma protein concentration (so-called physical factors).

The S_2 and S_3 portions of the proximal tubule also absorb fluid in an isosmotic fashion, but the net reabsorptive capacity of these segments is about one half to one third that of the S_1 segment. Moreover, these segments do not transport as much bicarbonate, glucose, and amino acids as the earlier segment. The epithelial cells of the S_2 and S_3 segments differ from those of the S_1 segment in that the brush borders are shorter, the basal cell invaginations are less prominent, and the mitochondria are fewer.

The proximal portions of the tubule play an important role in the maintenance of renal organic anion and cation homeostasis. These segments contain transporters primarily located in basolateral cell membranes that institute the initial step in the secretion of organic anions and cations into the urine. The organic anions include *p*-aminohippuric acid, uric acid, penicillin, certain cephalosporin antibiotics, and most of the diuretic drugs. Probenecid, which inhibits the secretion of some of these chemicals, slows the elimination and the natriuretic action of furosemide and other diuretics.

Organic cations are also secreted into the urine by the proximal

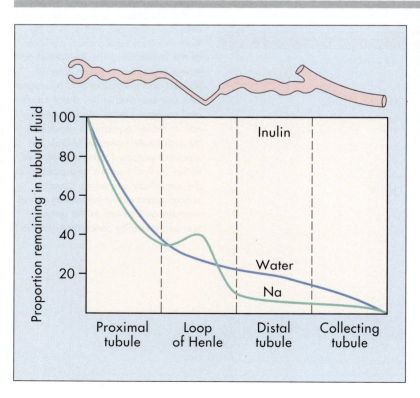

FIGURE 13.2 Quantitative view of tubule salt and water reabsorption. Most filtered salt and water is reabsorbed in the proximal tubule without developing appreciable transtubule osmotic gradients. Sodium is actually added to tubule fluid in the descending limb of Henle's loop, but there is absorption of sodium without water in the ascending portion (the diluting segment). Only a small fraction of filtered sodium is reabsorbed in the distal and collecting tubules. Inulin, a marker of glomerular filtration, is neither reabsorbed nor secreted.

segments, albeit to a lesser extent than for organic anions. Important cationic compounds that are secreted into the urine include creatinine, quinidine, quinine, trimethoprim, cimetidine, and ranitidine.

The thin descending limb of Henle's loop is highly permeable to water and relatively impermeable to solutes. Thus, water flows out of the tubule into the increasing osmotic gradient of the interstitium. Salt and urea are concentrated within the lumen osmotically. No active transport processes exist across this segment; diuretics appear to have no effect on this segment.

The thin ascending limb of Henle's loop is also composed of relatively simple epithelial cells with scant cytoplasm and organelles. In contrast to the descending limb, this segment is highly impermeable to water. However, sodium chloride is absorbed from tubule lumen into the interstitium, leading to dilution of the lumen contents.

The anatomical transition from the thin ascending limb to the medullary thick ascending limb is abrupt. The cells within this segment are cuboidal or columnar, lack brush borders, and contain plentiful basilar cell membrane invaginations and mitochondria. This segment is also relatively impermeable to water and reabsorbs sodium chloride against steep concentration gradients, thus diluting the urine. Sodium chloride transport across both the medullary and cortical thick ascending limb of Henle's loop is illustrated in Figure 13.1. A luminal membrane transporter carries two chloride ions from the lumen into the cell along with a sodium and a potassium ion. The energy for this transport is derived from the diffusion of sodium down its electrochemical gradient (i.e., outside the cell toward the cell interior), which, in turn, is established by the sodium pump (Na^+K^+-ATPase) located within the basolateral cell membranes.

The cortical portion of the thick ascending limb is characterized by thinner epithelial cells than those in the medullary portion. As in the other sections of the ascending limb, salt is reabsorbed but water is not, thus further diluting the urine. In normal humans the urine osmolality can be minimally lowered to about 50 mOsm/kg. The difference between the osmolality of the urine in the ascending limb and plasma osmolality represents the water in the glomerular filtrate that has been "freed" of solute. In other words, the ascending limb forms water that is "free" of solute.

Drugs that interfere with salt reabsorption in these segments prevent the achievement of minimally dilute urine and thus blunt the renal excretion of water. It is instructive to emphasize at this point that the ability to excrete water loads is importantly dependent on the function of the ascending limb. Malfunction in this segment can lead to retention of "free" water and to dilutional hyponatremia. As shown in Figure 13.2, approximately 20% of the filtered water and 10% of the filtered sodium remain at the end of the ascending limb of Henle. In other words, about 5% of the filtered water and about 25% of the filtered sodium are reabsorbed by the ascending limb of Henle.

The distal convoluted tubule is composed of several different types of epithelial cells. The "macula densa" is a specialized group of cells in the ascending limb–distal tubule junction that is in contact with the glomerular arterioles. This juxtaglomerular complex is the site of renin formation and release. The distal convoluted tubule is an important point for potassium entry into the urine, particularly the more distal portions of the segment called the connecting tubule. These cells, which incidentally are embryonically derived from the ureteric bud rather than the metanephros, increase sodium chloride absorption and potassium secretion in response to aldosterone in the plasma. Potassium, chloride, and bicarbonate can also be reabsorbed at this site under certain conditions. The tubule fluid is hypo-osmolar, just as in the terminal portions of the ascending limb of Henle's loop. These cells do not appear to be responsive to the effects of antidiuretic hormone (vasopressin).

The cortical collecting tubule begins at an ill-defined point at the end of the connecting tubule and extends to the first junction with another collecting tubule. The cortical collecting tubule actively reabsorbs sodium and chloride and actively secretes potassium. Aldosterone increases the transport of these ions, as does alkalinization of the urine and high urinary concentrations of sodium.

The cortical collecting tubules are exquisitely sensitive to antidiuretic hormone. This peptide increases the hydro-osmotic movement of water from the tubule lumen to the peritubular circulation and thus initiates the concentration of urinary solutes.

Collecting ducts make up the terminal segments of the renal tubules. Sodium is reabsorbed against steep gradients. In extreme states the urinary sodium level can be lowered to less than 1 mEq/liter in these segments. Urine is also maximally concentrated in collecting ducts in response to maximal plasma levels of antidiuretic hormone. Potassium is also secreted by the collecting ducts.

It is important to recognize that sodium and water excretion can be regulated by separate mechanisms. Sodium excretion is dependent on GFR, aldosterone, and atrial natriuretic factors (and other unknown natriuretic factors).[6] The osmotic concentration of the urine depends primarily on the GFR and the plasma antidiuretic hormone level. As shown in Figure 13.2, only about 1% of the filtered sodium and water normally remain at the end of the renal tubules.

PRINCIPLES OF DIURETIC ACTION
TYPES OF DIURESIS

There are two general types of diuresis: solute and water diuresis (Fig. 13.3). Solute diuresis develops when the transtubular reabsorption of solute is impaired and the solute entering the tubule lumen by glomerular filtration is not absorbed to a normal extent. Inhibition of salt transport in the renal tubule diminishes osmotic water absorption, and a solute diuresis ensues. Salt absorption can be inhibited in two ways. First, a substance such as mannitol may be freely filtered into the urine; however, mannitol is not absorbed by tubules and the impermeant solute reduces the osmotic absorption of water.[3,7] Agents that act principally as nonabsorbable filtered solutes are known collectively as osmotic diuretics. Solute diuresis can also result from inhibition of active salt reabsorption in the tubule cell (see Fig. 13.3). Pharmacologic agents interact with the machinery of transport to slow the absorption of solute and, secondarily, the osmotic absorption of fluid. Most potent diuretic drugs interfere with solute movement across urinary plasma membranes.

Water diuresis without a corresponding increase in solute loss may be induced by pharmacologic means (see Fig. 13.3). Agents that block the cellular action of vasopressin may cause water loss without a concurrent increase in solute excretion.

CELLULAR MECHANISMS OF DIURETIC ACTION

In general, sodium and chloride enter renal cells from the urine by association with special transport proteins in the urinary membrane. The movement of these ions is dissipative, that is, down electrochemical gradients. The gradient for the entry of sodium is established at the basolateral membrane where the cation is pumped out of the cells by the sodium pump, also known as the Na^+K^+-ATPase pump. Chloride appears to move into the cell coupled to the downhill movement of sodium and leaves the cells across the basolateral membrane down an electrochemical gradient.

Diuretics act primarily from the urine side to interfere with the coupling of sodium and other solute movement from urine to cytoplasm. It is clear that the loop diuretics (furosemide, ethacrynic acid, and bumetanide) act to block sodium, potassium, and chloride cotransport (Fig. 13.4). In the cortical distal tubule and collecting tubules amiloride and triamterene inhibit sodium entry into the cells from the lumen (Fig. 13.5).

Acetazolamide does not interact with sodium directly in the lumen membrane, but this carbonic anhydrase inhibitor effectively acts from the urinary side by diminishing first the absorption of bicarbonate from the urine, and secondarily that of sodium.[3,8]

Spironolactone acts primarily from the basolateral side of the tubule cells (see Fig. 13.5). It competes with aldosterone for cellular receptors, and in this way the effect of the hormone is diminished. Aldosterone potentiates sodium absorption by increasing the movement of sodium from urine to cytoplasm and by increasing the activity of the sodium pump.

There are several interesting consequences of the site and mechanism of action of phamacologic diuretics. Since most act primarily from the urine side, they must either be filtered or secreted into the urine to be effective. Many of the drugs are highly protein bound and are not filtered appreciably. The concentration of the diuretics in the urine by the combined processes of water absorption and tubular diuretic secretion leads to relatively high levels in the tubule fluid. This feature accounts for the apparent selective action within the kidney that spares other organs from the effects of the agents.

Recent work has revealed a powerful endogenous diuretic synthesized and stored in the atria of humans and other animals. This new diuretic is referred to as atrial natriuretic factor, cardionatrin, or atriopeptin, depending on the laboratory of record.[6] It is a polypeptide substance that is released from the atria in response to extracellular fluid volume expansion. The atrial factor decreases intrarenal vascular resistance and increases GFR. In addition, the peptide may decrease tubular sodium chloride reabsorption in the medullary collecting duct[9] The diuresis caused by the peptide is very impressive in experimental animals. The possible role of this substance in the regulation of body salt and water balance is under intensive study.

ACTION OF DIURETICS ON NEPHRON SEGMENTS

The nephron loci at which diuretic drugs exert their major inhibitory actions on salt and water transport are shown in Figures 13.4 through 13.6.

GLOMERULUS

Heretofore, it had been impossible to separate the glomerular from the tubular effects of diuretic drugs; however, Deen and associates[10] and Savin and Terreros[11] have devised experimental techniques that allow for a direct examination of glomerular filtration. From these studies, it appears that physiologic and pharmacologic substances may alter the GFR directly by changing either the rate of renal plasma flow, by means of afferent and efferent arteriolar constriction or dilation, or by changes in the ultrafiltration coefficient (K_f) of the filtration barrier. Diuretic drugs set into motion a cascade of secondary events such as renin release and in turn generation of angiotensin, aldosterone, antidiuretic hormone, and intrarenal prostaglandins. These substances may exert significant influences on the glomerular filtration barrier. There are currently no reports to indicate that diuretics have direct effects on the hydraulic permeability of the glomerular filtration barrier.

PROXIMAL TUBULE

The proximal tubule is a segment in which diuretics of even minor action could exert profound effects on urinary salt excretion since approximately 60% of the glomerular filtrate is reabsorbed here. Mannitol and other "osmotic" agents have only a small diuretic effect in the proximal tubule, and none of the clinically useful pharmacologic agents have a detectable effect in this segment.

Other diuretics (furosemide, ethacrynic acid, thiazides) can potentially inhibit salt and water absorption proximally, but in sustained states of plasma volume contraction caused by these agents, the proximal tubules absorb proportionately *more* salt and water than normal. This paradoxic feature of many diuretics is a reflection of the so-called braking phenomenon observed with the chronic use of diuretics.

Acetazolamide causes diuresis by inhibiting the absorption of bicarbonate from the proximal tubule fluid. When bicarbonate absorption is impaired this impermeant anion obligates sodium and water to be held in the urine. Acetazolamide is the drug with the most dependable proximal site of action, but its effect leads to metabolic acidosis due to bicarbonaturia.

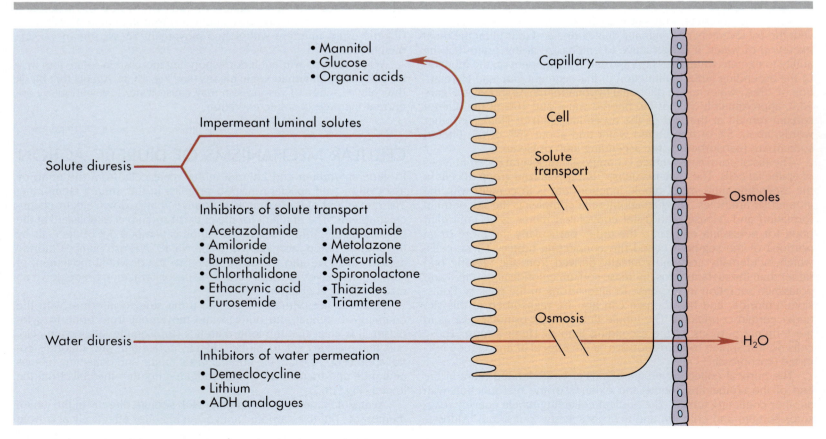

FIGURE 13.3 Principles of diuretic action. See text for details. (Modified from Grantham JJ, Chonko AM: Diuretics. In Brenner BM, Stein JH (eds): Topics in Nephrology, pp 178–209. New York, Churchill Livingstone, 1978)

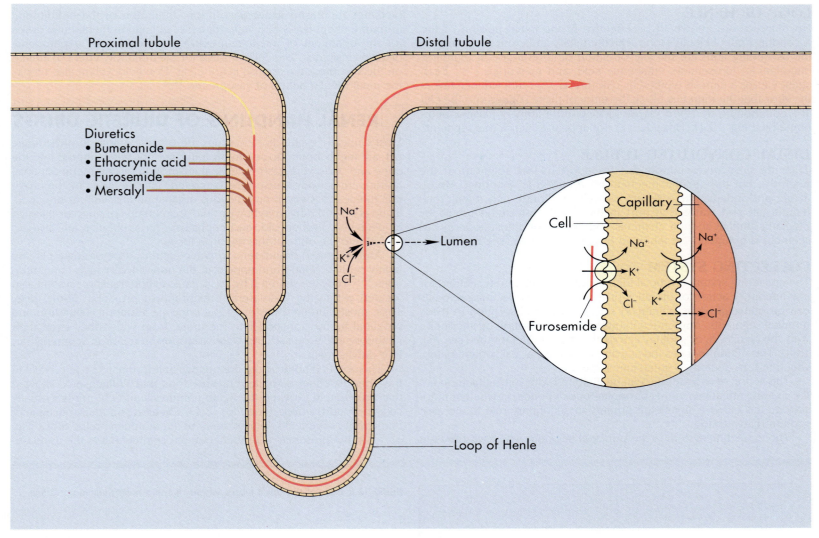

FIGURE 13.4 Mechanism of action of "loop" diuretics. The diuretics are secreted by proximal tubules and interfere with the luminal uptake of sodium, potassium, and chloride by cells of the ascending limb of Henle's loop. (Modified from Grantham JJ, Chonko AM: Diuretics. In Brenner BM, Stein JH (eds): Topics in Nephrology, pp 178–209. New York, Churchill Livingstone, 1978)

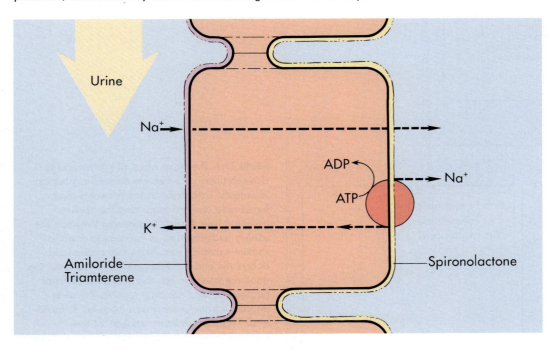

FIGURE 13.5 Mechanism of action of distal and collecting tubule diuretics. Spironolactone interferes with the effect of aldosterone to increase the rate of sodium–potassium exchange at the basolateral surface. Amiloride and triamterene interact with lumen membrane transporters to prevent the entry of urinary sodium into the cytoplasm. The net effect of all of these drugs is to decrease sodium absorption and potassium secretion.

LOOP OF HENLE

No diuretics are known to be effective in the initial portion of the ascending limb of Henle's loop. The medullary and cortical portions of the ascending limb are the site of action of several potent diuretics: bumetanide, furosemide, ethacrynic acid, and mercurials.[2,12,13] Each agent causes a diuresis typified by chloruresis. Current evidence favors the view that the diuretics block the entry of these solutes into the cell at a common co-transport carrier located at the urinary plasma membrane (see Fig. 13.4). Thiazides do not appear to act in this segment.

DISTAL CONVOLUTED TUBULE

Thiazide derivatives inhibit salt transport in this segment of the nephron, but the cellular mechanism of action is unknown. Metolazone and indapamide act here as well. Amiloride and triamterene inhibit salt and water transport in the distal convoluted tubule by blocking luminal sodium channels. The action of aldosterone in this segment is competitively inhibited by spironolactone (see Fig. 13.5).

COLLECTING SYSTEM

The collecting system is crucial in the context of all diuretic action, for any inhibitory action of diuretics proximal to the collecting segments can be outweighed by enhanced salt and water absorption in these terminal segments. Amiloride inhibits sodium absorption by interfering with the transport of sodium across the urinary membrane (see Fig. 13.5). This action reduces the activity of the basolateral sodium pump, which in turn decreases potassium secretion.

The action of aldosterone can be inhibited with spironolactone but the diuretic effectiveness of spironolactone depends on whether aldosterone has either a significant primary or secondary role to increase sodium reabsorption.

The collecting system is the principal segment where vasopressin mediates increased water absorption. Inhibition of the antidiuretic hormone effect leads to a water diuresis. Lithium in therapeutic doses for the treatment of manic-depressive illnesses causes nephrogenic diabetes insipidus. The cellular basis for the inhibitory effect of lithium on the vasopressin response is not clear. Demeclocycline also blocks the renal tubular action of vasopressin.[14,15]

RENAL HANDLING OF DIURETIC DRUGS

Most clinically useful diuretic drugs are organic anions at physiologic pH, are highly bound to serum proteins, are not freely filtered into the urine and, following gastrointestinal absorption or parenteral administration, are actively transported (secreted) into the urine by the proximal tubules.[2,16] Certain endogenous organic anions such as uric acid, lactic acid, and β-hydroxybutyric acid and certain common drugs such as penicillin, probenecid, and cephalosporin antibiotics are also secreted into the urine at this nephron locus.[17]

Amiloride and triamterene, organic cations at physiologic pH, are highly protein bound and appear in the urine in very high concentrations.[18,19] They are secreted by the organic cation transport system also located within the basolateral membrane of proximal tubule cells. Thus, most diuretic drugs enter the urine via glomerular filtration and proximal tubule transport into the urine, from which they exert their inhibitory effect on salt and water transport in nephron segments farther downstream.

The potent diuretic drugs are organic anions that must be present in the urine to effect a solute diuresis. Hook and Williamson[16] showed that probenecid blocked the acute natriuresis and chloruresis usually caused by furosemide (see Fig. 13.4). Chennavasin and colleagues[20] found that probenecid delayed entry of the diuretic into the urine (Fig. 13.7). In the presence of probenecid, furosemide enters the urine pri-

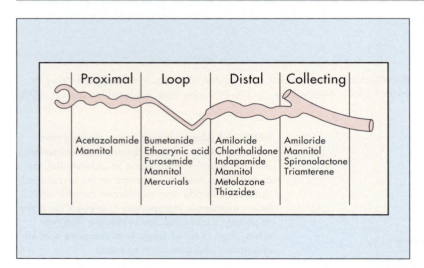

FIGURE 13.6 Sites of the renal tubule where diuretics have their major effect.

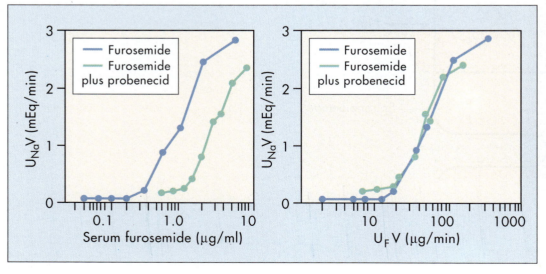

FIGURE 13.7 The acute effect of probenecid to diminish urinary furosemide excretion in human volunteers. **Left.** Relationship between serum furosemide concentrations and the sodium excretion rate. **Right.** Relationship between the urinary excretion rate of furosemide and the sodium excretion rate. Note that probenecid delays the entry of furosemide into the urine but does not interfere with the natriuretic effect of furosemide once the drug reaches the urine. (Modified from Chennavasin P, Seiwell R, Brater DC et al: Pharmacodynamic analysis of the furosemide-probenecid interaction in man. Kidney Int 16:187, 1979)

marily by filtration rather than by tubular secretion. Since furosemide is highly protein bound, glomerular filtration is a rather inefficient way to excrete the drug. Consequently, low levels of furosemide are excreted in the urine for longer periods in the presence than in the absence of probenecid. How furosemide recirculates in the renal plasma when its tubular secretion is blocked by probenecid is shown in Figure 13.8. The relatively short natriuresis and chloruresis caused by furosemide is prolonged by probenecid. Similar findings have been observed with probenecid and chlorothiazide in humans.[17,21]

Azotemic subjects are relatively resistant to diuretics. Furosemide is not excreted as promptly nor is the natriuresis as great in azotemic patients as in normal subjects, even though less of the drug is bound to plasma proteins in azotemia and a larger fraction of plasma furosemide is filtered into the urine.[22,23] The mechanism of impaired natriuresis in azotemia is unknown.

Inhibitors of prostaglandin synthesis (nonsteroidal anti-inflammatory drugs) may diminish the response to diuretics.[24,25] Indomethacin, a prototypical chemical, decreases the diuretic response to furosemide in humans without affecting the total amount or the rate of diuretic excretion in the urine. The inhibitors of prostaglandin synthesis may interfere with the tubular effects of urinary furosemide (and related "loop impairing" diuretics such as bumetamide or ethacrynic acid). Prostaglandin inhibitors also alter renal hemodynamics, and this effect may also play a role in the blunted natriuresis seen with these drugs.

RENAL COMPENSATORY RESPONSES TO DIURETICS: THE BRAKING PHENOMENON

Every perceptive clinician has noted that the diuresis induced by any drug is inherently self-limited. Diuresis sufficient to decrease the plasma volume causes the compensatory increase of solute and water absorption in portions of the nephron that are not pharmacologically inhibited by the drug. In other words, when a diuretic blocks solute and water transport across one particular nephron segment the fractional reabsorption of glomerular filtrate can increase across other segments of the nephron located proximal and/or distal to the inhibited segment.

Intrarenal adjustments in response to diuretics tend to slow down or "brake" the urinary excretion of salt. This "braking phenomenon" is illustrated schematically in Figure 13.9. A normal subject given a potent "loop diuretic" and a fixed daily salt intake quickly develops negative salt balance. During the first few days of diuretic administration body weight declines as the extracellular fluid volume decreases. After the initial diuresis the amount of salt appearing in the urine progressively diminishes so that within a few days the urinary salt losses fall to levels equal to the oral salt intake—a point of salt balance. At this point there is increased fractional reabsorption of salt in the proximal tubules and distal nephron sufficient to offset the saluretic action of the diuretic in the loop of Henle. The braking phenomenon to diminish the net excretion of salt in response to loop inhibition is mediated by increased absorption of salt proximally due to multiple factors that are operative at this nephron locus and by increased salt absorption in the distal nephron due to stimulation of aldosterone by volume contraction. The braking phenomenon conceptually appears to be the mirror image of the so-called escape phenomenon seen in patients on a high salt intake and exogenous mineralocorticoid.[3]

Recent work in normal humans has confirmed the braking phenomenon hypothesis.[26] Although furosemide is the only diuretic that has been tested experimentally in humans, it is reasonable to assume that the braking phenomenon plays a role in reestablishing salt and water balance in association with the use of most, if not all, clinically effective diuretics. The mechanism of the diuretic braking phenomenon with prolonged furosemide administration appears to be related to enhanced sodium reabsorption in the thiazide-sensitive nephron segment, most likely the distal convoluted tubule.[27]

The braking phenomenon has led to some misunderstanding among clinicians about the effectiveness of diuretics. Most clinicians judge the effectiveness of a diuretic by the volume of urine that is

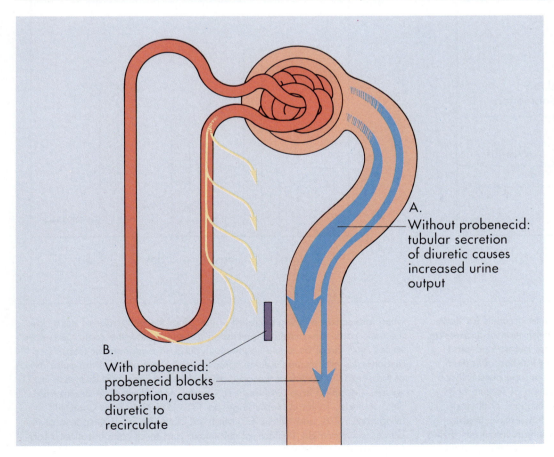

FIGURE 13.8 Schematic representation of the renal clearance of furosemide without (**A**) and with (**B**) probenecid administration. Furosemide is primarily secreted into the urine under normal conditions. When probenecid is administered, furosemide secretion is blocked and the diuretic recirculates in the plasma and enters the urine more slowly via glomerular filtration. (Modified from Chonko AM, Grantham JJ: Treatment of edema states. In Narins RG, Kleeman CR (eds): Clinical Disorders of Fluid and Electrolyte Metabolism, 4th ed. New York, McGraw-Hill, 1986)

excreted after the drug is given. If a drug is given in a dosage interval that ensures a persistent tubular effect, then the volume of urine and the amount of sodium excreted will fall to a level nearly equal to the oral intake in a few days. The patient will notice that the drug no longer causes an increase in urine formation, and the physician may conclude incorrectly that the drug is no longer effective. Very often this scenario leads to the physician choosing a drug with a short duration of action but one that causes an impressive urine response after each use. This, of course, simply leads to a "roller coaster ride" when one considers the fluctuations that will occur in the plasma volume in response to pulses of increased urine formation. The only way intermittent diuresis with a short-acting diuretic can cause persistent plasma volume contraction is for the patient to maintain a low dietary intake of sodium chloride (see Fig. 13.9).[26] Otherwise, the use of pulse doses of short-acting diuretics pleases the patient and the physician but not the cardiovascular system.

CLINICAL USE OF DIURETICS IN DISEASE STATES (TABLE 13.1)
CONGESTIVE HEART FAILURE

In congestive heart failure, it is the heart that fails not the kidneys. As shown in Figure 13.10, a failing heart has a higher left ventricular end-diastolic volume for a given ventricular performance than normal. The failure of cardiac output to increase with effort results in underperfusion of tissues, causing symptoms of increased fatigue and dyspnea on exertion. The initial response of the cardiovascular system to an added hemodynamic burden or insult to myocardial contractility is to recruit several compensatory mechanisms: an increase in catecholamine release, an increase in renal tubule sodium and water retention (designed to enhance the cardiac output via the Frank-Starling phenomenon), or development of myocardial hypertrophy. Thus, the renal response can be viewed as a protective mechanism in the course of pump failure (Figs. 13.10 and 13.11). As the cardiac output decreases, the kidney responds with increased retention of fluid. In consequence, the venous return to the heart is increased and the myocardium is stretched farther (*i.e.*, increased preload) to permit an increased stroke volume and cardiac output. Ultimately plasma volume expansion leads to pulmonary vascular congestion and translocation of fluid from the pulmonary capillaries into the alveoli (pulmonary edema).

Diuretics are beneficial by virtue of their ability to reduce both the plasma volume and the venous return to the heart (*i.e.*, decreased preload) so that the symptoms of dyspnea caused by pulmonary congestion are ameliorated. Diuretics do not necessarily improve myocardial performance by a direct mechanism (see Fig. 13.10); nevertheless, diuretics may improve myocardial performance indirectly by relieving pulmonary vascular congestion and improving blood oxygenation. Furosemide and ethacrynic acid are particularly useful in the treatment of acute pulmonary edema since these drugs cause augmented peripheral venous capacitance within minutes of intravenous administration independently of the diuretic effects of these agents (Fig. 13.12).[28,29] Diuretics may also lower arterial blood pressure and improve cardiac hemodynamics by lessening cardiac afterload. Diuretics should be used as adjunctive therapeutic agents in the treatment of chronic congestive heart failure. Therapeutic measures that directly improve myocardial performance should also be employed. Digitalis has a positive inotropic effect; vasodilators reduce left ventricular afterload and decrease pulmonary venous pressure.

Some patients with congestive heart failure appear to be refractory to the effects of furosemide. This may be due to impaired intestinal absorption, but refractoriness may be observed even when the drug is administered intravenously.[30,31] This "unresponsivity" is not due to lack of entry of furosemide into the urine; rather, the poor diuretic

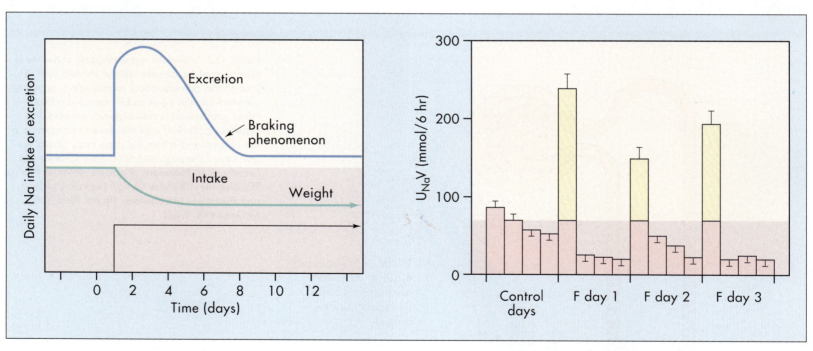

FIGURE 13.9 Illustration of the "braking phenomenon" that accounts for how salt (and fluid) balance is established during the administration of furosemide. **Left.** Relationship between sodium intake and excretion, before and after daily furosemide administration. Note that the urinary excretion of sodium exceeds dietary intake for several days during which time the person loses 1 to 2 kg of weight. After 7 to 8 days, the urinary excretion of sodium once again equals the daily intake of sodium as "hyperabsorption" of filtered sodium occurs across tubule segments not blocked by furosemide. **Right.** Relationship between sodium intake and excretion in human volunteers taking furosemide (F) and adhering to a constant intake of sodium. Note that the urine excretion of sodium exceeds intake only for several hours each day when furosemide is being excreted in the urine; the remainder of each day the urine sodium excretion is diminished to levels below the control excretory values (gray area) as tubule segments hyperabsorb glomerular filtrate in response to mild plasma volume contraction. The net effect of the pulse use of furosemide is to defeat the goal of producing a persistent decrease in ECF volume. (Modified from Grantham JJ, Chonko AM: Diuretics. In Brenner BM, Stein JH (eds): Topics in Nephrology, pp 178–209. New York, Churchill Livingstone, 1978; and Wilcox CS, Mitch WE, Kelly RA et al: Response of the kidney to furosemide: I. Effects of salt intake and renal compensation. J Lab Clin Med 102:450, 1983)

TABLE 13.1 COMPARISON OF VARIOUS DIURETICS

Drug	Protein Binding (%)	Major Excretory Routes	Normal Dose Interval (hr)	Dose Adjustment with Decrease GFR (ml/min)			Comments and Extrarenal Effects
				>50	10–50	<10	
Acetazolamide	90–95	Renal	6	6	12	Avoid	Decreases aqueous humor formation in the eye; diuresis ceases with development of metabolic acidosis
Amiloride	65–75	Renal	24	?	?	?	Blocks potassium excretion; tendency to induce hyperkalemia
Bumetanide	95–97	Renal/hepatic	6	6	Unchanged		Similar to furosemide except greater potency
Chlorthalidone	76	Renal/hepatic	24	24	24	48	Tendency for exaggerated urine potassium loss if patient fails to restrict sodium intake
Ethacrynic acid	90	Renal/hepatic	6	6	6	Avoid	Potential for ototoxicity due to effects on cochlear endolymph solute transport
Furosemide	91–99	Renal	6	6	6	6	Increases renal blood flow and increases peripheral venous capacitance
Indapamide	71–79	Renal	24	24	24	Avoid	Has direct arterial vasodilatory action
Mannitol	no	Renal	6	6	Avoid	Avoid	Avoid in renal failure
Mercurials		Renal	24	24	Avoid	Avoid	Relatively potassium sparing; replaced by newer drugs
Metolazone	95	Renal/hepatic	24	24	Unchanged		Appears to be useful when GFR < 30 ml/min
Spironolactone	98	Hepatic	6	6–12	12–24	Avoid	Blocks potassium excretion; tendency to induce hyperkalemia
Thiazides	65–95	Renal	12	12	12	Avoid	Usually not useful when GFR < 30 ml/min
Triamterene	70–80	Renal/hepatic	12	12	12	Avoid	Blocks potassium excretion; hyperkalemia; can cause nephrolithiasis; folic acid antagonist

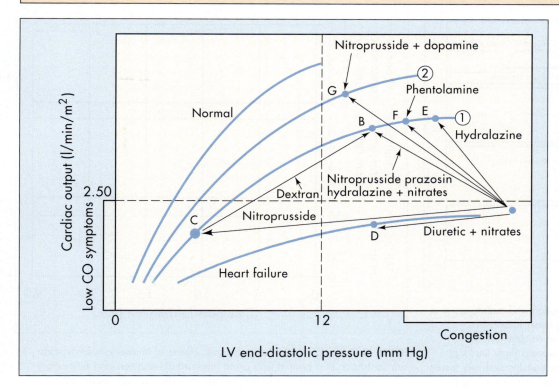

FIGURE 13.10 The relationship between cardiac output (CO) and left ventricular end-diastolic pressure (LVEDP) in a normal subject (*left curve*) and patients with congestive heart failure (*right curves*). The horizontal broken line indicates the lower limits of normal for CO and the vertical broken line indicates the upper limit of normal of LVEDP. Congestion indicates pulmonary venous congestion. Point A indicates the inefficient relationship between cardiac output and LVEDP ("cardiac preload") in a person with severe congestive heart failure. Intermediate curves (1) and (2) show the improved relationships between CO and LVEDP after administration of various vasodilator drugs such as hydralazine, nitrates plus hydralazine, prazosin, nitroprusside, and nitroprusside plus dopamine (an inotropic drug). Note that diuretic therapy alone (point D) or in combination with venodilators such as nitroglycerin relieves pulmonary venous congestion but does not usually improve the cardiac output significantly. (Modified from Mason DT, Awan NA, Joye JA et al: Treatment of acute and chronic congestive heart failure by vasodilator-afterload reduction. Arch Intern Med 140:1577, 1980)

response is more likely related to avid absorption of glomerular filtrate at nephron sites not blocked by furosemide (probably the proximal tubule and the late portions of the nephron). An inappropriate braking phenomenon is likely operative in this state (see Fig. 13.9). Although combined therapy with multiple diuretic drugs that work at several loci within the nephron (for instance combining furosemide with thiazide derivatives concomitantly blocks the loop of Henle and distal convoluted tubule) may be useful, often it is more beneficial to use vasodilator drug therapy (e.g., hydralazine) to effect an enhanced cardiac output and renal blood flow. The addition of the angiotensin-converting enzyme inhibitor captopril to the therapeutic regimen may be beneficial, but caution with this drug is indicated. Reports of a sudden fall in creatinine clearance following institution of captopril therapy in patients with bilateral renovascular disease and diffuse renal ischemia lend a cautionary note to the use of this drug in states of severe congestive heart failure.[32,33]

CIRRHOSIS AND ASCITES

Diuretics must be used cautiously to treat edema and ascites in cirrhotic patients who are highly susceptible to vascular collapse. The cornerstone of therapy is sodium restriction. Modest diuresis can be accomplished without complications in seriously ill patients with abdominal discomfort due to tense ascites. The rate of maximal ascites reabsorption is about 900 ml/day. Therefore, in patients with ascites and no peripheral edema, a diuresis that exceeds a net fluid loss of 900 ml/day may lead to rapid depletion of the plasma volume, vascular collapse, and renal hypoperfusion. Functional acute renal failure, the so-called hepatorenal syndrome, has resulted from the overaggressive use of diuretic agents in cirrhotic patients.[34,35]

Physicians favor spironolactone in the initial therapy of the cirrhotic patient who continues to accumulate ascites and edema while adhering to a sodium-restricted diet. Up to 75% of patients respond to spironolactone without other diuretic intervention.[36] Daily doses of 100 to 200 mg are usually successful with an upper limit of 400 mg/day. In refractory cases furosemide can be added in stepwise increased doses of 40 mg every 2 to 3 days, to a maximum dose of 120 mg/day.

NEPHROTIC SYNDROME

Generalized edema is a cardinal feature of the nephrotic syndrome. Intrarenal factors unrelated to the systemic development of hypoalbuminemia may contribute to enhanced salt and water retention by the kidneys.[37] Of interest, the tubule hyperabsorption of glomerular filtrate appears to take place beyond the distal convolution. Thus, there may be several mechanisms operative in the pathogenesis of avid renal salt and water retention in the nephrotic syndrome. In this condition the arterial circulation is perceived by the kidney as "ineffective," and enhanced tubule absorption of glomerular filtrate occurs even when the creatinine clearance is normal.

It appears that patients with edema formation due to nephrotic proteinuria represent a heterogeneous population in regard to the "adequacy of filling" of their plasma volumes.[38,39] In one study the relationship between plasma renin activity and urine sodium excretion in nephrotics suggested two different pathophysiologic forms.[39] One group had persistently elevated plasma renin and aldosterone levels and appeared "vasoconstricted." These persons had normal creatinine clearance rates, were normotensive, and often achieved complete remission with corticosteroid therapy. A second group had decreased plasma renin and aldosterone levels and appeared "hypervolemic." These persons had decreased creatinine clearance rates, were hypertensive, and did not respond to corticosteroids. The former, as opposed to the latter group, would probably be more prone to vascular collapse if aggressive pharmacologic diuresis were instituted.

Dietary limits are important in the management of the nephrotic syndrome. Sodium restriction, preferably to 40 to 60 mEq/day (1000

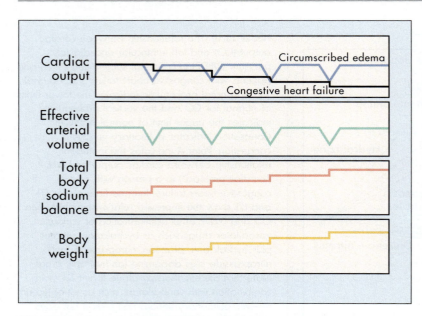

FIGURE 13.11 The authors' hypothesis for edema formation and maintenance in conditions of circumscribed edema versus congestive heart failure. In congestive heart failure (heavy line, top) a decrease in cardiac output decreases effective arterial volume; in circumscribed edema (light line, top) effective arterial volume is decreased because fluid is translocated into tissues as a result of venous or lymphatic obstruction or a local increase in capillary hydrostatic pressure. In both cases the renal response of increased sodium (and water) retention restores effective arterial volume at the expense of net increases in total body sodium and body weight. (Modified from Chonko AM, Grantham JJ: Treatment of edema states. In Narins RG, Kleeman CR (eds): Clinical Disorders of Fluid and Electrolyte Metabolism, 4th ed. New York, McGraw-Hill, 1986)

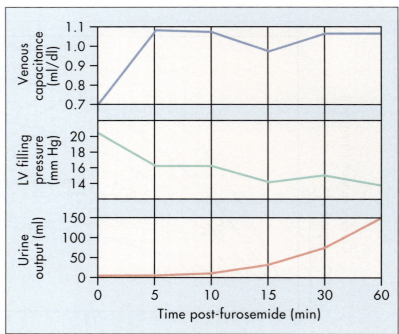

FIGURE 13.12 The beneficial hemodynamic effects of intravenous furosemide administration in a patient with acute myocardial infarction and pulmonary edema. Temporal changes in calf venous capacitance (top), mean left ventricular filling pressure (middle), and urine output (bottom) are illustrated. Note that the decrease in left ventricular filling pressure and the simultaneous increase in calf venous capacitance preceded significant increased urine output during the initial 15-minute interval after furosemide. (Modified from Dikshit K, Vyden JK, Forrester JS et al: Renal and extrarenal hemodynamic effects of furosemide in congestive heart failure after acute myocardial infarction. N Engl J Med 288:1087, 1971)

mg to 1500 mg), is effective in arresting or slowing the rate of edema formation in most persons and, in conjunction with cautious use of diuretics, can often lead to resolution of edema. Protein supplementation to intakes of 2 to 3 g/kg/day, particularly with proteins of high biologic quality (*i.e.*, rich in essential amino acids), can induce a positive nitrogen balance and support hepatic albumin synthesis. As an initial diuretic, a thiazide is a safe choice. If the edema is massive and resistant to therapy, and the patient does not have a symptomatic reduction in plasma volume, bumetanide, furosemide, or ethacrynic acid may be substituted or added to the thiazide. In hypokalemic patients, amiloride, triamterene, or spironolactone may be added to the diuretic regimen.

Some nephrotics are resistant to the effects of potent diuretic drugs. The natriuretic response to appropriate urinary levels of furosemide may be reduced in comparison to normal persons. An exaggerated braking phenomenon probably accounts for the hyperabsorption of glomerular filtrate across noninhibited portions of the nephron.

In refractory patients, combination therapy with metolazone and spironolactone has been useful.[40] Infusion of colloid ("salt-poor" albumin) in combination with diuretic agents is beneficial in mobilizing huge collections of edema. Unfortunately, such measures provide only temporary benefit since the infused protein is rapidly lost into the urine.

IDIOPATHIC EDEMA

Idiopathic edema is a common disorder of women characterized by cyclical episodes of sodium retention and edema formation in the absence of cardiac, endocrine, hepatic, or renal disease.[41,42] The etiology of this disorder remains unclear. Exaggerated orthostatic pooling of blood, exaggerated renal response to estrogen or to sympathetic nerve discharge, hypoalbuminemia, or alteration in peripheral capillary permeability have each been proposed to explain the tendency to retain salt. It has been suggested that the major cause of idiopathic edema is prolonged use of diuretics (and perhaps laxatives).[43,44] The intermittent use of potent loop-acting diuretics in the setting of wide variations in daily sodium, water, and carbohydrate intake may be particularly responsible. Many women with idiopathic edema appear to be extraordinarily conscious of their appearance and exhibit a dietary pattern of intermittent "starvation" followed by salt and carbohydrate "refeeding"; this sequence of events is known to precipitate the renal retention of sodium and water. The initial edema formation in this syndrome may be "refeeding" edema, which then is exacerbated by diuretic intake. In patients who have intermittent reductions in potassium intake and continue to take diuretic drugs chronically, potassium depletion may develop. Potassium depletion can potentiate the common clinical symptoms of this syndrome, which include weakness, malaise, irritability, abdominal bloating, and increased thirst. Idiopathic edema may be treated most effectively by withdrawing all diuretics and instituting a moderate dietary sodium and water restriction (87 mEq sodium and 1500 ml water per day). Dietary counseling to avoid a pattern of intermittent starvation and gluttony and the institution of an exercise program (daily swimming or bicycling) are also important therapeutic measures. Patients who stop diuretics and follow the dietary restrictions but do not become edema free within 4 weeks should be reexamined for the presence of occult thyroid or cardiac disease. Cautious use of angiotensin–converting enzyme inhibitors has been associated with weight loss and symptomatic improvement in patients with idiopathic edema.[45]

ESSENTIAL HYPERTENSION

Diuretics are useful drugs for the treatment of hypertension.[46,47] The major mechanism by which diuretics lower the mean arterial blood pressure in patients with hypertension is related to the contraction of the extracellular fluid volume induced by these drugs, particularly when the patient adheres to a sodium-restricted diet (about 2 g of sodium or 87 mEq of sodium per day).[46,47] It is common for persons to lose 1 to 2 liters of extracellular fluid (about 300 ml of plasma) in response to the start of therapy with a thiazide diuretic. Of interest, the patient's peripheral vascular resistance often rises in response to the initial plasma volume depletion. However, a major decrease in venous return to the heart (decreased preload) leads to a decreased cardiac output such that the net effect of the diuretic therapy is to lower the net product of cardiac output and the peripheral vascular resistance, the mean arterial blood pressure.

It appears that over the long term, continued diuretic therapy in conjunction with moderate dietary salt restriction produces a favorable readjustment in the basic hemodynamic relationships in persons with hypertension; namely, the peripheral resistance falls and the cardiac output rises, but the former more so than the latter so that the arterial blood pressure falls toward the normal range. The mechanisms responsible for the significant fall in peripheral vascular resistance induced in patients who take diuretic drugs for several months remains to be elucidated. Several hypotheses have been advanced, including readjustment of baroreceptor sensitivity, depletion of sodium from critical peripheral vascular receptor sites for endogenous vasopressors, such as angiotensin II and norepinephrine, and redistribution of calcium ions to critical intracellular sites within vascular smooth muscle cells.[48] There is little evidence in support of the notion that thiazide or loop diuretics have direct vasodilatory actions on the peripheral arterial vasculature. For instance, the blood pressure does not fall in nephrectomized patients taking thiazide or loop diuretics who are maintained on dialysis. An exception to this rule is indapamide, a new thiazide derivative that clearly possesses direct arteriolar vasodilating properties.[49]

We favor the use of long-acting thiazide (or related) diuretics to reduce elevated blood pressure unless the patient's GFR is below 40 to 50 ml/min, a point where a "loop diuretic" is indicated in order to induce and maintain a diuresis. Shorter-acting "loop diuretics" are potent agents, but they are excreted rapidly from the body and produce a sawtoothed pattern of natriuresis and antinatriuresis as the braking phenomenon supervenes in persons with a normal GFR. A long-acting diuretic such as trichlormethiazide or metolazone can be taken once per day, which enhances patient compliance and provides a smoother course of natriuresis and diuresis since the drug is slowly excreted into the urine over the course of the day.

Another potential benefit of thiazide diuretics in hypertensive patients relates to their effect to lower the urine calcium level and place the patient in a favorable calcium balance provided that calcium intake is adequate (800 to 1000 mg/day). Resnick and co-workers[50] and McCarron[51] have found that certain populations with "essential hypertension," particularly black persons and elderly persons, may ingest lower amounts of calcium in their diets and have lower amounts of serum ionized calcium (and presumably intracellular calcium) than nonhypertensive age-matched controls. Thiazide diuretics may be particularly useful as therapy for hypertension in these persons owing to the anticalciuric effects of these agents. Since loop diuretics such as bumetanide, ethacrynic acid, and furosemide all enhance calciuria, it may not be wise to use these diuretics as first-step agents for the treatment of hypertension, particularly if the patient has a normal GFR.

Since potent diuretics can cause renal magnesium and potassium wasting and induce carbohydrate intolerance and hyperlipidemia, some investigators have questioned whether diuretic drugs should be instituted as first-step therapy for patients with mild or borderline hypertension (systolic BP 140–150 mm Hg and diastolic BP 90–100 mm Hg), particularly since these patients often respond to monotherapy with β- or α-adrenergic blocking drugs, angiotensin–converting enzyme inhibitors or calcium channel blocking drugs that do not cause kaliuresis or magnesiuresis (and may not cause hyperlipidemia as consistently as potent diuretics).[52,53] However, persons who do not favorably respond to monotherapy with adrenergic blockade (*i.e.*, do not normalize their blood pressure) can be given diuretics as a second step since subtle plasma volume expansion often occurs with the adrenergic blockers and negates their antihypertensive effects.[53] Direct vasodilators such as hydralazine and minoxidil consistently induce renal salt retention and necessitate the addition of a diuretic drug in order to maintain blood pressure control.[54]

Recent concerns about the unfavorable impact of left ventricular cardiac hypertrophy on the survival of patients with essential hypertension has led to a further reevaluation of the general use of diuretic drugs as first-line therapy for all patients with hypertension. Diuretic drugs in general (with the possible exception of indapamide) do not show a beneficial effect to reverse left ventricular cardiac hypertrophy in clinical trials and animal experiments despite their beneficial effects on arterial blood pressure reduction. In contrast, calcium channel blockers, angiotensin–converting enzyme inhibitors, and centrally acting adrenergic inhibitors (α-methyldopa having been the first drug to display this property) have been shown to reverse left ventricular hypertrophy in clinical trials and animal experiments. These latter drugs may offer an important advantage over diuretics in the treatment of the patient with hypertension and left ventricular cardiac hypertrophy.[55-57]

CLINICAL COMPLICATIONS OF DIURETIC DRUGS (TABLE 13.2)

An understanding of the braking phenomenon is important when one considers the clinical complications commonly induced by diuretic drugs. Many of these complications derive from the increased absorption of glomerular filtrate mediated by plasma volume contraction in portions of the nephron not affected directly by the diuretic. The absorption of most filtered solutes is affected by the state of expansion or contraction of the extracellular fluid (ECF) volume. Therefore, most of the important complications of diuretics can be explained within the framework of our understanding of segmental nephron absorptive characteristics.

ECF volume depletion is a common complication of the potent loop-acting diuretics.[3-5] Patients are protected to some extent against ECF volume depletion by the braking phenomenon. Those patients most prone to develop ECF volume depletion have gastrointestinal tract complications such as nausea, vomiting, or diarrhea and are unable to ingest appropriate amounts of salt and water to correct the major portion of the ongoing daily urinary losses. In patients with underlying renal insufficiency, ECF volume depletion can lead to the development of overt uremia, although in many persons a picture of prerenal azotemia results.

Recent experiments in rodents indicate that 30% to 60% of the elevated plasma urea concentration that occurs in the animal during diuretic induced sodium depletion is accounted for by an enhanced urea appearance rate. Thus, both plasma volume contraction and enhanced urea production combine to produce a "prerenal" azotemic picture in patients who are too vigorously treated with diuretic drugs.[58]

ECF volume contraction is important in maintaining another complication of diuretic treatment, the genesis and maintenance of metabolic alkalosis. Both ECF volume depletion and the metabolic alkalosis respond to replenishment of the ECF with isotonic saline and/or discontinuation or dose reduction of the diuretic drugs.

Potassium depletion has received extensive attention in the recent medical literature.[59-65] Some investigators believe that concern about this complication is exaggerated.[61,62] Certainly severe potassium depletion may cause malfunction of other organ systems, including cardiac muscle irritability, particularly in conjunction with digitalis therapy[66]; decreased striated muscle blood flow and predisposition to rhabdomyolysis[67]; and sluggish pancreatic insulin release and carbohydrate intolerance.[68] Inhibition of potassium absorption in the proximal tubule may contribute to urinary potassium loss, but most diuretics promote urinary potassium loss by an indirect action on the distal convoluted and cortical collecting tubules. Urinary potassium secretion is strongly dependent on the rate of urine flow, high levels of sodium in the final urine, high levels of impermeant anions in urine (*i.e.*, carbenicillin), and elevated plasma levels of aldosterone.

In patients taking diuretics, exaggerated kaliuresis usually does not occur if an appropriate decrease in volume of the ECF compartment is achieved. Urinary potassium loss and potassium depletion are most pronounced in those patients who take diuretics and ingest large loads of solute and water! In these patients supplemental intake of potassium chloride may be necessary, although restriction of dietary sodium intake (about 87 mEq/day) is the most appropriate way to abolish excessive urinary potassium wasting.

Spironolactone, triamterene, and amiloride block potassium secretion in the distal and collecting tubules. These agents are effective when used in combination with the more potent agents that act in the loop of Henle and distal tubule in order to reduce the urinary loss of potassium.[69] Antikaliuretic drugs should not be used routinely in patients with renal insufficiency since life-threatening hyperkalemia and metabolic acidosis may develop.[70,71]

Metabolic alkalosis is often seen in the setting of total body potassium depletion during the use of diuretics.[72,73] Potassium depletion causes increased secretion of hydrogen ion by renal tubules together with an increased excretion of ammonium as the chloride salt. Consequently, for each equivalent of ammonium excreted one equivalent of bicarbonate is "generated" for the plasma compartment in place of chloride. Owing to contraction of the ECF volume the metabolic alkalosis is "maintained" by increased reabsorption of sodium bicarbonate. "Contraction" metabolic alkalosis can also result from the intense renal loss of sodium chloride caused by potent loop diuretics. In most cases of diuretic-induced metabolic alkalosis, reduction of the dose of diuretic will correct the alkalosis, although potassium supplementation in excess of normal dietary intake is sometimes required.[74]

Hyponatremia is seen relatively frequently in patients taking diuretics. Fichman and co-workers[75] studied ten patients with severe, symptomatic hyponatremia due to thiazides. All of the patients were potassium depleted. The plasma antidiuretic hormone activity was paradoxically elevated, and this may have contributed to the hyponatremic state.

Diuretics active in the ascending loop of Henle impair the generation of dilute urine by blocking sodium chloride absorption. Hyponatremia develops in patients who drink water at a rate faster than the ascending limb can generate dilute urine. Potent loop diuretics also cause contraction of the extracellular fluid compartment and the release of antidiuretic hormone to further the development of hyponatremia.[76]

Captopril, an oral drug that inhibits the enzyme responsible for the conversion of angiotensin I to angiotensin II, has been shown to correct the hypotonic, hyponatremic state that often develops in patients with severe congestive heart failure who require potent diuretic ther-

TABLE 13.2 COMPLICATIONS OF DIURETIC THERAPY

Fluid, Electrolyte, and Acid–Base Disorders
    Extracellular fluid volume depletion
    Potassium depletion
    Metabolic alkalosis
    Hyponatremia
    Hypercalcemia
    Metabolic acidosis
Metabolic Disorders
    Hyperuricemia
    Hyperglycemia
    Hyperlipidemia
    Gynecomastia/sexual dysfunction
    Osteomalacia
Toxic Disorders
    Ototoxicity
    Hypersensitivity

apy.[77,78] A combination of captopril and furosemide was superior to either drug used alone for the production of a sustained diuresis, which led to a rise in the serum sodium concentration in most patients.

Most diuretics acutely increase the renal excretion of calcium, phosphorus, and magnesium. In general, the increased rate of elimination reflects the natriuretic or chloruretic potency of the particular diuretic. The chronic administration of diuretics causes the calciuria and phosphaturia to return to (or fall below) the control values. There have been no reports of sustained diuretic-induced phosphaturia or calciuria that have resulted in overt phosphate or calcium depletion syndromes. On the contrary, long-term thiazide administration may lead to overt hypercalcemia.[79] Thus, it would seem that compensatory mechanisms, perhaps related to increased proximal tubule reabsorption due to ECF volume contraction, may counteract the acute phosphaturic and calciuric effects of certain diuretics.

There are a few important exceptions to these general rules. Thiazide diuretics decrease calcium excretion with acute and chronic use by augmenting calcium reabsorption in the distal tubule.[80,81] This property of the thiazides is central to their use in the treatment of calcium renal lithiasis.[82,83] By contrast, furosemide and ethacrynic acid increase calcium excretion on acute and chronic administration and are useful in the treatment of acute hypercalcemic conditions. Since overt calcium depletion has not resulted with long-term therapy with these drugs, it is likely that extrarenal mechanisms such as increased gastrointestinal calcium absorption must compensate for the increased calcium losses into the urine. When using furosemide to induce calciuresis in the treatment of hypercalcemia, isotonic saline solution must be given in generous amounts to match or slightly exceed the urine loss of sodium chloride.[84]

Thiazides and furosemide chronically increase renal magnesium wasting; however, the long-term consequences of this effect remain uncertain. Some investigators suggest that occult magnesium depletion accounts for a significant percentage of diuretic-related cardiac arrhythmias.[66]

Metabolic acidosis may occur as a complication of acetazolamide or spironolactone therapy. Acetazolamide induces renal sodium bicarbonate wasting, which halts when the plasma bicarbonate level falls to 18 to 19 mEq/liter. Amiloride, spironolactone, and triamterene may also produce hyperchloremic metabolic acidosis.[70,71] The elevated potassium levels reduce ammonia extraction by renal tubules and decrease net ammonium chloride excretion into the urine. Reducing body potassium stores (with polystyrene sulfonate resin [Kayexalate] may improve the acidosis.[88]

Hyperuricemia is common in patients treated with diuretics. Plasma uric acid is filtered by the glomeruli. Uric acid also enters the urine by secretion in proximal tubules. Urinary uric acid is also reabsorbed by these same proximal segments and in the last analysis an amount of uric acid equal to 8% to 12% of the filtered uric acid appears normally in the final urine.[17] The renal excretion of uric acid is decreased by plasma volume contraction and increased by plasma volume expansion. Diuretics elevate plasma uric acid levels by increasing tubular reabsorption of the anion in consequence of plasma volume contraction. Simultaneous replacement of urinary salt losses during the administration of a diuretic prevents the fall in uric acid clearance that occurs when volume contraction is allowed to develop, proving that the hyperuricemia is secondary to ECF volume contraction.[86]

Reduction in diuretic dose often corrects the hyperuricemia. However, such a reduction in dose may not be feasible in certain patients with avid salt retention. We find that addition of a uricosuric drug, such as probenecid, is beneficial since the diuretic effect is delayed when probenecid diminishes the rapid excretion of the diuretic into the urine (see Figs. 13.7 and 13.8). Both the natriuretic effect of the diuretic and the uricosuric effect of the probenecid are preserved when these drugs are administered together. An alternative strategy is to use the xanthine oxidase inhibitor allopurinol to reduce the plasma uric acid level. Because this drug may cause hepatitis, exfoliative dermatitis, and cataracts, it seems prudent to use allopurinol only in those patients with gouty arthritis or nephropathy. Sustained plasma uric acid elevations up to 10 mg/dl have no apparent deleterious effects on renal function[87]; however, levels higher than this may warrant treatment, particularly if the GFR is greater than 50 ml/min.

Hyperglycemia has been reported with the use of chlorothiazide, furosemide, and ethacrynic acid.[88-90] The mechanism(s) by which the thiazide derivatives and the loop of Henle agents induce glucose intolerance remains controversial, but potassium loss may be the most important factor relating the development of overt glucose intolerance with the use of potent diuretic drugs. Long-term studies of nondiabetic hypertensive patients taking diuretics indicate that less than 5% have overt glucose intolerance.[91] There may be more risk of decreasing glucose control, however, in insulin-dependent diabetics who require potent diuretics to control hypertension or edema formation. Hyperglycemia has not been reported with use of potassium-sparing diuretics.

During the past few years several investigators have found that glucose intolerance and/or hyperinsulinemia are commonly present in persons with high blood pressure.[92,93] More recently, it has also been demonstrated that resistance to insulin-stimulated glucose uptake is present in patients with hypertension. Moreover, hypertensive persons treated with hydrochlorothiazide, in contrast to those treated with the angiotensin–converting enzyme inhibitor captopril, had increased basal insulin concentration and an enhanced late insulin response to a glucose challenge.[94] Hydrochlorothiazide therapy was also associated with an adverse effect on blood lipids, whereas captopril therapy was not found to adversely affect blood lipids in the short term. These findings have led several investigators to recommend that diuretics be used in low dose for the treatment of hypertension.[95]

Hyperlipidemia is observed with the use of diuretics. Grimm and associates[96] reported that hydrochlorothiazide or chlorthalidone increased plasma total cholesterol, very low density and low density lipoprotein cholesterol, and plasma triglyceride concentrations, with triglyceride concentrations showing the largest increase. High-density lipoprotein cholesterol remained stable during thiazide diuretic treatment. Although the magnitude of the increase in plasma lipid content appears to be related to the dose of the thiazide diuretic drugs, the mechanism responsible for the increased lipid levels remains unclear. Furosemide and spironolactone administered under similar conditions also increase serum cholesterol and triglyceride levels.[97] The clinical significance of these observations remains controversial at present. Indapamide does not alter lipids in an unfavorable manner.[98]

Gynecomastia, irregular menses, and impotence have been associated with the use of spironolactone.

Ototoxicity has been reported following use of furosemide and ethacrynic acid; reversible hearing loss associated with high-dose therapy has been reported in patients with renal insufficiency.[99]

Hypersensitivity reactions also have been reported with diuretic drug use, particularly the thiazides and furosemide. These reactions include rash, leukopenia, thrombocytopenia, necrotizing vasculitis, and acute hypersensitivity pneumonitis. The common ground for these reactions may be the presence of sulfur within the ring structure of the thiazides and furosemide. Amiloride, triamterene, and ethacrynic acid do not contain sulfur and can be substituted for the former drugs when an idiosyncratic reaction develops.

Transient hemodynamic deterioration in chronic heart failure has been reported following intravenous administration of furosemide in patients with chronic heart failure.[100] An increase in mean arterial pressure, systemic vascular resistance, and left ventricular filling pressure, along with decreased cardiac output, were observed. The precise mechanism for this transient increase in left ventricular outflow resistance, which causes worsening of left ventricular pump function, remains unclear; however, there was evidence for activation of the neurohumoral axis as plasma renin activity, plasma norepinephrine, and arginine vasopressin levels increased concomitantly. Further studies will be required to delineate the clinical relevance of these hemodynamic and neurohumoral changes following intravenous administration of furosemide in patients with severe chronic heart failure.

REFERENCES

1. Sullivan LP, Grantham JJ: Physiology of the Kidney, 2nd ed. Philadelphia, Lea & Febiger, 1982
2. Chonko AM, Grantham JJ: The use of the isolated tubule preparation for the investigation of diuretics. In Martinez-Maldonado M (ed): Methods in Pharmacology, pp 47–71. New York, Plenum Press, 1976
3. Grantham JJ, Chonko AM: Diuretics. In Brenner BM, Stein JH (eds): Topics in Nephrology, pp 178–209. New York, Churchill Livingstone, 1978
4. Chonko AM, Grantham JJ: Treatment of edema states. In Narins RG, Kleeman CR (eds): Clinical Disorders of Fluid and Electrolyte Metabolism, 4th ed. New York, McGraw-Hill, 1986
5. Suki WN, Ng RCK: Renal actions and uses of diuretics. In Massry SG, Glassock RJ (eds): Textbook of Nephrology, vol 1. Baltimore, Williams & Wilkins, 1983
6. Grantham JJ, Edwards RM: Natriuretic hormones: At last, bottled in bond? J Lab Clin Med 103:333, 1984
7. Gennari FJ, Kassirer JP: Osmotic diuresis. N Engl J Med 291:714, 1974
8. Maren TH: Use of inhibitors in physiological studies of carbonic anhydrase. Am J Physiol 232:F291, 1977
9. Sonnenberg H, Honrath U, Chong CK, Wilson DR: Atrial natriuretic factor inhibits sodium transport in medullary collecting duct. Am J Physiol 250:F963, 1986
10. Deen WM, Troy JL, Robertson CR et al: Dynamics of glomerular ultrafiltration in the rat: IV. Determination of the ultrafiltration coefficient. J Clin Invest 52:1500, 1973
11. Savin VJ, Terreros DA: Filtration in single isolated mammalian glomeruli. Kidney Int 20:188, 1981
12. Burg M, Stoner L, Cardinal J et al: Furosemide effect on isolated perfused tubules. Am J Physiol 225:119, 1973
13. Koechel DA: Ethacrynic acid and related diuretics: Relationship of structure to beneficial and detrimental actions. Ann Rev Pharmacol Toxicol 21:265, 1981
14. Cherrill DA, Stote RM, Birge JR et al: Demeclocycline treatment in the syndrome of inappropriate antidiuretic hormone secretion. Ann Intern Med 83:654, 1975
15. Singer I, Forrest JN Jr: Drug-induced states of nephrogenic diabetes insipidus. Kidney Int 10:82, 1976
16. Hook JB, Williamson HE: Influence of probenecid and alterations in acid-base balance of the saluretic activity of furosemide. J Pharmacol Exp Ther 149:404, 1965
17. Chonko AM, Grantham JJ: Renal handling of organic anions and cations; metabolism and excretion of uric acid. In Brenner BM, Rector FC (eds): The Kidney, 3rd ed, pp 663–703. Philadelphia, WB Saunders, 1986
18. Baer JE, Jones CB, Spitzer SA et al: The potassium-sparing and natriuretic activity of N-amidino-3,5-diamino-6-chloropyrazine-carboxamide hydrochloride dihydrate (amiloride hydrochloride). J Pharmacol 157:472, 1967
19. Gussin RZ: Potassium-sparing diuretics. J Clin Pharmacol 17:651, 1977
20. Chennavasin P, Seiwell R, Brater DC et al: Pharmacodynamic analysis of the furosemide-probenecid interaction in man. Kidney Int 16:187, 1979
21. Brater DC: Increase in diuretic effect of chlorothiazide by probenecid. Clin Pharmacol Ther 23:259, 1978
22. Porter RD, Cathcart-Rake WF, Wan SH et al: Secretory activity and aryl acid content of serum, urine, and cerebrospinal fluid in normal and uremic man. J Lab Clin Med 85:723, 1975
23. Rose HJ, Pruitt AW, McNay JL: Depression of renal clearance of furosemide in man by azotemia. Clin Pharmacol Ther 21:141, 1976
24. Brater DC: Analysis of the effect of indomethacin on the response to furosemide in man: Effect of dose of furosemide. J Pharmacol Exp Ther 201:386, 1978
25. Chennavasin P, Seiwell R, Brater DC: Pharmacokinetic-dynamic analysis of the indomethacin–furosemide interaction in man. J Pharmacol Exp Ther 215:77, 1980
26. Wilcox CS, Mitch WE, Kelly RA et al: Response of the kidney to furosemide: I. Effects of salt intake and renal compensation. J Lab Clin Med 102:450, 1983
27. Loon NR, Wilcox CS, Unwin RJ: Mechanism of impaired natriuretic response to furosemide during prolonged therapy. Kidney Int 36:682, 1989
28. Dikshit K, Vyden JK, Forrester JS et al: Renal and extrarenal hemodynamic effects of furosemide in congestive heart failure after acute myocardial infarction. N Engl J Med 288:1087, 1971
29. Schuster C-J, Weil MH, Besso J et al: Blood volume following diuresis induced by furosemide. Am J Med 76:585, 1984
30. Brater DC, Chennavasin P, Seiwell R et al: Furosemide in patients with heart failure: Shift in dose-response curves. Clin Pharmacol Ther 28:182, 1980
31. Brater DC, Day B, Burdette A et al: Bumetanide and furosemide in heart failure. Kidney Int 26:183, 1984
32. Edwards RM: Segmental effects of norepinephrine and angiotensin II on isolated renal microvessels. Am J Physiol 244:F526, 1983
33. Hricik DE, Browning PJ, Kopelman R et al: Captopril-induced functional renal insufficiency in patients with bilateral renal-artery stenoses or renal-artery stenosis in a solitary kidney. N Engl J Med 308:373, 1983
34. Shear L, Kleinerman J, Gabuzda GJ: Renal failure in patients with cirrhosis of the liver: I. Clinical and pathologic characteristics. Am J Med 39:184, 1965
35. Shear L, Ching S, Gabuzda GJ: Compartmentalization of ascites and edema in patients with hepatic cirrhosis. N Engl J Med 282:1391, 1970
36. Eggert RC: Spironolactone diuresis in patients with cirrhosis and ascites. Br Med J 4:401, 1970
37. Ichikawa I, Rennke HG, Hoyer JR et al: Role for intrarenal mechanisms in the impaired salt excretion of experimental nephrotic syndrome. J Clin Invest 71:91, 1983
38. Chonko AM, Bay WH, Stein JH et al: The role of renin and aldosterone in the salt retention of edema. Am J Med 63:881, 1977
39. Meltzer JI, Keim HJ, Laragh JH et al: Nephrotic syndrome: Vasoconstriction and hypervolemic types indicated by renin-sodium profiling. Ann Intern Med 91:688, 1979
40. Lang GR, Westenfelder C, Nascimento L et al: Metolazone and spironolactone in cirrhosis and the nephrotic syndrome. Clin Pharmacol Ther 21:234, 1976
41. Edwards OM, Bayliss RIS: Idiopathic edema of women. Q J Med 177:125, 1976
42. Ferris TF, Bay WH: Idiopathic edema. In Brenner BM, Stein JH (eds): Sodium and Water Homeostasis, pp. 131–153. New York, Churchill Livingstone, 1978
43. MacGregor GA, Tasker PRW, deWardener HE: Diuretic-induced edema. Lancet 1:489, 1975
44. deWardener HE: Idiopathic edema: Role of diuretic abuse. Kidney Int 19:881, 1981
45. Docci D, Turci F, Salvi G: Therapeutic response of idiopathic edema to captopril. Nephron 34:198, 1983
46. Mroczek WJ, Davidov M, Finnerty FA Jr: Large dose furosemide therapy of hypertension: Long-term use in 22 patients. Am J Cardiol 33:546, 1974
47. Gifford RW Jr: The role of diuretics in the treatment of hypertension. Am J Med 77:102, 1984
48. Kaplan NM: The therapy of hypertension. In Clinical Hypertension, 4th ed, pp. 187–204. Baltimore, Williams & Wilkins, 1986
49. Noveck RJ, McMahon FG, Quiros A et al: Extrarenal contributions to indapamide's antihypertensive mechanism of action. Am Heart J 106:221, 1983
50. Resnick LM, Laragh JH, Sealey JE et al: Divalent cations in essential hypertension. N Engl J Med 309:888, 1983
51. McCarron DA: Calcium and magnesium nutrition in human hypertension. Ann Intern Med 98:800, 1983
52. Kaplan NM: New approaches to the therapy of mild hypertension. Am J Cardiol 51:621, 1983
53. The 1988 Report of the Joint National Committee on Detection, Evaluation, and Treatment of High Blood Pressure. The Joint Committee on Detection, Evaluation, and Treatment of High Blood Pressure. Arch Intern Med 148:1023, 1988
54. Koch-Weser J: Vasodilator drugs in the treatment of hypertension. Arch Intern Med 148:1023, 1988
55. Mace PJE, Littler WA, Glover DR et al: Regression of left ventricular hypertrophy in hypertension: Comparative effects of three different drugs. J Cardiovasc Pharmacol 7(2):S52, 1985
56. Frohlich ED: Reversal of target-organ involvement in systemic hypertension: A pharmacologic expeience. Am J Cardiol 60:31, 1987
57. Messerli FH, Nunez BD, Nunez MN et al: Hypertension and sudden death. Arch Intern Med 149:1263, 1989
58. Kamm DE, Wu L, Kuchmy BL: Contribution of the urea appearance rate to diuretic-induced azotemia in the rat. Kidney Int 32:47, 1987
59. Morgan DB, Davidson C: Hypokalaemia and diuretics: An analysis of publications. Br Med J 280:905, 1980
60. Holland OB, Nixon JV, Kuhnert L: Diuretic-induced ventricular ectopic activity. Am J Med 70:762, 1981
61. Harrington JT, Isner JM, Kassirer JP: Our national obsession with potassium. Am J Med 73:155, 1982
62. Freis ED: Critique of the clinical importance of diuretic-induced hypokalemia and elevated cholesterol level. Arch Intern Med 149:2640, 1989
63. Struthers AD, Whitesmith R, Reid JL: Prior thiazide diuretic treatment increases adrenaline-induced hypokalaemia. Lancet 1:1358, 1983
64. Kaplan NM: Our appropriate concern about hypokalemia. Am J Med 77:1, 1984
65. Knochel JP: Diuretic-induced hypokalemia. Am J Med 77:18, 1984
66. Hollifield JW: Potassium and magnesium abnormalities: Diuretics and arrhythmias in hypertension. Am J Med 77:28, 1984
67. Knochel JP, Schlein EM: On the mechanism of rhabdomyolysis in potassium depletion. J Clin Invest 51:1750, 1972
68. Fajans S, Floyd JC, Knopf RF et al: Benzothiadiazine suppression of insulin release from normal and abnormal islet cell tissue in man. J Clin Invest 45:481, 1966
69. Schnaper HW, Freis ED, Friedman RG et al: Potassium restoration in hypertensive patients made hypokalemic by hydrochlorothiazide. Arch Intern Med 149:2677, 1989
70. Gabow PA, Moore S, Schrier RW: Spironolactone-induced hyperchloremic acidosis in cirrhosis. Ann Intern Med 90:338, 1979
71. Greenblatt DJ, Koch-Weser J: Adverse reactions to spironolactone. JAMA 225:40, 1973
72. Seldin DW, Rector FC Jr: The generation and maintenance of metabolic

alkalosis. Kidney Int 1:306, 1972
73. Kurtzman NA, White MG, Rogers PW: Pathophysiology of metabolic alkalosis. Arch Intern Med 131:702, 1973
74. Garella S: Saline-resistant metabolic alkalosis or "chloride-wasting nephropathy." Ann Intern Med 73:31, 1970
75. Fichman MP, Vorherr H, Kleeman CR et al: Diuretic-induced hyponatremia. Ann Intern Med 75:853, 1971
76. Ashraf N, Locksley R, Arieff AI: Thiazide-induced hyponatremia associated with death or neurologic damage in outpatients. Am J Med 70:1163, 1981
77. Dzau VJ, Hollenberg NK: Renal response to captopril in severe heart failure: Role of furosemide in natriuresis and reversal of hyponatremia. Ann Intern Med 100:777, 1984
78. Packer M, Medina N, Yushak M: Correction of dilutional hyponatremia in severe chronic heart failure by converting-enzyme inhibition. Ann Intern Med 100:782, 1984
79. Higgins BA, Nassim JR, Collins J et al: The effect of bendrofluazide on urine calcium excretion. Clin Sci 27:457, 1964
80. Breslau N, Moses AM, Weiner IM: The role of volume contraction in the hypocalciuric action of chlorothiazide. Kidney Int 10:164, 1976
81. Costanzo LS, Windhager EE: Calcium and sodium transport by the distal convoluted tubule of the rat. Am J Physiol 235:F492, 1978
82. Yendt ER, Gagne RJA, Cohanim M: The effects of thiazides in idiopathic hypercalciuria. Am J Med Sci 251:449, 1966
83. Yendt ER, Guay GF, Garcia DA: The use of thiazides in the prevention of renal calculi. Can Med Assoc J 102:614, 1970
84. Suki WN, Yium JJ, VonMinden M et al: Acute treatment of hypercalcemia with furosemide. N Engl J Med 283:836, 1970
85. Szylman P, Better OS, Chaimowitz C et al: Role of hyperkalemia in the metabolic acidosis of isolated hypoaldosteronism. N Engl J Med 294:361, 1976
86. Steele TH, Oppenheimer S: Factors affecting urate excretion following diuretic administration in man. Am J Med 47:564, 1969
87. Berger L, Yu T: Renal function in gout: IV. An analysis of 524 gouty subjects including long-term follow-up studies. Am J Med 59:605, 1975
88. Wilkins RW: New drugs for the treatment of hypertension. Ann Intern Med 50:1, 1959
89. Wolff FW, Parmley WW, White K et al: Drug-induced diabetes. JAMA 185:568, 1963
90. Weller JM, Borondy M: Effect of furosemide on glucose metabolism. Metabolism 16:532, 1967
91. Berglund G, Andersson O: Beta blockers or diuretics in hypertension? A six year follow-up of blood pressure and metabolic side-effects. Lancet 1:744, 1971
92. Ferrannini E, Buzzigoli G, Bonadonna R et al: Insulin resistance in essential hypertension. N Engl J Med 317:350, 1987
93. Swislocki ALM, Hoffman BB, Reaven GM: Insulin resistance, glucose intolerance and hyperinsulinemia in patients with hypertension. Am J Hypertens 2:419, 1989
94. Pollare T, Lithell H, Berne C: A comparison of the effects of hydrochlorothiazide and captopril on glucose and lipid metabolism in patients with hypertension. N Engl J Med 321:868, 1989
95. Kaplan N: How bad are diuretic-induced hypokalemia and hypercholesterolemia? Arch Intern Med 149:109, 1989
96. Grimm RH, Leon AS, Hunninghake DB et al: Effects of thiazide diuretics on plasma lipids and lipoproteins in mildly hypertensive patients. Ann Intern Med 94:7, 1981
97. Ames RP: The influence of non-beta-blocking drugs on the lipid profile: Are diuretics outclassed as initial therapy for hypertension? Am Heart J 114:998, 1987
98. Meyer-Sabellek W, Gotzen R, Heitz J et al: Serum lipoprotein levels during long-term treatment of hypertension with indapamide. Hypertension 7:170, 1985
99. David DS, Hitzig P: Diuretics and ototoxicity. N Engl J Med 284:1328, 1971
100. Francis GS, Siegel RM, Goldsmith SR et al: Acute constrictor response to intravenous furosemide in patients with chronic congestive heart failure. Ann Intern Med 103:1, 1985

DIGITALIS, CATECHOLAMINES, AND OTHER POSITIVE INOTROPIC AGENTS

Kanu Chatterjee

It is now generally agreed that augmented contractility usually results from the increased availability of intracellular free calcium to the myocardial contractile proteins. Increased sensitivity of the filaments to calcium may also be associated with enhanced contractile force. The number of crossbridges formed between actin and myosin myofilaments appears to determine the amount of force developed during contraction. A regulating protein, tropomyosin, normally prevents interaction of actin and myosin. Binding of calcium to the subunit, troponin C of another regulatory protein, troponin, allows interaction of the myofilaments by reversing the inhibiting action of tropomyosin. The magnitude of developed force appears to depend on the number of troponin C subunits of troponin bound to calcium, which, in turn, is related to the intracellular free calcium concentration.[1-3]

Although the precise mechanism of increased intracellular calcium concentration necessary for increased contractility has not been totally clarified, it appears that a number of different mechanisms can enhance calcium concentration.[4] A transient increase in intracellular sodium is associated with increased calcium entry or calcium retention through the sodium–calcium exchange mechanism. Increased intracellular sodium concentration may result from inhibition of sodium efflux or enhanced sodium influx through the fast sodium channel. Higher extracellular concentration may promote calcium influx across the sarcolemmal membrane and enhance contractility. Increased calcium influx via the slow (calcium) channel, or due to increased sarcolemmal permeability to calcium, may also increase intracellular calcium concentration. Cytosolic calcium content may also increase from an augmented release of calcium from the sarcoplasmic reticulum or decreased calcium uptake by the sarcoplasmic reticulum.

Myocardial cyclic AMP (adenosine 3'5'-cyclic monophosphate) exerts an important regulatory influence on intracellular calcium concentration and contractile state. Cyclic AMP production is mediated by the membrane-bound enzyme adenylate cyclase, the activity of which is regulated by both stimulatory and inhibitory protein subunits.[5] The mechanism of action of the various agonists of the surface receptors to activate the adenylate cyclase appears to be mediated through these regulatory subunits.

Increased intracellular cyclic AMP content is associated with increased activation of the cyclic AMP–dependent protein kinase, which catalyzes the phosphorylation of proteins that regulate calcium fluxes across the sarcolemma, apparently through the slow calcium channels.[6] An increased release of calcium from the sarcoplasmic reticulum and augmented reuptake and storage of calcium in the sarcoplasmic reticulum may also occur as a result of increased intracellular cyclic AMP concentration.[7] Calcium flux into or out of the sarcoplasmic reticulum is partly mediated by the phosphorylation of a protein, phospholamban, which appears to regulate an adenosine triphosphate (ATP)–dependent calcium pump in the sarcoplasmic reticulum.[8]

Increased cyclic AMP concentration may also result from its decreased degradation, which is primarily mediated by the enzyme phosphodiesterase.[9] Thus, inhibition of the activity of phosphodiesterase enhances cyclic AMP content, which in turn is associated with increased intracellular calcium concentration. Furthermore, the inhibition of phosphoprotein phosphatase necessary for dephosphorylation of the phosphorylated proteins may produce similar effects to those of increased cyclic AMP.[10]

Although an increase in intracellular calcium content is the final mechanism for a positive inotropic effect of most pharmacologic agents, evidence exists that enhanced contractility may also occur from the increased sensitivity of contractile elements to calcium, without an increase in intracellular concentration. The classification of inotropic drugs based on the potential mechanisms as proposed by Katz[4] is shown in Table 14.1.

DIGITALIS GLYCOSIDES

In 1785, William Withering, in his accounts of foxglove, reported the beneficial effects of digitalis in dropsy, although apparently he did not recognize that dropsy might have resulted from heart failure.[11] In 1911, McKenzie observed that digitalis can slow the ventricular response in the presence of atrial fibrillation.[12] Thus, the potential beneficial cardiovascular effects of digitalis have long been acknowledged. However, the drug's physiologic and pharmacologic effects, and its pharmacokinetics and potential clinical applications, have only recently been elucidated.

PHARMACOLOGY

A number of cardiac glycosides are presently in clinical use. Digitoxin, gitalin, and digitalis are derived from the leaves of the foxglove plant (*Digitalis purpurea*); digoxin, lanatoside C, and deslanoside from *Digitalis lanata;* and ouabain from seeds of *Strophanthus gratus*. Presently, however, digoxin is the most commonly used cardiac glycoside.

Cardiac glycosides combine a steroid nucleus with an unsaturated lactose ring at the 17 position with a series of sugars attached to carbon 3 of the nucleus (Fig. 14.1).[13] The steroid and lactose part without the sugars, which appears essential for the activity, is called genin or aglycone. The sugar molecules influence the pharmacokinetic properties, including absorption, half-life, and metabolism.

DIGOXIN

Digoxin (12-hydroxydigitoxin) is relatively well absorbed from the gastrointestinal tract. However, its absorption may be influenced by a number of factors. Altered gastrointestinal motility due to foods or drugs may cause variable absorption. In general, decreased motility is associated with enhanced absorption, and increased motility with reduced absorption. Concurrent administration of nonabsorbable substances, such as cholestyramine, colestipol, kaolin, pectin, and antacids, retards absorption of digoxin from the gastrointestinal tract.[14] Antacids containing magnesium trisilicate may bind digoxin and prevent its absorption. Sulfasalazine and neomycin also interfere with the absorption of digoxin. Absorption of digoxin is passive and primarily occurs in the small intestine and colon; minimal absorption has been observed in the stomach.[15] Cardiac glycosides with a greater number of hydroxyl groups are less well absorbed.[16] Hydrolysis of digoxin and its derivatives is nearly complete at a pH of 1, but these drugs are stable above pH 3. Digoxin may, therefore, be hydrolyzed to a considerable extent into its active and inactive metabolites in patients with peptic ulcer with high gastric acidity and markedly delayed gastric emptying.

Although decreased plasma digoxin levels following oral administration have occasionally been observed in patients with congestive heart failure,[17] pharmacokinetic studies with the use of tritiated digoxin have failed to demonstrate any decrease in bioavailability and absorption of digoxin solution or digoxin tablets, even in patients with severe right-sided heart failure.[18] No significant differences in the plasma concentration curves were observed either before or after treatment of severe right-sided heart failure, suggesting that absorption of digoxin is not retarded in the presence of congestive heart failure.

Different preparations of digoxin tablets were reported to have dis-

TABLE 14.1 CLASSIFICATION OF INOTROPIC DRUGS BASED ON THEIR MECHANISM OF ACTION

Drugs That Increase Cytosolic Calcium
Drugs that, by increasing intracellular sodium, promote calcium entry or retention by sodium/calcium exchange.
    Drugs that inhibit sodium efflux (digitalis)
    Drugs that promote sodium influx via the fast (sodium) channel (veratrum alkaloids)
Drugs that directly increase calcium influx across the sarcolemma
    Drugs that increase extracellular calcium (parathyroid hormone)
    Drugs that promote calcium influx via the slow channel (calcium) (Bay-K-8644, possibly α-adrenergic agonists)
    Drugs that increase sarcolemmal calcium permeability (ionophores, e.g., A23187)
Drugs that inhibit calcium efflux across the sarcolemma (hypothetical)
Drugs that increase the movement of calcium from the sarcoplasmic reticulum into the cytosol
    Drugs that increase calcium efflux from the sarcoplasmic reticulum
    Drugs that decrease calcium uptake from the sarcoplasmic reticulum

Drugs That Increase Cyclic AMP Levels
Drugs that increase cyclic AMP production (β-adrenergic agonists, glucagon)
Drugs that decrease cyclic AMP breakdown (methylxanthines, bipyridines)

Drugs That Modify Myofibrillar Proteins
Drugs that increase calcium sensitivity of the contractile proteins (AR-L 115 BS, possibly α-adrenergic agonists)
Drugs that modify myosin isozyme composition (thyroxine)

(Reproduced by permission from Katz AM: Discussion section. Article by Endoh M, Yanagisawa T, Taira N, Blinks JR: Effects of new inotropic agents on cyclic nucleotide metabolism and calcium transients in canine ventricular muscle. Circulation 73(Suppl III):III-117, 1986)

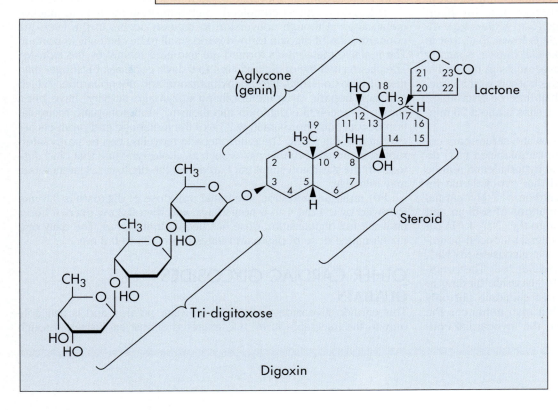

FIGURE 14.1 Structure of digoxin (glycoside). (Modified from Katzung BG, Parmley WW: Cardiac glycosides and the drugs used in treatment of congestive heart failure. In Katzung BG (ed): Basic and Clinical Pharmacology, p 144. Los Altos, CA, Lange Publications, 1984)

similar bioavailability (the percentage of orally administered drug entering the systemic circulation unaltered).[19] Dissolution rate of digoxin appears to be the major determinant of bioavailability. Digoxin solution (elixir) is better absorbed than tablets. However, digoxin tablets with a dissolution rate of greater than 65% have an absorption equivalent to that of oral solution.[20] The bioavailability of the presently available digoxin tablets is more predictable, due to the Food and Drug Administration's implementation of minimal dissolution rates of 55% or greater at 1 hour. The new gelatin capsule of digoxin (Lanoxicaps) increases bioavailability to 90% to 95%.[21] The absolute bioavailability is the percentage of the unchanged drug that is absorbed after oral administration, compared with the same dose of the drug administered intravenously. The average absolute bioavailability of digoxin tablets appears to be between 60% and 80%. With absorption of 70%, a 0.5-mg oral dose of digoxin is equivalent to 0.35 mg of digoxin given intravenously. This ratio of 1.5 to 1 between oral and intravenous digoxin is similar to that reported after biologic titration.[22]

Clinical response is an important consideration in determining the dose and route of administration in individual patients. In addition, abnormalities in absorption and concomitant drug therapy should be taken into account during oral digoxin therapy. Absorption characteristics of digoxin in patients with malabsorption syndromes have not been clarified. It appears, however, that when the dissolution rate of digoxin at 1 hour is high (greater than 65%), absorption of digoxin is adequate even in the presence of malabsorption states.[23]

Digoxin can be detected in plasma within 30 minutes following oral administration, but the peak levels occur between 30 and 60 minutes and a plateau is observed within 6 hours.[24] When digoxin tablets are given after meals, the peak plasma concentrations occur approximately 45 minutes later without significantly affecting the total bioavailability or the peak concentrations. When digoxin is administered in solution, absorption is not affected by food.[25] After intravenous injection, the pharmacologic effects of digoxin occur within 15 to 30 minutes and reach a peak within 1 to 5 hours.[26]

Digoxin is not extensively metabolized in humans. After absorption, digoxin is bound to plasma proteins to only a modest extent (approximately 25% or less). Plasma protein binding is even less in the presence of renal impairment.[27] Tissue proteins also bind digoxin; the concentration of the glycoside in human cardiac tissue may be as high as 30 times that in the plasma.[26] The plasma-to-myocardial ratio is remarkably constant; thus, the pharmacodynamic effects can generally be predicted from the serum concentrations. Digoxin is also readily bound to skeletal muscle, but adipose tissue contains little digoxin. Thus, lean body weight provides a more appropriate basis for determining its volume of distribution, which is large (5 to 8 liters/kg). Although digoxin concentration in skeletal muscle is lower than that in kidney or heart, the total digoxin content of skeletal muscle is significantly greater because of its proportionately larger mass in the body.

The time course of digoxin distribution in the body is well characterized by a two-compartment model.[28] The half-time of distribution from the vascular compartment to the peripheral sites is about 30 minutes.

Myocardial uptake of digoxin is influenced by the serum concentrations of sodium and potassium. Studies with radiolabeled (^{3}H) digoxin have demonstrated that hyponatremia and hyperkalemia reduce the myocardial concentration of digoxin and that hypokalemia increases the digoxin concentration in the myocardium.[29,30] Myocardial uptake during alterations in the serum concentrations of sodium and potassium correlates with the binding of digoxin to the (Na^+, K^+)ATPase and provides an explanation for the hypokalemia-induced potentiation of digitalis toxicity. The binding of digitalis glycoside to (Na^+, K^+)ATPase in intact cells is stimulated by intracellular Na^+. The conditions that enhance sodium influx also promote glycoside binding to (Na^+, K^+)ATPase. Concomitant administration of quinidine not only increases the serum digoxin concentration but also enhances the myocardial concentration of digoxin; however, the myocardial concentration of digoxin remains proportional to the serum digoxin concentrations.[31]

Digoxin is eliminated primarily by renal excretion; 60% to 90% of the administered dose is excreted unchanged in the urine and only a small fraction (15%–20%) appears in the stool. Renal elimination of digoxin is primarily by glomerular filtration, although the saturable tubular secretion process also contributes.[32] That digoxin serum levels may rise when tubular secretion is blocked by concomitant administration of spironolactone has been demonstrated.[22] The rate of digoxin excretion appears to be independent of the route of administration. The elimination half-life of digoxin in healthy persons with normal renal function is approximately 36 hours. Tubular reabsorption of digoxin has also been demonstrated. Tubular reabsorption can reduce renal clearance of digoxin in patients with cardiovascular disorders and prerenal azotemia.[27] Intestinal reabsorption of digoxin via the enterohepatic circulation is limited and represents approximately 6.5% of the administered dose.[33]

To initiate digitalization, an initial loading dose of 0.5 to 0.75 mg can be administered; this is followed by 0.25 to 0.5 mg at 6-hour intervals until digitalization is achieved. When *rapid digitalization* is required, digoxin is administered intravenously, with an initial 0.5- to 1.0-mg dose followed by 0.25 to 0.5 mg at 6-hour intervals until digitalization is achieved. If rapid digitalization is not required, one does not need to administer a loading dose; daily oral administration of 0.25 to 0.5 mg of digoxin produces digitalization of most adult patients within 7 to 10 days. The usual oral maintenance dose is 0.125 to 0.25 mg daily; however, the dose needs to be adjusted according to renal function. When gelatin capsules (Lanoxicaps) are used, rapid digitalization can be obtained by administering 0.4 mg orally initially, then four doses of 0.2 mg every 4 hours, not exceeding a total of 1.6 mg. For slow digitalization, 0.1 to 0.4 mg is administered daily for 7 days. The oral maintenance dose of gelatin capsules is 0.1 to 0.2 mg daily.

DIGITOXIN

Digitoxin is almost completely absorbed from the gastrointestinal tract. Since it is less polar than other glycosides, binding to plasma proteins is very high and almost 97% of digitoxin is bound to plasma albumin.[34] Consequently, the renal clearance of digitoxin is lower and the half-life of elimination of digitoxin (4–6 days) is very little influenced by renal function. Displacement of digitoxin from its binding sites with plasma proteins can occur with the concomitant use of a number of drugs[35]; however, the clinical relevance of such interactions remains unclear.

Digitoxin is almost completely metabolized in the liver to inactive metabolites. Although conversion to digoxin occurs in the liver, the concentration of digoxin formed is too small to be clinically important. The inactive metabolites formed are excreted mainly by the kidneys. The plasma half-life of digitoxin is 4 to 6 days, considerably longer than that of digoxin. Drugs like phenylbutazone and phenobarbital, which enhance hepatic drug-metabolizing enzymatic activity, have been shown to accelerate digitoxin metabolism.[36] Enterohepatic recirculation occurs and approximately 25% of the metabolic end-products are excreted in the feces. The enterohepatic recycling can be partly interrupted by nonabsorbable resins such as cholestyramine that bind digitoxin in the gastrointestinal tract, and thus the digitoxin clearance rate may increase.

For rapid digitalization, the initial oral dose of digitoxin is 0.6 mg, followed by 0.4 mg 4 to 6 hours later, and then 0.2 mg every 6 hours until the full digitalization dose has been administered. The daily oral maintenance dose of digitoxin ranges from 0.05 to 0.2 mg.

OTHER CARDIAC GLYCOSIDES
OUABAIN
This cardiac glycoside possesses very high polarity and is available only in the injectable form. It is excreted almost exclusively through

the kidney. The onset of action is within 5 to 10 minutes, and the peak effect is observed within 30 minutes to 2 hours. The plasma half-life is approximately 21 hours when renal function is normal; impaired renal function, however, will retard the excretion of ouabain. When very rapid pharmacohemodynamic effects are desired, ouabain is used occasionally in preference to other glycosides. The digitalizing dose is between 0.25 and 0.5 mg.

DESLANOSIDE

Deslanoside (Cedilanid-D) is structurally similar to digoxin, but its gastrointestinal absorption is unreliable and less than that of digoxin because of additional glucose residue attached to the terminal sugar. The onset of action when the drug is administered intravenously is within 10 to 30 minutes, and the peak effect tends to occur within 1 to 2 hours. Renal excretion is the principal means of elimination, and the plasma half-life is approximately 36 hours. Elimination of deslanoside is also influenced by renal function; slower elimination occurs with depressed renal function. Clinical use of deslanoside is extremely limited except for occasional emergency digitalization, when it can be administered intravenously in two doses of 0.6 to 0.8 mg each.

The pharmacokinetics of the cardiac glycosides are summarized in Table 14.2.

MECHANISMS OF ACTION OF CARDIAC GLYCOSIDES: POSITIVE INOTROPIC EFFECT

An increase in the amount of intracellular calcium available to react with the contractile proteins appears to be essential for the positive inotropic effect of the cardiotonic digitalis glycosides. However, the precise mechanism governing the increased availability of intracellular calcium still remains controversial. Using the photoactive calcium-sensitive protein, aequorin, an increase in the intracellular calcium transient, in response to acetylstrophanthidin, has been demonstrated.[37] It is generally accepted that the cardiac glycosides interact with the (Na^+, K^+)ATPase and that this enzyme represents the receptor for the cardiac glycosides; however, subsequent mechanisms for raising the intracellular calcium level are still in question. Various potential reactions that might contribute to increased intracellular calcium are illustrated in Figure 14.2.[13] Inhibition of (Na^+, K^+)ATPase may reduce the transport of sodium out of the cell (1, Fig. 14.2), resulting in an increase in

TABLE 14.2 THE PHARMACOKINETIC VALUES, DIGITALIZING AND MAINTENANCE DOSES OF CARDIAC GLYCOSIDES

	Digoxin	Digitoxin	Ouabain	Deslanoside
Gastrointestinal absorption	60%–85%	90%–100%	Unreliable	Unreliable
Onset of action	15–30 min	½–2 hr	5–10 min	10–30 min
Peak effect	1–5 hr	4–12 hr	½–2 hr	1–2 hr
Plasma half-life	36 hr	5–7 days	21 hr	36 hr
Plasma concentration (ng/ml)				
Therapeutic	0.8–1.6	14–26		
Toxic	>2.4	>34		
Principal elimination route	Renal	Hepatic–renal	Renal	Renal
Total digitalizing dose (mg)				
Oral	1.0–1.5	1.3–1.6		
Intravenous	0.75–1.5	1.2–1.6	0.25–0.5	1.2–1.6
Daily oral maintenance dose (mg)	0.125–0.5	0.05–0.2		

(Modified from Moe GK, Farah AE: Digitalis and allied cardiac glycosides. In Goodman LS, Gilman A (eds): The Pharmacological Basis of Therapeutics, 5th ed, p 653. New York, Macmillan, 1975)

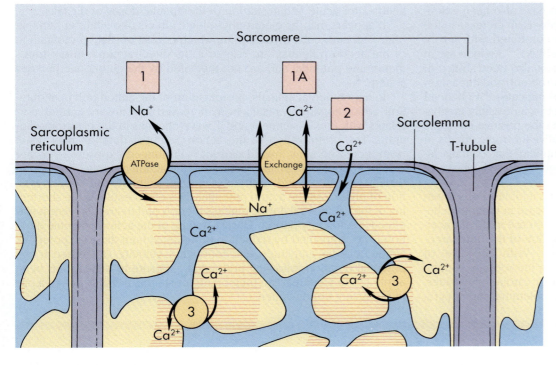

FIGURE 14.2 Schematic diagram to illustrate the possible sites of action of digitalis. The potential mechanisms are inhibition of sodium pump (1) and activation of the Na^+/Ca^{2+} exchanger (1a). It may also act on the ionic channel permeable to calcium (2) and the sarcoplasmic reticulum (SR; 3). (Modified from Katzung BG, Parmley WW: Cardiac glycosides and the other drugs used in the treatment of congestive heart failure. In Katzung BG (ed): Basic and Clinical Pharmacology, p 145. Los Altos, CA, Lange Publications, 1984)

intracellular sodium. This increase in sodium may retard the normal release of calcium from the cell via the Na^+/Ca^{2+} exchange mechanism (*1a*, Fig. 14.2), which results in an increase in intracellular calcium. Facilitation of the entry of calcium into the cell through the voltage-dependent calcium channel during the plateau phase of the action potential is another possibility (*2*, Fig. 14.2). A third potential mechanism for increased intracellular calcium is the enhanced release of stored calcium from the sarcoplasmic reticulum (*3*, Fig. 14.2). Substantial evidence now exists for the inhibition by cardiac glycosides of the sarcolemmal sodium pump, the magnesium (Mg^{2+}) and ATP-dependent, sodium- and potassium-activated transport enzyme complex, known as $(Na^+, K^+)ATPase$.[30] The effects on the sodium pump of therapeutic doses of cardiac glycosides, which only increased contractility without inducing toxic arrhythmias, were evaluated by measuring isotonic fluxes.[29,30] The uptake of the K^+ analog, rubidium-86 ($^{86}Rb^+$), as a measure of monovalent cation transport, was determined in the myocardial biopsy specimens before and after administration of cardiac glycosides. Contractile state was assessed by measuring the maximum rise of left ventricular pressure at the onset of systole left ventricular maximal rate of rise of pressure ($LVdP/dt_{max}$), which increased by 29% ± 3% after the administration of a subtoxic dose of ouabain. It was accompanied by a 21% ± 6% reduction of $^{86}Rb^+$ uptake (sodium pump inhibition). Toxic doses of digoxin caused a greater reduction of rubidium uptake, by 59%, at the onset of digoxin-toxic arrhythmias. The relative sensitivities of canine Purkinje fibers and myocardial cells to inhibition of the sodium pump after acute toxic doses of digoxin have been evaluated.[30] At the onset of overt toxicity, the reduction in $^{86}Rb^+$ uptake in myocardial tissue was 44% ± 0%, and in Purkinje fibers 76% ± 3%, suggesting a greater inhibition of the sodium pump by digoxin in Purkinje fibers. Studies using synchronously beating monolayers of cultured chick embryo ventricular cells have demonstrated sodium pump inhibition by cardiac glycosides.[30] Inhibition of $^{42}K^+$ or $^{86}Rb^+$ uptake associated with inhibition of sodium efflux was observed concurrently with an increase in inotropy, following exposure to ouabain. It has been suggested that mechanisms other than sodium pump inhibition may be involved in producing the positive inotropic effects of cardiac glycosides at low doses.[38–40] Indeed, with a very low dose of ouabain, positive inotropic effects associated with stimulation of the sodium pump have been observed.[38] It has been suggested that a stimulatory effect on the sodium pump is mediated by endogenous catecholamines.[30] Ouabain increases endogenous norepinephrine release in perfused organ preparations,[41] and with low concentrations it inhibits norepinephrine reuptake in guinea pig myocardium.[42] Sodium pump stimulation, as evidenced by rubidium uptake, is not observed in the presence of propranolol.

The potential mechanisms for increased intracellular calcium concentration following inhibition of sodium pump have also been extensively investigated. Most studies indicate that there is an increase in the "rapidly exchangeable calcium pool," often combined with an increase in both calcium "influx" and calcium "efflux."[30] An increase in the intracellular calcium transient by digitalis has also been shown in studies using the aequorin method,[37,43] microelectrode measurements,[44,45] and the intracellular calcium optical indicator.[46] Enhanced inward calcium current via the calcium channels is a potential mechanism for the increased intracellular calcium and the positive inotropic effect. However, such mechanisms for the positive inotropic effects of digitalis have not been established. It does appear that digitalis increases intracellular calcium directly or through increased release of catecholamines.[47–49]

Considerable evidence now suggests that the inhibition of sodium transport out of the cells, associated with an increase in the intracellular sodium concentration, causes a secondary increase in the intracellular pool. This apparently is mediated by activation of the transsarcolemmal sodium–calcium exchange system. With the use of sodium-sensitive microelectrodes, an increase in intracellular sodium concentration has been reported in response to cardiac glycosides, which increased contractility.[44,50,51] The transsarcolemmal sodium gradient has marked effects on the rapidly exchangeable component of the intracellular calcium pool.[29,30] Thus, it appears that the positive inotropic effects of cardiac glycosides are related to the inhibition of the sodium pump, which causes a transient increase in intracellular sodium.[52] The increase in intracellular sodium results in enhanced calcium exchange, leading to a positive inotropic effect. However, other mechanisms such as increased release or decreased uptake of endogenous norepinephrine might also be contributory.

ELECTROPHYSIOLOGIC EFFECTS

The electrophysiologic effects of digitalis have been reviewed in a number of recent publications.[29,30,53–56] Digitalis exerts its electrophysiologic effects directly, as well as through interaction with the autonomic nervous system. Direct actions initially cause a prolongation of the cellular action potential, with an increase in membrane resistance. This is followed by a period of shortening of the action potential, accompanied by a decrease in membrane resistance, probably due to increased intracellular calcium, which increases membrane potassium conductance. Reduction of the action potential duration may contribute to the shortening of atrial and ventricular refractoriness.

Indirect actions of cardiac glycosides on the cardiac conduction system appears to be mediated through the autonomic nervous system. In patients with heart failure, digitalis occasionally slows the sinus rate, presumably because of decreased sympathetic tone resulting from improved cardiac function. In the absence of heart failure, however, digitalis usually does not produce any change or may even cause a slight increase in the sinus rate. Therapeutic doses of digitalis appear to exert a predominant vagotonic effect on the atrial myocardium and specialized conduction tissues.[30,57] In the intact animal with preserved autonomic function, these indirect cholinergic effects are manifested by abbreviation of the atrial refractory period and enhanced conduction.[48] In conscious humans, however, no change, or even an increase in atrial refractory period, has been observed following intravenous administration of digitalis.[57] Atrial conduction velocity may not change or may not even increase.

Reduction of atrioventricular (AV) nodal conduction is one of the major therapeutic effects of digitalis. In both experimental animals and in human subjects, digitalis decreases AV nodal conduction and prolongs the nodal effective refractory period. AV nodal effects of digitalis appear to result primarily from its cholinergic and antiadrenergic actions, although a slight direct depression of the AV nodal conduction has been demonstrated in transplanted denervated hearts.[58] However, neither a significant reduction in conduction nor an increase in refractoriness of the AV node occur after vagal blockade or in transplanted hearts after acute administration of therapeutic doses of digitalis.

It appears that the electrophysiologic effects of digitalis in Purkinje fiber and ventricular myocardium, which consist of slight prolongation of the action potential, are related to its direct actions on the transmembrane potential and are not mediated by the autonomic nervous system.[30]

In experimental animals, prolongation of the action potential duration, which apparently results from increased slow inward current, correlates with the ST segment and T wave changes in the electrocardiogram. The prolongation of the action potential duration may result from increased slow inward current.[58] Prolonged exposure to higher concentrations of digitalis may shorten the action potential duration of the Purkinje fibers and ventricular muscle, primarily due to abbreviation of phase 2 of the action potential. This effect explains the shortening of the QT interval during digitalis therapy and decreased ventricular effective refractory period. The shortening of the action potential duration is accompanied by reduction of the maximum diastolic potential, action potential amplitude, and conduction velocity. Decreased action potential duration following prolonged exposure to digitalis has been attributed to a decrease in membrane resistance, possibly due to a rise in potassium conductance.

INTERACTION WITH THE AUTONOMIC NERVOUS SYSTEM

With the therapeutic concentrations of digitalis, the predominant effect is activation of the parasympathetic nervous system, and with toxic concentrations there also may be stimulation of the sympathetic system. Digitalis may increase vagal activity by several mechanisms. The therapeutic concentration of digitalis can modify the activity of the arterial baroreceptors, the cardiopulmonary receptors, the efferent vagal nerve pathways, and the end-organ responses to vagal stimulation.[56] Digitalis can activate arterial baroreceptors and chemoreceptors and other afferent nerve fibers in the nodose ganglion. Experiments using isolated carotid sinus or aortic arch and monitoring changes in hemodynamic and electrical activity have indicated that digitalis causes excitation of baroreceptors in the carotid sinus and aortic arch. Direct application of digitalis to the epicardium or selective injection into the left anterior descending coronary artery causes hypotension and bradycardia. In normal subjects, decreases in forearm blood flow and increases in forearm vascular resistance in response to lower body negative pressure were significantly greater after administration of lanatoside C, suggesting that digitalis augmented the tonic inhibitory influence of the cardiopulmonary receptors.[59] Thus, it appeared that digitalis sensitizes baroreceptors and cardiopulmonary receptors so that the afferent input to the central nervous system is enhanced. This results in increased vagal activity and possibly withdrawal of sympathetic activity.

Digitalis also influences the effects of the sympathetic nervous system. However, higher concentrations of digitalis are required to produce sympathetic effects than parasympathetic effects. Various experiments have shown that with high concentrations of digitalis in the brain, the efferent sympathetic outflow is increased.[49] A relatively large concentration of digitalis can induce neuronal release of catecholamines and prevent catecholamine reuptake. These peripheral effects and effects on the central nervous system may result in increased cardiac and systemic sympathetic tone.

The interactions of digitalis with the autonomic nervous system are important in determining its clinical effects. With therapeutic levels of digitalis, parasympathetic effects dominate; with larger toxic concentrations, sympathetic effects may be manifest.

Enhanced parasympathetic activity can potentially produce negative inotropic effects and decrease the cardiac response to its direct positive inotropic effects. Furthermore, the magnitude of increase in cardiac output due to the positive inotropic effects may be curtailed due to a concomitant reduction in heart rate. In patients with heart failure, vagal tone is reduced and the sympathetic tone is enhanced. Thus, direct actions of digitalis may be more prominent in the presence of heart failure. Reduction of the ventricular response in atrial flutter or fibrillation results primarily from its parasympathetic nervous system-mediated effects on the AV node. Conversion of supraventricular tachycardia to sinus rhythm by digitalis alone is in some instances most likely related to its vagotonic effect. The electrophysiologic effects of digitalis are influenced by end-organ autonomic tone. In patients with atrial fibrillation, the ventricular response following digitalis is slower at rest, when vagal tone is high; during exercise, when vagal tone is decreased and sympathetic activity is increased, the ventricular response is considerably faster.

Physiologic, biochemical, and histochemical studies have provided evidence for the vagal innervation of the ventricles, particularly in the interventricular septum in the region of the bundle branches.[60-62] Experimental studies have also suggested that vagal stimulation decreases β-adrenergic–mediated cardiac catecholamine release from the heart.[63,64] Such vagally mediated antiadrenergic effects have the potential to exert beneficial antiarrhythmic effects.

Interaction with the autonomic nervous system may also contribute to the development of digitalis-induced arrhythmias. Large concentrations of digitalis enhance sympathetic tone, both by effects on the central nervous system, which increase efferent nerve activity, and by increasing catecholamine release or decreasing catecholamine reuptake. However, antiadrenergic drugs are usually not very effective in the control of arrhythmias resulting from digitalis toxicity.

CLINICAL APPLICATIONS

The management of heart failure and the management of arrhythmias are the two major indications for digitalis therapy. Changes in cardiac function and systemic hemodynamics are related to the positive inotropic and peripheral vascular effects of digitalis. That digitalis augments myocardial contractility has been demonstrated in a number of experimental and clinical studies.[65] In isolated papillary muscle preparations, changes in contractility were assessed by determining the velocity of muscle shortening at varying loads, that is, the force-velocity curve, which shifted upward and to the right after strophanthidin.[66] The maximum velocity of shortening as well as the maximum developed isometric force increased. The time required to develop peak tension also decreases following digitalis. In papillary muscles obtained from cats with experimentally produced heart failure, similar changes in indices of contractility have been reported after digitalis.[67]

Chronic digoxin therapy increases the left ventricular rate of rise of pressure (dP/dt), velocity of circumferential fiber shortening, and excursion of left ventricular systolic diameter in normal, conscious, chronically instrumented dogs.[68] Echocardiographic studies in normal subjects have also demonstrated increased ejection fraction and mean rate of shortening of left ventricular dimensions after chronic digitalis administration.[69] The force-velocity curve in human subjects shifts upward and to the right, as in papillary muscle preparations after ouabain.[66] In both normal subjects and in patients with heart failure, digitalis decreases the $Q-S_2$ interval, left ventricular ejection time, and pre-ejection period. These findings suggest that digitalis enhances contractility of both normal and failing myocardium.

In normal subjects, and in the absence of depressed ventricular systolic function, cardiac output may not increase, despite an increased contractility, because of the counterbalancing effects of digitalis on the other determinants of cardiac output. A reduction in heart rate and the vagally mediated negative inotropic effects may potentially curtail the expected increase in cardiac output resulting from its direct positive inotropic effect. The most important counteracting mechanism, however, is the increase in systemic vascular resistance, which increases the resistance to left ventricular ejection and decreases stroke volume.

Digitalis-induced constriction of isolated arterial and venous segments, increased arterial and venous tone in intact animals, and increased systemic vascular resistance in normal humans have been demonstrated.[70,71] Increased systemic vascular tone results from its direct effects on the smooth muscle of peripheral vascular beds and also from activation of the sympathetic nervous system. Increased mesenteric vascular resistance, which may decrease splanchnic blood flow, constriction of hepatic veins leading to the pooling of blood in the portal venous system, and decreased venous return to the heart have been reported.[71,72] Increased coronary vascular tone in response to digitalis has been observed both in experimental animals and in patients with coronary artery disease.[73,74]

Activation of the sympathetic nervous system is an important mechanism of digitalis-induced peripheral vasoconstriction. Stimulation of the α-receptors, mediated through the central nervous system, appears to be the predominant mechanism.[75] Digitalis-induced vasoconstriction is blocked by the α-blocking agent phenoxybenzamine, providing evidence for the participation of α-receptors in promoting peripheral vascular tone.[73]

Systemic and regional vasoconstriction appears to be more pronounced after a rapid bolus injection of digitalis.[74] Clinical studies have demonstrated that a 10-second infusion of digitalis increased systemic and coronary vascular resistance significantly and caused transient deterioration of myocardial lactate metabolism. A 15-minute infusion of the same dose of digitalis was not associated with any significant change in systemic or coronary vascular resistance or in myocardial lactate metabolism. Thus, when intravenous administration of digitalis is required, a slow infusion is preferable to avoid these potentially deleterious peripheral vascular effects.

In patients with chronic heart failure associated with depressed left ventricular systolic function, cardiac output generally increases. Peripheral vascular responses to digitalis in heart failure also appear to be different from those in normal subjects. Reduction in both arteriolar and venous tone, instead of an increase, has been observed in heart failure.[70] In patients with chronic heart failure, systemic vascular resistance may remain unchanged in response to either acute or chronic administration of digitalis.[76] A lack of increase in peripheral vascular tone in heart failure may be secondary to improved cardiac output and a reflex decrease in sympathetic activity.

Increased cardiac output in patients with heart failure following digitalis therapy may be accompanied by improved renal hemodynamics and increased diuresis. However, digitalis has been shown to inhibit renal tubular reabsorption of sodium. A direct infusion of ouabain into the renal artery has been reported to inhibit renal (Na^+, K^+)ATPase and impair concentrating and diluting function.[77] Suppression of the renin-angiotensin system consequent on an increase of intracellular calcium by digitalis may have an important influence on renal hemodynamics.[78] However, the major mechanism for increased diuresis after digitalis in heart failure appears to be an improvement in cardiac function and increased cardiac output.

ACUTE MYOCARDIAL INFARCTION

Despite the demonstration in experimental and clinical studies that digitalis may increase myocardial contractility in the acute phase of myocardial infarction, the role of digitalis therapy in the management of pump failure in patients with acute myocardial infarction in sinus rhythm is extremely limited. Increased contractility of the nonischemic and border zones following digitalis has been reported after coronary artery ligation in the dog.[79,80] Systolic shortening of ischemic epicardial and endocardial myocardial layers in dogs increases after ouabain; however, systolic shortening of the infarcted segments remains unchanged. Increases in left ventricular dP/dt, stroke work index, and a reduction in left ventricular filling pressure have also been observed in patients with acute myocardial infarction.[81] In most investigations, however, no significant increase in cardiac output or decrease in left ventricular filling pressure occurred, suggesting that despite enhanced contractile function, overall cardiac pump function remained unchanged.[82,83] In patients with heart failure, variable and inconsistent changes in cardiac output and left ventricular filling pressure have been observed (Fig. 14.3).[84,85] Although a significant increase in left ventricular stroke work index was reported in the majority of these clinical studies, cardiac output and stroke volume usually remained unchanged. Similarly, inconsistent changes in pulmonary capillary wedge pressure and left ventricular end-diastolic pressure have been observed in response to digitalis.

It has also been demonstrated that in patients with acute myocardial infarction, when hemodynamic improvement occurs with digitalis, its magnitude is inversely related to the severity of heart failure.[86] Patients without heart failure responded with a significant increase in cardiac output; in patients with heart failure or shock, there was no change in either cardiac output or left ventricular filling pressure. Stroke work index also increased significantly only in those patients who had no clinical heart failure. Therefore, in patients with severe pump failure or cardiogenic shock, digitalis does not appear to produce any beneficial hemodynamic effects.[86-88] Digitalis also appears to be a relatively weaker inotropic agent compared with others presently available. Dobutamine, a β-receptor agonist, produces a much greater increase in cardiac output and a greater reduction in pulmonary capillary wedge pressure than digitalis (see Fig. 14.3).[85] The onset of the hemodynamic response of intravenous digitalis is also considerably slower than that of dobutamine.

Increased contractility and systemic vascular resistance following digitalis can potentially increase myocardial oxygen requirements. A concomitant increase in coronary vascular tone may decrease coronary blood flow; thus, the potential exists for precipitation or enhancement of myocardial ischemia with digitalis. In patients with chronic coronary artery disease without heart failure, coronary blood flow and myocardial oxygen consumption usually remain unchanged despite increased contractility.[89,90] However, coronary blood flow and myocardial oxygen consumption increase after intravenous ouabain in patients with acute myocardial infarction (Fig. 14.4).[86] In some patients angina and myocardial lactate production developed after ouabain, implying anaerobic metabolism and ischemia. In patients with chronic coronary artery disease, the left ventricular diastolic volume may decrease after digitalis; thus, decreased wall tension may prevent the expected increase in myocardial oxygen consumption. In the majority of patients with acute myocardial infarction and heart failure, left ventricular filling pressure and presumably left ventricular diastolic volume remain unchanged, providing a possible explanation for a net increase in myocardial oxygen consumption in these patients.

Whether digitalis, given in the acute phase of myocardial infarction, extends myocardial injury or not remains controversial. In experimental uncomplicated myocardial infarction, digitalis has been shown to

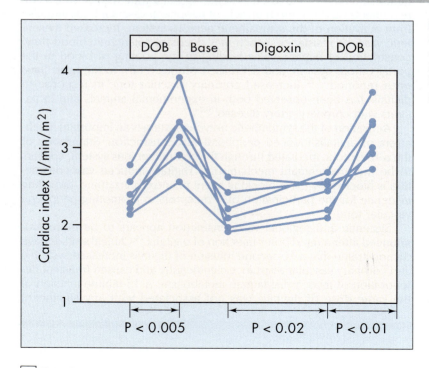

FIGURE 14.3 Changes in cardiac index in response to intravenous dobutamine (DOB) and digoxin in patients with acute myocardial infarction. With dobutamine there was a substantial increase in cardiac index; digoxin, however, produced insignificant changes. (Modified from Goldstein RA, Passamani ER, Roberts R: A comparison of digoxin and dobutamine in patients with acute infarction and cardiac failure. N Engl J Med 303:846, 1980)

increase the extent of myocardial injury.[91] Similarly, in patients without heart failure, increased creatine phosphokinase efflux, suggesting increased infarct size, has been observed after digoxin therapy.[92] However, in patients with heart failure and an elevated pulmonary capillary wedge pressure, decreased infarct size determined by creatine kinase (CK) curves has been reported.[93] Thus, the effects of digitalis on coronary hemodynamics, myocardial oxygen consumption, and extent of myocardial injury are likely to be variable and influenced both by the presence or absence of heart failure and by the magnitude of changes in the determinants of myocardial oxygen requirements and myocardial perfusion. Because of the lack of consistent beneficial hemodynamic effects, a slower onset of action, and the availability of more potent inotropic agents, digitalis is not the drug of choice for inotropic therapy of pump failure complicating acute myocardial infarction.

In some retrospective nonrandomized studies, continued digitalis therapy following acute myocardial infarction has been reported as an independent adverse risk factor for long-term survival.[94,95] During 3 years of follow-up, the cumulative survival rate for patients treated with digitalis was 66%, compared with 87% for those not treated.[94] This adverse influence on late survival has been considered a result of increased arrhythmogenicity with digitalis in the presence of healed myocardial infarction. In canine hearts, the healed infarcted myocardium was found to be the site of origin of ventricular tachycardia due to digitalis toxicity.[96] However, several clinical studies have suggested that digitalis is well tolerated by patients with myocardial infarction and that they are not more susceptible to arrhythmias. Digitalis therapy is usually instituted for the management of supraventricular arrhythmias or heart failure—the complications of acute myocardial infarction that are associated with a worse prognosis with or without digitalis therapy.[97] When the risks related to atrial arrhythmias and left ventricular failure are adjusted, no significant independent adverse influence of digitalis therapy is observed.[98] Thus, no conclusive evidence presently exists to suggest withholding long-term digitalis therapy if indicated in patients with healed myocardial infarction.

CHRONIC HEART FAILURE

That acute digitalis therapy increases contractile function in patients with chronic heart failure in sinus rhythm has been demonstrated in clinical studies.[99] Increased contractile function was evident from the shortening of Q-A$_2$ intervals and the ratio of pre-ejection period to left ventricular ejection time.[99] An increase in the mean velocity of circumferential fiber shortening was also observed; the increase in fiber shortening occurred without any change in end-diastolic volume and despite an increase in arterial pressure and a decrease in heart rate.[100] An increase in the maximum velocity of fiber shortening (V_{max}) has been reported in patients with overt heart failure.[89] Thus, it seems well established that acute digitalis therapy enhances contractile function, and the positive inotropic effect appears to be more pronounced when left ventricular function is depressed. In patients in sinus rhythm, variable changes in left ventricular function have been reported during maintenance digoxin therapy. In some studies, an abbreviation of systolic time intervals, decreased heart size, and improvement in left ventricular segmental wall motion were observed during oral digoxin therapy.[101,102] A sustained increase in the velocity of fiber shortening and ejection fraction has been reported during maintenance digoxin therapy.[100] Even in normal subjects, a persistent improvement in left ventricular performance has been reported during long-term oral administration of digoxin.[103] However, other similar uncontrolled studies have failed to establish long-term beneficial effects of digoxin in patients in sinus rhythm; there were no significant changes in systolic time intervals.[103] Radionuclide angiographic studies also failed to demonstrate any sustained improvement in resting left ventricular function after maintenance digoxin therapy.[104]

Hemodynamic studies have demonstrated that, after acute administration of digitalis, cardiac output does not always increase. In an earlier review of the response of acute digitalis therapy in 117 patients, it was found that about 65% of patients had a significant increase in cardiac output and a decrease in left atrial and pulmonary arterial pressures.[103] Another 20% of patients had a modest increase in cardiac output. Systemic vascular resistance may increase in some patients after bolus intravenous administration of digoxin.[105] Slow infusion of digoxin, however, does not change systemic vascular resistance, and cardiac output tends to increase in most patients.[76] Changes in left ventricular function during exercise were assessed after acute and chronic digitalis therapy; in general, an improvement in exercise hemodynamics and left ventricular performance was observed.[76,106] Withdrawal of chronic digoxin therapy has been shown to cause deterioration in hemodynamics and left ventricular function, both at rest and during exercise (Fig. 14.5). Hemodynamic improvement, however, is unlikely to occur in patients with severe chronic congestive heart failure (*e.g.*, New York Heart Association [NYHA] Class IV),[106] since the response to inotropic stimulation depends on the relative quantities of damaged myocardium devoid of contractile reserve.

Withdrawal of digitalis in patients with compensated heart failure causes variable changes in the clinical status.[107] Digitalis therapy could be discontinued without clinical deterioration in many patients: 48% to 100% of patients did not experience any symptomatic deterioration after withdrawal of digitalis. Results of diuretic therapy alone were compared with those of digoxin and diuretics, and no benefit of the addition of digoxin to diuretics was observed.[108-110] All these studies, however, were uncontrolled and frequently contained a smaller sample size. Furthermore, heterogeneous patient populations were investigated, and frequently the appropriateness of digitalis therapy was not specified.

Placebo-controlled studies, however, have suggested that chronic digoxin therapy is likely to produce clinical improvement in most pa-

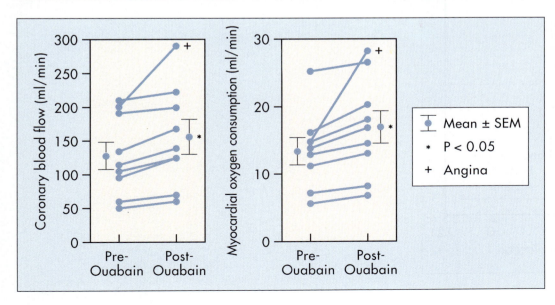

FIGURE 14.4 Ouabain-induced changes in coronary blood flow and myocardial oxygen consumption in patients with acute myocardial infarction. In most patients, coronary sinus blood flow and myocardial oxygen consumption increased, and occasionally the patient developed angina. (Modified from Forrester J, Chatterjee K: Preservation of ischemic myocardium. In Vogel JHK (ed): Advances in Cardiology, Vol II, p 158. Basel, S Karger, 1974)

tients with congestive heart failure who have depressed left ventricular systolic function and an S_3 gallop (Fig. 14.6).[111,112] Clinical deterioration occurred in most patients when placebo was substituted for digoxin. In patients with normal systolic function or in those without S_3 gallop, maintenance digoxin therapy was not associated with any improvement. In one placebo-controlled study, chronic digoxin therapy was found to be of no clinical benefit in patients with stable chronic congestive heart failure. However, in this study most patients were elderly and only one patient had an S_3 gallop.[113]

Withdrawal of digoxin was also associated with a significant increase in left ventricular end-diastolic dimension and left ventricular ejection time and pre-ejection period and a decrease in the velocity of circumferential fiber shortening, indicating deterioration of left ventricular function.

In another prospective but nonrandomized study,[114] withdrawal of maintenance digoxin therapy did not result in any change in symptoms, exercise tolerance, radiologic or clinical findings of heart failure, or the radionuclide left ventricular ejection fraction. The effect of chronic digoxin therapy on exercise performance has been compared with that of xamoterol, a partial β_1-receptor agonist in a prospective randomized, controlled study in patients with mild chronic heart failure.[115] Compared with placebo, exercise performance improved with xamoterol but not with digoxin. Lack of improvement in exercise duration with chronic digoxin therapy has been reported in other prospec-

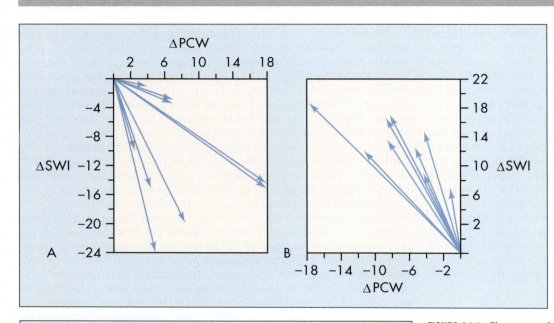

FIGURE 14.5 Changes in pulmonary capillary wedge pressure (ΔPCW) and stroke work index (ΔSWI) following withdrawal (**A**) and after rapid administration (**B**) of digoxin in patients with chronic heart failure in sinus rhythm. Discontinuation of chronic digoxin therapy was associated with decreased SWI and increased PCW pressure, and readministration of digoxin caused a decrease in PCW pressure and an increase in SWI. (Modified from Arnold S et al: Long-term digitalis therapy improves left ventricular function in heart failure. N Engl J Med 303:1443, 1980)

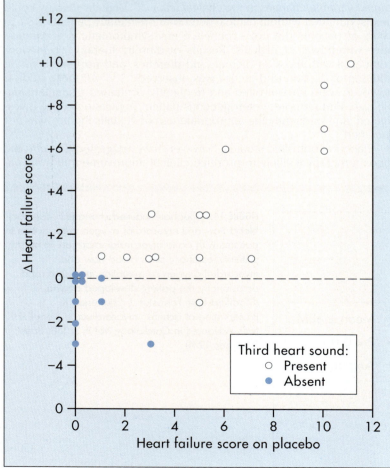

FIGURE 14.6 Changes in heart failure score while on maintenance digoxin treatment compared with while on placebo in a group of patients with chronic heart failure. Heart failure scores were determined based on the results of clinical, radiologic, and noninvasive investigations. Patients with a third heart sound had improvement while on digoxin therapy. (Modified from Lee DC, Johnson RA, Bingham JB: Heart failure in outpatients: A randomized trial of digoxin versus placebo. N Engl J Med 306:699, 1982)

tive randomized, placebo-controlled studies.[116] The Captopril-Digoxin Multicenter Research Group compared the effects of captopril with those of digoxin in patients with mild to moderate heart failure in a double-blind, placebo-controlled study. Compared with placebo, the magnitude of increase in exercise duration with digoxin was not statistically significant and also there was no improvement in clinical class in the digoxin-treated patients. Captopril therapy resulted in significantly improved exercise duration and clinical class. Digoxin, however, increased left ventricular ejection fraction significantly compared with captopril and placebo. Furthermore, the incidence of treatment failure, increased requirements of diuretic therapy, and hospitalizations was lower compared with placebo in both digoxin- and captopril-treated groups. The relative effectiveness of digoxin and enalapril, another converting enzyme inhibitor, in improving clinical class and exercise duration in patients with mild to severe congestive heart failure has also been studied in a randomized double-blind trial.[117] Both enalapril and digoxin therapy resulted in a significant improvement in clinical class and in exercise tolerance. In another double-blind, placebo-controlled trial, digoxin was found to cause a significant improvement in dyspnea, left ventricular fractional shortening as measured by M-mode echocardiography, heart failure score, and cardiothoracic ratio.[118] Unlike many other studies, in this study, digoxin doses were titrated to a therapeutic level.

Clinical efficacy, potential to improve ventricular function, arrhythmogenicity, and the impact on survival of digoxin therapy were compared with those of oral milrinone, a phosphodiesterase inhibitor, in a prospective randomized double-blind trial.[119] Exercise duration on a treadmill increased by similar magnitude with both digoxin and milrinone. Digoxin reduced the frequency of decompensation from heart failure from 47% with placebo to 15%; with milrinone, the frequency of decompensation decreased to 34%. However, clinical conditions deteriorated in a greater number of patients treated with milrinone (20%) than with digoxin (3%). Three-month mortality from all causes (according to the intention to treat) tended to be higher in patients treated with milrinone. Furthermore, increased ventricular arrhythmias occurred more frequently in patients receiving milrinone. Left ventricular ejection fraction increased with digoxin but remained unchanged with milrinone. Thus, digoxin therapy was as effective, if not more effective, than milrinone in these patient populations.

Concomitant digoxin and vasodilator therapy appears to be more effective than either therapy alone. In the Veterans Administration Heart Failure Trial,[120] the addition of hydralazine and isosorbide dinitrate to conventional treatment consisting of digitalis and diuretic therapy was associated with an improved survival. Similarly, in the CONSENSUS Trial,[121] combined enalapril and digitalis and diuretic therapy was more effective in causing symptomatic improvement and improvement in survival in patients with severe chronic congestive heart failure than when only conventional therapy (digitalis and diuretics) was employed. The comparative hemodynamic and neurohormonal effects of captopril and digoxin, given both separately and in combination, have been studied in patients with chronic heart failure.[122] Although both captopril and digoxin decreased pulmonary capillary wedge pressure and systemic vascular resistance significantly, only digoxin increased cardiac index and stroke work index. During maximal exercise, a significant reduction in systemic vascular resistance, and an increase in cardiac index were observed with captopril alone, whereas digoxin alone decreased pulmonary capillary wedge pressure and increased the stroke work index. The combination of captopril and digoxin caused a substantial reduction in pulmonary capillary wedge pressure and systemic vascular resistance, and an increase in the cardiac index both at rest and during exercise. A significant reduction in serum norepinephrine concentrations was observed with digoxin. Although in this study circulating norepinephrine levels remained unchanged with captopril, a significant reduction of norepinephrine has been observed during acute and chronic angiotensin converting enzyme inhibitor therapy.[123,124]

It is apparent that digoxin usually improves left ventricular function in patients with chronic congestive heart failure, although significant symptomatic improvement may not be obvious in many patients. Digoxin appears to be more effective in patients with overt heart failure with significantly impaired left ventricular systolic function. In patients with very mild heart failure with relatively preserved systolic function, digoxin therapy is less likely to produce sustained benefit. Digoxin therapy, however, is likely to be beneficial in symptomatic patients with more than very mild heart failure, and should be considered in conjunction with vasodilators or angiotensin-converting enzyme inhibitors and diuretics. Digoxin therapy is of particular benefit in the treatment of heart failure associated with atrial fibrillation. Presently, available data suggest that vasodilators and angiotensin-converting enzyme inhibitors improve the prognosis of patients concurrently treated with digitalis and diuretics; thus, digitalis and diuretic therapy alone should not be considered sufficient in the management of patients with chronic heart failure and vasodilators or angiotensin converting enzyme inhibitors should be added whenever feasible and tolerated.

In isolated mitral stenosis with normal sinus rhythm, digitalis is of little value. However, digitalis is clearly indicated in the presence of atrial fibrillation and produces its salutary effect by decreasing the ventricular response, which allows decompression of the left atrium. Hypertrophic cardiomyopathy is another relative contraindication for digitalis therapy; left ventricular systolic function is normal or supernormal, and a further increase in contractile state with digitalis may be associated with increased left ventricular outflow obstruction. In occasional patients with hypertrophic cardiomyopathy, left ventricular systolic function declines and congestive symptoms develop; in these patients digitalis can be used to improve left ventricular performance. When atrial fibrillation develops, digitalis can be used cautiously to decrease the ventricular response, provided the presence of accessory pathways is excluded. However, β-adrenergic blocking agents or calcium channel blocking drugs (verapamil or diltiazem) are preferable in these patients to control the ventricular response.

Clinical experience suggests that patients with restrictive cardiomyopathy also do not derive significant benefit from digitalis therapy. Amyloid heart disease appears to predispose to digitalis intoxication. Little benefit is also expected in patients with cardiac tamponade or constrictive pericarditis.

ANGINA PECTORIS

Although in patients with cardiomegaly, digoxin can decrease myocardial oxygen consumption by decreasing left ventricular volume, digoxin therapy is seldom indicated for treatment of angina pectoris. In patients with depressed left ventricular function, but without overt heart failure, the addition of digitalis to β-blocking drugs may improve exercise tolerance.[125] In patients with cardiomegaly and symptoms of heart failure, digoxin therapy occasionally decreases the frequency of angina.[111] However, nitrates and calcium channel blocking drugs are more appropriate pharmacologic agents for the treatment of angina in these patients.

In the absence of heart failure and depressed left ventricular function, digitalis does not produce any beneficial effects and may increase the frequency of anginal attacks.[126,127]

CHRONIC OBSTRUCTIVE PULMONARY DISEASE

Although digitalis exerts a positive inotropic effect in experimental animals with right-sided heart failure,[128] its role in the management of cor pulmonale secondary to obstructive lung disease has not been clarified. In the absence of right-sided heart failure, digitalis does not produce any beneficial effects.[129] Hemodynamic improvement can occur in some patients with overt heart failure due to cor pulmonale.[130] Acute digitalization, however, may increase pulmonary vascular resistance and cause deterioration of right ventricular performance. Furthermore, pulmonary disease may predispose to the development of digitalis toxicity. Patients with cor pulmonale with hypercapnia and hypoxemia appear to be more sensitive to digitalis during a strophanthidin test.[131] Arrhythmias suggestive of digitalis intoxication can develop in these patients with subtoxic serum concentrations of digoxin. Catecholamine release from cardiac adrenergic receptors and the adrenal glands in response to acute hypoxemia lowers the threshold for digitalis-induced arrhythmias.[132,133] Such mechanisms may explain the clinical observation that when systemic sympathomimetic amines are used for the treatment of chronic pulmonary disease, the addition of digitalis enhances the propensity to develop arrhythmias.

It appears that digitalis should be used with caution in patients with pulmonary disease who are hypoxemic. Furthermore, the hemodynamic and clinical benefits are marginal even in patients with right-sided heart failure. Thus, digitalis should be reserved only for those patients with cor pulmonale and right-sided heart failure unresponsive to alternative therapies (vasodilators and diuretics).

PROPHYLACTIC DIGITALIZATION

The value of long-term digitalis therapy in patients with aortic or mitral valve disease before the development of heart failure has not been established. In view of the potential risk of developing digitalis toxicity, prophylactic digitalis therapy is not indicated in these patients. Preoperative prophylactic digitalization has been advocated in patients undergoing aortocoronary bypass or major thoracoabdominal surgery to decrease the incidence of postoperative supraventricular tachyarrhythmias.[134] No conclusive evidence exists, however, for such beneficial effects; on the contrary, an increased incidence of tachyarrhythmias has been reported after coronary artery bypass surgery in digitalized patients.[135] Thus, there is little justification for routine preoperative digitalis therapy.

CARDIAC ARRHYTHMIAS

ATRIAL FIBRILLATION. Atrial fibrillation with a rapid ventricular response is the most common indication for the use of digitalis. Decreased atrioventricular conduction resulting from the vagotonic effect of digitalis is associated with a decreased ventricular response. Increased ventricular filling associated with a slower ventricular rate improves hemodynamics. Conversion of atrial fibrillation to sinus rhythm with digitalis alone is not expected. In certain clinical circumstances (e.g., postoperative atrial fibrillation), addition of β-adrenergic blocking or calcium channel blocking drugs (verapamil or diltiazem) decreases the ventricular response more effectively because of the synergistic effects to decrease AV conduction. In atrial flutter, decreased AV conduction with digitalis is associated with increased AV block and a decreased ventricular response. Usually a relatively larger dose of digitalis is required to decrease AV nodal conduction in atrial flutter than in atrial fibrillation because of the relatively increased refractoriness of the AV node in the presence of atrial fibrillation. Digitalis may occasionally convert atrial flutter to fibrillation with a further decrease in ventricular rate. As in atrial fibrillation, the concomitant use of β-adrenergic blocking drugs or calcium antagonists may decrease the ventricular response more effectively. Digitalis is also effective in the control of paroxysmal atrial or AV nodal tachycardia. The oral or intravenous administration of digoxin may abruptly terminate such attacks, probably as the result of its vagotonic effect. However, the calcium channel blocking agents verapamil and diltiazem and adenosine, which are more effective than digitalis in terminating supraventricular tachycardia, are the agents of choice.

Although digitalis is occasionally effective in controlling supraventricular tachycardia associated with the Wolff-Parkinson-White syndrome, it is not the drug of choice. Types Ia, Ic, and III antiarrhythmic drugs are more effective to control supraventricular tachyarrhythmias associated with the pre-excitation syndrome. Digitalis is contraindicated for the treatment of atrial fibrillation associated with the Wolff-Parkinson-White syndrome, since the ventricular rate may increase markedly.

DIGITALIS TOXICITY

Toxicity, which is occasionally life-threatening, is the major concern during digitalis therapy in patients with cardiovascular disorders. Withering stated, "The fox-glove, when given in very large and quickly repeated doses, occasions sickness, vomiting, purging, giddiness, confused vision, objects appearing green or yellow, increased secretion of urine, with frequent motions to part with it, and sometimes inability to retain it; slow pulse, even as low as 35 in a minute, cold sweats, convulsions, syncope and death." These clinical manifestations of severe digitalis toxicity, as observed by Withering more than 200 years ago, precisely outline both the cardiac and extracardiac manifestations of digitalis toxicity.

The true prevalence of digitalis toxicity is difficult to estimate. In Withering's era, the reported incidence was between 18% and 25%.[136] In hospitalized patients, adverse effects were observed in 19.8% to 21% of patients receiving digitalis.[137,138] Beller and co-workers reported a 23% incidence of definite digitalis toxicity in hospitalized patients.[139] Another 6% of patients had possible digitalis toxicity. Recent assessments have revealed a lower incidence, between 6% and 18%.[136,140] The apparent decreased prevalence might have resulted from increased knowledge of the pharmacodynamics and pharmacokinetics of presently available digitalis preparations, and also from an increased awareness of the potential manifestations of digitalis toxicity.

MANIFESTATIONS OF DIGITALIS TOXICITY. Manifestations of digitalis toxicity may be either extracardiac or cardiac. The extracardiac manifestations are often nonspecific and may be similar to those of congestive heart failure, making the diagnosis of digitalis toxicity difficult. In as many as 28% of patients, extracardiac symptoms may remain unsuspected as manifestations of digitalis toxicity. In almost 50% of patients, extracardiac symptoms do not precede cardiac arrhythmias related to digitalis toxicity.[141]

EXTRACARDIAC MANIFESTATIONS. Gastrointestinal symptoms (anorexia, nausea, vomiting, and diarrhea) are relatively common extracardiac symptoms of digitalis toxicity. Anorexia is often the earliest symptom and is followed by nausea or vomiting. Abdominal pain and bloating may also occur. Digitalis administration has been associated with mesenteric infarction, which, in some instances, results in fatal hemorrhagic necrosis of the gut.[142] Additionally, the malabsorption syndrome has been reported in patients with heart failure treated with digitalis.[143] Neurologic manifestations are characterized by fatigue and by muscular weakness involving legs and arms. Visual disturbances usually manifest as hazy vision, difficulty in reading, alteration of the color of objects, photophobia, glittering moving spots, and flashes of yellow, red, green, or dark colors. Difficulties of red-green perception are more frequent visual disturbances. Ocular symptoms compatible with a diagnosis of retrobulbar neuritis have been reported as manifestations of digitalis toxicity. Transient psychosis, hallucinations, restlessness, insomnia, apathy, and drowsiness have also been observed. Frank delirium, often termed *foxglove frenzy* or *digitalis delirium*, may also occur. Digitalis therapy has been associated with painful gynecomastia in men and breast enlargement in women. Rarely, allergic skin lesions have been attributed to digitalis toxicity. Urticaria, scarlatiniform rash, papules, vesicles, purpura bullosa, and angioneurotic edema associated with eosinophilia or thrombocytopenia have been observed. The mechanisms of all extracardiac manifestations[143] of digitalis toxicity have not yet been totally clarified. Digitalis has been demonstrated to increase visceral smooth muscle tone and prolong the transit time through the gastrointestinal tract. Rectal smooth muscles appear to be the most affected, and gastric smooth muscles the least sensitive to a digitalis-induced increase in tone. Decreased intestinal blood flow, resulting from vasoconstriction of the mesenteric and splanchnic circulations, has been implicated in many of the gastrointestinal symptoms of digitalis toxicity.[51] It has been demonstrated, however, that the emetic effects of digitalis are mediated by the area postrema at the base of the fourth cerebral ventricle.[51] Many of the extracardiac toxic effects of digitalis glycosides, including neurologic manifestations, appear to result from the excitation effects of digitalis on nerve cells in the cortical and medullary regions of the central nervous system. Perfusion of the lateral ventricles in experimental animals with ouabain causes a marked release of 5-hydroxytryptamine, suggesting that this compound plays a role in the genesis of digitalis glycoside-induced neurotoxicity. Digitalis may also increase the dopamine content of the central nervous system, which might contribute to its toxic effects. Although these experimental studies suggest that the effects of digitalis glycosides on the central nervous system, mediated by an alteration in one or more neurotransmitters, may precipitate cardiac and noncardiac toxicity, further studies will be required to establish the precise mechanisms.

The mechanism for gynecomastia in men or breast enlargement in women is probably related to an elevation in the serum estrogen level and a decrease in serum luteinizing hormone and plasma testosterone. The structural similarity between estrogens and digitalis glycosides and their metabolites might explain these endocrine side effects. The various extracardiac manifestations of digitalis toxicity are summarized in Table 14.3.

CARDIAC ADVERSE EFFECTS. Cardiac arrhythmias are the most serious side effects of digitalis toxicity.[144,145] Almost all types of arrhythmias have been reported to occur with digitalis intoxication. It needs to be emphasized, however, that with rare exception arrhythmias identical to those induced by digitalis may also occur owing to underlying pathologic conditions. Digitalis-induced arrhythmias may not be clinically manifest and can remain "masked" until the dominant rhythm is slowed. Arrhythmias related to digitalis toxicity can be categorized according to the electrophysiologic mechanisms (Table 14.4).[144]

Digitalis-induced arrhythmias should be suspected "when there is the appearance of a slow heart rate in a patient with fast or normal heart rate, the appearance of a fast heart rate in a patient with a normal heart rate, the appearance of a regular rhythm in a patient with an irregular rhythm, and the appearance of a regularly irregular rhythm."[145] Arrhythmias considered most suggestive of digitalis toxicity are nonparoxysmal AV junctional tachycardia and paroxysmal atrial tachycardia with AV block. Bidirectional tachycardia, nonconducted premature atrial contractions, and double junctional rhythm are virtually diagnostic of digitalis toxicity. Regularization of rhythm in a patient with atrial fibrillation and ventricular tachycardia with exit block is also very suggestive of digitalis toxicity. Bigeminal ventricular rhythm and multiform premature ventricular contractions are quite common but are nonspecific.

Arrhythmias that are relatively unlikely to be due to digitalis toxicity are sinus tachycardia, paroxysmal AV junctional tachycardia without AV block, multifocal atrial tachycardia, parasystole, and nonparoxysmal ventricular (idioventricular) tachycardia. Mobitz type II AV block, complete infranodal AV block, bilateral bundle branch block, and atrial flutter or fibrillation with a rapid ventricular response are extremely rare manifestations of digitalis toxicity.

Sinoatrial (SA) and AV nodal block appear to result from the interaction of the "indirect" effects of digitalis mediated through the parasympathetic nervous system and its direct effects. Decreased conduction in the specialized conduction system may result not only in a bradyarrhythmia but also in a tachyarrhythmia.

Abnormal impulse initiation resulting from digitalis toxicity may also cause tachyarrhythmias. Depolarization during phase 4 of the ac-

TABLE 14.3 EXTRACARDIAC MANIFESTATIONS OF DIGITALIS TOXICITY

Gastrointestinal
Anorexia, nausea, vomiting, diarrhea, abdominal pain, bloating, malabsorption, mesenteric infarction

Neurologic
Fatigue, muscular weakness, visual disturbances, difficulties in red-green perception, symptoms of retrobulbar neuritis, insomnia, apathy, drowsiness, frank delirium ("foxglove frenzy," digitalis delirium)

Endocrine
Gynecomastia in men, enlargement of breasts in women

Dermatologic
Allergic skin lesions

TABLE 14.4 ARRHYTHMIAS CAUSED BY DIGITALIS TOXICITY

1. Ectopic rhythm (re-entry, enhanced automaticity, or both)
   Atrial tachycardia with block
   Nonparoxysmal junctional tachycardia
   Reciprocation
   Ventricular tachycardia, flutter, fibrillation
   Bidirectional tachycardia
   Parasystolic ventricular tachycardia
   Atrial flutter, fibrillation
2. Depression of pacemakers with or without accelerated subsidiary pacemaker
   Sinus slowing
   Sinoatrial arrest
3. Depression of conduction
   Sinoatrial block, atrioventricular, exit block in association with
      Sinus rhythm
      Atrial tachycardia
      Atrial flutter
      Junctional rhythm
      Ventricular tachycardia
4. Ectopic rhythm with simultaneous depression of conduction
   Junctional rhythm
   Ventricular tachycardia with decreased atrioventricular conduction
5. Atrioventricular dissociation with escape of subsidiary pacemaker
   Double junctional rhythm
6. Triggered automaticity
   Ventricular tachycardia triggered by supraventricular tachycardia
   Junctional tachycardia triggered by ventricular tachycardia

(Adapted from Fisch C, Knoebel SB: Digitalis cardiotoxicity. J Am Coll Cardiol 5:91A, 1985)

tion potential may enhance pulse initiation. The transient inward current induced by toxic concentrations of digitalis is oscillatory and causes the delayed afterdepolarization. The afterdepolarization, in turn, may induce a rate-dependent tachycardia referred to as a "triggered" arrhythmia.

Afterdepolarization occurs as a result of toxic inhibition of the "sodium pump." The accumulation of intracellular sodium is associated with increased intracellular calcium resulting from altered function of the Na^+-Ca^{2+} exchange mechanism and calcium release from intracellular stores. The increase in intracellular calcium triggers a transient inward current, the immediate cause of afterdepolarizations.

Experimental studies suggest that afterdepolarizations and triggered activity may be the basis of many digitalis-induced arrhythmias,[55] particularly repetitive ventricular responses and tachyarrhythmias.

PREDISPOSING FACTORS FOR DIGITALIS TOXICITY.[144-147] AGE. Clinical observations suggest that elderly patients tolerate digitalis relatively poorly and develop digitalis toxicity more rapidly; in contrast, digitalis is well tolerated by younger persons. In infants, serum concentrations of digoxin of 2 to 3 ng/ml are not usually associated with any manifestations of digitalis toxicity. In comparison with adults, the absorption of digoxin in the newborn is not different but the volume of distribution is increased. In the premature infant, the rate of urinary excretion is decreased and the half-life of digoxin is increased. Experimental studies in animal models indicate that in young hearts a higher concentration of digitalis is required to induce depolarization of the cell membrane and afterdepolarization.[55] It has been suggested that the age-related changes in the sodium pump and its binding capacity for digitalis may account for the differences in tolerance to digitalis between the young and the elderly. The manifestations of digitalis toxicity in children are different from those in adults; in children, sinus bradycardia, sinoatrial block, and atrial or AV junctional rhythm are more common than the ventricular tachyarrhythmias.

After the administration of a similar dose of digoxin, the serum concentration of digoxin is higher in elderly patients than it is in younger patients. The higher serum concentration of digoxin in the elderly patient results from a decreased glomerular filtration rate and renal clearance and also from the decreased volume of distribution due to smaller skeletal muscle mass.

CARDIAC DISEASE. Certain cardiac disorders have been suspected to predispose to cardiac digitalis toxicity. Patients with chronic obstructive pulmonary disease appear to be more susceptible to the development of arrhythmias due to ventricular automaticity. Hypoxia, hypokalemia, and therapy with sympathomimetic agents and methylxanthines contribute to increased sensitivity. Patients with amyloid heart disease also appear to be prone to develop arrhythmias during digitalis therapy. Increased sensitivity to digitalis in ischemia or infarcted myocardium has been demonstrated in animal models.[96] The site of initiation of digitalis-induced ventricular tachycardia has been localized to the infarcted and peri-infarction zones. Patients with recent myocardial infarction, however, appear to tolerate the usual therapeutic doses of digitalis without an increase in the incidence of arrhythmias. The effect of digitalis therapy on long-term survival after myocardial infarction remains controversial. Some uncontrolled studies have suggested that the digitalis therapy may be an independent adverse risk factor for survival;[94] others have failed to demonstrate any increased risk of mortality in digitalis-treated patients.[148] Rather, the severity of the hemodynamic abnormality and the degree of depression of cardiac function influence the prognosis adversely.

RENAL FAILURE. Decreased digitalis tolerance in patients with impaired renal function has been well documented. Serum digoxin level increases due to decreased renal excretion and volume of distribution. In the presence of renal failure, digoxin clearance parallels creatinine clearance. The precise mechanism for the decreased volume of distribution remains unclear; however a decrease in affinity of the receptor site for digoxin remains a possibility. In patients with severe renal failure, the loading and maintenance dose of digoxin should be reduced. In patients with end-stage renal disease, an intravenous dose of 0.7 mg resulted in a 24-hour level of digoxin ranging between 1.0 to 2.1 ng/ml, which did not produce digitalis toxicity.[147] Patients with severe renal failure with end-stage renal disease who weigh 40 kg need a maintenance dose of 0.0625 mg daily, while the 90-kg patient requires 0.1 mg daily to maintain a serum digoxin level in the therapeutic range. Hemodialysis removes only a small fraction of total body digoxin stores, about 4%. A supplemental digoxin dose after dialysis can increase the serum digoxin levels and cause toxicity. Elimination of digitoxin is less dependent on kidney function, since it is extensively metabolized in the liver.

SERUM POTASSIUM. Hypokalemia predisposes to the toxic effects of digitalis. Decreased serum potassium levels following diuretic therapy, after dialysis, after administration of glucose, or due to gastrointestinal loss of potassium may induce ectopic arrhythmias after administration of relatively smaller doses of digitalis. Increased automaticity due to enhanced phase 4 depolarization occurs more frequently in the presence of low potassium concentrations. In animal models, lower doses of digoxin induce ventricular tachycardia in the presence of hypokalemia. Hypokalemia increases the uptake and binding of glycosides to (Na^+, K^+)ATPase. However, direct membrane effects of hyperkalemia- and hypokalemia-induced decreased renal excretin of digoxin may also contribute to digitalis toxicity. A decreased serum potassium concentration may enhance digitalis-induced depression of AV nodal conduction. Hypokalemia might be contributory to digitalis-induced ectopic atrial tachycardia with block and nonparoxysmal AV junctional tachycardia, which result from increased automaticity of ectopic pacemakers and depressed AV conduction. Severe hyperkalemia also depresses AV conduction and potentiates the effects of digitalis on AV conduction. In patients with atrial fibrillation treated with digitalis, hyperkalemia may precipitate complete AV block. The presence of AV junctional disease and the synergistic effects of digitalis and hyperkalemia on AV conduction may produce severe bradycardia or asystole.

SERUM CALCIUM. That infusion of calcium in digitalized patients may induce ventricular tachycardia has been observed in clinical studies.[149] However, in experimental studies, no deleterious effects of hypercalcemia were observed in digitalized animals and there was no evidence for the additive effects of calcium and digitalis. Thus, unless the rate of infusion of calcium is very rapid or the serum concentration of calcium is very high, it is unlikely that moderate, transient hypercalcemia will enhance cardiac toxicity.

SERUM MAGNESIUM. Hypomagnesemia can increase myocardial digoxin uptake, decrease the sodium pump activity, and increase the amplitude of digoxin-induced afterdepolarizations.[150] Hypomagnesemia can exist with normal serum levels and can cause intracellular hypokalemia that is refractory to potassium replacement. Thus, decreased magnesium stores, like hypokalemia, can precipitate toxicity at therapeutic levels of digoxin. In experimental animals, hypomagnesemia enhances ouabain-induced automaticity in the presence of AV block and lowers the ouabain doses required to induce ventricular tachyarrhythmias.[151] Clinical studies, however, have failed to demonstrate any conclusive evidence for the relation between the hypomagnesemia and digitalis toxicity.[152] Nevertheless, arrhythmias attributable to digitalis toxicity may respond favorably to intravenous administration of magnesium,[153] which may result from its nonspecific antiarrhythmic effect.

ALKALOSIS. In patients with metabolic alkalosis and normal potassium concentrations, therapeutic concentrations of digoxin may be associated with a greater incidence of arrhythmias than seen in patients without alkalosis.[154] The mechanism for this apparent increased sensitivity to digitalis associated with alkalosis remains unclear.

HYPOTHYROIDISM. Decreased thyroid function increases serum digoxin levels by decreasing glomerular filtration rate and the volume of distribution of digoxin. The myocardium of the myxedematous patient appears to have reduced tolerance to digoxin, which is reversed with thyroid replacement.[155] Hyperthyroid patients tend to tolerate larger doses of digitalis and eliminate glycosides faster.

CARDIOPULMONARY BYPASS. Sensitivity to the toxic effects of digitalis appears to increase in the first 24 hours after cardiopulmonary bypass.[156] Toxicity is not related to blood gas changes or serum electrolyte concentrations and is manifest at a relatively lower serum digoxin concentration.

DIGITALIS AND ELECTRIC SHOCK. In animal studies, digitalis administration decreases the amount of electrical energy required to induce ventricular tachyarrhythmias. Synchronized direct-current shock frequently precipitates supraventricular and ventricular ectopic arrhythmias in digitalized patients. However, recent animal and clinical studies have documented that in the presence of therapeutic concentrations of digoxin, direct-current shock does not enhance the incidence of arrhythmias attributable to digitalis toxicity.[157,158] However, in patients with overt digitalis toxicity, electrical shocks at all energy levels may precipitate sustained ventricular tachycardia. Thus, the risk of arrhythmia after direct-current shock is increased only in the presence of overt digitalis toxicity and countershocks can be applied safely in therapeutically digitalized patients.

DRUG INTERACTION.[147,158,159] Changes in serum digoxin levels due to interaction with other drugs may predispose the patient to digitalis toxicity. Digitalis-drug interactions are described elsewhere in these volumes. Concurrent administration of antacids, bran, kaolin pectate, cholestyramine, colestipol, activated charcoal, sulfasalazine, neomycin, or p-aminosalicyclic acid can decrease digoxin absorption.[159] Sudden withdrawal of these drugs without decreasing the oral dose of digoxin may enhance its absorption and increase its serum level, resulting in toxicity. Administration of certain antibiotics (e.g., erythromycin) may increase serum digoxin levels due to increased bioavailability resulting from decreased metabolism. In clinical practice, interaction with certain antiarrhythmic drugs that increase serum digoxin levels appears to predispose to digitalis toxicity more frequently. Quinidine causes an increase in the serum digoxin level in over 90% of patients, and this can precipitate toxicity. The increase in digoxin level in individual patients is variable and ranges from none to sixfold, with an average increase of twofold. The magnitude of increase in the serum digoxin level is proportional to the quinidine dose. Both extracardiac toxicity and AV conduction delay may occur as a result of this interaction.[160] The mechanism for the increased serum digoxin level following quinidine therapy is not completely understood. A decrease in total body, renal, and nonrenal clearance, and decreased volume of distribution of digoxin, appear to occur after administration of quinidine. It has been proposed that the early rise in serum digoxin levels results from the displacement of digoxin from tissue stores.

The ratio of skeletal to serum digoxin concentration decreases, which suggests displacement of digoxin from skeletal muscle. The ratio of myocardial to serum digoxin, however, remains unchanged during this interaction. Studies in animals demonstrate that the increased serum digoxin level is not accompanied by a proportional increase in digoxin effect as measured by percent inhibition of rubidium myocardial uptake, implying that digoxin may be selectively displaced from active binding sites, since overall myocardial digoxin content increases appropriately.[161]

Since the digoxin blood level tends to increase with the first dose of quinidine, and a new digoxin steady state is achieved by the fifth day, it has been suggested that the dose of digoxin should be halved prior to the addition of quinidine.[159] It is, however, more important to assess the patient clinically and to monitor electrocardiographic changes until the new steady state is achieved during concurrent quinidine–digoxin therapy.

Serum levels of digitoxin may also increase when quinidine is added. Renal clearance of digitoxin declines and is accompanied by an increased serum level. The nonrenal clearance may also decrease, but the volume of distribution remains unchanged and the digitoxin half-life is lengthened.[158]

Amiodarone, another potent antiarrhythmic agent, increases serum digoxin levels by 25% to 70%, and this increase appears to be related to the dose of amiodarone administered.[159] Generally, toxic manifestations of this interaction consist of bradycardia and varying degrees of AV block, rather than tachyarrhythmia. Renal and nonrenal clearance is decreased without any significant change in the apparent volume of distribution of digoxin. Procainamide, disopyramide, mexiletine, flecainide, and ethmozine do not appear to change serum digoxin concentrations significantly.

The calcium channel blocking agent verapamil interacts with digoxin and increases its serum concentrations in approximately 90% of patients.[159] Decreased renal and nonrenal clearance and volume of distribution result in elevated serum digoxin levels; these mechanisms are very similar to the digoxin–quinidine interaction. An inhibition of the tubular secretion of digoxin appears to be the mechanism for decreased renal clearance, since creatinine clearance remains unchanged. The magnitude of increase in serum digoxin levels is related to the dose of verapamil. A marked increase in the serum level of digoxin with concomitant administration of verapamil may cause potentially fatal cardiac toxicity, usually in the form of bradycardia and asystole rather than tachyarrhythmias. Tiapamil, a congener of verapamil, causes an increase in serum digoxin levels similar to that of verapamil. Nifedipine and nicardipine, two related calcium channel blocking agents, do not appear to affect serum digoxin levels significantly, and diltiazem, with larger doses (180 mg/day), causes only a small (average 22%) and probably not clinically relevant increase. Similarly, little or no change in digoxin levels is observed with gallopamil and lidoflazine.[159] Other drugs that can increase serum digoxin levels are spironolactone (inhibition of active tubular digoxin secretion) and some antihypertensive agents (decreased renal blood flow and glomerular filtration rate).[29]

Thus, several commonly used drugs can raise the serum digoxin concentrations and predispose to toxicity, and drug interactions should always be considered in patients who are on digitalis therapy.

DIAGNOSIS. Digitalis toxicity should be suspected in any patient receiving digitalis who complains of new gastrointestinal, ocular, or central nervous system symptoms. The appearance of a new arrhythmia should also be considered a potential indication of digitalis toxicity. Some electrocardiographic changes are very suggestive of digitalis effect; frequently, there is ST segment sagging, most prominent in leads I, aV_L, V_5, and V_6. The T wave voltage is frequently reduced and because of accelerated repolarization, the QT interval may be shortened. These changes do not indicate toxicity and do not necessarily precede arrhythmias.

The serum digoxin level is often helpful in the diagnosis of suspected digitalis toxicity, although the level by itself does not confirm or exclude digitalis toxicity in individual patients. The digoxin concentrations are usually measured by the radioimmunoassay technique. The optimal time for measurement of serum digoxin is just prior to the next dose, or at least 6 hours after an oral dose and 4 hours after intravenous administration. False-positive assays can be encountered in certain clinical circumstances, which include spironolactone therapy, the presence of circulating, gamma-emitting radioimagers, hyperbilirubinemia, and renal failure. In as many as 60% of patients with chronic renal failure, false-positive results can be observed and appear to be due to an endogenous circulating digoxin-like substance.[162]

To determine the therapeutic and toxic concentration of digoxin, correlations between the therapeutic and toxic manifestations to serum digoxin levels have been determined in normal volunteers and in patients with various cardiac disorders.[29] The mean serum digoxin level, in the absence of toxicity, was 1.4 ng/ml; in patients with toxicity, it was twofold to threefold higher. The therapeutic range has been regarded at 0.5 to 2.0 ng/ml. However, considerable overlap exists between the digoxin levels in toxic and nontoxic patients. Approximately 10% of patients who have serum digoxin concentrations within the therapeutic range manifest cardiac toxicity; similarly, in about 10% of patients without toxicity, serum digoxin levels are between 2 and 4 ng/ml. Studies correlating noncardiac symptoms of toxicity and serum digoxin concentrations have also revealed considerable overlap among serum digoxin levels in patients with and without extracardiac manifestations of toxicity, even when the mean serum digoxin levels in the two groups differed significantly.[29] Nevertheless, the higher the serum digoxin levels, the higher is the likelihood of toxicity; the probability of toxicity with serum digoxin levels exceeding 3 ng/ml is 12-fold higher than when the level is between 0 and 0.99 ng/ml.[163]

Serum concentrations of digoxin in relation to its inotropic and hemodynamic effects have been determined and the inotropic effects do not appear to be greater with serum digoxin levels above 1 to 2 ng/ml.[29] Supplemental doses of digoxin given intravenously to patients on conventional maintenance digoxin doses do not cause any further hemodynamic improvement.[76] These findings suggest that doses sufficient to maintain digoxin concentrations in the range of 1 to 2 ng/ml may provide maximal or near-maximal therapeutic effects. As the risk of digitalis toxicity increases with higher serum digoxin concentrations, the risk-to-benefit ratio appears to be optimal, with digoxin levels ranging between 1 and 2 ng/ml.[29] Mean serum levels of digitoxin, as with digoxin, were considerably higher (34–96 ng/ml) in patients with toxicity than in patients without toxicity (16.6–31.8 ng/ml) in different studies,[29] but considerable overlap in digitoxin concentrations was also found between the two groups.

It is apparent that the determination of serum digitalis levels is useful in the diagnosis of digitalis toxicity. However, levels within the "therapeutic range" should not be considered to exclude toxicity when clinical suspicion is strong, particularly in the presence of circumstances that predispose to digitalis toxicity (e.g., hypokalemia, hypomagnesemia, and severe acid-base imbalance).

In addition, as an aid in the diagnosis of digitalis toxicity, monitoring serum digitalis concentrations may be helpful to ensure adequate digitalization in a patient with suboptimal clinical response. Digitalis assays are also useful in detecting noncompliance, malabsorption, drug interactions, or poor bioavailability in patients who do not demonstrate the expected clinical response while on maintenance digitalis therapy.

It has been suggested that the estimation of electrolyte contents of the saliva may be useful to determine the digitalis effect in individual patients.[164] Salivary potassium and calcium concentrations and the products of potassium and calcium concentrations in saliva were significantly higher in the presence of digitalis toxicity than in the absence of toxicity. The diagnostic value of this test was independent of the digitalis preparation used. It has been postulated that changes in the salivary electrolyte concentrations represent inhibition of monovalent cation transport. This test, however, has not been adequately evaluated, and its role in the diagnosis of digitalis toxicity remains uncertain presently.

Red blood cell sodium and potassium levels may also correlate with digitalis effect.[165] Digitalis-induced inhibition of the sodium pump of erythrocytes decreases the rate of potassium or rubidium uptake, decreases the intracellular potassium, and increases sodium concentrations. Thus, erythrocyte rubidium uptake or the measurements of the intracellular concentrations of sodium and potassium of erythrocytes may aid in the diagnosis of digitalis toxicity. However, these tests have not been adequately evaluated and their clinical value has not been established. The acetyl strophanthidin test has been advocated to predict whether a given patient is overdigitalized or underdigitalized.[166]

The appearance of arrhythmias following intravenous administration of acetyl strophanthidin, a short-acting digitalis-like drug, had been considered suggestive of cardiac toxicity; however, the predictive value of this test has not been determined.

MANAGEMENT. All patients with significant arrhythmias, with or without hemodynamic compromise, should be hospitalized for observation and electrocardiographic monitoring. Patients with minor noncardiac symptoms, or with insignificant arrhythmias (e.g., occasional ectopic beats or atrial fibrillation with a slow ventricular response) do not require hospitalization and can be managed effectively by stopping the drug. Depending on the initial serum concentration, discontinuing digoxin for 24 to 48 hours causes adequate reduction of digoxin level, with reversal of toxicity in patients with normal renal function. Digitoxin should be discontinued for several days because of its longer half-life. The electrocardiogram should be repeated to ensure disappearance of the arrhythmia.

GENERAL THERAPY. General therapy of significant digitalis toxicity should include bed rest to avoid sympathetic stimulation and exacerbation of arrhythmias and discontinuation of digitalis, diuretics, and drugs that can potentially increase the serum digoxin level. Constant monitoring of cardiac rhythm is essential because multiple arrhythmias with variable hemodynamic consequences may occur over time. Serum electrolytes and digoxin concentrations should be determined and renal and hepatic function, as well as blood gases and acid-base balance, assessed. In patients with massive digitalis overdose, either suicidal or accidental, activated charcoal (50–100 g initially, then 20 g every 6 hours) may be administered to retard glycoside absorption. The corticosteroid-binding resin cholestyramine (4–8 g every 6 hours) may decrease the serum half-life of digitoxin significantly because it undergoes considerable enterohepatic circulation.[167] Colestipol appears to have a similar effect.[168] Digoxin has only minimal enterohepatic circulation, but cholestyramine may retard its initial absorption.

ATROPINE AND PACING.[158] Rhythm disturbances that compromise cardiac function require immediate and active intervention. Sinus bradycardia, AV block, and sinoatrial exit block can often be treated effectively with atropine alone. However, atropine is not always effective, and transvenous ventricular endocardial pacing may be required. The risk of ventricular arrhythmias during placement or displacement of the pacemaker electrode catheter appears to be higher. In the presence of intact AV conduction, atrial pacing reduces the risk of pacemaker-induced ventricular tachyarrhythmias; however, digitalis increases AV nodal refractoriness and, hence, ventricular pacing is preferable. Overdrive pacing can occasionally result in "overdrive acceleration" of the underlying tachyarrhythmia.

ANTIARRHYTHMIC AGENTS.[158] Phenytoin suppresses digitalis-induced enhanced automaticity and delayed afterdepolarization. It may also reverse digoxin-induced depression of AV and sinoatrial conduction. Decreased sympathetic outflow mediated by its effects on the central nervous system is considered as the mechanism of action.[169] Ventricular arrhythmias are particularly responsive to phenytoin (the other arrhythmias that may also respond are atrial tachycardia with block and nonparoxysmal junctional tachycardia). The inotropic effect of digitalis does not appear to be affected. It should be administered by slow intravenous infusion of 50 to 100 mg over 5 minutes, up to 15 mg/kg. Intravenous therapy should be followed by oral therapy (5 mg/kg daily) if the arrhythmia is controlled. Hypotension is the major complication of intravenous phenytoin therapy.

LIDOCAINE. Lidocaine is useful for controlling digitalis-induced ectopic rhythms. It does not adversely affect sinus rate or atrial, AV nodal, or His-Purkinje conduction. It does not possess any significant myocardial depressant effect. Rarely, lidocaine can suppress the ectopic pacemaker focus in the presence of advanced AV block and precipitate ventricular standstill. Indications for lidocaine therapy are ventricular tachyarrhythmias and atrial tachycardia with block.[170]

β-ADRENERGIC BLOCKING AGENTS. β-Adrenergic blocking agents are occasionally useful in controlling certain ectopic arrhythmias resulting from digitalis toxicity. The antiadrenergic effects decrease the automaticity and the direct effects shorten the refractory period of atrial and ventricular muscles and of the His-Purkinje fibers.[171] These potential beneficial effects, however, must be carefully weighed against the adverse effects, which include depression, sinoatrial and junctional pacemakers, and AV conduction. Thus, marked bradycardia or even asystole may result following the use of β-adrenergic blocking agents. Furthermore, their negative inotropic effects may cause hemodynamic compromise. Thus, in the presence of bradycardia, AV conduction abnormality, and heart failure, β-adrenergic blocking agents should not be used.

QUINIDINE, PROCAINAMIDE, AND DISOPYRAMIDE. Quinidine, procainamide, and disopyramide should be avoided in the treatment of arrhythmias associated with digitalis toxicity. These agents can cause depression of AV and His-Purkinje conduction and precipitate asystole. Myocardial depressant effects may worsen heart failure.

BRETYLIUM. Bretylium is also relatively contraindicated in digitalis toxicity. Initially, it can worsen tachyarrhythmias owing to release of stored catecholamines, which can enhance automaticity and delayed afterdepolarization and worsen hypokalemia.[172]

AMIODARONE. Amiodarone has been effective, occasionally, in controlling digitalis-induced ventricular tachycardia. However, amiodarone given intravenously or orally decreases AV conduction and can induce advanced AV block in the presence of digitalis toxicity. It also increases the serum digoxin level; thus, amiodarone should be avoided in the treatment of digitalis toxicity.

VERAPAMIL. Verapamil, a calcium channel blocking agent with negative inotropic and chronotropic properties, can worsen digitalis-induced AV block while suppressing delayed afterdepolarizations and triggered ectopy. It increases serum digoxin levels and can cause deterioration in heart failure. Thus, verapamil should not be used for treating supraventricular tachyarrhythmias associated with digitalis toxicity.

ELECTROLYTE REPLACEMENT. Potassium replacement is often the initial therapy of choice for ectopic rhythms, particularly in the presence of hypokalemia. Potassium replacement is effective in treating ventricular ectopy and tachycardia, atrial tachycardia with block, and nonparoxysmal AV junctional tachycardia. Increased extracellular potassium following potassium replacement therapy enhances sodium pump activity, which is associated with decreased intracellular calcium and secondary afterpolarization. Potassium should be administered with caution in the presence of conduction disturbances and should not be used in the absence of hypokalemia. The actions of potassium and digitalis are additive on the conduction tissues, and marked conduction abnormalities may occur following potassium therapy in the presence of digitalis toxicity. Potassium therapy is also contraindicated in renal failure and in the presence of pre-existing hyperkalemia. Hyperkalemia decreases resting membrane potential and potentiates digoxin's effect on AV conduction. A given dose of potassium chloride can produce a greater than expected increase in serum potassium level in patients with digitalis toxicity due to inhibition of the sodium–potassium pump. When indicated, potassium can be administered intravenously at a rate of 0.5 mEq/min in a saline solution through a large vein.

Magnesium given intravenously suppresses digitalis-induced ventricular arrhythmias.[173] However, it may also induce advanced AV block, hypotension, and respiratory depression. It is contraindicated in patients with renal failure, hypermagnesemia, and AV block.

CAROTID SINUS MASSAGE. Carotid sinus massage should not be attempted for diagnostic or therapeutic purposes in patients with supraventricular tachyarrhythmias due to suspected digitalis toxicity. In patients with digitalis toxicity, carotid sinus massage can precipitate ventricular asystole, advanced atrioventricular block, and malignant ventricular arrhythmias.[174]

CARDIOVERSION. Cardioversion should be avoided, if possible, in patients with digitalis toxicity. Digitalis decreases the energy threshold for cardioversion-induced arrhythmias by severalfold, and cardioversion can precipitate refractory ventricular tachyarrhythmias.[175] Release of catecholamines from cardiac nerve endings and alteration of membrane function leading to intracellular potassium egress might be the mechanism for the cardioversion-induced arrhythmias. Cardioversion, however, is recommended despite an increased risk of arrhythmias in patients in whom pharmacotherapy is ineffective and hemodynamic instability exists. Cardioversion therapy should be initiated at lower energy levels, which reduce the risk of developing arrhythmias. It needs to be emphasized that cardioversion does not enhance arrhythmias in the absence of overt digitalis toxicity.[176]

DIALYSIS. Renal or peritoneal dialysis is ineffective in decreasing total body digoxin content. Adsorptive hemoperfusion has been reported to increase the rate of removal of digoxin in some patients with digoxin toxicity.[177] With adsorptive hemoperfusion, the patient's blood is passed over an adsorbing substance such as charcoal and the drug is directly bound to the absorbent, which removes the glycoside. However, it is less effective than other therapeutic measures, such as digoxin-specific antibodies.

DIGOXIN-SPECIFIC ANTIBODIES. Digoxin-immune Fab is an antigen-binding agent and has emerged as an effective treatment for digitalis toxicity. In 1966, Buller and Chen demonstrated antibodies to digoxin in rabbits in response to immunization with a digoxin-albumin conjugate, and rabbit antiserum reversed manifestations of digitalis intoxication in experimental animals.[178] Subsequently, purified digoxin-specific antibodies were isolated from sheep antisera.[179] The whole heterologous antibodies, without purification, are likely to induce immediate and late hypersensitivity in humans, because of the presence of such foreign proteins. Digestion of the intact immunoglobulin (IgG) with papain yields two antigen-binding fragments (Fab) and one crystalline fragment (Fc), which contains the complement binding site. Digoxin-specific Fab can be isolated and purified from the papain-digested hyperimmune animal serum by the process of immunoadsorption. The purified Fab appears to possess the same affinity as the IgG for binding digoxin. Fab is less immunogenic than the IgG due to the absence of the Fc fragment. Because of the smaller size, these fragments distribute more rapidly and into a larger distribution of volume. The Fab-digoxin complex is also more rapidly excreted by glomerular filtration where the IgG-digoxin complex is slowly degraded by the reticuloendothelial system.

Fab binds one molecule of digoxin, and the affinity of Fab for digoxin is greater than the affinity of digoxin for (Na^+, K^+)-ATPase. $F(ab)_2$, an antibody fragment that contains two Fab molecules held together by a disulfide bond also has similar digoxin binding affinity and has been used for the treatment of digitalis toxicity.[180] Because of the higher binding affinity of the cardiac glycosides digoxin and digitoxin for Fab fragments, free cardiac glycosides rapidly bind with Fab and the concentrations of free glycosides decrease. Since the receptor-glycoside interactions are reversible, a concentration gradient is established as extracellular free digoxin concentrations decrease, causing a progressive efflux of cellular digoxin from its binding sites, which then bind to Fab fragments and become inactivated.

Following intravenous infusion of Fab, serum concentration of free (unbound) digoxin decreases to almost undetectable levels within a few minutes. Total serum digoxin concentrations, however, increase rapidly, usually exceeding pretreatment serum concentration of these glycosides by 10- to 20-fold. Almost all of the glycosides in serum are inactive and bound to Fab during the first 12 hours after the administration of Fab. The onset of action of Fab is usually within 30 minutes. The elimination half-life is between 15 and 20 hours in patients with normal renal function. In patients with renal failure, the excretion of the Fab-digoxin complex is probably significantly delayed. In functionally anephric patients, the Fab-digoxin complex is cleared not by glomerular filtration and renal excretion, but probably by the reticuloendothelial system. In patients with normal renal function, reinstitution of digoxin therapy should be delayed for 2 to 3 days until the Fab fragments are eliminated. In patients with impaired renal function a delay of 1 week or longer may be necessary.

Pharmacodynamic studies in experimental animal preparations have documented the efficacy of digoxin-specific antibodies and antibody fragments in reversing the physiologic and toxic effects of digoxin. Digoxin-induced inhibition of sodium and potassium transport in erythrocytes is reversed with digoxin antibody and antibody fragments.[179] Increased developed tension in isolated guinea pig atrial muscle strips with digoxin is reversed by antibody fragments.[179] The electrical inexcitability of canine Purkinje fibers exposed to toxic levels of digoxin can be reversed with digoxin antibodies with return of normal membrane properties.[181] Digoxin-induced increase in AV nodal effective and functional refractory period and conduction time are also rapidly reversed by digoxin antibodies.[181] Intact animal studies have shown that advanced cardiac toxicity is rapidly reversed with antibody fragments even after the administration of what are usually lethal doses for the animals.[182] The inotropic effects of digoxin are also reversed by Fab fragments and digoxin-specific antibodies.[183]

Several clinical studies have reported the efficacy of Fab fragments in the management of acute and chronic digoxin intoxication.[184-188] Extracardiac manifestations of digitalis toxicity are relatively less than cardiac manifestations in patients with acute digoxin intoxication. Many patients, particularly without pre-existing cardiac disorder, tolerate acute overdoses of digoxin well. Usual cardiac manifestations are sinus bradycardia, junctional rhythm, and varying degrees of AV block. However, ventricular tachyarrhythmias can occur that appear to be associated with a worse prognosis. Acute digoxin intoxication may be associated with hyperkalemia resulting from inhibition of the membrane-bound (Na^+, K^+)-ATPase pump, causing a net efflux of intracellular potassium and a rise in extracellular potassium. A serum potassium concentration higher than 5.5 mEq/liter has been reported to be associated with a very poor prognosis (almost 100% mortality) in patients with acute digoxin intoxication treated conventionally.[189] It has also been reported that with supportive treatment, in patients with acute digoxin intoxication, the overall mortality is about 20%, irrespective of serum potassium concentrations.[190] Manifestations and diagnosis of chronic digoxin intoxication have been outlined previously. The cardiac and noncardiac manifestations of digitalis toxicity are reversed by Fab fragments in the vast majority of patients. Wenger and co-workers[188] reported a complete resolution of digitalis toxicity in 53 of 56 patients treated with Fab. Reversal of digitalis toxicity occurred even in patients with impaired renal function and in both hyperkalemic and normokalemic patients. Only 2 of 15 patients with pretreatment serum potassium concentrations higher than 5.0 mEq/liter died, despite Fab therapy. Serum potassium levels decreased significantly and digoxin-induced bradyarrhythmias and tachyarrhythmias reversed in almost all patients.

Treatment with digoxin-immune Fab should be considered in patients with potentially life-threatening digoxin or digitoxin intoxication. Digoxin overdose, with ingestion of 10 mg of digoxin by previously healthy adults or 4 mg by healthy children or when the steady-state serum digoxin concentrations are greater than 10 ng/ml, is often associated with cardiac arrest, and these patients should be considered for treatment with Fab. A serum potassium concentration exceeding 5 mEq/liter is another indication of Fab treatment. Life-threatening arrhythmias such as ventricular tachycardia or progressive bradyarrhythmias, particularly when associated with compromised hemodynamics, are another indication for Fab therapy.

Commercially available digoxin antibody consists of ovine digoxin-specific antibody fragments (Fab) provided as a sterile lyophilized powder; each vial contains 40 mg of ovine Fab, 75 mg of sorbitol, and 28 mg of sodium chloride.

The dose of Fab is calculated to equal, in moles, the amount of digoxin or digitoxin in the patient's body. An estimate of total body load is based either on the known ingested dose or is estimated using a steady-state serum concentration. For *toxicity from an acute ingestion*, the total body load of digoxin will be approximately equal to the dose ingested.

To estimate total load from the steady-state serum concentration, the patient's serum *digoxin* concentration (SDC) in nanograms per milliliter is multiplied by the mean volume of distribution of digoxin in the body (5.6 liters/kg times patient weight in kilograms) to give total body load in micrograms. This is divided by 1000 to obtain the estimated amount of digoxin in the body in milligrams. For *digitoxin* toxicity, total body load can be estimated by using the value 0.56 liter/kg volume in place of the 5.6 liters/kg for digoxin.

The dose of Fab (in milligrams) is calculated by multiplying the total body load (in milligrams) by 60 (approximate ratio of molecular weight of Fab to molecular weight of digoxin providing an equimolar dose of antibody fragments).

For digoxin:

$$\text{Fab dose in mg} = [(\text{SDC})(5.6)(\text{weight in kg}) - 1000)](60)$$

For digitoxin:

$$\text{Fab dose in mg} = [(\text{SDC})(0.56)(\text{weight in kg}) - 1000)](60)$$

The dose can be rounded to the nearest multiple of 40 mg so that the full contents of each vial are administered.

The contents of each of the required number of vials are initially dissolved in 4 ml of sterile distilled water, giving an isosmotic solution with a Fab concentration of 10 mg/ml. This solution of Fab should be further diluted with isotonic saline (0.9% sodium chloride) to give a final concentration of Fab of 5 mg/ml. The final diluted solution is administered through a 0.22-μm Millipore filter intravenously at a constant rate over 20 minutes. In life-threatening situations it may be administered via bolus injection without a filter. No obvious adverse reactions to Fab therapy have been observed in clinical studies. Some degree of deterioration in left ventricular function was suspected in some patients; however, no controlled hemodynamic studies are available to assess the results of Fab therapy on cardiac function. Deterioration of renal function, acute hypersensitivity reaction, or delayed serum sickness have not been observed in patients receiving Fab therapy.

Skin testing of patients has revealed an extremely low incidence of reactions, and skin testing is not routinely required. Skin testing may be appropriate for high-risk patients, that is, those with a previous history of known allergies or previous exposure to digoxin-specific antibodies. Injection of 0.1 ml of 1:100 Fab (prepared by diluting 0.1 ml of already prepared solution with 9.9 ml sterile isotonic saline) and observing for 20 minutes or alternatively injecting 0.1 ml (1 mg) of undiluted Fab and observing for 5 minutes will help screen for sensitivity to Fab. If no reaction occurs, then full treatment should be started. The therapeutic approach for the treatment of digitalis toxicity is outlined in Table 14.5.

CATECHOLAMINES

A number of sympathomimetic amines are in clinical use, most commonly to correct hypotension or to increase cardiac output. Drugs such as norepinephrine, epinephrine, and isoproterenol, which contain O-dihydroxy benzene, also known as catechol, are frequently termed *catecholamines*.

The pharmacophysiologic effects of the sympathomimetic amines are mediated through their interaction with the adrenergic receptors. The response of the effector cells to catecholamines is related to activation of one of the two major types of receptors, α and β, as classified initially by Ahlquist in 1948,[191] based on the response to a number of sympathomimetic amines. Since then, subtypes of both α (α_1, α_2) and β (β_1, β_2) receptors have been identified along with their specific agonists and antagonists.[192] The distribution of the adrenoceptors is widespread, and the effector cells may have α- or β-receptors or both. α_1-Adrenoreceptors are present in the postganglionic effector cells, and activation of α_1-receptors is associated with contraction of vascular and nonvascular smooth muscles. α_2-Adrenoreceptors were initially recognized only in prejunctional nerve terminals, where their stimulation causes inhibition of the neuronal release of the neurotransmitter.[193] Recently, however, it has been appreciated that in many tissues, including vascular smooth muscle, the α_2-receptors can also be postjunctional, and stimulation of these receptors is associated with vasoconstriction.[194] It appears that in various animal species α_1-receptors are present in the myocardium.[195] Subtypes of β-receptors have been recognized by the sensitivity of β-receptors of different organs to their agonists and antagonists; heart, small intestine, and pancreas contain β_1-receptors, and bronchi, vascular beds, and uterus contain β_2-receptors. β_2-Receptors are also found on prejunctional nerve terminals, where their activation facilitates the release of neurotransmitters.[193] The activation of cardiac β_1-receptors is associated with increased contractility (positive inotropic effect), cardioacceleration (positive chronotropic effect), and enhanced AV nodal conduction (positive dromotropic effect). Vasodilation and decreased peripheral vascular tone result when β_2-adrenoreceptors are stimulated. Studies have indicated that a small proportion of the β-receptors in human myocardium are of the β_2-subtype.[196]

Normally, the adrenergic nervous system exerts an important physiologic role in regulating myocardial inotropic state and peripheral vascular tone. The inotropic state is modulated through the interaction of the myocardial β-receptors and the endogenous catecholamines. Norepinephrine released from the cardiac sympathetic nerve endings is the principal endogenous catecholamine involved in regulating the inotropic state; the circulating epinephrine released from the adrenal medulla and the norepinephrine released from noncardiac nerve endings appear to be of less importance. The influence of circulating catecholamines may become more important in patients with heart failure in maintaining the inotropic state. Various abnormalities of catecholamine kinetics and metabolism, and of adrenoreceptors, have been recognized in heart failure. The arterial plasma norepinephrine concentrations are frequently elevated. In some patients, the dopamine level is also increased but the epinephrine level may remain within the normal range.[197] Although increased plasma norepinephrine concentrations result partly from decreased clearance, there is also increased "spill over" from the neuronal junctions, which suggests enhanced sympathetic activity in heart failure.[198] Changes in sympathetic activity, however, are not uniform in all vascular beds. Myocardial and renal norepinephrine release is significantly increased, despite decreased clearance, whereas pulmonary clearance and release may remain unchanged.[198,199] An increased concentration of circulating norepinephrine and increased myocardial norepinephrine release occur in the presence of depleted myocardial norepinephrine stores.[200] The ratio of tissue concentrations of dopamine/norepinephrine in the failing myocardium increases, and it has been suggested that in the failing heart the rate-limiting enzyme for norepinephrine synthesis may not be tyrosine hydroxylase, which is necessary for conversion of tyrosine to dopa, but is dopamine β-hydroxylase, which is required for conversion of dopamine to norepinephrine.[201,202] The activity of tyrosine hydroxylase, normally a rate-limiting enzyme for norepinephrine production, may not change in heart failure. Similarly, neuronal reuptake and the activity of the enzymes catecholamine-orthomethyltransferase and monoamine oxidase necessary for the metabolism of catecholamines appear to be unaltered in heart failure. The precise explanation for decreased myocardial norepinephrine stores remains unclear; however, chronically enhanced cardiac sympathetic activity, as evident from increased myocardial norepinephrine release, has been suggested as the possible mechanism.[199] Decreased catecholamine sensitivity and reduced β-adrenoreceptor density have also been documented in failing human hearts.[203,204]

Changes in myocardial adrenergic function in heart failure may have considerable pathophysiologic and therapeutic implications.[205,206] Human atria and ventricles contain both β_1- and β_2-adrenoreceptors. Nonfailing human ventricles contain primarily β_1-receptors. Of the total pool of β-adrenoreceptors, approximately 80% are of β_1 type and 20% are of β_2 type, although the range of the latter can vary from 0 to 35%. Atria compared with ventricles may contain proportionately higher percentage of β_2-receptors, particularly in the region of the SA node, and the β_2-selective agonists may exert more pronounced chronotropic response compared with β_1-selective agonists. Binding of both subtypes of β-adrenoreceptors with the neurotransmitters or hormones enhances inotropism via increasing the adenylate cyclase activity and generation of cyclic AMP. Generation of cyclic AMP following β_1-receptor activation is much less than after activation of β_2-receptors. Nevertheless, the increase in inotropism following β_1-receptor stimulation is far greater than after β_2-receptor stimulation, because the degree of inotropic stimulation is proportionate to the number of receptors present. Adrenergic function appears to be significantly altered in heart failure. Myocardial β-adrenergic receptors of failing human ventricles are subsensitive to stimulation by isoproterenol, a nonselective β-adrenergic agonist. Maximal stimulation of inotropism and stimula-

TABLE 14.5 MANAGEMENT OF DIGITALIS TOXICITY

General Therapy
Discontinue digitalis
Monitor cardiac rhythm
Determine electrolytes and serum digoxin concentration
Observe for hemodynamic compromise
In massive digitalis overdose, give activated charcoal or cholestyramine orally

Management of Arrhythmias
Potassium and magnesium replacement, indicated in the presence of hypokalemia and contraindicated in the presence of preexisting hyperkalemia, bradycardia, and atrioventricular block
Phenytoin and lidocaine in ventricular arrhythmias in the presence of atrioventricular block
Atropine for sinoatrial and atrioventricular conduction anomalies
Pacemaker therapy for persistent bradycardia and atrioventricular block
Cardioversion with lowest effective energy for immediate therapy for ventricular tachycardia and fibrillation
Drugs to be avoided: procainamide, quinidine, disopyramide, β-blocking agents, isoproterenol, bretylium, amiodarone, and verapamil
Fab-digoxin therapy
  Life-threatening arrhythmias (ventricular tachycardia)
  Hyperkalemia (serum K^+ > 5.5 mEq/liter)

Management of Hypotension and Low-Output State
Vasopressor to maintain arterial pressure
Fab-digoxin therapy
Control associated arrhythmias

tion of adenylate cyclase by isoproterenol decrease markedly, which is related to a decrease in the total pool of β-adrenergic receptors. Decreased β-receptor density in heart failure results primarily from decreased β_1-receptor subtype, which may be 60% to 70% lower than the β_1-receptor density of the nonfailing ventricles. In the failing human ventricles, β_2-adrenergic receptor density appears to remain relatively unchanged; thus, β_1/β_2 subtype ratio changes from approximately 80:20 in nonfailing heart to 60:40 in failing heart. Although β_2-receptor density is maintained in heart failure, the adenylate cyclase response to β_2-selective agonists is attenuated, probably due to "uncoupling" of β_2-receptors from their pharmacologic pathway.

It has also been observed that the other components of the β-adrenergic receptor density and adenylate cyclase complex might be abnormal in patients with congestive heart failure. Abnormalities in the quantity or function of the guanine-nucleotide proteins have been observed in heart failure. A substantial decrease in the stimulating guanosine triphosphate (GTP) binding protein Gs has been observed in dogs with ventricular failure due to pressure overload and in patients with advanced congestive heart failure.[206] An increase in activity of the inhibitory G protein (G1) has also been observed and has been proposed for the uncoupling of the β_2-receptor in the failing human heart.[205] Abnormalities of myocardial adrenergic function may have important therapeutic implications in the inotropic treatment of congestive heart failure. Because of the down-regulation of the β_1-receptors, the selective β_1-receptor agonists may be less effective in enhancing inotropism of the failing ventricles. Inotropic agents with β_2-agonist properties such as dobutamine may have an advantage in the inotropic treatment of heart failure, since β_2-receptor density tends to remain unchanged.

Although β-receptors are the predominant myocardial adrenoreceptors, α_1-adrenergic receptors have also been demonstrated in mammalian myocardium, including human myocardium. However, the ratio of α- to β-receptor density in human myocardium is low, between 0.13 and 0.19.[207] Although activation of myocardial α_1-receptors is associated with positive inotropic effects, its contribution compared with β-receptor activation for enhancing inotropy is likely to be minor because of its much lower density. The duration of action potential is prolonged and the development of contraction is relatively slow following α_1-receptor stimulation.[208] The duration of contraction following β_1-receptor stimulation is shorter and myocardial relaxation is faster.[209,210] α_1-Receptor stimulation does not produce any myocardial relaxant effects.[208] Activation of myocardial β-receptors increases intracellular cyclic AMP concentration by stimulating the adenylate cyclase enzyme system. Cyclic AMP leads to activation of protein kinases and to phosphorylation of several proteins that apparently promote slow Ca^{2+} inward current. This causes an increased release of Ca^{2+} from the sarcoplasmic reticulum, either because it triggers Ca^{2+}-dependent Ca^{2+} release or because a greater filling of the sarcoplasmic stores with Ca^{2+} occurs, which is then available for subsequent contractions.[209,210] In contrast to β-receptor stimulation, α_1-receptor stimulation does not produce any significant changes in cyclic AMP levels. Phosphodiesterase inhibition potentiates the effects of β-receptor agonists by raising cyclic AMP levels but has no effects on α_1-receptor agonists, providing further evidence for the noncyclic AMP–mediated mechanism of action of the myocardial α_1-receptor activation. It has been suggested that α_1-receptor stimulation results in hydrolysis or turnover of polyphosphoinositides (P1), which results in formation of inositol 1,4,5-triphosphate (IP3) and diacyl-glycerol (DAG).[211,212] It has been shown that IP3 increases cytosolic free calcium by triggering release of calcium from internal stores and is the proposed mechanism of the positive inotropic effect of the α_1-receptor activation.[211]

The cardiovascular effects of sympathomimetic drugs result from activation of the α- or β-receptors or both, and the net effects are determined by the predominance of α- or β-receptor stimulation, which varies with the type of sympathomimetic amine. It needs to be appreciated that most sympathomimetic drugs influence both α- and β-receptor activity, but relative activation of α- and β-receptors varies tremendously. Some drugs, such as phenylephrine, possess almost pure α-receptor stimulating activity, and others, such as isoproterenol, have almost pure β-receptor stimulating activity. Drugs such as dopamine stimulate dopaminergic receptors, in addition to α- and β-adrenergic receptors. Drugs with both α- and β-receptor activity may produce variable responses on blood pressure, depending on the magnitude of α- and β-receptor activity. Stimulation of α-receptors increases blood pressure, and stimulation of β_2-receptors decreases blood pressure owing to reduction of systemic vascular resistance. A concomitant increase in cardiac output due to β_1-receptor stimulation may also modify the blood pressure response. Augmented contractility, increased heart rate, and decreased systemic vascular resistance may all contribute to an increased cardiac output following the use of sympathomimetic drugs possessing predominantly β-activity. On the other hand, drugs with predominant α-activity may cause a reduction in cardiac output owing to increased systemic vascular resistance, which also raises the resistance to left ventricular ejection.

The electrophysiologic effects of β_1-receptor agonists mediate their chronotropic and dromotropic effects and also their arrhythmogenicity. The sinus node discharge rate (automaticity) increases, resulting in an increased heart rate. The refractory period of the action potentials is abbreviated, and there is enhanced spontaneous phase 4 depolarization of the Purkinje cells, contributing to ventricular arrhythmias.[213] The electrophysiologic effects of different sympathomimetic drugs vary, and therefore their relative potency to induce tachycardia or arrhythmias is also variable. The expected hemodynamic effects of the various catecholamines in clinical use are summarized in Table 14.6.

CLINICAL APPLICATIONS IN CARDIOLOGY
NOREPINEPHRINE
The use of norepinephrine is limited to correct severe hypotension in some patients with cardiogenic or septic shock usually when other vasopressor agents fail to maintain adequate arterial pressure. Its hemodynamic effects have been evaluated in patients with pump failure and shock complicating myocardial infarction.[214] In patients with cardiogenic shock, arterial pressure and systemic vascular resistance increase with little or no change in cardiac output. Although it has the potential to increase cardiac output by stimulating the β_1-adrenoreceptors, a concomitant increase in systemic vascular resistance resulting from α-receptor stimulation increases resistance to left ventricular ejection, which tends to decrease cardiac output. Furthermore, excessive tachycardia and ventricular arrhythmias may occur when larger doses are used. Renal, cerebral, hepatic, and skeletal muscle blood flow may decrease because of regional vasoconstriction.[215] Coronary blood flow and myocardial oxygen consumption may increase due to increased myocardial oxygen requirements resulting from increased afterload, inotropic state and heart rate, and the worsening myocardial oxygen balance may enhance ischemia and the extent of myocardial injury following acute myocardial infarction. This effect, however, may be partially offset by the increase in blood pressure and therefore coronary perfusion pressure with improved myocardial perfusion.

Norepinephrine is administered intravenously, and the infusion rate should be increased slowly, starting with a small dose, 0.025 to 0.1 μg/kg/min while monitoring changes in arterial pressure; the usual dose is 2 to 8 μg/kg/min. The half-life of norepinephrine is approximately 2 minutes, and its pressor response usually disappears within 1 to 2 minutes after discontinuation of the infusion. Most of the infused norepinephrine is metabolized by catecholamine-orthomethyl-transferase and monoamine oxidase and is excreted as inactive compounds. Only 4% to 16% of an administered dose is excreted unchanged in the urine.[215]

EPINEPHRINE
Epinephrine is a potent agonist at α_1, α_2, β_1, and β_2 adrenergic receptors. At all doses, heart rate and myocardial contractility increase due to direct activation of myocardial β_1- and possibly β_2-adrenoreceptors.

The changes in peripheral vascular resistance appear to be dose dependent. At low doses (less than 0.1 µg/kg/min), systemic vascular resistance tends to fall because its β_2-adrenoreceptor–mediated vasodilatory effects predominate. Blood flow to skeletal muscle and splanchnic bed may increase with decreased flow to cutaneous and renal vascular beds. Low doses of epinephrine increase myocardial blood flow presumably from autoregulation rather than due to its direct effect on the coronary circulation. Higher doses of epinephrine also increase heart rate and myocardial contractility. However, vasoconstrictor responses mediated by activation of vascular α_1- and α_2-receptors override β_2-receptor–mediated vasodilator responses, resulting in increased systemic vascular resistance and arterial pressure. Myocardial blood flow may also increase owing to augmented perfusion pressure.

The principal therapeutic use of epinephrine is during resuscitation from cardiac arrest. Administration of epinephrine is associated with increased systolic and diastolic pressure and improved cerebral and coronary perfusion. Epinephrine is occasionally used to restore an idioventricular rhythm in patients with the Stokes-Adams syndrome before an artificial pacemaker is installed. However, isoproterenol is more effective than epinephrine for this indication. In some patients with low cardiac output and hypotension following cardiac surgery, epinephrine infusion is useful. However, excessive vasoconstriction and increased systemic vascular resistance may be associated with a decrease or no change in cardiac output. Furthermore, excessive tachycardia and arrhythmias limit its use. The usual dose of epinephrine, when given by intravenous infusion, is 0.25 to 0.30 µg/kg/min. The infused epinephrine is metabolized and disposed in the same way as norepinephrine.[215]

ISOPROTERENOL

Isoproterenol is a potent β-adrenoreceptor agonist that stimulates β_1- and β_2-adrenoreceptors equally. Myocardial contractility and heart rate increase due to activation of β_1-receptors, and systemic vascular resistance falls due to β_2-receptor–mediated vasodilatation. Marked reduction in systemic vascular resistance can produce significant hypotension and compromise myocardial perfusion due to decreased perfusion pressure. Decreased diastolic perfusion time due to excessive tachycardia may also impair myocardial perfusion. Myocardial oxygen requirements also increase concurrently, and myocardial oxygen balance may worsen. Thus, the potential exists for an increase in ischemia and the extent of myocardial injury, despite improvements in cardiac performance. At low doses, isoproterenol may increase coronary blood flow to the subendocardium and subepicardium; but at higher doses, subendocardial and subepicardial perfusion may decrease owing to decreased perfusion pressure and diastolic perfusion time.

Isoproterenol is also a potent arrhythmogenic agent, and ventricular tachyarrhythmias are common with larger doses of isoproterenol. Augmented cardiac output is usually distributed to skeletal muscles. Renal blood flow tends to increase in patients with cardiogenic shock, but there may be a redistribution of flow from the renal cortex to the medulla, causing no improvement in or a deterioration of renal function. These undesirable hemodynamic and metabolic effects of isoproterenol, along with its arrhythmogenicity, have restricted its use in most clinical situations. It is usually used in patients with bradycardia or complete AV block before a temporary pacemaker can be inserted. In patients with low cardiac output resulting from or associated with increased pulmonary vascular resistance, as in some patients following

TABLE 14.6 HEMODYNAMIC EFFECTS OF SYMPATHOMIMETIC DRUGS

Drug	Receptor Activation			Hemodynamic Effects				
	α	β_1	β_2	SVR	MAP	CO	HR	PCWP
Norepinephrine	+++	+	−	↑↑↑	↑↑↑	↔↓	↔↑	↑↔
Isoproterenol	−	+++	+++	↓↓↓	↓↓	↑↑↑	↑↑↑	↓↓
Epinephrine	+++	+++	+++	↓	↑↔	↑↑	↑↑↑	↑↔
Dopamine	++	++	−	↓↔	↑↑	↑↑	↑	↑↔
(and DA_1 and DA_2 receptors)								
Dobutamine	+	+++	+	↓	↔↓	↑↑↑	↔↑	↓↔
Phenylephrine	+++	+	−	↑↑↑	↑↑	↔↓	↓↔	↑↔
Methoxamine	+++	−	−	↑↑↑	↑↑↑	↔↓	↓	↑↔
Metaraminol	++	−	−	↑↑	↑↑	↔↓	↔↑	↑↔
Salbutamol	−	+	+++	↓↓	↓↔	↑↑	↔↑	↓↔
Pirbuterol	−	+	+++	↓↓	↓↔	↑↑	↔↑	↓↔
Prenalterol	−	++	+	↓	↔↓	↑	↔↓	↓↔
TA-064	−	++	+	↓	↔	↑	↔↑	↓↔
Butopamine	−	++	+	↓	↔	↑	↑	↓↔
Levodopa	+	+	+	↓	↔	↑	↔↑	↔
(activation of DA_1 and DA_2 receptors)								
Ibopamine	−	+	+	↓	↔	↑	↑↔	↑↔
(DA_1 and DA_2 receptor activation)								
Dopexamine	−	+	+	↓	↔↓	↑	↔	↓
(DA_1 receptor agonist)								
Propylbutyl-dopamine	−	−	−	↓	↓	↑	↔	↓
(activation of DA_1 and DA_2 receptors)								
Fenoldopam	−	−	−	↓	↔	↑	↔↑	↓
(DA_1 agonist)								

(+, Activation; −, no effect; ↑ increase; ↓ decrease; ↔ no change; SVR, systemic vascular resistance; MAP, mean arterial pressure; CO, cardiac output; HR, heart rate; PCWP, pulmonary capillary wedge pressure)

mitral valve surgery, isoproterenol infusion may improve hemodynamics. Isoproterenol is used frequently to maintain adequate heart rate and inotropic state of the denervated transplanted heart. The usual dose of isoproterenol when given by intravenous infusion is 2 to 5 μg/min. Its metabolism and excretion are similar to those of epinephrine and norepinephrine.[215]

DOPAMINE

Systemic and regional hemodynamic effects of dopamine are mediated through a number of mechanisms: activation of dopaminergic α- and β₁-receptors and release of norepinephrine (tyramine-like effect). The subtypes of dopamine receptors, DA_1 and DA_2 (D_1 and D_2) have been identified by radioligand binding assays and by pharmacophysiologic studies. DA_1 receptors are postsynaptic, and their stimulation is associated with dilatation of the renal, mesenteric, coronary, and cerebrovascular beds. Activation of DA_2 receptors, which are located on postganglionic sympathetic nerves and autonomic ganglia, is associated with inhibition of norepinephrine release from the sympathetic nerve endings. The expected pharmacologic effects of activation of dopamine receptors are illustrated in Figure 14.7. The subtype DA_2 receptors are also present in the emetic center of the area postrema and in the anterior lobe of the pituitary gland. Stimulation of DA_2 receptors in these areas is associated with nausea and vomiting and decreased prolactin release, respectively.

The renal, peripheral vascular, and cardiac effects of dopamine appear to be dose related.[216-218] With a dose of 0.5 to 2 μg/kg/min given intravenously, dopamine receptors are activated and some peripheral vasodilation, along with increased renal flow, urine volume, and sodium excretion result. Dopamine-induced natriuresis has been observed in the absence of any increase in total renal blood flow, and a redistribution of medullary flow to the cortex has been proposed as the potential mechanism. If there is a reduction in arterial pressure, renal function may not improve because of reduced renal perfusion pressure. With a larger dose, 2 to 5 μg/kg/min, cardiac β₁-receptors are stimulated and positive inotropic and chronotropic effects are manifest by an increase in cardiac output. Pulmonary capillary wedge pressure may decrease slightly or may remain unchanged, and there may not be any increase in arterial pressure. A larger dose, exceeding 5 to 10 μg/kg/min, is associated with peripheral vasoconstriction and increased systemic vascular resistance resulting from activation of the α-receptors. There is no further change in cardiac output as arterial pressure increases. Pulmonary capillary wedge pressure, pulmonary artery pressure, and pulmonary vascular resistance tend to increase.

It should be noted that in individual patients the hemodynamic responses expected in response to a given dose of dopamine may not occur. In some patients, with a very low dose of dopamine (e.g., 2 μg/kg/min), an increase in cardiac output due to increased contractility may be observed. At intermediate infusion rates, arterial and venous constriction may result from activation of α-adrenergic receptors, leading to increases in arterial and ventricular filling pressures. Increased filling pressures result primarily from increased venous return to the heart.

In patients with hypotension and low cardiac output, the addition of dobutamine to dopamine may allow maintenance of arterial pressure and cardiac output; and it is possible to use relatively lower doses of both dopamine and dobutamine, so that the potential adverse effects resulting from the administration of higher doses of these agents can be prevented. The increase in pulmonary capillary wedge pressure that tends to occur with high doses of dopamine can be avoided with maintaining adequate arterial pressure and cardiac output.[219]

Compared with isoproterenol, dopamine possesses less positive inotropic, chronotropic, and arrhythmogenic properties; as a result, the magnitude of increase in cardiac output with dopamine is less than that with isoproterenol, but excessive tachycardia and ventricular tachyarrhythmias are also less frequent.[215] Vasoconstriction and augmentation of peripheral vascular resistance with dopamine are less than with norepinephrine, and the magnitude of increase in arterial pressure is also less. However, dopamine induces fewer arrhythmias

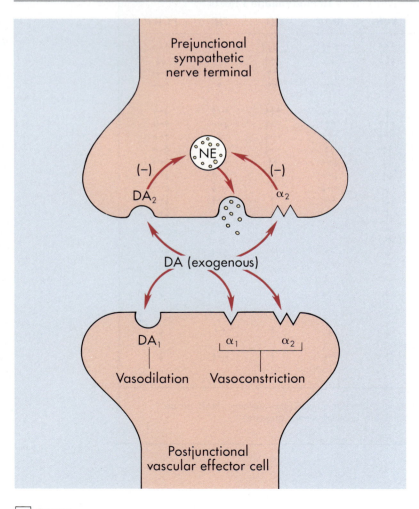

FIGURE 14.7 Location of the subtypes of dopamine and α receptors. DA_1 receptors, α₁-receptors, and α₂-receptors are located on postganglionic vascular effector cells and DA_2 receptors are on the prejunctional sympathetic nerve terminal. With dopamine infusion, activation of DA_1 receptors causes vasodilation and activation of DA_2 receptors causes inhibition of norepinephrine (NE) release. A higher dose of dopamine stimulates α₁- and α₂-receptors on the effector cells to cause vasoconstriction and prejunctional α₂-receptors to inhibit release of norepinephrine. (Modified from Goldberg LI, Razfers SI: Dopamine receptors: Applications in clinical cardiology. Circulation 72:245, 1985. Reprinted with permission of the American Heart Association, Inc)

and fewer adverse hemodynamic and metabolic effects compared with norepinephrine, and it is preferable to norepinephrine for the treatment of hypotension.

In certain clinical situations, the use of dopamine is preferable to the use of other catecholamines. In patients with decreased urine output with or without heart failure, an infusion of low-dose dopamine may augment urine output. When hypotension results primarily from low systemic vascular resistance, as in septic shock, dopamine is effective in maintaining arterial pressure. Dopamine is also useful for correcting the hypotension accompanying a reduced cardiac output, particularly when pulmonary capillary wedge pressure is not markedly elevated. A rise in pulmonary capillary wedge pressure can often be prevented by the concomitant use of a venodilator such as nitroglycerin. Excessive vasoconstriction with larger doses of dopamine may be associated with undesirable systemic hemodynamic effects, which can be reduced by the simultaneous administration of vasodilator-like sodium nitroprusside and nitroglycerin.[220,221]

In experimental animals with acute myocardial ischemia, dopamine increased blood flow in the normal and moderately ischemic myocardial segments; in the severely ischemic zones, blood flow remained virtually unchanged. However, if excessive tachycardia developed in response to dopamine, an increase in paradoxical systolic bulging of the ischemic myocardial segments along with decreased myocardial blood flow and endocardial/epicardial flow ratio to the severely ischemic zones were observed.[222] Thus, the potential benefits of dopamine on the mechanical and metabolic function of severely ischemic myocardium were offset by tachycardia. In the absence of cardiac acceleration, dopamine may not increase ischemic zone ST segment elevation, despite augmented contractility.[223] Increased arterial pressure and therefore coronary artery perfusion pressure may improve perfusion of the ischemic myocardial zones. An increment in myocardial blood flow in the territory of a narrowed coronary artery during dopamine infusion has been reported.[224] With higher doses of dopamine, increased arterial pressure, heart rate, systemic vascular resistance, and contractility augment myocardial oxygen requirements, and the potential exists for enhancement of myocardial ischemia in patients with coronary artery disease. Myocardial lactate production, indicating myocardial ischemia, has been observed in response to dopamine in patients with acute myocardial infarction and pump failure, despite improved systemic hemodynamics.[225] In these patients, left ventricular function may deteriorate during continued dopamine therapy. Thus, in patients with acute myocardial infarction and shock, a prolonged infusion of dopamine alone should be avoided and other measures, such as the concomitant use of vasodilators or intra-aortic balloon counterpulsation, or both, should be considered.

In addition to an increase in myocardial oxygen consumption and excessive vasoconstriction, dopamine may induce arrhythmias. Prolonged infusion has been reported to precipitate angina, nausea, vomiting, and peripheral gangrene. The duration of action of dopamine is brief, and its half-life of elimination is short. It is metabolized by monoamine oxidase.[215]

DOBUTAMINE

The synthetic sympathomimetic amine dobutamine is a potent β_1-receptor agonist. However, it also possesses β_2- and α-receptor agonist properties.[226] It does not cause neuronal norepinephrine release. Dobutamine is a racemic mixture of L-isomers and D-isomers. The L-isomer is an α_1-receptor agonist and a relatively weak β-receptor agonist. The D-isomer has pronounced effects on β-receptors and little effect on α-receptors. β_2-Receptor–mediated peripheral vasodilation is partly counteracted by the concomitant activation of vascular α_1-receptors. The positive inotropic effect of β_1-receptors is potentiated by simultaneous activation of the myocardial α-receptors. Unlike dopamine, the positive inotropic effect of dobutamine is not related to norepinephrine stores. The usual net hemodynamic effects are a substantial increase in cardiac output, with little or no change in arterial pressure and little or no increase in heart rate.[227] Systemic vascular and pulmonary vascular resistances decrease along with a modest decrease in pulmonary capillary wedge pressure.

In the experimental animals with acute ischemia, blood flow in the normal zones and in the moderately ischemic zones increases in response to dobutamine and the blood flow to the severely ischemic zones remains unchanged. However, if significant tachycardia developed, decreased blood flow and endocardial/epicardial blood flow ratio to the ischemic zone along with deterioration in regional myocardial mechanical function were observed.[222] In other experimental studies, in animals with acute or chronic myocardial ischemia, increased blood flow to all myocardial zones has been reported in response to dobutamine.[228] Intact autonomic nervous system activities may prevent tachycardia, and therefore the deleterious effects of dobutamine on myocardial ischemia may be avoided. In anesthetized open-chest dogs with acute myocardial infarction, the magnitude of ST segment elevation may increase, indicating an increase in infarct size probably related to excessive tachycardia frequently observed in these preparations.[228] Marked tachycardia-related increase in oxygen demand and concurrent impairment of myocardial perfusion due to shorter diastole might have been contributory to the deleterious effects on the ischemic injury in the presence of myocardial infarction.

In patients with acute myocardial infarction, dobutamine infusion does not appear to increase infarct size, the frequency of reinfarction, or the extension of infarction.[229] In patients with chronic, nonischemic congestive heart failure, improved coronary hemodynamics and myocardial energetics have been observed.[230] With lower (5 μg/kg/min) and higher doses (10 μg/kg/min) of dobutamine, myocardial oxygen consumption and coronary blood flow increased along with improvement in hemodynamics. However, myocardial oxygen/supply ratio remained unchanged and there was no clinical or biochemical evidence for myocardial ischemia. Comparative effects of dobutamine and dopamine on systemic and coronary hemodynamics have been evaluated in patients following cardiac surgery.[231] With similar increases in cardiac output and left ventricular dP/dt, myocardial oxygen consumption increased with both agents. With dobutamine, however, the increase in oxygen uptake was accompanied by a significantly greater increase in coronary blood flow, suggesting that dobutamine does not limit the increase in coronary blood flow associated with increased oxygen demand. In patients with chronic ischemic heart failure, dobutamine increases coronary blood flow and myocardial oxygen consumption (Fig. 14.8).[232] With increasing doses of dobutamine (5, 7.5, and 10 μg/kg/min) there was a progressively significant increase in coronary blood flow. Changes in myocardial oxygen consumption paralleled changes in coronary blood flow, and there was no change in myocardial oxygen extraction. An increase in coronary blood flow may result from decreased coronary vascular resistance secondary to increased metabolic demand. The direct coronary vasodilatory effect of dobutamine, mediated by activation of β_2-adrenergic receptors may also contribute to decreased coronary vascular resistance and increased coronary blood flow.[233] However, increased myocardial oxygen demands appear to be the important contributing factor for the increase in coronary blood flow in patients with ischemic heart failure. Larger doses of dobutamine (10 μg/kg/min) may cause a greater increase in myocardial oxygen demand than in coronary blood flow, thus enhancing the potential to induce myocardial ischemia.[234] A marked increase in heart rate contributes to an excessive increase in myocardial oxygen requirements. Changes in coronary hemodynamics in response to dobutamine may be influenced by the presence or absence of obstructive coronary artery disease. The increase in coronary blood flow may be substantially greater in patients without coronary artery disease than in patients with coronary artery disease, although changes in systemic hemodynamics and contractility were similar in both groups.[235] Differences in myocardial metabolic function between patients with and without coronary artery disease have been observed following infusion of dobutamine, despite similar improvement in systemic hemodynamics and cardiac performance.[236] In patients with primary dilated cardiomyopathy, myocardial lactate extraction remained unchanged.

However, in 11% of patients with coronary artery disease there was myocardial lactate production suggesting myocardial ischemia. About 17% of patients with coronary artery disease also develop angina. As larger doses of dobutamine infusion can induce myocardial ischemia in patients with obstructive coronary artery disease, dobutamine stress echocardiography is evolving as a method of evaluation of coronary artery disease by detecting reversible regional myocardial wall motion abnormalities.[237] With the therapeutic doses of dobutamine, however, myocardial ischemia is unlikely to develop, even in patients with obstructive coronary artery disease, provided excessive tachycardia does not occur. This is probably related to the maintenance of myocardial oxygen supply and demand balance.

Dobutamine, unlike dopamine, does not stimulate renal dopamine receptors and thus does not selectively increase renal blood flow. However, renal blood flow, urine volume, and sodium excretion may increase along with an increased cardiac output in patients with heart failure.

The hemodynamic effects of dobutamine have been compared with those of other catecholamines and vasodilators. The magnitude of the increase in cardiac output with dobutamine and isoproterenol was similar. Changes in mean arterial pressure, systemic vascular resistance, and mean pulmonary artery and pulmonary capillary wedge pressure were also similar.[238] The increase in heart rate, however, was considerably greater with isoproterenol than with dobutamine. The propensity to induce ventricular arrhythmias is also higher with isoproterenol.

The comparative hemodynamic effects of dobutamine and dopamine were determined in patients with chronic heart failure, cardiogenic shock, and following cardiac surgery.[239,240] Although both dobutamine and dopamine increase cardiac output, pulmonary capillary wedge pressure tends to increase with dopamine, whereas it decreases with dobutamine. Pulmonary artery pressure and pulmonary vascular resistance may also increase with dopamine. Although systemic vascular resistance may decrease with both agents, arterial pressure tends to increase with dopamine, but not with dobutamine, suggesting that for the same magnitude of increase in cardiac output, the relative reduction in systemic vascular resistance is less with dopamine than with dobutamine. Increase in cardiac output in response to dopamine is frequently due to an increase in heart rate, whereas dobutamine increases stroke volume consistently.[241]

Compared with nitroprusside, dobutamine causes less reduction in pulmonary capillary wedge pressure for a similar increase in cardiac output.[242] Myocardial oxygen consumption tends to decrease with nitroprusside while it increases with dobutamine. The magnitude of reduction in mean and diastolic arterial pressure is, however, more with nitroprusside than with dobutamine. Thus, in the presence of myocardial ischemia, nitroprusside has more potential to decrease coronary blood flow by reducing coronary artery perfusion pressure.

The systemic hemodynamic effects of dobutamine infusion and intravenous digoxin were evaluated in patients with mild to moderate heart failure complicating acute myocardial infarction.[85] Although dobutamine consistently increased cardiac output and decreased pulmonary capillary wedge pressure, hemodynamic changes following digoxin were variable and no improvement in left ventricular function was observed. Systemic vascular resistance fell with dobutamine but remained unchanged with digoxin.

Dobutamine is effective in the management of both acute and chronic heart failure. In patients with pump failure and low cardiac output, if inotropic support seems necessary, dobutamine is preferable to dopamine, particularly when the pulmonary capillary wedge pressure is elevated and the arterial pressure is adequate. When severe hypotension (mean arterial pressure < 60 mm Hg) accompanies low cardiac output, dobutamine should not be used initially and a vasopressor agent, such as dopamine, should be started to increase arterial pressure to the adequate range. For a further increase in cardiac output, dobutamine can then be added.[219] A combination of dopamine and dobutamine has also been shown to reduce the adverse hemodynamic effects of each. Dopamine in low doses may be added for its renal effects when urine output remains low, despite an increase in cardiac output with dobutamine. Dobutamine and nitroprusside can also be used concurrently because the combination may result in a higher cardiac output and lower pulmonary capillary wedge pressure than with either drug alone. In the presence of hypotension, however, this combination should be avoided, since further hypotension may ensue.

Dobutamine is effective in increasing cardiac output in patients with predominant right ventricular infarction. Right and left ventricular ejection fractions improve with little or no change in systemic and pulmonary venous pressure. The hemodynamic effects of dobutamine and nitroprusside have been compared in right ventricular infarction, and a greater increase in cardiac output with dobutamine has been observed.[243] Dobutamine is also effective in improving cardiac func-

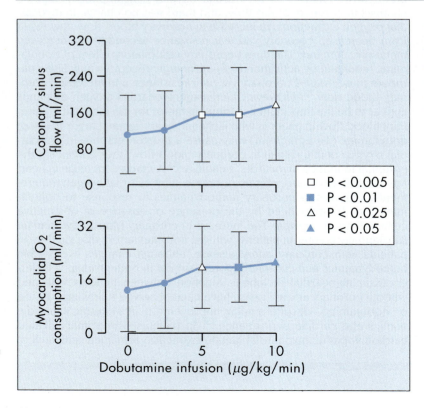

FIGURE 14.8 Changes in coronary sinus flow and myocardial oxygen consumption in response to dobutamine infusion in patients with ischemic heart failure. Both coronary sinus flow and myocardial oxygen consumption increased during the higher infusion rate. (Modified from Bendersky R, Chatterjee K, Parmley WW et al: Dobutamine in chronic ischemic heart failure: Alterations in left ventricular function and coronary hemodynamics. Am J Cardiol 48:554, 1981)

tion in patients following cardiac surgery; the indications for its use in these patients are similar to those for patients with acute myocardial infarction or chronic heart failure.

Dobutamine is frequently used for treating exacerbation of chronic heart failure. Chronic intermittent infusion of dobutamine has been found effective in maintaining clinical improvement.[244-246] Once-per-week dobutamine infusion for 24 weeks improved exercise tolerance and left ventricular function of patients with moderate to severe congestive heart failure.[244] A similar phenomenon was observed after a single 3-day infusion of dobutamine.[247] A double-blind placebo-controlled study has confirmed sustained improvement in exercise tolerance and left ventricular ejection fraction at 4 weeks after a single 3-day infusion of dobutamine in patients with severe chronic congestive heart failure.[246] The effects of intermittent administration of dobutamine to ambulatory patients, using a portable infusion pump, has been assessed for the long-term management of patients with severe chronic heart failure.[248-250] Although there was a tendency to clinical improvement in many patients, there was a strong tendency for a higher mortality rate in the dobutamine-treated patients. Many of the patients who died, died suddenly. Thus, dobutamine infusion is not recommended without supervision and monitoring for arrhythmias. The mechanism for improvement in left ventricular function and clinical improvement with intermittent dobutamine infusion remains unclear. Chronic dobutamine infusion into sedentary dogs has been reported to produce a "conditioning effect."[251] A similar conditioning effect has been proposed in patients with chronic heart failure receiving intermittent dobutamine infusions.[247] Myocardial biopsy of patients with chronic heart failure, before and after 3 days of infusion of dobutamine, demonstrated a decrease in mitochondrial size in the responders.[252] The significance of such findings, however, remains unclear.

The adverse effects are less frequent with dobutamine than with other catecholamines. Excessive tachycardia and ventricular tachyarrhythmias are less common, unless a very large dose is used, which may also induce hypotension. Increased myocardial oxygen consumption and the possibility of worsening myocardial ischemia remain potential disadvantages. The elimination half-life is short, only 2 to 3 minutes. The usual dose of dobutamine is 2.5 to 10 μg/kg/min. An excess of 10 μg/kg/min of dobutamine infusion is likely to induce undesirable tachycardia. The dose, however, should be titrated, starting with a lower infusion rate to obtain an adequate hemodynamic response.

EPHEDRINE[215]

Although some beneficial effects have been reported in patients with chronic heart failure, the use of ephedrine has not gained any popularity because of its unpredictable and inconsistent hemodynamic effects and because of the availability of more effective sympathomimetic amines that can also be administered orally. Similarly, its use has been abandoned for treatment of the Stokes-Adams syndrome since artificial pacemaker therapy has been available.

MEPHENTERMINE, METARAMINOL, AND PHENYLEPHRINE

The sympathomimetic amines with predominantly α-receptor stimulating properties are seldom used today, except occasionally to terminate supraventricular tachycardia. Verapamil, a calcium channel blocking agent, has almost totally replaced the vasopressor sympathomimetic amines in pharmacologic termination of supraventricular tachycardia. In experimental animals, reduction of infarct size has been reported to be significantly greater with the combined use of methoxamine or phenylephrine and nitroglycerin.[253] Such a beneficial response to phenylephrine in attenuating the adverse effects of nitroglycerin (reflex tachycardia) on infarct size has not been proven in patients with evolving myocardial infarction.

SALBUTAMOL AND PIRBUTEROL

Improvement in left ventricular function with these agents results primarily from a decrease in systemic vascular resistance due to activation of the β_2-receptors, although a modest increase in contractility may also be contributory. The systemic hemodynamic effects consist of an increase in cardiac output, a modest increase in heart rate, and a decrease in pulmonary capillary wedge pressure, along with a significant decrease in systemic vascular resistance.

Salbutamol has been used to treat left ventricular failure complicating acute myocardial infarction with some success.[254] However, the experience is limited and the incidence of adverse effects has not been determined. Salbutamol has also been used in the treatment of chronic heart failure, and some clinical benefit has been observed; the addition of isosorbide dinitrate to salbutamol was found to be more effective.[255-257] Without prospective, controlled studies, the potential benefit in the long-term management of chronic heart failure remains uncertain. The recommended oral dose of salbutamol is 4 to 8 mg three to four times daily.

The mechanism of action and hemodynamic effects of pirbuterol are similar to those of salbutamol. In experimental animals, left ventricular dP/dt increases in response to pirbuterol; however, whether the increased dP/dt results from increased contractility or from changes in ventricular loading conditions and heart rate has not been clarified.[258] Intravenous administration of pirbuterol to healthy volunteers has been associated with increased heart rate and stroke volume and decreased systemic vascular resistance.[259] In patients with chronic heart failure, however, the chronotropic effect is usually absent and a significant increase in cardiac output, along with a reduction in pulmonary capillary wedge pressure, may occur.[260,261] Myocardial oxygen and lactate extraction remain unchanged, suggesting that improved cardiac performance is not associated with increased metabolic cost.

Conflicting results have been reported regarding the efficacy of pirbuterol in the long-term management of patients with chronic heart failure. In some studies, improvement in treadmill exercise time following 6 weeks of chronic therapy has been observed.[261] A sustained increase in left ventricular ejection fraction also resulted from chronic maintenance therapy. However, in other studies there was no significant improvement in exercise tolerance or maximal oxygen consumption following chronic pirbuterol therapy.[262] A decline in ejection fraction after an initial increase has also been observed in some patients with chronic heart failure following maintenance therapy with pirbuterol.[263] This attenuation of the hemodynamic and clinical responses has been attributed to a down-regulation of β-receptor density in the myocardium and vascular beds following long-term treatment with pirbuterol.[263] The changes in β-receptor density were estimated in peripheral blood lymphocytes (β_2-receptors), which may not necessarily reflect changes in myocardial β_1-receptors.

Adverse effects such as ventricular tachyarrhythmias and fluid retention, nervousness, headache, tremors, dry mouth, palpitations, nausea, dizziness, fatigue, malaise, and insomnia have been observed during clinical trials. Because of these potential adverse effects and the uncertainty of clinical efficacy, the use of pirbuterol is usually not recommended for the long-term management of patients with chronic heart failure. After oral administration of pirbuterol, maximal plasma concentrations occur within 30 minutes to 4 hours, and the estimated half-life is 1 to 2 hours. It is readily metabolized following oral or intravenous administration, and in humans, biotransformation to the sulfate conjugate occurs extensively. Pirbuterol and its metabolites are primarily excreted via the kidney. In most clinical trials, a dose of 0.4 mg/kg or 10 mg three times daily has been used.

PARTIAL β_1-RECEPTOR AGONISTS

Prenalterol is a partial β_1-receptor agonist with minimal β_2-receptor stimulating effects. It has a more pronounced positive inotropic effect than chronotropic effect. In experimental animals, prenalterol increased left ventricular dP/dt, resulting from its positive inotropic effect.[264] Contractile force also increased in the nonischemic zones in myocardial infarction in experimental animals.[265] In normal volunteers, in patients with acute myocardial infarction, and in patients with chronic congestive heart failure, intravenous prenalterol increased cardiac output and decreased pulmonary capillary wedge pressure and systemic vascular resistance with little or no change in arterial pressure.[266,267] In normal volunteers, a considerable increase in heart rate may occur[267]; however, in patients with heart failure, there was usually little or no increase in heart rate.[268]

Systemic hemodynamic effects of both intravenous and oral prenalterol have been compared in patients with chronic congestive heart failure.[268] The magnitude of increase in cardiac index and the decrease in systemic vascular resistance were similar after intravenous and oral administration of prenalterol. The changes in heart rate, mean arterial pressure, stroke volume, stroke work, and pulmonary capillary wedge pressure were also similar.

Prenalterol, whether given orally or intravenously, tends to increase coronary blood flow and myocardial oxygen consumption.[268] Increased oxygen consumption occurs in the absence of any significant increase in the rate-pressure product, suggesting that the increased inotropic effect enhances myocardial oxygen consumption.

Although acute intravenous or oral prenalterol therapy is associated with hemodynamic improvement, clinical improvement during chronic therapy has not been established. In a double-blind, randomized trial, oral prenalterol therapy for 2 weeks did not improve exercise tolerance or maximal exercise following maintenance therapy.[269] The heart rate response during exercise was also attenuated. In some patients, relative bradycardia and evidence of a low cardiac output may develop during chronic oral prenalterol therapy. The mechanisms of these adverse effects remain unclear. In animal experiments, prenalterol was found to possess 70% of the sympathomimetic activity of isoproterenol and was classified as a partial agonist with some β-antagonistic effect. During acute prenalterol therapy, β-antagonist effects, such as a reduction in heart rate, may not be observed. During long-term therapy, it is possible that down-regulation of β-receptors occurs and the responsiveness to β_1-receptor activation declines. In these circumstances, the β-antagonist effect may be manifest. Since evidence for a long-term clinical benefit is lacking, and the adverse effects may be considerable, long-term prenalterol therapy cannot be recommended in patients with chronic heart failure. Xamoterol is another selective β_1-agonist that has been evaluated for the treatment of heart failure. In patients with mild to moderate heart failure, a positive inotropic effect with improved hemodynamics has been observed[271]; however, there was no improvement in cardiac function after its acute intravenous administration.[271] Lack of a beneficial response has also been observed in patients with acute myocardial infarction complicated by heart failure.[272]

The differences in the hemodynamic response to xamoterol in patients with mild and severe heart failure remain unexplained. Xamoterol is a partial agonist with approximately 43% of the inotropic/chronotropic response attainable with isoproterenol.[273] With this relatively modest β-agonist activity, significant inotropic stimulation would not be anticipated, particularly when the β-receptor density and myocardial responsiveness to catecholamines is diminished, as observed in patients with severe chronic heart failure. In these patients, a full agonist, such as dobutamine, is more likely to be effective. Xamoterol might still exert positive inotropic effects in patients with mild heart failure if myocardial responsiveness to β-receptor activation is relatively maintained. It is apparent that partial β-agonists are unlikely to be effective inotropic agents for the management of patients with more severe heart failure.

This may be because sympathetic tone is already markedly activated in severe heart failure, with an associated decrease in myocardial β-adrenoreceptor density. In mild or moderate heart failure there is a net stimulant (agonist) effect when sympathetic tone is low and a net blocking (antagonist) effect when the sympathetic tone is high. Consequently, xamoterol is believed to modulate the range over which sympathetic nervous activity can modulate cardiac function. Xamoterol has been shown to improve exercise tolerance and cardiac function, compared with digoxin, in patients with mild heart failure. The mechanism of such benefit is not fully understood but is probably not solely due to its β-agonist activity; it may also depend on the β-antagonist effect and improvements in ventricular diastolic function.[274]

OTHER β-RECEPTOR AGONISTS

A number of new sympathomimetic agents with varying degrees of β-receptor agonist properties have been developed. Most of these agents are undergoing clinical trials and their relative effectiveness, potential adverse effects, and clinical usefulness have not been delineated.

TA-064, (−)-(R)-L-(P-hydroxyphenyl)-2-(93,4-dimethoxyphenyl 6)-amino) ethanol, appears to possess selective β_1-receptor agonist properties, and its positive inotropic effect is greater than its chronotropic effect. In a limited number of patients with congestive heart failure, left ventricular dP/dt and cardiac output increased and this enhanced contractility was dose dependent.[274] TA-064 also causes dilatation of isolated vascular segments, especially the coronary arteries, but also the renal, mesenteric, and large intestinal arteries.[275] Peripheral vascular vasodilation has been believed to be mediated by β-receptor stimulation. TA-064 can be administered both intravenously and orally.

Butopamine, a synthetic sympathomimetic amine, is similar to dobutamine except that its molecules are resistant to O-methylation because of structural changes, and, thus, it can be administered orally.[276] In normal volunteers and in some patients with congestive heart failure, acute administration in doses of 0.08 to 1 μg/kg/min was associated with positive inotropic effects; however, it appeared to produce undesirable chronotropic effects that may limit its clinical usefulness.[277]

L-DOPA AND OTHER DOPAMINERGIC RECEPTOR AGONISTS

L-Dopa is a dopamine pro-drug that is converted to dopamine by the enzymatic aromatic amino acid decarboxylase in the liver and other tissues. After its oral administration, the peak blood levels of L-dopa and dopamine are attained in 1 to 3 hours. Previous studies in patients with Parkinson's disease have suggested that the cardiac effects of 1 to 1.5 g of L-dopa are similar to those of 2 to 4 μg/kg/min infusion of dopamine.[278] Based on this experience, the hemodynamic and clinical effects of 1 to 2 g of L-dopa given orally every 6 to 8 hours have been evaluated in patients with severe chronic congestive heart failure.[279,280] In the majority of patients, cardiac output increases without any significant change in arterial pressure or heart rate and pulmonary capillary wedge pressure also remains unchanged. In patients with an elevated pulmonary capillary wedge pressure, agents with the potential to decrease pulmonary capillary wedge pressure are preferable. A combination of L-dopa and captopril, an angiotensin-converting enzyme inhibitor, appears to produce a more advantageous hemodynamic effect than L-dopa alone.[281] This combination therapy maintained the augmented cardiac output by the L-dopa, and the pulmonary capillary wedge pressure decreased with the addition of captopril.

Despite the potential inotropic effect of L-dopa, myocardial oxygen consumption remained unchanged, presumably due to the concomitant reduction in systemic vascular resistance. With combined L-dopa and captopril, there was no significant change in coronary blood flow or myocardial oxygen consumption.[281] Following oral administration there was a significant increase in the level of arterial dopamine; however, there was no correlation between the magnitude of increase in the dopamine concentration and the hemodynamic response. Although without controlled studies the efficacy of long-term therapy cannot be established, uncontrolled studies suggest that in some patients clinical and hemodynamic improvement is maintained after chronic therapy with L-dopa.[279]

Intolerable side effects, particularly nausea, vomiting, lack of appetite, hallucinations, dyskinetic movement, nervousness, anxiety, and insomnia, limit the use of L-dopa in many patients. These symptoms are partly reduced if the dose is gradually increased from 250 mg four times daily to 1.5 to 2.0 g four times daily over 5 to 7 days. The concomitant daily administration of 50 mg of pyridoxine, which is required for the decarboxylation of L-dopa, has also been recommended.[279]

Approximately 95% of absorbed L-dopa is decarboxylated to dopamine by the aromatic L-amino acid, decarboxylase, in the peripheral tissues. A small amount is methylated to 3-O methyldopa. Rapid biotransformation of dopamine occurs to its principal metabolites, 3,4-dihydroxyphenylacetic acid (DOPAC) and 3-methoxy-4-hydroxyphenylacetic acid (homovanillic acid [HVA]), and these metabolites are rapidly excreted in the urine.[215]

IBOPAMINE

Ibopamine is an analogue of dopamine, and it undergoes hydrolysis to epinine (*N*-methyl dopamine), the active metabolite, which activates vascular α_1-adrenoreceptors, β-adrenoreceptors, and dopamine receptors.[282] In laboratory animals left ventricular dP/dt increases along with an increase in aortic blood flow, stroke volume, and arterial pressure.[282] In patients with heart failure, ibopamine increases cardiac index, stroke volume index, and stroke work index; heart rate, mean arterial pressure, and systemic and pulmonary venous pressures usually remain unchanged.[283] In some patients, a transient increase in right atrial and pulmonary capillary wedge pressures and total pulmonary resistance has been observed.[284] A few controlled studies have demonstrated hemodynamic and clinical improvement and increased exercise tolerance in ibopamine-treated patients compared with patients treated with either placebo or conventionally.[285] Improved left ventricular ejection fraction has also been observed, but the number of patients studied was small and the duration of therapy was short, not exceeding 30 days. Furthermore, after an initial improvement an attenuation of the hemodynamic response and maximal oxygen uptake during exercise has also been observed.[286] Ibopamine potentially may improve renal function, presumably due to activation of renal dopamine receptors. Urine output, urinary sodium and potassium clearance, renal blood flow, and creatinine clearance may also increase in some patients with heart failure associated with renal failure. Ibopamine may also reduce plasma norepinephrine concentrations either as a direct effect of DA_2 receptor stimulation or secondary to improved cardiac function. The recommended oral dose of ibopamine in congestive heart failure is 100 to 200 mg three times daily. Gastric paresis, increased frequency of premature ventricular beats, ventricular tachycardia, increased angina, and insomnia are the potential adverse effects of ibopamine.

Dopexamine hydrochloride is a short-acting dopamine analogue, with predominantly β_2-receptor and DA_1 receptor agonist activity. It has minimal or no β_1-agonist and α-agonist activity.[287] Dopexamine has also been shown to inhibit directly uptake of norepinephrine.[288] It can only be administered intravenously, and following an adequate dose there is usually a significant reduction in right atrial and pulmonary capillary wedge pressures and systemic vascular resistance. Mean arterial pressure and pulmonary artery pressure tend to decrease, and heart rate may increase slightly along with a significant increase in cardiac index and stroke volume index.[289]

The improvement in left ventricular function by dopexamine is likely to be caused, at least in part, by the reduction of left ventricular outflow resistance, as systemic vascular resistance falls consistently. Enhanced contractility mediated by activation of myocardial β_2-receptors may also be contributory. Increased contractility may partly be mediated through enhanced sympathoadrenergic activity as a result of norepinephrine uptake inhibition by dopexamine.[288]

Although dopexamine tends to increase heart rate and possibly contractility, the overall myocardial oxygen consumption remains unchanged. Concomitant reduction of left ventricular afterload, which decreases myocardial oxygen demand probably offsets the increased oxygen requirements owing to increased heart rate and contractility. Lack of increase in myocardial oxygen consumption may be an advantage of dopexamine over other catecholamines with positive inotropic effect. Dopexamine potentially can increase renal plasma flow and renal function in patients with congestive heart failure.

Propylbutyl dopamine is another parenteral dopaminergic receptor agonist with both DA_1 and DA_2 receptor activity.[290] In patients with severe congestive heart failure, a significant increase in cardiac output, along with a reduction in pulmonary capillary wedge pressure, was observed. There was no change in heart rate, but mean arterial pressure declined. The beneficial hemodynamic effects of propylbutyl dopamine result primarily from reduction of systemic vascular resistance, presumably due to activation of the DA_1 and DA_2 receptors.

Bromocriptine, an ergot derivative and a dopamine agonist, has been used in patients with severe congestive heart failure.[291] It has been shown to possess DA_2 agonist activity in peripheral nerves, but it also decreases sympathetic activity via a central nervous system mechanism. After its oral administration (2.5 mg), stroke volume increased, together with a reduction of heart rate and mean arterial, right atrial, and left ventricular end-diastolic pressures. Plasma norepinephrine concentrations decreased, suggesting that the withdrawal of sympathetic activity was contributory to its beneficial hemodynamic effects.

Fenoldopam is a selective DA_1 agonist, and after its oral administration (200 mg), the cardiac index increases along with a decrease in pulmonary capillary wedge pressure and systemic vascular resistance.[292] Increased renal blood flow and sodium excretion have been observed in hypertensive patients and normal volunteers. In patients with congestive heart failure, however, renal function may not improve despite increase in cardiac output and improved left ventricular function if arterial pressure falls concomitantly, which reduces renal perfusion pressure.

It is apparent that a number of new dopamine agonists are being developed and have the potential to improve cardiac function and hemodynamics in patients with heart failure; however, the safety and efficacy of these agents during long-term therapy remain to be determined. Further studies will be required to establish their clinical usefulness.

GLUCAGON

Glucagon is a pancreatic polypeptide, and it exerts its positive inotropic effects by stimulating myocardial glucagon receptors and activating the adenylate cyclase system. It is a relatively weak inotropic agent, and its clinical use is limited because of its high incidence of gastrointestinal side effects (nausea, vomiting) and rapid attenuation of its inotropic effect.[293] It is sometimes used to correct the low cardiac output resulting from β-blocker overdose. Glucagon is usually administered intravenously in a dose of 1 mg.

HISTAMINE

Stimulation of histamine-2 receptors in myocardial tissue by histamine is associated with positive inotropic effects.[294] Specific histamine-2 agonists, impromidine or dimaprit, exert a marked positive inotropic effect[295]; however, appropriate clinical studies will be required to determine their effectiveness in the management of heart failure. Furthermore, systemic administration of histamine is associated with severe adverse effects, and thus it is unlikely to be clinically useful.

FORSKOLIN

Forskolin, a diterpene compound, is derived from the extracts of an Indian coleus plant, and it exerts potent positive inotropic and vasodilating effects when given intravenously and orally.[296] In patients with congestive heart failure, a substantial increase in cardiac output and reduction in systemic vascular resistance have been reported. Marked tachycardia has been observed with high intravenous doses.

The mechanism of action of forskolin appears to be due to direct activation of the catalytic unit of the adenylate cyclase with a marked increase in cardiac cyclic AMP production.[297] Since its site of action is distal to the β-adrenergic receptor, attenuation of the positive inotropic effects due to desensitization, as occurs with β-adrenergic agonists, is not expected with forskolin. Further clinical studies are warranted to establish its value in the management of heart failure.

DIBUTYRYL-CYCLIC AMP

Dibutyryl-cyclic AMP is a phosphodiesterase-resistant cyclic nucleotide analogue, and it produces a prolonged positive inotropic effect in isolated papillary muscles. Exogenous cyclic AMP is rapidly metabolized and therefore cannot be used clinically, but its analogue, dibutyryl-cyclic AMP, is resistant to degradation by phosphodiesterase. Intravenous administration of dibutyryl-cyclic AMP in patients with chronic congestive heart failure has produced a significant increase in cardiac output and a decrease in systemic vascular resistance.[298] A modest decrease in left ventricular filling pressure was also noted. These hemodynamic effects, however, can result either from enhanced contractility or from cyclic AMP–mediated peripheral vasodilatation.

PHOSPHODIESTERASE INHIBITORS

The existence of several isozymes of cyclic nucleotide phosphodiesterase has been recognized in mammalian cells.[299] Although in cardiac muscle three distinct forms of phosphodiesterase isozymes designated as peak I, II, or III have been identified, peak III phosphodiesterase is the predominant form. A number of relatively specific peak III phosphodiesterase inhibitors have been developed that are undergoing clinical trials for the short-term and long-term treatment of congestive heart failure. Inhibition of peak III phosphodiesterase results in increased intracellular cyclic AMP in cardiac muscle and subsequent phosphorylation of cellular proteins by cyclic AMP–dependent protein kinase. Increased cyclic AMP in cardiac muscle leads to increased contractility and to enhanced rate of myocardial relaxation.

In contrast to cardiac muscle, both cyclic AMP and cyclic GMP have been identified as second messengers for relaxation of vascular smooth muscle.[300] However, peak III phosphodiesterase in vascular smooth muscle is pharmacologically similar to peak III phosphodiesterase in cardiac muscle.[301] Thus, peak III phosphodiesterase inhibitors not only enhance cardiac contractility but also promote vascular smooth muscle relaxation (Fig. 14.9).[299]

Theophylline and methylxanthine are nonspecific phosphodiesterase inhibitors, and their positive inotropic effects are partly related to inhibition of phosphodiesterase.[301] However, other mechanisms such as direct antagonism of the effects of adenosine, an endogenous nucleotide with negative inotropic actions, inhibition of calcium reuptake by the sarcoplasmic reticulum, and enhanced synthesis and release of endogenous catecholamines have also been believed to be contributory. Although theophylline and methylxanthine have been shown to exert positive inotropic effects in *in vitro* studies as well as in humans, these agents are seldom used as inotropic agents for the treatment of heart failure. Their inotropic potency is relatively weak, and undesirable gastrointestinal and central nervous system side effects are considerable. These agents are also prone to induce excessive tachycardia and arrhythmias. A number of other pharmacologic agents, including papaverine, isobutyl-methylxanthine, the piperidine derivatives, buquineran and carbazeran, and the coronary vasodilator trapidil, have been shown to exert positive inotropic effects by phosphodiesterase inhibition.[302-305] A number of other newer phosphodiesterase inhibitors are undergoing extensive clinical evaluation. These agents are structurally dissimilar from one another and from the methylxanthines but share similar pharmacophysiologic properties. These drugs, in general, do not inhibit Na^+-K^+ ATPase, and their actions are not blocked by histamine-2 antagonists or agents that block synthesis of prostaglandins. The principal mechanism of action of these agents is inhibition of peak III phosphodiesterase, which increases intracellular cyclic AMP concentrations.

The magnitude of response to peak III phosphodiesterase inhibitor is likely to be partly determined by the levels of cyclic AMP present in the tissue. The contractile response of the failing myocardium to the peak III phosphodiesterase inhibitors has been shown to be reduced compared with that of normal tissues,[307] presumably due to lower levels of cyclic AMP in the failing myocardium resulting from dysfunction of the β-adrenergic system. *In vitro* studies have demonstrated that pre-exposure of failing myocardium to low-dose dobutamine enhances myocardial contractile response to milrinone, a peak III phosphodiesterase inhibitor.[307] The cyclic AMP levels presumably increase in response to dobutamine, providing increased substrate for the peak III phosphodiesterase inhibitors. This provides the rationale for combination of a $β_1$-adrenoreceptor agonist and a peak III phosphodiesterase inhibitor for inotropic therapy of severe heart failure.

Amrinone, milrinone, and enoximone are three phosphodiesterase inhibitors that have been studied extensively for treatment of heart failure. Several other agents are also undergoing clinical trials. The

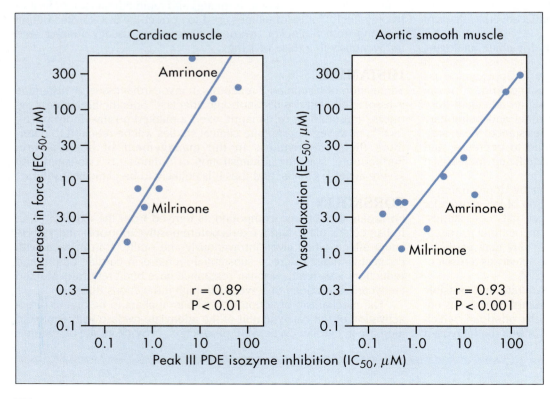

FIGURE 14.9 Enhanced inotropy (*left panel*) and vasorelaxation (*right panel*) as a function of peak III phosphodiesterase (PDE) inhibition in guinea pig (GP) cardiac and aortic smooth muscle. The potency (IC_{50}, μM) for isozyme inhibition as well as the potency (EC_{50}, μM) for increasing developed force in paced guinea pig papillary muscle or relaxation of phenylephrine-contracted aortic smooth muscle was determined for several PDE III inhibitors. (Modified from Silver PJ: Biochemical aspects of inhibition of cardiovascular low (Km) cyclic adenosine monophosphate phosphodiesterase. Am J Cardiol 63:2A, 1989)

relative efficacy of these various drugs and, in many instances, their long-term effects in the management of heart failure still need to be determined.

AMRINONE

Amrinone is a bipyridine derivative shown to have positive inotropic effects in *in vitro* studies. It increases peak development tension, maximal rate of tension development, and maximal rate of relaxation.[306] After acute administration of amrinone, either intravenously or orally, substantial improvement in hemodynamics, cardiac performance, and clinical status can occur, even in patients with severe refractory heart failure.[307-312] Cardiac output and stroke volume increase significantly, along with a reduction in right and left ventricular filling pressures. Pulmonary artery pressure and pulmonary vascular resistance also tend to decrease. A slight reduction in mean arterial pressure and a modest increase in heart rate may also be observed. Systemic vascular resistance decreases significantly. With larger doses, significant and undesirable hypotension and tachycardia may occur.

Although in *in vitro* studies, direct positive inotropic effects and primary peripheral vasodilation have been documented, the relative contributions of these two mechanisms in improving left ventricular function in patients with heart failure remain uncertain. In some studies, there was an increase in left ventricular dP/dt, despite no change in heart rate and a decrease in left ventricular filling pressure, indicating augmented contractility. There was also a significant reduction in systemic vascular resistance; thus, both positive inotropic and vasodilatory effects were evident.[309] In other studies, there were no changes in indices of contractility, such as dP/dt, contractile element velocity, and the end-systolic pressure–volume relation, although there was a significant reduction in systemic vascular resistance.[311] In some studies, intracoronary injections of amrinone were not associated with any evidence of enhanced myocardial contractility.[311] It appears, therefore, that the vasodilatory effect may be more pronounced than the inotropic effect in patients with chronic heart failure. Amrinone has been shown to produce direct smooth muscle relaxation in the coronary artery.[313,314] Changes in coronary hemodynamics and myocardial energetics have been assessed in a small number of patients with heart failure, and no significant changes in rate-pressure product, coronary blood flow, and myocardial oxygen consumption were observed.[315] In occasional patients, however, myocardial lactate production occurred, suggesting myocardial ischemia.

Intravenous administration of amrinone, followed by short-term oral therapy, is associated with both hemodynamic and clinical improvement in patients with severe refractory heart failure. In patients with acute myocardial infarction and pump failure, amrinone increases cardiac output and decreases systemic vascular resistance and pulmonary capillary wedge pressure, with little or no change in heart rate and blood pressure, when a low dose (200 μg/kg/hr) is infused.[316,317] With larger doses, although there is a greater decrease in pulmonary capillary wedge pressure, tachycardia and hypotension develop, which might be deleterious.

Intravenous amrinone has been found effective in the management of postoperative heart failure. Compared with dobutamine, amrinone appears to cause a greater reduction of systemic and pulmonary venous pressures.[318,319] In patients with severe postoperative pump failure or cardiogenic shock, refractory to catecholamines and intra-aortic balloon pump therapy, amrinone may cause a substantial increase in cardiac output and stroke volume and reduction of pulmonary capillary wedge pressure and systemic vascular resistance and improved tissue perfusion (Fig. 14.10).[320,321] The major indications for the use of amrinone in patients with postoperative pump failure are markedly elevated left ventricular filling pressures, low cardiac output, and poor peripleural perfusion, particularly when these hemodynamic abnormalities persist despite conventional therapy. The major undesirable effect in patients with acute heart failure is hypotension, which can be corrected by concomitant administration of norepinephrine.[321]

The efficacy of long-term oral amrinone therapy in the management of patients with chronic heart failure remains uncertain. In uncontrolled studies, amrinone has been shown to improve exercise tolerance both during short-term and long-term oral therapy.[322-324] An improvement in left ventricular pump function and maximal oxygen consumption during exercise has been noted after short-term and long-term therapy. Controlled studies, however, have failed to demonstrate any benefit during long-term therapy.[325,326] Compared with placebo, there was no improvement in the clinical status or exercise tolerance during maintenance amrinone therapy. Furthermore, some adverse effects were more frequently seen in the amrinone treated group. Thus, presently, amrinone therapy should be considered only for short-term therapy in patients with heart failure.

Gastrointestinal adverse effects, such as nausea, anorexia, abdominal pain, vomiting, and diarrhea occurred in 27% of patients receiving amrinone. Central nervous system complications, such as dizziness, headache, lightheadedness, and paresthesia, were also more frequent. Unexplained fever, abnormal liver function, and rash with pruritus may also occur. Thrombocytopenia is frequently seen with amrinone therapy, but clinically relevant (platelet counts < 50,000/mm^3) thrombocytopenia is uncommon. Thrombocytopenia appears to be dose related and is usually reversed by lowering the dose to 275 mg/day.[326]

Amrinone appears to cause an increase in maximal velocity, overshoot, and duration of the slow response action potential, resulting from its effects on the slow inward calcium current. Amrinone also shortens the atrio-His interval, AV nodal effective refractory period,

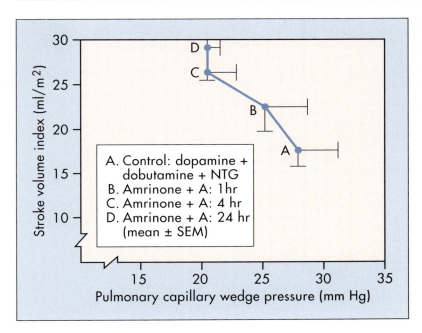

FIGURE 14.10 Improvement in left ventricular function in a patient with severe postoperative heart failure following the addition of a peak III phosphodiesterase inhibitor, amrinone, to initial combination therapy with dopamine, dobutamine, and nitroglycerin (NTG). (Modified from Goenen M et al: Heart failure after open heart surgery. In Perret C, Vincent JL (eds): Update in Intensive Care and Emergency Medicine, p 146. Berlin, Springer-Verlag, 1988)

and the maximal corrected sinus node recovery time. It does not appear to have any significant effect on ventricular arrhythmogenesis.[327,328]

However, clinical experience suggests that ventricular arrhythmias occur in up to 3% of patients receiving intravenous amrinone. Intravenous amrinone therapy is initiated with a 0.75 mg/kg bolus slowly over 2 to 3 minutes, and the infusion is then continued at a rate between 5 and 10 µg/kg/min. The total daily dose should not exceed 10 mg/kg. The oral dose should be less than 300 mg/day to avoid adverse effects, particularly thrombocytopenia.

Sudden withdrawal of amrinone therapy may be associated with rapid hemodynamic deterioration and should thus be avoided.[329,330] Deterioration of hemodynamics has been observed following withdrawal of amrinone after 2 to 10 weeks of oral therapy. The mechanisms for such deterioration after withdrawal of therapy remain unclear and speculative.

MILRINONE

Milrinone is also a bipyridine derivative and is closely related to amrinone; however, it is approximately 15 times more potent than amrinone.[331-333] Its positive inotropic effects have been well documented in papillary muscles, as evident from the increase in developed tension and the rate of tension development.[334,335] Intracoronary infusion of doses of milrinone that did not have any significant effects on arterial pressure and systemic vascular resistance was associated with an increase in left ventricular dP/dt, along with an increased stroke volume and decreased left ventricular end-diastolic pressure (Fig. 14.11).[336]

A substantial dose-dependent increase in left ventricular dP/dt along with an increase in stroke work index has been observed in response to intravenous milrinone.[337,338] In normal subjects, a dose-dependent increase in load-independent endsystolic indices of contractility in response to milrinone has been observed.[339] Milrinone administered orally also increased dP/dt, dP/dt/P, V_{max}, and left ventricular endsystolic pressure–volume ratio.[340,341] The direct vasodilatory effect of milrinone has also been demonstrated in isolated limb preparations. Intra-arterial injection of smaller doses of milrinone, which did not produce any significant change in systemic hemodynamics, decreased forearm vascular resistance and increased forearm blood flow.[342] Forearm venous capacitance increases substantially following intravenous administration of milrinone, and this venodilation appears to be due to both direct effect on the veins and an indirect effect due to withdrawal of vasoconstrictor tone.[343]

Milrinone may also improve left ventricular relaxation and diastolic distensibility.[344] A downward and rightward shift of the left ventricular diastolic pressure–volume curve has been observed. An increase in left ventricular negative dP/dt, the time constant for left ventricular relaxation, and the peak rate of diastolic filling also occurred. Increased left ventricular compliance is associated with a left and upward shift of the left ventricular function curve. The relative contributions of the positive inotropic effect, peripheral vasodilation, and improved left ventricular compliance to improved left ventricular function are difficult to determine.

Milrinone, like amrinone, does not appear to increase myocardial oxygen consumption.[345] Coronary sinus blood flow, however, tends to increase, together with a decrease in myocardial oxygen extraction. Since the heart rate–blood pressure product also remains unchanged, increased coronary blood flow appears to result from the primary decrease in coronary vascular resistance.

Such primary coronary arteriolar dilatation can result in redistribution of myocardial blood flow and may not contribute to improvement of myocardial ischemia. Comparative effects of milrinone, nitroprusside, and dobutamine on coronary hemodynamics and myocardial energetics have been evaluated.[346,347] Nitroprusside, a pure vasodilator, tends to decrease myocardial oxygen consumption more than by milrinone; while with dobutamine myocardial oxygen consumption increases consistently.

Oral milrinone therapy does not appear to increase renal blood flow or glomerular filtration rate despite a substantial increase in cardiac output. However, forearm blood flow increases proportionately with cardiac output, suggesting that milrinone preferentially increases skeletal muscle blood flow. Lack of increase in renal blood flow with milrinone may result from shunting of blood flow from the kidney or alternatively from activation of renal cellular mechanisms that might

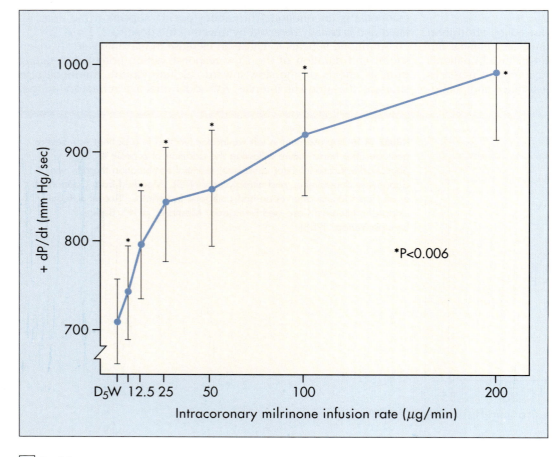

FIGURE 14.11 Dose-related increase in left ventricular + dP/dt caused by intracoronary infusion of milrinone. (Modified from Ludmer PL, Wright RF, Arnold MO et al: Separation of the direct myocardial and vasodilator actions of milrinone administered by an intracoronary infusion technique. Circulation 73:130, 1986)

offset the anticipated favorable renal response from increased cardiac output.[348]

Comparative effects of milrinone and captopril on renal and skeletal muscle blood flow have been evaluated in patients with chronic congestive heart failure after their acute administration.[349] Relative to the increase in cardiac output, the increase in renal blood flow with captopril was greater and there was no change in skeletal muscle blood flow, suggesting a direct effect of captopril on renovascular resistance. With milrinone, skeletal muscle flow increased but the increase in renal blood flow was relatively less (relative to the increase in cardiac output), indicating that milrinone probably does not exert a direct effect on renovascular resistance.

Electrophysiologic studies have demonstrated that milrinone improves conduction and reduces post-repolarization refractoriness in ischemic gap preparations. These findings suggest that milrinone may exert antiarrhythmic or arrhythmogenic effects by restoring or improving conduction in areas of depressed conductivity.[328] Although milrinone mildly improves AV nodal conduction, it does not change atrial, AV nodal, or ventricular refractoriness. Potential proarrhythmic effects of milrinone have not been substantiated during prospective Holter monitoring or electrophysiologic studies.[329]

Systemic hemodynamic effects of milrinone are similar to those of other phosphodiesterase inhibitors with combined inotropic and vasodilating properties. There is usually a significant increase in cardiac index, stroke volume, and stroke work index, along with a decrease in pulmonary capillary wedge and right atrial pressures (Fig. 14.12).[350] A significant decrease in mean arterial pressure and an increase in heart rate may also occur. Reduction in arterial pressure and systemic vascular resistance appears to be dose-dependent; a marked reduction in systemic vascular resistance with hypotension may be observed with larger doses.[351]

Short-term therapy with milrinone in uncontrolled studies has been reported to improve exercise tolerance and maximal oxygen consumption in patients with chronic heart failure.[352] However, some controlled studies have failed to demonstrate a sustained improvement in exercise tolerance during long-term oral therapy.[353]

In a large multicenter double-blind randomized controlled study, changes in exercise tolerance of patients with chronic congestive heart failure were assessed during 3 months of therapy with milrinone alone, digoxin alone, milrinone and digoxin, or placebo. All three treatment groups experienced better exercise performance than the placebo group, significantly so in the groups treated with milrinone alone and digoxin alone. Milrinone-treated patients also experienced better quality of life.[119] In another study, 155 patients with congestive heart failure, whose condition was stable on digitalis and diuretics, were randomized for 3 months to either milrinone, milrinone and digoxin, or digoxin alone[354] and the hemodynamic studies did not show any evidence for tolerance to milrinone. Although the quality of life was favorably influenced by milrinone therapy, clinical class was not affected.

Milrinone is usually well tolerated. Diarrhea or other gastrointestinal symptoms are uncommon. Rash, thrombocytopenia, and fever have not been observed. Fluid retention occurs in over 80% of patients, requiring increased diuretics during maintenance therapy.[351] Milrinone therapy did not improve survival in patients with severe heart failure. In one uncontrolled study, survival at 6 months was only 34%,[350] and in another similar study, 1-year survival was 39%.[355]

In the multicenter placebo-controlled milrinone-digoxin trial of 230 patients with chronic heart failure, during 3 months of therapy, 10 of 119 patients assigned to treatment with milrinone died, compared with only 6 of 111 patients assigned to the control group. These findings suggested an adverse influence of milrinone therapy on survival of patients with severe chronic congestive heart failure.[119]

ENOXIMONE[356–387]

Enoximone, an imidazole derivative, is also a peak III phosphodiesterase inhibitor and has been extensively evaluated for the management of patients with acute and chronic heart failure. Enoximone increases intracellular concentrations of cyclic AMP but not that of cyclic GMP. In experimental animals, it increases myocardial contractile force and the slope of the peak isovolumetric pressure–volume relation, which has been shown to represent the maximal elastance (E_{max}) of the ventricle for a given contractile state.[358,359] In patients with severe chronic heart failure, calculated E_{max} also tends to increase in response to intravenous enoximone.[359] In patients with impaired left ventricular function, peak dP/dt increases despite a decrease in left ventricular filling

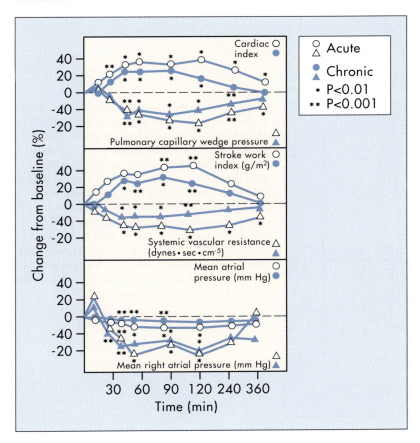

FIGURE 14.12 Acute and chronic hemodynamic effects of oral milrinone in 25 patients with severe congestive heart failure. Hemodynamic effects are expressed as percentage change from baseline (control). Chronic hemodynamic effects were determined after an average of 37 days (range 19 to 89 days) of therapy. (P values are compared with baseline.) There was no significant difference between acute and chronic responses. (Modified from Simonton CA, Chatterjee K, Cody RJ et al: Milrinone in congestive heart failure: Acute and chronic hemodynamic and clinical evaluation. J Am Coll Cardiol 6:453, 1985)

pressure and in the absence of any significant change in heart rate or blood pressure.[360] These findings suggest that enoximone exerts direct positive inotropic effect. Enoximone is also a potent vasodilator. In isolated canine hind limb preparation, enoximone produces direct relaxation of vascular smooth muscle.[357] A decrease in calculated systemic vascular resistance has also been observed in patients with chronic heart failure.[361] There is also evidence that enoximone increases left ventricular distensibility.[361] In some patients, left ventricular end-diastolic volume increases, despite a marked decrease in pulmonary capillary wedge pressure, which suggests a down and rightward shift of the left ventricular diastolic pressure volume curve (Fig. 14.13). Such a shift is associated with left and upward shift of the ventricular function curve. However, an increased left ventricular distensibility in response to enoximone is not a uniform finding.[362] In only approximately 30% of patients, a downward shift of the left ventricular pressure–volume curve occurred in response to enoximone. Furthermore, when the relationship between changes in transmural pressure (estimated by subtracting right atrial pressure from left ventricular diastolic pressure) and the changes in left ventricular diastolic volume were determined, no shift in left ventricular pressure-volume relation was found.[362]

Both intravenous and oral enoximone produce a marked increase in cardiac index, stroke volume, and stroke work index, and a significant decrease in pulmonary capillary, right atrial, and pulmonary artery pressures (Fig. 14.14). A slight increase in heart rate and a modest decrease in mean arterial pressure are frequently observed.[363,364]

In experimental animals, improved cardiovascular effects were not accompanied by any significant alterations in myocardial oxygen consumption.[357] Clinical studies on the effects of enoximone on myocardial energetics have suggested that there may be no change or modest increase in coronary blood flow with no change or decrease in myocardial oxygen consumption.[365,366] In one study, in which much larger doses of enoximone were used, a substantial increase in coronary blood flow and myocardial oxygen consumption was observed.[367] Coronary sinus venous oxygen content tends to increase and myocardial oxygen extraction tends to decrease, suggesting primary coronary vasodilatation by enoximone. Primary coronary vasodilatation may, however, be associated with shunting of blood to less metabolically active areas of the myocardium, which may induce myocardial ischemia.[366] Myocardial efficacy is usually estimated by computing the ratio of left ventricular stroke work to myocardial oxygen consumption. Following enoximone, myocardial efficiency usually increases, even when there is some increase in myocardial oxygen requirements.[365-367] Enoximone has also been shown to improve global ejection fraction and regional wall motion in patients after infarction.[368] There was marked improvement of regional wall motion of the noninfarcted segments, myocardial segments that were hypokinetic at control became normokinetic, and the extent of akinesis decreased by 40%.[368]

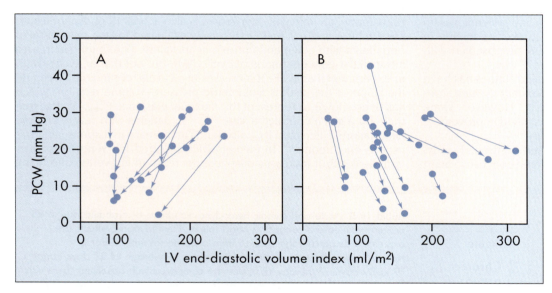

FIGURE 14.13 Relationship between changes in pulmonary capillary wedge pressure (PCW) and radioangiographically calculated left ventricular end-diastolic volume index in response to intravenous enoximone. In patients in **B**, a marked decrease in PCW was associated with an increase in EDVI. (Modified from Kereiakes DJ, Viquerat C, Lanzer P et al: Mechanisms of improved left ventricular function following intravenous MDL 17043 in patients with severe heart failure. Am Heart J 108:1278, 1984)

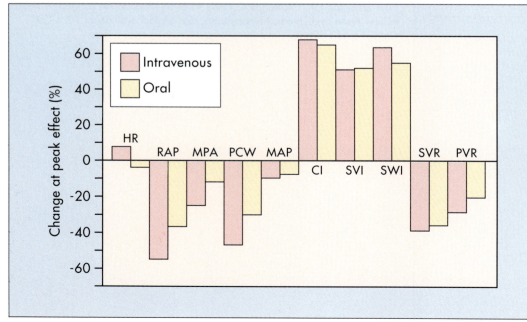

FIGURE 14.14 Comparative magnitude of the effect of intravenous and oral enoximone (MDL 17043) in 38 patients with congestive heart failure. The percentage change from baseline at peak drug effect of each hemodynamic variable is similar after either route of administration. Cardiac index (CI), stroke volume index (SVI), and stroke work index (SWI) increased markedly along with decreased systemic vascular resistance (SVR), pulmonary vascular resistance (PVR), pulmonary capillary wedge pressure (PCW), mean pulmonary artery pressure (MPA), and right atrial pressure (RAP). There was only a slight change in heart rate (HR) and mean arterial pressure (MAP).

Enoximone does not appear to change significantly the flow or resistance of renal or hepatic-splanchnic flow, although limb blood flow increases.[369] In normal volunteers, however, improved renal function has been observed with enoximone.[370] Electrophysiologic effects of enoximone have not been adequately evaluated. Like other phosphodiesterase inhibitors, it has little effect on His-Purkinje conduction but tends to shorten the atrio-His interval and ventricular refractoriness.[371]

Clinical improvement is observed during short-term therapy even in patients with severe refractory heart failure.[367] In patients with acute myocardial infarction complicated by left ventricular failure, improved clinical status and hemodynamics have been observed during short-term intravenous enoximone treatment.[372] In some patients with cardiogenic shock, refractory to dobutamine, intravenous enoximone treatment improved hemodynamics with resolution of signs of circulatory shock.[373] Intravenous enoximone therapy has also been found to be effective in the management of refractory low output state following cardiac surgery.[374] Rapid and sustained hemodynamic and clinical improvement have been observed in these patients.

Efficacy of long-term maintenance therapy on hemodynamics, exercise tolerance, and clinical status has been assessed mostly in uncontrolled studies. In some studies, no sustained improvement in hemodynamics or exercise tolerance was noted.[375,376] On the other hand, a number of other studies have reported sustained hemodynamic improvement and improvement in clinical status, exercise tolerance and maximal oxygen consumption in many patients with chronic heart failure during long-term maintenance therapy.[377-380]

A few controlled studies have indicated that during 12 weeks of enoximone therapy, a sustained improvement in exercise tolerance can be observed in patients with moderately severe chronic heart failure.[381-383] Some studies have noted a similar increase in exercise duration with captopril and enoximone.[379,383] These findings suggest that during relatively shorter periods of treatment with enoximone, sustained clinical improvement is expected in patients with moderately severe congestive heart failure.

No large-scale controlled long-term studies have been performed to assess survival rate in patients treated with enoximone. Results of an uncontrolled study suggest that the mortality of patients with severe chronic heart failure, particularly in patients refractory to vasodilator and angiotensin converting enzyme inhibitors, remains very high. The overall mortality at 6 months, in such patients, in one study was 55%.[367] In another study, mortality rates at 6 and 12 months were 50% and 58%, respectively. In patients who are dependent on intravenous inotropic drugs, the mortality was higher: 64% at 6 months and 73% at 1 year.[384] It is apparent that a significant improvement in survival is not expected in patients with severe refractory heart failure, particularly those who require intravenous inotropic supportive therapy. However, even in these patients, hemodynamic and clinical improvement can be expected for a shorter period with intravenous and oral enoximone therapy. Thus, enoximone therapy can be of use for stabilizing patients awaiting cardiac transplant and can be used as a pharmacologic bridge to cardiac transplantation.[385,386]

The major side effects are gastrointestinal: nausea, anorexia, vomiting, diarrhea, and abdominal bloating. Thrombocytopenia, rash, and altered taste sensation occur infrequently. Fluid retention and the need for increased diuretics are common. An increased incidence of ventricular arrhythmias, particularly during acute intravenous therapy, has also been suspected. Hypotension, insomnia, somnolence, agitation, anxiety, and headache have been reported.[387]

PIROXIMONE

Piroximone is also an imidazole derivative that has been demonstrated *in vitro* and in experimental animals to have direct positive inotropic and vasodilator actions.[388] After acute intravenous and oral administration in patients with chronic congestive heart failure, cardiac output, stroke volume, and stroke work increase, while pulmonary capillary wedge and right atrial pressures decrease.[389,390] Heart rate and blood pressure usually do not change, but systemic vascular resistance declines. Left ventricular dP/dt increases due to the drug's inotropic effects. Piroximone also tends to increase left ventricular distensibility in some patients.[390] Following acute intravenous therapy, a reduction in plasma norepinephrine levels and a tendency to increased plasma renin activity have been reported.[389]

Piroximone is effective when administered orally, and its inotropic potency appears to be five to ten times that of enoximone.[391] After an oral dose, the peak hemodynamic effects occur in about 30 minutes and the hemodynamic effects may last for 10 hours or longer. The effects of piroximone on regional blood flow have not been evaluated in patients with congestive heart failure. In experimental animals with heart failure, it does not appear to increase renal blood flow.[392] Clinical experience with piroximone is too limited to determine its long-term efficacy and side effect profile.

POSICOR (RO 13-6438)

Posicor is an imidazoquinazolinone derivative, which is also a peak III phosphodiesterase inhibitor. Its inotropic potency *in vitro* appears to be less than that of amrinone. Its inotropic effects are partially attenuated by pretreatment with reserpine and, like those of amrinone or milrinone, can be almost totally reversed by carbachol.[393]

Like other phosphodiesterase inhibitors, posicor increases cardiac output, stroke volume, and stroke work, while reducing right atrial and pulmonary capillary wedge pressure.[394] There is usually a slight increase in heart rate and a modest decrease in mean arterial pressure. Its vasodilatory action is evident from the marked reduction in systemic vascular resistance. The peak hemodynamic effects tend to occur within 1 hour, and the effects last for approximately 8 hours after a single oral dose.[394]

Posicor appears to produce primary coronary vasodilation as it decreases myocardial oxygen extraction and increases coronary sinus venous oxygen content.[394] Myocardial oxygen consumption does not increase, and the ratio of minute work/myocardial oxygen consumption, an index of left ventricular efficiency, tends to improve. Information regarding its clinical efficacy and side effects is not available to determine its role in the long-term management of patients with chronic heart failure.

SULMAZOLE (ARL 115BS)

Sulmazole is a phenylimidazopyridine derivative and also a phosphodiesterase inhibitor. It has been suggested that its positive inotropic effect may result, in part, from the release of endogenous catecholamines. It apparently also increases the sensitivity of myofibrils to calcium.[395,396] Its hemodynamic effects are similar to those of other phosphodiesterase inhibitors, and improvement in left ventricular function has been demonstrated in patients with severe congestive heart failure with sulmazole.[397,398] The long-term efficacy of this drug, however, has not been established. Serious gastrointestinal side effects, visual disturbances, and thrombocytopenia have been observed, even during short-term therapy. Hepatic neoplasms have developed in sulmazole-treated rodents.

OTHER INOTROPIC AGENTS[399-401]

CI-914 is an imidazolyphenyl pyridazinone that possesses phosphodiesterase-inhibiting properties. The benzimidazole derivatives UD-CG 212 and UD-CG 115, a quinolone derivative OPC 8212, and other phosphodiesterase inhibitors have been shown to possess positive inotropic properties. CI-914 improves hemodynamics in patients with chronic heart failure; however, mortality in patients treated with CI-914 appears to be higher compared with those treated with placebo.[402] OPC-8212 is an inotropic and vasodilator agent that increases contractility via an effect on ion channels and by increasing action potential duration. Randomized double-blind placebo controlled trial in patients with congestive heart failure indicated that patients treated with OPC-8212 have decreased morbidity and mortality.[403] Hemodynamic effects of OPC-8212 are similar to those of other phosphodiesterase inhibitors. Pimobendan (UD-CG-115), with specific phosphodiesterase inhibitory and calcium sensitizing properties, has also been shown to improve cardiac performance and exercise tolerance of patients with severe chronic congestive heart failure refractory to digitalis, diuretics, and angiotensin converting enzyme inhibitor therapy.[404] However, presently, the clinical experience with these newer inotropic vasodilator agents is too small to determine their potential roles in the management of heart failure.

Preliminary studies indicate that berberine, a plant alkaloid, and D13625, both orally active drugs, produce beneficial hemodynamic effects in patients with severe heart failure. Their mechanisms of action have not been clarified. The slow calcium channel agonist Bay K 8644 has been shown to exert positive inotropic effects by promoting calcium influx.[405] These agents also produce peripheral vasoconstriction and raise arterial pressure and coronary vascular tone. The co-enzyme Q_{10} is a mitochondrial respiratory chain redox component and reports suggest that it produces beneficial hemodynamic effects in patients with heart failure, both after intravenous and oral administration. Co-enzyme Q_{10} plays an important role in myocardial energy metabolism, and improvement in myocardial metabolic function has been believed to be the mechanism for hemodynamic improvement.[406] Intravenous administration of inosine and adenosine has been reported to improve left ventricular contractile function and to produce beneficial hemodynamic effects. It has been postulated that these agents facilitate myocardial adenine nucleotide repletion and augment myocardial metabolic and contractile function.[407] However, appropriate studies are lacking to demonstrate the clinical efficacy of these agents in the treatment of heart failure.

CLINICAL USE OF INOTROPIC AGENTS
ACUTE HEART FAILURE

It is apparent that a number of potent inotropic agents are now available that can be used clinically for the management of heart failure. The systemic hemodynamic effects of adrenergic agents are qualitatively similar, irrespective of their primary mechanisms of action. The acute hemodynamic effects of different phosphodiesterase inhibitors are also very similar, and the choice of a given agent should depend on its side effects and patient tolerance (Table 14.7). The systemic hemodynamic effects of most vasodilators are also qualitatively similar to those of the inotropic agents. However, adrenergic inotropic agents, in general, increase myocardial oxygen consumption, and with phosphodiesterase inhibitors, it may remain unchanged. In contrast, myocardial oxygen consumption tends to decrease in response to most vasodilators. Vasodilators can produce hypotension, which may preclude their use in relatively hypotensive patients. For the effective management of acutely decompensated patients and for appropriate selection of inotropic or vasodilator agents, hemodynamic monitoring is preferable, which also allows a change of therapy if response to a given agent is inadequate. The general guidelines for the use of inotropic

TABLE 14.7 RELATIVE CHANGES (COMPARED WITH CONTROL) IN SYSTEMIC HEMODYNAMICS AND OBSERVED SIDE EFFECTS DURING THERAPY WITH NEWER PHOSPHODIESTERASE INHIBITORS IN CHRONIC CONGESTIVE HEART FAILURE—EXPERIENCE AT THE UNIVERSITY OF CALIFORNIA, SAN FRANCISCO

Drug	Change in Systemic Hemodynamics (%)						Adverse Effects
	CI	PCWP	RAP	HR	MAP	SVR	
Milrinone (n = 37)	+49	−31	−39	+10	−13	−30	Fluid retention Ventricular arrhythmias Occasional gastrointestinal symptoms
Amrinone (n = 10)	+67	−36	−42	+3	−17	−48	Nausea Anorexia Loose bowel motions Fever Hepatic dysfunction Rash Ventricular arrhythmias Thrombocytopenia Fluid retention
Enoximone (n = 38)	+75	−42	−50	+9	−10	−42	Diarrhea Nausea Anorexia Fluid retention Hepatic dysfunction Ventricular arrhythmias Rarely thrombocytopenia
Piroximone (n = 15)	+53	−18	−43	+2	+3	−26	Nausea Anorexia Fluid retention Arrhythmia
Posicor	+58	−38	−45	+4	−10	−37	Fluid retention Arrhythmia Visual disturbances Nausea Anorexia

(CI, cardiac index; PCWP, pulmonary capillary wedge pressure; RAP, right atrial pressure; HR, heart rate; MAP, mean arterial pressure; SVR, systemic vascular resistance)

agents in the management of acutely decompensated heart failure patients are summarized in Table 14.8.

SEPTIC SHOCK

In patients with septic shock, hypotension is caused by marked peripheral vasodilatation and abnormally low systemic vascular resistance. Cardiac output may remain in the normal range or may be elevated. Right and left ventricular filling pressures may be normal, low, or elevated, depending on the degree of right and left ventricular dysfunction. Clinically, resuscitation from septic shock is usually initiated with repletion of a presumed volume deficit. However, frequently intravenous fluid therapy proves inadequate to correct hypotension and vasopressor agents need to be used. To increase systemic vascular resistance, the dose of dopamine that is likely to cause vasoconstriction due to activation of peripheral vascular α-receptors is frequently used. In some patients with severe hypotension, even large doses of dopamine may be ineffective in increasing systemic vascular resistance. It has been shown that the peripheral vasculature in patients with severe septic shock is relatively unresponsive to vasoconstricting effects of dopamine.[408] Norepinephrine, in these circumstances, may be effective in maintaining arterial pressure and cardiac performance and anticipated norepinephrine-induced renal insufficiency may not occur.[409] Improved renal function may occur due to decreased proximal tubular reabsorption with increased renal perfusion pressure with norepinephrine. Increased arterial pressure with norepinephrine may also improve right ventricular myocardial perfusion, which is dependant on the gradient from mean arterial pressure to right ventricular end-diastolic pressure.[410] Right ventricular dysfunction and pulmonary hypertension may complicate septic shock and adversely influence the prognosis.[411-413] Relative effects of norepinephrine and dopamine on hemodynamics and right ventricular performance in septic shock have been evaluated.[414] Dopamine infusion increased cardiac index, systemic oxygen delivery, and systemic oxygen consumption without any change in systemic and pulmonary vascular resistance and right ventricular volumes and right ventricular ejection fraction. With norepinephrine, there was also no change in right ventricular volumes and ejection fraction and cardiac index. Both systemic and pulmonary vascular resistance increased with norepinephrine. Thus, although norepinephrine may improve right ventricular oxygen supply–demand ratio, this potentially beneficial effect may be offset by a concomitant increase in right and left ventricular afterload that may prevent an increase in right and left ventricular stroke output. To increase cardiac output, dobutamine or a phosphodiesterase inhibitor can be added to norepinephrine.

In septic shock, increasing oxygen delivery by increasing cardiac output with the use of inotropic drugs has been found to be useful in some patients and has been reported to decrease mortality and morbidity in critically ill patients.[415,416] Critically ill patients suffering from sepsis syndrome, trauma, or acute respiratory failure or undergoing extended surgery have high oxygen requirements and need higher cardiac output to maintain adequate oxygen delivery and tissue perfusion. Frequently, blood lactate levels are determined to assess adequacy of cardiac output and tissue perfusion,[417] although measurements of lactate levels have limitations since concentration of lactate depends on its production as well as its elimination, which can also be altered in shock state.[418]

Inotropic drugs, particularly dobutamine, have been used for maximizing oxygen delivery in patients with septic shock, even in the presence of normal or high cardiac output.[419] Dobutamine infusion increased cardiac output, oxygen delivery, and oxygen consumption without any significant change in ventricular filling pressures.[420] Furthermore, hypotension did not result with the dose of dobutamine (5 μg/kg/min) used. It should be noted, however, that although dobutamine improves oxygen delivery, the impact of such therapy on the mortality and morbidity of septic shock remains to be established. Nevertheless, dobutamine therapy in addition to other supportive measurements deserves consideration in the presence of evidence for inadequate oxygen delivery. Phosphodiesterase inhibitors are also potentially useful in increasing cardiac output and oxygen delivery in these patients.

CHRONIC HEART FAILURE

In patients with overt chronic congestive heart failure, resulting from depressed left ventricular function, vasodilators, particularly angiotensin converting enzyme inhibitors, should be added to "digitalis and diuretic" therapy since these agents not only relieve symptoms and improve exercise tolerance and cardiac performance but also improve survival.[421-424] Long-term inotropic therapy with digoxin is indicated except in patients with significant renal failure or in those who are prone to develop digitalis toxicity. Patients who become refractory to vasodilators or angiotensin-converting enzyme inhibitors, or those patients who cannot tolerate vasodilators or angiotensin-converting en-

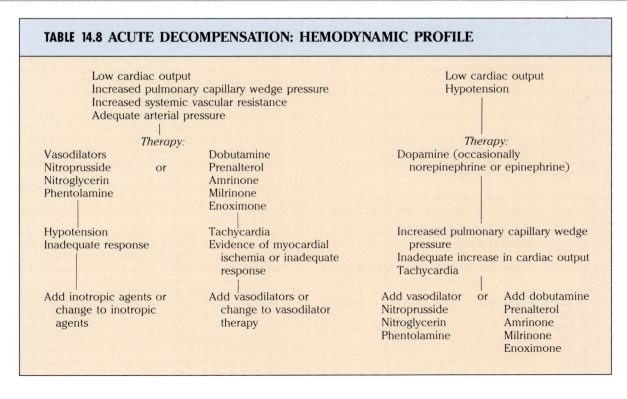

TABLE 14.8 ACUTE DECOMPENSATION: HEMODYNAMIC PROFILE

zyme inhibitors, are presently considered for long-term treatment with newer intropic agents. Patients with severe pump failure with low cardiac output and hypotension, particularly during exacerbation of chronic heart failure, are frequently treated with intermittent dobutamine and/or dopamine infusion or with intermittent parenteral phosphodiesterase inhibitors. Nonparenteral phosphodiesterase inhibitors are also effective in some patients. Such therapy is also frequently employed as a pharmacologic bridge to cardiac transplantation.

REFERENCES

1. Fabiato A, Fabiato F: Calcium and cardiac excitation-contraction coupling. Annu Rev Physiol 41:473, 1979
2. Wohlfart B, Noble MIM: The cardiac excitation-contraction coupling. Pharmacol Ther 16:1, 1982
3. Chapman RA: Control of cardiac contractility at the cellular level. Am J Physiol 245:H535, 1983
4. Katz AM: Discussion section. Article by Endoh M, Yanagisawa T, Taira N, Blinks JR: Effects of new inotropic agents on cyclic nucleotide metabolism and calcium transients in canine ventricular muscle. Circulation 73(Suppl III):III-117, 1986
5. Katz AM: Cyclic adenosine monophosphate effects on the myocardium: A man who blows hot and cold with one breath. J Am Coll Cardiol 2:143, 1983
6. Sperelakis N: Cyclic AMP and phosphorylation in regulation of Ca^{++} influx into myocardial cells and blockade by calcium antagonist drugs. Am Heart J 107:347, 1984
7. Kranias EG, Solaro J: Coordination of cardiac sarcoplasmic reticulum and myofibrillar function by protein phosphorylation. Fed Proc 42:33, 1983
8. Ikemoto N: Structure and function of the calcium pump protein of sarcoplasmic reticulum. Annu Rev Physiol 44:297, 1982
9. Strada SJ, Thompson WJ: Cyclic nucleotide phosphodiesterase. Adv Cyclic Nucleotide Protein Phosphorylation Res 16:1, 1984
10. Tada M, Kirchberger MA, Li H-C: Phosphoprotein phosphatase-catalyzed dephosphorylation of 22,000 dalton phosphoprotein of cardiac sarcoplasmic reticulum. J Cyclic Nucleotide Res 1:329, 1975
11. Withering W: An account of the foxglove and some of its medical uses with practical remarks on dropsy and other diseases. In Willius FA, Keys TE (eds): Classics of Cardiology, p 231. New York, Henry Schuman, 1941
12. McKenzie J: Digitalis. Heart 2:273, 1911
13. Katzung BG, Parmley WW: Cardiac glycosides and other drugs used in the treatment of congestive heart failure. In Katzung BG (ed): Basic and Clinical Pharmacology, p 143. Los Altos, Lange, 1984
14. Greenberger NJ, Caldwell JH: Studies on the intestinal absorption of 3H-digitalis glycosides in experimental animals and man. In Marks BH, Weissler A (eds): Basic and Clinical Pharmacology of Digitalis, p 15. Springfield, IL, Charles C Thomas, 1972
15. Caldwell JH, Martin JF, Dutta S, Greenberger NJ: Intestinal absorption of digoxin 3H in the rat. Am J Physiol 217:1747, 1969
16. Greenberger NJ et al: Intestinal absorption of six tritium labeled digitalis glycosides in rats and guinea pigs. J Pharmacol Exp Ther 167:265, 1969
17. Oliver GCH, Taxman R, Frederickson R: Influence of congestive heart failure on digoxin blood levels. In Stor-Stein O (ed): Digitalis Symposium, p 336. Oslo, Gyldenal Norsk Forlag, 1973
18. Ohnhaus EE, Vozel S, Nuesch E: Absorption of digoxin in severe right heart failure. Eur J Clin Pharmacol 15:115, 1979
19. Lindenbaum J, Mellow MH, Blackstone MO, Butler VP: Variation in biological availability of digoxin from four preparations. N Engl J Med 285:1344, 1971
20. Greenblatt DJ, Duhme DW, Koch-Wesser J, Smith TW: Equivalent bioavailability from digoxin elixir, and rapid dissolution tablets. JAMA 29:1774, 1974
21. Lindenbaum J: Greater bioavailability of digoxin solution in capsules. Clin Pharmacol Ther 21:278, 1977
22. Gold H, Catell M, Greiner T et al: Clinical pharmacology of digoxin. J Pharmacol Exp Ther 109:45, 1953
23. Marcus FI, Quinn EJ, Horton H et al: The effects of jejunoileal bypass on the pharmacokinetics of digoxin in man. Circulation 55(3):537, 1977
24. White RJ, Chamberlain DA, Howard M, Smith TW: Plasma concentrations of digoxin after oral administration in the fasting and postprandial state. Br Med J 1:380, 1971
25. Greenblatt DJ, Duhme DW, Koch-Wesser J, Smith TW: Bioavailability of digoxin tablets and elixir in the fasting and postprandial states. Clin Pharmacol Ther 16:444, 1974
26. Moe GK, Farah AE: Digitalis and allied cardiac glycosides. In Goodman LS, Gilman A (eds): The Pharmacologic Basis of Therapeutics, p 653. New York, Macmillan, 1975
27. Keys W: Digoxin. In Evans WE, Schentag JJ, Jusko WJ (eds): Applied Pharmacokinetics: Principles of Therapeutic Drug Monitoring, p 319. San Francisco, Applied Therapeutics, 1980
28. Doherty JE, deSoyza N, Kane JJ et al: Clinical pharmacokinetics of digitalis glycosides. Prog Cardiovasc Dis 21:141, 1978
29. Smith TW, Antman EM, Friedman PL et al: Digitalis glycosides: Mechanisms and manifestations of toxicity. Prog Cardiovasc Dis 26:413, 1984
30. Smith TW, Antman EM, Friedman PL et al: Digitalis glycosides: Mechanisms and manifestations of toxicity (Part III). Prog Cardiovasc Dis 27:21, 1984
31. Warner NJ, Barnard T, Bigger T: Tissue digoxin concentrations and digoxin effect during the quinidine-digoxin interaction. J Am Coll Cardiol 5:680, 1985
32. Steiner E: Renal tubular secretion of digoxin. Circulation 50:103, 1974
33. Beard OW, Perkins WH: Titrated digoxin XTL: Enterohepatic circulation, absorption and excretion studies in human volunteers. Circulation 42:867, 1970
34. Lukas DS, DeMartino AG: Binding of digitoxin and some related cardenolides to human plasma proteins. J Clin Invest 48:1041, 1969
35. Solomon HM, Abrams WB: Interactions between digitoxin and other drugs in man. Am Heart J 83:277, 1972
36. Bigger JT, Strauss HC: Digitalis toxicity: Drug interactions promoting toxicity and the management of toxicity. Seminars in Drug Treatment 2:147, 1972
37. Allen DG, Blinks JR: Calcium transients in aquorin-injected frog cardiac muscle. Nature 273:509, 1978
38. Lullman H, Peters T: Action of cardiac glycosides on the excitation-contraction coupling in heart muscle. Prog Pharmacol 2:5, 1979
39. Ghysel-Barton J, Godfraind T: Stimulation and inhibition of the sodium pump by cardioactive steroids in relation to their binding sites and their inotropic effect on guinea-pig isolated atria. Br J Pharmacol 66:175, 1979
40. Cohen I, Daut J, Noble D: An analysis of the actions of low concentrations of ouabain on membrane currents in Purkinje fibers. J Physiol 260:75, 1976
41. Sharma VK, Banerjee SP: Regeneration of $[^3H]$ ouabain binding to (Na^+-K^+)-ATPase in chemically sympathectomized cat peripheral organs. Mol Pharmacol 15:35, 1979
42. Sharma VK, Banerjee SP: Ouabain stimulation of adrenalin transport in guinea pig heart. Nature 286:817, 1980
43. Wier WG, Hess P: Excitation-contraction coupling in cardiac Purkinje fibers: Effects of cardiotonic steroids on the intracellular $[Ca^{2+}]$ transient, membrane potential and contraction. J Gen Physiol 83:395, 1984
44. Sheu S-S, Fozzard HA: Transmembrane Na^+ and Ca^{2+} electrochemical gradients in cardiac muscle and their relationship to force development. J Gen Physiol 80:325, 1982
45. Lee CO, Dagostine M: Effects of strophanthidin on intracellular Na ion activity and twitch tension of constantly driven canine cardiac Purkinje fibers. Biophys J 40:185, 1982
46. Sheu S-S, Sharma VK, Banerjee SP: Measurement of cytosolic free calcium concentration in isolated rat ventricular myocytes with Quin 2. Circ Res 55:830, 1984
47. Weingart R, Kass RS, Tgien RW: Is digitalis inotropy associated with enhanced slow inward calcium current? Nature 273:389, 1978
48. Marban E, Tgien RW: Enhancement of calcium current during digitalis inotropy in mammalian heart; positive feedback regulation by intracellular calcium? J Physiol (Lond) 329:589, 1982
49. Gillis RA, Quest JA: The role of the nervous system in the cardiovascular effects of digitalis. Pharmacol Rev 31:19, 1980
50. Ellis D: The effects of external cations and ouabain on the intracellular sodium activity of sheep heart Purkinje fibers. J Physiol (Lond) 273:211, 1977
51. Warserstrom JA, Schwartz DJ, Fozzard HA: Relation between intracellular sodium and twitch tension in sheep cardiac Purkinje strands exposed to cardiac glycosides. Circ Res 52:697, 1983
52. Katz AM: Effects of digitalis on cell biochemistry: Sodium pump inhibition. J Am Coll Cardiol 5:16A, 1985
53. Hoffman BF: Effects of digitalis on electrical activity of cardiac membranes. In Marks BH, Weissler AM (eds): Basic and Clinical Pharmacology of Digitalis, p 118. Springfield, IL, Charles C Thomas, 1972
54. Rosen MR, Wit AL, Hoffman BF: Electrophysiology and pharmacology of cardiac arrhythmias: Cardiac antiarrhythmic and toxic effects of digitalis. Am Heart J 89:391, 1975
55. Rosen MR: Cellular electrophysiology of digitalis toxicity. J Am Coll Cardiol 5:22A, 1985
56. Watanabe AM: Digitalis and the autonomic nervous system. J Am Coll Cardiol 5:35A, 1985
57. Dhingra RC, Amat-y-Leon F, Wyndham C et al: The electrophysiologic effects of ouabain on sinus node and atrium in man. J Clin Invest 56:555, 1975
58. Goodman DJ, Rossen RM, Cannon DS et al: Effect of digoxin on atrioventricular conduction. Studies in patients with and without cardiac autonomic innervation. Circulation 51:251, 1975
59. Nakamura M: Digitalis induced augmentation of cardiopulmonary baroreflex control of forearm vascular resistance. Circulation 71:11, 1985
60. Kent FM, Epstein SE, Cooper T, Jacobowitz DM: Cholinergic innervation of the canine and human ventricular conducting system: Anatomic and electrophysiologic correlations. Circulation 23:1197, 1974
61. Schmid PG, Greif B, Lund DD, Roskoski T: Regional choline acetyl transferase activity in the guinea pig heart. Circ Res 42:657, 1976

62. Brown OM: Cat heart acetylcholine structural proof and distribution. Am J Physiol 231:781, 1976
63. Vatner SF, Rutherford JD, Ochs HR: Baroreflux and vagal mechanisms modulating left ventricular contractile response to sympathetic amines in conscious dogs. Circ Res 44:195, 1979
64. Levy MN, Blattberg B: Effect of vagal stimulation on the outflow of norepinephrine into the coronary sinus during cardiac sympathetic nerve stimulation in the dog. Circ Res 38:81, 1976
65. Braunwald E: Effects of digitalis on the normal and failing heart. J Am Coll Cardiol 5:51A, 1985
66. Sonnenblick EH, Williams JF Jr, Glick G et al: Studies on Digitalis XV: Effects of cardiac glycosides on myocardial force-velocity relations in the now failing human heart. Circulation 34:532, 1966
67. Spann JF Jr, Buccino RA, Sonnenblick EH, Braunwald E: Contractile state of cardiac muscle obtained from cats with experimentally produced ventricular hypertrophy at heart failure. Circ Res 21:341, 1967
68. Mahler F, Karliner JS, O'Rourke RA: Effects of chronic digoxin administration on left ventricular performance in the normal conscious dog. Circulation 50:720, 1974
69. Crawford MH, Karliner JS, O'Rourke RA, Amon KW: Effects of chronic digoxin administration on left ventricular performance in normal subjects. Echocardiographic study. Am J Cardiol 38:843, 1976
70. Mason DT, Braunwald E: Studies on digitalis X: Effects of ouabain on forearm vascular resistance and venous tone in normal subjects and in all patients in heart failure. J Clin Invest 43:532, 1964
71. Shanbour LL, Jacobson ED: Digitalis and the mesenteric circulation. Am J Dig Dis 17:826, 1972
72. Ross J Jr, Braunwald E, Waldhausen JA: Studies of digitalis. II: Extracardiac effects on venous return and on the capacity of peripheral vascular bed. J Clin Invest 39:936, 1960
73. Sugar KB, Hanson EC, Powell WJ: Neurogenic vasoconstrictor effects during acute global ischemia in dogs. J Clin Invest 60:1248, 1977
74. DeMots H, Rahimtoola SH, McAnulty JH, Porter GA: Effects of ouabain on coronary and systemic vascular resistance and myocardial oxygen consumption in patients without heart failure. Am J Cardiol 41:88, 1978
75. Garan H, Smith TW, Powell WJ Jr: The central nervous system as a site of action for the coronary vasoconstrictor effect of digoxin. J Clin Invest 54:1365, 1974
76. Arnold SB, Byrd RC, Meister W et al: Long-term digitalis therapy improves left ventricular function in heart failure. N Engl J Med 303:1443, 1980
77. Torretti J, Hendler E, Weinstein E: Functional significance of Na-K-ATPase in the kidney: Effects of ouabain inhibition. Am J Physiol 222:1398, 1972
78. Covit AB, Schaer GL, Sealy JE et al: Suppression of the renin-angiotensin by intravenous digoxin in chronic congestive heart failure. Am J Med 75:445, 1983
79. Banka VS, Schadda KD, Bodenheimer MM et al: Digitalis in experimental acute myocardial infarction. Am J Cardiol 35:801, 1975
80. Hood WB Jr, McCarthy B, Lown B: Myocardial infarction following coronary ligation in dogs. Hemodynamic effects of isoproterenol and acetyl strophanthidin. Circ Res 21:191, 1967
81. Rahimtoola SH, Sinno MZ, Chuquimia R et al: Effects of ouabain on impaired left ventricular function in acute myocardial infarction. N Engl J Med 287:527, 1972
82. Forrester J, Bezdek W, Chatterjee K et al: Hemodynamic effects of digitalis in acute myocardial infarction. Ann Intern Med 76:863, 1972
83. Cohn JN, Tristani FE, Khatri IM: Cardiac and peripheral vascular effects of digitalis in clinical cardiogenic shock. Am Heart J 78:318, 1969
84. Lipp H, Denes P, Gametta M et al: Hemodynamic response to acute intravenous digoxin in patients with recent myocardial infarction and coronary insufficiency with and without heart failure. Chest 63:862, 1972
85. Goldstein RA, Passamani ER, Roberts R: A comparison of digoxin and dobutamine in patients with acute infarction and cardiac failure. N Engl J Med 303:846, 1980
86. Forrester JS, Chatterjee K: Preservation of ischemic myocardium. In Vogel JHK (ed): Advances in Cardiology, p 158. Basel, S Karger, 1974
87. Gunner RM, Loeb HS, Pietras RJT: Hemodynamic measurements in the coronary care unit. Prog Cardiovasc Dis 11:29, 1968
88. Gander MP, Kazamias TM, Henry P et al: Serial determinations of cardiac output and response to digitalis in patients with acute myocardial infarction. Circulation 42(Suppl 3):155, 1970
89. DeMots H, Rahimtoola SH, Kremkau EL et al: Effects of ouabain on myocardial oxygen supply and demand in patients with chronic coronary artery disease: A hemodynamic, volumetric and metabolic study in patients without heart failure. J Clin Invest 58:312, 1976
90. Kotter V, Schurer K, Schroder R: Effect of digoxin on coronary blood flow and myocardial oxygen consumption in patients with coronary artery disease. Am J Cardiol 42:563, 1978
91. Watanabe T, Covell JW, Maroko PR et al: Effects of increased arterial pressure and positive inotropic agents on the severity of myocardial ischemia in the acutely depressed heart. Am J Cardiol 30:371, 1972
92. Varomkov Y, Shell WE, Smirnov V et al: Augmentation of serum CPK activity in digitalis in patients with acute myocardial infarction. Circulation 55:719, 1977
93. Morrison J, Pizzarello R, Reduto L, Gulotta S: Effects of digitalis on predicted myocardial infarct size in man (abstr). Clin Res 23:198, 1975
94. Moss AJ, Davis HT, Conard DL et al: Digitalis associated cardiac mortality after myocardial infarction. Circulation 64:1150, 1981
95. Bigger JT, Fleiss JL, Rolnitsky LAM et al: Effect of digitalis treatment on survival after acute myocardial infarction. Am J Cardiol 55:629, 1985
96. Iesaka Y, Aonuma K, Gosselin AJ et al: Susceptibility of infarcted canine hearts to digitalis-toxic ventricular tachycardia. J Am Coll Cardiol 2:45, 1983
97. Chatterjee K, Parmley WW: Therapy of acute myocardial infarction. In Cohn PF (ed): Diagnosis and Therapy of Coronary Artery Disease, p 357. The Hague, Martinus Nijhoff Publishers, 1985
98. Ryan TJ, Baily KR, McCabe CH et al: The effects of digitalis treatment on survival after acute myocardial infarction. Circulation 67:735, 1983
99. Davidson C, Gibson D: Clinical significance of positive inotropic action of digoxin in patients with left ventricular disease. Br Heart J 35:970, 1973
100. Goldman RH: Left ventricular dynamics during long term digoxin treatment in patients with stable coronary artery disease. Am J Cardiol 41:937, 1978
101. Carliner NH, Gilbert CA, Puritt AW, Goldberg LI: Effects of maintenance digoxin therapy on systolic time intervals and serum digoxin concentrations. Circulation 50:94, 1974
102. Hoeschen RJ, Cuddy TE: Dose-response relation between therapeutic levels of serum digoxin and systolic time intervals. Am J Cardiol 35:469, 1975
103. Selzer A, Malmborg RO: Hemodynamic effects of digoxin in latent cardiac failure. Circulation 25:695, 1962
104. Vogel R, Frischknecht J, Stelle P: Short and long term effects of digitalis on resting and post-handgrip hemodynamics in patients with coronary heart disease. Am J Cardiol 40:171, 1977
105. Cohn K, Selzer A, Kersh ES et al: Variability of hemodynamic responses to acute digitalization in chronic cardiac failure due to cardiomyopathy and coronary artery disease. Am J Cardiol 35:461, 1975
106. Murray RG, Tweddel AC, Martin W et al: Evaluation of digitalis in cardiac failure. Lancet 1:1526, 1982
107. Murlow CD, Feussner JR, Velez R: Re-evaluation of digitalis efficacy. New light on old leaf. Ann Intern Med 101:113, 1984
108. Rader BR, Smith WW, Berger AR, Eichna LW: Comparison of the hemodynamic effects of mercurial diuretics and digitalis in congestive heart failure. Circulation 29:328, 1964
109. McHaffie D, Purcell H, Mitchell-Heggs P, Guz A: The clinical value of digoxin in patients with heart failure and sinus rhythm. Q J Med 47:401, 1978
110. Hutcheon D, Nemeth E, Quinland D: The role of furosemide alone and in combination with digoxin in the relief of symptoms of congestive heart failure. J Clin Pharmacol 20:59, 1980
111. Dobbs SM, Kenyon WI, Dobbs RJ: Maintenance digoxin after an episode of heart failure: Placebo-controlled trial in outpatients. Br Med J 1:749, 1977
112. Lee DC, Johnson RA, Bingham JB: Heart failure in outpatients: A randomized trial of digoxin versus placebo. N Engl J Med 306:699, 1982
113. Fleg JL, Gottlieb SH, Lakatia EG: Is digoxin really important in treatment of compensated heart failure: A placebo-controlled crossover study in patients with sinus rhythm. Am J Med 73:244, 1983
114. Gheorghiade M, Beller GA: Effects of discontinuing maintenance digoxin therapy in patients with ischemic heart disease and congestive heart failure in sinus rhythm. Am J Cardiol 51:1243, 1983
115. German and Austrian Xamoterol Study Group: Double-blind placebo-controlled comparison of digoxin and xamoterol in chronic heart failure. Lancet 1:489, 1988
116. The Captopril-Digoxin Multicenter Research Group: Comparative effects of therapy with captopril and digoxin in patients with mild to moderate heart failure. JAMA 259:539, 1988
117. Beaune J: For the enalapril versus digoxin French Multicenter Study Group: Comparison of enalapril versus digoxin for congestive heart failure. Am J Cardiol 63:22D, 1989
118. Guyatt GH, Sullivan MJJ, Fallen EL et al: A controlled trial of digoxin in congestive heart failure. Am J Cardiol 62:372, 1988
119. DiBianco R, Shabetai R, Kostruk W et al: For the milrinone Multicenter Trial Group: A comparison of oral milrinone, digoxin, and their combination in the treatment of patients with chronic heart failure. N Engl J Med 320:677, 1989
120. Cohn JN, Archibald DG, Ziesche S et al: Effect of vasodilator therapy on mortality in chronic congestive heart failure: Results of a Veterans Administration Cooperative Study. N Engl J Med 314:1547, 1988
121. CONSENSUS Trial Study Group: Effects of enalapril on mortality in severe congestive heart failure: Results of the Cooperative North Scandinavian Enalapril Survival Study (CONSENSUS). N Engl J Med 316:1429, 1987
122. Gheorghiade M, Hall V, Lakier JB, Goldstein S: Comparative hemodynamic and neurohormonal effects of intravenous captopril and digoxin and their combinations in patients with severe heart failure. J Am Coll Cardiol 13:134, 1989
123. DiCarlo L, Chatterjee K, Parmley WW et al: Enalapril: A new angiotensin-converting enzyme inhibitor in chronic heart failure: Acute and chronic hemodynamic evaluations. J Am Coll Cardiol 2:865, 1983
124. Mettauer B, Rouleau JL, Bichet D et al: Differential long-term intrarenal and neurohumoral effects of captopril and prazosin in chronic heart failure:

Importance of initial plasma renin activity. Circulation 73:492, 1986
125. Crawford MH, LeWinter MM, O'Rourke RA et al: Combined propranolol and digoxin therapy in angina pectoris. Ann Intern Med 83:449, 1975
126. Harding PR, Aronow WS, Eisenman J: Digitalis as an antianginal agent. Chest 64:439, 1973
127. Nederberger M, Bruce RA, Frederick R et al: Reproduction of maximal exercise performance in patients with angina pectoris despite ouabain treatment. Circulation 49:309, 1974
128. Vatner SF, Braunwald E: Effects of chronic heart failure on the inotropic response of the right ventricle of the conscious dog to a cardiac glycoside and to tachycardia. Circulation 50:728, 1974
129. Berglund E, Widimsky J, Malmberg R: Lack of effect of digitalis in patients with pulmonary disease with and without heart failure. Am J Cardiol 11:477, 1963
130. Ferrer MI, Harvey RM, Cathcart RT et al: Some effects of digoxin upon the heart and circulation in man: Digoxin in chronic cor pulmonale. Circulation 1:161, 1950
131. Baum GL, Dick MM, Schotz S, Gumpel RC: Digitalis toxicity in chronic cor pulmonale. South Med J 49:1037, 1956
132. Williams JF Jr, Boyd DC, Border JF: Effects of acute hypoxia and hypercapnic acidosis on the development of acetyl strophanthidin induced arrhythmias. J Clin Invest 47:1885, 1968
133. Goldman RH, Harrison DC: The effect of hypoxemia and hypercapnia on myocardial catecholamines. J Pharmacol Exp Ther 307:174, 1970
134. Johnson LW, Dickstein RA, Fruehass CT et al: Prophylactic digitalization for coronary artery bypass surgery. Circulation 53:819, 1976
135. Tyras DH, Stothert JC Jr, Kaiser GC et al: Supraventricular tachyarrhythmias after myocardial revascularization: A randomized trial of prophylactic digitalization. J Thorac Cardiovasc Surg 77:310, 1979
136. Aronson JK: Digitalis intoxication. Clin Sci 64:253, 1983
137. Ogilvie RJ, Ruedy J: Adverse drug reactions during hospitalization. Can Med Assoc J 97:1450, 1967
138. Hurwitz N, Wade OL: Intensive hospital monitoring of adverse reaction to drugs. Br Med J 1:531, 1969
139. Beller GA, Smith TW, Abelmann WH et al: Digitalis intoxication: Prospective clinical study with serum level correlations. N Engl J Med 284:989, 1971
140. Carter BL, Small RE, Garnett WR: Monitoring digoxin therapy in two long-term facilities. J Am Geriatr Soc 29:263, 1981
141. Lely AH, VanEnter CHJ: Noncardiac symptoms of digitalis intoxication. Am Heart J 83:149, 1972
142. Gazes P, Holmes CR, Mosely V, Pratt-Thomas HR: Acute hemorrhage and necrosis of the intestine associated with digitalization. Circulation 23:358, 1961
143. Longhurst JC, Ross J: Extracardiac and coronary vascular effects of digitalis. J Am Coll Cardiol 5:99A, 1985
144. Fisch C, Knoebel SB: Digitalis cardiotoxicity. J Am Coll Cardiol 5:91A, 1985
145. Wellens HJJ: The electrocardiogram in digitalis intoxication. In Yu PN, Goodwin JF (eds): Progress in Cardiology, vol 5, chap 10, p 271. Philadelphia, Lea & Febiger, 1976
146. Surawicz B: Factors affecting tolerance to digitalis. J Am Coll Cardiol 5:69A, 1985
147. Marcus FI: Current status of therapy with digoxin. In Proctor HW (ed): Current Problems in Cardiology, vol III, no 5, p 1. Chicago, Year Book Medical Publishers, 1978
148. Madsen EB, Oilpin E, Henning H et al: Prognostic importance of digitalis after acute myocardial infarction. J Am Coll Cardiol 3:681, 1984
149. Surawicz B: Use of the chelating agent EDTA in digitalis intoxication and cardiac arrhythmias. Prog Cardiovasc Dis 2:432, 1960
150. Goldman RH, Kleiger RE, Schweizer E, Harrison DC: The effect on myocardial 3-H digoxin of magnesium deficiency. Proc Exp Biol Med 136:747, 1971
151. Tackett RL, Holl JE: Increased automaticity and decreased inotropism of ouabain in dogs with furosemide-induced hypomagnesemia. J Cardiovasc Pharmacol 3:1269, 1981
152. Storstein O, Hansteen V, Hatle L et al: Studies on digitalis: XIV. Is there any correlation between hypomagnesemia and digitalis intoxication? Acta Med Scand 202:445, 1977
153. Cohen L, Kitzres R: Magnesium sulfate and digitalis-toxic arrhythmias. JAMA 249:2808, 1973
154. Brater DC, Morelli HF: Systemic alkalosis and digitalis-related arrhythmias. Acta Med Scand (Suppl) 647:79, 1981
155. Doherty JE, Perkins WH: Digoxin metabolism in hypo- and hyperthyroidism: Studies with titrated digoxin in thyroid disease. Ann Intern Med 64:489, 1966
156. Ebert PA, Morerow AG, Austen WG: Clinical studies of the effect of extracorporeal circulation on myocardial digoxin concentration. Am J Cardiol 11:201, 1963
157. Ditchey RV, Curtis GP: Effects of apparently nontoxic doses of digoxin on ventricular ectopy after direct-current electrical shocks in dogs. J Pharmacol Exp Ther 218:212, 1981
158. Doherty JE: Conventional drug therapy in the management of heart failure. In Cohn JN (ed): Drug Treatment of Heart Failure, p 91. New York, Yorke Medical Books, 1983
159. Marcus FI: Pharmacokinetic interactions between digoxin and other drugs. J Am Coll Cardiol 5:82A, 1985
160. Bigger JT, Leahey EB: Quinidine and digoxin—an important interaction. Drugs 24:229, 1982
161. Warner NJ, Barnard JT, Bigger JT: Tissue digoxin concentrations and digoxin effect during the quinidine-digoxin interactions. J Am Coll Cardiol 5:680, 1985
162. Graves SW, Brown B, Valdes R: An endogenous digoxin like substance in patients with renal impairment. Ann Intern Med 99:604, 1983
163. Eraker SA, Sasse L: The serum digoxin test and digoxin toxicity: A Bayesian approach to decision making. Circulation 2:409, 1981
164. Wotman S, Bigger JT Jr, Mandel ID et al: Salivary electrolytes in the detection of digitalis toxicity. N Engl J Med 285:871, 1971
165. Aronson JK, Grahame-Smith DG, Hallis KF et al: Monitoring digoxin therapy: I. Plasma concentrations and *in vitro* assay of tissue response. Br J Clin Pharmacol 4:213, 1977
166. Klein MD, Lown B, Barr I et al: Comparison of serum digoxin level measurement with acetyl strophanthidin tolerance testing. Circulation 49:1053, 1974
167. Caldwell JH, Bush CA, Greenberger NJ: Interruption of the enterohepatic circulation of digitoxin by cholystyramine: II. Effect on metabolic disposition of tritium-labeled digitoxin and cardiac systolic intervals in man. J Clin Invest 50:2638, 1971
168. Bazzano G, Bazzano GS: Digitalis intoxication: Treatment with new steroid-binding resin. JAMA 220:828, 1972
169. Garan H, Ruskin JN, Powell WJ: Centrally mediated effect of phenytoin on digoxin induced ventricular arrhythmias. Am J Physiol 241:H67, 1981
170. Castellanos A, Ferreiro J, Pefkaros K et al: Effects of lidocaine on bidirectional tachycardia and on digitalis induced atrial tachycardia with block. Br Heart J 48:27, 1982
171. Davis LD, Temte JV: Effects of propranolol on the transmembrane potentials of ventricular muscle on Purkinje fibers of the dog. Circ Res 22:261, 1968
172. Gillis RA, Clancy MM, Anderson RJ: Deleterious effects of bretylium in cats with digitalis induced ventricular tachycardia 57:974, 1973
173. Cohen L, Kitzes R: Magnesium sulfate and digitalis toxic arrhythmias. JAMA 249:2808, 1983
174. Lown B, Levine SA: The carotid sinus. Circulation 23:766, 1961
175. Lown B, Kleiger R, Williams J: Cardioversion and digitalis drugs: Changes in threshold to electric shock in digitalized animals. Circ Res 57:519, 1965
176. Ditchey RV, Karliner JS: Safety of electrical cardioversion in patients without digitalis toxicity. Ann Intern Med 95:676, 1981
177. Gilfrich HJ, Kasper W, Meinertz T et al: Treatment of massive digitoxin overdose by charcoal hemoperfusion. Lancet 1:505, 1978
178. Buller VP, Chen JP: Digoxin specific antibodies. Proc Natl Acad Sci USA 57:71, 1967
179. Curd J, Smith TW, Jaton J, Haber E: The isolation of digoxin specific antibody and its use in reversing the effects of digoxin. Proc Natl Acad Sci USA 68:2401, 1971
180. Haber E: Antibodies and digitalis: The modern revolution in the use of an ancient drug. J Am Coll Cardiol 5:111A, 1985
181. Mandel WJ, Bigger JT Jr, Butler VP Jr: The electrophysiologic effects of low and high digoxin concentrations on isolated mammalian cardiac tissue reversal by digoxin-specific antibody. J Clin Invest 51:1378, 1972
182. Lloyd BL, Smith TW: Contrasting rates of reversal of digoxin toxicity by digoxin-specific IgG and Fab fragments. Circulation 58:280, 1978
183. Ochs HR, Vatner SF, Smith TW: Reversal of inotropic effects of digoxin by specific antibodies and their Fab fragments in the conscious dog. J Pharmacol Exp Ther 207:64, 1978
184. Clarke W, Ramoska EA: Acute digoxin overdose: Use of digoxin-specific antibody fragments. Am J Emerg Med 6:465, 1988
185. Erdmann E, Mair W, Knedel M, Schaumann W: Digitalis intoxication and treatment with digoxin antibody fragments in renal failure. Klin Wochenschr 67:16, 1989
186. Schaumann W, Kaufmann B, Neubert P, Smolarz A: Kinetics of the Fab fragments of digoxin antibodies and of bound digoxin in patients with severe digoxin intoxication. Eur J Clin Pharmacol 30:527, 1986
187. Smith TW, Butler VP Jr, Haber E et al: Treatment of life threatening digitalis intoxication with digoxin-specific Fab antibody fragments: Experience in 26 cases. N Engl J Med 307:1357, 1982
188. Wenger TL, Butler VP, Haber E, Smith TW: Treatment of 63 severely digitalis-toxic patients with digoxin-specific antibody fragments. J Am Coll Cardiol 5:118A, 1985
189. Bismuth C, Gautlier M, Corso F, Efehymiou ML: Hyperkalemia in acute digitalis poisoning: Prognostic and therapeutic implications. Clin Toxicol 6:153, 1973
190. Ekins BR, Watanabe AS: Acute digoxin poisoning: Review of therapy. Am J Hosp Pharm 35:268, 1978
191. Ahlquist RP: A study of adrenotropic receptors. Am J Physiol 153:586, 1948
192. Watanabe AM: Recent advances in knowledge about beta-adrenergic receptors: Application to clinical cardiology. J Am Coll Cardiol 1:82, 1983
193. Langer SZ: Presynaptic regulation of catecholamine release. Biochem Pharmacol 23:1793, 1974
194. Goldberg M, Robertson D: Evidence for the existence of vascular alpha$_2$ adrenoreceptors in humans. Hypertension 6:551, 1984
195. Colucci WS: Alpha-adrenergic receptors in cardiovascular medicine. In Karliner JS, Haft JI (eds): Receptor Science in Cardiology, p 43. Mt Kisco,

NY, Futura Publications, 1984
196. Lefkowitz RJ, Stadel JM, Caron MG: Adenylate cyclase-coupled beta adrenergic receptors: Structure and mechanisms of activation and desensitization. Annu Rev Biochem 52:159, 1983
197. Viquerat CE, Daly P, Swedberg K et al: Endogenous catecholamines in chronic heart failure: Relation to the severity of hemodynamic abnormalities. Am J Med 78:455, 1985
198. Hasking GJ, Esler MD, Jennings GL et al: Norepinephrine spillover to plasma in patients with congestive heart failure: Evidence of increased overall and cardiorenal sympathetic nervous activity. Circulation 73:615, 1986
199. Swedberg K, Viquerat C, Rouleau J-L et al: Comparison of myocardial catecholamine balance in chronic congestive heart failure and in angina pectoris without failure. Am J Cardiol 54:783, 1984
200. Chidsey CA, Braunwald EB, Morrow AG, Mason DT: Myocardial norepinephrine concentration in man: Effects of reserpine and of congestive heart failure. N Engl J Med 269:653, 1963
201. Pierpont GL, Francis GS, DeMaster EG et al: Elevated left ventricular myocardial dopamine in preterminal idiopathic dilated cardiomyopathy. Am J Cardiol 52:1033, 1983
202. Sole MJ, Helke CJ, Jascobowitz DM: Increased dopamine in the failing hamster heart: Transvesicular transport of dopamine limits the rate of norepinephrine synthesis. Am J Cardiol 49:1682, 1982
203. Bristow MR: Myocardial beta-adrenergic receptor down regulation in heart failure. Int J Cardiol 5:648, 1984
204. Bristow MR, Ginsburg R, Minobe W et al: Decreased catecholamine sensitivity and beta-adrenergic receptor density in failing human hearts. N Engl J Med 307:205, 1982
205. Bristow MR, Port JD, Sandoval AB et al: β-Adrenergic receptor pathways in the failing human heart. Heart Failure 5:77, 1989
206. Karliner JS: Myocardial adrenergic function in heart failure. In Chatterjee K (ed): Dobutamine: A Ten Year Review, pp 5–31. New York, NCM Publishers, 1989
207. Lee HR: α_1-Adrenergic receptors in heart failure. Heart Failure 5:62, 1989
208. Scholz H: Effects of beta- and alpha-adrenoreceptor activators and adrenergic transmitter releasing agents on the mechanical activity of the heart. In Szekeres L (ed): Handbook of Experimental Pharmacology, Part 1, Adrenergic Activators and Inhibitors, vol 54, pp 651–733. Berlin, Springer-Verlag, 1980
209. Reuter H: Localization of beta adrenergic receptors and effects of noradrenaline and cyclic nucleotides on action potentials, ionic currents and tension in mammalian cardiac muscle. J Physiol (London) 242:429, 1974
210. Reiter M: Drugs and heart muscle. Annu Rev Pharmacol 12:111, 1972
211. Berridge MJ, Irvine RF: Inositol triphosphate, a novel second messenger in cellular signal transduction. Nature 312:315, 1984
212. Kikkawa U, Nishizuka Y: The role of protein kinase in transmembrane signaling. Annu Rev Cell Biol 2:149, 1986
213. Aronson RS, Gelles JM: Electrophysiologic effects of dopamine on sheep cardiac Purkinje fibers. J Pharmacol Exp Ther 188:595, 1974
214. Abrams E, Forrester JS, Chatterjee K et al: Variability in response to norepinephrine in acute myocardial infarction. Am J Cardiol 32:919, 1973
215. Innes IR, Nickerson M: Norepinephrine, epinephrine and the sympathomimetic amines. In Goodman LS, Gilman A (eds): Pharmacological Basis of Therapeutics, 5th ed, p 477. New York, Macmillan, 1975
216. Goldberg LI, Rafzer SI: Dopamine receptors. Applications in clinical cardiology. Circulation 72:245, 1985
217. Goldberg LI: Cardiovascular and renal actions of dopamine. Potential applications. Pharmacol Rev 24:1, 1972
218. Goldberg LI, Hsieh YY, Resnekov L: Newer catecholamines for treatment of heart failure and shock: An update on dopamine and a first look at dobutamine. Prog Cardiovasc Dis 4:327, 1977
219. Richard C, Ricome JL, Rimailho A et al: Combined hemodynamic effects of dopamine and dobutamine in cardiogenic shock. Circulation 67:620, 1983
220. Miller RR, Awan NA, Joye JA et al: Combined dopamine and nitroprusside therapy in congestive heart failure: Greater augmentation of cardiac performance by addition of inotropic stimulation to afterload reduction. Circulation 55:881, 1977
221. Loeb HS, Ostrenga JP, Gaul W et al: Beneficial effects of dopamine combined with intravenous nitroglycerin on hemodynamics in patients with severe left ventricular failure. Circulation 68:813, 1983
222. Vatner SF, Baig H: Importance of heart rate in determining the effects of sympathomimetic amines on regional myocardial function and blood flow in conscious dogs with acute myocardial ischemia. Circ Res 45:793, 1979
223. Ramanathan KB, Bodenheimer MM, Banka VS et al: Contrasting effects of dopamine and isoproterenol in experimental myocardial infarction. Am J Cardiol 39:413, 1977
224. McClenathan JH, Guyton RA, Breyer RH et al: The effects of isoproterenol and dopamine on regional myocardial blood flow after stenosis of circumflex coronary artery. J Thorac Cardiovasc Surg 73:431, 1977
225. Mueller HS, Evans R, Ayers SM: Effect of dopamine on hemodynamics and myocardial metabolism in shock following acute myocardial infarction in man. Circulation 57:361, 1978
226. Ruffolo RR Jr, Spradlin TA, Pollock GD et al: Alpha and beta adrenergic effects of the stereoisomers of dobutamine. J Pharmacol Exp Ther 219:447, 1981
227. Chatterjee J, Bendersky R, Parmley WW: Dobutamine in heart failure. Eur Heart J 3:107, 1982
228. Willerson JT, Hutton I, Watson JT et al: Influence of dobutamine on regional myocardial blood flow and ventricular performance during acute and chronic myocardial ischemia in dogs. Circulation 53:828, 1976
229. Gillespie TA, Ambos HD, Sobel BE et al: Effects of dobutamine in patients with acute myocardial infarction. Am J Cardiol 39:588, 1977
230. Magotrien RD, Unverferth DV, Brown GP et al: Dobutamine and hydralazine: Comparative influences of positive inotropy and vasodilation on coronary blood flow and myocardial energetics in nonischemic congestive heart failure. J Am Coll Cardiol 1:499, 1983
231. Fowler MB, Alderman EL, Oesterle SN et al: Dobutamine and dopamine after cardiac surgery: Greater augmentation of myocardial blood flow with dobutamine. Circulation 70(Suppl 1):1103, 1984
232. Bendersky R, Chatterjee K, Parmley WW et al: Dobutamine in chronic ischemic heart failure: Alterations in left ventricular function and coronary hemodynamics. Am J Cardiol 48:554, 1981
233. Hamilton FN, Feigl ED: Coronary vascular sympathetic β-receptor innervation. Am J Physiol 230:1569, 1976
234. Kupper W, Waller D, Hanrath P et al: Hemodynamic and cardiac metabolic effects of inotropic stimulation with dobutamine in patients with coronary artery disease. Eur Heart J 3:29, 1982
235. Meyer SL, Curry GC, Donsky MS et al: Influence of dobutamine on hemodynamics and coronary blood flow in patients with and without coronary artery disease. Am J Cardiol 38:103, 1976
236. Pozen RG, DiBianco R, Katz RJ et al: Myocardial metabolic and hemodynamic effects of dobutamine in heart failure complicating coronary artery disease. Circulation 63:1279, 1981
237. Sawada SG, Segar DS, Brown SE et al: Dobutamine stress echocardiography for evaluation of coronary disease (abstr). Circulation 80:II-66, 1989
238. Loeb HS, Khan M, Saudeye A, Gunnar RM: Acute hemodynamic effects of dobutamine and isoproterenol in patients with low output heart failure. Circ Shock 3:55, 1976
239. Leier CV, Heban PT, Huss P et al: Comparative systemic and regional hemodynamic effects of dopamine and dobutamine in patients with cardiomyopathic heart failure. Circulation 58:466, 1978
240. Loeb HS, Bvedakis J, Gunnar RM: Superiority of dobutamine over dopamine in patients with low output cardiac failure. Circulation 55:375, 1977
241. Stoner JD III, Bolen JL, Harrison DC: Comparison of dobutamine and dopamine in treatment of severe heart failure. Br Heart J 39:536, 1977
242. Berkowitz C, McKeever L, Croke RP et al: Comparative responses to dobutamine and nitroprusside in patients with chronic low output cardiac failure. Circulation 56:918, 1977
243. Dell'Italia LJ, Starling MR, Blumhardt R et al: Comparative effects of volume loading, dobutamine and nitroprusside in patients with predominant right ventricular infarction. Circulation 72:1327, 1985
244. Unverferth DV, Magorien RD, Lewis RP, Leier CV: Long-term benefit of dobutamine in patients with congestive cardiomyopathy. Am Heart J 100:622, 1980
245. Unverferth DV, Magorien RD, Altschuld R et al: The hemodynamic and metabolic advantages gained by a three-day infusion of dobutamine in patients with congestive cardiomyopathy. Am Heart J 106:29, 1983
246. Liang C, Sherman LG, Doherty JU et al: Sustained improvement of cardiac function in patients with congestive heart failure after short-term infusion of dobutamine. Circulation 69:113, 1984
247. Leier CV, Huss P, Lewos RP, Unverferth DV: Drug-induced conditioning in congestive heart failure. Circulation 65:1382, 1981
248. Applefeld MM, Newman KA, Grove WR et al: Intermittent continuous outpatient dobutamine infusion in the management of congestive heart failure. Am J Cardiol 51:455, 1983
249. Krell MJ, Kline EM, Bates ER et al: Intermittent ambulatory dobutamine infusions in patients with severe congestive heart failure. Am Heart J 112:787, 1986
250. Dies F: Intermittent dobutamine in ambulatory patients with chronic cardiac failure. Br J Clin Pract 45:37, 1986
251. Liang C, Tuttle RR, Hood WB Jr, Gavras H: Conditioning effects of chronic infusions of dobutamine: Comparison with exercise training. J Clin Invest 64:613, 1979
252. Unverferth DV, Leier CV, Magorien RD et al: Improvement of human myocardial mitochondria after dobutamine: A quantitative ultrastructural study. J Pharmacol Exp Ther 215:527, 1980
253. Hirshfeld JW Jr, Borer JS, Goldstein RE et al: Reduction in severity and extent of myocardial infarction when nitroglycerin and methoxamine are administered during coronary occlusion. Circulation 49:291, 1974
254. Timmis AD, Strak SK, Chamberlin PA: Hemodynamic effects of salbutamol in patients with acute myocardial infarction and severe left ventricular dysfunction. Br Med J 2:1101, 1979
255. Sharma B, Goodwin JF: Beneficial effect of salbutamol on cardiac function in severe congestive cardiomyopathy: Effect on systolic and diastolic function of the left ventricle. Circulation 58:449, 1978
256. Bourdillon PDV, Dawson JR, Foale RA et al: Salbutamol in the treatment of

257. Mifune J, Kuramoto K, Ueda K et al: Hemodynamic effects of salbutamol, an oral long-acting beta stimulant in patients with congestive heart failure. Am Heart J 104:1011, 1982
258. Gold FL, Horwitz LD: Hemodynamic effects of pirbuterol in conscious dogs. Am Heart J 102:591, 1981
259. Leier CV, Nelson S, Huss P et al: Intravenous pirbuterol. Clin Pharmacol Ther 31:89, 1982
260. Rude RE, Turi Z, Brown EJ et al: Acute effects of oral pirbuterol on congestive heart failure. Circulation 64:139, 1981
261. Awan NA, Needham K, Evenson MK et al: Therapeutic efficacy of oral pirbuterol in severe chronic congestive heart failure: Acute hemodynamic and long-term ambulatory evaluation. Am Heart J 102:555, 1981
262. Weber KT, Andrews V, Janicki JS: Pirbuterol in the long-term treatment of congestive heart failure. Circulation 65(Suppl 4):307, 1981
263. Colucci WS, Alexander RW, Williams GH et al: Decreased lymphocyte beta-adrenergic–receptor density in patients with heart failure and tolerance to the beta-adrenergic agonist pirbuterol. N Engl J Med 305:185, 1981
264. Manders WT, Watner SF, Braunwald E: Cardio-selective beta adrenergic stimulation with prenalterol in the conscious dog. J Pharmacol Exp Ther 215:266, 1980
265. Kirlin PC, Pitt B, Lucchesi BR: Comparative effects of prenalterol and dobutamine in a canine model of acute ischemic heart failure. J Cardiovasc Pharmacol 3:896, 1981
266. Kirlin PC, Pitt B: Hemodynamic effects of intravenous prenalterol in severe heart failure. Am J Cardiol 47:670, 1981
267. Wahr D, Swedberg K, Rabbino M et al: Intravenous and oral prenalterol in congestive heart failure. Effects on systemic and coronary hemodynamics and myocardial catecholamine balance. Am J Med 76:999, 1984
268. Svendsen TL, Harling OJ, Tap-Jensen J: Immediate haemodynamic effects of prenalterol, a new adrenergic beta-1 receptor agonist, in healthy volunteers. Eur J Clin Pharmacol 18:219, 1980
269. Roubin GS, Choong CVP, Devenish-Meares S et al: β-Adrenergic stimulation of the failing ventricle: A double-blind, randomized trial of sustained oral therapy with prenalterol. Circulation 69:955, 1984
270. Simonsen S: Hemodynamic effects of ICI 118,587 in cardiomyopathy. Br Heart J 51:654, 1984
271. Bhatia JSS, Swedberg K, Chatterjee K: Acute hemodynamic and metabolic effects of ICI 118,587 (Corwin), a selective partial beta agonist, in patients with dilated cardiomyopathy. Am Heart J 111:692, 1986
272. Svensson G, Rehnqvist N, Sjogren A, Erhardt L: Hemodynamic effects of ICI 118,587 (Corwin) in patients with mild cardiac failure after myocardial infarction. J Cardiovasc Pharmacol 7:97, 1985
273. Nuttal A, Snow HM: The cardiovascular effects of ICI 118,587: A beta-1 adrenoreceptor partial agonist. Br J Pharmacol 77:381, 1982
274. Kino M, Hirota Y, Yamamoto S et al: Cardiovascular effects of a newly synthesized cardiotonic agent (TA-064) on normal and diseased hearts. Am J Cardiol 51:802, 1983
275. Ozaki N, Bito K, Kinoshita M, Kawakita S: Effects of a cardiotonic agent, TA-064, on isolated canine cerebral, coronary, femoral, mesenteric and renal arteries. J Cardiovasc Pharmacol 5:818, 1983
276. Thompson MJ, Huss P, Unverferth DV et al: Hemodynamic effects of intravenous butopamine in congestive heart failure. Clin Pharmacol Ther 28:324, 1980
277. Nelson S, Leier CV: Butopamine in normal human subjects. Curr Ther Res 30:405, 1981
278. Goldberg LI: Cardiovascular and renal actions of dopamine: Potential clinical applications. Pharmacol Rev 24:1, 1972
279. Rajfer SI, Anton AH, Rossen J, Goldberg LI: Beneficial hemodynamic effects of oral levodopa in heart failure: Relationship to the generation of dopamine. N Engl J Med 310:1357, 1984
280. Chatterjee K, De Marco T: Central and peripheral adrenergic receptor agonists in heart failure. Eur Heart J 10(Suppl B):55, 1989
281. Daly PA, Curran D, Chatterjee K: Effects of L-dopa and captopril on resting neurodynamics and coronary blood flow (abstr). Circulation 72(Suppl III):406, 1985
282. Harvey CA, Owen DAA: Hemodynamic responses to ibopamine, an orally active dopamine analogue, in anesthetized cats. Br J Pharmacol 78:127P, 1983
283. Dei Cas L, Manca C, Bermardini B et al: Noninvasive evaluation of the effects of oral ibopamine (SB 7505) on cardiac and renal function in patients with congestive heart failure. J Cardiovasc Pharmacol 4:436, 1982
284. Leier CV, Ren JH, Huss P et al: The hemodynamic effects of ibopamine, a dopamine congener in patients with congestive heart failure. Pharmacotherapy 6:35, 1986
285. Cantelli I, Lolli C, Bomba E et al: Sustained oral treatment with ibopamine in patients with chronic heart failure. Curr Ther Res 39:900, 1986
286. Rajter SI, Rossen JD, Douglas FL et al: Effects of long-term therapy with oral ibopamine on resting hemodynamics and exercise capacity in patients with heart failure: Relationship to the generation of N-methyldopamine and to plasma norepinephrine levels. Circulation 73:740, 1986
287. Brown RA, Dixon J, Farmer JB et al: Dopexamine: A novel agonist at peripheral dopamine receptors and beta$_2$ adrenoreceptors. Br J Pharmacol 85:599, 1985
288. Bass AS, Kohli JD, Lubbers NL et al: Potentiation of cardiovascular effects of norepinephrine by dopexamine. Fed Proc 46:205, 1987
289. De Marco T, Kwasman M, Lau D et al: Dopexamine hydrochloride improved cardiac performance without increased metabolic cost. Am J Cardiol 62:57C, 1988
290. Fennell WH, Taylor AA, Young JB et al: Propylbutyldopamine: Hemodynamic effects in conscious dogs, normal human volunteers and patients with heart failure. Circulation 67:829, 1983
291. Francis GS, Parks R, Cohn JN: The effects of bromocriptine in patients with congestive heart failure. Am Heart J 106:100, 1983
292. Leon CA, Suarez JM, Aranoff RD et al: Fenoldopam: Efficacy of a new orally active dopamine analog in heart failure. Circulation 70(Suppl II):II-307, 1984
293. Goldstein RE, Skelton CL, Levey GS et al: Effects of chronic heart failure on the capacity of glucagon to enhance contractility and adenyl cyclase activity of human papillary muscles. Circulation 44:638, 1971
294. Bristow MR, Cubicciotti R, Ginsburg R et al: Histamine-mediated adenylate cyclase stimulation in human myocardium. Mol Pharmacol 21:671, 1982
295. Baumann G, Felix SB, Riess G et al: Effective stimulation of cardiac contractility and myocardial metabolism by impromidine and dimaprit—two new H$_2$-agonist compounds—in the surviving catecholamine-insensitive myocardium after coronary occlusion. J Cardiovasc Pharmacol 4:542, 1982
296. Linderer T, Biamino G, Bruggeman T et al: Hemodynamic effects of forskolin, a new drug with combined positive inotropic and vasodilating properties (abstr). J Am Coll Cardiol 3:562, 1984
297. Daly JW: Forskolin, adenylate cyclase, and cell physiology: An overview. Adv Cyclic Nucleotide Protein Phosphorylation Res 17:81, 1984
298. Matsue S, Murakami E, Takekoshi N et al: Hemodynamic effects of dibutyryl cyclic AMP in congestive heart failure. Am J Cardiol 51:1364, 1983
299. Silver PJ, Harris AL: Phosphodiesterase isozyme inhibitors and vascular smooth muscle. In Halpern W, Pegram B, Brayden J et al (eds): Proceedings of the Second International Symposium on Resistance Arteries, pp 284–291. Ithaca, Perinatology Press, 1988
300. Silver PJ, Hamel LT, Perrone MH et al: Differential pharmacologic sensitivity of cyclic nucleotide phosphodiesterase isozymes isolated from cardiac muscle, arterial and airway smooth muscle. Eur J Pharmacol 150:85, 1988
301. Stirt JA, Sullivan SF: Aminophylline. Anesth Analg 60:587, 1981
302. Chasin M, Harris D: Inhibitors and activators of cyclic nucleotide phosphodiesterase. Adv Cyclic Nucleotide Res 7:225, 1976
303. Endoh M, Sato K, Yamashita S: Inhibition of cyclic AMP phosphodiesterase activity and myocardial contractility: Effects of cilostamide, a novel PDE inhibitor, and methylisobutylxanthine on rabbit and canine ventricular muscle. Eur J Pharmacol 66:43, 1980
304. Hutton I, Hillis WS, Langhan CE et al: Cardiovascular effects of a new inotropic agent, UK 14275, in patients with coronary heart disease. Br J Clin Pharmacol 4:513, 1977
305. Azuma J, Harada H, Sawamura A et al: Concentration-dependent effect of trapidil on slow action potentials in cardiac muscle. J Mol Cell Cardiol 15:43, 1983
306. Endoh M, Yamashita S, Taira N: Positive inotropic effect of amrinone in relation to cyclic nucleotide metabolism in the canine ventricular muscle. J Pharmacol Exp Ther 221:775, 1982
307. Mancini D, LeJemtel T, Sonnenblick E: Intravenous use of amrinone for the treatment of the failing heart. Am J Cardiol 56:8B, 1985
308. Likoff M, Weber KT, Andrews V et al: Amrinone in the treatment of chronic heart failure. J Am Coll Cardiol 3:1281, 1984
309. Benotti JR, Grossman W, Braunwald E et al: Hemodynamic assessment of amrinone: A new inotropic agent. N Engl J Med 299:1373, 1978
310. LeJemtel TH, Keung E, Sonnenblick EH et al: Amrinone: A new non-glycosidic, non-adrenergic cardiotonic agent effective in the treatment of intractable myocardial failure in man. Circulation 59:1098, 1979
311. Wilmshurst PT, Thompson DS, Juul SM et al: Comparison of the effects of amrinone and sodium nitroprusside on haemodynamics, contractility, and myocardial metabolism in patients with cardiac failure due to coronary artery disease and dilated cardiomyopathy. Br Heart J 52:38, 1984
312. Firth B, Ratner AV, Grassman ED et al: Assessment of the inotropic and vasodilator effects of amrinone versus isoproterenol. Am J Cardiol 54:1331, 1984
313. Millard RW, Dube G, Grupp G et al: Direct vasodilator and positive inotropic actions of amrinone. J Mol Cell Cardiol 12:647, 1980
314. Toda N, Nakajima M, Nishimura K, Miyazaki M: Responses of isolated dog arteries to amrinone. Cardiovasc Res 18:174, 1984
315. Benotti JR, Grossman W, Braunwald E, Carabello BA: Effects of amrinone on myocardial energy metabolism and hemodynamics in patients with severe congestive heart failure due to coronary artery disease. Circulation 62:28, 1980
316. Baim DS: Effects of amrinone on myocardial energetics in severe congestive heart failure. Am J Cardiol 56:16B, 1985
317. Taylor SH, Verma SP, Hussain M et al: Intravenous amrinone in left ventricular failure complicated by acute myocardial infarction. Am J Cardiol 56:29B, 1985
318. Klein M, Siskind S, Frishman W et al: Hemodynamic comparison of intravenous amrinone and dobutamine in patients with chronic congestive heart failure. Am J Cardiol 48:160, 1981
319. Goener M, Pedemonte O, Baele P et al: Amrinone in the management of low

cardiac output after open heart surgery. Am J Cardiol 56:33B, 1985
320. Goener M: Severe perioperative cardiogenic shock in open heart surgery: Benefits of combined therapy. In Unger F (ed): Coronary Artery Surgery in the Nineties. Berlin, Springer, 1987
321. Robinson RJJ, Tehervenkov C: Treatment of low cardiac output after aortocoronary bypass surgery using a combination of norepinephrine and amrinone. J Cardiothorac Anesth 1:229, 1987
322. Weber KT, Andrews V, Janicki JS et al: Amrinone and exercise performance in patients with chronic heart failure. Am J Cardiol 48:164, 1981
323. Siegel LA, LeJemtel TH, Strom J et al: Improvement in exercise capacity despite cardiac deterioration: Noninvasive assessment of long-term therapy with amrinone in severe heart failure. Am Heart J 106:1042, 1983
324. Leier CV, Dalpiaz K, Huss P et al: Amrinone therapy for congestive heart failure in outpatients with idiopathic dilated cardiomyopathy. Am J Cardiol 52:304, 1983
325. DiBianco R, Shabetai R, Silverman BD et al (with the Amrinone Multicenter Study Investigators): Oral amrinone for the treatment of chronic congestive heart failure: Results of a multicenter randomized double-blind and placebo-controlled withdrawal study. J Am Coll Cardiol 4:855, 1984
326. Massie B, Bourassa M, DiBianco R et al: Long-term oral administration of amrinone for congestive heart failure: Lack of efficacy in a multicenter controlled trial. Circulation 71:963, 1985
327. Naccarelli GV, Gray EL, Dougherty AH et al: Amrinone: Acute electrophysiologic and hemodynamic effects in patients with congestive heart failure. Am J Cardiol 54:600, 1984
328. Naccarelli GV, Goldstein RA: Electrophysiology of phosphodiesterase inhibitors. Am J Cardiol 63:35A, 1989
329. Maskin CS, Forman R, Klein NA et al: Long-term amrinone therapy in patients with severe heart failure: Drug-dependent hemodynamic benefits despite progression of disease. Am J Cardiol 72:113, 1982
330. Packer M, Medina N, Yushak M: Hemodynamic and clinical limitations of long-term therapy with amrinone in patients with severe chronic heart failure. Circulation 70:1038, 1984
331. Alousi AA, Canter JM, Montenaro MJ et al: Cardiotonic activity of milrinone, a new and potent cardiac bipyridine on the normal and failing heart of experimental animals. J Cardiovasc Pharmacol 5:792, 1983
332. Alousi AA, Canter JM, Cicero F et al: Pharmacology of milrinone. In Braunwald E, Sonnenblick EH, Chakrin LW, Schwartz RP Jr (eds): Milrinone: Investigation of New Inotropic Therapy for Congestive Heart Failure, p 21. New York, Raven Press, 1984
333. Alousi AA, Stankus GP, Stuart JC, Walton LH: Characterization of the cardiotonic effects of milrinone, a new and potent cardiac bipyridine, on isolated tissues from several animal species. J Cardiovasc Pharmacol 5:804, 1983
334. Alousi AA, Iwan T, Edelson J, Biddlecome C: Correlation of the hemodynamic and pharmacokinetic profile of intravenous milrinone in anesthetized dog. Arch Int Pharmacodyn Ther 267:59, 1984
335. Harris AL, Wassey ML, Grant AM, Alousi AA: Direct vasodilating effect of milrinone and sodium nitrite in the canine coronary artery (abstr). Fed Proc 43:938, 1984
336. Ludmer PL, Wright RF, Arnold MO et al: Separation of the direct myocardial and vasodilator actions of milrinone administered by an intracoronary infusion technique. Circulation 73:130, 1986
337. Baim DS, McDowell AV, Chernileo J et al: Evaluation of a new bipyridine inotropic agent—milrinone—in patients with severe congestive heart failure. N Engl J Med 309:748, 1983
338. Jaski BE, Fifer MA, Wright RF et al: Positive inotropic and vasodilator actions of milrinone in patients with severe heart failure. J Clin Invest 75:643, 1985
339. Borow KM, Come PC, Neumann et al: Physiologic assessment of the inotropic, vasodilator and afterload reducing effects of milrinone in subjects without cardiac disease. Am J Cardiol 55:1204, 1985
340. Timmis AD, Smyth P, Monaghan M et al: Milrinone in heart failure: Acute effects on left ventricular systolic function and myocardial metabolism. Br Heart J 54:36, 1985
341. Piscione F, Serruys PW, Hugenholtz PG: Left ventricular function after oral milrinone in patients with congestive heart failure: A hemodynamic and angiographic study. In Erdmann E, Greef K, Skou JC (eds): Cardiac Glycosides 1785–1985, pp 237–244. New York, Springer, 1986
342. Cody RJ, Muller FB, Kubo SH et al: Identification of the direct vasodilator effect of milrinone with an isolated limb preparation in patients with chronic congestive heart failure. Circulation 73:124, 1986
343. Arnold JM, Ludmar PL, Wright RF et al: Role of reflex sympathetic withdrawal in the hemodynamic response to an increased inotropic state in patients with severe heart failure. J Am Coll Cardiol 8:413, 1986
344. Monrad ES, McKay RG, Baim DS et al: Improvement in index of diastolic performance in patients with congestive heart failure treated with milrinone. Circulation 70:1030, 1984
345. Monrad ES, Baim DS, Smith HS et al: Effects of milrinone on coronary hemodynamics and myocardial energetics in patients with congestive heart failure. Circulation 71:972, 1985
346. Grose R, Strain J, Greenberg M et al: Systemic and coronary effects of intravenous milrinone and dobutamine in congestive heart failure. J Am Coll Cardiol 7:1107, 1986
347. Monrad ES, Baim DS, Smith HS et al: Milrinone, dobutamine and nitroprusside: Comparative effects on hemodynamics and myocardial energetics in patients with severe congestive heart failure. Circulation 73(Suppl III):III-168, 1986
348. Cody RJ: Renal and hormonal effects of phosphodiesterase III inhibition in congestive heart failure. Am J Cardiol 63:31A, 1989
349. LeJemtel TH, Maskin CS, Mancini D et al: Systemic and regional effects of captopril and milrinone administration alone and concomitantly in patients with heart failure. Circulation 72:364, 1985
350. Simonton CA, Chatterjee K, Cody RJ et al: Milrinone in congestive heart failure: Acute and chronic hemodynamic and clinical evaluation. J Am Coll Cardiol 6:453, 1985
351. Kubo SH, Cody RJ, Chatterjee K et al: Acute dose-range study of milrinone in congestive heart failure. Am J Cardiol 55:726, 1985
352. White HD, Ribeiro JP, Hartley LH, Colucci WS: Immediate effects of milrinone on metabolic and sympathetic response to exercise in severe congestive heart failure. Am J Cardiol 56:93, 1985
353. Schoeller R, Bruggemann T, Vohringer H et al: Long-term oral administration of milrinone for dilated cardiomyopathy (abstr). J Am Coll Cardiol 7:180A, 1986
354. Chesbro JH, Browne KF, Fenster PE et al: The hemodynamic effects of oral milrinone therapy: A multicenter controlled trial (abstr). J Am Coll Cardiol 11:144A, 1988
355. Baim DS, Colucci WS, Monrad SE et al: Survival of patients with severe congestive heart failure treated with oral milrinone. J Am Coll Cardiol 7:661, 1986
356. Kariya T, Wille LJ, Dage RC: Biochemical studies on the mechanism of cardiotonic activity of MDL 17043. J Cardiovasc Pharmacol 4:509, 1982
357. Roebel LE, Dage RC, Cheng HC, Woodward JK: Characterization of the cardiovascular activities of a new cardiotonic agent, MDL 17043 (1,3-dihydro-4-methyl-5 4-(methylthio)-benzoyl)-2H-imidazole-2-one). J Cardiovasc Pharmacol 4:721, 1982
358. Dage RE, Kariya T, Hsieh CP et al: Pharmacology of enoximone. Am J Cardiol 60:10C, 1987
359. Janicki JS, Shnoff SG, Weber KT: Physiologic response to the inotropic and vasodilator properties of enoximone. Am J Cardiol 60:15C, 1987
360. Crawford MH, Richards KL, Sodums MT, Kennedy GT: Positive inotropic and vasodilator effects of MDL 17043 in patients with reduced left ventricular performance. Am J Cardiol 53:1051, 1984
361. Kereiakes DJ, Viquerat C, Lanzer P et al: Mechanisms of improved left ventricular function following intravenous MDL 17043 in patients with severe chronic heart failure. Am Heart J 108:1278, 1984
362. Herman HC, Ruddy TD, Dee GW et al: Diastolic function in patients with severe heart failure: Comparison of the effects of enoximone and nitroprusside. Circulation 75:1214, 1987
363. Kereiakes D, Chatterjee K, Parmley WW et al: Intravenous and oral MDL 17043 (a new inotrope-vasodilator agent) in congestive heart failure: Hemodynamic and clinical evaluation in 38 patients. J Am Coll Cardiol 4:884, 1984
364. Uretsky BF, Generalovich T, Reddy PS et al: Acute hemodynamic effect of oral MDL 17043: A new inotropic vasodilator agent in patients with severe heart failure. J Am Coll Cardiol 5:326, 1985
365. Amin DK, Shah PK, Hulse S et al: Myocardial metabolic and hemodynamic effects of intravenous MDL-17043, a new cardiotonic drug in patients with chronic, severe heart failure. Am Heart J 108:1285, 1984
366. Martin JL, Likoff MJ, Janicki JS et al: Myocardial energetics and clinical response to the cardiotonic agent MDL 17043 in advanced heart failure. J Am Coll Cardiol 4:875, 1984
367. Viquerat CE, Kereiakes D, Morris DL et al: Alterations in left ventricular function, coronary hemodynamics, and myocardial catecholamine balance with MDL 17043: A new inotropic vasodilator agent in patients with severe heart failure. J Am Coll Cardiol 5:326, 1985
368. Rigaud M, Benit E, Castadot M et al: Comparative effects of enoximone and nitroglycerin on left ventricular performance and regional wall motion in ischemic cardiomyopathy. Br J Clin Pract 42(Suppl 64):26, 1988
369. Leier CV, Meiler SEL, Mathews S et al: A preliminary report of the effects of orally administered enoximone on regional hemodynamics in congestive heart failure. Am J Cardiol 60:27C, 1987
370. Clifton GG, Macmahon FG, Ryan FR et al: Effects of enoximone on renal function and plasma volume in normal volunteers. Curr Ther Res 39:436, 1986
371. Miles WM, Heger JJ, Minardo JD et al: Electrophysiologic and hemodynamic effects of intravenous enoximone (abstr). Circulation 74(Suppl II):II-38, 1986
372. Renard M, Dereppe H, Henuzet C et al: Effects of enoximone in patients with cardiac failure after myocardial infarction. Br J Clin Pract 42(Suppl 64):37, 1988
373. Vincent JL, Carlier E, Berre J et al: Administration of enoximone in cardiogenic shock. Am J Cardiol 62:419, 1988
374. Gonzales M, Desager JP, Jacquemart JL et al: Efficacy of enoximone in the management of refractory low output states following cardiac surgery. Br J Clin Pract 42(Suppl 64):53, 1988
375. Shah PK, Amin DK, Hulse S et al: Inotropic therapy for refractory congestive heart failure with oral enoximone (MDL-17,043): Poor long-term results despite early hemodynamic and clinical improvement. Circulation 71:326, 1985
376. Rubin SA, Tabak L: MDL 17,043: Short and long-term cardiopulmonary and

clinical effects in patients with heart failure. J Am Coll Cardiol 5:1422, 1985
377. Weber KT, Janicki JS, Jain MC: Enoximone (MDL 17,043) for stable chronic heart failure secondary to ischemic or idiopathic cardiomyopathy. Am J Cardiol 58:589, 1986
378. Maskin CS, Weber KT, Janicki JS: Long-term oral enoximone therapy in chronic cardiac failure. Am J Cardiol 60:63C, 1987
379. Schriven AJI, Lipkin DP, Anand IS et al: A comparison of hemodynamic effects of one-month oral captopril and enoximone treatment for severe congestive heart failure. Am J Cardiol 60:68C, 1987
380. Triese N, Erbel R, Pilcher J et al: Long-term treatment with oral enoximone for chronic congestive heart failure: The European Experience. Am J Cardiol 60:85C, 1987
381. Khalife K, Zannad F, Brunotte F et al: Placebo-controlled study of oral enoximone in congestive heart failure with initial and final intravenous hemodynamic evaluation. Am J Cardiol 60:75C, 1987
382. Narahara K and Western Enoximone Study Group: Enoximone versus placebo: A double-blind trial in chronic congestive heart failure (abstr). Circulation 80(Suppl II):II-175, 1989
383. Crawford MH, Deedwania P, Massie B et al: Comparative efficacy of enoximone versus captopril in moderate heart failure. Circulation 80(Suppl II):II-175, 1989
384. Jessup M, Ulrich S, Samaha J et al: Effects of low dose enoximone for chronic congestive heart failure. Am J Cardiol 60:80C, 1987
385. Dubois-Rande JL, Loisance D, Duval AM et al: Enoximone, a pharmacological bridge to transplantation. Br J Clin Pract 42(Suppl 64):73, 1988
386. Bristow MR, Lee HE, Gilbert EM et al: Use of enoximone in patients awaiting cardiac transplant. Br J Clin Pract 42(Suppl 64):69, 1988
387. Crawford MH: Intravenous use of enoximone. Am J Cardiol 60:42C, 1987
388. Okerholm RA, Keeley FJ, Weiner DL, Spangenberg RB: The pharmacokinetics of a new cardiotonic agent, MDL 19205, 4-ethyl-1,3-dihydro-5-(4-pyridinyl)-2H-imidazol-2-one (abstr). Fed Proc 42:1131, 1983
389. Petein M, Levine B, Cohn JN: Hemodynamic effects of a new inotropic agent, piroximone (MDL 19,205) in patients with chronic heart failure. J Am Coll Cardiol 4:364, 1984
390. Axelrod RJ, De Marco T, Dae M et al: Hemodynamic and clinical evaluation of piroximone, a new intrope-vasodilator agent in severe congestive heart failure. J Am Coll Cardiol 9:1124, 1987
391. Dage RC, Roebel LE, Hsieh CP, Woodward JK: Cardiovascular properties of a new cardiotonic agent, MDL 19,205. J Cardiovasc Pharmacol 6:35, 1984
392. Petein M, Pierpont GL, Heppner B et al: Hemodynamic and regional blood flow response to MDL-19205 in dogs: A comparison with dobutamine (abstr). Circulation 68(Suppl III):III-128, 1983
393. Holck M, Thorens S, Muggli R, Eigenmann R: Studies on the mechanism of positive inotropic activity: RO13-6438, a structurally novel cardiotonic agent with vasodilating properties. J Cardiovasc Pharmacol 6:520, 1984
394. Daly PA, Chatterjee K, Viquerat CE et al: RO13-6438, a new inotrope-vasodilator: Systemic and coronary hemodynamic effects in congestive heart failure. Am J Cardiol 55:1539, 1985
395. Pouleur H, Marechal G, Balasim H et al: Effects of dobutamine and sulmazol (AR-L 115BS) on myocardial metabolism and coronary, femoral, and renal blood flows: A comparative study in normal dogs and in dogs with chronic volume overload. J Cardiovasc Pharmacol 5:861, 1983
396. Pouleur H, Rousseau MF, VanMechelen H et al: Cardiovascular effects of AR-L 115BS in conscious dogs with and without chronic congestive heart failure. J Cardiovasc Pharmacol 4:409, 1982
397. Renard M, Jacobs P, Dechamps P et al: Hemodynamic and clinical response to three-day infusion of sulmazol (AR-L 115BS) in severe congestive heart failure. Chest 84:408, 1983
398. Thormann J, Schlepper M, Kramer W et al: Effects of AR-L 115BS (sulmazol), a new cardiotonic agent in coronary artery disease: Improved ventricular wall motion, increased pump function and abolition of pacing induced ischemia. J Am Coll Cardiol 2:332, 1983
399. Evans DB, Potoczak RE, Newton RS et al: Preclinical cardiovascular pharmacology of CI-914, a novel pyridiazinone cardiotonic (abstr). Circulation 70(Suppl II):II-307, 1984
400. Mancini D, Sonnenblick EH, Latts JR et al: Hemodynamic and clinical benefits of CI-914, a new cardiotonic agent. Circulation 70(Suppl II):II-307, 1984
401. Colucci WS, Wright RF, Braunwald E: New positive inotropic agents in the treatment of congestive heart failure. N Engl J Med 314:349, 1986
402. Packer M: Effects of phosphodiesterase inhibitors on survival of patients with chronic congestive heart failure. Am J Cardiol 63:41A, 1989
403. Feldman AM, Baughman KL, Lee WK et al: Randomized double-blind placebo trial of OPC-8212 in patients with heart failure: Morbidity/mortality in 80 patients (abstr). Circulation 80(Suppl II):II-176, 1989
404. Katz SD, Kubo SH, Jessup M et al: Pimobendan improves exercise capacity in digitalized patients with severe congestive heart failure (abstr). Circulation 80(Suppl II):II-176, 1989
405. Gross R, Schramm M, Thomas G, Toward R: Bay K8644, a positive inotropic dihydropyridine with Ca^{++} agonist properties. J Mol Cell Cardiol 15(Suppl 4):29, 1983
406. Judy WV, Hall JH, Toth PD, Fokers K: Influence of coenzyme Q10 on cardiac function in congestive heart failure (abstr). Fed Proc 43:358, 1984
407. Smiseth OA: Inosine infusion in dogs with acute ischemic left ventricular failure: Favorable effects on myocardial performance and metabolism. Cardiovasc Res 17:192, 1983
408. Chernow B, Roth BL: Pharmacologic manipulation of the peripheral vasculature in shock: Clinical and experimental approaches. Circ Shock 18:141, 1986
409. Deojars P, Pinaud M, Potel G et al: Reappraisal of norepinephrine therapy in human septic shock. Crit Care Med 15:134, 1987
410. Vlahakes GJ, Turley K, Hoffman JIE: The pathophysiology of failure in right ventricular hypertension: Hemodynamic and biochemical correlations. Circulation 63:87, 1981
411. Hoffman MJ, Greenfield LJ, Sugarman HJ et al: Unsuspected right ventricular dysfunction in shock and sepsis. Ann Surg 198:307, 1983
412. Kimchi A, Ellrodt AG, Berman DS et al: Right ventricular performance in septic shock: A combined radionuclide and hemodynamic study. J Am Coll Cardiol 4:945, 1984
413. Sibbald WJ, Driedger AA: Right ventricular function in acute disease states: Pathophysiologic considerations. Crit Care Med 11:339, 1983
414. Schreuder WO, Schneider AJ, Groeneveld ABJ et al: Effect of dopamine vs. norepinephrine on hemodynamics in septic shock: Emphasis on right ventricular performance. Chest 95:1282, 1989
415. Shoemaker WC, Appel PL: Pathophysiology of adult respiratory distress syndrome after sepsis and surgical operations. Crit Care Med 13:166, 1985
416. Shoemaker WC: A new approach to physiology, monitoring and therapy of shock states. World J Surg 11:113, 1987
417. Gilbert EM, Haupt MT, Mandanas RY et al: The effect of fluid loading, blood transfusion and catecholamine infusion on oxygen delivery and consumption in patients with sepsis. Am Rev Respir Dis 134:873, 1986
418. Vincent JL, Dufaye P, Berre J et al: Serial lactate determinations during circulatory shock. Crit Care Med 11:449, 1983
419. Shoemaker WC, Appel PL, Kramm HB: Hemodynamic and oxygen transport effects of dobutamine in critically ill general surgical patients. Crit Care Med 14:1032, 1986
420. Vincent JL, Roman A: Dobutamine infusion in septic shock: Effects on arterial pressure (abstr). Chest 94(Suppl):75, 1988
421. Cohn JN, Archibald DG, Ziesche S et al: Effect of vasodilator therapy on mortality in chronic congestive heart failure: Results of Veterans Administration Cooperative Study. N Engl J Med 134:1547, 1986
422. Chatterjee K, Parmley WW, Cohn JN et al: A cooperative multicenter study of captopril in congestive heart failure: Hemodynamic effects and long-term response. Am Heart J 110:439, 1985
423. Consensus Trial Study Group: Effects of enalapril on mortality in severe congestive heart failure: Results of the Cooperative North Scandinavian Enalapril Survival Study (CONSENSUS). N Engl J Med 316:1429, 1987
424. Newman TJ, Maskin CS, Dennick LG et al: Effects of captopril on survival in patients with heart failure. Am J Med 84(Suppl 3A):140, 1988

NITRATES

Jonathan Abrams

The use of nitroglycerin (NTG) and other organic nitrate esters in cardiovascular medicine has increased substantially during the past decade. These drugs, once used only for the treatment of angina pectoris, are playing an increasing role in the management of patients with unstable angina and acute myocardial infarction, as well as in vasodilator therapy for acute and chronic congestive heart failure. Nitrates represent one of the oldest cardiac therapies; an oral solution of NTG was first employed in the treatment of angina over 100 years ago.

Vasodilatation of arteries and veins is the major physiologic characteristic of organic nitrates. These drugs are classified as direct-acting vasodilators; they act on vascular smooth muscle to induce vasodilatation throughout the body. Nitrates have potent venodilating activity, a unique feature compared with most vasodilators; their effect on veins is more prominent than on arteries and arterioles. Nitrates have no direct action on cardiac contractility or electrophysiologic properties of the heart.

NTG and other nitrates may induce reflex sympathetic nervous system discharge. Resultant vasoconstriction in the various regional circulations may counteract the vasodilating actions of nitrates. Vascular beds that have dense sympathetic innervation are particularly likely to respond to nitrate-induced hypotension with arterial and venous vasoconstriction. Reflex tachycardia is commonly seen when central aortic pressure falls following nitrate administration. Activation of baroreceptor reflexes is prominent in individuals with normal cardiac function. However, when nitrates are given to patients with impaired left ventricular contractility or overt congestive heart failure, the vasodilating actions of these drugs are not usually accompanied by reflex sympathetic discharge. It is important to keep in mind the differences in the hemodynamic effects of nitrates in the normal and failing circulations.

The mechanisms of actions and clinical pharmacology of nitrates are reviewed in this chapter, and the efficacy of nitrate therapy in the various ischemic syndromes as well as in vasodilator therapy of congestive heart failure will be discussed.

MECHANISMS OF ACTION OF NITROGLYCERIN AND ORGANIC NITRATES

Nitrates produce vascular smooth muscle relaxation through a direct action on blood vessels. Their vasodilating effects are not modulated through neurohumoral mechanisms such as is seen with the angiotensin-converting enzyme inhibitors (captopril, enalapril) or sympatholytic agents (prazosin, trimazosin). The precise cellular mode of action of nitrates remains controversial. Some years ago Needleman proposed that nitrates induce vascular relaxation by interacting with a sulfhydryl group on a putative "nitrate receptor" on the surface of vascular smooth muscle cells.[1] More recent evidence indicates that organic nitrates are converted to S-nitrosothiols within the smooth muscle cell (Fig. 15.1). These short-lived compounds stimulate cyclic guanosine monophosphate (GMP) production through the activation of guanylate cyclase.[2] The resultant increase in intracellular cyclic GMP initiates vasodilatation. Recent observations indicate that organic nitrates may be directly converted to nitric oxide (NO), the compound necessary for stimulation of guanylate cyclase. The issue of an obligatory role for S-nitrosothiols is unresolved; there may be an extracellular pathway for nitrosothiol formation as well.[3] Sodium nitroprusside also induces vascular relaxation by conversion to S-nitrosothiols with subsequent stimulation of the enzyme guanylate cyclase. Thus, it appears that cyclic GMP is the final common pathway for these two vasodilators, although intracellular metabolism of these two drugs is different.[2] Figure 15.1 represents a current hypothesis regarding the cellular mechanism of action of the organic nitrates and nitroprusside.

It has been suggested that NTG and other nitrates may act by stimulation of prostaglandins.[4] NTG induces prostacyclin production by smooth muscle endothelial cells; at high nitrate concentrations thromboxane A_2 production is inhibited. However, recent work suggests that the prostaglandin system is not an important modulator of nitrate effects.[5]

Of great importance has been the discovery that nitric oxide is one of the main endothelial relaxant factors (EDRF), if not EDRF itself. Nitroglycerin and the organic nitrates act on vascular tissue independently of intact endothelial function, and along with molsidomine and nitroprusside, are known as nitro-vasodilators. These compounds are all endothelium-independent relaxers of vascular smooth muscle. Thus, the nitrates are capable of dilating the coronary arteries when endothelial function is impaired, as is often the case in coronary atherosclerosis.

Although an antiaggretory action of the organic nitrates has been previously documented *in vitro*, this phenomenon has not been felt to be clinically relevant because such platelet effects were only demonstrable at very high (*i.e.*, pharmacologic) concentrations. Recent work from a number of centers has suggested that nitrates, particularly intravenous NTG, may have significant antiplatelet activity in humans at readily obtainable plasma nitrate concentrations.[6–8] If the nitrates do have significant antiplatelet and antithrombotic actions, these drugs would have a potentially important additional role in the treatment of acute ischemic syndromes, such as unstable angina and acute myocardial infarction. Antiplatelet and antithrombotic effects would help explain the demonstrated efficacy of these drugs in these major ischemic conditions.

NITRATE TOLERANCE

The clinical aspects of this important subject are discussed later in the chapter. It is presently believed that intracellular events involved in nitrate metabolism are critical to the development of tolerance. Specifically, the relative unavailability of reduced sulfhydryl (—SH) moieties within vascular smooth muscle cells limits organic nitrate conversion to nitric oxide (see Fig. 15.1) and subsequent vasodilatation. The sulfhydryl groups are "depleted" during the conversion of the organic nitrate to nitric oxide.

HEMODYNAMIC EFFECTS OF NITRATES

Nitrates induce vasodilatation of veins, arteries, and arterioles. Responsiveness to nitrates varies according to the type of vascular tissue. Differing vascular nitrate metabolism and kinetics may account for the differences in response of various vascular beds to NTG. For instance, following systemic NTG administration veins have a higher concentration of NTG per weight than arteries.[9]

VENODILATION

Nitrates induce venodilation at very low doses. The venous dose-response curve is relatively flat; as NTG plasma concentration increases there is little additional venous vasodilation, which is near maximal at low plasma concentrations (Fig. 15.2). Both regional and systemic venous beds dilate following nitrate administration.

In the normal subject, venodilation results in pooling or sequestration of blood in the venous or capacitance circulation. Seventy to 75% of the circulating blood volume is stored in the veins. Nitrates shift the distribution of blood into the central venous circulation at a reduced venous pressure; this results in decreased return of blood to the right side of the heart. Intracardiac pressures and volumes decrease and are accompanied by a fall in stroke volume and cardiac output. Reflex tachycardia, if marked, may limit or even prevent a decrease in cardiac output.

Some experts believe that the pronounced systemic venodilation is responsible for much of the beneficial effects of nitrates in ischemic heart disease. These potent venodilating actions result in a decrease in myocardial oxygen requirements owing to a reduction in cardiac pre-load accompanying the decrease in ventricular volumes and intracardiac filling pressures. Nitrate venodilation is extremely important in producing beneficial effects in patients with congestive heart failure and contributes to the decrease in signs and symptoms of pulmonary

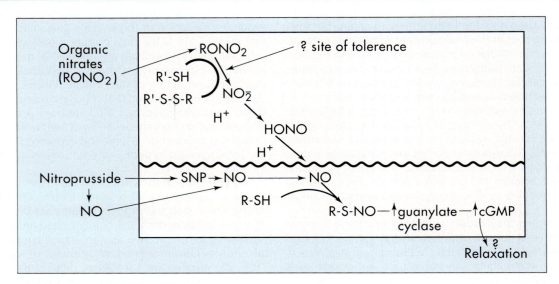

FIGURE 15.1 Current hypothesis of intracellular events leading to vascular smooth muscle relaxation following organic nitrate or nitroprusside administration. Both compounds are metabolized within the cell and result in the formation of S-nitrosothiols, which in turn stimulate the production of cyclic GMP, believed to be a common mediator of smooth muscle relaxation. This schematic diagram also indicates a possible site for the development of nitrate tolerance, shown here at the conversion of nitroglycerin to nitrogen dioxide. Both organic nitrates and nitroprusside are metabolized to nitric oxide prior to conversion to S-nitrosothiols. Sulfhydryl groups are necessary for nitrate metabolism and their relative availability appears to be related to the development of nitrate tolerance. More recent work suggests that organic nitrate ($RONO_2$) may be converted directly to NO without initial transformation to NO_2^- or HONO. The role of S-nitrosothiols (R-S-NO) is unclear; this compound may not be necessary for activation of guanylate cyclase. (Modified from Armstrong PW, Moffat JA: Tolerance to organic nitrates: Clinical and experimental perspectives. Am J Med 74(suppl):73, 1983)

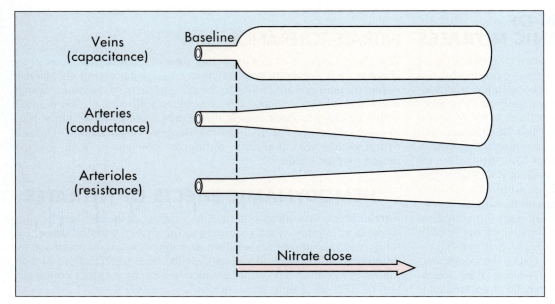

FIGURE 15.2 Actions of organic nitrates on the major vascular beds and relationship of vasodilatation to the size of the administered dose. The venous or capacitance system dilates maximally with very low doses of organic nitrates. Increasing the amount of drug does not cause appreciable additional venodilatation. Arterial dilation and enhanced arterial conductance begins at low doses of nitrates with further vasodilation appearing as the dosage is increased. With high plasma concentrations of nitrates the arteriolar or resistance vessels dilate, resulting in a decrease in systemic and regional vascular resistance. (See text.) (Modified from Abrams J: Hemodynamic effects of nitroglycerin and long-acting nitrates. Am Heart J 110(part 2):216, 1985)

congestion. In normal subjects nitrates substantially reduce left ventricular chamber size (Fig. 15.3), although this effect is not consistently observed in patients with congestive heart failure.

ARTERIAL VASODILATATION

At low doses nitrates have an effect on large arteries,[10] manifested by an increase in arterial conductance and distensibility and an augmented rate of rise of the arterial pulse upstroke. These effects are seen even when systemic blood pressure is not altered. In larger doses nitrates induce more pronounced arterial vasodilatation (see Fig. 15.2). It is not known if minor changes in arterial compliance in the absence of a significant fall in systemic vascular resistance or systolic blood pressure have any positive clinical effect, although it is likely that arterial vasodilatation of various regional circulations, particularly the limbs, may reduce left ventricular afterload in the absence of a change in arterial pressure.[10]

A recent observation suggests that brachial artery or routine arm cuff measurements of blood pressure may *underestimate* the actual effect of administered nitrate on lowering central aortic pressure.[11] Thus, standard blood pressure determinations may not accurately reflect the maximal effect of nitrates on the arterial system.

ARTERIOLAR VASODILATATION

Large doses of nitrates that produce high plasma and tissue nitrate concentrations induce arteriolar or resistance vessel dilatation (see Fig. 15.2). Systemic vascular resistance falls. Nitrates also decrease resistance in the regional circulations, such as the coronary, splanchnic, and renal beds.

The combination of vasodilatation of the systemic arterioles and generalized venodilatation resulting in decreased return of blood to the central circulation can reduce central aortic pressure, often excessively. Tachycardia is common after nitrate administration. Increased sympathetic tone may attenuate or even prevent nitrate-induced decreases in systolic blood pressure; such reflex adrenergic responses occasionally produce untoward reactions to nitrate administration, such as palpitations and rare episodes of angina pectoris.

Nitrate-induced arteriolar vasodilatation appears to be an important component of the beneficial response of the failing circulation to nitrate administration. A decrease in regional bed and systemic vascular resistance improves the efficiency of left ventricular emptying in congestive heart failure.

MODULATORS OF NITRATE ACTION (TABLE 15.1)
SYMPATHETIC NERVOUS SYSTEM

It has already been stressed that sympathetic activation following nitrate administration plays an important role in modulating the effects of NTG and other nitrates on the systemic and regional circulations. Reflex tachycardia and vasoconstriction may counteract the desired effects of nitrates in patients with ischemic heart disease. These responses may also prevent or limit adverse sequelae relating to marked nitrate hypotension.

STATUS OF LEFT VENTRICULAR FUNCTION

Nitrates produce a different hemodynamic profile depending on whether cardiac function is normal or abnormal. The classic circulatory response to nitrates in an individual with normal ventricular function consists of a pronounced fall in systolic blood pressure and a reduction in cardiac output and an increase in heart rate. On the other hand, in the presence of congestive heart failure or significant left ventricular dysfunction, nitrates do not usually decrease cardiac output. In fact, if arteriolar vasodilatation occurs, cardiac performance may actually be enhanced with an increase in stroke volume and cardiac output, usually in the absence of reflex tachycardia. In addition, blood pressure responses to nitrates in patients with congestive heart failure are much less prominent than in patients with normal left ventricular function. Because cardiac output is maintained or even augmented in congestive heart failure after nitrate administration, reflex sympathetic vasoconstriction is uncommon. In addition, the biphasic response of

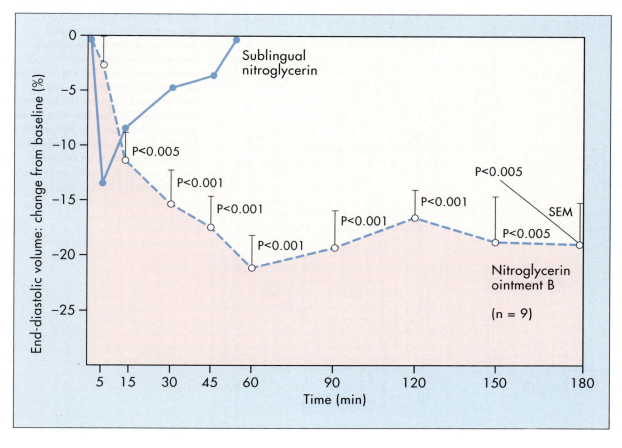

FIGURE 15.3 Reduction in left ventricular end-diastolic volume following administration of sublingual nitroglycerin or 2% nitroglycerin ointment in normal subjects. The data represent calculations derived from measurements of left ventricular diameter obtained by M-mode echocardiography in nine normal subjects. Similar reductions in left ventricular end-systolic diameter and volume were observed. (Modified from Abrams J: Pharmacology of nitroglycerin and long-acting nitrates and their usefulness in the treatment of congestive heart failure. In Gould L, Reddy CVR (eds): Vasodilator Therapy for Cardiac Disorders, pp 129–167. Mt. Kisco, NY, Futura Publishing, 1979)

various regional circulations to nitrates (initial vasodilation followed by reflex vasoconstriction) is less likely to occur.

PRESENCE OR ABSENCE OF NITRATE TOLERANCE

There is no longer any doubt that inappropriate dosing with organic nitrates will induce attenuation or tolerance to the hemodynamic and clinical actions of nitrates in many individuals (see below). If a state of partial or complete vascular tolerance exists, the expected response to nitrates will be diminished or absent.

SIZE OF DOSE

Small doses of nitrates will induce systemic venodilatation with relatively little arteriolar effects. Large doses will produce a greater fall in arterial pressure and a decrease in systemic vascular resistance. Regional circulatory responses probably share the systemic vascular dose-response relationship to nitrate administration, with regional bed venous capacitance changes occurring at lower nitrate concentrations than will induce vasodilatation of the arteriolar resistance vessels.

SYSTEMIC RESPONSES TO NITRATES

In an individual with a normal circulation, nitrate administration produces a fall in systolic blood pressure and an increase in heart rate, more pronounced in the upright position. Stroke volume and cardiac output usually decrease, although reflex tachycardia may prevent cardiac output from declining excessively. Systemic venous and right-sided heart pressures are decreased. Cardiac chamber volumes become smaller (Fig. 15.3), and left and right ventricular filling pressures decrease.

REGIONAL CIRCULATORY RESPONSES TO NITRATES

LIMB

Nitrates induce vasodilatation of the arm and leg vasculature, accompanied by a fall in limb vascular resistance and an increase in limb blood flow. Limb venous tone decreases (Fig. 15.4).[12]

SPLANCHNIC AND MESENTERIC

The effects of nitrates on the splanchnic and mesenteric circulations have not been well studied. These drugs appear to induce initial vasodilatation associated with a decrease in splanchnic and mesenteric vascular resistance and an increase in regional blood flow. In dogs without heart failure this effect is short-lived and is followed by reflex vasoconstriction.[13] It is not clear if this also occurs in humans, and the data are conflicting.[14,15] In patients with congestive heart failure, splanchnic and mesenteric vasodilation results in a sustained sequestration of blood in the splanchnic circulation, which is probably an important component of the beneficial response to nitrates.[16] Hepatic blood flow decreases or remains unchanged after nitrate administration.

TABLE 15.1 IMPORTANT MODULATORS OF NITRATE ACTIVITY

Reflex sympathetic nervous system discharge
Status of left ventricular function
  The normal left ventricle
  Congestive heart failure and/or dilated ventricle
Presence or absence of nitrate tolerance
Size of administered dose

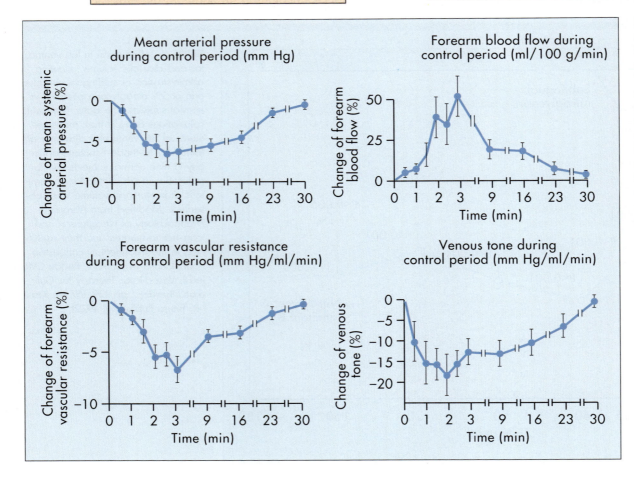

FIGURE 15.4 Nitroglycerin-induced changes in arterial pressure, forearm blood flow and resistance, and venous tone in normal subjects. Values are expressed as percent changes from control. Eight normal subjects were given 0.6 mg to 0.9 mg of sublingual nitroglycerin. (MAP, mean arterial pressure; FBF, forearm blood flow; FVR, forearm vascular resistance) (Modified from Mason DT, Braunwald E: The effects of nitroglycerin and amyl nitrite on arteriolar and venous tone in the human forearm. Circulation 32:755, 1965)

PULMONARY

Nitrates cause marked vasodilatation of the pulmonary vascular bed and probably dilate the pulmonary veins as well. Pulmonary artery and right ventricular filling pressures fall after nitrate administration. These effects are of value in the treatment of congestive heart failure and pulmonary hypertension.

RENAL

Nitrates produce direct vasodilatation of the renal arteries, although reflex constriction may occur if cardiac output falls.[13] In patients with congestive heart failure, renal circulatory effects parallel the central circulatory responses to nitrate administration; secondary renal artery vasoconstriction is not uncommon.[17] In general, nitrates do not importantly influence renal blood flow in patients with congestive heart failure.

EFFECTS OF NITRATES ON THE CORONARY CIRCULATION (TABLE 15.2)

Nitrates dilate the coronary arterial bed. It was initially believed that coronary arterial dilation was responsible for the beneficial actions of nitrates in patients with angina. This theory was subsequently abandoned because of experiments indicating that other potent coronary vasodilators, such as dipyridamole, can induce substantial coronary bed vasodilatation without any improvement in angina. When given in doses that cause systemic arterial vasodilatation NTG relieves pacing-induced angina yet fails to do so when administered directly into the coronary bed.[18] Recently, however, the direct actions of nitrate on the coronary circulation have again been emphasized as being of potential importance for the relief of myocardial ischemia.[10,19]

CORONARY BLOOD FLOW

Nitroglycerin induces a short-lived increase in coronary flow followed by a fall in global myocardial blood flow below baseline that parallels nitrate-modulated decreases in myocardial oxygen requirements. Failure to document a sustained increase in overall myocardial perfusion after NTG administration has led some investigators to conclude that direct coronary actions of nitrates do not represent a viable means whereby these drugs produce their salutory effects in ischemic heart disease. Nitrates dilate coronary collateral vessels and augment coronary collateral blood flow. Smaller coronary vessels dilate to a relatively greater degree than larger vessels.[19,20]

It has long been believed that coronary atherosclerotic disease is "fixed" and that coronary obstructive lesions cannot change diameter. However, recent work using quantitative angiography demonstrates unequivocally that nitrates can induce stenosis dilatation of some coronary atherosclerotic obstructions (Fig. 15.5).[19,20] Not all coronary arterial stenoses dilate after NTG administration. More eccentric lesions have a greater tendency to dilate than those with concentric narrowing.

NITRATE EFFECTS DURING MYOCARDIAL ISCHEMIA

A variety of experiments in animals and in humans dating back to the late 1960s indicate that nitrates have a beneficial action on ischemic zones of myocardium.[10,16,21] The subendocardial-subepicardial blood flow ratio in ischemic myocardium is improved following nitrate administration. Subendocardial oxygenation increases. Although global myocardial blood flow may not change after NTG administration, many studies have shown that perfusion to regional zones of ischemia often improves.

TABLE 15.2 EFFECTS OF NITROGLYCERIN AND ORGANIC NITRATES ON THE CORONARY CIRCULATION

- Brief increase in global coronary blood flow followed by late reduction in blood flow as myocardial oxygen requirements decrease
- Dilatation of epicardial (conduit) coronary arteries
- Dilatation of smaller coronary arteries proportionately more than larger ones
- Dilatation of small (resistance) coronary arterioles with large doses of nitrate
- Dilatation of coronary collateral arteries and enhanced collateral blood flow
- Dilatation of atherosclerotic coronary artery stenoses (eccentric lesions)
- Reversal and prevention of coronary spasm and vasoconstriction
- Improvement of ischemic zone subendocardial and regional nutrient myocardial blood flow

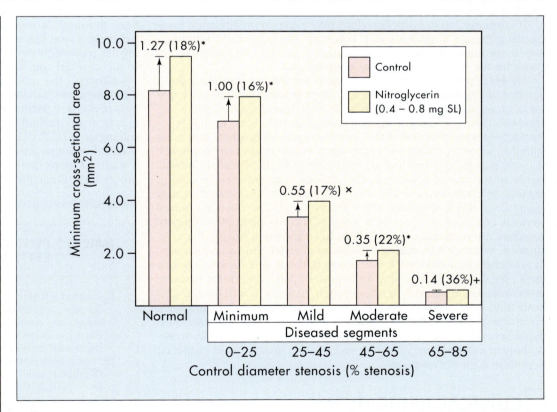

FIGURE 15.5 Nitroglycerin-induced increases in luminal cross-sectional area of coronary arteries and coronary atherosclerosis stenoses. Each bar represents the average increase in cross-sectional area for the group before and after the sublingual nitroglycerin. The calculated percent increase in area was greater in smaller coronary arteries and in the more severe coronary narrowings. (Modified from Brown G, Bolson E, Petersen RB et al: The mechanisms of nitroglycerin action: Stenosis vasodilatation as a major component of drug response. Circulation 64:1089, 1981)

The precise mechanism(s) of action for these positive effects remains unclear. Many believe that the direct vasodilating effects of nitrates on coronary arteries, coronary arterioles, or coronary collaterals, or on the coronary stenosis itself, may be important in reversing or preventing myocardial ischemia.[11,19-21] Reduced left ventricular diastolic compressive forces may be beneficial in some patients, particularly in those who have very high left ventricular diastolic pressure and reduced ventricular compliance in response to acute ischemia.

Other experts continue to believe that the dominant action of nitrates in myocardial ischemia is unrelated to these various coronary effects and that the major beneficial effects are modulated through peripheral mechanisms, resulting in decreased myocardial oxygen requirements.[12,18] These include decreased blood pressure and systemic vascular resistance, a reduction of left ventricular diastolic and systolic volumes, and a fall in intraventricular filling pressures.

Possible mechanisms whereby nitrates may be beneficial in patients with myocardial ischemia are listed in Table 15.3.

CORONARY VASOMOTION

In recent years the potential adverse consequences of coronary vasoconstriction or overt spasm in patients with underlying coronary atherosclerosis have been emphasized and the concept of "mixed angina" or dynamic coronary obstruction has been given considerable attention. This view supports a major role for coronary vasoconstriction superimposed on underlying coronary atherosclerosis, leading to the precipitation of ischemic events. Thus, any coronary artery narrowing would become more obstructive if local or generalized coronary arterial tone increased; a reversible total coronary obstruction is possible in such circumstances. It has been demonstrated that exertion can induce coronary vasoconstriction or spasm in some patients; this observation lends credence to the hypothesis that changes in vasomotor tone may play a role in precipitating angina at rest as well as during physical activity.

If coronary vasoconstriction does play a role in precipitating myocardial ischemia in patients with coronary atherosclerosis, nitrate-induced coronary vasodilatation is another potential mechanism to account for the beneficial effects of these drugs.

Of great potential importance has been the observation from a number of laboratories that coronary atherosclerotic lesions are capable of changing diameter in response to various endogenous and exogenous stimuli.[19,22,23] Such responses are often paradoxic in that coronary arterial vasodilatation is the normal consequence of the particular stimulus, whereas constriction may occur in diseased vessel segments. If there is sufficient residual smooth muscle in the coronary arterial media at the site of a stenosis, the stenotic segment may be able to enlarge or constrict (see Fig. 15.5). Transient total obstruction may even occur; this is reversible with nitroglycerin.[23] The phenomenon of stenosis constriction offers new insights into the pathophysiology of coronary artery disease. Nitrates have been shown to reverse this constriction, whether it be during exercise or acetylcholine administration or is cold-pressor-induced. Enlargement of the atherosclerotic stenosis itself (see Fig. 15.5) may play an important part in the relief of acute myocardial ischemia with nitrates in some patients. It is of interest that both mild and severe coronary stenoses are capable of paradoxic constriction, lending further evidence that the coronary circulation is dynamic even in the setting of advanced atherosclerosis. NTG, an endothelium-independent coronary vasodilator, should be of particular benefit in such circumstances.

☐ CLINICAL INDICATIONS FOR NITRATE USE

ISCHEMIC HEART DISEASE

NTG and nitrates remain a mainstay for the treatment for coronary heart disease. Many consider these drugs to be the first-line agents for use in patients with stable or unstable angina pectoris. There is a considerable amount of evidence that nitrates may reduce infarct size in acute myocardial infarction. Recent data suggest that nitrates may have a "protective" action in the post–myocardial infarction patient.[24] It has been demonstrated that infusion of intravenous NTG for 48 hours beginning early in the acute infarct period may protect the left ventricle from the deleterious effects of infarct expansion, wall thinning, and left ventricular cavity dilatation in the weeks to months following transmural myocardial infarction.[25]

STABLE ANGINA PECTORIS

Sublingual NTG remains the primary therapy for acute episodes of angina pectoris. Long-acting nitrate formulations are extremely effective in the treatment of chronic effort-induced angina pectoris. In my opinion, nitrates should be the initial therapy for most patients with untreated angina pectoris.[21,26] There is an extensive worldwide experience with long-acting nitrates in patients with angina pectoris.[21]

The use of long-acting nitrates in ischemic heart disease has had a checkered history; during the 1960s and early 1970s most physicians believed that these drugs were of little benefit in the treatment of angina pectoris. It was widely thought that orally administered nitrates could not be effective because of extensive hepatic nitrate metabolism. This hypothesis, promulgated by Needleman and others, was extremely influential in convincing clinicians that these drugs were of no value in clinical practice.[27] In addition, the quality of much of the early published investigations using nitrates in angina pectoris was uneven, lending considerable uncertainty as to the efficacy of these agents. By the mid to late 1970s, however, the use of nitrate formulations in angina pectoris became increasingly widespread as much new favorable clinical data convinced physicians that these drugs have major benefits.

Many well-designed double-blind randomized trials using a variety of nitrate compounds have shown unequivocally positive effects.[21,26,27] Decreased angina attacks and reduced NTG consumption rates have been reported. More importantly, objective assessment of myocardial ischemia during placebo-controlled treadmill or bicycle exercise testing has repeatedly documented that nitrates improve exercise duration to the onset of angina.

Although the other two major classes of antianginal agents, the β-blockers and calcium channel antagonists, are also effective in angina pectoris, it seems reasonable to initiate therapy with a long-acting nitrate in any patient with angina pectoris shown to be responsive to sublingual NTG.[26] Classic improvement of chest pain, that is, relief of discomfort within 3 to 10 minutes after sublingual NTG, should prompt a trial of nitrate therapy in patients who require chronic antianginal prophylaxis. Some patients cannot tolerate nitrates because of adverse

---

TABLE 15.3 POTENTIAL MECHANISMS OF NITRATE EFFICACY IN ANGINA PECTORIS

Decreased left ventricular preload
   Systemic venous dilatation
   Pulmonary venous dilatation
   Decrease in left ventricular diastolic compressive forces
   Decreased left ventricular volume and filling pressure
Decreased left ventricular afterload
   Decreased aortic impedance
   Decreased systolic arterial pressure
   Decreased systemic vascular resistance
   Decreased left ventricular end-diastolic volume
Coronary circulation
   Coronary artery and arteriolar dilatation
   Spasm reversal or prevention
   Stenosis dilatation
   Increased collateral flow
   Improvement of regional subendocardial ischemia

side effects, and in such instances excellent alternative therapy is available. Reflex increase in sympathetic activity resulting in excessive tachycardia and contractility may blunt the efficacy of nitrates. Concomitant administration of β-adrenergic blocking agents prevents these undesirable effects and produces beneficial synergetic effects for the treatment of angina.

Nitrates are particularly indicated in patients with angina who have impaired left ventricular function or in those in whom it is believed that an element of coronary vasoconstriction or spasm plays a role in the ischemic syndrome. In several double-blind studies nitrates have been shown to be equally effective as calcium channel blockers for patients with variant or Prinzmetal's angina.[28] There are no available data to indicate which class of drugs is more effective in "mixed angina," and in fact there is no evidence demonstrating that nitrates are less effective than β-blockers or calcium channel blocking agents in any anginal syndrome.

Table 15.4 lists angina patient subsets who should be preferentially considered for nitrate therapy.

UNSTABLE ANGINA PECTORIS

Nitrates are appropriate first-line therapy in patients with unstable angina. This syndrome, while variably defined, consists of accelerating angina and/or the onset of episodes of rest pain with objective evidence for myocardial ischemia. Such patients should be promptly hospitalized, usually in an intensive care unit. In this setting, the administration of NTG in intravenous or ointment form is usually beneficial.[29] Many of these patients may require an additional class of antianginal medication.

A variety of clinical investigations have demonstrated the benefits of nitrates when used aggressively in hospitalized patients with unstable angina.[30,31] It is possible that the antiplatelet actions of these compounds (see above) provide additional benefit in this syndrome. Most experts agree that an intravenous NTG infusion is a mainstay of therapy in severe unstable angina.

ACUTE MYOCARDIAL INFARCTION

The use of NTG and long-acting nitrates in the setting of acute myocardial necrosis has been the subject of numerous animal and human investigations. A variety of earlier studies indicated that nitrate administered early during acute myocardial infarction may reduce infarct size and decrease complications of acute myocardial infarction.[32] Nevertheless, until recently nitrate therapy in acute infarction has been limited to those patients with continuing or recurrent ischemic pain, acute heart failure, or hypertension. New data, however, suggest a more expanded role for nitrate therapy in acute infarction.[25,33]

A recent meta-analysis of a number of clinical trials employing intravenous nitroglycerin suggested a substantial mortality benefit over placebo-treated subjects when the drug was administered within the first 48 hours after admission.[34] More recently, an important trial from Canada demonstrated a major reduction of both early and late (1 year) mortality in patients with anterior wall myocardial infarction given intravenous NTG for 48 hours or more (Fig. 15.6).[25,33] Not only was mortality reduced, but many serious complications of acute infarction were decreased in the NTG-treated cohort; in addition, late postinfarction remodeling was prevented in the nitrate-treated patients.

Thus, it can now be suggested that routine (albeit careful) administration of nitroglycerin for 24 to 48 hours in the early hours of the post-infarction period may be appropriate in Q wave infarcts, particularly anterior. Such a recommendation may be premature, but the available data are most encouraging.[25,32–34] It had been previously suggested that patients who have had a myocardial infarction and who continue to take nitrates may have a better long-term prognosis than individuals who do not use nitrates.[24]

Nitrates are indicated in certain clinical situations following acute myocardial infarction. Recurrent episodes of chest pain may be effectively treated with intravenous or topical NTG. Patients with persistent hypertension represent another indication for nitrate therapy. In such cases intravenous NTG should be carefully administered to lower systolic blood pressure. Persistent hypertension may also be treated with sodium nitroprusside. The use of sodium nitroprusside in acute myocardial infarction may be deleterious in some patients,[32] particularly in those who are normotensive and do not show evidence of congestive heart failure.[35] For this reason some advocate that administration of intravenous NTG for complications of acute myocardial infarction may be a better initial choice than nitroprusside, although this remains controversial.

Patients with pump failure are definite candidates for nitrate administration. The beneficial effects of these drugs in individuals with depressed left ventricular function, particularly when ischemic, is often striking. NTG usually results in an improvement in left ventricular regional wall motion and global ejection fraction as well as a decrease in cardiac dimensions and left ventricular filling pressure. Nitrates may normalize ventricular dyssynergy.

The clinical indications for nitrate therapy in acute myocardial infarction are listed in Table 15.5. It is important to ensure that the systolic arterial pressure and left ventricular filling pressure are adequate before using intravenous NTG. Invasive monitoring is essential in patients with complicated conditions.

CORONARY VASOSPASM

Organic nitrates are effective in reversing coronary vasospasm. This has been shown repeatedly in the cardiac catheterization laboratory. Sublingual NTG remains the drug of choice for acute episodes of chest

---

TABLE 15.4 GUIDELINES FOR SELECTION OF ANGINA PATIENTS FOR LONG-ACTING NITRATE THERAPY

Demonstrated responsiveness to sublingual or oral NTG spray
Any normotensive subject with typical angina pectoris
Symptoms suggestive of intermittent increases in coronary vasomotor tone:
    Variable angina threshold
    Common occurrence of episodes of pain at rest or during slight physical activity
    Early morning angina
    Cold induced angina
    Emotion-induced angina
Overt vasospastic anginal attacks
History or evidence of congestive heart failure
Depressed LV ejection fraction (<0.40) and/or major cardiomegaly
Presence of mitral regurgitation
Postinfarction angina
Relative or absolute contraindications of β-adrenergic blockers and/or calcium channel antagonists

pain in patients who have documented variant angina. In addition, long-acting nitrate therapy has been shown to be beneficial in this syndrome. Some experts believe that patients with documented coronary spasm should preferentially receive a calcium channel blocker, either alone or in combination with a long-acting nitrate. Nevertheless, available data at this time do not clearly indicate that calcium channel blockers are more effective than nitrates.

CONGESTIVE HEART FAILURE

Nitrates are one of the major classes of drugs that have been successfully employed for vasodilator treatment of congestive heart failure.[17,36,37] These agents have been repeatedly shown to be effective in Class III–IV patients with heart failure. Several well-designed double-blind studies indicate that nitrates have sustained beneficial actions over a period of months.[37,38]

The concept of vasodilator therapy is reviewed elsewhere. This therapeutic approach is based on the beneficial hemodynamic response of the failing or impaired left ventricle to afterload reduction. Afterload, defined as ventricular wall stress in early systole, is increased in patients with congestive heart failure. Left ventricular dilatation, an abnormal cavity–wall thickness ratio, and systemic arterial vasoconstriction all contribute to an increase in left ventricular wall stress. A reduction of afterload produced by an arteriolar vasodilator will result in improved left ventricular emptying with an augmented ejection fraction.[36]

Nitrates have a modest effect in increasing cardiac output in congestive heart failure compared with more potent arterial vasodilators, such as hydralazine. However, the action of nitrates in reducing left ventricular preload by systemic and regional bed venodilatation gives these drugs a unique advantage over relatively pure arterial vasodilators. Nitrates reduce pulmonary capillary wedge pressure and right heart filling pressures owing to a redistribution of circulating blood volume and increase in systemic venous pooling. At the same time the arteriolar vasodilating actions of these drugs helps in "unloading" the left ventricle and result in enhanced systolic performance; left ventricular function improves and stroke volume usually rises. In patients with heart failure, nitrate-induced arteriolar vasodilatation results in enhanced left ventricular performance, and this prevents the decrease in cardiac output that typically accompanies the reduction in left ventricular preload occurring in normal subjects after nitrate administration.

It is difficult to demonstrate that nitrates significantly reduce left ventricular cavity size in patients with severe heart failure. Nitrates may decrease left ventricular compliance by reducing intrapericardial pres-

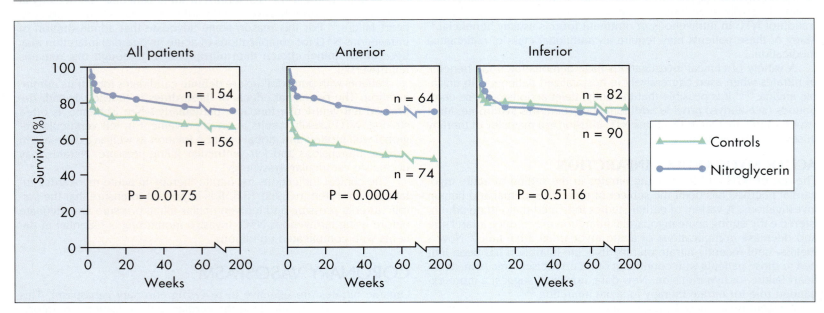

FIGURE 15.6 Improved mortality with the use of a 48-hour infusion of intravenous nitroglycerin in acute myocardial infarction. In this protocol, 310 patients, immediately after hospitalization, were randomized to begin an infusion of low-dose intravenous NTG or placebo. Mortality, both early and late, was decreased in the NTG group due to a marked reduction in early deaths in the anterior wall myocardial infarction cohort. There was a 46% reduction in hospital deaths up to 38 days from admission in the NTG patients, with the benefit mainly seen in the anterior Q wave infarction group. Note that the curves remain parallel for 43 months of follow-up. In addition, Killip score, infarct expansion and extension, left ventricular thrombus, and cardiogenic shock were all considerably reduced in the NTG group. (Modified from Jugdutt BI, Warnica JW: Intravenous nitroglycerin therapy to limit myocardial infarct size, expansion, and complications. Effect of timing, dosage, and infarct location. Circulation 78:706, 1988)

TABLE 15.5 INDICATIONS FOR NITRATES IN ACUTE MYOCARDIAL INFARCTION

Persistent and recurrent chest pain
Sustained hypertension (BP > 140/90 mm Hg)
Major left ventricular dysfunction: acute pulmonary edema or congestive heart failure
Papillary muscle dysfunction with mitral regurgitation (potential indication only)
Potential role for careful routine administration of intravenous NTG during the first 24–48 hours of acute Q wave infarction (see text)

sure.[40] In patients with ischemic heart disease nitrates may have an additional beneficial effect if nutrient myocardial blood flow is increased. Nitrates usually improve mitral regurgitation, a common accompaniment of severe left ventricular decompensation.

ACUTE CONGESTIVE HEART FAILURE

Nitrates, particularly the rapid-acting formulations such as intravenous, sublingual, oral spray, or buccal NTG, are very effective in decreasing the elevated left ventricular filling pressure of acute pulmonary edema. At the same time, the arteriolar vasodilating effects of nitrates reduce left ventricular work and improve forward cardiac output. Although there are limited published data on nitrate therapy in pulmonary edema or acute congestive heart failure, clinical experience indicates that these drugs are very useful adjunctive agents in reducing the signs and symptoms of severe pulmonary congestion.

CHRONIC CONGESTIVE HEART FAILURE

Numerous studies have shown that long-acting nitrates are beneficial for patients with chronic congestive heart failure.[36] Pulmonary capillary wedge and pulmonary artery pressure are reduced at rest and during exercise; stroke volume may increase modestly or remain unchanged but rarely falls after nitrate administration. Systemic and pulmonary vascular resistance decrease.

Several long-term trials indicate that nitrates maintain their effectiveness in reducing pulmonary capillary wedge pressure during chronic therapy.[37,38] Exercise performance in patients with congestive heart failure treated with isosorbide dinitrate (ISDN) increases over time when compared with placebo treatment.[38] Present evidence indicates that ISDN and captopril are the only vasodilator drugs that have been consistently shown to produce beneficial effects in patients with chronic congestive heart failure over a period of months.[37,38]

In summary, nitrates are an excellent choice for patients with symptoms of pulmonary venous congestion, such as orthopnea, paroxysmal nocturnal dyspnea, and dyspnea on exertion. Evidence of pulmonary congestion on radiography, the presence of rales on physical examination, and an elevated jugular venous pressure are all clues that nitrate administration will be beneficial. Patients with congestive heart failure typically require larger doses of nitrates than those with normal ventricles.

Of major importance have been the results of the Veterans Administration Cooperative Trial of Congestive Heart Failure[39] that demonstrated a significant long-term reduction in mortality in patients with heart failure treated with the combination of isosorbide dinitrate and hydralazine for several years (Fig. 15.7). This trial has provided the first evidence that any pharmacologic intervention in congestive heart failure can exert a positive benefit on mortality. Although it is not known for certain which drug (or both) provided the protective benefit, it is likely that isosorbide dinitrate played an important role. This study suggests that long-term administration of nitrates in subjects with heart failure may be truly cardioprotective.

ADDITIONAL USES FOR NITROGLYCERIN AND LONG-ACTING NITRATES

PULMONARY HYPERTENSION

Nitrates are effective pulmonary vasodilators. They reduce pulmonary vascular resistance and pulmonary artery pressure in a variety of conditions. Several studies indicate that intravenous NTG is quite effective in lowering pulmonary artery pressure after open heart surgery. Long-acting nitrates have been used successfully in occasional patients with chronic severe pulmonary hypertension.

HYPERTENSION

During the 1940s and 1950s the organic nitrates were used for the treatment of hypertension. Although it is true that acute nitrate administration decreases systolic blood pressure, particularly in the upright position, tolerance to the hypotensive effects of these drugs rapidly occurs; after 1 or more weeks of therapy a given dose of nitrate no

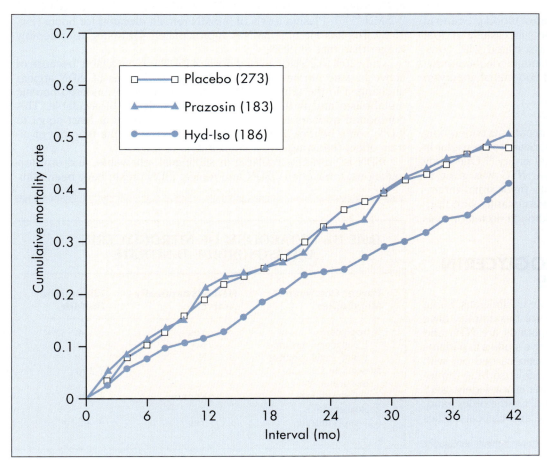

FIGURE 15.7 Improvement in mortality in the VA Cooperative Trial of Congestive Heart Failure. In this multicenter trial of patients with class II-III heart failure, individuals were treated with placebo, prazosin, or the combination of hydralazine, 75 mg qid, and isosorbide dinitrate, 40 mg qid (Hyd-Iso). There was a reduction of mortality seen at 1, 2, and 3 years after onset of the study; the major benefits were derived in the first year. This study was the first to document that medical therapy for congestive heart failure can impart an improvement in longevity. Subsequent analysis demonstrated that only persons with an increase in ejection fraction enjoyed a mortality benefit. (Modified from Leier CV, Huss P, Magorien RP et al: Improved exercise capacity and differing arterial and venous tolerance during chronic isosorbide dinitrate therapy for congestive heart failure. Circulation 67:817, 1983)

longer has the same effect on systemic arterial pressure as it does initially. Thus, these drugs are not appropriate choices for the outpatient treatment of hypertension. Nevertheless, a recent report suggests that oral ISDN has a favorable effect on systolic hypertension in the elderly.[41]

Acute administration of intravenous NTG, on the other hand, is a safe and effective mode of therapy for lowering blood pressure in the intensive care unit setting. Intravenous NTG infusion usually results in a gradual decline in blood pressure. The hypotensive effects are directly related to the infusion rate. With moderate to high concentrations of NTG, arteriolar vasodilatation occurs and the drug achieves a hypotensive potency comparable to sodium nitroprusside. Intravenous NTG does not lower blood pressure as rapidly as nitroprusside, diazoxide, or sublingual nifedipine. The magnitude and response time of blood pressure lowering may be greater with these other vasodilators, but this has not been subjected to rigorous clinical testing.

MITRAL REGURGITATION

Nitrates reduce the degree of the mitral regurgitation; the height of the left atrial v wave and mean atrial pressure fall after nitrate administration.[42] Stroke volume is often augmented. Nitrates are probably not as effective as are pure arterial vasodilators (such as hydralazine) in reducing the regurgitant fraction in mitral or aortic regurgitation. These drugs are particularly useful if there is underlying left ventricular dysfunction or in subjects with ischemic heart disease with papillary muscle dysfunction.

ESOPHAGEAL SPASM

Nitrates have potent relaxant effects on smooth muscle throughout the body, including the esophagus, gallbladder, and uterus. These actions have been used to prevent or reverse esophageal spasm in patients who have motility disorders of the esophagus.[43] In addition, efforts have been made to use nitrates to lower portal venous pressure in individuals with cirrhosis of the liver.

CONTROLLED ARTERIAL PRESSURE DURING SURGICAL PROCEDURES

Intravenous NTG has been effectively used to control blood pressure in a variety of surgical procedures. It has been used successfully to treat intraoperative and postoperative hypertension associated with coronary bypass grafting and has been employed to induce deliberate hypotension during neurosurgery, hip surgery, and abdominal aneurysm repair.[44,45]

INTERVENTIONAL CARDIOLOGY

The use of intravenous NTG has been increasing in patients undergoing percutaneous coronary angioplasty. This drug appears to be useful in preventing early spasm or reclosure of the target artery.[46] One study suggested a benefit in ventricular function when NTG was given in addition to intracoronary streptokinase in acute myocardial infarction.[47] It is likely that intravenous NTG given concomitantly with fibrinolytic therapy would have beneficial effects, although no major trials have been reported to date.

PHARMACOLOGY OF NITROGLYCERIN AND LONG-ACTING NITRATES

A wide variety of organic nitrate esters are available to clinicians. Some agents, such as erythrityl tetranitrate and mannitol hexanitrate, have fallen into disuse. The most widely used compounds are NTG and ISDN. The majority of published clinical investigative studies in patients with angina and congestive heart failure have been carried out with these two agents. Pentaerythritol tetranitrate and 5-isosorbide mononitrate (5-ISMN) are currently available. The former is not widely used, and clinical data supporting its efficacy are limited. On the other hand, 5-ISMN enjoys considerable popularity in Europe and clinical studies are currently being carried out in North America. This interesting compound is one of the two major metabolites of ISDN and has a longer duration of action.[48,49]

METABOLISM OF NITROGLYCERIN AND ISOSORBIDE DINITRATE (TABLE 15.6)

NITROGLYCERIN

The half-life of NTG is very short (*e.g.*, less than 5 minutes). NTG is rapidly converted into two inactive metabolites, the 1,2- and 1,3-glyceryl dinitrates. Both metabolites are found in the urine after oral administration. These compounds have little hemodynamic activity. Because of the large amounts of the enzyme glutathione organic nitrate reductase in the liver, it has been assumed that hepatic metabolism is solely responsible for NTG degradation. This led to the hypothesis that orally administered nitrates could not produce clinically useful effects because of potent hepatic first-pass metabolism. It is now recognized that the blood vessels of the body directly metabolize nitrates and appear to be responsible for considerable degradation of these compounds,[9,49] particularly after systemic (nonoral) administration. After intravenous administration of NTG there is a large systemic arteriovenous NTG gradient with higher arterial than venous NTG concentrations.[50] This observation is consistent with substantial vascular uptake of NTG.

NTG is available in the United States in sublingual, intravenous, oral spray, buccal, oral, ointment, and transdermal disc or patch formulation.

ISOSORBIDE DINITRATE

ISDN has theoretic advantages over NTG because of its much longer half-life and higher plasma levels. This compound is converted to two active metabolites, the 2- and 5-isosorbide mononitrate. Both metabolites have vasodilatory activity; 2-ISMN is less active than 5-ISMN. The latter appears to be an effective drug for the treatment of angina and congestive heart failure. Metabolism and clearance of the parent compound ISDN is more rapid than that of the metabolites; after oral dosing, plasma concentrations of ISDN are lower than those of ISMN and 2-ISMN.[48,49,51] Plasma levels of 5-ISMN remain elevated for hours (Fig. 15.8). The half-life of 5-ISMN is approximately 4½ hours, considerably longer than that of ISDN.

Only 20% to 25% of an oral dose of ISDN is bioavailable because of active hepatic nitrate metabolism.[51] The metabolites of ISDN appear unchanged in the urine. 5-ISMN, however, does not undergo hepatic metabolism and is therefore virtually completely bioavailable. This compound appears to have a vasodilating potency at least equal to ISDN; some believe that 5-ISMN is responsible for the majority of nitrate effect following oral administration of ISDN.

ISDN is currently available in sublingual, chewable, and oral formulations. Intravenous ISDN and topical ISDN cream have been clini-

TABLE 15.6 METABOLISM OF NITROGLYCERIN AND ISOSORBIDE DINITRATE

Parent Compound/ Metabolites	Hemodynamically Active	Elimination Half-life
Nitroglycerin	Yes	1.5–4.5 min
1,2-glyceryl dinitrate	No	
1,3-glyceryl dinitrate	No	
Isosorbide Dinitrate	Yes	1.2 hr
Isosorbide-2-mononitrate	Possible	1.8 hr
Isosorbide-5-mononitrate	Yes	4–4.5 hr

cally tested and are used in other countries. An oral ISDN spray is available in West Germany, and a new translucent plastic wrap impregnated with ISDN may undergo clinical trials in the future.

NITRATE PLASMA CONCENTRATIONS

There is considerable uncertainty and controversy regarding the value of nitrate blood levels. It is not easy to obtain accurate and reliable measurements of NTG and ISDN, although the latter is more readily assayed because of its higher plasma concentrations and longer half-life. Gas chromatographic techniques for nitrate measurement have become available in recent years, but these assays are performed in only a very few laboratories because of technical difficulties in obtaining reliable and reproducible data.

In acute dosing studies, NTG plasma nitrate concentrations bear a proportional relationship to the hemodynamic effects of the administered drug. However, with chronic dosing, plasma nitrate concentrations no longer are predictive of the hemodynamic effects (Fig. 15.9).[52] It has been observed that plasma nitrate concentrations tend to increase with chronic dosing (Fig. 15.9).[52,53] This appears to result from a decreased clearance of the parent nitrate compound apparently due to a reduction of vascular nitrate metabolism.[9,49] Alterations in nitrate vascular kinetics with chronic dosing may be related to the development of nitrate tolerance.[49] Uptake and metabolism of organic nitrate by veins and arteries is diminished in the presence of nitrate tolerance; tolerance is associated with higher plasma nitrate levels (see Fig. 15.9) and decreased clearance of the drug from the systemic circulation.[9]

FACTORS INFLUENCING NITRATE PHARMACOKINETICS

Data have become available evaluating potential alterations of nitrate metabolism during varying physiologic states. It is difficult to demonstrate any significant impact on nitrate metabolism during differing clinical conditions. Plasma ISDN levels are not affected by whether the dose is taken before or after a meal; cigarette smoking does not alter ISDN pharmacokinetics.[54] Nitrate levels do not appear to be affected by the presence of reduced renal function.[55] Limited data do suggest that in cirrhotic patients plasma ISDN concentrations may be higher after oral dosing.[55] Congestive heart failure does not appear to affect nitrate kinetics.[54] β-Blockers and cimetidine, drugs that are known to alter hepatic enzymatic function and thus potentially alter the metabolism of other drugs, do not influence nitrate metabolism (see Fig. 15.8).[55]

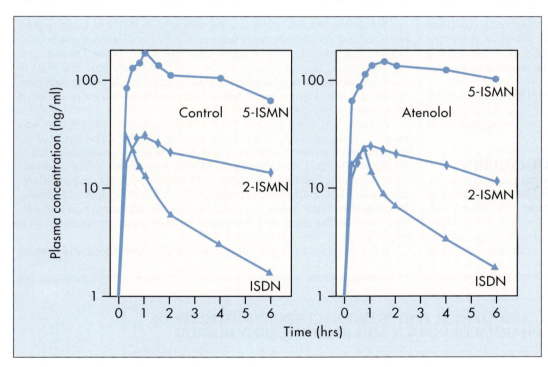

FIGURE 15.8 Plasma concentrations of isosorbide dinitrate (ISDN), isosorbide 2-mononitrate (2-ISMN), and isosorbide 5-mononitrate (5-ISMN) following administration of 10 mg of oral ISDN before and after treatment with 100 mg of atenolol. Note that the plasma concentration of 5-ISMN is substantially higher than that of the parent compound ISDN and that 5-ISMN persists in the plasma at a constant level for several hours longer than ISDN. β-Blocker administration did not alter ISDN pharmacokinetics. (Modified from Bogaert MG, Rosseel MT: Fate of orally given isosorbide dinitrate in man: Factors of variability. Z Kardiol 72(suppl 3):11, 1983)

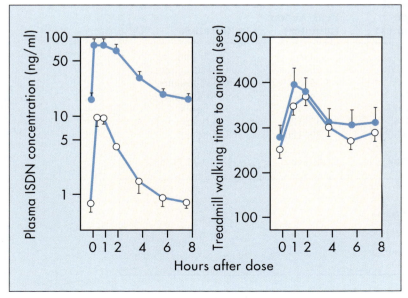

FIGURE 15.9 Relationship of plasma isosorbide dinitrate (ISDN) concentration to improvement in treadmill walking time in a double-blind, placebo-controlled study of patients with angina. These data from the study of Thadani and co-workers[52] compare plasma ISDN concentrations and treadmill walking time in patients who took 15 mg of ISDN four times daily for 1 week (open circles) and 120 mg of ISDN four times daily for 1 week (closed circles). In the acute dosing study (not illustrated) there was a dose–response relationship between the amount of administered ISDN and improvement in treadmill walking time. However, after chronic short-term therapy the small dose of 15 mg produced the same improvement as the large dose of 120 mg; both resulted in marked attenuation of exercise improvement at 4, 6, and 8 hours, a finding indicative of nitrate tolerance. During the acute dosing study, exercise performance was improved over a placebo from 4 to 8 hours (not shown). Plasma ISDN concentrations were higher after chronic therapy than with acute dosing. (Modified from Fung H-L: Pharmacokinetic determinants of nitrate action. Am J Med 76:22, 1984)

NITRATE DELIVERY SYSTEMS

A wide variety of nitrate formulations are presently available.[56] Nitrates are well absorbed across the skin and mucosal surfaces, and the diverse dosing forms take advantage of this characteristic. When a sufficient amount of oral nitrate is given, hepatic metabolism is readily bypassed and "therapeutic" concentrations of nitroglycerin and ISDN appear in the blood.

The currently available nitrate delivery systems, dose recommendations, the time to peak effect, and the total duration of activity of each compound are listed in Table 15.7. Nitrate pharmacokinetics in a given patient are not predictable; the pharmacokinetic information listed in Table 15.7 represents averages of many studies.

RAPID-ONSET FORMULATIONS
SUBLINGUAL NITRATES

The gold standard of therapy for angina attacks is sublingual NTG, an extremely effective formulation. Sublingual or chewable ISDN tablets are also useful for acute therapy, but their onset of action is somewhat slower than that of sublingual NTG. Sublingual ISDN has a longer duration of activity than sublingual NTG and may be desirable for patients who need sustained protection after an episode of angina. Neither of these formulations represent practical therapy for long-term angina prophylaxis in individuals who have frequent attacks of chest pain.

It is important for patients with angina to be instructed to use sublingual NTG or ISDN prophylactically *prior to* activities or situations that are likely to induce chest pain. If this is done, potential angina attacks can be prevented and patients may be able to conduct normal activities without interruption.

Oral NTG and ISDN sprays have been evaluated that appear to be effective in aborting episodes of angina. An oral NTG spray has recently become available in the United States. It acts comparably to sublingual NTG.

BUCCAL OR TRANSMUCOSAL NITROGLYCERIN

A buccal tablet of NTG has been available for several years, consisting of NTG dispersed in a special cellulose matrix.[56,57] The unique property of buccal NTG is its extremely rapid onset of action combined with sustained hemodynamic and clinical effects. The medication is placed in the buccal pouch between the upper lip and teeth. A gel or seal rapidly forms and the tablet subsequently adheres to the mucosa. Most patients find that they can eat, drink, and talk without difficulty once the medication is in place. NTG is released immediately across the mucosal membranes into the rich capillary bed of the mouth; the onset of NTG effect is as rapid as with sublingual NTG.[57] Thus, this drug can be used for acute prophylaxis of anginal attacks instead of sublingual NTG or ISDN. NTG is absorbed at a constant rate while the buccal tablet remains intact in the mouth. Studies have indicated that the average duration of availability of the tablet ranges between 3 and 6 hours. NTG plasma concentrations are well in the therapeutic range after buccal NTG administration.[57]

LONG-ACTING NITRATES
ORAL NITRATES

Both NTG and ISDN have been available for many years. These drugs are manufactured in standard formulation and as sustained-action tablets or capsules.

Oral nitrates produce prolonged hemodynamic effects that last from 3 to 8 hours with acute dosing. Therapeutic plasma concentrations are sustained for many hours. Unfortunately, gastrointestinal absorption of oral nitrates is variable and unpredictable from one patient to the next. Thus, a fixed oral dose of NTG or ISDN should not be employed; rather, patients should be given oral nitrates in increasing amounts until the clinical syndrome is well controlled and/or side-effects occur.

Numerous studies attest to the efficacy of ISDN in both angina pectoris and congestive heart failure.[21,26-28,36,38,52] This compound has been investigated more thoroughly than any other nitrate. Data on oral NTG are more limited. It is probable that when sufficient oral NTG is given its effects are similar to that of ISDN, although direct comparative studies are few. Many experts believe that oral ISDN is a more effective formulation than oral NTG.

Patients too often receive smaller doses of oral nitrates than are optimal. Although high-dose nitrate therapy may be more likely to induce nitrate tolerance, it is important that a dose be established that is clinically effective. Physicians should follow patients closely when nitrate therapy is instituted. In those with angina pectoris, angina attack rates should be markedly decreased with an effective dosing regimen. In congestive heart failure, it is best to carefully assess clinical parameters, such as the signs and symptoms of pulmonary congestion, as a rough guide to dose adequacy.

It is important to begin nitrate therapy with low doses and then to

TABLE 15.7 SUBLINGUAL AND LONG-ACTING NITROGLYCERIN AND ISOSORBIDE DINITRATE: PHARMACOKINETICS AND RECOMMENDED DOSAGE

Medication	Recommended Dosage (mg)	Onset of Action (minutes)	Peak Action (minutes)	Duration
Sublingual NTG	0.3–0.8	2–5	4–8	10–30 minutes
Sublingual ISDN	2.5–10	5–20	15–60	45–120 minutes*
Oral NTG spray	0.4	2–5	4–8	10–30 minutes
Buccal NTG	1–3	2–5	4–10	30–300 minutes
Oral ISDN	10–60	15–45	45–120	2–6 hours
Oral NTG	6.5–19.5	20–45	45–120	2–6 hours
NTG ointment (2%)	½–2 inches	15–60	30–120	3–8 hours
NTG discs (transdermal)	10–20 mg†	30–60	60–180	Up to 24 hours‡

* Up to 3 to 4 hours in some studies.

† Higher doses may be needed, especially in congestive heart failure.

‡ Clinical effects may not persist for 24 hours.

(NTG, nitroglycerin; ISDN, isosorbide dinitrate)

increase the dosage to reach an effective dosing regimen. At the same time, one should always attempt to use as little nitrate as possible because of the possibility that higher doses will more readily induce nitrate tolerance. The physician must strike a balance in prescribing a nitrate dosing regimen that ensures nitrate efficiency while minimizing the likelihood of tolerance.

NITROGLYCERIN OINTMENT

A 2% NTG ointment formulation has been available for many years. In 1974 Reichek and co-workers published the results of a double-blind, placebo-controlled study that demonstrated a prolonged (3-hour) protective action of 2% NTG ointment in patients with angina.[58] Numerous other investigations in patients with angina and heart failure have demonstrated the effectiveness of NTG ointment. The effects of this compound last 4 to 6 hours or longer in acute dosing trials.

As with oral nitrates the effective dosage of NTG ointment is variable and unpredictable. There is some argument about the size of the skin area over which the ointment should be spread; some believe that a 6 × 6-inch area is necessary, while others believe that a smaller surface area is satisfactory. It is best to spread the NTG ointment on the chest or arms. This formulation is relatively messy and readily soils clothes. It is particularly useful for patients in intensive care units who require the long-acting nitrates. A recently developed adhesive unit that prevents leakage of the ointment from the bandage has made NTG ointment more practical for active patients.

NTG ointment should also be considered in patients who have nocturnal symptoms of chest pain or those with congestive heart failure who have orthopnea and paroxysmal nocturnal dyspnea.

TRANSDERMAL NITROGLYCERIN PATCHES

The NTG disc or patch units were introduced in 1982 and have received an enthusiastic welcome by patients and physicians. The NTG discs consist of NTG impregnated into a silicone gel or matrix. The discs provide a constant NTG delivery across the skin barrier for 24 to 48 hours, at a release rate of approximately 0.5 mg NTG per square centimeter of disc area. New FDA guidelines require manufacturers to list the actual NTG release rate per hour for each size of dosing unit.

A number of investigations indicate that lower doses of the disc (5–10 mg/day) are not very effective in many patients with angina.[59,60] One should begin with a minimum of 10 mg/day and increase the NTG dose to 20–30 mg/day in patients who continue to have the symptoms of angina or heart failure. In the latter situation, particularly large doses are usually necessary.

The NTG patches have stimulted a considerable amount of controversy since their introduction. Early studies suggested less than optimal efficacy in "standard" doses (e.g., 5–10 mg per 24 hours). It is now clear that a predictable and classic nitrate effect can be obtained with higher doses; in general, a minimum of 10–15 mg per 24 hours is necessary, and often more, especially in heart failure patients.

The more important aspect of the patch controversy was stimulated by early observations that classic nitrate effects appeared in many studies to wane by 24 hours in angina and congestive heart failure.[59-62] A subsequent major investigation has confirmed this phenomenon in a large number of patients.[63] Although not every subject will become tolerant to continuous patch administration, this is likely to occur in the majority of individuals. Many clinical investigations of tolerance have confirmed that dosing regimens designed to provide sustained nitrate exposure to the vasculature will readily induce some degree of attenuation of nitrate activity. The NTG patches have been a pharmacologic innovation that has elucidated much information about tolerance.

It is now well established that an intermittent or on-off dosing strategy can maintain responsiveness to NTG patches.[64-66] (Fig. 15.10). Thus, removing the unit nightly for 10 to 12 hours is a reasonable strategy that will provide continued nitrate efficacy during the patch-on period.

INTRAVENOUS NITROGLYCERIN

Intravenous NTG has been commercially available in the United States since the early 1980s. This formulation has achieved widespread popularity in intensive care units. It is an excellent drug for patients with acute myocardial infarction complicated by hypertension, recurrent chest pain, or pump failure. Intravenous NTG is also useful in acute pulmonary edema or severe congestive heart failure.

Intravenous NTG has a rapid onset of action; similarly, its effects quickly disappear when the infusion is discontinued. At low NTG con-

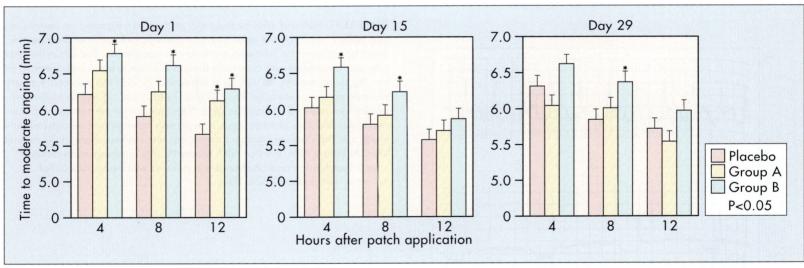

FIGURE 15.10 Efficacy of intermittent nitroglycerin patch administration to avoid tolerance in angina pectoris. The results are from a multicenter placebo-controlled trial involving 215 randomized patients. The groups included placebo, low-dose transdermal NTG (10–20 cm², group A) and high-dose transdermal NTG (30–40 cm², group B). Patients wore a placebo or active patch for 12 hours each day for a total of 29 days. Treadmill time to angina of moderate intensity is shown in the vertical column for each group at 4, 8, and 12 hours on the three testing days: days 1, 15, and 29. An antianginal response was seen in the high-dose group on day 1 and day 15 (except at 12 hours); after 1 month, exercise duration was longer than placebo at all testing intervals but reached statistical significance only at hour 8 on day 29. There was a reduction in anginal attacks and sublingual NTG consumption per week in both groups, although the frequency of angina was low in this study. A retrospective analysis of the 20-cm² group indicated that there was a similar trend toward improvement of angina, compared with placebo, at this dosage strength. Attenuation or tolerance seemed to be more of a problem after 4 weeks of long-term therapy compared with day 15 in both dosing groups. (Modified from DeMots H, Glasser SP. Intermittent transdermal nitroglycerin therapy in the treatment of chronic stable angina. J Am Coll Cardiol 13:786, 1989)

centrations venodilatation is dominant, but as the infusion rate increases arterial and arteriolar vasodilatation occur and systemic vascular resistance decreases (Fig. 15.2).

It is not necessary to use specialized polyethylene tubing and infusion sets when administering intravenous NTG. This has been suggested because NTG is readily absorbed onto conventional polyvinyl chloride (PVC) tubing. In one study it was demonstrated that the benefits of using polyethylene tubing instead of PVC tubing were insignificant.[67]

Intravenous NTG infusion should begin at a rate 5 µg to 20 µg/min and be increased by 5 µg to 10 µg/min every 5 to 10 minutes until the desired clinical or hemodynamic effect is achieved. Hypotension, tachycardia, nausea, and headache are potential complications. Particular care should be used in hypovolemic patients.

PROBLEMS WITH NITRATE THERAPY

The two major areas of difficulty resulting from nitrate administration are the acute side effects and the potential for induction of nitrate tolerance.

ADVERSE EFFECTS

Classic nitrate side effects include headache and dizziness. Headaches are the most debilitating feature relating to nitrate administration and preclude continuation of long-acting nitrates in approximately 20% of patients. The headache may be mild or intense; it may consist of a throbbing sensation or a severe generalized headache. Nitrate headaches frequently attenuate or completely disappear after several days to 2 weeks of daily therapy. If patients take mild analgesics concomitantly with nitrates for several days they will often be able to tolerate nitrates on a long-term basis when the headaches disappear. Some subjects, however, refuse to use sublingual NTG or other nitrates because of an unhappy experience with initial doses. It is important for the physician to inform patients in advance that headache is to be expected and to encourage the short-term use of analgesics.

Nausea and vomiting occasionally result from nitrate therapy, but these symptoms are not usually serious or persistent. Acute hypotensive reactions to sublingual NTG or other nitrates may cause dizziness and even syncope. These reactions tend not to persist, since the blood pressure and heart rate responses following nitrate administration rapidly become attenuated with chronic dosing.

Topical nitrates may cause skin irritation and dermatitis. The adhesive or metallic components of the NTG discs may result in erythema and occasional skin reactions.

Paradoxic bradycardia and hypotension may follow sublingual or intravenous nitrate administration (Fig. 15.11).[68] Such reactions usually occur when sublingual NTG is given to a patient with acute myocardial infarction or ischemia. This paradoxic response to nitroglycerin appears to result from reflex activation of afferent cardiac mechanoreceptors (Bezold-Jarisch reflex) and can be promptly reversed by administration of atropine.

NTG has been shown to reduce systemic oxygen saturation in patients with chronic obstructive lung disease. In patients with right ventricular dysfunction related to pulmonary hypertension, NTG has been shown to decrease right ventricular stroke work as well as right ventricular diastolic dimensions. Thus, in patients with significant chronic lung disease the use of nitrates might be deleterious, although the clinical significance of these observations remains to be elucidated. In patients with right ventricular infarction, cardiac output and blood pressure may decrease markedly following administration of NTG and nitrates and therefore these drugs should be avoided.

Several investigators have measured elevated methemoglobin levels in patients receiving large amounts of nitrates.[69] The clinical significance of this problem is minimal. It is not necessary to monitor methemoglobin levels in patients on chronic nitrate therapy, although this might be a consideration in a subject receiving enormous doses of NTG who develops unexplained cyanosis.[45]

NITRATE TOLERANCE

Tolerance to NTG and long-acting nitrates is a controversial problem that has been argued for many years.[4,70-73] The development of nitrate vascular tolerance occurs rapidly in experimental animals given frequent doses of NTG. It has long been known that the blood pressure reduction following acute nitrate administration rapidly becomes attenuated. Decreased blood pressure and heart rate responses as well as the loss of headaches during chronic therapy certainly represent

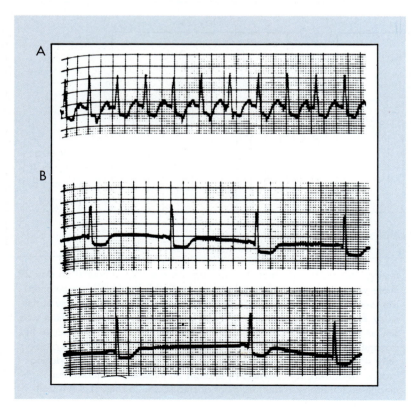

FIGURE 15.11 Profound sinus bradycardia and arterial hypotension developing in a patient with an acute anteroseptal myocardial infarction and congestive heart failure given an intravenous infusion of nitroglycerin. The fall in the heart rate was associated with a marked decline in mean arterial pressure from 84 mm Hg to 36 mm Hg, as well as a substantial drop in the pulmonary artery diastolic pressure, which fell from 23 mm Hg to 7 mm Hg. All hemodynamic parameters returned to baseline after administration of intravenous atropine and discontinuation of intravenous nitroglycerin. Reinfusion of nitroglycerin at a lower rate than before produced similar but less marked changes 30 minutes later. **A.** Before NTG. **B.** After NTG. (Come PC, Pitt B: Nitroglycerin-induced severe hypotension and bradycardia in patients with acute myocardial infarction. Circulation 54:624, 1976)

manifestations of nitrate tolerance. Until recently, however, it had not been demonstrated unequivocally that the desired clinical actions of these drugs become less effective during chronic therapy.

Many studies, particularly from Europe and Canada, indicate that clinically relevant tolerance to nitrates is a real phenomenon and is more common than previously thought.[2,52,72,73] In one early investigation in patients with angina pectoris it was demonstrated that the duration of effect of ISDN shortened considerably and the dose–response relationship between the amount of administered ISDN and the resultant beneficial effects on treadmill walking time disappeared after several weeks of ISDN therapy.[52] As discussed previously, many additional reports have documented the development of partial or complete nitrate tolerance in angina pectoris and congestive heart failure with various dosing regimens and nitrate compounds.

Parker and colleagues have shown that "chronic therapy" with NTG discs and a long-acting ISDN cream resulted in complete attenuation of nitrate effect at all testing intervals in patients with angina.[53,62] These data suggest that any nitrate formulation providing 12 or more hours of sustained nitrate availability may induce a more complete form of tolerance than intermittent nitrate dosing regimens.

Tolerance is not related to a specific formulation. Large doses, frequent dosing schedules, and sustained-acting formulations are all pro-tolerant; conversely, small doses, less frequent dosing, and shorter-acting compounds may avoid the induction of tolerance. Of great importance is the presence or absence of a *nitrate-free interval* each day. Thus, a designated period of no nitrate exposure each day for at least 10 to 12 hours should be part of each patient's dosing program. Fewer doses, *e.g.*, two to three times daily for oral nitrates, have been associated with less tolerance.[74,75] Twelve to 14 hours of NTG patch application, with removal on a daily basis, are also recommended.[64-66] It is important for the vasculature to be exposed to declining nitrate plasma levels for a protracted period each day; the longer the better.

GUIDELINES FOR NITRATE THERAPY. Current recommendations for nitrate therapy should take into account the newer data regarding nitrate tolerance (Table 15.8). Nitrates are best administered using the smallest effective dose and in the least number of doses that control the clinical syndrome. Sustained-action formulations, transdermal NTG discs, and large or frequent nitrate doses may quickly induce a hyporeactive state in blood vessels. Intermittent nitrate therapy employing a nitrate-free interval of at least 6 to 10 hours may avoid or delay the development of nitrate tolerance. Many patients treated with nitrates do not need "around the clock" protection; clinicians should give serious consideration to having patients take the last daily dose of nitrates in the late afternoon or early evening, including the NTG patches.

CLINICAL IMPLICATIONS

Nitrate therapy represents one of the oldest forms of treatment for cardiovascular diseases. Physicians have had extensive experience with these agents, which are relatively safe and well tolerated. Side effects are circumscribed and predictable. These drugs are not costly, although the NTG disc systems are expensive.

Nitrates have important actions in patients with ischemic heart disease. These compounds lower the preload and afterload of the heart and result in a reduction in myocardial energy requirements and an increased efficiency of left ventricular ejection. Nitrates have direct effects on the coronary circulation, such as increasing coronary collateral flow, stenosis dilatation, and enhancement of nutrient subendocardial perfusion during myocardial ischemia. These actions may be important in relieving chest pain in a variety of anginal syndromes. Nitrates are beneficial in acute myocardial infarction complicated by hypertension, recurrent chest pain, or congestive heart failure. Routine administration of these compounds in acute myocardial infarction is not indicated. There are suggestive data that long-term nitrate administration in patients who have chronic coronary heart disease may improve longevity.

Nitrates are useful in congestive heart failure. These drugs lower intracardiac filling pressures and improve exercise capacity when taken for several weeks or months. They are particularly indicated in patients who have signs and symptoms of an elevated pulmonary capillary wedge pressure, pulmonary hypertension, or associated with right ventricular failure.

Nitrate side effects of headache and transient hypotension are common with initial therapy but usually attenuate over time. Some patients cannot be maintained on long-term nitrate administration because of adverse effects. Nitrate tolerance remains a problem, but its clinical implications are still unclear. It is prudent to use the least amount of nitrate that controls the clinical syndrome.

Patients with angina, acute myocardial infarction, and congestive heart failure can derive important clinical benefits from the proper use of nitrate therapy. When used intelligently these drugs provide consistent and effective cardiovascular therapy at low cost and with rare serious side effects.

TABLE 15.8 CURRENT RECOMMENDATIONS FOR NITRATE THERAPY

1. Begin with small dose.
2. Establish a dose threshold that achieves the desired clinical effect.
3. Use the least amount of nitrate that provides continued symptomatic benefit.
4. Avoid use of sustained-action formulations; these preparations may more readily induce nitrate tolerance.
5. Establish a dosing regimen that provides a nitrate-free interval of at least 10–12 hours.

REFERENCES

1. Needleman P, Johnson EM: The pharmacological and biochemical interaction of organic nitrates with sulfhydryls: Possible correlations with the mechanism for tolerance development, vasodilation and mitochondrial and enzyme reactions. In Needleman P (ed): Organic Nitrates. Handbook of Experimental Pharmacology, vol 40, pp 97–114. New York, Springer Verlag, 1975
2. Armstrong PW, Moffat JA: Tolerance to organic nitrates: Clinical and experimental perspectives. Am J Med 74(suppl):73, 1983
3. Kowaluk E, Fung HL: Pharmacology and pharmacokinetics of organic nitrates. In Abrams J, Pepine C, Thadani V (eds): Medical Therapy of Ischemic Heart Disease. Boston, Little, Brown, in press.
4. Levin RI, Jaffe EA, Weksler BB et al: Nitroglycerin stimulates synthesis of prostaglandin by cultured human endothelial cells. J Clin Invest 67:762, 1981
5. Rehr RB, Jackson JA, Winniford MD et al: Mechanism of nitroglycerin-induced coronary dilatation: Lack of relations to intracoronary thromboxane concentrations. Am J Cardiol 54:971, 1984
6. Lam JYT, Chesebro JH, Fuster V: Platelets, vasoconstriction and nitroglycerin during arterial wall injury. Circulation 78:712, 1988
7. Diodati J, Theroux P, Latour J-G, et al: Nitroglycerin at therapeutic doses inhibits platelet aggregation in man. JACC 11:54A, 1988
8. Johnstone M, Lam JYT, Waters D: The antithrombotic action of nitroglycerin: cyclic GMP as a potential mediator. JACC 13:231A, 1989
9. Fung H-L, Sutton SC, Kamiya A: Blood vessel uptake and metabolism of organic nitrates in the rat. J Pharmacol Exp Ther 228:334, 1984
10. McGregor M: Pathogenesis of angina pectoris and role of nitrates in relief of myocardial ischemia. Am J Med 74(suppl):21, 1983
11. Kelly R, Gibbs R, Morgan J, et al: Brachial artery pressure measurements underestimate beneficial effects of nitroglycerin on left ventricular afterload. JACC 13:231A, 1989
12. Mason DT, Braunwald E: The effects of nitroglycerin and amyl nitrite on

arteriolar and venous tone in the human forearm. Circulation 32:755, 1965

13. Vatner SF, Pagani M, Rutherford JD et al: Effects of nitroglycerin on cardiac performance and regional blood flow distribution in conscious dogs. Am J Physiol 234(3):H244, 1978
14. Ferrer MI, Bradley SE, Wheeler HO et al: Some effects of nitroglycerin upon the splanchnic, pulmonary and systemic circulations. Circulation 33:357, 1966
15. Manyari DE, Smith ER, Spragg J: Isosorbide dinitrate and glyceryl trinitrate: Demonstration of cross tolerance in the capacitance vessels. Am J Cardiol 55:927, 1985
16. Abrams J: Hemodynamic effects of nitroglycerin and long-acting nitrates. Am Heart J 110 (part 2):216, 1985
17. Leier CV, Magorien RD, Desch CE et al: Hydralazine and isosorbide dinitrate: Comparative central and regional hemodynamic effects when administered alone or in combination. Circulation 63:102, 1981
18. Ganz W, Marcus HS: Failure of intracoronary nitroglycerin to alleviate pacing-induced angina. Circulation 46:880, 1972
19. Brown G, Bolson E, Petersen RB et al: The mechanisms of nitroglycerin action: Stenosis vasodilatation as a major component of drug response. Circulation 64:1089, 1981
20. Conti CR, Feldman RL, Pepine CJ et al: Effect of glyceryl trinitrate on coronary and systemic hemodynamics in man. Am J Med 74(suppl):28, 1984
21. Abrams J: The role of nitroglycerin and long-acting nitrates in the treatment of angina. In Weiner DA, Frishman W (eds): Therapy of Angina, pp 53–81. New York, Marcel Dekker, 1986
22. Gage JE, Hess OM, Murakami T, et al: Vasoconstriction of stenotic coronary arteries during dynamic exercise in patients with classic angina pectoris: reversibility by nitroglycerin. Circulation 73:865, 1986
23. Ludmer PL, Selwyn AP, Shook TL, et al: Paradoxical vasoconstriction induced by acetylcholine in atherosclerotic coronary arteries. N Engl J Med 1986; 315:1046
24. Rapaport E, Remedios P: The high risk patient after recovery from myocardial infarction: Recognition and management. J Am Coll Cardiol 1:391, 1983
25. Jugdutt BI, Warnica JW: Intravenous nitroglycerin therapy to limit myocardial infarct size, expansion, and complications. Effect of timing, dosage, and infarct location. Circulation 78:706, 1988
26. Hoekenga D, Abrams J: Rational medical therapy for stable angina pectoris. Am J Med 76:309, 1984
27. Abrams J: Usefulness of long-acting nitrates in cardiovascular disease. Am J Med 64:183, 1978
28. Hill JA, Feldman RL, Pepine CJ et al: Randomized double-blind comparison of nifedipine and isosorbide dinitrate in patients with coronary arterial spasm. Am J Cardiol 49:431, 1982
29. Curfman GD, Heinsimer JA, Lozner EC et al: Intravenous nitroglycerin in the treatment of spontaneous angina pectoris: A prospective randomized trial. Circulation 67:276, 1983
30. Conti CR: Use of nitrates in unstable angina pectoris. Am J Cardiol 60:31H, 1987
31. Horowitz JD, Henry CA, Syranen ML, et al: Combined use of nitroglycerin and N-acetylcysteine in the management of unstable angina pectoris. Circulation 77:787, 1988
32. Flaherty JT: Comparison of intravenous nitroglycerin and sodium nitroprusside in acute myocardial infarction. Am J Med 74(suppl):53, 1983
33. Jugdutt BI: Nitroglycerin in acute myocardial infarction. Can J Cardiol 5:110, 1989
34. Yusuf S, Collins R, MacMahon S, Peto R: Effect of intravenous nitrates on mortality in acute myocardial infarction: an overview of the randomized trials. Lancet I:1088–1092, 1988
35. Cohn JN, Franciosa JA, Francis GA: Effect of short-term infusion of sodium nitroprusside on mortality rate in acute myocardial infarction complicated by left ventricular failure. N Engl J Med 306:1129, 1982
36. Abrams J: Pharmacology of nitroglycerin and long-acting nitrates and their usefulness in the treatment of congestive heart failure. In Gould L, Reddy CVR (eds): Vasodilator therapy for cardiac disorders, pp 129–167. Mt Kisco, NY, Futura Publishing, 1979
37. Packer M: New perspectives on therapeutic application of nitrates as vasodilator agents for severe chronic heart failure. Am J Med 74(suppl):61, 1983
38. Leier CV, Huss P, Magorien RP et al: Improved exercise capacity and differing arterial and venous tolerance during chronic isosorbide dinitrate therapy for congestive heart failure. Circulation 67:817, 1983
39. Cohn JN, et al: Effect of vasodilator therapy on mortality in chronic congestive heart failure. Results of a Veterans Administration cooperative study. N Engl J Med 374:1547, 1986
40. Smith ER, Smiseth OA, Kingma I et al: Mechanisms of action of nitrates: Role of changes in venous capacitance and in the left ventricular diastole pressure-volume relation. Am J Med 76(6A):14, 1984
41. Duchier J, Iannoscoli F, Safar M: Antihypertensive effect of sustained-release isosorbide dinitrate for isolated systolic systemic hypertension in the elderly. Am J Cardiol 60:99–102, 1987
42. Chatterjee K, Parmley WW, Swan HJC et al: Beneficial effects of vasodilator therapy in severe mitral regurgitation due to dysfunction of subvalvular apparatus. Circulation 48:684, 1973
43. Swamy N: Esophageal spasm: Clinical and manometric response to nitroglycerine and long-acting nitrates. Gastroenterology 72:23, 1977
44. Hill NS, Antman EM, Green LH et al: Intravenous nitroglycerin: A review of pharmacology, indications, therapeutic effects and complications. Chest 79:69, 1981
45. Herling IM: Intravenous nitroglycerin: Clinical pharmacology and therapeutic considerations. Am Heart J 108:141, 1984
46. Margolis JR, Chen C: Coronary artery spasm complicating PTCA: role of intracoronary nitroglycerin. Z Kardiol 78 (suppl 2):41, 1989
47. Rentrop KP, Feit F, Sherman W et al: Late thrombolytic therapy preserves left ventricular function in patients with collateralized total coronary occlusion primary and point findings of the Second Mount Sinai-New York University Reperfusion Trial. JACC 14:58, 1989
48. Abrams J: Pharmacology of nitroglycerin and long-acting nitrates. Am J Cardiol 56:12A, 1985
49. Fung H-L: Pharmacokinetic determinants of nitrate action. Am J Med 76(6A):22, 1984
50. Armstrong PW, Moffat JA, Marks GS: Arterial-venous nitroglycerin gradient during intravenous infusion in man. Circulation 66:1273, 1982
51. Chasseaud LF: Newer aspects of the pharmacokinetics of organic nitrates. Z Kardiol 72(suppl 3):20, 1983
52. Thadani U, Fung H-L, Darke AC et al: Oral isosorbide dinitrate in angina pectoris: Comparison of duration of action and dose response relationship during acute and sustained therapy. Am J Cardiol 49:411, 1982
53. Parker JO, Van Koughnett KA, Fung H-L: Transdermal isosorbide dinitrate in angina pectoris: Effect of acute and sustained therapy. Am J Cardiol 54:8, 1984
54. Fung H-L, Ruggirello D, Stone JA et al: Effects of disease, route of administration, cigarette smoking, food intake on the pharmacokinetics and circulatory effects of isosorbide dinitrate. Z Kardiol 72(suppl 3):5, 1983
55. Bogaert MG, Rosseel MT: Fate of orally given isosorbide dinitrate in man: Factors of variability. Z Kardiol 72(suppl 3):11, 1983
56. Abrams J: Nitrate delivery systems in perspective: A decade of progress. Am J Med 76:38, 1984
57. Abrams J: New nitrate delivery systems: Buccal nitroglycerin. Am Heart J 105:848, 1983
58. Reichek N, Goldstein RE, Redwood DR et al: Sustained effects of nitroglycerin ointment in patients with angina pectoris. Circulation 50:348, 1974
59. Abrams J: The brief saga of transdermal nitroglycerin discs: Paradise lost? Am J Cardiol 54:220, 1984
60. Abrams J: Transcutaneous nitroglycerin: Ointment or disc? Am Heart J 108:1597, 1984
61. Reichek N, Priest C, Zimrin D et al: Limited antianginal effects of nitroglycerin patches. Am J Cardiol 54:1, 1984
62. Parker JO, Fung H-L: Transdermal nitroglycerin in angina pectoris. Am J Cardiol 54:471, 1984
63. Multicenter Transdermal Nitroglycerin Trial (in press)
64. Schaer DH, Buff LA, Katz RJ: Sustained antianginal efficacy of transdermal nitroglycerin patches using an overnight 10-hour nitrate-free interval. Am J Cardiol 61:46, 1988
65. Sharpe N, Coxon R, Webster M, Luke R: Hemodynamic effects of intermittent transdermal nitroglycerin in chronic congestive heart failure. Am J Cardiol 59:895, 1987
66. DeMots H, Glasser SP: Intermittent transdermal nitroglycerin therapy in the treatment of chronic stable angina. JACC 13:786, 1989
67. Young JB, Pratt CM, Farmer JA et al: Specialized delivery systems for intravenous nitroglycerin: Are they necessary? Am J Med 76:27, 1984
68. Come PC, Pitt B: Nitroglycerin-induced severe hypotension and bradycardia in patients with acute myocardial infarction. Circulation 54:624, 1976
69. Arsura E, Lichstein E, Guadagnino V et al: Methemoglobin levels produced by organic nitrates in patients with coronary artery disease. J Clin Pharmacol 24:160, 1984
70. Abrams J: Nitrate tolerance and dependence. Am Heart J 99:113, 1980
71. Abrams J: Nitrate tolerance in angina pectoris. In Cohn J, Rittinghausen R (eds): Mononitrates, pp 154–170. Berlin, Springer-Verlag, 1985.
72. Blasini R, Froer KL, Blume I et al: Wirkungsverlust von Isosorbiddinitrat bei Lanzeitbetrandlung der chronischen Herzinsuffizienz. Herz 7:250, 1982
73. Armstrong PW, Moffat JA: Tolerance to organic nitrates: Clinical and experimental perspectives. Am J Med 74(suppl):73, 1983
74. Parker JO: Intermitent transdermal nitroglycerin therapy in the treatment of chronic stable angina. JACC 13:794, 1989
75. Elkayam U, Jamison M, Roth A et al: Oral isosorbide dinitrate in chronic heart failure: tolerance development to QID vs TID regimen. JACC 13:178A, 1989

THE α- AND β-ADRENERGIC BLOCKING DRUGS

William H. Frishman • Shlomo Charlap

CHAPTER 16 — VOLUME 1

Catecholamines are neurohumoral substances that mediate a variety of physiologic and metabolic responses in humans. The effects of the catecholamines ultimately depend on their physiologic interactions with receptors, which are discrete macromolecular components located on the plasma membrane. Differences in the ability of the various catecholamines to stimulate a number of physiologic processes were the criteria used by Ahlquist in 1948 to separate these receptors into two distinct types: α- and β-adrenergic.[1] Subsequent studies suggested that β-adrenergic receptors exist as two discrete subtypes called β_1 and β_2.[2] It is now also appreciated that there are two subtypes of α-receptors, designated α_1 and α_2.[3] Specific drugs are available that will inhibit or block these receptors. In this chapter we examine the adrenergic receptors and the drugs that can inhibit their function. The rationale for use and clinical experience with α- and β-adrenergic blocking drugs in the treatment of various cardiovascular and noncardiovascular disorders is also discussed.

α-ADRENERGIC BLOCKERS
CLINICAL PHARMACOLOGY

When a nerve is stimulated, catecholamines are released from their storage granules in the adrenergic neuron, enter the synaptic cleft, and bind to α-receptors on the effector cell.[4] A feedback loop exists by which the amount of neurotransmitter released can be regulated: accumulation of catecholamines in the synaptic cleft leads to stimulation of α-receptors in the neuronal surface and inhibition of further catecholamine release. Catecholamines from the circulation can also enter the synaptic cleft and bind to presynaptic or postsynaptic receptors.

Initially it was believed that α_1-receptors were limited to postsynaptic sites where they mediated vasoconstriction, whereas the α_2-receptors only existed at the prejunctional nerve terminals and mediated the negative feedback control of norepinephrine release. The availability of compounds with high specificity for either α_1- or α_2-receptors demonstrated that while presynaptic α-receptors are almost exclusively of the α_2-subtype, the postsynaptic receptors are made up of comparable numbers of α_1- and α_2-receptors.[4] Stimulation of the presynaptic α_2-receptors causes vasoconstriction. However, a functional difference does exist between the two types of postsynaptic receptors. The α_1-receptors appear to exist primarily within the region of the synapse and respond preferentially to neuronally released catecholamine, whereas α_2-receptors are located extrasynaptically and respond preferentially to circulating catecholamines in the plasma.

Drugs having α-adrenergic blocking properties are of several types (Fig. 16.1)[4–12]:

1. Nonselective α-blockers having prominent effects on both the α_1- and α_2-receptors (e.g., the older drugs such as phenoxybenzamine and phentolamine). Although virtually all of the clinical effects of phenoxybenzamine are explicable in terms of α-blockade, this is not the case with phentolamine, which also possesses several other properties, including a direct vasodilator action and sympathomimetic and parasympathomimetic effects.

2. Selective α_1-blockers having little affinity for α_2-receptors (e.g., prazosin, terazosin, and other quinazoline derivatives). Originally introduced as direct-acting vasodilators, it is now clear that these drugs exert their major effect by reversible blockade of postsynaptic α_1-receptors. Other selective α_1-blockers include indoramin, doxazosin, trimazosin, and urapadil (Table 16.1). Urapadil is of interest because of its other actions, which include stimulation of presynaptic α_2-adrenergic receptors and a central effect.

3. Selective α_2-blockers (e.g., yohimbine). The primary use of these drugs has been as tools in experimental pharmacology. Yohimbine is now marketed in the United States as an oral sympatholytic and mydriatic agent. Male patients with impotence from vascular or diabetic origins or from psychogenic origin have been treated successfully with yohimbine.

4. Blockers that inhibit both α- and β-adrenergic receptors (e.g., labetalol). Labetalol, like prazosin and terazosin, is a selective α_1-blocker. Since this agent is more potent as a β-blocker than an α-blocker, it is discussed in greater detail in the section on β-blockers.

5. Agents having α-adrenergic blocking properties but whose major clinical use appears unrelated to these properties (e.g., chlorpromazine, haloperidol, quinidine, bromocriptine, amiodarone, and ketanserin, a selective blocking agent of serotonin-2 receptors). It has been demonstrated that verapamil, a calcium channel blocker, also has α-adrenergic blocking properties. Whether this is a particular property of verapamil and its analogues or is common to all calcium channel blockers is not clear.[13] Also to be clarified is whether verapamil-induced α-blockade occurs at physiologic plasma levels and helps to mediate the vasodilator properties of the drug.

All the α-blockers in clinical use inhibit the postsynaptic α_1-receptor and result in relaxation of vascular smooth muscle and vasodilation. However, the nonselective α-blockers also antagonize the presynaptic α_2-receptors, allowing for increased release of neuronal norepinephrine. This results in attenuation of the desired postsynaptic blockade and spillover stimulation of the β-receptors and, consequently, in troublesome side effects such as tachycardia and tremulousness and increased renin release. The α_1-selective agents that preserve the α_2-mediated presynaptic feedback loop prevent excessive norepinephrine release and thus avoid these adverse cardiac and systemic effects.

Because of these potent peripheral vasodilatory properties, however, one would anticipate that even the selective α_1-blockers would induce reflex stimulation of the sympathetic and renin–angiotensin system similar to that seen with other vasodilators such as hydralazine and minoxidil. The explanation for the relative lack of tachycardia and renin release observed after prazosin and terazosin may, in part, be due to the drugs' combined action of reducing vascular tone in both resistance (arteries) and capacitance (veins) beds. Such a dual action may prevent the marked increases in venous return and cardiac output observed with agents that act more selectively to reduce vascular tone only in the resistance vessels. The lack of tachycardia with prazosin and terazosin use has also been attributed by some investigators to a significant negative chronotropic action of the drug independent of its peripheral vascular effect.[14]

USE IN CARDIOVASCULAR DISORDERS

HYPERTENSION

Increased peripheral vascular resistance is present in the majority of patients with long-standing hypertension. Since dilation of constricted arterioles should result in lowering of elevated blood pressure, interest has focused on the use of α-adrenergic blockers in the medical treatment of systemic hypertension. The experience with nonselective α-blockers in the treatment of hypertension was disappointing because of accompanying reflex stimulation of the sympathetic and renin–angiotensin system, resulting in frequent side effects and limited long-term antihypertensive efficacy. However, the selective α_1-blockers prazosin and terazosin have been shown to be effective antihypertensive agents.[4,5,12]

Prazosin and terazosin decrease blood pressure in both the standing and supine positions, although blood pressure decrement tends to be somewhat greater in the upright position. Because their antihypertensive effect is accompanied by little or no increase in heart rate, plasma renin activity, or circulating catecholamines, prazosin and terazosin have been found useful as first-step agents in hypertension.

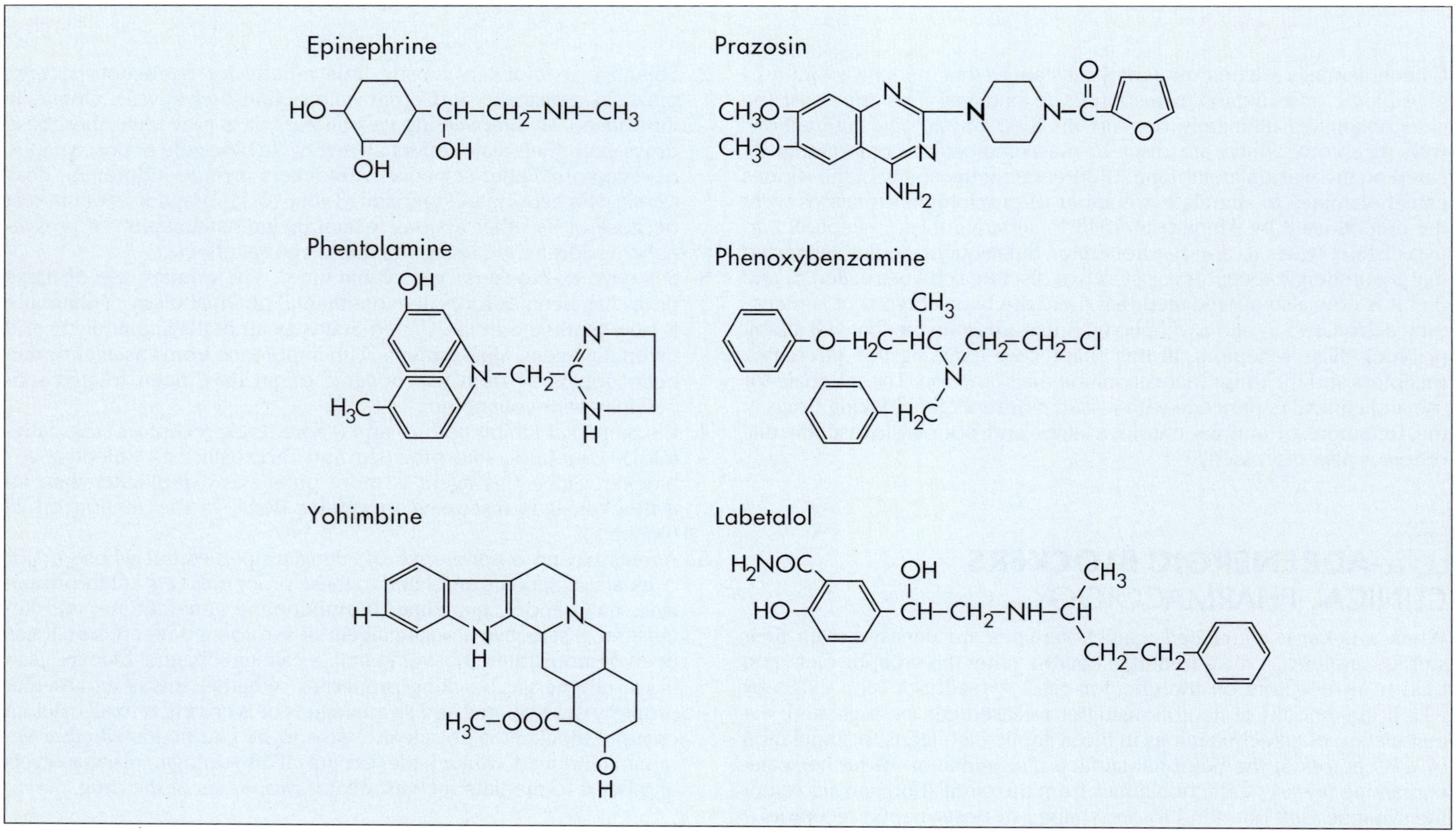

FIGURE 16.1 Molecular structure of the α-adrenergic agonist epinephrine and some α-blockers.

TABLE 16.1 PHARMACOKINETICS OF SELECTIVE α_1-ADRENERGIC BLOCKING DRUGS

Selective α_1-Blocker	Daily Dose (mg)	Frequency per Day	Bioavailability (% of Oral Dose)	Plasma Half-life	Urinary Excretion (% of Oral Dose)
Doxazosin*	1–16	1	65	10–12	NA
Indoramin*	50–125	2–3	NA	5.0	11
Prazosin	2–20	2–3	44–69	2.5–4	10
Prazosin GITS†	2.5–20	1			
Terazosin	1–20	1	90	12	39
Trimazosin*	100–900	2–3	61	2.7	NA

* Investigational drug

† Gastrointestinal therapeutic system

NA, Not available

(Adapted from Luther RR: New perspectives on selective α_1-blockade. Am J Hypertens 2:731, 1989)

Monotherapy with these agents, however, promotes sodium and water retention in some patients, although it is less pronounced than with other vasodilators. The concomitant use of a diuretic prevents fluid retention and in many cases markedly enhances the antihypertensive effect of the drugs. In clinical practice, prazosin and terazosin have their widest application as adjuncts to one or more established antihypertensive drugs in treating moderate-to-severe hypertension. Their effects are additive to those of diuretics, β-blockers, α-methyldopa, and the direct-acting vasodilators. The drugs cause little change in glomerular filtration rate or renal plasma flow and can be used safely in patients with severe renal hypertension. There is no evidence for attenuation of the antihypertensive effect of prazosin or terazosin during chronic therapy.

Selective α_1-blockers appear to have neutral or even favorable effects on plasma lipids and lipoproteins when administered to hypertensive patients. Investigators have reported mild reductions in levels of total cholesterol, low-density lipoprotein (LDL) and very-low-density lipoprotein (VLDL) cholesterol, and triglycerides and elevations in levels of high-density lipoprotein (HDL) cholesterol with prazosin, doxazosin, and terazosin.[15] With long-term use, selective α_1-blockers also appear to decrease left ventricular mass in patients with hypertension and left ventricular hypertrophy.[16]

A number of prazosin and terazosin analogues have been developed (e.g., trimazosin and doxazosin) that in preliminary clinical trials have also shown promise as antihypertensive agents.[9,10] Doxazosin and terazosin have a longer duration of action than prazosin and have been shown to produce sustained blood pressure reductions with single daily administration. Indoramin, also a selective α_1-blocker, has been found to be effective in the treatment of systemic hypertension, but it produces many unwanted effects, such as lethargy and impotence, which may limit its clinical value. In contrast to prazosin, the drug appears to have little dilative effect on the venous circulation. Only prazosin and terazosin are available for clinical use in the United States.

A new formulation of prazosin, prazosin GITS (gastrointestinal therapeutic system) is now undergoing clinical trials and may soon be released.[7] This is an extended once-daily formulation designed as an osmotic pump. Through this innovative delivery system, prazosin is released at an approximately steady rate over a 16-hour period, allowing once-daily clinical administration in hypertension.[7]

CONGESTIVE HEART FAILURE

α-Adrenergic blocking drugs appear particularly attractive for use in the treatment of heart failure because they hold the possibility of reproducing balanced reductions in resistance and capacitance beds. In fact, phentolamine was one of the earlier vasodilators to be shown effective in the treatment of heart failure.[17,18] The drug was infused into normotensive patients with persistent left ventricular dysfunction after a myocardial infarction and found to induce a significant fall in systemic vascular resistance accompanied by considerable elevation in cardiac output and a reduction in pulmonary artery pressure.[18] Because of its high cost and the frequent side effects that it produces, especially tachycardia, phentolamine is no longer used in the treatment of heart failure. Oral phenoxybenzamine has also been used as vasodilator therapy in heart failure; like phentolamine, it has been replaced by newer vasodilator agents.

Studies evaluating the acute hemodynamic effects of prazosin in patients with congestive heart failure consistently find significant reductions in systemic and pulmonary vascular resistances and left ventricular filling pressures associated with increases in stroke volume.[14] In most studies, there is no change or a decrease in heart rate. The response pattern seen with prazosin is similar to that observed with nitroprusside with the exception that the heart rate tends to be higher with the use of nitroprusside and, therefore, the observed increases in cardiac output are also higher.

Controversy still exists as to whether the initial clinical and hemodynamic improvements seen with prazosin are sustained during long-term therapy.[19] Whereas some studies have demonstrated continued efficacy of prazosin therapy after chronic use, others have found little hemodynamic difference between prazosin- and placebo-treated patients. Some investigators believe that whatever tolerance to the drug does develop is most likely secondary to activation of counterposing neurohumoral forces; if the dose is raised and the tendency toward sodium and water retention is countered by appropriate increases in diuretic dose, prazosin is likely to remain effective. Others argue that sustained increases in plasma renin activity or plasma catecholamines are not seen during long-term therapy and that tolerance is not prevented or reversed by a diuretic. Some clinical studies suggest that patients with initially high plasma renin activity experience attenuation of beneficial hemodynamic effects more frequently. What appears clear is the need to evaluate patients individually as to the continued efficacy of their prazosin therapy. Whether there are subgroups of patients with heart failure (e.g., those with highly activated sympathetic nervous systems) that are more likely to respond to prazosin or other α-blockers remains to be determined.

A multicenter study from the Veterans Administration Hospitals has shown that prazosin, when compared with placebo therapy, did not reduce mortality with long-term use in patients with advanced forms of congestive heart failure.[20] In the same study, a favorable effect on mortality was seen with an isosorbide dinitrate–hydralazine combination.[20]

There is increasing evidence that α_1-adrenergic receptors, different from those of other tissues, also exist in the myocardium and that an increase in the force of contraction may be produced by stimulation of these sites.[21] The mechanism of α-adrenergic positive inotropic response is unknown. What the biologic significance of α-adrenergic receptors in cardiac muscle is and whether these receptors play a role in the response to α-blocker therapy in congestive heart failure also remain to be determined.

ANGINA PECTORIS

α-Adrenergic receptors help mediate coronary vasoconstriction. It has been suggested that a pathologic alteration of the α-adrenergic system may be the mechanism of coronary spasm in some patients with variant angina.[22] In uncontrolled studies, the administration of α-adrenergic blockers, both acutely and chronically, has been shown effective in reversing and preventing coronary spasm. However, in a long-term randomized, double-blind trial prazosin was found to exert no obvious beneficial effect in patients with variant angina.[23] The demonstration of an important role for the postsynaptic α_2-receptors in determining coronary vascular tone may help explain prazosin's lack of efficacy. Further study in this area is anticipated.

ARRHYTHMIAS

It has been postulated that enhanced α-adrenergic responsiveness occurs during myocardial ischemia and that it is a primary mediator of the electrophysiologic derangements and resulting malignant arrhythmias induced by catecholamines during myocardial ischemia and reperfusion.[24] In humans, there have been favorable reports of the use of an α-blocker in the treatment of supraventricular and ventricular ectopy. Whether there is a significant role for α-adrenergic blockers in the treatment of cardiac arrhythmias will be determined through further clinical study.

USE IN NONCARDIOVASCULAR DISORDERS
PHEOCHROMOCYTOMA

α-Blockers have been used in the treatment of pheochromocytoma to control the peripheral effects of the excess catecholamines.[25] In fact, intravenous phentolamine was used as a test for this disorder but the test is now rarely done because of reported cases of cardiovascular collapse and death in patients who exhibited exaggerated sensitivity to the drug. The drug is still rarely used in cases of pheochromocytoma-related hypertensive crisis. However, for long-term therapy, oral phenoxybenzamine is the preferred agent. β-Blocking agents may also be needed in pheochromocytoma for control of tachycardia and arrhythmias. All β-blockers, but primarily the nonselective agents, should not be initiated prior to adequate α-blockade since severe hypertension may occur as a result of the unopposed α-stimulating activity of the circulating catecholamines.

SHOCK

In shock, hyperactivity of the sympathetic nervous system occurs as a compensatory reflex response to reduced blood pressure. Use of β-blockers in shock has been advocated as a means of lowering peripheral vascular resistance and increasing vascular capacitance while not antagonizing the cardiotonic effects of the sympathomimetic amines. Although investigated for many years for the treatment of shock, α-adrenergic blockers are still not approved for this purpose.[26] A prime concern when using α-blockers for shock is that the rapid drug-induced increase in vascular capacitance may lead to inadequate cardiac filling and profound hypotension, especially in the hypovolemic patient. Adequate amounts of fluid replacement prior to use of an α-blocker can minimize this concern.

LUNG DISEASE

PULMONARY HYPERTENSION. The part played by endogenous circulating catecholamines in the maintenance of pulmonary vascular tone appears to be minimal. Studies evaluating the effects of norepinephrine administration on pulmonary vascular resistance have found the drug to have little or no effect. The beneficial effects on the pulmonary circulation that phentolamine and other α-blockers have demonstrated in some studies is most likely primarily due to their direct vasodilative actions rather than to α-blockade.[27] Like other vasodilators, in patients with pulmonary hypertension due to fixed anatomical changes, α-blockers can produce hemodynamic deterioration secondary to their systemic vasodilative properties.[28]

BRONCHOSPASM. Bronchoconstriction is mediated in part through catecholamine stimulation of α-receptors in the lung. It has been suggested that in patients with allergic asthma, a deficient β-adrenergic system or enhanced α-adrenergic responsiveness could result in α-adrenergic activity being the mean mechanism of bronchoconstriction.[29] Several studies have shown bronchodilation or inhibition of histamine and allergen- or exercise-induced bronchospasm with a variety of α-blockers.[30] Additional studies are needed to define more fully the role of α-blockers for use as bronchodilators.

ARTERIOCONSTRICTION

Oral α-adrenergic blockers can produce subjective and clinical improvement in patients experiencing episodic arterioconstriction (Raynaud's phenomenon). α-Blockers may also be of value in the treatment of severe peripheral ischemia caused by an α-agonist (e.g., norepinephrine) or ergotamine overdose. In cases of inadvertent infiltration of a norepinephrine infusion, phentolamine can be given intradermally to avoid tissue sloughing.

BENIGN PROSTATIC OBSTRUCTION

α-Adrenergic receptors have been identified in the bladder neck and prostatic capsule of male patients. In clinical studies, use of α-blockers in patients with benign prostatic obstruction has resulted in increased urinary flow rates and reductions in residual volume and obstructive symptoms.[31] It would appear that α-blockers may have an important role in the medical treatment of patients with benign prostatic obstruction.

CLINICAL USE AND ADVERSE EFFECTS

Oral phenoxybenzamine has a rapid onset of action, with the maximal effect from a single dose seen in 1 to 2 hours.[32,33] The gastrointestinal absorption is incomplete, and only 20% to 30% of an oral dose reaches the systemic circulation in active form. The half-life of the drug is 24 hours, with the usual dose varying between 20 and 200 mg daily in one or two doses. Intravenous phentolamine is initially started at 0.1 mg/min and is then increased at increments of 0.1 mg/min every 5 to 10 minutes until the desired hemodynamic effect is reached. The drug has a short duration of action of 3 to 10 minutes. Little is known about the pharmacokinetics of long-term oral use of phentolamine. The main side effects of the drug include postural hypotension, tachycardia, gastrointestinal disturbances, and sexual dysfunction. Intravenous infusion of norepinephrine can be used to combat severe hypotensive reactions. Oral phenoxybenzamine is approved for use in pheochromocytoma.

Prazosin is almost completely absorbed following oral administration, with peak plasma levels achieved at 2 to 3 hours. The drug is 90% protein bound. Prazosin is extensively metabolized by the liver. The usual half-life of the drug is 2½ to 4 hours; in patients with heart failure, the half-life increases to the range of 5 to 7 hours.

The major side effect of prazosin is the first-dose phenomenon—severe postural hypotension occasionally associated with syncope seen after the initial dose or after a rapid dose increment.[4,5] The reason for this phenomenon has not been clearly established but may involve the rapid induction of venous and arteriolar dilatation by a drug that elicits little reflex sympathetic stimulation. It is reported more often when the drug is administered as a tablet rather than a capsule, possibly related to the variable bioavailability or rates of absorption of the two formulations.[4] (In the United States, the drug is available in capsule form.) The postural hypotension can be minimized if the initial dose of prazosin is not higher than 1 mg and if it is given at bedtime. In treating hypertension, a dose of 2 to 3 mg/day should be maintained for 1 to 2 weeks, followed by a gradual increase in dosage titrated to achieve the desired reductions in pressures, usually up to 20 to 30 mg/day, given in two or three doses. In treating heart failure, larger doses (2–7 mg) may be used to initiate therapy in recumbent patients, but the maintenance dose is also usually not more than 30 mg. Higher doses do not seem to produce additional clinical improvement.

Other side effects of prazosin include dizziness, headache, and drowsiness. The drug produces no deleterious effects on the clinical course of diabetes mellitus, chronic obstructive pulmonary disease, renal failure, or gout. It does not adversely affect the lipid profile. Prazosin is presently approved for use in hypertension. Prazosin GITS may soon become available for once-daily use in systemic hypertension. With this formulation, there are narrower peak-to-trough fluctuations in drug plasma levels, which may be associated with less postural hypotension.[7]

Terazosin, which has been approved for once-daily use in hypertension, may be associated with a lesser incidence of first-dose postural hypotension than prazosin.[12] The usual recommended dose range is 1 to 5 mg administered once a day; some patients may benefit from doses as high as 20 mg daily or from divided doses.

Doxazosin, another long-acting α_1-blocker, may soon become available.

The α_2-blocker yohimbine, 5.4 mg orally, is used three times daily to treat male impotence. Urologists have used yohimbine for the diagnostic classification of certain cases of male erectile impotence. Increases in heart rate and blood pressure, piloerection, and rhinorrhea are the most common adverse reactions. Yohimbine should not be used with antidepressant drugs.

β-ADRENERGIC BLOCKERS
CLINICAL PHARMACOLOGY

The β-adrenergic receptor blocking drugs (Fig. 16.2) differ from one another in respect to several pharmacodynamic and pharmacokinetic properties.[34–36] The properties considered here are potency, membrane stabilizing activity, selectivity, intrinsic sympathomimetic activity, and, finally, pharmacokinetic characteristics (Tables 16.2 and 16.3).

POTENCY

β-Adrenergic receptor blocking drugs are competitive inhibitors of catecholamine binding at β-adrenergic receptor sites. In the presence of a β-blocker, the dose-response curve of the catecholamine is shifted to the right; that is, a higher concentration of the catecholamine is required to provoke the response. The potency of a β-blocker tells us how much of the drug must be administered in order to inhibit the effects of an adrenergic agonist. Potency can be assessed by noting the dose of the drug that is needed to inhibit tachycardia produced by an agonist or by exercise. It has been found that potency differs from drug to drug, with pindolol being the most potent and esmolol the least potent. While differences in potency explain the different dosages needed to achieve effective β-adrenergic blockade, they have no therapeutic relevance, except when switching patients from one drug to another.

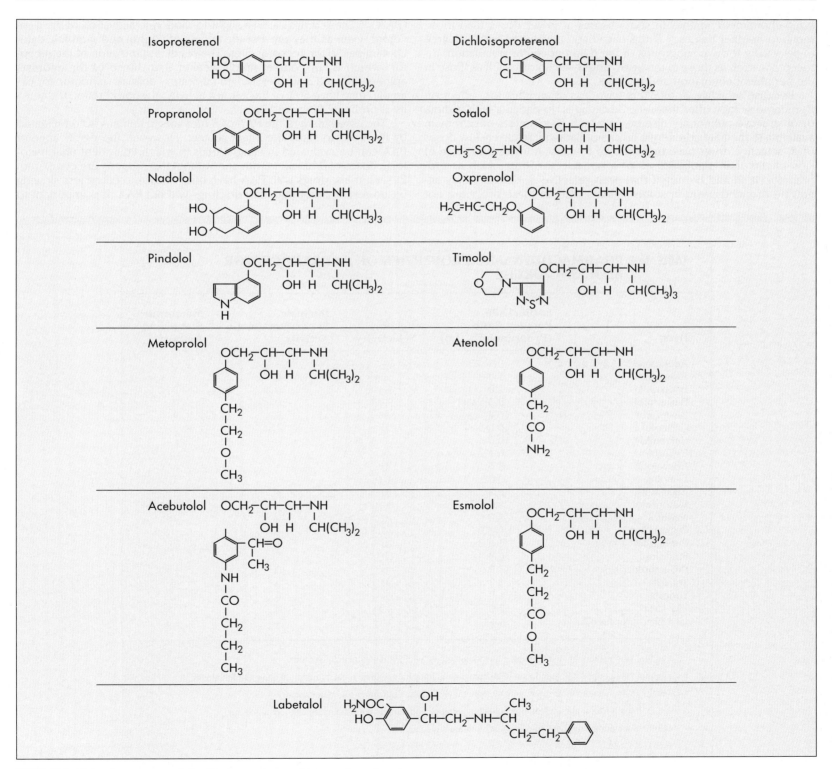

FIGURE 16.2 Molecular structure of the β-adrenergic agonist isoproterenol and some β-blockers.

MEMBRANE STABILIZING ACTIVITY

At very high concentrations, certain β-blockers have a quinidine or local anesthetic effect on the cardiac action potential. There is no evidence that membrane stabilizing activity is responsible for any direct negative inotropic effect of the β-blockers, since drugs with and without this property equally depress left ventricular function. In therapeutic situations, the concentration of the β-blocker is probably too small to produce the membrane stabilizing activity. Only during massive β-blocker intoxication is the activity manifested.

SELECTIVITY

The β-adrenoceptor blockers can be classified as selective or nonselective, according to their relative abilities to antagonize the actions of sympathomimetic amines in some tissues at lower doses than those required in other tissues.[37] Drugs have been developed with a degree of selectivity for two subgroups of the β-adrenoceptor population: β_1-receptors, such as those in the heart, and β_2-receptors, such as those in the peripheral circulation and bronchi.

Because selective β_1-blockers have less of an inhibitory effect on β_2-receptors, they offer theoretic advantages. In patients with asthma or obstructive pulmonary disease, in which β_2-receptors must remain available to mediate adrenergic bronchodilatation, relatively low doses of β_1-selective drugs have been shown to cause a lower incidence of side effects than similar doses of a nonselective drug, such as propranolol. It should be noted that even selective β_1-blockers may aggravate bronchospasm in some patients; and so these drugs are not generally recommended for patients with asthma and other bronchospastic disease.

Selective β_1-blockers also have less of an inhibitory effect on the β_2-receptors that mediate dilation of arterioles and are thus less likely to impair peripheral blood flow. In the presence of epinephrine, nonselective β-blockers can cause a vasopressor response by blocking β_2-receptor mediated vasodilation (since α-adrenergic vasoconstriction receptors remain operative). Selective β_1-blockers may not induce this effect. Whether this offers an advantage in treating hypertension is yet to be demonstrated.

INTRINSIC SYMPATHOMIMETIC ACTIVITY

Certain β-adrenoceptor blockers possess partial agonist activity (PAA).[38] These drugs cause a slight-to-moderate activation of the β-receptor, even as they prevent the access of natural and synthetic catecholamines to the receptor sites. The result is stimulation of the receptor, which is, of course, much weaker than those of the agonists epinephrine and isoproterenol. In laboratory animals, pindolol, for example, may have 50% of the agonist activity of isoproterenol; the activity is probably lower in humans.

The assessment of the PAA of β-blockers in humans is complicated by the need to study the intact subject. However, the significance of PAA can be evaluated in clinical trials in which equivalent pharmacologic doses of β-blockers with and without this property are compared. In such trials, drugs with PAA have been shown to cause less slowing of the resting heart rate than do drugs without PAA. It is important to

TABLE 16.2 PHARMACODYNAMIC PROPERTIES OF β-ADRENOCEPTOR BLOCKING DRUGS

Drug	β_1-Blockade Potency Ratio (Propranolol = 1.0)	Relative β_1 Selectivity	Intrinsic Sympathomimetic Activity	Membrane Stabilizing Activity
Acebutolol	0.3	+	+	+
Atenolol	1.0	++	0	0
Betaxolol	1.0	++	0	+
Bevantolol	0.3	++	0	0
Bisoprolol	10.0	++	0	0
Carteolol	10.0	0	+	0
Carvedilol*	10.0	0	0	++
Celiprolol†	0.4	+	+	0
Dilevalol‡	1.0	0	+	0
Esmolol	0.02	++	0	0
Labetalol§	0.3	0	+	0
Metoprolol	1.0	++	0	0
Nadolol	1.0	0	0	0
Oxprenolol	0.5–1.0	0	+	+
Penbutolol	1.0	0	+	0
Pindolol	6.0	0	++	+
Propranolol	1.0	0	0	++
Sotalol¶	0.3	0	0	0
Timolol	6.0	0	0	0
YM 151‖	1.0	++	0	0
Isomer: D-propranolol	—	—	—	++

* Carvedilol has additional α_1-adrenergic blocking activity without peripheral β_2 agonism.

† Celiprolol has peripheral β_2 agonism and may have additional α_2-adrenergic blocking activity at high doses.

‡ Dilevalol is an isomer of labetalol with peripheral β_2 agonism but no α_1-blocking activity.

§ Labetalol has additional α_1-adrenergic blocking activity and direct vasodilatory actions (β_2 agonism).

¶ Sotalol has an additional type of antiarrhythmic activity.

‖ YM 151 has additional dihydropyridine calcium channel blocker activity.

(Frishman WH: Clinical Pharmacology of the β-Adrenoceptor Blocking Drugs, 2nd ed. Norwalk, CT, Appleton-Century-Crofts, 1984)

note, by contrast, that both types of β-blockers similarly reduce the increases in heart rate that occur with exercise or isoproterenol. An explanation for these findings is that the importance of the PAA of pindolol, for example, relative to its β-blocker action, is greatest when sympathetic tone is low, as it is in the resting subject. During exercise, when sympathetic tone is high, the β-blocking effect of pindolol predominates over its PAA. It is for this reason that all β-blockers have been found to be equally effective in reducing the increases in heart rate and blood pressure that occur with exercise.

Whether PAA in a β-blocker offers an overall advantage in cardiac therapy remains a matter of controversy.[38] Some investigators suggest that drugs with this property may reduce peripheral vascular resistance and may depress atrioventricular conduction less than other β-blockers. Other investigators claim that PAA in a β-blocker protects against myocardial depression, bronchial asthma, and peripheral vascular complications in patients receiving therapy. However, these claims have not yet been substantiated by definitive clinical trials.

α-ADRENERGIC ACTIVITY

Labetalol is the first of a group of β-blockers that acts as comparative pharmacologic antagonist at both α- and β-adrenergic receptors.[39] Labetalol is 4 to 16 times more potent at β-adrenergic receptors than at α-adrenergic receptors. In a series of tests, the drug has been shown to be 6 to 10 times less potent than phentolamine at α-adrenergic receptors and 1½ to 4 times less potent than propranolol at β-adrenergic receptors.

Whether concomitant α-adrenergic activity is generally advantageous in a β-blocker is yet to be determined. In the case of labetalol, the additional α-adrenergic blocking action does result in a reduction of peripheral vascular resistance that may be useful in the treatment of hypertensive emergencies, and, unlike other β-blockers, the drug may maintain cardiac output. It has also been suggested that unlike other β-blockers, labetalol may be effective in the black patient with hypertension. Its overall efficacy in the treatment of arrhythmias, hypertension, and angina pectoris is similar to that of other β-blockers.[35,39]

An isomer of labetalol, dilevalol, a β-blocking drug that has direct vasodilating activity mediated by partial $β_2$-agonist activity but no α-adrenergic blocking effects, is being evaluated in clinical trials.

COMBINED β-ADRENERGIC AND CALCIUM CHANNEL BLOCKADE

An agent, YM 151, has been developed that demonstrates the pharmacologic properties of a $β_1$-selective adrenergic blocker and a dihydropyridine-like calcium channel blocker (see Table 16.2). This unique compound is now undergoing investigation in hypertension and angina pectoris.

PHARMACOKINETIC PROPERTIES

Although the β-adrenergic blocking drugs have similar therapeutic effects, their pharmacokinetic properties differ significantly (see Table 16.3),[35,40] that is, in ways that may influence their clinical usefulness in some patients. On the basis of their pharmacokinetic properties, the β-blockers can be classified into two broad categories: those eliminated by the hepatic metabolism and those eliminated unchanged by the kidney. Drugs in the first group, for example, propranolol and metoprolol, are lipid soluble, are almost completely absorbed by the small intestine, and are largely metabolized by the liver. They tend to have highly variable bioavailability and relatively short plasma half-lives. In contrast, drugs in the second category are more water soluble, are incompletely absorbed through the gut, and are eliminated unchanged by the kidney. They show less variable bioavailability and have longer half-lives.

Many of the β-blockers, including those with short plasma half-lives, can be administered as infrequently as once or twice daily. Of

TABLE 16.3 PHARMACOKINETIC PROPERTIES OF VARIOUS β-ADRENOCEPTOR BLOCKING DRUGS

Drug	Extent of Absorption (% of Dose)	Extent of Bioavailability (% of Dose)	Dose-Dependent Bioavailability (Major First-Pass Hepatic Metabolism)	Interpatient Variations in Plasma Levels	β-Blocking Plasma Concentrations	Protein Binding (%)	Lipid Solubility*
Acebutolol	≃70	≃40	No	7-fold	0.2–2.0 μg/ml	25	Moderate
Atenolol	≃50	≃40	No	4-fold	0.2–5.0 μg/ml	<5	Weak
Betaxolol	>90	≃80	No	2-fold	5–20 ng/ml	50	Moderate
Bevantolol	≃90	≃55	No	4-fold	0.13–3.0 μg/ml	95	Moderate
Carteolol	≃90	≃90	No	2-fold	40–160 ng/ml	20–30	Weak
Celiprolol	≃30	≃30	No	3-fold		≃30	Weak
Dilevalol	≃100	≃12	Yes	10-fold	5–15 ng/ml	62	Weak
Esmolol†	NA	NA	NA	5-fold	0.15–1.0 μg/ml	55	Weak
Labetalol	>90	≃33	Yes	10-fold	0.7–3.0 μg/ml	≃50	Weak
Metoprolol	>90	≃50	No	7-fold	50–100 ng/ml	12	Moderate
Nadolol	≃30	≃30	No	7-fold	50–100 ng/ml	≃30	Weak
Oxprenolol	≃90	≃40	No	5-fold	80–100 ng/ml	80	Moderate
Penbutolol	>90	≃90	No	4-fold		98	High
Pindolol	>90	≃90	No	4-fold	5–15 ng/ml	57	Moderate
Propranolol	>90	≃30	Yes	20-fold	50–100 ng/ml	93	High
Long-acting propranolol	>90	≃20	Yes	10- to 20-fold	20–100 ng/ml	93	High
Sotalol	≃70	≃60	No	4-fold	0.5–4.0 μg/ml	0	Weak
Timolol	>90	≃75	No	7-fold	5–10 ng/ml	≃10	Weak

* Determined by the distribution ratio between octanol and water.

† Ultra-short-acting β-blocker available only in intravenous form.

NA, Not applicable.

(Frishman WH: Clinical Pharmacology of the β-Adrenoceptor Blocking Drugs, 2nd ed. Norwalk, CT, Appleton-Century-Crofts, 1984)

course, the longer the half-life, the more useful the drug is likely to be for patients who experience difficulty in complying with β-blocker therapy. A recent addition to the list of available β-blockers is a long-acting, sustained-release preparation of propranolol that provides β-blockade for 24 hours. Studies have shown that this compound provides a much smoother curve of daily plasma levels than comparable divided doses of conventional propranolol and that it has fewer side effects.

Ultra-short-acting β-blockers, with a half-life of no more than 10 minutes, also offer advantages to the clinician, for example, in patients with questionable congestive heart failure in whom β-blockers may be harmful. Such drugs are now being tested, and one, esmolol, has already been approved for clinical use in patients with supraventricular tachycardias.[41] The short half-life of esmolol relates to the rapid metabolism of the drug by blood tissue and hepatic esterases.

In medical practice, the pharmacokinetic properties of the different β-adrenergic blockers become important. The dose of the drug, for example, depends on its first-pass metabolism; if the first-pass effect is extensive, not much of an orally administered drug will reach the systemic circulation and so dosage will have to be larger than the intravenous dose would be. Knowing if the drug is transformed into active metabolites as opposed to inactive metabolites is important in gauging the total pharmacologic effect. Finally, for some β-blockers, lipid solubility has been associated with the entry of these drugs into the brain, resulting in side effects that are probably unrelated to β-blockade, such as lethargy, mental depression, and even hallucinations. Whether drugs that are less lipid soluble cause fewer of these adverse reactions remains to be determined.

USE IN CARDIOVASCULAR DISORDERS
HYPERTENSION

It is now well recognized that β-adrenergic blockers are effective in reducing the blood pressure of many patients with systemic hypertension.[35,42] There is, however, no consensus as to the mechanism(s) by which these drugs lower blood pressure. It is probable that some, or all, of the following proposed mechanisms play a part.

NEGATIVE CHRONOTROPIC AND INOTROPIC EFFECTS. Slowing of the heart rate and some decrease in myocardial contractility with β-blockers lead to a decrease in cardiac output, which in the short term and long term may lead to a reduction in blood pressure. It might be expected that these factors would be of particular importance in the treatment of hypertension related to high cardiac output and increased sympathetic tone.

DIFFERENCES IN EFFECTS ON PLASMA RENIN. The relation between the hypotensive action of β-blocking drugs and their ability to reduce plasma renin activity remains controversial. There is no doubt that some β-blocking drugs can antagonize sympathetically mediated renin release. However, the important question remains whether there is a clinical correlation between the β-blocker effect on plasma renin activity and the lowering of blood pressure.

CENTRAL NERVOUS SYSTEM EFFECT. There is now good clinical and experimental evidence to suggest that β-blockers cross the blood–brain barrier and enter the central nervous system. Although there is little doubt that β-blockers with high lipophilicity enter the central nervous system in high concentrations, a direct antihypertensive effect mediated by their presence has not been well defined.

VENOUS TONE AND PLASMA VOLUME. Decreased plasma volume has been seen with use of β-blockers in hypertension. One would have expected the reduced cardiac output with β-blockade to have caused a reflex increase in plasma volume. These findings suggest that decreased plasma volume may play a role in the hypotensive action of β-blockers. Further study is anticipated.

PERIPHERAL RESISTANCE. Nonselective β-blockers have no primary action in lowering peripheral resistance and indeed may cause it to rise by leaving the α-stimulatory mechanisms unopposed. The vasodilating effect of catecholamines on skeletal muscle blood vessels is β_2-mediated, suggesting possible therapeutic advantages in using β_1-selective blockers, agents with PAA, and drugs with α-blocking activity when blood pressure control is desired. Since β_1-selectivity diminishes as the drug dosage is raised, and since hypertensive patients generally have to be given far larger doses than are required simply to block the β_1-receptors alone, β_1-selectivity offers the clinician little, if any, real specific advantage in antihypertensive treatment.

"QUINIDINE EFFECT." Some early clinical investigations indicated that the antihypertensive effect of propranolol paralleled that of quinidine, suggesting that the "membrane stabilizing" effect in the β-blocker might be important. Subsequent studies refuted these early findings. All β-blockers appear to reduce blood pressure, regardless of "membrane effects."

RESETTING OF BARORECEPTORS. In patients with long-standing hypertension, the baroreceptors may react less strongly to a reduction in blood pressure than they would in a normal subject. It may be that β-blockers achieve some of this antihypertensive effect by "resetting" or increasing the sensitivity of the baroreceptor. The clinical significance of this proposed mechanism is unknown.

EFFECTS ON PREJUNCTIONAL RECEPTORS. The stimulation of prejunctional β-receptors is followed by an increase in the quantity of norepinephrine released by the postganglionic sympathetic fibers. Blockade of prejunctional β-receptors should, therefore, diminish the amount of norepinephrine released, leading to a weaker stimulation of postjunctional α-receptors, an effect that would produce less vasoconstriction and lower blood pressure. Opinions differ, however, on the importance of the contribution of presynaptic β-blockade to the antihypertensive effects of β-blocker drugs.

ANGINA PECTORIS

Sympathetic innervation of the heart causes the release of norepinephrine, activating β-adrenergic receptors in myocardial cells. This adrenergic stimulation causes an increment in heart rate, isometric contractile force, and maximal velocity of muscle fiber shortening, all of which lead to an increase in cardiac work and myocardial oxygen consumption. The decrease in intraventricular pressure and volume caused by the sympathetic-mediated enhancement of cardiac contractility tends, on the other hand, to reduce myocardial oxygen consumption by reducing myocardial wall tension (Laplace's law). Although there is a net increase in myocardial oxygen demand, this is normally balanced by an increase in coronary blood flow. Angina pectoris is believed to occur when oxygen demand exceeds supply. Since cardiac sympathetic activity increases myocardial oxygen demand, it might be expected that blockade of cardiac β-adrenergic receptors would relieve the symptoms of the anginal syndrome. It is on this basis that the early clinical studies with β-blocking drugs in angina were initiated.

The reduction in heart rate effected by β-blockade has two favorable consequences: (1) a decrease in cardiac work, thus reducing myocardial oxygen needs, and (2) a longer diastolic filling time associated with a slower heart rate, allowing for increased coronary perfusion.[43,44] β-Blockade also reduces exercise-induced blood pressure increments, the velocity of cardiac contraction, and oxygen consumption at any patient workload. Concomitant with the decrease in myocardial oxygen consumption, β-blockers can cause a reduction in coronary blood flow and a rise in coronary vascular resistance. The reduction in myocardial oxygen demand may be sufficient cause for this decrease in coronary blood flow. Although there is a decrease in total coronary flow, animal studies have demonstrated that β-blocker–induced shunting occurs in the coronary circulation, maintaining blood flow to ischemic areas, especially in the subendocardial region.

Although exercise tolerance and work capacity improve with β-blockade, the rate-pressure product (systolic blood pressure × heart rate) achieved when pain occurs is lower than that reached during a control run. This effect may relate to the action of β-blockers to increase left ventricular size, causing increased left ventricular wall tension and an increase in oxygen consumption at a given blood pressure.

The therapeutic benefit of β-blockers in chronic stable angina is now established beyond question. Many double-blind studies of β-blockers in patients have demonstrated a significant reduction in the frequency of angina attacks. Observed improvement is dose related, and dosage must be titrated for each patient.

COMBINED USE WITH OTHER ANTIANGINAL THERAPIES IN STABLE ANGINA. NITRATES. Combined therapy with nitrates and β-blockers may be more efficacious for the treatment of angina pectoris than the use of either drug alone. The primary effect of β-blockers is to cause a reduction in both resting heart rate and the response of heart rate to exercise. Nitrates produce a reflex increase in heart rate and contractility, owing to a reduction in arterial pressure, and concomitant β-blocker therapy is extremely effective because it blocks this reflex increment in the heart rate. In patients with a propensity for myocardial failure who may have a slight increase in heart size with the β-blockers, the nitrates will counteract this tendency; the peripheral venodilatory effects of these drugs reduce the left ventricular volume. Similarly, the increase in coronary resistance associated with β-blocker administration can be ameliorated by the administration of nitrates.

CALCIUM CHANNEL BLOCKERS. Calcium channel blockers block transmembrane calcium currents in vascular smooth muscle to cause arterial vasodilatation. Some calcium channel blockers also slow the heart rate and reduce atrioventricular conduction. Combined therapy with β-adrenergic and calcium channel blockers can provide clinical benefits for patients with angina pectoris who remain symptomatic with either agent used alone.[44] Because adverse effects can occur (heart block, heart failure), however, patients being considered for such treatment must be carefully selected and observed.

ANGINA AT REST AND VASOSPASTIC ANGINA. Although β-blockers are effective in the treatment of patients with angina of effort, their use in angina at rest is not so well established. The rationale for therapy with β-blockers was based on the assumption that the pathogenesis of chest pain at rest is similar to that with exertion. However, angina pectoris can be caused by multiple mechanisms, and increased coronary vascular tone may be responsible for ischemia in a significant proportion of patients with angina at rest.[44] Therefore, β-blockers that primarily reduce myocardial oxygen consumption but fail to exert vasodilating effects on coronary vasculature may not be totally effective in patients in whom angina is caused or increased by dynamic alterations in coronary luminal diameter. Despite their theoretic dangers in rest and vasospastic angina, β-blockers have been successfully used alone and in combination with vasodilating agents in many patients.

ARRHYTHMIAS

β-Adrenergic receptor blocking drugs have two main effects on the electrophysiological properties of specialized cardiac tissue.[35] The first effect results from specific blockade of adrenergic stimulation of cardiac pacemaker potentials. By competitively inhibiting adrenergic stimulation, β-blockers decrease the slope of phase 4 depolarization and the spontaneous firing rate of sinus or ectopic pacemakers and thus decrease automaticity. Arrhythmias occurring in the setting of enhanced automaticity, as seen in myocardial infarction, digitalis toxicity, hyperthyroidism, and pheochromocytoma, would therefore be expected to respond well to β-blockade.[45] The second electrophysiologic effect of β-blockers involves membrane stabilizing activity, also known as "quinidine-like" or "local anesthetic" action. Characteristic of this effect is a reduction in the rate of rise of the intracardial action potential without an effect on the spike duration of the resting potential. This effect and its attendant changes have been explained by inhibition of the depolarizing inward sodium current.

Sotalol is unique among the β-blockers in that it possesses class III antiarrhythmic properties, causing prolongation of the action potential period and thus delaying repolarization.[35] Clinical studies have verified the efficacy of sotalol in control of arrhythmias,[46] but additional investigation will be required to determine whether its class III antiarrhythmic properties contribute significantly to its efficacy as an antiarrhythmic agent.

The most important mechanism underlying the antiarrhythmic effect of β-blockers, with the possible exclusion of sotalol, is believed to be β-blockade with resultant inhibition of pacemaker potentials. If this view is accurate, then one would expect all β-blockers to be similarly effective at a comparable level of β-blockade. In fact, this appears to be the case. No superiority of one β-blocking agent over another in the therapy of arrhythmias has been convincingly demonstrated.[35] Differences in overall clinical usefulness are related to their other associated pharmacologic properties.

SUPRAVENTRICULAR ARRHYTHMIAS. SINUS TACHYCARDIA. Sinus tachycardia usually has an obvious cause (e.g., fever, hyperthyroidism, congestive heart failure), and therapy should focus on correcting the underlying condition. If the rapid heart rate itself is compromising the patient, however, causing recurrent angina in a patient with coronary artery disease, for example, then direct intervention with a β-blocker may be effective. Patients with heart failure, however, should not be treated with β-blockers unless they have been placed on diuretic therapy and cardiac glycosides and even then only with extreme caution. Some patients with primary cardiomyopathy with congestive heart failure appear to benefit from prolonged very-low-dose β-blocker therapy; the mechanisms for such beneficial effect, however, remain unclear.

SUPRAVENTRICULAR ECTOPIC BEATS. As in sinus tachycardia, specific treatment of these extrasystoles is seldom required and therapy should be directed to the underlying cause. Although supraventricular ectopic beats often are the precursors to atrial fibrillation, there is no evidence that prophylactic administration of β-blockers can prevent the development of atrial fibrillation. Supraventricular ectopic beats due to digitalis toxicity generally respond well to β-blockade.

PAROXYSMAL SUPRAVENTRICULAR TACHYCARDIA. By delaying atrioventricular conduction (e.g., increased atrio-His interval in bundle of His electrocardiograms) and prolonging the refractory period of the reentrant pathways, β-blockers are effective in terminating many cases of paroxysmal supraventricular tachycardia. Vagal maneuvers after β-blockade may effectively terminate an arrhythmia when they previously may have been unsuccessful without β-blockade. Even when β-blockers do not convert an arrhythmia to sinus rhythm, by increasing atrioventricular nodal refractoriness they often will slow the ventricular rate. The use of β-blocking drugs also still allows the option of direct-current countershock cardioversion.

ATRIAL FLUTTER. β-Blockade can be used to slow the ventricular rate (by increasing atrioventricular block) and may restore sinus rhythm in a large percentage of patients. This is a situation in which β-blockade may be of diagnostic value; given intravenously, β-blockers slow the ventricular response and permit the differentiation of flutter waves, ectopic P waves, or sinus mechanism.

ATRIAL FIBRILLATION. The major action of β-blockers in rapid atrial fibrillation is the reduction in the ventricular response caused by increasing the refractory period of the atrioventricular node. Although β-blocking drugs have been effective in slowing ventricular rates in patients with atrial fibrillation, they are less effective than quinidine or direct-current cardioversion in changing atrial fibrillation to sinus rhythm.

β-Blockers must be used with caution when atrial fibrillation occurs in the setting of a severely diseased heart that depends on high levels of adrenergic tone to avoid myocardial failure. These drugs may be particularly useful in controlling the ventricular rate in situations in which this is difficult to achieve with maximally tolerated doses of digitalis (e.g., thyrotoxicosis, hypertrophic cardiomyopathy, mitral stenosis, and after cardiac surgery).

VENTRICULAR ARRHYTHMIAS. The response of ventricular arrhythmias to β-blockade appears to be comparable to that following therapy with quinidine. β-Blockers are particularly useful if these arrhythmias are related to excessive catecholamines (e.g., exercise, halothane anesthesia, pheochromocytoma, exogenous catecholamines), myocardial ischemia, or digitalis. Since β-blockers are effective in preventing ischemic episodes, arrhythmias generated by these episodes may be prevented. β-Blockers are also quite effective in controlling the frequency of premature ventricular contractions in hypertrophic cardiomyopathy and in mitral valve prolapse. In controlled studies, however, β-blocker therapy has not been found to be effective in controlling complex life-threatening arrhythmias.

VENTRICULAR TACHYCARDIA. β-Blocking drugs should not be considered agents of choice in the treatment of acute ventricular tachycardia. Cardioversion or other antiarrhythmic drugs should be the initial mode of therapy. β-Blockers have been shown to be of benefit for prophylaxis against recurrent ventricular tachycardia, particularly if sympathetic stimulation and/or myocardial ischemia appear to be precipitating causes. Several studies have been reported showing the prevention of exercise-induced ventricular tachycardia by β-blockers; in many previous cases they had been a poor response to digitalis or quinidine.[35]

PREVENTION OF VENTRICULAR FIBRILLATION. β-Blockade agents can attenuate cardiac stimulation by the sympathetic nervous system, and perhaps the potential for reentrant ventricular arrhythmias and sudden death.[47] Experimental studies have shown that β-blockers raise the ventricular fibrillation threshold in the ischemic myocardium.[47] Placebo-controlled clinical trials have shown that β-blockers reduce the number of episodes of ventricular fibrillation and cardiac arrest during the acute phase of myocardial infarction.[48] The long-term β-blocker postmyocardial infarction trials and other clinical studies with β-blockers have demonstrated that there is a significant reduction of complex ventricular arrhythmias.[49]

USE IN SURVIVORS OF ACUTE MYOCARDIAL INFARCTION

The results of placebo-controlled long-term treatment trials with some β-adrenergic blocking drugs in survivors of acute myocardial infarction have demonstrated a favorable effect on total mortality, cardiovascular mortality (including sudden and nonsudden cardiac deaths), and the incidence of nonfatal reinfarction.[50,51] These beneficial results with β-blocker therapy can be explained by both the antiarrhythmic and the anti-ischemic effects of these drugs. Two nonselective β-blockers, propranolol and timolol, have been approved by the Food and Drug Administration for reducing the risk of mortality in infarct survivors when started 5 to 28 days after an infarction. Metoprolol and atenolol, two $β_1$-selective blockers, are approved for the same indication and can be used in both intravenous and oral forms. β-Blockers have also been suggested as a treatment for reducing the extent of myocardial injury and mortality during the hyperacute phase of myocardial infarction with and without thrombolysis, but their exact role in this situation remains unclear.[52]

"SILENT" MYOCARDIAL ISCHEMIA

In recent years, investigators have observed that not all myocardial ischemic episodes detected by electrocardiography are associated with detectable symptoms.[53] Positron emission imaging techniques have validated the theory that these silent ischemic episodes are indicative of true myocardial ischemia.[54] The prognostic importance of silent myocardial ischemia occurring at rest and/or during exercise has not been determined. β-Blockers are successful in reducing the frequency of silent ischemic episodes detected by ambulatory electrocardiographic monitoring, as in reducing the frequency of painful ischemic events.[53]

HYPERTROPHIC CARDIOMYOPATHY

β-Adrenergic receptor blocking drugs have been proven efficacious in therapy for hypertrophic cardiomyopathy and idiopathic hypertrophic subaortic stenosis (IHSS).[55] These drugs are useful in controlling the dyspnea, angina, and syncope that occur with these disorders. β-Blockers have also been shown to lower the intraventricular pressure gradient both at rest and with exercise.

The outflow pressure gradient is not the only abnormality in hypertrophic cardiomyopathy; more important is the loss of ventricular compliance, which impedes normal left ventricular function. It has been shown that propranolol produces favorable changes in ventricular compliance in some patients with hypertrophic cardiomyopathy. The salutary hemodynamic and symptomatic effects produced by propranolol derive from its inhibition of sympathetic stimulation of the heart. However, there is no evidence that the drug alters the primary cardiomyopathic process; many patients remain in or return to their severely symptomatic state and some die despite its administration.

DILATED CARDIOMYOPATHY

The ability of intravenous sympathomimetic amines to effect an acute increase in myocardial contractility through stimulation of the β-adrenergic receptor has prompted hope that oral analogues may provide long-term benefit for patients with severe heart failure. Recent observations concerning the regulation of the myocardial adrenergic receptor and abnormalities of β-receptor–mediated stimulation in the failing myocardium have caused a critical reappraisal of the scientific validity of sustained $β_1$-adrenergic receptor stimulation, however.[56,57] New evidence suggests that $β_1$-receptor blockade may, when tolerated, have a favorable effect on the underlying cardiomyopathic process.[58,59]

The excessive catecholamine stimulation of the heart that occurs in chronic congestive heart failure can cause myocardial catecholamine depletion,[60,61] a direct toxic effect on the heart,[62–64] and down-regulation of β-adrenergic receptors.[56,57,65] It appears that β-adrenergic blockade can correct these abnormalities and possibly improve left ventricular function.[59]

Preliminary studies with chronic β-blockade have demonstrated improvement in left ventricular function in many patients with advanced cardiomyopathy.[66–69] These studies have included patients who showed dramatic improvement in their hemodynamic situations while awaiting cardiac transplantation.[70] A large, prospective, double-blind, multicenter study (Metoprolol in Dilated Cardiomyopathy [MIDIC]) is in progress, evaluating the efficacy of β-blocker therapy in patients with idiopathic cardiomyopathies. A similar pilot study using carvedilol and metoprolol is also in progress.

MITRAL VALVE PROLAPSE

Mitral valve prolapse, characterized by a nonejection systolic click, a late systolic murmur, or a midsystolic click followed by a late systolic murmur, has been studied extensively over the past 15 years. Atypical chest pain, malignant arrhythmias, and nonspecific ST and T wave abnormalities have been observed with this condition. By decreasing sympathetic tone, β-adrenergic blockers have been shown to be useful for relieving the chest pains and palpitations that many of these patients experience and for reducing the incidence of life-threatening arrhythmias and other electrocardiographic abnormalities.[71]

DISSECTING ANEURYSMS
β-Adrenergic blockade plays a major role in the treatment of patients with acute aortic dissection.[72] During the hyperacute phase, β-blocking agents reduce the force and velocity of myocardial contraction (dp/dt) and hence the progression of the dissecting hematoma. However, such administration must be initiated simultaneously with the institution of other antihypertensive therapy that may cause reflex tachycardia and increases in cardiac output, factors that can aggravate the dissection process. Initially, propranolol is administered intravenously to reduce the heart rate to below 60 beats per minute. Once a patient is stabilized and long-term medical management is contemplated, the patient should be maintained on oral β-blocker therapy to prevent recurrence.

TETRALOGY OF FALLOT
By reducing the effects of increased adrenergic tone on the right ventricular infundibulum in tetralogy of Fallot,[73] β-blockers have been shown to be useful for the treatment of severe hypoxic spells and hypercyanotic attacks. With long-term use, these drugs have also been shown to prevent prolonged hypoxic spells. These drugs should be looked at only as palliative, and definitive surgical repair of this condition is usually required.

QT INTERVAL PROLONGATION SYNDROME
The syndrome of electrocardiographic QT interval prolongation is usually a congenital condition associated with deafness, syncope, and sudden death.[74] Abnormalities in sympathetic nervous system functioning in the heart have been proposed as explanations for the electrophysiologic aberrations seen in these patients. Propranolol appears to be the most effective drug for treatment of this syndrome. It reduces the frequency of syncopal episodes in most patients and may prevent sudden death. This drug will reduce the electrocardiographic QT interval.

EPINEPHRINE-INDUCED HYPOKALEMIA
Experimental studies have established that the infusion of catecholamines decreases serum potassium levels. Recently, it was demonstrated that physiologic concentration of epinephrine, such as that which may be seen with a myocardial infarction, may also induce hypokalemia, primarily through stimulation of β_2-receptors.[75] Subsequent studies have found that only the nonselective β-blockers can completely block the hypokalemic effect of epinephrine.[76] Considering the importance given to avoiding hypokalemia in the patient with an acute myocardial infarction, further study in this area is anticipated.

REGRESSION OF LEFT VENTRICULAR HYPERTROPHY
Left ventricular hypertrophy induced by systemic hypertension is an independent risk factor for cardiovascular mortality and morbidity.[16] Regression of left ventricular hypertrophy with drug therapy is feasible and may improve patient outcome.[16] β-Adrenergic blockers can cause regression of left ventricular hypertrophy, as determined by echocardiography with or without an associated reduction in blood pressure.[16]

USE IN NONCARDIOVASCULAR DISORDERS
THYROTOXICOSIS
Despite the inability to define precisely the relationship between catecholamines and hyperthyroidism, certain antiadrenergic agents (*i.e.*, reserpine, guanethidine, and β-blockers) are capable of alleviating many of the sympathomimetic manifestations of the thyrotoxic state.[77] Because of their relative freedom from side effects, ease of administration, and rapid onset of action, β-blockers are the agents of choice.

The exact mechanism of β-blocker benefit in hyperthyroidism is not fully defined. It is not resolved whether the effects of β-blockade are mediated by adrenergic blockade or by blocking the peripheral conversion of triiodothyronine to thyroxine.

PROPHYLAXIS OF MIGRAINE
The use of β-adrenergic blocking drugs to prevent migraine headache first was suggested in 1966. Clinical trials confirmed the safety and efficacy of propranolol for the prophylaxis of common migraine.[78] Propranolol is approved by the Food and Drug Administration for the treatment of migraine headache.

OPEN ANGLE GLAUCOMA
As early as 1968, topical applications of propranolol were shown to reduce intraocular pressure but its mild local anesthetic properties made investigators reluctant to use it for treatment of glaucoma. Topical application of timolol, a nonselective β-blocker without this local anesthetic property or PAA, also reduced intraocular pressure.[79] The mechanism of its ocular hypotensive effect has not been firmly established, but it may reduce the pressure by decreasing the production of aqueous humor. Of note, aggravation or precipitation of certain cardiovascular and pulmonary disorders has been reported with topical application of the drug and is presumably related to the systemic effects of β-adrenergic receptor blockade. Recently, two new ophthalmic β-blocker solutions were approved for glaucoma. Betaxolol is a β_1-selective drug that is applied twice daily. Levobunolol is a nonselective drug that can be used once or twice daily. These new drugs do not provide any efficacy or side-effect advantage over timolol.

ESSENTIAL TREMOR
The β-blocker propranolol has been approved for treatment of benign essential tremor.

ADVERSE EFFECTS
MYOCARDIAL FAILURE
There are two circumstances by which blockade of β-receptors may cause congestive heart failure: (1) in an enlarged heart with impaired myocardial function in which excessive sympathetic drive is essential to maintain the myocardium on a compensated Starling curve and (2) in hearts in which the left ventricular stroke volume is restricted and tachycardia is needed to maintain cardiac output. In patients with impaired myocardial function who require β-blocking agents, digitalis and diuretics can be used, preferably with drugs having intrinsic sympathomimetic activity or α-adrenergic blocking properties.

SINUS NODE DYSFUNCTION AND ATRIOVENTRICULAR CONDUCTION DELAY
Slowing of the resting heart rate is a normal response to treatment with β-blocking drugs with and without PAA. In most cases, this does not present a problem; healthy persons can sustain a heart rate of 40 to 50 beats per minute without disability unless there is clinical evidence of heart failure. Drugs with PAA do not lower the resting heart rate to the same degree as propranolol.[38] However, all β-blocking drugs are contraindicated (unless an artificial pacemaker is present) in patients with sick sinus syndrome.

β-ADRENERGIC RECEPTOR BLOCKER WITHDRAWAL
Following abrupt cessation of chronic β-blocker therapy, exacerbation of angina pectoris and, in some cases, acute myocardial infarction and death have been reported.[80] The exact mechanism for this reaction is unclear. There is some evidence that the withdrawal phenomenon may be due to the generation of additional β-adrenergic receptors during the period of β-adrenergic receptor blockade (hyperadrenergic state). Other suggested mechanisms for the withdrawal reaction include heightened platelet aggregability, an elevation in thyroid hormone ac-

tivity, and an increase in circulating catecholamines. However, continuing the same level of activity as during β-blocker therapy appears to be the major contributing mechanism for the exacerbation of angina.

BRONCHOCONSTRICTION

The bronchodilator effects of catecholamines on the bronchial β-receptors (β_2) are inhibited by nonselective β-blockers. Comparative studies have shown that β-blocking compounds with PAA, β_1-selectivity, and α-adrenergic blocking actions are less likely to increase airway resistance in asthmatics than propranolol. β_1-Selectivity, however, is not absolute and may be lost with high therapeutic doses; therefore, all β-blockers should be avoided in patients with bronchospastic disease.

PERIPHERAL VASCULAR EFFECTS (RAYNAUD'S PHENOMENON)

Raynaud's phenomenon is one of the more common side effects of treatment with propranolol. Also, cold extremities and absent pulses have been reported to occur more frequently in patients receiving β-blockers for hypertension than in those receiving methyldopa. This is probably due to the reduction in cardiac output and blockade of β_2-adrenergic receptor–mediated vasodilation, resulting in unopposed α-adrenergic receptor vasoconstriction. β-Blocking drugs with β_1-selectivity or PAA will not affect peripheral vessels to the same degree as propranolol.

MISCELLANEOUS SIDE EFFECTS

Several authors have described severe hypoglycemic reactions during therapy with β-adrenergic blocking drugs. Studies of resting normal volunteers have demonstrated that propranolol produces no alteration in blood glucose values, although the hyperglycemic response to exercise is blunted. The enhancement of insulin-induced hypoglycemia and its hemodynamic consequences may be less with β_1-selective agents and agents with intrinsic sympathomimetic activity. There is also marked diminution in the clinical manifestations of the catechol-

TABLE 16.4 DRUG INTERACTIONS THAT MAY OCCUR WITH β-ADRENOCEPTOR BLOCKING DRUGS

Drug	Possible Effects	Precautions
Aluminum hydroxide gel	Decreased β-blocker adsorption and therapeutic effect	Avoid β-blocker–aluminum hydroxide combination.
Aminophylline	Mutual inhibition	Observe patient's response.
Amiodarone	May induce cardiac arrest	Combination should be used with extreme caution.
Antidiabetic agents	Enhanced hypoglycemia; hypertension	Monitor for altered diabetic response.
Calcium channel inhibitors (verapamil, diltiazem)	Potentiation of bradycardia, myocardial depression, and hypotension	Avoid use, although few patients show ill effects.
Cimetidine	Prolongs half-life of propranolol	Combination should be used with caution.
Clonidine	Hypertension during clonidine withdrawal	Monitor for hypertensive response; withdraw β-blocker before withdrawing clonidine.
Digitalis glycosides	Potentiation of bradycardia	Observe patient's response; interactions may benefit angina patients with abnormal ventricular function.
Epinephrine	Hypertension; bradycardia	Administer epinephrine cautiously; cardioselective β-blocker may be safer.
Ergot alkaloids	Excessive vasoconstriction	Observe patient's response; few patients show ill effects.
Glucagon	Inhibition of hyperglycemic effect	Monitor for reduced response.
Halofenate	Reduced β-blocking activity; production of propranolol withdrawal rebound syndrome	Observe for impaired response to β-blockade.
Indomethacin	Inhibition of antihypertensive response to β-blockade	Observe patient's response.
Isoproterenol	Mutual inhibition	Avoid concurrent use or choose cardiac-selective β-blocker.
Levodopa	Antagonism of levodopa's hypotensive and positive inotropic effects	Monitor for altered response; interaction may have favorable results.
Lidocaine	Propranolol pretreatment increases lidocaine blood levels and potential toxicity	Combination should be used with caution; use lower doses of lidocaine.
Methyldopa	Hypertension during stress	Monitor for hypertensive episodes.
Monoamine oxidase inhibitors	Uncertain, theoretical	Manufacturer of propranolol considers concurrent use contraindicated.
Phenothiazines	Additive hypotensive effects	Monitor for altered response, especially with high doses of phenothiazines.
Phenylpropanolamine	Severe hypertensive reaction	Avoid use, especially in hypertension controlled by both methyldopa and β-blockers.
Phenytoin	Additive cardiac depressant effects	Administer IV phenytoin with great caution.
Quinidine	Additive cardiac depressant effects	Observe patient's response; few patients show ill effects.
Reserpine	Excessive sympathetic blockade	Observe patient's response.
Rifampin	Increased metabolism of β-blockers	Observe patient's response.
Smoking	Increased metabolism of β-blockers	Observe patient's response.
Tricyclic antidepressants	Inhibits negative inotropic and chronotropic effects of β-blockers	Observe patient's response.
Tubocurarine	Enhanced neuromuscular blockade	Observe response in surgical patients, especially after high doses of propranolol.

(Frishman WH: Clinical Pharmacology of the β-Adrenoceptor Blocking Drugs, 2nd ed. Norwalk, CT, Appleton-Century-Crofts, 1984, and Missri JC: How do beta-blockers interact with other commonly used drugs? Cardiovasc Med 8:668, 1983)

amine discharge induced by hypoglycemia (tachycardia).[81] These findings suggest that β-blockers interfere with compensatory responses to hypoglycemia and can mask certain "warning signs" of this condition. Other hypoglycemic reactions, such as diaphoresis, are not affected by β-adrenergic blockade.

Dreams, hallucinations, insomnia, and depression can occur during therapy with β-blockers. These symptoms are evidence of drug entry into the central nervous system and are especially common with the highly lipid-soluble β-blockers.

Diarrhea, nausea, gastric pain, constipation, and flatulence have been noted occasionally with all β-blockers (2% to 11% of patients). Hematologic reactions are rare: purpura and agranulocytosis have been described with propranolol.

A characteristic immune reaction, the oculomucocutaneous syndrome, affecting singly or in combination the eyes, mucous and serous membranes, and the skin (often in association with a positive antinuclear factor), has been reported in patients treated with practolol and has led to the curtailment of this drug in clinical practice. Fears that other β-adrenergic receptor blocking drugs may cause this syndrome have not been substantiated.

DRUG INTERACTIONS

The wide diversity of diseases for which β-blockers are employed raises the likelihood of their concurrent administration with other drugs. It is imperative, therefore, that clinicians become familiar with the interactions of β-blockers with other pharmacologic agents. The list of commonly used drugs with which β-blockers interact is extensive (Table 16.4).[35,82] The majority of the reported interactions have been associated with propranolol, the best studied of the β-blockers, and may not apply to other drugs in this class.

CLINICAL USE

More than 15 β-adrenoceptor blocking drugs are now available worldwide. As of 1989, with the introduction of betaxolol,[83] carteolol, and penbutolol,[84] 12 β-blockers are marketed for approved uses in the United States. These are propranolol for angina pectoris, arrhythmia, systemic hypertension, essential tremor, prevention of migraine headache, and reducing the risk of mortality of survivors of acute myocardial infarction; atenolol and nadolol for angina pectoris and hypertension; timolol for hypertension, open angle glaucoma, and reducing the risk of mortality and reinfarction in survivors of acute myocardial infarction; metoprolol and atenolol for hypertension, angina pectoris, and reducing the risk of mortality in survivors of acute myocardial infarction; acebutolol for hypertension and ventricular arrhythmias; betaxolol, carteolol, penbutolol, and pindolol for hypertension; intravenous esmolol for supraventricular tachycardias; and labetalol for hypertension and hypertensive emergencies. Five β-blockers (bisoprolol, bevantolol, carvedilol, celiprolol, dilevalol) are now under consideration by the Food and Drug Administration for marketing approval or are being studied actively in clinical trials. Oxprenolol has been approved for use in hypertension but has not yet been marketed.

The various β-blocking compounds given in adequate dosage appear to have comparable antihypertensive, antiarrhythmic, and antianginal effects. Therefore, the β-blocking drug of choice in an individual patient is determined by the pharmacodynamic and pharmacokinetic differences between the drugs, in conjunction with the patient's other medical conditions (Table 16.5).

TABLE 16.5 CLINICAL SITUATIONS THAT WOULD INFLUENCE THE CHOICE OF A β-BLOCKING DRUG

Condition	Choice of β-Blocker
Asthma, chronic bronchitis with bronchospasm	Avoid all β-blockers if possible; however, small doses of β_1-selective blockers (e.g., acebutolol, atenolol, metoprolol) can be used; β_1-selectivity is lost with higher doses; drugs with partial agonist activity (e.g., pindolol, oxprenolol) and labetalol with α-adrenergic blocking properties can also be used.
Congestive heart failure	Drugs with partial agonist activity and labetalol might have an advantage, although β-blockers are usually contraindicated.
Angina	In patients with angina at low heart rates, drugs with partial agonist activity are probably contraindicated; patients with angina at high heart rates but who have resting bradycardia might benefit from a drug with partial agonist activity; in vasospastic angina, labetalol may be useful, but other β-blockers should be used with caution.
Atrioventricular conduction defects	β-Blockers are generally contraindicated by drugs with partial agonist activity and labetalol can be tried with caution.
Bradycardia	β-Blockers with partial agonist activity and labetalol have less pulse-slowing effect and are preferable.
Raynaud's phenomenon, intermittent claudication, cold extremities	β_1-Selective blocking agents, labetalol, and those with partial agonist activity might have an advantage.
Depression	Avoid propranolol; substitute a β-blocker with partial agonist activity.
Diabetes mellitus	β_1-Selective agents and partial agonist drugs are preferable.
Thyrotoxicosis	All agents will control symptoms, but agents without partial agonist activity are preferred.
Pheochromocytoma	Avoid all β-blockers unless an α-blocker is given; labetalol is the drug of choice.
Renal failure	Use reduced doses of compounds largely eliminated by renal mechanisms (nadolol, acebutolol, sotalol, atenolol) and of those drugs whose bioavailability is increased in uremia (propranolol); also consider possible accumulation of active metabolites (acebutolol, propranolol)
Insulin and sulfonyl urea use	Danger of hypoglycemia; possibly less using drugs with β_1-selectivity
Clonidine	Avoid sotalol (other nonselective β-blockers); severe rebound effects with clonidine withdrawal
Oculomucocutaneous syndrome	Stop drug; substitute any other β-blocker.
Hyperlipidemia	Avoid nonselective β-blockers; use agents with partial agonism, β_1-selectivity, or labetalol.

(Frishman WH: Clinical Pharmacology of the β-Adrenoceptor Blocking Drugs, 2nd ed. Norwalk, CT, Appleton-Century-Crofts, 1984)

REFERENCES

1. Ahlquist RP: Study of the adrenotropic receptors. Am J Physiol 153:486, 1948
2. Lands AM, Luduena FP, Buzzo HJ: Differentiation of receptor systems responsive to isoproterenol. Life Sci 6:2241, 1967
3. Berthelsen S, Pettinger WA: A functional basis for classification of alpha-adrenergic receptors. Life Sci 21:596, 1977
4. Frishman WH, Charlap S: α-Adrenergic blockers. Med Clin North Am 72:427, 1988
5. Luther RR: New perspectives on selective α_1-blockade. Am J Hypertens 2:729, 1989
6. Taylor SH: Clinical pharmacotherapeutics of doxazosin. Am J Med 87(2A):2S, 1989
7. Singleton W, Dix RK, Monsen L et al: Efficacy and safety of Minipress XL, a new once-a-day formulation of prazosin. Am J Med 87(2A):45S, 1989
8. Van Zwieten PA: Pharmacology profile of urapadil. Am J Cardiol 64:1D, 1989
9. Elliott HL, Meredith PA, Vincent J et al: Clinical pharmacological studies with doxazosin. Br J Clin Pharmacol 21:27S, 1986
10. Reid JL, Meredith PA, Elliot HL: Pharmacokinetics and pharmacodynamics of trimazosin in man. Am Heart J 106:1222, 1983
11. Archibald JL: Recent developments in the pharmacology and pharmacokinetics of indoramin. J Cardiovasc Pharmacol 8(suppl 2):516, 1986
12. Frishman WH, Eisen G, Lapsker J: Terazosin: A new long-acting α_1-adrenergic antagonist for hypertension. Med Clin North Am 72:441, 1988
13. Katz AM, Hager WD, Mesineo FC et al: Cellular actions and pharmacology of the calcium channel blocking drugs. Am J Med 77:2, 1984
14. Ribner HS, Bresnahan D, Hsieh AM: Acute hemodynamic responses to vasodilation therapy in congestive heart failure. Prog Cardiovasc Dis 25:1, 1982
15. Johnson BF, Danylchuk MA: The relevance of plasma lipid changes with cardiovascular drug therapy. Med Clin North Am 73:449, 1989
16. Hachamovitch R, Strom JA, Sonnenblick EH, Frishman WH: Left ventricular hypertrophy in hypertension and the effects of antihypertensive drug therapy. Curr Probl Cardiol 13:371, 1988
17. Gould L, Reddy CVR: Phentolamine. Am Heart J 92:392, 1976
18. Majid PA, Sharma B, Taylor SH: Phentolamine for vasodilator treatment of severe heart failure. Lancet 2:719, 1971
19. Packer M: Vasodilator and inotropic therapy for severe chronic heart failure: Passion and skepticism. J Am Coll Cardiol 2:841, 1983
20. Cohn JN, Archibald DG, Ziesche S et al: Effect of vasodilator therapy on mortality in chronic congestive heart failure: Results of a Veterans Administration Cooperative Study (V-Heft). N Engl J Med 314:1547, 1986
21. Scholz H: Inotropic drugs and their mechanism of action. J Am Coll Cardiol 4:389, 1984
22. Orlick AE, Ricci DR, Cipriano PR et al: The contribution of alpha-adrenergic tone to resting coronary vascular resistance in man. J Clin Invest 62:459, 1978
23. Winniford MD, Flipchuk N, Hillis DL: Alpha-adrenergic blockade for variant angina: A long-term double-blind randomized trial. Circulation 67:1185, 1983
24. Corr PB, Shayman JA, Kramer JB et al: Increased α-adrenergic receptors in ischemic cat myocardium: A potential mediator of electrophysiologic derangements. J Clin Invest 67:1232, 1981
25. Manger WM, Gifford RW: Pheochromocytoma. New York: Springer-Verlag, 1977
26. Honston MC, Thompson WL, Robertson D: Shock. Arch Intern Med 144:1433, 1984
27. Fein SA, Frishman WH: The pathophysiology and management of pulmonary hypertension. Cardiol Clin 5:563, 1987
28. Cohen ML, Kronzon I: Adverse hemodynamic effects of phentolamine in primary pulmonary hypertension. Ann Intern Med 95:591, 1981
29. Henderson WR, Shelhamer JH, Reingold DB et al: Alpha-adrenergic hyperresponsiveness in asthma. N Engl J Med 300:642, 1979
30. Barnes PJ, Wilson NM, Vickers H: Prazosin, an alpha$_1$-adrenoceptor antagonist, partially inhibits exercise-induced asthma. J Allergy Clin Immunol 68:411, 1981
31. Hedlund H, Andersson KE, Ek A: Effects of prazosin in patients with benign prostatic obstruction. J Urol 130:275, 1983
32. Oates JA, Robertson D, Wood AJJ: Alpha and beta-adrenergic agonists and antagonists. In Rosen MR, Hoffman BF (eds): Cardiac Therapy, p 145. Boston, Martinus Nijhoff, 1983
33. Westfall DP: Adrenoceptor antagonists. In Craig CR, Zitzel RE (eds): Modern Pharmacology, p 141. Boston, Little, Brown & Co, 1982
34. Frishman WH: β-Adrenoceptor antagonists: New drugs and new indications. N Engl J Med 305:500, 1981
35. Frishman WH: Clinical Pharmacology of the β-Adrenoceptor Blocking Drugs, 2nd ed. Norwalk, CT, Appleton-Century-Crofts, 1984
36. Frishman WH: β-Adrenergic blockers. Med Clin North Am 72:37, 1988
37. Koch-Weser J: Metoprolol. N Engl J Med 301:698, 1979
38. Frishman WH: Pindolol: A new β-adrenoceptor antagonist with partial agonist activity. N Engl J Med 308:940, 1983
39. Frishman W, Halprin S: Clinical pharmacology of the new beta-adrenergic blocking drugs: VII. New horizons in beta-adrenoceptor blocking therapy: Labetalol. Am Heart J 98:660, 1979
40. Johnsson G, Regardh CG: Clinical pharmacokinetics of β-adrenoceptor blocking drugs. Clin Pharmacokinet 1:233, 1976
41. Murthy VF, Frishman WH: Controlled beta-receptor blockade with esmolol and flestolol. Pharmacotherapy 8:168, 1988
42. Frishman W, Silverman R: Clinical pharmacology of the new beta-adrenergic blocking drugs: III. Comparative clinical experience and new therapeutic applications. Am Heart J 98:119, 1979
43. Frishman WH: Multifactorial actions of β-adrenergic blocking drugs in ischemia heart disease: Current concepts. Circulation 67(suppl 1):11, 1983
44. Frishman WH: Beta-adrenergic blockade in the treatment of coronary artery disease. In Hurst JW (ed): Clinical Essays on the Heart, vol 2, p 25. New York: McGraw-Hill, 1983
45. Singh BN, Jewitt DE: β-Adrenoceptor blocking drugs in cardiac arrhythmias. In Avery G (ed): Cardiovascular Drugs, vol 2, p 141. Baltimore, University Park Press, 1977
46. Fogelman F, Lightman SL, Sillett RW et al: The treatment of cardiac arrhythmias with sotalol. Eur J Clin Pharmacol 5:72, 1972
47. Pratt C, Lichstein E: Ventricular antiarrhythmic effects of beta-adrenergic blocking drugs: A review of mechanism and clinical studies. J Clin Pharmacol 22:335, 1982
48. Ryden L, Ariniego R, Arnman K et al: A double-blind trial of metoprolol in acute myocardial infarction: Effects on ventricular tachyarrhythmias. N Engl J Med 308:614, 1983
49. Lichstein E, Morganroth J, Harrist R et al: Effect of propranolol on ventricular arrhythmias: The beta-blockers: Preliminary data from the Heart Attack Trial Experience. Circulation 67(suppl I):I-32, 1983
50. Frishman WH, Furberg CD, Friedewald WT: β-Adrenergic blockade for survivors of acute myocardial infarction. N Engl J Med 310:830, 1984
51. Frishman WH, Skolnick AE, Lazar EJ: β-Adrenergic blockade and calcium channel blockade in myocardial infarction. Med Clin North Am 73:409, 1989
52. TIMI Study Group: TIMI II Comparison by Invasive and Conservative Strategies after Treatment with IV TPA in Acute MI Results of Thrombolysis in MI TIMI Phase II trial. N Engl J Med 320(10):618, 1989
53. Frishman WH, Teicher M: Antianginal drug therapy for silent myocardial ischemia. Am Heart J 114:140, 1987
54. Deanfield JE, Shea MJ, Selwyn AP: Clinical evaluation of transient myocardial ischemia during daily life. Am J Med 79(suppl 3A):18, 1985
55. Swan DA, Bell B, Oakley CM et al: Analysis of symptomatic course and prognosis in treatment of hypertrophic obstructive cardiomyopathy. Br Heart J 33:671, 1971
56. Bristow MR, Ginsberg R, Minobe W et al: Decreased catecholamine sensitivity and β-adrenergic receptor density in failing human hearts. N Engl J Med 307:205, 1982
57. Colucci WS, Alexander RW, Williams GH et al: Decreased lymphocyte beta-adrenergic receptor density in patients with heart failure and tolerance to the beta-adrenergic agonist parbuterol. N Engl J Med 305:185, 1981
58. Bristow MR: The adrenergic nervous system in heart failure. N Engl J Med 311:850, 1984
59. Shanes J, Kasabali B, Blend M: Beta-adrenergic blockade in heart failure: Potential mechanisms of action. Heart Failure 2:138, 1986
60. Rose CP, Burgess JH, Cousineau D: Reduced aortocoronary sinus extraction of epinephrine in patients with left ventricular failure secondary to long-term pressure or volume overload. Circulation 68:241, 1983
61. Sole MJ, Kamble AB, Hussain MN: A possible change in the rate-limiting step for cardiac norepinephrine synthesis in the cardiomyopathic Syrian hamster. Circ Res 41:814, 1977
62. Bloom S, Davis DL: Calcium as mediator of isoproterenol-induced myocardial necrosis. Am J Pathol 69:459, 1972
63. Kahn DS, Rona G, Chappel CI: Isoproterenol-induced cardiac necrosis. Ann NY Acad Sci 156:285, 1969
64. Simons M, Downing S: Coronary vasoconstriction and catecholamine cardiomyopathy. Am Heart J 109:297, 1985
65. Heinsimer JA, Lefkowitz RJ: The beta-adrenergic receptor in heart failure. Hosp Pract 18:103, 1983
66. Engelmeier RS, O'Connell JB, Walsh R et al: Improvement in symptoms and exercise tolerance by metoprolol in patients with dilated cardiomyopathy. A double-blind, randomized, placebo-controlled trial. Circulation 72:536, 1985
67. Swedberg K, Hjalmarson A, Waagstein F et al: Adverse effects of beta-blockade withdrawal in patients with congestive cardiomyopathy. Br Heart J 44:134, 1980
68. Swedberg K, Hjalmarson A, Waagstein F et al: Beneficial effects of long-term beta-blockade in congestive cardiomyopathy. Br Heart J 44:117, 1980
69. Waagstein F, Hjalmarson A, Swedberg K et al: Beta-blockers in dilated cardiomyopathies: They work. Eur Heart J 4:173, 1983
70. Fowler MB, Bristow MR, Laser JA et al: Beta-blocker therapy in severe heart failure: Improvement related to β_1-adrenergic receptor regulation? Circulation 70(suppl 2):112, 1984
71. Winkle RA, Lopes MG, Goodman DS et al: Propranolol for patients with mitral valve prolapse. Am Heart J 93:422, 1970
72. Slater EE, DeSanctis R: Dissection of the aorta. Med Clin North Am 63:141, 1979
73. Shah PM, Kidd L: Circulatory effects of propranolol in children with Fallot's

74. Vincent GM, Abildskov JA, Burgess MJ: Q-T interval syndromes. Prog Cardiovasc Dis 16:523, 1974
75. Brown MJ, Brown DC, Murphy MB: Hypokalemia from beta$_2$-receptor stimulation by circulating epinephrine. N Engl J Med 309:1414, 1983
76. Struthers AD, Reid JL, Whitesmith R et al: The effect of cardioselectivity and nonselective beta-adrenoceptor blockade on the hypokalemic and cardiovascular responses to adrenomedullary hormone in man. Clin Sci 65:143, 1983
77. Ingbar SH: The role of antiadrenergic agents in the management of thyrotoxicosis. Cardiovasc Rev Rep 2:683, 1981
78. Caviness VS Jr, O'Brien P: Headache. N Engl J Med 302:446, 1980
79. Heel RC, Brogden RN, Speight TM et al: Timolol: A review of its therapeutic efficacy in the topical treatment of glaucoma. Drugs 17:38, 1979
80. Frishman WH: Beta-blocker withdrawal. Am J Cardiol 59:26F, 1987
81. Lloyd-Mostyn RH, Oram S: Modification by propranolol of cardiovascular effects of induced hypoglycemia. Lancet 2:1213, 1975
82. Missri JC: How do beta-blockers interact with other commonly used drugs? Cardiovasc Med 8:668, 1983
83. Frishman WH, Tepper D, Lazar E, Behrman D: Betaxolol: A new long-acting β_1-selective adrenergic blocker. J Clin Pharmacol, 1990 (in press)
84. Frishman WH, Covey S: Carteolol and penbutolol, two new β-adrenergic blockers with partial agonist activity. J Clin Pharmacol, 1990 (in press)

CALCIUM CHANNEL BLOCKERS IN THERAPEUTICS

Bramah N. Singh • Martin A. Josephson
Koonlawee N. Nademanee

CHAPTER 17
VOLUME 1

It is now more than 20 years since the prototype of calcium antagonists, verapamil, was first introduced. Rapid advances in our understanding of the pharmacodynamics of these agents and their clinical applications followed only after the important conceptual framework was provided by Fleckenstein in the early 1970s.[1] The pioneering work focused attention on the selectivity of effects of calcium antagonists on the myocardial slow channel, and the electrophysiologic effects of agents such as verapamil and prenylamine[1] in cardiac muscle were found to be similar to those produced by calcium-free media. The slow channel could be blocked markedly with drug concentrations that had little or no effect on the fast sodium channel. Agents with this selectivity of myocardial action also had the propensity to block calcium fluxes in vascular smooth muscle; thus, they were all peripheral and coronary vasodilators. However, it soon became clear[2-5] that the so-called calcium antagonist compounds (defined primarily as those agents that produced excitation-contraction uncoupling in cardiac muscle by blocking the slow channel) manifested a bewildering heterogeneity in chemical structure and were not completely selective for the myocardial slow channel. Some agents were truly selective for the slow channel in extremely low concentrations (*e.g.*, the dihydropyridines), and others blocked the slow as well as the fast channel in approximately the same drug concentrations (*e.g.*, perhexiline). Recent approaches have focused attention on the development of agents either with a broad pharmacologic profile or with a particular tissue selectivity.[5] This has led to an increasing plethora of newer calcium antagonists or calcium channel blocking drugs, many still under investigation, while a number have been introduced into therapeutics.[2-5] Calcium antagonism as a therapeutic modality has been established in the treatment of various ischemic myocardial syndromes, hypertension, certain cardiac arrhythmias, and hypertrophic cardiomyopathies. Numerous lesser indications are under investigation.

In this chapter, the pharmacologic basis of the therapeutic actions of calcium antagonists is discussed with particular reference to their hemodynamic and electrophysiologic actions. Their expanding role in the management of various cardiocirculatory disorders is delineated in relation to the pharmacodynamic and pharmacokinetic properties of the individual agents.

PHARMACOLOGIC CONSIDERATIONS

The ubiquitous role of calcium in mediating numerous physiologic responses is now well recognized. In relation to the actions of calcium antagonists, the role of calcium in mediating excitation-contraction coupling in cardiac muscle[6,7] and in vascular smooth muscle[8] is of the greatest significance.

In the myocardium, the primary locus of action of these drugs is on the slow calcium channel.[7] The voltage clamp technique has established that the depolarizing current in cardiac muscle is mediated by two discrete components. The first current component ("fast response"), carried by sodium ions, is rapidly activated and inactivated and is blocked selectively by fast-channel blockers, which are essentially local anesthetics. The second current is the slow current ("slow response"), the charge carrier for which is calcium for the most part.[7] This current, which completes the terminal phase of depolarization, is slowly activated at more positive membrane voltages and is much more slowly inactivated than the fast sodium current. This leads to excitation-contraction uncoupling with little or no change in the gross electrophysiologic parameters of the action potential in fast-channel-dependent fibers. Particularly evident in isolated tissue is the striking reduction in contractility, the overall effect resembling that of calcium-free media.[1] These changes are evident especially in atrial and ventricular myocardium in which neither conduction nor refractoriness is altered. It is the blockade of the slow calcium current in cardiac muscle that constitutes the cardinal property of the so-called calcium antagonists or calcium channel blockers. The effects of myocardial calcium antagonism is thus minimal in fast-channel-dependent fibers (atria, ventricles, His–Purkinje system, and bypass tracts); they are most pronounced in slow-channel-dependent fibers (sinoatrial and atrioventricular nodes). In isolated preparation of smooth muscle cells, slow-channel blockers exert a much more complex effect, since the process of excitation-contraction coupling is not governed by a single process.[8] Calcium entry across smooth muscle membrane is regulated either by a voltage-dependent mechanism or by a receptor-mediated channel. These mechanisms may be affected by different slow-channel blockers, but the net effect is varying degrees of smooth muscle relaxation due to competitive inhibition of calcium influx.

A very heterogeneous group of compounds has been shown to exhibit the phenomenon of calcium antagonism. These compounds have varying potencies for blocking the myocardial slow channel and for inhibiting calcium fluxes in vascular smooth muscle cells. Furthermore, because of the structural heterogeneity, many of the agents have additional pharmacologic properties. For example, some of the compounds influence the autonomic nervous system by their propensity to noncompetitively inhibit catecholamine α- and β-receptors (e.g., verapamil and diltiazem). These properties therefore influence the balance of actions of these compounds between their direct myocardial effects on chronotropic, dromotropic, and inotropic actions and the reflex changes that occur from the activation of the sympathetic nervous system due to peripheral vascular dilatation. Some of the agents have additional electrophysiologic actions owing to their associated effects on the fast channel and on cardiac repolarization (e.g., bepridil, lidoflazine). It is clear that unlike β-blockers the net pharmacologic effects of individual calcium antagonists may not be predictable solely on the basis of their ability to competitively inhibit calcium fluxes in the myocardium or smooth muscle cells. The net effects may differ significantly *in vivo* when compared with those *in vitro*; these differences are of much clinical significance.

CLASSIFICATION OF CALCIUM ANTAGONISTS

Fleckenstein[1] recently suggested that calcium antagonists may be classified into two categories. He placed agents such as verapamil, diltiazem, and nifedipine with its derivatives, which have a marked selectivity for inhibiting the slow channel versus the fast sodium channel in the heart, into one group (group A) and those such as prenylamine, terodiline, fendiline, and perhexiline, which also inhibit the slow channel but have a broad array of other electrophysiologic actions, into another group (group B). However, the expanding knowledge of the electropharmacology of these and newer agents suggests a need for an alternative classification. The one proposed in Table 17.1, developed along clinical lines,[5] may also eventually need modification owing to the rapidly increasing clinical and experimental data relating to calcium antagonists.

TYPE I: CALCIUM ANTAGONISTS WITH *IN VIVO* MYOCARDIAL EFFECTS

The chemical structures of diltiazem, tiapamil, and gallopamil (D_{600}) are shown in Figure 17.1 relative to that of the reference calcium antagonist verapamil and are compared with that of nifedipine, the prototype dihydropyridine (see below). Except for diltiazem, there are structural similarities among the other three compounds. All four are moderately potent peripheral vasodilators and are effective in mild to

TABLE 17.1 CLINICAL CLASSIFICATION OF CALCIUM ANTAGONISTS

Type I.	Calcium antagonists with *in vivo* myocardial, electrophysiologic, and vascular effects
	Verapamil Diltiazem
	Gallopamil (D_{600}) Tiapamil
Type II.	Calcium antagonists with predominant vascular effects *in vivo*
	Nifedipine Nicardipine
	Nitrendipine Niludipine
	Nisoldipine Felodipine
	Nimodipine
Type III.	Calcium antagonists with selective vascular effects
	Cinnarizine
	Flunarizine
Type IV.	Calcium antagonists with complex pharmacologic profile
	Bepridil Perhexiline
	Lidoflazine

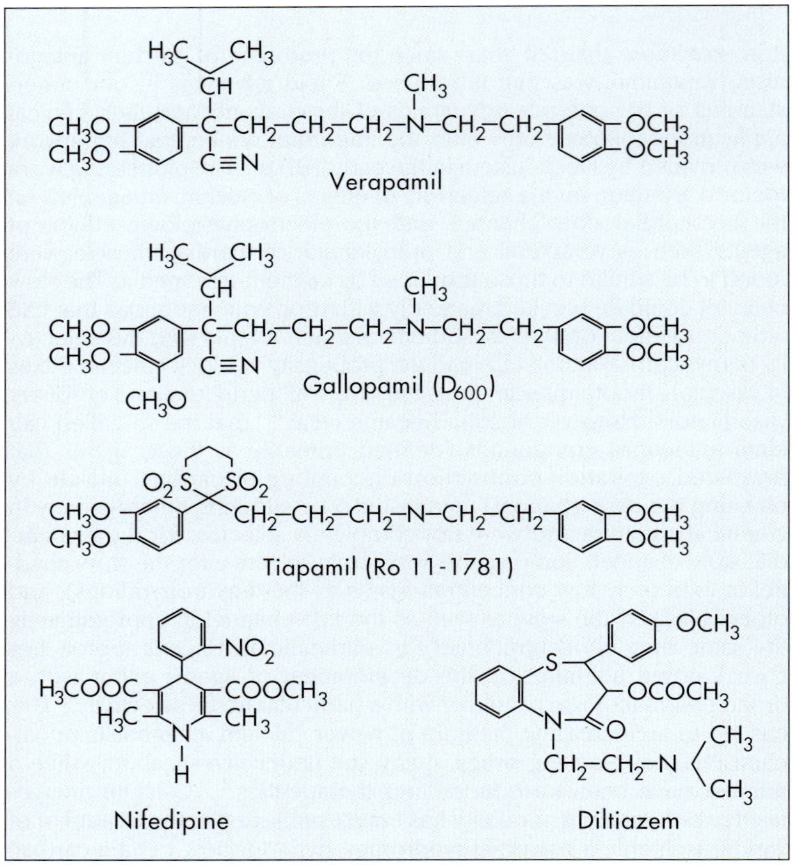

FIGURE 17.1 Structural formulas of certain calcium antagonists. Structurally, gallopamil (the methoxy derivative of verapamil) and tiapamil resemble verapamil. Diltiazem is a benzothiazepine derivative, and nifedipine is dihydropyridine. All compounds block the slow channel in the myocardium and relax smooth muscle in vascular and other tissues.

moderate hypertension. Their predominant electrophysiologic actions are lengthening conduction time and prolonging refractoriness in the atrioventricular node, properties that account for much of their known antiarrhythmic effects. The hemodynamic effects of verapamil in experimental animals and in patients with varying levels of ventricular function are reasonably well defined; there are modest data for diltiazem and very little for either tiapamil or gallopamil. There are preliminary data to indicate that gallopamil might be extremely effective in terminating supraventricular tachycardias and in controlling chronic stable angina; further data are needed to determine critically the comparative efficacy of tiapamil and gallopamil on the one hand and verapamil and diltiazem on the other.

TYPE II: THE DIHYDROPYRIDINE SUBGROUP OF CALCIUM ANTAGONISTS

Numerous dihydropyridine derivatives are currently under investigation for the control of a variety of cardiocirculatory disorders, depending on each drug's presumed specific pharmacologic properties. Of the newer compounds, these are the most closely related structurally. As a group, the potency of the dihydropyridines is much greater in relation to smooth muscle compared with cardiac muscle; these agents, *in vivo*, are nearly or completely devoid of clinically significant electrophysiologic properties, their overall hemodynamic effects being dominated by striking peripheral vasodilatation. From the therapeutic standpoint this may prove of particular value in the control of hypertensive emergencies as well as in the long-term management of essential hypertension, either as single agents or in combination with diuretics, β-adrenergic blocking drugs, or other hypotensive agents. Since all of these agents produce marked reflex increases in heart rate and contractility, angina may sometimes be aggravated in some patients with coronary artery disease if concomitant sympatholytic agents are not used. The cardioprotective effects of these agents in experimental animals appear to be less striking than those of type I agents.

The dihydropyridines may exert tissue selectivity.[9] At present, the dihydropyridine that has been approved for therapeutic use is nifedipine, but numerous others are likely to be introduced in the foreseeable future. Niludipine and nisoldipine are both more potent than nifedipine as vasodilators, but *in vitro* have the same cardiac activity. Preliminary data suggest that nimodipine might have selectivity of action in the cerebral vasculature.[9]

TYPE III: THE PIPERAZINE DERIVATIVES: FLUNARIZINE AND CINNARIZINE

The properties of the compounds in this type of calcium antagonist drug, namely, cinnarizine and its difluoro derivative, flunarizine, are highly selective for calcium channels in vascular smooth muscle relative to cardiac muscle.[10]

The properties and therapeutic uses of flunarizine have recently been reviewed by Holmes and co-workers.[10] Flunarizine has a much longer plasma elimination half-life than does cinnarizine. The majority of the therapeutic trials with flunarizine have been in the prophylaxis of migraine, in occlusive peripheral vascular disease, and in vertigo of central and peripheral origin. The preliminary data with the piperazine derivatives appear to offer potentially new and useful pharmacologic approaches to the control of a number of circulatory disorders, but the definition of the precise role of these compounds in the therapy of such conditions must await stringently controlled comparative studies.

TYPE IV: CALCIUM ANTAGONISTS WITH COMPLEX PHARMACOLOGIC PROFILE

Another group of pharmacologic agents may be categorized as calcium antagonists that have a selectivity of action either for vascular tissues (as in the case of lidoflazine)[11] or for both cardiac as well as smooth muscle (as in the case of perhexiline[12] and bepridil[13]) while also having the propensity to block the fast sodium channel in the heart to a variable degree. Some of these agents have yet other electrophysiologic properties. Thus, these agents not only are heterogeneous chemically but, by virtue of their overall complex pharmacologic properties, may exert a somewhat different spectrum of therapeutic effects. This pertains particularly to their cardiac electrophysiologic actions and to the control of cardiac arrhythmias; bepridil is the most important in this regard, having a long elimination half-life (almost 40 hours).

Electrophysiologically, bepridil blocks the slow calcium channel in the heart while also inhibiting the fast channel and lengthening the repolarization phase of the cardiac action potential in all myocardial tissues; bepridil shortens the repolarization phase in Purkinje's fibers. These data are consistent with clinical studies,[14] which have shown that intravenous bepridil prolongs the effective refractory period of atria, ventricles, and the atrioventricular node and lengthens the Wenckebach cycle length of the atrioventricular node during rapid atrial pacing. The spontaneous sinus cycle length is not significantly altered, nor is the sinus node recovery time in patients with normal sinus node function. The effects in patients with the sick sinus syndrome are not known. The AH interval is prolonged, with a trend toward an increase in the HV interval during electrophysiologic studies. The QTc interval is prolonged.

The available data suggest that, unlike most other calcium antagonists, bepridil is likely to be effective in ventricular as well as supraventricular tachyarrhythmias, although the relative potency of the compound in these two groups of dysrhythmias remains to be determined. However, there have been reports that the compound may produce *torsade de pointes* under certain clinical conditions, but the agent is of pharmacologic interest in exhibiting such a wide array of electrophysiologic properties.

From the standpoint of clinical utility, the most widely studied agents are verapamil, diltiazem, and nifedipine. Their electrophysiologic, pharmacokinetic, and systemic and coronary hemodynamic effects will be described before their role in the management of various cardiocirculatory disorders is discussed. The other calcium antagonists are mentioned briefly for completeness.

CLINICAL ELECTROPHYSIOLOGIC EFFECTS

The clinical and experimental electrophysiologic effects of verapamil and its congeners diltiazem and nifedipine are consistent.[14] The major effects are summarized in Table 17.2. The effects of tiapamil and gallopamil are qualitatively similar to those of verapamil or diltiazem and differ from those of the dihydropyridines.

As might be expected, none of the three best-known calcium antagonists affect the QRS duration or the QTc interval of the surface electrocardiogram. Nor do they alter the effective refractory period of the atria, bypass tracts, ventricles, or His–Purkinje system. They have no effect on infranodal conduction (*i.e.*, HV interval in the His-bundle electrograms). The QRS and QTc intervals are lengthened by bepridil and lidoflazine, both of which produce a corresponding prolongation of the effective refractory period in most cardiac tissues. The main electrophysiologic effect of conventional calcium antagonists in therapeutic doses is to influence the properties of myocardial cells which are dependent on the slow-channel function for depolarization (*e.g.*, sinoatrial and atrioventricular nodes). Thus, the most readily demonstrable effects are on the atrioventricular node (Figs. 17.2 and 17.3). Here, they increase the intranodal conduction (*i.e.*, AH interval) and prolong the effective and functional refractory periods in the antegrade and retrograde directions (see Table 17.2). They also reduce the Wenckebach periodicity during right atrial pacing. However, as already indicated, there are differences among various calcium antagonists in this regard. For example, whereas diltiazem and verapamil (and its congeners) do exert these effects *in vitro* and *in vivo*, the effects of the dihydropyridines are either reversed or nullified because of the potent reflex effects generated by their marked peripheral vasodilator actions.

Unlike verapamil and diltiazem, the dihydropyridines do not appear to exert sympatholytic effects. Thus, agents such as nifedipine have actions opposite to those of verapamil and diltiazem on the atrioventricular node, *reducing* rather than prolonging the effective refractory period and shortening the intranodal conduction (see Figs. 17.2 and 17.3). A depressant effect on the atrioventricular node may become apparent with the dihydropyridines if the sympathetic reflexes are blunted as might occur with substantial β-blockade or pathologically induced autonomic insufficiency.

In general, calcium antagonists have little or no effects on the maximum sinus node recovery time or in sinoatrial conduction in the setting of normal sinus nodal function. However, their depressant effect becomes evident in patients with conduction system disease, but it tends to be less pronounced with the dihydropyridines.

It should also be emphasized that while calcium antagonists as a class of agents exert little effect on the electrophysiologic parameters of normal fast-channel-dependent myocardial fibers, in the setting of ischemia they may increase the effective refractory period and improve conduction. This is not a primary effect but is likely related to the amelioration of ischemia and is of clinical relevance.

It will be evident that an appreciation of the electrophysiologic effects of calcium antagonists in humans allows the appropriate choice

TABLE 17.2 COMPARATIVE CLINICAL ELECTROPHYSIOLOGIC EFFECTS OF CALCIUM CHANNEL BLOCKERS

Electrophysiologic Parameter	Verapamil	Nifedipine	Diltiazem	Bepridil
RR interval				
QRS interval	0	0	0	+
QTc interval	0	0	0	++
PR interval	++	±	++	++
AH interval	+++	±	+	+++
HV interval	0	0	0	+
Atrial ERP	±	0	±	++
AV node ERP	++++	±	+++	+++
AV node FRP	++++	±	+++	+++
Ventricular ERP	0	0	0	++
His–Purkinje ERP	0	0	0	++
Bypass tract ERP	±	0	±	++
Sinus node recovery time	0*	0	0*	+
Ventricular atuomaticity	0	0	0	

* Prolonged in sick sinus syndrome.

(↓, decrease; ↑, increase; ↑↓, variable effect; +-++++, indicates graded increase in intensity of effect; *AV*, atrioventricular; *ERP*, effective refractory period; *FRP*, functional refractory period)

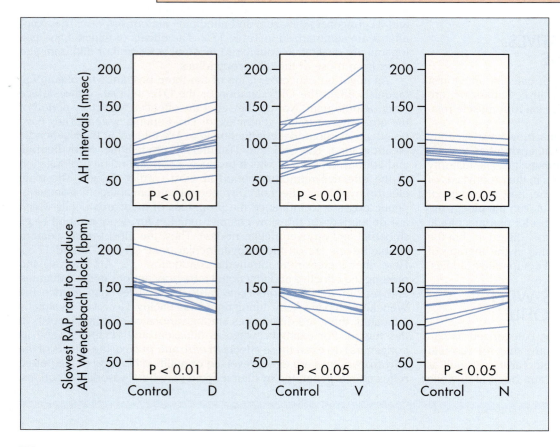

FIGURE 17.2 Effects of diltiazem (D), verapamil (V), and nifedipine (N) on AH intervals and slowest rate of right atrial pacing (RAP) to produce Wenckebach AH block (minimal RAP rate to reproduce Wenckebach in clinical cases). Thick lines represent mean values. (Modified from Kawai C, Tomotsuga K, Matsuyoma E et al: Comparative effects of three calcium antagonists, diltiazem, verapamil and nifedipine, on the sino-atrial and atrioventricular nodes: Experimental and clinical studies. Circulation 63:1035, 1981. By permission of the American Heart Association, Inc)

of an agent in the elective and prophylactic control of the arrhythmias in which these compounds are of value.

SYSTEMIC HEMODYNAMIC EFFECTS

The hemodynamic effects of calcium antagonists represent a complex interplay of simultaneous alterations in preload, afterload, contractility, and coronary blood flow.[3,4,15] The net effect is determined by the overall properties of individual calcium antagonists, the level of baseline ventricular function, the integrity of the autonomic nervous system, and the presence or absence of myocardial ischemia. To these must be added the route and dose of the antagonist used. In general, the net effect is largely determined by the degree to which the intrinsic negative inotropic effect of the individual agent (determined by its potency as an antagonist of the slow calcium channel in the heart) is offset by its peripheral dilator actions in vascular smooth muscle.[4]

VERAPAMIL

In healthy subjects verapamil exerts a trivial degree of negative inotropic effects, readily abolished with mild exercise. In patients with cardiac disease with relatively well-preserved ventricular function, when given intravenously, verapamil functions as a moderately potent peripheral vasodilator (Fig. 17.4). It reduces systemic arterial pressure and resistance, with a slight increase in cardiac output and with no fall in stroke volume. There is a mild but significant increase in pulmonary wedge pressure (and other right-sided pressures) accompanied by a decrease in contractility, although the left ventricular ejection fraction, determined either by contrast or radionuclide ventriculography, is not reduced. In some studies a mild increase has been reported.

While hemodynamic variables are not affected adversely by intravenous verapamil in patients with relatively preserved or moderately impaired ventricular function, deterioration may occur in those with severely impaired ventricular performance.[15,16] For example, in those with a left ventricular ejection fraction below 35% and filling pressures exceeding 18 mm Hg, the usual infusion regimen has been shown to induce marked clinical and hemodynamic exacerbation with steep increases in the left ventricular filling pressures.[16] This suggests caution in the use of the intravenous drug in patients with severe reduction in function. However, this does not preclude the use of the drug in the setting of myocardial ischemia and cardiac arrhythmias in patients with reduced ejection fraction, since the salutary effects of the drug in ischemia and in arrhythmias will offset the intrinsic depressant effect of the compound. The hemodynamic effects of intravenously administered gallopamil and tiapamil are likely to be similar to those of verapamil.

Relatively little data are available on the hemodynamic effects of orally administered verapamil in patients with cardiac disease. Single oral doses of the drug in patients with uncomplicated myocardial infarction have revealed no significant depressant effect,[17] but during long-term therapy with the agent (320 mg–480 mg/day) in patients with ischemic heart disease and in hypertrophic cardiomyopathy, verapamil has been reported to reduce left ventricular ejection fraction and to produce heart failure in a small number of cases.[18]

DILTIAZEM

Diltiazem appears to be a somewhat less potent peripheral vasodilator and with less negative inotropic effect than verapamil, although a direct comparison between the two agents in man has not been made. The mean hemodynamic effects of intravenous (0.16 mg–0.25 mg/kg) diltiazem in patients with coronary artery disease[19] with normal or near-normal ejection fraction are summarized in Figure 17.5. The drug produced a 22% decrease in systemic vascular resistance, a 12% decrease in mean arterial pressure, an 8% increase in cardiac index, and a 10% increase in mean pulmonary wedge pressure. A modest increase in left ventricular ejection fraction was also found. These overall effects are similar to those found with verapamil in a comparable group of patients with cardiac disease.

Recent studies with intravenous and oral diltiazem (360 mg/day) in patients with Class III-IV heart failure (New York Heart Association) and with dilated cardiomyopathy having a mean ejection fraction of 26% and wedge pressure of 29 mm Hg indicated that the drug does not produce an aggravation of heart failure in this subset of patients. In these patients, intravenous diltiazem increased cardiac index by 20%, stroke volume index by 50%, stroke work index by 20%, heart rate by 23%, mean arterial pressure by 18%, and pulmonary wedge pressure by

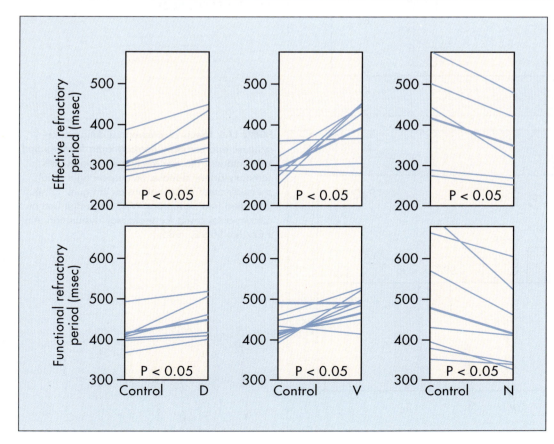

FIGURE 17.3 Effects of diltiazem (D), verapamil (V), and nifedipine (N) on effective and functional refractory periods in clinical cases. Thick lines denote mean values. (<, Cases in which failure of atrial capture by extrastimulus preceded—therefore, the actual value is lower than that shown in the figure) (Modified from Kawai C, Tomotsuga K, Matsuyoma E et al: Comparative effects of three calcium antagonists, diltiazem, verapamil and nifedipine on the sino-atrial and atrioventricular nodes: Experimental and clinical studies. Circulation 63:1035, 1981. By permission of the American Heart Association, Inc)

34% without a change in left ventricular dp/dt.[20] Equivalent hemodynamic alterations were produced by short-term oral diltiazem. These findings are in contrast to those reported for verapamil, but further studies are needed to substantiate the observations with diltiazem and to define the possible mechanisms for the differences. It must be emphasized, however, that while the short-term studies with diltiazem suggest that the drug can be used with impunity in patients with heart failure, long-term experience is not available, and it would not be prudent to advocate the use of the drug as an afterload-reducing agent in preference to the conventional vasodilators.

NIFEDIPINE AND OTHER DIHYDROPYRIDINES

When administered orally, sublingually, or intravenously, the hemodynamic effects of the drug are characterized by a profound fall in arterial pressure and systemic resistance with a corresponding reflex increase in heart rate. This leads to an increase in cardiac index and in many patients to a fall in the left ventricular filling pressure with an increase in cardiac contractility. A 20-mg dose of the drug may induce an 18% increase in cardiac index and about a 10% increase in the left ventricular ejection fraction. The effects of other dihydropyridines are directionally similar (see Figure 17.6 in the case of nicardipine). The intrinsic negative inotropic effects of these calcium antagonists are nullified or reversed by their reflex effects. However, if the reflex effects are attenuated or abolished by either disease or drugs (e.g., β-blockers), a frankly depressant effect may emerge.

The improvement in hemodynamic effects following the use of nifedipine and other dihydropyridines is particularly marked and of clinical utility in the setting of hypertensive crises and pulmonary edema.[21] In this setting the ventricular ejection fraction may increase, with a fall in the left ventricular end-diastolic pressure. However, the improved hemodynamic responses after nifedipine in cases of pulmonary edema are often striking only after the initial dose and are not sustained during long-term therapy. Significantly greater enhancement of left ventricular performance has been reported after equihypotensive doses of hydralazine than after nifedipine in patients with congestive heart failure.[22] Hemodynamic deterioration may also occur with nifedipine in a subset of such patients, especially in those in whom the drug does not produce increases in heart rate. This is consistent with the recent reports of cardiac failure occurring in patients given nifedipine in combination with β-blockade.[21] It is likely that in this respect the effects of other dihydropyridines are likely to be similar.

The hemodynamic effects of calcium antagonists summarized above suggest that while these drugs are safe in patients without cardiac failure, their use in failure may be attended by unpredictable effects, with an aggravation of decompensation in a subset of patients. The experience does not justify their use as afterload-reducing agents in preference to the conventional vasodilators (see below). However,

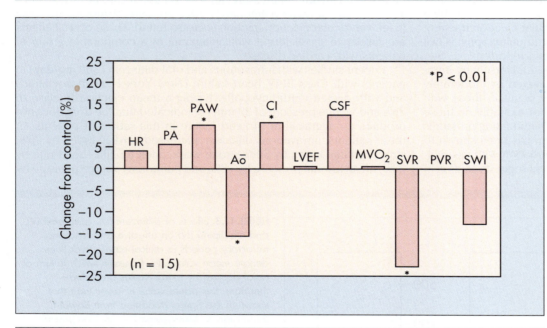

FIGURE 17.4 Effects of intravenous verapamil on systemic and coronary hemodynamics and left ventricular ejection fraction in 15 patients with coronary artery disease. (Ao, mean aortic pressure; C.I., cardiac index; CSF, coronary sinus flow; HR, heart rate; LVEF, left ventricular ejection fraction; MVO$_2$, myocardial oxygen consumption; PA, mean pulmonary artery pressure; PAW, mean pulmonary capillary wedge pressure; PVR, pulmonary vascular resistance; SVR, systemic vascular resistance; SWI, stroke work index). (Modified from Josephson MA, Singh BN: Use of calcium antagonists for ventricular dysfunction. Am J Cardiol 55:81B, 1985)

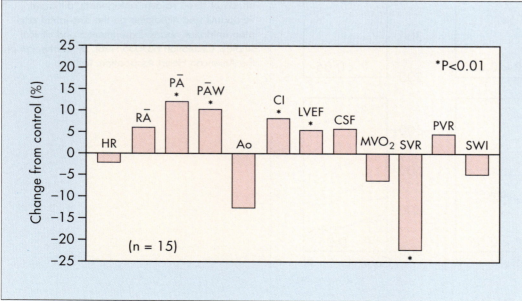

FIGURE 17.5 Effects of intravenous diltiazem on systemic and coronary hemodynamic features and left ventricular ejection fraction in patients with coronary artery disease. (RA, mean right atrial pressure; other abbreviations as in Figure 17.4) (Modified from Josephson MA, Singh BN: Use of calcium antagonists for ventricular dysfunction. Am J Cardiol 55:81B, 1985)

from the practical clinical standpoint, it is important to appreciate the differences in the hemodynamic effects among various calcium antagonists. Such differences permit the rational choice of an agent for a particular clinical indication, especially in relation to the varying spectrum of abnormality in ventricular performance.

EFFECTS ON THE CORONARY CIRCULATION

There are major similarities in the pharmacologic actions of these drugs in the coronary circulation with respect to their dilator actions in the resistance and capacitance vessels and in coronary sinus flow as measured by thermodilution in humans.[3,4,23] Although in experimental models, differences have been found in the potency of verapamil, diltiazem, and nifedipine for dilating coronary arteries, such differences are difficult to define in humans. Nor do they appear to be of clinical significance if present.

When nifedipine, verapamil, and diltiazem are given intravenously, they produce an increase in oxygen tension in the coronary sinus effluent with a small but significant dilatation of not only normal but also narrowed segments of the coronary arteries with a corresponding decrease in the estimated flow resistance when determined by computer-assisted angiographic techniques.[23] Such a vasodilatory response is accompanied by a fall in total coronary vascular resistance with a tendency for the coronary sinus flow to increase, indicating that these agents dilate resistance as well as capacitance segments of the coronary circulation. However, there is no significant decrease in myocardial oxygen consumption as determined by standard hemodynamic techniques.

Of particular clinical relevance is the finding that these drugs prevent coronary stenosis constriction provoked by α-adrenergic and serotonergic receptor stimulation.[23] For example, handgrip produces a constriction of 20% in the minimal luminal area; such an area may increase by 3% with handgrip during the continuous infusion of diltiazem. Stenosis dilatation is also produced by nitrates but not by such potent coronary arterial dilators as dipyridamole, which does not block handgrip-induced coronary vasoconstriction. It is now believed that stenosis dilatation may be an integral component of the anti-ischemic actions of calcium antagonists.[23] Calcium antagonists do not appear to have the potential to produce the coronary steal syndrome in humans.

PHARMACOKINETICS

The salient features of the pharmacokinetics of the three commonly used calcium antagonists are presented elsewhere[24] and are summarized in Table 17.3.

NIFEDIPINE

Over 90% of orally or buccally administered nifedipine is absorbed, with the drug appearing in the plasma within 3 minutes of buccal and 20 minutes of oral administration. The peak plasma concentrations are reached about 1 to 2 hours after an oral dose. The first-pass effect for nifedipine is low, and systemic bioavailability is over 65%. The drug is metabolized in the liver, but its metabolites are not pharmacologically active. A linear correlation between plasma drug levels and clinical effects for nifedipine has not been demonstrated.

Nifedipine does not appear to accumulate following long-term therapy, and its elimination half-life remains stable. A pharmacokinetic interaction has been suggested but is not confirmed. If it occurs, it is likely to be trivial. Nifedipine is available as a tablet and a liquid-filled capsule; its intravenous formulation is not stable. The dosage regimens are indicated in Table 17.3.

DILTIAZEM

Diltiazem is almost completely absorbed following oral administration. It appears in the plasma within 15 minutes of ingestion, and the peak concentration develops after 30 minutes. Diltiazem is subject to extensive hepatic metabolism; the major pathway of metabolism is deacetylation. Its metabolite, deacetyldiltiazem, is pharmacologically active, having approximately 40% the activity of the parent compound.

The bioavailability of diltiazem appears to increase with continued drug administration without a change in the elimination half-life, a phenomenon probably due to the saturation of the metabolic pathway of the compound in the liver. The elimination half-life of diltiazem is not altered by renal failure, and there is no known interaction with digoxin, hydrochlorothiazide, warfarin, or propranolol. However, a significant interaction has been demonstrated with cimetidine during the concomitant administration of which dose adjustment of diltiazem is required.

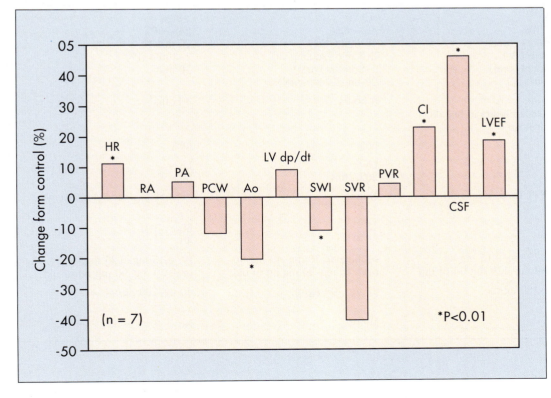

FIGURE 17.6 Effects of intravenous nicardipine on coronary and systemic hemodynamics in patients with coronary artery disease. Abbreviations as in Figures 17.4 and 17.5. (Modified from unpublished observation of Josephson MA, Singh BN, 1986)

VERAPAMIL

The elimination half-life of verapamil is similar after short-term intravenous or oral drug administration; however, during long-term drug administration, there is nonlinear accumulation of the drug with reduced clearance and prolongation of elimination half-life. This indicates that, as in the case of diltiazem, verapamil may be administered twice daily, although sustained release formulations of both drugs are becoming available.

The elimination of verapamil is essentially by hepatic metabolism by an enzyme that is inducible by phenobarbitone. Numerous metabolites are formed, but only nor-verapamil is active, having about 25% of the activity of the parent compound. Verapamil exhibits a marked first-pass effect in the liver; thus, its serum levels are likely to vary with hepatic disease, especially cirrhosis of the liver. Because of the first-pass effect, the serum concentrations of the drug are likely to vary tenfold or greater in different subjects at the same dosage regimens. Verapamil at the protein binding sites in the plasma may be displaced by lidocaine, diazepam, propranolol, and disopyramide, but the clinical significance of this effect is unclear. However, the pharmacokinetic interaction with digoxin is of clinical significance. The steady-state levels of digoxin may be elevated by over 50% by the concomitant administration of verapamil. In part, this may be due to reduced renal clearance, and dose adjustment is usually necessary when the two drugs are given together. It should also be emphasized that the electrophysiologic effects of the two drugs on the atrioventricular node may summate.

DRUG INTERACTIONS WITH CALCIUM ANTAGONISTS

Drug interactions may be pharmacokinetic (*e.g.*, diltiazem and cimetidine or verapamil and digoxin), hemodynamic, or electrophysiologic. For example, the potential negative inotropic effect of certain calcium antagonists (particularly type I) may summate with those of β-blockers and disopyramide; similarly, the electrophysiologic effects may be additive to those of β-blockers and amiodarone or other antiarrhythmic drugs that influence adrenergic and slow-channel functions in the heart. Such interactions are of the greatest importance in patients with overt or covert conduction system disease.

THERAPEUTIC APPLICATIONS OF CALCIUM CHANNEL BLOCKERS

Although a great deal has been learned about the pharmacodynamic effects of calcium antagonists recently, their complete spectrum of therapeutic applications is still not fully defined. The major established indications and the newer potential ones are listed in Table 17.4.

The role of these drugs is best established in ischemic myocardial syndromes, especially in Prinzmetal's angina, unstable angina, and chronic stable angina; their potential roles in myocardial protection in the context of cardiac surgery and in survivors of acute myocardial infarction remain to be established. Electrophysiologic studies have now established the role of this class of drugs in the control of certain supraventricular tachyarrhythmias, but their place in the treatment of ventricular arrhythmias is less well defined. In the past few years, perhaps the greatest promise that these agents have shown is in the control of mild to moderate essential hypertension and in the management of hypertensive emergencies. These aspects of their clinical applications in relation to the newer aspects of the pathophysiology of the various disorders in which calcium antagonists are of value are discussed below.

MYOCARDIAL ISCHEMIC SYNDROMES

Many observations from hemodynamic monitoring, radionuclide perfusion studies, metabolic investigations, and Holter recordings in ambulatory and hospitalized patients have now established two important findings about the nature of myocardial ischemia in the setting of coronary artery disease.[25] These findings have a bearing on the therapeutic

TABLE 17.3 CLINICAL PHARMACOKINETIC PARAMETERS OF THREE CALCIUM ANTAGONISTS

	Verapamil	Nifedipine	Diltiazem
1. Absorption	>79%	>90%	>90%
Bioavailability	10%–20%	45%–62%	24%–90%
Onset of action	1–2 hours (oral)	15 min (oral)	15 min (oral)
	½–1 min (IV)	2–3 min (sublingual)	2–3 min (IV)
Peak action	3–4 hours (oral)	1–2 hours (oral)	30 min
	2–5 min (IV)	20 min (sublingual)	
2. Elimination half-life	3–7 hours*	4 hours	4 hours
	(up to 26 hours in hepatic cirrhosis)		
3. Protein binding (approximately)	90%	90%	80%
4. Metabolism	Liver	Liver	Liver
First pass	85%	20%–30%	50%
5. Metabolites activity	20%–25% (nor-verapamil)	None	40%–50% (deacetyldiltiazem)
6. Excretion (%)			
Gastrointestinal	25	15	60
Renal	75	85	40
7. Dose	IV: 0.075 mg–0.15 mg/kg	sublingual: 10 mg–40 mg tid	IV: 0.15 mg–0.25 mg/kg
	oral: 80 mg–120 mg tid or qid	oral: 10 mg–40 mg tid or qid	oral: 30 mg–90 mg tid or qid
8. Therapeutic plasma concentration	80 ng–100 ng/ml	25 ng–100 ng/ml	40 ng–200 ng/ml
9. Interaction with digoxin	Yes	Minor	No

* Increases as a function of time.

effects of calcium antagonists. First, it is clear that over two thirds of the transient ischemic episodes detected by continuous monitoring in variant angina, unstable angina, and chronic stable angina are not associated with chest pain or equivalents (*i.e.*, they are "silent"). Second, a somewhat greater number, perhaps over 80%, of the episodes in unstable as well as chronic stable angina are not triggered by increases in heart rate or blood pressure. Thus, the majority of episodes of ischemia in coronary artery disease may be due to a primary reduction in myocardial flow as a result of intermittent arterial obstruction produced either by thrombus formation or by coronary vasoconstriction. These observations have an important bearing on the mechanism of action of calcium antagonists in the various syndromes of myocardial ischemia in patients with coronary artery disease. The human coronary artery is subject to numerous neurohumoral influences that may alter its caliber. If these were to occur in association with an eccentrically placed atherosclerotic plaque in juxtaposition to an arc of normal tissue, variation in the caliber of the coronary artery as little as 10% may lead to a critical reduction in coronary blood flow.[23] Calcium antagonists are coronary vasodilators and may antagonize such a tendency to vasoconstriction in various anginal syndromes. It has also been shown that these drugs reverse or negate the vasoconstrictive effects of ergonovine on the coronary arteries and prevent the sympathetically mediated vasoconstriction induced by handgrip or other physiological interventions.[23] Thus, unlike the effects of β-blockers, a significant action of calcium antagonists in ischemic syndromes may be mediated by their effects on coronary vessels over and above those on myocardial oxygen consumption. The potential mechanisms that determine the salutary effects of calcium antagonists in myocardial ischemia are summarized in Table 17.5.

It must be emphasized that the effects on myocardial oxygen consumption among various calcium antagonists may differ significantly. For example, type I calcium antagonists tend to lower heart rate, whereas the dihydropyridines (*e.g.*, nifedipine and nicardipine) may induce significant tachycardia at least during the early stages of therapy. In a proportion of such patients this may lead to an increase in oxygen demand and aggravation of ischemia; rarely, myocardial infarction may be precipitated in the early stages of therapy. Thus, the dihydropyridines are best used in combination with β-blockers in patients with chronic stable angina, although the aggravation of heart rate has not been shown to be of much clinical significance in either variant angina or unstable angina or during chronic therapy with the dihydropyridines in chronic stable angina. This suggests that an adaptation in the reflex responses may occur during protracted therapy.

At present, the effects of calcium antagonists on silent myocardial ischemia occurring in various subsets of coronary artery disease are not clearly defined but may be of therapeutic significance.

VARIANT OR PRINZMETAL'S ANGINA. The advent of calcium antagonists has constituted a major advance in the control of variant angina. All the available agents (*e.g.*, verapamil, diltiazem, nifedipine, and those currently under investigation) have been found to reverse coronary artery spasm and reduce the frequency (Fig. 17.7) of ischemic episodes as judged by symptoms, nitroglycerin consumption, and ST segment deviations documented on Holter recordings.[26] No significant differences in efficacy have been established among the different agents, and although excellent theoretical reasons may be cited to support the use of combination therapy with different calcium antagonists, at present there is no decisive evidence that combination therapy is superior to the maximally tolerated doses of a single agent. Similarly, it is not certain whether these agents have a greater efficacy compared with nitrates. The available data suggest that the overall efficacy of the two classes of compounds may be comparable. However, because of the more predictable half-life and easier dosing schedules with less likelihood of tolerance developing during continuous drug therapy, calcium antagonists are now used increasingly in most cases of Prinzmetal's angina in conjunction with nitrates. On pharmacologic grounds, combination therapy of nitrates and calcium antagonists appears rational and should always be considered in recalcitrant cases. The role of β-blockers in this setting when compared with that of calcium antagonists is less well established. In vasotonic angina with normal coronary arteries, β-blockers have been shown to increase the duration of ischemic episodes when compared with the effects of placebo.[27] However, the precise clinical significance of this observation is unclear.

The overall clinical impression is that over 80% of patients with Prinzmetal's angina respond to calcium antagonism. However, it remains uncertain whether the continuous prophylactic therapy of variant angina with calcium antagonists, while being effective in relieving symptoms, leads to enhanced survival. The drugs are nevertheless effective in preventing recurrent ventricular arrhythmias complicating ischemic episodes, the primary effect being on ischemia rather than on the arrhythmia in this setting.

UNSTABLE ANGINA. At present the exact mechanisms underlying the development of the unstable angina syndrome are uncertain.[28] It is known that the rate of progression of the atherosclerotic disease may

---

TABLE 17.4 THERAPEUTIC APPLICATIONS OF CALCIUM ANTAGONISTS

Established Clinical Indications
Ischemic myocardial syndromes
    Prinzmetal's angina
    Unstable angina
    Chronic stable angina
Cardiac arrhythmias
Hypertension and hypertensive emergencies
Hypertrophic cardiomyopathies

Potential Indications
Cardioprotection
Pulmonary hypertension and afterload reduction
Migraine and cluster headaches
Cerebral insufficiency
Raynaud's phenomenon
Disorders of gastrointestinal motility
Exercise-induced bronchospasm
Prevention of atherosclerosis

TABLE 17.5 POTENTIAL MECHANISMS OF ACTION OF CALCIUM ANTAGONISTS IN CHRONIC STABLE ANGINA*

Increased Myocardial Oxygen Supply
Increased coronary blood flow (all agents)
    Coronary arterial dilatation including lesion dilatation
    Improved subendocardial perfusion
    ? Decreased platelet aggregability

Decreased Myocardial Oxygen Demand
Decreased peripheral vascular resistance afterload (all agents)
Decreased myocardial contractility (verapamil, bepridil)
Decreased heart rate (verapamil, diltiazem, bepridil)
Decreased intracellular metabolism

* Not all the postulated mechanisms have been verified in patients. They have been extrapolated from findings in experimental models of myocardial ischemia.

(Adapted from Singh BN, Ellrodt G, Nademanee K: Calcium antagonists: Cardiocirculatory effects and therapeutic applications. In Hurst JW (ed): Clinical Essays on the Heart, vol 2, pp 65–98. New York, McGraw-Hill, 1984)

be accelerated in patients with unstable angina; it is also known that in some of them there is evidence of coronary vasospasm and in others, especially those who die, evidence of antemortem clot formation is convincing. Experimental data (see below) have indicated a beneficial effect of calcium antagonism in atherosclerosis, and *in vitro* data involving human platelets have documented significant effects of calcium antagonists on platelet aggregability (see below). Which of these potential mechanisms that are affected by calcium antagonists lead to their salutary effects in unstable angina remains uncertain, although the short-term effects of these drugs in alleviating the symptoms and electrocardiographic abnormalities have been well documented in the case of verapamil, diltiazem, and nifedipine.[3,21]

However, there is no systematic experience on the effects of intravenously administered calcium antagonists in the rapid and effective control of ischemia in unstable angina. For example, it is not known whether these agents have efficacy comparable to that of intravenous nitrates in unstable angina, although short-term oral therapy with calcium antagonists and with nitrates appears to be equally effective. Nor is it known whether the combination of nitrates and calcium antagonists is superior to the use of individual agents alone in the control of unstable angina.

Nearly all cases of unstable angina occur in the setting of advanced coronary artery disease, and, as indicated above, there may be a significant incidence of abnormal coronary vasomobility in these patients. Therefore, it has been felt that β-blockers might aggravate the development of ischemia in this context. At present, this possibility is no more than a theoretical one, there being no controlled observations that β-blockade might exert a deleterious influence on the clinical course of unstable angina. In fact, a recent controlled study comparing the effects of propranolol and diltiazem revealed no differences in morbidity and mortality in unstable angina.[29] Whether combination therapy consisting of β-blockers and calcium antagonists might be more effective than either modality alone in unstable angina is not known.

As far as the role of calcium channel blockers is concerned, numerous studies have established the effectiveness of these drugs in relieving symptoms of unstable angina and reducing the electrocardiographic abnormalities that accompany symptomatic ischemia. Whether these drugs may reduce the incidence of silent ischemic episodes in unstable angina and thereby prolong survival has not been established for any of the antianginal agents, including β-blockers, nitrates, and calcium channel blockers.

CHRONIC STABLE ANGINA. The role of calcium antagonists in chronic stable angina is now well defined.[3,21] Numerous studies with verapamil and its congeners nifedipine and diltiazem, using blinded placebo-controlled protocols, have shown that these drugs reduce the frequency of angina and the number of sublingual nitroglycerin tablets consumed, increase exercise capacity during a treadmill test, and delay the onset of ischemia as judged by electrocardiographic parameters. These drugs also elevate anginal threshold and attenuate the ischemic manifestations during rapid atrial pacing in patients with coronary artery disease undergoing cardiac catheterization.[30] They also reduce the extent of fall in left ventricular ejection due to ischemia induced either by exercise or by rapid atrial pacing.[19,30]

It is of interest that the heart rate and blood pressure product, an index of oxygen demand, tends to be lower at any given work load

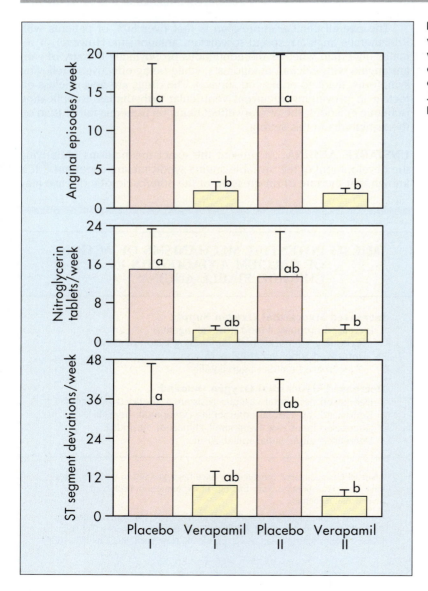

FIGURE 17.7 Double-blind placebo-controlled study of the effects of oral verapamil in Prinzmetal's angina. Each phase shown contains the mean of weekly data over 2 months. Verapamil had a significant effect on ST segment deviations recorded on 24-hour Holter recordings, nitroglycerin consumption, and anginal episodes. (Modified from Johnson SM, Mauritson DR, Willerson JT et al: A controlled trial of verapamil in Prinzmetal's variant angina. Reprinted by permission of the New England Journal of Medicine 306:862, 1981)

under the influence of calcium antagonism, although it is not as low as that found with β-blockers (Fig. 17.8). However, it is known that the peak heart rate and blood pressure during exercise is not significantly different during treadmill exercise when a patient is on or off calcium antagonists, although the peak effect on these variables is delayed when the patient is taking calcium channel blockers.[21]

The data thus suggest that the effects of calcium antagonists in chronic stable angina differ in terms of mechanisms when compared with those of β-blockers, which appear to produce their salutary effects essentially by reducing myocardial oxygen demand. In the case of calcium antagonists, the possibility cannot be excluded that these agents act, at least in part, by augmenting regional blood flow by altering coronary vasomobility, even though the precise measurements of regional flow in humans are rarely possible. The possibility also exists that part of the anti-ischemic effect of calcium antagonists may be mediated through an effect on platelet adhesiveness, since many of these agents exert significant effects on platelet aggregability, an effect that has also been shown to hold for propranolol and other β-blockers. Furthermore, it is not clear whether, as a class, calcium antagonists influence survival in patients with chronic stable angina.

CALCIUM ANTAGONISTS AND OTHER ANTIANGINAL AGENTS

An appreciation of the pharmacodynamic effects of the three classes of antianginal drugs (Table 17.6) allows one to predict their overall effects in angina especially during combination therapy. Since the fundamental mechanisms of action of β-blockers, nitrates, and calcium antagonists differ somewhat, there exists a rationale for combining these drugs in what has become a "step-care" approach to the therapy of angina pectoris. However, there are a number of limitations to this approach. First, there are multiple objectives in the treatment of angina, and the three classes of agents are not equally effective in this regard. For example, to date only β-blockers have been demonstrated to reduce the incidence of sudden death and reinfarction during chronic prophylactic therapy of survivors of acute myocardial infarction,[31] although all three classes of agents have been shown to reduce infarct size in experimental animals and in man. Second, not all patients can tolerate β-blockers (*e.g.*, these agents are contraindicated,

relatively or absolutely, in insulin-dependent diabetes, bronchospastic disease, and peripheral vascular disease). These are not influenced adversely by calcium antagonists. Third, in certain subsets of patients combination therapy might be deleterious. For instance, in patients with impaired ventricular function, heart failure might be precipitated, and in patients with conduction system disease, serious lapses of conduction might develop if β-blockers and certain calcium antagonists are combined. The combination of nitrates and large doses of the dihydropyridine type of calcium antagonists might produce significant hypotension, which may also lead to potentially serious cardiovascular complications. Thus, in the treatment of chronic stable angina, an individualized approach rather than a simple step-care approach is desirable if combination therapy is contemplated. For patients with impaired ventricular performance or those with conduction system disease, a combination of β-blockers with either verapamil or diltiazem is likely to be more hazardous than with the dihydropyridines (although cases have been reported documenting deleterious effects even with nifedipine in this context).

CARDIOPROTECTION

The experimental data have suggested that the administration of calcium antagonists to experimental animals with coronary artery occlusion leads to smaller infarct size, less histologic and ultrastructural damage, increased collateral blood flow to ischemic areas, and less severe electrocardiographic and enzymatic evidence of ischemic damage.[32] These findings are consistent with the intracellular overload hypothesis of ischemic damage following coronary occlusion. A reduction in myocardial enzyme release has also been demonstrated in humans with acute myocardial infarction when a calcium antagonist is given in the early stages of acute myocardial infarction.[33] The addition of calcium antagonists to cardioplegic solutions during cardiopulmonary bypass surgery has been shown to reduce systolic and diastolic abnormalities during protracted total myocardial ischemia; in humans a reduction in myocardial enzyme release with a decrease in the severity of myocardial ischemic injury as detected by technetium pyrophosphate scintigraphy has also been demonstrated.[34] At present it remains uncertain whether infarct size reduction in the case of calcium antagonists (as with other agents such as nitrates and β-blockers) will go

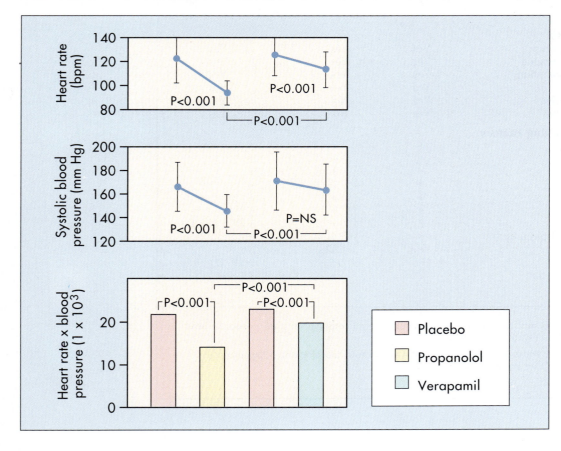

FIGURE 17.8 Comparative effects of long-term administration of propranolol and verapamil on heart rate, systolic blood pressure, and rate–pressure product at rest and during exercise on supine bicycle exercise. β-Blockade has a greater depressant effect than calcium antagonism on these variables.

beyond the experimental laboratory, and clinical investigation is unclear. Perhaps the same holds true for protection of ischemic myocardium during cardiac surgery.

Thus, whether the experimental and preliminary observations on cardioprotection will eventually be translated into routine clinical indications remains to be established. The role of focal spasm in mediating coronary obstruction in the setting of infarction now appears to be unlikely in most patients. However, a clear rationale exists for these agents to be used to control persistent or recurrent myocardial ischemia or supraventricular tachyarrhythmias in the early stages of acute myocardial infarction.[3] Both oral and intravenous agents may be used for this purpose.

EFFECT OF CALCIUM ANTAGONISM ON SURVIVAL AND REINFARCTION IN SURVIVORS OF ACUTE MYOCARDIAL INFARCTION

There is compelling evidence that β-adrenergic blocking drugs given prophylactically to survivors of acute myocardial infarction reduce the incidence of sudden death and reinfarction.[31] To date there are no studies that have indicated that the prophylactic administration of calcium antagonists has such a salutary effect on mortality or reinfarction rate in the survivors of acute myocardial infarction. The reported results[35,36] have either been negative (nifedipine) or equivocal (verapamil). The trials have not been stringently controlled and have suffered from flaws in protocol design. The ongoing trials (e.g., diltiazem, verapamil) in this context may, however, provide decisive answers that are needed to establish or deny the role of calcium antagonism in altering mortality and morbidity in the survivors of acute infarction.

CALCIUM ANTAGONISM AND ATHEROSCLEROSIS

It has been recognized for some time that calcium may have a significant role in a number of steps such as aggregation of platelets, release of platelet-derived growth factor, smooth muscle cell replication, protein synthesis, and lipid binding of the macromolecules involved in atherogenesis. It might therefore be expected that inhibition of intracellular calcium influx might reduce calcification and atherosclerosis. Fleckenstein[1] and others[35,36] have indeed provided experimental evidence that this might be so. For example, experimental studies have suggested that prophylactic administration of calcium antagonists delays or reduces the tendency for atherosclerosis to develop in animals fed a high cholesterol diet.[37,38] While these animal studies are of major clinical interest, there are at present no controlled studies in humans to confirm or deny such a possibility.

CARDIAC ARRHYTHMIAS

The role of calcium antagonists in the treatment of cardiac arrhythmias is reasonably well defined, especially in supraventricular tachycardias.[39] The spectrum of clinical activity is in line with the electrophysiologic effects (see Table 17.2) and is summarized in Table 17.7. The major effects are those related to the propensity of these agents to predictably inhibit or completely but transiently block the anterograde

TABLE 17.6 COMPARISON OF ANTIANGINAL DRUGS

	Nitrate Therapy	β-Blocking Drugs	Calcium Blocking Agents	
Physiological Effects				
Heart rate	↑	↓	↓ (V, D)	N↑
AV conduction	—	↓	↓	N↑
Systemic resistance	↓	↑ (acutely)	↓	N↓
Coronary resistance	↓	↑	↓	N↓
Contractility	↑	↓	↓	N±
Therapeutic effects				
Reduce angina frequency	Yes	Yes	Yes	
Improve exercise tolerance	Yes	Yes	Yes	
Decrease TNG consumption	Yes	Yes	Yes	
Decrease MVO$_2$	Yes	Yes	Yes	
Dilate coronary arteries	Yes	No	Yes	
Reduce silent ischemia	Yes	No	Yes	
Favorable and Limiting Factors				
Exertional angina	+	+	+	
Variant angina	+	—	+	
Once-a-day therapy	—	+	+	
Partial tolerance	+	—	—	
Side effects	+	+	+	
Drug interactions	+	+	+	
May worsen CHF	—	+	+ (V > N > D)	
May worsen bronchospasm and claudication	—	Yes	No	
Bradyarrhythmias	—	+	+ (V, D)	
Reduce sudden death and reinfarction	?	+	?	

(*AV*, atrioventricular; *TNG*, nitroglycerin; *MVO*$_2$, myocardial oxygen consumption; *CHF*, congestive heart failure; *V*, verapamil; *D*, diltiazem; *N*, nifedipine)

(Adapted from McCall D, Walsh RA, Frohlich ED et al: Calcium entry blocking drugs: Experimental studies and clinical uses. Curr Probl Cardiol 10:1, 1985)

impulses across the atrioventricular node and to lengthen its effective and functional refractory periods. The bulk of the experience relates to the effects of verapamil, but the effects of diltiazem and the congeners of verapamil such as tiapamil or gallopamil (*i.e.*, type I calcium antagonists) are qualitatively similar.

SUPRAVENTRICULAR ARRHYTHMIAS

When these agents are given intravenously, paroxysmal reentrant supraventricular tachycardia (PSVT) is promptly terminated in most cases (especially after verapamil). In the acute conversion of PSVT, intravenous verapamil is now thought to be the agent of choice once the commonly used vagal maneuvers fail. The termination is usually prompt (within 2 minutes of a bolus injection of the calcium antagonist); often the conversion is preceded by ventricular ectopic beats, atrial fibrillation, or transient atrioventricular dissociation with a junctional escape rhythm. The conversion of PSVT following intravenous verapamil is undoubtedly related to high initial serum drug levels (Fig. 17.9). In case of the orthodromic tachycardia complicating the Wolff-Parkinson-White syndrome, cycle length alternation may occur before conversion occurs. Calcium antagonists are generally ineffective in antidromic tachycardias, although controlled observations have not been made. It is conceivable that they may terminate the tachycardia by blocking the retrograde conduction in the atrioventricular node. Whether intravenous calcium antagonists also terminate PSVT involving sinus or intra-atrial preentry is not certain.

While the role of intravenous calcium antagonists for the treatment of PSVT is well established, the precise role of the oral drugs in the prophylaxis of recurrent arrhythmia is less clear. However, if the intravenous drug is effective in preventing the reinduction of the PSVT in the electrophysiologic laboratory, subsequent oral therapy may be highly effective in preventing arrhythmia recurrences. At present, there is little experience in which the issue of efficacy of verapamil and other calcium antagonists versus other agents has been systematically addressed.

ATRIAL FLUTTER AND FIBRILLATION

Short-term intravenous injections of type I calcium antagonists predictably reduce the ventricular rate in atrial flutter and fibrillation, with rare cases converting to sinus rhythm, especially if the arrhythmias are of short duration and the heart is not large. In a small number of cases regularization of the ventricular response is seen. Oral verapamil (and presumably other type I calcium antagonists) is highly effective in reducing the ventricular response in atrial flutter and fibrillation at rest, as well as during exercise, in contrast to the effect of digoxin, which lowers the ventricular response essentially at rest. They are effective alternatives to β-blockers and digoxin in this setting. Neither the electrophysiologic effects nor the clinical experience suggest that these drugs are likely to be effective in preventing relapses of atrial flutter-fibrillation following chemical or electrical conversion of these arrhythmias. Calcium antagonists are contraindicated in patients with atrial flutter and fibrillation complicating the Wolff-Parkinson-White syndrome (Fig. 17.10), since they aggravate the ventricular response and precipitate ventricular fibrillation.

MULTIFOCAL ATRIAL TACHYCARDIA

The effects of calcium antagonists in multifocal atrial tachycardia are poorly defined. They are sometimes of value especially in the case of orally or intravenously administered verapamil. Their role in ectopic atrial tachycardia is poorly defined. Reports of anecdotal cases suggest that calcium antagonists produce transient atrioventricular block without terminating the tachycardia.

VENTRICULAR ARRHYTHMIAS

As a class of agents, calcium antagonists have a limited role in the control of ventricular tachyarrhythmias except in cases in which ventricular tachycardia or fibrillation is due to coronary artery spasm. These drugs are weak suppressants of premature ventricular contractions in either normal subjects or those with organic cardiac disease; they rarely suppress ventricular tachycardia inducible by programmed

TABLE 17.7 ANTIARRHYTHMIC EFFECTS OF CALCIUM ANTAGONISTS

Arrhythmia	Response to Parenteral Administration	Response During Long-term Prophylaxis
1. Sinus tachycardia	Variable	Of little value
2. Paroxysmal supraventricular tachycardia		
a. Atrioventricular (AV) node reentrant	90–100% conversion	Modest effect in preventing recurrence
b. Circus movement (orthodromic) with bypass tract (overt or concealed)	80–90% conversion	Modest effect in preventing recurrence
c. Circus movement (antidromic) with bypass tract	No effect	Of little value
d. Sinus node or intra-atrial reentrant	Probably effective	Effect uncertain
e. Ectopic atrial tachycardia	Produces AV block without conversion	Of little value
3. Paroxysmal atrial tachycardia with AV block (with or without digitalis toxicity)	May convert to sinus rhythm (? mechanism)	Effect uncertain
4. Multifocal atrial tachycardia	Variable	Variable (more data needed)
5. Atrial fibrillation	Slows ventricular response (conversion to sinus rhythm rare)	Control of ventricular response at rest and with exercise excellent
6. Atrial flutter	Slows ventricular response (conversion to sinus rhythm rate)	Control of ventricular response at rest and with exercise good
7. Atrial flutter and fibrillation with Wolff-Parkinson-White syndrome (wide QRS)	May accelerate ventricular response	Contraindicated
8. Ventricular tachyarrhythmias (including *torsade de pointes*)	Generally low rate of conversion except when due to coronary artery spasm	Rarely successful except secondarily by preventing myocardial ischemia and exercise-induced tachycardia
9. Ventricular tachycardia with right bundle branch block and left axis deviation	Effective in producing conversion	Effective in prophylaxis

(Adapted from Singh BN, Ellrodt G, Nademanee K: Calcium antagonists: Cardiocirculatory effects and therapeutic applications. In Hurst JW (ed): Clinical Essays on the Heart, vol 2, pp 65–98. New York, McGraw-Hill, 1984)

electrical stimulation. There is, however, preliminary experience to suggest that calcium antagonists are effective in controlling ventricular tachycardia induced by exercise in patients with coronary artery disease; they appear to be effective also in young patients without organic heart disease having ventricular tachycardia with the right bundle branch block morphology associated with left axis deviation. The nature of this arrhythmia is uncertain, but it may be due to triggered automaticity responsive to calcium antagonism.

CONTROL OF SYSTEMIC HYPERTENSION

Although the vasodilator properties of calcium antagonists have been recognized for many years, it is only in the past 5 years that numerous reports have suggested a significant role of these drugs in the control of hypertensive emergencies and in the control of mild to moderate essential hypertension. Interest in these drugs as hypotensive agents has grown *pari passu* with the developing concept implicating the role of calcium in the pathogenesis of hypertension.[40,41]

When calcium antagonists are given orally or intravenously in patients with hypertension, they reduce systemic vascular resistance, increase cardiac output, and increase stroke volume index. These properties have been used in the treatment of hypertensive emergencies with or without encephalopathy. In this context, the dihydropyridines (*e.g.*, nifedipine and nitrendipine) have been shown to be markedly effective in most patients; the most extensive experience has been with sublingual nifedipine. The usual dose of nifedipine for this purpose is 10 mg to 20 mg. The hypotensive response is attained rapidly within 30 to 60 minutes and may be maintained with 6-hourly dosage schedules.

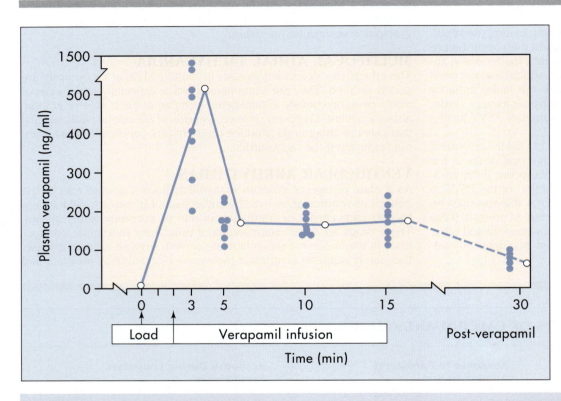

FIGURE 17.9 The time course of serum drug level changes following a rapid bolus injection and a constant infusion regimen of verapamil. The initial bolus ("load") was 0.145 mg/kg, followed by 0.005 mg/kg/min. Note the high serum levels of the drug attained following the bolus injection. In the case of PSVT, conversion occurs in nearly all patients at the time serum levels are high.

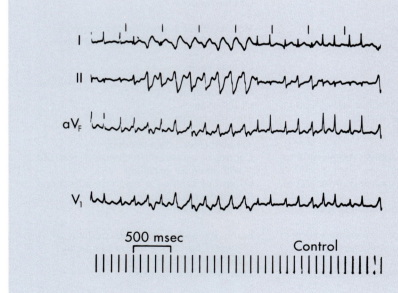
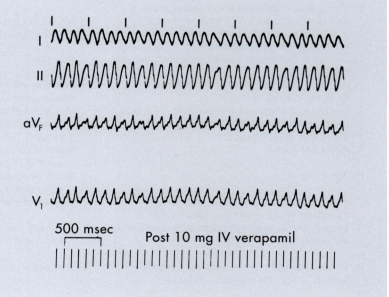

FIGURE 17.10 Effects of intravenously administered verapamil in a patient with atrial fibrillation complicating the Wolff-Parkinson-White syndrome. *Control:* Note that some fibrillatory impulses are conducted antegradely over the atrioventricular node and others over the bypass tract. *Post 10 mg IV verapamil:* All impulses are transmitted over the bypass tract at a much more rapid rate. (Unpublished observations of Dr. K. Nademanee and Dr. B. N. Singh)

This modality of therapy may obviate the necessity for the use of parenteral therapy with nitroprusside and other agents in most patients, but further controlled studies are needed to validate this approach.

Numerous studies, many blinded as well as placebo controlled, have indicated that verapamil, nifedipine, and diltiazem are as potent as β-blockers or diuretics in the control of mild to moderate systemic hypertension.[40,41] For example, in the case of verapamil and propranolol, in their commonly used dosage regimens, the hypotensive effects of the two compounds were comparable.[42] Most studies have used thrice-daily regimens, but the increasing availability of long-acting formulations of these agents is likely to make them of increasing appeal for the control of systemic hypertension.

In the case of verapamil and other calcium antagonists, these drugs are equally effective in patients with low-renin as well as high-renin status. Furthermore, unlike β-blockers, these drugs do not alter blood lipids adversely and may be used with impunity in patients with diabetes mellitus, peripheral vascular disease, and, above all, bronchospastic disorders. Unlike diuretics, calcium antagonists do not adversely affect numerous metabolic functions, nor do they deplete body stores of potassium. Thus, it is likely that, as a class, calcium antagonists will be used increasingly as the initial agents not only for the immediate control of hypertensive emergencies but also in the long-term treatment of mild to moderate essential hypertension as monotherapy or in combination with other hypotensive compounds. As in the case of β-blockers, they are likely to be of particular value in patients with combined ischemic heart disease and systemic hypertension, particularly if the ongoing clinical trials establish the cardioprotective effects of calcium antagonists in the survivors of acute myocardial infarction.

HYPERTROPHIC CARDIOMYOPATHY

Patients with hypertrophic cardiomyopathy are known to have both systolic and diastolic abnormalities of ventricular function.[43] The degree of dynamic obstruction to left ventricular ejection is directly related to the inotropic state, and for this reason β-blockers have long been used in this context with a variable degree of success. They increase exercise capacity and decrease the incidence of angina pectoris. Propranolol and other β-blockers, however, may reduce neither the incidence of serious ventricular arrhythmias nor the risk of sudden death. Because of their intrinsic negative inotropic activity, calcium channel blockers might be expected to exert a salutary effect in hypertrophic cardiomyopathy. It has been found that calcium antagonists prevent the development of hereditary cardiomyopathy in hamsters, a disorder akin to hypertrophic obstructive cardiomyopathy and possibly related to abnormal calcium flux across myocardial cell membranes. These observations have formed the basis for the clinical evaluation of calcium antagonists in hypertrophic cardiomyopathy.

The most extensive data are available for verapamil. Early studies with the drug (480 mg daily) demonstrated significant improvement in symptoms compared to β-blockers. In uncontrolled clinical studies involving verapamil therapy, reductions in electrocardiographic signs of left ventricular hypertrophy and heart size assessed radiographically were observed. Follow-up catheterization studies have also demonstrated a decline in the resting outflow tract obstruction in 50% of patients, with decrease in left ventricular mass in 70% of patients. Extensive studies by Rosing and associates[43] have shown that an improvement in basal and provoked left ventricular outflow gradients is significant in most patients and is dependent on dose. Cardiac output remains unchanged or increases slightly, without significant increases in left ventricular end-diastolic pressure.

A direct but uncontrolled comparison of verapamil and propranolol at varying doses has shown that both produce a short-term increase in exercise tolerance of about 20% to 25%. However, with long-term therapy exercise capacity deteriorates more frequently with propranolol and may actually increase with verapamil (120 mg qid). Patients symptomatically prefer verapamil. Unfortunately, a large number of patients develop significant side effects with long-term verapamil use, including sinoatrial and atrioventricular node dysfunction and occasionally severe myocardial dysfunction and heart failure. These adverse reactions may be accentuated when propranolol and verapamil are combined, although some refractory cases may respond satisfactorily to the combination therapy. As in the case of β-blockers, calcium antagonists do not appear to reduce the incidence of life-threatening ventricular arrhythmias and have no effect on survival. There are preliminary echocardiographic data that indicate verapamil may reduce the degree of hypertrophy during chronic therapy.

Whether other type I calcium antagonists or the dihydropyridines may also be of value in the treatment of hypertrophic cardiomyopathy is unclear at present. The precise mechanism mediating the salutary effects of these drugs in hypertrophic cardiomyopathy is also uncertain. However, it is known that abnormalities of diastolic function in patients with hypertrophic cardiomyopathy may be improved by calcium antagonists, an action that correlates with the evidence of objective symptomatic improvement.[44] For example, verapamil has been shown to shorten the abnormally prolonged, isovolumic relaxation time in such patients. Nifedipine has also been demonstrated to favorably modify abnormal left ventricular relaxation and diastolic filling rates in hypertrophic cardiomyopathy.[43] This effect does not appear to be related to the depression of left ventricular systolic function. Administration of nifedipine alone could be deleterious through its potent vasodilator effects with reflex sympathetic discharge. The combined administration of nifedipine and propranolol may be superior to the use of the calcium channel blocker alone. The combination reduces left ventricular peak systolic pressure, total peripheral resistance, and resting left ventricular outflow gradient without altering cardiac index or pulmonary capillary wedge pressure or inducing conduction defects. In hypertrophic cardiomyopathy, diltiazem exerts effects similar to those of verapamil and attenuates the exercise-induced elevation of pulmonary artery diastolic pressure, suggesting an improvement in left ventricular diastolic function.[43]

Thus, calcium antagonists, alone or in combination with β-blockers, appear to improve both systolic and diastolic function in hypertrophic cardiomyopathy. Long-term follow-up studies and determination of comparative efficacy of the various calcium antagonists and combination regimens may further define the role of these agents in hypertrophic cardiomyopathy. However, there are no definitive data to indicate that these drugs may reduce sudden death or the incidence of symptomatic arrhythmias or induce regression of hypertrophy in this form of cardiomyopathy. When used in combination with β-blockers they may, in a proportion of patients, produce sinus arrest, atrioventricular block, and cardiac failure.

PULMONARY HYPERTENSION

Although promising from a theoretical and experimental standpoint, the efficacy of calcium channel blockers in the various forms of pulmonary hypertension appears to be limited.[45] The effects of intravenous verapamil (mean dose 9.6 mg), reported[46] in 12 patients with a mean pulmonary artery pressure of 57 mm Hg due to pulmonary fibrosis, congenital heart disease, or primary pulmonary hypertension, showed a slight decrease in mean pulmonary artery pressure and right ventricular performance in several patients, while in others it had a marked negative inotropic effect with an increase in pulmonary arteriolar resistance. Overall, right atrial pressure, right ventricular end-diastolic pressure, pulmonary arteriolar resistance, and cardiac index were unchanged. Perhaps because of nifedipine's less inherent negative inotropic properties in humans, preliminary studies have suggested that the drug may be considered to be effective in some patients in specific clinical settings. For example, in one case of primary pulmonary hypertension, nifedipine produced a 54% decrease in pulmonary vascular resistance, a 49% decrease in systemic vascular resistance, and a 90% increase in cardiac output.[47] The improvement was maintained over a 3-month period. In another study of patients with acute respiratory failure and chronic airways obstruction, nifedipine dilated pulmonary vessels constricted by hypoxemia but had no further vasodilatory effect when hypoxemia was corrected. No adverse effects on arterial oxygenation were noted. Experience with diltiazem and other calcium antagonists is still limited, but effects similar to those after verapamil and nifedipine are likely.

It is apparent that although available data concerning calcium antagonists in pulmonary hypertensive states are encouraging in individual patients, they are preliminary and essentially anecdotal. In addition, adverse effects have been noted probably due to inherent myocardial depressant properties and possibly due to differential vasodilatation of the pulmonary and systemic vascular beds. Such adverse effects are most likely in patients in whom right ventricular function has been severely impaired by chronic pressure load. In these cases, markedly depressant effects on right ventricular function may outweigh the hemodynamic improvement resulting from a reduction in pulmonary vascular resistance. For this reason it is unlikely that calcium antagonists will make a major impact on the chronic prophylactic therapy of pulmonary hypertension. Deterioration of right ventricular function may occur in a significant number of patients, limiting the utility of this class of drugs in pulmonary hypertension.

ACUTE AND CHRONIC CONGESTIVE HEART FAILURE

While calcium antagonists are potent vasodilators and may function as agents to ameliorate heart failure by impedance reduction, it must be emphasized that as a class these compounds are unlikely to be the first-line therapy in this regard. Their effects in this setting are often unpredictable and variable and sometimes depressant even with the dihydropyridines. However, they may be of value in patients who have myocardial ischemia in the setting of cardiac decompensation. Available data suggest that nifedipine and other dihydropyridines may be effective preload- and afterload-reducing agents in the setting of acute pulmonary edema. The administration of 10 mg to 20 mg of nifedipine sublingually may improve congestive heart failure secondary to hypertensive, rheumatic, or primary heart disease.[48] The drug induces a sustained decrease in preload and afterload and appears to enhance contractility. Compared to nitrates, nifedipine has a greater tendency to increase cardiac output without inducing venous pooling. In patients with advanced chronic congestive heart failure the short-term administration of nifedipine (20 mg sublingually) may increase cardiac index and stroke work index, while decreasing preload significantly. These changes appear to be due to decreased systemic vascular resistance. However, sustained hemodynamic improvement has been noted in less than 50% of patients at 24 hours with continuous therapy, suggesting tolerance or possible sodium retention. Deterioration of ventricular function may also occur in some patients. The role of the other calcium antagonists in this setting is unexplored, but that of the newer dihydropyridines such as nitrendipine and nicardipine will be of therapeutic interest. The dihydropyridines may also be of value as afterload-reducing agents in patients with aortic and mitral regurgitation. It is possible that some of the newer dihydropyridines such as nicardipine may produce a more consistent hemodynamic improvement in patients with cardiac decompensation. However, it is rarely if ever justified to use calcium antagonists as first-line afterload-reducing agents.

MISCELLANEOUS DISORDERS

Numerous studies in a wide variety of cardiovascular and noncardiovascular conditions have suggested that the overall spectrum of therapeutic utility of calcium antagonists is exceedingly wide. It may be wider than that of β-adrenergic blocking drugs. Calcium antagonists may be effective in the control of migraine and cluster headaches,[49] but their efficacy in relation to that of β-blockers and conventional regimens remains unclear. Calcium antagonists may prevent or minimize cerebral damage in cases of developing strokes by reversing cerebral vasoconstriction[9]; they have been shown to be efficacious in preventing the development of exercise-induced bronchial asthma,[50,51] in disorders of esophageal motility,[52,53] and in Raynaud's phenomenon.[54]

CEREBRAL VASOCONSTRICTION

The rationale for the use of prophylactic calcium antagonistic therapy in evolving cerebral stroke relates to the supposition that the initial event in the development of cerebral arterial spasm is the contraction of smooth muscle cells in the large cerebral arteries. Thus, an agent that inhibits such contractions may prevent spasm as well as the resulting neurologic damage. Experimental data have indicated that certain dihydropyridines may be selective in their action with respect to regional circulatory beds. Thus, they may have the potential to dilate cerebral vessels without producing severe hypotension. This appears to be most striking in the case of nimodipine. Preliminary clinical trials have suggested that prophylactic administration significantly decreases the occurrence of severe neurologic deficits.[9] However, further vindication of these data is needed before the routine clinical use of calcium antagonists in this setting can be established.

EXERCISE-INDUCED ASTHMA AND CALCIUM ANTAGONISM

Recent studies[50] have emphasized the role of calcium in the control of smooth muscle tone in bronchial tissue. This has provided the basis for clinical trials of calcium antagonists in bronchial asthma. Although experience is limited, it appears that these agents are weak bronchodilators for symptomatic bronchial asthma, but they may be of therapeutic utility in instances of exercise-induced bronchoconstriction.[51] This has been demonstrated for nifedipine and verapamil. The drugs may be of value as tools to determine the role of calcium in bronchial physiology and in the pathophysiologic mechanism of asthma.

GASTROINTESTINAL TRACT DISORDERS AND CALCIUM CHANNEL BLOCKERS

Calcium channel blockers have the potential to alter secretory and motility processes in the gastrointestinal tract.[52] In both experimental animals and humans, diltiazem, verapamil, and nifedipine have been found to decrease contractions in smooth muscle, decreasing peristalsis and sphincter pressures.[53] Thus, a rational basis exists for the role of this class of drugs for the amelioration of symptoms referable to upper gastrointestinal tract motility. Their precise role, however, remains to be defined.

RAYNAUD'S PHENOMENON

Since calcium channel blockers are often powerful peripheral arterial dilators, they have been used in Raynaud's phenomenon.[54] Their role in this setting is under clinical evaluation.

SIDE EFFECTS

The major side effects of verapamil, nifedipine, and diltiazem are generally predictable from their inherent vasodilatory and relatively negative inotropic and chronotropic properties (see Table 17.6). Their side effects may also vary in relation to the route of administration. The nature and incidence of side effects following oral therapy are shown in Table 17.8.

Although the safety of nifedipine and other dihydropyridines has not been thoroughly studied, a recent review of the records of over 3000 patients treated with the drug provides valuable basic information.[55] In this review of patients with various anginal syndromes, some complicated by congestive heart failure and many studied for longer than 6 months, about 60% of the patients reported no adverse side effects. Dizziness and light-headedness were reported in 12.1% of the total population but were more frequent in patients with congestive heart failure and in those on long-term therapy. Edema, swelling, and fluid retention occurred in 7.7% of the population and were also more common in patients with congestive heart failure and during long-term therapy. Disturbances of upper gastrointestinal tract function and headaches occurred in about 7% of patients, and flushing or burning or a general or specific feeling of weakness was reported in 7.4% and 5.9% of cases, respectively. Less commonly reported side effects related to cardiovascular function included hypotension, precipitation of angina, preinfarction angina or myocardial infarction, and congestive heart failure in less than 4% of patients. The total percentage of patients in whom therapy was discontinued owing to an adverse experience was 5%, but the overall incidence of side effects may be higher and has been estimated to be about 17%. The overall side effects of other dihydropyridines are likely to be similar, being dominated by a striking degree of peripheral vasodilatation.

Following intravenous verapamil the adverse effects reported have been those expected from the drug's known pharmacologic properties. Perhaps the most common is a transient fall in blood pressure. More serious side effects, including hypotension, bradycardia, and rarely ventricular asystole, have been observed, however. In general, these latter occurred in patients receiving concomitant β-blocking drugs. Suicidal overdose with verapamil, manifested by unconsciousness, hypotension, anuria, and atrioventricular block, has been reported. These severe side effects of verapamil can be successfully treated with intravenous atropine (partially effective), catecholamines (particularly isoproterenol), and intravenous calcium gluconate. Occasionally temporary transvenous ventricular pacing may be necessary. The effects of intravenous diltiazem, gallopamil, tiapamil, and bepridil are likely to be qualitatively similar to those of intravenous verapamil.

Overall, oral verapamil is well tolerated. The most common side effects include constipation, dizziness, nausea, headache, and ankle edema. In general, these symptoms are relatively mild and can be managed symptomatically. Less common side effects include galactorrhea and reversible hepatic toxicity. Prolongation of first degree atrioventricular block occurs in a proportion of patients given chronic oral verapamil therapy, but in the absence of antecedent conduction system disease more advanced grades of heart block are unusual. In patients with normal ventricular function the precipitation of clinically evident cardiac failure is very uncommon. The overall incidence of side effects following oral verapamil therapy is about 9%.

Experience with diltiazem is more limited in terms of side effects, and data are derived from studies in angina. Dizziness, headache, fatigue, blurred vision, flushing, and minor degrees of atrioventricular block have been reported when the drug is administered in daily doses of 240 mg to 360 mg. Overall, however, diltiazem appears to have the lowest incidence of side effects, with estimates of about 4%.

CHOICE OF A CALCIUM ANTAGONIST IN THERAPY

With the increasing number of calcium antagonists becoming available for use in a wide variety of clinical disorders, the question has arisen as to which agent should be used for a particular clinical indication.[3] Unlike the β-blockers, which exert the bulk of their therapeutic effects by their propensity to block β-receptors, the overall electrophysiologic and hemodynamic effects of various calcium channel blockers may differ markedly. Thus, guidelines can be suggested only on the basis of a thorough knowledge of the pharmacology (including the side-effect profile) of the individual agents relative to the pathophysiology of the clinical entity under consideration. For example, it is known that in the case of Prinzmetal's angina, unstable angina, or chronic stable angina all calcium antagonists are perhaps equally effective if the dosage regimen is appropriate; the choice of one compound over another is likely to depend on the side-effect profile and on the presence of associated features in the patient. Thus, the presence of conduction system disease, bradycardia, or ventricular dysfunction may warrant the use of a dihydropyridine rather than diltiazem or verapamil and its congeners. On the other hand, it is known that since the dihydropyridines may produce reflex tachycardia, they may aggravate angina or ischemia in a proportion of patients with chronic stable angina; the efficacy of the dihydropyridines in this setting may be limited. Thus, a rate-lowering calcium antagonist might be preferred for monotherapy. Similarly, in the case of hypertrophic cardiomyopathy, it is likely that a rate-lowering and less potent vasodilator calcium antagonist and one that exerts a modest negative inotropic effect is preferable. In the case of hypertensive emergencies, dihydropyridines may be preferred because of their rapid onset of action and potent vasodilator effects. On the other hand, in the long-term treatment of mild to moderate hypertension, most calcium antagonists are effective. The choice of an individual agent will be dictated by the pharmacokinetic features and the side-effect profiles of various agents. Whether striking differences may exist in the efficacy of individual agents with respect to other conditions in which these drugs may be effective as a class needs further critical evaluation.

TABLE 17.8 ADVERSE EFFECTS OF CALCIUM CHANNEL BLOCKERS

Nifedipine (17%)*	Verapamil (9%)*	Diltiazem (4%)*
Ankle edema	Constipation	Dizziness
Headache	Headache	Headache
Dizziness	Dizziness	Fatigue
Tinnitus	Nausea	Blurred vision
Flushing	Galactorrhea	Flushing
Hypotension	Hepatotoxicity	Atrioventricular block/ bradycardia
Aggravation of angina (occasionally)	Atrioventricular block/ bradycardia	
Nasal congestion	Congestive heart failure	

* Estimated overall incidence of side effects in therapeutic doses. It should be emphasized that under certain clinical circumstances, all three agents may aggravate cardiac failure.

(Adapted from Singh BN, Ellrodt G, Nademanee K: Calcium antagonists: Cardiocirculatory effects and therapeutic applications. In Hurst JW (ed): Clinical Essays on the Heart, vol 2. New York, McGraw-Hill, 1984)

REFERENCES

1. Fleckenstein A: History of calcium antagonists. Circ Res 52(Suppl II):1, 1983
2. Epstein SE, Rosing DR, Conti CR: Calcium-channel blockers: Present status and future directions. Am J Cardiol 55:1B, 1985
3. Singh BN, Ellrodt G, Nademanee K: Calcium antagonists: Cardiocirculatory effects and therapeutic applications. In Hurst JW (ed): Clinical Essays on the Heart, vol 2, pp 65–98. New York, McGraw-Hill, 1984
4. Singh BN, Hecht HS, Nademanee K et al: Electrophysiologic and hemodynamic effects of slow-channel blocking drugs. Prog Cardiovasc Dis 5:103, 1982
5. Singh BN, Baky S, Nademanee K: Second generation calcium antagonists: Search for greater selectivity and versatility. Am J Cardiol 55:214B, 1985
6. Fozzard HA: Cardiac muscle: Excitability and passive electrical properties. Prog Cardiovasc Dis 19:343, 1977
7. Tsien RW: Calcium channels in excitable cell membranes. Ann Rev Physiol 45:341, 1983
8. Johnsson B: Processes involved in vascular smooth muscle contraction and relaxation. Circ Res 43:14, 1978
9. Allen GS, Ahn HS, Preziosi TJ et al: Cerebral arterial spasm—a controlled trial of nimodipine in patients with subarachnoid hemorrhage. N Engl J Med 308:619, 1983
10. Holmes B, Brogden RN, Heel RG et al: Flunarizine: A review of its pharmacodynamic and pharmacokinetic properties and therapeutic use. Drugs 22:6, 1984
11. Shapiro W, Narahara KA, Park J: The effects of lidoflazine on exercise performance and thalium stress scintigraphy in patients with angina pectoris. Circulation 65(suppl II):1–43, 1982
12. Vaughan Williams EM: Antiarrhythmic Action and the Puzzle of Perhexiline, pp 1–143. London, Academic Press, 1980
13. Bianco R, Albert J, Katz RJ et al: Bepridil for chronic stable angina pectoris: Results of a prospective multicenter, placebo-controlled, dose-ranging study in 77 patients. Am J Cardiol 33:35, 1984
14. Singh BN, Nademanee K, Feld G et al: Comparative electrophysiologic profiles of calcium antagonists with particular reference to bepridil. Am J Cardiol 55:14C, 1985
15. Josephson MA, Singh BN: Use of calcium antagonists for ventricular dysfunction. Am J Cardiol 55:81B, 1985
16. Chew CYC, Hecht HS, Collett JT et al: Influence of the severity of ventricular dysfunction in hemodynamic responses to intravenously administered verapamil in ischemic heart disease. Am J Cardiol 47:917, 1981
17. Theroux P, Waters DD, Debaisieux JC et al: Hemodynamic effects of calcium ion antagonists after acute myocardial infarction. Clin Invest Med 50:689, 1982
18. Bonow R: Effects of calcium-channel blocking agents on left ventricular diastolic function in hypertrophic cardiomyopathy and in coronary artery disease. Am J Cardiol 55:172B, 1985
19. Josephson MA, Hopkins J, Singh BN: Hemodynamic and metabolic effects of diltiazem during coronary sinus pacing with particular reference to left ventricular ejection fraction. Am J Cardiol 55:286, 1985
20. Walsh RA, Porter CB, Starling MR et al: Beneficial hemodynamic effects of intravenous and oral diltiazem in severe congestive heart failure. J Am Coll Cardiol 3(4):1044, 1984
21. McCall D, Walsh RA, Frohlich ED et al: Calcium entry blocking drugs: Experimental studies and clinical uses. Curr Probl Cardiol 10:1, 1985
22. Elkayam U, Weber L, McKay CR et al: Differences in hemodynamic response to vasodilatation due to calcium channel antagonism with nifedipine and direct-acting agonism with hydralazine in chronic refractory congestive heart failure. Am J Cardiol 54:126, 1984
23. Brown BG, Bolson EL, Dodge HT: Dynamic mechanisms in human coronary stenosis. Circulation 10:917, 1984
24. McAllister RG, Hamann SR, Blouin RA: Pharmacokinetics of calcium-entry blockers. Am J Cardiol 55:30B, 1985
25. Singh BN (ed): Detection, quantification and clinical significance of silent myocardial ischemia in coronary artery disease. Am J Cardiol 15(4):1B, 1986
26. Johnson SM, Mauritson DR, Willerson JT et al: A controlled trial of verapamil in Prinzmetal's variant angina. N Engl J Med 306:862, 1981
27. Robertson RH, Wood AJJ, Vaughan WK et al: Exacerbation of vasotonic angina pectoris by propranolol. Circulation 65:281, 1982
28. Falk E: Unstable angina with fatal outcome: Dynamic coronary thrombosis leading to infarction and/or sudden death. Circulation 71:699, 1985
29. Theroux P, Taeymans Y, Morissette D et al: A randomized study comparing propranolol and diltiazem in the treatment of unstable angina. J Am Coll Cardiol 5:717, 1985
30. Hecht HS, Chew CYC, Burnam M et al: Radionuclide ejection fraction and regional wall motion during atrial pacing in stable angina pectoris: Comparison with metabolic and hemodynamic parameters. Am Heart J 101:726, 1981
31. Singh BN, Venkatesh N: Prevention of myocardial reinfarction and sudden death in survivors of acute myocardial infarction: Role of prophylactic β-adrenoceptor blockade. Am Heart J 107:189, 1984
32. Hamm CV, Opie LH: Protection of infarcting myocardium by slow channel inhibitors. Circ Res (Suppl 1) 54:129, 1983
33. Bussman WD, Seher W, Gruengras M: Reduction of creative kinase-MB indexes of infarct size by intravenous verapamil. Am J Cardiol 54:1224, 1984
34. Clark RE, Christlieb IY, Vanderwonder JC et al: Use of nifedipine to decrease ischemic-reperfusion injury in the surgical setting. Am J Cardiol 55:125B, 1985
35. Earle DL: Nifedipine in acute myocardial infarction. Am J Cardiol 54:21E, 1984
36. Hansen JA: Verapamil in acute myocardial infarction. Eur Heart J 5:516, 1984
37. Parmley WW, Blumlein S, Sievers R: Modification of experimental atherosclerosis by calcium-channel blockers. Am J Cardiol 55:165B, 1985
38. Henry PD, Bentley KI: Suppression of atherogenesis in cholesterol-fed rabbit treated with nifedipine. J Clin Invest 68:1366, 1981
39. Singh BN, Nademanee K, Baky S: Calcium antagonists: Uses in the treatment of cardiac arrhythmias. Drugs 25:125, 1983
40. Buhler FR, Hulthen L: Calcium channel blockers: A pathophysiologically based antihypertensive treatment concept for the future. Eur J Clin Invest 2:1, 1982
41. Frohlich ED: Calcium channel blockers: A new dimension in antihypertensive therapy. Am J Med 77(2B):1, 1984
42. Singh BN, Rebanal P, Piontek M et al: Comparative hypotensive actions of calcium antagonists and β-blockers: Evaluation of the efficacy of verapamil and propranolol in mild to moderate hypertension. Am J Cardiol 57:990, 1986
43. Rosing DR, Idanpaan-Heikkila U, Maron BJ et al: Use of calcium-channel blocking drugs in hypertrophic cardiomyopathy. Am J Cardiol 55:185B, 1985
44. Bonow RO, Dilsizian V, Rosing DR et al: Verapamil-induced improvement in left ventricular diastolic filling and increased exercise tolerance in patients with hypertrophic cardiomyopathy. Circulation 71:853, 1985
45. Packer M: Therapeutic application of calcium-channel antagonists for pulmonary hypertension. Am J Cardiol 55:196B, 1985
46. Landmark K, Refsum AM, Simonsen S et al: Verapamil and pulmonary hypertension. Acta Med Scand 204:299, 1978
47. Camerini F, Alberti E, Klugmann S et al: Primary pulmonary hypertension: Effect of nifedipine. Br Heart J 44:352, 1980
48. Polese A, Fiorentini C, Olvari MT et al: Clinical use of a calcium antagonist agent (nifedipine) in acute pulmonary edema. Am J Med 66:145, 1979
49. Gelmer HJ: Nimodipine: A new calcium antagonist in the prophylactic treatment of migraine. Headache 23:106, 1983
50. Triggle DJ: Calcium in the control of smooth muscle function and bronchial hyper-reactivity. Allergy 38:1, 1983
51. Fanta CH: Calcium-channel blockers in the prophylaxis and treatment of asthma. Am J Cardiol 55:202B, 1985
52. Fox J, Daniel E: Role of Ca^{++} ions on genesis of lower esophageal sphincter tone and other active contractions. Am J Physiol 237:E163, 1979
53. Castell DO: Calcium-channel blocking agents for gastrointestinal disasters. Am J Cardiol 55:210B, 1985
54. Rodeheffer RJ, Rommer JA, Wigley F: Controlled double-blind trial of nifedipine in the treatment of Raynaud's phenomenon. N Engl J Med 308:880, 1983
55. Terry RW: Nifedipine therapy in angina pectoris: Evaluation of safety and side effects. Am Heart J 104:681, 1982

Supported in part by grants from the Medical Research Service of the Veterans Administration and the American Heart Association, the Greater Los Angeles Affiliate.

Vasodilator Drugs in the Treatment of Heart Failure

William W. Parmley

The general approach to the management of congestive heart failure is outlined elsewhere in this volume. This chapter discusses the principal vasodilator drugs that have been used in the treatment of acute and chronic heart failure. Although vasodilation has been used as a treatment of heart failure for more than three decades, it is clear that appreciation of its beneficial effects has occurred only within the past 15 years, and relatively routine use of this form of therapy has taken place only in the past 5 years. In general, vasodilator drugs have been used in patients who are relatively unresponsive to standard therapy with digitalis and diuretics.

Current ongoing studies are investigating whether vasodilators might be considered as first-line therapy, instead of digitalis. In most patients with congestive heart failure, diuretics will always be a part of the medical regimen irrespective of other drugs that are used. There are some circumstances, however, in which vasodilators may be good candidates for first-line therapy. For example, in patients with severe regurgitant lesions such as mitral or aortic regurgitation (in whom surgical therapy is not a current consideration), vasodilator drugs are extremely beneficial in reducing regurgitant fraction and increasing forward cardiac output. Under these circumstances they produce greater beneficial hemodynamic effects than digitalis and could be considered as first-line therapy. Consider, for example, patients with severe aortic or mitral regurgitation in whom ventricular contractility is preserved and there is no immediate consideration of valve replacement. Although unproven as yet, the rationale for the use of these drugs would be to reduce regurgitant fraction and thus reduce the diastolic volume load on the heart. This might attenuate the rate of gradual cardiac dilation and irreversible decline in cardiac contractility. One might thus be able to treat the patient medically for a longer period until surgical therapy is required to replace the defective valve. It should be emphasized, however, that vasodilator therapy should not be used as a substitute for surgery under these circumstances. When an intrinsic decline in myocardial contractility is recognized, it is important to consider surgical therapy before further reductions in myocardial contractility occur. Vasodilators can also be considered if the heart failure is so severe that surgical therapy is not felt to be a reasonable option.

PATHOPHYSIOLOGIC BASIS FOR THE USE OF VASODILATOR DRUGS

The neurohumoral response that accompanies congestive heart failure leads to peripheral vasoconstriction and an increase in calculated systemic vascular resistance. Many factors contribute to this increase in resistance.[1] These include an increase in sympathetic tone and circulating catecholamines, an increase in arginine vasopressin (ADH), and activation of the renin–angiotensin–aldosterone system. The arteriolar constriction thus produced is helpful in maintaining arterial pressure in the face of a fall in cardiac output. As Figure 18.1 suggests, however, this sets up a vicious cycle that can be deleterious to the patient with congestive heart failure. The increased systemic vascular resistance and increased impedance to ejection of blood may further reduce cardiac output by the afterload principle. Thus, patients spiral down this vicious cycle until they reach a new, low, steady-state level at which cardiac output is lower and systemic vascular resistance is higher than is optimal for the patient. Under these circumstances, the use of arteriolar vasodilator drugs can reduce resistance and improve forward cardiac output.

The rationale for the use of venodilators is closely related to the above argument. Venoconstriction is also produced by a marked increase in sympathetic tone and circulating catecholamines. Initially, this may help increase venous return and partially preserve cardiac output by the Frank-Starling mechanism. The peripheral veins serve as the capacitance reservoir of the circulation. Venoconstriction, therefore, will tend to shift more blood to the chest and, thus, increase right and left atrial filling pressures. Venodilators can attenuate this venoconstriction and redistribute blood away from the chest into the peripheral circulation. This produces a reduction in right and left atrial filling pressures and can help relieve the signs and symptoms of pulmonary and systemic congestion. It should be apparent from the above that in selecting vasodilators for the management of heart failure, it is frequently advisable to combine arteriolar and venodilators or to select therapy that will produce this combined effect.

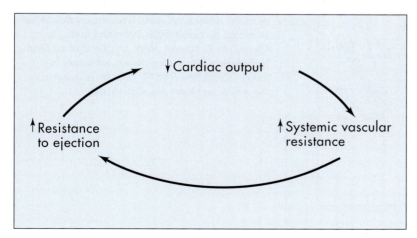

FIGURE 18.1 Vicious cycle in congestive heart failure. The decrease in cardiac output leads to a neurohumoral reflex increase in systemic vascular resistance. In turn, this further reduces ejection and leads to an additional reduction in cardiac output. Patients spiral down this cycle to a new steady-state level, where cardiac output is lower and systemic vascular resistance is higher than is optimal for the patient.

The following discussion focuses on those drugs with arteriolar dilating properties, those with venodilating properties, and drugs with mixed effects, including the angiotensin–converting enzyme inhibitors. The α-adrenergic blocking drugs and the nitrates are discussed in more detail elsewhere in these volumes.

Although the classification of drugs as arteriolar or venodilators has a theoretical basis, its pragmatic value has been questioned.[2] Nevertheless, this classification will generally be followed in this chapter.

ARTERIOLAR VASODILATORS

HYDRALAZINE

Hydralazine is a potent, direct-acting vasodilator that causes smooth muscle relaxation of arteriolar resistance vessels.[3] It produces effective vasodilation of the renal and peripheral vasculature with little change in liver blood flow. It also has no major direct effect on coronary blood flow. Changes in coronary blood flow parallel changes in myocardial oxygen demand. Hydralazine has essentially no effect on the venous capacitance bed. In patients with hypertension and normal ventricular function, reflex tachycardia is frequent. In patients with hypertension and coronary artery disease, but normal ventricular function, hydralazine may worsen angina, presumably because of the reflex increase in heart rate and cardiac contractility produced by lowering the blood pressure. Although hydralazine has been alleged to have direct positive inotropic effects on the heart, it appears that its effects are mostly mediated by a reflex increase in sympathetic tone. In isolated heart muscle, hydralazine releases myocardial norepinephrine, but at doses that far exceed usual therapeutic doses.[4] With the depletion of myocardial norepinephrine stores and the blunted baroreceptor response in patients with congestive heart failure, it is less likely that hydralazine has a major impact on cardiac contractile state.

Although hydralazine is rapidly and almost completely absorbed from the gastrointestinal tract, its bioavailability depends on the degree of acetylation in the liver, which is an inherited trait. The United States population, in general, has about 50% rapid acetylators and 50% slow acetylators. Slow acetylators are more prone to develop the lupus syndrome and require lower doses for a pharmacologic effect. On the other hand, rapid acetylators have minimal risks for the lupus syndrome and require higher doses. Peak serum concentration is attained 30 minutes to 2 hours after an oral dose, which corresponds with its hemodynamic effects. Hydralazine is about 90% protein bound, and 2% to 15% of an administered dose is excreted unchanged in the urine.

In patients with chronic congestive heart failure,[3,5] hydralazine produces a marked decrease in systemic vascular resistance, with an approximate 50% or more increase in forward cardiac output (Fig. 18.2). In general, arterial pressure and heart rate are little altered. Pulmonary artery pressure and left ventricular filling pressure are little altered or in some cases may decrease slightly. Pulmonary vascular resistance decreases somewhat but generally less than with the nitrates. In patients with chronic mitral and aortic regurgitation, regurgitant fraction is reduced and forward stroke volume and cardiac output are increased.[6,7]

The usual administration of oral hydralazine is 200 mg to 400 mg daily in divided doses. In some patients, particularly those who are rapid acetylators, doses up to 1200 mg/day have been used. The lupus syndrome is seen in 15% to 20% of patients receiving more than 400 mg/day. Fluid retention is very common with hydralazine and must be treated with increased doses of diuretics or antialdosterone agents. The most frequent and troublesome side effects are nausea and other gastrointestinal symptoms. Rarely, polyneuropathy due to pyridoxine deficiency has been reported. Other very rare side effects include fever or a syndrome of flushing, sweating, and urticaria, perhaps secondary to inhibition of histamine.

Despite acute beneficial hemodynamic effects, there is usually no immediate increase in exercise tolerance. Chronic studies are more variable in attesting to the efficacy of hydralazine. Some studies suggest benefit with long-term administration,[8] while others have shown no sustained increase in exercise tolerance.[9] As is true of all vasodilators, tolerance may develop to the beneficial effects of hydralazine therapy in some patients. Hydralazine is usually combined with a vasodilator such as isosorbide dinitrate, which will reduce pulmonary capillary wedge pressure.

Endralazine is a structural analogue of hydralazine; it has the advantage that its metabolism is independent of the patient's acetylator status and the lupus syndrome has not been observed.[10] Furthermore, the duration of action is longer and the hemodynamic effects appear to be similar. In 12 patients followed for an average of 3 months, there appeared to be sustained hemodynamic and functional improvement.[11]

MINOXIDIL

Minoxidil is a potent arteriolar vasodilator whose hemodynamic effects are quite similar to those of hydralazine. Minoxidil is almost completely absorbed after an oral dose, reaching a peak plasma concentration in 1 hour with a plasma half-life of 4 hours. About 10% of a dose is excreted unchanged in the urine. The usual dose is 10 mg to 20 mg twice daily.

Minoxidil produces an increase in stroke volume and cardiac output (Fig. 18.3) with a striking reduction in systemic vascular resistance. In general, however, there is no change in arterial or pulmonary pres-

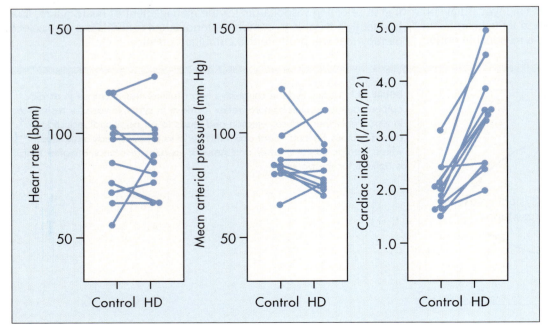

FIGURE 18.2 The hemodynamic effects of hydralazine (HD) in a group of patients with New York Heart Association Class III and IV heart failure who are doing poorly on digoxin and diuretics. Although there is some variability in response, there is no major change in heart rate or mean arterial pressure, whereas cardiac index increases by about 50%. (Modified from Chatterjee K, Parmley WW, Massie B et al: Oral hydralazine therapy for chronic refractory heart failure. Circulation 54:879, 1976. By permission of the American Heart Association, Inc)

sures or in heart rate.[12] Gastrointestinal symptoms are a limiting side effect of minoxidil. In addition, there is significant fluid retention, which almost invariably requires an increase in the dose of diuretics. Hair growth may be troublesome in female patients. Minoxidil is best considered as an alternative drug to hydralazine, perhaps in those who develop the lupus syndrome or intolerable side effects. It will also be more tolerable in patients who do not have considerable edema and can thus be appropriately controlled with increased doses of diuretics. A recent study did not show any improvement in exercise tolerance in a placebo-controlled trial of minoxidil, despite improved acute and chronic hemodynamics.[13] Data in general suggest that arteriolar vasodilators have far less beneficial effects on exercise tolerance than drugs with venodilating effects, such as the nitrates and angiotensin–converting enzyme inhibitors.

CALCIUM ENTRY BLOCKERS

Calcium entry blocking agents have potent peripheral arteriolar vasodilating effects by interfering with calcium entry into peripheral smooth muscle. This reduction in systemic vascular resistance is effective in increasing cardiac output in patients with moderate congestive heart failure. Three calcium entry blockers are currently available in the United States: nifedipine, verapamil, and diltiazem. Nifedipine is the most potent arteriolar vasodilator and is associated with the greatest tendency for reflex tachycardia. Verapamil has the greatest negative inotropic effect on the myocardium, and nifedipine, the least. Both verapamil and diltiazem depress atrioventricular conduction, while nifedipine has essentially no effect. Thus, nifedipine appears to have the most favorable profile for use in heart failure. Studies have been done with all three agents.[14–16] Representative effects with nifedipine are shown in Figure 18.4. There is a modest increase in stroke volume and cardiac output; arterial pressure decreases slightly, and there is no significant change in heart rate and pulmonary capillary wedge pressure. Right atrial pressure is unchanged or slightly reduced. An appropriate dose of nifedipine is 10 mg to 20 mg three times daily. The dose of diltiazem is 60 mg three times daily, and the dose of verapamil is 80 mg to 120 mg three times daily. Nicardipine is a new calcium entry blocker that is primarily an arteriolar vasodilator. Preliminary studies suggest that it may be effective in increasing cardiac output in patients with moderate heart failure.[17] Because of the potential for negative inotropic effects, it is unclear whether the calcium entry blockers will have a primary role in the treatment of congestive heart failure as arteriolar vasodilators. In patients with hypertension or associated angina, they may play a greater role. Adverse effects include hypotension, headache, flushing, palpitations, peripheral edema, and gastrointestinal side effects.[18] Increased atrioventricular block occurs with diltiazem and with verapamil; flushing, hypotension, and ankle edema are more common with nifedipine. Patients with the sick sinus syndrome may also be at risk for bradycardia, especially with verapamil or diltiazem. Along with other arteriolar vasodilators, the calcium entry blockers have been used occasionally in the therapy of primary pulmonary hypertension.[19] Some patients may benefit from the calcium blockers or other arteriolar vasodilators, but the response to all vasodilator agents has been generally disappointing.[20]

VENODILATORS

Nitroglycerin and all the other nitrates are the prototype venodilator drugs.[21] The relative magnitude of their vasodilating effects is venous ≥ large arteries ≥ arterioles. Since the different nitrates are discussed in detail elsewhere in this volume, only pertinent facts related to the management of heart failure are discussed here. It appears that the mechanism of smooth muscle relaxation with the nitrates is due to an increase in cyclic guanosine monophosphate (GMP).[22] The nitrate ester is hydrolyzed (—SH dependent), and mononitrate stimulates the enzyme guanylate cyclase, perhaps through an intermediary (S-nitrosothiol), which increases cyclic GMP synthesis. Cyclic GMP in turn appears to decrease available calcium for smooth muscle contraction. This may occur through reduction of calcium release from intracellular stores and a decrease in the influx/efflux ratio across the cell membrane. The predominant effect of the nitrates is on venous capacitance,[23] with a striking reduction in systemic and pulmonary venous pressures (Fig. 18.5). In general, there is no major increase in cardiac output, although following high doses, especially with intravenous nitroglycerin,[24] the arteriolar vasodilating effect may become more prominent.

The duration of effect depends on the preparation used. Following sublingual nitroglycerin, the onset occurs within 2 to 3 minutes and lasts for about 20 to 30 minutes. Sublingual isosorbide dinitrate may last between 2 and 3 hours; topical nitroglycerin ointment may last for 4 to 6 hours; and orally administered isosorbide dinitrate may last up to 6 hours. Because oral nitrates are rapidly inactivated by first-pass metabolism in the liver, much larger doses must be given orally as compared with sublingual or transdermal preparations. Isosorbide dinitrate

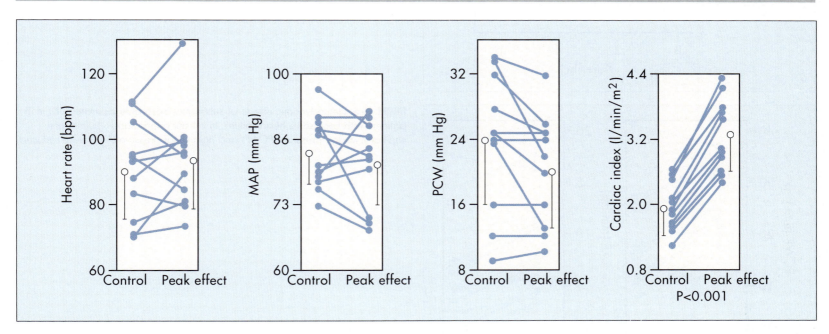

FIGURE 18.3 Peak hemodynamic effects of 10 mg to 30 mg of minoxidil in 11 patients with congestive heart failure. There are minimal effects on heart rate, mean arterial pressure (MAP), and pulmonary capillary wedge pressure (PCW), but a substantial increase in cardiac index. (Modified from McKay C, Chatterjee K, Ports TA et al: Minoxidil in chronic congestive heart failure: A hemodynamic and clinical study. Am Heart J 104:575, 1982)

is metabolized more slowly than glycerol trinitrate. Its primary metabolites include mononitrates, which exhibit a half-life of about 2½ to 5 hours and markedly reduced potencies compared with the dinitrate. They may contribute, however, to the prolonged duration of action.[25] Usual therapeutic doses of oral isosorbide dinitrate are 20 mg to 80 mg, three or four times a day.

Preliminary studies suggest that nitroglycerin patches are ineffective at usual doses in chronic congestive heart failure. Large doses up to 60 mg (six standard 10-mg patches) are required to produce a reduction in pulmonary capillary wedge pressure.[26] Recent information also suggests that tolerance to nitrates can develop with continuous exposure. There appears to be some correlation between the potency of nitrates and their ability to induce tolerance. The development of tolerance is assumed to be caused by conversion of SH to SS bonds, thus decreasing the available SH groups.[27] Therefore, a dose-free interval may be required for the vasculature to regain responsiveness. Thus, intermittent dosing may be more effective than continuous nitrate delivery.

A continuous infusion of nitroglycerin can be effective, however, in certain clinical circumstances. When infused intravenously at the usual therapeutic doses of 10 μg to 100 μg/min, it has more pronounced arteriolar dilating effects and thus may increase cardiac output.[24] It generally is less effective than nitroprusside, however, in increasing cardiac output.[28] It is an effective drug in relieving ischemic pain, presumably by reducing blood pressure and pulmonary capillary wedge pressure, relieving vasoconstriction, and enhancing collateral flow. Although there is suggestive evidence that nitroglycerin might slightly reduce infarct size[29] and mortality[30] in patients with acute myocardial infarction, this remains unproven, and it should not be given routinely for this purpose. Its major hemodynamic benefit is the lowering of

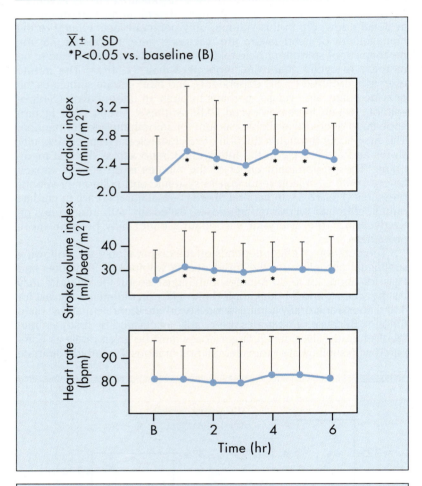

FIGURE 18.4 Hemodynamic effects of nifedipine (0.2 mg/kg orally) in 11 patients with congestive heart failure. There is a moderate increase in stroke volume and cardiac index in the supine position. (Modified from Leier CS, Patrick TS, Hermiller J et al: Nifedipine in congestive heart failure: Effects on resting and exercise hemodynamics and regional blood flow. Am Heart J 108:1461, 1984)

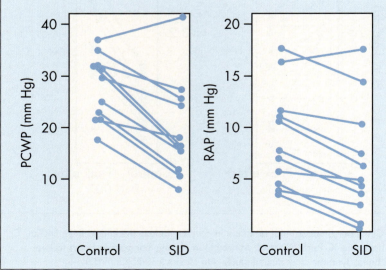

FIGURE 18.5 Hemodynamic effects of sublingual isosorbide dinitrate (*SID*) in 11 patients with congestive heart failure. In all but one instance, pulmonary capillary wedge pressure (*PCWP*) and right atrial pressure (*RAP*) were reduced.

pulmonary capillary wedge pressure, and its major symptomatic benefits are the relief of dyspnea and rest angina.

Although oral nitrates can produce a striking reduction in pulmonary capillary wedge pressure, there may be no change in acute exercise tolerance. After several weeks of continued therapy with isosorbide dinitrate, however, exercise tolerance has improved in patients with chronic congestive heart failure.[31]

Since nitrates have little effect on cardiac output, they are frequently combined with an arteriolar vasodilator such as hydralazine.[32] This combined therapy can increase forward cardiac output and reduce pulmonary capillary wedge pressure, thus relieving the two major hemodynamic abnormalities in patients with chronic heart failure (Fig. 18.6). Nitrates may also produce beneficial hemodynamic effects in patients with mitral regurgitation, resulting in an increase in forward cardiac output and a decrease in regurgitant volume.[33]

The most common side effect of nitrate therapy is headache, to which tolerance frequently develops over a period of days. In some patients postural dizziness, hypotension, and weakness may occur, presumably because of too great a reduction in pulmonary capillary wedge pressure. Patients who are relatively hypovolemic because of high-dose diuretic therapy may be at risk for this hemodynamic side effect. Methemoglobinemia is a rare complication with long-term treatment using large doses of nitrates.

Molsidomine (N-ethoxycarbonyl-3-morpho-linosydnonimine) belongs to the class of sydnonimines and has actions similar to the nitrates.[34] Thus, it is predominantly a venodilator and has been effective in angina pectoris and in heart failure with elevated atrial pressures. Its active metabolite (SIN-1A) presumably depends on the presence of a free nitroso group, which stimulates guanylate cyclase, increases cellular levels of cyclic GMP, and initiates relaxation by removal of free calcium ions from smooth muscle cells. Although its side effect profile is similar to that of nitrates, it has been said to exhibit little or no tolerance during chronic administration, which may be an advantage over nitrates. It is not yet approved for use in the United States.

DRUGS WITH MIXED EFFECTS ON VEINS AND ARTERIES

PRAZOSIN

Prazosin is a quinazoline derivative that is a relatively selective α_1 (postsynaptic)-blocker, which produces vasodilation.[35] It also can inhibit phosphodiesterase and cause smooth muscle relaxation. Prazosin produces a decrease in limb vascular resistance and hepatic resistance (at low doses) but does not influence renal vascular resistance significantly. Prazosin is rapidly and almost completely absorbed from the gastrointestinal tract, with a bioavailability ranging from 44% to 70%. About 6% of the drug is excreted unchanged in the urine, and the majority of the drug is excreted in the feces. The drug is more than 90% protein bound, with a mean elimination half-life of about 2½ hours. Hemodynamic effects last approximately 6 hours. The usual dose is 3 mg to 5 mg administered three to four times daily.

The hemodynamic effects are relatively balanced between arteriolar dilation and venodilation. Thus, there is an increase in cardiac output associated with a decrease in systemic vascular resistance and arterial pressure. Venodilation produces a reduction in atrial pressures and in pulmonary artery pressure with some decline in pulmonary vascular resistance. Controlled studies have noted an increase in exercise tolerance after long-term therapy with prazosin hydrochloride.[36,37]

Despite these demonstrated long-term beneficial effects, however, there appears to be a rapid attenuation of its hemodynamic effects with long-term therapy.[38,39] The first dose produces the most dramatic ef-

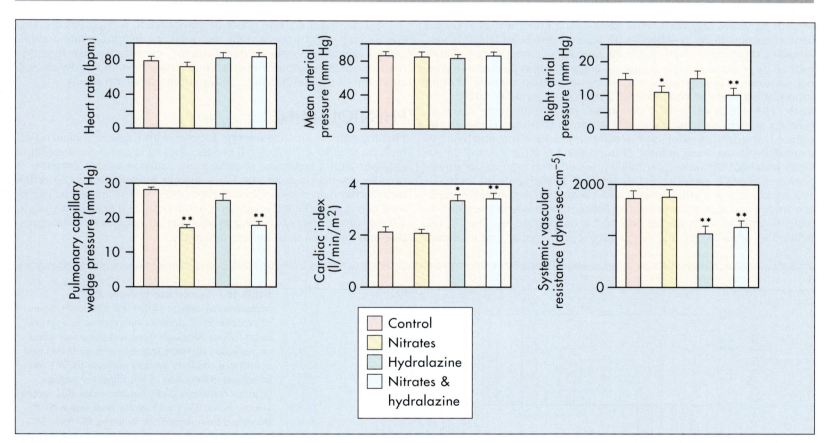

FIGURE 18.6 Hemodynamic effects of nitrates, hydralazine, and combination of nitrates plus hydralazine as compared with control in 12 patients with chronic congestive heart failure. Nitrates reduced right atrial and pulmonary capillary wedge pressures, and hydralazine decreased systemic vascular resistance and increased cardiac output. The combination of the two produced combined effects on filling pressures and cardiac output. (Modified from Massie B, Chatterjee K, Werner J et al: Hemodynamic advantage of combined oral hydralazine and nonparenteral nitrates in the vasodilator therapy of chronic heart failure. Am J Cardiol 40:794, 1977)

fects, and subsequent doses show a marked attenuation (Fig. 18.7). Although the mechanism for this attenuation is unclear, plasma norepinephrine has been shown to increase during chronic therapy.[40] The increased vasoconstriction might therefore counteract some of the vasodilating effects of prazosin. Severe hypotension after a first dose is a potential problem, and 1.0 mg should be used as the first dose. Other side effects, such as gastrointestinal symptoms, palpitations, drowsiness, depression, and nervousness, are infrequent. Because of this hemodynamic attenuation of its effects in congestive heart failure, prazosin has been used less frequently than other vasodilator agents.

TRIMAZOSIN

Trimazosin is closely related to prazosin and appears to produce similar hemodynamic effects. Exercise tolerance has been reported to increase with long-term trimazosin therapy.[41] Another study produced beneficial hemodynamic effects during exercise but no change in resting hemodynamics or in exercise tolerance.[42] In some cases increased doses of diuretics have been required. The beneficial hemodynamic dose varies between 25 mg and 100 mg three times daily. At this writing, trimazosin has not yet been approved by the Food and Drug Administration, and data are too limited to determine its potential role in the management of chronic congestive heart failure.

TERAZOSIN

Terazosin is another α_1-adrenoreceptor with hemodynamic effects similar to trimazosin. An increase in cardiac output and a decrease in atrial pressures occur both at rest and following exercise.[43] More data are required to assess its potential role in chronic heart failure.

SODIUM NITROPRUSSIDE

Sodium nitroprusside is available intravenously and is a potent relaxant of both arterioles and veins. This direct-acting effect results in potent hemodynamic effects in patients with acute severe heart failure. These include a significant reduction of systemic vascular resistance together with an increase in cardiac output. In general, some decrease in arterial pressure accompanies the increase in cardiac output.[44] Potent venodilation leads to reduction of atrial and pulmonary artery pressures. The effects on renal function are variable. In some cases increased sodium and potassium excretion may occur, although decreased arterial pressure may worsen renal function and lead to increased plasma renin activity. Nitroprusside is most valuable in patients with high left ventricular filling pressures and reasonable arterial pressures (systolic pressure $\geq$ 100 mm Hg). In such patients there is a striking increase in cardiac output and a reduction in pulmonary capillary wedge and right atrial pressures. Nitroprusside is best given only in patients with an intra-arterial line and a balloon tip catheter in the pulmonary artery. Thus, one can avoid excessive reductions in arterial pressure while at the same time measuring the reduction in pulmonary capillary wedge pressure. The drug is initially administered at a dose level of about 15 μg/min, with a gradual titration upward until pulmonary capillary wedge pressure is reduced and cardiac output increased. At the same time, the fall in arterial pressure must be minimized. In patients with significant mitral or aortic regurgitation, sodium nitroprusside is effective in increasing forward cardiac output and reducing regurgitant volume.[45,46] In general, it is used in patients with acute severe heart failure who have a reasonable blood pressure and a high filling pressure. It might also be helpful in patients with acute severe mitral or aortic regurgitation or for the short-term therapy of patients with severe chronic heart failure in whom oral therapy is going to be subsequently initiated.

The effects of nitroprusside in patients with acute severe heart failure following myocardial infarction[47] are shown in Figure 18.8. Group II and III patients with the most severe heart failure following myocardial infarction showed an increase in stroke volume together with a decrease in left ventricular filling pressure. Group I patients, who had an initial left ventricular filling pressure less than 15 mm Hg, had a reduction in stroke volume as they moved down the ascending limb of their ventricular function curve. This was accompanied by hypotension and tachycardia. Thus, nitroprusside should be limited to patients with a high left ventricular filling pressure, and care should be taken not to reduce filling pressure much below the optimal range of 15 mm Hg to 18 mm Hg. If this occurs, volume loading to bring the filling pressure up to a higher level can still retain the beneficial effects of nitroprusside. In two controlled studies in patients with acute myocardial infarction, nitroprusside reduced mortality in one study[48] and had no effect in the other.[49] In the latter study, it was most beneficial several hours after the infarct and in patients with high filling pressures. Some studies have suggested that nitroprusside may cause a coronary steal syndrome[50] and thus be less beneficial than intravenous nitroglycerin. No significant deleterious effects of nitroprusside have been found in other studies.[51]

The most serious side effect of nitroprusside is hypotension. This can be managed by temporarily discontinuing the drug. Rare complications include decreased arterial oxygen, cyanide toxicity, hypothyroidism, methemoglobinemia, lactic acidosis, vitamin B_{12} deficiency, inhibition of platelet function, and gastrointestinal symptoms.

PHENTOLAMINE

Phentolamine is an α-adrenergic blocker with relatively balanced effects on arteries and veins.[52] It produces an increase in cardiac output together with a reduction in pulmonary capillary wedge pressure. It reduces arterial pressure and has a greater tendency to cause reflex tachycardia than does sodium nitroprusside. It is restricted to parenteral administration and is infused continuously at a dose of 0.1 mg to 2.0 mg/min. It does not appear to have any advantages over nitroprusside and has been used far less frequently.

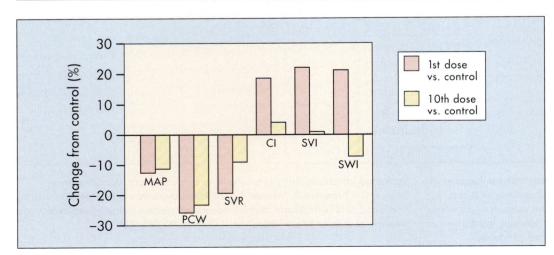

FIGURE 18.7 Comparison between the hemodynamic effects of the first and tenth doses of prazosin in 12 patients with chronic congestive heart failure. Although there is a persistent effect on reduction of mean arterial pressure (MAP) and pulmonary capillary wedge pressure (PCW), there is marked attenuation of the effect on systemic vascular resistance (SVR), cardiac index (CI), stroke volume index (SVI), and stroke work index (SWI). (Modified from Arnold SB, Williams RL, Ports TA et al: Attenuation of prazosin effect on cardiac output in chronic heart failure. Ann Intern Med 91:345, 1979)

ANGIOTENSIN–CONVERTING ENZYME INHIBITORS

CAPTOPRIL

The renin–angiotensin–aldosterone system is activated in chronic congestive heart failure.[1] Decreased perfusion pressure, adrenergic stimulation, and reduced sodium all stimulate the juxtaglomerular apparatus around the afferent arteriole in the renal glomerulus to release renin. Renin converts angiotensinogen (which is produced in the liver) to angiotensin I, an inactive decapeptide. Angiotensin I is then changed by converting enzyme to angiotensin II, a potent vasoconstrictor. Angiotensin II has three effects that may be deleterious to the patient with heart failure. First of all, it is a potent vasoconstrictor that can directly increase systemic vascular resistance. Second, it facilitates sympathetic outflow and may worsen the sympathetic-mediated increase in systemic vascular resistance. Third, it stimulates the production and release of aldosterone, which leads to further sodium retention. Theoretically, therefore, if one could prevent the formation of angiotensin II, one might benefit patients with heart failure.

Converting enzyme, which alters angiotensin I to angiotensin II, is located everywhere in the body, but appears to predominate in pulmonary capillary endothelial cells. Inhibition of this enzyme leads to reduced levels of angiotensin II, even though there is a feedback increase in renin levels. Converting enzyme is also responsible for the degradation of bradykinin, a potent vasodilator.[53] Thus, inhibition of converting enzyme may produce vasodilation both by decreasing angiotensin II levels and increasing bradykinin levels. Captopril is the first orally available angiotensin converting enzyme inhibitor to be used in chronic congestive heart failure. Its hemodynamic effects[54] include a substantial fall in systemic vascular resistance with a fall in arterial pressure. Despite the fall in arterial pressure, there may be a slight decrease in heart rate (Fig. 18.9). Presumably this occurs because of a reduction in sympathetic tone to the sinoatrial node. After a single oral dose, these effects last for up to 8 hours. Together with the decrease in systemic resistance, there is an increase in forward cardiac output (Fig. 18.10). There is also considerable venodilation, with a reduction in pulmonary capillary wedge pressure and right atrial pressure. The precise reason for a decrease in pulmonary capillary wedge pressure is unclear. Angiotensin II is not a potent venoconstrictor. It is more likely that withdrawal of sympathetic tone plays a more prominent role in the venodilation than does a reduction in angiotensin II levels. Furthermore, a reduction in arterial pressure enhances ejection of blood and in and of itself can reduce end-diastolic volume. There is frequently a concordant change in arterial pressure and pulmonary capillary wedge pressure.[55]

Vasodilators also increase the apparent compliance of the left ventricle. This is not due to a change in the intrinsic stiffness properties of the myocardium, but rather to a reduction in intrapericardial pressure, due to a reduction in the intrapericardial volume.[56] All of these effects may contribute to the fall in diastolic pressures of the heart.

There are important dose response considerations[57] to the use of captopril in chronic congestive heart failure. In general, there may be a potent first-dose hypotensive effect, so it is wise to begin at an extremely low dose. One can begin with 6.25 mg three times a day and gradually work up to a dose of 25 mg to 50 mg three times a day, or 50 mg twice a day. Since the major effect of captopril is to block converting enzyme, when that has occurred higher doses produce no greater effect (Fig. 18.11). In general, 25 mg three times a day is an effective dose in approximately 90% of patients with chronic congestive heart failure. The responsiveness to captopril depends on several factors. In patients with a low serum sodium, there is a more dramatic response to captopril, presumably because of the increased renin levels.[58] There is a generally increased response in patients with higher renin levels and a clear-cut increased response in patients with higher systemic vascular resistance.

Controlled randomized clinical trials have shown that captopril causes an improvement in exercise tolerance.[59,60] In addition, there appears to be a sense of well-being associated with the administration of captopril, which is maintained despite low arterial pressures.

A number of side effects have been noted. Severe hypotension is the most important hemodynamic effect, particularly following the first dose. Skin rash is relatively common, but may go away with continued use of captopril. A change in taste, nausea, anorexia, or diarrhea may occur in some patients. Proteinuria, neutropenia, and hemolytic anemia are very infrequent side effects. Since smaller doses have been used in the treatment of heart failure as compared with the treatment of hypertension, it appears that the side effect profile in patients with congestive heart failure may not be as high as those treated for hypertension.

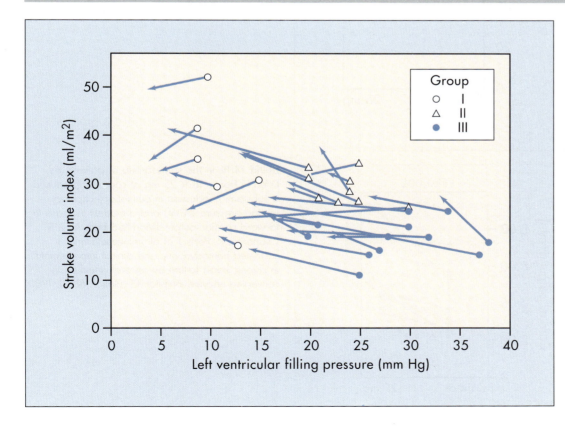

FIGURE 18.8 Hemodynamic effects of nitroprusside on left ventricular function in patients with acute myocardial infarction. Group I patients had an initial filling pressure less than 15 mm Hg. Group II and III patients had left ventricular failure with filling pressures greater than 15 mm Hg. In Group III, the stroke work index was less than 20 g-m/m^2, and in Group II it was greater than 20 g-m/m^2. In Groups II and III, nitroprusside produced an increase in stroke volume, together with a reduction in left ventricular filling pressure. In Group I patients, the effects on stroke volume were more variable, but tended to decrease because of the reduction in filling pressure down the ascending limb of the ventricular function curve. (Modified from Chatterjee K, Parmley WW: The role of vasodilator therapy in heart failure. Prog Cardiovasc Dis 19:301, 1977)

The effects on renal function are variable.[61] In some cases there is direct improvement in renal function. At the same time, renal function may deteriorate in some patients, perhaps related to the reduction in blood pressure. The counterbalancing of these two adverse effects will tend to have variable effects on renal function in individual patients. In a double-blind study of the effects of captopril on renal function, modest reductions in renal function occurred despite improvement in the symptoms of congestive heart failure.[62] It was postulated that loss of the direct compensatory effects of angiotensin II led to the decline in renal function. Angiotensin–converting enzyme inhibitors tend to increase serum potassium levels. This presumably occurs because of the reduction in angiotensin II and aldosterone levels and the resultant reduction in renal potassium excretion. Thus, one should not combine these drugs with potassium-sparing diuretics, since serious hyperkalemia may result.

ENALAPRIL

Enalapril is a longer-acting angiotensin–converting enzyme inhibitor that may have fewer side effects than captopril. It can be administered twice daily, with a usual dose of 5 mg to 10 mg. It appears to be devoid of problems with skin rash, proteinuria, and metallic taste. Further experience is needed with this angiotensin–converting enzyme inhibitor, although it appears to be a promising drug for the management of patients with chronic congestive heart failure. Preliminary data suggest that the hemodynamic and clinical profiles are similar to those of captopril.[63] A multicenter study of 73 patients showed improved exercise capacity and hemodynamics with chronic treatment. The dose used was 10 mg to 20 mg/day in either single or divided doses.[64] A direct comparison of captopril and enalapril suggested that the longer-acting enalapril could produce more hypotension and syncope or near-syncope than captopril.[65] Because large fixed doses of enalapril (40 mg/day) were used, however, it is probable that enalapril and captopril can produce similar beneficial effects at appropriate doses.

COMBINATION THERAPY

In considering the application of vasodilator drugs for the management of heart failure, it is clear that combination therapy may be more valuable than any single drug alone. For example, the combination of hydralazine and nitrates has been very effective in producing the desired hemodynamic effects of both arteriolar dilation and venodilation.[32] In

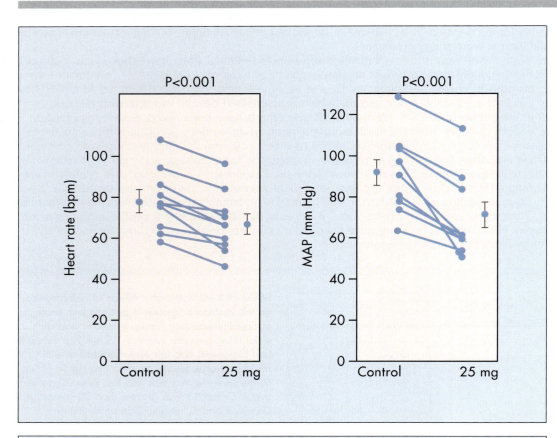

FIGURE 18.9 Effects of 25 mg of captopril on the hemodynamics of 9 patients with congestive heart failure. Despite a reduction in mean arterial pressure (*MAP*), there is no reflex increase in heart rate. In fact, heart rate tends to slow slightly. (Modified from Ader R, Chatterjee K, Ports T et al: Immediate and sustained hemodynamic and clinical improvement in chronic heart failure by an oral angiotensin converting enzyme inhibitor. Circulation 61:931, 1980)

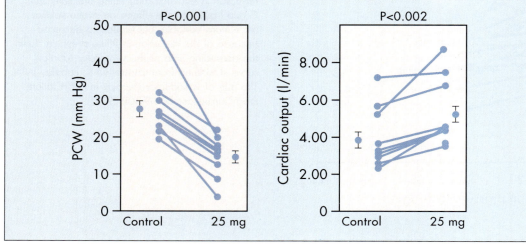

FIGURE 18.10 In the same group of patients as listed in Figure 18.9, 25 mg of captopril produced a substantial reduction in pulmonary capillary wedge pressure (*PCW*) and a modest increase in forward cardiac output. (Modified from Ader R, Chatterjee K, Ports T et al: Immediate and sustained hemodynamic and clinical improvement in chronic heart failure by an oral angiotensin converting enzyme inhibitor. Circulation 61:931, 1980)

a similar fashion, combinations of hydralazine and captopril are useful in individual patients.[66] Although captopril is effective in reducing pulmonary capillary wedge pressure, its arteriolar dilating effects are relatively modest, resulting in only minor increases in forward cardiac output. The addition of hydralazine can dramatically increase forward cardiac output in patients already on captopril. These two combinations of vasodilator drugs appear to be the most effective ones studied, although other combinations will undoubtedly emerge in the future that may be useful in the management of patients with chronic heart failure.

It should also be noted that vasodilators and inotropic agents are generally synergistic in their hemodynamic effects.[67,68] This occurs because they work by different mechanisms. Inotropic agents increase the contractility of the myocardium, while vasodilators reduce the load against which the heart works. Several combinations of these two classes of drugs can be helpful in individual patients.

EFFECTS ON LEFT VENTRICULAR COMPLIANCE

All vasodilators that lower atrial pressures appear to increase the compliance of the left ventricle in patients with congestive heart failure. That is, the passive pressure–volume relationship is shifted downward.[69] An example of this phenomenon is seen in Figure 18.12.[70] When the left ventricular diastolic pressure is displayed on a log scale, the exponential passive pressure–volume relationship becomes a straight line. The top line represents early and late diastolic pressure and volume in a patient with heart failure. Following sublingual nitroglycerin, the passive pressure–volume relationship is shifted downward. In particular, note that there is a reduction in left ventricular end-diastolic pressure, with no change in end-diastolic volume.

Several mechanisms have been postulated to explain this phenomenon. Since ischemia can stiffen muscle and decrease left ventricular compliance, one could speculate that relief of ischemia with vasodilator therapy might be responsible.[71] Although this hypothesis might explain changes in some instances of ischemia, it can't explain similar changes in patients without ischemic heart disease. It seems clear that the usual cause of this change in compliance is not relief of ischemia. In addition, vasodilators apparently do not have a direct significant effect on the diastolic properties of heart muscle.

Two other effects appear to account for this phenomenon: the influence of a stiff pericardial sac and the interaction of the left and right heart chambers.[72] The pericardium has a stiff passive pressure–volume relationship, which becomes manifest in heart failure as a restraining influence on the dilated heart. The transmural pressure, which fills the left ventricle, is the left ventricular diastolic pressure minus the intrapericardial pressure (assuming the intrathoracic pressure is near zero). When one gives a vasodilator drug that lowers right and left atrial pressures by decreasing heart volume, there is a decrease in intrapericardial pressure. Because the pericardium is such a stiff structure, it takes very little reduction in intrapericardial volume to produce a substantial fall in intrapericardial pressure. If there is a similar fall in left ventricular diastolic and intrapericardial pressures, there is little change in the transmural filling pressure of the left ventricle. Hence, diastolic pressure falls with little change in left ventricular volume. It is obviously not possible to measure intrapericardial pressure in the routine clinical situation. However, experimental studies have shown that under most circumstances, mean right atrial pressure is a reasonable approximation of intrapericardial pressure.[73] Thus, one can quantitate the potential importance of this mechanism by noting changes in right atrial pressure produced by vasodilator drugs.

The second mechanism responsible for this shift in the left ventricular pressure–volume relationship is closely related. Within the pericardial sac are the four heart chambers, which can interact with each other.[74] As one decreases intrapericardial pressure and volume, it appears that left ventricular volume increases in relation to the other chambers. Perhaps the decrease in right-sided pressures diminishes the potential interactive effect of the right ventricle on the left ventricle.

Overall, it is clear that the pericardium has an important effect on the diastolic properties of the failing left ventricle and that vasodilator drugs produce beneficial effects on left ventricular compliance. By lowering diastolic pressures, there is a reduction in pulmonary congestion. Preservation of end-diastolic volume preserves stroke volume at a given ejection fraction. Reduction of systemic vascular resistance then enhances stroke volume at a given end-diastolic volume.

This phenomenon probably occurs with any intervention that reduces atrial pressures. It has also recently been noted with the new potent inotropic–vasodilator drugs, which can dramatically alter resting hemodynamics.[75]

VASODILATOR DRUGS AND MECHANICAL LESIONS

In patients with acute myocardial infarction and acute severe mitral regurgitation due to papillary muscle dysfunction, vasodilators such as nitroprusside can be dramatic in reversing the deleterious hemodynamic consequences (Fig. 18.13). When this was first described, it wasn't clear whether or not the beneficial effect was due only to relief

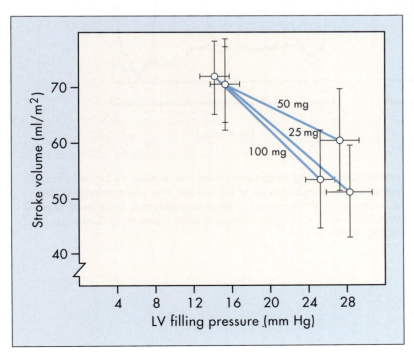

FIGURE 18.11 In the same group of patients listed in Figure 18.9, the sequential effects of 25 mg, 50 mg, and 100 mg of captopril are illustrated. Patients were allowed to return to control levels between doses. The shift up and to the left produced by captopril, with an increase in stroke volume and reduction in left ventricular filling pressure, was similar with each of the three doses. At this dose range, therefore, patients were on the plateau of responsiveness, presumably due to maximal inhibition of converting enzyme. (Modified from Ader R, Chatterjee K, Ports T et al: Immediate and sustained hemodynamic and clinical improvement in chronic heart failure by an oral angiotensin converting enzyme inhibitor. Circulation 61:931, 1980)

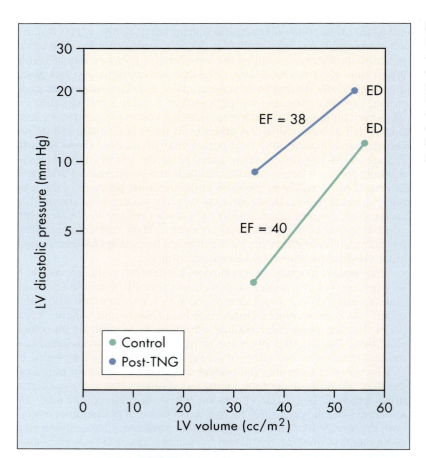

FIGURE 18.12 Representative changes in passive pressure–volume relationship in the left ventricle following nitroglycerin in a patient with chronic coronary artery disease and congestive heart failure. Early and late diastolic pressure and volume points are plotted on a log scale, such that the exponential passive–pressure volume relationship tends to become a straight line. Following the administration of 0.4 mg of nitroglycerin sublingually, there was a reduction in end-diastolic pressures at approximately the same end-diastolic volume. There was no change in ejection fraction. (Modified from Parmley WW, Chuck L, Chatterjee K et al: Acute changes in the diastolic pressure-volume relationship of the left ventricle. Eur J Cardiol 4:105, 1976)

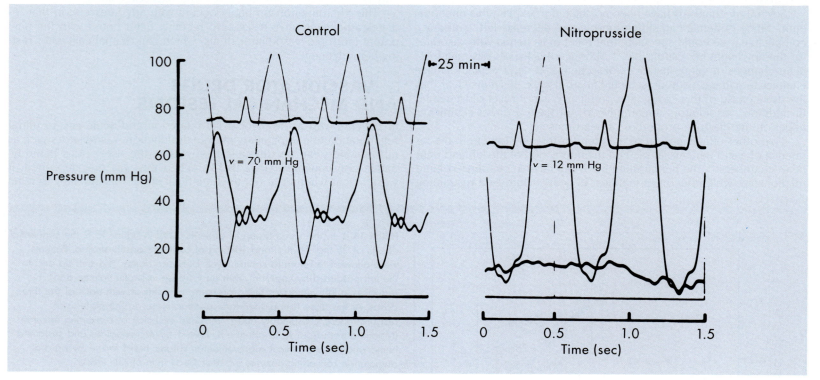

FIGURE 18.13 Hemodynamic effects of sodium nitroprusside in a patient with acute, severe mitral regurgitation following acute myocardial infarction. Pulmonary capillary wedge pressure and left ventricular pressure are illustrated before and after nitroprusside infusion. Note the large v waves, up to 70 mm Hg, and elevated diastolic pressures prior to nitroprusside administration. During nitroprusside there is a dramatic reduction in diastolic pressures and disappearance of the v waves. This was accompanied by disappearance of the murmur of mitral regurgitation. (Chatterjee K, Parmley WW: The role of vasodilator therapy in heart failure. Prog Cardiovasc Dis 19:301, 1977)

of ischemia.[76] Subsequent studies in patients with chronic mitral regurgitation unrelated to ischemia[45] demonstrated similar beneficial effects: decreased pulmonary capillary wedge pressure and regurgitant fraction and increased cardiac output (Fig. 18.14). The beneficial effect of arteriolar dilation is the enhancement of forward output. The beneficial effect of venodilation is probably a reduction in left ventricular size with an improvement in mitral valve competence.

It should be noted that vasoconstrictor drugs can potentially worsen mitral regurgitation. In the setting of acute heart failure and severe mitral regurgitation, preference should be given to vasodilator drugs. This problem is compounded because in very low flow states in acute heart failure, there may not be a characteristic murmur,[77] and the mitral regurgitation can then be detected only by abnormal v waves in the pulmonary capillary wedge pressure trace.

Aortic regurgitation is a clinical situation in which arteriolar vasodilators such as hydralazine can enhance forward cardiac output and decrease regurgitant volume.[7] There are several clinical situations in which they might be useful. In the patient with severe acute aortic regurgitation, due for example to a ruptured cusp, hydralazine can help stabilize the hemodynamics while more definitive surgical therapy is being considered. In patients with chronic aortic regurgitation and heart failure in whom surgical therapy is considered inadvisable because of high risk or other problems, vasodilator therapy would be extremely important. A more difficult clinical question concerns the asymptomatic patient with moderately severe aortic or mitral regurgitation. An attractive hypothesis is that vasodilator therapy might be able to unload the left ventricle and reduce the rate of cardiac dilatation.[78] This might retard the rate at which cardiac contractility declines and thus delay surgical replacement of the valve. There are no firm data to support this hypothesis, but it appears physiologically sound.

Another mechanical lesion that can be helped with vasodilator therapy is a ruptured interventricular septum following acute myocardial infarction. The degree of left-to-right shunting in this circumstance depends on the size of the defect and the relative magnitude of pulmonary and systemic vascular resistance. A drug such as sodium nitroprusside usually decreases systemic vascular resistance more than pulmonary vascular resistance and thus decreases the magnitude of the left-to-right shunt.[79] In some cases, however, the reverse can occur and the shunt will worsen. With a balloon-tip catheter in the pulmonary artery, one can measure the step-up in oxygen content of blood from the right atrium to the pulmonary artery. Changes in the oxygen content reflect changes in the degree of shunting. For example, a decrease in oxygen content following nitroprusside administration reflects a decrease in the left-to-right shunt. In children with a congenital ventricular septal defect, data suggest that vasodilator therapy can worsen the shunting owing to a greater reduction in pulmonary vascular resistance, especially with a low baseline systemic vascular resistance.[80]

Another potential adverse effect of vasodilator therapy is a reduction in arterial oxygen in patients with initially high filling pressures.[81] This occurs because of a ventilation–perfusion mismatch. With high filling pressures, perfusion is preferentially shifted toward the upper lobes where ventilation is also better. Vasodilators that lower left ventricular filling pressure lead to better perfusion of the lower lobes in areas of poor ventilation. Thus, shunting of poorly oxygenated blood across the lungs leads to a reduction in arterial oxygen content. This is rarely deleterious and in fact is generally accompanied by clinical im-

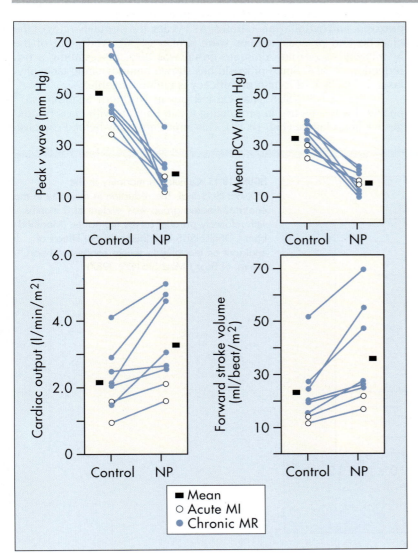

FIGURE 18.14 Hemodynamic effects of sodium nitroprusside (NP) in 8 patients with mitral regurgitation. Two patients had mitral regurgitation on the basis of acute myocardial infarction (acute MI), and 6 patients had chronic mitral regurgitation. A. Note that sodium nitroprusside (NP) produced a dramatic reduction in peak v wave and mean pulmonary capillary wedge (PCW) pressure in all patients. B. Similarly, nitroprusside produced an increase in cardiac output and forward stroke volume. (Modified from Chatterjee K, Parmley WW, Swan HJC et al: Beneficial effects of vasodilator agents in severe mitral regurgitation due to dysfunction of subvalvar apparatus. Circulation 48:684, 1973)

provement in dyspnea due to a reduction in pulmonary capillary wedge pressure.

SELECTION OF A VASODILATOR IN CHRONIC CONGESTIVE HEART FAILURE

In general, vasodilator drugs have been used after patients have failed to respond to "standard therapy" with digitalis and diuretics. In patients with moderately severe heart failure but reasonably preserved arterial pressure, the angiotensin converting enzyme inhibitors are the next class of agents that should be considered. Their ability to improve clinical class and exercise tolerance is well documented. They will be especially beneficial in patients who have a low serum sodium and a high renin level.[78] If blood pressure is too low to consider initiating angiotensin–converting enzyme inhibitors, hydralazine or hydralazine plus nitrates can be considered in such patients. Minoxidil can be considered as an alternative to hydralazine if the lupus syndrome develops and if potential problems with edema formation and hypertrichosis are not an issue. The calcium blockers and captopril can be considered in patients with hypertension and heart failure. These agents might also be effective in patients with associated coronary artery disease and angina pectoris. The ability of the calcium blockers and captopril to reduce myocardial oxygen consumption should be effective in this setting.

One difficulty in patients with chronic heart failure is assessing the chronic response to vasodilators. Studies have noted that the acute hemodynamic response will not necessarily correlate with the chronic clinical response.[82] Similarly, there has been great difficulty in using objective measures, such as echocardiography or radionuclide angiography, to follow the response to vasodilator therapy.[83] Clinical response and an increase in exercise tolerance are the most important markers of improvement in patients treated for congestive heart failure. Several ways of monitoring this improvement have been used. Increase in exercise time on a treadmill is useful, but also depends considerably on the motivation of the patient and the interaction with the physician conducting the test. Total body oxygen consumption (VO_2) provides useful quantitative information, although it is also subject to the same pitfalls as time on the treadmill.

"Anaerobic threshold," as monitored by a rise in lactate and an alteration in the respiratory exchange ratio, provides important biochemical information about the adequacy of oxygen delivery to exercising skeletal muscles.[84] It appears that limited flow to skeletal muscle is extremely important as a mechanism for producing fatigue in heart failure patients.

Some improvement in exercise tolerance in such patients can be achieved by exercise conditioning. Although the degree of such exercise training is obviously limited in symptomatic patients, it may be an important factor in the beneficial long-term response to vasodilator drugs. Such drugs may increase the cardiovascular capacity and thus allow patients to exercise more and benefit from the training effects thus obtained.

Although many of these drugs can be started in outpatients, it appears prudent to hospitalize patients with severe heart failure and use invasive hemodynamic monitoring to select an appropriate dose. Although the acute response may not necessarily predict the chronic clinical response of the patient, it is helpful in selecting an appropriate dose of the drug and documenting a beneficial hemodynamic effect. Furthermore, one can avoid hypotensive effects and avoid lowering left ventricular filling pressure too much. Tolerance may potentially develop with all of the drugs that have been mentioned,[85] although it probably is least common with the angiotensin–converting enzyme inhibitors.

Besides improving symptoms, there is evidence that vasodilators have a favorable effect on long-term survival. Furberg and Yusuf[86] analyzed evidence from a number of short-term studies using different vasodilator drugs. They noted some favorable trends, especially with the angiotensin–converting enzyme inhibitors. More importantly, the multicenter Veterans Administration cooperative trial (VHEFT) provided direct evidence of benefit.[87] Heart failure patients on digitalis and diuretics were randomized into three treatment groups: placebo, prazosin, and hydralazine–nitrates. At 3 years, the mortality rates of the placebo and prazosin groups were similar (47%), while that of the hydralazine–isosorbide dinitrate group was 36%, representing a risk reduction of 36%. Since prazosin has shown hemodynamic tachyphylaxis,[38,39] its lack of long-term efficacy is understandable.

In the CONSENSUS Trial carried out in Northern Scandinavia,[88] enalapril was effective in prolonging life in patients with class IV congestive heart failure (Fig. 18.15). This important study helped establish

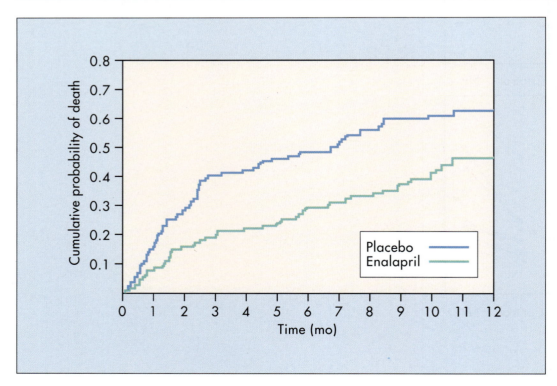

FIGURE 18.15 Cumulative mortality in the CONSENSUS Trial. The reduction in mortality in the enalapril-treated group was evident at 3 months, with relatively parallel curves thereafter. (Modified from CONSENSUS Trial Study Group: Effects of enalapril on mortality in severe congestive heart failure. N Engl J Med 316:1429, 1987)

angiotensin–converting enzyme inhibitor therapy as the premier vasodilator therapy for patients with congestive heart failure. Not only does this therapy increase exercise tolerance and prolong life, it also appears to improve well-being and the quality of life better than other vasodilator drugs. Whether angiotensin–converting enzyme inhibitors prolong life more than hydralazine-isosorbide dinitrate is unclear at this time. The VHEFT 2 trial is underway to answer that question by comparing enalapril to hydralazine–isosorbide dinitrate.

REFERENCES

1. Chatterjee K, Parmley WW: Vasodilator therapy for acute myocardial infarction and chronic heart failure. J Am Coll Cardiol 1:133, 1983
2. Packer M: Conceptual dilemmas in the classification of vasodilator drugs for severe chronic heart failure. Advocacy of a pragmatic approach to the selection of a therapeutic agent. Am J Med 76:3, 1984
3. Chatterjee K, Parmley WW, Massie B et al: Oral hydralazine therapy for chronic refractory heart failure. Circulation 54:879, 1976
4. Koch-Weser J: Myocardial inactivity of therapeutic concentrations of hydralazine and diazoxide. Experientia 30:170, 1974
5. Franciosa JA, Pierpont G, Cohn J: Hemodynamic improvement after oral hydralazine in left ventricular failure. Ann Intern Med 86:388, 1977
6. Greenberg BH, Massie BM, Brundage BH et al: Beneficial effects of hydralazine in severe mitral regurgitation. Circulation 58:273, 1978
7. Greenberg B, DeMot H, Murphy E et al: Beneficial effects of hydralazine on rest and exercise hemodynamics in patients with severe aortic insufficiency. Circulation 62:49, 1980
8. Chatterjee K, Ports TA, Brundage BH et al: Oral hydralazine in chronic heart failure: Sustained beneficial hemodynamic effects. Ann Intern Med 92:600, 1980
9. Franciosa JA, Weber KT, Levine TB et al: Hydralazine in the long term treatment of chronic heart failure: Lack of difference from placebo. Am Heart J 104:587, 1982
10. Quyyumi AA, Wagstaff D, Evans TR: Acute hemodynamic effects of endralazine: A new vasodilator for chronic refractory congestive heart failure. Am J Cardiol 51:1353, 1983
11. Quyyumi AA, Wagstaff D, Evans TR: Long-term beneficial effects of endralazine, a new arteriolar vasodilator at rest and during exercise capacity in chronic congestive heart failure. Am J Cardiol 54:1020, 1984
12. McKay C, Chatterjee K, Ports TA et al: Minoxidil in chronic congestive heart failure: A hemodynamic and clinical study. Am Heart J 104:575, 1982
13. Franciosa JA, Jordan RA, Wilen MM et al: Minoxidil in patients with chronic left heart failure: Contrasting hemodynamic and clinical effects in a controlled trial. Circulation 70:63, 1984
14. Leier CS, Patrick TS, Hermiller J et al: Nifedipine in congestive heart failure: Effects on resting and exercise hemodynamics and regional blood flow. Am Heart J 108:1461, 1984
15. Ferlinz J, Citron PD: Hemodynamic and myocardial performance characteristics after verapamil use in congestive heart failure. Am J Cardiol 51:1339, 1983
16. Walsh RW, Porter CB, Starling MR et al: Beneficial hemodynamic effects of intravenous and oral diltiazem in severe congestive heart failure. J Am Coll Cardiol 3:1044, 1984
17. Ryman KS, Kubo SH, Lystash J et al: The effect of nicardipine on rest and exercise hemodynamics in chronic congestive heart failure. Am J Cardiol 58:583, 1986
18. McAllister RG Jr: Clinical pharmacology of slow channel blocking agents. Prog Cardiovasc Dis 25:83, 1982
19. Camerini F, Alberti E, Klugmann S et al: Primary pulmonary hypertension: Effects of nifedipine. Br Heart J 44:352, 1980
20. Packer M, Medina N, Yushak M: Adverse hemodynamic and clinical effects of calcium channel blockade in pulmonary hypertension secondary to obliterative pulmonary vascular disease. J Am Coll Cardiol 4:890, 1984
21. Packer M: New perspectives on therapeutic application of nitrates as vasodilator agents for severe chronic heart failure. Am J Med (Suppl)74:61, 1983
22. Ignarro LJ, Lippton H, Edwards JC et al: Mechanism of vascular smooth muscle relaxation by organic nitrates, nitrites, nitroprusside and nitrate oxide: Evidence for the involvement of S-nitrothols as active intermediates. J Pharmacol Exp Ther 218:739, 1981
23. Franciosa JA, Nordstrom LA, Cohn JN: Nitrate therapy for congestive heart failure. JAMA 240:443, 1978
24. Herling IM: Intravenous nitroglycerin: Clinical pharmacology and therapeutic considerations. Am Heart J 108:141, 1984
25. Bogaert MG: Clinical pharmacokinetics of organic nitrates. Clin Pharmacokinet 8:410, 1983
26. Rajfer S, Demma FJ, Goldberg LI: Sustained beneficial hemodynamic responses to large doses of transdermal nitroglycerin in congestive heart failure, and comparison with intravenous nitroglycerin. Am J Cardiol 54:120, 1984
27. Needleman P, Johnson EM Jr: Mechanism of tolerance development to organic nitrates. J Pharmacol Exp Ther 184:709, 1973
28. Armstrong PW, Walker DC, Burton JR et al: Vasodilator therapy in acute myocardial infarction: A comparison of sodium nitroprusside and nitroglycerin. Circulation 52:1118, 1975
29. Flaherty JT, Becker LC, Bulkley BH et al: A randomized prospective trial of intravenous nitroglycerin in patients with acute myocardial infarction. Circulation 68:576, 1983
30. Derrida JR, Sal R, Chiche P: Effects of prolonged nitroglycerin infusion in patients with acute myocardial infarction. Am J Cardiol 41:407, 1978
31. Franciosa JA, Goldsmith SR, Cohn JN: Contrasting immediate and long-term effects of isosorbide dinitrate on exercise capacity in congestive heart failure. Am J Med 69:559, 1980
32. Massie B, Chatterjee K, Werner J et al: Hemodynamic advantage of combined oral hydralazine and nonparenteral nitrates in the vasodilator therapy of chronic heart failure. Am J Cardiol 40:794, 1977
33. Sniderman AD, Marpole DGT, Palmer WH et al: Response of the left ventricle to nitroglycerin in patients with and without mitral regurgitation. Br Heart J 36:357, 1974
34. Denolin H (ed): International symposium on Molsidomine. Am Heart J 109:625, 1985
35. Miller RR, Awan NA, Maxwell KS et al: Sustained reduction of cardiac impedance and preload in congestive heart failure with the antihypertensive vasodilator, prazosin. N Engl J Med 297:303, 1977
36. Markham RV, Corbett JR, Gilmore R et al: Efficiency of prazosin in the management of chronic congestive heart failure: A six month randomized double blind placebo controlled study. Am J Cardiol 51:1346, 1983
37. Colucci WS, Wynne J, Holman BL et al: Long-term therapy of heart failure with prazosin: A randomized double blind trial. Am J Cardiol 45:337, 1980
38. Packer M, Meller J, Gorlin R et al: Hemodynamic and clinical tachyphylaxis to prazosin-mediated afterload reduction in severe chronic congestive heart failure. Circulation 59:531, 1979
39. Arnold SB, Williams RL, Ports TA et al: Attenuation of prazosin effect on cardiac output in chronic heart failure. Ann Intern Med 91:345, 1979
40. Colucci WS, Williams GH, Braunwald E: Increased plasma norepinephrine during prazosin therapy for severe congestive heart failure. Ann Intern Med 93:452, 1980
41. Weber KT, Kinasewitz GA, West JS et al: Long term vasodilator therapy with trimazosin in chronic cardiac failure. N Engl J Med 303:242, 1980
42. Kirlin PC, Das S, Pitt B: Chronic alpha-adrenoreceptor blockade with trimazosin in congestive heart failure. Int J Cardiol 8:89, 1985
43. Leier CV, Patterson SE, Huss P et al. The hemodynamic and clinical responses to terazosin, a new alpha blocking agent in congestive heart failure. Am J Med Sci 292:128, 1986
44. Franciosa JB, Guiha NM, Limas CJ et al: Improved left ventricular function during nitroprusside infusion in acute myocardial infarction. Lancet 1:650, 1972
45. Chatterjee K, Parmley WW: The role of vasodilator therapy in heart failure. Prog Cardiovasc Dis 19:301, 1977
46. Bolen JL, Alderman EL: Hemodynamic consequences of afterload reduction in patients with chronic aortic regurgitation. Circulation 53:879, 1976
47. Chatterjee K, Parmley WW, Ganz W et al: Hemodynamic and metabolic responses to vasodilator therapy in acute myocardial infarction. Circulation 48:1183, 1973
48. Durrer JD, Lie KL, VanCapelle FRJ et al: Effect of sodium nitroprusside on mortality in acute myocardial infarction. N Engl J Med 306:1121, 1982
49. Cohn JN, Franciosa JA, Francis CS et al: Effect of short term infusion of sodium nitroprusside on mortality rate in acute myocardial infarction complicated by left ventricular failure. N Engl J Med 306:1129, 1982
50. Chiarello M, Gold HK, Leinbach RC et al: Comparison between the effects of nitroprusside and nitroglycerin on ischemic injury during acute myocardial infarction. Circulation 54:766, 1976
51. daLuz PL, Forrester JS, Wyatt LH et al: Hemodynamic and metabolic effects of sodium nitroprusside on the performance and metabolism of regional ischemic myocardium. Circulation 52:400, 1975
52. Walinsky P, Chatterjee K, Forrester JS et al: Enhanced left ventricular performance with phentolamine in acute myocardial infarction. Am J Cardiol 33:37, 1974
53. Witzball H, Hirsch F, Scherer B et al: Acute hemodynamic and hormonal effects of captopril are diminished by indomethacin. Clin Sci 62:611, 1982
54. Ader R, Chatterjee K, Ports T et al: Immediate and sustained hemodynamic and clinical improvement in chronic heart failure by an oral angiotensin converting enzyme inhibitor. Circulation 61:931, 1980
55. Franciosa JA, Guiha NH, Limas CJ et al: Arterial pressure as a determinant of left ventricular filling pressure after acute myocardial infarction. Am J Cardiol 34:506, 1974
56. Glantz SA, Parmley WW: Factors which affect the diastolic pressure-volume curve. Circ Res 32:171, 1978
57. Chatterjee K, Rouleau JL, Parmley WW: Hemodynamic and myocardial metabolic effects of captopril in chronic heart failure. Br Heart J 47:233, 1982

58. Packer M, Medina N, Yushak M: Relation between serum sodium concentration and the hemodynamic and clinical responses to converting enzyme inhibition with captopril in severe heart failure. J Am Coll Cardiol 3:1035, 1984
59. Kramer BL, Massie BM, Topic N: Controlled trial of captopril in chronic heart failure: A rest and exercise hemodynamic study. Circulation 67:807, 1983
60. Captopril Multicenter Research Group: A placebo controlled trial of captopril in refractory chronic congestive heart failure. J Am Coll Cardiol 2:755, 1983
61. Dzau VJ, Colucci WS, Williams GH et al: Sustained effectiveness of converting-enzyme inhibition in patients with severe congestive heart failure. N Engl J Med 302:1373, 1980
62. Cleland JG, Dargie HJ, Gillen G et al: Captopril in heart failure: A double blind study of the effects on renal function. J Cardiovasc Pharmacol 8:700, 1986
63. DiCarlo L, Chatterjee K, Parmley WW et al: Enalapril: A new angiotensin-converting enzyme inhibitor in chronic heart failure: Acute and chronic hemodynamic evaluations. J Am Coll Cardiol 2:865, 1983
64. Gomez HJ, Cirillo VJ, Davies RO et al: Enalapril in congestive heart failure: Acute and chronic invasive hemodynamic evaluation. Int J Cardiol 1:37, 1986
65. Packer M, Lee WH, Yushak M, Medina N: Comparison of captopril and enalapril in patients with severe chronic heart failure. N Engl J Med 315:847, 1986
66. Massie BM, Packer M, Hanlon JT et al: Hemodynamic responses to combined therapy with captopril and hydralazine in patients with severe heart failure. J Am Coll Cardiol 2:338, 1983
67. Parmley WW, Chatterjee K: Combined vasodilator and inotropic therapy: A new approach in the treatment of heart failure. In Mason D (ed): Advances in Heart Disease, p 45. New York, Grune & Stratton, 1977
68. Verma SP, Silke B, Nelson GF et al: Hemodynamic advantages of a combined inotropic/venodilator regimen over inotropic monotherapy in acute heart failure. J Cardiovasc Pharmacol 7:943, 1985
69. Alderman EL, Glantz SA: Acute hemodynamic interventions shift the diastolic pressure-volume curve in man. Circulation 54:662, 1976
70. Parmley WW, Chuck L, Chatterjee K et al: Acute changes in the diastolic pressure-volume relationship of the left ventricle. Eur J Cardiol 4:105, 1976
71. Mann T, Goldberg S, Mudge GH et al: Factors contributing to altered left ventricular diastolic properties during angina pectoris. Circulation 59:14, 1979
72. Tyberg JV, Misbach GA, Glantz SA et al: The mechanism for shifts in the diastolic left ventricular pressure-volume curve: The role of the pericardium. Eur J Cardiol (Suppl)7:1963, 1978
73. Smith ER, Smiseth OA, Kingma I et al: Mechanism of action of nitrates: Role of changes in venous capacitance and in the left ventricular diastolic pressure-volume relation. Am J Med 76(6A):14, 1984
74. Visner MS, Araentzen CE, O'Connor MJ et al: Alterations in left ventricular three-dimensional dynamic geometry and systolic function during acute right ventricular hypertension in the conscious dog. Circulation 67:353, 1983
75. Kereiakes DJ, Viquerat C, Lanzer P et al: Mechanisms of improved left ventricular function following intravenous MDL in 17,043 patients with severe chronic heart failure. Am Heart J 108:1278, 1984
76. Chatterjee K, Parmley WW, Swan HJC et al: Beneficial effects of vasodilator agents in severe mitral regurgitation due to dysfunction of subvalvar apparatus. Circulation 48:684, 1973
77. Forrester JS, Diamond G, Freedman S et al: Silent mitral insufficiency in acute myocardial infarction. Circulation 44:877, 1971
78. Greenberg BH, Rahimtoola SH: Usefulness of vasodilator therapy in acute and chronic valvular regurgitation. Curr Probl Cardiol 9:1, 1984
79. Tecklenberg PL, Fitzgerald J, Allaire BI et al: Afterload reduction in the management of postinfarction ventricular septal defect. Am J Cardiol 38:956, 1976
80. Zakazawa M, Atsuyoshi T, Chon T et al: Significance of systemic vascular resistance in determining the hemodynamic effects of hydralazine on large ventricular septal defects. Circulation 68:420, 1983
81. Benowitz HZ, LeWinter M, Wagner PD: Effect of sodium nitroprusside on ventilation-perfusion mismatching in heart failure. J Am Coll Cardiol 4:918, 1984
82. Franciosa JA, Dunkman B, Leddy CL: Hemodynamic effects of vasodilators and long-term response in heart failure. J Am Coll Cardiol 3:1521, 1984
83. Franciosa JA, Park M, Levine B: Lack of correlation between exercise capacity and indices of resting left ventricular performance in heart failure. Am J Cardiol 47:33, 1981
84. LeJemtel TH, Mancini D, Gumbardo D et al: Pitfalls and limitations of maximal oxygen uptake as an index of cardiovascular functional capacity in patients with chronic heart failure. Heart Failure 1:112, 1985
85. Packer M: Tolerance to vasodilator therapy. Cardiovasc Rev Rep 4:903, 1983
86. Furberg CD, Yusuf S: Effect of vasodilators on survival in chronic congestive heart failure. Am J Cardiol 55:1110, 1985
87. Cohn JN, Archibald DG, Ziesche S et al: Effect of vasodilator therapy on mortality in chronic congestive heart failure. N Engl J Med 314:1547, 1986
88. CONSENSUS Trial Study Group. Effects of enalapril on mortality in severe congestive heart failure. N Engl J Med 316:1429, 1987

HYPOLIPIDEMIC AGENTS

Mary J. Malloy • John P. Kane

The rationale for the prevention of atherosclerotic disease by diet and drugs rests primarily on the epidemiologic identification of atherogenic classes of lipoproteins in plasma. These lipoproteins have been shown to carry cholesterol and cholesteryl esters into the artery wall. Rational therapy would dictate that the diet and drug combinations that are most effective in reducing circulating levels of these lipoproteins should be employed. In this respect, the maximum advantage in retarding the progression of or even inducing regression of existing lesions should be obtained by reducing these offending lipoproteins to the lowest levels that are observed in healthy humans. Potent combined drug regimens are being developed that will permit intervention studies to determine the validity of this concept.

Among the lipoproteins of plasma, low density lipoproteins (LDL) and the structurally related Lp(a) lipoproteins as well as intermediate density lipoproteins (IDL) have been demonstrated immunochemically in atheromatous lesions. Studies in which lipoprotein particles resembling very low density lipoproteins (VLDL) have been extracted from human arterial plaques suggest that VLDL may also play a direct role in atherogenesis. Because some large epidemiologic studies have identified VLDL as a moderate risk factor for atherosclerosis,[1,2] it would appear reasonable to attempt to normalize VLDL levels, especially in a patient with known coronary disease or in whose kindred early coronary artery disease is present. The hypertriglyceridemias in general show greater response to diet than other forms of hyperlipidemia. Hence, an aggressive approach to diet should be pursued. Drug therapy should be considered in those patients whose plasma triglyceride levels cannot be maintained below 300 to 500 mg/dl with diet. An exception would be those patients with lipoprotein lipase deficiency or related disorders in whom diet is the only appropriate treatment.

Abundant evidence has been accumulated from studies in animals to support the basic concept that significant reduction in the levels of circulating atherogenic lipoproteins can retard the development of atherosclerosis. Furthermore, very conclusive evidence has been adduced in the rhesus monkey that profound reduction of levels of atherogenic lipoproteins, achieved by diet, can result in reversal of atherosclerotic lesions in which lipid-filled macrophages are the predominant element.[3] Because of possible species differences and because many human atherosclerotic lesions involve extracellular deposition of cholesterol and cholesteryl esters, tests of the "lipid hypothesis" in humans are of great importance. Several intervention studies have now yielded evidence that moderate lowering of blood levels of LDL is associated with retarded progression of coronary lesions.[4-7] Likewise, multifactor intervention has been shown to reduce the severity of lesions in the femoral arteries, as evidenced by a quantitative angiographic technique.[8,9] Whether reversal of human coronary arteriosclerosis is possible awaits the application of quantitative angiography in studies in which the powerful new combined drug regimens are employed.

A contemporary model of atherogenesis also must consider the retrieval processes by which cholesterol is removed from peripheral sites. This is collectively referred to as the *centripetal transport system*. In this light, hypertriglyceridemia assumes new importance with the demonstration of impaired acceptor properties for centripetally generated cholesteryl esters in certain patients with primary and secondary hypertriglyceridemia.[10] Future assessments of hypolipidemic regimens will have to take into account potential effects on this system. Likewise, certain subspecies of high density lipoproteins (HDL) that are now being identified and characterized also play critical roles in centripetal transport of cholesterol. The influence of treatment on these elements is therefore of additional importance in emerging strategies of intervention.

Severe hypertriglyceridemia is also an important cause of acute pancreatitis. Because the risk of pancreatitis appears to be related to levels of circulating triglyceride-rich lipoproteins, aggressive treatment of the hyperlipidemia by diet, abstinence from alcohol, and the application, if necessary, of drug treatment can be expected to effect material reduction in risk.

Before treatment with any drug is initiated in the management of hyperlipidemia, modification of diet should be attempted. Successful dietary control often makes the use of drugs unnecessary. The recommended diet, which restricts the patient's intake of saturated fat and cholesterol and controls calories and alcohol consumption in selected persons, is outlined elsewhere in these volumes. Although patients vary with respect to the degree of effect of cholesterol and saturated fat intake on levels of LDL, both tend to raise LDL. Excess caloric intake increases synthesis and secretion of VLDL, especially in obese persons. Alcohol tends to increase levels of HDL cholesterol, but it appears, from ultracentrifugal analysis at least, that the species of HDL affected are not those associated with the greatest inverse risk relationship with respect to coronary heart disease. Because it is a major determinant of secretion rates of VLDL triglycerides, alcohol should be avoided by patients with hypertriglyceridemia.

Formal guidelines have been developed by a panel of experts sponsored by the National Institutes of Health[11] for treatment of patients with elevated levels of LDL, based either on total cholesterol or on LDL-cholesterol level in serum. By using diet first and then diet plus drugs if necessary, the goal is to reduce total cholesterol to below 240 mg/dl (LDL cholesterol of 160 mg/dl) in the absence of coronary disease or in the absence of at least two defined risk factors. If coronary disease or two or more additional defined risk factors are present, the goal is a total serum cholesterol level at or below 200 mg/dl (LDL cholesterol level of 130 mg/dl or less).

If drug therapy is prescribed, the diet should be continued. It has been observed that, at least in the majority of patients, hyperlipidemia is better controlled, and sometimes at lower drug dosage, when the patient also follows the suggested diet.

Drugs used to treat hyperlipidemia should not be used in women who are pregnant or likely to become pregnant or during lactation. Familial hypercholesterolemia is the only primary hyperlipidemia for which drug treatment should be considered in children. Persons homozygous for this disease should be treated early and aggressively. Drug treatment of heterozygous children, however, remains experimental and should probably not be started before age 7 or 8, at which time myelination of the central nervous system is nearly complete. Such factors as the level of LDL in plasma, the child's special circumstances, and the family history should be considered before initiating drug treatment. The drug of choice is a bile acid binding resin.

AVAILABLE AGENTS
BILE ACID BINDING RESINS

MECHANISM OF ACTION. The two available resins, colestipol and cholestyramine, are high molecular weight polymers that bind the anionic bile acids in the intestinal lumen.[12] The resins are not absorbed from the intestine and hence carry the bile acids out into the stool. They are capable of binding some nonionic hydrophobic substances, but apparently do not interfere significantly with the absorption of fat-soluble vitamins in persons with a normal gastrointestinal tract. Binding of some cationic molecules, such as iron, probably involves bridging with a polyanion, such as the phosphate ion. Again, this is not of clinical significance in patients with a normal iron economy.

The bile acids, which are formed from cholesterol, are normally reabsorbed from the intestine with over 95% efficiency. The blockade of reabsorption results in up to tenfold increase in the rate of bile acid synthesis by liver from cholesterol via the 7α-hydroxylase reaction and subsequent steps. This draft on cholesterol pools results in increased expression of high-affinity LDL receptors on hepatocyte membranes, drawing on circulating LDL for cholesterol to meet the increased requirements of bile acid production. However, *de novo* synthesis of cholesterol in the liver also occurs. Suppression of this compensatory increase in sterol biosynthesis is an important site of action for agents that afford complementariness to the bile acid binding resins.

The bile acid sequestrants are of use only in those forms of hyperlipidemia involving elevations of LDL. Hypertriglyceridemia, if present in addition to elevated LDL levels, may be aggravated significantly by resin therapy. The addition of another agent, such as nicotinic acid, is indicated in such situations. Bile acid binding resins are contraindicated in treatment of primary hypertriglyceridemias without elevated LDL levels.

SIDE EFFECTS. Most patients complain of constipation and bloating, both of which are easy to control if adequate amounts of bran are eaten. Psyllium seed preparations, which may be mixed with the resin, are also useful. Occasionally, diarrhea or even steatorrhea occurs. The latter and rare cases of bowel obstruction have only been reported in patients who have cholestasis or preexisting bowel disease. Prothrombin time should be measured more frequently in patients who are also taking coumarin or indandione anticoagulants. There is a theoretical risk of increased formation of gallstones, particularly in obese patients, although this risk appears to be very small in practice. The resins may impair the absorption of other drugs. Some known to be affected are digitalis glycosides, thiazide diuretics, warfarin, thyroxine, iron salts, folic acid, phenylbutazone, and tetracyclines. Hence, it is recommended that any medication except nicotinic acid be given 1 hour before or at least 2 hours after the resin is given.

DOSAGE. Colestipol is available in 5-g packets or in bulk. Most patients tolerate the drug better if the dose is increased over several weeks from 5 g three times daily to the maximum dose of 10 g three times daily. Some of the milder forms of hypercholesterolemia respond well to a total dose of 15 g to 20 g daily. The granules are mixed with water or juice and should hydrate for at least 10 seconds. Colestipol is preferably taken with meals in three daily doses. To avoid irritation of the pharynx by residual granules, it is advisable to follow the medication with a small amount of soft food. Cholestyramine is available in 4-g packets, has a usual maximum dose of 24 g to 32 g/day, and should be taken in similar fashion.

USES. The resins are used to treat patients with heterozygous familial hypercholesterolemia, in whom a reduction in LDL of about 20% may be expected in compliant patients. In combination with nicotinic acid, however, levels of LDL are normalized in most of these patients. Greater reductions, often at lower dosages, are seen in persons with milder forms of hypercholesterolemia. They are also useful drugs in patients with familial combined hyperlipidemia (familial multiple lipoprotein-type hyperlipidemias). If hypertriglyceridemia is also present, the resins often cause further increases in VLDL that require the addition of a second agent, such as nicotinic acid or perhaps one of the fibric acid derivatives.

NICOTINIC ACID (NIACIN)

MECHANISM OF ACTION. Nicotinic acid, which decreases levels of both LDL and VLDL, is a water-soluble B vitamin. Although the amide of nicotinic acid (nicotinamide) functions normally in the role of vitamin cofactor, it completely lacks effect on lipid metabolism. Physicians should thus be alert to substitution of nicotinamide for nicotinic acid, a frequent error in dispensing the medication. Nicotinic acid probably acts primarily by inhibiting secretion of VLDL, thus decreasing production of LDL as well.[13] There is also increased clearance of VLDL via the lipoprotein lipase pathway, and cholesterogenesis is inhibited.[14] Excretion of neutral sterols in bile is increased, but that of bile acids is not.[15] Catabolism of HDL is decreased, and concentrations of HDL, chiefly HDL_2 and apolipoprotein A-I, the chief protein species of HDL, rise in plasma.[16] Levels of circulating fibrinogen are reduced, and levels of tissue plasminogen activator rise, perhaps influencing thrombogenesis or atherogenesis. Nicotinic acid may reduce VLDL production through its potent inhibitory effect on the intracellular lipase system of adipose tissue. The inhibition results in a decreased flux of free fatty acid precursors to liver, but it has not been established that this effect is sustained during long-term treatment.

SIDE EFFECTS. When nicotinic acid treatment is begun and when dosage is increased, almost all patients complain of a warm sensation, usually accompanied by a flush. This prostaglandin-mediated phenomenon, a harmless vasodilation, can be blunted if the patient takes 0.3 g of aspirin 20 to 30 minutes before the nicotinic acid. Itching and a transient rash are also common. Liver function should be assessed prior to starting the drug and at regular intervals thereafter, since nicotinic acid may cause mild-to-moderate elevations of transaminase levels. This effect is reversible and is minimized if the dose is increased slowly. It is probably due in most cases to microsomal enzyme induction rather than to hepatic parenchymal toxicity. Serious hepatic toxicity occurs rarely. However, if transaminase levels exceed three to four times normal, the drug should be discontinued or the dose reduced. Such patients require careful observation. More severe pruritus, prolonged rash, dry skin, and acanthosis nigricans have been observed. Nausea and abdominal discomfort are experienced by some patients. These symptoms are minimized by taking the medications with meals and by the use of antacids, if necessary. These symptoms are rarely encountered if nicotinic acid is taken at the same time as colestipol or cholestyramine because of the buffering properties of the resins. The drug should not be given to persons with severe peptic disease, however. Moderate impairment of carbohydrate tolerance has occurred, but is reversible except in some patients who appear to have latent diabetes. Hyperuricemia is a relatively common side effect, but is unlikely to become symptomatic unless the patient has preexisting gout. Arrhythmias have been encountered rarely. Another, very rare, toxic effect is macular edema, which is usually first manifested by blurring of vision. Again, if medication is stopped in timely fashion, this lesion is completely reversible.

DOSAGE. The starting dose should be 100 mg three times daily with meals. The patient should be told to expect the common side effects and warned not to take the drug on an empty stomach. The dose should be increased slowly by 100-mg increments as tolerated. The daily dose should not exceed 2.5 g by the end of the first month. The maximum dose should never exceed 7.5 g. Patients with heterozygous familial hypercholesterolemia or familial combined hyperlipidemia vary greatly in the dose of nicotinic acid required in combination with a resin to normalize their levels of LDL. The usual range, however, is 4 g to 6 g daily. Patients with other forms of hypercholesterolemia or with hypertriglyceridemia may require much lower doses (1.5 g–3.5 g daily).

USES. Nicotinic acid, in combination with a bile acid binding resin,[17] normalizes levels of LDL in most patients with heterozygous familial hypercholesterolemia and familial combined hyperlipidemia. Also, in combination with the resin, it is useful in the treatment of some patients with the hyperlipidemia of nephrosis. In patients with severe mixed lipemias who have incomplete response to diet therapy, and in those with familial dysbetalipoproteinemia, very small doses are often effective. Follow-up of the patients who had taken niacin in the Coronary Drug Project revealed a significant reduction in total mortality compared to patients who received other therapies or placebo.[18]

CLOFIBRATE

MECHANISM OF ACTION. Clofibrate is a fibric acid derivative that decreases plasma levels of VLDL. Although LDL levels are also decreased in some patients, they often tend to increase in hypertriglyceridemic patients who are receiving clofibrate. This drug appears to increase the activity of lipoprotein lipase, thus increasing the clearance of triglyceride-rich lipoproteins. The resulting flux of LDL precursor may explain the often observed increase of LDL levels in plasma as triglyceride levels decline. Fecal and biliary excretion of cholesterol[19] are enhanced and hepatic cholesterol biosynthesis is inhibited, resulting in decreased body pools of cholesterol. Concomitant with the decrease in VLDL levels, total HDL concentration often increases slightly while triglycerides in HDL are reduced.

SIDE EFFECTS. Patients taking this drug may complain of nausea and abdominal discomfort. Elevated levels of creatinine phosphokinase, which are more likely to occur in nephrotic patients or those with azotemia, may be associated with myalgia.[20] Involvement of the myocardium has been described. A twofold to fourfold increased incidence of cholelithiasis and a slightly increased risk of gastrointestinal tract cancer were reported in some clinical trials. In general, the effects of clofibrate on the progression of coronary artery disease appear equivocal.[21,22] Activity of coumarin and indanedione anticoagulants may be potentiated, and doses of these drugs should be reduced by 30% to 50% when treatment with clofibrate is initiated. Rashes, liver toxicity, bone marrow depression, brittle hair, alopecia, and decreased libido in men have been reported.

DOSAGE. The usual dose is 1 g twice daily. In patients with dysbetalipoproteinemia, however, as little as 0.5 g daily may suffice.

USES. Marked reduction of triglyceride-rich lipoproteins in patients with familial dysbetalipoproteinemia can often be achieved. In cases of moderately severe endogenous hypertriglyceridemia, moderate amelioration of lipemia is often achieved with clofibrate. It has no value in patients with primary chylomicronemia or in the treatment of familial hypercholesterolemia. In some patients with milder forms of hypercholesterolemia, it may effect moderate decreases in levels of LDL.

GEMFIBROZIL

MECHANISM OF ACTION. Gemfibrozil is a fibric acid derivative that closely resembles clofibrate in action and side effects. It decreases levels of VLDL in plasma. There is a decreased flux of free fatty acids to the liver since the drug decreases lipolysis in adipose tissue. LDL levels may be reduced, but only modestly, and levels of HDL cholesterol are moderately increased.[23] There is apparently a moderate increase in HDL protein.

SIDE EFFECTS. Like clofibrate, this drug may cause muscular, gastrointestinal, and cutaneous side effects. It has been implicated in the development of elevated levels of liver enzymes and decreases in white blood cell count and hematocrit in a few patients. Doses of coumarin and indanedione anticoagulants should be reduced and monitored closely when gemfibrozil is prescribed. The likelihood of myopathy with increased plasma levels of creatine kinase is increased if gemfibrozil is given with lovastatin. If this combination is used, the dosage of lovastatin must be limited to 20 mg to 40 mg per day and the patients creatine kinase level monitored closely.

DOSAGE. Although the usual dose is 600 mg twice daily, some patients have a good lipid-lowering effect with half this amount.

USES. Gemfibrozil is useful in the same conditions as is clofibrate and, in some patients, may be more effective in lowering levels of triglycerides. Men who took gemfibrozil in the Helsinki Heart Study had a 34% decrease in the incidence of coronary events compared to those taking placebo.[24]

OTHER FIBRIC ACID DERIVATIVES

Other, somewhat more potent, congeners are available in Europe. One is fenofibrate, given in doses of 100 mg three times a day. It is secreted virtually entirely as the anion by the kidneys. Another is bezafibrate, given in doses of 200 mg three times daily.

NEOMYCIN

Neomycin has been used for 20 years for treatment of hypercholesterolemia. Although very useful as a secondary therapeutic choice in certain instances, it has not yet been approved by the Food and Drug Administration for this indication.

MECHANISM OF ACTION. Levels of LDL in serum are reduced by this aminoglycoside antibiotic. Poorly absorbed itself, it inhibits absorption of cholesterol, increases excretion of bile acids, and decreases the total body pool of cholesterol.[25]

SIDE EFFECTS. Even low doses of neomycin may occasionally cause nausea, cramping, diarrhea, and malabsorption. Enterocolitis has occurred secondary to overgrowth of resistant bacteria. Patients with preexisting bowel disease may have enhanced absorption of the drug and a greater incidence of the well-known otic, nephric, hematopoietic, and hepatic toxicity. These effects are otherwise extremely rare when the daily dose is no greater than 2 g. Neomycin should be avoided in patients with kidney disease and is known to decrease absorption of digitalis glycosides. Because high-frequency hearing loss is the earliest manifestation of neomycin ototoxicity, patients with previous high-frequency loss should probably not be treated with this drug.

DOSAGE. The usual dose is 0.5 g to 2 g daily. It should be given with meals in two divided doses.

USES. Neomycin alone can achieve approximately a 20% reduction in cholesterol levels in patients with familial hypercholesterolemia when they are unable to tolerate other agents.[26,27] It is also likely to be beneficial in other disorders with elevated levels of LDL. Its complementarity with bile acid binding resins is variable and limited, probably because the principal modes of action of the drugs, interference with bile acid reabsorption, are redundant. However, complementarity with nicotinic acid appears to exist. Neomycin has no value in the treatment of isolated hypertriglyceridemia.

PROBUCOL

MECHANISM OF ACTION. Probucol treatment is associated with increased fractional clearance of LDL[28] and increased excretion of bile acids.[29] Some inhibition of cholesterol biosynthesis also occurs. Unlike the time course of most other agents, probucol causes LDL levels in plasma to decrease continuously for 4 months or more, achieving a reduction of 15% to 20% in most cases. Decreases of up to 27% have been described in patients with homozygous familial hypercholesterolemia, a more striking effect than that obtained with most agents. Impressive decreases in the diameters of tendon xanthomas have been observed in patients with homozygous and heterozygous familial hypercholesterolemia and in the corresponding animal model, the Watanabe heritable hyperlipidemic (WHHL) rabbit. This suggests that the most important action of probucol may be at the level of the uptake of LDL by the macrophage. Reports of amelioration of atheromatous disease in patients homozygous for familial hypercholesterolemia and in homozygous WHHL rabbits suggest that this effect extends to arterial plaques as well.[30,31] Potent inhibition of the endothelial cell-mediated oxidation of LDL resulting in decreased uptake of LDL by the scavenger pathway of macrophages is consistent with such an effect on both tendons and atherosclerotic plaques.[32] Thus, probucol may inhibit atherogenesis by a mechanism independent of its ability to lower LDL levels.

Levels of HDL in plasma are frequently decreased proportionately even more than those of LDL.[33] This effect includes levels of apolipoprotein A-I as well as the lipid constituents of HDL. Because low HDL-cholesterol levels are correlated epidemiologically with an increased risk of coronary heart disease, it remains to be determined whether decreases in plasma levels of HDL resulting from treatment with probucol are inimical. However, preliminary results suggest that centripetal transport of cholesterol may be enhanced by probucol. This hydrophobic drug partitions into adipose tissue from which it reenters plasma slowly after treatment is stopped. Thus, substantial plasma levels of the drug may be present for up to several months.

SIDE EFFECTS. Serious ventricular arrhythmias and prolonged QT intervals have been reported in animals receiving high doses of probucol. Increases in the QT interval of 20 msec to 25 msec are commonly observed in humans treated with probucol. This is apparently unassociated with increased frequency of premature ventricular contractions. It remains unknown whether more serious problems with cardiac rhythmicity might occur in the presence of acid–base or electrolyte disturbances or during myocardial ischemia in humans. Patients may experience diarrhea, nausea, and abdominal pain.

DOSAGE. The usual dose is 500 mg twice daily.

USES. The inhibition of foam cell formation with its attendant impact on atherogenesis provides an attractive potential rationale for the use of this agent. The available data suggest that it may be the most useful drug available for treatment of patients with homozygous familial hypercholesterolemia. However, further evidence of its safety and a better understanding of its effects on HDL will be required before broad application in the prevention of atherosclerosis is warranted.

DEXTROTHYROXINE

MECHANISM OF ACTION. Dextrothyroxine is a synthetic isomer of thyroxine that is alleged to have little of the calorigenic property of its naturally occurring isomer, levothyroxine, while retaining the effects of thyroid hormone on lipid metabolism. However, it appears that substantial calorigenic activity remains. Thyroxine appears to exert its primary influence on lipid metabolism by stimulating the conversion of cholesterol to bile acids[34] and by increasing the number of high-affinity LDL receptors on cell membranes.[35] Neutral sterol excretion in the stool is increased, and a modest decrease in circulating levels of LDL is observed.

SIDE EFFECTS. Because some of the calorigenic and related adrenergic effects of levothyroxine are retained, arrhythmias and increased angina are frequently encountered.

DOSAGE. The usual dose is 4 mg to 8 mg daily.

USES. Because other agents are more effective in lowering levels of LDL cholesterol, and because of the apparent risk of ventricular arrhythmia, there is no current indication for use of this drug.

HMG-CoA REDUCTASE INHIBITORS

MECHANISM OF ACTION. HMG-CoA reductase inhibitors are structural analogs of hydroxymethylglutaryl CoA, an obligatory intermediary in the biosynthesis of sterols and other isoprenoid substances.[12] These agents act by competitive inhibition of HMG-CoA reductase, leading to reduced production of mevalonic acid. The original compounds, compactin (released abroad) and its methylated derivative mevinolin (more recently given the generic name lovastatin), are soluble products formed by species of *Penicillium* and *Aspergillus*, respectively. A number of synthetic congeners are now being developed. These compounds apparently do not significantly suppress synthesis of nonsterol isoprenoids, such as ubiquinone and dolichol, because the enzymes in the initial reactions leading to these products have a high affinity for mevalonate.[36]

In humans, the primary effect of lovastatin is induction of increased numbers of LDL receptors, leading to increased fractional clearance of LDL[37] and a decrease of 20% to 50% in levels of LDL cholesterol in plasma. A decrease in the production rate of LDL may also result from an increased endocytotic flux of VLDL remnants into liver via the LDL receptor, resulting in diminished conversion of these precursor lipoproteins to LDL. Slight increases in total HDL cholesterol also occur.

SIDE EFFECTS. A number of minor side effects of lovastatin, such as minimal gastroenteric symptoms, rash, muscle cramps, and insomnia, have been described that do not frequently preclude use of the drug. Two potentially serious side effects have appeared in clinical experience: a myopathic syndrome and a chemical hepatitis. The lovastatin myopathy is characterized by painful, tender muscles, high levels of serum creatine kinase, and, in extreme cases, myolysis with myoglobinemia, myoglobinuria, and the risk of renal shutdown. Marked elevations of creatine kinase can occur in the absence of painful muscles. When lovastatin is used as a single agent, this complication occurs in less than 1% of patients and is completely reversible on cessation of the drug but tends to recur with resumption of treatment. It can appear with doses as small as 20 mg/day. Risk of the myopathy is increased by the concomitant administration of drugs that compete with lovastatin for catabolism. The most important of these is cyclosporin. Research in progress suggests that very small doses of lovastatin (10 mg or less a day) may be compatible with this drug. However, the combination of these agents must be monitored with extreme care. Other drugs that may increase the incidence of myopathy when given with lovastatin include the fibric acid derivatives gemfibrozil and clofibrate, erythromycin, and, to a lesser extent, niacin. In all cases, it is important to follow creatine kinase levels closely when these agents are used with lovastatin. In practice, modest elevations of creatine kinase activity, up to two times the upper limit of normal, may occur in some patients, particularly after strenuous exercise, without signaling a significant myopathy.

The hepatitis associated with lovastatin occurs in about 2% of patients and may accompany the myopathic syndrome. It is characterized by marked elevations in transaminase enzymes in serum, often with symptoms of malaise and nausea. It is reversible on cessation of lovastatin, but tends to recur if the drug is reinstituted. In practice, many patients on lovastatin have elevations of serum transaminase levels up to three times the upper limit of normal with no apparent deleterious effect in contrast to the marked elevations encountered in the chemical hepatitis described above. Current experience suggests that therapy may be continued with frequent monitoring of liver function in the patients with the lesser elevations of transaminase activity. In all patients, transaminase levels should be monitored at 4- to 6-week intervals during the first year of therapy and at about 3-month intervals thereafter. HMG-CoA reductase inhibitors should not be given to persons with overt hepatic dysfunction.

DOSAGE. Dosage ranges, according to the biological response, are between 20 and 80 mg/day. The drug may be given in one evening dose or twice daily. Diminished dosage and close monitoring are required if lovastatin is given with agents that may precipitate the myopathic syndrome.

USES. HMG-CoA reductase inhibitors are primarily used in disorders involving elevated levels of LDL in serum. There is no indication for their use in severe forms of hypertriglyceridemia, despite the fact the serum cholesterol levels may be elevated, because LDL levels tend to be low in these disorders. In patients with mild elevations of LDL, lovastatin in doses of 20 to 40 mg/day may reduce serum cholesterol levels from 20% to 40%. In patients with heterozygous familial hypercholesterolemia, similar decreases in levels of LDL cholesterol may be achieved with doses of 40 to 60 mg/day.[38,39] Usually there is a diminished incremental effect with increases to 80 mg/day. The effectiveness of lovastatin in severe primary hypercholesterolemia is greatly increased when it is combined with other agents (see later). Lovastatin is effective in treating familial dysbetalipoproteinemia in some persons. It is also effective in familial combined hyperlipoproteinemia, especially when combined with niacin and bile acid sequestrants.

DRUG COMBINATIONS

Treatment with two or more drugs in combination may be necessary in the following circumstances: (1) when a bile acid binding resin fails to normalize levels of LDL, (2) when both VLDL and LDL are elevated, and (3) when levels of VLDL increase significantly during treatment of hypercholesterolemia with a resin.

Those combinations that have been found to offer significant complementarity are nicotinic acid with resin, nicotinic acid with neomycin, and combinations of niacin, bile acid sequestrant, or neomycin with HMG-CoA reductase inhibitors. The neomycin with resin combination lowers serum cholesterol by only about 35%, but may afford some additional effect for patients with familial hypercholesterolemia who are taking bile acid binding resin, but are unable to tolerate nicotinic acid.

The combination of bile acid binding resin with nicotinic acid is the first combination of choice for treatment of heterozygous familial hypercholesterolemia,[17,40] reflecting the combined effects of the individual drugs. A significant increase in levels of HDL due to the nicotinic acid is also observed. This may prove to be of additional benefit if centripetal transport of cholesterol is shown to be enhanced. There are no additional toxic effects and, in fact, the acid-neutralizing property of the resin relieves the gastric irritation experienced by some patients who take nicotinic acid. The absorption of nicotinic acid is not impeded by the resin so the drugs may be taken together. To achieve normalization of LDL in heterozygous familial hypercholesterolemia, the full dose of resin with 4 g to 7.5 g of nicotinic acid is usually required. A few patients with this disorder do not normalize their LDL while taking nicotinic acid with resin.

The combination of a resin with an HMG-CoA reductase inhibitor may prove to be as effective as the resin with nicotinic acid regimen in lowering LDL levels, although the former does not appear to raise HDL-cholesterol levels substantially.[37,41]

The combination of nicotinic acid and neomycin offers an alternative treatment for patients with severe hypercholesterolemia who cannot take bile acid binding resins. It appears to be somewhat less effective than the nicotinic acid with resin combination, but is usually more effective than any agent used alone.

Maximum effectiveness in treatment of hypercholesterolemia is afforded by the ternary regimen consisting of lovastatin, colestipol, and niacin.[41] In patients with severe heterozygous familial hypercholesterolemia, total serum cholesterol levels were reduced from a mean of 433 mg/dl on diet alone to 183 mg/dl on the ternary regimen.

Drug combinations also may be of use in treating severe endogenous or mixed hypertriglyceridemia in which the combination of niacin and gemfibrozil appears to be more effective than either agent alone.

TREATMENT OF HOMOZYGOUS FAMILIAL HYPERCHOLESTEROLEMIA

Patients with homozygous familial hypercholesterolemia are rare, but the fulminant nature of the atherosclerosis demands the most aggressive treatment regimens. In the totally receptor-negative patient, bile acid binding resins have essentially no effect. Many patients have some residual receptor activity, however, affording the opportunity for a small effect of resins. The most effective means of lowering levels of LDL appears to be extracorporeal immunophoresis. When niacin, probucol, or neomycin are used in concert with this approach, reaccumulation of LDL is significantly delayed. Patients with severe hypercholesterolemia due to various genetic compound states are much more common than those with homozygous hypercholesterolemia. Often they have combinations of tuberous or planar cutaneous xanthomas with tendinous xanthomas. Because many of these patients tend to develop atherosclerotic lesions at a very rapid rate, they, too, should receive aggressive multiple drug therapy.

REFERENCES

1. Carlson LA, Bottinger LE, Ahfeldt PE: Risk factors for myocardial infarction in the Stockholm prospective study: A 14-year followup focusing on the role of plasma triglycerides and cholesterol. Acta Med Scand 206:351, 1979
2. Kannel WB, Castelli WP, Gordon T: Cholesterol in the prediction of atherosclerotic disease: New perspectives based on the Framingham Study. Ann Intern Med 90:85, 1979
3. Armstrong ML, Warner ED, Connor WE: Regression of coronary atheromatosis in rhesus monkeys. Circ Res 27:59, 1970
4. The Lipid Research Clinics Coronary Primary Prevention Trial Results. JAMA 251:351, 365, 1984
5. Brensike JF, Levy RI, Kelsey SF et al: Effects of therapy with cholestyramine on progression of coronary arteriosclerosis: Results of the NHLBI type II coronary intervention study. Circulation 69:313, 1984
6. Blankenhorn DH, Nessim SA, Johnson RL et al: Beneficial effects of combined colestipol–niacin therapy on coronary atherosclerosis and coronary venous bypass grafts. JAMA 257:3233, 1987
7. Frick MH, Elo O, Haapa K et al: Helsinki Heart Study: Primary prevention trial with gemfibrozil in middle-aged men with dyslipidemia. N Engl J Med 317:1237, 1987
8. Barndt R, Blankenhorn DH, Crawford DW, Brooks SH: Regression and progression of early atherosclerosis in treated hyperlipoproteinemic patients. Ann Intern Med 86:139, 1977
9. Blankenhorn DH: Reversibility of latent atherosclerosis: Studies by femoral angiography in humans. Mod Concepts Cardiovasc Dis 47:79, 1978
10. Fielding PE, Fielding CJ, Havel RJ et al: Cholesterol net transport, esterification and transfer in human hyperlipidemic plasma. J Clin Invest 71:449, 1983
11. Report of the National Cholesterol Education Program Expert Panel on Detection, Evaluation and Treatment of High Blood Cholesterol in Adults. Arch Intern Med 146:36–69
12. Kane JP, Havel RJ: Treatment of hypercholesterolemia. Annu Rev Med 37:427, 1986
13. Grundy SM, Mok HYI, Zech L, Berman M: Influence of nicotinic acid on metabolism of triglycerides and cholesterol in man. J Lipid Res 22:24, 1981
14. Miettinen TA: Effect of nicotinic acid on catabolism and synthesis of cholesterol in man. Clin Chim Acta 20:43, 1968
15. Einarsson K, Hellstrom K, Leijd B: Bile acid kinetics and steroid balance during nicotinic acid therapy in patients with hyperlipoproteinemia types II and IV. J Lab Clin Med 90:618, 1977
16. Shepherd J, Packard CJ, Patsch JR et al: Effects of nicotinic acid therapy on plasma high density lipoprotein subfraction distribution and composition and on apolipoprotein A metabolism. J Clin Invest 63:858, 1979
17. Kane JP, Malloy MJ, Tun P et al: Normalization of low density lipoprotein levels in heterozygous familial hypercholesterolemia with a combined drug regimen. N Engl J Med 304:251, 1981
18. Canner PL, Berge KG, Wenger NK et al: Fifteen-year mortality in Coronary Drug Project patients: Long term benefit with niacin. J Am Coll Cardiol 8:1245, 1986
19. Grundy SM, Ahrens EH Jr, Salen G et al: Mechanisms of action of clofibrate on cholesterol metabolism in patients with hypertriglyceridemia. J Lipid Res 13:531, 1972

20. Langer T, Levy RI: Acute muscular syndrome associated with administration of clofibrate. N Engl J Med 279:856, 1968
21. The Coronary Drug Project Research Group: Clofibrate and niacin in coronary heart disease. JAMA 231:360, 1975
22. World Health Organization: Cooperative trial on primary prevention of ischemic heart disease using clofibrate to lower serum cholesterol. Lancet 2:379, 1980
23. Lewis JE: Long term use of gemfibrozil (Lopid) in the treatment of dyslipidemia. Angiology 33:603, 1982
24. Frick MH, Elo O, Haapa K et al: Helsinki Heart Study: Primary prevention trial with gemfibrozil in middle-aged men with dyslipidemia. N Engl J Med 317:1237, 1987
25. Thompson GR, Barrowman J, Gutierrez L: Action of neomycin on the intraluminal phase of lipid absorption. J Clin Invest 50:319, 1971
26. Miettinen TA: Effects of neomycin alone and in combination with cholestyramine on serum cholesterol and fecal steroids in hypercholesterolemic subjects. J Clin Invest 64:1485, 1979
27. Samuel P: Treatment of hypercholesterolemia with neomycin—a time for reappraisal. N Engl J Med 301:595, 1979
28. Kesaniemi YA, Grundy SM: Influence of probucol on cholesterol metabolism in man. J Lipid Res 25:780, 1984
29. Nestel PJ, Billington T: Effects of probucol on low density lipoprotein removal and high density lipoprotein synthesis. Atherosclerosis 38:203, 1981
30. Kita T, Nagano Y, Yokode M et al: Probucol prevents the progression of atherosclerosis in Watanabe heritable hyperlipidemic rabbit: An animal model for familial hypercholesterolemia. Proc Natl Acad Sci USA 84:5928, 1987
31. Yamamoto A, Matsuzawa Y, Yokoyama S et al: Effects of probucol on xanthomata regression in familial hypercholesterolemia. Am J Cardiol 57:29H, 1986
32. Parthasarathy S, Young SG, Witztum JL et al: Probucol inhibits oxidative modification of low density lipoprotein. J Clin Invest 77:641, 1986
33. Mellies MJ, Gartside PS, Glatfelter L et al: Effects of probucol on plasma cholesterol high and low density lipoprotein cholesterol and apolipoproteins A-I and A-II in adults with primary hypercholesterolemia. Metabolism 29:956, 1980
34. Myant NG: The thyroid and lipid metabolism. In Paoletti R (ed): Lipid Pharmacology, pp 229–323. New York, Academic Press, 1964
35. Chait A, Bierman EL, Albers JJ: Regulatory role of triiodothyroxine in the degradation of low density lipoproteins by cultured human skin fibroblasts. J Clin Endocrinol Metab 49:877, 1979
36. Brown MS, Goldstein JL: Multivalent feedback regulation of HMG CoA reductase, a control mechanism coordinating isoprenoid synthesis and cell growth. J Lipid Res 21:505, 1980
37. Bilheimer DW, Grundy SM, Brown MS et al: Mevinolin and colestipol stimulate receptor mediated clearance of low density lipoprotein from plasma in familial hypercholesterolemia heterozygotes. Proc Natl Acad Sci USA 80:4124, 1983
38. Illingworth DR, Sexton GJ: Hypocholesterolemic effects of Mevinolin in patients with heterozygous familial hypercholesterolemia. J Clin Invest 74:1972, 1984
39. Havel RJ, Hunninghake DB, Illingworth DR et al: Lovastatin (Mevinolin) in the treatment of heterozygous familial hypercholesterolemia: A multicenter study. Ann Intern Med 107:609–615, 1987
40. Illingworth DR, Phillipson BE, Rapp JH et al: Colestipol plus nicotinic acid in treatment of heterozygous familial hypercholesterolemia. Lancet 1:296, 1981
41. Malloy MJ, Kane JP, Kunitake ST, Tun P: Complementarity of colestipol, niacin, and lovastatin in treatment of severe familial hypercholesterolemia. Ann Intern Med 107:616–623, 1987

Antithrombotic Therapy in Cardiac Disease

John H. Ip • Valentin Fuster
William P. Fay • James H. Chesebro

Thrombosis within the circulatory system has been recognized as the principal mechanism responsible for cardiovascular morbidity and mortality.[1,2] The pathogenic process leading to thrombosis in various disease states such as in the coronary arteries, cardiac chambers, and prosthetic heart valves appear to be different.[3–5] Thrombosis in the coronary arteries depends on the activation of both the platelets and the clotting system. On the other hand, thrombus formation in dilated cardiac chambers depends mainly on the clotting system and platelets may play a minor role, whereas dilated cardiac chambers depend on the activation, primarily, of the coagulation system and, secondarily, of the platelets. Thus, understanding of these pathogenic mechanisms is essential in the formulation of therapeutic and preventive strategies in these disease entities.

In this chapter we address the role of platelet activation and fibrin formation in thrombogenesis; the pharmacology of the antithrombotic agents; the pathogenesis and the risk of thrombosis and embolism in coronary arteries, cardiac chambers, and prosthetic valves; and the role of antithrombotic therapy in cardiac disease.

ROLE OF PLATELET ACTIVATION AND FIBRIN FORMATION IN THROMBOGENESIS

Platelets are fragments of membrane-enclosed megakaryocytic cytoplasm that travel in the periphery of the circulating mass and do not adhere to intact endothelium. When endothelial injury is superficial, only a monolayer of platelets adheres to the exposed subendothelium. When endothelial damage is more severe, exposure of collagen and other elements of the vessel wall stimulates the activation of platelets and coagulation system leading to thrombus formation. In this section, we will examine the processes of platelet adhesion, platelet aggregation and activation of the clotting system, as well as endogenous inhibitors of thrombosis.

PLATELET ADHESION: ROLE OF COLLAGEN FIBERS AND VON WILLEBRAND FACTOR

Platelets do not attach to the intact endothelium but firmly adhere to a disrupted or damaged endothelial surface.[6] After removal of the endothelial lining of a normal blood vessel by a mild or superficial injury, the subendothelium becomes coated by a layer of adherent platelets.[6] Platelet receptors are essential in the process of adhesion and aggregation (Fig. 20.1). Glycoprotein Ib in the platelet membrane appears to be important for normal initial contact of platelets with von Willebrand factor in the subendothelial surface. Glycoprotein Ia, which binds directly to exposed subendothelial collagen, may also be important. Glycoprotein IIb/IIIa in the platelet membrane is the receptor for a variety of circulating proteins, including von Willebrand factor and fibronectin and, aside from being important in platelet aggregation (see later), also favors platelet adhesion.[6] In the clinical context, subtle injury of the endothelial cell layer, for example that produced by flowing blood at arterial branch points or through stenoses, may trigger platelet adhesion. The release of platelet and endothelial cell growth factors may contribute to the early process of atherogenesis. On the other hand, in the acute coronary syndromes, severe vascular injury (plaque rupture) exposes components of the arterial media, particularly fibrillar collagen (with type I being more prevalent in diseased vessels and type III in normal vessels), which in addition to other mediators discussed later, induce platelet adhesion, aggregation, and thrombus formation.[6–8]

Platelet adhesion is determined not only by the degree of vascular injury as described previously but also by transport of the platelets to the injured area. This transport is determined by the wall shear rate, which is a measure of the difference in blood velocity between the center of the vessel and along the wall. At higher wall shear rates, characteristic of medium-sized stenotic arteries, initial platelet deposition rate and maximum extent of deposition are significantly higher.[9,10]

On artificial surfaces, the process of platelet adhesion is less understood. A film of adsorbed plasma proteins forms immediately after exposure of the surface to blood, and apparently different surfaces become coated with different proteins, which, by means of their surface charge, react differently with platelets.[11] Among the adsorbed plasma proteins that have been studied are fibrinogen, which tends to increase platelet adherence, and albumin, which tends to have the opposite effect.

PLATELET AGGREGATION AND RELEASE: ROLE OF COLLAGEN, THROMBIN, THROMBOXANE A_2, ADENOSINE DIPHOSPHATE, AND SEROTONIN

In this second stage, platelets adhere to each other and the platelet mass builds. This platelet aggregation seems to depend primarily on an increase in cytoplasmic calcium, which appears to be mediated by three pathways. First, concomitant with the process of platelet adhesion there is an activation of platelets by extrinsic stimuli, specifically collagen and thrombin; second, during such platelet activation there is the release of platelet intracytoplasmic granule constituents, particularly adenosine diphosphate (ADP), which further activate neighboring platelets, causing aggregation; and third, also during such platelet activation there is synthesis and release of the platelet prostanoid thromboxane A_2 (TXA_2), which also activates neighboring platelets, causing aggregation.

In certain pathologic situations, such as when an atherosclerotic plaque ruptures, there are extrinsic factors that may be very potent in triggering calcium release and platelet aggregation, specifically exposed collagen from the vessel wall and thrombin generated from the activation of the intrinsic and extrinsic clotting systems (Figs. 20.1 and 20.2). Through the actions of these extrinsic activators, calcium is then released from the dense tubular system into the cytoplasm, which in turn is associated with the activation of the actin–myosin system. These reactions in the adherent platelets and in the circulating neighboring platelets cause platelet contraction and the release of ADP and serotonin (see second pathway); also, TXA_2 synthesis then takes place followed by its release (see third pathway).[6,12] In addition, collagen and thrombin may also have a direct effect on platelets, possibly through a platelet-activating factor (PAF; see Fig. 20.2) which may expose the platelet membrane receptor IIb-IIIa to fibrinogen and von Willebrand factor, thus promoting aggregation.[6,12-15] For the purpose of this discussion, these reactions, which are dependent on collagen and thrombin, constitute the first pathway of platelet activation and aggregation.

After the adherent platelets and circulating neighboring platelets have been exposed to collagen and thrombin, the second pathway may be activated. This pathway is mediated by ADP and serotonin, which are released from the platelet-dense granules after contraction (see Figs. 20.1 and 20.2). ADP is a potent inducer of platelet aggregation in the presence of calcium and fibrinogen. It stimulates neighboring platelets and, most importantly, exposes their binding sites IIb-IIIa to fibrinogen and von Willebrand factor,[6,12-15] thus promoting aggregation. Furthermore, the turbulence present in stenotic areas and at branching points within the arterial tree promotes red blood cell lysis, with the subsequent release of ADP, which in turn activates platelets and promotes their aggregation.

Again, after the adherent platelet and neighboring platelets have been exposed to collagen and thrombin, a third pathway of TXA_2 synthesis may be activated (see Figs. 20.1 and 20.2). This pathway is mediated by arachidonic acid, which is released from the platelet membrane by the action of phospholipase A_2 on phosphatidylcholine.[16] Cyclo-oxygenase converts arachidonic acid into the proaggregating prostaglandin endoperoxide intermediates (prostaglandins G_2 and H_2); TXA_2 is formed by the action of thromboxane synthetase, particularly on prostaglandin H_2. TXA_2 is both a potent platelet aggregating substance and a vasoconstrictor. It stimulates platelet aggregation by promoting the mobilization of intracellular calcium and, most importantly, causes a conformational change in the glycoprotein IIb/IIIa complex, which results in the exposure of previously occult fibrinogen and von Willebrand factor binding sites, thus promoting aggregation.[6,12-15]

In summary, collagen that becomes exposed after vessel injury, thrombin generated by activation of the coagulation system, and products of platelet secretion such as ADP and TXA_2 can enhance the thrombotic process by stimulating adjacent platelets and also facilitating the exposure of their membrane receptors to fibrinogen and von Willebrand factor. These reactions, in turn, promote further platelet aggregation and thrombus growth.

ACTIVATION OF THE CLOTTING MECHANISM: ROLE OF THROMBIN AND FIBRIN FORMATION

In addition to adhering to the injured vessel wall, activated platelets markedly accelerate the generation of thrombin.[16] Perhaps by rear-

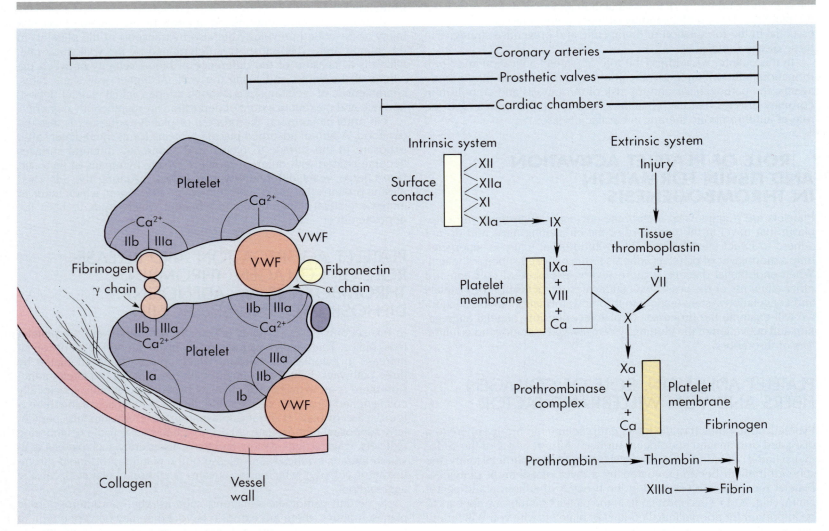

FIGURE 20.1 Left. Schematic representation of the interactions among platelet membrane receptors (glycoproteins Ia, Ib, and IIb/IIIa), adhesive macromolecules, and the disrupted vessel wall. Numbers indicate the different pathways of platelet activation, dependent on (1) collagen, (2) thrombin, (3) adenosine diphosphate (*ADP*) and serotonin, and (4) thromboxane A_2 (*TXA₂*).

Right. The intrinsic and extrinsic systems of the coagulation cascade. Note the interaction between clotting factors and the platelet membrane. (*Ca*, calcium; *VWF*, von Willebrand factor) (Modified from Fuster V, Stein B, Badimon L, Chesebro JH: Antithrombotic therapy after myocardial reperfusion in acute myocardial infarction. J Am Coll Cardiol 12(Suppl A): 78A-8XA, 1988)

ranging their surface lipoproteins during contraction, activated platelets promote the interaction of clotting factors.[16] It is on the platelet surface that the interactions between factors IX and VIII and factors X and V occur.[16]

Classic and didactic schematization requires a division to be made between the intrinsic and extrinsic pathways of activation (see Fig. 20.1).[17] In the intrinsic pathways, all necessary factors are present in the circulating blood itself and the initial reaction is set off by contact of the blood with a negatively charged surface (e.g., subendothelial collagen) or with a foreign surface (e.g., the glass wall of a test tube). In the extrinsic activation pathway it is not a plasma component but tissue fluid that initiates the blood coagulation process; following vessel damage, this tissue factor, called tissue thromboplastin, mixes with the blood and starts the coagulation process. After activation of factor X, the two pathways merge into one. In addition, both appear to be equally necessary to ensure normal hemostasis. More specifically, and as outlined in Figure 20.2, in the intrinsic system, coagulation is initiated by the adsorption of factor XII onto a foreign surface or collagen. Both kallikrein and high-molecular-weight kininogen are required for the rapid surface activation of factor XII. In addition, high-molecular-weight kininogen increases the reactivity of factor XIIa in the conversion of factor XI to XIa. Factor XIa converts factor IX to the activated protease factor IXa, whereupon factors VIII and IXa form a complex, activating factor X. Both platelet phospholipid, made available by aggregated platelets, and calcium are essential for maximal activation of factor X. In the presence of factor V, calcium, and platelet phospholipid, factor Xa subsequently converts prothrombin (factor II) to thrombin. As mentioned, the extrinsic system is triggered by the release of the tissue thromboplastin, a protein–phospholipid mixture that activates factor VII or VIIa. Together they serve as cofactors for the

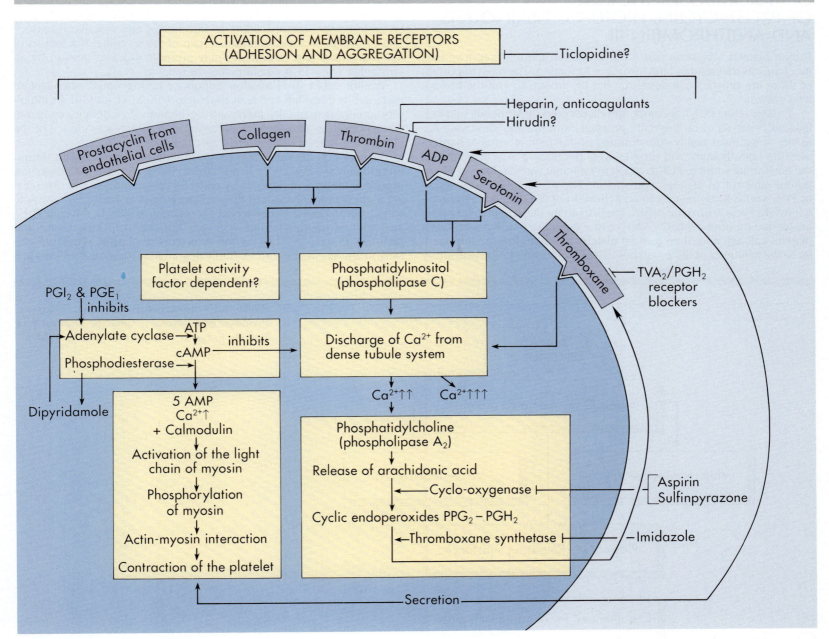

FIGURE 20.2 Mechanisms of platelet activation and presumed sites of action of various platelet inhibitor agents. Platelet agonists lead to the mobilization of calcium (Ca^{++}), which functions as a mediator of platelet activation through metabolic pathways dependent on adenosine diphosphate (ADP), thromboxane A_2 (TXA_2), thrombin, and collagen. Cyclic adenosine monophosphate (cAMP) inhibits calcium mobilization from the dense tubular system. Note that thrombin and collagen may independently activate platelets by means of platelet activating factor. Asterisk indicates a platelet inhibitor. Dashed line indicates a presumed site of drug action. (ATP, adenosine triphosphate; EPA, eicosapentaenoic acid; PGE_1, prostaglandin E_1; PGH_2, prostaglandin H_2; PGI_2, prostaglandin I_2) (Modified from Fuster V, Stein B, Badimon L, Chesebro JH: Antithrombotic therapy after myocardial reperfusion in acute myocardial infarction. J Am Coll Cardiol 12(Suppl A): 78A-8XA, 1988)

activation of both factor IX and factor X. Once factor Xa is formed, thrombin production proceeds as described previously. Thrombin cleaves fibrinogen to fibrin, activates factor XIII, which stabilizes fibrin, and also, as previously mentioned, induces platelet aggregation.

It should be emphasized that platelet aggregation and the subsequent generation of thrombin may be activated by circulating catecholamines. This may be of major importance because it may be a link between conditions of stress and the development of arterial thrombosis. Of no less importance is the increasing evidence of an enhanced thrombogenicity in cigarette smokers and in patients with a strong family history of coronary disease,[1,18] as well as in patients with hyperlipidemia and in patients with diabetes mellitus.[1]

ENDOGENOUS INHIBITORS OF THROMBOSIS: THE ROLE OF PROSTACYCLIN, PROTEIN C FIBRINOLYSIS, AND ANTITHROMBIN III

During platelet activation and fibrin formation there are endogenous mechanisms that tend to limit thrombus formation. The most important of these are prostacyclin, antithrombin III, protein C, and the fibrinolytic system.

Prostacyclin (PGI_2), a compound discovered by Moncada and colleagues,[19] seems to be the main prostaglandin metabolite in vascular tissue, being most highly concentrated on the intimal surface, particularly the endothelium, and progressively decreasing in activity toward the adventitial surface. PGI_2 is a potent systemic vasodilator and also a potent inhibitor of platelet aggregation. The platelet-inhibitory action of PGI_2 seems to be related to an activation of the platelet membrane adenylate cyclase enzyme, which leads to an increase in platelet cyclic adenosine monophosphate (AMP) and a decrease in the activation of platelet calcium and, therefore, of platelet function. Presumably, similar to the synthesis of the prostanoid TXA_2 by the platelet, as previously discussed, the vessel wall synthesizes PGI_2 from its own precursors (Fig. 20.3). That is, arachidonic acid is converted into cyclic endoperoxides by means of the cyclo-oxygenase enzyme, and such endoperoxides are subsequently converted into PGI_2 synthetase enzyme. It has been claimed that PGI_2 can be produced by the cells of the vessel wall in response to stimulation by endothelial injury or thrombin; most importantly, the platelets adhering to sites of vascular damage not only release TXA_2, which promotes the aggregation of platelets, but also concomitantly release endoperoxides, which potentiate PGI_2 synthesis by the arterial wall. Thus, the process of platelet aggregation and thrombosis may tend to be limited or prevented. In this context, Greenland Eskimos, who have a bleeding tendency but in whom thrombosis or atherosclerosis does not develop, seem to have little platelet TXA_2 (or rather a biologically low active TXA_3) and a substantial amount of a prostacyclin-type substance (prostaglandin I_3), all of these factors presumably related to diet.[20,21] Indeed, it has been suggested that an imbalance between platelet proaggregating and disaggregating activity of both prostaglandin systems (TXA_2 and PGI_2) may be an important factor leading to thrombosis and vascular disease.[16] Thus, it has been suggested that certain of the so-called risk factors of atherosclerosis and thrombosis may promote vascular disease by altering this TXA_2–PGI_2 equilibrium system.[1]

Antithrombin III is another important endogenous anticoagulant that inhibits thrombin and activated factors IX, X, XI, and XII. Its inhibitory action is markedly increased by heparin.[22] A deficiency in antithrombin III is associated with thrombosis, which is evidence of the clinical relevance of this control mechanism.[23]

Protein C is activated by the association of thrombin with thrombomodulin (see Fig. 20.3). In addition to being a potent anticoagulant, protein C initiates fibrinolysis by activating plasminogen and neutralizing a circulating inhibitor of tissue plasminogen activator.[24] Once activated, plasminogen is converted to plasmin, which hydrolyzes fibrin into soluble fragments and degrades fibrinogen, prothrombin, and factors VIII and V.[25] The proteolytic activity of plasmin remains localized to the fibrin surface; as fibrin degradation proceeds to comple-

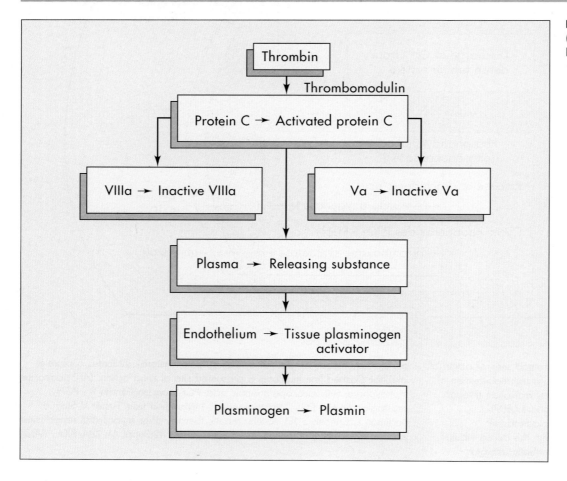

FIGURE 20.3 Activation of protein C and fibrinolysis. (Modified from Wessler S, Gitel SN: Warfarin from bedside to bench. N Engl J Med 311:645, 1984)

tion, plasmin is rapidly inactivated by α_2 plasmin inhibitor. A specific plasminogen activator inhibitor has been identified in human platelets[26] and in the extracellular matrix of cultured endothelial cells.[27] Recent findings underscore the importance of the fibrinolytic system in maintaining normal hemostasis and suggest that the balance between plasminogen activators and inhibitors may be important in both arterial and venous thrombotic disorders. Indeed, patients who are congenitally deficient in protein C and persons who have low fibrinolytic response are prone to recurrent thrombosis.[28,29]

PHARMACOLOGY OF THE ANTITHROMBOTIC AGENTS

In this section we present a review of the pharmacology of platelet inhibitors, heparin, oral anticoagulants, and thrombolytic agents.

PLATELET INHIBITORS

Assessment of the pharmacologic actions that inhibit platelet function can be considered in three broad categories: drugs that inhibit the platelet arachidonate pathway; drugs that increase platelet cyclic AMP levels; and drugs that specifically block thrombin-mediated platelet activation.

INHIBITORS OF ARACHIDONIC ACID PATHWAY
INHIBITORS OF PLATELET CYCLO-OXYGENASE–ASPIRIN.
MECHANISM OF ACTION. The cyclo-oxygenase enzyme, which is important in the conversion of arachidonic acid into the cyclic endoperoxides prostaglandin G_2 and prostaglandin H_2, can be blocked by numerous nonsteroidal anti-inflammatory drugs such as aspirin, indomethacin, ibuprofen, and naproxen. Acetylsalicylic acid, or aspirin (Fig. 20.4), inhibits cyclo-oxygenase in platelets by acetylating it, which inhibits the formation of TXA_2. Aspirin only partially inhibits platelet aggregation induced by ADP, collagen, or thrombin (at low concentrations). The adherence of the initial layer of platelets to the subendothelium and the release of granule contents are not inhibited by aspirin.[30] Consequently, the effects of platelet-derived growth factor and other mitogens on smooth muscle cell proliferation may still occur in the presence of cyclo-oxygenase inhibitors.[31] In contrast, these drugs inhibit platelet aggregate formation of the layer of adherent platelets, presumably by blocking TXA_2 synthesis.

The acetylation of cyclo-oxygenase on platelets exposed to aspirin is permanent,[32] and thus the effects of the drug persist for the life of the platelets. The long-term administration of 1 mg/kg/day of aspirin effectively inhibits platelet cyclo-oxygenase and TXA_2 formation. In contrast, aspirin inhibition of vascular endothelial cyclo-oxygenase is not reversible because these cells are capable of synthesizing new enzyme, although they may require several hours to do so. Although earlier studies suggested that platelet cyclo-oxygenase was more sensitive to the inhibitory effects of low-dose aspirin than was vascular wall cyclo-oxygenase, more recent experimental data[33] challenge this concept.

IDEAL DOSE. Beneficial effects of aspirin on cyclo-oxygenase–dependent platelet aggregation may be approximately equivalent over a dose range of at least 100 to 1500 mg daily. Numerous clinical studies have demonstrated the protective effects of aspirin in this dose range in patients with unstable angina and acute myocardial infarction, as well as in primary and secondary prevention of cardiovascular disease.[34-38] For example, two recent randomized clinical trials[34,35] using aspirin in doses of 324 and 1300 mg daily in patients with unstable angina showed similar reduction in mortality and nonfatal myocardial infarction. Similarly, in a recent overview of 25 clinical trials[38] using antiplatelet agents in the secondary prevention of cardiac disease, it was shown that aspirin used in doses ranging from 100 to 1500 mg per day reduced vascular mortality by 13%, nonfatal myocardial infarction by 31%, nonfatal stroke by 42%, and all important vascular events by 25%. There was no evidence that doses of 900 to 1500 mg of aspirin daily were any more effective in avoiding cardiovascular events than a lower dose of 300 mg, or one standard aspirin tablet, per day. This observation is pharmacologically plausible because doses lower than 300 mg/day would have been sufficient to produce virtually complete inhibition of cyclo-oxygenase–dependent platelet aggregation. However, direct evidence of the effects of aspirin in doses lower or less frequent than 300 mg/day is not available from these trials of secondary prevention. At present, the best studied, most inexpensive, and least toxic dose range is of 160 to 325 mg/day.

SIDE EFFECTS. Aspirin side effects are mainly gastrointestinal and dose related.[39] Aspirin rarely causes significant generalized bleeding unless it is combined with anticoagulant therapy. There is evidence that aspirin affects the gastric mucosa by inhibiting synthesis of prostaglandins.[40] The effect of aspirin on gastric mucosa is reduced by treatment with cimetidine or antacid and by the use of enteric-coated aspirin.[41] Most of the side effects of aspirin are dose related. The recently completed UK-TIA trial tested two daily dosages of aspirin versus placebo among 2,345 patients with a history of transient ischemic attacks or mild ischemic stroke.[42] It was, therefore, possible to compare directly the frequencies of side effects reported at 300 mg/day and at 1200 mg/day. For each category of symptom, including indigestion, nausea or heartburn, constipation, any gastrointestinal hemorrhage, and serious gastrointestinal hemorrhage, the percentage of participants reporting it was lowest in the placebo group, somewhat higher in the group receiving 300 mg/day, and highest of all among those receiving 1200 mg/day. Moreover, for symptoms of gastrointestinal distress as well as for any gastrointestinal hemorrhage, the differences between the low- and high-dose group were statistically significant. Since there is no evidence that the higher doses are any more effective than the lower doses, an aspirin dose of 160 to 325 mg/day for the prevention of thromboembolic disease is currently recommended.

OTHER INHIBITORS OF PLATELET CYCLO-OXYGENASE. Although nonsteroidal anti-inflammatory drugs reversibly inhibit cyclo-oxygenase, the antithrombotic activity of these compounds has not been properly tested in large randomized trials and therefore their use cannot be recommended.[43] Furthermore, one of the nonsteroidal anti-inflammatory agents, indomethacin, has been found to increase coronary vascular resistance and exacerbate ischemic attacks in patients with coronary disease.[44]

DRUGS THAT ALTER PLATELET MEMBRANE PHOSPHOLIPIDS (OMEGA-3-FATTY ACIDS). Both eicosapentaenoic acid and docosahexaenoic acid are present in high concentration in most saltwater fish and may account for the lower incidence of coronary heart disease in Greenland Eskimos and populations who consume large amounts of fish.[45,46] Eicosapentaenoic acid competes with arachidonic acid for platelet cyclo-oxygenase. This leads to the formation of two endoperoxidases (prostaglandins G_3 and H_3) and TXA_3, which have minimal biologic activity.[47] Furthermore, eicosapentaenoic acid not only does not inhibit endothelial cell prostacyclin production but also stimulates the formation of prostaglandin I_3, which has antiplatelet activity. The net result is a shift in the hemostatic balance toward an antiaggregative and vasodilative state. Docosahexaenoic acid also has platelet inhibitory effects and undergoes retroconversion to eicosapentaenoic acid.[48] Although fish consumption may decrease the incidence of coronary artery disease, fish oils are associated with some potentially adverse events, such as increased bleeding diathesis and reduced inflammatory and immune responses.[48] Before fish oils are recommended for the prevention of atherosclerosis, more properly designed and controlled human trials are necessary.[47] The role of fish oils in the prevention of restenosis after coronary angioplasty is reviewed later in this chapter.

INHIBITORS OF THROMBOXANE SYNTHETASE. Imidazole analogue thromboxane synthetase inhibitors have been developed with the expectation of not only suppressing TXA_2 biosynthesis but also sparing or even enhancing the formation of prostacyclin by the vascular endothelium.[49] The rationale behind this hypothesis was that, in the presence of a thromboxane synthetase inhibitor, platelet-derived prostaglandin G_2 would be transferred to the endothelial cells and used in the production of prostacyclin. Although thromboxane synthetase inhibitors have shown some benefits in experimental models,[50] their effects in clinical trials[51,52] in patients with coronary artery disease have been controversial. This may be a result of two factors: (1) TXA_2 may not be completely suppressed by the available compounds, and (2) the prostaglandin endoperoxide intermediates that result from thromboxane synthetase inhibition have themselves significant proaggregating effects.

BLOCKERS OF THROMBOXANE AND PROSTAGLANDIN ENDOPEROXIDE RECEPTORS. A promising approach to the inhibition of the proaggregating and vasoconstrictive effects of TXA_2 is the pharmacologic blockade of the receptors for both TXA_2 and the prostaglandin endoperoxidases.[53] However, it remains to be demonstrated that such agents will offer an advantage over aspirin in suppressing TXA_2-dependent platelet function. The combination of a thromboxane synthetase inhibitor (which potentiates prostacyclin synthesis) and a TXA_2–prostaglandin H_2 receptor blocker (which prevents the proaggregative effects of these compounds) may offer a unique approach to platelet inhibition[54] but requires further testing.

DRUGS THAT INCREASE PLATELET CYCLIC AMP LEVELS

DIPYRIDAMOLE. MECHANISM OF ACTION. Dipyridamole (see Fig. 20.4) increases platelet cyclic AMP by three mechanisms: (1) it blocks its breakdown by inhibiting phosphodiesterase; (2) it activates adenylate cyclase by a prostacyclin-mediated effect on the platelet membrane[55]; and (3) it increases the levels of plasma adenosine by inhibiting its uptake by vascular endothelium and red blood cells.[56,57] Adenosine, in turn, enhances platelet adenylate cyclase activity. In addition, the vasodilative effects of dipyridamole also appear to be related to the elevation in plasma adenosine levels. Although there are *in vitro* data to support dipyridamole's mechanisms of action on the platelet, there is no firm clinical evidence that such mechanisms contribute to a significant antithrombotic effect in humans.[57]

In contrast to aspirin, the antithrombotic effects of dipyridamole are more evident on prosthetic materials (artificial heart valves[58,59] and arteriovenous cannulas) than on biologic surfaces. Although one study[60] showed that aspirin potentiates the efficacy of dipyridamole in experimental thromboembolism on prosthetic surfaces, other studies[57] have shown conflicting results with regard to the pharmacologic interaction between these two agents. Furthermore, aspirin alone was as effective as the combination of aspirin and dipyridamole in recent antithrombotic trials[61-65] in patients with myocardial infarction, saphenous vein graft disease, and stroke. On the basis of these findings, there is little evidence to support the use of dipyridamole as an antithrombotic agent except in combination with warfarin in high-risk patients with a mechanical prosthesis[66-70] and perhaps in the preoperative period in patients with coronary artery bypass surgery[71,72] by preventing platelet activation by the extracorporeal pump; however this last indication has not been properly tested.

SIDE EFFECTS. Epigastric discomfort or nausea occurs in more than 10% of patients; however, these symptoms tend to subside after a few days, particularly if a low dose is used initially and is given with meals. In addition, and in contrast with aspirin, when dipyridamole is given alone or in combination with anticoagulants, it does not seem to increase the incidence of gastritis, gastroduodenal ulcer, or the tendency to bleed. Because dipyridamole is a vasodilator, headaches occur in almost 10% of patients, but they become major problems in only 3% of those patients. Allergy, particularly skin rash, occurs infrequently.

PROSTAGLANDIN E_1 AND PROSTACYCLIN (PGI_2). Prostaglandin E_1 and prostacyclin are powerful systemic vasodilators and inhibitors of platelet aggregation by virtue of their ability to increase platelet cyclic AMP. Intravenous infusions of prostaglandin E_1 are commonly used in neonates with congenital heart disease, who are dependent on

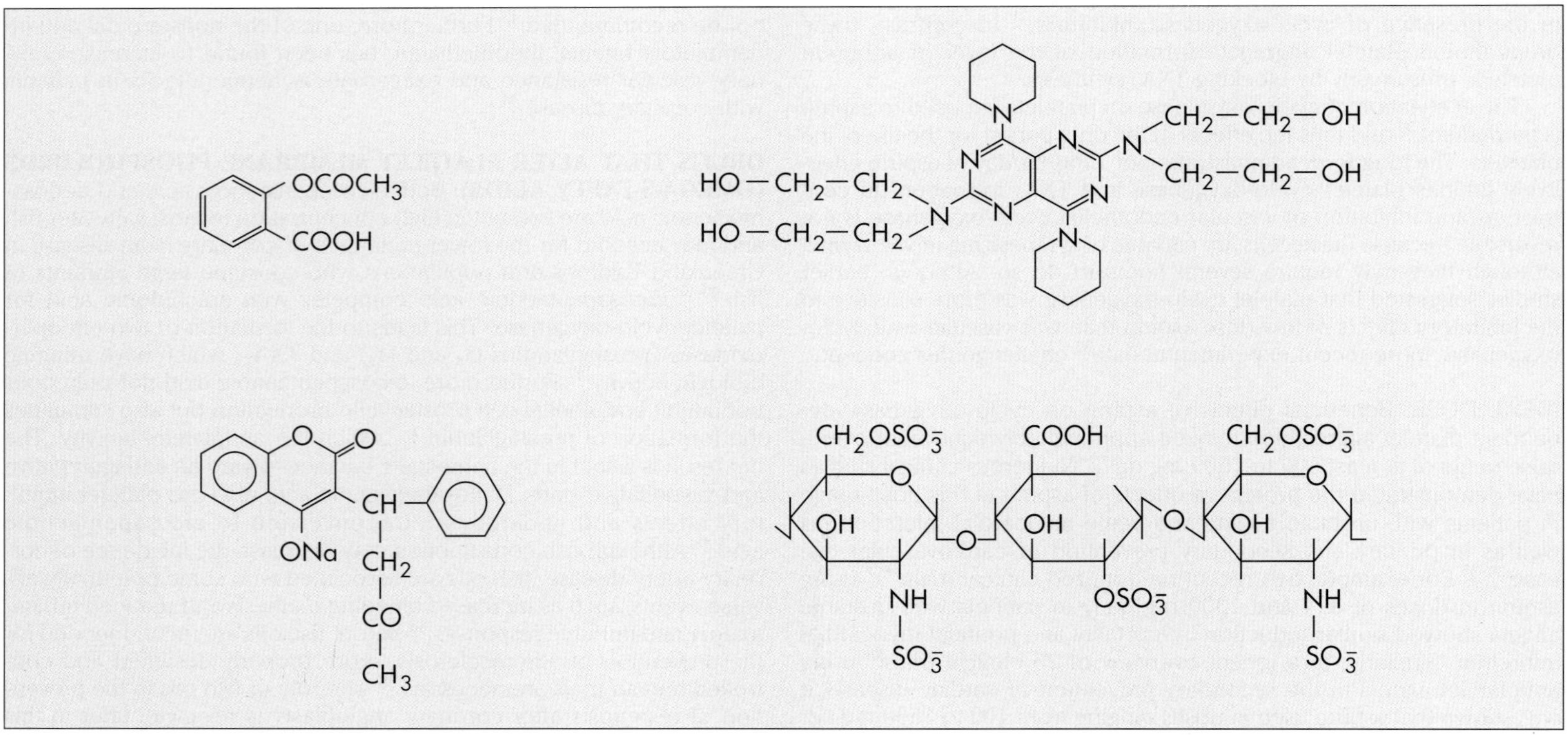

FIGURE 20.4 Chemical structure of the antithrombotic agents most commonly used in the United States: (clockwise) Acetylsalicylic acid (aspirin), dipyridamole (Persantine), heparin, and warfarin sodium.

the persistence of a patent ductus arteriosus until surgical correction is done. These agents have also been used to improve myocardial function in patients with acute myocardial infarction and to treat peripheral vascular disease.[73]

Prostacyclin is a potent, naturally occurring platelet inhibitor. Its clinical use has been limited by its instability at neutral pH and its propensity to cause significant systemic hypotension at the doses required for platelet inhibition. Its duration of action is very short, and the pharmacologic effects disappear in 30 minutes. Infusion of prostacyclin strongly limits platelet interaction with artificial surfaces and preserves platelet number and function during cardiopulmonary bypass.[74,75] The effects of prostacyclin in patients with ischemic heart disease and peripheral vascular insufficiency are controversial.[73] Emerging data, however, suggest that these prostanoids may improve the results of intracoronary thrombolysis in acute myocardial infarction.[76,77] Further research in this area is needed.

PROSTACYCLIN ANALOGUES. Iloprost, a new synthesized prostacyclin analogue, is chemically stable at neutral pH. In an *in vitro* comparison with equimolar concentrations of prostaglandin E_1 and prostacyclin, iloprost was found to be more potent in increasing the levels of cyclic AMP and inhibiting platelet aggregation by various agonists, particularly thrombin.[78] Another prostacyclin analogue, ciprostene, was found to reduce the rate of ischemic events in patients after coronary angioplasty and was associated with a beneficial trend toward a lower rate of restenosis.[79] Therefore, clinically stable analogues of prostacyclin may be effective for temporary control of platelet activity in the management of thromboembolic disorders. These compounds are undergoing clinical testing.

OTHER PLATELET INHIBITORS

TICLOPIDINE. Ticlopidine hydrochloride is a novel platelet anti-aggregant that functions primarily as an inhibitor of the adenosine diphosphate pathway of platelet aggregation.[80] In contrast to aspirin, ticlopidine inhibits most of the known stimuli to platelet aggregation when they are tested at physiologic concentrations. Ticlopidine does not inhibit the cyclo-oxygenase pathway, nor does it block the production of thromboxane by platelets or the production of prostacyclin by endothelial cells. Like aspirin, ticlopidine alters platelet function for the normal life span of the platelet.[81] Optimal efficacy is reached only after 3 days after its administration, and its effects last for several days after administration of the drug has been stopped.

Clinical evaluation of this drug is now underway. Preliminary evidence from an Italian multicenter trial[82] suggests that it is effective in patients with unstable angina for the prevention of myocardial infarction and cardiovascular death. Another recent study[83] showed a reduction in the incidence of acute occlusion and thrombosis after coronary angioplasty in patients treated with ticlopidine. In addition, this agent was found to be effective in reducing vein graft closure in patients after aortocoronary bypass surgery.[84] Recent published data[85,86] suggest that ticlopidine reduces cardiovascular morbidity and mortality in patients with stroke and appears more effective than aspirin in patients with transient ischemic attacks. However, ticlopidine is associated with occasional side effects, including rash and neutropenia.

SULFINPYRAZONE. Sulfinpyrazone is structurally related to phenylbutazone but has minimal anti-inflammatory activity. In contrast to aspirin, sulfinpyrazone is a competitive inhibitor of platelet cyclo-oxygenase, but the exact mechanism of its antithrombotic activity is not well understood.[60] It inhibits the formation of thrombus on the subendothelium and protects the endothelium from chemical injury *in vitro* and possibly *in vivo*. In addition, sulfinpyrazone produces a dose-dependent inhibition of experimental thromboembolism in artificial cannulas,[60] reduces the rate of thrombotic events in patients with arteriovenous cannulas,[87] and normalizes platelet survival in patients with artificial heart valves.[88] Overall, beneficial effects have been more consistent on prosthetic than biologic surfaces. Thus, despite a beneficial trend in decreasing vascular events after myocardial infarction[89] and reducing the occlusion rates in saphenous vein coronary grafts,[65,90] sulfinpyrazone was found to have no additional benefit in unstable angina[35] and stroke.[91] Side effects of sulfinpyrazone include increased sensitivity to warfarin, hypoglycemia when combined with sulfonylureas, exacerbation of peptic ulcer, and precipitation of uric acid stones.

DEXTRAN. Dextran of a molecular weight of 65,000 to 80,000 daltons prolongs the bleeding time after intravenous infusion of more than 1 liter. Its mechanism of action is unclear. It may involve some alteration on platelet membrane function[92] or interference with factor VIII–von Willebrand factor complex.[93] Although some experimental studies[94] have shown an antithrombotic effect of dextran, no effect was found in a randomized trial[95] in patients undergoing coronary angioplasty. Furthermore, dextran has been associated with a low but disturbing incidence (0.6%) of anaphylactoid reactions.[96] Data supporting the role of dextran as an antithrombotic agent on foreign materials (*i.e.*, arterial stents and vascular grafts) are emerging.

PLATELET THROMBIN INHIBITORS

By inhibiting thrombin formation with heparin, oral anticoagulant agents or other thrombin inhibitors, the effects of thrombin on platelet activation can be partially prevented.

PEPTIDE BLOCKERS OF THROMBIN. An emerging strategy in antithrombotic therapy involves the synthesis of peptides that specifically block thrombin-mediated platelet activation.[97] A number of these agents have been studied *in vitro* and in experimental animals; however, no clinical experience is yet available. Another potent selective thrombin inhibitor, hirudin, initially isolated from the salivary secretions of the medicinal leech, was recently synthesized by deoxyribonucleic acid recombinant technology. Hirudin prevents the activation of clotting factors V, VIII and XIII. In addition, by being a powerful thrombin inhibitor, it blocks the metabolic pathway of platelet activation dependent on thrombin. Hirudin has been shown to prevent thrombosis in an animal model of carotid angioplasty and was found to have a more potent antithrombotic effect than heparin.[98] Because these agents may effectively inhibit platelet activation by blocking thrombin, their potential for clinical use is enormous. Intensive research in this area is underway.

HEPARIN
MECHANISMS OF ACTION

Heparin is a complex mucopolysaccharide of variable molecular weight (Fig. 20.4). The term *heparin* refers not to a single structure but rather to a family of mucopolysaccharide chains of varying length and composition. The heparin used clinically is derived from porcine intestinal mucosa or bovine lung and is composed of molecules of molecular weights ranging from 4,000 to 40,000 daltons. The effect of heparin as an anticoagulant is essentially direct and immediate and depends on its ability to accelerate the action of the naturally occurring plasma inhibitor antithrombin III; indeed, the absence or near absence of antithrombin III renders heparin useless for antithrombotic therapy. Antithrombin III inhibits thrombin as well as several of the proteases of the coagulation cascade, including factors Xa, IXa, XIa, and XIIa by the formation of 1:1 protease–inhibitor complexes. The interaction of heparin with antithrombin III leads to a conformational change in the inhibitor, which greatly accelerates its interaction with coagulation proteases, particularly thrombin and factor Xa.[99] For example, the inactivation of thrombin by antithrombin III is accelerated approximately 1,000-fold by heparin. However, the efficiency of antithrombin III in inhibiting blood clotting may be more dependent on inhibition of factor Xa activity than on inhibition of thrombin.[100] This is because inhibition of earlier steps in the blood coagulation system (see Fig. 20.1) should have a more potent antithrombotic effect than inhibition of subsequent steps, owing to the amplification process inherent in the coagulation cascade; that is, a single factor Xa molecule can lead to the generation of multiple thrombin molecules.[101,102] Heparin-enhanced inactivation of factor Xa by antithrombin III is believed to be the mechanism by which relatively low doses of subcutaneous heparin prevent venous thrombosis in high-risk patients.

Pharmaceutical-grade heparin preparations can be fractionated into distinct subpopulations on the basis of either molecular weight or affinity for antithrombin III. Low-molecular-weight heparin (molecular weight 5,000 to 7,000 daltons) effectively catalyzes the inactivation of factor Xa by antithrombin III, yet does not prolong the activated partial thromboplastin time (APTT) (*i.e.*, less antithrombin effect) nor interact with platelets to the extent that high-molecular-weight heparin does.[103,104] Therefore, it has been suggested that low-molecular-weight heparin may be an effective antithrombotic agent with a relatively low risk of hemorrhagic side effects.[105]

DOSE, ADMINISTRATION, AND CONTROL OF THERAPY

The major aim of heparin administration is to prevent both the formation and extension of thrombi while minimizing the risk of bleeding. Since even at low plasma concentration heparin is antithrombotic, the appropriate amount of anticoagulation depends on the intensity of the thrombogenic stimulus. Heparin is not absorbed by the gastrointestinal mucosa and must be given parenterally. It may be given continuous intravenously, intermittent intravenously, or subcutaneously into the fat of the subcutaneous tissue over the lower abdominal wall near the iliac crest or into the chest wall below the clavicle. Absorption from these depot sites is erratic, and hematomas are common at sites of intramuscular injection; hence, the intramuscular route should be avoided. Both calcium and sodium salts of heparin seem to be equally safe and effective. The volume of distribution of heparin seems largely confined to the intravascular space, reflecting its strong binding to protein. After intravenous injection, the average half-life in humans is about 90 minutes when average doses are used (5,000 units every 4 hours).[106] After subcutaneous injection, half-life values are longer. Heparin half-life is, however, variable, and clinicians must be aware that dose requirements are not identical for all patients. In addition, correlation between heparin anticoagulant effect and heparin dose is poorer in patients with disease states than in normal volunteers. For example, in patients with pulmonary embolism, heparin clearance is accelerated, which necessitates higher dosage early in the treatment course.

At present there is no test that is completely satisfactory for monitoring heparin effect. What is needed is a test that directly monitors the generation of thrombin as well as the blood levels of antithrombin III. In the absence of such information at this time, only general guidelines can be recommended. The most commonly used test to monitor heparin therapy is the APTT,[107,108] which measures the effect of heparin on the intrinsic and common coagulation pathways (see Fig. 20.1). The protamine sulfate neutralization assay, which measures the amount of protamine sulfate (a heparin inactivator) necessary to normalize the thrombin clotting time, can also be used to monitor heparin therapy.[109,110] The anticoagulation effect of heparin should be maintained at a level that is equivalent to 0.1 to 0.5 unit of heparin per milliliter (using protamine sulfate titration standard curve). This heparin level corresponds to an APTT of one and one-fourth to two and one-half times control. The activated clotting time (ACT), which measures the effect of heparin on whole blood clotting, allows rapid determination of the anticoagulant effect of heparin and has been used to regulate heparin therapy during cardiopulmonary bypass and percutaneous transluminal coronary angioplasty.[111,112]

When used to treat patients with active thrombosis, heparin should be administered in a dose sufficient to prolong an appropriate coagulation test to within a defined level. In most cases, it is desirable to achieve an anticoagulant effect rapidly and to sustain it throughout the period of treatment. This is achieved by an initial intravenous bolus injection of heparin, which can be followed either by continuous infusion or by intermittent intravenous injections. A moderately large bolus dose of heparin of between 5,000 and 10,000 units is injected intravenously, producing heparin levels immediately after injection considerably higher than the therapeutic range. This is followed by a dose between 20,000 and 40,000 units of heparin over 24 hours (depending on the patient's response), which maintains the majority of patients with a therapeutic range (Table 20.1).[113] If a patient with active thrombosis is at risk of bleeding (*e.g.*, early postoperative period), heparin should be given by continuous intravenous infusion; and if the degree of risk is very high, a lower dose of heparin may be used. If patients are not at high risk of bleeding, heparin can be administered by 4-hourly intermittent intravenous injections in full therapeutic doses. Therapeutic levels of heparin can also be achieved with subcutaneous injections. In addition, subtherapeutic levels of heparin achieved by injecting a low dose subcutaneously may be used in prophylaxis of venous thrombosis.

CONTINUOUS INFUSION. Continuous heparin infusion (Fig. 20.5, Table 20.1) is commonly used in patients with acute coronary syndromes, cardiac-chamber thrombosis, and ongoing venous thrombosis. Heparin is given as an initial bolus injection followed by a maintenance infusion with an automatic infusion pump.[113] The laboratory test used for monitoring heparin is performed approximately 6 hours after the bolus injection and then at least once more in the first 24 hours. Monitoring is continued twice daily until the desired effect is achieved and the dose–response relationship is stable. Monitoring is then continued on a once-daily basis.

TABLE 20.1 HEPARIN REGIMENS

Dosage (units/24 hr)	Route	Clinical Indications	Therapeutic Range (APTT Ratio)
Low (10,000)	Subcutaneous (continuous intravenous)	Elective general surgery (not including major orthopedic procedures)	
Intermediate (20,000)	Subcutaneous (continuous intravenous)	Orthopedic procedures Acute myocardial infarction, heart failure, and immobilization Post acute venous thromboembolism	1½
Average or "therapeutic" (20,000–50,000)	Intravenous (continuous or intermittent, or subcutaneous)	Acute thromboembolism	1½–2
High (40,000–60,000)	Intravenous (continuous or intermittent)	Massive acute venous thromboembolism	2–2½

An initial bolus injection of 5,000 units should be followed by a maintenance infusion of 24,000 units/24 hr, which can then be adjusted according to the results of the test used to monitor heparin therapy. In patients with major pulmonary embolism, an initial bolus dose of 10,000 units of heparin should be given, both because of the urgency of obtaining a marked anticoagulant effect and because heparin clearance is accelerated in patients with pulmonary embolism. The anticoagulant effect of heparin should then be maintained at a level that is equivalent to 0.3 to 0.4 unit of heparin per milliliter (using protamine sulfate titration), since this is the heparin concentration that prevents the extension of experimental thrombi. This heparin level corresponds to an APTT of one and one-half to two times control. In patients with pulmonary embolism, it is most desirable that the regimen used achieves levels of about 0.4 to 0.5 unit of heparin per milliliter, corresponding to an APTT of two to two and one-half times control; this may require infusion of near 50,000 units of heparin/24 hr. If the APTT (or corresponding test) is above the therapeutic range, the dose of heparin should be reduced, usually between 2,000 and 4,000 units/24 hr, and the APTT be repeated 4 to 6 hours later. If the results of the monitoring test are below the therapeutic range, a second bolus of 2,000 units can be given and the dose of heparin increased by 3,000 units/24 hr. It should be noted that the dosage requirements may change after the first 2 to 3 days of treatment, but thereafter the dose–response relationship in any patient is usually stable.

Lower doses of heparin may be given in a patient with calf vein or even proximal vein thrombi in the early postoperative period or in a patient who has a hemostatic defect. In these patients, the initial bolus dose should be 2,000 units followed by a maintenance dose of 15,000 to 20,000 units for 24 hours, and the laboratory effect of heparin should be monitored more frequently than usual to maintain the heparin level at between 0.1 and 0.2 unit/ml.[113] This corresponds to an APTT of one and one-fourth to near one and one-half times control.

INTERMITTENT INTRAVENOUS INJECTION. When infusion pumps are not readily available or cannot be adequately supervised or early ambulation is desired, there are some practical advantages to using a heparin lock with an intermittent intravenous protocol (see Fig. 20.5 and Table 20.1). In addition, with such intermittent intravenous injection the need for careful monitoring is less important. For these reasons many physicians prefer separate intravenous injection of 5,000 units intravenously every 4 hours or 10,000 units intravenously every 6 hours. However, this approach has been reported to produce more bleeding in patients who have a high risk of hemorrhage.[114,115] Nevertheless, it should be noted that in these studies about 25% higher daily doses of heparin were used in the groups given intermittent intravenous injections, so that the increased rate of bleeding could have been related to the dose rather than the method of administration. Although it is sometimes recommended that the dose be adjusted to produce an APTT of approximately one and one-half times control immediately before the next injection is due, in practice, laboratory monitoring with intermittent heparin is difficult and is not performed routinely in many institutions.

SUBCUTANEOUS INJECTION. Subcutaneous heparin can be given in either low, intermediate, or full therapeutic doses (see Fig. 20.5 and Table 20.1).[113] When heparin is used prophylactically in patients subjected to elective abdominal or thoracic surgery, it is usually given by subcutaneous injection in doses of 5,000 units every 8 or 12 hours.[116-118] The first dose is given 2 hours preoperatively and thereafter every 8 or 12 hours for the first 7 days, preferably until 2 days after complete mobilization.[102] For this purpose, 0.2 ml of concentrated heparin containing 5,000 units is used. Monitoring is not required provided that the patient does not have a history of abnormal bleeding.

An intermediate heparin regimen of about 10,000 units given every 12 hours is of prophylactic value in patients at very high risk of venous thromboembolism and can also be used for the secondary prevention of venous thrombosis after a 7- to 10-day course of full-dose heparin.[118] A dose of 10,000 to 12,000 units given every 12 hours has been successful in acute myocardial infarction for prevention of recurrence[119] and for prevention of left ventricular thrombi.[120] The dosage requirement should first be determined by adjusting the APTT for 2 or 3 days, and then outpatient laboratory monitoring is no longer required. The dose is adjusted so that the APTT 6 hours after injection is about one and one-half times control (heparin level, 0.2 to 0.3 units/ml). In general, heparin should not be used in patients with a hemorrhagic diathesis, hypertension (diastole blood pressure persistently greater than 105 mm Hg), cerebrovascular hemorrhage, major trauma, acute ulceration, or overt bleeding from the gastrointestinal, genitourinary, or respiratory tracts.[121]

HEPARIN NEUTRALIZATION AND HEPARIN SIDE EFFECTS

Many reported episodes of major bleeding are related to risk factors for hemorrhage more overriding than dose or route administration. These risk factors include lack of hemostatic competence prior to heparinization, invasive procedures, aspirin use, bodily trauma, and recent surgery while on therapy. In general, heparin should not be used in patients with hemorrhagic diathesis, hypertension with a diastolic pressure persistently over 105, cerebrovascular hemorrhage, major trauma, acute ulceration, or overt bleeding from gastrointestinal, genitourinary, or respiratory tracts.

With continuous infusion, the anticoagulant effect of heparin is

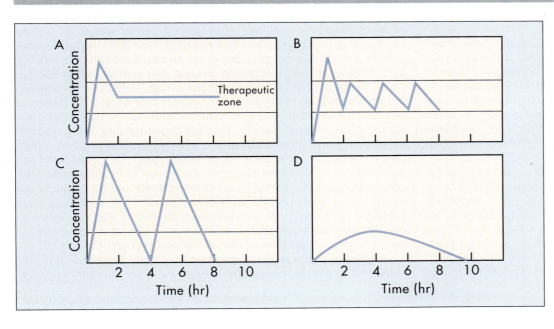

FIGURE 20.5 Blood concentration of heparin after **(A)** bolus injection followed by continuous intravenous infusion, **(B and C)** intermittent intravenous injections, and **(D)** subcutaneous injection. The risk of bleeding is higher when high-dose intermittent intravenous injection **(C)** is used and lower with subcutaneous injection **(D)**. (Modified from Verstraete M, Vermylen J: Antithrombotic and fibrinolytic agents and substances which lower blood viscosity. In Thrombosis, pp 76–112. New York, Pergamon Press, 1985)

gone within hours of discontinuing of the drug, so minor bleeding is not a threat. When heparin is given as a bolus dose, the duration of the effect depends on dose size (*i.e.*, 3 to 4 hours with 5,000 units and 6 hours with 15,000 units). Heparin given subcutaneously produces low peak blood levels of the drug but sustains these for up to 12 hours. When bleeding is more severe, protamine sulfate (1% solution) is the drug of choice to neutralize heparin. The protamines are low-molecular-weight proteins rich in arginine and therefore strongly basic; they combine quickly with heparin to form salts devoid of anticoagulant activity. One milligram of protamine sulfate neutralizes about 100 units of heparin. Only 50% of the calculated protamine sulfate dose should be administered, and only 25% of the calculated dose should be given if it has been 2 hours since heparin was administered. No more than 50 mg of protamine sulfate should be given in any 10-minute period, since severe toxic reactions, including hypotension and anaphylaxis, may occur (epinephrine and corticosteroids should be available when protamine is used).

Heparin can cause thrombocytopenia (platelet count < 100,000/mm^3) in 3% to 10% of patients.[122,123] This appears to be an immune-mediated phenomenon that typically occurs from 6 to 12 days after initiation of heparin therapy and is unique among the drug-induced thrombocytopenias in that it can be complicated by arterial thromboembolism. The diagnosis of heparin-induced thrombocytopenia is confirmed by rapid normalization of the platelet count on discontinuation of heparin.

Other complications of heparin therapy include osteoporosis, urticaria, alopecia, elevation of hepatic transaminases, and development of painful nodules at sites of subcutaneous injection.

OVERLAPPING OF COUMARIN WITH HEPARIN

When patients are being converted from heparin to warfarin, heparin should be continued for at least 24 hours after a therapeutic prothrombin time has been achieved since the anticoagulant effect of warfarin can be delayed relative to its effect on prothrombin time. This is because factor VII has a half-life (5 hours) that is shorter than the other vitamin K–dependent clotting factors (factors II, IX, and X). Consequently, early in the course of coumarin therapy the prothrombin time, which assesses the extrinsic coagulation pathway (see Fig. 20.1), can be prolonged while the intrinsic and common coagulation pathways are still "intact." In addition, the half-life of protein C, an endogenous vitamin K–dependent anticoagulant, is similar to that of factor VII, and antithrombin III levels are transiently depressed after a course of heparin therapy. Therefore, a relative prothrombotic state due to protein C and antithrombin III deficiency could potentially be created by discontinuing heparin as soon as the prothrombin time becomes therapeutic.

ORAL ANTICOAGULANTS
MECHANISM OF ACTION

Coagulation factors II, VII, IX, and X, protein C, and protein S are vitamin K–dependent proteins that are synthesized in hepatocytes. Post-translational modification of these proteins is necessary in order to yield biologically active molecules and involves the γ-carboxylation of glutamic acid residues located near the carboxy terminus of each protein. Coumarin anticoagulants inhibit vitamin K-2,3-epoxide reductase within hepatic microsomes and thus prevent recycling of vitamin K, which is necessary for the synthesis of γ-carboxyglutamic acid (Gla) residues.[124]

The clotting factors in blood are normally in a state of dynamic equilibrium, with the level of each individual factor not changing much over time. With a dose of coumarin sufficiently large to completely block hepatic synthesis, each factor disappears from the blood in accord with its half-life. With discontinuance of the drug, the clotting factors return to normal depending on their intrinsic synthesis rates. Thus, after a latent period peculiar to each type of oral anticoagulant, the prothrombin time becomes prolonged, mainly from the effect of lowering of the concentration of factor VII, the vitamin K–dependent factor with the shortest half-life (5 hours). Plasma concentration of the other vitamin K–dependent coagulation factors will decrease more slowly because their half-life is longer (20 to 60 hours for factor IX and X, and 80 to 100 hours for prothrombin). After 3 to 5 days of coumarin treatment, the lowered blood levels of the affected coagulation factors become virtually uniform. For effective treatment of thrombosis, the levels of factors II, VII, IX, and X should remain at approximately 25% of normal.

In North America, warfarin sodium is preferred among the coumarin drugs and the indanedione drugs are seldom used for oral anticoagulant therapy since they are more prone to side effects and more difficult to control. Although the various coumarin congeners do differ in speed of induction of effect and in their individual metabolism, they all induce quantitatively similar effects on the clotting mechanism. Warfarin is extremely soluble in an aqueous medium and is completely absorbed from the gastrointestinal tract. It is almost totally bound to plasma proteins, which may be partially responsible for its long plasma half-life. The biologic half-life of warfarin ranges from 35 to 45 hours and is independent of the size of the dose.[106] Warfarin is metabolized by hepatic microsomal enzymes. It can cross the placental barrier, but there is no firm evidence that the drug appears in breast milk in significant amounts. In one study involving mothers and infants, no warfarin was found either in the mother's milk or in the plasma of the breast-fed infant.[125]

DOSE, ADMINISTRATION, AND CONTROL OF THERAPY

Treatment with warfarin is usually begun by the oral route. O'Reilly and Aggeler were the first to suggest that in order to decrease the danger of hemorrhage in sensitive patients, warfarin therapy should be started without large loading doses.[126] As suggested by the guidelines of the American Heart Association, warfarin therapy can be instituted with daily doses of 10 to 15 mg/day for the first 2 to 3 days.[101] Subsequent doses can be tailored according to the prothrombin time. Maintenance doses are usually less than 10 mg/day. To establish the optimum regimen for each patient, the prothrombin time should be monitored two to three times each week during the first several weeks of therapy. After the therapeutic range is achieved, the frequency of prothrombin time determinations may be decreased to every 2 weeks. In some patients this interval may be decreased to 3 or 4 weeks, but it is inadvisable to obtain a prothrombin time assay at intervals of more than 1 month.

Oral anticoagulants are contraindicated in patients with a hemorrhagic diathesis, poorly controlled hypertension, cerebrovascular hemorrhage, major trauma, active peptic ulcer disease, or overt bleeding from the gastrointestinal, genitourinary, or respiratory tracts. Inadequate laboratory facilities or unsatisfactory patient cooperation should also be considered as contraindications. Relative contraindications to oral anticoagulation include concomitant use of aspirin in a dose causing gastric erosion (over 325 mg/day), vasculitis, bacterial endocarditis, pericarditis complicating acute myocardial infarction, renal or liver disease, and thyrotoxicosis treated with radioactive iodine because of the possibility of gland hemorrhage. Adequate preparation before administration of oral anticoagulants may reduce the hazard of bleeding in disorders such as ulcerative colitis, sprue, steatorrhea, and pancreatitis. Among diabetic patients requiring long-term warfarin therapy, the question often arises whether anticoagulation would create the risk of vitreous or retinal hemorrhage.[101,127] Advanced age has been considered a relative contraindication to long-term oral anticoagulation due to potentially lethal side-effects and the frequent use of other drugs that may interact with warfarin.[127,128] Nevertheless, clear evidence concerning the risk–benefit ratio of oral anticoagulation in elderly patients is not available, and age alone should not proscribe the use of warfarin in patients at high risk of thromboembolism.[129-131]

Numerous medications interact with warfarin. Therefore, it is vital to instruct all patients on warfarin therapy to report promptly when any drug is deleted from or added to their therapeutic regimen, including nonprescription compounds. Frequent prothrombin time determinations will permit dose adjustments that can prevent either underanticoagulation or overanticoagulation. Similarly, any major change in diet (*e.g.*, leafy vegetables, green beans, and liver contain large amounts of vitamin K) should be reported so that drug dosage can be adjusted based on more frequent determinations of the prothrombin time. Drugs that interact with warfarin can do so by altering warfarin absorption, plasma protein binding, and metabolism, consequently causing significant potentiation or inhibition of the drug's anticoagulant effect. A list of the more important interactions is presented in Table 20.2.

The prothrombin time is the test most frequently used to monitor warfarin therapy. It is performed by adding calcium and thromboplastin to citrated plasma and then measuring the time to fibrin formation. Thromboplastin is an extract of brain, lung, or placenta that contains tissue factor and phospholipid, which are necessary for the activation of factor X by factor VII.[132] Thromboplastins extracted from different organs or species can vary significantly in their sensitivity to reductions in levels of vitamin K–dependent factors; that is, a single plasma sample from a patient on coumarin could yield significantly different prothrombin times if assayed in two different laboratories that used different commercial thromboplastins. Approximately 90% of the thromboplastins used in North America are extracted from rabbit brain. Therefore, major variations in prothrombin times between laboratories are unlikely to occur. However, thromboplastins used in the United Kingdom are significantly more sensitive to reductions in vitamin K–dependent factors than North American thromboplastins. Therefore, in order to properly interpret the clinical literature concerning oral anticoagulation, the reader must bear in mind the thromboplastin used (Table 20.3).

In an effort to standardize prothrombin time determinations and thus allow direct comparison of assays performed with different thromboplastins, the World Health Organization (WHO) has recommended the use of an internal normalized ratio (INR), which is defined as the prothrombin time (PT) ratio (*i.e.*, PT observed/PT control) results that would be obtained if WHO primary international reference thromboplastin (IRP) were used to test the plasma sample.[132] This is based on the determination of the international sensitivity index (ISI) of the thromboplastin used in the local laboratory. The ISI is a measure of the responsiveness of a given thromboplastin to reduction of the vitamin K–dependent coagulation factors. For a PT ratio with a thromboplastin with an ISI value of C, INR = (observed ratio)^C. For example, for a thromboplastin with an ISI of 1.4, a PT ratio of 2.5 is equivalent to $2.5^{1.4} = 3.6$ with the IRP.

The intensity of oral anticoagulation necessary to properly treat or present intravascular thrombosis varies depending on the clinical situation. The American College of Chest Physicians Conference on Antithrombotic Therapy has offered the following recommendations concerning oral anticoagulant therapy[132]:

1. A less intense degree of oral anticoagulation (INR 2.0 to 3.0, corresponding to a PT ratio of 1.3 to 1.5 using a typical North American thromboplastin with an ISI = 2.4) should be used in the following clinical situations:
   a. Prevention of venous thromboembolism in high-risk patients
   b. Treatment of venous thrombosis and pulmonary embolism (after an initial course of heparin)
   c. Prevention of systemic embolism in patients with tissue cardiac valve prostheses and in selected patients with atrial fibrillation, acute transmural anterior wall myocardial infarction, or valvular heart disease
2. A more intense degree of oral anticoagulation (INR = 3.0 to 4.5, corresponding to a PT ratio of 1.5 to 2.0 using a typical North American thromboplastin with an ISI = 2.4) should be used in patients with mechanical cardiac valve prostheses and in patients with recurrent systemic thromboembolism.

SIDE EFFECTS

The most important side effect of oral anticoagulation is bleeding. The risk of bleeding varies from patient to patient depending on the intensity of anticoagulation, the indication for its use, and the presence of co-morbid conditions. Hull and colleagues have shown that in patients with venous thrombosis, those randomized to more intense anticoagulant therapy (INR 2.5 to 4.5) have an over fivefold greater risk of bleeding (22% *vs.* 4%) than those randomized to less intense anticoagulation (INR 2.0).[133] Levine and colleagues pooled data from 171 studies dealing with rates of bleeding in patients on long-term oral anticoagulant therapy.[134] The risk of major bleeding (intracranial or retroperitoneal bleeding or bleeding leading directly to death, hospitalization, or transfusion) was 8.1% in patients anticoagulated because of venous thromboembolism, 7% in ischemic cerebrovascular disease,

TABLE 20.2 DRUGS AFFECTING ANTICOAGULANT ACTIVITY

Enhanced Effect	Decreased Effect
Chloramphenicol	Vitamin K
Cimetidine	Oral contraceptives
Anabolic steroids	Rifampin
D-Thyroxine	Griseofulvin
Clofibrate	Glutethimide
Metronidazole	Cholestyramine
Phenylbutazone	Barbiturates
Sulfinpyrazone	Phenytoin
Quinidine	
Disulfiram	
Sulfonamides	
Chloral hydrate	
Alcohol (abuse only)	
Allopurinol	
Amiodarone	
Antibiotics	
Methyldopa	
Aspirin (in high doses)	

TABLE 20.3 THERAPEUTIC RANGES FOR VARIOUS THROMBOPLASTINS EQUIVALENT TO THE CONVENTIONAL RANGE WITH THE BRITISH COMPARATIVE THROMBOPLASTIN (RATIO 2.0–4.0)

Reagent	Range of Ratios
British Comparative Thromboplastin	2.0–4.0
Thrombotest	2.0–3.5
Rabbit Thromboplastin (brain–lung)	1.5–2.0
Rabbit Thromboplastin (brain)	1.3–1.7

4.7% in ischemic heart disease, and 2.4% in patients with prosthetic cardiac valves. The incidence of major bleeding is best expressed in terms of rate per 100 patient-years of therapy. It ranges from 2 to 22/100 patient-years in ischemic cerebrovascular disease and from 0 to 7.7/100 patient-years in myocardial infarction and is 0.8/100 patient-years in patients with prosthetic cardiac valves. Levine and colleagues[134] concluded that the reason for the relatively high incidence of bleeding complications in patients with ischemic cerebrovascular disease and venous thromboembolism is the frequent presence of co-morbid conditions such as hypertension, malignancy, and recent surgery.

Bleeding in patients on oral anticoagulants may occur at unusual sites. Hemorrhage into the bowel lumen, the intestinal wall, the mesentery, the rectus muscle, or the corpus luteum may simulate an acute abdominal crisis. Similar conditions apply to genitourinary bleeding, which may mimic a renal tumor. Hematomas may cause carpal tunnel compression, and, rarely, there may be pericardial, adrenal, or retroperitoneal hemorrhage. When to search for the cause of an episode of spontaneous bleeding, such as from the genitourinary or gastrointestinal tracts, can be decided if the prothrombin time is obtained within 24 hours of hemorrhage. Experience has shown that when the prothrombin time ratio is in the range of 1.5 to 2.0, the likelihood of finding a localized lesion is less than if the prothrombin time is in excess of 2.5. In the former situation, further efforts to identify the bleeding source should be undertaken promptly.

Minor bleeding in patients with prolonged prothrombin times can be treated by withholding warfarin temporarily. Major bleeding will necessitate discontinuing the drug and administration of vitamin K_1 or blood products, when appropriate. The dose of vitamin K_1 depends not only on the endpoint desired but also on the intensity of warfarin effect. A common mistake is the administration of a high dose of vitamin K_1 in an effort to return the prothrombin time to normal more rapidly. Larger doses of vitamin K_1 do not increase the rate of synthesis of the individual vitamin K–dependent clotting factors; rather, vitamin K_1 restores extrinsic synthesis rates for a period that is dose dependent. The route of vitamin K_1 administration may be intravenous, subcutaneous, or oral, depending on the nature and urgency of the clinical situation. Some correction of the prothrombin time is noted within 6 hours, and full correction occurs within 24 hours. If the patient is to remain on warfarin, the dose should be limited to 0.5 to 1.0 mg. Higher amounts, up to 10 mg, may be indicated if the patient is not to be maintained on therapy after the hemorrhage is controlled. Large doses of vitamin K_1 may make the patient resistant to warfarin for many days, preventing effective anticoagulant therapy for that time period. An immediate reversal of the clotting defect can be achieved by transfusion of blood, plasma, or plasma concentrates rich in the vitamin K–dependent clotting factors. Because these factors are relatively stable, they remain fully potent in ordinary banked blood or lyophilized plasma. Three units or 15 ml/kg of blood or plasma should suffice for an initial effect, providing time for concomitant vitamin K_1 administration to exert its action.[101] In patients with limited cardiac reserve, the recommended volumes of blood or plasma may precipitate pulmonary edema unless significant blood loss has occurred. Plasma concentrates rich in factors II, VII, IX, and X obviate the hazard of hypervolemia but carry with them the risk of thrombosis and hepatitis.

Nonhemorrhagic side effects of warfarin include coumarin embryopathy and coumarin-induced skin necrosis. Coumarin readily crosses the placenta and has been found to be teratogenic, particularly during the first trimester of pregnancy.[135] Fetal bone and cartilage development appear sensitive to warfarin, as evidenced by the best described abnormalities of coumarin embryopathy: nasal deformity and stippling of the bony epiphyses. This effect may be mediated by deficiency of osteocalcin, a vitamin K–dependent protein.[136] An increased incidence of fetal wastage and central nervous system defects has also been observed with exposure to warfarin during pregnancy.[137] For this reason, the majority of experts advise substitution of subcutaneous heparin (e.g., approximately 12,500 units subcutaneously every 12 hours with target APTT one and one-half to two times control) for coumarin at least during the first trimester of pregnancy as well as for several weeks prior to delivery.[138] Indeed, high-dose subcutaneous heparin has been advocated all throughout the pregnancy by many. Therefore, fertile women receiving warfarin must be warned of the risks of teratogenicity and should be advised to notify their physicians at the earliest suspicion of pregnancy.

Coumarin-induced necrosis of the skin and subcutaneous tissues is a rare but striking complication of warfarin therapy that has been associated with hereditary protein C deficiency.[139] The lesion appears within 3 to 10 days of drug administration, usually in the lower half of the body. It occurs particularly in women and in areas of abundant subcutaneous fat, such as the buttocks, breasts, thighs, and abdomen. The initial manifestation of coumarin-induced skin necrosis is an erythematous patch. Frank hemorrhagic necrosis may develop within 24 hours. Coumarin necrosis should not be confused with purple toes syndrome,[140] in which painful, blue toes develop, often with livedo reticularis to the knees or to the iliac crest; this is believed to represent atheromatous embolization to the extremities, perhaps accentuated by warfarin.[141] When coumarin-induced necrosis occurs, warfarin should be discontinued. If further anticoagulation is indicated, heparin therapy should be initiated.[101]

THROMBOLYTIC AGENTS

The acute coronary syndromes including acute myocardial infarction, unstable angina, and sudden death are caused by thrombotic occlusion of critically situated blood vessels. Timely pharmacologic dissolution of blood clots therefore might abort the evolution of these syndromes with preservation of the myocardium and reduction of mortality. This can be achieved with intravenous infusion of thrombolytic agents, which convert plasminogen, the inactive proenzyme of the fibrinolytic system, to the proteolytic enzyme plasmin, which lyses the fibrin of blood clots (see Fig. 20.3). The fibrinolytic system contains a proenzyme, plasminogen, which can be converted to the active enzyme plasmin by the action of several different types of plasminogen activator.[142,143] Plasmin is a serine protease that digests fibrin to soluble degradation products. Natural inhibition of the fibrinolytic system occurs both at the level of the plasminogen and also at the level of the plasmin. Plasminogen is a single-chain glycoprotein consisting of 790 amino acids that is converted to plasmin by cleavage of the Arg560–Val561 peptide bond. The plasminogen molecule contains structures, called lysine-binding sites, that mediate its binding to fibrin and accelerate the interactions between plasmin and its physiological inhibitor α_2-antiplasmin. The lysin binding plays a critical role in the regulation of fibrinolysis. Plasminogen activators are serine proteases with a high specificity for plasminogen, which hydrolyzes the Arg560–Val561 peptide bond, yielding the active enzyme plasmin.

Currently, five thrombolytic agents are either approved for clinical use or under clinical investigation in patients with acute myocardial infarction: streptokinase, recombinant tissue-type plasminogen activator (rt-PA), acylated plasminogen streptokinase activator complex (APSAC), urokinase, and single-chain urokinase-type plasminogen activator (scu-PA, prourokinase).[143,144] Readers should bear in mind that the field of thrombolysis is progressing rapidly and the goal of this section is to present a brief overview of the current status of thrombolysis.

STREPTOKINASE
MECHANISM OF ACTION. Streptokinase is a nonenzymatic antigenic protein produced by Lancefield group-C strains of beta-hemolytic streptococci. It forms a 1:1 stoichiometric complex with plasminogen, a process that exposes the active site of the light chain of plasminogen. This complex is converted spontaneously to a streptokinase-plasmin complex, which is a powerful activator of plasminogen. Streptokinase, however, does not discriminate between circulating and fibrin-bound plasminogen. Circulating plasmin is initially neutralized by

alpha-antiplasmin, but when the antiplasmin level is significantly reduced, plasmin exerts its proteolytic effects on several plasma proteins, including fibrinogen and factors V and VIII; this last reaction contributes to the bleeding risk of streptokinase. The half-life of streptokinase in the blood is approximately 30 minutes.[143-146]

REPERFUSION. Many factors influence the success of thrombolytic therapy: some relate to the nature of the occlusion, such as the age, location, and concentration of plasminogen and plasmin inhibitors on the thrombus, and others relate to the therapeutic regimen, such as the dosage of the agent used, the duration of the therapy, and the speed with which treatment is begun.[143-146] Rentrop and co-workers pioneered the use of intracoronary streptokinase in patients with acute myocardial infarction.[147] The enthusiasm stemmed in part from the anticipated greater incidence of thrombolysis with the drug delivered directly in the vicinity of the clot, the potential for efficacy with a lower dose, and the advantage of confirmation of the presence of an occlusive thrombus prior to treatment and angiographic assessment of its response to lytic therapy. Although these advantages are real, the delay associated with intracoronary administration and the relatively limited immediate availability of cardiac catheterization facilities for most patients presenting with acute infarction have led to virtual abandonment of the intracoronary route as the primary or sole approach for most patients. The collective experience from numerous earlier studies of intracoronary streptokinase with a dose of 250,000 units in patients with acute myocardial infarction indicates that thrombolysis with reperfusion occurs in about 85% of patients.[148-150]

The reported patency rate of intravenous streptokinase in patients with acute myocardial infarction is much lower than that achieved with intracoronary streptokinase. The cumulative database from 13 angiographic studies indicates that infarct vessel patency rate at 60 to 120 minutes was approximately 48% with the use of 1.5 million units infused over 1 hour.[151-163] However, a definite "catch-up" phenomenon for streptokinase has been documented by serial angiography performed up to 24 hours after symptom onset.[163] By the time of late follow-up cardiac catheterization, the patency rate of arteries treated with streptokinase approaches 80%.[163]

COMPLICATIONS. The complications of administration of intracoronary streptokinase are related to the catheterization and angiographic procedures, the thrombolytic agent, the adverse effects of reperfusion, and the consequences of reocclusion. The major risk of either intracoronary or intravenous streptokinase is hemorrhage.[164] A systemic lytic state with fibrinogenolysis is induced even when the subtherapeutic or low dose intracoronary streptokinase is administered. Bleeding occurs most frequently at the site of vascular puncture. However, systemic hemorrhage, including cerebral, gastrointestinal, mediastinal, and urinary tract bleeding, may be encountered, particularly when occult predisposing causes are present. The reported prevalence of hemorrhage requiring transfusion after intracoronary or intravenous streptokinase has ranged from 1.3% to 18%, but most studies report an incidence of 10% or less. Fortunately, the incidence of intracerebral bleeding is rare, occurring in fewer than 1% of patients.[144-146] Transient hypotensive episodes have also been reported in approximately 9% of patients given intracoronary streptokinase and in 17% of patients given intravenous streptokinase.[164] However, hypotension has generally responded to transient interruption of the infusion of streptokinase and administration of fluids or atropine. Another side effect of streptokinase is related to its antigenicity. Overt allergic reactions are not common. Frank anaphylaxis is extremely rare, and rash, swollen lips, and urticaria occur in less than 2% of patients.[164]

RECOMBINANT TISSUE-TYPE PLASMINOGEN ACTIVATORS

MECHANISM OF ACTION. Native tissue-type plasminogen activator (t-PA) is a trypsin-like serine protease composed of 527 amino acids and produced by recombinant DNA technology.[144-146] As a consequence of limited plasmin action on the fibrin surface, native t-PA is rapidly converted to a two-chain activator. The heavy chain (A) of this molecule contains two regions that share a high degree of homology with the five kringles of plasminogen, while the catalytic site is located on the light chain (B).[144-146] The one-chain and two-chain forms of t-PA have different amidolytic activities in vitro, but have virtually the same fibrinolytic activity. t-PA is a poor plasminogen activator in the absence of fibrin, but it binds specifically to fibrin and activates plasminogen at the fibrin surface several hundredfold more efficiently than in the circulation. The underlying principle of this phenomenon is that both plasminogen and t-PA bind to fibrin and form a cyclic ternary complex. Thus, fibrin serves as a cofactor for plasminogen activation by lowering the Km of t-PA for plasminogen. As a consequence of these kinetic characteristics, plasmin is predominantly generated on the fibrin surface.[144-146] This in turn results in a relative sparing of circulating fibrinogen and other plasma proteins to plasmin-mediated degradation. Recombinant tissue-type plasminogen activator (rt-PA) is produced through complex biologic techniques and is predominantly single-chain t-PA and the only one currently on the market for clinical use.

The optimal regimen of rt-PA has not yet been established. Because of its relatively short half-life (2–7 minutes), current practice uses a 10-mg initial bolus injection, followed by 50 mg in 1 hour and 40 mg in the subsequent 2 hours. The use of a higher dosage (150 mg) appears to yield a higher patency rate but is associated with a significantly higher incidence of intracerebral hemorrhage. Thus, a dose of 100 mg is currently recommended.[144-146]

REPERFUSION. The cumulative data from numerous angiographic studies[151-163] in patients with acute myocardial infarction indicates that the infarct vessel patency rate is approximately 80% at 120 minutes following 100 mg of rt-PA. Controversy exists as to whether the fibrin specificity of rt-PA would confer advantage over streptokinase in terms of reperfusion and myocardial salvage. As discussed previously, although the patency rate at early phase appears to be higher in patients receiving rt-PA, a "catch-up" phenomenon has been demonstrated for streptokinase.[163] At 24 hours after thrombolytic therapy, the patency rate of arteries treated with agents lacking fibrin selectivity is similar to that of patients treated with rt-PA. Thus, although rt-PA holds promise for improved early coronary thrombolytic action, it has not yet been demonstrated whether this effect translates into superior preservation of left ventricular function or a reduction of mortality.[165] Several ongoing large clinical trials will address this question.

COMPLICATIONS. Speculation has ranged from a prediction that rt-PA would be associated with less bleeding because of the absence of a systemic lytic state[166,167] to fear that it would result in an increased risk of bleeding secondary to augmented fibrinolytic potency.[145,168] Direct comparative trial data with streptokinase showed little difference in extracranial bleeding complications, except for a slight advantage with rt-PA in two of the four trials.[151,169-171] In the largest study of rt-PA in terms of patients treated, the recently completed Thrombolysis in Myocardial Infarction-II (TIMI-II) trial,[172] the incidence of intracranial hemorrhage was 0.5% in 2,742 patients treated with 100 mg. As opposed to other large mortality trials,[173-176] this overall low frequency was established with detailed data collection and routine computed axial tomographic scanning for any new neurologic deficit. In contrast to streptokinase, rt-PA is nonantigenic and lacks hypotensive effect.

ACYLATED PLASMINOGEN STREPTOKINASE ACTIVATOR COMPLEX

MECHANISM OF ACTION. Acylated plasminogen-streptokinase-activator complex (APSAC) is an equimolar complex of streptokinase and Lys-plasminogen that is rendered inactive by acylation of the catalytic center of the plasminogen portion.[144-146,177] When introduced in the systemic circulation, APSAC can attach itself to fibrin-bound plasminogen without being inactivated by alpha 2-antiplasmin. Deacylation occurs spontaneously and results in sustained activity. Activation of

APSAC bound to the fibrin of clot theoretically confers a fibrin specificity to the drug. In fact, when the drug is administered intravenously to patients in therapeutic dose (30 units), systemic fibrinogenolysis is constant. Progressive deacylation after injection confers a prolonged half-life to the drug, averaging 90 minutes compared with 23 minutes with streptokinase. This prolonged half-life results in long-lasting thrombolytic effects. Because the intravenous injection of the complex does not cause profound hemodynamic effects, the drug can be administered in a bolus injection.[144–146,177]

REPERFUSION. Results of several clinical studies[176–179] indicate that the patency rate of infarct-related artery at 90 minutes following intravenous APSAC (30 units) is approximately 69%. A direct comparison of intravenous APSAC and streptokinase was made in a French randomized, open-designed multicenter study and demonstrated a slightly higher patency rate in patients receiving APSAC as compared with streptokinase (72% vs. 55%).[179] A larger, more definitive trial of intravenous APSAC versus streptokinase has just been completed in the United States, but the results have not yet been presented.

COMPLICATIONS. The bleeding complication rate produced by APSAC is remarkably similar to that of other thrombolytic agents with or without fibrin specificity. In a French multicenter trial involving 231 patients, a bleeding complication was observed in 6.5% of the APSAC-treated patients, and only half of these patients required blood transfusion.[179]

UROKINASE AND SINGLE-CHAIN UROKINASE-TYPE PLASMINOGEN ACTIVATOR

MECHANISM OF ACTION. Urokinase is a double-chain glycoprotein that acts as a trypsin-like protease.[143,144] It may occur in two molecular forms—S1 (32kd) and S2 (54kd)—the former being a proteolytic degradation product of the latter. Urokinase isolated from human urine or cultured embryonic kidney cells is nonantigenic. It is a direct activator of plasminogen and generates plasmin by cleaving the Arg560-Val 561 bond of the plasminogen molecule. Urokinase does not have fibrin specificity and activates fibrin-bound as well as circulating plasminogen; therefore, it also induces a systemic activation of the fibrinolytic system as soon as the alpha 2-antiplasmin level is reduced. The half-life of urokinase is about 10 minutes, and thus the persistence of thrombolysis may be less than with streptokinase. Single-chain urokinase-type plasminogen activator (scu-PA) or prourokinase is a single-chain glycoprotein containing 411 amino acids, which is converted to urokinase by hydrolysis of the Lys158–Ile159 peptide bond. scu-PA has very little activity toward low-molecular-weight substrate but has intrinsic plasminogen-activating potential, but with a catalytic efficiency that is two orders of magnitude lower than that of urokinase. The half-life of scu-PA is about 8 minutes.[143,144]

REPERFUSION. Two reports[180,181] have indicated that the patency rate at 60 minutes in patients with acute myocardial infarction given either intracoronary or intravenous urokinase is about 60%. This moderately fibrin-selective thrombolytic agent can be given intravenously with a reduced systematic lytic state and predictably lower bleeding risk than intravenous streptokinase. The recanalization rate of scu-PA in patients with acute myocardial infarction is about 78% as reported by Van der Werf and co-workers[182] using 70 mg of scu-PA infused over 1 hour. The potential value of these two agents appears to relate to the fact that they may provide synergistic effects on clot lysis and reperfusion when combined with other thrombolytic agents. The recently completed TIMI-II study[183] demonstrated that although the patency rates in patients with acute myocardial infarction given the combination of t-PA and urokinase were not significantly higher than those achieved by t-PA alone, the reocclusion rate was substantially lower. Similarly, some beneficial effects in terms of bleeding complications and reocclusion were observed when the combination of t-PA and scu-PA was used.[184] Other combinations such as t-PA and streptokinase are currently being evaluated. These synergistic combinations of thrombolytic agents may offer better cost–benefit and risk–benefit ratios than obtainable with single-agent therapy. However, in order to reach valid conclusions, continued investigation of synergism should be carried out with the use of adequate investigational procedures with respect to both experimental design and data analysis.

PATHOGENESIS OF THROMBOSIS AND EMBOLISM IN CORONARY ARTERIES, CARDIAC CHAMBERS, AND PROSTHETIC VALVES

The pathogenic mechanisms leading to thrombosis and embolism in coronary arteries, cardiac chambers, and prosthetic heart valves appear to be different. The pathogenesis of arterial thrombosis involves damage to the vessel wall and exposure of a thrombogenic substrate, leading to platelet activation and fibrin formation. Intracavitary thrombosis mainly occurs in situations of blood stasis, which favor the activation of the coagulation system and the generation of fibrin. Platelet activation may play a role in the presence of endocardial injury. Prosthetic heart valves mainly promote activation, primarily of the coagulation system and secondarily of the platelets.

CORONARY ARTERIES: PLATELETS AND FIBRIN

THE CONCEPT OF VASCULAR INJURY: PLATELETS AND FIBRIN

Vascular injury and thrombus formation represent the key events in the progression of atherosclerosis, in the pathogenesis of acute coronary syndromes, and in various vascular diseases. We have previously proposed a pathologic classification of vascular injury and its pathophysiologic cellular responses in an attempt to help understanding of the pathogenesis of various vascular diseases and formulate therapeutic strategies in the prevention of these diseases.[185] We proposed the classification of vascular injury into three types (Fig. 20.6):

Type I: functional alterations of endothelial cells without significant morphologic changes
Type II: endothelial denudation and intimal injury but with intact internal elastic lamina and media
Type III: endothelial denudation with damage of intima and media

In type I endothelial injury no significant platelet deposition or thrombus formation can be demonstrated, although there is some recent evidence that few platelets interact with such subtle injured endothelium and contribute, by the release of growth factors, to some intimal hyperplasia; this may be the basis of the initiation of the atherosclerotic process. In contrast, with type II injury, an obvious monolayer of a few layers of platelets with or without thrombus formation can be seen; the release of platelet growth factors may contribute to an accelerated intimal hyperplasia as it occurs in the coronary vein graft within the first postoperative year. In type III injury with exposure of components of the medial layer, particularly the fibrillar collagen, marked platelet aggregation with mural thrombus formation follows. Vascular injury of this magnitude also stimulates thrombin formation through both the intrinsic (surface-activated) and extrinsic (tissue factor–dependent) coagulation pathways, in which the platelet membrane facilitates interactions between clotting factors (see Fig. 20.1). And as discussed above, thrombin promotes the formation and polymerization of fibrin, which is responsible for stabilization of the expanding thrombotic mass, allowing it to resist dislodgement by the forces of arterial blood flow. Like collagen, thrombin is also a powerful activator of platelet aggregation. Platelets and the coagulation system are therefore clearly interrelated in the genesis of arterial thrombosis following deep type III injury as it is seen in the acute coronary syndromes or following coronary angioplasty.

LABILE VERSUS FIXED THROMBUS

Delivery and activation of platelets at the site of vascular injury are dependent both on shear rate, which is a measure of the difference in blood velocity between the center and the periphery of the vessel,[186] and on the degree of vessel injury (type II vs. type III). In areas of luminal stenosis, high shear rate promotes contact between blood elements and the vessel wall[10] and favors platelet activation. Most importantly, the influence of the severity of vascular injury on thrombus formation has been demonstrated in perfusion chamber experiments[9] in which different tissue substrates were exposed to blood at various shear rates. With type II vascular injury, platelet deposition and thrombus formation may occur, but the phenomenon is usually transient; with type III injury, platelet aggregation is considerably increased, leading to fixation of thrombus and persistent vascular occlusion.

CLINICAL CORRELATIONS OF VASCULAR INJURY AND THROMBOSIS

The concepts of vascular injury and thrombosis are important in the understanding of the pathogenesis of various vascular diseases, including the initiation and progression of atherosclerosis, the acute coronary syndromes, vein graft disease, and restenosis following coronary angioplasty.

INITIATION AND PROGRESSION OF ATHEROSCLEROSIS. The process of type I vascular injury followed by intermittent deposition of few platelets and monocytes, lipid accumulation, smooth muscle cell proliferation, and resultant plaque formation represents the prevalent view of the initiation of spontaneous atherogenesis.[187] However, the precise nature of the injury remains unknown; that is, whether it is the turbulence of blood flow that injures the endothelium or whether it is injured from inside the vessel wall by means of toxic lipids (oxidized cholesterol) is controversial.

Accumulating evidence suggests that repetitive type II injury of soft fatty plaques (see later in section on acute coronary syndromes) with thrombus formation and incorporation represents a major mechanism for the progression of atherosclerosis.[188,189] In an autopsy study[190] of coronary arteries of 129 patients with atheromatous disease who died of noncardiac causes, Davies and co-workers demonstrated that 16% of the arteries studied revealed the presence of fissure in atherosclerotic plaque (type II injury) and, in some cases, overlying thrombi. This degree of frequency of plaque fissure (type II injury) in a static patho-

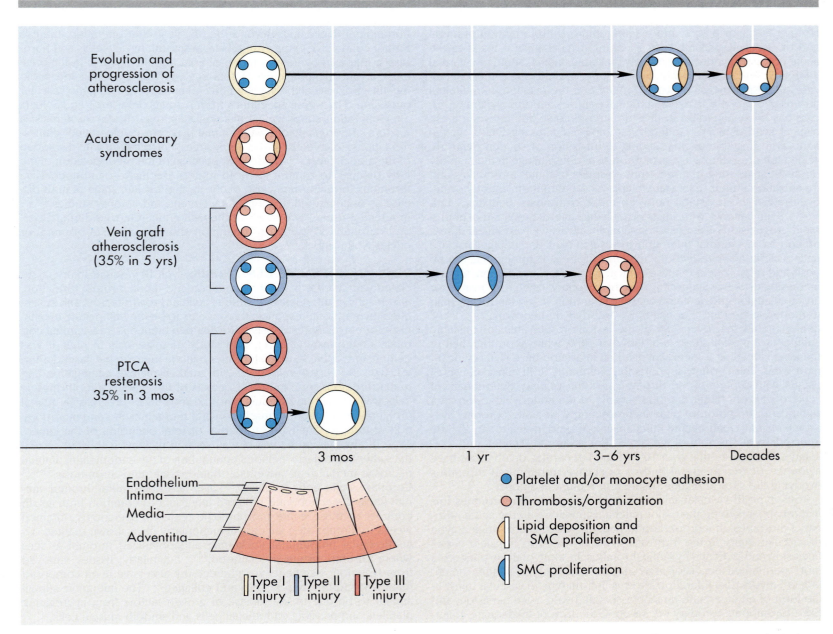

FIGURE 20.6 The role of vascular injury and various cellular interactions in the pathogenesis of atherosclerosis, acute coronary syndromes, acute and chronic vein graft occlusion, and PTCA restenosis. (PTCA, percutaneous transluminal coronary angioplasty; SMC, smooth muscle cells)

logic evaluation probably suggests that a single plaque may undergo many fissures, with subsequent thrombus formation and organization, during the evolution and progression into an advanced lesion. Indeed, analysis of coronary trees in patients dying of ischemic heart disease showed morphologic appearance consistent with previously healed fissures with various stages of thrombus incorporation and organization to be almost ubiquitous and suggest that most fissures probably reseal with incorporation of overlying thrombus without manifestation of clinical symptoms.[8,189] Further evidence for supporting thrombosis and thrombus incorporation as part of plaque progression is provided by a study using monoclonal antibodies in identifying fibrin, fibrinogen, and fibrin(ogen) degradation products.[191] It was demonstrated that in advanced fibrous plaque, fibrin and fibrin-related products were detected in the intima, neointima, and subintima and even in the deeper medial layer, especially around thrombus, collagen, and smooth muscle cells; on the other hand, these fibrin and fibrin-related products were found in small quantities in early lesions and normal arteries. Although it is as yet unknown how prevalent this process is, its clinical significance is potentially enormous because mural thrombi in the region of fissures may be prevented by platelet inhibitors or anticoagulant agents.

ACUTE CORONARY SYNDROMES. Pathologic,[8,192] angioscopic,[193] and angiographic[194,195] data have firmly established that type III vascular injury—major plaque and plaque rupture, with formation of mural and or occlusive thrombus as a common mechanism—leads to the acute coronary syndromes, namely, unstable angina, acute myocardial infarction, and sudden death. In addition, accumulating evidence indicates that the process of type III injury and the resulting intraluminal thrombotic process is dynamic and repetitive, and this dynamic process has been suggested to provide a physiologic link between these clinical syndromes.[7,196] Indeed, pathologic studies by Falk[192] in patients with unstable angina leading to infarction or sudden death revealed the presence of layers of thrombi of different age in the majority of cases, suggesting that recurrent episodes of mural thrombosis and organization, rather than a single episode of abrupt thrombotic event, occurred in the transition between these syndromes. Similarly, studies[195,197] in patients with unstable angina have demonstrated both a rapid progression of stenosis angiographically as well as clinical deterioration to myocardial infarction in a significant percentage of these patients. This again reflects the dynamic process of intraluminal thrombosis and organization in these clinical syndromes. In addition, there is increasing evidence suggesting that the coronary lesion responsible for unstable angina and acute myocardial infarction is frequently only mild to moderate stenotic. For example, Ambrose and co-workers[195,197,198] demonstrated that over 70% of the lesions responsible for unstable angina have a prior stenosis of less than 50%, while about one half of the lesions leading to acute myocardial infarction have nonsignificant narrowing. This strongly supports the fact that type III injury of a small plaque with superimposed thrombosis is the primary determinant of acute occlusion, rather than the severity of the underlying lesion, in a significant proportion of patients presenting with acute coronary syndromes. Similar pathogenic mechanisms of sudden death can also be inferred from the pathologic data. For example, Davies and colleagues[190] reported that over 70% of sudden cardiac death cases have evidence of recent mural and/or occlusive intraluminal thrombus overlying the sites of plaque fissure and rupture at autopsy.

Thus, type III vascular injury—plaque rupture—with thrombus formation appears to be the major mechanism leading to the acute coronary syndromes. In a proportion of patients with unstable angina, type III vascular injury in the form of fissure may lead to transient vessel occlusion and ischemia by labile thrombus; in some of these patients, a more permanent occlusion may lead to infarction or sudden death. Indeed, myocardial infarction may result from type III vascular injury in the form of an ulcer, and thus be associated with more persistent and fixed thrombotic coronary occlusion in the face of inadequate collateral flow. In addition, spontaneous or pharmacologic lysis of thrombus occurs in some patients, placing them at high risk of reocclusion.[7,196] Why a plaque ruptures, then leading to the growing of the atherosclerotic plaque or acute coronary syndromes, is unclear. Thus far, it appears that small plaques that rupture are soft because they have a high content of fat (vulnerable plaques); in addition they contain numerous macrophages, which favors the formation of an abscess.[7,199]

VEIN GRAFT DISEASE. Vascular injury also appears to be the critical initiating event in coronary vein graft disease. Vein grafts are subject to mechanical injury, which may occur when the veins are harvested and by handling during the operation, resulting in a transient predominantly type III injury; this injury may lead to acute thrombotic occlusion, but in most cases the vessel wall heals quickly.[200,201] With the exposure of the vein grafts to a relatively high pressure flow and the presence of various biologic risk factors such as hypercholesterolemia and smoking, this may induce and perpetuate type II injury and hinder the process of reendothelialization, which might otherwise occur under normal conditions. During the first postoperative year, the most notable and consistent histologic change in the vein graft is marked intimal thickening characterized by smooth muscle cell proliferation and an increase in hyaline matrix.[201] Lie and associates[202] reported that even within 3 weeks after the operation, smooth muscle cells appear in the subendothelial portion of the intima, followed by proliferation and fibrointimal thickening. Beyond the first year after operation, there is further connective tissue synthesis from smooth muscle cells and fibroblasts, followed by incorporation of lipid into the lesions. In the presence of various biologic risk factors, such as hyperlipidemia and smoking, this process can be accelerated and enhanced, leading to vascular occlusion. Thus, graft specimens from patients between 1 and 5 years after operation show typical histologic features of atherosclerosis: a mixture of fibrous plaque with intimal hyperplasia, ulceration, cholesterol clefts, foam cells, and in some areas, calcification with disruption of the medial layer.[203] In addition, because of the predisposition of the fatty plaques to rupture (type III injury), occlusive or nonocclusive thrombus formation may also occur during this late stage of graft disease as documented in surgical specimens and autopsy studies.[202,203] In a recent report, two thirds of the vein grafts removed during a second coronary artery bypass operation showed evidence of mural or occlusive thrombus.[204]

POST ANGIOPLASTY RESTENOSIS. Type III vascular injury, associated with intense platelet aggregation and mural thrombi formation, also results in the release of various cellular growth factors and subsequent hyperplastic response; this appears to be the pathogenic mechanism for coronary restenosis following percutaneous transluminal coronary angioplasty (PTCA). In a study of restenosis in pigs, it was demonstrated that immediately after balloon injury to the carotid arteries, type III injury was induced with marked platelet aggregation and mural thrombus formation.[205] Necrosis of the medial smooth muscle cells was evident at 24 hours, and the process of progressive intimal proliferation of smooth muscle cell and reorganization and incorporation of thrombi finally led to partial or total occlusion of the lumen. Type III changes in the vessel wall seen in patients who died several days after angioplasty included denudation of the endothelium, intimal necrosis, medial tear, adventitial hemorrhage, and thrombosis.[206-208] Coronary angioscopy studies[209,210] also described mural thrombi, intimal flaps, dissection, and ruptured atheroma as common findings. In contrast to these acute morphologic features, specimens obtained weeks to months after successful angioplasty have shown marked circumferential fibrointimal thickening and organized thrombi at sites where chronic restenosis occurred.[206-208] Similarly, tissues removed from restenotic segments via atherectomy also have been composed mainly of smooth muscle cells and collagen.[211] The mitogenic stimuli appear to be due to the release of growth factors from aggregating platelets and possibly endothelial cells and smooth muscle cells.

CARDIAC CHAMBERS: PREDOMINANCE OF FIBRIN COMPONENT

Intracavitary mural thrombi develop frequently in patients with acute myocardial infarction, chronic left ventricular aneurysm, dilated cardiomyopathy, and atrial fibrillation. The pathogenesis of thrombosis may be outlined along the lines established more than a century ago by the pathologist Rudolf Virchow, who defined a triad of precipitating factors: (1) endothelial injury, (2) a zone of circulatory stasis, and (3) a hypercoagulable state.[212] In addition to these factors, the clinical significance derives from the potential for systemic embolism, which also depends on dynamic forces of the circulation.

ENDOTHELIAL INJURY

In the first few days after acute myocardial infarction, leukocytic infiltration separates endothelial cells from their basal lamina.[213] The resulting exposure of subendothelial tissue to intracavitary blood serves as the nidus for thrombus development. Specific endocardial abnormalities have also been identified histologically in surgical and postmortem specimens from patients with left ventricular aneurysms[214] and at autopsy in patients with idiopathic dilated cardiomyopathy.[215]

BLOOD STASIS

Both experimental[216] and clinical studies[217,218] have emphasized the importance of wall motion abnormalities in the development of left ventricular thrombi, and it seems clear that stasis of blood in regions of akinesis or dyskinesis is the essential factor. Similarly, stasis is important in the development of atrial thrombi,[219] when effective mechanical atrial activity is impaired, as occurs in atrial fibrillation, atrial enlargement, mitral stenosis, and cardiac failure. Stasis is paramount to conditions of low shear rate, in which activation of the coagulation system rather than of platelets leads to fibrin formation and constitutes the predominant pathogenetic mechanism in the development of intracavitary thrombi (see Fig. 20.1).

HYPERCOAGULABLE STATE

One study of patients with acute myocardial infarction found a significantly greater incidence of thromboembolism in cases of elevated serum fibrinogen levels,[220] suggesting a hypercoagulable tendency in this condition. Although this limb of Virchow's triad is controversial, it is conceivable that a systemic procoagulant tendency arises during the acute stage of myocardial infarction and predisposes to thromboembolic events. More relevant is experimental evidence that suggests that the surface of a fresh thrombus is itself highly thrombogenic, producing, at least, a local if not a systemic hypercoagulable state.[7]

DYNAMIC FORCES OF THE CIRCULATION

The problems of thromboembolism originating from the cardiac chambers prompt consideration of the balance between the effects of regional injury, stasis, and procoagulant factors, which favor thrombus formation, and dynamic forces of the circulation, which are responsible for the migration of thrombotic material into the systemic circulation. Even though stasis favors thrombus formation within the sac of a left ventricular aneurysm, isolation from dynamic circulatory forces protects against embolic migration.[221,222] In diffusely dilated cardiomyopathy, on the other hand, mural thrombus is not isolated from the circulation and the embolic risk is higher. Thus, factors leading to thrombus formation are not the same as those that produce systemic embolism, and this paradox must not be neglected in the selection of therapeutic options.

PROSTHETIC VALVES: FIBRIN AND PLATELETS

MECHANICAL PROSTHESIS

Once circulation is restored after implantation of a prosthetic cardiac valve, platelet deposition begins almost immediately both on the prosthetic surface itself-particular on the endocardium-suture-prosthesis interfaces—and on damaged perivalvular tissues.[223,224] The prosthetic surface area exposed to the circulation is the major factor leading not only to platelet deposition but, more importantly, to activation of factor XII, initiating the coagulation cascade.[225] In addition, the flow stasis and abnormal hemodynamic characteristic of the prosthetic devices promote mainly fibrin generation and, less importantly, platelet activation (see Fig. 20.1). Finally, the process of fibrin thrombus formation can be facilitated in areas with stasis and decreased blood flow, such as in the left atrium during atrial fibrillation and in the left ventricle during low cardiac output state secondary to left ventricular dysfunction.

BIOLOGIC PROSTHESIS

Bioprosthetic valves are considerably less thrombogenic,[226] mainly because of the natural or biologic properties of the material used in their construction and also because of their characteristic axial flow profile, leaflet pliability, and cyclic sinusoidal washout.[227]

ROLE OF ANTITHROMBOTIC THERAPY IN CARDIAC DISEASE

We established in the foregoing sections the importance of pathogenesis at the site of thrombosis: platelet and fibrin components in arterial disease, predominance of fibrin in cardiac chambers, and predominance of fibrin over platelet component in prosthetic valves. We can also classify the various clinical heart disease syndromes according to absolute and relative risk of developing thromboembolic events (Table 20.4).[228] We shall discuss three general risk categories: the highest involving more than six episodes per 100 patients per year, a medium risk range of 2% to 6% annually, and a lower risk rate of less than two events per 100 patients per year. Persons without overt evidence of heart disease have a comparable annual event rate below 1%. The concept of pathogenesis and the concept of risk stratification are conclusive toward the therapeutic role and intensity of the various antithrombotic strategies in preventing thromboembolism in coronary arteries, cardiac chambers, and prosthetic heart valves.

CORONARY ARTERIES
ACUTE CORONARY SYNDROMES

Type III vascular injury with recurrent thrombosis is the major mechanism linking the acute coronary syndromes. During the early phase of the acute coronary syndromes of unstable angina and acute myocardial infarction, the risk of developing thrombotic occlusion (or reocclusion after vessel reperfusion) is substantial, varying between 5% and 20%.[168] This high risk of thrombotic occlusion or reocclusion makes antithrombotic therapy mandatory in patients with unstable angina and myocardial infarction.

UNSTABLE ANGINA. There have been three large, randomized, placebo-controlled, double-blind studies of aspirin in unstable angina. In the Veterans Administration Cooperative Study,[34] 1266 men with unstable angina were randomized to buffered aspirin (324 mg/day) or placebo for 12 weeks. During the treatment period, the incidence of death and acute myocardial infarction was reduced from 10.1% to 5.0% in the treated group (P = 0.0005). More importantly, the benefits of aspirin were maintained in the 1 year followup period. No increase in the gastrointestinal side effects were seen. In the Canadian Multicenter trial,[35] 555 patients (73% men) with unstable angina were randomized to receive aspirin (1,300 mg/day), sulfinpyrazone (800 mg/day), a combination of both, or placebo. After 2 years, the incidence of death and myocardial infarction was reduced in the aspirin-treated groups from 17% to 8.6%, a risk reduction of 51% (P = 0.008). Sulfinpyrazone conferred no benefit and did not interact with aspirin. Gastrointestinal side effects were more frequently seen in the aspirin-treated groups, probably related to the high dosages used.

In the recently published Montreal Heart Institute Study,[229] 479 patients with unstable angina were randomized to aspirin (325 mg twice daily), intravenous heparin, a combination of both, or placebo. The study was ended after a mean of 6 days, when a final therapeutic decision for the individual patient was made. Aspirin significantly reduced the rate of myocardial infarction, by 72% compared with placebo. Further support for the use of antiplatelet agents in unstable angina comes from the recently completed Italian Study of Ticolpidine in Unstable Angina (STAI).[82] Preliminary evidence from this study showed that the ticlopidine, at a dose of 250 mg twice daily for 6 months, reduced the incidence of mortality and myocardial infarction by greater than 50%.

ANTICOAGULANTS. Evidence of the beneficial effects of heparin in unstable angina was suggested by Telford and Wilson,[230] who demonstrated an 80% reduction in the incidence of myocardial infarction in patients with unstable angina treated with heparin for 7 days. Deficiencies in patient recruitment, however, left the conclusions of this study less convincing. The strongest support for immdiate anticoagulation in unstable angina comes from the Montreal Heart Institute Study.[229] Heparin decreased the rate of infarction by 89% and the incidence of refractory angina by 50%. Although no statistically significant difference among aspirin, heparin, or their combination was found, there was a trend favoring heparin over aspirin.

There is already strong evidence supporting the use of either intravenous heparin or aspirin in the management of patients with unstable angina beginning as soon as after onset. Because a substantial proportion of these patients develops myocardial infarction despite treatment with one agent or the other, there is a pressing need to test combinations of low-dose aspirin and heparin in larger clinical trials. Indeed, preliminary reports from a randomized, placebo-controlled trial in patients with unstable angina demonstrated the combination use of intravenous heparin and aspirin significantly reduced the risk of myocardial infarction during the followup period of 90 days.[230a] Further clinical trials and longer term followup are needed to confirm the beneficial effects. Otherwise, beyond the acute phase, we recommend aspirin in a dose of 325 mg/day.

THROMBOLYTIC THERAPY. The role of thrombolytic therapy in unstable angina is uncertain.[231] As of the time of this writing, there are nine reported studies using thrombolytic therapy in patients with unstable angina. All nine studies[232-240] were small, containing 5 to 41 patients, and the data were inconclusive. As yet, there is no consensus on which patients with unstable angina will have clinical or angiographic benefit from thrombolytic therapy. Part of the problem in reaching a consensus is that these studies have differed in patient populations, timing of angiography after episodes of rest pain, baseline medications, dose, route and duration of thrombolytic therapy, angiographic endpoints, and use of control groups for analysis of clinical outcome after thrombolytic therapy. More importantly, significant differences in coronary substrates leading to unstable angina as compared with those leading to acute myocardial infarction probably explain why the success in thrombolytic therapy in myocardial infarction cannot be duplicated in unstable angina.[231] First, of patients present with an acute myocardial infarction with ST segment elevation, 70% to 90% have total occlusion

TABLE 20.4 EMERGING ANTITHROMBOTIC APPROACH TO CARDIAC DISEASE BASED ON PATHOGENESIS AND THROMBOEMBOLIC RISK

Pathogenesis	Thromboembolic Risk		
	High (>6% per year)	*Medium (2%–6% per year)*	*Low (<2% per year)*
Arterial System	Unstable angina Acute MI MI: after thrombolysis PTCA: early phase SVBG: early phase	Chronic stable angina Chronic phase after MI PTCA: chronic phase SVBG: chronic phase	Primary prevention of cardiovascular disease
Platelets = Fibrin	Platelet inhibitor plus anticoagulant*	Platelet inhibitor or anticoagulant (INR 2.0–3.0)†	Platelet inhibitor‡
Cardiac Chambers	A-fib: prior embolism A-fib: mitral stenosis	A-fib: other forms of organic heart disease Early phase after anterior MI Dilated cardiomyopathy	A-fib: idiopathic Chronic LV aneurysm
Fibrin > Platelets	Anticoagulant (INR 3.0–4.5 in prior embolism or 2.0–3.0 in mitral stenosis)	Anticoagulant (INR 2.0–3.0) Platelet inhibitor	Usually no need for therapy
Prosthetic Valves	Old mechanical prostheses Mechanical prostheses: prior embolism	Recent mechanical prostheses Bioprostheses: A-fib	Bioprostheses: normal sinus rhythm
Fibrin > Platelets	Anticoagulant (INR 3.0–4.5) plus platelet inhibitor	Anticoagulant (INR 3.0–4.5 in mechanical prostheses or 2.0–3.0 in bioprostheses)	Usually no need for therapy

MI, myocardial infarction; PTCA, percutaneous transluminal coronary angioplasty; SVBG, saphenous vein bypass graft; INR, international normalized ratio of prothrombin suppression; A-fib, atrial fibrillation; LV, left ventricular

* Heparin may be used in acute phase (APTT: 1.5–2.0 × control)

† Although both are beneficial, platelet inhibitor therapy is recommended based on lower toxicity, cost, and ease of administration.

‡ Only to be considered for persons at high risk for coronary disease.

of the infarct-related artery on angiography. In unstable angina, the frequency of total occlusion of the ischemic-related artery is significantly less and as low as 8%.[197] Second, the thrombus formation in unstable angina develops slowly after type III injury and much of the thrombus present in these lesions may be partially organized by the time of clinical presentation. This partial organization may explain the pathologic finding by Falk,[192] who showed layering of thrombus in most of the patients who died after an episode of unstable angina. Therefore, in such patients only small amounts of thrombus would be present and amenable to thrombolysis. In addition, thrombus formation in patients with unstable angina may occur not within the lumen but beneath the fibrous cap of the plaque. Moreover, after type III injury, there may be a geometric change in the shape of the plaque without significant intraluminal thrombus formation. In both situations, little thrombus would be available for thrombolysis.[231] Finally, the extent of type III injury in unstable angina is probably less than in acute myocardial infarction and may thus result in a smaller amount of intraluminal thrombus formation.[231]

Thus, at present, the data are insufficient to reach a definite conclusion. The future of thrombolysis in unstable angina is dependent on the results of large randomized trials similar to those in acute myocardial infarction. Both angiographic and clinical trials are required to assess the efficacy. The risks and benefits of thrombolysis will also need to be determined.

ACUTE MYOCARDIAL INFARCTION. As in unstable angina, type III vascular injury and superimposed thrombotic occlusion play major roles in the development of acute myocardial infarction.[8] In some patients, particularly those with non–Q wave infarction, spontaneous early vessel reperfusion occurs as a result of thrombus lysis or resolution of vasospasm, limiting myocardial necrosis[241,242] but setting the stage for subsequent ischemic events. The more extensive necrosis, which occurs in Q wave infarction, probably results from persistent thrombotic coronary occlusion in the face of inadequate collateral flow. In addition, because spontaneous vessel recanalization seems to occur in both non–Q and Q wave infarction, an aggressive antithrombotic approach using thrombolytic agents and antithrombotic drugs to these patients is beginning to emerge for achieving both successful lysis and the prevention of thrombotic reocclusion.

THROMBOLYTIC THERAPY AND RETHROMBOSIS. The use of thrombolytic therapy in acute myocardial infarction is discussed in a separate chapter. We therefore will concentrate on one of the major problems we face currently in patients following successful thrombolytic therapy: rethrombosis.

Reocclusion after successful recanalization is a frequent problem that precludes improvement in left ventricular function and increases mortality.[243] Serial coronary angiography is necessary before, during, and after therapy to assess the reperfusion of the artery. Thus, few studies have systemically determined the incidence of reocclusion. Some studies have defined nonangiographic clinical reperfusion and reocclusion, which is unreliable because of spasm or silent reocclusion with or without collaterals. In this context, early reocclusion is defined as the angiographic closure of a reperfused or patent artery within the first 24 hours of thrombolytic therapy and late occlusion as angiographic closure usually assessed just before hospital discharge. The rate of early reocclusion is quite variable[243]; it ranges from 0% to 45% and usually is 6% to 18%. Late reocclusion ranges from 11% to 24%. Both processes are due to rethrombosis, which in turn appears to depend on two main factors[243]: (1) the pathologic substrate, namely, type III vascular injury with exposure of collagen and lipid gruel and the thrombogenic surface of the residual thrombus on the atherosclerotic plaque, and (2) the rheologic factors or the increase in shear rate and turbulent flow created by the residual stenosis.[9-11]

As discussed in the previous section, type III vascular injury with the exposure of various thrombotic elements creates a strong stimulus for thrombosis. Potent thrombotic stimuli include the release of tissue thromboplastin, depletion of factors that inhibit tissue factor, and the activation of platelets by collagen, fatty gruel, and smooth muscle cells.[7,243] In addition, deep medial structures such as the fibrillar collagen can activate the coagulation system. The intrinsic pathway is activated by the negatively charged collagen, while the extrinsic pathway is activated by the thromboplastin released from the damaged tissue. This leads to mural thrombosis. Furthermore, during lysis (endogenous or exogenous) there is release of active thrombin from within the dissolving thrombus and activation of platelets by the active surface of the thrombus. Thus, theoretically, the use of both an antiplatelet agent and an anticoagulant following thrombolysis appears to be advisable.

Thus, prevention of reocclusion requires inhibition of mechanisms involved in rethrombosis and includes two basic principles: (1) thorough lysis and (2) antithrombotic therapy. The first principle involves the use of the newer generation of, and synergistic combination of, thrombolytic agents. This area is under active investigation. Preliminary results with scu-PA[182-184] seem to be promising, especially in reducing the reocclusion rate. In addition, studies using a combined infusion of rt-PA and urokinase[183] appear to reduce the reocclusion rate as compared with that of rt-PA alone. Similarly, the use of streptokinase and half the usual dose of rt-PA revealed a late reocclusion rate of only 6%.[143,144] However, the data are still insufficient to conclude which combinations will provide the best therapeutic results; large randomized clinical trials are currently underway. The role of antiplatelet therapy and anticoagulant is discussed below.

ANTIPLATELET THERAPY. The strongest evidence supporting the use of platelet inhibitors in the acute stage of myocardial infarction comes from the recently published Second International Study of Infarct Survival (ISIS-2).[36] Patients with suspected myocardial infarction treated within 24 hours had a 23% reduction in 5-week vascular mortality compared with those given placebo. This dramatic benefit was possibly related to prevention of reinfarction in patients with spontaneous vessel recanalization. Indeed, aspirin reduced the rate of nonfatal reinfarction by almost half.[36]

As discussed previously, patients with acute myocardial infarction treated with thrombolytic agents are at high risk of early reocclusion, which approaches 5% to 20%.[244] The importance of concomitant platelet inhibitor therapy in patients undergoing thrombolysis was emphasized by the results of the ISIS-2 trial,[36] in which streptokinase alone decreased early cardiovascular mortality by 25%, while the combination of aspirin and streptokinase decreased the death rate by 42% compared with placebo. The benefits of these agents appeared independent of one another, and the addition of aspirin to streptokinase reduced the clinical reinfarction rate by 50%. Thus, we advocate aspirin (160–325 mg daily) as early as possible in the treatment of acute myocardial infarction, whether or not thrombolytic agents are given. Daily aspirin therapy should be continued on discharge.

ANTICOAGULANT THERAPY. The role of anticoagulants in patients with acute infarction for the prevention of coronary rethrombosis, infarct extension, and death has not been settled. Of the large number of studies conducted, only three randomized trials[245-247] have been large enough to be able to detect a significant effect of therapy. Although all three studies showed a beneficial trend toward reduced incidence of death and reinfarction, only the Bronx Municipal Hospital trial[246] found a significant reduction (30%) in the case fatility rate. In addition, anticoagulation therapy has been clearly shown to reduce pulmonary and systemic embolism after myocardial infarction.[245-247] When the results of the only six published randomized trials were pooled,[248] a significant 21% reduction in mortality in treated patients emerged. Despite the limitation inherent in retrospective meta-analysis of heterogeneous trials, short-term anticoagulation in acute myocardial infarction appears to provide a modest reduction in early mortality. Because of the high risk of reinfarction, however, the combination of aspirin and an anticoagulant may prove beneficial and deserves clinical testing. The role of heparin in patients with acute myocardial infarction treated with thrombolytic therapy is unresolved. The preliminary report from the International TPA versus Streptokinase Mortality Trial, which involved more than 20,000 patients, demonstrated no significant improvement in mortality and reinfarction rate in patients treated with both thrombolytic therapy and high-dose subcutaneous heparin compared to patients treated with thrombolytic therapy only. In addition, the bleeding complication was significantly higher in the heparin group. The administration of heparin subcutaneously began 12 hours after thrombolysis, however, so it is possible adequate anticoagulation was not achieved during the acute period of clot lysis. Thus, given the marked thrombogenicity of residual thrombus following vessel recanalization, and while awaiting results of further clinical trials, heparin therapy is sensible for a period of 3 to 7 days after thrombolysis.[249]

CHRONIC PHASE AFTER MYOCARDIAL INFARCTION

Survivors of acute myocardial infarction are at medium risk of recurrent infarction or cardiac death.[250] Because cardiac morbidity and mortality during the period may be related to a number of factors, including left ventricular dysfunction, ventricular arrhythmias, and recurrent myocardial infarction, proving that antithrombotic therapy is beneficial in these patients has been difficult and has generated controversy for several decades.

PLATELET INHIBITORS. With respect to the use of antiplatelet agents for secondary prevention of vascular events, no less than 10 randomized, placebo-controlled, double-blind trials in postmyocardial infarction patients have been conducted.[38] Despite the large total number of patients studied (>17,000), no clear evidence of benefit from therapy was shown in any single study. Reduction in cardiac mortality rate varied from 12% to 57%. An extensive meta-analysis of these studies was recently published.[38] Despite the inherent problems of pooled data, this overview concluded that among survivors of myocardial infarction, platelet inhibitors reduced vascular mortality by 13%, nonfatal reinfarction by 31%, nonfatal stroke by 42%, and all important vascular events by 25%. Aspirin alone was at least as effective as the combination of aspirin and dipyridamole and more effective than sulfinpyrazone. Available data do not justify the additional cost and frequency of administration of drugs other than aspirin in this group of patients.[38]

ANTICOAGULANTS. Numerous studies have assessed the usefulness of long-term anticoagulation in the secondary prevention of cardiovascular disease after myocardial infarction, but only four randomized controlled trials[249-252] were large enough to be able to detect a significant effect from therapy. Only one study[252] showed a trend toward lower case-fatality rate; all suggested a reduction in reinfarction of 25% to 50%, but it was statistically significant in one trial. A pooled analysis[253] of nine trials of anticoagulation in postinfarction patients showed that this therapy decreased overall mortality by about 20%. However, because not all trials were properly controlled, the conclusion of this collective analysis must be interpreted with caution. Emerging evidence from a Norwegian trial[254] supports the use of warfarin after myocardial infarction for the prevention of reinfarction and reduction of mortality.

Considering the above data, the evidence supporting the use of aspirin in the secondary prevention of cardiovascular morbidity and mortality beyond the acute phase of myocardial infarction is at least as strong as that supporting anticoagulation. At a daily dose of 325 mg, aspirin offers several advantages over long-term anticoagulants in cost, ease of administration, and side effects. Thus, to survivors of myocardial infarction, daily aspirin is recommended.

CHRONIC STABLE CORONARY ARTERY DISEASE

Patients with a remote history of myocardial infarction (beyond 2 years) and those with chronic stable angina are at medium risk of coronary ischemic events, which varied between 2.5% and 5% per year.[250] In patients with remote myocardial infarction, recurrent thrombotic events are probably the main cause of mortality. Most studies of platelet inhibitors in survivors of myocardial infarction have shown a beneficial trend toward lower mortality and reinfarction, which became significant only when the data derived from all available trials were pooled.[38]

For anticoagulant therapy, in the Sixty-Plus Reinfarction Study,[255] patients older than 60 and treated for a median of 6 years with warfarin after myocardial infarction were randomly assigned to continue anticoagulant or substitute placebo. The design was double blinded, and anticoagulant dosage was tightly controlled for a period of 2 more years, at which point anticoagulated patients had a 26% lower mortality rate ($P = 0.07$) and 55% lower incidence of reinfarction ($P = 0.0005$) when compared with patients treated with placebo. It appears, therefore, that both aspirin and anticoagulants are effective in prevention of reinfarction and reduction in mortality in asymptomatic patients after remote myocardial infarction, but the former is associated with lower cost and risk.

Although no randomized trial of antithrombotic therapy in chronic stable angina has been published, the sustained beneficial effects of aspirin after initial therapy for patients with unstable angina suggest a role for aspirin in stable coronary disease.[34,35] A dose of 325 mg daily is associated with minimal gastrointestinal toxicity and should be considered in these patients.

PRIMARY PREVENTION OF CORONARY EVENTS

Results from a double-blind, placebo-controlled trial[37] of more than 22,000 male physicians in the United States assigned to receive aspirin (325 mg every other day) for 5 years revealed a 44% reduction in the incidence of myocardial infarction from approximately 0.4% to 0.2% per year ($P = <0.00001$). Before advising the widespread use of aspirin in apparently healthy people, three issues need to be addressed. First, there was a slight increase in the incidence of hemorrhagic stroke in the aspirin-treated group. Secondly, in a randomized British primary prevention trial[256] involving more than 5,000 male physicians, the use of aspirin (500 mg/day) did not reduce the rate of myocardial infarction, but did increase the incidence of disabling stroke. Finally, the long-term effects of aspirin blockade of the prostaglandin system in various tissues, particularly the central nervous system, are unknown.

Even though these studies were done in healthy volunteers and, admittedly, their conclusions should be applied only to "healthy individuals," the increased incidence of hemorrhagic stroke is disconcerting. Aspirin therefore should be recommended for primary prevention only to individuals at high risk for coronary artery disease, those for whom the benefits of therapy outweigh its risks. Further analysis of the United States Physicians' Health Study[257] suggests that aspirin exerts a greater impact on patients at higher risk for coronary events, namely those with cardiovascular risk factors or evidence of cerebral or peripheral vascular disease.

PROGRESSION OF ATHEROSCLEROSIS

As discussed earlier, repetitive type II injury of soft fatty plaques with thrombus formation and incorporation represents a major mechanism for the progression of atherosclerosis.[188,189] This concept is based on the pathologic finding of old, organized coronary thrombi difficult to distinguish from atherosclerotic changes in the arterial wall. A more recent study[191] demonstrated the presence of fibrinogen, fibrin, and their degradation products in areas of advanced atherosclerotic plaques. On the basis of these observations, recurrent episodes of plaque disruption and thrombosis may lead not necessarily to acute ischemic syndromes but to progressive narrowing of the coronary arteries. Although it is still unclear how prevalent this process is, its clinical significance is enormous because thrombotic episodes may be prevented by platelet inhibitors or anticoagulants. In this context, a 5-year trial of platelet-inhibitor therapy in the angiographic progression of coronary disease in patients with stable angina was recently completed at the Mayo Clinic. Preliminary evidence suggests that platelet inhibitors reduce the incidence of myocardial infarction and new lesion formation.[258]

CORONARY INTERVENTIONS

VEIN GRAFT DISEASE FOLLOWING BYPASS SURGERY. Coronary vein graft disease is the most important contributor to cardiac mortality and morbidity after coronary artery surgery. Occlusion rates are 8% to 18% per distal anastomosis at 1 month postoperatively, and 16% to 26% at 1 year. At the end of 5 years, up to 35% of vein grafts will be occluded.[200,201] Vein graft disease can be divided into 3 stages: an early postoperative stage of thrombotic occlusion related to type III injury; a second stage of intimal hyperplasia that occurs within the first year and is probably due to repetitive type II injury, platelet aggregation, and mitogen release. Beyond the first year, lipid accumulation, further smooth-muscle cell proliferation, and thrombus incorporation resembling that of spontaneous atherosclerosis, constitute the final stage of atheroma formation.[200,201]

EARLY GRAFT OCCLUSION. As discussed in previous sections, early occlusion seems to be related to a type III vascular injury caused by surgical manipulation and exposure of the graft to high rates of arterial blood flow.[200] This process is mainly thrombotic in origin, and platelets play a major pathogenetic role. Antithrombotic therapy is most effective in reducing the rate of early postoperative thrombotic occlusion.

PLATELET INHIBITORS. Several trials[259-261] have documented that aspirin, with or without dipyridamole, or ticlopidine reduces the incidence of early vein graft occlusion. Antiplatelet therapy should be instituted preoperatively or in the immediate postoperative period, because benefit is lost if therapy is initiated more than 3 days after surgery. Administration of aspirin before surgery carries the risk of increased postoperative bleeding,[261] so we prescribe dipyridamole preoperatively, followed by aspirin alone (325 mg daily) beginning immediately after surgery. Whether the addition of preoperative dipyridamole offers any real value over postoperative aspirin alone is unknown. Because extracorporeal circulation activates the coagulation system and platelets, the routine use of heparin intraoperatively may be important in the prevention of thrombus formation and early graft occlusion. Thus, the combination of intraoperative heparin and perioperative platelet inhibitor drugs effectively reduces the incidence of graft occlusion in this high-risk population.

ANTICOAGULANTS. Two studies[262,263] have addressed the effect of anticoagulation on vein graft patency. In one,[262] there was a trend toward higher patency rate with warfarin, started 3 to 4 days postoperatively. In another,[263] this drug offered no advantage over placebo. These studies were compromised by incomplete angiographic follow-up, small sample size, or late implementation of antithrombotic therapy. Although no comparative studies have been published, it is difficult to advocate the use of anticoagulants because of the impressive success of aspirin after saphenous vein graft surgery.

LATE GRAFT OCCLUSION. The beneficial effect of antiplatelet therapy is less apparent, however, in late graft occlusion as a different pathologic process supervenes. This process includes smooth muscle cell proliferation, lipid accumulation, and recurrent thrombus formation and organization, a process similar to that of spontaneous atherosclerosis.[200] Although the beneficial effects of antiplatelet agents in reducing late occlusion are less striking, these patients are at a medium risk of developing thrombotic and ischemic events and long-term aspirin therapy appears sensible.

CORONARY ANGIOPLASTY. Coronary angioplasty has been an important alternative to surgical revascularization in suitable patients with coronary artery disease since its introduction by Andreas Gruntzig in 1977,[264] and its use has been greatly expanded in the last few years. Despite improvement in equipment and technique, however, acute reocclusion after successful angioplasty occurs in about 5% of patients, whereas late restenosis, generally within 3 to 6 months, occurs in 25% to 35% of patients.[185,265] As discussed in previous sections, acute occlusion appears to be secondary to a type III vascular injury with resultant thrombus formation, while the process of late restenosis is due to intimal hyperplasia and thrombus organization.

ACUTE OCCLUSION. Several studies[266-269] have clearly shown that pretreatment of patients with aspirin, aspirin plus dipyridamole, or ticlopidine (all in association with heparin) significantly reduces the rate of acute thrombotic complications after angioplasty. The role of heparin alone in prevention of acute vessel occlusion during angioplasty has not been properly tested clinically, but there is experimental evidence that suggests an inverse relation between the dose of heparin and both platelet deposition and mural thrombosis.[270] In addition, uncontrolled preliminary studies in patients with unstable angina have demonstrated that pretreatment with heparin for 1 to 8 days reduces the incidence of acute thrombotic occlusion during and after angioplasty.[271-273] Therefore, high-dose heparin is widely used during this intervention. Given the substantial risk of acute thrombotic complication associated with angioplasty, pretreatment with aspirin combined with adequate heparization throughout the procedure is strongly recommended. The angiographic appearance of intraluminal thrombus or vessel dissection usually dictates the duration of heparin therapy on completion of the procedure.

LATE RESTENOSIS. The effects of antithrombotic therapy on late restenosis have been disappointing. Clinical trials[267-269] using different platelet-inhibiting regimens have shown no impact on the restenotic rate. Similarly, anticoagulation with heparin[274] or warfarin[275] was of no benefit when compared with aspirin. However, long-term aspirin therapy is recommended to these patients, on the basis of favorable experience in chronic coronary artery disease for secondary prevention of ischemic complications.[258]

CARDIAC CHAMBERS
ATRIAL FIBRILLATION

Systemic embolism is a common and potentially devastating complication of atrial fibrillation associated with both mitral valve disease and certain other forms of organic heart disease. Blood stasis appears to play a predominant pathogenetic role in thrombus formation in patients with atrial fibrillation. Patients at highest risk are those with a history of systemic embolism in the previous 2 years; in this group, the embolic risk approaches 10% to 20% in the first 1 or 2 years.[276] Although no prospective randomized trials of anticoagulants are available, the current recommendation is for long-term anticoagulant therapy aimed at prolonging prothrombin time to one and one-half to two times control (standard INR of prothrombin suppression 3.0–4.5) in these patients.

Patients at somewhat lower but nevertheless substantial risk of embolism (which approaches 6% per year) are those with atrial fibrillation associated with mitral stenosis. Data from numerous nonrandomized and uncontrolled trials have suggested that anticoagulation reduces the rates of embolism and death in patients with rheumatic valvular disease by 25%.[277] Based on known embolic risk and on results of clinical trials, chronic anticoagulation to prolong prothrombin time to one and one-third to one and one-half times control (INR 2.0–3.0) is recommended for these patients. In addition, patients with uncontrolled hyperthyroidism and heart failure appear to be at increased risk of embolism.[277] Although anticoagulation in these patients has not been evaluated by prospective randomized trials, this therapy is recommended until the patients become euthyroid and reversion to sinus rhythm has been achieved.

At the lower end of the spectrum of embolic risk in patients with atrial fibrillation are those without evidence of associated organic heart disease. The natural history of lone atrial fibrillation was addressed by the Framingham investigators,[278] who followed 30 of these patients for more than 10 years and found a fourfold increase in the incidence of stroke as compared with matched controls. Aside from the small sample size, other limitations of the analysis were the relatively advanced age of the subjects (mean, 70 years) and the inclusion of patients with hypertension. In another study,[279] 97 normotensive patients younger than 60 years with lone atrial fibrillation were followed for a mean of 17 years at the Mayo Clinic. Anticoagulants were used in just a few subjects. Only eight embolic events were identified, an overall incidence well below 1% per year. These data suggest that for patients younger than 60 years with atrial fibrillation but no evidence of organic heart disease, the hazards of chronic anticoagulation outweigh its potential benefits.

Between these two poles exists a large group of patients with an intermediate but incompletely defined risk of embolism: those with nonvalvular atrial fibrillation associated with various forms of cardiovascular disease. The embolic risk in these patients lies between 4% and 6% per year[276,280] and accounts for almost one half of cardioembolic strokes. Given the severe functional deficits that often follow embolic stroke and the fact that these events are usually unheralded by warning signs, preventive therapy is the only rational approach. In a retrospective study at the Montreal Heart Institute,[280] nonanticoagulated patients had a incidence of systemic embolism of 5.5% per year, whereas anticoagulated patients had a significantly lower embolic rate of 0.7% per year.

In a recently completed Danish trial,[281] patients with nonvalvular atrial fibrillation were randomized to receive warfarin, aspirin, or placebo. The total incidence of stroke and transient ischemic attacks was reduced nearly 75% with warfarin adjusted to maintain the prothrombin time to 1.5 to 2 times control (INR 3.0–4.5). The incidence of severe and fatal stroke, however, was similar in both treatment groups. This study suggests that chronic anticoagulation with warfarin may be beneficial for prevention of embolic stroke in patients with constant, nonvalvular atrial fibrillation, although a high proportion of anticoagulated patients were withdrawn from active treatment. The warfarin dose used in this trial was higher than the one recommended by a consensus of investigators,[277] who proposed that prolonging the prothrombin time to one and one-third to one and one-half times control (INR 2.0–3.0) is sufficient for patients without prior history of embolism. In the Danish trial,[281] no advantage of aspirin over placebo for embolism prevention was identified. Although the results of this study support the use of warfarin, the differentiation of subgroups in the broad category of nonvalvular atrial fibrillation that stand to gain most from anticoagulation remained to be accomplished.

ACUTE MYOCARDIAL INFARCTION

Approximately one third of patients with acute anterior myocardial infarction and less than 5% of those with inferior infarction develop left ventricular mural thrombi.[282] These thrombi tend to occur in the first week and particularly in the first 2 days. Thrombi are more likely to form in cases of large infarcts (peak serum creatine kinase > 2,000 units/liter). Systemic embolism, which occurs in about 10% of cases in which left ventricular thrombi are echocardiographically apparent, is the most important complication, affecting 2% to 5% of victims of myocardial infarction.[282] Echocardiographically, thrombi that protrude into the left ventricular cavity and have increased mobility are more likely to embolize than those without these characteristics.[282]

Because the incidence of embolism is highest in the first 1 to 3 months after myocardial infarction and short-term anticoagulation has been demonstrated to reduce the embolic rate by 25% to 75%,[245-247] the following approach is recommended: Patients with increased embolic risk, namely, those with large anterior infarcts, congestive heart failure, or atrial fibrillation, should receive heparin on admission (aimed at prolonging the APTT to one and one-half to two times control). A study by Turpie and colleagues[283] demonstrated that high-dose subcutaneous heparin (12,500 units every 12 hours) significantly reduced the incidence of mural thrombosis in patients with anterior infarcts as compared with low-dose heparin (5,000 units twice daily). Heparin therapy may be followed by warfarin to prolong the prothrombin time to 1.3 to 1.5 times control (INR 2.0–3.0) in patients with echocardiographic evidence of mural thrombi or large akinetic regions. Warfarin may be stopped after 1 to 3 months unless there is the risk of heart failure or impaired left ventricular function or persistent echocardiographic evidence of mural thrombi. The optimal duration of anticoagulation in this group has not been determined.

CHRONIC LEFT VENTRICULAR ANEURYSM

In contrast to the prevalence of thromboembolism in acute myocardial infarction, the incidence of embolism in chronic left ventricular aneurysm is significantly lower (0.35% per year).[284] The reason for this difference is probably twofold. First, thrombi formed after acute myocardial infarction are usually mobile, are friable, and protrude into the ventricular cavity, whereas thrombi in chronic aneurysms are laminated and more adherent to the endocardium.[214,282] Second, thrombi located within an aneurysmal sac, which is devoid of contractile fibers, are less prone to propulsion into the left ventricular outflow tract.[222] Although some investigators have found a persistent risk of embolism in postinfarction patients, it was not the presence of an aneurysm but rather the mobility and protrusion of thrombus that predicted embolic events. Given available data, patients with remote infarction and chronic left ventricular aneurysm are at low risk of embolism and need not receive anticoagulants. Whether these drugs should be given to patients with echocardiographic evidence of mobile and protruding thrombi, however, remains to be established.

DILATED CARDIOMYOPATHY

Pathologic studies[215] have found a high prevalence of right and left ventricular mural thrombi in patients with idiopathic dilated cardiomyopathy. Blood stasis and low shear rate present in a dilated, hypocontractile ventricle lead to activation of coagulation processes. Because the mural thrombus is not mechanically isolated, as occurs in a ventricular aneurysm, embolism of thrombotic materials may occur. In a retrospective study,[285] patients treated with anticoagulants had no evidence of systemic embolism, whereas those not anticoagulated had an embolic rate of 3.5% per year. Lacking any prospective trial of antithrombotic therapy in these patients at medium risk for embolism, this evidence supports chronic warfarin administration,[285] particularly in those with overt heart failure or atrial fibrillation.

PROSTHETIC VALVES
MECHANICAL PROSTHESES

Prosthetic surfaces are thrombogenic by virtue of their ability to activate both the intrinsic coagulation system and platelets. Increased shear rate, blood stasis (particularly in high-profile prosthetic devices), and associated disturbances of the cardiac chambers predispose to thromboembolism.[225] Patients with history of embolism and valves manufactured before the mid 1970s are at highest risk, which exceeds six events per 100 patients per year.[226,227] Atrial fibrillation and left ventricular thrombus contribute additional risk. Patients with newer mechanical valves have a risk of thromboembolism that ranges between 1% and 5% per year despite anticoagulation.

ANTICOAGULANTS. Warfarin, at a dose sufficient to prolong the prothrombin time to one and one-half to two times control (INR 3.0–4.5), is the most important agent for prevention of thromboembolism.[226,286] Studies in patients with mechanical prostheses have consistently shown that anticoagulation significantly reduces the incidence of valvular thrombosis and embolism.[227,286] In fact, inadequate anticoagulation increases the thromboembolic risk twofold to sixfold,[226,227] whereas excessive anticoagulation (prothrombin time more than two and one-half times control) increases the risk of bleeding complications fourfold to eightfold.

ANTICOAGULANTS PLUS PLATELET INHIBITORS. Platelet inhibitors alone have not been found to confer protection against embolism in patients with mechanical prostheses. Indeed, studies of aspirin plus dipyridamole in these patients have shown an incidence of thromboembolism as high as 10% per year.[287,288] Patients with mechanical valves treated with warfarin had significantly fewer thromboembolic events compared with those treated with aspirin combined with either dipyridamole or pentoxifylline.[288] It seems clear, therefore, that patients with mechanical prostheses should receive anticoagulant therapy indefinitely, aimed at a prothrombin time of one and one-half to two times control (INR 3.0–4.5).[226,286] However, the addition of a platelet inhibitor such as dipyridamole (300–400 mg daily) to warfarin may reduce the thromboembolic risk below that of warfarin alone. Indeed, the antithrombotic effects of dipyridamole are more evident on prosthetic materials such as artificial heart valves than on biologic surfaces; in patients with mechanical prostheses, the combination of warfarin and aspirin is questionable and, in addition, the risk of gastrointestinal bleeding is increased when aspirin is given in daily doses of 500 mg or more.[226] Therefore, we suggest supplementing warfarin with dipyridamole (300–400 mg/day) in patients with mechanical valves and prior embolism and in those with older prosthetic devices. In patients who are intolerant of dipyridamole, the addition of sulfinpyrazone (800 mg/day in four divided doses) to warfarin therapy may be recommended.[226] This therapy is empirically based, since no randomized prospective trial has been carried out; uncontrolled studies, however, do suggest that the agent is effective; the prothrombin time, which may be prolonged by sulfinpyrazone, should be checked frequently after such therapy is started.

BIOLOGICAL PROSTHESES

Although bioprosthetic valves are less thrombogenic than mechanical valves, thromboembolism may occur with an incidence of two to three per 100 patients per year, particularly in the first 3 months after surgery, and more often in those patients with mitral than aortic prostheses and in those with atrial fibrillation or prior embolism.[226,227,286] Patients with mitral bioprostheses should receive warfarin postoperatively, aimed at a prothrombin time of one and one-third to one and one-half times control (INR 2.0–3.0) for 1 to 3 months, unless atrial fibrillation persists, in which case warfarin should be used indefinitely.[226,286] Although aortic bioprostheses are associated with a lower incidence of embolism, the concomitant presence of atrial fibrillation may warrant the use of chronic warfarin therapy in these patients as well.

Patients who maintain normal sinus rhythm postoperatively without left ventricular dysfunction or prior embolism are at low risk. In these patients there may be no need for sustained anticoagulant therapy. This is particularly true for patients with aortic bioprostheses, in whom even platelet inhibitor may be unnecessary.[226,286] No randomized, controlled studies of platelet inhibitors in patients with bioprostheses have been reported. In an uncontrolled trial, long-term aspirin therapy was associated with a low incidence of embolism in these patients.

SPECIAL SITUATIONS

Four special situations should be considered in prescribing anticoagulant therapy for patients with prosthetic heart valves[226]: noncardiac surgery, prosthetic valve endocarditis, anticoagulation after a thromboembolic event, and anticoagulation during pregnancy.

NONCARDIAC SURGERY. Temporary discontinuation of anticoagulation for 7 to 10 days appears to be of minimal risk for patients undergoing a noncardiac operation. To keep this risk to a minimum and unless contraindicated, however, it is recommended to discontinue the warfarin 4 to 5 days before operation and to start heparin administration (to maintain the activated partial thromboplastin time at two times control, and dipyridamole 300 to 400 mg/day). The heparin infusion should be continued 4 to 5 hours before the operation. Subcutaneous heparin (15,00 units/day given in two or three divided doses) can be considered during and early after operation. Warfarin therapy should be restarted as soon as safe after the operation.

PROSTHETIC VALVE ENDOCARDITIS. Of patients with prosthetic valve endocarditis who are not receiving anticoagulant therapy, thromboembolism to the central nervous system occurs in about 50%. Three nonrandomized clinical trials[289–291] in patients with prosthetic valve endocarditis who were receiving anticoagulant therapy suggest that the thromboembolic rate can be decreased six-to ninefold with adequate anticoagulation. It should be noted, however, that the risk of intracranial hemorrhage is substantial and may approach 14%.[290,291] Although the benefits and the risks of anticoagulation in patients with native or bioprosthetic valve endocarditis are not well defined, it is currently recommended that anticoagulant therapy not be given to patients with uncomplicated infective endocarditis involving a native valve or a bioprosthetic valve in patients with normal sinus rhythm. This is based on the increased incidence of hemorrhage in these patients and the lack of demonstrated efficacy and anticoagulance in this setting.

ANTICOAGULATION AFTER THROMBOEMBOLIC EVENT. The appropriate time to start anticoagulation after thromboembolism to the brain has been controversial. A second embolism can occur early after the initial event, so that immediate anticoagulation appears rational. Caution should be exercised, however, because anecdotal reports and experimental studies suggest that immediate anticoagulation, especially in patients with a large embolic infarct, can result in secondary hemorrhage with increased morbidity. Data from 15 prospective and retrospective studies[292] suggest that approximately 12% of patients with aseptic embolism to the brain from a cardiac source experience a second embolic event within 2 weeks. Immediate anticoagulation with heparin appears to decrease the risk of recurrent embolism. Several nonrandomized studies suggested that there was a reduction in early recurrent embolism within 14 days to about one-third of that in patients who did not receive anticoagulation.[292]

There are wide variations in the reported risk of symptomatic brain hemorrhage after immediate anticoagulation for embolic stroke. One group of studies showed no hemorrhage worsening in 162 patients who received anticoagulation immediately, but others have reported hemorrhage worsening in 1% to 24% of these patients.[292] A lack of reporting about the details of anticoagulant administration does not allow analysis of these discrepant results.

Patients with a large infarct appear to be at greater risk of hemorrhagic worsening after immediate anticoagulation of embolic stroke. Spontaneous hemorrhagic transformation may be delayed for several days, but appears most likely to occur within 48 hours. Thus, it is recommended that immediate anticoagulation be started in patients who are nonhypertensive and have small and moderately sized embolic strokes in whom a CT scan of the head can be done within 48 hours after the stroke to exclude hemorrhagic transformation. The same principles appear to apply for the continuation of anticoagulant therapy in patients with a prosthetic valve who experience an embolic stroke during long-term anticoagulant therapy. Because patients with a large embolic infarct or severe hypertension appear to be at special risk for delayed hemorrhagic transformation, anticoagulation should be postponed for 5 to 7 days. This allows time to document that a repeat tomographic scan of the head does not show hemorrhagic transformation. In patients with hemorrhagic complications, anticoagulation should be postponed 8 to 10 days.

ANTITHROMBOTIC THERAPY DURING PREGNANCY. For pregnant patients with prosthetic heart valves, the use of heparin and oral anticoagulation is problematic because neither the safety of oral anticoagulant therapy during pregnancy nor the efficacy of heparin therapy for prophylaxis of systemic embolism is established. Patient education is critical for women of childbearing age who have a prosthetic cardiac valve. Ideally pregnancy should be well planned and the regimen of anticoagulant therapy should be modified to avoid the teratogenic effects of warfarin, since fetal wastage is approximately 60% in women who receive warfarin therapy at the time of conception and during the first trimester. In addition, warfarin exposure in the first trimester and possibly thereafter may predispose to congenital anomalies, especially nasal hypoplasia, stippling of bones, mental retardation, optic atrophy, and microcephally. Furthermore, because the coumarin derivative cross the placental barrier, hemorrhagic complications can occur in the fetus, especially at the time of delivery. In contrast, heparin does not cross the placental barrier.

Two approaches have been recommended: The first is to use heparin therapy throughout pregnancy, administered every 12 hours by subcutaneous injection in doses adjusted to keep APTT at 1½ times control. This regimen should be continued until 1 week before delivery when the patients should be hospitalized and switched to heparin infusion, which is continued until the induction of labor. Since the beneficial effect of subcutaneous heparin with mechanical prosthetic valves during pregnancy is not fully proven, however, a bioprosthetic heart valve is preferred for women of childbearing age, because many of them do not need chronic anticoagulation. Nevertheless, the risk of bioprosthetic calcification and need for reoperation in very young women has to be kept in mind.

The second approach is to use heparin until the 13th week, change to warfarin until the middle of the third trimester, then restart heparin therapy until delivery. Although the latter approach might avoid warfarin embryopathy, other fetopathic effects (e.g., central nervous system abnormalities) are still possible. Before this approach is recommended, therefore, the potential risks should be explained to the patient. In addition, the use of warfarin at any time during pregnancy carries significant medicolegal implications, because the manufacturer explicitly states that warfarin usage in pregnancy is contraindicated. Thus, this approach is not recommended in the United States.

Antiplatelet agents should be avoided during pregnancy because aspirin may cause premature closure of the ductus arteriosus, and dipyridamole and sulfinpyrazone have indeterminate effects on the fetus and are not approved for use during pregnancy. In addition, platelet-inhibitor drugs do not appear to offer significant protection against thromboembolism during pregnancy.

In summary, activation of the coagulation system and, secondarily, of platelets occurs in patients with prosthetic valves. For those at high risk, combination of anticoagulation and a platelet inhibitor is suggested. Medium-risk patients can be managed with an anticoagulant alone and those at low risk may not require antithrombotic treatment.

CONCLUSIONS

An approach to antithrombotic therapy in various cardiovascular diseases has emerged based on the evolving concept of vascular injury and thrombosis, and with the knowledge of pathophysiology and an appreciation of differential clinical features determining morbid risk. The essential parameters of this approach form the framework of Table 20.4.

In the arterial circulation, type II and III injury leads to both platelet activation and production of thrombin and fibrin, suggesting a combined therapeutic approach with a platelet inhibitor, an anticoagulant, or a combination of both (acutely and short term). The propensity to thrombosis determines the intensity of antithrombotic therapy. High-risk patients with unstable angina and evolving acute myocardial infarction should be treated aggressively with a platelet inhibitor and perhaps acutely with an anticoagulant as well, although the final recommendation awaits the results of several ongoing clinical trials. Patients undergoing coronary angioplasty or saphenous bypass surgery should receive platelet inhibitors and adequate anticoagulation during the procedure. Coronary disease patients are at more moderate risk in the chronic phase of stable angina, post myocardial infarction, of angioplasty, and of bypass surgery; such patients are best managed with a platelet inhibitor rather than an anticoagulant for reasons of convenience, safety, and economy. In low-risk patients in whom prevention of complications of atherosclerosis is desired, aspirin may be prescribed to those with certain risk factors, such as diabetes, family history, tobacco exposure, and hypercholesterolemia. However, a hint that long-term aspirin administration may be associated with an escalated chance of intracerebral hemorrhage militates against its indiscriminate use; furthermore, the long-term effects (benefits or risks) of aspirin therapy are unknown.

Within the cardiac chambers, stasis of blood flow causes coagulation to predominate over platelet activation as the principal mechanism of thrombus formation, and anticoagulant therapy alone seems most appropriate in management of these patients. At highest risk are patients with atrial fibrillation and prior embolism; at somewhat lower but yet substantial risk are those patients with atrial fibrillation associated with mitral stenosis or uncontrolled hyperthyroidism. In all of such patients at high risk, high-intensity anticoagulation is recommended. Patients at medium risk are those immediately after large anterior myocardial infarction and uncompensated dilated cardiomyopathy; for these patients, there is sufficient evidence to suggest the need for moderately intense chronic anticoagulation. Some patients with nonvalvulopathic atrial fibrillation associated with other forms of cardiac disease benefit from warfarin therapy, but subgroups in this population have not yet been identified. At lowest risk are patients with lone atrial fibrillation without overt heart disease and those with chronic left ventricular aneurysm in whom anticoagulants are not required.

The thrombogenicity of prosthetic heart valves involves both fibrin formation and, to a lesser extent, platelet activation and is considerably greater for mechanical than biologic devices. Patients at highest risk—those with older mechanical prostheses or prior embolism—should be treated with a combination of an anticoagulant and a platelet inhibitor; while either dipyridamole or, to a lesser extent, aspirin may be beneficial, dipyridamole has the advantage of not potentiating bleeding. At medium risk are patients with modern mechanical valves and those with bioprostheses in the presence of atrial fibrillation, who can be successfully managed with an anticoagulant alone. When bioprostheses are in place along with normal sinus rhythm, the embolic risk is low enough that antithrombotic therapy may not be needed.

Sections of this chapter are a modification of Antithrombotic Agents in Cardiac Disease: Platelet inhibitors, anticoagulants, and fibrinolytics. In Giuliani ER, Fuster V, Gersh B et al (eds): Cardiology: Fundamentals and Practice. Chicago, Year Book Medical Publishing, 1990. By permission of the Mayo Foundation.

REFERENCES

1. Fuster V, Chesebro JH: Current concepts of thrombogenesis: Role of platelets. Mayo Clin Proc 56:102, 1981
2. Baumgartner HR: The role of blood flow in platelet adhesion, fibrin deposition and formation of mural thrombi. Microvasc Res 5:167, 1973
3. Davies MJ, Thomas T: The pathological basis and microanatomy of occlusive coronary thrombi formation in human coronary arteries. Philos Trans Soc Lond 294:225, 1981
4. Fuster V, Chesebro JH: Pharmacologic effects of platelet-inhibitor drugs. Mayo Clin Proc 56:185, 1981
5. Fuster V, Chesebro JH: Role of platelet-inhibitor drugs in the management of arterial thromboembolic and atherosclerotic disease. Mayo Clin Proc 56:265, 1981
6. Hawiger J: Formation and regulation of platelet and fibrin hemostatic plug. Hum Pathol 18:111, 1987
7. Fuster V, Badimon L, Cohen M et al: Insights into the pathogenesis of acute ischemic syndromes. Circulation 77:1213, 1988
8. Davies MJ, Thomas AC: Plaque fissuring—the cause of acute myocardial infarction, sudden ischemic death and crescendo angina. Br Heart J 53:363, 1985
9. Badimon L, Badimon JJ, Galvez A et al: Influence of arterial damage and wall shear rate on platelet deposition: *Ex vivo* study in a swine model. Arteriosclerosis 6:312, 1986

10. Badimon L, Badimon JJ: Mechanism of arterial thrombosis in nonparallel streamlines; platelet thrombi grew on the apex of stenotic severely injured vessel wall: Experimental study in the pig model. J Clin Invest 84:1134, 1989
11. Lindon JN, Collins REC, Coe NP et al: In vivo assessment in sheep of thromboresistant materials by determination of platelet survival. Circ Res 46:83, 1971
12. Stein B, Fuster V, Israel DH et al: Platelet inhibitor agents in cardiovascular disease: An update. J Am Coll Cardiol 14:813, 1989
13. Peerschke EB: The platelet fibrinogen receptor. Semin Hematol 22:241, 1985
14. Shattil SJ, Brass LP: Induction of the fibrinogen receptor on human platelets by intracellular mediators. J Biol Chem 262:992, 1987
15. Coller BS: Activator effects access to the platelet receptor for adhesive glycoproteins. J Cell Biol 103:451, 1986
16. Moncada S, Vane JR: Arachidonic acid metabolite and the interactions between platelet and vessel wall. N Engl J Med 300:1142, 1979
17. Verstraete M, Vermylen J: Cellular, chemical and rheological factors in thrombosis and fibrinolysis. In Thrombosis, pp 1–54. New York, Pergamon Press, 1985
18. Fuster V, Chesebro JH, Frye RL et al: Platelet survival and the development of coronary artery disease in the young: The effects of cigarette smoking, strong family history, and medical therapy. Circulation 63:546, 1981
19. Moncada S, Gryglewski R, Bunting S et al: An enzyme isolated from arteries transforms prostaglandin endoperoxides to an unstable substance that inhibits platelet aggregation. Nature 263:1976
20. Dyerberg J, Bang HO, Stoffersen E et al: Eicosapentaenoic acid and prevention of thrombosis and atherosclerosis. Lancet 2:117, 1978
21. Kromhout D, Bosschieter EB, Coulander CDL: The inverse relation between fish consumption and 20-year mortality from coronary heart disease. N Engl J Med 312:1205, 1985
22. McNeely TB, Griffith MJ: The anticoagulant mechanism of actin of heparin in contact-activated plasma: Inhibition of factor X activation. Blood 65:1226, 1985
23. Egeberg O: Inherited antithrombin deficiency causing thrombophilia. Thromb Haemost 13:516, 1965
24. van Hinsberg VWM, Bertina RM, van Wijingaraden A et al: Activated protein C decreases plasminogen activator-inhibitor activity in endothelial cell conditioned media. Blood 65:444, 1985
25. Collen D: On the regulation and control of fibrinolysis. Thromb Haemost 43:77, 1980
26. Erikson LA, Ginsberg MH, Loskutoff DJ: Detection and partial characterization of an inhibitor of plasminogen activator in human platelets. J Clin Invest 74:1465, 1984
27. Minuro J, Schleef RR, Loskutoff DJ: Extracellular matrix of cultured bovine aortic endothelial cells contain functionally active type 1 plasminogen activator inhibitor. Blood 70:721, 1987
28. Griffin JH, Evatt B, Zimmerman TS et al: Deficiency of protein C in congenital thrombotic disease. J Clin Invest 68:1370, 1981
29. Dreyer NA, Pizzo SV: Blood coagulation and idiopathic thromboembolism among fertile women. Contraception 22:123, 1980
30. Tschopp TB: Aspirin inhibits platelet aggregation, but not adhesion to, collagen fibrils: An assessment of platelet adhesion and platelet deposited mass by morphometry and ^{51}Cr-labelling. Thromb Res 11:619, 1977
31. Clowes AW, Karnovsky MJ: Failure of certain antiplatelet drugs to affect myointimal thickening following arterial endothelial injury in the rat. Lab Invest 36:452, 1977
32. Roth GL, Majerus PW: The mechanism of the effects of aspirin on human platelets: I. Acetylation of a particulate fraction protein. J Clin Invest 56:624, 1975
33. Kyrle PA, Eichler HG, Jagh V, Lechner K: Inhibition of prostacyclin and thromboxane A_2 generation by low-dose aspirin at the site of plug formation in man in vivo. Circulation 75:1025, 1987
34. Lewis HD, Davies JW, Archibald DG et al: Protective effects of aspirin against acute myocardial infarction and death in man with unstable angina, results of a Veterans Administration Cooperative Study. N Engl J Med 309:396, 1983
35. Cairns JA, Gent M, Singer J et al: Aspirin, sulfinpyrazone, or both in unstable angina. N Engl J Med 313:1369, 1985
36. ISIS-2 (Second International Study of Infarct Survival) Collaborative Group: Randomized trial of intravenous streptokinase, oral aspirin, both or neither among 17,187 cases of suspected acute myocardial infarction: ISIS-2. Lancet 2:349, 1988
37. Final report of the aspirin component of the ongoing Physician Health Study. N Engl J Med 321:129, 1989
38. Antiplatelet Trialists' Collaborative: Secondary prevention of vascular disease by prolonged antiplatelet treatment. Br Med J 296:320, 1988
39. Graham DY, Smith LJ: Aspirin and the stomach. Ann Intern Med 104:390, 1986
40. Ali M, Zamecnik J, Cerskus AL et al: Synthesis of thromboxane A_2 and prostaglandins by bovine gastric mucosa microsomes. Prostaglandins 14:819, 1977
41. MacKerchner PA, Ivery KL, Baskin WN et al: Protective effects of cimetidine on aspirin-induced gastric mucosal damage. Ann Intern Med 87:676, 1977
42. UK-TIA Study Group: United Kingdom Transient Ischemic Attack (UK-TIA) aspirin trial: Interim result. Br Med J 296:316, 1988
43. Neri Serneri GG, Castellani S: Platelet and vascular prostaglandins: Pharmacological and clinical implication. In Born GVR, Neri Serneri GG (eds): Antiplatelet Therapy, Twenty Years' Experience, pp 37–51. Amsterdam, Elsevier, 1987
44. Friedman PL, Brown EJ, Gunther S et al: Coronary vasoconstrictor effect of indomethacin in patients with coronary artery disease. N Engl J Med 305:1171, 1981
45. Kromhout D, Bosschieter EB, Coulander CDL et al: The inverse relation between fish consumption and 20-year mortality from coronary heart disease. N Engl J Med 312:1205, 1985
46. Shekelle RB, Missel L, Paul O et al: Letter: Fish consumption and mortality from coronary heart disease. N Engl J Med 313:549, 1985
47. Von Schacky C: Prophylaxis of atherosclerosis with marine omega-3 fatty acids: A comprehensive strategy. Ann Intern Med 107:890, 1987
48. Leaf A, Weber PC: Cardiovascular effects of n-3 fatty acids. N Engl J Med 318:549, 1988
49. Fitzgerald GA, Reilly LA, Perderson AK: The biochemical pharmacology of thromboxane synthetase inhibition in man. Circulation 72:1194, 1985
50. Mullane KM, Fornabaio D: Thromboxane synthetase inhibitors reduce infarct size by a platelet-dependent, aspirin-sensitive mechanism. Circ Res 62:668, 1988
51. Rueben SR, Kuan P, Cairns T, Gysle OH: Effects of dazoxiben and exercise performance in chronic stable angina. Br J Clin Pharmacol 15(Suppl):83, 1983
52. Thaulow E, Dale J, Myhre E: Effects of a selective thromboxane synthetase inhibitor, dazoxiben, and of acetylsalicylic acid on myocardial ischemia in patients with coronary artery disease. Am J Cardiol 53:1255, 1984
53. Saussy DL Jr, Mais DE, Knapp DR et al: Thromboxane A_2 and prostaglandin endoperoxide receptors in platelets and vascular smooth muscle. Circulation 72:1202, 1985
54. Gresele P, Van Houtte E, Arnout J et al: Thromboxane synthetase inhibition combined with thromboxane receptor blockade: A step forward in antithrombotic therapy. Thromb Haemost 52:364, 1984
55. Moncada S, Korbut R: Dipyridamole and other phosphodiesterase inhibitors act as antithrombotic agents by potentiating endogenous prostacyclin. Lancet 1:1286, 1978
56. Crutchley DJ, Ryan US, Ryan JW: Effects of aspirin and dipyridamole on the degradation of adenosine diphosphate by cultured cells derived from bovine pulmonary artery. J Clin Invest 66:29, 1980
57. Fitzgerald GA: Dipyridamole. N Engl J Med 316:1247, 1987
58. Harker LA, Slichter SJ: Studies of platelet and fibrinogen kinetics in patients with prosthetic heart valves. N Engl J Med 283:1302, 1970
59. Weily HS, Steele PP, Davies H et al: Platelet survival in patients with substitute heart valves. N Engl J Med 290:534, 1974
60. Hanson SR, Harker LA, Bjornsson TD: Effects of platelet-modifying drugs of arterial thromboembolism in baboons: Aspirin potentiates the antithrombotic effects of dipyridamole and sulfinpyrazone by mechanisms independent of platelet cyclo-oxygenase inhibition. J Clin Invest 75:1591, 1985
61. The Persantine-Aspirin Reinfarction Study Group: Persantine and aspirin in coronary artery disease. Circulation 62:449, 1980
62. Bousser MG, Eschwege E, Haugenau M et al: "AICLA" controlled trial of aspirin and dipyridamole in the secondary prevention of atherothrombotic cerebral ischemia. Stroke 14:5, 1983
63. American-Canadian Cooperative Study Group: Persantine–aspirin trial in cerebral ischemia: II. Endpoint results. Stroke 16:406, 1985
64. Brown BG, Cukingnan RA, DeRouen T et al: Improved graft patency in patients treated with platelet-inhibiting therapy after coronary bypass surgery. Circulation 72:138, 1985
65. Goldman S, Copeland J, Mortiz T et al: Improvement in early saphenous vein graft patency after coronary artery bypass surgery with antiplatelet therapy: Results of a Veterans Administration Cooperative Study. Circulation 77:1324, 1988
66. Sullivan JM, Harken DE, Gorlin R: Pharmacologic control of thromboembolic complications of cardiac valve replacement. N Engl J Med 284:1391, 1971
67. Kasahara T: Clinical effect of dipyridamole ingestion after prosthetic heart valve replacement—especially on the blood coagulation system. J Jpn Assoc Thorac Surg 25:1007, 1977
68. Groupe de Recherche PACTE: Prevention des accidents thromboemboliques systemiques chez les porteurs de prosthesis valvulaires artificielles: Essai cooperatif controle du dipyridamole. Coeur 9:915, 1978
69. Rajah SM, Sreeharan N, Joseph A et al: A prospective trial of dipyridamole and warfarin in heart valve patients (abstr). Acta Ther 6(Suppl 93):54, 1980
70. Chesebro JH, Fuster V, Elveback LR et al: Trial of combined warfarin plus dipyridamole or aspirin therapy in prosthetic heart valve replacement: Danger of aspirin compared with dipyridamole. Am J Cardiol 51:1537, 1983
71. Chesebro JH, Clements IP, Fuster V et al: A platelet-inhibitor drug trial in coronary artery bypass operation: Benefit of perioperative dipyridamole and aspirin therapy on early postoperative vein graft patency. N Engl J Med 307:73, 1982
72. Chesebro JH, Fuster V, Elveback LR et al: Effect of dipyridamole and aspirin

in late vein graft patency after coronary artery bypass surgery. N Engl J Med 310:209, 1984
73. Weksler BB: Prostaglandin and vascular function. Circulation 70(Suppl III):III-63, 1984
74. Coppe D, Sobel M, Seavans L et al: Preservation of platelet function and number by prostacyclin during cardiopulmonary bypass. J Thorac Cardiovasc Surg 81:274, 1981
75. Smith MC, Danviriyasup K, Crow JW et al: Prostacyclin substitution for heparin in long-term hemodialysis. Am J Med 81:274, 1982
76. Uchida Y, Hanai T, Hasewaga K et al: Recanalization of obstructed coronary artery by intracoronary administration of prostacyclin in patients with acute myocardial infarction. Adv Prostaglandin Thromboxane Leukotriene Res 11:377, 1983
77. Sharma B, Wyeth RP, Heinemann FM, Bissett JK: Addition of intracoronary prostaglandin E_1 to streptokinase improves thrombolysis and left ventricular function in acute myocardial infarction (abstr). J Am Coll Cardiol 11(Suppl A):104A, 1988
78. Fisher CA, Kappa JR, Sinha AK et al: Comparisons of equimolar concentrations of iloprost, prostacyclin, and prostaglandin E_1 on human platelet function. J Lab Clin Med 109:184, 1987
79. Raizner A, Hollman J, Demke D, Wakefield L: Beneficial effects of ciprostene in PTCA: A multicenter, randomized, controlled trial (abstr). Circulation 78(Suppl II):II-290, 1988
80. Lee H, Paton RC, Ruan C: The in vivo effect of ticlopidine on fibrinogen and factor VIII binding to human platelets (abstr). Thromb Haemost 46:67, 1981
81. O'Brien JR: Ticlopidine, a promise for the prevention and treatment of thrombosis and its complications. Haemostasis 13:1, 1983
82. Violi F, Scrutini D, Cimminielli C et al: STAI (Study of Ticlopidine in Unstable Angina) (abstr). J Am Coll Cardiol 13(Suppl A):238A, 1989
83. White CA, Chaitman B, Lasser TA et al: Antiplatelet agents are effective in reducing the immediate complications of PTCA: Results from the multicenter trial of ticlopidine (abstr). Circulation 76(Suppl IV):IV-400, 1987
84. Limet R, David JL, Magotteaux P et al: Prevention of aorto-coronary bypass graft occlusion. J Thorac Cardiovasc Surg 94:773, 1987
85. Gent M, Blakeley JA, Easton JD et al: The Canadian American Ticlopidine Study (CATS) in thromboembolic stroke. Lancet 1:1215, 1989
86. Hass WK, Easton JD, Adams HP et al: A randomized trial comparing ticlopidine hydrochloride with aspirin for the prevention of stroke in high risk patients. N Engl J Med 321:501, 1989
87. Kaegi A, Pineo GF, Shimizu A et al: Arteriovenous venous shunt thrombosis: Prevention by sulfinpyrazone. N Engl J Med 290:304, 1974
88. Steele PP, Rainwater J, Vogel R: Platelet suppressant therapy in patients with prosthetic heart valves: Relationship of clinical effectiveness to alteration of platelet survival time. Circulation 60:910, 1979
89. Report from the Anturane Reinfarction Italian Study: Sulfinpyrazone in post-myocardial infarction. N Engl J Med 290:304, 1974
90. Baur HR, Van Tassel RA, Pierach CA, Gobel RL: Effects of sulfinpyrazone on early graft occlusion after myocardial revascularization. Am J Cardiol 49:420, 1982
91. Canadian Cooperative Study Group: A randomized trial of aspirin and sulfinpyrazone in threatened stroke. N Engl J Med 299:53, 1978
92. Harker LA, Fuster V: Pharmacology of platelet inhibitors. J Am Coll Cardiol 8(Suppl B):21B, 1986
93. Oberg M, Hedner U, Bergentz SE: Effect of dextran 70 on factor VIII and platelet function in von Willebrand's disease. Thromb Res 12:629, 1978
94. Weiss HJ: The effect of clinical dextran on platelet aggregation, adhesion and ADP release in man: In vivo and in vitro studies. J Lab Clin Med 69:37, 1967
95. Swanson KT, Vlietstra RE, Holmes DR et al: Efficacy of adjunctive dextran during PTCA. Am J Cardiol 54:447, 1984
96. Brown RIG, Aldridge HE, Schwartz L et al: The use of dextran-40 during PTCA: A report of three cases of anaphylactoid reactions—one near fatal. Cathet Cardiovasc Diagn 11:591, 1985
97. Hanson SR, Harker LA: Interruption of acute platelet-dependent thrombosis by the synthetic antithrombin D-phenylalanyl-L-prolyl-L-arginyl-chloromethyl ketone. Proc Natl Acad Sci USA 85:3184, 1988
98. Heras M, Chesebro JH, Penny WJ et al: Effects of thrombin inhibition on the development of acute platelet–thrombus deposition during angioplasty in pigs. Circulation 79:657, 1989
99. Rosenberg RD: Biochemistry of heparin antithrombin interactions and the physiologic role of this natural anticoagulant mechanism. Am J Med 87:3, 1989
100. Yin ET: Effect of heparin on the neutralization of Factor Xa and thrombin by the plasma α_2 globulin inhibitor. Thromb Haemost 33:43, 1974
101. Wessler S: A Guide to Anticoagulant Therapy, pp 1–28. Washington, DC American Heart Association, 1984
102. Verstraete M, Vermylen J: Antithrombotic and fibrinolytic agents and substances which lower blood viscosity. In Thrombosis, pp 76–112. New York, Pergamon Press, 1985
103. Carter CJ, Kelton JG, Hirsh J et al: The relationship between the hemorrhagic and antithrombotic properties of low molecular weight heparin in rabbits. Blood 59:1239, 1982
104. Salzman EW, Rosenberg RD, Smith MH et al: Effect of heparin and heparin fractions on platelet aggregation. J Clin Invest 65:64, 1980

105. Samama B, Boissel JP, Combe-Tazali S, Leizorovicz A: Clinical studies with low molecular weight heparins in the prevention and treatment of venous thromboembolism. Ann NY Acad Sci 556:386, 1989
106. Wessler S, Gitel SN: Pharmacology of heparin and warfarin. J Am Coll Cardiol 8:10B, 1986
107. Basu D, Gallus A, Hirst J et al: A prospective study of the value of monitoring heparin treatment with the activated partial thromboplastin time. N Engl J Med 287:324, 1972
108. Schriever HG, Epstein SE, Mintz MD: Statistical correlation and heparin sensitivity of activated partial thromboplastin time, whole blood coagulation time and automated coagulation time. Am J Clin Pathol 60:323, 1973
109. Perkins HA, Osborn JJ, Hurt R et al: Neutralization of heparin in vivo with protamine: A simple method of estimating the required dose. J Lab Clin Med 48:223, 1956
110. Chiu HM, Hirsh J, Yung WL et al: Relationship between anticoagulant and antithrombotic effects of heparin in experimental venous thrombosis. Blood 49:171, 1977
111. Esposito RA, Culliford AT, Colvin SB et al: The role of the activated clotting time in heparin administration and neutralization for cardiopulmonary bypass. J Thorac Cardiovasc Surg 85:174, 1983
112. Ogilby JD, Kopelman HA, Klein LW, Agarwal JB: Adequate heparinization during PTCA: Assessment using activated clotting time. J Am Coll Cardiol 11:237A, 1988
113. Hirsch J: Pharmacology, monitoring and administration of heparin: Proceedings of the ACCP-NHLBI International Conference on Antithrombotic Therapy. Chest 89:26S, 1986
114. Salzman EW, Deykin D, Shapiro RM et al: Management of heparin therapy: Controlled prospective trial. N Engl J Med 292:1046, 1975
115. Glazier RL, Crowell EB: Randomized prospective trial of continuous vs intermittent heparin therapy. JAMA 236:1365, 1976
116. Salzman EW: Heparin for prophylaxis of venous thromboembolism. Ann NY Acad Sci 556:371, 1989
117. Kakkar VV: Current recommendations in prevention of thrombosis in surgery. Lancet 1:237, 1987
118. Gold EW: Prophylaxis of deep venous thromboembolism: Literature review. Orthopedics 11:1197, 1988
119. The SCATI Group: Randomized controlled trial of subcutaneous calcium-heparin in acute myocardial infarction. Lancet 2:182, 1989
120. Turpie AGG, Robinson JG, Doyle DJ et al: Comparison of high-dose with low-dose subcutaneous heparin to prevent left ventricular mural thrombosis in patients with acute transmural anterior myocardial infarction. N Engl J Med 320:352, 1989
121. Levine MN, Hirsh J, Kelton JG: Hemorrhagic complications of antithrombotic therapy. In Colman RW, Hirsh J, Marder VJ, Salzman EW (eds): Hemostasis and Thrombosis, Basic Principles and Clinical Practice, pp 873–885. Philadelphia, JB Lippincott, 1987
122. Miller ML: Heparin-induced thrombocytopenia. Cleve Clin J Med 56:483, 1989
123. Warkentin TE, Kelton JG: Heparin-induced thrombocytopenia. Annu Rev Med 40:31, 1989
124. Olson RE: Vitamin K. In Colman RW, Hirsh J, Marder VJ, Salzman EW (eds): Hemostasis and Thrombosis, Basic Principles and Clinical Practice, pp 846–860. Philadelphia, JB Lippincott, 1987
125. Batty JD, Breckenridge A, Lewis PJ et al: May mothers taking warfarin breast feed their infants? Br J Clin Pharmacol 3:969, 1976
126. O'Reilly RA, Aggeler PM: Studies on coumarin anticoagulant drugs: Initiation of warfarin therapy without a loading dose. Circulation 47:2657, 1968
127. Scott PJW: Anticoagulant drugs in the elderly: The risks usually outweigh the benefits. Br Med J 297:1261, 1988
128. Wintzen AR, deJonge H, Loeligar EA, Bots GTAM: The risk of intracerebral hemorrhage during oral anticoagulant treatment: A population study. Ann Neurol 16:553, 1984
129. Second Report of the Sixty Plus Reinfarction Study Research Group: Risks of long-term anticoagulant therapy in elderly patients after myocardial infarction. Lancet 1:64, 1982
130. Joglerkar M, Mohanaruban K, Bayer AJ, Pathy MSJ: Can old people on oral anticoagulants be safely managed as outpatients? Postgrad Med J 64:775, 1988
131. Lowe GD: Anticoagulant drugs in the elderly: Valuable in selected patients. Br Med J 297:1261, 1988
132. Hirsh J, Poller L, Deykin D et al: Optimal therapeutic range from oral anticoagulants. Chest 95:5S, 1989
133. Hull R, Hirsh J, Jay R et al: Different intensities of oral anticoagulant therapy in the treatment of proximal-vein thrombosis. N Engl J Med 307:1676, 1982
134. Levine MN, Raskob G, Hirsh J: Hemorrhagic complications of long-term anticoagulant therapy. Chest 95:26S, 1989
135. Salazar E, Zajarias A, Gutierrez N et al: The problem of cardiac valve prostheses, anticoagulants, and pregnancy. Circulation 70(Suppl I):I-69, 1984
136. O'Reilly RA: Vitamin K antagonists. In Colman RW, Hirsh J, Marder VJ, Salzman EW (eds): Hemostasis and Thrombosis, Basic Principles and Clinical Practice, pp 1367–1372. Philadelphia, JB Lippincott, 1987
137. Sareli P, England MJ, Berk MR et al: Maternal and fetal sequelae of anticoagulation during pregnancy in patients with mechanical heart valve prosthe-

ses. Am J Cardiol 63:1462, 1989
138. Howie PW: Anticoagulants in pregnancy. Clin Obstet Gynecol 13:349, 1986
139. McGehee WG, Klotz TA, Epstein DJ, Rappaport SI: Coumarin necrosis associated with hereditary protein C deficiency. Ann Intern Med 101:59, 1984
140. Feder W, Auerback R: "Purple toes": An uncommon sequela of oral coumarin drug therapy. Ann Intern Med 55:911, 1976
141. Kazmier FJ, Sheps SG, Bernatz PE et al: Livedo reticularis and digital infarcts: A syndrome due to cholesterol emboli arising from atheromatous abdominal aortic aneurysm. Vasc Dis 3:12, 1966
142. Bachman F: Fibrinolysis. In Verstrate M, Vermylen J, Lyner R, Arnout J (eds): Thrombosis and Haemostasis, pp 227–265. Leuven, Belgium, Leuven University Press, 1987
143. Collen D, Gold HK: Fibrin specific thrombolytic agents and new approaches to coronary arterial thrombolysis. In Julian D, Kubler W, Norris RM et al (eds): Thrombolysis in Cardiovascular Disease, pp 45–67. New York, Marcel Dekker, 1989
144. Collen D, Stump DC, Gold HK: Thrombolytic therapy. Ann Rev Med 39:405, 1988
145. Marder VT, Sherry S: Thrombolytic therapy: Current status: Part I. N Engl J Med 318:1512, 1988
146. Marder VT, Sherry S: Thrombolytic therapy: Current status: Part II. N Engl J Med 318:1585, 1988
147. Rentrop KP, Feit F, Blanke H et al: Effects of intracoronary streptokinase and intracoronary nitroglycerin on coronary angiographic patterns and mortality in patients with acute myocardial infarction. N Engl J Med 319:1457, 1984
148. Feldman RL, Crick WF, Conti CR, Pepine CJ: Quantitative coronary angiography during intracoronary streptokinase in acute myocardial infarction: How long to continue thrombolytic therapy. Cathet Cardiovasc Design 9:9, 1983
149. Simoons ML, Serruys PW, Band MVD et al: Improved survival after thrombolysis in acute myocardial infarction: A randomized trial conducted by the ICI in the Netherlands. Lancet 1:578, 1985
150. Rentrop KP: Thrombolytic therapy in patients with acute myocardial infarction. Circulation 71:627, 1985
151. Verstraete M, Bory M, Collen D et al: Randomized trial of intravenous recombinant tissue type plasminogen activator resists intravenous streptokinase in acute myocardial infarction. Lancet 1:842, 1985
152. Verstraete M, Brower RW, Collen D et al: Double-blind randomized trial of intravenous tissue type plasminogen activator versus placebo in acute myocardial infarction. Lancet 2:965, 1985
153. Verstraete M, Arnold AER, Brower RW et al: Acute coronary thrombolysis with recombinant tissue type plasminogen activator: Initial patency and influence of maintained infusion on reocclusion rate. Am J Cardiol 60:231, 1987
154. Simoons ML, Arnold AER, Betriu W et al: Thrombolysis with rt-PA in acute myocardial infarction: No beneficial effects of immediate PTCA. Lancet 1:197, 1988
155. Topol EJ, Morris DC, Smalling RW et al: A multicentered, randomized, placebo-controlled trial of a new form of intravenous rt-PA (Activase) in acute myocardial infarction. J Am Coll Cardiol 9:1205, 1987
156. Topol EJ, Califf RM, George BS et al: A randomized trial of immediate versus delayed elective angioplasty after intravenous TPA in acute myocardial infarction. N Engl J Med 317:581, 1987
157. Topol EJ, George BS, Kereiakes DJ et al: A randomized controlled trial of intravenous TPA and early intravenous heparin in acute myocardial infarction. Circulation 79:281, 1989
158. Gold HK, Leinbach RC, Garabedian HD et al: Acute coronary reocclusion after thrombolysis with recombinant human tissue type plasminogen activator: Prevention using a maintenance infusion. Circulation 73:347, 1986
159. TIMI Research Group: Immediate versus delayed catheterization and angioplasty following thrombolytic therapy for acute myocardial infarction. JAMA 260:2849, 1988
160. Johns JA, Gold HK, Leinbach RC et al: Prevention of coronary artery occlusion and reduction in late coronary artery stenosis after thrombolytic therapy in patients with acute myocardial infarction. Circulation 78:546, 1988
161. Stack RS, O'Conner CM, Mark DB et al: Coronary perfusion during acute myocardial infarction with a combined therapy of coronary angioplasty and high dose intravenous streptokinase. Circulation 77:151, 1988
162. Brochier ML, Quillet L, Kulbertus H et al: Intravenous anisoylated plasminogen streptokinase in evolving myocardial infarction. Drugs 3(Suppl 3):140, 1987
163. Meyer J, Bar F, Barth H et al: International double blind randomized trial of intravenous r-scu-PA vs streptokinase in acute myocardial infarction (PRIMI) (abstr). Circulation 78(Suppl II):II-303, 1988
164. Bono DD: Problems with thrombolysis. In Julian D, Kubler W, Norris RM (eds): Thrombolysis in Cardiovascular Disease, pp 279–292. New York, Marcel Dekker, 1989
165. Topol E, Califf RM: Tissue type plasminogen activator: Why the backlash. J Am Coll Cardiol 13:1477, 1989
166. Collen D, Topol E, Tiefenbrumd AJ et al: Coronary thrombolysis with r-TPA: A prospective randomized controlled trial. Circulation 70:1012, 1984
167. Collen D: Human tissue type plasminogen activator: From the laboratory to the bed side. Circulation 72:18, 1985
168. Pitt B: Clot specific thrombolytic agents: Is there an advantage. J Am Coll Cardiol 12:588, 1988
169. Magnani B, for the PAIMS investigators. Plasminogen Activator Italian Multicenter Study (PAIMS): Comparison of intravenous rt-PA with intravenous streptokinase in acute myocardial infarction. J Am Coll Cardiol 13:19, 1989
170. White HD, Rivers JT, Maslowski AH et al: Effects of intravenous streptokinase as compared with that of tissue type plasminogen activator on left ventricular function after first myocardial infarction. N Engl J Med 320:817, 1989
171. Chesebro JH, Knatterud G, Roberts R et al: Thrombolysis in myocardial infarction (TIMI) trial, phase I: A comparison between intravenous tissue type plasminogen activator and intravenous streptokinase. Circulation 76:142, 1987
172. TIMI Study Group: Comparison of invasive and conservative strategies after treatment with intravenous tissue type plasminogen activator in acute myocardial infarction: Results of the TIMI-II trial. N Engl J Med 320:618, 1989
173. Gruppo Italiano per lo studio della streptochinasé nell unfarto, miocardio: Effectiveness of intravenous thrombolytic therapy in acute myocardial infarction. Lancet 1:397, 1986
174. ISIS-2 Collaborative Group: Randomized trial of intravenous streptokinase, oral aspirin, both, or neither among 17,187 cases of suspected myocardial infarction. Lancet 2:349, 1988
175. Wilcox RG, von der Lippe G, Olsson CG et al: Trial of tissue plasminogen activator for mortality reduction in acute myocardial infarction. Lancet 2:525, 1988
176. AIMS Trial Study Group: Effects of intravenous APSAC on mortality after myocardial infarction: Preliminary report of a placebo-controlled clinical trial. Lancet 1:545, 1988
177. Monk JP, Heel RC: Anisoylated plasminogen streptokinase activator complex (APSAC): A review of its mechanism of action, clinical pharmacology and therapeutic use in acute myocardial infarction. Drugs 34:25, 1987
178. Anderson JL, Rothbard RL, Hackworthy RA et al: Multicenter reperfusion trial of intravenous anisoylated streptokinase activator complex (APSAC) in acute myocardial infarction: Controlled comparison with intracoronary streptokinase. J Am Coll Cardiol 12:561, 1988
179. Bassand JP, MacheCourt J, Cassagnes J et al: Multicenter trial of intravenous anisoylated activator complex (APSAC) in acute myocardial infarction: Effects on infarct size and left ventricular function. J Am Coll Cardiol 13:988, 1989
180. Mathey DG, Schofer J, Sheehan EH et al: Intravenous urokinase in acute myocardial infarction. Am J Cardiol 55:878, 1985
181. Tennant SN, Dixon J, Venable TC et al: Intracoronary thrombolysis in patients with acute myocardial infarction: Comparison of the efficacy of urokinase with streptokinase. Circulation 69:756, 1984
182. Van der Werf F, Vanhaecke J, de Grost H et al: Coronary thrombolysis with recombinant single chain urokinase-type plasminogen activator in patients with acute myocardial infarction. Circulation 74:1066, 1986
183. Topol EJ, Califf RM, George BS et al: Coronary arterial thrombolysis with combined infusion of r-TPA and urokinase in patients with acute myocardial infarction. Circulation 77:1100, 1988
184. Collen D, Van der Werf F: Coronary thrombolysis with low dose synergistic combinations of r-TPA and recu-PA in man. Am J Cardiol 60:431, 1987
185. Ip JH, Fuster V, Badimon L et al: Syndromes of accelerated atherosclerosis: Role of vascular injury and smooth muscle cell proliferation. J Am Coll Cardiol 15:1667, 1990
186. Goldsmith HL, Turitto VT: Rheological aspects of thrombosis and haemostasis: Basic principles and implications. Thromb Haemost 55:415, 1986
187. Ross R: The pathogenesis of atherosclerosis: An update. N Engl J Med 314:488, 1986
188. Schwartz CJ, Valente AJ, Kelly JL et al: Thrombosis and the development of atherosclerosis: Rokitanski revisited. Semin Thromb Hemost 14:189, 1988
189. Davies MJ: Thrombosis and coronary atherosclerosis. In Julian D, Kubler WS, Norris RM et al (eds): Thrombolysis in Cardiovascular Disease, pp 25–44. New York, Marcel Dekker, 1989
190. Davies MJ, Bland MJ, Hartgartner WR et al: Factors influencing the presence or absence of acute coronary thrombi in sudden ischemic death. Eur Heart J 10:203, 1989
191. Bini A, Fenoglia JJ, Mesa-Tejada R et al: Identification and distribution of fibrinogen, fibrin and fibrin degradation products in atherosclerosis: Use of monoclonal antibody. Atherosclerosis 1:109, 1989
192. Falk E: Unstable angina with fatal outcome, dynamic coronary thrombosis leading to infarction and/or sudden death: Autopsy evidence of recurrent mural thrombosis with peripheral embolization culminating in total vascular occlusion. Circulation 71:699, 1985
193. Sherman CT, Litvak F, Grundfest W et al: Coronary angioscopy in patients with unstable angina. N Engl J Med 315:913, 1986
194. Levin DC, Fallon JT: Significance of the angiographic morphology of localized coronary stenosis: Histopathological correlates. Circulation 66:316, 1982
195. Ambrose JA, Winters SL, Stern A et al: Angiographic morphology and the pathogenesis of unstable angina. J Am Coll Cardiol 5:609, 1985
196. Gorlin R, Fuster V, Ambrose JA: Anatomic-physiologic link between the

197. Ambrose JA, Tennebaum MA, Alexopoulos D et al: Angiographical progression of coronary artery disease and the development of myocardial infarction. J Am Coll Cardiol 12:256, 1988
198. Ambrose JA, Hjendale-Monsen CE, Borrico S et al: Angiographic demonstration of a common link between unstable angina pectoris and non Q wave myocardial infarction. Am J Cardiol 61:244, 1988
199. Richardson PD, Davies MJ, Born GVR: Influence of plaque configuration and stress distribution on fissuring of coronary atherosclerotic plaques. Lancet 2:941, 1989
200. Fuster V, Chesebro JH: Role of platelets and platelet inhibitor in coronary artery vein graft bypass disease. Circulation 73:227, 1986
201. Ip JH, Fuster V, Badimon L, Chesebro JH: Interactions between blood and coronary arterial wall. Curr Opin Cardiol 4:0772, 1989
202. Lie JT, Lawrie WM, Morris GC: Aortocoronary bypass saphenous vein graft atherosclerosis. Am J Cardiol 40:906, 1977
203. Atkinson JB, Forman BB, Vaugh WK et al: Morphologic changes in long term saphenous vein bypass grafts. Chest 88:341, 1985
204. Solymoss BC, Nadeau P, Millette D, Campeau L: Late thrombosis of saphenous vein coronary bypass graft related to risk factors (abstr). Circulation 78(Suppl II):II-140, 1988
205. Steele PM, Chesebro JH, Stanson AW et al: Balloon angioplasty in natural history of pathophysiological responses to injury in a pig model. Circ Res 57:105, 1985
206. Waller BF, Gorfinkel HJ, Rogers FJ et al: Early and late morphological changes in major epicardial coronary arteries after PTCA. Am J Cardiol 53(Suppl):42C, 1984
207. Wallers BF: "Crackers, breakers, stretchers, drillers, scrapers, shavers, welders and melters": The future treatment of atherosclerotic coronary artery disease? A clinical-morphological assessment. J Am Coll Cardiol 13:969, 1989
208. O'Hara J, Nanto S, Asada S et al: Ultrastructural study of proliferating and migrating smooth muscle cells at the site of PTCA as an explanation for restenosis (abstr). Circulation 78(Suppl II):290, 1988
209. Uchida Y, Kawamura K, Shibuya I, Hasegawa P: Percutaneous angioscopy of the coronary luminal changes induced by PTCA (abstr). Circulation 78(Suppl):II-84, 1988
210. Mizuno K, Mugamoto A, Shibuya T et al: Changes in angioscopic macromorphology following coronary angioplasty (abstr). Circulation 78(Suppl II):II-289, 1988
211. Johnson DE, Robertson G, Simpson SB: Coronary atherectomy: Light microscopic and immunohistochemical study of excised tissues (abstr). Circulation 78(Suppl II):II-82, 1988
212. Virchow R: Gesammelte Abhandluinger zum Wissenschaftlichen Medicine, pp 219–732. Frankfurt, Medinger Son & Co, 1856
213. Johnson RC, Crissman RS, Didio LA: Endocardial alteration in myocardial infarction. Lab Invest 40:183, 1979
214. Hochman JJ, Platia EB, Bulkley BH: Endocardial abnormalities in left ventricular aneurysm: A clinical pathologic study. Ann Intern Med 100:29, 1984
215. Roberts WC, Seigel RJ, McNanus BM: Idiopathic dilated cardiomyopathy: Analysis of 152 necrosy patients. Am J Cardiol 60:1340, 1987
216. Mikell FL, Asinger RW, Elsperger KJ et al: Regional stasis of blood in the dysfunctional left ventricle: Echocardiographic detection and differentiation from early thrombosis. Circulation 66:755, 1982
217. Asinger RW, Mikell FL, Elsperger KJ, Hodges M: Incidence of left ventricular thrombosis after acute myocardial infarction: Serial evaluation by two-dimension echocardiogram. N Engl J Med 305:297, 1981
218. Weinrich DJ, Burke JF, Pauletto FJ: Left ventricular mural thrombi complicating acute myocardial infarction: Long term follow-up with serial echocardiography. Ann Intern Med 100:789, 1984
219. Shresta NK, Moreno FL, Narciso FV et al: Two-dimensional echocardiographic diagnosis of left atrial thrombus in rheumatic heart disease: A clinicopathologic study. Circulation 67:341, 1983
220. Fulton RM, Duckett K: Plasma-fibrinogen and thromboemboli after myocardial infarction. Lancet 2:1161, 1976
221. Fuster V, Halperin JL: Left ventricular thrombi and cerebral embolism. N Engl J Med 320:392, 1989
222. Cabin HS, Roberts WC: Left ventricular aneurysm, intra-aneurysmal thrombus and systemic embolus in coronary heart disease. Chest 320:392, 1980
223. Dewanjee MK, Fuster V, Rao SA et al: Noninvasive radioisotopic technique for detection of platelet deposition in mitral valve prosthesis and quantification of visceral microembolism in dogs. Mayo Clin Proc 58:307, 1983
224. Acar J, Vahanian V, Fauchet M et al: Detection of prosthetic valve thrombosis using indium III platelet imaging (abstr). Eur Heart J 20:261, 1989
225. Chesebro JH, Adams PC, Fuster V: Antithrombotic therapy in patients with valvular heart disease and prosthetic heart valves. J Am Coll Cardiol 8(Suppl):42B, 1986
226. Fuster V, Badimon L, Badimon JJ, Chesebro JH: Prevention of thromboembolism induced by prosthetic heart valves. Semin Thromb Hemost 14:50, 1988
227. Edmunds HC Jr: Thrombosis and bleeding complications of prosthetic heart valves. Ann Thorac Surg 44:430, 1987
228. Stein B, Fuster V, Halperin JL, Chesebro JH: Antithrombotic therapy in cardiac disease: An emerging approach based on pathogenesis and risk. Circulation 80:1501, 1989
229. Theroux P, Ouimet H, McCanu T et al: Aspirin, heparin or both to treat acute unstable angina. N Engl J Med 319:1105, 1988
230. Telford AM, Wilson C: Trial of heparin versus atenolol in prevention of myocardial infarction in intermediate coronary syndrome. Lancet 1:1225, 1981
230a. Wallentine L for the Risk Study Group in South East Sweden: Aspirin 75 mg and/or Heparin after an episode of unstable coronary artery disease—risk for myocardial infarction and death in a radiologic placebo-controlled study. (abstract) Circulation 80(Suppl II):II-1664, 1989
231. Ambrose JA, Alexoupoulous D: Thrombolysis in unstable angina: Will the beneficial effects of thrombotic therapy in myocardial infarction apply to patients with unstable angina? J Am Coll Cardiol 13:1666, 1989
232. Lawrence JR, Shephard JT, Bone I et al: Fibrinolytic therapy in unstable angina: A controlled clinical trial. Thromb Res 17:767, 1980
233. Rentrop P, Blanke H, Karsch KP et al: Selective intracoronary thrombolysis in acute myocardial infarction and unstable angina. Circulation 63:307, 1981
234. Vetrovec GW, Leinbach RC, Gold HK, Crowley MJ: Intracoronary thrombolysis in syndromes of unstable ischemia: Angiographic and clinical results. Am Heart J 104:946, 1982
235. Mandelkorn JB, Wolf NM, Singh S et al: Intracoronary thrombus in nontransmural myocardial infarction and in unstable angina pectoris. Am J Cardiol 52:1, 1983
236. Ambrose JA, Hjemdahl-Monsen C, Borrico S et al: Quantitative and qualitative effects of intracoronary streptokinase in unstable angina and non-Q wave myocardial infarction. J Am Coll Cardiol 9:1156, 1987
237. Gold HK, Johns JA, Leinbach RC et al: A randomized, blinded placebo-controlled trial of recombinant human TPA in patients with unstable angina. Circulation 9:1156, 1987
238. Gotoh K, Minamino T, Katoh O et al: The role of intracoronary thrombus in unstable angina: Angiographic assessment and thrombolytic therapy during ongoing angina attacks. Circulation 77:526, 1988
239. DeZwaan C, Bar FW, Janssen JHA et al: Effects of thrombolytic therapy in unstable angina: Clinical and angiographic results. J Am Coll Cardiol 12:301, 1988
240. Topol EJ, Nicklas JM, Kandler NH et al: Coronary revascularization after intravenous TPA for unstable angina pectoris: Results of a randomized double-blind, placebo-controlled trial. Am J Cardiol 62:368, 1988
241. Gibson RS, Beller GA, Gheorghiade M et al: The prevalence and clinical significance of residual myocardial ischemia 2 weeks after uncomplicated non-Q wave infarction: A prospective natural history study. Circulation 73:1186, 1986
242. Timmis AD, Griffin B, Crick JCP et al: The effects of early coronary patency on the evolution of myocardial infarction: A prospective arteriographic study. Br Heart J 58:345, 1987
243. Heras M, Chesebro JH, Thompson PL, Fuster V: Prevention of early and late rethrombosis and further strategies after coronary reperfusion. In Julian D, Kubler W, Norris M et al (eds): Thrombolysis in Cardiovascular Disease, pp 203–229. New York, Marcel Dekker, 1989
244. Fuster V, Stein B, Badimon L, Chesebro JH: Antithrombotic therapy after myocardial reperfusion in acute myocardial infarction. J Am Coll Cardiol 12(Suppl A):78A, 1988
245. Report of the Working Party on Anticoagulation Therapy in Coronary Thrombosis to the Medical Research Council: Assessment of short term anticoagulation administration after cardiac infarction. Br Med J 1:335, 1969
246. Drapkin A, Merskey C: Anticoagulation therapy after myocardial infarction: Relation of therapeutic benefit to patient's age, sex and severity of infarction. JAMA 222:541, 1977
247. Veterans Administration Hospital Investigators: Anticoagulation in acute myocardial infarction: Results of a cooperative clinical trial. JAMA 225:724, 1973
248. Chalmers TC, Matta RJ, Smith H, Kunzler AM: Evidence favoring the use of anticoagulation in the hospital phase of acute myocardial infarction. N Engl J Med 297:1091, 1977
249. Second Report of the Working Party on Anticoagulation in Coronary Thrombosis to the Medical Council: An assessment of long term anticoagulant administration after acute myocardial infarction. Br Med J 2:2263, 1964
250. Kannel WB, Wolf PA, Garrison RJ: Survival following initial cardiovascular events: Framingham Study: Section 35, publication No. PB 88-204049. US Department of Health and Human Services, National Institutes of Health, US Department of Commerce. Washington, DC, US Government Printing Office, 1988
251. Ebert RV, Borden CW, Hipp HR et al: Long-term anticoagulant therapy after myocardial infarction: Final report of the Veterans Administration Cooperative Study. JAMA 207:2263, 1969
252. Breddin K, Loew D, Lechner K et al: The German-Austrian Aspirin trial: A comparison of acetylsalicylic acid, placebo and phenprocoumon in secondary prevention of myocardial infarction. Circulation 62(suppl V):62, 1980
253. International Anticoagulation Review Group: Collaborative analysis of long-term anticoagulation administration after acute myocardial infarction. Lancet 1:203, 1970

254. Smith P, Arnesen H: Oral anticoagulant reduces mortality, reinfarction and cerebral vascular event after myocardial infarction: WARIS study (abstr). Eur Heart J 30:264, 1989
255. Report of the Sixty-Plus Reinfarction Study Research Group: A double-blind trial to assess long-term oral anticoagulation therapy in elderly patients after myocardial infarction. Lancet 2:989, 1980
256. Peto R, Gray R, Collins R et al: A randomized trial of the effects of prophylactic daily aspirin among British male doctors. Br Med J 296:313, 1988
257. Fuster V, Cohen M, Halperin J: Aspirin in the prevention of coronary disease. N Engl J Med 321:129, 1989
258. Chesebro JH, Webster MW, Smith HC et al. Antiplatelet therapy in coronary disease progression-reduced infractions and even lesion progression (abstr) Circulation 80(Suppl II):II–266, 1989
259. Chesebro JH, Clements IP, Fuster V et al: A platelet inhibitor trial in coronary artery bypass operations: Benefit of perioperative dipyridamole and aspirin therapy on early postoperative vein-graft patency. N Engl J Med 307:73, 1982
260. Limet R, David JL, Magotteauz P et al: Prevention of aorta-coronary bypass graft occlusion. J Thorac Cardiovasc Surg 94:773, 1987
261. Goldman S, Copeland J, Mortiz T et al: Improvement in early saphenous vein graft surgery with antiplatelet therapy: Results of a Veterans Administration Cooperative Study. Circulation 77:1324, 1988
262. McEnany MT, Salzman EW, Mundth ED et al: The effect of antithrombotic therapy on the patency rates of saphenous vein bypass grafts. J Thorac Cardiovasc Surg 83:81, 1982
263. Pantley GA, Goodnight SH, Rahimtoola SH et al: Failure of antiplatelet and anticoagulant therapy to improve patency of grafts after coronary artery operation: A controlled randomized study. N Engl J Med 301:962, 1979
264. Gruntzig AR, Senning A, Suganthalan WE: Nonoperative dilation of coronary artery stenosis: Percutaneous transluminal coronary angioplasty. N Engl J Med 301:61, 1979
265. McBride W, Lange RA, Hillis DC: Restenosis after successful coronary angioplasty: Pathophysiology and prevention. N Engl J Med 318:1734, 1988
266. Barnathan ES, Schwartz JS, Taylor L et al: Aspirin and dipyridamole in the prevention of acute coronary thrombosis complicating coronary angioplasty. Circulation 76:125, 1987
267. Schwartz L, Bourassa MG, Lesperance J et al: Aspirin and dipyridamole in the prevention of restenosis after percutaneous transluminal coronary angioplasty. N Engl J Med 318:1714, 1988
268. White CW, Chaitman B, Lassar TA et al: Antiplatelet agents are effective in reducing the immediate complication of PTCA: Results from the Ticlopidine Multicenter Trial. Circulation 76(Suppl IV):400, 1987
269. White CW, Knudson M, Schmidt D et al: Neither ticlopidine nor aspirin-dipyridamole prevents restenosis post PTCA: Results from a randomized placebo controlled multicenter trial (abstr). Circulation 76:IV-213, 1987
270. Heras M, Chesebro JH, Penny WJ et al: Importance of adequate heparin dosage in arterial angioplasty in a porcine model. Circulation 78:654, 1988
271. Lukas MA, Deutsch E, Laskey WK: Beneficial effect of heparin therapy on PTCA outcome in unstable angina (abstr). J Am Coll Cardiol 11(Suppl A):132A, 1988
272. Douglas JS, Lutz JF, Clements SD et al: Therapy of large intracoronary thrombi in candidates for PTCA (abstr). J Am Coll Cardiol 11(Suppl A):238A, 1988
273. Pow TK, Varricchione TR, Jacobs AK et al: Does pretreatment with heparin prevent abrupt closure following PTCA (abstr). J Am Coll Cardiol 11(Suppl A):A238, 1988
274. Ellis SG, Roubin GS, Wilente J et al: Results of a randomized trial of heparin and aspirin versus aspirin alone for prevention of acute closure and restenosis after PTCA (abstr). Circulation 76(suppl):IV-213, 1987
275. Thorton MA, Gruntzig AR, Hollman J et al: Coumadin and aspirin in the prevention of restenosis after PTCA: A randomized study. Circulation 69:721, 1984
276. Halperin JL, Hart RG: Atrial fibrillation and stroke: New ideas and persisting dilemmas. Stroke 19:937, 1988
277. Dunn M, Alexander J, deSilva R, Hildner F: Antithrombotic therapy in atrial fibrillation. Chest 95(Suppl):118S, 1989
278. Brand FN, Abbott RD, Kannel WB, Wolf PA: Characteristic and prognosis of lone atrial fibrillation: 30-year follow-up in the Framingham Study. JAMA 254:3449, 1985
279. Kopecky SL, Gersh BJ, McGoon MD et al: The natural history of lone atrial fibrillation: A population-based study over three decades. N Engl J Med 317:669, 1987
280. Roy D, Marchand E, Gagne P et al: Usefulness of anticoagulation therapy in the prevention of embolic complications of atrial fibrillation. Am Heart J 112:1039, 1986
281. Peterson P, Godtfredsen J, Boysen G et al: Placebo-controlled, randomized trial of warfarin and aspirin for prevention of thromboembolic complications in chronic atrial fibrillation: The Copenhagen AFASAK Study. Lancet 1:175, 1989
282. Meltzer RS, Visser CA, Fuster V: Intracardiac thrombi and systemic embolization. Ann Intern Med 104:689, 1986
283. Turpie AGG, Robinson JG, Doyle DJ et al: Comparison of high dose and low dose subcutaneous heparin to prevent left ventricular mural thrombosis in patients with acute transmural myocardial infarction. N Engl J Med 320:352, 1989
284. Lapeyre AC, Steele PP, Kazmier FJ et al: Systemic embolism in chronic left ventricular aneurysm: Incidence and role of anticoagulation. J Am Coll Cardiol 6:534, 1985
285. Fuster V, Gersh BJ, Giuliani ER et al: The natural history of idiopathic dilated cardiomyopathy. Am J Cardiol 47:525, 1981
286. Stein P, Kantrowitz A: Antithrombotic therapy in mechanical and biological prosthetic heart valves and saphenous vein bypass graft. Chest 95:107S, 1989
287. Meyers ML, Lawrie GM, Crawford ES et al: The St. Jude valve prosthesis: Analysis of the clinical results in 815 implants and the need for systemic anticoagulation. J Am Coll Cardiol 13:57, 1989
288. Mok CY, Boey J, Wang R et al: Warfarin versus dipyridamole-aspirin and pentoxylline-aspirin for the prevention of prosthetic valve thromboembolism: A prospective randomized clinical trial. Circulation 72:1059, 1985
289. Wilson WR, Geraci JE, Danielson GK et al: Anticoagulation therapy and central nervous system complications in patients with prosthetic valve endocardites. Circulation 57:1004, 1978
290. Garvey GJ, Neu HC. Infective endocarditis—An evolving disease. A review of endocardites at the Columbia Presbyterian Medical Center Medicine 57:105, 1978
291. Karchmer AW, Dismukes WE, Buckley MJ, et al: Late prosthetic valve endocarditis—clinical features influencing therapy. Am J Med 64:199, 1978
292. Sherman DG, Dyken ML, Fisher M, Hanison MJG, Hart RG. Antithrombotic therapy for cerebrovascular disorders. Chest 95:140, 1989

CARDIOVASCULAR DRUG INTERACTIONS

Neal L. Benowitz

GENERAL CONSIDERATIONS

Multiple drug therapy is common in patients with cardiovascular disease. In one teaching hospital survey[1] the median number of drugs administered to hospitalized patients was 12 (range 8–25). A patient receiving ten drugs simultaneously is exposed to approximately 10 million possible interactions. Most of these interactions are inconsequential. Some interactions are beneficial and are used to therapeutic advantage. Other drug interactions may have adverse or even lethal consequences. These are the subject of this chapter. Physicians can and should be able to anticipate significant adverse drug interactions and adjust the types or doses of medications so as not to injure the patient.

Characteristics of drug interactions that are likely to lead to significant consequences include (1) an interaction of substantial magnitude and (2) a steep dose-response relationship so that slight or moderate decrease in drug action leads to therapeutic failure or (3) a narrow therapeutic index such that a small or moderate increase in drug action leads to toxicity. Many of the drugs fitting this description are those used in treating patients with cardiovascular disease. Adverse drug interactions in such patients are often not recognized because it is difficult to distinguish adverse drug effects from worsening of the underlying disease. Awareness of the potential for drug interactions combined with an understanding of the pharmacology of the agents and careful observation when new drugs are started are the key elements to preventing adverse drug interactions.

Drug interactions may occur because of altered pharmacokinetics or pharmacodynamics. Examples of various mechanisms of interaction are given in discussion of individual drugs. Case examples are presented to place interactions in a clinical context.

CARDIAC GLYCOSIDES (TABLE 21.1)
INTERACTIONS AFFECTING BIOAVAILABILITY

Case Example A 71-year-old woman with chronic congestive heart failure developed a respiratory tract infection associated with cough and wheezing. To her customary drug regimen of hydralazine, furosemide, isosorbide dinitrate, and digoxin, 0.25 mg/day, erythromycin and theophylline were added. Her usual serum di-

TABLE 21.1 DRUG INTERACTIONS AFFECTING DIGOXIN

Interacting Drug	SDC	Type of Interaction	Possible Mechanism	Recommendations
Amiodarone	↑	Decreased clearance	Inhibits metabolism or renal excretion	Decrease digoxin dose; monitor SDC
Antacids	↓	Decreased absorption		Do not give antacids within 1 hour of digoxin
Cholestyramine	↓	Decreased absorption, increased clearance	Binds digoxin in intestine; interferes with enterohepatic recirculation	Do not give cholestyramine within 1 hour of digoxin; monitor SDC
Diltiazem	↑	Decreased clearance	Inhibits metabolism and renal excretion	Reduce digoxin dose; monitor SDC
Erythromycin	↑	Increased bioavailability, decreased clearance	Decreases gut metabolism (significant in only small % of patients)	Monitor SDC; adjust dose in affected patients
Furosemide (and other diuretics)	↑	Decreased renal clearance, increased toxicity	Overdiuresis reduces tubular secretion; hypokalemia, hypomagnesemia	Observe carefully; monitor SDC; monitor potassium and magnesium levels
Hydralazine	↓	Increased renal clearance	Increases filtration and secretion (heart failure patients)	Uncertain
Nitroprusside	↓	Increased renal clearance	Increases filtration and secretion (heart failure patients)	Uncertain
Rifampin	↓	Increased clearance	Accelerates metabolism or biliary secretion	Monitor SDC; increase dose as necessary
Quinidine	↑	Decreased clearance, reduced distribution volume	Inhibits metabolism and renal excretion; displacement from tissue binding sites	Reduce dose by 50%; monitor SDC
Spironolactone	↑	Decreased clearance	Inhibits renal tubular secretion	Monitor SDC; decrease dose as necessary
Tetracycline	↑	Increased bioavailability, decreased clearance	Decreases gut metabolism (significant in only small % of patients)	Monitor SDC; adjust dose in affected patients
Verapamil	↑	Decreased clearance	Inhibits metabolism and renal excretion	Reduce digoxin dose; monitor SDC

(*SDC*, serum digoxin concentration)

goxin concentration was 1.4 ng/ml. Four days later she developed nausea and vomiting with an atrioventricular junctional rhythm. The serum digoxin concentration was 2.6 ng/ml.[2]

Digoxin tablets, because of slow absorption, are variably absorbed; absorption is more complete from elixir (capsule) preparations. Absorption from tablets may be reduced in patients with rapid gastrointestinal transit. Accelerating gastrointestinal transit with metoclopramide may decrease and slowing transit with propantheline (and other drugs with anticholinergic activity) may increase bioavailability, leading to significant changes in digoxin levels.[3] Such interactions are not usually seen when patients are taking elixir preparations because absorption is more rapid.

Digoxin that is not absorbed in the upper gastrointestinal tract or that is excreted into the bile may be reductively metabolized by anaerobic bacteria (*Eubacterium alantum*) in the colon. Reduced digoxin metabolites such as dihydrodigoxin, which are not believed to be pharmacologically active, may account for up to 40% of eliminated digoxin in a minority (about 10%) of patients. In such patients administration of antibiotics such as erythromycin or tetracycline can lead to substantially increased bioavailability of digoxin and may result in clinical toxicity as illustrated in the case example.[4] Patients who excrete a major fraction of digoxin as reduced metabolites are typically those who require a higher than usual daily digoxin dose. This is an example of an uncommon but potentially predictable interaction.

Cholestyramine and colestipol, drugs used in treating hypercholesterolemia, as well as some antacids and kaolin-pectin, may bind digoxin in the gut and reduce absorption. The magnitude of the effect when digoxin is given with cholestyramine is a 20% to 30% reduction in bioavailability, but can be minimized by spacing digoxin dosing at least an hour before that of the resins.[5] Enterohepatic recirculation occurs to a small extent with digoxin and to a much larger extent for digitoxin. Cholestyramine or charcoal binds cardiac glycosides in the gut and reduces the extent of enterohepatic recycling. As a consequence, elimination half-life may be substantially shortened.[6,7] This interaction has been used successfully in the therapy of digitoxin poisoning.[8]

INTERACTIONS RESULTING IN ALTERED DISTRIBUTION

Case Example A 50-year-old man was taking digoxin, 0.25 mg/day, and quinidine sulfate, 300 mg every 6 hours. The morning predosing serum digoxin concentration was 1 ng/ml. Two hours after the afternoon quinidine dose, PR interval prolongation was noted and the serum digoxin concentration was 2.5 ng/ml.

Cardiac glycosides are extensively distributed to body tissues. There appear to be both specific and nonspecific digitalis binding sites. Quinidine and some of the calcium entry blockers may displace digoxin from nonspecific binding sites (Fig. 21.1). This displacement results in transient elevation of serum digoxin concentrations, so that digoxin levels rise and fall in parallel with rising and falling quinidine concentrations.[9] The transient rise in serum digoxin concentration may be associated with manifestations of digitalis toxicity, although the overall clinical significance of this phenomenon is unknown. Alteration in distribution kinetics *per se* does not affect steady state digoxin levels and does not require dosage adjustment.

INTERACTIONS RESULTING IN ALTERED ELIMINATION

Case Example A 74-year-old woman was hospitalized with new-onset atrial fibrillation. On digoxin, 0.25 mg/day for 8 days, serum digoxin concentration was 0.8 ng/ml and she had a ventricular response rate of 80 beats per minute. The following day she was started on quinidine, 300 mg every 6 hours, and discharged in hope of pharmacologic cardioversion. Five days later she developed abdominal pain and nausea. One week later she was admitted with high-degree atrioventricular block and frequent premature ventricular contractions. Serum digoxin concentration was 5.8 ng/ml and quinidine, 2.2 μg/ml.

Digoxin and quinidine have been used together for more than 60 years, yet it was not until 1978 that the significant interaction between the two was noted.[10] A clinical presentation such as that described in the case above would have been attributed in past years to spontaneous changes in the severity of disease. With the availability of serum digoxin assays and the knowledge of how to conduct pharmacokinetic studies, we now know that quinidine, amiodarone, and some of the calcium entry blockers significantly influence digoxin elimination.

Digoxin is eliminated by both metabolism (about 40%) and renal excretion (about 60%). Metabolism of digoxin is inhibited by quinidine, verapamil, and, possibly, diltiazem and amiodarone.[11-14] There is controversy about whether nifedipine influences digoxin metabolism.[15,16] These same drugs, as well as spironolactone, inhibit tubular secretion of digoxin, resulting in reduced renal elimination as well.[17] Rifampin, in contrast, accelerates the elimination of digoxin, either by increased metabolism or by increased biliary secretion.[18] The magnitude of effect of drugs on digoxin elimination varies considerably from drug to drug and may be dose related. Quinidine and spironolactone together have additive effects on digoxin elimination.[19]

Drug-related changes in hemodynamics such as in the therapy of cardiac failure patients may influence digoxin renal excretion. Hydralazine and nitroprusside acutely increase the filtration and secretion of digoxin,[20] although the relevance of this observation to long-term therapy is as yet undefined. In contrast, excessive diuresis results in re-

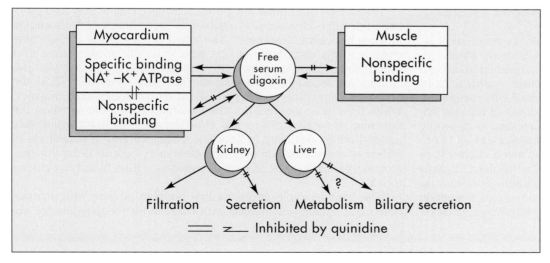

FIGURE 21.1 Mechanism of digoxin–quinidine interaction.

duced renal as well as nonrenal clearance of digoxin and may result in toxicity if the dose is not changed.[21]

Assuming an unchanged dosing regimen, changes in drug clearance or elimination rate result in a new steady state concentration. This effect can result in toxicity as illustrated by the case example. There has been debate as to whether quinidine and other drugs might block the action of digoxin at the cardiac receptor. However, most animal studies and clinical observations indicate that quinidine and other drugs that increase digoxin levels may result in increased digoxin action and, presumably, toxicity. Therefore, adjustments in the maintenance dose should be made. For example, when adding quinidine to a stable dose of digoxin, a 50% reduction in clearance should be anticipated. Thus, the digoxin dose should be reduced by 50%. Since the magnitude of the effect is variable from person to person, final dose adjustments need to be made on the basis of repeated drug level determinations or on the basis of clinical response, such as ventricular response rate in atrial fibrillation.

The time course of rise of digoxin levels when clearance is reduced by an interacting drug needs to be considered in planning dosing. Because of the long half-life of digoxin, it takes at least 1 week and maybe as long as several weeks to reach a new plateau level. Patients need to be carefully monitored for development of toxicity for this period.

Whereas digoxin is primarily excreted by the kidney and secondarily metabolized, digitoxin is primarily metabolized. Metabolism of digitoxin is accelerated by drugs such as phenobarbital, phenytoin, rifampin, and phenylbutazone. Accelerated metabolism can reduce steady state serum digitoxin concentrations, requiring increased dosage to maintain a desired level. Quinidine inhibits digitoxin clearance; interactions between calcium entry blockers and digitoxin have not yet been reported.

PHARMACOLOGIC INTERACTIONS

Digitalis actions and toxicity are exaggerated in the presence of hypokalemia or hypomagnesemia. Deficiencies of both electrolytes may occur during treatment with diuretics. Serum potassium or magnesium levels do not necessarily reflect whole-body concentrations. For example, digitalis toxicity responsive to magnesium may occur in the presence of normal serum but reduced lymphocyte magnesium and potassium levels. Guidelines for magnesium therapy in patients taking diuretics have not been established.

Case Example A 66-year-old man with chronic heart failure, chronic obstructive lung disease, and a history of peptic ulcer disease who was regularly taking digoxin and theophylline developed burning epigastric pain. Antacids and cimetidine were initiated, with relief of symptoms. Five days later he presented with atrial flutter with a rapid ventricular response rate. Theophylline was stopped, and he was treated with extra doses of digoxin until the ventricular rate decreased. Three days later digitalis-toxic cardiac rhythms, including ventricular tachycardia, were noted. Theophylline and digoxin levels were 19.2 μg/ml and 3.4 ng/ml, respectively.

This case illustrates a complex but predictable sequence of pharmacodynamic drug interactions. Cimetidine inhibits theophylline metabolism (see section on theophylline), which then resulted in theophylline toxicity. This was manifested as atrial flutter with a rapid ventricular response rate. Digoxin was used to treat this rhythm, although successful treatment required very high doses of digoxin. Digoxin toxicity was not seen despite high levels because of opposing effects of digoxin and theophylline on cardiac automaticity and conduction. However, the half-life of theophylline is much shorter than that of digoxin. As the toxic effects of theophylline resolved, digitalis toxicity became apparent. Similar pharmacologic interactions may be observed with digoxin and other sympathomimetic or anticholinergic drugs. Such an interaction is used to therapeutic advantage when digoxin is given prior to quinidine therapy in patients with atrial fibrillation, to prevent anticholinergic-mediated increases in ventricular response rate.

Conversely, sympatholytic drugs, such as β-blockers, or drugs that depress cardiac conduction, such as calcium entry blockers, may interact with digitalis to produce additive atrioventricular block or bradyarrhythmias. Such interactions are used therapeutically when used for control of ventricular response rate in atrial fibrillation. Adverse interactions due to combination therapy are discussed in later sections.

ANTIARRHYTHMIC DRUGS (TABLES 21.2 AND 21.3)
LIDOCAINE

Case Example A 75-year-old woman with chronic congestive heart failure and peptic ulcer disease was admitted with dyspnea and somnolence. Chest films showed pulmonary edema. Drug treatment included oxygen, digoxin, furosemide, cimetidine, and intravenous theophylline. Eighteen hours after admission she developed frequent premature ventricular beats. A 75-mg bolus of lidocaine was administered, followed by a 2-mg/min infusion. Twelve hours later she had generalized seizures. The following drug concentrations were noted: lidocaine, 14 μg/ml; theophylline, 17 μg/ml; and digoxin, 2.5 ng/ml.

Lidocaine is usually administered by bolus and then constant intravenous infusion. Slow distribution from the vascular system to tissues may result in unexpectedly high blood lidocaine concentrations and possibly toxicity in the few minutes after a bolus loading injection. The usual circumstance in which this occurs is severe cardiac failure or shock states. Slowed distribution to tissues is thought to be a consequence of intense sympathetic nervous stimulation and low cardiac output, resulting in reduced flow to organs such as muscle and adipose tissue, which are important reservoirs for lidocaine uptake. Although not well documented, coadministration of sympathomimetic drugs such as norepinephrine or dopamine could reduce the distribution volume of lidocaine. The result could be toxicity following bolus injection of a usual dose of lidocaine. This type of interaction can be avoided by slowly administering loading doses.

During constant infusion the level of lidocaine is determined primarily by clearance. Most drug interactions with lidocaine involve alterations in lidocaine clearance. Lidocaine is extensively metabolized, being extracted to a high degree by the liver. Clearance of lidocaine is roughly proportional to liver blood flow. Drugs such as β-blockers, which decrease liver blood flow, decrease clearance, and drugs such as isoproterenol, which increase hepatic blood flow, increase clearance of lidocaine.[21,22] In contrast to propranolol, pindolol, a β-blocker with sympathetic agonist activity that does not decrease cardiac output or presumably hepatic blood flow, does not affect lidocaine clearance.[23]

Alterations of intrinsic drug-metabolizing capacity may also influence lidocaine clearance. Phenobarbital accelerates and cimetidine reduces lidocaine clearance.[24] The effect of cimetidine on lidocaine clearance was considered at one time to be due to decreased liver blood flow; however, ranitidine, another H_2-blocker that also decreases liver blood flow, does not alter lidocaine clearance.[25] Thus, the action of cimetidine appears to be on drug-metabolizing enzymes. When there is a potential drug interaction it is prudent to adjust the lidocaine infusion by 25% to 50%. However, since there is considerable interindividual variability in lidocaine clearance and in magnitude of effects of other drugs on lidocaine clearance, optimal doses for prolonged infusion therapy may require guidance from blood level monitoring.

The case example illustrates two possible adverse drug interactions. The patient was treated with intravenous theophylline for obstructive lung disease and with cimetidine for peptic ulcer disease. The patient ultimately had near-toxic theophylline levels, which were probably the result of cimetidine inhibition of theophylline metabolism. For treatment of ventricular ectopy, which may have been related to theophylline toxicity, lidocaine infusion was started. However, in determining the dose of lidocaine that was given the predictable effects of severe cardiac failure or of cimetidine on lidocaine clearance were not considered. Assuming multiplicative reductions of clearance by cardiac failure and cimetidine, and assuming the infusion should be reduced by 50% for each factor, then 25% of the usual dose, or 0.5 mg/min, would have been more appropriate. This dose reduction would have prevented the development of lidocaine toxicity with associated seizures. Few pharmacodynamic interactions involving lidocaine have been reported. A likely interaction is additive central nervous system toxicity with tocainide, a drug with similar pharmacologic and toxic actions.

QUINIDINE

Case Example A 38-year-old man with epilepsy and valvular heart disease was receiving long-term therapy with primidone. Because of recurrent atrial arrhythmias he was begun on quinidine sulfate. Despite a quinidine dose of 300 mg every 4 hours, plasma levels were less than 1 μg/ml.[26]

Absorption of quinidine may be reduced by antacids and probably by drugs such as cholestyramine and colestipol. Such drugs should always be spaced at least an hour following the quinidine dose. As mentioned previously, quinidine may interact significantly with digoxin.

Quinidine is extensively metabolized. Several drugs have been shown to influence the rate of quinidine metabolism. Phenobarbital, phenytoin, and rifampin accelerate and cimetidine and amiodarone inhibit quinidine metabolism.[26-28] When these drugs are added or deleted from a patient's drug regimen, the quinidine dose should be appropriately adjusted. In the illustrative case, phenobarbital, a major metabolite of primidone, accelerated the rate of quinidine metabolism threefold. Thus, much higher doses of quinidine were required to achieve therapeutic concentrations in this patient. Conversely, had the patient stopped his primidone but continued the quinidine dose, quinidine intoxication would be predicted.

Quinidine is excreted to a small degree (20%) unchanged by the kidney. Since quinidine is a weak base, its renal excretion may be influenced by urinary pH. With alkaline urine, as might occur with intensive antacid therapy (such as might be used to treat quinidine-induced gastric upset), renal clearance will be reduced. For most patients this will not have a significant effect on total clearance. Possibly in individual patients with relatively high renal and low metabolic clearance, such an interaction could result in quinidine toxicity.

Several pharmacodynamic interactions with quinidine have been described. Quinidine may increase the anticoagulant action of warfarin, believed to be by direct inhibition of synthesis of clotting factors.[29] Hypotension has been described in patients receiving oral quinidine and intravenous verapamil.[30] This appears to be a result of additive α-adrenoceptor blocking actions. Quinidine weakly inhibits neuromuscular transmission. The duration of muscular paralysis after the use of curare or succinylcholine during anesthesia may be prolonged.[31] Quinidine and other type Ia antiarrhythmic drugs slow ventricular repolarization, associated with QT interval prolongation. This is occasionally associated with reentry ventricular tachycardias of the polymorphous or *torsade de pointes* type. QT interval prolongation may be additive with other type Ia antiarrhythmic drugs or amiodarone, resulting in an increased risk of *torsade de pointes*.[32] Similar interactions may occur with psychotropic drugs such as tricyclic antidepres-

TABLE 21.2 PHARMACOKINETIC DRUG INTERACTIONS AFFECTING ANTIARRHYTHMIC DRUGS

Antiarrhythmic Drug	Interacting Drug	Change in Blood Level	Type of Interaction	Probable Mechanism	Comments
Lidocaine	Cimetidine	↑	Reduced clearance	Inhibits metabolism	Reduce lidocaine infusion rate
	Phenobarbital	↓	Increased clearance	Accelerates metabolism	Uncertain
	Propranolol (and other β-blockers except pindolol)	↑	Reduced clearance	Reduces liver blood flow	Reduce lidocaine infusion rate
Quinidine	Antacids	↑	Reduced clearance	Alkalinizes urine, reduces renal clearance	Monitor quinidine levels; in some but not all patients dose may need to be reduced
	Amiodarone	↑	Reduced clearance	Inhibits metabolism	Reduce quinidine dose
	Cimetidine	↑	Reduced clearance	Inhibits metabolism	Reduce quinidine dose
	Phenobarbital (and other barbiturates, primidone)	↓	Increased clearance	Accelerates metabolism	Increase quinidine dose; when these drugs are stopped, quinidine dose should be reduced
	Rifampin	↓	Increased clearance	Accelerates metabolism	Increase quinidine dose; when rifampin is stopped, quinidine dose should be reduced
Procainamide	Amiodarone	↑	Reduced clearance	Inhibits metabolism	Reduce procainamide dose, monitor levels
	Cimetidine	↑	Reduced clearance	Competes for tubular secretion	Monitor levels
Mexiletine	Phenytoin	↓	Increased clearance	Accelerates metabolism	Increase mexiletine dose
	Rifampin	↓	Increased clearance	Accelerates metabolism	Increase mexiletine dose

sants or phenothiazines. In management of poisoning involving the latter drugs, quinidine and other type I antiarrhythmics are absolutely contraindicated.

PROCAINAMIDE

Procainamide and its active metabolite N-acetyl procainamide (NAPA) are excreted unchanged to a considerable extent (60% and 80%, respectively) by the kidney. Renal excretion of these basic compounds is influenced by urinary pH. Clearance may be reduced when antacids or other drugs that alkalinize the urine are administered. The magnitude of the pH effect on renal clearance is small, suggesting that tubular secretion is the major determinant of renal clearance, with relatively little passive reabsorption.[33] Cimetidine, another basic drug excreted by renal tubular secretion, inhibits renal excretion of procainamide.[34] The mechanism is primarily competition for active secretion. The result is a 35% decrease in procainamide clearance. Reduction of glomerular filtration rate, which occasionally occurs during therapy with β-blockers or nonsteroidal anti-inflammatory drugs, is also expected to reduce the clearance of procainamide and NAPA. However, the clinically significant drug interactions involving changes in renal clearance are not well established. This is probably because of a relatively high toxic/therapeutic ratio, at least during short-term administration of procainamide.

Additive effects of procainamide and other type I antiarrhythmic drugs, as discussed with quinidine, are expected for procainamide.

AMIODARONE

Although amiodarone has only recently been used in the United States, a number of significant interactions have been reported.[35] A major action of amiodarone is to reduce the rate of metabolism of other drugs. Amiodarone enhances the anticoagulant response to warfarin.[36] In anticipation of this effect the warfarin dose should be halved. Onset of the inhibition of warfarin metabolism may be from 3 to 4 days up to several weeks, presumably reflecting the time required for buildup of

TABLE 21.3 DRUG INTERACTIONS IN WHICH ANTIARRHYTHMIC DRUGS INFLUENCE OTHER DRUG ACTIONS

Antiarrhythmic Drug	Interacting Drug	Effect	Probable Mechanism	Comments
Quinidine	Amiodarone, type I antiarrhythmic drugs	Marked QT prolongation, ventricular arrhythmias (*torsade de pointes*)	Additive slowing of repolarization	Use combinations cautiously
	Digoxin	Increased digoxin levels, digoxin toxicity	Quinidine reduces metabolism and renal excretion of digoxin	Reduce digoxin dose by 50%; monitor SDC
	Neuromuscular blocking agents (curare, succinylcholine, and others)	Prolonged muscular paralysis, postoperative respiratory arrest	Additive neuromuscular blockade	Intensively monitor respiratory function
	Verapamil (IV)	Hypotension	Additive α-adrenergic blocking effect	Use cautiously in combination
	Warfarin	Excessive anticoagulation, bleeding	Quinidine inhibits clotting factor synthesis, augments warfarin action	Reduce warfarin dose; monitor prothrombin time
Amiodarone	Digoxin	Increased digoxin levels	Reduces digoxin metabolism or renal excretion	Reduce digoxin dose; monitor SDC
	Procainamide	Increased procainamide levels, potential toxicity	Inhibits procainamide and N-acetyl procainamide (NAPA) metabolism	Reduce procainamide dose; monitor levels
	Quinidine	Increased quinidine levels, potential toxicity	Inhibits quinidine metabolism	Reduce quinidine dose; monitor levels
	Quinidine and other type I antiarrhythmic drugs	Ventricular arrhythmias (*torsade de pointes*)	Additive slowing of ventricular repolarization	Use cautiously in combination
	Warfarin	Excessive anticoagulation, bleeding	Inhibits warfarin metabolism	Reduce warfarin dose; monitor prothrombin time
	Propranolol and other β-blockers	Hypotension, bradyarrhythmias, sinus arrest, asystole	Additive depression of myocardial contractility, sinus and AV node conduction	Use cautiously in combination, particularly in patients with cardiac failure or sinus/AV nodal disease
	Calcium entry blockers	Hypotension, bradyarrhythmias, sinus arrest, asystole	Additive depression of myocardial contractility, sinus and AV node conduction	Use cautiously in combination, particularly in patients with cardiac failure or sinus/AV nodal disease

(*SDC*, serum digoxin concentration; *AV*, atrioventricular)

amiodarone concentrations adequate to inhibit warfarin metabolism. Since amiodarone has an extremely long half-life, the effect on warfarin metabolism may persist for up to 4 months after amiodarone is discontinued.

Amiodarone consistently elevates digoxin concentrations, on average about twofold.[14] Amiodarone also elevates blood levels of quinidine, procainamide, N-acetyl procainamide, and phenytoin.[28,35] These metabolic interactions plus the expected pharmacodynamic interaction with type I antiarrhythmic drugs may explain marked QT prolongation and the development of *torsades de pointes* observed after combined therapy with amiodarone and quinidine, disopyramide, propafenone, or mexiletene.[32]

Pharmacodynamic interactions have been reported between amiodarone and β-blockers or calcium entry blockers.[37,38] Amiodarone decreases sinus node automaticity, increases atrioventricular nodal refractoriness, and depresses myocardial contractility. Combining amiodarone with other drugs with similar effects may result in excessive bradycardia, sinus arrest, asystole, or low output states. This is most likely to occur in patients with underlying sinus or atrioventricular node or myocardial disease. Because of the long half-life of amiodarone, such interactions might occur following treatment with β-blockers or calcium entry blockers weeks or even months after discontinuation of amiodarone.

MEXILETINE AND TOCAINIDE

Mexiletine is extensively metabolized and is subject to the metabolic influences of other drugs.[39] Phenytoin and rifampin have been shown to accelerate mexiletine metabolism; phenobarbital would be expected to do so as well. Renal elimination of mexiletine is influenced by urinary pH. However, because only about 10% is excreted unchanged, changes in renal clearance have relatively little clinical significance.

Tocainide is both metabolized and excreted unchanged by the kidney. Renal clearance is pH dependent, ranging from 35% to 40% of total clearance of uncontrolled or acid pH to 15% at alkaline pH.[40] Thus alkali therapy has the potential to significantly influence tocainide levels, although the clinical significance of this interaction is not established.

β-BLOCKERS (TABLE 21.4)
PHARMACOKINETIC INTERACTIONS

Although many pharmacokinetic interactions involving β-blockers have been described, they are not perceived as creating a substantial therapeutic problem. This is because of difficulty in appreciating inadequate dosing in patients with dynamic diseases such as angina or hy-

TABLE 21.4 DRUG INTERACTIONS INVOLVING β-BLOCKERS

Drug	Interacting Drug	Effects	Probable Mechanism	Comments
All β-blockers	Verapamil and possibly other calcium entry blockers	Excessive bradycardia, complete heart block, asystole,* cardiac failure	Additive depression of myocardial conduction and contractility	Primarily seen in patients with preexisting left ventricular dysfunction or conduction disturbance
	Amiodarone	Same as calcium entry blockers	Additive myocardial depressant and sympathetic blocking actions	
	Epinephrine, insulin or oral hypoglycemic agents (hypoglycemia, epinephrine release)	Hypertension (stroke)	Unopposed α-adrenergic vasoconstriction	Primarily seen with nonselective β-blockers; possibly also with high doses of selective blockers
	Antacids, cholestyramine, colestipol	Reduced absorption	Binding in gut	Separate dosing by at least 1 hour
Propranolol and metoprolol	Phenytoin, phenobarbital, rifampin	Reduced bioavailability	Accelerated metabolism, increased first pass metabolism	May need higher doses of propranolol
	Cimetidine	Increased bioavailability	Decreased first pass metabolism	May need to decrease propranolol dose
	Hydralazine	Increased bioavailability; increased systemic clearance; variable effect on propranolol blood levels	Accelerated systemic metabolism; ? saturation of presystemic metabolism	Interaction is probably of hemodynamic nature; fixed relationship between propranolol and hydralazine dosing desirable
	Lidocaine	Propranolol may reduce lidocaine clearance, resulting in higher than expected levels	Reduced liver blood flow; ? direct inhibition of metabolism	Reduce lidocaine infusion rate; may occur with other β-blockers as well
Propranolol and pindolol	Indomethacin, possibly other NSAIDs	Reduced antihypertensive action of β-blockers	Inhibition of prostaglandin synthesis	Avoid combination if possible; if NSAIDs are necessary, monitor BP closely

* After IV verapamil

pertension, the high toxic/therapeutic ratio, and the intrinsic wide individual variability in the pharmacokinetics of many of the β-blockers. However, pharmacokinetic interactions can be of a substantial magnitude and should be considered when there is toxicity or unexpected failure to respond.

β-Blockers fall into two broad pharmacokinetic classes. Propranolol and metoprolol are highly lipophilic and are rapidly and extensively metabolized. Absorption is complete, but bioavailability is relatively low owing to extensive first-pass metabolism. In contrast, atenolol, nadolol, and pindolol are less lipophilic and are eliminated primarily unchanged by the kidney. Absorption may be incomplete, but because there is little first-pass metabolism, bioavailability is less variable than for the more lipophilic β-blockers.

Absorption of all β-blockers is potentially interfered with by coingestion of antacids or bile-acid-binding resins. Aluminum hydroxide antacids, cholestyramine, and colestipol have specifically been shown to decrease bioavailability of propranolol.

For drugs with high presystemic (first-pass) metabolism, interacting drugs that affect rate of metabolism will influence both bioavailability and systemic clearance. When bioavailability is low owing to extensive first-pass metabolism, small changes in clearance may have large effects on bioavailability. For example, phenytoin, phenobarbital, and rifampin accelerate propranolol and metoprolol metabolism, resulting in reduced bioavailability.[41,42] Half-life after absorption may or may not be shortened owing to concomitant increase in systemic clearance. Conversely, cimetidine decreases the metabolism and increases the bioavailability of propranolol and metoprolol.[43] As a clinical consequence, excessive bradycardia associated with high levels of propranolol has been reported in a patient in whom cimetidine was added to propranolol therapy.[44]

Hydralazine has unusual affects on propranolol kinetics. Both systemic clearance and bioavailability increase.[45] Extraction of propranolol by the liver is high such that propranolol clearance is regarded as being dependent on hepatic blood flow. Hydralazine increases systemic clearance of propranolol by increasing cardiac output and hepatic blood flow. However, hydralazine may also increase bioavailability due to rapid delivery of drug to the liver and saturation of metabolic pathways. The magnitude of the increased bioavailability far exceeds the change in systemic clearance. As a result, propranolol levels increase in the presence of hydralazine (and presumably other vasodilators).

The magnitude of drug interaction effects on bioavailability of propranolol and metoprolol may be large, requiring substantial dosage adjustment to maintain constant blood levels or effects. For vasodilators the interaction appears to be of a hemodynamic nature, so the magnitude of effect may be related to the temporal relationship between dosing of the two drugs. To reduce dose-to-dose variability in blood levels of the β-blockers, vasodilators and propranolol should be given on a fixed relative dosing schedule.

The β-blockers that are eliminated by renal excretion are not subject to metabolic interactions but are sensitive to changes in renal function. Drugs that might affect renal function, such as nonsteroidal anti-inflammatory drugs, could therefore influence elimination rate.

β-Blockers can affect the pharmacokinetics of other drugs. Propranolol has been shown to reduce the clearance of antipyrine and may result in increased blood levels of chlorpromazine. The effect on antipyrine metabolism is a direct metabolic effect rather than due to β-blockade. By reducing hepatic blood flow, β-blockers can slow the metabolism of other rapidly metabolized drugs, such as lidocaine.

PHARMACODYNAMIC INTERACTIONS

Myocardial depression, cardiac failure, hypotension, bradycardia, and atrioventricular block are the most significant adverse effects of β-blockers as a drug class. Such adverse reactions generally occur in people who have underlying myocardial or conduction disease or who are taking other myocardial depressant drugs. Among these are the calcium entry blockers and type I antiarrhythmic drugs, particularly disopyramide. Of the calcium entry blockers, verapamil has been implicated in adverse interactions with β-blockers most often, presumably because it has the greatest myocardial depressant activity at usual therapeutic doses. Most instances of hypotension or asystole have occurred in patients on β-blockers following intravenous verapamil, possibly related to high circulating levels of verapamil after rapid administration.[46,47] Nifedipine and diltiazem combined with β-blockers are usually well tolerated. However, in patients with depressed cardiac function, hypotension or cardiac failure may occur with these combinations as well.[48,49] In high-risk patients on β-blockers, verapamil is best avoided; other calcium entry blockers should be administered initially in low doses and with careful observation. Amiodarone has sympathetic blocking activity and may also have additive myocardial depressant effects with β-blockers.[37]

All β-blockers inhibit reflex tachycardia. This property is used therapeutically in combining β-blockers with vasodilators in the therapy of hypertension. However, instances of profound hypotension in patients receiving β-blockers and then parenteral vasodilators, such as intravenous hydralazine or diazoxide, and potentiation of postural hypotension due to prazosin have been reported.

Case Example A 57-year-old woman taking propranolol, 60 mg/day, for palpitations visited an emergency room for treatment of urticaria. Two minutes after receiving 0.3 ml 1:1000 epinephrine subcutaneously, blood pressure rose from 120/70 to 220/110. The patient developed headache, right-sided weakness, and aphasia. Computed tomographic scan of the head showed a left parietal hematoma with associated subdural hematoma.[50]

Most β-blockers nonselectively antagonize, that is, they act on both cardiac and vascular β-adrenergic receptors. The cardioselective β-blockers such as metoprolol and atenolol are cardioselective only in low doses. At higher doses commonly used for many patients cardioselectivity is lost. A consequence of mixed nonselective blockade is the epinephrine reversal phenomenon. In the absence of β-blockers, epinephrine increases systolic blood pressure slightly and decreases diastolic blood pressure. After pretreatment with propranolol, epinephrine produces marked systolic and diastolic hypertension.[51] Epinephrine alone constricts and dilates resistance blood vessels by stimulation of α_1- and β_2-receptors, respectively. These actions counterbalance one another. Blocking β_2-receptors, as occurs with nonselective β-blockade, results in unopposed α_1-stimulation and therefore hypertension. In patients receiving β-blockers, epinephrine administered therapeutically, such as in the case example, or released endogenously, as in association with insulin-induced hypoglycemia or an epinephrine-secreting pheochromocytoma, may result in severe hypertension with cerebral vascular accident or myocardial injury or infarction. Similar interactions between β-blockers and sympathomimetic drugs, which act by releasing catecholamines, might also be expected. Chronic β-blockade has been shown to increase twofold the pressor sensitivity to norepinephrine and angiotensin.[52] (See also the section on sympathomimetic and antihypertensive drugs.) The mechanism for this interaction has not been defined. The antihypertensive effects of β-blockers may be antagonized by addition of nonsteroidal anti-inflammatory drugs. This interaction is discussed in further detail in the section on nonsteroidal anti-inflammatory drugs.

CALCIUM ENTRY BLOCKERS (TABLE 21.5)
PHARMACOKINETIC INTERACTIONS

Verapamil, diltiazem, and nifedipine are rapidly and extensively metabolized by the liver such that metabolism is dependent upon liver blood flow.[53] Drugs such as β-blockers, which decrease liver blood flow, may decrease the clearance of verapamil, resulting in higher than expected verapamil concentrations during constant dosing. That interaction might aggravate the pharmacodynamic interaction between calcium entry blockers and β-blockers as discussed below. Verapamil, diltiazem, and nifedipine undergo considerable first-pass metabolism. Thus, the bioavailability of these drugs is relatively low (20%–50%). Phenobarbital, phenytoin, and rifampin would be expected to accelerate the clearance and decrease the bioavailability of calcium entry blockers; conversely, cimetidine would be expected to decrease clearance and increase bioavailability.[54]

Verapamil and diltiazem reduce the metabolism or renal clearance of digoxin, resulting in increased digoxin levels (see digoxin section).

Although not well studied, calcium entry blockers clearly have the potential to influence the disposition of other drugs by way of hemodynamic mechanisms. For example, these drugs decrease liver blood flow,[55] which could affect the rate of metabolism of drugs such as lidocaine or propranolol, whose metabolism is dependent on liver blood flow. Reversible deterioration of renal function following nifedipine treatment in patients with chronic renal insufficiency, presumably due to intrarenal hemodynamic effects, has been described.[56] Impaired excretion of other drugs could be a consequence.

PHARMACODYNAMIC INTERACTIONS

Case Example A 54-year-old man presented with new-onset angina. He had been treated with metoprolol, 100 mg twice a day for 16 days, without complete control of pain. Verapamil, 120 mg every 8 hours, was added. The following day the patient developed confusion, sweating, nausea, and vomiting, with findings of pulmonary edema, hypotension, and bradycardia with a junctional rhythm at 56 per minute. There were no electrocardiographic or enzyme changes indicating acute myocardial infarction. Medications were stopped, and he recovered fully. Subsequent coronary angiography showed triple-vessel coronary disease with a normal ejection fraction.[47]

Cardiac toxicity from calcium entry blockers includes sinus bradycardia or arrest, high-grade atrioventricular block, asystole, hypotension, and cardiac failure. These toxic reactions have occurred most often in patients receiving other drugs that depress cardiac conduction or contractility. For example, asystole following intravenous administration of verapamil has been seen in patients taking β-blockers or digitalis.[46,57] Excessive hypotension, worsening angina, or cardiac failure following administration of nifedipine has been observed in patients receiving β-blockers.[48,49,58] Verapamil, because it has the greatest effects on cardiac conduction and contractility, has been the most often implicated in such drug interactions. Nifedipine and diltiazem also depress myocardial function, but these drugs produce more vasodilation, activating sympathetic reflexes, so that heart rate, cardiac output, and atrioventricular conduction are usually minimally affected. Blocking sympathetic reflexes with β-blockers may unmask the myocardial depressant actions of calcium entry blockers.

Identifying persons who are at risk for adverse drug interactions is important because combination therapy with calcium entry blockers and β-blockers is effective and often desirable therapy for anginal syndromes. Likewise calcium entry blockers and antiarrhythmic drug combinations are often required for patients with coronary artery disease and chronic ventricular arrhythmias. Laboratory studies indicate that verapamil decreases cardiac performance in patients on β-blockers, but if left ventricular function is normal or only moderately depressed and if there are no conduction abnormalities, verapamil is well tolerated.[59,60] However, occasionally severe left ventricular dysfunction or conduction disease is not apparent on routine evaluation or, as in the case illustrated, patients may appear to have normal left ventricular function but are particularly sensitive to drug effects, and unpredictable interactions may develop. Because of its myocardial effects, it is most prudent (when possible) to avoid combining verapamil with β-blockers or antiarrhythmic drugs such as disopyramide, which strongly depress myocardial functions. Alternative calcium blockers should be selected. However, because of the unpredictability of interactions when starting any calcium blockers in patients taking β-blockers or antiarrhythmic drugs, the possible development of cardiac failure, hypotension, or bradyarrhythmias (including unexplained syncopal episodes) should be considered.

Verapamil and digitalis are frequently used together. The combination is tolerated well by most patients. However, there is concern

TABLE 21.5 DRUG INTERACTIONS INVOLVING CALCIUM ENTRY BLOCKERS

Drug	Interacting Drug	Effect	Probable Mechanism	Comments
Verapamil (other calcium entry blockers possible but less likely)	β-blockers	Heart block, cardiac failure, asystole (after IV verapamil)	Additive depression of AV conduction, myocardial contractility	Primarily seen with verapamil; should be used with caution in patients on β-blockers
	Digitalis (toxicity)	Aggravates heart block; asystole	Additive depression of cardiac conduction	Avoid use of calcium blockers in patients with digitalis toxicity
Verapamil Diltiazem	Digoxin	Reduced digoxin clearance, increased digoxin levels	Inhibition of metabolism and renal excretion of digoxin	Reduce digoxin dose after starting verapamil or diltiazem; monitor SDC
Verapamil	Quinidine	Hypotension (after IV verapamil)	Additive α-adrenergic blockade	Use IV verapamil cautiously in patients taking quinidine or other drugs with α-blocking activity
All calcium entry blockers	Oral hypoglycemic agents	Hyperglycemia	Inhibition of insulin release by sulfonylurea drugs	May need to increase oral hypoglycemic or insulin doses to maintain control; caution about hypoglycemia when calcium blockers are stopped

(*AV*, atrioventricular; *SDC*, serum digoxin concentration)

about serious adverse interaction if digitalis toxicity develops. Patients have developed high-degree heart block or asystole after receiving intravenous verapamil with possible coexisting digitalis toxicity. Verapamil is contraindicated in the presence of digitalis toxicity. Caution is particularly necessary when adding verapamil (or diltiazem) to a stable digoxin regimen because these calcium blockers increase digoxin levels and could themselves induce digitalis toxicity, which would lead to a catastrophic drug interaction.

Case Example A 62-year-old man developed recurrent supraventricular arrhythmias following coronary artery bypass surgery. He was treated with digoxin and a quinidine gluconate, 320 mg three times a day. Four days later he developed atrial fibrillation with a ventricular rate of 140. Verapamil, 5 mg, was given by intravenous injection. Within 2 minutes blood pressure fell from 130/70 to 80/50; heart rate fell to 50. Two days later, after quinidine had been stopped, the patient was rechallenged with the same dose of verapamil without adverse consequence.[30]

In addition to direct effects on myocardial function or vascular tone, verapamil has α-adrenergic blocking activity. This is seen in concentrations associated with therapeutic use and is particularly evident after rapid intravenous injection when blood levels are high. The case example as well as other case reports describe hypotension following combination therapy with quinidine and verapamil, presumably due to additive α-blocking effects. Hypotension might also be anticipated after rapid injections of verapamil in any patient whose blood pressure is dependent on increased α-adrenergic tone or who is receiving other drugs with α-blocking activity.

Calcium may antagonize the action of calcium entry blockers. Calcium infusion has been used to manage overdoses and untoward cardiovascular reactions to calcium entry blockers.[61,62] Animal studies indicate that calcium will reverse negative inotropic effects and partially reverse depressed atrioventricular conduction, but will not reverse sinus node depression or vasodilation.[63] Substantial increases in calcium levels are required to reverse calcium blocker effects; in most patients oral calcium supplements or antacids are unlikely to raise calcium concentrations sufficiently to influence calcium blocker action.

Calcium entry blockers inhibit glucose or sulfonylurea-induced insulin release by interfering with calcium entry into beta islet cells.[64] Deterioration of carbohydrate tolerance in diabetics may occur after calcium entry blockers are initiated.[65] Blood glucose should be monitored carefully when calcium blockers are given to diabetics. Doses of insulin or oral hypoglycemic drugs may need to be increased. Conversely, when calcium blockers are stopped in patients under good control with hypoglycemic medications, the possible development of hypoglycemia should be anticipated.

DIURETICS

Pharmacokinetic interactions involving diuretics do not have major clinical significance. A few pharmacodynamic interactions can result in substantial changes in diuretic efficacy or toxicity (Table 21.6). The combination of loop and thiazide-type diuretics, used in some patients with refractory heart failure, may result in massive fluid and electrolyte losses and circulatory collapse.[66] The efficacy of loop diuretics in sodium-retaining states, such as severe cardiac failure, in which renal blood flow and glomerular filtration rate are depressed, is limited by avid distal tubular sodium reabsorption. Thiazide-type diuretics will inhibit distal tubular reabsorption of sodium, resulting in marked natriuresis and kaliuresis. This combination must be used judiciously, beginning with low doses of thiazide (2.5 mg of metolazone or 12.5 mg of hydrochlorothiazide), with careful monitoring for development of hypokalemia and azotemia. When diuresis is excessive, thiazide may be given every other day. Similarly, theophylline may act synergistically with loop diuretics, presumably by increasing renal blood flow and glomerular filtration rate.[67]

Natriuretic and antihypertensive actions of loop diuretics may be inhibited by indomethacin or other nonsteroidal anti-inflammatory drugs.[68] Loop diuretics appear to work in part producing renal vasodilation by stimulation of renal prostaglandin synthesis, an effect that is blocked by indomethacin. Other adverse interactions involving diuretics and nonsteroidal anti-inflammatory drugs on renal function are discussed in the next section.

Ototoxicity is a well-described side effect of loop diuretics. It is most commonly seen with high-dose administration in patients with diminished renal function. The risk of ototoxicity may be increased in patients receiving aminoglycoside antibiotics. Doses of loop diuretics should be kept to a minimum in such patients, and hearing should be appropriately monitored.

Diuresis itself may result in hemodynamically mediated changes in the elimination of other drugs. For example, tubular secretion and total renal clearance of digoxin may be reduced in patients who are diuresed to the point of prerenal azotemia in therapy of heart failure.[21]

TABLE 21.6 DRUG INTERACTIONS INVOLVING DIURETICS

Drug	Interacting Drug	Effect	Mechanism	Comments
Loop diuretics	Thiazides, metolazone	Marked natriuresis and diuresis	Inhibition of sodium reabsorption at multiple sites within nephron	May result in severe dehydration, circulatory collapse; start thiazide or metolazone at low doses
	Theophylline	Marked natriuresis and diuresis	Increased renal blood flow and glomerular filtration rate	Observe carefully when adding theophylline
	Indomethacin and other nonsteroidal anti-inflammatory drugs	Inhibition of diuretic and antihypertensive actions	Inhibition of prostaglandin-mediated renal vasodilation	Avoid NSAIDs, or if necessary use lowest doses possible; may need to increase diuretic dose
	Aminoglycosides	Ototoxicity	Additive injury to vestibular or cochlear sensory cells	Use lowest possible dose of loop diuretics; monitor for ototoxicity
All diuretics	Digitalis	Ventricular arrhythmias	Potassium or magnesium depletion	Monitor potassium and magnesium levels; supplement as necessary
	Lithium	Increased lithium levels, lithium toxicity	Sodium depletion reduces renal clearance of lithium	Decrease lithium dose 25% to 50%; monitor lithium levels

Any drug whose clearance is primarily by the kidney may be subject to similar interactions. A common diuretic-drug interaction is diuretic-induced hypokalemia or hypomagnesemia with digitalis, resulting in ventricular arrhythmias. This interaction was discussed in the section on cardiac glycosides.

Diuretic use, even without excessive diuresis, reduces the renal excretion of lithium, which may lead to lithium toxicity.[69] In a state of even mild sodium depletion, tubular reabsorption of lithium increases. Lithium dose should be reduced by 25% to 50% when diuretics are added, with the ultimate maintenance dose determined by serum level monitoring.

NONSTEROIDAL ANTI-INFLAMMATORY DRUGS

Case Example A 64-year-old man with a history of hypertension, angina, and hyperuricemia was taking Dyazide (25 mg of hydrochlorothiazide and 50 mg of triamterine), 3 per day, propranolol, and nitroglycerine. He was hospitalized for an acute myocardial infarction, which was uncomplicated. On the third hospital day, prodagra of the right great toe developed, and the patient was treated with indomethacin, 50 mg every 6 hours, for seven doses. Within 12 hours of initiation of treatment the patient became oliguric and subsequently anuric. Serum creatinine rose from 1.1 mg to 14.0 mg/dl over 6 days, and intermittent hemodialysis was required. Sixty days later renal function returned to normal.[70]

Nonsteroidal anti-inflammatory drugs (NSAIDs) are among the most widely prescribed class of drugs, particularly in treatment of chronic arthritis in the elderly, a population with a high prevalence of heart disease. The potential for adverse drug interactions, although only recently recognized, is believed to be highly significant (Table 21.7). Pharmacokinetic interactions resulting in changes in blood levels of NSAIDs are not usually clinically significant. NSAIDs may influence the kinetics and effects of other drugs, particularly warfarin. For example, diflunisal, mefenamic acid, phenylbutazone, and possibly other NSAIDs, which are highly protein bound, displace warfarin from protein binding sites and transiently increase free warfarin concentrations and its hypoprothrombinemic effects. Conversely, when NSAID therapy is stopped, free warfarin levels and anticoagulant efficacy decrease. Phenylbutazone also inhibits warfarin metabolism, resulting in substantially and sustained increased anticoagulant action.[71] Ibuprofen, naproxen, and tolmetin appear not to affect the hypoprothrombinemic action of warfarin.

Indomethacin decreases renal clearance of lithium, resulting in 30% to 50% increased plasma lithium levels.[72] The mechanism of interaction is uncertain, but may be linked to the increased sodium reabsorption associated with NSAID action on renal tubular function.

The most important interactions involving NSAIDs relate to their inhibition of cyclo-oxygenase and prostaglandin synthesis. Inhibition of prostaglandin synthesis in platelets results in a reduced platelet aggregation response. Hypoprothrombinemia, abnormal platelet function, and the potential for gastrointestinal irritation due to NSAIDs, in combination with warfarin or heparin therapy, predispose to hemorrhagic complications. Combined use of NSAIDs with anticoagulants is best avoided if possible. If NSAIDs are necessary in such patients, the safest are those that least potentiate warfarin action, as described above.

There has been much recent concern about adverse effects of NSAIDs on renal function. Renal effects are also a source of significant adverse drug interactions. Renal prostaglandins play an important role in autoregulation of renal blood flow and glomerular filtration rate (GFR), particularly in situations in which the renal circulation is threatened by hypovolemia, hypotension, or intrinsic kidney disease[73] (Fig. 21.2). Indomethacin, the prototypic NSAID, reduces renal blood flow and creatinine clearance in sodium-depleted persons but not sodium-replete healthy persons. Indomethacin reduces creatinine clearance and has resulted in acute renal failure in patients with hypovolemia, cardiac failure, cirrhosis, and intrinsic renal disease. Diuretic therapy is an important determinate of sodium and volume status. A person on diuretics, particularly if in treatment of congestive heart failure, is at risk

TABLE 21.7 DRUG INTERACTIONS INVOLVING NONSTEROIDAL ANTI-INFLAMMATORY DRUGS

Drug	Interacting Drug	Effect	Probable Mechanism	Comments
Diflunisal	Warfarin	Transient excessive hypoprothrombinemia	Displacement from protein binding sites	Transient action—no dose adjustment necessary
Phenylbutazone	Warfarin	Excessive hypothrombinemia	Inhibition of drug metabolism	Reduce warfarin dose
All NSAIDs	Warfarin and other anticoagulants	Bleeding complications	Additive effects of hypoprothrombinemia and inhibition of platelet aggregation	Avoid combination when possible
All NSAIDs (except maybe sulindac)	Diuretics	Decreased creatinine clearance; acute renal failure (sodium-depleted patients)	Inhibition of prostaglandin-mediated vasodilation of renal blood vessels	Use NSAIDs cautiously in patients on diuretics (or in cardiac failure)
Indomethacin (? all NSAIDs)	Furosemide	Antagonizes diuretic action, worsening of heart failure, edema	Reduced renal blood flow, increased tubular reabsorption of sodium	Carefully monitor after adding NSAIDs
	Potassium supplements, potassium-sparing diuretics; captopril	Hyperkalemia	NSAIDs inhibit renin release and create a state of hyporeninemic hypoaldosteronism	Monitor (K$^+$) closely when using these combinations
	β-blockers	Reverse antihypertensive actions; uncontrolled blood pressure	Unknown	Monitor blood pressure closely when using the combination
	Captopril	Reverse antihypertensive actions; uncontrolled blood pressure	Inhibition of prostaglandin-mediated vasodilator action of bradykinin	Monitor blood pressure closely when using the combination

for an adverse renal effect of NSAIDs, as illustrated in the case example. Although any diuretic that causes hypovolemia might increase the hazards of NSAIDs, triamterene in particular has been implicated in cases of indomethacin-induced acute renal failure.[70,74] Whether this is a coincidence or whether triamterene in particular presents a high risk for interactions with NSAIDs is not known. Aspirin has been shown to antagonize spironolactone-induced natriuresis in healthy volunteers; however, the clinical significance of this observation has not been established. It is prudent to carefully monitor renal function in any high-risk patient after initiation of NSAID therapy.

Case Example A 63-year-old man was treated for severe congestive heart failure with digoxin, furosemide, spironolactone, and isosorbide dinitrate. He developed acute gout, which was treated with indomethacin, 50 mg four times a day. Signs of cardiac failure increased, and he developed anasarca. The dose of furosemide was increased, with little improvement. The indomethacin was discontinued, and a brisk diuresis ensued. The cardiac failure resolved rapidly with a loss of 9 kg over 4 days.[75]

Renal prostaglandins play a role in sodium and water homeostasis. Prostaglandins increase renal blood flow and inhibit tubular reabsorption of sodium and chloride. Conversely, treatment with NSAIDs results in reduced renal blood flow and increased tubular reabsorption of sodium and chloride, resulting in reduced sodium excretion, sodium retention, and in some cases edema. These actions of NSAIDs directly oppose the therapeutic effects of diuretics. Experimental and clinical studies indicate that indomethacin antagonizes the natriuretic effects of furosemide and other diuretics.[76] The clinical consequence of such interactions may be the development or worsening of heart failure, as in the case example. Patients should be carefully monitored after initiation of NSAID therapy, and appropriate changes in NSAID or diuretic doses should be made if necessary.

Renal prostaglandins antagonize the effects of antidiuretic hormone and redistribute medullary blood flow such as to increase the ability of the kidney to produce dilute urine and excrete water. Therapy with NSAIDs results in impaired diluting ability and increased susceptibility to hyponatremia. Ibuprofen-induced hyponatremia in a patient with renal insufficiency has been reported.[77] One would predict a greater risk of hyponatremia in patients on combination therapy with NSAIDs and thiazides, since both drugs impair free water clearance.

Renal prostaglandins promote and NSAIDs inhibit renin release. NSAID therapy may result in a state of hyporeninemic hypoaldosteronism. The consequence, particularly in diabetics or patients with renal insufficiency, is impaired tolerance to potassium and increased susceptibility to hyperkalemia.[78,79] This represents a potentially serious drug interaction with potassium supplements, potassium-sparing diuretics, or captopril, the latter of which also inhibits angiotensin-mediated aldosterone release.

Not surprisingly from the above discussion, NSAIDs may influence blood pressure control in patients treated for hypertension. The evidence concerning effects of indomethacin on blood pressure control in hypertensive patients is conflicting.[80] Several studies have found increased blood pressure; a few have found no effect. In addition to general effects on sodium balance and the renin–aldosterone system, indomethacin has also been reported to inhibit the blood-pressure-lowering effects of β-blockers and captopril.[81,82] The precise role of prostaglandins in the action of these drugs and the clinical significance of the interaction have not been established. One might expect that hypertensive patients whose hypertension is volume dependent might experience worse hypertension on NSAIDs owing to sodium retention, but those with renin-dependent hypertension might have reduction of

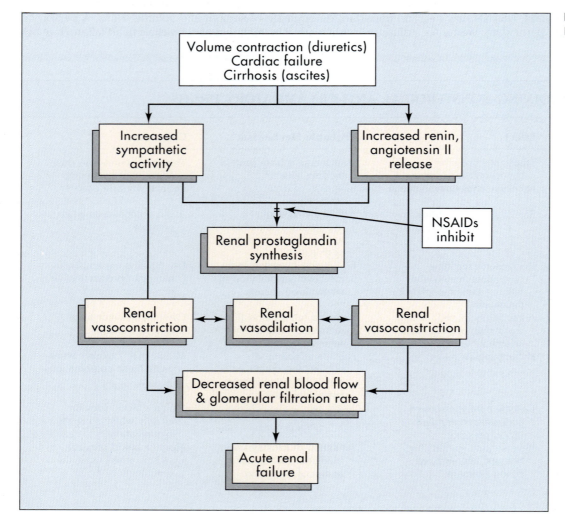

FIGURE 21.2 Mechanism of diuretic-cardiac failure-NSAID interaction.

blood pressure due to suppression of renin. Although the response of hypertensive patients to NSAIDs is not at present predictable, the possibility of an interaction should be anticipated, and the patient's blood pressure should be monitored more frequently in the period after initiation of NSAID treatment. Since vasodilation with captopril is partly mediated by increased synthesis and release of vasodilator prostaglandins, consequent on angiotensin-converting enzyme inhibition, concomitant administration of indomethacin may curtail the beneficial effects of captopril in treatment of heart failure and hypertension.

Although all NSAIDs seem to act by inhibition of prostaglandin synthesis, there may be differences among the drugs in the risk of adverse effects on the kidney. Sulindac has been shown in several studies to have less effect on renal production of prostaglandin E_2 and renal hemodynamics in chronic renal disease, despite the same magnitude of inhibition of platelet cyclo-oxygenase as ibuprofen or indomethacin.[83,84] Sulindac may also be less likely to aggravate hypertension.[85] Sulindac itself is a pro-drug, which is converted from the inactive sulfoxide to the active sulfide, primarily in the liver.[86] The kidney interconverts the sulfide and sulfoxide forms. On balance, the equilibrium favors the sulfoxide, so that in effect the kidney is detoxifying the active sulfide. Since relatively little of the active sulfide is present in the kidney parenchyma, there is little inhibition of cyclo-oxygenase, and renal prostaglandin synthesis is minimally affected. Although experimental studies suggest that sulindac is the NSAID of choice in chronic renal failure and probably in cardiac failure, the safety advantage of sulindac over other NSAIDs in populations of high-risk patients remains to be demonstrated.

SYMPATHOMIMETIC AND ANTIHYPERTENSIVE DRUGS (TABLE 21.8)

SYMPATHOMIMETIC DRUGS

Adverse reactions to sympathomimetic drugs resulting in excessive adrenergic stimulation usually occur as a consequence of unsuspected drug interactions. The epinephrine reversal phenomenon as discussed previously (see under β-blockers) is an important example. Since so many people take propranolol and other nonselective β-blockers for therapy of hypertension, coronary heart disease, migraine headache, and other indications, the potential for an interaction involving epinephrine comes up commonly in the therapy of anaphylactic or anaphylactoid reactions to drugs or insect bites. For such patients it is probably better to use β_2-agonists such as metaproterenol, terbutaline, or albuterol to treat bronchoconstriction and to titrate α-agonists such as dopamine or norepinephrine separately for management of vascular collapse. In people who have a history of anaphylactic reactions it is best to use relatively cardioselective β-blockers, although in usual therapeutic doses cardioselectivity is only partial and epinephrine reversal might still be observed.

The pressor sensitivity to some sympathomimetic drugs is increased by other drugs that retard the removal of catecholamines from the circulation. Tricyclic antidepressants, guanethidine, and bretylium are examples of drugs that inhibit uptake of catecholamines by adrenergic neurons. The result is a significant increase in sensitivity to pressor effects of norepinephrine, epinephrine, and other direct-acting sympathomimetic drugs such as phenylephrine and phenylpropranolamine found in over-the-counter (OTC) preparations.[87,88] If pressor drugs are required for such patients, therapy should be initiated with low doses and gradually increased to the desired end point. Patients taking inhibitors of catecholamine uptake should be advised about the risks of using over-the-counter sympathomimetic preparations.

Severe hypertension and other catastrophic reactions have occurred after the use of sympathomimetic drugs in patients receiving monoamine oxidase inhibitors. These are discussed in the next section.

Hypertension has been reported in one patient following indomethacin ingestion during long-term therapy with phenylpropanolamine, taken as an appetite suppressant.[89] While taking phenylpropanolamine the patient was normotensive. Following ingestion of 25 mg of indomethacin, blood pressure rose to 200/150. The mechanism of this interaction is unknown but may represent prostaglandin synthesis as a homeostatic response in moderating phenylpropanolamine-induced vasoconstriction.

Vagal reflexes resulting in bradycardia represent another important homeostatic response to drug-induced hypertension. Atropine therapy doubles the pressor sensitivity to infused phenylephrine.[90] A number of over-the-counter antihistaminic and sedative drugs, as well as some tricyclic antidepressants, have strong anticholinergic activity, which could contribute to excessive hypertension following sympathomimetic drug treatment.

Anesthetic drugs, particularly cyclopropane and the halogenated anesthetics such as halothane, enflurane, and isoflurane, sensitize the heart to the arrhythmogenic actions of catecholamines. In experimental animals the threshold dose of epinephrine required to induce ventricular fibrillation is lowered. Post-operative patients may be high risk for malignant cardiac arrhythmias during therapy with pressor drugs or bronchodilators, which have significant β-adrenergic activity.

MONOAMINE OXIDASE INHIBITORS

Fortunately very few patients are currently receiving monoamine oxidase (MAO) inhibitors for therapy of hypertension. However, these drugs are still widely used in psychiatric practice, particularly as the availability of electroconvulsive therapy for depression becomes more limited. Drug interactions involving monoamine oxidase inhibitors continue to occur and should be understood by the cardiologist. MAO is responsible for intraneuronal oxidation of amines. MAO is also present in the liver and the gastrointestinal tract, where it metabolizes amines before they reach the systemic circulation. The consequences of inhibition of MAO is to increase the neuronal content of catecholamines and serotonin and to reduce the presystemic metabolism of dietary amines such as tyramine. Sympathomimetic drugs, such as amphetamines, ephedrine or pseudoephedrine, or phenylpropranolamine, which release catecholamines, can produce severe hypertension in persons taking MAO inhibitors.[91] Ingestion of foods high in tyramine content results in higher-than-usual blood levels of tyramine (due to reduced presystemic metabolism) and a greater magnitude of catecholamine release from neurons. As a result, hypertension, as well as flushing, headache, sweating, anxiety, and palpitations, occurs, presumably a combined effect of release of catecholamines, serotonin, and other vasoactive amines. Other drugs, such as meperidine and, rarely, tricyclic antidepressants, have been reported to cause a syndrome of excitement, delirium, hyperpyrexia, and convulsions, as well as hypertension. The mechanism of this interaction is unknown.

Hypertension occurring in the context of MAO inhibitor drug therapy is catecholamine mediated and is treated similarly to therapy for pheochromocytoma. α-Adrenergic blockers (such as phentolamine), combined α- and β-blockers (labetalol), or parenteral nitroprusside is most appropriate.

ANTIHYPERTENSIVE DRUGS

Drug interactions are commonly employed in combination antihypertensive drug regimens. These therapeutic interactions are not the focus of this chapter except to mention a few cases in which significant untoward reactions have occurred. For example, first-dose hypotension following prazosin or hypotension following intravenous diazoxide is more profound in patients who are hypovolemic due to prior diuretic therapy or who are receiving β-blockers, thereby blunting homeostatic responses. Tricyclic antidepressant therapy is associated with significant orthostatic hypotension. Compensation for orthostatic hypotension occurs in part by sodium and fluid retention. Patients on

TABLE 21.8 DRUG INTERACTIONS INVOLVING SYMPATHOMIMETIC AND ANTIHYPERTENSIVE DRUGS

Drug	Interacting Drug	Effect	Probable Mechanism	Comments
Epinephrine, indirect sympathomimetic agents	Propranolol and other non-selective β-blockers	Hypertension	Propranolol antagonizes $β_2$-vasodilation, leaving unopposed α-vasoconstriction	Particular problem in treating anaphylaxis. In patients on β-blockers, titrate $β_1$-bronchodilators and α-adrenergic vasoconstrictors separately
Sympathomimetic drugs (such as phenylephrine, phenylpropranolamine)	Tricyclic antidepressants	Hypertension	Blockade of neuron uptake of amines	Avoid these combinations; warn patients about OTC sympathomimetics
	Anticholinergic drugs (including OTC antihistamines)	Hypertension	Blunting of vagal reflex compensation for drug-induced vasoconstriction	Primarily of concern with excessive doses of sympathomimetic drugs; do not use atropine in such patients
Sympathomimetic pressor drugs (such as dopamine, norepinephrine)	Anesthetics	Arrhythmias	Sensitization of heart to actions of catecholamines	Use pressor drugs cautiously in postoperative patients; monitor heart
Monoamine oxidase inhibitors	Indirect sympathomimetic drugs	Hypertension	Excessive intraneuronal stores and release of catecholamines	Avoid the combination; warn patients about OTC sympathomimetics
	Tyramine-containing foods	Hypertension	Decreased presystemic metabolism and increased bioavailability of tyramine	Avoid the combination; warn patients about tyramine-containing food
	Meperidine; rarely tricyclic antidepressants	Hypertension, excitement, delirium, hyperpyrexia	Unknown	Avoid meperidine; begin tricyclics in low doses with careful monitoring
Methyldopa	Digoxin	Sinus bradycardia	Additive sympatholytic and vagal actions	Primarily seen in patients with sinus node diseases
	Haloperidol	Delirium	Unknown	Unclear clinical significance
Clonidine	Propranolol, sotolol	Hypertension	Possibly due to unopposed α-vasoconstrictor action of clonidine	Uncommon, but should be considered as possible explanation for treatment failure
	Tricyclic antidepressants	Reversal of hypotensive actions	Blockade of central α-receptors	Avoid the combination
Guanethidine, bethanidine, debrisoquin	Tricyclic antidepressants, chlorpromazine, amphetamine	Reversal of hypotensive actions	Blockade of neuronal uptake of guanethidine and related drugs	Avoid the combination
	Catecholamines, direct sympathomimetic drugs	Hypertension	Increased adrenergic receptor sensitivity	Avoid OTC sympathomimetics; begin pressor drugs in low doses
Captopril	Potassium supplements, potassium-sparing diuretics	Hyperkalemia	Inhibition of aldosterone release; inability to excrete potassium	Use potassium very cautiously; monitor potassium levels frequently
	Indomethacin (and possibly other NSAIDs)	Reversal of hypotensive action	Inhibition of kinin-mediated prostaglandin synthesis	Avoid combination if possible; if necessary, monitor blood pressure closely

diuretics or other antihypertensive drugs are more likely to experience more severe orthostatic hypotension, which may result in vascular accidents, especially in the elderly.

A number of adverse interactions involving specific antihypertensive drugs have been described. Those involving diuretics and β-blockers are discussed in other sections.

METHYLDOPA AND CLONIDINE

Methyldopa has been associated with development of sinus bradycardia in patients receiving digoxin.[92] This may occur, although rarely, even in patients with normal sinus node function, presumably on the basis of additive sympatholytic and vagal effects of the two drugs. Clonidine and other central-acting sympatholytic drugs would be expected to have similar interactions.

Clonidine has been reported to aggravate hypertension in some patients receiving propranolol or sotalol.[93,94] This is hypothesized to result from unmasking the intrinsic α-agonist vasoconstrictor activity of clonidine in the presence of β_2 (vasodilator)-antagonism. Why this interaction occurs only rarely is unclear.

The antihypertensive action of clonidine is inhibited by prior treatment with tricyclic antidepressant drugs.[95] Clonidine exerts its hypotensive action by stimulating central nervous system α_2-receptors. Tricyclic antidepressants are α-adrenergic antagonists and by that mechanism antagonize the central actions of clonidine. Tricyclics do not inhibit the hypotensive action of methyldopa, which also acts on central system α-receptors. Maprotiline, a tetracyclic antidepressant, does not antagonize clonidine effects and may be used when antidepressant drug therapy is required in patients receiving clonidine.

GUANETHIDINE, BETHANIDINE, AND DEBRISOQUIN

Case Example A 47-year-old man with chronic hypertension was taking guanethidine, 75 mg/day; methyldopa, 750 mg/day; and trichlormethazine, 8 mg/day. Blood pressure was 118/80 mm Hg supine and 118/96 mm Hg standing. Because of depression he was referred to a psychiatrist who prescribed amitriptyline, 25 mg three times a day. One month later his blood pressure was 190/122 mm Hg supine and 160/115 mm Hg standing.[96]

To exert their antihypertensive action, guanethidine and related compounds bethanidine and debrisoquin must be taken up by adrenergic nerve terminals. Drugs that block uptake of amines inhibit the uptake and action of guanethidine and related drugs, resulting in loss of blood pressure control.[97] Many of the tricyclic antidepressants, as well as chlorpromazine, may reverse guanethidine action.[97,98] Tricyclic antidepressant reversal of guanethidine action occurs slowly, requiring more than 12 hours. In contrast, the reversal occurs quickly after bethanidine. The kinetics of the reversal is consistent with the idea that the rate of loss of antihypertensive action is related to rate of exit of drug from the neuron after reuptake is inhibited. Guanethidine is slowly but bethanidine rapidly eliminated from the neuron. Amphetamines and related over-the-counter sympathomimetic drugs may also reverse guanethidine action, both by blocking uptake and by causing release of intraneuronal guanethidine.[99]

Guanethidine competes with norepinephrine and related amines for neuronal uptake. Long-term therapy reduces endogenous adrenergic activity, resulting in enhanced receptor sensitivity. One or both of these actions may explain the pressor supersensitivity to exogenously administered or released norepinephrine in patients receiving guanethidine.[97] Similarly, hypertensive interactions are expected with over-the-counter sympathomimetic drugs. It is best to avoid the use of these drugs in patients taking guanethidine or related drugs.

CAPTOPRIL

Case Example A 58-year-old woman with ischemic cardiomyopathy was hospitalized for treatment of refractory cardiac failure. Therapy included digoxin, furosemide, hydrochlorothiazide, nitroglycerin ointment, and captopril. Admission electrolytes included sodium, 128 mEq/liter; potassium, 3.0 mEq/liter; chloride, 88 mEq/liter; carbon dioxide, 26 mEq/liter; blood urea nitrogen (BUN), 19 mg/dl; and creatinine, 0.7 mg/dl. Because of hypokalemia, potassium chloride, 40 mEq/day, was added. Over the first 48 hours the patient diuresed briskly, losing 4 kg in weight. She subsequently became oliguric. BUN and creatinine rose to 36 and 1.2, respectively. On the third hospital day, serum potassium was 4.9. On the fourth hospital day, 2 hours after the morning potassium dose, the patient had a cardiac arrest. The laboratory later reported the serum potassium prior to the potassium dose had been 6.5 mEq/liter.

This case illustrates the most important drug interaction involving captopril, that is, hyperkalemia during therapy with potassium or potassium-sparing diuretics. Captopril inhibits the formation of angiotensin II and therefore the release of renin and aldosterone. Inhibition of aldosterone release results in diminished potassium excretion and enhanced susceptibility to hyperkalemia. Patients are particularly susceptible when the glomerular filtration rate is reduced, as in patients with cardiac failure after vigorous diuresis. As in the case illustration, rapid and marked increases in serum potassium can be observed with even modest potassium supplementation. To avoid hyperkalemia, potassium supplementation should be ordered on a day-by-day basis after reviewing that day's potassium level.

Although the primary antihypertensive action of captopril appears to be by inhibition of angiotensin II, inhibition of metabolism of kinins also appears to contribute to captopril action. Kinins exert a hypotensive action in part by increasing prostaglandin synthesis. Indomethacin inhibits prostaglandin synthesis and antagonizes the antihypertensive actions of captopril.[82] Other nonsteroidal anti-inflammatory drugs, although not explicitly studied, could presumably interact in a similar fashion.

THEOPHYLLINE

Case Example A 71-year-old woman had a history of chronic obstructive lung disease, coronary heart disease, and peptic ulcer disease. She was hospitalized for worsening of bronchospasm for which she was treated with theophylline. On 300 mg every 6 hours the serum theophylline level was 15 μg/ml. She developed midepigastric burning pain and was treated with cimetidine, 300 mg four times a day. Four days later she experienced a grand mal seizure. Serum theophylline concentration 8 hours after the last dose was 29 μg/ml.

Theophylline is commonly prescribed to cardiac patients. It has a low toxic/therapeutic ratio and is one of the most common drugs causing adverse reactions. Many adverse reactions to theophylline occur because of interactions with other drugs (Table 21.9). Theophylline is almost exclusively (90%) metabolized. The rate of metabolism is variable and influenced by age, liver disease, cardiac failure, smoking history, and diet. Most drug interactions are pharmacokinetic and as a consequence result in reduced or accelerated theophylline metabolism.[100]

Drugs that accelerate theophylline metabolism include phenobarbital, phenytoin, carbamazepine, rifampin, and sulfinpyrazone. Theophylline toxicity is observed when these drugs are stopped while the patient continues to take an unchanged dose of theophylline. Drugs that inhibit theophylline metabolism include erythromycin, triacetyloleandomycin (troleandomycin), cimetidine, oral contraceptives, and, possibly, allopurinol in high doses (600 mg/day). Commonly, adverse drug interactions occur in patients receiving theophylline for treatment of chronic obstructive lung disease, who develop a respiratory tract infection for which they are prescribed erythromycin, or who develop abdominal symptoms (which may be a side effect of theophylline itself) and are prescribed cimetidine. It is best in patients receiving theophylline to use antibiotics such as ampicillin or tetracycline or cephalosporins and to use antiulcer therapies such as ranitidine, sucralfate, or antacids, which do not inhibit theophylline metabolism.

Influenza vaccination is given routinely to patients with severe cardiac and pulmonary disease. Vaccination results in formation of interferon, which potentially may inhibit cytochrome P-450 drug oxidation. Several reports have indicated an inhibitory effect of influenza vaccination on theophylline clearance, including a few cases of apparent clinical toxicity.[101] However, other researchers have not been able to confirm depression of theophylline clearance.[102,103] Although the clinical significance of this interaction is not confirmed, it is prudent to consider the possibility, particularly for patients whose usual theophylline concentrations are at the high end of the therapeutic range.

Pharmacodynamic interactions involving theophylline may occur in combination with diuretics, as discussed in the diuretic section. Theophylline toxicity may present as the development of tachyarrhythmias, the treatment of which with digoxin may result in subsequent digitalis intoxication, as described in the cardiac glycosides section.

When drug therapy that is known to change theophylline kinetics is required, dosage adjustments should be anticipated. However, because the magnitude of interaction is variable, adjustments should be guided by measurements of serum theophylline concentrations.

ANTICOAGULANTS

Case Example A 71-year-old man with an aortic valve prosthesis, placed for rheumatic heart disease and coronary artery disease, had been taking warfarin, 5 mg/day, for 10 years. Because of ventricular arrhythmias refractory to other medications he was begun on amiodarone, 600 mg/day. Two weeks later he presented with bruising and easy bleeding. Prothrombin time had gone from its usual 20 seconds to 85 seconds. On a warfarin dose of 2.5 mg/day, prothrombin time again returned to the therapeutic range.[36]

Oral anticoagulants are typically taken over long periods, and concurrent administration of cardiovascular and other drugs is common. Many drug interactions involving anticoagulants have been described and have been known to physicians for many years (Tables 21.10 and 21.11).[71] Yet in most hospitals adverse drug interactions involving anticoagulants continue to occur. The consequences of such interactions, excessive bleeding or thrombosis, are potentially life-threatening. Nearly all are avoidable. Most of the interactions described in this section refer to warfarin (Coumadin). Pharmacokinetic interactions may not necessarily be the same for bishydroxycoumarin (dicumarol); pharmacodynamic interactions are similar.

DRUGS THAT ENHANCE RESPONSES TO ORAL ANTICOAGULANTS

Initiation of drugs that enhance responses to anticoagulants in patients who have been stabilized on a particular dose of an oral anticoagulant requires reduction in that dose. Cessation of therapy requires increasing the anticoagulant dose to maintain the same degrees of anticoagulation.

PHARMACOKINETIC INTERACTIONS

Pharmacokinetic interactions are those that result in increased concentrations of unbound warfarin in plasma. Most commonly the interacting drug slows the metabolism of warfarin. This type of interaction persists as long as the interacting drug is administered. Drugs that have been clearly shown to inhibit the metabolism of warfarin include allopurinol, chloramphenicol (inhibits dicumarol), cimetidine, disulfiram, metronidazole, oxyphenbutazone, phenylbutazone, trimethoprim-sulfamethoxazole and other sulfonamides, and possibly amiodarone and erythromycin.[71,104] Warfarin is a racemic mixture of equal amounts of two optical isomers. S-Warfarin is four times more potent than R-warfarin. This is significant because some warfarin-drug interactions

TABLE 21.9 DRUG INTERACTIONS INVOLVING THEOPHYLLINE

Interacting Drug	Serum Theophylline Concentration	Typical % Change in Clearance	Mechanism	Comments
Carbamazepine	Decreased		Acceleration of metabolism	When drugs are added to stable theophylline dose, monitor theophylline levels and increase dose as necessary. Discontinuation of interacting drug may lead to theophylline toxicity. Decrease theophylline dose when or before other drug is stopped
Phenobarbital	Decreased	30	Acceleration of metabolism	
Phenytoin	Decreased	40–70	Acceleration of metabolism	
Rifampin	Decreased	20	Acceleration of metabolism	
Sulfinpyrazone	Decreased	20	Acceleration of metabolism	
Allopurinol (high doses)	Increased	20	Inhibition of metabolism	When drugs are added decrease theophylline dose (in proportion to typical change in clearance), monitor levels to optimal dose. Discontinuation of interacting drugs may result in subtherapeutic levels and require an increased theophylline dose
Cimetidine	Increased	30–40	Inhibition of metabolism	
Erythromycin	Increased	20–30	Inhibition of metabolism	
Oral contraceptives	Increased	30	Inhibition of metabolism	
Triacetyloleandomycin	Increased	50	Inhibition of metabolism	

involve stereoselective alterations in warfarin metabolism. Phenylbutazone, sulfinpyrazone, and metronidazole, as well as trimethoprim-sulfamethoxazole, primarily inhibit S-warfarin metabolism.

Warfarin is highly (99%) bound to plasma proteins, predominantly albumin. Drugs that displace warfarin from protein binding sites increase the unbound warfarin concentration and potentially cause a greater hypoprothrombinemic action. However, the unbound concentration also determines the rate of metabolism of warfarin. Increased unbound warfarin results in an increased rate of metabolism, which ultimately results in return of the unbound drug concentration to its original level, despite the persistence of the interacting drug. Thus, transient enhancement of anticoagulant action is observed. Since the fraction unbound is increased, but the steady state concentration of the unbound drug is held constant by metabolism, the total plasma concentration of warfarin decreases. Chloral hydrate, diflunisal, mefenamic acid, oxyphenbutazone, phenylbutazone, and possibly clofibrate interact with warfarin by displacing it from plasma proteins.

The time course of drug interactions involving warfarin may be complex. It depends on the kinetics of the interacting drug, the kinetics of the interacting event, the kinetics of warfarin, and the kinetics of the clotting factors. For example, cimetidine has a half-life of 2 to 3 hours. With constant dosing, steady state levels of cimetidine occur within 24 hours. Inhibition of metabolism occurs rapidly and becomes maximal in a day or two.[105] Increased prothrombin time is observed within 2 or 3 days. In contrast, amiodarone has a half-life of a month or more. Many days or weeks of constant dosing may be necessary before

TABLE 21.10 DRUGS INCREASING RESPONSES TO WARFARIN

Interacting Drug	Mechanism	Comments
Allopurinol Amiodarone Cimetidine Disulfiram Metronidazole Oxyphenbutazone Phenylbutazone Sulfonamides	Inhibition of warfarin metabolism	Requires reduction in warfarin dose
Trimethoprim-sulfamethoxazole Chloral hydrate Diflunisal Mefenamic acid	Displacement of warfarin from plasma proteins	Transient increase in hypoprothrombinemic action; warfarin dose does not need adjustment
Erythromycin, 3rd generation cephalosporin, and other broad-spectrum antibiotics	Reduction in vitamin K availability	Primarily in malnourished patients
Salicylate (high doses) Quinidine	Depression of clotting synthesis	May need to adjust warfarin dose
Thyroid hormones Clofibrate Anabolic steroids	Accelerated catabolism of vitamin K–dependent clotting factors	May need to adjust warfarin dose
Salicylates and other nonsteroidal anti-inflammatory drugs Carbenicillin Cefamandole Cefoperazone Moxalactam	Interference with platelet function	Avoid combination when possible; if necessary, monitor closely for bleeding complications

TABLE 21.11 DRUGS DECREASING RESPONSES TO WARFARIN

Interacting Drug	Mechanism	Comments
Barbiturates Carbamazepine Glutethimide Griseofluvin Phenytoin Rifampin	Accelerated warfarin metabolism	Warfarin dose needs to be increased to maintain hypoprothrombinemic effect. Caution concerning excessive anticoagulation when interacting drugs are discontinued—reduce warfarin dose at time of or prior to discontinuation of interacting drug
Cholestyramine Colestipol	Decreased absorption; possibly interfere with enterohepatic recycling of warfarin	Warfarin dose needs to be increased to maintain hypoprothrombinemic effect. Caution concerning excessive anticoagulation when interacting drugs are discontinued—reduce warfarin dose at time of or prior to discontinuation of interacting drug
Vitamin K	Antagonizes action of warfarin	Avoid combination
Oral contraceptives	Increased synthesis of Factors VII and X	Increase warfarin dose as necessary

amiodarone blood levels accumulate to the point where a significant interaction occurs. The effects of amiodarone on warfarin metabolism may persist for months after amiodarone is discontinued.

The half-life of warfarin averages 35 hours. If an interacting drug suddenly changes the rate of warfarin metabolism, it takes three half-lives, or 105 hours (longer if half-life is prolonged), to reach a new steady state level of warfarin. When a displacing drug is administered, there is an immediate change in protein binding, but the return to the original unbound concentration requires metabolism and the same 100 hours (three half-lives). Changes in the hypoprothrombinemic action of warfarin depend on changes in the synthesis of clotting factors, each of which has its own characteristic kinetics. The half-lives of Factor VII, IX, X, and II are approximately 6, 20, 40, and 60 hours, respectively. Thus, it may take 180 hours, or a little more than 1 week, to reach a steady state effect when the blood level of warfarin changes.

Because of the complexities of simultaneous kinetic processes it is impossible to predict exactly the time course of warfarin drug interaction effects on coagulation. For most drugs interactions start and become manifest within 2 or 3 days and become maximal at 1 to 2 weeks. Drug displacement interactions are maximal at 3 to 5 days and return to baseline by 2 weeks.

PHARMACODYNAMIC INTERACTIONS

Drugs may enhance warfarin action by increasing the hypoprothrombic response to a given unbound warfarin concentration. This may occur by reducing the availability of vitamin K, by inhibiting the synthesis or accelerating catabolism of clotting factors, or by affecting nonprothrombin-dependent hemostatic mechanisms.

Vitamin K is primarily obtained from food. Intestinal bacteria synthesize small quantities of vitamin K, which becomes important when dietary intake is poor. Sensitivity to warfarin is increased in patients who are deficient in vitamin K owing to starvation or malabsorption. In such patients therapy with antibiotics may result in a critical reduction in vitamin K availability, resulting in an enhanced warfarin response.[106]

Drugs that depress clotting factor synthesis include salicylate in high doses (>3 g/day) and quinidine. Accelerated catabolism of vitamin K–dependent clotting factors may be seen in treatment with thyroid hormones, clofibrate, and possibly anabolic steroids.

The most significant pharmacodynamic interactions involve additive effects of drugs that affect hemostasis by another mechanism. This may result in excessive bleeding without alteration in prothrombin time. Drugs such as salicylates and other nonsteroidal anti-inflammatory drugs, clofibrate, carbenicillin, and some of the third-generation cephalosporins (cefamandole, cefoperazone, and moxalactam), which affect platelet function, or drugs such as heparin, which affect other clotting factors, are most commonly implicated. When possible these drugs should not be administered in patients receiving oral anticoagulants.

DRUGS THAT DECREASE RESPONSES TO ORAL ANTICOAGULANTS

Initiation of drugs that decrease responses to oral anticoagulants in patients stabilized on oral anticoagulants may result in inadequate anticoagulation and thrombosis. To avoid this possibility an increase in the anticoagulant dose should be anticipated. Cessation of therapy with the same drug may result in excessive anticoagulation if the dose of warfarin is not adjusted. The latter is the source of many adverse drug interactions.

PHARMACOKINETIC INTERACTIONS

Most drugs that antagonize anticoagulant responses to warfarin do so by decreasing warfarin concentrations. Several do so by accelerating warfarin metabolism. These include barbiturates, carbamazepine, glutethimide, griseofulvin, phenytoin, and rifampin. Other drugs, such as cholestyramine and colestipol, may decrease warfarin concentrations by binding warfarin in the gut. This is an obvious problem when the drugs are given in temporal proximity.

There may also be an element of enterohepatic recirculation of warfarin such that warfarin clearance is accelerated in patients taking repeated doses of cholestyramine.

PHARMACODYNAMIC INTERACTIONS

Pharmacodynamic interactions that antagonize the effects of warfarin include administration of vitamin K analogues (vitamin K_1 and vitamin K_2), which directly antagonizes the actions of warfarin, and the administration of oral contraceptives, which increases the synthesis of Factors VII and X.

REFERENCES

1. Koch-Weser J: Drug interactions in cardiovascular therapy. Am Heart J 90:93, 1975
2. Friedman HS, Bonventre MV: Erythromycin-induced digoxin toxicity. Chest 82:202, 1982
3. Manninen V, Melin J, Apajalahti A et al: Altered absorption of digoxin in patients given propantheline and metoclopramide. Lancet 1:398, 1981
4. Lindenbaum J, Rund DG, Butler VP et al: Inactivation of digoxin by gut flora. N Engl J Med 305:789, 1981
5. Brown DD, Juhl RP, Warner SL: Decreased bioavailability of digoxin due to hypocholesterolemic interventions. Circulation 58:164, 1978
6. Caldwell J, Bushe A, Greenberger NJ: Interruption of the enterohepatic circulation of digitoxin by cholestyramine: II. Effect on metabolic disposition of tritium-labeled digitoxin and cardiac systolic intervals in man. J Clin Invest 50:2638, 1971
7. Lalonde RL, Deshpande R, Hamilton PP et al: Acceleration of digoxin clearance by activated charcoal. Clin Pharmacol Ther 37:367, 1985
8. Pond S, Jacobs M, Marks J et al: Treatment of digitoxin overdose with oral activated charcoal. Lancet 2:1177, 1981
9. Powell JR, Fenster PE, Hager WD et al: Quinidine-digoxin interaction. N Engl J Med 302:176, 1980
10. Leahy EB, Reiffel JA, Drusin RE et al: Interaction between quinidine and digoxin. JAMA 533, 1978
11. Hagar WD, Fenster P, Mayernsohn M et al: Digoxin-quinidine interaction. N Engl J Med 300:1238, 1979
12. Klein HO, Lang R, Weiss E et al: The influence of verapamil on serum digoxin concentration. Circulation 65:998, 1982
13. Rameis H, Magometschnigg D, Ganzinger U: The diltiazem-digoxin interaction. Clin Pharmacol Ther 36:183, 1984
14. Moysey JO, Jaggarao NSV, Grundy GN et al: Amiodarone increases plasma digoxin concentrations. Br Med J 282:272, 1981
15. Belz GG, Doering W, Munkes R et al: Interaction between digoxin and calcium antagonists and antiarrhythmic drugs. Clin Pharmacol Ther 33:410, 1983
16. Schwartz JB, Raizner A, Akers S: Effects of nifedipine on serum digoxin concentrations in patients. Am Heart J 107:669, 1984
17. Waldorff S, Andersen JD, Heebøll-Nielsen N et al: Spironolactone-induced changes in digoxin kinetics. Clin Pharmacol Ther 24:162, 1978
18. Gault H, Longerich L, Dawe M et al: Digoxin-rifampin interaction. Clin Pharmacol Ther 35:750, 1984
19. Fenster PE, Hagar WD, Goodman MM: Digoxin-quinidine-spironolactone interaction. Clin Pharmacol Ther 36:70, 1984
20. Cogan JJ, Humphreys MH, Carlson J et al: Acute vasodilator therapy increased renal clearance in patients with congestive heart failure. Circulation 64:973, 1981
21. Benowitz NL: Effects of cardiac disease on pharmacokinetics: Pathophysiologic considerations. In Benet LZ, Massoud N, Gambertoglio JG (eds): Pharmacokinetic Basis for Drug Treatment, pp 89–103. New York, Raven Press, 1984
22. Ochs HR, Carstens G, Greenblatt DJ: Reductions in lidocaine clearance during continuous infusion and by coadministration of propranolol. N Engl J Med 303:373, 1980
23. Svendsen TL, Tangø M, Waldorff S et al: Effects of propranolol and pindolol on plasma lignocaine clearance in man. Br J Clin Pharmacol 13:223S, 1982
24. Knapp AB, Maguire W, Keren G et al: The cimetidine-lidocaine interaction. Ann Intern Med 98:174, 1983
25. Jackson JE, Bentley JB, Glass SJ et al: Effects of histamine-2 receptor blockade on lidocaine kinetics. Clin Pharmacol Ther 37:544, 1985
26. Data JL, Wilkinson DR, Nies AS: Interaction of quinidine with anticonvulsant drugs. N Engl J Med 294:699, 1976
27. Twum-Barima Y, Carruthers SG: Quinidine-rifampin interactions. N Engl J Med 304:1466, 1981
28. Saal AK, Werner JA, Greene HL et al: Effects of amiodarone on serum quinidine and procainamide levels. Am J Cardiol 53:1264, 1984
29. Koch-Weser J: Quinidine-induced hypoprothrombinemic hemorrhage in patients on chronic warfarin therapy. Ann Intern Med 68:511, 1968
30. Maisel AS, Motulsky HJ, Insel PA: Hypotension after quinidine plus verap-

31. Argov Z, Mastaglia FL: Disorders of neuromuscular transmission caused by drugs. N Engl J Med 301:409, 1979
32. Tartini R, Steinbrunn W, Kappenberger L et al: Dangerous interaction between amiodarone and quinidine. Lancet :1327, 1982
33. Galeazzi RL, Sheiner LB, Lockwood T et al: The renal elimination of procainamide. Clin Pharmacol Ther 19:55, 1976
34. Somogyi A, McLean A, Heinzow B: Cimetidine-procainamide pharmacokinetic interaction in man: Evidence of competition for tubular secretion of basic drugs. Eur J Clin Pharmacol 25:339, 1983
35. Marcus Fl: Drug interactions with amiodarone. Am Heart J 106:924, 1983
36. Hamer A, Peter T, Mandel WJ et al: The potentiation of warfarin anticoagulation by amiodarone. Circulation 65:1025, 1982
37. Derrida JP, Ollagnier J, Benaim R et al: Amiodarone et propranolol: Une association dangereus? Nouv Presse Med 8:1429, 1979
38. Lee TH, Friedman PL, Goldman L et al: Sinus arrest and hypotension with combined amiodarone-diltiazem therapy. Am Heart J 109:163, 1985
39. Bigger T: The interaction of mexiletine with other cardiovascular drugs. Am Heart J 107:1079, 1984
40. Lalka D, Meyer MB, Duce BR et al: Kinetics of oral antiarrhythmic lidocaine congener, tocainide. Clin Pharmacol Ther 19:757, 1976
41. Wood AJJ, Feely J: Pharmacokinetic drug interactions with propranolol. Clin Pharmacokinet 8:253, 1983
42. Bennett PN, John VA, Whitmarsh VB: Effects of rifampin on metoprolol and antipyrine kinetics. Br J Clin Pharmacol 13:387, 1982
43. Heagerty AM, Donovan MA, Castleden CM et al: Influences of cimetidine on pharmacokinetics of propranolol. Br Med J 282:1917, 1981
44. Donovan MA, Heagerty AM, Patel L et al: Cimetidine and bioavailability of propranolol. Lancet 1:164, 1981
45. McLean AJ, Skews H, Bobik A et al: Interaction between oral propranolol and hydralazine. Clin Pharmacol Ther 27:726, 1980
46. Benaim ME: Asystole after verapamil. Br Med J 15:169, 1972
47. Wayne VS, Harper RW, Laufer E et al: Adverse interaction between beta-adrenergic blocking drugs and verapamil: Report of three cases. Aust NZ J Med 12:285, 1982
48. Anastassiades CJ: Nifedipine and beta-blocker drugs. Br Med J 281:1251, 1980
49. Opie LH, White DA: Adverse interaction between nifedipine and beta-blockade. Br Med J 281:1462, 1980
50. Hansbrough JF, Near A: Propranolol-epinephrine antagonism with hypertension and stroke. Ann Intern Med 92:717, 1980
51. van Herwaarden CLA, Fennis JFM, Binkhort RA et al: Haemodynamic effects of adrenaline during treatment of hypertensive patients with propranolol and metoprolol. Eur J Clin Pharmacol 12:397, 1977
52. Reeves RA, Boer WH, DeLeve L et al: Nonselective beta-blockade enhances pressor responsiveness to epinephrine, norepinephrine and angiotensin II in normal man. Clin Pharmacol Ther 35:461, 1984
53. McAllister RG, Hamann SR, Blouin RA: Pharmacokinetics of calcium entry blockers. Am J Cardiol 55:30B, 1985
54. Loi CM, Rollins DE, Dukes GE et al: Effect of cimetidine on verapamil disposition. Clin Pharmacol Ther 37:654, 1985
55. Hamann SR, Blouin RA, Chang SL et al: Effects of hemodynamic changes on the elimination kinetics of verapamil and nifedipine. J Pharmacol Ther 231:301, 1984
56. Diamond JR, Cheung JY, Fang LS: Nifedipine-induced renal dysfunction. Am J Med 77:905, 1984
57. Kounis NG: Asystole after verapamil and digoxin. Br J Clin Pract 34:57, 1980
58. Boden WE, Korr KS, Bough GW: Nifedipine-induced hypotension and myocardial ischemia in refractory angina pectoris. JAMA 253:1131, 1985
59. Reddy RS, Uretsky BF, Steinfield M: The hemodynamic effects of intravenous verapamil in patients on chronic propranolol therapy. Am Heart J 107:97, 1984
60. Packer M, Meller J, Medina N et al: Hemodynamic consequences of combined beta-adrenergic and slow calcium channel blockade in man. Circulation 65:660, 1982
61. Zoghbi W, Schwartz JB: Verapamil overdose: Report of a case and review of the literature. Cardiovasc Rev Rep 5:355, 1984
62. Morris DL, Goldschlager N: Calcium infusion for reversal of adverse effects of intravenous verapamil. JAMA 249:3211, 1983
63. Harriman RJ, Mangiardi LM, McAllister RG et al: Reversal of the cardiovascular effects of verapamil by calcium and sodium: Differences between electrophysiologic and hemodynamic responses. Circulation 59:797, 1979
64. Devis G, Somers G, VanObberghen E et al: Calcium antagonists and islet function: I. Inhibition of insulin release by verapamil. Diabetes 24:547, 1975
65. Bhatnagar SK, Amin MMA, Al-Yusuf AR: Diabetogenic effects of nifedipine. Br Med J 289:19, 1984
66. Oster JR, Epstein M, Smoller S: Combined therapy with thiazide-type and loop diuretic agents for resistant sodium retention. Ann Intern Med 99:405, 1983
67. Sigurd B, Olesen KH: The supra-additive natriuretic effect addition of theophylline ethylenediamine and bumetanide in congestive heart failure. Am Heart J 94:168, 1977
68. Chennavasin P, Seiwell R, Brater DL: Pharmacokinetic-dynamic analysis of the indomethacin-furosemide interaction in man. J Pharmacol Exp Ther 215:77, 1980
69. Himmelhoch JM, Poust RI, Mallinger AG et al: Adjustment of lithium dose during lithium-cholothiazide therapy. Clin Pharmacol Ther 22:225, 1977
70. McCarthy JT, Torres VE, Ramero JC et al: Acute intrinsic renal failure induced by indomethacin. Mayo Clin Proc 57:289, 1982
71. Koch-Weser J, Sellers EM: Drug interactions with coumarin anticoagulants. N Engl J Med 285:487, 1971
72. Frolich JC, Leftwich R, Ragheb M et al: Indomethacin increases plasma lithium. Br Med J 1:1115, 1979
73. Clive DM, Stoff JS: Renal syndromes associated with nonsteroidal antiinflammatory drugs. N Engl J Med 310:563, 1984
74. Lavre L, Glasson P, Vallotton MB: Reversible acute renal failure from combined triamterene and indomethacin. Ann Intern Med 96:317, 1982
75. Allan SG: Interaction between diuretics and indomethacin. Br Med J 283:1611, 1981
76. Favre L, Glasson PH, Riondel A et al: Interaction of diuretics and nonsteroidal antiinflammatory drugs in man. Clin Sci 64:407, 1983
77. Blum M, Aviram A: Ibuprofen induced hyponatremia. Rheumatol Rehabil 19:258, 1980
78. Berioniade V, Corneille L, Haraoui B: Indomethacin-induced inhibition of prostaglandin with hyperkalemia. Ann Intern Med 91:499, 1979
79. Tan SY, Shapiro R, Franco R et al: Indomethacin-induced prostaglandin inhibition with hyperkalemia: A reversible cause of hyporeninemic hypoaldosteronism. Ann Intern Med 90:783, 1979
80. Gerber JG: Indomethacin-induced rises in blood pressure. Ann Intern Med 99:555, 1983
81. Durao V, Prata MM, Guncalves LMD: Modification of antihypertensive effect of beta-adrenoreceptor-blocking agents by inhibition of endogenous prostaglandin synthesis. Lancet 2:1005, 1977
82. Moore TJ, Crantz FR, Hollenberg NK et al: Contribution of prostaglandins to the antihypertensive action of captopril in essential hypertension. Hypertension 3:168, 1981
83. Ciabattoni G, Cinotti GA, Pierucci A et al: Effects of sulindac and ibuprofen in patients with chronic glomerular disease. N Engl J Med 310:279, 1984
84. Berg KJ, Talseth T: Acute renal effects of sulindac and indomethacin in chronic renal failure. Clin Pharmacol Ther 37:447, 1985
85. Steiness E, Waldroff S: Different interactions of indomethacin and sulindac with thiazides in hypertension. Br Med J 285:1702, 1982
86. Miller MJS, Bednar MM, McGiff JC: Renal metabolism of sulindac: Functional implications. J Pharmacol Exp Ther 231:449, 1984
87. Boakes AJ, Laurence DR, Teoh PC et al: Interaction between sympathomimetic amines and antidepressant agents in man. Br Med J 1:311, 1973
88. Muelheims GH, Entrup RW, Paiewonsky D et al: Increased sensitivity of the heart to catecholamine-induced arrhythmias following guanethidine. Clin Pharmacol Ther 6:757, 1965
89. Lee KY, Beilin LJ, Vandongen R: Severe hypertension after ingestion of an appetite suppressant (phenylpropanolamine) with indomethacin. Lancet 1:1110, 1979
90. Goldstein DS, Keiser HR: Pressor and depressor responses after cholinergic blockade in humans. Am Heart J 107:974, 1984
91. Cuthbert MF, Greenberg MP, Morley SW: Cough and cold remedies: A potential danger to patients on monoamine oxidase inhibitors. Br Med J 1:404, 1969
92. Davis JC, Reifeel JA, Bigger JT: Sinus node dysfunction caused by methyldopa and digoxin. JAMA 245:1241, 1981
93. Warren SE, Ebert E, Swerdlin A et al: Clonidine and propranolol paradoxical hypertension. Arch Intern Med 139:253, 1979
94. Saarimaa H: Combination of clonidine and sotalol in hypertension. Br Med J 1:810, 1976
95. Briant RH, Reid JL, Dollery CT: Interaction between clonidine and desipramine in man. Br Med J 1:522, 1973
96. Meyer JF, McAllister K, Goldberg LI: Insidious and prolonged antagonism of guanethidine by amitriptyline. JAMA 213:1487, 1970
97. Mitchell JR et al: Guanethidine and related agents: III. Antagonism by drugs which inhibit the norepinephrine pump in man. J Clin Invest 49:1596, 1970
98. Stafford JR, Fann WE: Drug interactions with guanidinium antihypertensives. Drugs 13:57, 1977
99. Gulati OD, Dave BT, Gokhale SD et al: Antagonism of adrenergic neuron blockade in hypertensive subjects. Clin Pharmacol Ther 7:510, 1965
100. Jonkman JHG, Upton RA: Pharmacokinetic drug interactions with theophylline. Clin Pharmacokinet 9:309, 1984
101. Renton KW, Gray JD, Hall RI: Decreased elimination of theophylline after influenza vaccination. Can Med Assoc J 123:288, 1980
102. Bukowsky M, Mont PW, Wigle R et al: Theophylline clearance: Lack of effect of influenza vaccination and ascorbic acid. Am Rev Respir Dis 129:672, 1984
103. Meredith CG, Christian CD, Johnson RF et al: Effects of influenza virus vaccine on hepatic drug metabolism. Clin Pharmacol Ther 37:396, 1985
104. Standing Advisory Committee for Haematology of the Royal College of Pathologists: Drug interaction with coumarin derivative anticoagulants. Br Med J 285:274, 1982
105. Serlin MJ, Mossman S, Sibeon RG et al: Cimetidine: Interaction with oral anticoagulants in man. Lancet 2:317, 1979
106. Sato RI, Gray DR, Brown SE: Warfarin interaction with erythromycin. Arch Intern Med 144:2413, 1984

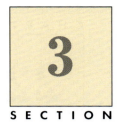

Section Editor
Kanu Chatterjee, MB, FRCP

BEDSIDE EVALUATION OF THE PATIENT

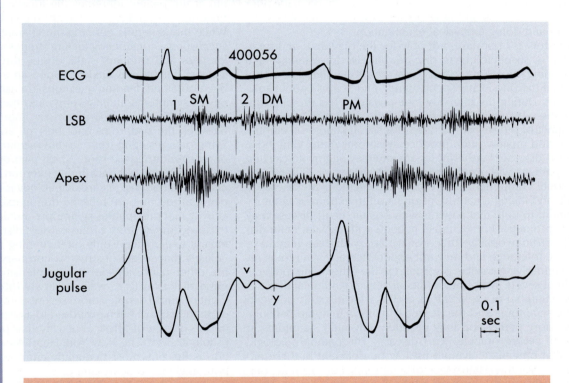

THE HISTORY

Kanu Chatterjee

Despite the availability of a large number of investigative procedures, the history and physical examination still remain the initial methods of evaluating patients with cardiovascular disorders. In many instances, the history alone provides the diagnosis, which is only confirmed by subsequent noninvasive or invasive tests. Careful analysis of symptoms is essential in assessing the severity of cardiac illness. In certain disorders, such as valvular heart disease, clinical examination may frequently establish the diagnosis, obviating the need for further diagnostic investigation. Also, intelligent selection of specialized tests for the diagnosis and management of a given disorder can only be made after one suspects the diagnosis and assesses the severity of the illness by taking a history and doing a physical examination.

Taking a history is important, not only for the diagnosis and treatment of known or suspected heart disease, but also for establishing a rapport and gaining the patient's trust. Total care is enhanced when the patient feels that the physician "spends time" and "cares" about solving the problem. During the interview, the physician has the opportunity to assess the personality and attitude of the patient as well as the emotional impact of the suspected heart disease. It should be emphasized that fear and anxiety often produce symptoms mimicking those of organic heart disease. Furthermore, anxiety may aggravate existing symptoms in patients with established cardiac disorders. Differentiating the functional components from those of organic heart disease is often difficult, and taking a careful history is often extremely helpful.

It is important to note that patients with organic heart disease may be totally asymptomatic. For example, patients with valvular heart disease, dilated cardiomyopathy, or coronary artery disease may have normal exercise tolerance and may not experience any symptoms referable to the underlying cardiac disorder. On the other hand, patients may complain of severe symptoms in the presence of minimal disease. There may be a number of explanations for this wide disparity between the severity of symptoms and the degree of illness. In some patients, inadequate sensory perception may produce only mild symptoms in the presence of severe organic heart disease. The pathophysiologic mechanisms that precipitate symptoms may be deficient in these patients, accounting for the relative lack of symptoms. For example, diabetic patients with severe coronary artery disease may sustain myocardial infarction without experiencing pain. Patients with even severe valvular heart disease or coronary artery disease may complain of few, if any, symptoms if physical activity remains at the subthreshold level; many patients unconsciously reduce their physical activity and never perceive any significant symptoms. The importance of inquiring about exercise habits and physical activity to assess the severity of symptoms while taking the history is apparent. Some patients may deny, minimize, or ignore symptoms because they cannot believe that they could be afflicted with heart disease or because they are reluctant to accept further investigations. Low threshold to symptoms and high sensitivity to minor problems are also observed. Patients with mitral valve prolapse may complain of severe chest pain or dyspnea and may be very sensitive to benign premature beats. During the interview, the physician should attempt to form an impression about the psychological make-up of the patient.

APPROACH

The standard approach to taking a history is to allow the patient to describe his or her symptoms first. It is desirable not to interrupt frequently by asking leading questions during the patient's spontaneous description of symptoms. During this period the physician can observe concurrently the manner in which the patient describes the symptoms and the overall emotional state and mood. Simple observation while the patient relates the history can provide diagnostic clues. For example, if the patient identifies the location of chest pain with only one fingertip, it is unlikely that the chest pain is due to myocardial ischemia. While the patient is defining the character of the chest pain, gestures suggesting a constricting feeling strengthen a suspicion of angina. Restlessness and frequent sighs during the narration of symptoms may suggest heightened anxiety. Once an account of the symptoms has been obtained, leading questions are asked to determine the chronology of symptoms, their severity, and their relation to potential cardiovascular disorders. It is extremely important to seek the association between the symptoms and the type and degree of physical activity. Symptoms resulting from cardiovascular disorders, in general, appear or worsen during exertion. Chest pain or discomfort and shortness of breath experienced only during exertion are more likely due to cardiac disease; in contrast, a cardiac etiology is unlikely if the same symptoms occur at rest and are relieved during exertion. The degree of physical activity that precipitates symptoms should also be determined in order to assess the severity of the cardiac disorder. For example, when angina is experienced only after running or jogging several miles, it is unlikely that severe obstructive coronary artery disease is present. On the other hand, angina of any intensity that occurs during minimal physical activity (*e.g.*, walking slowly 100 yards or climbing slowly up a flight of stairs) denotes more severe coronary artery disease. A number of methods have been proposed to assess functional impairment based on the degree of physical activity that precipitates cardiac symptoms (Table 22.1).[1,2] The New York Heart Association Functional Classification is the one most frequently employed to evaluate the severity of both angina and heart failure.

Although the New York Heart Association Classification has been found useful to assess prognosis and results of therapy, particularly in patients with heart failure,[3,4] its limitations must be recognized. "Usual" physical activity is difficult to define and varies considerably from patient to patient. Patients may be symptomatic at rest on occasion and yet may be able to tolerate moderate physical activity. Paroxysmal nocturnal dyspnea or nocturnal angina can be encountered in the absence of symptoms during moderate exertion. Thus, a considerable overlap should be expected between these different functional classes (see Table 22.2).

Goldman and co-workers[5] noted that the New York Heart Association estimation of the functional classes had a reproducibility of only 56%, and only 51% of the estimates agreed with treadmill exercise performances. The reproducibility and validity of the Canadian Cardiovascular Society system were 73% and 59%, respectively. Other methods of classification have been proposed[6,7] based on the patient's

TABLE 22.1 FUNCTIONAL CLASSIFICATION BASED ON THE DEGREE OF PHYSICAL ACTIVITY PRECIPITATING CARDIAC SYMPTOMS

Functional Class	New York Heart Association Functional Classification	Canadian Cardiovascular Society Functional Classification
I	Patients with cardiac disease but without resulting limitations of physical activity. Ordinary physical activity does not cause undue fatigue, palpitations, dyspnea, or anginal pain.	Ordinary physical activity does not cause angina, such as walking and climbing stairs. Angina occurs with strenuous or rapid or prolonged exertion at work or recreation.
II	Patients with cardiac disease resulting in slight limitations of physical activity. They are comfortable at rest. Ordinary physical activity results in fatigue, palpitations, dyspnea, or anginal pain.	Slight limitation of ordinary activity. Walking or climbing stairs rapidly, walking uphill, walking or stair climbing after meals, or in cold, or in wind, under emotional stress or only during the first few hours after awakening. Walking more than 2 blocks on the level and climbing more than one flight of ordinary stairs at a normal pace in normal conditions.
III	Patients with cardiac disease resulting in marked limitation of physical activity. They are comfortable at rest. Less than ordinary physical activity causes fatigue, palpitation, dyspnea, or anginal pain.	Marked limitations of ordinary physical activity. Symptoms occur after walking one to two blocks on the level and climbing one flight of stairs in normal conditions and at normal pace.
IV	Patients with cardiac disease resulting in inability to carry on any physical activity without discomfort. Symptoms of cardiac insufficiency or of the anginal syndrome may be present even at rest. If any physical activity is undertaken, discomfort is increased.	Inability to carry on any physical activity without discomfort; anginal syndrome may be present at rest.

(Adapted from Goldman L et al: Comparative reproducibility and validity of symptoms for assessing cardiovascular functional class: Advantages of a new specific activity scale. Circulation 64:1227, 1981. Reproduced by permission of the American Heart Association, Inc.)

TABLE 22.2 THE CRITERIA FOR SPECIFIC ACTIVITY SCALE CLASSIFICATION

Functional Class	Criteria
I	Patient can perform to completion any activity requiring ≥7 metabolic equivalents (shovel snow, spade soil, skiing, basketball, touch football, squash, handball, jog/walk 5 miles per hour, carry 80-lb objects, carry 24 pounds up 8 steps).
II	Patient can perform to completion any activity requiring ≥5 metabolic equivalents but can not or does not perform to completion activity requiring ≥7 metabolic equivalents (rake garden, weed, roller skate, dance foxtrot, walk at a 4-mile-per-hour rate on level ground, sexual intercourse without stopping, carry anything up a flight of 8 steps without stopping).
III	Patient can perform to completion any activity requiring ≥2 metabolic equivalents but cannot or does not perform to completion any activity requiring ≥5 metabolic equivalents (shower without stopping, strip and make bed, mop floors, hang washed clothes, walk 2.5 miles per hour, bowl, play golf, push power lawn mower).
IV	Patient cannot or does not perform to completion activity requiring ≥2 metabolic equivalents.

(Adapted from Goldman L et al: Comparative reproducibility and validity of symptoms for assessing cardiovascular functional class: Advantages of a new specific activity scale. Circulation 64:1227, 1981. Reproduced by permission of the American Heart Association, Inc.)

occupation, customary and sporadic activities, the amount of therapeutic intervention, and the intensity of the symptoms. These methods have not gained popularity because of the cumbersome and complicated nature of the systems.

Treadmill exercise tests are occasionally employed to assess functional capacity because they provide an approximate estimate of oxygen consumption. Furthermore, exercise duration also correlates significantly with oxygen consumption during exercise. An approximate assessment of the metabolic equivalents is possible by inquiring about the nature and duration of the physical activity that the patient can perform. Based on the nature of the physical activity that can be performed without experiencing undue symptoms, Goldman and coworkers have proposed a classification of the assessment of the functional capacity (Table 22.2). The reproducibility and validity of the criteria of the Specific Activity Scale Classification were 73% and 68%, respectively. Although this method of classification was based on the performance on treadmill, further experience will be required to establish this classification in clinical practice.

In addition to cardiac history, a detailed general medical history including past history, occupational history, family history, and review of symptoms should be obtained. A history of rheumatic fever, chorea, streptococcal infections, venereal disease, and thyroid disease should be obtained. When bacterial endocarditis is suspected, inquiry should be made for prior dental, oral, or genitourinary surgery and intravenous drug abuse. In patients with suspected coronary artery disease, it is important to ask for a history of risk factors for atherosclerosis, particularly cigarette smoking, hypertension, diabetes, and hyperlipidemia. Controversy exists regarding the positive family history as an independent risk factor for atherosclerotic coronary artery disease.

Aggregation of coronary risk factors and a higher incidence of coronary heart disease in families have been well recognized.[8,9] Whether a positive family history of coronary artery disease is an independent risk factor or not has not been established. Conroy and associates failed to confirm positive family history as an independent risk factor in individuals 60 years of age or younger.[10] The Western Collaborative Study reported that a positive family history was independently predictive of coronary heart disease only in men aged less than 50 years.[11]

Inquiries should be made for a history of familial hyperlipidemia and leg claudication in patients with suspected coronary artery disease. In very young individuals with established angina or myocardial infarction, it is relevant to take a history of chest trauma and "mucocutaneous lymph node syndrome" (Kawasaki's syndrome).[12]

When one suspects hypertrophic cardiomyopathy, and in patients with congenital long QT syndrome, it is important to inquire about the occurrence of syncope and "sudden death" among family members; a positive family history appears to have adverse prognostic influence. Hypertrophic cardiomyopathy is generally transmitted as an autosomal dominant trait; therefore, inquiries for the presence of this condition in other members of the family are relevant.

When the physician entertains the possibility of congenital heart defects, it is prudent to ask about a history of maternal rubella and the presence of congenital heart disease in siblings and other members of the family. Certain types of congenital heart defects are more likely to occur in the rubella syndrome (patent ductus arteriosus, atrial and ventricular septal defects, supravalvular aortic stenosis, peripheral pulmonary artery branch stenosis). Familial incidence of the secundum type of atrial septal defect associated with congenital anomalies of the upper extremities (Holt-Oram syndrome) has been observed.

ANALYSIS OF SYMPTOMS

The major symptoms associated with cardiovascular disease are chest pain, dyspnea, palpitations, dizziness and syncope, edema, cough, hemoptysis, and fatigue and tiredness. However, the same symptoms may occur from noncardiac disorders and careful analysis during history taking is therefore required to ascertain the etiology of these symptoms.

CHEST PAIN OR DISCOMFORT

Chest pain or discomfort associated with cardiovascular disorders can be of various types. The characteristics of anginal pain are different from those of chest pain produced by pleuropericarditis. Patients with marked left ventricular hypertrophy (*e.g.*, aortic regurgitation, hypertrophic cardiomyopathy) may complain of chest discomfort that may be prolonged in duration, throbbing in character, and worse in the left lateral decubitus position. The pathogenesis of such types of chest pain in these patients remains unclear. Chest pain originating from noncardiac structures such as the mediastinum, esophagus, cervicothoracic spine, costochondral junctions, pleura, lungs, stomach, duodenum, pancreas, and gallbladder may mimic angina. Severe prolonged chest pain that occurs during acute myocardial infarction can be qualitatively similar to that observed in other pathologic conditions. The important differential diagnoses are (1) pericarditis, (2) extracardiac but intrathoracic lesions such as thoracic aortic dissection, acute massive pulmonary embolism, acute mediastinitis, ruptured esophagus, and left-sided tension pneumothorax; and (3) extrathoracic conditions such as acute cholecystitis, pancreatitis, and perforating peptic ulcers. Acute myocarditis may also be occasionally associated with severe chest pain similar to that of acute myocardial infarction.[13]

History is the most important clinical tool for the differential diagnosis of chest pain. The character, location, duration, radiation, and the factors which precipitate or relieve chest pain need careful analysis to determine its pathogenesis.

ANGINA

Angina is chest pain that results from myocardial ischemia. The meaning of angina, however, is "choking." Indeed, many patients do not complain of pain but of a "discomfort" that is "difficult to describe." The discomfort may be "heaviness," a "sense of pressure," "tightness or band across the chest," or "weight on the chest," or it may actually be pain. The other descriptions that patients frequently volunteer when asked to characterize their discomfort are "strangling," "constricting," "squeezing," "pressing," "bursting," and "burning." Occasionally patients describe the discomfort only as an unpleasant sensation. A sensation of fluttering, tingling, or emptiness is unlikely to be due to myocardial ischemia.

The character of ischemic pain is almost always "dull and deep," and not "sharp and superficial." Initial location of pain or discomfort is frequently in the central chest and retrosternal. However, the left pectoral region, arms and hands, root of the neck (throat), epigastrium, and infrequently the right side of the chest may be initial sites. Occasionally patients may complain of only interscapular or left infrascapular back pain as manifestations of myocardial ischemia. Lower abdominal pain, low back pain, or pain starting at the back of the neck is usually not angina. When chest pain is sharply demarcated and localized over small areas that can be indicated with one or two fingers it is unlikely to result from myocardial ischemia.

Radiation of pain also should be analyzed to determine the etiology. It should be recognized that anginal pain might occur without radiation. Radiation most frequently occurs peripherally along the medial side of the left arm or both arms (centripetal). Radiation of angina along the lateral sides of the arms is uncommon. However, occasionally patients may complain that "the whole arm aches." One or both sides of the neck, lower jaw, back (infrascapular region), left shoulder or both shoulders, armpits, and epigastrium are frequent sites of angina radiation. Radiation to suprascapular regions, particularly to the left, is more characteristic of pericardial pain than of angina. Anginal pain does not radiate to the upper jaw, the lower abdomen, or the lower back alongside the spine. Very rarely pain may start in the periphery and then radiate to the central chest (centrifugal).

The intensity of angina increases slowly and attains its peak and plateau in minutes rather than in seconds. Relief is also relatively gradual. Chest pain, which attains its maximum intensity instantaneously and is relieved abruptly, is unlikely to be angina pectoris. Duration of pain also provides an important clue in the diagnosis of angina; it usually lasts for 2 to 15 minutes. However, duration varies in the different anginal syndromes. For example, in patients with unstable or variant (Prinzmetal's) angina, chest discomfort may last as long as 30 minutes. Very brief chest pain, lasting for a few seconds, is unlikely to be angina pectoris. Similarly, constant severe chest pain lasting for several hours does not result from myocardial ischemia and almost always evidence for myocardial necrosis is present.

Precipitating and aggravating factors should be assessed to determine the etiology of chest discomfort. Angina of effort or "classic" angina is characteristically induced by physical activity such as hurrying or walking up an incline. Angina pectoris is frequently worse or precipitated more easily in cold weather, while walking against the wind, or after eating heavy meals. Some patients experience angina more frequently in the morning, despite less physical activity at this time than during the rest of the day. Exercising the upper extremities above the level of the head precipitates angina pectoris more easily than exercising with the inferior extremities. Emotional stress may also precipitate angina. In patients with stable "classic" exertional angina, the level of exercise that precipitates chest discomfort is usually predictable. Thus, the severity of the coronary artery disease can be generally inferred from the degree of physical activity that induces angina. Angina occurring during minimal physical activity, such as walking slowly for a few yards, is likely to be associated with severe coronary artery stenosis. On the other hand, when angina is precipitated during prolonged running or jogging, the presence of severe coronary artery stenosis is unlikely. An occasional patient only experiences angina at the beginning of physical activity (*e.g.*, walking), and angina is not experienced later, despite continuation of the same physical activity ("walk-through angina"). The precise pathophysiologic mechanism of "walk-through angina" remains unclear, although coronary artery spasm has been implicated.[14] It needs to be emphasized, however, that in the majority of patients with obstructive atherosclerotic coronary artery disease, the intensity of angina increases with continued physical activity.

Angina occurring after meals (postprandial angina) can be experienced without any other physical activity and during the process of eating. Postprandial angina can also occur only during physical activity following meals. It is likely that the mechanisms of "spontaneous" and "exercise-related" postprandial angina are different; the former is more likely to be due to an inappropriate increase in coronary vascular tone[15] and the latter to an exercise-induced increase in myocardial oxygen requirements. Postprandial angina is almost always associated with significant atherosclerotic coronary artery disease.

The relief of "classic angina" characteristically occurs with cessation of the activity that induces angina. Prompt relief is also achieved with the use of sublingual nitroglycerin. Amelioration of angina *following nitroglycerin* does not occur instantaneously or within a few seconds of administration of nitroglycerin. Hemodynamic effects of sublingual nitroglycerin usually begin within one to three minutes, and the angina is also relieved within three to four minutes. Thus, chest pain that is instantaneously relieved by nitroglycerin is unlikely to be angina pectoris. If chest discomfort abates 10 to 15 minutes or longer after sublingual nitroglycerin, it is unlikely to be stable angina; unstable angina or chest pain of noncardiac origin is a more plausible diagnosis. It needs to be recognized that nitroglycerin relieves not only angina but also pain associated with esophageal spasm. Thus, "relief by nitroglycerin" is not pathognomonic evidence of angina pectoris.

Nocturnal angina is defined as angina that occurs after lying in bed in a supine position. Instead of pain, patients may complain of "dyspnea," a so-called angina equivalent. Some patients experience angina within one to two hours after retiring; others, several hours after going to bed or early in the morning. The mechanism of angina in the former group of patients is likely to be due to increased intracardiac volume, which increases myocardial oxygen requirements. The supine position is associated with increased intravascular volume due to fluid shifts from the extravascular space. When angina occurs much later or in the early hours of the morning, a primary decrease in coronary blood flow due to increased coronary vascular tone (vasospastic angina) is the more probable mechanism.[16]

The character, location, and radiation of variant angina are similar to those of classic angina; however, the duration may be longer and the intensity more severe, and it is accompanied by ST segment elevation in the electrocardiogram. Variant angina frequently occurs at rest and may not be precipitated by physical activity. Not uncommonly, angina recurs more or less at the same time of day or night (cyclic phenomenon). Some patients give a history of migraine headache or Raynaud's phenomenon, or both. However, these characteristics may not be present and considerable variation in the clinical presentation can be observed. The duration of angina may be brief, without any cyclic phenomenon. Some patients may also experience angina more frequently in the morning and during strenuous physical activity. History is the most important clue in the diagnosis of "mixed angina"—a newly proposed angina syndrome.[17] Dynamic vasoconstriction superimposed on fixed atherosclerotic coronary artery lesions has been postulated as the mechanism for the variable threshold of chest discomfort, the essential clinical feature of "mixed angina." A significant variation in the degree of physical activity that induces angina is an important diagnostic feature. Furthermore, these patients may experience rest or nocturnal angina on certain occasions, and also exertional angina, with varying degrees of physical activity, at other times. Angina may also occur on exposure to cold, during emotional stress, or after meals.

The duration of chest discomfort in patients with unstable angina is usually longer than in patients with stable angina. A sudden change in the character, location, radiation, and duration in the stable angina pattern may herald the onset of unstable angina. The precipitating factors, particularly the level of exercise that induces angina, may also change. Angina that worsens with decreasing physical activity may precede the onset of rest angina. In patients with "new onset angina," this clinical profile also suggests unstable angina.

The location, character, and radiation of chest discomfort associated with evolving myocardial infarction are similar to angina pectoris; however, the intensity is usually (but not always) more severe and the duration much longer. Very frequently, the precipitating factors are not discernible. The discomfort may develop when the patient is doing very little or is at rest. It may awaken the patient from sleep. In patients with angina pectoris, the onset of myocardial infarction during physical activity is relatively uncommon. Prompt relief of pain in response to nitroglycerin usually does not occur in patients with evolving myocardial infarction. The usual history is that the patients cannot get "comfortable." The intensity of the chest pain associated with prolonged myocardial ischemia is not influenced by breathing or movement. Profuse sweating, dizziness, dyspnea, and nausea and vomiting may accompany chest pain due to prolonged myocardial ischemia and evolving myocardial infarction.

The quality, location, and radiation of postinfarction angina (angina recurring within 30 days of infarction) are similar to those of other types of angina. However, it may occur at rest or with minimal physical activity. As the prognosis of patients who develop angina at rest or with minimal physical activity appears to be less favorable, it is desirable to take a history of the precipitating factors. Postmyocardial infarction syndrome and episternal pericarditis are also associated with chest pain in patients with recent myocardial infarction. However, the pain of pericarditis is qualitatively different from that of angina, and the distinction can usually be made from the history and physical examination.

The pain of acute pericarditis is sharper and more superficial, and is usually located in the left pectoral region. It may radiate to both shoulders, the back, flanks, or sides of the neck. Radiation to the left suprascapular region is very suggestive of pericarditis. However, the location and radiation of pain due to pericarditis may be similar to those of prolonged myocardial ischemia. The pain of pericarditis is frequently aggravated by deep breathing, by movement of the body (twisting or turning), and by swallowing. Occasionally, the intensity of pain may fluctuate with the heart beat (e.g., it may worsen with tachycardia). Pericardial pain is frequently worse while lying flat on the back and is partially relieved while leaning forward. The pain lasts for hours and is usually of constant intensity that does not vary with physical activity. Nitroglycerin does not relieve the pain of pericardial origin.

Chest pain associated with aortic dissection is usually excruciating, and the initial sites may be the thoracic portion of the back or the anterior chest. The pain is usually prolonged, lasting for hours. Most frequently, it starts abruptly, with maximum intensity at the onset. Radiation tends to follow the course of progression of the dissection, to the arms, neck, lower back, abdomen, and even to the inferior extremities. It should be recognized, however, that radiation of pain may be absent in aortic dissection. The intensity of pain resulting from aortic dissection is not influenced by breathing or movement. The pain is not relieved by nitroglycerin, and more than the usual amount of analgesics may be needed for amelioration. The pain associated with chronic thoracic aortic aneurysm results from erosion of the vertebral bodies. It is usually localized, with a dull, boring quality, and it may be worse at night.

Chest pain is occasionally associated with acute massive pulmonary embolism, and may be severe and similar to that of myocardial infarction. Acute distressing dyspnea accompanying chest pain, in the absence of clinical and radiologic evidence of pulmonary venous hypertension, is an important clue in the diagnosis of massive pulmonary embolism. Submassive or minor pulmonary emboli may not cause any chest pain. When pulmonary infarction develops, pleuritis may cause pain, usually in the lateral portion of the chest, which is aggravated by breathing and coughing and may by accompanied by hemoptysis. Patients with chronic pulmonary hypertension may experience chest discomfort similar to that of typical angina pectoris. The mechanism of chest pain in these patients remains unclear; dilatation of the pulmonary artery and right ventricular ischemia have been postulated.

Chest wall pain due to costochondritis or myositis, or following herpes zoster or chest trauma, is superficial and usually sharper in quality. It should not be confused with the pain of angina pectoris. Tietze's syndrome,[18] caused by swelling of the costochondral and costosternal joints, also produces superficial chest wall pain. Chest pain associated with these conditions is commonly intensified by coughing, deep breathing, and movements of the chest. Localized tenderness can usually be elicited by palpation.

Functional chest pain associated with anxiety (Da Costa's syndrome or neurocirculatory asthenia) frequently creates a dilemma in the diagnosis of angina pectoris.[19] Chest pain in patients with mitral valve prolapse is most commonly precipitated by anxiety. Anxiety-related chest discomfort differs considerably from angina in its clinical profile. It is usually localized over the left inframammary region near the area of the cardiac apex and may be very sharp, like lancinating stabs, or dull, like an ache or pressure. On occasion, it may last only for a few seconds; on other occasions it may be constant and last for several hours. Emotional stress and fatigue frequently precipitate the attacks and the intensity of chest pain not influenced by physical activity. Other manifestations of anxiety, such as palpitations, hyperventilation, a sense of inability to take deep breaths (perceived as dyspnea), and deep sighing respirations, may accompany chest pain. The relief of pain is also unsatisfactory, despite a myriad of interventions, and patients may demonstrate signs of emotional instability and depression.

Chest pain can be associated with esophageal dysfunction, gallbladder disease, gastroduodenal disorders, diseases of the pleura, lung, and mediastinum, and hand–shoulder syndrome. These conditions should be considered in the differential diagnosis of angina.

DYSPNEA

Dyspnea is an uncomfortable awareness of breathing and is an important symptom of many cardiac disorders. The history and physical examination provide the most important clues for the diagnosis of the etiology of dyspnea. It should be recognized that even healthy individuals may experience uncomfortable breathing during very strenuous activity. Subjects unaccustomed to exercise may be aware of the discomfort at a lower level of physical activity. Thus, dyspnea, to be pathologic, has to occur at rest or with a degree of physical activity not expected to cause breathing difficulty in individual subjects.

Exertional dyspnea is an important symptom of chronic heart failure, but it also occurs in chronic pulmonary disease. Exertional dyspnea in chronic heart failure usually progresses slowly. Dyspnea at rest indicates severe heart failure. In patients with organic heart disease with rest dyspnea, even minimal physical activity worsens the symptoms. Some patients with obstructive coronary artery disease may experience exertional dyspnea instead of angina as a manifestation of myocardial ischemia (angina equivalent). Shortness of breath during physical activity, however, may occur in noncardiac conditions: obesity, pregnancy, pleural effusion, chronic pulmonary disease, and musculoskeletal disorders of the thoracic cage. Dyspnea-like chest pain may also be caused by anxiety. When dyspnea occurs only at rest and not during exertion, or when physical activity relieves dyspnea, a functional etiology such as anxiety is the likely cause. Dyspnea of functional origin is frequently associated with other manifestations of anxiety: stabbing, sharp left pectoral pain, restlessness, and sighing respirations. These patients frequently say that they "can't get enough air in the lungs." This symptom is not uncommonly relieved by taking deep breaths or by physical activity.

Wheezing associated with dyspnea does not always imply lung disease; it may also occur as a manifestation of heart failure (cardiac asthma). When wheezing accompanies dyspnea in an adult over the age of 40, a cardiac cause should be suspected. However, if there is a history of wheezing since childhood, bronchial asthma and lung disease are more probable causes.

Orthopnea implies that the patient has less dyspnea when the upper part of the torso is elevated to the sitting position than when lying flat. Although this symptom is a manifestation of congestive heart failure, it also occurs in patients with chronic lung disease. Patients with severe congestive heart failure frequently give histories of an inability to lie down and of sleeping in a sitting position with three or four pillows.

Paroxysmal nocturnal dyspnea is a specific type of shortness of breath that occurs at night, usually one to two hours after the patient goes to sleep in a recumbent position. Characteristically, the patient is awakened from sleep with the sudden onset of dyspnea. Dyspnea is relieved by assuming an upright or sitting position. Some patients may prefer standing for a few minutes to get relief. Usually a longer time is required for relief of paroxysmal nocturnal dyspnea than for cardiac orthopnea. Left ventricular failure is the most important and almost specific cause of paroxysmal nocturnal dyspnea, and results from interstitial pulmonary edema, primarily due to increased pulmonary venous pressure. Patients with chronic pulmonary disease may also awaken at night complaining of dyspnea. However, in these patients paroxysms of coughing usually precede dyspnea. The condition is usually relieved by expectorating the secretions and not specifically by sitting up.

Cheyne-Stokes respiration is a type of periodic breathing in which phases of hyperpnea and apnea alternate. During the hyperpneic phase, even minimal physical activity worsens the symptoms. During hyperpnea, a progressive decrease in Pco_2 inhibits the respiratory drive; during the apneic phase, a progressive accumulation of CO_2 stimulates the respiratory center and initiates the breathing. Dyspnea is experienced during the hyperpneic phase of Cheyne-Stokes respiration. Cheyne-Stokes breathing tends to occur more commonly in relatively elderly patients with depressed central nervous system function. However, this altered respiratory pattern is also frequently observed in patients with severe left ventricular failure associated with low cardiac output.[20] Cheyne-Stokes breathing is occasionally relieved following an increase in cardiac output. Biot respiration, a type of periodic breathing, is characterized by irregular respiratory periods with four or five breaths during each period with identical depth of each respiration. Biot respiration is seen in patients with increased intracranial pressure and not in patients with heart failure.

The hemodynamic determinant of cardiac dyspnea is the increased Starling gradient, primarily due to elevation of pulmonary venous and capillary pressures. Exertional dyspnea results from an exercise-induced increase in pulmonary capillary wedge pressure. In patients with dyspnea at rest, the pulmonary capillary wedge pressure is already excessively elevated, usually higher than 25 mm Hg. Paroxysmal nocturnal dyspnea results from an increased pulmonary capillary wedge pressure associated with increased intravascular and intracardiac volumes in the recumbent position.

The sudden onset of acute dyspnea can be caused by both cardiac and noncardiac disorders. Acute myocardial ischemia or infarction should always be considered in the differential diagnosis in patients without prior history of heart failure. Other cardiac causes of acute dyspnea are severe mitral regurgitation due to ruptured chordae or papillary muscle dysfunction, acute aortic regurgitation, and the onset of atrial fibrillation in the presence of mitral valve obstruction. Ventricular tachycardia rarely precipitates acute dyspnea. The noncardiac causes include pulmonary embolism, pneumothorax, pneumonia, and obstruction of a major airway.

The sudden onset of severe dyspnea, with or without wheezing, may indicate pulmonary embolism. Tachypnea, palpitations, pleuritic chest pain, and hemoptysis may be associated with the dyspnea of pulmonary embolism. Patients with massive pulmonary embolism usually prefer the recumbent position, despite dyspnea, because they may feel faint in an upright sitting position. In contrast, patients with cardiac dyspnea prefer the upright position, which decreases shortness of breath. Pulmonary embolism should be suspected when sudden, unexpected dyspnea develops during the postsurgical or postpartum period, or in a patient with heart failure.

Some patients give a history of episodic, severe dyspnea due to pulmonary edema without a history of chronic heart failure. These patients may be relatively asymptomatic and may have reasonable exercise tolerance between episodes of acute dyspnea. A few cardiac disorders should be considered in the differential diagnosis in these patients (Table 22.3). Left atrial myxoma may cause intermittent dyspnea due to obstruction of the mitral valve, which suddenly increases pulmonary venous pressure. Dyspnea may be positional and associated with syncope. Intermittent papillary muscle ischemia may produce severe mitral regurgitation and episodic dyspnea. These patients usually have significant coronary artery disease and angina. Episodic dyspnea resulting from severe myocardial ischemia is a rare clinical entity that only occurs in the presence of severe coronary artery disease. In patients with markedly abnormal left ventricular diastolic function with decreased left ventricular distensibility (stiff heart syndrome), a slight increase in intracardiac volume elevates pulmonary capillary wedge pressure and precipitates dyspnea.[21] A history of diabetes, hypertension, and coronary artery disease is usually present in these patients. Fluid retention, either from the lack of use of diuretics or from dietary indiscretion, precedes episodes of dyspnea. Atrial or ventricular tachycardia does not usually produce pulmonary edema in the absence of valvular or myocardial disease. However, paroxysmal tachyarrhythmias can be associated with episodic dyspnea in the presence of mild to moderate left ventricular dysfunction or mild to moderate mitral valve stenosis. Patients with a right-to-left shunt usually experience exertional dyspnea due to hypoxia. However, these patients may also develop episodes of breathlessness and increased cyanosis with or without syncope.

CYANOSIS

Cyanosis is the bluish discoloration of the skin and mucous membranes due to an abnormal amount of reduced hemoglobin or methemoglobin in the capillary vascular bed of these areas. Cyanosis does not appear if the absolute amount of reduced hemoglobin is less than 4 g/dl. A methemoglobin concentration of 1.5 g/dl or 0.5 g/dl of sulfhemoglobin also causes cyanosis. When the hemoglobin is normal, about one third of hemoglobin has to be in the reduced form for cyanosis to develop. Since the absolute amount of reduced hemoglobin determines the presence or absence of cyanosis, cyanosis is more likely to be observed in patients with increased hemoglobin, as in polycythemia. For the same reason, cyanosis does not occur in patients with severe anemia with a markedly reduced hemoglobin.

Two types of cyanosis are usually recognized. Central cyanosis is characterized by decreased arterial saturation and results from intracardiac (right-to-left), intrapulmonary, or certain vascular shunts. Central cyanosis is noticed in the buccal mucous membrane and in the mucous membrane of the soft palate and tongue. Peripheral cyanosis, on the other hand, is frequently localized in the extremities (hands and fingers), nose, lips, and earlobes. The buccal mucous membranes, tongue, and soft palate are not affected. Peripheral cyanosis results from cutaneous vasoconstriction and is frequently associated with reduced cardiac output. Peripheral cyanosis may also occur due to vasoconstriction in response to exposure to cold (*e.g.*, Raynaud's phenomenon).

A history of cyanosis restricted to one extremity suggests local vascular disease. Cyanosis due to intracardiac right-to-left shunt usually worsens during exertion. Central cyanosis since infancy suggests right-sided obstructive lesions with intracardiac communications. Development of cyanosis later in life may result from Eisenmenger's syndrome, Ebstein's anomaly, or severe pulmonary arterial hypertension with a patent foramen ovale. In patients with Eisenmenger's syndrome associated with patent ductus arteriosus, the cyanosis is more pronounced in the feet than in the hands (differential cyanosis). It needs to be recognized that the bluish discoloration of the skin may result from argyria and methemoglobinemia. Hereditary methemoglobinemia is a rare disorder in which there is a history of bluish discoloration of the skin since infancy. In acquired methemoglobinemia, drug overdose (nitrates, nitrites, nitroprusside) should be considered. Slate blue discoloration of the skin in argyria results from the deposition of melanin stimulated by silver iodide.[22]

PALPITATION

This symptom is perceived as an uncomfortable sensation associated with the heartbeat. When it is felt intermittently and irregularly and lasts for a second or fraction of a second, premature beats should be suspected. It is frequently described as "skipped" beats. When it is described as "the heart stops" or "stopped beating," it frequently correlates with the compensatory pause following premature beats. When premature beats produce palpitations, patients are usually aware of the postextrasystolic beat, not the premature beat. Slow regular palpitations may result from sinus bradycardia, junctional rhythm, or complete atrioventricular block. When the onset and termination of fast palpitations are abrupt, the most likely diagnosis is paroxysmal supraventricular tachycardia. Atrial fibrillation, on the other hand, is associated with fast, irregular palpitations. A gradual onset and cessation of

TABLE 22.3 CARDIAC CAUSES OF EPISODIC SEVERE DYSPNEA

1. Intermittent mitral valve obstruction—left atrial myxoma, ball valve thrombus
2. Intermittent severe mitral regurgitation—intermittent papillary muscle ischemia
3. Intermittent ischemic paralysis
4. "Stiff heart syndrome"
5. Paroxysmal tachyarrhythmias
6. Congenital heart disease with right-to-left shunt

fast palpitations suggests sinus tachycardia, which may be caused by an anxiety state. Fast, sustained palpitations due to supraventricular tachycardia may be associated with other symptoms: dizziness, dyspnea, sweating, and chest discomfort. Some patients also give a history of polyuria during prolonged attacks of palpitation. The mechanism for polyuria is unclear, although reflex suppression of antidiuretic hormone and release of atrial natriuretic peptide have been postulated.

Increased stroke volume due to the hyperkinetic heart syndrome, high output state (thyrotoxicosis, anemia), and valvular regurgitation may be associated with palpitation. Patients with severe aortic or tricuspid regurgitation may feel the forceful heartbeat along with a throbbing sensation in the neck. Some patients can hear the heartbeats along with palpitations while lying in the left lateral decubitus position.

The history of how the palpitations terminate may also provide clues about the cause. When palpitation stops abruptly, it is more likely due to supraventricular tachycardia. Some patients give a history that they can stop their palpitations by breath holding, induced gagging, or vomiting—maneuvers associated with vagal stimulation. Such a history also suggests supraventricular tachycardia as the cause of palpitation. A history of presyncope or syncope immediately after the cessation of fast palpitations (not during palpitation) strongly suggests the brady-tachy syndrome.

Anxiety-induced palpitation is usually due to sinus tachycardia and is frequently associated with other symptoms such as atypical chest pain, hyperventilation, tingling of the hands, and circumoral paresthesias. The onset and offset of palpitation due to sinus tachycardia are gradual rather than abrupt. The onset of palpitations resulting from ventricular tachycardia may be either sudden or relatively gradual; the termination may also be abrupt or gradual. Associated symptoms are nausea, sweating, chest discomfort, dizziness, and syncope.

SYNCOPE

Syncope is transient loss of consciousness associated with weakness and inability to maintain an upright position. Near syncope or presyncope is the clinical situation in which the patient feels dizzy or weak and "as if he is going to faint." Syncope caused by cardiovascular disorders results from decreased cerebral blood flow and reduced perfusion of the brain. Sudden reduction of cerebral blood flow is precipitated by a fall in cardiac output and arterial pressure. Reduction of cardiac output and hypotension can result from a number of pathologic conditions, including dysrhythmias, abnormalities of the autonomic nervous system, right and left ventricular outflow obstructions, and pulmonary and systemic vascular disorders. Cardiovascular syncope must be distinguished from other causes of loss of consciousness, such as seizure disorders, hypoglycemia, hyperventilation, anxiety, and hysterical fainting.

A careful history provides important diagnostic clues for the etiology of cardiac syncope. During history taking, inquiry should be made regarding the mode of onset and the circumstances under which syncope occurred (at rest or during exertion), body position (supine or upright), and symptoms preceding and following recovery from the attacks. An interview with witnesses is extremely helpful in determining the underlying mechanism of syncope. Changes in a patient's appearance during and after recovery from the syncopal attacks, observed by witnesses, may aid in the diagnosis of the cause of syncope. Some observers may be trained to examine the arterial pulse; the presence or absence of the arterial pulse during the attacks is obviously a very important finding in the differential diagnosis of syncope. Inquiry should be made about a family history of syncope and sudden death.

A history of abrupt onset of syncope suggests the Stokes-Adams-Morgagni syndrome, in which loss of consciousness results from transient ventricular asystole or ventricular tachyarrhythmias in the presence of atrioventricular block. Syncopal attacks occurring independent of body position, at rest or during exertion, during sleep or while awake, and without any preceding symptoms, also suggest Stokes-Adams attacks. A history of prolonged periods of unconsciousness is not the usual feature of Stokes-Adams syndrome. Patients regain consciousness quite promptly, become aware of their surroundings almost instantaneously, and do not remain confused after recovery. Witnesses to the event frequently observe sudden facial flushing with the onset of recovery. Generalized convulsive movements, although relatively uncommon, may occur either during or after recovery from unconsciousness.

A history of presyncope or syncope during rapid palpitation suggests supraventricular or ventricular tachycardia as the underlying arrhythmia and the onset of syncope is more gradual in these patients. A history of dizziness and syncope occurring immediately after termination of, and not during, the rapid palpitation is strongly suggestive of the brady-tachy syndrome (sick sinus syndrome). A history of fainting during rapid palpitation that is precipitated by assuming an upright position suggests orthostatic tachycardia.

A history of syncope of more gradual onset that usually occurs in the upright position suggests vasodepressor syncope. Following recovery, the patients are usually pale and diaphoretic, and the heart rate may be slow. Similarly, a history of dim vision, nausea, yawning, sweating, and dizziness, suggesting autonomic hyperactivity preceding loss of consciousness, may be obtained in patients with vasodepressor syncope. Syncope precipitated by sudden movement of the head, rubbing or shaving the neck, or wearing a tight collar suggests carotid sinus syncope. A history of syncope while swallowing or drinking cold liquids may suggest glossopharyngeal syncope. It is usually caused by bradycardia or asystole and severe hypotension and may be accompanied by paroxysms of neuralgic pain.[23] Postmicturition syncope usually occurs during or immediately after voiding and appears to be caused by a reflex precipitous fall in systemic vascular resistance.[24] Patients with micturition syncope may give histories of nocturia and consuming large amounts of alcoholic beverage. Patients with "cough syncope," also known as laryngeal vertigo and tussive syncope, give characteristic histories of losing consciousness immediately following paroxysms of vigorous coughing. These patients are usually smokers and may suffer from chronic bronchitis. The mechanism underlying the decreased cerebral blood flow in patients with cough syncope remains unclear. A marked decrease in cardiac output due to increased intrathoracic pressures, reflex peripheral vasodilation following coughing, compression of intracranial vascular beds resulting from increased cerebrospinal fluid pressure, and increased cerebrovascular resistance due to hypocapnea resulting from coughing have been postulated.[25,26]

Syncope in patients with orthostatic hypotension occurs in an upright position and is relatively gradual in onset. Inquiries should be made about antihypertensive drug therapy, neurologic disorders, diabetes, and the manifestations of autonomic dysfunction, such as impotence, sphincter disturbances, and anhydrosis.

The syncope of cerebrovascular disturbances is also usually of gradual onset and is often preceded by manifestations of neurologic deficits, such as loss of vision, aphasia, muscular weakness, or confusion. A history of impairment or loss of consciousness during exercise of the upper extremities is very suggestive of subclavian "steal" syndrome.[27]

Seizure disorders can produce sudden loss of consciousness; again, the history is very valuable in distinguishing neurologic disorders from cardiac syncope. Although the loss of consciousness may be sudden and can occur in any body position, a history of prodromal aura preceding the seizure is frequently obtained. Furthermore, a history of urinary and fecal incontinence and biting the tongue and other injuries supports the diagnosis of epilepsy. Regaining of consciousness is also gradual and is frequently followed by a confusional state, headache, and drowsiness.

Patients with right or left ventricular outflow obstruction, mitral valve obstruction, and precapillary pulmonary hypertension can also experience syncopal attacks. A history of syncope occurring in a certain body position, or during bending or leaning, suggests intermittent mitral valve obstruction by left atrial myxoma or ball valve thrombus. Syncope occurring during or immediately after exertion suggests left ventricular outflow obstruction (aortic stenosis and hypertrophic cardiomyopathy) or precapillary pulmonary hypertension. In patients with hypertrophic cardiomyopathy, syncope may occur during the Valsalva maneuver or after paroxysms of coughing. A family history of syncope and sudden death appears to exert an adverse prognostic influence in patients with hypertrophic cardiomyopathy. Exertional syncope associated with worsening cyanosis suggests Eisenmenger's syndrome or right ventricular outflow tract obstruction with a right-to-left shunt. It needs to be recognized that spontaneous syncopal attacks unrelated to exertion may occur in patients with left ventricular outflow obstruction, aortic stenosis and regurgitation, and precapillary pulmonary hypertension. Nonexertional syncope in these patients presumably results from dysrhythmias. Children with cyanotic congenital heart disease may also develop spontaneous syncope due to cerebral anoxia, resulting either from increased right-to-left shunt caused by enhanced right ventricular outflow obstruction or a decrease in systemic vascular resistance. Syncope at the onset of myocardial infarction is uncommon; however, prolonged angina preceding the onset of unconsciousness supports the diagnosis. On rare occasions, syncope may be the first manifestation of acute myocardial infarction. Hypoglycemia, hyperventilation, or blood loss may also precipitate syncope. A history of diabetes and insulin use, sweating and palpitations preceding syncope, and relatively gradual onset suggest hypoglycemia. Hypovolemia due to blood loss should be suspected when a history of melena, anemia, menorrhagia, or trauma precedes syncopal attacks. Hysterical fainting is frequently associated with atypical chest pain, sweating, hyperventilation, paresthesias of the hands or face, and sighing respiration.

EDEMA

Edema can be caused by both cardiac and noncardiac conditions. Inquiries should be made about the initial site of edema, nature of progression, and associated symptoms to determine its etiology. Dependent edema (in ankles, feet, and legs), which is worse toward the end of the day, suggests right heart failure or chronic venous insufficiency. Edema, along with a history of dyspnea, orthopnea, and paroxysmal nocturnal dyspnea, is most commonly due to left heart failure or mitral valve obstruction. In patients with primary right heart failure or constrictive pericarditis, a history of orthopnea or paroxysmal nocturnal dyspnea is usually absent. Patients with severe tricuspid regurgitation may give a history of fullness in the neck and abdominal tenderness.

With progressively worsening cardiac edema the legs, thighs, genitalia, and the abdominal wall can be involved, but the face is usually spared. Localization of edema around the eyes and face occurs in the nephrotic syndrome, angioneurotic edema, glomerulonephritis, hypoproteinemia, and myxedema. Edema localized in the lower extremities and abdomen may also result from cirrhosis of the liver.

A history of edema confined to the upper extremities, face, and neck suggests the superior vena caval syndrome; in these patients inquiry should be made about symptoms suggestive of carcinoma of the lung or lymphoma. Angioneurotic edema occurs intermittently, and a history of exposure to allergens is usually obtained.

COUGHING AND HEMOPTYSIS

Coughing is not an uncommon symptom in patients with cardiac disease; however, it is more commonly encountered in various tracheobronchial and pulmonary diseases. Pulmonary venous hypertension, irrespective of its etiology, may induce coughing, which is usually dry, irritating, and unproductive, and worse at night. A history of associated exertional and nocturnal dyspnea suggests elevation of the pulmonary venous pressure. The paroxysm of cough may precede paroxysmal nocturnal dyspnea and may be associated with a frothy pink sputum. The paroxysms of cough can indicate an adverse drug reaction and have been noted to occur with angiotensin-converting enzyme inhibitor enalapril therapy.

Coughing, expectoration, and exertional dyspnea are also observed in patients with chronic obstructive lung disease. A long history of coughing, expectoration, and chronic bronchitis may be elicited. White mucoid sputum or thick yellowish sputum usually accompany coughing due to chronic pulmonary disease.

Hoarseness may occur in some patients with mitral stenosis, with a markedly enlarged left atrium and pulmonary artery (Ortner's syndrome), in the absence of any tracheobronchial disease.[28,29] The compression of the recurrent laryngeal nerve by both left atrium and enlarged pulmonary artery has been thought to be contributory.

Hemoptysis in cardiovascular disease may result from pulmonary edema, rupture of bronchopulmonary venous anastomatic vessels, pulmonary infarction, and erosion of the tracheobronchial tree by the vascular bed. The history is extremely useful in the differential diagnosis of hemoptysis associated with cardiovascular disease. Frank hemoptysis of large volumes is extremely rare with pulmonary edema. Frothy pink blood-tinged sputum is more characteristic. In patients with mitral stenosis, recurrent episodes of limited hemoptysis are more common. Hemoptysis associated with pulmonary venous hypertension is frequently accompanied by dyspnea. In rare patients with severe mitral stenosis associated with pulmonary hypertension, profuse hemoptysis (pulmonary apoplexy), resulting from the rupture of bronchopulmonary venous anastomotic vessels, can occur. Massive hemoptysis may also result from rupture of a pulmonary arteriovenous aneurysm or from erosion of the tracheobronchial tree by an aortic aneurysm. Profuse, frank hemoptysis, however, is uncommon in cardiac patients, and primary bronchopulmonary disease is more likely the cause.

When acute pleuritic chest pain accompanies hemoptysis, pulmonary infarction from pulmonary embolism should be suspected. Pneumonia may also cause pleuritic chest pain and hemoptysis, but it is usually associated with rusty sputum and significant temperature elevation. Patients with cyanotic congenital heart disease, precapillary pulmonary hypertension, Eisenmenger's syndrome, or Osler-Weber-Rendu disease with pulmonary arteriovenous malformations may also develop hemoptysis; chest pain is usually absent. In patients with congenital cyanotic heart disease or Eisenmenger's syndrome, hemoptysis is usually associated with marked polycythemia and may result from thrombosis *in situ* of the pulmonary vessels.

Patients on anticoagulation and antiplatelet therapy may also complain of hemoptysis; thus, inquiry should be made about drug ingestion in any patient who develops hemoptysis. Bleeding from other organs suggests a generalized coagulation abnormality.

REFERENCES

1. The Criteria Committee of the New York Heart Association: Diseases of the Heart and Blood Vessels: Nomenclature and Criteria for Diagnosis, 6th ed. Boston, Little, Brown & Co, 1964
2. Campeau L: Grading of angina pectoris (letter). Circulation 54:522, 1975
3. Wilson JR, Schwartz S, St John Sutton M et al: Prognosis in severe heart failure: Relation to hemodynamic measurements and ventricular activity. J Am Coll Cardiol 2:403, 1983
4. Kereiakes D, Chatterjee K, Parmley WW et al: Intravenous and oral MDL 17043 (a new inotrope-vasodilator agent) in congestive heart failure: Hemodynamic and clinical evaluation in 38 patients. J Am Coll Cardiol 4:884, 1984
5. Goldman L, Hashimoto B, Cook EF et al: Comparative reproducibility and validity of systems for assessing cardiovascular functional class: Advantages of a new specific activity scale. Circulation 64:1227, 1981
6. Feinstein AR, Wells CK: A new clinical taxonomy for rating change in functional activities of patients with angina pectoris. Am Heart J 93:172, 1977
7. Peduzzi P, Hultgren HN: Effect of medical versus surgical treatment on symptoms in stable angina pectoris. The Veterans Administration cooperative study of surgery for coronary arterial occlusive disease. Circulation 60:888, 1979
8. Rissanen AM: Family aggregation of coronary risk factors in families of men with fatal and non-fatal coronary heart disease. Br Heart J 42:373, 1979
9. Rissanen AM: Family aggregation of coronary heart disease in a high incidence area (North Karelia, Finland). Br Heart J 42:294, 1979
10. Conroy RM, Mulcahy R, Hickey N, Daly L: Is a family history of coronary

heart disease an independent coronary risk factor? Br Heart J 53:378, 1985
11. Sholtz RI, Rosenman RH, Brand RJ: The relationship of reported parental history to the incidence of coronary heart disease in the Western Collaborative Group Study. Am J Epidemiol 102:350, 1975
12. Kawasaki T: Acute febrile mucocutaneous syndrome with lymphoid involvement with specific desquamation of the fingers and toes in children: Clinical observation of 50 cases. Japanese J Allergol 16:178, 1967
13. Costanzo-Nordin MR, O'Connell JB, Subramanian R et al: Myocarditis confirmed by biopsy presenting as acute myocardial infarction. Br Heart J 53:25, 1985
14. Sturzenhofecker PK, Peter S, Gornandt L et al: Coronary artery spasm combined with walk-through phenomenon. A special type of Prinzmetal angina. Symposium on coronary arterial spasm. Lille, November, 1979
15. Figueras J, Singh BN, Ganz W et al: Hemodynamics and electrocardiographic accompaniments of resting postprandial angina. Br Heart J 42:402, 1979
16. Figueras J, Singh BN, Ganz W et al: Mechanisms of rest and nocturnal angina: Observations during continuous haemodynamic and electrocardiographic monitoring. Circulation 59:955, 1979
17. Maseri A: Pathogenetic mechanisms of angina pectoris: Expanding views. Br Heart J 43:648, 1980
18. Karon EH, Achor RWP, Janes JM: Painful nonsuppurative swelling of costochondral cartilages (Tietze's syndrome). Proc Staff Meetings Mayo Clinic 33:45, 1958
19. Cohen ME, White PD, Johnson RE: Neurocirculatory asthenia, anxiety neurosis or the effort syndrome. Arch Intern Med 81:260, 1948
20. Gottlieb SS, Kessler P, Lee WH et al: What is the significance of Cheyne-Stokes respiration in severe chronic heart failure? Hemodynamic and clinical correlates in 167 patients. J Am Coll Cardiol 7:43A, 1986
21. Dode KA, Kassebaum DG, Bristow JD: Pulmonary edema in coronary artery disease without cardiomegaly. Paradox of the stiff heart. N Engl J Med 286:1347, 1972
22. Rich LL, Epinette WW, Nasser WK: Argyria presenting as cyanotic heart disease. Am J Cardiol 30:20, 1972
23. Kong Y, Heyman A, Entman ML et al: Glossopharyngeal neuralgia associated with bradycardia, syncope and seizures. Circulation 30:109, 1964
24. Lyle CB Jr, Monroe JT Jr, Flinn DE et al: Micturition syncope: Report of 24 cases. N Engl J Med 265:982, 1961
25. McIntosh HD, Estes EH, Warren JV: The mechanisms of cough syncope. Am Heart J 52:70, 1956
26. Kerr A Jr, Eich RH: Cerebral concussion as a cause of cough syncope. Arch Intern Med 108:138, 1961
27. Mannick JA, Suter CG, Hume DG: The "subclavian steal" syndrome: A further documentation. JAMA 182:254, 1962
28. Fetterolf G, Norris GW: The anatomical explanation of the paralysis of the left recurrent laryngeal nerve found in certain cases of mitral stenosis. Am J Med Sci 141:625, 1911
29. Wood P: Chronic rheumatic heart disease. In Diseases of the Heart and Circulation, 2nd ed, p 502. London, Eyre & Spottiswoode, 1956

GENERAL REFERENCES

Braunwald E: The history. In Braunwald E (ed): Heart Disease: A Textbook of Cardiovascular Medicine, 2nd ed, pp 3–13. Philadelphia, WB Saunders, 1984

Fowler NO: The history in cardiac diagnosis. In Fowler NO (ed): Cardiac Diagnosis and Treatment, 3rd ed, p 23. Hagerstown, MD, Harper & Row, 1980

Hurst JW: A history, symptoms due to diseases of the heart and blood vessels. In Hurst JW, Logue RB, Schlant RS, Kasswenger N (eds): The Heart, 4th ed, p 153. New York, McGraw-Hill, 1978

Wood P: The chief symptoms of heart failure. In Diseases of the Heart and Circulation, 3rd ed, pp 1–25. Philadelphia, JB Lippincott, 1968

Bedside Evaluation of the Heart: The Physical Examination

Kanu Chatterjee

Like history taking, detailed examination of the cardiovascular and other organ systems is an integral step in the initial evaluation of a patient with suspected or established cardiovascular disease. Physical examination alone establishes the diagnosis of several valvular and cardiomyopathic disorders. Furthermore, the need and choice of appropriate tests for confirmation of the diagnosis and for assessment of the severity of an underlying disorder can be established only after careful physical examination. General inspection of the patient, which includes overall assessment of the general appearance and the symptomatic status, can be done while the history is being obtained.

INSPECTION

If the patient is complaining of chest pain, the physician should observe the general expression, the skin color, and the posture, which may provide diagnostic clues. Pale skin, sweating, restlessness, and inability to find a more comfortable position during pain are more frequent in patients with evolving acute myocardial infarction. In contrast, patients having angina usually remain still and avoid any physical activity. Patients with angina pectoris also frequently clench the fist over the sternum while describing the location of pain (Levine's sign). Attempts to suppress a normal breathing pattern may indicate pain originating from the pleura or thoracic cage. Pericardial pain is usually less intense while leaning forward, and such posture may suggest pericarditis.

Labored and uncomfortable breathing may be obvious during general inspection. Inability to lie down or a dry, irritating cough with dyspnea may signal pulmonary venous congestion. Increased respiratory rate, which may result from a variety of cardiopulmonary disorders, and slow and deep respiration, which may accompany metabolic disorders, are evident during general inspection. Patients with primary pulmonary disease and pulmonary embolism usually prefer the supine position, despite dyspnea. Frequent sighing respirations and a restless, anxious look are suggestive of an anxiety state or neurocirculatory asthenia. Respiratory distress resulting from chronic obstructive pulmonary disease can also be suspected from the general appearance (the blue bloater and the pink puffer).

During general inspection, the nutritional status of the patient should be observed. Marked obesity, which may be associated with a high cardiac output and biventricular hypertrophy, is easily recognized. Severe obesity with dusky skin color and somnolence are suggestive of the pickwickian syndrome. Truncal obesity, buffalo hump, or moon facies should raise the suspicion of Cushing's syndrome, particularly in the hypertensive patient. Marked weight loss and cachexia may result from severe chronic heart failure, bacterial endocarditis, and systemic diseases (neoplastic), which may involve the cardiovascular system secondarily.

Edema, when generalized and severe, is easily detected and usually results from the nephrotic syndrome and also from severe sepsis due to the accumulation of fluid in extravascular compartments. It is rarely seen in patients with severe heart failure. Edema of the legs and thighs, including the genitalia, with or without ascites (protuberant abdomen), may, however, occur in patients with severe, chronic right-sided heart failure and constrictive pericarditis. Edema of the face, neck, upper extremities, and trunk, with prominent veins in the same regions, raises the possibility of superior vena caval obstruction. When swelling and induration involve the face, neck, thorax, and upper extremities, but spares the hands, scleredema should be suspected. Scleredema is a rare connective tissue disease that develops following respiratory streptococcal or other infections and rarely may be associated with transient myocardial and pericardial disease.[1] Localized and asymmetric edema involving one extremity usually results from local venous or lymphatic obstruction.

An unusual appearance and abnormal gait provide clues in the diagnosis of certain systemic disorders, which may also involve the cardiovascular system. Subjects with Marfan's syndrome have long extremities with the arm span exceeding the height, a longer upper segment (head to pubis) than lower segment (pubis to feet), kyphoscoliosis, and pectus deformities. A tall stature, long extremities, and eunuchoid appearance is observed in Klinefelter's syndrome, which can be associated with congenital heart disease. Congenital heart disease occurs, although infrequently, in association with dwarfism resulting from various musculoskeletal disorders.

Abnormal gait due to a prior stroke may suggest a thromboembolic cause associated with valvular heart disease, atrial fibrillation, myocardial infarction, left atrial myxoma, or bacterial endocarditis. Also, prior stroke should alert the physician to search for the presence of hypertension and atherosclerotic cardiovascular complications. An abnormal gait suggesting a parkinsonism disorder with bradykinesia, coarse tremor and rigidity, and symptoms and signs of autonomic insufficiency should raise the possibility of Shy-Drager syndrome in a patient with a history of orthostatic hypotension.[2] An ataxic broad-based gait associated with Argyll Robertson pupils and Charcot's joints indicates syphilis, which may involve the cardiovascular system. Aortic valvular regurgitation, aortitis, ascending aortic aneurysm, coronary arterial ostial stenosis, and conduction disturbances are important manifestations of cardiovascular syphilis. Dysrhythmias and hypertrophic cardiomyopathy are observed in Friedreich's ataxia, in which musculoskeletal abnormalities such as kyphoscoliosis and abnormal gait also occur. Pseudohypertrophic muscular dystrophy may be associated with cardiomyopathy and mitral valve prolapse and can be suspected from the characteristic gait. Certain metabolic disorders, which may also cause cardiovascular complications, may alter the general appearance. Exophthalmos, lid lag, tremor, and perspiration suggest hyperthyroidism; enlarged skull, jaws, and extremities, along with a coarse facial appearance, occur in acromegaly. Dull facial appearance, periorbital puffiness, dry, sparse hair, a large tongue, and generalized sluggish appearance suggest myxedema.

Examination of the head, neck, face, and extremities occasionally provides important clues in the diagnosis of various congenital and acquired cardiovascular disorders. Down's syndrome (mongolism, trisomy 21), which is often associated with congenital heart disease (*e.g.*, ventricular septal defect, atrioventricular canal defects), can be recognized from the presence of prominent medial epicanthus, a large protruding tongue, low-set ears, depressed nasal bridge, and hypoplastic mandible with a small head and orbit. Simian palmar creases and an inwardly curved short fifth finger also occur in Down's syndrome. A long narrow head, high-arched palate, ectopia lentis, and tremulous iris may suggest Marfan's syndrome or homocystinuria. Arachnodactyly and lax joints also occur in these conditions.

In patients with Turner's syndrome, coarctation of the aorta is the major cardiovascular complication. A low hairline, a short, webbed neck, a small jaw, along with epicanthal folds, a high-arched palate, hypertelorism and ptosis, low-set ears, and pigmented moles may also be present in patients with Turner's syndrome.

In some patients with congenital supravalvular aortic stenosis, the external facial appearance is quite distinctive. A broad, high forehead, hypertelorism, low-set ears, upturned nose, wide mouth with a large upper lip, hypoplastic mandible with pointed chin, small teeth, strabismus, and epicanthal folds characterize the facial appearance. The important abnormalities of the musculoskeletal system and the type of cardiovascular involvements in some systemic disorders are summarized in Table 23.1.

A bluish discoloration of the lips, nose, and earlobes suggests peripheral cyanosis, which frequently results from low cardiac output. A malar flush with cyanotic lips, and occasionally slight jaundice, is seen in patients with severe mitral stenosis. Malar flush, however, can also occur in patients with severe precapillary pulmonary hypertension. The presence of transverse earlobe creases in a relatively young person (under 45 years of age) may suggest the possibility of coronary artery disease. Telangiectasia of the lips, tongue, and buccal mucosa may be associated with pulmonary arteriovenous fistula (Osler-Weber-Rendu disease). A bluish discoloration of the tongue, uvula, and buccal mucous membrane suggests central cyanosis, which results from intrapulmonary or intracardiac right-to-left shunt. Bobbing of the head coincident with each heart beat (de Musset's sign) occurs in severe aortic regurgitation, whereas lateral movements of the earlobes with each cardiac cycle suggest severe tricuspid regurgitation.

The most common cause of bilateral exophthalmos is hyperthyroidism, which may be associated with high output cardiac failure. In occasional patients, with chronic congestive heart failure, with severe pulmonary and systemic venous hypertension, exophthalmos and lid retraction may be observed; lid retraction probably results from heightened sympathetic activity, which is a frequent neurohumoral change in heart failure. Pulsatile bilateral exophthalmos is a rare manifestation of severe tricuspid regurgitation. When arcus, a circumferential light ring around the iris that begins inferiorly, occurs in a relatively young person, it may suggest premature atherosclerosis. Arcus is frequently associated with hypercholesterolemia and xanthelasma (deposits of cholesterol on the eyelids). The physician should look for a variety of abnormalities of the sclera, cornea, or iris that accompany systemic and musculoskeletal disorders (see Table 23.1) that also involve the cardiovascular system.

Fundoscopic examination provides useful information regarding certain cardiovascular disorders. Careful examination of the fundi is essential during evaluation of a patient with suspected or established hypertension. The degree of narrowing or irregularities of arterioles, the presence of arteriovenous defects (nicking or nipping), hemorrhages, exudates, and papilledema should be searched for to assess the severity of vascular complication of hypertension. The classification of retinal changes introduced by Keith and co-workers[3] in 1939 is still widely used:

KWI: Minimal irregularity of the arteriolar lumen and narrowing with increased light reflex.
KWII: Arteriovenous nicking, more marked narrowing and irregularity of the arterioles, distention of the veins.
KWIII: Flame-shaped hemorrhages and fluffy "cotton wool" exudates, in addition to arteriolar changes. Hard exudates may be present.
KWIV: Papilledema and any of the changes seen in I to III.

Generally, KWI and KWII changes are present in benign hypertension, whereas KWIII or KWIV changes are seen in accelerated or malignant hypertension. It needs to be emphasized that it is difficult to differentiate between hypertensive and atherosclerotic changes when KWII changes are recognized. Grade IV changes are urgent indications for immediate and vigorous antihypertensive therapy. In patients with suspected bacterial endocarditis, vascular occlusions, in addition to conjunctival petechial hemorrhages, indicate systemic embolization. Hemorrhagic areas with white centers (Roth spots) result from emboli in the nerve fiber retinal layer in bacterial endocarditis. Roth spots, however, are not diagnostic of bacterial endocarditis and can be seen in other conditions, such as leukemia. Mycotic aneurysms resulting from large emboli may be occasionally discovered in the retinal vessels. Embolic retinal vascular occlusions should lead to the search for the source of emboli: rheumatic heart disease, bacterial endocarditis, calcific aortic valve disease, mitral valve prolapse, left atrial myxoma, dilated cardiomyopathy, left ventricular aneurysm, and atherosclerosis of the aorta or arch vessels.

Examination of the fundi may reveal other findings relevant to the diagnosis of cardiovascular pathology. Beading of the retinal artery may suggest hypercholesterolemia. Microinfarction in the peripheral retina is seen in sickle cell disease. Angioid streaks may suggest pseudoxanthoma elasticum, which may be associated with hypertension, intermittent claudication, angina (coronary artery calcification), and arrhythmias. In Takayasu's syndrome, characteristic, wreathlike arteriovenous anastomoses around the disk can be identified.

In addition to examining the jugular venous and carotid artery pulse, evidence for thyroid gland enlargement and abnormal pulsation should be searched for while examining the neck. Suprasternal pulsation may indicate aortic arch aneurysm. The most common cause of a pulsatile mass at the root of the right side of the neck, however, is a kinked, tortuous right carotid artery. The presence of discoloration of the skin and some skin lesions occasionally provides diagnostic clues. Peripheral cyanosis, which indicates reduced peripheral blood flow, is detected in the skin of the hands, fingers, toes, earlobes, nose, lips, and nail beds. Central cyanosis, however, is detected in warm sites: conjunctiva, tongue, buccal mucous membrane, soft palate, and uvula. Central cyanosis results from intracardiac or intrapulmonary right-to-left shunting. Slate or bronze pigmentation of the skin may suggest hemochromatosis, which may be associated with restrictive cardiomyopathy. Marked jaundice is not caused solely by cardiovascular pathology; however, mild jaundice may be observed in patients with heart failure, with congestive hepatopathy in cardiac cirrhosis, and with pulmonary embolism. Prosthetic valve malfunction should be suspected if jaundice is detected in a patient with artificial heart valves. A blotchy cyanotic discoloration of the skin in a patient with a history of episodic flushing should raise the suspicion of carcinoid heart disease. Livedo reticularis, with cyanosis of the toes and preserved peripheral pulses, suggests cholesterol emboli (blue toes syndrome), particularly in patients undergoing left-sided heart catheterization or descending aorta surgery.[4] Acrosclerosis (i.e., taut, thickened, or edematous skin bound tightly to subcutaneous tissue in the hands and fingers) may suggest systemic sclerosis, which may be associated with several cardiac complications: right-sided heart failure secondary to pulmonary hypertension, fibrous replacement of myocardium (sclerodermal heart disease), conduction defects and arrhythmias, and angina and sudden death due to Raynaud's phenomenon in the heart. Ochronosis, which can produce valvular lesions, is associated with blue-black pigmentation of the ear and nose. Vitiligo is an occasional cutaneous manifestation of hyperthyroidism and Addison's disease. Exfoliative dermatitis, purpura, and petechial lesions can be manifestations of many commonly used cardiovascular drugs (e.g., quinidine, captopril, dyazide). Although erythema marginatum is characteristic of acute rheumatic fever, erythema nodosum is an entirely nonspecific finding and occurs in many systemic diseases. Café au lait spots occur in neurofibromatosis, which occasionally is associated with hypertrophic cardiomyopathy.

Cutaneous and subcutaneous nodular lesions are present in a number of systemic and metabolic diseases, which may also involve the cardiovascular system. Rheumatic nodules of acute rheumatic fever are

TABLE 23.1 ABNORMALITIES OF THE MUSCULOSKELETAL SYSTEM ASSOCIATED WITH CARDIOVASCULAR INVOLVEMENT

Disorders with Musculoskeletal Abnormalities	Anomalies of Appearance	Important Cardiovascular Lesions
Hurler's syndrome	Large, boat-shaped head, small and widely spaced teeth, broad nose, flaring nostrils, large lips, protuberant tongue, cloudy cornea, deafness, short neck, kyphoscoliosis, pigeon breast, barrel chest	Ischemic heart disease, endocardial fibroelastosis, nodular valve lesions
Marquio's syndrome	Large, boat-shaped head, broad nose, large lips, protuberant tongue, kyphoscoliosis, pigeon breast, barrel chest	Primary myocardial disease, aortic regurgitation
Down's syndrome (trisomy 21)	Prominent medial epicanthus, large protruding tongue, low-set ears, depressed nasal bridge, hypoplastic mandible, small head and orbits, hypertelorism, cataracts, simian palmar crease, inwardly curved, short fifth fingers	Atrioventricular canal defects, ventricular septal defect, atrial septal defect, patent ductus arteriosus, tetralogy of Fallot
Trisomy 13-15	Cleft palate, cleft lip, low-set, malformed ears, small head and jaw, slanted forehead	Ventricular septal defect, patent ductus arteriosus, atrial septal defect, dextrocardia, pulmonary valve stenosis
Trisomy 18	Triangular mouth, low-set, malformed ears, hypoplastic mandible with a receding chin, high-arched palate, webbed neck, stubby fingers, a tightly clenched fist, an index finger overlapping the third finger and a fifth finger overlapping the fourth finger	Ventricular septal defect, patent ductus arteriosus, atrial septal defect, pulmonary stenosis, coarctation of the aorta
Marfan's syndrome	Long narrow head, high-arched palate, arachnodactyly, kyphoscoliosis, ectopia lentis, increased arm span, lax joints, pectus deformities	Aortic regurgitation, aortic aneurysm and dissection, mitral valve prolapse and regurgitation (redundant chordae), dilated mitral annulus, primary myocardial disease, hypertensive heart disease, pulmonary artery dilatation, tricuspid regurgitation
Homocystinuria	Kyphoscoliosis, long extremities, pectus carinatum	Thrombosis of the intermediate-sized arteries, myocardial infarction, claudication
Klinefelter's syndrome	Tall stature, eunuchoid appearance, long extremities	Ventricular septal defects, patent ductus arteriosus, tetralogy of Fallot
Ellis van Creveld syndrome	Dwarfism, lip tie, polydactyly, hypoplastic fingernails	Atrial septal defect, ventricular septal defect, atrioventricular canal defect
Osteogenesis imperfecta	Short stature, bowed legs, saber shins, pseudoarthroses, blue scleras	Aortic and mitral regurgitation, calcification of the arteries
Friedreich's ataxia	Kyphoscoliosis, hammer toe, equinovarus, nystagmus	Hypertrophic cardiomyopathy, myocardial disease, arrhythmias
Refsum's disease	Deafness, ichthyosis, cataracts, polyneuropathy, cerebellar ataxia, night blindness	Myocardial disease, conduction abnormalities
Pseudohypertrophic muscular dystrophy (Duchenne)	Lordosis, protruding abdomen, pseudohypertrophy of the calves, waddling gait	Myocardial disease, mitral valve prolapse, tall R in ECG leads V_1, V_2 (simulate true posterior wall myocardial infarction)
Cornelia de Lange syndrome	Bushy, confluent eyebrows, low-set ears, hypoplastic mandible, arched palate, flat upturned nose	Ventricular septal defect
Werner's syndrome	Beaked nose, premature graying of the hair, premature balding, cataracts, proptosis	Premature coronary arterial atherosclerosis and myocardial infarction
Rubinstein-Taybi syndrome	Prominent forehead, beaked nasal bridge, large, low-set ears, antimongoloid slant of the eyes, high-arched palate	Atrial septal defect, patent ductus arteriosus
Klippel-Feil syndrome	Low hair line, low-set ears, small jaw, webbed neck, facial asymmetry, cleft palate, torticollis, deafness, strabismus, hydrocephaly	Ventricular septal defect
Noonan's syndrome	Short stature, webbed neck, dental malocclusion, antimongoloid slanting of the eyes, mental retardation, hypogonadism	Pulmonary valve stenosis, obstructive and nonobstructive cardiomyopathy
Mulibrey nanism	Triangular face, bulging forehead, low nasal bridge, retarded growth, hemangiomas, retinal pigmentary changes	Constrictive pericarditis
Myotonia dystrophilia	Masklike facial expression, drooping eyelids, receding hairline, sunken cheeks, cataracts	Dysrhythmias, myocardial disease
Facioscapulohumeral muscular dystrophy	Grimacing facial expression, atrophy of the shoulder girdle muscles	Silent atrium
Cardiofacial syndrome	Unilateral lower facial weakness	Ventricular septal defect
Progeria	Small face, bulging eyes, beaked nose, minimal subcutaneous fat with prominent scalp veins, premature aged appearance	Severe premature atherosclerosis with myocardial infarction
Pierre Robin syndrome	Cleft palate, hypoplastic mandible with shrewlike face	Patent ductus arteriosus, atrial septal defect, dextrocardia, coarctation of the aorta
Rubella syndrome	Cataracts, deafness, nystagmus	Peripheral pulmonary artery stenosis, patent ductus arteriosus
Ehler-Danlos syndrome	Hyperelastic velvety skin, "cigarette paper" scars, hyperextensible joints	Mitral regurgitation, dissection of the aorta, arterial rupture
Holt-Oram syndrome	Thumb with extra phalanx (fingerized thumb), deformities of the radius and ulna	Atrial septal defect

(Adapted from Silverman ME, Hurst JW: Inspection of the heart. In Hurst JW (ed): The Heart, 4th ed, p 162. New York, McGraw-Hill, 1978)

small and not tender. These most frequently occur on the knuckles, extensor surface of the elbows, and suboccipital regions. Rheumatoid nodules are large and characteristically localized over points of pressure or friction, most commonly the extensor surfaces of the proximal forearms. Pericarditis, conduction disturbances, and valvular regurgitation are the cardiovascular complications of rheumatoid arthritis. Xanthomas, cholesterol-filled nodules, occur in different types of abnormalities of lipoprotein metabolism, and the recognition of the distribution of xanthomas aids in the diagnosis of these disorders. Tendon xanthomas and xanthomas occurring on planar, patellar, and digital extensors, as well as tuberous xanthomas, occur in familial hypercholesterolemia (type II hyperbetalipoproteinemia), which is associated with premature atherosclerosis. Planar xanthomas, particularly in the palmar and digital creases, are peculiar to familial dysbetalipoproteinemia, but tuberous, tuberoeruptive, and tendinous lesions also occur. Premature coronary and peripheral vascular atherosclerotic diseases are quite common. Eruptive xanthomas (small yellow papules in the skin that are surrounded by an erythematous halo) are the charcateristic cutaneous lesions of primary hypertriglyceridemia (familial lipoprotein lipase deficiency), which is associated with pancreatitis and usually not premature coronary atherosclerosis. Eruptive xanthomas also occur in patients with endogenous and mixed hypertriglyceridemia (types IV and V hyperlipoproteinemia), and ischemic vascular disease is observed.

Various congenital and acquired cardiovascular disorders are associated with a variety of changes in the chest, abdomen, and extremities, as summarized in Table 23.1. A barrel-shaped chest with low diaphragm suggests emphysema, which can be associated with cor pulmonale. A right parasternal or upper sternal bulge may be observed in patients with chronic thoracic aortic aneurysm. Prominent tortuous veins in the upper part of the trunk may result from superior vena caval obstruction. A prominent left precordial bulge is occasionally seen in patients with congenital cyanotic heart disease.

Hepatomegaly frequently results from systemic venous hypertension: systolic pulsation of the liver is diagnostic of severe tricuspid regurgitation, and presystolic hepatic pulsation indicates significant tricuspid stenosis. An abdominal aortic pulsation is present with aortic aneurysm, but this is also frequently palpated in normal, young individuals with relatively shallow abdominal cavities. To differentiate between hepatic pulsation and abdominal aortic pulsation, palpation should be done laterally over the right hypochondrium, preferably during held inspiration. Splenomegaly rarely occurs in patients with severe right-sided heart failure, cardiac cirrhosis, and bacterial endocarditis. Similarly, obvious ascites is infrequently observed in patients with congestive heart failure but may result from constrictive pericarditis. In patients with hypertension, palpable bilateral, nonpulsatile abdominal masses should raise the possibility of polycystic disease of the kidneys. In hypertensive patients, auscultation over the subcostal regions and renal angles may reveal a systolic bruit when hypertension is caused by renal artery stenosis. A systolic bruit over the lower left posterior subcostal region may suggest splenic artery aneurysm, and the bruit originating from the splenic artery shifts location with inspiration.

While examining extremities, the physician should look for clubbing of the fingers and toes. The important cardiovascular causes of clubbing are cyanotic congenital heart disease, Eisenmenger's syndrome, and subacute or chronic bacterial endocarditis. Concomitant cyanosis is observed in patients with cyanotic heart disease. Differential cyanosis and clubbing, in which toes and feet are involved and hands and fingers are spared, suggest Eisenmenger's syndrome with patent ductus arteriosus. Reversed differential cyanosis and clubbing, in which fingers and hands are involved and lower extremities are spared, may be seen in patients with transposition of the great vessels, pulmonary hypertension, preductal coarctation of the aorta, and reversal of flow through a patent ductus arteriosus.

Splinter hemorrhages in the nail beds may suggest bacterial endocarditis; however, splinter hemorrhages can occur in normal subjects following mild trauma and also in patients with trichinosis. Osler's nodes are tender nodular, erythematous skin lesions that are most frequently observed in the palms, soles of the feet, and pads of the fingers or toes, resulting from emboli in bacterial endocarditis. Janeway lesions are nontender, raised hemorrhagic nodules usually occurring in the palms of the hands and soles of the feet and are also cutaneous manifestations of bacterial endocarditis.

Edema of the ankles and feet is a common finding of systemic venous hypertension, which is a frequent hemodynamic abnormality of congestive heart failure. However, edema is a nonspecific finding and occurs in several noncardiac disorders. Concomitant elevation of systemic venous pressure strongly supports congestive heart failure. Localized and unilateral edema of the extremities frequently results from local vascular or lymphatic disease. Unilateral or bilateral leg edema are not infrequently observed after the leg veins have been harvested for coronary artery bypass surgery.

EXAMINATION OF THE JUGULAR VENOUS PULSE

Analysis of the jugular venous pressure and pulse provides information regarding hemodynamic changes in the right side of the heart. It is preferable to examine the internal jugular, rather than the external jugular, veins. The presence of valves between the superior vena cava and the external jugular veins interferes with pressure transmission. The external jugular venous bulb is also a site for thrombus formation, which causes partial obstruction of the external jugular veins. Thus, assessment of right atrial pressure by estimating the jugular venous pressure is frequently inaccurate. Partial obstruction of the left innominate vein from compression by the aorta, particularly in relatively elderly patients, impairs transmission of right atrial pressure to the left internal jugular vein. This is also the most common cause of unequal pressures between right and left internal jugular veins. During modest inspiration, partial compression of the left innominate vein is usually relieved as the diaphragm and the aorta descend and the pressure in the two internal jugular veins becomes equal. The right innominate and internal jugular veins are in a direct line with the superior vena cava, allowing better transmission of right atrial pressures and pulses to the right internal jugular vein. Thus, examination of the right internal jugular venous pulse is preferable, while assessing the hemodynamic changes in the right side of the heart.

Examination of the neck veins should be performed in adequate light, keeping the head of the patient in the midline position at 30° to 45°. When the venous pulse is not easily recognized, the venous pressure may be either too high or too low. The position of the neck and trunk should be elevated or lowered accordingly. When the venous pressure is high, the venous pulsations are best seen when the trunk is elevated to 90°. In the presence of normal or low venous pressure, examination is performed with the patient in the supine position. It is apparent that the neck and trunk position for maximum venous pulsation varies from patient to patient and should be determined for each person. Raising of the legs or abdominal compression increases venous pressure and facilitates analysis of the jugular venous pulse. The hepatojugular or abdominojugular reflux is assessed by applying firm, sustained pressure over the upper abdomen while the patient is breathing quietly. This maneuver increases jugular pressure only transiently in normal subjects about 1 cm; in patients with right ventricular failure, however, sustained elevation of venous pressure is observed during continued compression. The mechanisms for positive hepatojugular reflux have not been clearly elucidated. Increased venous return to the right side of the heart from increased intra-abdominal pressure increases right ventricular preload during abdominal compression. It is assumed that the failing right ventricle is unable to respond normally to this increased preload. However, a raised diaphragm during abdominal compression compromises cardiac filling by decreasing intrathoracic and mediastinal volume available for cardiac expansion. Abnormal elevation of systemic venous pressure may be the consequence of volume expansion and raised diaphragm during abdominal compression.[5] It is to be noted that until this maneuver is performed correctly, the significance of the hepatojugular reflux is liable to misinterpretation. Furthermore, the sensitivity and specificity of this maneuver in the diagnosis of right ventricular failure is low.

Differentiation of the venous from the arterial pulse is sometimes difficult but can be made by the following distinguishing features:

1. During inspection, the venous pulse is recognized by its double undulation, frequently associated with relatively sharper inward movement, unlike the single, sharp outward movement of the carotid pulse. The carotid pulse is more easily visible medially and higher in the neck in the submandibular region. The dominant movement in the venous pulse is always inward, the y descent, and is caused by the opening of the tricuspid valve. In the presence of atrial fibrillation, the double undulation character of the venous pulse is lost due to the absence of an a wave associated with atrial systole. The venous pulse still can be recognized from its dominant inward movement.
2. The venous pressure and, hence, the amplitude of the venous pulse can be manipulated; it can be decreased by raising the level of the head and trunk above the level of the right atrium (e.g., sitting or standing) or increased by enhancing the venous return to the right side of the heart (raising the legs or compressing the abdomen).
3. During inspiration, pressure in the neck veins decreases appreciably, giving the impression of "inspiratory collapse." Arterial pulse amplitude does not change significantly during inspiration. It is to be noted that in certain conditions the "inspiratory collapse" of the jugular venous pulse does not occur; indeed, venous pressure may increase (Kussmaul's sign) in constrictive pericarditis, massive pulmonary embolism, and right ventricular infarction.[6]
4. Gentle to moderate compression (by the fingers or by stethoscope tubes) at the root of the neck obliterates the venous pulse in the neck above the level of compression, but the arterial pulsation remains visible. This maneuver is extremely useful in separating a very prominent venous pulsation from the carotid artery pulsation. It is to be noted that compression at the root of the neck may cause distention of the veins by impeding flow of blood to the heart, but pulsation will be absent due to blockade of the retrograde transmission of the pulse wave from the right atrium.
5. The arterial pulse is more easily palpable than the venous pulse. Occasionally, the venous pulse also becomes palpable when venous pressure is extremely high and the veins are distended.

Once the venous pulse is recognized, the venous pressure is estimated by noting the height of the oscillating top of the venous pulse above the sternal angle. Right atrial pressure is then approximated by adding 5 cm to the height of the venous column since it is assumed that the right atrium is located about 5 cm below the sternal angle. The normal right atrial pressure should not exceed 9 cm H_2O. In the horizontal position, the venous pulsation is usually visible in the neck when the right atrial pressure is normal; if the neck veins collapse in the horizontal position, subnormal right atrial pressure is suspected. Elevated jugular venous pressure with pulsation only indicates increased right atrial pressure, which can be caused by various pathologic conditions, such as functional and organic obstruction of the tricuspid valve, tricuspid valve incompetence, right ventricular failure, and restriction of right atrial and right ventricular filling. The cause of elevated right atrial pressure cannot be determined by simply noting the height of the jugular venous pulse; the character of the venous pulse and other physical findings need to be incorporated.

The normal jugular venous pulse wave or right atrial pressure wave recordings usually consist of three positive waves, a, c and v, and two negative waves, x and y (Fig. 23.1). The positive a wave is caused by transmitted right atrial pressure to the jugular veins during right atrial systole. The peak of the a wave is reached just before or during the first heart sound (S_1) and before the onset of ventricular ejection (carotid pulse upstroke). At the bedside the a wave can be identified by timing with the carotid pulse upstroke or the S_1; the a wave precedes the carotid pulse upstroke and precedes or coincides with S_1.

Atrial relaxation initiates the descent of the a wave. Rarely, when the PR interval is markedly prolonged, the descent may continue until a plateau is reached (the z point, which occurs just prior to the ventricular systole). However, the descent is usually interrupted by the c wave. In the right atrial pressure tracing, the c wave is recognized with the onset of right ventricular systole and presumably occurs from bulging of the tricuspid valve into the right atrium. During atrioventricular dissociation, dissociation of the a and c waves also occurs. The c wave in the jugular venous pulse probably results from transmission of the adjacent carotid artery pulsation and transmission of the right atrial c wave caused by right ventricular systole. Generally, the c wave of the jugular venous pulse cannot be identified separately by clinical examination and the recording of the jugular venous pulse is required.

Following the c wave, the negative x wave is recognized, both in the jugular venous pulse and in the right atrial pressure tracing. The initial portion of this wave is termed the x descent. Right atrial relaxation appears to be the primary mechanism for the x wave, although the downward displacement of the tricuspid valve during right ventricular ejection, which causes a fall in right atrial pressure, is also contributory. Normally, the x wave is lower than the y wave during inspiration. In the right atrial pressure tracing, the x wave occurs during early or mid systole; in the jugular venous pulse, it occurs in late systole due

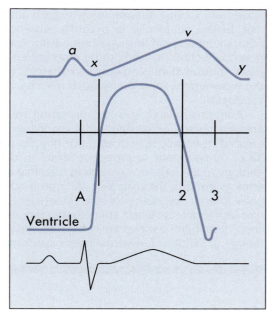

FIGURE 23.1 Schematic diagrams of jugular venous pulse, heart sounds, ventricular pressure pulse, and electrocardiogram. The a wave in the jugular venous pulse occurs before S_1 and before ventricular ejection begins. Ventricular ejection coincides with the upstroke of the carotid pulse. (a, a wave; x, x descent; v, v wave; y, y descent; A, atrial sound; 1, first heart sound; 2, second heart sound; 3, third heart sound) (Leatham A: An Introduction to the Examination of the Cardiovascular System, p 10. Oxford, Oxford University Press, 1967)

to the delay in transmission of the pulse. Clinically, the x wave is recognized by first identifying the a wave, which is followed by the x wave.

The mechanism of the v wave is the rise in right atrial and jugular venous pressure due to continued inflow of blood to the venous system during late ventricular systole when the tricuspid valve is still closed. The peak of the normal v wave is immediately after ventricular systole. At the bedside, when one uses the carotid pulse as the reference, the normal v wave coincides with the downslope of the carotid pulse, after the peak amplitude is felt. The v wave of tricuspid regurgitation (regurgitant wave), however, occurs earlier and in patients with severe tricuspid regurgitation; the v wave may occur with the carotid pulse upstroke.

The descending limb of the v wave, termed the y descent (occasionally the v descent) is caused by the opening of the tricuspid valve and the rapid inflow of blood to the right ventricle from the right atrium and the venous system. The initial y descent occurs during the rapid filling phase of the right ventricle, and the right ventricular third heart sound (S_3) corresponds to the nadir of the y wave. The ascending limb of the y wave (y ascent) occurs during continued inflow of blood to the venous system and right ventricle after the rapid filling phase. In the jugular venous pulse, the y wave is recognized by identifying the v wave first, which is then followed by the y descent. During longer ventricular diastole, as in bradycardia, the y wave may be occasionally followed by a brief positive wave, called the l wave, preceding the a wave. It is to be noted that the l wave can only be identified in the jugular venous pulse or right atrial pressure tracings and cannot be recognized clinically at the bedside.

During tachycardia, it is often difficult to identify a and v waves or x and y descents separately. Not infrequently, only one positive and one negative wave are recognized. Occasionally, simultaneous carotid massage to slow the heart rate is necessary for better analysis of the jugular venous pulse. In patients with atrial fibrillation, the jugular venous pulse is irregular and usually only v and y waves are appreciated. In atrial flutter, occasionally flutter waves are recognized, and the frequency of the flutter waves are higher than the arterial pulse rate.

ABNORMALITIES OF THE VENOUS PULSE AND THEIR SIGNIFICANCE

ELEVATION OF THE MEAN SYSTEMIC VENOUS PRESSURE

An elevation of the mean systemic venous pressure with bilateral distention of the neck veins and without venous pulsation should raise the suspicion of superior vena cava obstruction. Prominent distended veins in the upper extremities and in the upper torso, with lateral thoracic veins draining caudally to the veins below the umbilicus, also suggest superior vena caval obstruction, and the presence of these findings should initiate further investigations (chest film, chest computed tomography, magnetic resonance imaging, and angiography).

An elevated venous pressure with venous pulsation indicates that the mean right atrial pressure is higher than normal, which may result from a number of pathologic processes: (1) impaired emptying of the right atrium due to obstruction of the tricuspid valve; (2) incompetent tricuspid valve; (3) primary right ventricular failure; (4) right ventricular failure secondary to precapillary or postcapillary pulmonary hypertension; (5) increased intrapericardial and intrapleural pressure; (6) decreased right ventricular compliance; (7) constrictive pericarditis; and (8) volume overload. The differential diagnosis at the bedside depends on the presence of abnormal physical findings resulting from the specific hemodynamic abnormalities in the various disorders.

Once it is established that the systemic venous pressure is elevated, it is important to assess the changes in pressure during normal respiration. Normally, the mean level of venous pressure declines during inspiration but the amplitude of the a wave increases. Lack of decrease or increase in jugular venous pressure during inspiration is abnormal (Kussmaul's sign) and observed in a number of conditions, including (1) constrictive pericarditis, (2) restrictive cardiomyopathy, (3) predominant right ventricular infarction, (4) massive pulmonary embolism, (5) partial obstruction of the venae cavae, (6) right atrial and right ventricular tumors, (7) occasionally in tricuspid stenosis, (8) sometimes in congestive heart failure, and (9) rarely in cardiac tamponade.

The mechanism of Kussmaul's sign in these conditions is not entirely clear; however, increased resistance to right atrial filling during inspiration appears to be a common contributory factor. It is to be noted that Kussmaul's sign is seen more frequently in certain conditions than in others. In patients with inferior or inferoposterior acute myocardial infarction, the presence of Kussmaul's sign almost invariably indicates predominant right ventricular infarction.[6] Indeed, the sensitivity and specificity of Kussmaul's sign for the diagnosis of right ventricular infarction in patients with inferior myocardial infarction exceeds 90%.[6] In chronic situations, Kussmaul's sign is more frequently present in constrictive or effusive constrictive pericarditis. Chronic isolated right ventricular failure may be associated with an inspiratory increase of jugular venous pressure. Once constrictive pericarditis is suspected, other findings suggestive of chronic pericardial constriction (sharp y descent, diastolic left parasternal impulse, and pericardial knock) should be searched for and subsequent investigations should be planned accordingly. It is to be noted that Kussmaul's sign is rare in cardiac tamponade; the presence of Kussmaul's sign in a patient with known pericardial effusion should raise the possibility of effusive constrictive pericarditis.

ABNORMALITIES OF THE A WAVE IN THE JUGULAR VENOUS PULSE

In atrial fibrillation, the a wave is absent, whereas flutter waves can be occasionally recognized in atrial flutter. The a wave may also be absent when the right atrium is dilated and does not possess effective mechanical systole, as in severe Ebstein's anomaly and in the presence of giant silent right atrium. A number of dysrhythmias can be suspected at the bedside by analysis of the character of the venous pulse. In the presence of a regular, slow pulse, irregular cannon waves suggest complete atrioventricular block. A cannon wave is a large positive venous pulse wave produced by atrial contraction during ventricular systole when the tricuspid valve is closed. In complete atrioventricular block, atrial systole occurs randomly during ventricular diastole and systole, explaining irregular cannon waves. The most common cause of irregularly occurring cannon waves, however, is atrial, ventricular, or junctional premature beats; in these circumstances, the pulse is also irregular. Regular cannon waves occur in junctional rhythm, slow ventricular tachycardia, 2:1 atrioventricular block, and bigeminy. Regular cannon waves may also occur in first-degree atrioventricular block with a markedly prolonged PR interval and atrial systole occurring during the preceding ventricular systole. Analysis of the venous pulse and the intensity of S_1 are occasionally helpful in the differential diagnosis of wide complex tachycardia. Irregularly occurring cannon waves and varying intensity of S_1 suggest atrioventricular dissociation and, hence, ventricular tachycardia. Absence of cannon waves and constant intensity of S_1 suggest supraventricular tachycardia with aberrant conduction. It needs to be emphasized, however, that the diagnosis of dysrhythmia can only be suspected from the abnormalities of the venous pulse, and its diagnosis must be confirmed by the electrocardiogram.

Abnormally large a waves occurring with each beat indicate increased resistance to right atrial emptying during atrial systole. Increased resistance may occur at or beyond the tricuspid valve (Table 23.2). A systematic approach is useful in determining the potential etiology of the large a wave and in selecting the appropriate investigations to confirm the diagnosis. A large a wave in the jugular venous pulse is more likely to occur in the absence of interatrial or interventricular septal defects when atrial contraction can generate higher pressure. Prominent a waves are, therefore, uncommon in trilogy and tetralogy of Fallot or in Eisenmenger's syndrome.

ABNORMAL V WAVES

The diagnosis of tricuspid regurgitation can be made frequently by observing the amplitude of the *v* wave and the character of the *y* descent. Severe tricuspid regurgitation produces an early large *v* wave (regurgitant wave) followed by a steep *y* descent. With the onset of right ventricular systole, regurgitation to the right atrium ensues, explaining the early onset of the *v* wave. The amplitude of the *v* wave depends on the regurgitant volume and right atrial compliance. A steep *y* descent results from the increased pressure gradient across the tricuspid valve, which allows rapid inflow to the right ventricle and decompression of the right atrium in early diastole. The regurgitant wave of significant tricuspid regurgitation occurs concurrently with the carotid pulse and can be easily recognized when one times the onset with the carotid pulse upstroke. If tricuspid regurgitation is suspected from the presence of an early *v* wave in the jugular venous pulse, a search for other corroborative findings, such as a pansystolic murmur along the lower right and left sternal border, which increases in intensity during inspiration, and systolic pulsation of the liver, should be made. It is to be noted that severe tricuspid regurgitation may be present without any obvious *v* wave in the jugular venous pulse, particularly in patients with a markedly dilated right atrium. In atrial fibrillation, the *a* wave is absent and thus it is difficult to determine the relative amplitude of the *v* wave (compared with the *a* wave) from analysis of the jugular venous pulse alone. In patients with mild tricuspid regurgitation, there may not be any alternation in the jugular venous pulse.

A prominent *v* wave is occasionally detected in patients with atrial septal defect without significant pulmonary arterial hypertension and in the absence of tricuspid regurgitation. The mechanism remains unclear; however, concomitant systemic venous return and left-to-right shunt during ventricular systole may cause a rapid increase in right atrial pressure and, hence, a prominent *v* wave.

ABNORMALITIES OF THE Y DESCENT

A slow *y* descent may suggest tricuspid valve obstruction, which can be confirmed by auscultatory findings of tricuspid stenosis (Fig. 23.2). A slow *y* descent, however, may also occur in the presence of severe right ventricular hypertrophy, as in pulmonary valve or infundibular stenosis when resistance to early right ventricular filling is increased. The presence of a steep *y* descent is strong evidence against significant tricuspid valve obstruction. A rapid *y* descent following a large *v* (regurgitant) wave is characteristic of tricuspid regurgitation.

A sharp *y* descent without a prominent *v* wave occurs in constric-

---

TABLE 23.2 DIFFERENTIAL DIAGNOSIS OF THE LARGE A WAVE IN THE JUGULAR VENOUS PULSE

Increased Resistance at the Tricuspid Valve	Increased Resistance Distal to the Tricuspid Valve

Tricuspid valve obstruction:
  1. Rheumatic tricuspid stenosis
  2. Right atrial myxoma
  3. Carcinoid heart disease
  4. Lupus endocarditis
  5. Right atrial thrombus
  6. Congenital tricuspid stenosis
  7. Tricuspid atresia
 	
Important physical findings, except in tricuspid atresia:
  1. Along the left lower sternal border, a mid-diastolic rumble, which increases in intensity during inspiration
  2. Tricuspid opening snap
  3. Slow *y* descent in the jugular venous pulse
  4. Presystolic hepatic pulsation
	Right ventricular outflow obstruction (*e.g.*, pulmonary valve stenosis, hypertrophic cardiomyopathy)
	
	Important physical findings:
	  1. Long ejection systolic murmur that increases in intensity along the left sternal border
	  2. Widely split S_2 with decreased intensity of the pulmonary component
	  3. Sustained left parasternal impulse
	
	Right ventricular hypertrophy without outflow obstruction: precapillary pulmonary arterial hypertension, including peripheral pulmonary artery branch stenosis; postcapillary pulmonary artery hypertension
	
	Important physical findings:
	  1. Sustained left parasternal impulse
	  2. Narrowly split S_2 with P_2 louder than A_2 and P_2 transmitted to the mitral area

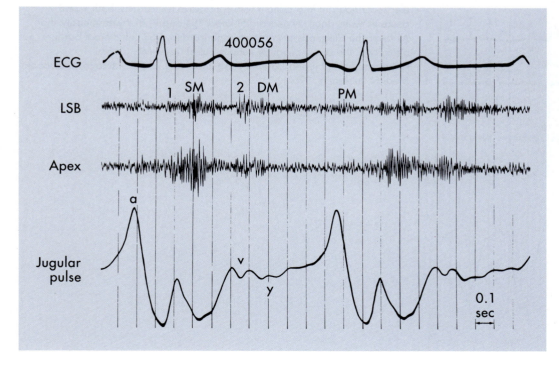

FIGURE 23.2 Jugular venous pulse tracing, electrocardiogram, and phonocardiographic recordings in a patient with tricuspid stenosis in normal sinus rhythm. A prominent *a* wave with a markedly attenuated *y* descent is apparent. A diastolic murmur (*DM*) with presystolic accentuation (*PM*) was recorded along the left sternal border (*LSB*). A systolic murmur (*SM*) was also recorded. (*1*, first heart sound; *2*, second heart sound) (Tavel ME: Clinical Phonocardiography and External Pulse Recording, p 184. Chicago, Year Book Medical Publishers, 1967)

tive pericarditis, in restrictive cardiomyopathy, or in severe right-sided heart failure with a markedly elevated systemic venous pressure. In constrictive pericarditis and restrictive cardiomyopathy, the mean jugular venous pressure is elevated and the amplitudes of the a and v waves are usually similar. Thus, the striking movement in the jugular venous pulse is the sharp inward y descent. It is difficult to differentiate between constrictive pericarditis and restrictive cardiomyopathy at the bedside; however, the presence of a left parasternal diastolic impulse and pericardial "knock" favors constrictive pericarditis, and physical findings indicating significant right ventricular systolic and pulmonary arterial hypertension are more common in restrictive cardiomyopathy. The presence of a relatively prominent v wave (Lancisi's sign), presumably due to associated tricuspid regurgitation, favors the diagnosis of severe right-sided heart failure.

In some patients with constrictive pericarditis, a steeper x descent may be present instead of a sharp y descent (Fig. 23.3). The mechanism of a sharp x descent is not clear; however, it is more likely to occur in effusive, constrictive pericarditis. In cardiac tamponade, the mean jugular venous pressure is elevated and x and y descents are not prominent. An elevated mean jugular venous pressure with a quiet precordium and the absence of any physical findings of pulmonary arterial hypertension should initiate a search for pericardial effusion. It needs to be emphasized that the analysis of the jugular venous pulse alone at the bedside does not provide the diagnosis. Nevertheless, careful analysis of the jugular venous pulse and pressure is necessary to decide what other physical findings one should look for to determine the diagnosis.

EXAMINATION OF THE ARTERIAL PRESSURE AND PULSE

Although some idea about the level of arterial systolic pressure can be obtained by gauging the amount of compressive pressure required to obliterate the arterial pulse, arterial pressure should be routinely measured at the bedside with the use of a sphygmomanometer. Appropriate selection of cuff size and proper application of the cuff are required for accurate determination of blood pressure. For adults with average arm size, the standard 5-inch wide cuff is used. For infants a 1½-inch cuff is used, and for young children a 3-inch cuff is required. In obese persons with large arms, an 8-inch wide cuff is preferable. A large cuff size is also required to determine the lower extremity pressures in adults, when the cuff is applied to the thighs. When the cuff size is inappropriately small for the arm or thigh size, arterial pressure is overestimated, and when the cuff is too large, pressure is underestimated.

The cuff should be applied snugly around the limb, and the bag should be long enough to extend at least halfway around the limb. The lower edge of the cuff should be at least 1 inch above the antecubital space, and the diaphragm of the stethoscope should be applied on the arterial pulse, close to the lower edge of the cuff. To determine lower extremity blood pressure, the patient should lie in the prone position and the cuff should be applied over the thigh with the compression bag placed on the posterior aspect, above the popliteal fossa. Lower leg pressure is measured by applying the cuff over the calf and auscultating over the posterior tibial artery.

The limb is placed at the level of the heart, and the cuff is inflated to 20 mm Hg to 30 mm Hg pressure above the level required to obliterate the arterial pulse. The cuff is then deflated slowly, listening for the Korotkoff sounds at the same time. Five phases of Korotkoff sounds are recognized when blood flow is allowed into the constricted artery as the cuff pressure is released: Phase I is when a clear tapping sound first appears, which represents systolic blood pressure. During phase II, the discrete sounds are replaced by soft murmurs. During phase III, the murmurs are louder. Phase IV is recognized when the sounds and murmurs suddenly become muffled, and phase V is when the Korotkoff sounds just disappear. Phase IV pressure overestimates intra-arterial diastolic pressure. If a significant difference exists between phase IV and V pressures (>10 mm Hg), it is preferable to record both pressures. In certain conditions with marked "diastolic runoff" (e.g., aortic regurgitation, arteriovenous fistula, large patent ductus arteriosus, extreme bradycardia), phase V pressure may be very low, often 0 mm Hg, and in these circumstances phase IV pressure is recorded as the diastolic pressure. The intensity of the phase I Korotkoff sounds appears to be influenced by the level of the distal arterial pressure and the slope of the pressure pulse at the time of reestablishing flow through the compressed artery. The slower the slope of the pressure pulse, and the higher the distal arterial pressure, the softer is the Korotkoff sound. The opposite effects are noted with increased slope and decreased distal pressure. In patients with severe aortic stenosis, and in patients with marked peripheral vasoconstriction or a low output state with elevated systemic vascular resistance, the Korotkoff sounds may be very soft or even inaudible. In shock states, therefore, measurement of cuff pressure by sphygmomanometer is unreliable and direct measurement of the arterial pressure by inserting an intra-arterial cannula is preferable.

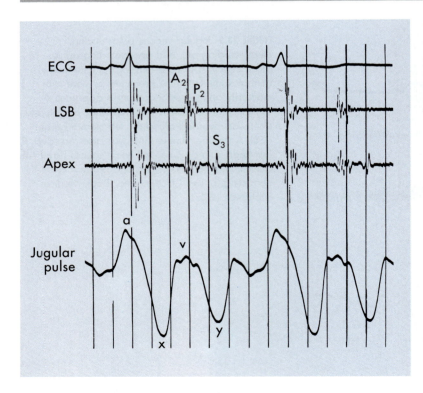

FIGURE 23.3 Jugular venous pulse tracing, phonocardiograms, and electrocardiogram in a patient with constrictive pericarditis. Both x and y descents were deep. A pericardial knock (S_3) and P_2 of lower intensity than A_2 favor the diagnosis of constrictive pericarditis. (LSB, left sternal border; apex, over the apex; j, jugular venous pulse) (Tavel ME: Clinical Phonocardiography and External Pulse Recording, p 183. Chicago, Year Book Medical Publishers, 1967)

In patients with a slow heart rate, atrial fibrillation, and other dysrhythmias, the cuff should be deflated very slowly, otherwise phase I sounds (systolic blood pressure) can be missed and the recorded systolic blood pressure will be erroneously lower. Unawareness of an auscultatory gap may also cause falsely low systolic blood pressure readings. The auscultatory gap is a relatively long period of silence between the Korotkoff phases I and II and tends to occur when the velocity of arterial flow is decreased.

During initial evaluation, blood pressure should be recorded in both arms and normally the difference in pressure in the two arms is usually less than 10 mm Hg. A pressure difference exceeding 15 mm Hg should initiate a search for obstructive lesions of the aorta or often brachiocephalic arteries (*e.g.*, atherosclerotic obstruction, extrinsic compression, aortic dissection, pre-subclavian coarctation, Takayasu's disease, aortic aneurysm, and embolic obstruction). In congenital supravalvular aortic stenosis, a blood pressure difference between the right and left arms (usually the right is greater than the left) exceeding 20 mm Hg is found in more than 50% of patients. In the subclavian steal syndrome, which may be associated with symptoms of cerebrovascular insufficiency, a lower blood pressure may be found in the ipsilateral arm.

Direct and indirect measurements of brachial and popliteal pressures, both in adults and children, usually demonstrate no significant differences. Significantly lower pressures in the inferior extremities compared with those of the arms may occur in post-subclavian coarctation of the aorta, aortic dissection, descending thoracic and abdominal aortic aneurysm, saddle embolus of the aorta, isolated aortoiliac disease (Leriche's syndrome), and extrinsic aortic compression. A difference between the right and left lower extremity pressures may occur in thromboembolic disease of the iliofemoral arteries, aortic dissection, and atherosclerotic peripheral vascular disease. In Takayasu's disease (pulseless disease), hypertension in the inferior extremities may occur with absent superior extremity pulses. It is apparent that blood pressure should be recorded both in the superior and inferior extremities when these disorders are suspected.

In patients with suspected orthostatic hypotension, blood pressure should be recorded both in the supine and upright positions. Assumption of the upright posture by normal adults is usually associated with a fall in systolic blood pressure of about 10 mm Hg and a rise in diastolic blood pressure of about 5 mm Hg. This is usually associated with an increase in heart rate by 5 to 20 beats. Any fall in diastolic blood pressure associated with symptoms of cerebral hypoperfusion constitutes orthostatic hypotension. In patients on antihypertensive drug therapy, it is also essential to record blood pressure in the upright posture.

Examination of the arterial pulse is an integral part of the cardiovascular examination and provides important diagnostic information. Carotid, radial, brachial, femoral, posterior tibial, and dorsalis pedis pulses should be examined bilaterally routinely to ascertain any differences in the pulse amplitude. When lower extremity arterial disease is suspected, popliteal pulses should also be examined. The carotid pulse contour is very similar to that of the central aortic pulse, and a delay in the onset of the ascending limb of the carotid pulse, compared with the central aortic pulse, is only about 20 msec. Thus, examination of the carotid pulse provides the most accurate representation of changes in the central aortic pulse. The brachial arterial pulse is examined to assess the volume and consistency of the peripheral vessels.

Inequality in the amplitude of the peripheral pulses may result from obstructive arterial diseases (atherosclerosis is the most common), aortic dissection, aortic aneurysm, and Takayasu's disease. Simultaneous palpation of the radial and femoral pulses may demonstrate a delay in the onset of the femoral pulse, which may suggest coarctation of the aorta. In normal adults, the pulse transmission delay in the radial artery is about 75 msec, and in the femoral artery it is about 70 msec. Thus, normally, the upstrokes of the radial and femoral pulses appear simultaneously. In coarctation of the aorta, the amplitude of the femoral pulse is also diminished. In supraventricular aortic stenosis, the right carotid, brachial, and radial pulses are larger in amplitude and volume than those on the left side. This is because of the preferential streaming of the jet toward the innominate artery.

PULSUS ALTERNANS

A search for the presence of pulsus alternans should be made while examining the peripheral pulses. The variation in pulse amplitude occurring with alternate beats, due to changing systolic pressure, is best appreciated by applying light pressure on the arterial pulse. Pulsus alternans is frequently precipitated by ectopic beats. The most important cause of pulsus alternans is left ventricular failure. Pulsus alternans is rarely encountered in patients with cardiac tamponade. In the presence of marked tachypnea, and when the respiratory rate is half of the heart rate, pulsus alternans may occur; however, when respiration is held transiently, pulsus alternans resulting from an inspiratory decrease in the pulse amplitude is no longer appreciated. Apparent pulsus alternans may also be observed in bigeminal rhythm. In bigeminy, the premature beats are usually out of phase with the normal beats and the postectopic pauses are generally appreciated.

Simultaneous auscultation of the sequence of the heart sounds and palpation of the arterial pulse can differentiate between true pulsus alternans and apparent pulsus alternans due to bigeminy. It is to be noted that pulsus alternans should not be diagnosed when cardiac rhythm is irregular.

Pulsus alternans can be confirmed by measuring blood pressure by sphygmomanometer. When the cuff pressure is slowly released, phase I Korotkoff sounds are initially heard only during the alternate strong beats; with further release of cuff pressure, the softer sounds of the weak beat also appear. The degree of pulsus alternans can be quantitated by measuring the difference in systolic pressure between the strong and the weak beat. The precise mechanism for pulsus alternans remains unclear. Alternating preload (Frank-Starling mechanism) and incomplete relaxation have been proposed as the potential mechanisms.[7] Changes in afterload (lower after preceding the strong beat) have also been thought to be contributory. However, it has also been suggested that a change in ventricular contractility is the primary mechanism and that changes in end-diastolic volume and pressure are secondary to changes in contractility. In experimental animals, acute myocardial ischemia can be associated with regional pulsus alternans, and it has been suggested that alternating potentiation and attenuation or deletion of contraction accounts for pulsus alternans.[8] In isolated canine heart preparations, the slope of the end-systolic pressure–volume relationship of the strong beats was significantly greater than those of weak beats. These studies suggest that pulsus alternans results primarily from an alternating contractile state of the ventricle. However, the magnitude of the alteration of pressure and stroke volume (indices of pump function) during pulsus alternans reflects the interaction of alternating contractile state with the alterations in preload and afterload. In clinical practice, true pulsus alternans is rarely seen in the absence of significant left ventricular myocardial failure; thus, recognition of pulsus alternans at the bedside should initiate further investigation to determine the severity and cause of left ventricular myocardial dysfunction. In patients with hypertrophic cardiomyopathy with significant rest or provocable outflow gradient, left ventricular pulsus alternans without systemic arterial pulsus alternans has been observed.[9] The mechanism remains unclear. Abolition of left ventricular alternans occurs after successful myomectomy.

PULSUS PARADOXUS

Respiratory variation of pulse amplitude should be observed during examination of the arterial pulse. Systolic arterial pressure normally falls during inspiration; however, the magnitude of decrease usually does not exceed 8 mm Hg to 12 mm Hg and the changes in pulse amplitude are not usually appreciated by palpation. A more marked inspiratory decrease in arterial pressure (exceeding 20 mm Hg) is termed *pulsus paradoxus* and is easily detectable by palpation. Pulsus paradoxus is readily recognized with the sphygmomanometer. When the cuff pressure is slowly released, the systolic pressure at expiration is first noted. With further slow deflation of the cuff, the systolic pressure during inspiration can also be detected. The difference between the pressures during expiration and inspiration is the magnitude of pulsus paradoxus. During very deep inspiration or Valsalva maneuver, the inspiratory decrease in systolic pressure is accentuated; thus, assessment of pulsus paradoxus should be made only during normal respiration.

Pulsus paradoxus is an important physical finding for the diagnosis of cardiac tamponade. The mechanism for the marked inspiratory decrease in arterial pressure appears to be related to the marked inspiratory decline of left ventricular stroke volume due to a decreased end-diastolic volume. In cardiac tamponade, the interventricular septum shifts toward the left ventricular cavity during inspiration (reverse Bernheim's effect), thereby decreasing left ventricular preload.[10] An inspiratory decrease in pulmonary venous return to the left side of the heart has also been thought to contribute to decreased left ventricular preload. In patients with hemodynamically significant aortic regurgitation and atrial septal defect, pulsus paradoxus may not occur, despite cardiac tamponade. In patients with suspected cardiac tamponade, echocardiography should be performed, not only to detect pericardial effusion but also to detect right ventricular diastolic collapse, which appears to be more specific and sensitive than pulsus paradoxus for the diagnosis of tamponade.[11] Besides tamponade, pulsus paradoxus occurs in chronic obstructive pulmonary disease, in hypovolemic shock, and infrequently in constrictive pericarditis and restrictive cardiomyopathy. Pulsus paradoxus is rarely observed in pulmonary embolism, pregnancy, marked obesity, and partial obstruction of the superior vena cava.

In hypertrophic obstructive cardiomyopathy, arterial pressure occasionally rises during inspiration (reversed pulsus paradoxus); the precise mechanism for this phenomenon remains unclear.[12]

In addition to changes in the amplitude, configurational changes of the carotid pulse may occur, which when appreciated help in suspecting certain disease states (Fig. 23.4).

PULSUS BISFERIENS

Pulsus bisferiens is characterized by two peaks during left ventricular ejection separated by a midsystolic dip. The carotid arterial pulse tracing and the central aortic pulse waveform normally consist of an earlier peak, the percussion wave, resulting from the rapid left ventricular ejection, and a second smaller peak, the "tidal wave," presumed to represent a reflected wave from the periphery. In hypertensive patients, or when the systemic vascular resistance is elevated, the tidal wave may increase in amplitude. Radial and femoral pulse tracings usually demonstrate a single sharp peak in normal circumstances. In pulsus bisferiens, both percussion and tidal waves are accentuated. It is apparent that at the bedside one cannot recognize with certainty (by simple palpation) that the two peaks are occurring in systole (pulsus bisferiens) and not one peak in systole and the other peak in diastole (dicrotic pulse). When a double-peaked pulse is appreciated, a search should be made for the conditions that can be associated with pulsus bisferiens or dicrotic pulse.

Pulsus bisferiens is frequently observed in patients with hemodynamically significant aortic regurgitation and usually is not appreciated in patients with mild or trivial aortic regurgitation. In patients with mixed aortic stenosis and aortic regurgitation, bisferiens pulse occurs when regurgitation is the predominant lesion. It is to be noted that the absence of pulsus bisferiens does not exclude significant aortic regurgitation. The mechanism of pulsus bisferiens is not clear; however, this waveform appears to be related to a large, rapidly ejected left ventricular stroke volume associated with increased left ventricular and aortic dp/dt. Thus, pulsus bisferiens can be occasionally felt in patients with a large patent ductus arteriosus or arteriovenous fistula. In chronic, hemodynamically significant aortic regurgitation, the Corrigan or water-

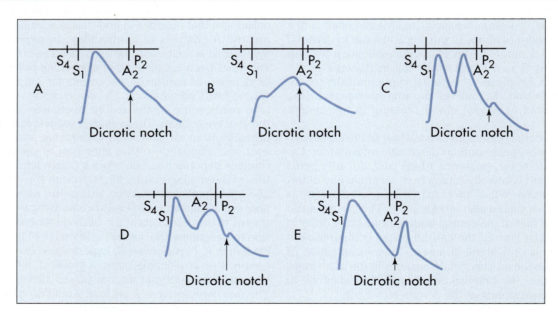

FIGURE 23.4 Schematic diagrams of the configurational changes in the carotid pulse and their differential diagnosis. Heart sounds are also illustrated. **A.** Normal. **B.** Anacrotic pulse with slow initial upstroke. The peak is close to the second heart sound. These features suggest fixed left ventricle outflow obstruction. **C.** Pulsus bisferiens with both percussion and tidal waves occurring during systole. This type of carotid pulse contour is most frequently observed in patients with hemodynamically significant aortic regurgitation or combined aortic stenosis and regurgitation with dominant regurgitation. It is rarely observed in mitral valve prolapse, in normal individuals. **D.** Pulsus bisferiens in hypertrophic obstructive cardiomyopathy. It is rarely appreciated at the bedside by palpation. **E.** Dicrotic pulse results from an accentuated dicrotic wave and tends to occur in sepsis, severe heart failure, hypovolemic shock, cardiac tamponade and also after aortic valve replacement. (S_4, atrial sound; S_1, first heart sound; A_2, aortic component of the second heart sound; P_2, pulmonary component of the second heart sound)

hammer pulse is frequently appreciated. The water-hammer pulse is characterized by an abrupt, very rapid upstroke of the peripheral pulse (percussion wave), followed by rapid collapse. The water-hammer pulse is better appreciated by raising the arm abruptly and feeling for the characteristics in the radial pulse. The Corrigan or water-hammer pulse probably results from very rapid ejection of a large left ventricular stroke volume into a low resistance arterial system.

In acute aortic regurgitation, left ventricular stroke volume may not increase appreciably and the systemic vascular resistance may not be low; the left ventricle is not dilated. Thus, changes in arterial pulse that are observed in chronic aortic regurgitation, such as bounding pulse, pulsus bisferiens, Corrigan's pulse, or increased pulse pressure, are not observed in acute aortic regurgitation, even when the regurgitation is severe.

A bounding arterial pulse is not diagnostic of aortic regurgitation and can occur in many conditions associated with increased stroke volume, as in patent ductus arteriosus, large arteriovenous fistulas, hyperkinetic states, thyrotoxicosis anemia, and extreme bradycardia.

In hypertrophic obstructive cardiomyopathy, pulsus bisferiens is rarely palpable but often recorded. In most patients with hypertrophic cardiomyopathy, the carotid pulse upstroke is sharp and the amplitude is normal. The rapid upstroke and prominent percussion wave result from rapid left ventricular ejection into the aorta during early systole. This is followed by a rapid decline as left ventricular outflow tract obstruction ensues, and the second peak is related to the tidal wave. Occasionally, a bisferiens quality can be precipitated by Valsalva maneuver or by inhalation of amyl nitrite. A bisferiens quality of the arterial pulse is rarely noted in patients with significant mitral valve prolapse and very rarely in normal individuals.

DICROTIC PULSE

A dicrotic pulse is frequently confused with pulsus bisferiens at the bedside; indeed, without a pulse recording it is almost impossible to distinguish between these two types of pulse configurations. A dicrotic pulse results from the accentuated dicrotic wave that follows the dicrotic notch. It tends to occur when the dicrotic notch is low, as in patients with decreased systemic arterial pressure and vascular resistance (*e.g.*, fever). However, a dicrotic pulse is also noted in patients with severe heart failure, hypovolemic shock, or cardiac tamponade and also with conditions associated with a decreased stroke volume and elevated systemic vascular resistance.

A dicrotic pulse can also occur in patients following aortic valve replacement during the immediate postoperative period.[13] The precise mechanism for a dicrotic pulse in these patients is not clear, but it is more frequently observed in patients with pump failure postoperatively. A dicrotic pulse may be confused with pulsus bisferiens, and a potential exists for mistaken diagnosis of aortic regurgitation due to malfunction of the prosthetic valve. Appropriate investigations, including detailed clinical evaluation and echocardiography, are required to establish the diagnosis. Dicrotic pulse is occasionally noted in normal individuals, particularly after exercise.

ARTERIAL PULSE IN AORTIC STENOSIS

In the presence of fixed left ventricular outflow tract obstruction, characteristic changes in the morphology of the arterial pulse may occur and careful examination of the arterial pulse provides useful information in the diagnosis and assessment of the severity of aortic stenosis. Increased resistance to left ventricular ejection due to fixed obstruction prolongs left ventricular total ejection time and retards the rate of initial stroke output into the aorta and distal arterial system. As a result, the carotid pulse tracing demonstrates an abnormally slow initial upstroke and a delayed peak, indicating increased left ventricular ejection time. Several systolic time intervals can be measured from the carotid pulse tracings to determine changes in left ventricular ejection character and to assess the severity of aortic stenosis (Fig. 23.5). Left ventricular ejection time (LVET) is measured as the period from the initial rise of the ascending limb of the carotid pulse to the dicrotic notch or incisura. LVET is inversely related to heart rate and, therefore, it is corrected for heart rate, using the following formula:

$$\text{corrected LVET} = \frac{\text{observed LVET}}{\text{preceding RR cycle length}}$$

The upstroke time (U time) is the period from the initial rise of the carotid upstroke to the peak of the carotid pulse and is also corrected for heart rate. The t time represents the rate of the carotid pulse upstroke and is equal to the time required for the carotid pulse to reach one half of its peak amplitude. The systolic time intervals determined from the carotid pulse tracings in normal individuals and in patients with aortic stenosis are summarized in Table 23.3.[14-20]

In general, the systolic time intervals determined from the carotid pulse tracings are abnormal in patients with hemodynamically significant aortic stenosis. However, no single measurement appears to be sensitive or specific enough for the precise estimation of the severity of aortic stenosis. A prolonged corrected t time exceeding 0.046 second occurs in approximately 70% of patients with aortic stenosis; a normal t time, however, does not exclude severe aortic stenosis. Similarly, a corrected U time is usually prolonged (exceeding 0.17 second) in severe aortic stenosis; however, the U time may be normal in many patients with significant aortic stenosis, particularly when left ventricular systolic function is depressed. Furthermore, U time is frequently overestimated when the tidal wave is incorporated as the peak of the carotid pulse. When the corrected left ventricular ejection time is longer than 0.36 second, aortic stenosis is usually hemodynamically signifi-

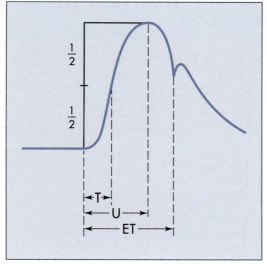

FIGURE 23.5 Measurement of systolic time intervals from the carotid pulse tracing. The t time (T) is the time required for the pulse to reach half of its total height. The U time (U) is the time required for the pulse to reach maximum height. Ejection time (ET) is the time between the onset of the pulse and the dicrotic notch. (Tavel ME: Clinical Phonocardiography and External Pulse Recording, p 144. Chicago, Year Book Medical Publishers, 1967)

cant, with a peak transvalvular gradient exceeding 45 mm Hg. However, the left ventricular ejection time may remain normal in many patients with severe aortic stenosis, particularly when the stroke volume is markedly decreased or when myocardial function is depressed. It is apparent that systolic time intervals alone cannot be relied on in individual patients to assess the severity of aortic stenosis, particularly when a decision needs to be made regarding surgical therapy. The presence of left ventricular outflow tract obstruction, however, should be suspected when abnormalities of systolic time intervals are detected.

At the bedside, one relies on changes in configuration of the arterial pulse to detect the presence of aortic stenosis and for the approximate assessment of its severity. The presence of aortic stenosis can be suspected from a number of abnormalities of arterial pulse: delayed upstroke of the ascending limb (pulsus tardus), anacrotic character (anacrotic pulse), delayed peak, small amplitude (pulsus parvus), and shudder (thrill) on the ascending limb. These abnormalities are best appreciated in the central pulse.

In the central aortic pulse there is a notch (anacrotic notch) on the ascending limb; however, on the upstroke of the carotid pulse, the anacrotic notch is rarely palpable in the absence of aortic stenosis. An anacrotic pulse gives the impression of interruption of the upstroke of the carotid pulse. When the anacrotic notch is felt immediately after the onset of the upstroke, aortic stenosis is likely to be hemodynamically significant. An anacrotic radial pulse also suggests moderate to severe aortic stenosis. Normally, the anacrotic notch is absent in the radial pulse. In the presence of severe aortic stenosis, an anacrotic notch occurs very early on the ascending limb of the arterial pulse and, therefore, can be appreciated in the radial pulse.

A delayed peak and slower upstroke of the carotid pulse suggest a prolonged left ventricular ejection time, which, however, cannot be estimated precisely at the bedside. By simultaneous palpation of the carotid pulse and auscultation of the interval between S_1 and S_2 (duration of systole), one can appreciate the delay in the peak of the carotid pulse. Normally, the peak of the carotid pulse occurs closer to S_1; in the presence of severe aortic stenosis, it is usually closer to S_2. In the presence of fixed outflow obstruction, the central aortic pulse demonstrates a progressively slower rise of the ascending limb, a lower anacrotic shoulder, and a peak closer to the incisura as the severity of obstruction increases. With a decreasing stroke volume, the pulse amplitude also decreases (pulsus parvus). These changes in the central aortic pulse are reflected in the carotid pulse. Frequently a thrill (carotid shudder) is also palpable on the ascending limb of the pulse. It needs to be emphasized that the diagnosis of the presence and severity of aortic stenosis should not be based on changes in the carotid pulse configuration alone; the auscultatory findings of aortic stenosis and evidence for left ventricular hypertrophy should be sought. In elderly patients, carotid arteries may become rigid and less compliant owing to arteriosclerosis, and the usual changes in the carotid pulse due to aortic stenosis are modified, particularly the amplitude, which may not decrease even in the presence of severe aortic stenosis. In these patients, any clinical evidence of aortic stenosis (e.g., a slower initial upstroke of the carotid pulse or carotid shudder) should prompt further evaluation, such as an echocardiogram-Doppler study to estimate the left ventricular outflow gradient and fluoroscopy of the aortic valve to detect calcification.

EXAMINATION OF THE PRECORDIAL PULSATIONS

Inspection and palpation of precordial cardiovascular pulsations is best performed with patients supine and with a modest elevation of the head and chest (not over 45°), not only by looking down at the chest but also looking from the side. Normally, a slight abrupt inward pulsation can be seen over to the left parasternal area, particularly in children and thin-chested subjects. Epigastric and subxiphoid pulsations are usually abnormal and are related to right ventricular hypertrophy and dilation or to abdominal aortic aneurysm. However, in patients with emphysema, subxiphoid pulsations may not always indicate right ventricular hypertrophy. In children and in persons with a scaphoid abdomen, an abdominal aortic pulsation is frequently visible over the epigastrium. Pulsation over the right second intercostal space or right sternoclavicular joint may indicate aneurysm of the ascending aorta; aneurysm of the arch of the aorta is occasionally associated with suprasternal pulsation. The most common cause of right supraclavicular pulsation, however, is a kinked tortuous carotid artery. Occasionally, a pulsation is visible over the left second or third interspace, which is usually due to a dilated pulmonary artery. Systolic outward parasternal and left ventricular outward movements are better appreciated by palpation than by inspection. A hyperdynamic left ventricular impulse associated with severe aortic or mitral regurgitation is frequently visible and can cause occasional shaking of the entire precordium. Cardiac pulsations, when visible lateral to the left midclavicular line, usually suggest cardiac enlargement. Leftward cardiac displacement due to left pulmonary fibrosis, right-sided tension pneumothorax or massive pleural effusion, absent left pericardium, and thoracic deformity may also cause visible pulsation beyond the midclavicular line. Retraction of the chest wall anteriorly with each cardiac cycle may occur in patients with biventricular hypertrophy or constrictive pericarditis. Retraction of the ribs in the left axilla (Broadbent's sign) usually indicates adhesive pericarditis, rather than constrictive pericarditis. In patients

TABLE 23.3 SYSTOLIC TIME INTERVALS DETERMINED FROM THE CAROTID PULSE TRACINGS IN NORMAL INDIVIDUALS AND IN PATIENTS WITH AORTIC STENOSIS

Study	LVET (sec)		U Time (sec)		t time (sec)	
	N	AS	N	AS	N	AS
Duchosal and co-workers					0.04–0.06	0.06–0.14
Donoso and co-workers	0.24–0.34	0.26–0.44	0.05–0.15	0.06–0.28		
Benchimol and co-workers*	0.28–0.34	0.31–0.41	0.06–0.11	0.08–0.29	0.02–0.04	0.02–0.10
Daoud and co-workers					0.04–0.09	0.06–0.11
Robinson	0.22–0.34	0.29–0.37	0.12–0.25	0.10–0.32		
Braunwald	0.257 (avg)	0.340 (avg)	0.051 (avg)	0.15 (avg)	0.025 (avg)	0.055 (avg)
Epstein and Coulshed*	0.26–0.34	0.30–0.48	0.05–0.11	0.08–0.33	0.02–0.046	0.025–0.11

* All measurements corrected for heart rate. (LVET, left ventricular ejection time; avg, average; N, normal; AS, aortic stenosis)
(Adapted from Tavel ME: Clinical Phonocardiography and External Pulse Recordings. Chicago, Year Book Medical Publishers, 1967)

with severe dilated congestive cardiomyopathy, occasionally a double impulse is visible over the apical region, usually due to a sustained left ventricular impulse and a prominent early diastolic filling impulse.

PALPATION

Palpation of the precordium should include the apical, midprecordial, lower left and right parasternal, pulmonary, aortic, suprasternal, and epigastric areas. The primary objective of palpation of the precordium is to detect the character of the right and left ventricular impulse, which is helpful to assess changes in cardiac dynamics and function.

LEFT VENTRICULAR IMPULSE

The apex impulse (left ventricular thrust or apex beat) is the outward movement of the left ventricular apical region and is normally localized; its extent does not exceed more than 2 to 3 cm in diameter and is situated in the fourth or fifth left intercostal space, just medial to the left midclavicular line. Generally, the apex beat is the point of maximal impulse, but occasionally right parasternal pulsation or pulsation associated with a dilated pulmonary artery and aortic aneurysm may be more forceful than the left ventricular impulse. When the right ventricle is markedly dilated, as in some patients with a large atrial septal defect or severe mitral stenosis, the left ventricular apical impulse may not be palpable because of the posterior displacement of the left ventricle.

The apex impulse is best palpated when the patient lies in a partial left lateral decubitus position. Both the systolic and diastolic portions of the apex impulse should be analyzed. Pathophysiologic information that can be obtained by palpation of the apex impulse at the bedside stems from the knowledge of apex cardiograms in normals and in patients with various cardiovascular disorders. The physiologic correlations between the various components of the apex cardiogram and the left ventricular dynamic events have been studied both in experimental animals and in humans.[21-24] The onset of the upstroke of the apex cardiogram coincides with the onset of the isovolumic phase of left ventricular systole, and the upstroke phase is usually completed before left ventricular ejection begins. During the isovolumic phase, the intraventricular pressure rises, which is associated with increased external cardiac circumference and alterations in ventricular shape. The upstroke portion of the apex cardiogram in normal subjects terminates with the E point, which usually coincides with the beginning of the ejection phase. Normally, the apex impulse on palpation corresponds to the E point of the apex cardiogram. During isovolumic systole, there is a counterclockwise rotation of the heart in normal subjects, which brings the lower anterior portion of the left ventricle in close proximity to the anterolateral chest wall and causes an outward motion. The normal outward motion of the apex impulse during palpation, or when recorded, is very brief. In the normal apex cardiogram, a gradual inward movement is recorded after the E point, resulting from a decreasing ventricular volume during the ejection phase of systole. A more rapid inward movement begins just before S_2 and continues up to the O point, which coincides approximately with mitral valve opening; thus, this portion of the apex cardiogram corresponds to the left ventricular isovolumic relaxation phase. After the O point, a rapid filling wave, followed by a slow filling wave, corresponding to the rapid and slow ventricular filling phases, are described. With atrial systole, an a wave is recorded after the slow filling wave in the later part of diastole. Normally, the a wave is relatively small and its height usually does not exceed 15% of the total height of the outward movement (Fig. 23.6).

The outward movement (systolic portion) in the apex cardiogram can be classified as normal, hyperdynamic, or sustained. The hyperdynamic apex impulse, when recorded, shows an outward movement of increased amplitude but of normal configuration. It is frequently associated with an accentuated rapid-filling wave. At the bedside, the hyperdynamic apex impulse is appreciated as a thrust of large amplitude that immediately disappears from the palpating fingers. When one estimates the duration of the ejection phase from the carotid pulse upstroke, or from the interval between S_1 and S_2, the hyperdynamic apex impulse does not extend throughout systole. It is found in conditions associated with an increased stroke volume or volume overload but in the absence of significant left ventricular hypertrophy or depressed ejection fraction. In patients with a hyperdynamic impulse, increased end-diastolic volume is usually associated with a proportional increase in total stroke volume.[25] Thus, in normal subjects after exercise, in hypermetabolic states (thyrotoxicosis, anemia), in primary mitral regurgitation, in aortic regurgitation with normal systolic function, and in some patients with a large patent ductus arteriosus and ventricular septal defect, the hyperdynamic apex impulse can be appreciated.

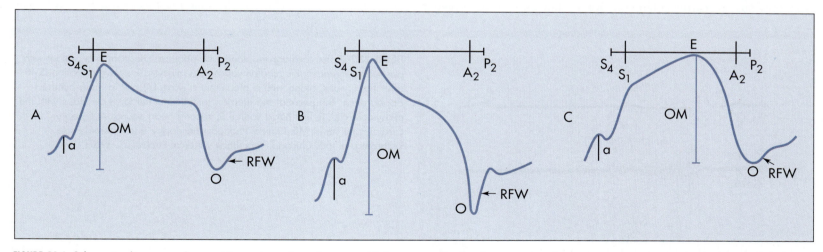

FIGURE 23.6 Schematic diagrams of normal hyperdynamic and sustained left ventricular impulse. Heart sounds are also illustrated. **A.** Normal apex cardiogram. The a wave, related to ventricular filling during atrial systole, usually does not exceed 15% of the total height. E point usually coincides with the beginning of left ventricular ejection. Following E point, there is a gradual inward movement explaining the brief duration of the normal left ventricular impulse. The O point approximately coincides with the mitral valve opening. **B.** Hyperdynamic left ventricular impulse is usually seen in left ventricular volume overloaded conditions such as primary mitral regurgitation and aortic regurgitation. Left ventricular ejection fraction is usually normal. Increased amplitude of a wave may be associated with palpable a waves, which are usually associated with increased left ventricular end diastolic pressure. Accentuated rapid filling wave is frequently associated with audible S_3. **C.** Sustained left ventricular impulse (outward movement continued during ejection phase) is usually seen in the presence of decreased ejection fraction or when left ventricle is markedly hypertrophied. (S_4, atrial sound; S_1, first heart sound; A_2, aortic component of the second heart sound; P_2, pulmonary component of the second heart sound; a, a wave; E, E point beginning of ejection; OM, outward movement; O, O point; RFW, rapid filling wave)

In the apex cardiogram, the sustained outward movement is characterized by a plateau or a dome-shaped or rising curve after the E point in contrast to the systolic decline after the E point seen in normal or hyperdynamic impulse curves. At the bedside, a sustained apical impulse is felt as a heave; however, it is preferable to assess the duration of the apex impulse (outward movement) by timing with the duration of the carotid pulse upstroke or with the interval between S_1 and S_2 (duration of the systolic phase). The sustained apex impulse is prolonged and is felt by the palpating fingers throughout the systolic phase.

A sustained apex impulse is usually found when there is significant left ventricular hypertrophy, as in patients with left ventricular outflow obstruction or systemic hypertension. A sustained impulse is also appreciated when left ventricular systolic function (ejection fraction) is depressed, as in patients with dilated cardiomyopathy, those with ischemic heart disease, and patients with aortic regurgitation with a reduced ejection fraction.[25] If one can exclude conditions that can be associated with left ventricular hypertrophy, a sustained apex impulse should raise the suspicion of a depressed ejection fraction. In patients with chronic coronary artery disease, cardiomegaly on the chest film is usually associated with a reduced left ventricular ejection fraction. The presence of a Q wave myocardial infarction on the electrocardiogram and history and physical findings of congestive heart failure, in addition to displacement of the left ventricular impulse, have a predictive accuracy of 81% in the assessment of the presence of a normal or depressed left ventricular ejection fraction.[26] It is to be noted that, at the bedside, it is only possible to approximate the left ventricular ejection fraction.

In hypertrophic cardiomyopathy with left ventricular outflow obstruction, a midsystolic bulge during the systolic portion of the apex cardiogram may produce a bifid outward movement.[27,28] Along with a prominent *a* wave, a triple-humped appearance may be observed (Fig. 23.7). At the bedside, a triple impulse may also be felt; however, most frequently a double impulse, consisting of a palpable *a* wave and a sustained outward movement, is appreciated. A midsystolic bulge has been thought to be due to midsystolic left ventricular outflow obstruction.

In patients with angina pectoris and coronary artery disease, various abnormalities in the graphic records of precordial motion (kinetocardiography) have been described.[29] Early systolic, late systolic, or combined early and late systolic bulges have been recorded. These abnormal systolic motions were more frequently present in patients with previous myocardial infarction. Systolic bulges were also noted in the absence of infarction, presumably resulting from myocardial ischemia, particularly when such abnormal motion appeared during stress or anginal pain. At the bedside, however, these abnormal systolic motions are difficult to appreciate. In most patients with previous myocardial infarction with a reduced left ventricular ejection fraction, a sustained apex impulse is observed. In the presence of normal left ventricular function, the left ventricular apex impulse is also normal; however, in occasional patients, a transient sustained impulse can be precipitated during stress, such as hand grip.

In patients with mitral valve prolapse, occasionally a deep notch in the systolic portion of the left ventricular impulse, which coincides with the midsystolic click, is recorded in the apex cardiogram. At the bedside, such a bifid impulse is almost never palpable and in the vast majority of patients with the mitral valve prolapse syndrome, the apex impulse is normal in character.

An accentuated rapid-filling wave with a sharper configuration (rapid-filling spike) in the apex cardiogram can be recorded in a number of conditions associated with augmented early diastolic filling, such as mitral regurgitation, patent ductus arteriosus, and ventricular septal defect. A prominent rapid-filling wave is also observed in normal, young subjects. Thus, a prominent rapid-filling wave recorded in the apex cardiogram is not a pathologic finding by itself. At the bedside, a palpable rapid filling wave, however, is always abnormal and the most consistent hemodynamic association is an elevated left ventricular diastolic pressure.

A prominent *a* wave in the apex cardiogram, with an amplitude exceeding 15% of the total height, is seen when left ventricular compliance is decreased,[30] which includes conditions associated with left ventricular hypertrophy (aortic stenosis, systemic hypertension, and hypertrophic cardiomyopathy), myocardial disease (cardiomyopathy), ischemic heart disease, and chronic left ventricular aneurysm. In patients with angina pectoris, an accentuated *a* wave can occur during angina pectoris or stress. It needs to be emphasized that the absence of a prominent *a* wave or normal *a*/OM ratio in the apex cardiogram does not exclude conditions with decreased left ventricular compliance. Furthermore, a proportionate accentuation of the outward movement may be associated with a normal *a*/OM ratio, even in the presence of decreased left ventricular compliance. At the bedside, the *a* wave is not palpable until it is markedly accentuated. A palpable *a* wave is always an abnormal physical finding, and the most common hemodynamic association is an elevated left ventricular end-diastolic pressure. The absence of a palpable *a* wave, however, does not exclude an abnormal left ventricular end-diastolic pressure. An *a* wave is usually

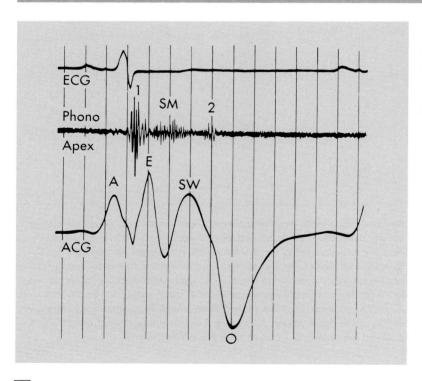

FIGURE 23.7 Apex cardiogram along with phonocardiogram in a patient with obstructive hypertrophic cardiomyopathy. A midsystolic outward motion (SW) after the E point, along with a prominent *a* wave (A) give a triple-humped appearance. The peak of the ejection systolic murmur (SM) coincides with the midsystolic dip. (1, first heart sound; 2, second heart sound; ACG, apex cardiogram) (Tavel ME: Clinical Phonocardiography and External Pulse Recording, p 166. Chicago, Year Book Medical Publishers, 1967)

absent in conditions associated with marked restriction of inflow to the left ventricle, such as mitral valve obstruction or constrictive pericarditis. A palpable *a* wave or an accentuated *a* wave in the apex cardiogram in a patient with mitral stenosis usually signifies insignificant mitral valve obstruction. In patients with acute, severe aortic regurgitation, premature closure of the mitral valve can occur due to a rapid increase in left ventricular diastolic pressure exceeding aortic diastolic pressure; in these circumstances also, the *a* wave may be absent.[31]

RIGHT VENTRICULAR IMPULSE

Normally, an inward movement (systolic retraction) is appreciated by palpation of the lower left parasternal area. In children, or in occasional adults with thin chest walls, a brief, gentle thrust may be palpable over the left third and fourth interspaces. Graphic recordings at these locations are qualitatively similar to the apex cardiogram. The amplitudes of the waveforms, however, are smaller. A prolonged left parasternal or upward or outward movement is distinctly abnormal. One can assess the duration of the left parasternal lift by timing it with the duration of the carotid pulse upstroke or with the interval between S_1 and S_2. A sustained left parasternal outward movement is palpable throughout systole.

A sustained systolic left parasternal lift is most frequently appreciated in the presence of significant right ventricular hypertrophy. Longstanding, severe pulmonary arterial hypertension, whether it is precapillary (*e.g.,* primary pulmonary hypertension) or postcapillary (*e.g.,* mitral stenosis, cardiomyopathy), produces right ventricular hypertrophy and a sustained lower left parasternal lift. It may also be associated with a palpable presystolic *a* wave preceding the right ventricular lift (heave). In patients with mitral stenosis, the left ventricular apex impulse remains brief and has a tapping quality. In the right apex cardiogram, the accentuated *a* wave is frequently recorded in patients with right ventricular hypertrophy, suggesting decreased compliance. Similar sustained left lower sternal systolic movement and an accentuated right-sided *a* wave are observed in patients with significant pulmonary valve stenosis. Pulmonary hypertension and pulmonary valve stenosis, however, can be easily differentiated at the bedside: the former is associated with a narrowly split S_2 with a markedly accentuated intensity of P_2 (pulmonary component), and the latter has a long ejection systolic murmur over the left second and third interspaces and a widely split S_2 and reduced intensity of P_2.

In patients with tetralogy of Fallot, the lower left sternal impulse may not be prominent or sustained and no right-sided *a* wave is palpable, despite right ventricular hypertrophy, probably due to the presence of a ventricular septal defect, which allows right-to-left shunting and decompression of the right ventricle.

In patients with significant mitral regurgitation, a left parasternal and midprecordial systolic outward impulse, similar to that associated with right ventricular hypertrophy, can be palpable. The systolic pulsation appears to result from left atrial expansion due to mitral regurgitation pressing the anterior structures forward toward the anterior chest wall. Right ventricular apex cardiographic and kinetocardiographic tracings usually reveal a late systolic bulge, coincident with the incisura of the carotid pulse tracing, a configuration that is different from that associated with right ventricular hypertrophy.[32] At the bedside, however, one cannot easily differentiate between the left parasternal systolic impulses owing to right ventricular hypertrophy and mitral regurgitation. If a subxiphoid epigastric pulsation is also present, right ventricular hypertrophy should be suspected.

In atrial septal defect, right ventricular volume is increased and a hyperdynamic, but not markedly prolonged, left parasternal systolic impulse may be palpable. When pulmonary arterial hypertension is also present, the left parasternal impulse becomes sustained during systole. In tricuspid regurgitation secondary to pulmonary hypertension, a right ventricular heave is palpable and a sustained left parasternal systolic motion is recorded. In primary severe tricuspid regurgitation without pulmonary hypertension, however, a left parasternal lift occurs in diastole and an inward movement occurs during systole.[33] The value of timing the impulse with the carotid pulse upstroke is apparent. One should also search for the other findings of pulmonary arterial hypertension. An inward systolic movement and an outward movement during diastole are also palpable and recorded in some patients with constrictive pericarditis (Fig. 23.8).[34] The diastolic movement usually coincides in timing with the pericardial knock. The precise explanation for this unusual precordial impulse in constrictive pericarditis remains unknown; however, it has been suggested that the usual outward movement during isovolumic systole is inhibited by the constriction and the outward movement during early diastole becomes accentuated.[34] It is to be noted, that in patients with severe, longstanding constrictive pericarditis, the precordium may be quiet and no precordial impulse may be palpable or recorded. In patients with Ebstein's anomaly, the precordium may also be quiet. In some patients, a right parasternal systolic outward movement, presumably due to a large ventricularized right atrium, is appreciated.

A chronic left ventricular aneurysm can produce systolic motion in unusual locations, such as over the midprecordium. An apex cardiogram frequently records a late systolic bulge and an accentuated *a* wave.[35] If the electrocardiogram demonstrates an old anteroseptal myocardial infarction, with or without ST segment elevation in the precordial leads, left ventricular aneurysm should be suspected. This abnormal precordial motion indicates decreased systolic function and compliance of the left ventricle. Pulsation in the left second interspace is usually associated with an enlarged pulmonary artery resulting from severe pulmonary arterial hypertension. Precordial records reveal a delayed upstroke of this pulsation in relation to the Q wave of the electrocardiogram. Pulmonary artery pulsation is also palpable when the pulmonary artery is dilated from a marked increase in pulmonary flow, as in patients with atrial septal defect. In such patients, the intensity of P_2 may not be increased.

AUSCULTATION

Cardiac auscultation is one of the most useful investigative tools that the physician can use at the bedside to detect alterations in cardiovascular anatomy and physiology. It is preferable to adopt a systematic approach for auscultation, although the approach may vary according to an individual's perference. Repeated and routine use of the same methods help synthesis of the auscultatory findings and understanding of their significance.

Adequate exposure of the areas of auscultation are essential, and auscultation should be carried out whenever possible with the patient in the left lateral decubitus, supine, and sitting positions. When a certain diagnosis is suspected, auscultation should be done with patients in additional positions, such as leaning forward (in aortic regurgitation), standing and squatting (hypertrophic cardiomyopathy), and standing (mitral valve prolapse). Routine auscultation can begin over the cardiac apex (mitral area), and then one can proceed counterclockwise to the left fourth interspace (tricuspid area), left third interspace, left second interspace (pulmonic area), right second interspace (aortic area), right fourth interspace adjacent to the sternal borders, and then over the epigastrium. The terms *mitral, tricuspid, pulmonary,* and *aortic* areas should be discarded because these terms denote that the sounds and murmurs heard over these areas originate from these structures. In addition to the principal sites, auscultation should be done over other areas, particularly when certain diagnoses are suspected. For example, areas of auscultation should include the left axilla, thoracic spine and vortex of the head (in mitral regurgitation), axilla and back (in atrial septal defect and pulmonary branch stenosis), posterior chest (coarctation of the aorta), left infraclavicular region (patent ductus arteriosus), and sternoclavicular joints (venous hum).

Both the bell and the diaphragm of the stethoscope should be used, particularly in the principal areas of auscultation. For auscultation of the low- and medium-frequency heart sounds and murmurs (S_3 and S_4, diastolic rumble of mitral and tricuspid valve stenosis), the bell should be used; high-frequency heart sounds (S_1 and S_2, opening snap) and murmurs (regurgitant murmurs) are better heard with the diaphragm of the stethoscope. The bell should be applied lightly over the skin for detection and analysis of low-frequency sounds. Application of firm pressure with the bell makes the underlying skin taut, which, in essence, forms a diaphragm and defeats the purpose of using the bell. To differentiate between the low- and high-frequency sounds and murmurs, one can use the bell, initially applying light pressure and then firm pressure to convert the bell to a diaphragm; with lighter pressure, low-frequency sounds appear more distinct, and with conversion of the bell to a diaphragm, these sounds become muffled and distant. It needs to be emphasized that a stethoscope suitable for everybody and ideal for all types of heart sounds and murmurs has not been developed. One should use a stethoscope that is comfortable and practical. It has been recommended, however, that a stethoscope should have both bell and diaphragm, the earpieces should be large enough to fit snugly into the external auditory meatus, and the long axes of the earpieces should be parallel to the long axes of the external auditory canals. The tubes connecting the earpieces and the chest pieces should be fairly rigid and 10 to 12 inches long with an internal diameter of ⅛ inch. The diaphragm should be fairly large (diameter of approximately 1½ inches). The bell should be relatively shallow with a diameter of approximately 1 inch. It is to be noted that these specifics for a stethoscope are less important than the understanding of the significance of the auscultatory findings elicited by the stethoscope.

HEART SOUNDS

The genesis of heart sounds continues to be a subject of debate, and the precise mechanisms of their production have not been identified with certainty. Regarding S_1, arguments have continued in relation to the contributions of the atrioventricular valves in the origin of the sound. One hypothesis suggests that the principal high-frequency elements of S_1 are related to the movement and acceleration of blood in early systole and influenced by left ventricular dp/dt and ejection of blood into the root of the aorta.[36] The classic hypothesis, on the other hand, relates the high-frequency components of S_1 to mitral and tricuspid valve closure.[37] The first component of S_1 is attributed to mitral valve closure (M_1) and the second to tricuspid valve closure (T_1). Studies with the use of catheter-tipped micromanometers, echophonocardiography, intracardiac phonocardiography, and high-speed cineangiography support the classic theory that the atrioventricular valves contribute significantly to the genesis of S_1.[38-40] If one supports the classic hypothesis, analysis of the behavior and character of S_1 at the bedside provides useful information regarding cardiac hemodynamics.

INTENSITY OF S_1

S_1 is best heard with the diaphragm of the stethoscope, and its intensity is normally maximum over the cardiac apex. At the bedside, S_1 is identified by timing with the carotid pulse upstroke; S_1 occurs just before or coincident with the upstroke of the carotid pulse. Simultaneous recordings of the phonocardiogram and indirect carotid pulse tracings reveal that M_1 precedes the upstroke of the carotid pulse because the mitral valve closure occurs before left ventricular ejection begins. However, the delay between M_1 and the upstroke of the carotid pulse normally is too short to be appreciated at the bedside. Normally T_1 tends to coincide with the upstroke of the carotid pulse in phonocarotid pulse recordings.

In most clinical conditions, the intensity of S_1 is primarily determined by the intensity of M_1. Several factors contribute to the intensity of M_1: mitral valve position at the onset of systole, the rate of mitral valve closure, the mobility of the mitral valve, the PR interval, and the strength of the ventricular systole.[41-43] Some of these factors, such as the rate of mitral valve closure and the strength of ventricular systole, are interrelated, and more than one factor may contribute to the altered intensity of S_1.

The position of the atrioventricular valves at the beginning of ven-

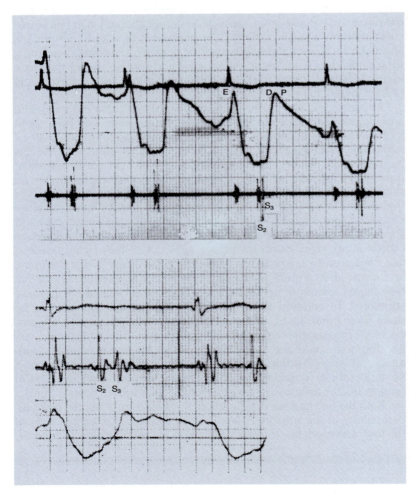

FIGURE 23.8 Precordial displacement record along with phonocardiograms in patients with constrictive pericarditis. A downward movement during systole and an outward movement during diastole were recorded in both upper and lower panel. (E, E point; DP, diastolic pulsation; S_2, second heart sound) (El-Sherif A, El-said G: Jugular, hepatic and precordial pulsations in constrictive pericarditis. Br Heart J 33:305, 1971)

tricular systole and the velocity of closure appear to be important determinants of the intensity of S_1. It is to be noted that the mitral valve closure begins a few milliseconds before the onset of the rise of the left ventricular pressure pulse. When the mitral valve remains wide open at end-diastole and then closes rapidly, the intensity of M_1 is increased. The greater distance of travel of the leaflets from the open to the closed position and the increased velocity of closure contribute to the increased intensity of M_1. In clinical situations, where there is an increased transvalvular gradient (mitral valve obstruction), increased transvalvular flow (left-to-right shunt in patent ductus arteriosus, ventricular septal defect, and high output state), shortened diastole (tachycardia), and short PR intervals (pre-excitation syndrome), the mitral valve remains open in end-diastole and the intensity of M_1 is increased. The relative contribution of the distance of travel and the velocity of closure of the mitral valve to increased intensity of S_1 is difficult to determine, but both factors are likely to play a role. When mitral valve closure occurs on the steeper part of the left ventricular pressure pulse, the intensity of S_1 increases, and this phenomenon may also be contributory to an accentuated S_1, as observed in patients with extremely short PR intervals and left atrial myxoma.[44]

The increased intensity of T_1 in atrial septal defect and tricuspid valve obstruction (tricuspid stenosis, right atrial myxoma) can also be explained by the same phenomenon, that is, the tricuspid valve is held open by the increased transvalvular flow and transvalvular gradient, respectively, until final closure with increased velocity occurs with right ventricular systole. A decrease in the intensity of S_1 can be observed in a number of conditions. Since the mobility and degree of anatomical apposition of the atrioventricular valve leaflets are important determinants of the intensity of S_1, restricted valve mobility and lack of apposition of the valve leaflets decrease the intensity of S_1. Thus, when the mitral valve is calcified and fibrosed and, consequently, immobile, S_1 is soft, despite a significant transvalvular gradient. When mitral regurgitation results from fibrosis and destruction of the valve leaflets, which prevent effective mitral valve closure, as in patients with rheumatic valve disease, S_1 is very soft or absent. Decreased intensity of S_1, however, does not occur in mitral regurgitation of any etiology. Mitral regurgitation resulting from perforation of the valve leaflets due to bacterial endocarditis may not be associated with a reduced intensity of S_1. Similarly, in patients with mitral valve prolapse with late systolic regurgitation, S_1 is normal or even accentuated. Increased intensity of S_1 in some patients with the mitral valve prolapse syndrome may be caused by an increased strength of ventricular systole (hyperkinetic).[45]

Reduced intensity of S_1 may also occur when the mitral valve remains in the semiclosed position before the onset of ventricular systole and when the distance of travel and the velocity of valve closure are decreased. When the PR interval is prolonged, exceeding 0.2 second, S_1 is usually soft, because semiclosure of the mitral valve occurs following atrial systole and before ventricular systole begins. In patients with severe acute aortic regurgitation, premature closure of the mitral valve may occur due to a rapid rise in left ventricular diastolic pressure, and the mitral valve may be virtually closed at the onset of systole, resulting in a markedly decreased intensity of S_1 or even an absent S_1.[46]

In some patients with left bundle branch block, and without any other obvious abnormality, S_1 may be soft, the precise mechanism of which remains unclear. Decreased velocity of valve closure resulting from myocardial dysfunction remains a possibility. Hemodynamically significant aortic stenosis may be associated with a soft S_1, which may occur in the absence of spreading calcification to the mitral valve and in the presence of a normal PR interval.[44] Semiclosure of the mitral valve, resulting from a powerful atrial contraction and from an abnormally elevated left ventricular diastolic pressure before the onset of ventricular systole, is the most likely explanation. In patients with dilated cardiomyopathy, S_1 is frequently soft, even in the absence of a prolonged PR interval or bundle branch block. A decreased S_1 in these patients is almost invariably associated with a significantly reduced left ventricular ejection fraction and elevated pulmonary capillary wedge pressure. The mechanism for a soft S_1 in these patients remains unclear; however, semiclosure of the mitral valve due to an elevated left ventricular diastolic pressure and decreased velocity of valve closure due to myocardial dysfunction might be contributory.

Varying intensity of S_1 is a frequent feature of atrial fibrillation, and the mechanism appears to be a variation in the velocity of valve closure related to changes in the RR cycle length. The intensity of S_1 also varies in the presence of premature beats. Changing intensity of S_1 also occurs in atrioventricular dissociation, whether the heart rate is fast or slow, and results from the random variation of the PR interval; the short PR interval is associated with an increased intensity, and the long PR interval has a decreased intensity of S_1. It is to be noted that the pulse is regular in atrioventricular dissociation; thus, the varying intensity of S_1 in a patient with a regular pulse almost always suggests atrioventricular dissociation. Auscultatory alternans, in which S_1 is soft and loud with alternate beats, is a rare finding in severe cardiac tamponade, and is almost always associated with electrical alternans and pulsus paradoxus. Although the pulse is regular, changes in the intensity of S_1 occur regularly with the alternate beats and not randomly as in atrioventricular dissociation.

Decreased conduction of sounds through the chest wall reduces the intensity of S_1 in patients with chronic obstructive pulmonary disease, obesity, and pericardial effusion. In these circumstances, however, all heart sounds appear soft and distant.

One of the practical difficulties in assessing the intensity of S_1 at the bedside is the lack of any objective method to standardize its intensity. One usually uses one's subjective impression to determine whether S_1 is normal, soft, or loud. Even during phonocardiographic recordings, precise assessment of the intensity of S_1 is not possible because of the difficulty in calibration. S_1 normally is louder than S_2 over the apex and along the lower left sternal border. If S_1 is softer than S_2 over these areas, one is certainly dealing with a reduced intensity of S_1. On the other hand, if S_1 is much louder than S_2 over the left or right second interspace, the intensity of S_1 is likely to be accentuated.

SPLITTING OF S_1

Phonocardiographic recordings in most normal subjects reveal two high-frequency components of S_1: the mitral component, M_1, precedes the carotid pulse upstroke, and the second component, T_1, occurs later. The interval between M_1 and T_1 is 0.02 to 0.03 second and can be appreciated with the use of the diaphragm of the stethoscope along the lower left sternal border.[37] M_1 is much louder than T_1 and is normally heard widely; T_1 being of low intensity is not transmitted and is best heard over the left third and fourth interspaces close to the sternal border.

A relatively loud atrial sound (S_4) preceding S_1 may be confused with a split S_1. The left ventricular S_4 is usually localized over the cardiac apex and is best heard with the bell of the stethoscope. If one starts auscultation with the bell over the apex, both S_4 and S_1 are heard easily. When the bell is moved gradually to the left sternal edge ("inching" method of auscultation), S_4 becomes softer. Furthermore, when the bell is converted to the diaphragm by applying firm pressure over the underlying skin, S_4 decreases in intensity or disappears, whereas splitting of S_1 becomes more obvious.

The combination of a systolic ejection sound (also a high-frequency sound) and S_1 may appear as split S_1; the S_1 and ejection sound interval is usually greater than the normal M_1 and T_1 interval. Furthermore, an aortic ejection sound is heard over the cardiac apex, along the left sternal border and over the right second interspace. T_1, however, is usually heard along the left lower sternal border and, therefore, splitting of S_1 is not heard over the right or left second interspace. Pulmonary ejection sounds can be easily distinguished from T_1. Pulmonary ejection sounds are usually localized and best heard over the left second interspace; more importantly, pulmonary ejection sounds decrease in intensity during inspiration, whereas the intensity of T_1 remains unchanged or increases following inspiration.

A combination of S_1 and a midsystolic click is rarely confused with a split S_1. The interval between S_1 and a midsystolic click is usually far greater than that between M_1 and T_1. Furthermore, the S_1–click interval can be changed by maneuvers like standing and squatting. With these maneuvers, no significant changes in the normal splitting of S_1 can be appreciated.

The combination of a pacemaker sound and S_1 should not be confused with the splitting of S_1. The "pacemaker sound" that results from the stimulation of the intercostal muscles during pacing, has a very high frequency and precedes S_1 and thus occurs well before the upstroke of the carotid pulse.[47] Furthermore, the pacemaker sound disappears with discontinuation of pacing.

Abnormal splitting of S_1 can result either from conduction disturbances or mechanical causes. A widely split S_1 occurs in complete right bundle branch block, during left ventricular pacing, with ectopic beats of left ventricular origin, and in ventricular tachycardia and idioventricular rhythm when the QRS complex morphology is of right bundle branch block configuration. When wide splitting of S_1 occurs due to conduction abnormalities, S_2 is also widely split, with a further increase in the splitting of S_2 during inspiration. A widely split S_1 in conduction anomalies results from a delay in the onset of the right ventricular pressure pulse.

Delayed closure of the tricuspid valve may occur in patients with atrial septal defect with large left-to-right shunting, resulting in a delayed closure of the tricuspid valve and, therefore, a widely split S_1. Wide splitting of S_1 also occurs in patients with significant tricuspid stenosis due to a similar mechanism as in atrial septal defect. Wide splitting of S_1 with increased intensity of the second component is a feature of Ebstein's anomaly.[48] It is partly related to the commonly associated right bundle branch block (Fig. 23.9). In patients with right atrial myxoma, a delay in closure of the tricuspid valve also causes wide splitting of S_1. Wide splitting of S_1 resulting from hemodynamic causes may not be associated with wide splitting of S_2 (except atrial septal defect), and other physical findings characteristic of each anomaly are usually present for the differential diagnosis.

Reversed splitting of S_1 (i.e., T_1 preceding M_1) is seldom recognized at the bedside, although it can be occasionally recorded in the phonocardiogram in patients with severe mitral valve stenosis, in whom mitral valve closure can be markedly delayed. In left atrial myxoma, mitral valve closure occurs after the tumor is expelled from the left ventricle to the left atrium, resulting in wide and reversed splitting of S_1. With premature beats arising from the right ventricle (left bundle branch block pattern), reversed splitting of both S_1 and S_2 occurs and occasionally can be recognized at the bedside. In most patients with left bundle branch block, however, reversed splitting of S_1 is not appreciated, suggesting that no significant delay in the onset of left ventricular mechanical systole occurs due to this conduction anomaly. The causes and the differential diagnosis of abnormalities of S_1 are summarized in Tables 23.4 and 23.5.

S_2

The genesis of S_2 appears to be related to aortic and pulmonary valve closure and, thus, S_2 consists of two components, traditionally designated as A_2 and P_2,[37] related to aortic and pulmonary valve closure sounds, respectively. Both *in vitro* and *in vivo* studies, using various techniques, including high-speed cinematography, high-fidelity aortic root pressure recordings, and echophonocardiography, clearly have demonstrated the simultaneous occurrence of the onset of A_2, aortic valve closure, and the dicrotic notch of the aortic root pressure pulse.[49,50] Echocardiographic studies have indicated that there may be a variable degree of delay between pulmonary valve closure and the onset of P_2.[51] However, phonocardiographic studies suggest that P_2 is likely to be related to pulmonary valve closure.[37] The two components of S_2 are best heard with the diaphragm of the stethoscope and over the left second interspace close to the sternal border. In relation to the carotid pulse, it occurs after the peak and coincides with its downslope. Simultaneous recordings of phonocardiograms and the indirect carotid pulse tracing show that normally A_2 precedes the incisura of the carotid pulse tracing by usually not more than 0.02 second, and it is widely transmitted to the right second interspace, along the left and right sternal border, and to the cardiac apex. Normally, P_2 is best heard and recorded over the upper left sternal border and is poorly transmitted.

INTENSITY OF S_2

The major determinants of the intensity of A_2 are the aortic pressure, the relative proximity of the aorta to the chest wall, the size of the aortic root, and the degree of apposition of the valve leaflets and their mobility. Increased intensity of A_2 is frequently appreciated in systemic hypertension, coarctation of the aorta, and ascending aortic aneurysm, and not uncommonly, a "tambour" quality of A_2 is observed. When the aortic root is relatively anterior and closer to the anterior chest wall, as in tetralogy of Fallot and transposition of the great arteries, the intensity of A_2 is significantly increased.

Decreased intensity of A_2 occurs where there is lack of apposition of the valve leaflets, as in severe luetic aortic regurgitation. Decreased arterial diastolic pressure is also contributory to the decreased intensity of A_2, as in significant aortic regurgitation. The presence of a relatively immobile aortic valve due to calcification decreases the intensity of A_2 in patients with calcific aortic stenosis. Relatively lower arterial pressure in hemodynamically significant aortic stenosis also contributes to the reduced intensity of A_2. It needs to be noted that the increase in intensity of A_2 cannot be quantitated objectively at the bedside by auscultation or by phonocardiography, and one has to rely on one's subjective impression. On the other hand, when the intensity of A_2 is less than that of P_2 over the left second interspace, this suggests an increased intensity of P_2.

The intensity of P_2 is determined by the pulmonary arterial pres-

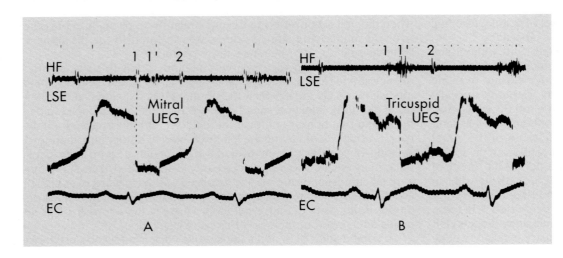

FIGURE 23.9 Wide splitting of S_1 due to delayed closure of the tricuspid valve that coincides with T_1 in Ebstein's anomaly. Associated right bundle branch block also contributes to the wide splitting. (**A**, mitral valve ultrasound; **B**, tricuspid valve ultrasound; HF, high frequency; LSE, left sternal edge; 1 and 1', mitral and tricuspid valve closure sounds; 2, second heart sound) (Crews TL, Pridie RB, Benham R et al: Auscultatory and phonocardiographic findings in Ebstein's anomaly: Correlation of first heart sound with ultrasonic records of tricuspid valve movement. Br Heart J 34:681, 1972)

TABLE 23.4 CAUSES OF FIRST HEART SOUND (S₁) ABNORMALITIES

Abnormality	Causes
Increased intensity	
Atrioventricular valve obstruction	
Mitral	Mitral stenosis and left atrial myxoma
Tricuspid	Tricuspid stenosis and right atrial myxoma
Increased transvalvular flow	
Mitral	Patent ductus arteriosus; ventricular septal defect; atrial septal defect
Tricuspid	
Forceful ventricular systole	Hyperkinetic heart syndrome; tachycardia (after exercise); mitral valve prolapse
Short PR interval	Pre-excitation syndrome
Decreased intensity	
Immobility of mitral valve	Calcific mitral stenosis
Lack of apposition of the mitral leaflets	Rheumatic mitral regurgitation
Presystolic semiclosure of the atrioventricular valves	Long PR interval; acute aortic regurgitation; significant aortic stenosis; dilated cardiomyopathy
Conduction anomaly	Left bundle branch block
Wide splitting of S₁	
Conduction abnormalities	Complete right bundle branch block; left ventricular pacing; pre-excitation syndrome (left ventricular connection); Ebstein's anomaly
Mechanical	Tricuspid stenosis; atrial septal defect; Ebstein's anomaly
Reversed splitting of S₁	
Arrhythmia	Premature beats (right ventricular origin)
Mechanical	Severe mitral stenosis and left atrial myxoma

TABLE 23.5 DIFFERENTIAL DIAGNOSIS OF PHYSIOLOGIC SPLITTING OF S₁

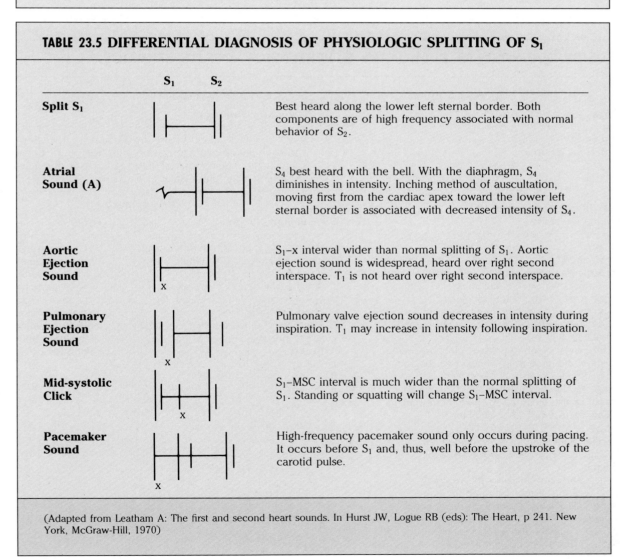

Split S₁	Best heard along the lower left sternal border. Both components are of high frequency associated with normal behavior of S₂.
Atrial Sound (A)	S₄ best heard with the bell. With the diaphragm, S₄ diminishes in intensity. Inching method of auscultation, moving first from the cardiac apex toward the lower left sternal border is associated with decreased intensity of S₄.
Aortic Ejection Sound	S₁–x interval wider than normal splitting of S₁. Aortic ejection sound is widespread, heard over right second interspace. T₁ is not heard over right second interspace.
Pulmonary Ejection Sound	Pulmonary valve ejection sound decreases in intensity during inspiration. T₁ may increase in intensity following inspiration.
Mid-systolic Click	S₁–MSC interval is much wider than the normal splitting of S₁. Standing or squatting will change S₁–MSC interval.
Pacemaker Sound	High-frequency pacemaker sound only occurs during pacing. It occurs before S₁ and, thus, well before the upstroke of the carotid pulse.

(Adapted from Leatham A: The first and second heart sounds. In Hurst JW, Logue RB (eds): The Heart, p 241. New York, McGraw-Hill, 1970) sure, particularly the diastolic pressure, the size of the pulmonary artery, and the degree of apposition of the pulmonary valve leaflets.

The intensity of P_2 is determined at the bedside and by phonocardiography by comparing its intensity with that of A_2. In normal subjects, S_2 is usually single during expiration, particularly when auscultation or recordings are performed with subjects in the semirecumbent position. During the inspiratory phase of continuous respiration, however, the separation of A_2 and P_2 occurs, which allows comparison of the relative intensities of these two components of S_2. Simultaneous phonocardiographic recordings from the second left interspace and cardiac apex, and other areas, reveal that A_2 is the louder component, even in pulmonary areas (left second interspace), and it is the only component recorded over the cardiac apex in almost all normal subjects.[52] P_2 is much softer than A_2, and although it can be heard or recorded over the right second interspace and along the left sternal border, it is extremely rare for P_2 to be transmitted to the cardiac apex. In only about 5% of normal subjects, and only when they are young (under 20 years old), can P_2 be recorded over the cardiac apex. The relative intensity of A_2 is almost always greater than P_2 over the left second interspace in normal subjects, and in only approximately 2% of normal subjects is the intensity of A_2 equal to that of P_2 in this area. Normally, A_2 is almost never of lower intensity than P_2. Thus, a P_2 of louder intensity than A_2 over the left second interspace or transmission of P_2 to the cardiac apex, either demonstrated by auscultation or by phonocardiographic recordings, signifies an increase in intensity of P_2.

The most common cause of the increased intensity of P_2 is pulmonary arterial hypertension, irrespective of etiology.[53] Although an increased intensity of P_2 ($P_2 > A_2$ in pulmonary areas) is the most important physical finding for diagnosing pulmonary arterial hypertension, other physical findings that support the diagnosis and provide clues to the etiology of pulmonary hypertension should be searched for at the bedside. A prominent *a* wave in the jugular venous pulse, a sustained left parasternal outward impulse, epigastric pulsation, a palpable P_2 over the left second interspace, and clinical features of tricuspid regurgitation and secondary pulmonary insufficiency all support the diagnosis of significant pulmonary arterial hypertension. It is to be noted that all these secondary findings result as the consequences of severe pulmonary hypertension and are not present in all patients. Furthermore, other noninvasive tests, such as the electrocardiogram (right ventricular hypertrophy), chest film, and echo-Doppler studies should be performed in all patients with suspected pulmonary arterial hypertension to investigate the etiology and severity of pulmonary hypertension. Invasive investigations, including right- and left-sided heart catheterization, are frequently required to estimate the severity of pulmonary arterial hypertension and to establish its etiology. However, at the bedside, certain physical findings provide important clues in the diagnosis of the severity and etiology of pulmonary hypertension, if one follows a systematic and logical approach (Table 23.6). Once pulmonary arterial hypertension is suspected, the physician should assess the severity of pulmonary hypertension from the physical findings that indicate right ventricular hypertension and right ventricular hypertrophy and failure, secondary tricuspid regurgitation, and pulmonary insufficiency. Significant pulmonary arterial hypertension may result primarily from an elevation of the pulmonary venous pressure (postcapillary) or from increased pulmonary vascular resistance (precapillary). Evidence of increased pulmonary venous pressure is ob-

---

TABLE 23.6 BEDSIDE DIAGNOSIS OF PULMONARY HYPERTENSION AND ITS ETIOLOGY

Increased Intensity of P_2 (Pulmonary Arterial Hypertension)

Primary Findings	*Secondary Findings*
$P_2 > A_2$, P_2 transmitted to cardiac apex, pulmonary ejection sound, pulmonary sufficiency murmur	Right ventricular failure, tricuspid regurgitation, increased jugular venous pressure with prominent *a* wave, right ventricular S_4 and S_3 gallop, pansystolic murmur that increases in intensity during inspiration, systolic hepatic pulsation

Postcapillary (Evidence for Increased Pulmonary Venous Pressure)	**Precapillary**	
	Eisenmenger Complex	*Others*
1. Pulmonary venous occlusive disease: (special investigations required)	1. Patent ductus arteriosus: differential cyanosis, physiologic splitting of S_2; chest film, echo-Doppler	1. Cor pulmonale: evidence for primary pulmonary disease
2. Mitral valve obstruction: mitral stenosis, left atrial myxoma, mild diastolic rumble over the cardiac apex, electrocardiogram, chest film, echo-Doppler	2. Atrial septal defect: cyanosis, widely split S_2 with increased P_2; chest film, echo-Doppler	2. Thromboembolic: ventilation–perfusion; scan, computed tomography, magnetic resonance imaging
3. Mitral regurgitation: cardiac enlargement, pansystolic murmur over the apex, left-sided S_3; electrocardiogram, chest film, echo-Doppler	3. Ventricular septal defect: cyanosis, single loud S_2; chest film, echo-Doppler	3. Primary pulmonary hypertension: by exclusion of other causes
4. Aortic stenosis: delayed carotid upstroke, ejection systolic murmur, left ventricular hypertrophy; electrocardiogram, chest film, echo-Doppler		
5. Aortic regurgitation: cardiac enlargement, early diastolic murmur, increased pulse pressure, Austin-Flint murmur; electrocardiogram, chest film, echo-Doppler		
6. Cardiomyopathy: a) Dilated: cardiac enlargement, S_3, sustained left ventricular impulse; chest film, echocardiogram, radioangiogram b) Hypertrophic: sharp carotid pulse, left ventricular hypertrophy, ejection systolic murmur increased intensity with Valsalva maneuver; echocardiogram, echo-Doppler c) Restrictive: pulmonary and systemic venous hypertension, relatively normal cardiac size; electrocardiogram, chest film, radioangiogram		

tained from symptoms suggestive of cardiac dyspnea, the presence of rales (pulmonary congestion), and the radiologic findings of pulmonary venous hypertension. If increased pulmonary venous pressure is suspected, one is obliged to search for its cause. There are rare conditions, such as pulmonary venous occlusive disease and pulmonary venous obstruction from extrinsic compression of the pulmonary veins, in which pulmonary venous pressure is elevated in the presence of normal left atrial and left ventricular diastolic pressures. These conditions are not associated with any characteristic physical findings, and other noninvasive and invasive investigations are essential to establish the diagnosis. In some patients with total anomalous pulmonary venous drainage (infracardiac variety), pulmonary venous pressure may be high in the presence of a relatively normal left atrial pressure, and this anomaly can be suspected in infants from the abnormal radiologic findings. These conditions, however, are rarely encountered in adult patients, and postcapillary pulmonary hypertension almost always results from an increased left atrial pressure.

Left atrial pressure is elevated without a concomitant increase in left ventricular diastolic pressure in patients with mitral valve obstruction (mitral stenosis, left atrial myxoma) and must always be excluded whenever pulmonary hypertension is diagnosed. The most frequent causes of mitral valve obstruction are surgically correctible. Mitral valve obstruction is suspected at the bedside from the presence of an accentuated S_1 and a mid-diastolic rumble over the cardiac apex. An echocardiographic study is always indicated to diagnose the presence and etiology of mitral valve obstruction.

If mitral valve obstruction is excluded, the other remaining hemodynamic cause of postcapillary pulmonary hypertension is increased left ventricular diastolic pressure, which causes an increase in left atrial and pulmonary venous pressures. Mitral regurgitation, fixed left ventricular outflow obstruction (*e.g.*, aortic valve stenosis), and aortic regurgitation can cause postcapillary pulmonary hypertension and can be suspected at the bedside from the presence of specific physical findings, which are fairly characteristic of each valvular lesion. A palpable S_4, a loud, audible S_4, a soft S_1, and a sharp and loud S_3 may all indicate elevated left ventricular diastolic pressure. In addition to the electrocardiogram (left atrial enlargement) and chest film, an echo-Doppler study is indicated to detect aortic and mitral valve disease as the cause of pulmonary hypertension. If left-sided valvular heart lesions are excluded, primary myocardial disease (*i.e.*, dilated, hypertrophic, or restrictive cardiomyopathy) should be suspected as the potential cause for postcapillary pulmonary hypertension. A carotid pulse with a normal or sharp upstroke, an ejection systolic murmur along the left sternal border and over to the cardiac apex, which increases in intensity during the Valsalva maneuver, and clinical and electrocardiographic findings for left ventricular hypertrophy strongly suggest obstructive hypertrophic cardiomyopathy. An elevated jugular venous pressure with a sharp *y* descent in the jugular venous pulse and a relatively normal heart size should raise the suspicion of restrictive cardiomyopathy. Evidence of cardiac enlargement (laterally displaced apical impulse) in the absence of valvular heart disease indicates dilated congestive cardiomyopathy. It needs to be emphasized that other ancillary investigations (electrocardiogram, chest film, echocardiography) are almost always indicated to establish the diagnosis.

When the causes of postcapillary pulmonary hypertension are not present, a search should be made to identify any cause associated with a markedly elevated pulmonary vascular resistance as the principal mechanism for pulmonary arterial hypertension. An underlying anatomical lesion causing Eisenmenger's syndrome (resulting from a markedly elevated pulmonary artery pressure and pulmonary vascular resistance equal to or greater than the systemic vascular resistance) can be suspected at the bedside.[53] Patent ductus arteriosus with Eisenmenger's changes causes cyanosis of the inferior extremity, sparing the superior extremities (differential cyanosis), and narrow physiologic splitting of S_2 with a markedly accentuated P_2. Eisenmenger's syndrome associated with an atrial septal defect is characterized by wide splitting of S_2 with a markedly increased intensity of P_2 and other findings indicating right-to-left shunt. In Eisenmenger's ventricular septal defect, S_2 is genuinely single and the physical findings of severe right ventricular hypertrophy and of a right-to-left shunt are also present. In the adult population, chronic obstructive and other pulmonary disease, and pulmonary embolism, are more frequent causes of precapillary pulmonary hypertension than is Eisenmenger's syndrome. Primary pulmonary hypertension is also infrequently encountered. Besides the physical findings of pulmonary hypertension and its consequences, there are no characteristic cardiac findings that are helpful to distinguish between the various causes of cor pulmonale and primary pulmonary hypertension.

In atrial septal defect, even with a normal or slightly elevated pulmonary artery pressure, the intensity of P_2 is increased considerably and frequently greater than A_2 over the left second interspace.[54] In about 50% of patients, P_2 is heard over the cardiac apex. The mechanism for this increased intensity of P_2, despite low pulmonary artery diastolic pressure and pulmonary vascular resistance, remains unclear. A dilated pulmonary artery and considerable right ventricular dilatation might be contributory.

In patients with mitral regurgitation, A_2 is soft and, thus, P_2 might appear to be of increased intensity. In these circumstances, one cannot rely on the relative intensity of P_2 for the diagnosis of pulmonary hypertension and other corroborative evidence should be sought.

A decreased intensity of P_2 occurs whenever there is a lower pulmonary artery diastolic pressure; the exception, however, is atrial septal defect. In the presence of significant right ventricular outflow obstruction, such as in patients with pulmonary valve stenosis, P_2 is soft and delayed. In patients with severe pulmonary insufficiency due to a congenitally absent pulmonary valve, P_2 is also absent. In pulmonary insufficiency secondary to pulmonary hypertension, P_2 is markedly accentuated.

SPLITTING OF S_2

Inspiratory splitting of S_2 can be appreciated and recorded in normal subjects 24 to 48 hours after birth, when the pulmonary vascular resistance is considerably lower than at birth. In normal adult subjects, A_2 and P_2 are usually fused during the expiratory phase of continuous respiration. Occasionally, a slight expiratory splitting is heard in normal subjects in the recumbent position. When auscultation is performed in the semirecumbent position (30° to 40° from the horizontal), S_2 almost always appears single during the expiratory phase. During the inspiratory phase, however, separation of A_2 and P_2 occurs and the degree of splitting varies from 0.02 to 0.06 second.[55] The splitting of S_2 is best heard with the diaphragm of the stethoscope over the left second interspace.

Multiple mechanisms contribute to the normal inspiratory splitting of S_2. Simultaneous recordings of high-fidelity pressures from the right and left ventricles and from the pulmonary artery and aorta demonstrate that A_2 (coincident with the incisura of the aortic pressure pulse) occurs on the average 0.02 second after the left ventricular systolic pressure falls below the aortic pressure. On the other hand, P_2 (pulmonary arterial incisura) occurs 0.03 to 0.09 second after the crossover point of right ventricular and central pulmonary arterial pressure.[56,57] The interval between the pressure crossover point and the incisura (the onset of A_2 or P_2) has been termed *hangout time*. The hangout time is inversely proportional to the impedance to blood flow in the systemic arterial and pulmonary arterial systems. Normally, systemic vascular resistance is considerably higher than pulmonary vascular resistance and systemic arteries are less compliant than the pulmonary arteries. These differences account for the shorter hangout time in the aorta than in the pulmonary artery. During inspiration, pulmonary vascular impedance declines with a further increase in the pulmonary hangout time, which appears to be the principal mechanism for inspiratory splitting of S_2 (Fig. 23.10).

The other contributions to a normal inspiratory splitting of S_2 result from an increased right ventricular ejection time. More negative intrathoracic pressure during inspiration is associated with an increased venous return to the right ventricle and an increased right ventricular stroke volume, which increases its ejection time and delays the P_2. Inspiratory delay of aortic valve closure is minimal[58,59] probably due to a much shorter aortic hangout time compared with that of pulmonary hangout time. It needs to be appreciated that the immediate inspiratory increase in right ventricular stroke volume is followed after one to three cardiac cycles by a similar increase in stroke volume of the left ventricle associated with increased left ventricular ejection time.[60] During normal respiration, prolongation of left ventricular ejection time and delayed A_2 usually occur during the expiratory phase, whereas lengthening of the right ventricular ejection time and delayed pulmonary valve closure coincide with the inspiratory phase. The relative contributions of these different mechanisms to the normal inspiratory splitting of S_2 are difficult to determine. Traditionally, it has been thought that prolongation of the right ventricular ejection time accounts for a major part of the normal inspiratory separation of A_2 and P_2. Recent studies, however, suggest that the increase in pulmonary hangout time is the major contribution to normal inspiratory splitting of S_2.

WIDE SPLITTING OF S_2

As has been mentioned earlier, in normal adult subjects, A_2 and P_2 are fused and S_2 appears single during the expiratory phase of respiration, particularly in the semirecumbent, sitting, and standing positions. If the A_2-P_2 separation is appreciated in these positions during expiration, wide splitting of S_2 should be suspected. The A_2-P_2 interval needs to be 0.03 second or more to be appreciated by auscultation at the bedside. A wide splitting of S_2 can result either from conduction disturbances or from hemodynamic causes. Conduction anomalies that cause wide splitting of S_2 include complete right bundle branch block, artificial pacing from the left ventricle, and the Wolff-Parkinson-White syndrome with left ventricular pre-excitation. Premature beats and an idioventricular rhythm of left ventricular origin (QRS complex of right bundle branch block morphology) are also associated with wide splitting of S_2. Wide splitting of S_2 due to conduction disturbances results from delayed activation of the right ventricle and, consequently, delayed completion of right ventricular ejection. Widened splitting of S_2 during inspiration and concomitant splitting of S_1 occur in these circumstances.

Increased resistance to right ventricular ejection and prolongation of right ventricular ejection time are other important causes of wide expiratory splitting of S_2. Pulmonary valve and infundibular stenosis, supravalvular and pulmonary branch stenoses, and pulmonary arterial hypertension of any etiology lengthen right ventricular ejection time and cause relatively wide splitting of S_2. The intensity of P_2 is related to the pulmonary arterial diastolic pressure; a lower pressure is associated with a reduced intensity and a higher pressure with increased intensity. Thus, in patients with pulmonary valve and infundibular stenoses, wide splitting of S_2 is associated with reduced intensity of P_2, whereas in pulmonary hypertension and pulmonary branch stenosis, P_2 is accentuated. In pulmonary valve stenosis, the degree of expiratory splitting of S_2 (i.e., the A_2-P_2 interval) is directly related to the severity of stenosis and right ventricular systolic hypertension; the wider is expiratory splitting of S_2, the higher the right ventricular systolic pressure.[61] Further splitting of S_2 during inspiration usually occurs in these conditions, but wide splitting of S_1 is not observed.

In pulmonary hypertension, although the expiratory splitting is obvious, the degree of splitting is much less than in other conditions, which also increase the resistance to right ventricular ejection. This is because of a significant reduction in pulmonary hangout time due to decreased pulmonary vascular compliance in pulmonary hypertension.[56] For the same reason, the magnitude of inspiratory widening of the splitting of S_2 is smaller. Thus, in patients with chronic pulmonary arterial hypertension, a relatively narrow expiratory splitting of S_2, with only a slight inspiratory increase, is expected.

Isolated reduction of the left ventricular ejection time may also cause wide splitting of S_2 due to the early occurrence of A_2. The best example of such a mechanism is significant mitral regurgitation, which decreases impedance to left ventricular ejection and also forward stroke volume.[62] In some patients with a ventricular septal defect with increased pulmonary flow and decreased pulmonary vascular resistance, wide splitting of S_2 can occur due to the same mechanism, although a delay in the onset of right ventricular mechanical systole has

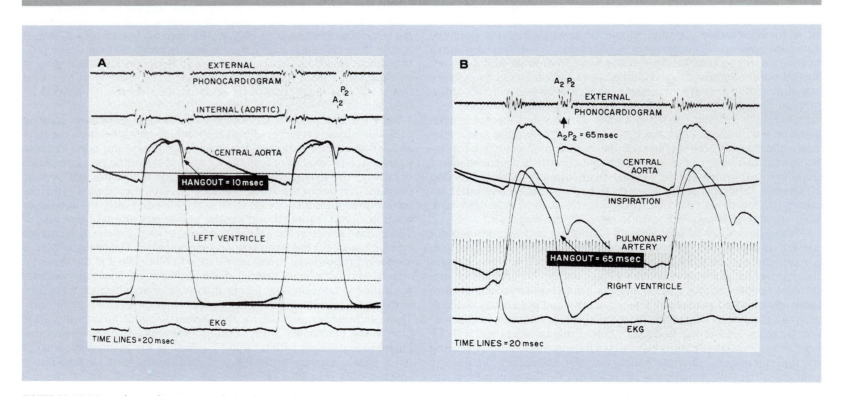

FIGURE 23.10 Normal sound–pressure relationships in the systemic (**A**) and pulmonary (**B**) circulations. Equisensitive micromanometers were used to record left ventricular and central aortic pressure. Hangout time in aorta was much shorter than the pulmonary hangout time, and the normal inspiratory splitting of S_2 could be explained by the increased pulmonary hangout time. (A_2, aortic component of the second heart sound; P_2, pulmonic component of the second heart sound) (Curtiss EI, Mathews RC, Shaver JA: Mechanism of normal splitting of the second heart sound. Circulation 51:157, 1975)

also been observed.[63] Inspiratory widening of S_2 is maintained in patients in this category, and S_1 usually remains normal. Inspiratory reduction in left ventricular ejection time may also occur in constrictive pericarditis, which may account for the wide inspiratory splitting of S_2 that occasionally is observed in these patients.[64]

WIDE AND "FIXED" SPLITTING OF S_2

Fixed splitting of S_2 occurs when the A_2–P_2 interval does not vary more than 0.1 second during the inspiratory and expiratory phases of respiration.

In most patients with a relatively large interatrial communication (atrial septal defect, common atrium) and left-to-right or bidirectional shunt, respiratory variations of the A_2–P_2 intervals are minimal or absent and abnormally wide splitting of S_2 occurs. The mechanism of wide expiratory splitting of S_2 in atrial septal defect appears to be due to isolated shortening of the ejection time of the left ventricle while the right ventricular ejection time remains normal and to an increase in pulmonary hangout time resulting from the decreased pulmonary vascular impedance.[54,65] During inspiration, P_2 is delayed, as in normal subjects, due to prolongation of the right ventricular ejection time, but unlike in normal subjects, A_2 does not occur earlier, suggesting the absence of inspiratory shortening of left ventricular ejection time. Lack of shortening of left ventricular ejection time may result from the transient increase in venous return to the left ventricle due to a reduction in the magnitude of the left-to-right shunt. Thus, the A_2–P_2 interval remains relatively constant during normal, continuous respiration. In patients with partial anomalous venous return, or with the sinus venosus type of atrial septal defect in which interatrial communication is small, there is usually respiratory variation in the splitting of S_2.

The other cause of fixed splitting of S_2 is right ventricular failure, when the right ventricle is unable to vary its stroke volume during inspiration and, therefore, inspiratory prolongation of its ejection time and delay of P_2 does not occur. Any condition that induces severe right ventricular failure, such as right ventricular outflow obstruction, pulmonary hypertension, and primary right ventricular dysfunction can be associated with fixed splitting of S_2.

REVERSED (PARADOXIC) SPLITTING OF S_2

When aortic closure (A_2) follows pulmonary closure (P_2) during the expiratory phase of respiration, the normal sequence of A_2 preceding P_2 is reversed. The splitting of S_2 is then maximal during expiration and the splitting is less, or S_2 becomes single, during inspiration with the normal inspiratory delay of P_2.[37,66]

Reversed splitting of S_2 may result from either conduction disturbances or hemodynamic causes. Left bundle branch block, artificial right ventricular pacing, pre-excitation of the right ventricle (Wolff-Parkinson-White syndrome), and premature beats of right ventricular origin are examples of conduction disturbances associated with reversed splitting of S_2. Delayed activation of the left ventricle and, consequently, delayed completion of left ventricular ejection causes a delayed A_2 and reversed splitting of S_2. In left bundle branch block or the pre-excitation syndrome, splitting of S_1 does not usually occur. Splitting of S_1, however, may accompany splitting of S_2 with right ventricular pacing or ectopic beats. With a lesser degree of left bundle branch block or right ventricular pre-excitation, the P_2–A_2 interval during expiration may be very short (reversed splitting), and normal splitting may occur during inspiration.

Markedly prolonged left ventricular ejection time may delay A_2 sufficiently to cause reversed splitting of S_2. With fixed left ventricular outflow tract obstruction, such as in patients with aortic valve stenosis, left ventricular ejection time is lengthened and reversed splitting of S_2 usually indicates hemodynamically significant outflow obstruction. In these conditions, however, P_2 can be inaudible due to the long ejection systolic murmur of aortic stenosis, making recognition of the reversed splitting of S_2 by auscultation difficult. The differential diagnosis between hypertrophic cardiomyopathy and mitral regurgitation or ventricular septal defect (the character and locations of the systolic murmur may appear similar on auscultation in these conditions) is facilitated if one can recognize the character of the splitting of S_2. If reversed splitting of S_2 is present, the diagnosis is likely to be hypertrophic cardiomyopathy; physiologic splitting of S_2, on the other hand, favors mitral regurgitation or ventricular septal defect. In some patients with hypertension, reversed splitting of S_2 is observed; however, the P_2–A_2 interval in expiration is usually short and normal inspiratory splitting may occur. Prolongation of left ventricular ejection time and reversed splitting of S_2 can occur with myocardial dysfunction, as during myocardial ischemia.[67] In severe heart failure, however, reversed splitting is rarely observed because of the concomitant decrease in stroke volume, which is an important determinant of left ventricular ejection time. A selective increase in left ventricular forward stroke volume may prolong left ventricular ejection time sufficiently to cause reversed splitting of S_2; such a mechanism explains reversed splitting of S_2 in some patients with patent ductus arteriosus with a large left-to-right shunt and in patients with significant chronic aortic regurgitation. Reversed splitting of S_2 is often difficult to recognize at the bedside by auscultation because the inspiratory noise frequently obscures the relatively soft P_2.

SINGLE S_2

A single S_2 may result from the absence of either of the two components of S_2 or from the fusion of A_2 and P_2 without the inspiratory splitting.

Absence of A_2 is occasionally observed in severe calcific aortic stenosis with an immobile aortic valve. In some patients with severe aortic regurgitation due to destruction of the valve leaflets, A_2 may be absent. P_2 is absent in the congenital absence of the pulmonary valve, pulmonary atresia, and truncus arteriosus. In severe pulmonary valve stenosis or in tetralogy of Fallot, P_2 may be markedly attenuated and escapes recognition, both by auscultation and phonocardiography. Fusion of A_2 and P_2 without inspiratory splitting occurs in Eisenmenger's syndrome with ventricular septal defect and in single ventricle. It is to be noted that truly single S_2 is rare. An apparently single S_2 usually results from the inability to hear or record P_2 due to emphysema, obesity, or pericardial effusion. The abnormalities of S_2 and their potential mechanisms are summarized in Table 23.7.

S_3 AND S_4

S_3 and S_4 are low-frequency diastolic sounds that appear to originate in the ventricles. Although the precise mechanism of the genesis of these sounds has not been identified with certainty, the sounds are associated with ventricular filling and are heard and recorded during rapid filling and atrial filling phases of the ventricle, respectively.[68] S_3 occurs as the passive ventricular filling begins after the actual relaxation is completed.[69] It appears to be related to a sudden limitation of the movement during ventricular filling along its long axis.[70] It coincides with the y descent of the atrial pressure pulse and the end of the rapid filling phase of the apex cardiogram, occurring usually 0.14 to 0.16 second after S_2. S_4 occurs after the P wave in the electrocardiogram and coincides with the *a* waves of the atrial pressure pulse and the apex cardiogram. It is generally agreed that both S_3 and S_4, occasionally termed *ventricular filling sounds* are associated with ventricular filling and an increase in ventricular dimensions. S_3 and S_4 are best heard with the bell of the stethoscope. Auscultation over the cardiac apex in the left lateral decubitus position is preferable for identification of left ventricular S_3 and S_4. Right ventricular S_3 and S_4 are best heard along the lower left sternal border; occasionally right-sided filling sounds are also heard over the lower right sternal border and over the epigastrium. During inspiration, the intensity of S_3 and S_4 of right ventricular origin usually increases, whereas that of left ventricular origin remains unchanged. S_3 is closer to S_2 and S_4 occurs prior to S_1.

S_3 can be heard and recorded in healthy young adults; however, when it is heard in subjects over the age of 40 years, it is usually abnormal. Owing to decreased ventricular compliance with increasing age, S_4 can be heard, as well as recorded, in many older adults without any other cardiac abnormality. When S_4 is heard in young adults and children, it is usually abnormal. An abnormal S_3 and S_4 tend to be louder and of higher pitch (sharper) and are frequently referred to as gallops; S_3 is the ventricular gallop, and S_4 is the atrial gallop sound. During tachycardia, S_3 and S_4 can be fused to produce a loud diastolic filling sound, which is termed a *summation gallop*.[71] At the bedside, carotid massage can cause separation of S_3 and S_4 as the heart rate slows. S_3 and S_4 can occasionally be intensified or precipitated by exercise or by sustained hand grip. Occasionally, gallops can be seen and palpated.

LEFT VENTRICULAR GALLOPS. S_3 is almost always present in patients with hemodynamically significant chronic mitral regurgitation. Thus, the absence of S_3 is an important finding to exclude severe chronic mitral regurgitation. An S_3 gallop in patients with chronic aortic regurgitation is frequently associated with a decreased left ventricular ejection fraction and increased diastolic volume; its recognition should prompt further evaluation.[72] An S_3 gallop is an important and frequently early finding of heart failure in dilated cardiomyopathy, and it occurs with equal frequency in patients with or without coronary artery disease. The hemodynamic correlates of an S_3 gallop have been evaluated in patients with aortic valve disease, coronary artery disease, and congestive cardiomyopathy. An S_3 gallop in these patients was associated with left atrial pressures exceeding 20 mm Hg; absence of an S_3 gallop usually indicated normal left atrial pressure.[71] Clinical benefits from chronic digitalis therapy in patients with chronic heart failure in sinus rhythm have been reported to occur generally in those patients with an S_3 gallop.[73] Recognition of an S_3 gallop, therefore, becomes important before institution of long-term digitalis therapy in these patients. In high-output states, such as thyrotoxicosis or pregnancy, S_3 occurs frequently but does not necessarily indicate left ventricular dysfunction.[74]

S_4 can be recorded by phonocardiography in about 50% of patients who are relatively older, healthy subjects, but because of its decreased intensity, it is usually not audible. An audible S_4 is abnormal in younger subjects and children, and when it is palpable, it is always abnormal, irrespective of the age of the subject. With a prolonged PR interval, S_4 may become audible in otherwise healthy subjects due to the separation of S_4 from S_1. In patients with complete atrioventricular block, S_4 is heard at a faster rate than S_1 and S_2 and may not indicate any hemodynamic abnormality.

An abnormal S_4 is most frequently observed in patients with decreased left ventricular distensibility.[75] Thus, S_4 is common in hypertensive heart disease, aortic stenosis, and hypertrophic cardiomyopathy. Left ventricular hypertrophy, which is present in all these conditions, contributes to decreased left ventricular distensibility and, therefore, an S_4. In aortic stenosis, the presence of an S_4 has been reported to indicate hemodynamically significant left ventricular outflow obstruction (the peak transvalvular gradient is 70 mm Hg or more) and an elevated left ventricular end-diastolic pressure.[76] It should be noted, however, that in patients over 40 years of age, S_4 can occur due to myocardial disease in the absence of significant aortic stenosis; thus, in elderly patients, the presence of an S_4 cannot be used to assess the severity of aortic stenosis. Associated coronary artery disease may also cause an S_4 in patients with mild to moderate aortic stenosis.

During the acute phase of myocardial infarction, S_4 is heard in the vast majority of patients.[77] Although pulmonary venous pressure may also be elevated concurrently, a poor correlation exists between the presence and absence of an S_4 and hemodynamic abnormalities. Thus, at the bedside, S_4 is a poor guide to assess the severity of left ventricular dysfunction in patients with acute myocardial infarction. Audible and/or palpable atrial gallops are a frequent finding in chronic left ventricular aneurysm and are usually associated with left ventricular dyskinesia and also elevated end-diastolic pressures. In patients with chronic coronary artery disease, the transient appearance of an S_4, particularly during chest pain, is a strong indication of transient myocardial ischemia.

In patients with acute and severe mitral or aortic regurgitation, a loud S_4 is a frequent finding and it is also usually palpable. It is almost always associated with an increased left ventricular end-diastolic pressure.[78]

RIGHT VENTRICULAR GALLOPS. An S_3 gallop of right ventricular origin frequently occurs in patients with significant tricuspid regurgitation, whether it is primary or secondary to pulmonary hypertension and right ventricular failure. An S_3 gallop is also heard in right ventricular failure in the absence of tricuspid regurgitation. An S_4 of right ventricu-

---

TABLE 23.7 ABNORMALITIES OF THE SECOND HEART SOUND (S_2) AND THEIR MECHANISMS

Wide Splitting of S_2 with Maintained Inspiratory Delay of P_2
Delayed activation and completion of right ventricular ejection
   Complete right bundle branch block
   Artificial left ventricular pacing
   Pre-excitation of the left ventricle (Wolff-Parkinson-White syndrome)
   Premature beats and idioventricular rhythm originating from the left ventricle
Prolonged right ventricular ejection time
   Pulmonary hypertension due to any cause
   Right ventricular outflow obstruction (*e.g.*, pulmonary stenosis)
Increased pulmonary hangout time
   Idiopathic dilatation of the pulmonary artery
   Mild pulmonary stenosis
   Postoperative atrial septal defect
Decreased left ventricular ejection time (early A_2)
   Mitral regurgitation
   Ventricular septal defect with low pulmonary vascular resistance
   Constrictive pericarditis

Fixed Splitting of S_2
Unchanged right ventricular stroke volume during respiration; severe right ventricular failure due to any cause
Interatrial communication; atrial septal defect; common atrium

Reversed Splitting of S_2
Delayed left ventricular activation and completion of ejection
   Left bundle branch block
   Artificial right ventricular pacing
   Pre-excitation of the right ventricle
   Premature beats of right ventricular origin
Prolonged left ventricular ejection time
   Increased resistance to left ventricular ejection (aortic stenosis, obstructive hypertrophic cardiomyopathy, hypertension)
   Isolated increase in left ventricular forward stroke volume (aortic regurgitation, patent ductus arteriosus)
   Myocardial dysfunction (mild to moderate left ventricular failure, myocardial ischemia or infarction)
Increased aortic hangout time (not the sole cause)
   Aortic regurgitation
   Patent ductus arteriosus
   Aortic stenosis

Single S_2
Apparent: obesity, emphysema, pericardial effusion
Absent A_2: severe aortic stenosis, severe aortic regurgitation
Absent P_2: absent pulmonary valve, pulmonary atresia, tetralogy of Fallot, truncus arteriosus
Fusion of A_2 and P_2: Eisenmenger's ventricular septal defect, common ventricle

lar origin is most frequently heard in patients with right ventricular outflow obstruction (pulmonary valve stenosis) and pulmonary arterial hypertension.[79] Presumably, it denotes decreased right ventricular distensibility due to hypertrophy.

At the bedside, it is often difficult to distinguish between gallop sounds of right and left ventricular origin when they are present in the same patient; however, if one follows the "inching" method of auscultation (*i.e.*, auscultation starting over the cardiac apex and then gradually moving the stethoscope inch-by-inch to the left lower sternal border), one can appreciate the decreasing intensity of gallops of left ventricular origin and the increasing intensity of gallops of right ventricular origin. Furthermore, the intensity of the right-sided gallop sounds increase during inspiration.

It is to be noted that effective atrial contraction and ventricular filling are both required for production of atrial gallop sounds, which therefore are usually absent in atrial fibrillation and in significant atrioventricular valve stenosis.

PERICARDIAL KNOCK

In constrictive pericarditis, ventricular filling is confined to early diastole and terminates with a sharp S_3, which is usually termed *pericardial knock*. Its timing, however, is earlier than a normal S_3 and usually occurs 0.10 to 0.12 second after S_2. It is a very frequent finding in constrictive pericarditis and can occur with or without pericardial calcification.[80] It is occasionally heard only during inspiration and along the lower right sternal border, suggesting an early manifestation of right ventricular constriction. A loud early diastolic sound of relatively low frequency, in the absence of an obvious parasternal impulse, should always raise the question of the presence of pericardial constriction, and other physical findings suggestive of constrictive pericarditis (elevated jugular venous pressure with Kussmaul's sign) should be investigated.

EJECTION SOUNDS

An aortic ejection sound is a high-frequency "clicky," early systolic sound, usually recorded 0.12 to 0.14 second after the Q wave on the electrocardiogram. It is best heard with the diaphragm of the stethoscope. It is widely transmitted and heard at the cardiac apex and also over the right second interspace. Its intensity does not vary with respiration. Aortic ejection sounds occur in association with a deformed but mobile aortic valve and with aortic root dilatation. Thus, it is present in aortic valve stenosis, bicuspid aortic valve, aortic regurgitation, and with aneurysm of the ascending aorta. In some patients with systemic hypertension, an aortic ejection sound is heard, probably due to associated aortic root dilatation.

Aortic ejection sounds are heard frequently in patients with mild to moderate aortic valve stenosis and may be absent in severe calcific aortic stenosis, presumably due to the loss of valve mobility.[81] Since ejection sounds are usually absent in subvalvular and supravalvular aortic stenosis, the presence of an ejection sound helps to identify the site of obstruction at the level of the aortic valve. An ejection sound also does not favor the diagnosis of hypertrophic cardiomyopathy.

At the bedside, identification of the aortic ejection sound is the most important clue for the diagnosis of an uncomplicated bicuspid aortic valve.[82] A normal carotid pulse upstroke, a short ejection systolic murmur, and a normal S_2, with or without a short early diastolic murmur, constitute the physical findings of bicuspid aortic valve. Of these, an aortic ejection sound is the most consistent finding, and if it is present in the absence of hypertension, a bicuspid aortic valve should always be suspected. The clinical relevance of an uncomplicated bicuspid aortic valve lies in the fact that once the diagnosis is made, these patients should be given antibiotic prophylaxis to protect against bacterial endocarditis, and then they should be followed for the future development of calcific aortic stenosis. In patients with coarctation of the aorta, an aortic ejection sound usually signifies the presence of an associated bicuspid aortic valve and similar evaluations are recommended.

A pulmonary ejection sound occurs earlier than an aortic ejection sound and is recorded 0.09 to 0.11 second after the Q wave on the electrocardiogram. It is also a "clicky" sound of high frequency and is best heard with the diaphragm of the stethoscope. It is, however, not widely transmitted and usually best heard at the left second interspace and along the left sternal border; it is not usually heard over the cardiac apex or right second interspace. The most helpful distinguishing feature of a pulmonary ejection sound, however, is its decreased intensity, or even its disappearance during the inspiratory phase of respiration. A pulmonary valve ejection sound begins at the time of maximal opening of the pulmonary valve. During expiration, the valve opens rapidly from its fully closed position, and sudden "halting" of this rapid opening movement is associated with a maximal intensity of the ejection sound. With inspiration, the increased venous return to the right ventricle augments the effect of right atrial systole and causes partial opening of the pulmonary valve prior to ventricular systole. The lack of a sharp opening movement of the pulmonary valve explains the decreased intensity of the pulmonary ejection sound during inspiration. The tricuspid closure sound (T_1) should not be confused with the pulmonary ejection sound, because the intensity of T_1 tends to increase rather than decrease during inspiration. Pulmonary ejection sounds tend to be present in clinical conditions associated with a deformed pulmonary valve and pulmonary artery dilatation.[83-86] Thus, they are frequently heard in pulmonary valve stenosis, idiopathic dilatation of the pulmonary artery, and chronic pulmonary arterial hypertension of any etiology. The interval between the S_1 and the pulmonary ejection sound is directly related to the right ventricular isovolumic contraction time, which usually is prolonged in pulmonary hypertension, explaining a relatively late occurrence of the ejection sound in these patients. With increasing severity of pulmonary valve stenosis, the isovolumic systolic interval shortens and, therefore, the pulmonary ejection sound tends to occur soon after S_1. In patients with very severe pulmonary valve stenosis, the ejection sound may be fused with S_1 and may not be recognized.

When ejection sounds, whether aortic or pulmonary, occur in the presence of normal semilunar valves, it has been thought that these sounds originate in the proximal aortic or pulmonary artery segments, hence the term, *vascular ejection* sound, has been suggested. These sounds, in general, tend to occur later and are not associated with "doming" of the semilunar valves, which is characteristic of a valvular ejection sound. The mechanism of the vascular ejection sound remains unclear.

NON-EJECTION SYSTOLIC CLICKS

The non-ejection systolic clicks are also high-frequency sounds that occur much later after S_1 and are also best heard with the diaphragm of the stethoscope. These sounds are not widely transmitted and not usually heard over the right or left second interspace. It has been demonstrated that the non-systolic ejection click occurs in most instances owing to prolapse of the mitral valve, and the timing coincides with maximal prolapse of the mitral valve into the left atrium.[87-90] It may or may not be associated with a late systolic murmur. When a click associated with mitral valve prolapse occurs early in systole, it can be confused with the ejection sound or the second component of a widely split S_1; however, a number of bedside maneuvers can be performed to confirm the presence of a midsystolic click (MSC) (Table 23.8). The systolic dimension or volume at which mitral valve prolapse, and therefore MSC, occurs tends to remain fixed in the same patient.[91] In other words, whenever the "click" volume or dimension is reached following the onset of ventricular ejection (corresponding roughly to S_1), an MSC occurs. The S_1–MSC interval, therefore, can vary according to the pre-ejection (end-diastolic) ventricular volume and the rate of ejection. The S_1–MSC interval will increase (late MSC) whenever there is an increase in end-diastolic volume (supine position, squatting, hand grip). A reduction in end-diastolic volume (standing, phase 2 Valsalva maneuver, amyl nitrite) is associated with a decreased S_1–MSC interval (*i.e.*, early occurrence of mitral valve prolapse and MSC). With the postectopic beat, the S_1–MSC interval usually shortens and the click tends to occur earlier, due to postectopic potentiation, which enhances the rate of ejection. Once the MSC is recognized, it is important to identify the other cardiovascular anomalies that may accompany mitral valve prolapse. These conditions include Marfan's syndrome, atrial septal defect (secundum or primum), musculoskeletal abnormalities, systemic lupus erythematosus, hypertrophic cardiomyopathy, and pseudohypertrophic muscular dystrophy. When no obvious association is identified, the idiopathic mitral valve prolapse syndrome is diagnosed, which has been variously termed as *Barlow's syndrome, billowing mitral valve,* or *floppy valve*.[87]

The systolic "whoop" or "precordial honk" are short musical systolic murmurs often preceded by a click and occurring in mid or late systole. These sounds can be transient, can occur only in certain positions, or can be precipitated by exercise. The "whoop" or "honk" have been found to be caused by mitral valve prolapse in most instances,[92,93] and these patients should be managed in the same manner as patients with the "click-murmur" syndrome.

Tricuspid valve prolapse also produces high-frequency midsystolic, "clicky" sounds, and these are best heard with the diaphragm of the stethoscope over the lower left sternal border and occasionally over the lower right sternal border. The interval between S_1 and the tricuspid valve click tends to increase following inspiration and after raising the legs and other maneuvers that increase right ventricular volume. Isolated tricuspid valve prolapse occurs only rarely, and in most instances it accompanies mitral valve prolapse. Tricuspid valve prolapse, however, may occur in the absence of mitral valve prolapse in patients with Ebstein's anomaly.

In some patients with hypertrophic cardiomyopathy, a non-ejection sound has been observed to occur associated with the systolic anterior motion of the anterior mitral leaflet.[94] This sound, termed *pseudo-ejection sound*, begins, unlike the ejection click of aortic stenosis, considerably after the upstroke of the carotid pulse. The precise mechanism of the pseudo-ejection sound in hypertrophic cardiomyopathy remains unclear. It may either result from the contact of the anterior leaflet with the septum or from the deceleration of blood flow in the left ventricular outflow tract.

EARLY DIASTOLIC HIGH-FREQUENCY SOUNDS

The opening snap is a high-frequency, early diastolic sound associated with mitral or tricuspid valve opening (Table 23.9). This opening of the atrioventricular valves is normally silent but becomes audible in the presence of pathologic conditions. The most common cause of a mitral opening snap is mitral valve stenosis, and it is best heard with the diaphragm of the stethoscope, medial to the cardiac apex. It is usually widely transmitted and can be easily heard over the left second interspace and along the left sternal border. In phonoechocardiographic recordings, the opening snap coincides with the full opening of the mitral valve and it usually occurs 0.04 to 0.12 second after S_2.[95] Since the opening snap is frequently transmitted to the left second interspace, it can be easily confused with a split S_2; however, careful auscultation over the left second interspace, in the supine position and during both phases of respiration, reveals three high-frequency sounds in close proximity to each other during inspiration; the initial two are the two components of S_2, and the third is the opening snap. The recognition of these three sounds during inspiration helps to differentiate mitral stenosis, as seen in mitral valve obstruction, from atrial septal defect, which may also be associated with a mid-diastolic rumble. In atrial septal defect, only the two components of the S_2 are heard during expiration and inspiration. The opening snap results from rapid opening of the mitral valve to its maximal open position and, thus, the mobility of the valve contributes to its genesis. It is absent when the mitral valve is heavily calcified and immobile; however, the opening snap is heard in the vast majority of patients with mitral stenosis, and along with an accentuated S_1, frequently provides the first clue to the diagnosis.

The severity of mitral stenosis can be assessed at the bedside by noting the interval between A_2 and the opening snap. The shorter the A_2-opening snap interval, the more severe is the mitral stenosis. The A_2-opening snap interval is related to the difference in pressures at the time of aortic valve closure and the opening of the mitral valve, which occurs during the isovolumic relaxation phase, when the left ventricular pressure falls below the left atrial pressure. When mitral stenosis is severe, left atrial pressure is higher and the pressure crossover point between the left ventricle and left atrium is closer to A_2, which reduces the A_2-opening snap interval. At the bedside, the shorter A_2-opening snap interval sounds like a widely split S_2. Recordings of the phonocardiogram and indirect cardiac pulse tracings provide a more accurate estimation of the A_2-opening snap interval and, hence, the severity of mitral stenosis; however, echo-Doppler evaluation appears to be a better noninvasive technique to assess the severity of mitral stenosis.

It needs to be emphasized that the A_2-opening snap interval is not only related to the height of the left atrial pressure but also to aortic valve closing pressure. Thus, with a higher aortic valve closing pressure (systemic hypertension), the A_2-opening snap interval may be longer with the same degree of elevation of left atrial pressure. Similarly, when

TABLE 23.8 ALTERATIONS IN S_1–CLICK INTERVAL AND THE CHARACTER OF THE LATE SYSTOLIC MURMUR DURING PHYSIOLOGIC AND PHARMACOLOGIC MANEUVERS IN MITRAL VALVE PROLAPSE

Maneuvers	S_1–Click Interval	Onset of Late Systolic Murmur in Relation to S_1	Duration of Late Systolic Murmur in Relation to Total Duration of Systole
Supine position	Increased	Late	Shorter
Standing position	Decreased	Early	Longer
Squatting	Increased	Late	Shorter
Valsalva (phase 2)	Decreased	Early	Longer
Hand grip	Increased	Late	Shorter
Postectopic beat	Usually decreased	Usually late	Usually longer
Amyl nitrite	Decreased	Early	Longer
Phenylephrine	Increased	Late	Shorter

TABLE 23.9 CAUSES OF A HIGH FREQUENCY SOUND IN EARLY DIASTOLE

Mitral opening snap
   Organic mitral stenosis
   Rarely, pure mitral regurgitation
Tricuspid opening snap
   Organic tricuspid stenosis
   Functional tricuspid stenosis (rare)
   Atrial septal defect
"Tumor plop"
   Left atrial myxoma
   Right atrial myxoma
Opening clicks of mitral stenosis
Mitral valve prolapse
Ebstein's anomaly

the aortic valve closing pressure is lower (aortic regurgitation and aortic stenosis), the A_2-opening snap interval becomes shorter with the same degree of mitral stenosis. When mitral stenosis is associated with mitral regurgitation with a large v wave, the A_2-opening snap interval becomes shorter. Tachycardia also decreases the A_2-opening snap interval as the left atrial pressure increases with increasing heart rate in mitral stenosis. Thus, assessment of the severity of mitral stenosis by estimating the A_2-opening snap interval alone should be done with caution in the presence of tachycardia, hypertension, mitral regurgitation, and aortic valve disease. Although mitral stenosis is the most frequent and important cause of an opening snap, it can occur rarely in patients with pure mitral regurgitation.[78,96]

Tricuspid valve stenosis may also be associated with a tricuspid valve opening snap, which is not widely transmitted and can be heard best over the lower left sternal border. The tricuspid opening snap may also be heard in some patients with an atrial septal defect and a large left-to-right shunt.[54] A high-frequency, diastolic sound can be heard in other conditions and should be differentiated from the opening snap. In some patients with mitral valve prolapse, a high-frequency sound is heard in early diastole, which appears to be related to the rapid inward movement of the prolapsed mitral valve toward the left ventricular cavity before the opening of the mitral valve.[97] In patients with the click-murmur syndrome, therefore, mitral stenosis should not be diagnosed, confusing this early diastolic sound with the opening snap.

In atrial myxoma, early diastolic sounds (tumor "plop") can be heard occasionally, and these sounds appear to occur when tumors move into the ventricle and come to a sudden halt.[98] In patients with hypertrophic cardiomyopathy with a decreased left ventricular cavity, early diastolic, high-frequency sounds are heard in some patients and these sounds coincide with the time of contact of the anterior leaflet of the mitral valve to the interventricular septum.[99] In severe mitral regurgitation due to ruptured chordae, high-frequency early diastolic sounds, similar to the opening snap, can be heard in some patients. It is apparent that the conditions associated with a high-frequency, early diastolic sound cannot be diagnosed based on the presence of this sound alone; other physical findings must be incorporated.

ARTIFICIAL VALVE SOUNDS

The various types of prosthetic and tissue valves that are in use for valve replacement produce both opening and closing sounds. The relative intensity of the opening and closing sounds vary according to the type and design of the prosthetic valve used. In general, with the disk valve, the closing sound is louder than the opening sound. With the ball and cage type of valve, however, both the opening and closing sounds are loud. The closing sounds of the porcine valve are much louder than the opening sounds. The usual auscultatory findings of the normally functioning valve prosthesis in mitral and aortic prostheses are summarized in Table 23.10.[100] The artificial valve sounds are of high frequency, are much louder than normal valve sounds, and are of a "clicky" character. The opening or closing sound may consist of multiple clicks, which do not necessarily indicate valve malfunction. *Ball variance* is a term used to describe certain physical changes in a caged ball and is associated with changes in the intensity of opening and closing sounds.[101] Ball variance was related to a specific model of the caged ball type of prosthetic valve, which is rarely used at the present time. Since the closing sound is usually louder than the opening sound, irrespective of the type of prosthetic valve used, a decreased intensity of the closing sound should raise the possibility of malfunction of the artificial valve. The absence of an opening click has been found in dehiscence of the mitral valve prosthesis.[102] Obstruction of a prosthetic valve in the mitral position may be associated with a markedly decreased A_2-opening sound interval. Echophonocardiographic studies have demonstrated that a marked variation in the A_2-mitral prosthesis opening sound may indicate malfunction of the Bjork-Shiley mitral prosthesis. With a normal functioning prosthesis, the variation in this interval usually does not

---

TABLE 23.10 NORMAL AUSCULTATORY FINDINGS OF PROSTHETIC VALVES ACCORDING TO TYPE AND LOCATION

	Auscultatory Findings	
Valve Prosthesis	*Mitral*	*Aortic*
Ball valves (e.g., Starr-Edwards)	A_2–MO interval 0.07–0.11 second MO louder than MC Soft systolic murmur No diastolic murmur	S_1–AO interval 0.07 second AO louder than AC Soft, harsh systolic ejection murmur "Seating puff"—diastolic rumble
Disc valves (e.g., Bjork-Shiley)	A_2–MO interval 0.05–0.09 second MO is soft or may not be audible Soft systolic murmur Soft and short diastolic rumble	S_1–AO interval 0.04 second AC louder than AO Soft systolic ejection murmur "Seating puff"—diastolic rumble
Tissue valves (e.g., Hancock)	A_2–MO interval 0.1 second MC louder than MO MO is audible in approximately 50% Soft apical systolic murmur Soft diastolic rumble	S_1–AO interval 0.03–0.08 second AC louder than AO AO may be absent Soft systolic ejection murmur No diastolic rumble
Bi-leaflet valves (e.g., St. Jude)		Loud AO and AC Soft systolic ejection murmur

(A_2, aortic valve closure sound; MO, mitral prosthesis opening sound; MC, mitral prosthesis closing sound; S_1, first heart sound; AO, aortic prosthesis opening sound; AC, aortic prosthesis closing sound)

(Data from Smith ND, Raizada V, Abrams J: Auscultation of the normally functioning prosthetic valve. Ann Intern Med 95:594, 1981)

exceed 25 msec.[103] It should be noted that malfunction of an artifical valve may exist despite a normal intensity or character of the opening or closing sounds. Echo-Doppler studies have been found more useful for diagnosing malfunctioning prosthetic valves.[104] Cardiac catheterization is also frequently required to confirm an abnormally functioning artificial valve.

MURMURS

A cardiovascular murmur should be assessed in relation to its location and radiation, timing (systolic or diastolic), intensity (loudness), frequency (pitch), configuration (shape), quality, and duration. Once the character of a murmur is recognized, its diagnostic and pathophysiologic significance can be determined when interpreted in association with other physical findings.

The intensity of a murmur is primarily determined by the quantity and the velocity of blood flow at the site of its origin, the transmission characteristic of the tissues between the site of origin, the site of auscultation or recording, and the distance of transmission. In general, the intensity declines in the presence of obesity, emphysema, and pericardial effusion. Murmurs are usually louder in children and in thin individuals. Conventionally, six grades are used to classify the intensity of a murmur:

Grade I/VI is the faintest murmur that can be heard (with difficulty).
Grade II/VI murmur is also a faint murmur but can be identified immediately.
Grade III/VI murmur is moderately loud.
Grade IV/VI murmur is loud.
Grade V/VI murmur is very loud but cannot be heard without the stethoscope.
Grade VI/VI murmur is the loudest and can be heard without a stethoscope.

The gradation of intensity is purely subjective; however, it allows recognition of changes in the intensity of the murmur, which does have diagnostic relevance. The frequency determines the pitch, which may be high or low. The shape of a murmur is recognized from the phonocardiographic recordings; however, one can form a mental image about the configuration of the murmur during auscultation. A number of configurations are recognized: crescendo (increasing), decrescendo (diminishing), crescendo-decrescendo (increasing-decreasing or diamond shaped), and plateau (unchanged in intensity). The quality of a murmur can be described only by auscultation, such as harsh, rumbling, scratchy, grunting, blowing, squeaky, and musical. The quality of a murmur may also change and, if recognized, can be helpful in the diagnosis of an anomaly. The duration of a murmur is assessed by determining the length of systole or diastole that the murmur occupies. The murmur can be long (*i.e.*, it occupies most of systole or diastole), or it can be brief. The direction of radiation of a murmur follows the direction of blood flow and can provide information regarding the origin of the murmur.

Determination of the timing of the murmur in relation to the cardiac cycle is the initial step in identifying the cause and significance of the murmur. A murmur can be systolic, diastolic, or continuous (Fig. 23.11); both systolic and diastolic murmurs can be either left sided or right sided.

A systolic murmur starts with or after S_1 and terminates before or at S_2. A diastolic murmur starts with or after S_2 and ends at or before S_1. A continuous murmur begins in systole and continues to diastole without interruption, encompassing the S_2. Systolic murmurs are further classified according to the time of onset and termination in systole: an ejection systolic murmur (midsystolic) begins after the S_1 and ends before A_2 (left-sided) or P_2 (right-sided); a holosystolic murmur starts with S_1 and extends up to A_2 (left-sided) or P_2 (right-sided); an early systolic murmur starts with S_1 and extends for a variable length in systole but does not extend up to S_2; a late systolic murmur starts after S_1 and extends to A_2 (left-sided) or P_2 (right-sided).

Diastolic murmurs are also classified according to the time of onset and termination of the murmur in diastole. An early diastolic murmur starts with A_2 (left-sided) or P_2 (right-sided) and extends into diastole for a variable duration. A mid-diastolic murmur starts after S_2 and ter-

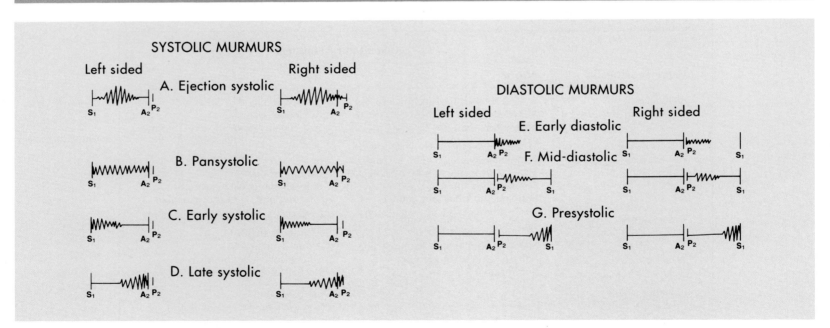

FIGURE 23.11 Schematic diagrams of the various types of systolic and diastolic murmurs. An ejection systolic murmur (**A**) starts after the first heart sound (S_1) and ends before the aortic component of the second heart sound (A_2) when left sided, and before the pulmonary component of the second heart sound (P_2) when right sided. A pansystolic murmur (**B**) starts with S_1 and terminates at A_2 when left sided and at P_2 when right sided. An early systolic murmur (**C**) starts with the S_1 and does not extend up to A_2 or P_2. A late systolic murmur (**D**) starts after S_1 and extends up to A_2 when left sided and up to P_2 when right sided. An early diastolic murmur (**E**), when left sided starts with A_2 and when right sided starts with P_2. A mid-diastolic murmur (**F**) starts after A_2 when left sided and after P_2 when right sided and does not extend up to S_1. A presystolic murmur (**G**) starts before S_1 and terminates at S_1. (Adapted from Perloff JK: Systolic, diastolic and continuous murmur. In Hurst JW (ed): The Heart, 4th ed, p 268. New York, McGraw-Hill, 1978)

minates before S_1; a late diastolic (presystolic) murmur starts well after S_2 and extends up to the mitral component (left-sided) or to the tricuspid component (right-sided) of S_1.

SYSTOLIC MURMURS

At the bedside, systolic murmurs are recognized by identifying S_1 and S_2 and timing them with the carotid pulse. In patients with marked tachycardia, a long diastolic murmur can be occasionally confused with a systolic murmur and timing with the carotid pulse upstroke avoids an incorrect diagnosis.

The ejection or midsystolic murmur is related to flow of blood across the semilunar valves, and the onset of the murmur coincides with the beginning of ejection and the termination with the cessation of forward flow. The S_1 occurs at the onset of isovolumic systole during which ventricular pressure rises and ejection begins at the end of isovolumic systole, when the ventricular pressures exceed the semilunar valve opening pressure. It is apparent why the onset of an ejection systolic murmur is separated from S_1. The interval between S_1 and the onset of the murmur is proportional to the duration of the isovolumic systole. During the initial rapid ejection phase, the intensity of the ejection murmur also increases (crescendo), and with the later slow ejection, intensity declines (decrescendo). The configuration of most ejection systolic murmurs is crescendo-decrescendo. The forward flow from the ventricle stops when ventricular pressure falls below the aortic or pulmonary artery pressures, before the closure of the semilunar valves. With cessation of flow, the murmur terminates before A_2 or P_2, depending on whether the murmur is left or right sided, respectively. The interval between the termination of the murmur and A_2 or P_2 is proportional to the aortic or pulmonary hangout time, respectively.

The important causes of ejection systolic murmurs are outflow tract obstruction, increased flow across normal semilunar valves, dilatation of the aortic root or pulmonary trunk, and anatomical changes in the semilunar valves without obstruction. An ejection systolic murmur is frequently the first clue at the bedside for diagnosing left ventricular outflow tract obstruction, whether fixed or dynamic. An ejection systolic murmur associated with fixed obstruction is crescendo-decrescendo and harsh and rough. The time of peaking of the murmur after its onset bears some correlation to the severity of the obstruction. In patients with aortic stenosis, the longer and later peaking murmur is usually associated with hemodynamically significant obstruction. A brief and early peaking murmur indicates less severe stenosis. The intensity of the murmur is variable and may not correlate with the severity of aortic stenosis. It should be emphasized that in the presence of heart failure and a reduced stroke volume, the duration, configuration, and intensity bear a poor correlation to the degree of obstruction.

The site of maximum intensity and direction of radiation of the murmur are related to the site of obstruction and the direction of the jet in the aortic root. In valvular aortic stenosis, the maximum intensity is appreciated over the right second interspace and a thrill may also be palpable over the same area. The murmur radiates up into the neck and over both carotid arteries. In supravalvular aortic stenosis, the murmur may be loudest at a slightly higher location and the intensity of the radiated murmur over the right carotid may be greater than over the left carotid artery. In subvalvular left ventricular outflow obstruction (hypertrophic cardiomyopathy), the maximum intensity of the murmur is usually located along the lower left sternal border or over the cardiac apex and it radiates poorly to the base and neck. In older patients with calcific tri-leaflet aortic valve stenosis, an ejection systolic murmur with a musical quality is frequently heard over the cardiac apex or along the lower left sternal border, in addition to a harsh murmur over the right second interspace. A musical murmur appears to originate from the vibration of the valve and subvalvular structures and can be recorded in the left ventricular cavity (Gallavardin phenomenon); a harsh murmur originates in the aortic root and is related to the high-velocity ejection jet.

It is to be noted that the site of the left ventricular outflow obstruction cannot be identified with certainty by the location, radiation, and character of the ejection systolic murmur. An ejection sound at the onset of the murmur indicates aortic valve stenosis; however, in severe aortic valve stenosis, the ejection sound is usually absent. For determination of the site of a fixed obstruction, other noninvasive and invasive investigations are frequently required.

It is, however, not difficult to distinguish between fixed (aortic stenosis) and dynamic (obstructive hypertrophic cardiomyopathy) left ventricular outflow obstruction. The character of the carotid pulse provides important clues for the differential diagnosis. In aortic valve stenosis, the initial upstroke and the peak of the carotid pulse are delayed and the volume may be reduced. In obstructive hypertrophic cardiomyopathy, the initial upstroke of the carotid pulse is usually sharp and the volume is normal. The changes in intensity of the ejection systolic murmur in response to different maneuvers should be determined for the differential diagnosis. Assumption of a standing position increases the intensity of the murmur in hypertrophic cardiomyopathy, whereas it is decreased in aortic valve stenosis. A Valsalva maneuver is relatively simple to apply at the bedside, and during phase 2 (straining phase) the murmur of hypertrophic cardiomyopathy increases in intensity along with a decreased or unchanged carotid pulse volume. In aortic stenosis, both the intensity of the murmur and the carotid pulse volume decline. Another helpful maneuver that can also be performed at the bedside is amyl nitrite inhalation. Along with an increased heart rate and fall in arterial pressure, the murmur of hypertrophic cardiomyopathy increases in intensity and the carotid pulse volume decreases or remains unchanged. In aortic stenosis, the intensity of the murmur also increases; however, the carotid pulse volume increases as well. It is apparent that it is more difficult to interpret the responses to amyl nitrite than to standing up or to a Valsalva maneuver in distinguishing hypertrophic cardiomyopathy from aortic valve stenosis.

In certain clinical situations, considerable difficulties might be encountered at the bedside in distinguishing between a long ejection systolic murmur and a holosystolic regurgitant murmur. In dynamic or fixed left ventricular outflow obstruction, the ejection systolic murmur transmitted to the cardiac apex may appear on auscultation, similar to the murmur of mitral regurgitation or ventricular septal defect. When S_1 is soft (which may occur in aortic stenosis or mitral regurgitation), it is often difficult to appreciate the onset of the murmur. When A_2 is soft, determination of the timing of the termination of the murmur may also be difficult. There are a number of distinguishing features that can be elicited by auscultation or by phonocardiographic recording. If A_2 is clearly audible over the cardiac apex, the murmur is likely to be ejection or midsystolic. If A_2 is heard over the right and left second interspaces, but not over the apex, it is likely that A_2 is "drowned" by the holosystolic murmur of mitral regurgitation. If the patient is in atrial fibrillation with a varying RR cycle, or with premature beats, the variation in the intensity of the murmur with variation in the RR interval or during the postectopic beat may distinguish an ejection systolic murmur from a holosystolic regurgitant murmur. The intensity of the ejection systolic murmur increases with a longer RR cycle and with the postectopic beat, whereas that of regurgitant murmur usually remains unchanged. At the bedside, one can note changes in the intensity of the murmur in response to hand grip, which increases the intensity of a mitral regurgitation murmur (increased afterload effect) and usually decreases the intensity of an aortic stenosis murmur. The physiologic responses to hand grip are complex. In addition to an increase in systemic vascular tone and arterial pressure, a reflex increase in contractility may also occur, which tends to increase the intensity of the stenotic murmur. Amyl nitrite inhalation is a very helpful bedside pharmacologic intervention to distinguish between an ejection systolic murmur and a holosystolic regurgitant murmur of left ventricular origin. The intensity of the ejection systolic murmur increases, whereas that of the regurgitant holosystolic murmur decreases. Amyl nitrite inhalation is associated with decreased systemic vascular resistance and arterial pressure, which decreases the severity of the regurgitation and, hence, the intensity of the regurgitant murmur. In aortic stenosis, the intensity of the ejection systolic murmur increases because of the increased flow across the stenotic aortic valve. In hypertrophic cardiomyopathy, the intensity of the murmur increases due to an accentuated left ventricular outflow obstruction. The effects of different pharmacologic and nonpharmacologic interventions on systolic murmurs of fixed and dynamic left ventricular outflow obstruction and of mitral regurgitation are summarized in Table 23.11. It should be noted that only infrequently does one need to perform all these maneuvers, and much less frequently does one have to record phonocardiograms and indirect carotid pulse tracings to distinguish between an ejection systolic murmur and a regurgitant murmur.

The murmur of valvular pulmonary stenosis is also harsh and is best heard over the left second interspace; when loud, this murmur radiates to the left side of the neck and is frequently accompanied by a palpable thrill. A pulmonary ejection sound at the onset of the murmur may be heard, and S_2 is widely split with a decreased intensity of P_2. The duration of the murmur correlates reasonably well with the severity of stenosis.[105] At the bedside, one can roughly estimate the duration by determining the timing of the termination of the murmur in relation to A_2. A murmur terminating before A_2 (relatively short) is usually associated with mild to moderate stenosis. If the murmur drowns A_2 (terminating after A_2), the stenosis is likely to be more severe. Occasionally, the long, harsh ejection systolic murmur of pulmonary stenosis can be confused with the holosystolic murmur of a ventricular septal defect. This is more likely to occur with infundibular than valvular stenosis because of the lower location of the murmur. Careful attention to the behavior of S_2 helps in the differential diagnosis. S_2 is usually normal in ventricular septal defect, whereas in pulmonary stenosis it is widely split and the intensity of P_2 is decreased. Amyl nitrite inhalation is sometimes helpful, which usually decreases the intensity of the ventricular septal defect murmur but not that of the pulmonary stenosis murmur (which may be accentuated). Echo-Doppler evaluation is very helpful in the differential diagnosis.

A bicuspid aortic valve is another frequent cause of an ejection systolic murmur, and this diagnosis should always be entertained if the murmur is brief. This murmur is best heard over the right second interspace with little or no radiation. If it is accompanied by an aortic ejection sound and a short early diastolic murmur, but with normal carotid pulse upstroke and normal S_2, the diagnosis is virtually confirmed.

Aortic root dilatation or dilatation of the proximal pulmonary artery may be associated with an ejection systolic murmur. The usual findings of idiopathic dilatation of the pulmonary artery are a pulmonary ejection sound, a short ejection systolic murmur, a relatively widely split S_2 with normal intensity of P_2, and occasionally a short pulmonary insufficiency murmur. There is no hemodynamic abnormality. It is to be noted that the auscultatory findings are very similar in pulmonary hypertension, except S_2 is narrowly split with P_2 markedly accentuated and the pulmonary ejection sound relatively late. Hemodynamic abnormalities are always evident in pulmonary hypertension.

An ejection systolic murmur also occurs in the presence of normal valves when the flow across the semilunar valve is significantly increased, as in anemia, pregnancy, or thyrotoxicosis. In patients with pure aortic regurgitation, an ejection systolic murmur may result simply from the markedly increased flow and should not be considered as evidence for aortic stenosis in the absence of other findings indicative of aortic valve obstruction. An example of an ejection systolic murmur resulting from increased flow across the pulmonary valve is atrial septal defect. These murmurs do not indicate associated pulmonary stenosis.

The murmur of so-called aortic sclerosis is also a midsystolic ejection murmur. It is benign, since it is not associated with hemodynamic consequences. It must be considered in the differential diagnosis of aortic stenosis in elderly patients. This benign aortic systolic murmur results from stiffening and degenerative fibrous thickening of the roots of the aortic cusps at the site of their insertions. These morphologic changes do not cause any impairment of mobility of the valve and, hence, no obstruction. The murmur of aortic sclerosis is usually best heard over the right second interspace. In some patients, a musical high-frequency murmur of brief duration can be heard along the lower left sternal border and cardiac apex. In general, the murmur of aortic sclerosis is of brief duration and not very loud. A normal carotid pulse and normal S_2 also confirm the absence of aortic stenosis.

TABLE 23.11 DIFFERENTIATION OF MURMURS DUE TO FIXED LEFT VENTRICULAR OUTFLOW OBSTRUCTION, OBSTRUCTIVE HYPERTROPHIC CARDIOMYOPATHY, AND MITRAL REGURGITATION OR VENTRICULAR SEPTAL DEFECT BY PHYSIOLOGIC AND PHARMACOLOGIC MANEUVERS

Maneuvers	Fixed Left Ventricular Outflow Obstruction Ejection Systolic Murmur Intensity	Obstructive Hypertrophic Cardiomyopathy Ejection Systolic Murmur Intensity	Mitral Regurgitation Pansystolic Murmur Intensity
Leg raising	Increased	Decreased	Increased
Standing	Decreased	Increased	Decreased
Squatting	Decreased	Decreased	Increased
Hand grip	Decreased	Decreased	Increased
Supine position	Usually no change	Decreased	Usually no change
Postectopic beat	Increased	Increased	Usually no change
Valsalva (phase 2)	Decreased	Increased	Decreased
Amyl nitrite	Increased	Increased	Decreased
Phenylephrine	Decreased	Decreased	Increased
Nitroglycerin	Usually decreased	Usually increased	Usually decreased

Note: Assessment of changes in carotid pulse volume, along with changes in the intensity of the ejection systolic murmur simultaneously, is desirable to distinguish between aortic stenosis and obstructive hypertrophic cardiomyopathy (see text). Increased intensity of the ejection systolic murmur in obstructive hypertrophic cardiomyopathy is usually associated with decreased or unchanged carotid pulse volume. In fixed aortic stenosis, carotid pulse volume usually increases as the intensity of the murmur increases. Furthermore, a slow initial upstroke and delayed peak of the carotid pulse distinguishes fixed aortic stenosis from obstructive hypertrophic cardiomyopathy.

Innocent murmurs are, by and large, ejection type and midsystolic in timing.[106] In children, a short, vibrating murmur can be heard over the midprecordium, and it is not accompanied by any other abnormality. This murmur, termed *Still's murmur*, is thought to arise from vibrations of the attachments of the leaflets of the pulmonary valve. Another type of innocent systolic ejection murmur that is heard in children and young adults has a blowing quality and is best heard over the left second interspace. It is thought to originate from vibrations of the pulmonary trunk. In patients with the straight back syndrome, with a decreased anteroposterior diameter of the chest, a superficial ejection systolic murmur is heard over the left second interspace.[107] The mechanism of this murmur remains unclear. It should be emphasized that whether an ejection systolic murmur is "innocent" or not should not depend on the duration or intensity of the murmur but on whether any other abnormal finding is present. If any abnormal finding coexists, such as an abnormality of S_2, even a short, grade I/VI ejection systolic murmur should not be considered innocent. The bedside diagnosis of the various causes of ejection systolic murmurs is summarized in Tables 23.12 and 23.13.

HOLOSYSTOLIC (PANSYSTOLIC) MURMURS. Holosystolic, or pansystolic, murmurs are physiologically regurgitant murmurs and occur when blood flows from a chamber whose pressure throughout systole is higher than pressure in the chamber receiving the flow. Essentially, there are three causes of holosystolic murmurs: (1) mitral regurgitation, (2) tricuspid regurgitation, and (3) ventricular septal defect (Fig. 23.12). The timing and duration of the holosystolic murmurs are best explained by the hemodynamic changes of mitral regurgitation. In hemodynamically significant mitral insufficiency, regurgitant flow from the left ventricle to the left atrium begins with the onset of isovolumic systole when the pressure in the left ventricle just exceeds the pressure in the left atrium. This pressure crossover point also marks

---

TABLE 23.12 BEDSIDE DIAGNOSIS OF THE PRINCIPAL CAUSES OF EJECTION SYSTOLIC MURMURS (ESM) IN ADULT PATIENTS

Identification
Begins after S_1, terminates before A_2 and/or P_2. A_2 clearly heard over the cardiac apex, usually crescendo-decrescendo configuration.
Useful maneuvers to differentiate from regurgitant murmur:
  Hand grip usually decreases the intensity of the ejection murmur
  Amyl nitrite usually increases the intensity of the ejection murmur

Examination of the Carotid Pulse Character
Slow Initial Upstroke
Delayed Peak
Small Volume
Anacrotic Character
Thrill
  ↓
Fixed left ventricular outflow obstruction (aortic stenosis):
  Aortic ejection sound indicates valvular aortic stenosis.
  Soft S_1 in the absence of prolonged PR interval; reversed splitting of S_2 in the absence of left bundle branch block; audible or palpable atrial sounds in young patients; soft sustained left ventricular impulse suggests hemodynamically significant aortic stenosis.
Normal or Sharp Initial Upstroke
  ↓
Suspected hypertrophic cardiomyopathy
  Pulsus bisferiens may be present.
  Aortic ejection sound and aortic regurgitation murmur are absent.
  Sustained left ventricular impulse with palpable a wave (presystolic impulse)
  Reversed splitting of S_2 may be present.
  Valsalva maneuver, amyl nitrite, and standing increase the intensity of the murmur.
Suspected right ventricular outflow obstruction (pulmonary stenosis)
  Long systolic murmur along the left sternal border
  Sustained left parasternal impulse may be present.
  Widely split S_2 with reduced intensity of P_2 and an inspiratory increase in A_2–P_2 interval
  Audible or palpable right-sided atrial gallop may be present.
  Pulmonary ejection sound indicates pulmonary valve stenosis.

TABLE 23.13 BEDSIDE DIAGNOSIS OF THE PRINCIPAL CAUSES OF EJECTION SYSTOLIC MURMUR (ESM) IN ADULT PATIENTS (FLOW AND INNOCENT MURMURS)

Identification
Begins after S_1, terminates before A_2 and/or P_2. A_2 clearly heard over the cardiac apex, usually crescendo-decrescendo configuration.
Useful maneuvers to differentiate from regurgitant murmur:
  Hand grip usually decreases the intensity of the ejection murmur
  Amyl nitrite usually increases the intensity of the ejection murmur

Normal Carotid Pulse
Increased flow across the aortic valve
  Aortic regurgitation: aortic diastolic murmur and other features of aortic regurgitation
  Hypermetabolic state: hyperdynamic cardiac impulse
Aortic sclerosis
  Elderly patients
  Short and soft ESM
  Normal S_1 and S_2
  Normal cardiac impulse
  "Grunting" quality of the murmur may be present.
Suspected uncomplicated bicuspid aortic valve
  Short and soft ESM
  Normal S_1 and S_2
  Aortic ejection sound in the absence of aortic aneurysm, hypertension
  Short, early aortic diastolic murmur may be present.
  Normal cardiac impulse
Suspected atrial septal defect
  Short and soft ESM
  Wide and fixed splitting of S_2
  Wide splitting of S_1; tricuspid opening snap; mid-diastolic rumble over the lower left sternal border may be present.
  Hyperdynamic left parasternal impulse
Suspected idiopathic dilatation of the pulmonary artery
  Short and soft ESM
  S_1 normal; S_2 may be widely split; normal inspiratory increase in A_2–P_2 interval
  Pulmonary ejection sound
  Short, early pulmonary diastolic murmur may be present.
  Normal cardiac impulse
Innocent murmur
  Short and soft ESM
  Normal S_1 and S_2
  Normal cardiac impulse
  No evidence for any hemodynamic abnormality

the S_1, explaining the onset of the holosystolic murmur with S_1. Throughout systole, and extending to the early part of the isovolumic relaxation phase, the left ventricular pressure remains higher than the left atrial pressure. Thus, the regurgitant flow continues throughout systole, and even after aortic valve closure, explaining the holosystolic character of the regurgitant murmur and also why A_2 is frequently drowned out by the murmur over the cardiac apex. The holosystolic murmur of mitral regurgitation is high pitched and is best heard with the diaphragm of the stethoscope with the patient in the left lateral decubitus position. The radiation depends on the intensity of the murmur, which may be variable. The direction of radiation follows the direction of the regurgitant jet into the left atrium. When the jet is directed posterolaterally, the apical holosystolic murmur radiates toward the left axilla and inferior angle of the left scapula and over the thoracic spine.[108] If the regurgitant stream is directed anteromedially, against the interatrial septum near the base of the aorta, the radiation of the murmur occurs toward the base and root of the neck. Thus, it can be confused with the murmur of aortic stenosis or obstructive hypertrophic cardiomyopathy. The character of the carotid pulse and the behavior of S_2, as described earlier, provide important clues at the bedside for differential diagnosis. Once mitral regurgitation is diagnosed, an attempt should be made to assess its severity. The absence of an S_3 and cardiac enlargement usually indicate hemodynamically insignificant, chronic mitral regurgitation. Clinical evidence of pulmonary hypertension (accentuated P_2, right ventricular systolic hypertension) and right-sided heart failure are almost always associated with significant mitral regurgitation, provided no other cause of pulmonary hypertension coexists. Electrocardiographic and radiologic evidence of left atrial and left ventricular enlargement support the diagnosis. If signs of pulmonary venous and arterial hypertension are present on the chest film in a patient with chronic mitral regurgitation, mitral regurgitation is likely to be severe. It needs to be emphasized that the absence of clinical or radiologic findings of pulmonary venous or arterial hypertension does not exclude significant chronic mitral regurgitation. Left ventricular function should also be assessed by determining the character of the left ventricular apical impulse. A normal or hyperdynamic apical impulse suggests a normal left ventricular ejection fraction and, therefore, primary mitral regurgitation. A displaced and sustained apical impulse is usually associated with a decreased left ventricular ejection fraction, which, of course, can result from long-standing, severe mitral regurgitation, or it may indicate secondary mitral regurgitation due to dilated cardiomyopathy. Thus, evidence of a normal ejection fraction and not of a reduced ejection fraction is helpful in the differential diagnosis of primary and secondary mitral regurgitation. In dilated cardiomyopathy, S_3 and findings of pulmonary hypertension may be present without significant mitral regurgitation.

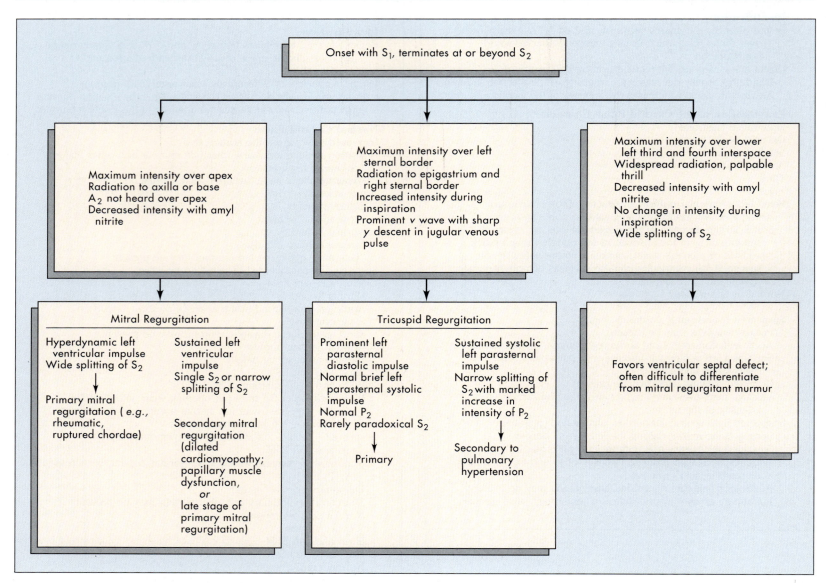

FIGURE 23.12 Differential diagnosis of pansystolic murmur (regurgitant). (S_1, first heart sound; S_2, second heart sound; A_2, aortic component of the second heart sound; P_2, pulmonary component of the second heart sound [echo-Doppler evaluation should be considered for differential diagnosis].)

Thus, differentiation between primary and secondary mitral regurgitation, in the presence of depressed left ventricular systolic function, cannot be made at the bedside, and noninvasive and invasive investigations are necessary.

Acute primary mitral regurgitation (*i.e.* ruptured chordae) may also be associated with a holosystolic murmur (Fig. 23.13). The murmur is frequently very loud and may be accompanied by a palpable thrill. Occasionally, a crescendo-decrescendo configuration is appreciated and widespread radiation both toward the base and posteriorly is frequent.[109] Sudden onset and rapidly progressing symptoms, sinus rhythm, lack of significant cardiac enlargement, a prominent left parasternal impulse, a hyperdynamic apical impulse, a palpable and/or audible atrial gallop, and a wide splitting of S_2 with accentuated P_2 are other findings that suggest acute, severe primary mitral regurgitation due to ruptured chordae. A high-frequency, early diastolic sound, and a short mid-diastolic flow rumble may be present. Lack of electrocardiographic evidence for left atrial and left ventricular enlargement and a relatively normal heart size with evidence of pulmonary venous hypertension on the chest film also support the diagnosis of hemodynamically significant acute mitral regurgitation. In severe mitral regurgitation, an early systolic murmur can occur, instead of a holosystolic murmur.

Tricuspid regurgitation is another valvular lesion that may be associated with a holosystolic murmur. It is also best heard with the diaphragm of the stethoscope over the left second and third interspaces along the left sternal border. With a dilated right ventricle, the location of maximum intensity may be shifted toward the cardiac apex and, thus, can be misdiagnosed as a murmur of mitral regurgitation. Radiation and respiratory changes in the intensity of the murmur are the two important distinguishing features. If the murmur is heard along the right sternal border or over the epigastrium, it is very likely due to tricuspid regurgitation. During the inspiratory phase of respiration, the intensity of the murmur of tricuspid regurgitation increases (Carvallo's sign), provided severe right ventricular failure is not present. A right ventricular S_3 gallop and a mid-diastolic flow murmur, which also increase in intensity with inspiration, suggest more severe tricuspid regurgitation. It is to be noted that the increase in intensity of the murmur does not occur immediately with the onset of inspiration but after one or two cardiac cycles. The mechanism for the increase in intensity of the murmur appears to be due to augmented regurgitant flow following the inspiratory increase in right ventricular volume. It is apparent that in the presence of severe right ventricular failure, when right ventricular volume may not change appreciably, the intensity of the murmur also does not change. Indeed, in the presence of severe right-sided heart failure, the murmur may be absent, or only an early systolic murmur can be recognized. In these circumstances, the bedside diagnosis of tricuspid regurgitation relies on the presence of other physical findings, such as a prominent v wave in the jugular venous pulse and systolic hepatic pulsation.

Tricuspid regurgitation is most often secondary to pulmonary arterial hypertension, and thus a prominent left parasternal impulse and narrow splitting of S_2 with an accentuated P_2 suggest secondary tricuspid regurgitation. Theoretically, severe tricuspid regurgitation may produce reversed splitting of S_2 due to shortened right ventricular ejection time; in practice, it is a rare finding. Primary tricuspid regurgitation is much less common but can occur following bacterial endocarditis in patients indulging in intravenous drug abuse or in patients with Ebstein's anomaly, carcinoid heart disease, or prior right ventricular infarction. A hyperdynamic left parasternal impulse and normal or only slightly accentuated P_2 may suggest primary tricuspid regurgitation, but its diagnosis primarily depends on the elimination of pulmonary hypertension and left-sided disorders, such as mitral and aortic valve disease and cardiomyopathy. In primary tricuspid regurgitation, the murmur, instead of holosystolic, may be early systolic and may have a decrescendo shape in the phonocardiographic recording.

Ventricular septal defect may also be associated with a holosystolic murmur, if pressure in the right ventricle is lower than that in the left ventricle throughout systole.[110,111] This hemodynamic profile is present in small ventricular septal defects and is associated with normal pulmonary artery pressure and pulmonary vascular resistance. Thus, S_2 is

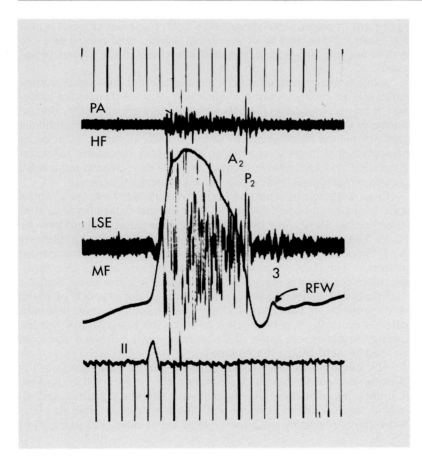

FIGURE 23.13 Phonocardiographic and apex cardiographic recordings in a patient with ruptured chordae. The murmur along the left sternal border (LSB) starts with S_1 and extends beyond the aortic component of S_2 (A_2). The pulmonary component of S_2 (P_2) is accentuated, indicating pulmonary hypertension. The normal character of the left ventricular impulse suggests normal left ventricular ejection fraction. The rapid filling wave (RFW) is pronounced and coincides with S_3 (3). (PA, pulmonary area; HF, high frequency; MF, medium frequency; LSE, left sternal edge) (Sutton GC, Chatterjee K, Caves PK: Diagnosis of severe mitral regurgitation due to nonrheumatic chordal abnormalities. Br Heart J 35:877, 1973)

normal and the findings of pulmonary hypertension are absent. The murmur is usually loud and may be accompanied by a thrill. The left-to-right shunt is directed to the right ventricular cavity, and the murmur is maximal over the third and fourth interspaces along the sternal border when the ventricular septal defect is below the crista supraventricularis. When the defect is above the crista, the shunt is directed toward the pulmonary trunk. The maximal intensity of the murmur then may be in the left second interspace, and it can be confused with the murmur of pulmonary valve stenosis.[105] The changes in S_2 help in the differential diagnosis: a wide splitting of S_2 with reduced intensity of P_2 is present in pulmonary stenosis, and a normal S_2 favors ventricular septal defect. With increased right ventricular and pulmonary artery pressure, as well as an elevated pulmonary vascular resistance in a large ventricular septal defect, the character and timing of the systolic murmur change. Instead of being holosystolic, it becomes early systolic and the peak of the murmur also occurs earlier. The physical findings of pulmonary arterial hypertension and right ventricular hypertrophy are present. In Eisenmenger's complex, when the shunt is reversed, the murmur through the ventricular septal defect may be absent and an ejection systolic murmur due to dilatation of the pulmonary trunk appears. S_2 is markedly accentuated and single.[53] Murmurs of tricuspid pulmonary regurgitation may also be present. It is apparent that a holosystolic murmur in a patient with a ventricular septal defect usually indicates favorable hemodynamics (*i.e.*, relatively normal right-sided pressures).

EARLY SYSTOLIC MURMURS. These murmurs begin with S_1, do not extend to S_2, and generally have a decrescendo configuration. Early systolic murmurs may result from mitral regurgitation, tricuspid regurgitation, or ventricular septal defect.

Either severe or mild mitral regurgitation can be associated with an early systolic murmur. Acute severe mitral regurgitation causes a rapid increase in left atrial pressure and a giant regurgitant wave (*v* wave) during the latter part of ventricular systole. An equalization of left atrial and left ventricular pressure may occur, preventing the regurgitant flow during this part of systole. Thus, the regurgitant murmur terminates before A_2. Since the regurgitant flow is maximal at the beginning of systole and decreases with increasing left atrial pressure, a decrescendo configuration of this early systolic murmur is frequent.[112-114] Findings of pulmonary hypertension, hyperdynamic apical impulse, a late systolic left parasternal impulse, and atrial and ventricular gallops are recognized at the bedside and can be recorded in the phonocardiograms and apex cardiograms.

In some patients with mitral stenosis, an early systolic murmur is heard and probably represents mild mitral regurgitation. Secondary mitral regurgitation in dilated cardiomyopathy is usually mild and may be early systolic in timing. Mitral annular calcification may be associated with an early systolic murmur and indicates trivial mitral regurgitation. Ineffective reduction of the circumference of the annulus at the beginning of systole, due to calcification, is probably the underlying mechanism for mild mitral regurgitation and the early systolic murmur.[113]

Primary tricuspid regurgitation, with normal right ventricular systolic pressure, as seen with infective endocarditis in drug addicts, may be associated with an early systolic murmur with a decrescendo configuration. The mechanism is similar to that in acute, severe mitral regurgitation. A rapid increase in right atrial pressure and an accentuated *v* wave in the later part of systole decreases the regurgitant flow. The frequency of these murmurs is usually lower than the murmurs associated with an elevated right ventricular systolic pressure, presumably due to a lower rate of regurgitation. In addition to a relatively normal S_2, palpation and recording of the left parasternal impulse may reveal a systolic inward movement and a diastolic outward movement reflecting right ventricular volume changes in systole and diastole.

As described earlier, in a large ventricular septal defect with pulmonary hypertension, the murmur may be early systolic in timing, since the increasing right ventricular pressure during late systole decreases the left-to-right shunt. Findings of pulmonary hypertension are always present. An early systolic murmur may also occur in some patients with ventricular septal defect in the absence of pulmonary hypertension or increased pulmonary vascular resistance. These murmurs are more frequently localized and of shorter duration. They tend to occur not uncommonly in those ventricular septal defects that later close spontaneously.[115] Small muscular ventricular septal defects may also cause an early systolic murmur, since the defect closes soon after the onset of systole. Evidence of pulmonary hypertension is obviously absent, and the electrocardiograms and chest film do not reveal any abnormality.

LATE SYSTOLIC MURMURS. A late systolic murmur starts after S_1 and, if left-sided, extends to A_2, usually in a crescendo manner. Mitral valve prolapse is the most common cause of a late systolic murmur. It is best heard with the diaphragm of the stethoscope and over, or just medial to, the cardiac apex. It is usually preceded by single or multiple clicks.[116,117] Mitral valve prolapse can occur from disorders of the mitral annulus, redundancy of the leaflets, abnormalities of the chordae, or contraction abnormalities of the left ventricular wall. Mitral regurgitation occurs when prolapse is sufficient to cause a lack of apposition of the leaflets. The most common type of mitral valve prolapse syndrome ("floppy" valve or Barlow's syndrome) is thought to occur because of redundancy of valve tissue with respect to the valve ring. This disparity increases with a decreased left ventricular volume, which is associated with an earlier onset of prolapse and, therefore, the late systolic murmur occupies a relatively greater portion of systole. Standing, sitting, Valsalva's maneuver (phase 2), and amyl nitrite inhalation, all decrease left ventricular volume and cause an earlier onset of the clicks and murmurs, which also appear longer. The intensity, however, becomes softer. Conversely, squatting, elevation of the legs, isometric exercise (hand grip), and infusion of phenylephrine, which increases left ventricular volume, delay the onset of the clicks and murmurs, the intensity of which may increase. A "whoop" or "honk," which is a high-frequency, musical, loud, and widely transmitted murmur, can appear intermittently in some patients with mitral valve prolapse and can be precipitated by a change of posture.

In general, mitral valve prolapse with a late systolic murmur is only associated with mild mitral regurgitation and is not accompanied by an S_3 or signs of pulmonary hypertension. Left ventricular function is normal. Apex cardiograms in some patients reveal a bifid configuration in systole and the notch coincides with the clicks in the phonocardiogram.

A late systolic murmur is also a manifestation of mild mitral regurgitation due to papillary muscle dysfunction in acute myocardial infarction. It may also occur in patients with chronic coronary artery disease during an episode of myocardial ischemia, presumably due to ischemic papillary muscle dysfunction. In these patients, isometric exercise or maneuvers that increase ventricular volume may precipitate mitral regurgitation and late systolic murmur because of increased myocardial oxygen requirements, which may induce myocardial ischemia.

In patients with pseudohypertrophic muscular dystrophy, mitral valve prolapse and a late systolic murmur are manifestations of cardiac involvement. These may or may not be associated with midsystolic clicks. The electrocardiogram almost always demonstrates a relatively tall R wave in leads V_1, and V_2, simulating true posterior myocardial infarction. The mechanism of mitral valve prolapse and its electrocardiographic changes is fibrosis of the posterior left ventricular wall.

Tricuspid valve prolapse is uncommon in the absence of mitral valve prolapse. It also causes a late systolic murmur that, however, extends up to P_2. It is best heard over the left lower sternal border. During inspiration, the onset of the murmur may be delayed due to an increase in right ventricular volume.

The diagnosis of mitral valve prolapse can be easily made at the bedside in most instances. Auscultation for clicks and late systolic murmurs should be done with the patient in different positions, particularly in the recumbent position and then immediately after standing. When the auscultatory manifestations of mitral valve prolapse are not obvious, an echocardiogram and auscultation should be performed following pharmacologic and physiologic maneuvers, which almost always establish or exclude the diagnosis (see Table 23.8).

DIASTOLIC MURMURS

EARLY DIASTOLIC MURMURS. These murmurs typically start at the time of closure of the semilunar valves and their onset coincides with S_2. Phonocardiographic recordings and the carotid pulse demonstrate that an aortic regurgitation murmur begins with the A_2 of the S_2, while that of pulmonary regurgitation begins with the P_2. The configuration of the aortic regurgitation murmur is usually decrescendo, because the magnitude of regurgitation progressively declines, the maximal being at the onset of diastole. These are high-frequency murmurs and have a "blowing" character. Occasionally these murmurs can be musical in quality (diastolic whoop), and the "whoop" can be mid, late or pansystolic.[118] They are best heard with the diaphragm of the stethoscope. Occasionally the murmur of aortic regurgitation may have a musical quality, and this has been attributed to a flail everted aortic cusp. The duration of the murmur is variable but usually terminates before S_1. The duration of the murmur does not always correlate with the severity of aortic regurgitation. Mild aortic regurgitation may be associated with a murmur of brief duration. In acute severe aortic regurgitation, the murmur may also be short because of a rapid increase in left ventricular diastolic pressure, which equalizes with aortic diastolic pressure soon after the onset of diastole. If the aortic pressure remains higher than left ventricular pressure throughout diastole, a pandiastolic murmur may be present, even when the severity of aortic regurgitation is only moderate. Low-intensity, high-pitched aortic regurgitation murmurs may not be easily heard until one applies firm pressure with the diaphragm of the stethoscope over the left sternal border or over the right second interspace while the patient sits and leans forward, with the breath held in full expiration. The radiation of an aortic regurgitation murmur is toward the cardiac apex, and the location of maximum intensity may vary considerably. It can be best heard in some patients over the midprecordium, along the lower left sternal border, or even over the cardiac apex. Radiation of the murmur to the right sternal border is more frequent in aortic regurgitation caused by aortic root or aortic cusp anomalies.[119] Bedside evaluation of the severity is based on a determination of the hemodynamic consequences of aortic regurgitation. In patients with chronic aortic regurgitation, arterial diastolic pressure progressively declines and the pulse pressure increases with increasing severity. An arterial diastolic pressure higher than 60 mm Hg and a normal pulse pressure are uncommon in chronic, severe aortic regurgitation. A water-hammer pulse, Corrigan's pulse, or a bisferiens quality of the carotid pulse usually indicate hemodynamically significant aortic regurgitation. Determination of cardiac size at the bedside and by chest film is important to assess the severity of aortic regurgitation, since chronic aortic regurgitation of any severity increases left ventricular volume. Lack of displacement of the cardiac apex and normal heart size on the chest film suggest insignificant chronic aortic regurgitation. The duration of the regurgitant murmur correlates poorly with the severity; however, an Austin Flint murmur is more likely to be associated with significant aortic regurgitation. Similarly, a decreased intensity of S_2 does not necessarily suggest significant aortic regurgitation; however, reversed splitting of S_2, in the absence of left bundle branch block, which usually results from increased left ventricular forward stroke volume, indirectly suggests significant aortic regurgitation. Changes in the intensity of S_1 should be noted, since its reduced intensity is usually associated with an elevated left ventricular end-diastolic pressure, which is more likely to occur in severe aortic regurgitation. Physical findings of pulmonary venous and arterial hypertension and right-sided heart failure, if related to aortic regurgitation, clearly indicate hemodynamically significant aortic regurgitation. Assessment of left ventricular function is important, particularly with respect to the timing of surgery. A hyperdynamic left ventricular impulse is associated with a relatively normal ejection fraction; a sustained impulse and S_3 gallop, on the other hand, may indicate a reduced ejection fraction, and further evaluation to assess left ventricular function is indicated. The onset of heart failure can modify many of the physical findings that indicate significant aortic regurgitation. The pulse pressure that was initially high may decrease, and the arterial diastolic pressure that was low may increase. The duration of the regurgitant murmur may decrease as the left ventricular diastolic pressure increases. Thus, serial evaluations are helpful to assess changes in the hemodynamics, left ventricular function, and severity of the aortic regurgitation.

The hemodynamic consequences of acute, severe aortic regurgitation differ considerably from those of chronic aortic regurgitation, explaining the differences in physical findings. Sudden severe volume overload in a nondilated left ventricle causes a rapid increase in diastolic pressure and often equalization of left ventricular and aortic root pressures in mid-diastole. Thus, the regurgitant murmur can be of short duration. The S_1 is soft or absent. Phonoechocardiographic recordings demonstrate a reduced intensity of the mitral component of S_1 and premature closure of the mitral valve.[46] The P_2 of S_2 is frequently accentuated owing to postcapillary pulmonary hypertension. A marked increase in left ventricular end-diastolic pressure may prevent effective left ventricular filling during left atrial systole, and thus an atrial gallop may be absent. Since left ventricular forward stroke volume may not increase, or may even decrease, the carotid pulse may appear small, although the character remains normal. As the systemic vascular resistance either increases or remains normal and the arterial diastolic pressure does not fall, the pulse pressure may become narrow, if the forward stroke volume declines concomitantly. A lack of left ventricular dilation and hypertrophy is recognized by the relatively normal position of the left ventricular impulse. The chest film reveals little or no cardiac enlargement, normal left atrial size, and usually pulmonary venous congestion. Evidence of left atrial or left ventricular enlargement is usually absent on the electrocardiogram.

Diastolic murmurs, similar to those of aortic regurgitation, can be heard in some patients with left anterior descending coronary artery stenosis (Dock's murmur).[120] The murmur, however, is not widespread like that of aortic regurgitation and usually is best heard over the left second or third interspace, a little lateral to the left sternal border. The murmur is caused by turbulent flow across the coronary artery stenosis, and its duration may be short or long (Fig. 23.14). Dock's murmur usually indicates moderately severe stenosis of the left anterior descending coronary artery. Coronary artery bypass surgery abolishes the murmur. Aortic regurgitation and its causes need to be excluded before the diagnosis of Dock's murmur can be established.

Pulmonary regurgitation is another cause of an early diastolic murmur, and in the adult patient it is most frequently a result of pulmonary hypertension (Graham Steell murmur).[109] This is a high-pitched, "blowing" murmur that starts with an accentuated P_2 of S_2 and can be of variable duration. It may occupy the whole of diastole if there is a pandiastolic gradient between the pulmonary artery and right ventricular diastolic pressure. The murmur has a decrescendo configuration like that of aortic regurgitation; differentiation is difficult if not impossible by auscultation alone. The murmur may increase in intensity during inspiration and may be more localized. It is best heard over the left second and third interspaces. Pulmonary regurgitation is suspected when other findings of pulmonary hypertension are present and peripheral signs of aortic regurgitation are absent. Phonocardiographic recordings may be of help in distinguishing it from aortic regurgitation, since it starts with P_2 of S_2; however, echo-Doppler studies are more revealing and sensitive and demonstrate diastolic tricuspid valve fluttering and a regurgitant jet into the right ventricular cavity.

Pulmonary regurgitation can occur in the absence of pulmonary hypertension, as in patients with idiopathic dilatation of the pulmonary artery, after pulmonary valvulotomy, with right-sided endocarditis, and with congenital absence of the pulmonary valve. In these conditions, the pulmonary artery diastolic pressure is normal or low, which is associated with a lower rate of regurgitant flow, so that the regurgitant murmur is of low to medium pitch. The murmur usually begins after and not with the P_2 of S_2. The delayed onset of the murmur is related to the minimal pulmonary artery–right ventricular pressure gradient at the time of pulmonary valve closure. Regurgitation increases as the right ventricular pressure declines rapidly after the pulmonary valve closure, increasing the pressure gradient. The murmur does not extend to S_1 because the relatively low pulmonary artery pressure equilibrates with that of right ventricular pressure at the latter part of diastole. P_2 is absent, and there is a silent interval between A_2 and the onset of the regurgitant murmur in congenital absence of the pulmonary valve. A loud to-and-fro murmur may be heard in these patients.

MID-DIASTOLIC MURMURS. Mid-diastolic murmurs result from turbulent flow across the atrioventricular valves during the rapid filling phase because of mitral or tricuspid valve stenosis and an abnormal pattern of flow across these valves.

The mid-diastolic murmur of mitral stenosis has a rumbling character and is best heard with the bell of the stethoscope and over the left ventricular impulse with the patient in the left lateral decubitus position. The murmur originates in the left ventricular cavity, explaining its location of maximum intensity. The murmur is present both in sinus rhythm and in atrial fibrillation. It characteristically starts with an opening snap, and its duration is a reasonably good guide to assess the severity of mitral stenosis.[121] The longer the duration of the murmur, the more severe is the mitral stenosis, provided the diastolic interval is not too short (absence of tachycardia). The duration of the murmur correlates with the duration of the diastolic pressure gradient across the mitral valve. If the murmur extends up to S_1 during a longer diastolic interval, it can be assumed that the pressure gradient is still present at end-diastole, which implies severe mitral stenosis. It needs to be emphasized that when the flow across the mitral valve is markedly reduced, which may result from associated right-sided heart failure and pulmonary hypertension, the murmur may be of very brief duration or even absent (so-called silent mitral stenosis), even in the presence of severe mitral stenosis. Conversely, with enhanced flow across the valve, as in the high-output state of pregnancy, the intensity and duration of the murmur increase even with less severe stenosis. In these circumstances, one cannot rely on the duration of the murmur to assess the severity of mitral stenosis, and other ancillary investigations, particularly echocardiographic studies, are necessary.

TRICUSPID STENOSIS. Tricuspid stenosis may also be associated with a mid-diastolic rumble, which is best heard along the left sternal border. The most characteristic feature is the increase in intensity of the murmur with inspiration (Carvallo's sign).[122] Tricuspid stenosis most frequently occurs in association with mitral stenosis, and most patients are in atrial fibrillation. The murmur in these patients is mid-diastolic when the transvalvular pressure gradient is maximum. In sinus rhythm, the murmur may occur only in late diastole, resulting from an increased flow due to right atrial systole. Isolated tricuspid stenosis is uncommon, but when suspected, carcinoid heart disease and right atrial myxoma should be investigated as possible etiologies. A prominent a wave and a relatively slow y descent in the jugular venous pulse, presystolic hepatic pulsation, and the absence of a right atrial gallop should strengthen the suspicion of tricuspid stenosis. The mid-diastolic rumble may be associated with a tricuspid opening snap and wide splitting of S_1 due to delayed closure of the tricuspid valve.

ATRIAL MYXOMA. Atrial myxoma may cause obstruction of the atrioventricular valves and, therefore, a mid-diastolic murmur. In left atrial myxoma, the auscultatory findings may be similar to those of mitral stenosis; however, the character and the intensity of the murmur may change with alterations of position.[123] The murmur is frequently presystolic and crescendo in configuration, which appears to occur with the onset of ventricular systole when the tumor is moved toward the left atrium through the mitral orifice, and when the flow across the

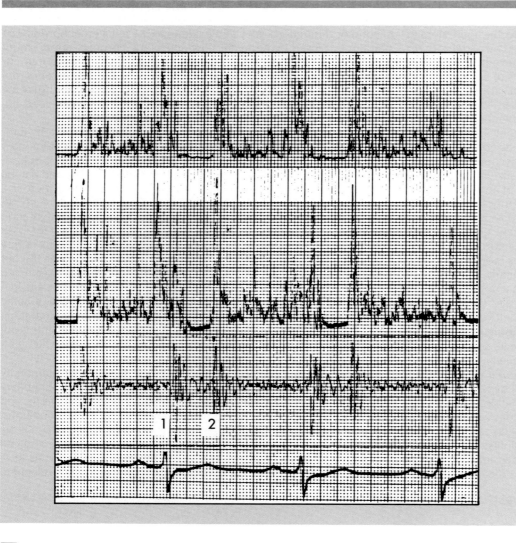

FIGURE 23.14 Diastolic murmur associated with left anterior descending coronary artery stenosis (Dock's murmur). This murmur can be similar to that of aortic regurgitation. (1, first heart sound; 2, second heart sound) Dock W, Zoneraich S: A diastolic murmur arising in a stenosed coronary artery. Am J Med 742:617, 1967)

valve is still continuing. It is difficult to distinguish between a left atrial myxoma and mitral stenosis at the bedside. Sinus rhythm, changing intensity and character of the murmur, and a "tumor plop" sound favor the diagnosis of left atrial myxoma; however, echocardiographic evaluation is necessary and is always recommended in a patient with suspected mitral stenosis. Right atrial myxoma is far less common than left atrial myxoma. Auscultatory findings may be similar to those of tricuspid stenosis.

Mid-diastolic murmurs may occur in the presence of normal atrioventricular valves when the flow across the valve is markedly increased in mid-diastole (flow murmurs). In pure severe, mitral regurgitation, a larger volume of blood (due to the regurgitant volume) moves from the left atrium to the left ventricle during diastole. Echophonocardiographic studies have demonstrated that a partial closing movement of the mitral valve occurs after it opens widely at the beginning of diastole. The rapid flow to the left ventricle continues, and thus "functional mitral stenosis" occurs, explaining the mid-diastolic rumble. A mid-diastolic pressure gradient has been demonstrated in some patients.[124-126]

In left-to-right shunt, antegrade blood flow across the mitral valve increases during diastole, which may be associated with a mid-diastolic murmur; the mechanism may be similar to that seen in mitral regurgitation. In atrial septal defect or anomalous pulmonary venous drainage, a tricuspid flow murmur can be heard along the lower left sternal border (Fig. 23.15). The intensity of the tricuspid flow murmur tends to increase during inspiration. In atrial septal defect, an echocardiogram also demonstrates a partial closing movement of the tricuspid valve after its full opening in early diastole and functional tricuspid stenosis occurs at mid diastole—the timing of the tricuspid flow murmurs.[127]

In pure aortic regurgitation, an apical diastolic rumbling murmur was first described by Austin Flint in 1876.[128,129] Several mechanisms have been proposed to explain the genesis of this murmur. Fluttering of the mitral valve from the impingment by the aortic regurgitant jet, diastolic mitral regurgitation, and relative mitral stenosis have been suggested. The murmur originates in the left ventricular cavity and, therefore, is not due to diastolic mitral regurgitation. Echocardiographic studies have demonstrated that a premature, partial closing movement of the mitral valve occurs at mid diastole and also during left atrial systole. As the antegrade flow continues across the mitral valve, functional mitral stenosis occurs and a mid-diastolic rumble and presystolic murmur can occur. Mitral fluttering is not the mechanism of the Austin Flint murmur, since fluttering occurs in early diastole with the onset of regurgitation, whereas the rumble occurs in mid or late diastole.

The Austin Flint murmur, if not recognized, may lead to a mistaken diagnosis of organic mitral stenosis. The presence of an opening snap suggests organic mitral stenosis. Amyl nitrite inhalation is a helpful method of differentiation; an Austin Flint murmur tends to decrease in intensity and duration as the severity of the aortic regurgitation decreases with decreased left ventricular afterload. In contrast, the murmur of mitral stenosis increases in intensity and duration with an increased heart rate and increased antegrade flow across the mitral valve; however, echocardiographic studies are recommended for a more definitive diagnosis.

In acute rheumatic fever, a mid-diastolic murmur over the left ventricular impulse (Carey-Coombs murmur) has been attributed to acute mitral valvulitis; however, first-degree atrioventricular block (prolonged PR interval) is frequent in rheumatic carditis, and an increased flow due to earlier atrial systole coinciding with the rapid filling phase might be contributory to a Carey-Coombs murmur.

LATE DIASTOLIC (PRESYSTOLIC) MURMURS. These murmurs occur in late diastole and extend up to S_1. They usually have a crescendo configuration (presystolic). The murmurs result from increased flow across the mitral or tricuspid valve and are most frequently observed in the presence of normal sinus rhythm.

In mitral stenosis, atrial contraction increases the pressure gradient and flow at end-diastole, generating the presystolic murmur. When a mid-diastolic rumble accompanies a presystolic murmur, frequently the intensity of the mid-diastolic murmur decreases before the onset of the presystolic murmur. The presence of only a presystolic murmur associated with increased intensity of S_1 implies mild mitral stenosis. Crescendo presystolic murmurs can occur in the presence of atrial fibrillation; mitral valve closure begins before the onset of isovolumic systole and during this period antegrade flow across the mitral valve continues.[130] Thus, presystolic murmurs can occur even in the absence of atrial systole because of the reduction of an effective mitral orifice before the onset of S_1.

In tricuspid stenosis with sinus rhythm, the murmur is usually presystolic because the transvalvular gradient is maximum during this period.[122] The intensity of the presystolic murmur of tricuspid stenosis also increases during inspiration, which is associated with an increased venous return to the right atrium. Increased right atrial volume is associated with more forceful right atrial contraction and, therefore, an

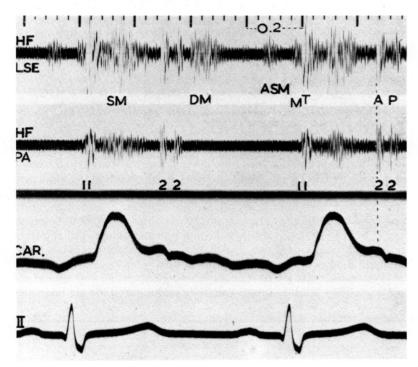

FIGURE 23.15 Phonocardiographic findings in atrial septal defect with a large left-to-right shunt. Wide fixed splitting of S_2 (2 2) along with an ejection systolic murmur and mid-diastolic murmur were present. Tricuspid component of the first heart sound (T) was prominent. (LSE, left sternal edge; HF, high frequency; PA, pulmonary area; CAR, indirect carotid pulse tracing; SM, ejection systolic murmur; DM, diastolic murmur; ASM, atrial systolic murmur; M, mitral component of the first heart sound; T, tricuspid component of the first heart sound; A, aortic component of the second heart sound; P, pulmonary component of the second heart sound; 1 1, two components of the first heart sound) (Leatham A, Gray I: Auscultatory and phonocardiographic signs of atrial septal defect. Br Heart J 18:193, 1956)

increased pressure gradient during this interval and the accentuation of the murmur.

In left or right atrial myxoma, presystolic murmurs may also occur due to obstruction of the atrioventricular valves. Flow murmurs due to a large left-to-right shunt are usually mid-diastolic in location but occasionally can extend to late diastole.

In complete atrioventricular block with a slow idioventricular rhythm, a short mid-diastolic murmur can occasionally be heard and recorded (Rytand's murmur). The precise mechanism of Rytand's murmur has not been elucidated, but diastolic mitral regurgitation has been postulated.[131] Doppler echocardiography has demonstrated intermittent mid- or late-diastolic mitral regurgitation in patients with advanced atrioventricular block.[132] Diastolic mitral regurgitation appears to depend on the position of the P wave and atrial systole in ventricular diastole.[132]

CONTINUOUS MURMURS

Continuous murmurs are defined as murmurs that begin in systole and extend up to diastole without interruption and do not necessarily need to occupy the total duration of systole and diastole. Continuous murmurs result from blood flow from a higher pressure chamber or vessel to a lower system associated with a persistent pressure gradient between these areas during systole and diastole. These murmurs may occur due to aortopulmonary connections, arteriovenous communication, and disturbances in the flow patterns in the arteries or veins.[133-136]

Patent ductus arteriosus is one relatively common cause of a continuous murmur in an adult population. In patent ductus arteriosus, aortic pressure is higher than pulmonary artery pressure, both during systole and diastole, and the blood flow from the high-pressure descending thoracic aorta to the low-pressure pulmonary artery causes the continuous murmur (Gibson's murmur, machinery murmur). The maximum intensity of the murmur usually occurs at S_2. The duration of the murmur depends on the pressure difference between aorta and pulmonary artery. With pulmonary hypertension, pulmonary artery diastolic pressure increases, and when it approaches systemic level, the diastolic portion of the continuous murmur becomes shorter and ultimately absent.[137] With more severe pulmonary hypertension, pulmonary artery systolic pressure may equalize with aortic systolic pressure and the systolic component of the murmur may also be absent (silent ductus). Differential cyanosis due to the reversal of the shunt and signs of pulmonary hypertension with or without evidence of right-sided heart failure are the only physical findings that are recognizable at the bedside in these circumstances.

Continuous murmurs may also be present in aortopulmonary window; however, because of the large size of the communication, pulmonary vascular resistance and pulmonary artery diastolic pressure tend to be higher, which is associated with a shorter duration of the diastolic component of the continuous murmur. A left-to-right shunt through a small atrial septal defect in the presence of mitral valve obstruction (Lutembacher's syndrome) may occasionally cause a continuous murmur.[138] Total anomalous pulmonary venous drainage, a small atrial septal defect without mitral valve obstruction, and mitral stenosis with a persistent left superior vena cava are very rare causes of continuous murmurs.

Congenital or acquired arteriovenous fistulas also cause continuous murmurs. Coronary artery venous fistulas should be considered in the differential diagnosis.

The location, duration, and character of the continuous murmur due to a coronary arteriovenous communication depends on the anatomical type of coronary arteriovenous fistulas. For example, the right coronary and right atrial, or coronary sinus, communication produces continuous murmurs that are usually located along the parasternal areas. The murmur of a circumflex coronary artery and coronary sinus communication are usually located in the left axilla. The configuration of the murmur and the intensity of the systolic and diastolic components are variable. Marked systolic compression of the abnormal vessels reduces the systolic flow; therefore, the systolic component of the murmur may be very soft. On the other hand, an increased systolic gradient may result from the partial compression of the intramural communication, which will tend to increase the intensity of the systolic portion of the murmur.

A communication between the sinus of Valsalva and the right atrium or right ventricle produces continuous murmurs, which may appear as to-and-fro murmurs due to the increased intensity of both the systolic and diastolic components and a softer intensity around S_2.

Systemic and pulmonary arteriovenous fistulas are also associated with continuous murmurs. Although a systemic arteriovenous communication usually produces loud murmurs, the murmurs of pulmonary arteriovenous fistulas are softer and may be primarily systolic. The major pressure gradient occurs in systole, and the diastolic gradient is usually very small. Pulmonary arteriovenous fistulas usually involve the lower left or right middle lobe, and the location of the murmurs is also over these areas.

Constriction in the systemic or pulmonary arteries can be associated with continuous murmurs due to a persistent pressure gradient across the narrowed segment of the vessel. In coarctation of the aorta, a continuous murmur can be heard in the back overlying the area of constriction. Continuous murmurs may originate in large tortuous collateral arteries in coarctation of the aorta, which are also heard in the back over the interscapular regions. Sometimes large, tortuous intercostal vessels are visible when the shoulders are rotated medially and forward to separate the scapulas (Suzman's sign).[139] Pulmonary artery branch stenosis and a partial occlusion of the pulmonary artery due to pulmonary embolism may also cause continuous murmurs.

Rapid flow through tortuous collateral vessels, as in coarctation of the aorta, may cause a continuous murmur. Bronchial arterial collateral vessels develop in certain types of cyanotic congenital heart disease (tricuspid atresia, pulmonary atresia with ventricular septal defect), and loud continuous murmurs may be heard along the parasternal area.

The "mammary souffle" associated with pregnancy may be systolic or continuous. These innocent murmurs are usually of higher frequency (high-pitched) and louder in systole. Another innocent continuous murmur that should be recognized at the bedside is a venous hum, which results from altered flow in the veins. The venous hum is heard with the patient in the sitting position (usually in the supraclavicular fossa) and frequently disappears when the patient moves to the supine position. The hum tends to be louder in diastole and can be completely abolished by compression of the ipsilateral internal jugular vein. A loud, left-sided venous hum transmitted below the clavicle should not be mistaken for the murmur of patent ductus arteriosus. Venous hum is not heard in the supine position, and pressure on the internal jugular vein abolishes the venous hum. The murmur of patent ductus arteriosus persists in the supine position and despite pressure on the internal jugular vein.

PERICARDIAL FRICTION RUBS AND OTHER ADVENTITIOUS SOUNDS

A pericardial rub is generated by the friction of two inflamed layers of the pericardium and occurs during the maximal movement of the heart within its pericardial sac. Thus, the rub can be heard during atrial systole, ventricular systole, and the rapid-filling phase of the ventricle (three-component rub); however, the rub may be present only during one (one component) or two phases (two components) of the cardiac cycle. In episternopericarditis following transmural myocardial infarction, a one-component rub, usually during ventricular systole, is more frequent than two- or three-component rubs.

Pericardial rubs are of scratching or grating quality and appear superficial. They are best heard with the diaphragm of the stethoscope.

The intensity frequently increases after application of firm pressure with the diaphragm and during held inspiration and with the patient leaning forward. The rub may be localized or widespread but usually is heard over the left sternal border.

Pericardial rubs should be distinguished from the other superficial "scratchy" sounds. In patients with thyrotoxicosis, a to-and-fro, high-pitched sound may be heard over the left second interspace, which may simulate a pericardial friction rub (Means-Lerman scratch). Acute mediastinal emphysema, usually a benign, relatively common complication of open heart surgery, may be associated with a "crunching" noise over the precordium that is coincident with ventricular systole (mediastinal crunch). In patients with Ebstein's anomaly, the sail sound may be of a scratchy quality and may simulate a pericardial friction rub. The movement of the balloon flotation catheter or the transvenous pacing catheter across the tricuspid valve may cause an early systolic superficial scratchy sound that may also simulate a soft, one-component friction rub. These sounds frequently disappear with the alteration of patient position.

A pleuropericardial rub results from the friction between the inflamed pleura and the parietal pericardium, and can be heard only during the inspiratory phase of respiration. Twitching of the intercostal muscles, or of the diaphragm during artificial pacing, may cause a superficial scratchy and high-frequency sound unrelated to the cardiac cycle. These sounds are not to be confused with a pericardial friction rub. Inadvertent entry of air into the right ventricular cavity via the systemic venous system may occur during placement of catheters or pacemakers in the right side of the heart or as a complication of needle aspiration biopsy of the lungs. The movement of air in the right ventricular cavity with systole and diastole may produce peculiar "slushing" or crunching sound ("mill wheel" murmur) over the entire precordium, which may occasionally resemble pericardial friction rub.[140]

PHYSIOLOGIC AND PHARMACOLOGIC MANEUVERS IN THE DIFFERENTIAL DIAGNOSIS OF MURMURS AND HEART SOUNDS

Physiologic maneuvers and administration of vasoactive drugs may alter systemic hemodynamics sufficiently to change the character, behavior, and intensity of the heart sounds and murmurs and, therefore, can be applied for their diagnosis.

ABRUPT STANDING

Abrupt standing from the supine position decreases venous return to the heart and, consequently, right and left ventricular diastolic volumes and stroke volumes decline, along with some fall in arterial pressure and a reflex increase in heart rate. These hemodynamic changes are associated with a decreased intensity of the murmurs of pulmonary and aortic stenosis and of mitral and tricuspid regurgitation. In ventricular septal defect without significant pulmonary hypertension, the intensity of the systolic murmur tends to decrease. In hypertrophic cardiomyopathy, a decrease in left ventricular outflow size is associated with an increase in the intensity of the ejection systolic murmur along with a decrease or unchanged carotid pulse volume. In mitral valve prolapse, an earlier onset of the click and of the late systolic murmur are recognized.

SQUATTING

Squatting from a standing position is associated with a simultaneous increase in venous return and systemic vascular resistance and a rise in arterial pressure. Increased systemic vascular resistance and arterial pressure enhance mitral regurgitation and the magnitude of the left-to-right shunt in ventricular septal defect with an increased intensity of the systolic murmur in these conditions. In patients with tetralogy of Fallot, a decreased left-to-right shunt and increased pulmonary flow are associated with an increased intensity of the pulmonary ejection systolic murmur. The intensity of the diastolic murmur of aortic regurgitation also increases due to augmented regurgitation, and the intensity of the Austin Flint murmur may also increase. Squatting is a useful bedside maneuver for diagnosing hypertrophic cardiomyopathy, in which the intensity of the ejection systolic murmur promptly declines owing to an increased left ventricular volume and arterial pressure, which increase the effective orifice size of the outflow tract. The carotid pulse upstroke remains sharp, and the volume may increase. The intensity of the murmur of aortic stenosis, however, shows variable changes, depending on the type of hemodynamic response. A significant increase in systemic vascular resistance is associated with a decreased intensity and an increased left ventricular volume with increased intensity of the murmur. In patients with mitral valve prolapse, squatting delays the onset of the click and of the late systolic murmur.

VALSALVA MANEUVER

The hemodynamic changes resulting from a Valsalva maneuver are different in its different phases. During phase 1, with the onset of the maneuver, there is a transient increase in left ventricular output. During the straining phase (phase 2), with a decrease in venous return, right and left ventricular volumes, stroke volumes, mean arterial pressure, and pulse pressure decline with a reflex increase in heart rate. During phase 3 (release of Valsalva), which only lasts for a few cardiac cycles, there is a further reduction in left ventricular volume. Phase 4 is characterized by an increase in stroke volume and in arterial pressure and reflex slowing of heart rate (the overshoot).

Analysis of changes in the intensity and character of the murmur during phase 2 of the Valsalva maneuver is most useful and practical for the differential diagnosis. The intensity of flow murmurs, murmurs of aortic and pulmonary stenosis, tricuspid and mitral regurgitation, aortic and pulmonary regurgitation, and mitral and tricuspid stenosis decreases. The volume of the carotid pulse also decreases. In contrast, the murmur of hypertrophic cardiomyopathy increases in intensity as the left ventricular outflow size decreases with a decreased venous return. The carotid pulse volume also declines. For the same reasons, an early onset of the click and the murmur occur in mitral valve prolapse. During phase 4, the opposite effects are observed.

HAND GRIP

Hand grip (isovolumic exercise), another physical maneuver, can be applied at the bedside to distinguish murmurs of different etiology. During sustained hand grip for 20 to 30 seconds, systemic vascular resistance, arterial pressure, and cardiac output increase, along with an increase in left ventricular volume and filling pressure. These hemodynamic changes are associated with an increased severity of aortic and mitral regurgitation and increased left-to-right shunt in ventricular septal defect. The intensity of the murmurs in these conditions also increases. The intensity of the murmur of aortic stenosis tends to decrease, along with a decreased transvalvular pressure gradient. The diastolic murmur of mitral stenosis becomes accentuated because of an increased heart rate and cardiac output. In hypertrophic cardiomyopathy, the intensity of the ejection systolic murmur softens due to an increased left ventricular volume. For a similar reason, the click and the murmur of mitral valve prolapse are delayed. Hemodynamic changes during hand grip are variable and not always similar in all patients. For example, the increase in arterial pressure may be relatively greater than the increase in heart rate or cardiac output; thus, the changes in intensity of the murmur in these different conditions are not always predictable. This maneuver is most useful in differentiating between the ejection systolic murmur of aortic stenosis and the regurgitant murmur of mitral insufficiency.

POSTECTOPIC POTENTIATION

If premature beats occur during clinical examination, analysis of the changes in intensity and character of the murmur during the postectopic beat can provide clues to the diagnosis of valvular heart disease.

Following a premature beat, the postectopic pause is associated with an increased ventricular volume; however, myocardial contractility also increases due to postectopic potentiation. In most circumstances, the effect of increased contractility supercedes the effect of an increased ventricular volume. Both in aortic stenosis and in hypertrophic cardiomyopathy the intensity of the ejection systolic murmur increases; however, the carotid pulse volume increases in aortic stenosis and decreases or remains unchanged in hypertrophic cardiomyopathy. The murmur of aortic regurgitation may also increase due to an increased arterial pressure, which augments the regurgitant flow. Tricuspid regurgitation murmurs also increase due to an increased right ventricular volume. The pansystolic murmur of mitral regurgitation, particularly of rheumatic origin, does not usually change. In mitral valve prolapse, postectopic potentiation causes a rapid rate of ejection and, therefore, an earlier onset of the click and the murmur.

AMYL NITRITE

Inhalation of amyl nitrite is the most practical pharmacologic maneuver that can be applied at the bedside.[141-144] Amyl nitrite is predominantly an arteriolar dilator and initially produces marked vasodilation and reduction in arterial pressure, and then a reflex increase in heart rate, which is followed by increased venous return, stroke volume, and cardiac output. Decreased systemic vascular resistance and arterial pressure reduce mitral regurgitation and left-to-right shunts in ventricular septal defect, and the systolic murmurs in these conditions also soften. The ejection systolic murmur of aortic and pulmonary stenosis, hypertrophic cardiomyopathy, and innocent systolic flow murmurs are all accentuated. In aortic stenosis, carotid pulse volume increases, but in hypertrophic cardiomyopathy it decreases or remains unchanged.

Decreased arterial pressure is associated with an increased right-to-left shunt and reduced pulmonary flow in tetralogy of Fallot; the systolic ejection murmur, therefore, becomes softer.

Amyl nitrite inhalation also can differentiate between an Austin Flint murmur and the murmur of mitral stenosis. The duration and intensity of the Austin Flint murmur diminishes as the regurgitant flow of aortic insufficiency declines due to decreased systemic vascular resistance and arterial pressure. The murmur of aortic regurgitation also becomes softer. The murmur of mitral stenosis becomes louder because of tachycardia and an increased cardiac output. The A_2-opening snap interval decreases concurrently. In mitral valve prolapse, the click and late systolic murmur occur earlier following inhalation of amyl nitrite.

METHOXAMINE

An increase in systemic vascular resistance and arterial pressure following administration of methoxamine or phenylephrine produce effects opposite to those of amyl nitrite. Both agents cause reflex bradycardia and a lower cardiac output. The murmur of aortic regurgitation (diastolic), mitral regurgitation, ventricular septal defect, and tetralogy of Fallot increase in intensity. The murmurs of aortic stenosis and hypertrophic cardiomyopathy become softer, and the click and murmur of mitral valve prolapse are delayed. The A_2-opening snap interval in mitral stenosis becomes longer as a result of increased arterial pressure. Occasionally, isoproterenol infusion is used for diagnosing hypertrophic cardiomyopathy, and it increases the intensity of the murmur with little or no change in the carotid pulse volume. Of all the pharmacologic agents, amyl nitrite is the easiest to use at the bedside and provides adequate information for the differential diagnosis of the cause of a murmur.

TABLE 23.14 BEDSIDE DIAGNOSIS OF CARDIOMYOPATHY

Hypertrophic Cardiomyopathy	Dilated Cardiomyopathy	Restrictive Cardiomyopathy
Ejection systolic murmur with normal or sharp carotid pulse upstroke	Displaced and sustained left ventricular impulse in the absence of causes of volume-loaded left ventricle (aortic or mitral regurgitation, ventricular septal defect)	Elevated jugular venous pressure; sharp *y* descent; manifestations of systemic venous hypertension (peripheral edema) with normally located or only slightly displaced cardiac impulse
Sustained, normally located or slightly displaced left ventricular impulse with or without palpable *a* wave in the absence of systemic hypertension or aortic stenosis	*or*	*or*
Giant T wave inversion with left ventricular hypertrophy by voltage in the electrocardiogram without apparent cause	Displaced and sustained left ventricular impulse in the absence of causes for left ventricular hypertrophy (systemic hypertension, left ventricular outflow obstruction)	Other findings of constrictive pericarditis, such as Kussmaul's sign
Simultaneous palpation of the carotid pulse and auscultation of the character of the ejection systolic murmur and the behavior of S_2 during maneuvers	Evaluation of left ventricular systolic function and left ventricular cavity size	Evaluation for pulmonary hypertension and atrioventricular valvular regurgitation
Example: Increased intensity of the ejection systolic murmur with decreased or unchanged carotid pulse volume and reversed splitting of S_2 in the absence of left bundle branch block during standing, Valsalva maneuver, or amyl nitrite inhalation	*Example:* Sustained left ventricular impulse and reversed S_2 in the absence of left bundle branch block suggest decreased ejection fraction and displaced left ventricular impulse-dilatation of the left ventricle.	*Example:* Loud P_2, prominent and sustained left parasternal lift, parasternal systolic impulse, and tricuspid and/or mitral regurgitation murmurs favor restrictive cardiomyopathy.

Note: The purpose of bedside evaluation in diagnosing various types of cardiomyopathy is to discover the manifestations of their important pathophysiologic characteristics. Hypertrophic cardiomyopathy is characterized by normal systolic function and left ventricular hypertrophy without cavitary dilatation. Left ventricular outflow obstruction is frequently present and can be recognized at the bedside. Increased left ventricular cavity size with depressed left ventricular systolic function without massive left ventricular hypertrophy are the usual pathologic features of dilated cardiomyopathy. Thus, a displaced and sustained left ventricular impulse are the usual physical findings. Restriction of ventricular filling, normal or only slightly increased ventricular cavity size, and normal or only slightly decreased ventricular systolic function are the pathophysiologic features in restrictive cardiomyopathy. Thus, manifestations of abnormally elevated ventricular diastolic pressures in the presence of a relatively normal cardiac size dominate the clinical picture.

CONCLUSIONS

Clinical assessment should begin with a careful history, which provides important information regarding the underlying cardiovascular pathology and, more importantly, about the functional status of the patient, which directly reflects the severity of the disease. A systematic approach to the physical examination should follow: inspection, palpation, and auscultation. Careful physical examination and attention to the details of the findings are often rewarding, not only for the diagnosis of cardiac abnormalities but also for the assessment of associated hemodynamic abnormalities. In adult patients, it is often possible to suspect primary myocardial or pericardial disease at the bedside from abnormal findings, and the appropriate investigations can then be performed to confirm the diagnosis (Table 23.14). Detection of a murmur is usually the first indication of the presence of valvular heart disease. An analysis of the murmurs, heart sounds, ejection and non-ejection sounds, jugular venous and arterial pulse, and precordial impulse, coupled with information obtained from the electrocardiogram and chest film provide clues to the nature of the valvular heart disease. It needs to be emphasized that history and physical examinations can only furnish the physician with qualitative information. For quantitative assessments, other noninvasive and frequently invasive tests are required. Furthermore, the abnormalities specific to a cardiovascular problem may not always be present or detected at the bedside. Nonetheless, bedside clinical examination should be considered as the most important initial investigation in all patients with suspected cardiovascular abnormalities, and subsequent investigations should be formulated based on the results of an initial clinical evaluation.

REFERENCES

1. Greenberg LM, Geppert C, Worthen HG et al: Scleredema "adultorium" in children. Rev World Lit Pediatr 32:1044, 1963
2. Shy GM, Drager GA: A neurologic syndrome associated with orthostatic hypotension: A clinical-pathologic study. Arch Neurol 2:511, 1960
3. Keith NM, Wagener HP, Barker ND: Some different types of essential hypertension: Their course and prognosis. Am J Med Sci 197:332, 1939
4. Holdveen-Geronimus M, Merriam JC Jr: Cholesterol embolization: From pathological curiosity to clinical entity. Circulation 35:946, 1967
5. Cohn J, Hamosh P: Experimental observations on pulsus paradoxus and hepatojugular reflux. In Reddy PS (ed): Pericardial Disease, p 249. New York, Raven Press, 1982
6. Dell'Italia LJ, Starling MR, O'Rourke RA: Physical examination for exclusion of hemodynamically important right ventricular infarction. Ann Intern Med 99:608, 1983
7. Gleason WL, Braunwald E: Studies on Starling's law of the heart: VI. Relationships between left ventricular end-diastolic volume and stroke volume in man with observations on the mechanism of pulsus alternans. Circulation 25:841, 1962
8. Parmley W, Tomoda H, Fujimura S et al: Relation between pulsus alternans and transient occlusion of the left anterior descending coronary artery. Cardiovasc Res 6:709, 1972
9. McGaughey MD, Maughan L, Sunagawa K et al: Alternating contractility in pulsus alternans studied in the isolated canine heart. Circulation 71:357, 1985
10. Donhurst AL, Howard P, Leathart GL: Pulsus paradoxus. Lancet 1:746, 1952
11. Singh S, Wann LS, Klopfenstein HS et al: Usefulness of right ventricular diastolic collapse in diagnosing cardiac tamponade and comparison to pulsus paradoxus. Am J Cardiol 57:652, 1986
12. Massumi RA, Mason DT, Zakuddin V et al: Reversed pulsus paradoxus. N Engl J Med 289:1272, 1973
13. Orchard RC, Craig E: Dicrotic pulse after open heart surgery. Circulation 62:1107, 1980
14. Duchosal PW, Ferrero C, Lupin A et al: Advances in the clinical evaluation of aortic stenosis by arterial pulse recording of the neck. Am Heart J 51:861, 1956
15. Donoso E, Sapin SO, Kuhn LA et al: Use of indirect arterial pulse tracings in the diagnosis of congenital heart disease: Congenital subaortic and aortic stenosis. Pediatrics 18:205, 1956
16. Benchimol A, Dimond EG, Yen Shen: Ejection time in aortic stenosis and mitral stenosis. Am J Cardiol 5:728, 1960
17. Daoud G, Reppert EH, Butterworth JS: Basal systolic murmurs and carotid pulse curve in the diagnosis of calcareous aortic stenosis. Ann Intern Med 50:323, 1959
18. Robinson B: The carotid pulse: I. Diagnosis of aortic stenosis by external recordings. Br Heart J 25:51, 1963
19. Braunwald E, Roberts WC, Goldblatt A et al: Aortic stenosis: Physiological, pathological and clinical concepts. Ann Intern Med 58:494, 1963
20. Epstein EJ, Coulshed N: Assessment of aortic stenosis from the external carotid pulse wave. Br Heart J 26:84, 1964
21. Agress CM, Fields LG: New method for analyzing heart vibrations. Am J Cardiol 4:184, 1959
22. Deliyannis AA, Gillam PMS, Mounsey JPD et al: The cardiac impulse and the motion of the heart. Br Heart J 26:393, 1964
23. Benchimol E, Dimond EG: The normal and abnormal apex cardiogram. Am J Cardiol 12:368, 1963
24. Sutton GC, Craige E: Quantitation of precordial movement: I. Normal subjects. Circulation 35:476, 1967
25. Sutton GC, Prewitt TA, Craige E: Relationship between quantitated precordial movement and left ventricular function. Circulation 31:179, 1970
26. Mattleman SJ, Hakki AH, Iskandrian AS et al: Reliability of bedside evaluation in determining left ventricular function: Correlation with left ventricular ejection fraction determined by radionuclide ventriculography. J Am Coll Cardiol 1:417, 1983
27. Braunwald E, Lambrew CT, Rockoff SD et al: Idiopathic hypertrophic subaortic stenosis: I. A description of the disease based upon an analysis of 64 patients. Circulation 30(suppl IV):IV-3, 1964
28. Tafur E, Cohen LS, Levine HD: The apex cardiogram in left ventricular outflow tract obstruction. Circulation 30:392, 1964
29. Eddleman EE Jr, Harrison TR: The kinetocardiogram in patients with ischemic heart disease. Prog Cardiovasc Dis 6:189, 1963
30. Voigt GC, Friesinger GC: The use of apex cardiogram in the assessment of left ventricular diastolic pressure. Circulation 41:1015, 1970
31. Fortuin NJ, Craige E: On the mechanism of the Austin-Flint murmur. Circulation 45:558, 1972
32. Tucker WT, Knowles JL, Eddelman EE Jr: Mitral insufficiency: Cardiac mechanics as studied with the kinetocardiogram and ballisto cardiogram. Circulation 12:278, 1955
33. Armstrong TG, Gotsman MS: The left parasternal lift in tricuspid incompetence. Am Heart J 88:183, 1974
34. El-Sherif A, El-said G: Jugular, hepatic and precordial pulsations in constrictive pericarditis. Br Heart J 33:305, 1971
35. Craige E, Fortuin NJ: Noninvasive measurement of ventricular function in chronic ischemic heart disease. In Likoff W, Segal BL, Insull W et al (eds): Atherosclerosis and Coronary Heart Disease, p 221. New York, Grune & Stratton, 1972
36. Luisada AA, MacCanon DM, Kumar S et al: Changing views on the mechanism of the first and second heart sounds. Am Heart J 88:503, 1974
37. Leatham A: Splitting of the first and second heart sounds. Lancet 267:607, 1954
38. O'Toole JD, Reddy PS, Curtiss EL et al: The contribution of tricuspid valve closure to the first heart sound: An intracardiac micromanometer study. Circulation 53:752, 1976
39. Warder W, Craig E: The first heart sound and ejection sounds: Echo-phonocardiographic correlation with valvular events. Am J Cardiol 35:346, 1975
40. Laniado S, Yellin EL, Miller H et al: Temporal relation of the first heart sound to closure of the mitral valve. Circulation 47:1006, 1973
41. Millis P, Craige E: Echocardiography. Prog Cardiovasc Dis 20:337, 1978
42. Kostis JB: Mechanisms of heart sounds. Am Heart J 89:546, 1975
43. Shah PM, Kramer DH, Gramiak R: Influence of the timing of atrial systole in mitral valve closure and on the first heart sound in man. Am J Cardiol 26:231, 1970
44. Leatham A: Auscultation of the Heart and Phonocardiography, 2nd ed. London, J and A Churchill, 1975
45. Dashkoff N, Fortuin NJ, Hutchins GM: Clinical features of severe mitral regurgitation due to floppy mitral valve. Circulation 50(suppl 3):60, 1974
46. Mann T, McLaurin L, Grossman W et al: Acute aortic regurgitation due to infective endocarditis. N Engl J Med 293:108, 1975
47. Harris A: Pacemaker "heart sound." Br Heart J 29:608, 1967
48. Crews TL, Pridie RB, Benham R et al: Auscultatory and phonocardiographic findings in Ebstein's anomaly: Correlation of first heart sound with ultrasonic records of tricuspid valve movement. Br Heart J 34:681, 1972
49. Sabbah HN, Stein PD: Investigation of the theory and mechanism of the origin of the second heart sound. Circ Res 29:874, 1976
50. Hirschfeld S, Liebman J, Borkat G et al: Intracardiac pressure–sound correlates of echocardiographic aortic valve closure. Circulation 55:602, 1977
51. Chandraratna A, Lopez J, Cohen L: Echocardiographic observations on the

mechanism of production of the second heart sound. Circulation 51:292, 1975
52. Harris A, Sutton G: The normal second heart sound. Br Heart J 30:739, 1968
53. Harris A, Leatham A, Sutton G: The second heart sound in pulmonary hypertension. Br Heart J 30:743, 1968
54. Leatham A, Gray I: Auscultatory and phonocardiographic signs of atrial septal defect. Br Heart J 18:193, 1956
55. Leatham A, Towers M: Splitting of the second heart sound in health. Br Heart J 13:575, 1951
56. Curtiss EI, Mathews RG, Shaver JA: Mechanism of normal splitting of the second heart sound. Circulation 51:157, 1975
57. Shaver JA, O'Toole JD, Curtiss E et al: Second heart sound. In Physiological Principles of Heart Sounds and Murmurs, monograph No. 46, p 58. New York, American Heart Association, 1975
58. Boyer SH, Chisholm AW: Physiologic splitting of the second heart sound. Circulation 18:1010, 1958
59. Castle FR, Jones KL: The mechanism of respiratory variations in splitting of the second heart sound. Circulation 24:180, 1961
60. Dornhorst AC, Howard P, Leathart GL: Respiratory variations in blood pressure. Circulation 6:553, 1952
61. Leatham A, Weitzman DW: Auscultatory and phonocardiographic signs of pulmonary stenosis. Br Heart J 19:303, 1957
62. Brigden W, Leatham A: Mitral incompetence. Br Heart J 15:55, 1953
63. Leatham A, Segal B: Auscultatory and phonocardiographic signs of ventricular septal defect with left to right shunt. Circulation 25:318, 1962
64. Beck W, Schrire V, Vogelpoel L: Splitting of the second heart sound in constrictive pericarditis with observations on the mechanism of pulsus paradoxus. Am Heart J 64:765, 1962
65. Damore S, Murgo JP, Bloom KR et al: Second heart sound dynamics in atrial septal defect. Circulation 64(suppl IV):28, 1981
66. Gray I: Paradoxical splitting of the second heart sound. Br Heart J 18:21, 1956
67. Yurchak PM, Gorlin R: Paradoxical splitting of the second heart sound in coronary heart disease. N Engl J Med 269:741, 1963
68. Abrams J: The third and fourth heart sounds. Primary Cardiol 8:47, 1982
69. Ozawa Y, Smith D, Craige E: Origin of the third heart sound: II. Studies in human subjects. Circulation 67:399, 1983
70. Ozawa Y, Smith D, Craige E: Localization of the origin of the third heart sound. Circulation 66(suppl II):210, 1982
71. Shah PM, Jackson D: Third heart sound and summation gallop. In Leon DF, Shaver JA (eds): Physiological Principles of Heart Sounds and Murmurs, monograph No. 46, p 79. New York, American Heart Association, 1975
72. Abdulla AM, Frank MJ, Erdin RA Jr et al: Clinical significance and hemodynamic correlates of the third heart sound gallop in aortic regurgitation. A guide to optimal timing of cardiac catheterization. Circulation 64:463, 1981
73. Lee DC-S, Johnson RA, Bingham JB et al: Heart failure in outpatients: A randomized trial of digoxin versus placebo. N Engl J Med 306:699, 1982
74. Nixon PGF: The genesis of the third heart sound. Am Heart J 65:712, 1963
75. Gibson TC, Madry R, Grossman W et al: The A wave of the apex cardiogram and left ventricular diastolic stiffness. Circulation 49:441, 1974
76. Goldblatt A, Aygen MM, Braunwald E: Hemodynamic phonocardiographic correlations of the fourth heart sound in aortic stenosis. Circulation 26:92, 1962
77. Hill JL, O'Rourke RA, Lewis RP et al: The diagnostic value of the atrial gallop in acute myocardial infarction. Am Heart J 78:194, 1969
78. Sutton GC, Chatterjee K, Caves PK: Diagnosis of severe mitral regurgitation due to nonrheumatic chordal abnormalities. Br Heart J 35:877, 1973
79. Kesteloot H, Willems J: Relationship between the right apex cardiogram and the right ventricular dynamics. Acta Cardiol 22:64, 1967
80. Dayem MKA, Wasfi RM, Bentall HH et al: Investigation and treatment of constrictive pericarditis. Thorax 22:242, 1967
81. Hancock EW: The ejection sound in aortic stenosis. Am J Med 40:569, 1966
82. Leech G, Millis P, Leatham A: The diagnosis of a nonstenotic bicuspid aortic valve. Br Heart J 40:941, 1978
83. Leatham A, Vogelpoel L: Early systolic sound in dilatation of the pulmonary artery. Br Heart J 16:21, 1954
84. Hultgren HN, Reeve R, Cohn K et al: The ejection click of valvular pulmonic stenosis. Circulation 40:631, 1969
85. Curtiss EI, Reddy PS, O'Toole JD et al: Alterations of right ventricular systolic time intervals by chronic pressure and volume overloading. Circulation 53:997, 1976
86. Millis P, Amara I, McLaurin LP et al: Noninvasive assessment of pulmonary hypertension from right ventricular isovolumic contraction time. Am J Cardiol 46:272, 1980
87. Barlow JB, Bosman CK: Aneurysm protrusion of the posterior leaflet of the mitral valve: An auscultatory-electrocardiographic syndrome. Am Heart J 71:166, 1966
88. Roman JA, Perloff JK, Harvey WP: Systolic clicks and the late systolic murmur: Intracardiac phonocardiographic evidence of their mitral valve origin. Am Heart J 70:319, 1965
89. Leon DF, Leonard JJ, Kroetz FW et al: Late systolic murmurs, clicks and whoops arising from the mitral valve: Transseptal intracardiac phonocardiographic analysis. Am Heart J 72:325, 1966
90. Criley JM, Lewis KB, Humphries JO et al: Prolapse of the mitral valve: Clinical and cine-angiocardiographic findings. Br Heart J 28:488, 1966
91. Mathey DG, DeCoodt PR, Allen HN et al: The determinants of onset of mitral valve prolapse in the systolic click-late systolic murmur syndrome. Circulation 53:872, 1976
92. Behar VS, Whalen RE, McIntosh HD: Ballooning mitral valve in patients with the "precordial honk" or "whoop." Am J Cardiol 20:789, 1967
93. Rackley CE, Whalen RE, Floyd WL et al: Precordial Honk. Am J Cardiol 17:609, 1966
94. Sze KC, Shah PM: Pseudoejection sound in hypertrophic subaortic stenosis: An echocardiographic correlative study. Circulation 54:504, 1976
95. Craige E: Editorial on the genesis of heart sounds: Contribution made by echocardiographic studies. Circulation 53:207, 1976
96. Millward DK, McLaurin LP, Craige E: Echocardiographic studies to explain opening snaps in the presence of nonstenotic mitral valves. Am J Cardiol 31:64, 1973
97. Wei J, Fortuin NJ: Diastolic sounds and murmurs associated with mitral valve prolapse. Circulation 63:559, 1981
98. Millis P, Craige E: Echocardiography. Prog Cardiovasc Dis 20:337, 1978
99. Spodick DH: Hypertrophic obstructive cardiomyopathy of the left ventricular (idiopathic hypertrophic subaortic stenosis). In Burch GE, Brest AN (eds): Cardiovascular Clinics, vol 4, p 156. Philadelphia, FA Davis, 1972
100. Smith ND, Raizada V, Abrams J: Auscultation of the normally functioning prosthetic valve. Ann Intern Med 95:594, 1981
101. Dayem MKA, Raftery EB: Phonocardiogram of the ball-and-cage aortic valve prosthesis. Br Heart J 29:446, 1967
102. Leachman RD, Cokkinos DVP: Absence of opening click in dehiscence of mitral valve prosthesis. N Engl J Med 281:461, 1969
103. Assanelli D, Aquilina M, Marangoni S et al: Echo-phonocardiographic evaluation of the Bjork-Shiley mitral prosthesis. Am J Cardiol 57:165, 1986
104. Sagar KB, Wann LS, Paulsen WHJ et al: Doppler echocardiographic evaluation of Hancock and Bjork-Shiley prosthetic valves. J Am Coll Cardiol 7:681, 1986
105. Perloff JK: The Clinical Recognition of Congenital Heart Disease. Philadelphia, WB Saunders, 1970
106. Perloff JK: Innocent or normal murmurs. In Russek HI (ed): Cardiovascular Problems: Perspectives and Progress. Baltimore, University Park Press, 1976
107. DeLeon AC Jr, Perloff JK, Twigg H et al: The straight back syndrome: Clinical cardiovascular manifestations. Circulation 32:193, 1965
108. Perloff JK, Harvey WP: Auscultatory and phonocardiographic manifestations of pure mitral regurgitation. Prog Cardiovasc Dis 5:172, 1962
109. Perloff JK: Auscultatory and phonocardiographic manifestations of pulmonary hypertension. Prog Cardiovasc Dis 9:303, 1967
110. Craige E: Phonocardiography in interventricular septal defects. Am Heart J 60:51, 1960
111. Hollman A, Morgan JJ, Goodwin JF et al: Auscultatory and phonocardiographic findings in ventricular septal defect. Circulation 28:94, 1963
112. Cheng TO: Some new observations on the syndrome of papillary muscle dysfunction. Am J Med 47:924, 1969
113. Roberts WC, Perloff JK: Mitral valvular disease: A clinicopathologic survey of the conditions causing the mitral valve to function abnormally. Ann Intern Med 77:939, 1972
114. Ronan JA, Steelman RB, DeLeon AC et al: The clinical diagnosis of acute severe mitral insufficiency. Am J Cardiol 27:284, 1971
115. Perloff JK: Therapeutics of nature: The invisible sutures of spontaneous closure. Am Heart J 82:581, 1971
116. Devereux RB, Perloff JK, Reichek N et al: Mitral valve prolapse. Circulation 54:3, 1976
117. Hutter AM, Dinsmore RE, Willerson JT et al: Early systolic clicks due to mitral valve prolapse. Circulation 40:516, 1971
118. Suwa M, Hirota Y, Kino M et al: Late diastolic whoop in severe aortic regurgitation. Am J Cardiol 57:699, 1986
119. Harvey WP, Corrado MA, Perloff JK: "Right-sided" murmurs of aortic insufficiency. Am J Med Sci 245:533, 1963
120. Dock W, Zoneraich S: A diastolic murmur arising in a stenosed coronary artery. Am J Med 742:617, 1967
121. Wood P: An appreciation of mitral stenosis. Br Med J 1:1051, 1954
122. Perloff JK, Harvey WP: Clinical recognition of tricuspid stenosis. Circulation 22:346, 1960
123. Nasser WK, Davis RH, Dillon JC et al: Atrial myxoma: I. Clinical and pathologic features in nine cases. Am Heart J 83:694, 1972
124. Fortuin NJ, Craige E: Echocardiographic studies of genesis of mitral diastolic murmurs. Br Heart J 35:75, 1973
125. Hubbard TF, Dunn FL, Neis DD: A phonocardiographic study of apical diastolic murmurs in pure mitral insufficiency. Am Heart J 57:223, 1959
126. Nixon PGF, Wooler GH: Left ventricular filling pressure gradient in mitral incompetence. Br Heart J 25:382, 1963
127. Wooley CF, Levin HS, Leighton RF et al: Intracardiac sound and pressure

128. Fortuin NJ, Craige E: On the mechanism of the Austin-Flint murmur. Circulation 45:558, 1972
129. Reddy PS, Curtiss EI, Salerni R et al: Sound pressure correlates of the Austin-Flint murmur: An intracardiac sound study. Circulation 53:210, 1976
130. Criley JM, Hermer AJ: Crescendo presystolic murmur of mitral stenosis with atrial fibrillation. N Engl J Med 285:1284, 1971
131. Rutishauser W, Wirz P, Gander M et al: Atriogenic diastolic reflux in patients with atrioventricular heart block. Circulation 34:807, 1966
132. Panidis IP, Ross J, Munley B et al: Diastolic mitral regurgitation in patients with atrioventricular conduction abnormalities: A common finding by Doppler echocardiography. J Am Coll Cardiol 7:768, 1986
133. Craige E, Milward DK: Diastolic and continuous murmurs. Prog Cardiovasc Dis 14:38, 1971
134. Neil C, Mounsey P: Auscultation in patent ductus arteriosus with a description of two fistulae simulating patent ductus. Br Heart J 20:61, 1958
135. Gasul BM, Arcilla RA, Fell EH et al: Congenital coronary arteriovenous fistula. Pediatrics 25:531, 1960
136. Harris A, Jefferson K, Chatterjee K: Coronary arteriovenous fistula with aneurysm of coronary sinus. Br Heart J 31:400, 1969
137. Myers GS, Scannel JG, Wyman JM et al: Atypical patent ductus arteriosus with absence of the usual aortic pressure gradient and the characteristic murmur. Am Heart J 41:819, 1951
138. Steinbrunn W, Cohn KE, Selzer A: Atrial septal defect associated with mitral stenosis: The Lutembacher syndrome revisited. Am J Med 48:295, 1970
139. Campbell M, Suzman SS: Coarctation of the aorta. Br Heart J 9:185, 1947
140. Gottlieb JD, Ericsson JA, Sweet RB: Venous air embolism. Anesth Analg 44:773, 1965
141. Beck W, Schrire V, Bogelpoel L et al: Hemodynamic effects of amyl nitrite and phenylephrine on the normal human circulation and their relative changes in cardiac murmur. Am J Cardiol 8:341, 1961
142. Perloff JK, Calvin J, DeLeon AC et al: Systemic hemodynamic effects of amyl nitrite in normal man. Am Heart J 66:460, 1963
143. DeLeon AC, Perloff JK: The pulmonary hemodynamic effects of amyl nitrite in normal man. Am Heart J 72:337, 1966
144. Epstein SE, Henry WL, Clark CE et al: Asymmetric septal hypertrophy. Ann Intern Med 81:650, 1974

GENERAL REFERENCES

Braunwald E: The history. In Braunwald E (ed): Heart Disease: A Textbook of Cardiovascular Medicine, p 3. Philadelphia, WB Saunders, 1984

Braunwald E: The physical examination in heart disease. In Braunwald E (ed): Heart Disease: A Textbook of Cardiovascular Medicine, p 14. Philadelphia, WB Saunders, 1984

Constant J: Bedside Cardiology, 2nd ed. Boston, Little, Brown & Co, 1976

Craige E: Echocardiography and other noninvasive techniques to elucidate heart murmur and to solve diagnostic problems. In Braunwald E (ed): Heart Disease: A Textbook of Cardiovascular Medicine, p 70. Philadelphia, WB Saunders, 1980

Craige E: Heart sounds: Phonocardiography, carotid, apex, and jugular venous pulse tracings, systolic time intervals. In Braunwald E (ed): Heart Disease: A Textbook of Cardiovascular Medicine, p 40. Philadelphia, WB Saunders, 1984

Eddleman EE Jr: Inspection and palpation of the precordium. In Hurst JW (ed): The Heart, p 192. New York, McGraw-Hill, 1970

Harvey PW: Gallop sounds, clicks, snaps, whoops, honks, and other sounds. In Hurst JW (ed): The Heart, 4th ed, p 255. New York, McGraw-Hill, 1978

Leatham A: Auscultation of the Heart and Phonocardiography, 2nd ed. London, JI Churchill, 1975

Leatham A: An Introduction to the Examination of the Cardiovascular System. Oxford, Oxford University Press, 1977

Leatham A: The first and second heart sounds. In Hurst JW (ed): The Heart, 4th ed, p 237. New York, McGraw-Hill, 1978

Millis P, Craige E: Echophonocardiography. Prog Cardiovasc Dis 20:337, 1978

Perloff JK: Systolic, diastolic and continuous murmurs. In Hurst JW (ed): The Heart, 4th ed, p 268. New York, McGraw-Hill, 1978

Silverman ME, Hurst JW: Inspection of the heart. In Hurst JW (ed): The Heart, 4th ed, p 162. Philadelphia, McGraw-Hill, 1978

Tavel ME: Clinical Phonocardiography and External Pulse Recording. Chicago, Year Book Medical Publishers, 1967

Wood P: The chief symptoms of heart disease. In Wood P (ed): Diseases of the Heart and Circulation. London, Eyre & Spottiswoode, 1956

Wood P: Physical signs. In Wood P (ed): Diseases of the Heart and Circulation. London, Eyre and Spottiswoode, 1956

EXAMINATION OF THE LUNGS

Thomas Killip

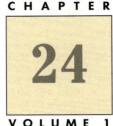

CHAPTER 24
VOLUME 1

Diseases of the heart and lung are both clinically and physiologically intertwined. The lung sits astride the circulation, receiving venous blood from the right heart and delivering oxygenated blood to the left heart. Disease of the heart affects the lungs; disease of the lung influences cardiac function. Thus, in the patient with heart disease, careful examination of the chest and the lungs may provide important clues about the status of the cardiovascular system. Furthermore, symptoms such as chest pain, dyspnea, or shortness of breath on exertion may reflect either cardiac or pulmonary disorder. Examination of the chest may provide the evidence to pinpoint the cause of the complaints.

LUNG FUNCTION

Normally the lungs and the chest are in a state of dynamic tension. The elastic recoil of the lungs tends toward collapse, whereas the configuration of the chest tends toward expansion. If the chest is incised, producing a pneumothorax, the lungs retract and reduce in volume yet the hemithorax freed from the elastic recoil expands. Thus, in the patient with pneumothorax, the hemithorax on the afflicted side has a greater volume than the uninvolved side.

Ventilation, an act usually below the level of consciousness, increases thoracic volume by elevation of the ribs, contraction of the scalene and intercostal muscles, and descent of the diaphragm. Intrathoracic pressure is reduced, and the respiratory tidal volume fills the increased thoracic space. In the absence of airway obstruction, expiration is passive. Throughout the ventilatory cycle of inspiration–expiration, intrathoracic pressure is negative. In the presence of airway obstruction, however, as in cardiac asthma, for example, expiration requires muscular work, air flow becomes turbulent, and intrathoracic pressure reverses from negative to positive.

In the normal chest, the ratio of anteroposterior to lateral diameter is about 0.8 to 1.0. The anteroposterior diameter is measured at the level of T-8; the lateral measurement is taken at the level of the right diaphragm. Changes in chest configuration due to skeletal or muscular abnormality may be associated with secondary cardiac disease. A well-known example is the development of cor pulmonale in severe kyphoscoliosis. The phenotype of the straight back syndrome may be recognized by simple frontal and lateral inspection.

A cardinal symptom of pulmonary or cardiac disease is *dyspnea*. Strictly speaking, dyspnea is defined as a subjective sensation of difficulty in breathing. The physiologist emphasizes that in dyspnea, breathing has reached a level of conscious awareness, while the clinician emphasizes apparent shortness of breath or breathlessness.[1] Clinicians frequently make the statement that a patient is dyspneic, equating dyspnea with the bedside observation that respirations appear to be labored, difficult, or associated with air hunger. Whether dyspnea is normal or abnormal depends on the circumstances. An awareness of forceful breathing is perfectly normal following vigorous physical exercise. Unusual breathlessness upon minimal or moderate exertion, and especially at rest, is cause for clinical concern and is usually but not always an indication of cardiopulmonary disease. Exercise-induced dyspnea and hence limitation of exertion is a cardinal symptom of heart or lung disease.

Physiologic studies have shown that dyspnea is closely correlated with a measurable excess ventilation for the level of physical activity. Respiratory rate is increased, and the oxygen cost of breathing is above normal. Dyspnea has been correlated with reduced vital capacity, encroachment of minute ventilation on possible maximal voluntary ventilation, and increased work of breathing. Since dyspnea involves a conscious awareness, it is generally agreed that the brain must be receiving messages from thoracic structures.[1,2] It is not certain where these thoracic structures are located, although reduction in pulmonary compliance and increased work of breathing have been well correlated with the sensation of dyspnea in many subjects, suggesting that the chest wall is involved. Other studies have pointed to the J receptors, located near the pulmonary capillaries and the alveoli, which transmit impulses centrally by way of unmyelinated vagal fibers.[3]

In many patients with heart disease, symptoms may be minimal or absent at rest. It is characteristic of most cardiac disorders, however, that symptoms reflecting abnormal response of the heart to stress are made worse by exercise. Thus, dyspnea may be absent at rest but may appear dramatically during and following exertion. In left ventricular dysfunction (or mitral valve abnormality) exercise induces pulmonary congestion secondary to increased pulmonary venous pressure, edema of pulmonary structures, and consequent increased resistance to air flow in the small airways of the lung. The condition may be permanent or reversible, depending on etiology and acuteness of onset. Dyspnea may be marked in pulmonary edema, for example, when lung compliance is reduced to as much as one tenth of normal, but following successful treatment, pulmonary function can return to near normal and the sensation completely disappear.

Orthopnea, a special case of dyspnea when the patient is prone, has been extensively studied.[1] The sensation appears well correlated with changes in pulmonary compliance associated with disease of the left side of the heart. The lungs are stiffest with the patient lying flat. Compliance is increased in the upright position. The most reasonable explanation for the changes relates the position of the lung and its blood volume to the position of the heart. With the patient supine, most of the lung is below the heart, thus hydraulic pressures in the pulmonary venous circuit are increased. With the patient upright, major portions of the lung are above the heart and the distending vascular pressures within the lung are decreased, with consequent reduction in stiffness and a fall in the work and oxygen cost of breathing. With left ventricular failure and consequent high filling pressure, these changes are exaggerated. In patients with fluid retention, mobilization of extravascular fluid into the circulation contributes to left ventricular overload when the patient has been lying down for a time, thus contributing to nocturnal orthopnea.

In *cardiac asthma*, increased pulmonary venous pressure is associated with a reduction of the lumen of the small intrapulmonary airways and thickening of the bronchiolar walls by secretions and edema. High intrathoracic pressure is required to overcome the obstructed airways. Resistance is high during expiration, turbulent flow ensues, and the narrow small bronchioles may narrow even further and collapse during forced expiration. Expiration is prolonged, and a characteristic wheezing is audible at the bedside, which can be confirmed by auscultation.

Abnormality of lung function may often be recognized by two simple observations. A normal person can exhale all available air in 6 seconds. In patients with chronic obstructive pulmonary disease, the exhalation is excessively prolonged or is interrupted because of fatigue. Another test is the ability to blow out a paper match held 3 inches from the mouth without pursing the lips. Failure to snuff out the match suggests serious reduction of exhaled air velocity. Of course, false-positive and false-negative results occur, and interpretation of this test depends on proper evaluation of all relevant clinical factors.

APPROACH TO THE PATIENT

Maximum information is gained during physical examination of the chest from an organized approach to the patient. If the deliberate stepwise approach of first *inspection*, then *palpation* and *percussion*, followed by *auscultation* is followed, data will be obtained in an orderly manner and the ramifications of each observation will be fully realized. Of course, the patient is not examined without first obtaining a careful clinical history.

The wise clinician obtains the clinical data base sequentially. During the creation of the history and the performance of the physical examination, the physician should be sorting out the clinical priorities of the presenting illness. Is the patient sick or not sick? Does the illness appear to be organic, behavioral, or a combination? If organic, which organ systems are probably involved? How seriously ill is the patient? Is the condition acute and possibly life-threatening? Is it chronic, of long duration? Has there been recent, sudden change in the severity of illness? Careful questioning and evaluation of the history obtained from the patient or other observers will provide much information to answer these questions.

As the history is developed, the practitioner should consciously create a series of hypotheses as a preliminary attempt to explain the patient's illness. It is important not only to identify the problem but also to explain its pathogenesis and establish one or more diagnostic entities. In general, effective treatment demands accurate diagnosis. Hypotheses formulated from the history may guide the practitioner to focus greater attention than usual on some aspect of the physical examination. Additionally, the physical examination may buttress or refute earlier hypotheses or generate additional postulates. The history and physical examination may be viewed as a dynamic evaluation of the patient's problems, which should be actively synthesized into a tentative explanation of the patient's illness. Laboratory data and additional observation will confirm, deny, or extend the initial hypotheses.

Some argue that x-ray examination of the chest is so revealing that physical examination of the lungs, especially percussion and auscultation, is no longer necessary. There is no doubt that careful radiographic examination of the lungs reveals abnormalities that cannot be detected by physical examination. In many instances, however, there is a good correlation between the inference from an abnormal physical examination and the findings on chest film. Furthermore, an abnormal finding on physical examination is often the stimulus to closely examine some portion of the radiograph, and vice versa.

Several studies of health care practices have suggested that the routine chest film in the healthy, asymptomatic person without undue risk factors does not provide useful information, needlessly exposes the patient to radiation, albeit a small dose, and is not cost-effective. It has recently been suggested that routine chest film on admission to the hospital be abandoned. Careful physical examination of the chest and the demonstration of an abnormal finding can provide solid indication for radiography. Furthermore, the recognition of a new finding on serial physical examination of the chest in the acutely ill patient may be the clue that helps explain a change in clinical status, as in the postoperative patient, for example. Thus, the ability to perform a careful examination of the chest, lungs, and heart is an important skill for all practitioners.

INSPECTION

Observation of the respiratory pattern may provide important clues. If the patient is agitated, unable to lie still, unable to lie flat, and tachypneic, acute possible life-threatening illness may be likely. Respirations may be rapid and shallow or rapid and deep, demonstrating air hunger or Kussmaul's respiration. Extreme air hunger suggests metabolic acidosis with marked increase in plasma hydrogen ion (H^+) concentration, since H^+ is one of the most potent respiratory stimulants. An altered pattern of respiration as in Cheyne-Stokes or Biot's respiration may suggest marked circulatory insufficiency, possibly associated with central nervous system disorder.

Careful inspection of the chest with the patient undressed during quiet breathing provides important information. The use of accessory muscles of respiration, retraction of the lower costal margins, and poor excursion of the diaphragm are often suggestive of chronic obstructive pulmonary disease. Unilateral signs suggest localized infiltrative or obstructive lesions.

A variety of abnormal chest configurations are associated with heart disease. Longstanding ventricular enlargement leads to precordial chest wall prominence, due to local protrusion of the chest wall. This may be particularly prominent in congenital disorders such as ventricular septal defect, pulmonic stenosis, or tetralogy of Fallot in the area around the anterior left second and third ribs. Modest precordial prominence may be difficult to assess if the patient is left-handed. Asymmetry of the anterior chest is best appreciated if, with the patient supine and flat, the observer views the chest from the foot of the bed.

Straight back syndrome, or pectus excavatum, may be associated with apparent increase in cardiac volume on the standard anteroposterior chest film because of a narrow anteroposterior diameter. Cardiac width is often impressively reduced in the lateral view, but overall heart volume and function are usually normal. Additionally, pulmonic systolic ejection clicks or mitral valve prolapse may be present. A variety of chest deformities, including pectus carinatum, occur in Marfan's syndrome. Abnormalities of cardiac pulsation are discussed in the section on examination of the heart.

PALPATION

Asymmetrical chest wall movement may be recognized by, with the patient sitting, placing the hands palm down symmetrically on the lower portion of the chest with the thumbs pointing toward the midline. Pleural rubs and sonorous rhonchi may be appreciated by simple palpation with the fingers or palm over the afflicted area. When a major bronchus is severely obstructed, yet permits the passage of some air with each breath, the entire hemithorax may vibrate.

Patients with chest pain may describe the symptoms in such detail that it appears obvious that the origin is the chest wall itself. In others, the description of chest discomfort is confusing, imprecise, and not helpful. It is most important, in such circumstances, to determine whether the complaint originates in the chest wall or from the structures underneath. It is surprising how often the discomfort of a traumatized or fractured rib or a costochondral separation cannot be localized by the patient, yet careful palpation pinpoints the source of discomfort.

Recognition of a costochondral separation may be especially difficult. In most persons, firm palpation with the tip of the thumb over the anterior costochondral junctions is uncomfortable. In the patient with a costochondral separation, however, such palpation is exquisitely tender. The area of discomfort is usually sharply localized. It is important to compare the discomfort of palpation of the adjacent costochondral junctions with the area in question. Always palpate the uninvolved or normal region first. Not infrequently, especially after moderate chest trauma, more than one junction is painful. Because twisting or turning of the thorax may exacerbate the pain, an occasional patient with a suspected diagnosis of exercise-induced angina pectoris is found to have only chest wall discomfort due to costochondral separation. In the patient with atypical complaints of chest pain, careful palpation of the chest may reveal a local, not a cardiac, cause.

Changes in vocal *fremitus* may reflect differences in aeration or density of the tissue beneath the palpating hand on the affected side.[4] (*Fremitus* from the Latin, a murmuring or roaring, means a vibration.) It is important to compare the fremitus symmetrically on the two sides of the thorax over the two lungs. The palm of the hand is placed in various areas of the chest, and the patient is instructed to repeat a phrase, such as "ninety-nine," at each palpation with the same intensity of speech. In the lower parts of the thorax posteriorly, the ulnar surface of the palm is used to determine at which point the fremitus is lost as the hand has moved from underlying lung tissue to nonconducting substance.

PERCUSSION

Two forms of thoracic percussion are generally applied.[5] In *direct percussion,* the examiner elicits the sound resonating from the underlying structures when the tips of the fingers or the palm of the hand is struck in a reproducible manner on the chest wall. With practice, direct percussion with the fingertips can be most informative. The observer notes the resonance of the chest following each strike but is also aware of the density of the chest wall under the fingers. A chest mass or fluid in the lung is associated with loss of resonance and a sense of firmness. In hyperinflation, the normal resonance is increased and a drumlike sensation of hollowness may be appreciated. I have used direct percussion with the fingertips for many years and have found it most useful. There is seldom the need to employ other techniques.

In *indirect percussion,* the palmar surface of the second finger (the pleximeter) is firmly pressed onto an intercostal space and is struck sharply by the tip of the same finger from the other hand (the plexor), producing a resonating note. In this maneuver, the arm should be held rather stiffly and flexed at the elbow; the blow is delivered by flexion at the wrist. Thus, the weight of the hand forces the plexor to strike the pleximeter. It is important also that the blow be sharply done and that the plexor be lifted quickly after the blow. Skillful performers may produce rather loud notes, but appreciation of the substance of the chest wall and the structures beneath may not be as discriminating or as subtle with each blow as with direct percussion. Maximum information is obtained from both the sound and the touch during percussion.

The feedback to the observer from percussion is influenced by structures beneath the surface of the pleura to the depth of a few centimeters. Thus, unless an abnormality is close to the pleural surface, it may be missed. Mediastinal masses are usually not detected by this technique. However, peripheral areas of consolidation, lobar pneumonia, fluid in the chest, and other abnormalities are often readily detected by evaluation of vocal fremitus and percussion.

Percussion of the cardiac silhouette is discussed in another chapter. However, it is worth reiterating that one of the most useful measures for evaluating cardiac size is palpation of the apical impulse. The observer notes the location, the area occupied by the impulse, the degree of thrust, and whether there are diastolic as well as systolic components. Percussion of the edge of cardiac dullness usually provides little additional information after the apical impulse has been palpated and its character analyzed. Precise determination of the shape and size of the heart is best determined by other techniques such as chest roentgenography or echocardiography.

AUSCULTATION

Sounds produced by the movement of air through the bronchial columns are altered by changes in density of the surrounding tissue, swelling or obstruction of the airway, or sudden opening of previously closed bronchial passages. Normally, inspiration is longer than expiration in the ratio of 3:1. Disease of the lungs is often associated with prolongation and intensity of the expiratory phase.

Normal sounds of quiet breathing have been termed vesicular, but are best called "*normal*."[4] *Bronchial,* or tubular, breathing is louder and more intense, usually with some prolongation of expiration. Bronchial breathing is abnormal and indicates consolidation or compression around the bronchial tree; it has the same significance as the air bronchogram seen on chest film. Auscultation over the normal trachea produces a sound similar to bronchial breathing. Markedly prolonged expiration, as in asthmatic breathing or wheezing, is a sign of high-grade, diffuse airway obstruction due to mucosal edema, accumulation of secretions, or spasm.

The invention of the stethoscope by Laennec was a singular achievement in the development of medicine as we know it today. "The stethoscope drew the physician into the private world in which signs were directly communicated to him from the patient's body."[6] Using his new invention, Laennec undertook a remarkable clinicopathologic correlation of the sounds heard in the chest in pulmonary disease.

Laennec devised the term *rale,* which he applied to a variety of sounds, including the "death rattle." He postulated that the bubbling, gurgling sounds heard on inspiration during auscultation reflected air passing through fluid-filled airways. The term *rale* has since been extended to describe any of the plethora of inspiratory sounds that can be heard in abnormality of the respiratory system. A complex terminology describing breath sounds as vesicular or bronchovesicular and classifying rales as wet, dry, crepitant, subcrepitant, and so forth has developed over the years. Generations of students have struggled through physical diagnosis of the chest, attempting to understand the meaning of these differences. Even more difficult has been the challenge to the student or physician in training to convince himself that the sounds described by this arcane terminology actually existed in the patients being examined!

Recently, the American Thoracic Society and others have moved to simplify terminology.[7] The explosive sounds heard over the lung fields during auscultation in inspiration are termed *crackles* (formerly rales) (Table 24.1). There are basically two kinds of crackles: *fine* and *coarse*. The sound of fine crackles may be simulated by moistening the

TABLE 24.1 CLASSIFICATION OF LUNG SOUNDS

American Thoracic Society Nomenclature	Synonym	Acoustic Characteristics
Fine crackle	Fine rale, crepitation	Short duration, not loud, high pitch, discontinuous, interrupted explosive sounds
Coarse crackle	Coarse rale	Louder and lower in pitch than above
Rhonchus	Sonorous rhonchus	Continuous sounds > 250 msec, a snoring sound
Wheeze	Sibilant rhonchus	High-pitched continuous sound, >250 msec, with musical components

TABLE 24.2 CLINICAL DIAGNOSIS AND TIMING OF INSPIRATORY CRACKLES

Early	Late
Asthma	Alveolitis (fibrosing)
Chronic bronchitis	Asbestosis
	Heart failure
Emphysema	Pulmonary fibrosis
	Sarcoidosis
	Scleroderma
	Rheumatoid lung

palmar surfaces of the index finger and thumb and, in a quiet room, pressing the tips together and pulling them apart close to the ear. Rolling a hank of hair between the fingertips close to the ear produces a similar sound.

It has been taught for decades that fine crackles represent the movement of air through fluid-filled small bronchial passages. Forgacs has argued convincingly that this is untenable.[8,9] He suggests that the change in auscultatory findings with position, their location generally at the base of the lungs, and their occurrence during inspiration but not expiration supports the argument that crackles represent the sudden opening of small airways as thoracic volume increases during inspiration. High fidelity recordings of pulmonary crackles demonstrate their sudden explosive nature.[10]

More important than the nature of the pulmonary crackles is their timing. Nath and Capel recorded inspiratory crackles simultaneously with inspiratory flow rates in patients with airway obstruction and those with restrictive defects.[11] On the basis of extensive studies, they concluded that early inspiratory crackles are associated with airway obstruction, whereas late inspiratory crackles are reflective of restrictive defects. Thus, early crackles occur in chronic bronchitis, asthma, and various forms of chronic obstructive pulmonary disease. Late inspiratory crackles are found in the pulmonary congestion of heart failure, alveolitis, asbestosis, sarcoidosis, and so forth (Table 24.2).

Auscultation of whispered and spoken voice sounds is useful in detecting areas of pulmonary consolidation. Normally, whispered words are faint and indistinct when the stethoscope is applied to the lung. Spoken words are louder but lack distinctness. When the surrounding pulmonary parenchyma is consolidated yet the airways remain open, transmission of sound is altered. Whispered words are well conducted through the stethoscope. The resultant change in intensity is termed *whispered pectoriloquy*. Spoken words are also heard crisply and distinctly; this is called *bronchophony*. When the lung is compressed, as in a narrow strip above a pleural effusion, spoken words have a peculiar nasal or bleating quality, termed *egophony*. All of these findings have the same physiological meaning: compression of lung from a contiguous mass or fluid.

In the patient suspected of pulmonary or cardiac disease, careful examination for *post-tussic crackles* may be rewarding. The patient is instructed to breathe quietly in, then exhale and cough at the end of the exhalation. This technique may detect crackles when examination during quiet breathing is unrevealing.

A variety of other abnormal sounds may be heard on auscultation of the chest in various clinical situations. A pleural friction rub, which may or may not be associated with the searing pain of pleurisy, is appreciated as a dry, leathery, scratching sound associated with the chest movement of inspiration. It is characteristic of the pain of pleurisy that if the patient stops breathing, the pain is no longer present. Wheezes are characteristic of asthma or discrete bronchial obstruction. A rhonchus may be a localized finding in bronchial obstruction, as with tumor or associated with mucus plugs.

Mediastinal emphysema is appreciated as crunching, popping, or clicking sounds heard with inspiration–expiration and occasionally timed with the cardiac cycle. Often subcutaneous crepitation in the neck accompanies mediastinal emphysema. A peculiar, coarse, loud crunch of mediastinal emphysema heard over the anterior chest and precordium is termed Hamman's crunch. Occasionally, in fractured rib or costochondral separation, crackling sounds can be heard with respiratory movement or chest wall pressure as the separated parts rub together, usually coincident with significant discomfort on the part of the patient.

A century and a half of clinical analysis of the findings on physical examination of the chest in a variety of conditions has produced an extensive terminology and classification of abnormality. With the availability in today's practice of radiography of the chest, ultrasound, and computed tomography, much of this has become less useful. But physical examination of the chest is not a dead art, nor is the stethoscope a useless instrument. The presence of an altered respiratory pattern of breathing, evidence of pulmonary consolidation, detection of crackles suggesting airway obstruction, or excessive secretions documented on physical examination indicate objective evidence of pulmonary or cardiac abnormality. The wise use of modern medical technology in the diagnosis of disease demands discrimination on the part of the physician. The clinical hypotheses developed to explain the problem and identify the cause of disease during the performance of the history and physical examination allow the physician to focus logically on clinical decision making to determine which test or tests will be most useful to confirm the original postulates. Competency in the physical diagnosis of the chest is an essential skill for the practicing physician. This simple truth is confirmed repeatedly in everyday practice in the office or at the bedside.

REFERENCES

1. Fishman AP: Manifestations of respiratory disorders. In Fishman AP (ed): Pulmonary Diseases and Disorders, pp 3–28. New York, McGraw-Hill, 1980
2. The enigma of breathlessness. Lancet 1:891, 1986
3. Paintal AS: Thoracic receptors connected with sensation. Br Med Bull 33:169, 1977
4. George RF: History and physical examination. In George RB, Light RW, Matthay RA (eds): Chest Medicine, pp 123–134. New York, Churchill Livingstone, 1983
5. DeGowen EL, DeGowen RL: Bedside Diagnostic Examination, pp 224–459. New York, Macmillan, 1976
6. Reiser SJ: The medical influence of the stethoscope. Sci Am 240:148, 1979
7. Loudon R, Murphy RL Jr: Lung sounds. Am Rev Respir Dis 130:663, 1984
8. Forgacs P: The functional basis of pulmonary sounds. Chest 73:399, 1978
9. Cugell DW: Editorial: Sounds of the lungs. Chest 73:311, 1978
10. Forgacs P: Crackles and wheezes. Lancet 2:203, 1977
11. Nath AR, Capel LH: Inspiratory crackles: Early and late. Thorax 29:223, 1974

GENERAL REFERENCE

Bates B: A Guide to Physical Examination, 3rd ed, chap 6, pp 125–156. Philadelphia, JB Lippincott, 1983

BEDSIDE DIAGNOSIS OF CONGENITAL HEART DISEASE

Alvin J. Chin • William F. Friedman

Relatively few patients with congenital heart lesions present initially to the cardiologist in adulthood, since most lesions become apparent early in life, often coincident with the rapid transition from the fetal to the adult circulatory pattern. For example, patients with malformations creating severe or complete obstruction to antegrade pulmonary blood flow require for survival that the pulmonary circulation be supplied by way of a patent ductus arteriosus. Since the ductus arteriosus closes normally within days or months of birth, prolonged survival depends on the presence of aortopulmonary collaterals or the surgical creation of a systemic arterial–pulmonary arterial shunt. Thus, unoperated patients with severe pulmonary stenosis or pulmonary atresia do not live into adulthood unless they have significant aortopulmonary collaterals. In contrast, pulmonary stenosis of initially mild or moderate severity is compatible with long-term survival.

Similarly, congenital heart lesions causing moderate or severe obstruction to systemic blood flow do not present initially in adulthood. Systemic blood flow is also dependent on patency of the ductus arteriosus in patients with severe left-sided obstruction. Even moderate left ventricular outflow tract obstruction is often progressive and leads to rapid decompensation of the systemic ventricle. In general, left-sided obstructive lesions that present clinically for the first time in adulthood are those that are initially mild or relatively slow to progress.

Left-to-right shunt lesions, while presenting later in the newborn period than ductal-dependent lesions, still usually become apparent in the first few months of life. Pulmonary vascular resistance and impedance fall normally during the first few months after birth, allowing left-to-right shunting to increase. Large communications between the left and right sides of the heart are not associated with a pressure gradient across the defect and are termed nonrestrictive. Such defects at the ventricular or great arterial levels almost always result in congestive heart failure and require surgical repair in the first few years of life. Those patients with large ventricular septal defects who survive without operation have developed either subpulmonary stenosis or pulmonary vascular obstructive disease. Patients with a small or moderate-sized, "restrictive," ventricular septal defect, for example, can survive until adulthood without surgical intervention.

Only 5% of patients with atrial septal defect (even if large) develop heart failure in infancy.[1,2] Thus, atrial septal defects are among the more common left-to-right congenital cardiac lesions that present to the cardiologist in adulthood.

PULMONARY VASCULAR OBSTRUCTIVE DISEASE

Increased pulmonary blood flow may interfere with the normal growth and multiplication of the intra-acinar pulmonary arteries[3] and may also cause anatomical changes in pulmonary vessels. Heath and Edwards[4] observed a gradation of structural changes: muscular extension in arterioles and medial thickening, intimal proliferation, intimal fibrosis, plexiform lesions, medial fibrosis, and necrotizing arteritis. The number and structure of peripheral pulmonary arterioles are major determinants of pulmonary vascular impedance, and abnormalities of either increase the impedance and thus reduce the magnitude of any left-to-right shunt. If the pulmonary vascular disease is severe, the shunt may actually become bidirectional or right-to-left.

The physical findings of pulmonary vascular obstructive disease include cyanosis and digital clubbing, the intensity of which depends on the reduction in oxygen saturation and the increase in hemoglobin concentration, both of which are related to the magnitude of the right-to-left shunt. The jugular venous waveform usually shows a normal mean atrial pressure unless there is superimposed right ventricular failure or tricuspid regurgitation. Tricuspid regurgitation is associated with accentuated v waves and with systolic hepatic pulsations. The right ventricular impulse is increased in both parasternal and epigastric locations, and systolic expansion of the proximal main pulmonary artery is often palpable. A loud, early systolic to mid-systolic pulmonary ejection sound is followed by little or no systolic murmur. Commonly, little or no inspiratory splitting is detected of the second heart sound; there is marked accentuation of the pulmonic component. The presence of a high-frequency, diastolic decrescendo pulmonary regurgitation murmur usually indicates that pulmonary vascular impedance is at or above systemic levels.

The chest film reveals a very large proximal main pulmonary artery and much smaller peripheral pulmonary arteries; the overall heart size is generally normal or only minimally enlarged. The electrocardiogram shows hypertrophy of the pulmonary ventricle and, sometimes, right atrial enlargement.

OBSTRUCTION TO PULMONARY BLOOD FLOW

VALVAR PULMONARY STENOSIS

Usually there is commissural fusion with thickening of the pulmonary valve leaflets (patients with dysplastic valves present in childhood).

Most patients are symptom free, although occasionally dizziness or syncope can occur with exercise, presumably when the right ventricle can no longer augment its stroke volume.

Cyanosis is absent unless there is an associated patent foramen ovale allowing right-to-left shunting. The a wave in the jugular and hepatic venous waveforms is increased in severe cases. The parasternal right ventricular impulse is increased in amplitude and duration. An early systolic ejection sound, closely following the first heart sound, is almost always heard over the second left interspace,[5] moving closer to the first heart sound with increasingly severe stenosis.[6] Characteristically, the ejection sound decreases with inspiration and may even disappear, but it is heard easily with expiration; an inspiratory increase in right atrial contraction transmits to the pulmonary valve cusps before the onset of right ventricular contraction, reducing the systolic excursion of the valve and diminishing the loudness of the ejection sound. An early systolic murmur is heard in the second left interspace, usually radiating well to the left side of the neck and left shoulder. If there is an associated thrill, it is palpated best in the second left interspace. The greater the obstruction, the longer the duration of right ventricular ejection and the longer the murmur. With moderate or severe stenosis, the systolic murmur peaks later and lengthens to envelop the aortic component of the second sound.[7,8] At the lower left sternal border, the murmur is less intense and the aortic component of the second heart sound is often audible. With increasing stenosis, pulmonary valve closure becomes delayed and fainter.

The chest film usually shows a normal overall heart size and peripheral pulmonary vascularity; enlargement of the proximal main pulmonary artery due to post-stenotic dilatation is common (Fig. 25.1). The electrocardiogram shows right axis deviation and right ventricular hypertrophy in cases of moderate or severe stenosis. Right atrial enlargement is associated with severe stenosis. When obstruction is mild, the electrocardiogram is often normal.

Two-dimensional echocardiographic visualization of pulmonary valve morphology is usually possible from the parasternal window. Now that catheter techniques are available for therapeutic balloon valvuloplasty,[9-11] accurate measurements of pulmonary valve annulus size are helpful in selecting the balloon catheter of proper size. Doppler ultrasound assessment of the right ventricle–pulmonary artery peak systolic pressure gradient has been validated,[12] and, like the electrocardiogram, may be useful to determine whether invasive investigation is necessary.

TETRALOGY OF FALLOT

The basic malformation results from anterior, superior, and leftward displacement of the infundibular septum away from its normal position between the two limbs of the septal band (septomarginal trabecula).[13,14] This displacement causes subpulmonary obstruction, aortic "override," and a large, nonrestrictive, malalignment-type ventricular septal defect. Valvar pulmonary stenosis, usually a bicuspid pulmonary valve, typically coexists[15]; stenosis or atresia of the origin of a branch pulmonary artery is also common.[16]

Cyanosis is the principal symptom dating from early childhood. The degree of cyanosis depends on the severity of the subvalvar and valvar pulmonary stenosis. The right ventricular impulse is often normal. A systolic ejection murmur of turbulent flow across the right ventricular outflow tract is usually grade 3/6 and heard best over the third left interspace. A systolic thrill is rare; its presence signifies that the valvar component of the pulmonary stenosis is most significant hemodynamically. Likewise, a pulmonary systolic ejection sound is rare, except in cases with predominant valvar stenosis. The aortic component of the second heart sound is usually accentuated; pulmonary valve closure is faint or inaudible.[17,18]

The chest film shows a normal-sized, boot-shaped heart (*coeur en sabot*) with a concavity in the region of the main pulmonary artery. The pulmonary vascular markings are diminished in those patients with a significant right-to-left shunt. The aortic arch is right sided, and the thoracic aorta descends on the right in 25% of patients.

Two-dimensional echocardiography from the parasternal window demonstrates the malalignment ventricular septal defect and the subpulmonary stenosis, although this is easier to display from the subcostal window. The presence or absence of stenoses at the origins of the branch pulmonary arteries can also be assessed with magnetic resonance imaging.[19]

TETRALOGY OF FALLOT WITH PULMONARY ATRESIA AND AORTOPULMONARY COLLATERALS

The most severe anatomical form of tetralogy of Fallot has subvalvar pulmonary atresia,[20] usually coexisting with atresia of the pulmonary valve and proximal main pulmonary artery. Aortopulmonary collateral arteries[21] or, rarely, a persistent ductus arteriosus supplies the distal pulmonary arterial flow. If the blood flow in the collateral arteries is exceptionally high, a large left-to-right shunt may result in the symptoms of congestive heart failure.

Cyanosis is invariably present, the degree of which depends on the number and size of aortopulmonary collaterals, which often develop stenoses along their length. In some patients, a short mid-systolic murmur may be heard at the left sternal border, presumably representing the increased aortic flow in cases with large collateral arterial flow. A prominent, early systolic ejection sound is heard along the upper right sternal border.[22] The ejection sound is aortic in origin and does not vary with respiration. Continuous murmurs are heard over the anterior chest and back as a result of blood flow through the systemic collateral vessels. A diastolic decrescendo murmur is heard in those patients with acquired aortic regurgitation.[23]

The chest film shows a normal heart size or mild cardiomegaly with a concavity in the region of the proximal main pulmonary artery. The systemic collateral arteries are often visible (Fig. 25.2); sometimes one notes a reticular pattern to the peripheral pulmonary vascular markings. The aortic arch is right sided in approximately 25%. The electrocardiogram usually demonstrates only right ventricular hypertrophy, but, in cases of markedly increased pulmonary blood flow, can show biventricular hypertrophy.

Two-dimensional echocardiography demonstrates the large malalignment-type ventricular septal defect and the level(s) of pulmonary outflow atresia, but cannot display the distal branch pulmonary arteries or the course of most types of aortopulmonary collateral vessels.[24] Doppler echocardiography accurately detects aortic regurgitation.[25]

ANOMALOUS MUSCLE BUNDLE OF THE RIGHT VENTRICLE AND DOUBLE-CHAMBERED RIGHT VENTRICLE

Patients with large ventricular septal defects do not present initially in adulthood unless they have developed subpulmonary stenosis[26-29] or pulmonary vascular obstructive disease. Within the former group, there are several subsets: (1) patients who have a malalignment-type ventricular septal defect, and initially little subpulmonary stenosis (and who develop more severe outflow tract obstruction owing to progressive hypertrophy of the malaligned infundibular septum, evolving into typical tetralogy of Fallot[30,31]); (2) patients with either a malalignment or a large perimembranous type of ventricular septal defect who have a superiorly displaced, hypertrophied, and obstructive moderator band,[32] the muscle which usually runs from the apical aspect of the septal band (septomarginal trabecula) to the anterior papillary muscle of the right ventricle; (3) patients with either a malalignment-type or large perimembranous ventricular septal defect who have a normally situated moderator band, but who have an anomalous muscle bundle within the right ventricle causing subpulmonary obstruction,[33,34] and (4) patients who would belong to the first subset but who have, *in addition*, either a displaced obstructive moderator band or an anomalous muscle bundle.[32] Obviously, patients with a small or moderate-sized perimembranous ventricular septal defect, or even those with an intact ventricular septum, may also have a displaced moderator band or an anomalous muscle bundle in the right ventricle.

The anomaly in the second subset has been classified as "double-chambered right ventricle" and should be distinguished from classic tetralogy of Fallot and from those described in the first subset who progress to tetralogy anatomy. The double-chambered right ventricle differs not only in intracardiac anatomy but also in a lower incidence of branch pulmonary stenosis and right aortic arch. The incidence of coexistent valvar pulmonary stenosis is also much lower, whereas the incidence of discrete fibrous subaortic stenosis is higher.[35,36]

Patients with double-chambered right ventricle and those with anomalous muscle bundle of the right ventricle have similar clinical manifestations. The presence of cyanosis and clubbing depends on the severity of the subpulmonary stenosis. The jugular venous waveform is usually normal. The parasternal right ventricular impulse is accentuated; a systolic thrill is often present. The first heart sound is normal; systolic ejection sounds are absent. The second heart sound is single if the subpulmonary stenosis is severe; otherwise, it is physiologically split with a soft pulmonic component. There is a harsh systolic ejection murmur at the mid to lower left sternal border.

The chest film is indistinguishable from tetralogy of Fallot, except that the concavity is usually absent in the region of the proximal main pulmonary artery because it is usually normal in size.

The electrocardiogram often demonstrates increased right-sided forces only in lead V_{4R}.

In adults with double-chambered right ventricle or anomalous muscle bundle, two-dimensional echocardiography is of most use in making the distinction from tetralogy of Fallot. The anatomy of the ventricular septal defect and subaortic stenosis (if present) can usually be appreciated (Fig. 25.3).

Magnetic resonance imaging, with its wide field of view, is probably the technique of choice in adults.

EBSTEIN'S ANOMALY OF THE TRICUSPID VALVE

Ebstein's malformation is characterized by the distal displacement of part of the line of proximal attachment of the tricuspid leaflets.[37,38] The displacement extends maximally to the junction of the inlet and trabecular zones of the right ventricle.[39]

Patients with relatively severe anatomical abnormalities usually have predominant tricuspid stenosis and present clinically as neonates with marked cyanosis. Adults have milder anatomical malformations and present with arrhythmias or with exercise intolerance.

Cyanosis depends on the severity of the tricuspid stenosis or regurgitation, the patency of the foramen ovale, and the presence or absence of associated subvalvar or valvar pulmonary stenosis. The jugular venous waveform is often normal, probably because increased compliance of the right atrium blunts the v waves of tricuspid regurgitation. An undulant or rippling motion during held expiration can occasionally be seen over the left lower sternal border, representing the systolic motion of the "atrialized" portion of the right ventricle.[40a]

The first heart sound is usually widely split[41] with a loud second component, caused by delayed closure of the large anterior tricuspid leaflet. The second sound may be normal or widely split, but in cases with severe tricuspid stenosis or with associated valvar pulmonary stenosis, the pulmonary component may not be audible. Both third and fourth heart sounds are frequently present and can produce triple or quadruple rhythms.

The systolic murmur of tricuspid regurgitation (regurgitation from the trabecular portion of the right ventricle to the atrialized portion) varies from a soft, early systolic short murmur to a pansystolic murmur with a palpable thrill. It is usually maximal at the lower left sternal border. Inspiratory augmentation of the murmur is not always present, since the small trabecular and outflow portions of the right ventricle cannot increase their share of stroke volume with inspiration.[40b]

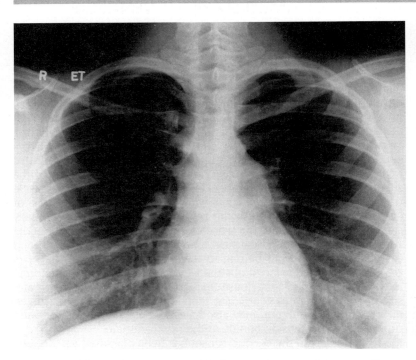

FIGURE 25.1 Valvar pulmonic stenosis. The heart size is normal; however, there is post-stenotic dilatation of the main pulmonary artery.

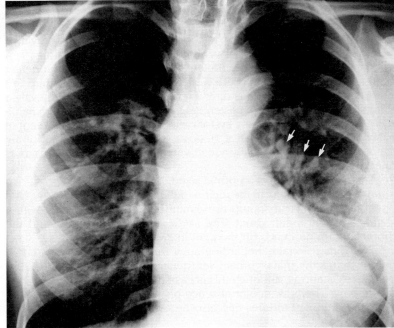

FIGURE 25.2 Tetralogy of Fallot with pulmonary atresia. The ascending aorta and descending aorta are both dilated; there is a concavity in the region of the main pulmonary artery. The lungs are supplied by aortopulmonary collaterals. Arrows show collaterals to the left lung; some collaterals to the right lung are also visible.

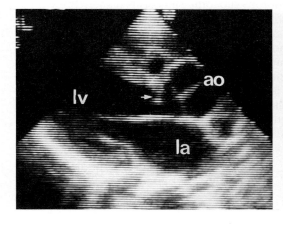
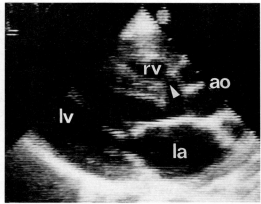

FIGURE 25.3 Two-dimensional echocardiograms of a double-chambered right ventricle. (Left) Parasternal long axis view of left ventricular outflow tract obstruction due to discrete fibrous subaortic stenosis (arrow). (Right) Slight angulation from the above view reveals a perimembranous ventricular septal defect (arrowhead). (ao, aorta; la, left atrium; lv, left ventricle; rv, right ventricle)

A diastolic murmur of augmented antegrade flow from the right atrium may be present as well, depending on the magnitude of tricuspid regurgitation.[42]

The typical chest film shows convexity of the borders of both right and left sides of the heart, leading to a "boxlike" silhouette (Fig. 25.4). The convex border of the left side of the heart is due to displacement of the outflow portion of the right ventricle superiorly by the large inflow portion. The prominent border of the right side of the heart is due to the dilated right atrium. Distal pulmonary vascular markings are normal unless pulmonary blood flow is reduced by right-to-left shunting across a patent foramen ovale.

The electrocardiogram usually shows sinus rhythm, although atrial fibrillation or flutter may also be observed. The PR interval is prolonged in patients without Wolff-Parkinson-White syndrome. The P waves demonstrate right atrial enlargement. The QRS shows a right bundle branch block pattern and abnormally low R waves in the right precordial leads (Fig. 25.5). Wolff-Parkinson-White syndrome occurs in at least 10% of patients with Ebstein's anomaly[43] and is associated often with supraventricular tachyarrhythmias. The accessory atrioventricular pathways are right-sided, either in the posterior septum or the posterolateral free wall.[44]

Two-dimensional echocardiography is used currently as the primary tool for diagnosis, since ultrasound provides unique assessment of the malformation's morphologic features.[45] Shiina and co-workers have suggested that patients with elongated, mobile anterior leaflets may have competent "unicusp" valves created by a surgical plastic repair, whereas those with pronounced tethering of leaflets cannot.[46] The abnormalities of the left side of the heart associated with Ebstein's anomaly (e.g., mitral valve prolapse and left ventricular dyskinesis) may also be assessed noninvasively.[47,48]

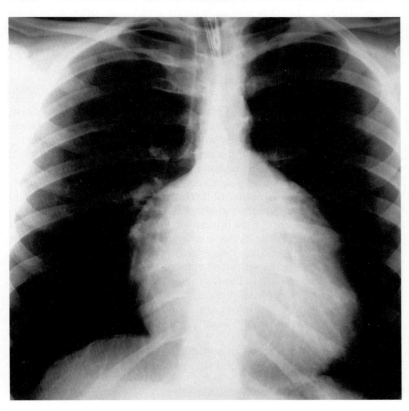

FIGURE 25.4 Ebstein's anomaly of the tricuspid valve. The characteristic "boxlike" cardiac silhouette is evident.

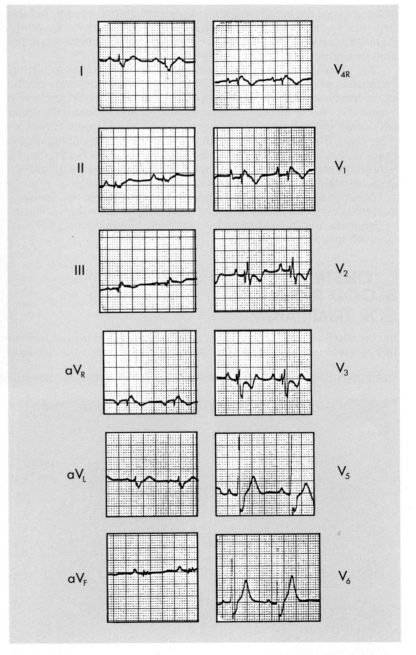

FIGURE 25.5 Ebstein's anomaly of the tricuspid valve. There is borderline first degree atrioventricular block. The P waves are enlarged in the right precordial leads. There is right bundle branch block.

COMPLEX CONOTRUNCAL ANOMALIES WITH PULMONARY STENOSIS WITH OR WITHOUT SINGLE VENTRICLE

Other than tetralogy of Fallot and truncus arteriosus, there are four conotruncal anomalies: double outlet right ventricle, transposition of the great arteries, anatomically corrected malposition, and double outlet left ventricle; all can have associated pulmonary stenosis. Furthermore, all conotruncal anomalies can occur in hearts with both ventricles of normal size, as well as in those designated single ventricle, with hypoplasia of one ventricular chamber. Virtually all patients presenting initially in adulthood with conotruncal anomalies have large malalignment-type ventricular septal defects. Therefore, the functional consequences reflect the severity of the pulmonary stenosis.

The patient will show varying degrees of cyanosis, depending on the degree of pulmonary stenosis. The jugular venous waveform is usually normal. The first heart sound is normal, and the pulmonic component of the second heart sound is often faint. A systolic ejection murmur is usually heard best at the upper left sternal border, but this depends on the anatomical location of the main pulmonary artery. Pulmonary ejection sounds are rare because the predominant component of pulmonary stenosis is almost always subvalvar.

The chest film shows mild cardiomegaly and normal to slightly increased pulmonary vascularity. The heart contour depends on the exact anatomical lesion. For example, in cases of single ventricle with a subaortic "outlet chamber" situated anterior and leftward, the upper left border shows a prominent convexity denoting the outlet chamber (Fig. 25.6). The electrocardiogram is also variable, depending on the exact defect. Patients with left-sided subaortic outlet chamber and a right-sided morphologic left ventricle have Q waves in V_{4R} and V_1, demonstrating an inverted pattern of septal depolarization.

Two-dimensional echocardiography demonstrates the ventriculoarterial connections and the type and severity of pulmonary stenosis.

Magnetic resonance imaging is extremely helpful in the adult with complex malformations.

OBSTRUCTION TO SYSTEMIC BLOOD FLOW
COR TRIATRIATUM

In cor triatriatum, the left atrium is partially partitioned into a chamber that receives the pulmonary veins and one that contains the left atrial appendage and empties through the mitral valve. The communication between the proximal chamber into which the pulmonary veins drain and the remainder of the left atrium can be of varying size.[49-51] If the communication is initially nonrestrictive but progressively grows smaller, the onset of pulmonary venous hypertension is delayed. The functional consequences are usually shortness of breath with exertion and fatigue.

The right ventricular impulse is increased. The second heart sound is single or narrowly split with an accentuated, often palpable, pulmonic component. Diastolic murmurs of flow across the obstructing membrane are usually heard.[51,52] A continuous murmur is heard only when the communication is severely restrictive.

The chest film often shows a normal heart size or mild cardiomegaly with a large main pulmonary artery. There is pulmonary venous congestion.[40c] The electrocardiogram shows right axis deviation, right atrial enlargement, and right ventricular hypertrophy.

Two-dimensional echocardiography, in addition to showing dilatation of the right ventricle and pulmonary artery, can often detect the atrial partitioning.[53,54]

This anomaly can also be identified with magnetic resonance imaging.[55,56]

VALVAR AORTIC STENOSIS

Most adults will have bicuspid bicommissural valves,[57] since patients with a unicommissural valve virtually always present in infancy. Occasionally a trileaflet valve is seen with marked disparity in cusp size.

Dizziness or syncope with exertion and chest pain are the most common symptoms, although many patients are asymptomatic.

A left ventricular lift is palpable when the stenosis is significant. Palpable presystolic distention of the left ventricle suggests severe stenosis. A loud, harsh, diamond-shaped systolic ejection murmur is heard best in the second right interspace. A thrill may be palpable over both carotid arteries and in the suprasternal notch. In older patients with calcific trileaflet aortic stenosis, the murmur in the second right interspace is harsh, whereas the murmur at the cardiac apex is typically musical. The dissociation in the characteristics of these two murmurs is called the Gallavardin phenomenon.[58a] Those patients whose murmur peaks in the last 60% of systole are likely to have severe obstruction. The pulse pressure is small; there is usually a slow upstroke and a sustained peak.

In patients whose stenotic aortic valves are not yet calcified, the aortic component of the second heart sound is heard easily. With in-

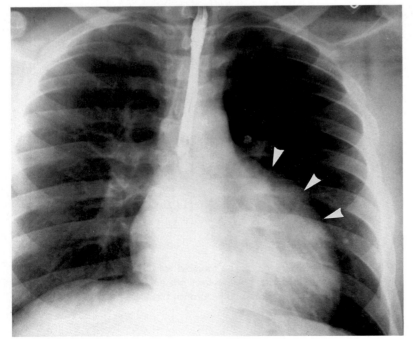

FIGURE 25.6 Single ventricle with a leftward anterior subaortic outlet chamber (arrowheads).

creasingly severe stenosis, aortic closure may be delayed so that it occurs paradoxically after pulmonary valve closure. An important auscultatory finding is a systolic ejection sound heard at the apex or second right interspace; in contrast to the ejection sound of valvar pulmonary stenosis, there is no respiratory variation. The presence of a fourth heart sound in the absence of PR interval prolongation suggests severe aortic stenosis,[59] arbitrarily defined as a peak systolic pressure gradient from left ventricle to aorta of 80 mm Hg or greater in association with a normal cardiac index, or an effective aortic orifice area of 0.5 cm^2/m^2 or less.[60]

The chest film typically shows post-stenotic dilatation of the ascending aorta and a normal or minimally enlarged heart. The electrocardiogram usually reveals left ventricular hypertrophy; ST segment depression and T-wave inversion indicate subendocardial ischemia (Fig. 25.7).

Two-dimensional echocardiography often demonstrates the aortic valve morphology[61]; annulus size can be assessed if balloon valvuloplasty is contemplated.[62-64] Predicting the severity of aortic stenosis by assuming constant end-systolic meridional or circumferential wall stress and then estimating left ventricular pressure is not reliable.[65] Doppler echocardiography is the most accurate means for noninvasively assessing the magnitude of obstruction.[66-68]

SUBVALVAR AORTIC STENOSIS

The most common form of congenital subaortic stenosis is hypertrophic cardiomyopathy (discussed elsewhere in these volumes). The second most common form is the discrete subaortic membrane, consisting of fibrous tissue just beneath the aortic valve.

The physical findings are difficult to distinguish from valvar aortic stenosis, although the absence of a systolic ejection sound suggests subaortic obstruction. In addition, some patients who have been followed for years as examples of a small ventricular septal defect prove ultimately to have discrete subaortic stenosis. Aortic regurgitation is presumed to result from trauma to the valve leaflets from the high-velocity jet, although it may, in fact, be caused by extensions of the subaortic fibroelastic tissue to the aortic cusps.[69]

The chest film usually demonstrates less post-stenotic dilatation of the aorta than in patients with valvar obstruction. The heart size and pulmonary vascular markings are usually normal. The electrocardiogram is similar to that of valvar stenosis.

Two-dimensional echocardiography is diagnostic; the subaortic membrane is demonstrable from both apical and parasternal windows.

The aortic valve leaflets may appear slightly thickened.[70] Doppler echocardiography demonstrates turbulence proximal to the aortic valve and may also detect aortic regurgitation.[71]

COARCTATION OF THE AORTA

This malformation consists of a thickening and infolding of the posterior wall of the aorta opposite the ligamentum arteriosum.[72]

Major symptoms are related to four complications: congestive heart failure, aortic rupture, bacterial endocarditis, and cerebral hemorrhage.[73,74]

The diagnosis is generally suspected on the basis of two abnormal findings: upper extremity hypertension and a basal mid-systolic murmur. Often a soft, mid-systolic murmur is most easily appreciated over the back. Thrills are generally absent in the absence of significant aortic valve stenosis. Continuous murmurs are audible if aortic collaterals are prominent. The first heart sound is generally normal. An early systolic ejection sound is often present, owing to the bicuspid aortic valve present in at least 50% of patients. Absent or diminished pulsations in the femoral arteries with a diminished lower extremity systolic blood pressure are the diagnostic signs.

The electrocardiogram usually reveals left ventricular hypertrophy, but may be normal. The chest film commonly reveals a normal heart size. Dilatation of the ascending aorta may occur from coexistent valvar aortic stenosis. Indentation of the descending aorta at the site of coarctation occurs with prestenotic and post-stenotic dilatation (the "3" sign) (Fig. 25.8). Rib notching is due to erosion of bone by dilated intercostal arteries.

Two-dimensional echocardiography (parasternal or suprasternal windows) can usually identify the site and length of coarctation in the adult. It is also useful in ruling out coexistent aortic valve or mitral valve disease (Fig. 25.9).[75,76] Doppler echocardiography can be used to assess the severity of not only the coarctation,[77] but also aortic and mitral disease, if present.[78,79]

Spin echo or cine[80] magnetic resonance imaging can yield useful information in coarctation.

☐ LEFT-TO-RIGHT SHUNT LESIONS
ATRIAL SEPTAL DEFECT

There are three types of atrial septal defects. Ostium secundum defects result from deficiencies of the septum primum, the flap valve of the foramen ovale. Ostium primum defects are a subtype of atrioventricu-

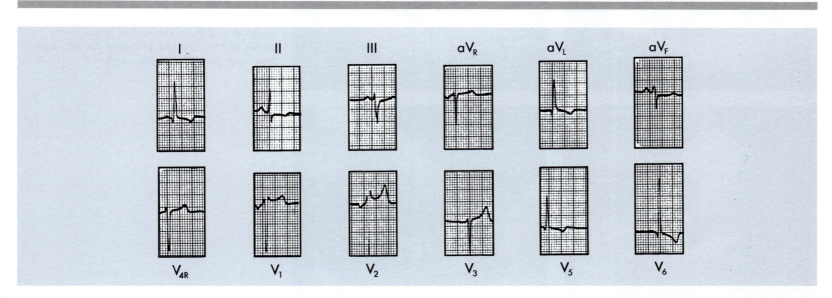

FIGURE 25.7 Valvar aortic stenosis. This patient had a 140-mm-Hg peak systolic ejection gradient. The T-wave inversion in the left precordial leads developed over the course of 2 years.

lar canal (atrioventricular septal) defects, in which the malformed atrioventricular valves attach to the ventricular septal crest, obliterating any communication between the left and right ventricle. Sinus venosus defects typically occur high in the atrial septum near the superior vena cava orifice and are usually associated with anomalous connection of the right superior pulmonary vein to the right atrium or superior vena cava. Sinus venosus defects may also occur low in the atrial septum (near the inferior vena cava orifice), associated with anomalous connection of the right inferior pulmonary vein to the right atrium.[81]

The so-called "coronary sinus atrial septal defect" (coronary sinus septal defect or unroofed coronary sinus)[82,83] is a defect in the wall between the coronary sinus and the left atrium. Thus, although it produces the identical physiologic consequences, it is not classified as an anatomic type of atrial septal defect.

The magnitude of the left-to-right shunt depends on the size of the atrial defect, the diastolic properties of both ventricles,[84] and the relative impedance in the systemic and pulmonary circulations. Symptoms are usually trivial or absent, but congestive heart failure may develop if

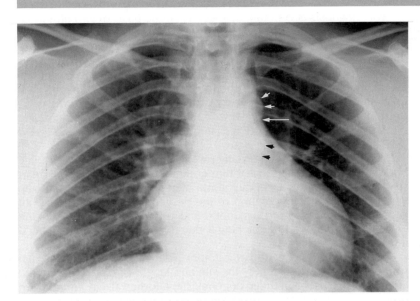

FIGURE 25.8 Coarctation of the aorta. The "3" sign (*long arrow*) is produced by prestenotic (*short white arrows*) and post-stenotic (*black arrows*) dilatation of the descending aorta.

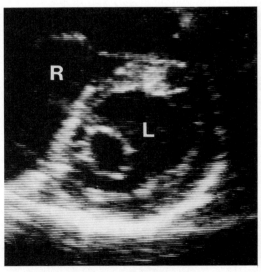
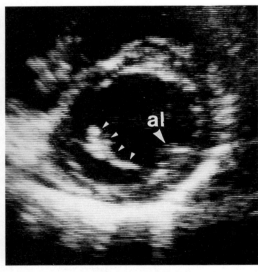
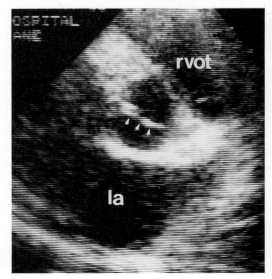
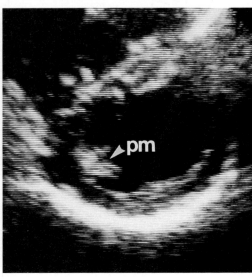

FIGURE 25.9 Two-dimensional echocardiographic demonstration of parachute mitral valve and bicuspid aortic valve in a patient with coarctation of the aorta. (*Upper left*) Parasternal short axis view, diastole. (R, right ventricle; L, left ventricle) (*Upper right*) Systole. The small arrows point to the line of coaptation of the mitral leaflet tissue. The anterolateral (*al*) papillary muscle is hypoplastic, and none of the chordae attach to it. (*Lower right*) A short axis cut somewhat closer to the apex than in the picture at upper right. The posteromedial (*pm*) papillary muscle is slightly larger than usual, and all of the mitral chordae attach to it. (*Lower left*) High parasternal short axis view. The line of coaptation of the aortic leaflets (*arrowheads*) shows that this is a bicuspid valve. (*la*, left atrium; *rvot*, right ventricular outflow tract)

the left ventricular compliance decreases, resulting in a progressively larger left-to-right shunt.

The jugular venous waveform shows a conspicuous x descent and a tall v wave, so that a and v waves appear equal.[58b] The right ventricular impulse is usually increased and the pulmonary artery pulsation palpable. A pulmonary mid-systolic ejection murmur is often soft and generally heard best over the second left interspace. A precordial thrill is rare. There is usually wide splitting of the second heart sound, which is "fixed" in most patients. A short, mid-diastolic, tricuspid flow rumble at the lower right and left sternal borders is heard in patients with a large left-to-right shunt. A pansystolic murmur is heard at the apex in some cases of ostium secundum defect with mitral valve prolapse[85] and in ostium primum defect with a regurgitant mitral valve. A mid-systolic click in the patients with mitral prolapse is often difficult to hear, and left ventricular precordial hyperactivity is commonly absent because mitral regurgitation is usually mild in these patients. In approximately 5% of patients, even with a large atrial septal defect, the physical findings are unimpressive.

In ostium secundum defects, the chest film shows right atrial and right ventricular enlargement and increased pulmonary vascularity. The superior vena cava shadow is often "absent" (hidden behind the sternal shadow) owing to leftward rotation of the heart caused by the right ventricular volume overload. The electrocardiogram usually shows sinus rhythm, although a small number of patients have atrial fibrillation or flutter. The P-wave axis is normal, but there is a rightward deviation of the QRS axis and a right ventricular conduction delay, especially when the left-to-right shunt is large (pulmonary/systemic blood flow ratio greater than 2.0).[86]

In ostium primum defects, the chest film may show considerable right atrial or left atrial enlargement, depending on the magnitude and direction of the mitral regurgitant jet (Fig. 25.10). The electrocardiogram shows a superior and leftward QRS axis in over 95% of cases. Left ventricular hypertrophy may coexist with right ventricular hypertrophy in patients with significant mitral regurgitation.

In sinus venosus defects of the superior vena cava type, the electrocardiogram often shows an abnormal P-wave axis, directed leftward and superiorly instead of rightward and inferiorly.

Noninvasive assessment seeks direct visualization of the defect from subcostal, right parasternal, or apical windows. Transesophageal imaging with color Doppler flow mapping can be of use in patients with poor transthoracic windows. Radionuclide angiographic analysis of pulmonary/systemic blood flow ratio is an alternative confirmatory test.[87,88] Indirect echocardiographic signs of an atrial defect are right ventricular dilatation and paradoxical ventricular septal motion. In ostium primum defects, the characteristic "cleft" (trileaflet) mitral valve can be visualized in the parasternal short-axis view.[89] Double-orifice mitral valve is a common associated anomaly.[90,91] Solitary left ventricular papillary muscle[90,91] is important to detect preoperatively;[92] plastic surgical repair can produce mitral stenosis in such patients. Doppler assessment of the severity of mitral regurgitation, if present, is also useful.

PARTIAL ANOMALOUS PULMONARY VENOUS CONNECTION

If the right-sided pulmonary veins are involved, common sites of connection are to the right atrium (as part of a sinus venosus defect—discussed in the section on atrial septal defect), superior vena cava, coronary sinus, and inferior vena cava. If the left-sided pulmonary veins are involved, the common sites of connection are to a left anterior cardinal vein or the coronary sinus.

The symptoms, physical findings, and electrocardiograms are similar to those in patients with atrial septal defect, except that in cases of partial anomalous pulmonary venous connection with intact atrial septum, there is respiratory variation of second sound splitting.

The chest film is also similar to atrial septal defect except in the subset of patients with "scimitar syndrome,"[93] who demonstrate anomalous connection of the right pulmonary veins to the inferior vena cava, and often, right lung hypoplasia, dextrocardia, and anomalous systemic arterial supply to the right lower lobe from the descending aorta. The characteristic sickle-like shadow produced by the anomalous pulmonary vein is present in the right lower lung field (Fig. 25.11).

Computed tomography[94,95] and magnetic resonance imaging are probably easier to use than echocardiography in the adult with this malformation.

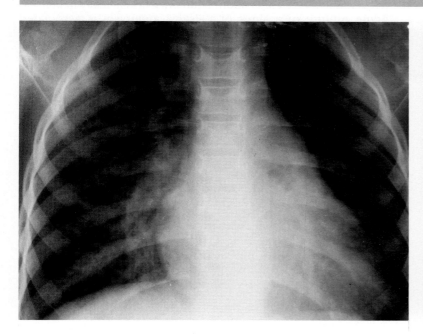

FIGURE 25.10 Ostium primum atrial septal defect. Contributing to the cardiomegaly was moderate mitral regurgitation associated with a "cleft" (trileaflet) mitral valve.

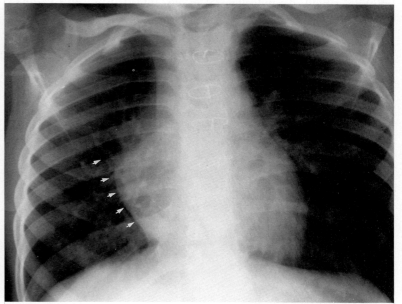

FIGURE 25.11 Scimitar syndrome. The arrows denote the right-sided pulmonary veins draining caudad into the inferior vena cava. This patient did not have dextrocardia. Repair was performed by creating a tunnel within the inferior vena cava and right atrium to direct pulmonary venous blood from the anomalous entrance through the atrial septum into the left atrium.

VENTRICULAR SEPTAL DEFECT

Only small or moderate-sized defects are seen initially in adulthood, since the vast majority of patients with an isolated large (nonrestrictive) ventricular septal defect present in the first few months of life. Even anatomically small ventricular septal defects can result in large left-to-right shunts. Small or moderate-sized ventricular septal defects are almost always defects in the membranous or muscular portions of the septum.

Depending on the size of the shunt there may be cardiomegaly and a forceful left ventricular impulse. The usual auscultatory finding is a loud pansystolic murmur at the lower left sternal border. There is often a palpable thrill at the lower left sternal edge. The very small ventricular septal defect (in which the communication is obliterated in late systole) may produce a short early systolic murmur, occasionally associated with an early systolic ejection sound from an accessory tricuspid valve partially closing the defect tissue.[96,97] Patients with a pulmonary/systemic blood flow ratio greater than 2.0 usually have a short mid-diastolic rumble at the apex of flow across the mitral valve. The second heart sound is usually split physiologically, but, rarely, splitting may be fixed.[98] The pulmonic component of the second heart sound is normal in intensity.

The chest film shows left atrial and left ventricular enlargement with increased pulmonary vascularity in patients with a pulmonary/systemic blood flow ratio of 2.0 or greater (Fig. 25.12). The electrocardiogram in patients with an anatomically small ventricular septal defect is normal, unless the left-to-right shunt is large, resulting in left ventricular hypertrophy. In moderate-sized defects there may be some degree of right ventricular hypertrophy, as well as a right ventricular conduction delay.

Approximately 5% of patients with ventricular septal defect develop aortic regurgitation, although this usually has occurred by age 10 years.[99] In contrast to patients with a patent ductus arteriosus, in whom the murmur is continuous and peaks in late systole, the systolic component of the to-and-fro murmur in patients with ventricular septal defect and aortic regurgitation peaks in mid-systole and is heard better at the lower left sternal border.

Noninvasive diagnostic identification of the small ventricular septal defect is best accomplished with cine magnetic resonance imaging. Detection of the jet by color Doppler ultrasound is possible in many patients. Again, a pulmonary/systemic blood flow ratio estimate can be obtained by standard pulsed Doppler[87] or by radioisotope angiography.

PATENT DUCTUS ARTERIOSUS

Symptoms in the adult presenting initially with persistence of a small (restrictive) ductus arteriosus are rare and are often related to the complication of infective endocarditis.

The right ventricular impulse is normal; the left ventricular impulse may be normal or increased, depending on the magnitude of the left-to-right shunt. The peripheral pulses are usually increased in amplitude owing to the diastolic aortic runoff. There is a continuous murmur typically peaking near the second heart sound. It is loudest in the second left interspace. The second heart sound is split normally. In the presence of a large left-to-right shunt, the second heart sound may be paradoxically split.

The chest film and electrocardiographic findings reflect the size of the left-to-right shunt. Patients with a pulmonary/systemic blood flow ratio of 2.0 or greater usually have left atrial and left ventricular enlargement.

Color Doppler echocardiography can frequently demonstrate the ductus arteriosus; pulsed Doppler echocardiographic interrogation of the main pulmonary artery shows pandiastolic retrograde flow. If the sample volume is placed within the ductus, continuous flow can be displayed from the aorta toward the pulmonary artery.

☐ LESIONS SIMULATING VALVAR AORTIC REGURGITATION
AORTIC SINUS OF VALSALVA ANEURYSM

There is a separation or lack of fusion between the media of the aorta and the annulus fibrosus of the aortic valve.[100] Aneurysms of the left sinus of Valsalva are rare and cause narrowing of the left coronary artery or rupture into the pericardial cavity. Aneurysms of the noncoronary sinus generally rupture into the right atrium, whereas those of the right sinus usually rupture into the right atrium or right ventricular outflow tract[101] or dissect the interventricular septum.[102] Aortico–left ventricular tunnel is distinct from aortic sinus of Valsalva aneurysm with fistula; it is a congenital vessel that originates above the coronary ostia, enters the infundibular septum, bypasses the aortic valve, and enters the left ventricle.[101,103] The malformation presents clinically in infancy.

Acute rupture of a sinus of Valsalva aneurysm is associated with chest pain, dyspnea, congestive failure, and rarely acute renal failure.[104]

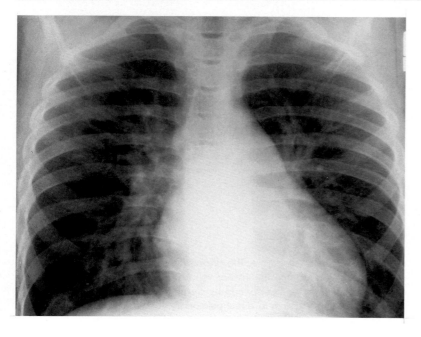

FIGURE 25.12 Ventricular septal defect, moderate-sized, with a pulmonary/systemic blood flow ratio of 2.5. There is left ventricular and mild left atrial enlargement and increased pulmonary vascularity.

A loud, superficial continuous murmur is present that usually peaks in diastole when the sinus of Valsalva aneurysm with fistula enters the right ventricle; it is often associated with a thrill along the right or left lower sternal borders.[40d] The pulses are increased as a result of the aortic runoff. The electrocardiogram shows left ventricular or biventricular hypertrophy. The chest film shows cardiomegaly and pulmonary venous congestion.

Two-dimensional echocardiography may demonstrate the anomaly, and Doppler ultrasound may show the disturbed flow pattern.[105-108]

CORONARY ARTERIOVENOUS FISTULA, CORONARY ARTERIOCAMERAL FISTULA

A coronary arteriovenous fistula consists of a communication between one of the coronary arteries and the coronary sinus, whereas in patients with a coronary arteriocameral fistula, the coronary artery drains into a cardiac chamber (most commonly the right ventricle).

Both ventricular impulses are increased. A continuous murmur is present, the location of which depends on the site of drainage.[40e]

The electrocardiogram may show biventricular hypertrophy. The chest film shows cardiomegaly and increased pulmonary blood flow.

Doppler echocardiography can demonstrate the site of drainage[109-111]; if the site of origin is relatively proximal, it may be detectable by two-dimensional echocardiography.

CONGENITALLY CORRECTED TRANSPOSITION OF THE GREAT ARTERIES

In this lesion, the right-sided ventricle has the morphologic characteristics of a left ventricle (*i.e.*, the septal surface is finely trabeculated and does not contain a septal band—septomarginal trabecula). This chamber ejects blood into the pulmonary artery, which lies posteriorly and to the right of the aorta. The left-sided ventricle has the morphologic characteristics of a right ventricle (*i.e.*, the septal surface displays a septal band and coarse trabeculations); it ejects blood into the aorta. This arrangement of the great arteries and ventricles permits functional correction of the circulation, since systemic venous blood passes into the pulmonary artery and pulmonary venous blood passes into the aorta. When congenitally corrected transposition occurs in isolated form or with a small ventricular septal defect, patients have no symptoms unless they have third degree atrioventricular block, a finding present in 22%[112] and attributed to the abnormal course of the conduction system.[113] In such patients, exertional or nocturnal dyspnea may develop.[114]

The majority of patients with corrected transposition also have a ventricular septal defect (usually a malalignment-type or atrioventricular canal-type) and subpulmonary stenosis (due either to malalignment of the infundibular septum or to accessory atrioventricular valve tissue). Anomalies of the left-sided (morphologically tricuspid) atrioventricular valve are frequent, ranging from atresia to Ebstein's anomaly.[115,116]

The morphologic left ventricle can be palpated as lying to the right by noting its anterior systolic movement. The plane of the interventricular sulcus can be detected by observing the retraction of the left-sided morphologic right ventricle laterally. The second heart sound is often single (with an inaudible pulmonary component due to both subpulmonary stenosis and the posterior position of the pulmonary valve) and accentuated because the aorta lies closer to the chest wall.

The chest film is very helpful, demonstrating a convexity of the upper left cardiac border produced by the leftward-situated aorta (Fig. 25.13). The electrocardiogram reveals an inverted relationship of the precordial QRS pattern (Fig. 25.14).

Two-dimensional echocardiography best demonstrates the inverted relationship of the ventricles, coexistent subpulmonary stenosis, and the anomalies of the left-sided atrioventricular valve; often, the ventricular septal defect can be visualized as well. Color Doppler echocardiography can be used to detect left atrioventricular valve regurgitation.

POSTOPERATIVE CONGENITAL HEART DISEASE

We have chosen in this chapter to discuss only those congenital cardiac anomalies that can present initially in adulthood. However, with the rapid improvement in cardiovascular surgical techniques that have occurred in the past 15 years, cardiologists may expect to see many long-term survivors of corrective operation in infancy. These patients often prove to be challenging to the bedside diagnostician because of the variety of hemodynamic and electrophysiologic sequelae of cardiac operations.[117] The use of prosthetic material in corrective surgery hampers two-dimensional and Doppler echocardiographic imaging. Therefore, the cardiologist must pay meticulous attention to the details of the operative procedure (*e.g.*, size and type of valved conduits, precise location of anastomoses) to optimize the yield from palpation, auscultation, chest roentgenography, electrocardiography, and echocardiography in postoperative adult patients.

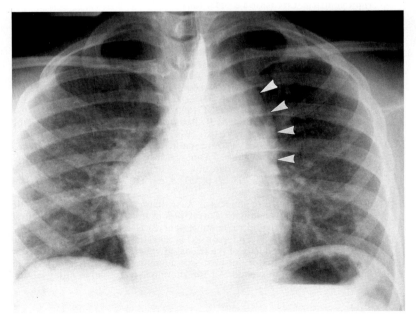

FIGURE 25.13 Corrected transposition of the great arteries. The aorta arises to the left of the pulmonary artery and, in this patient, ascends nearly vertically (*arrowheads*).

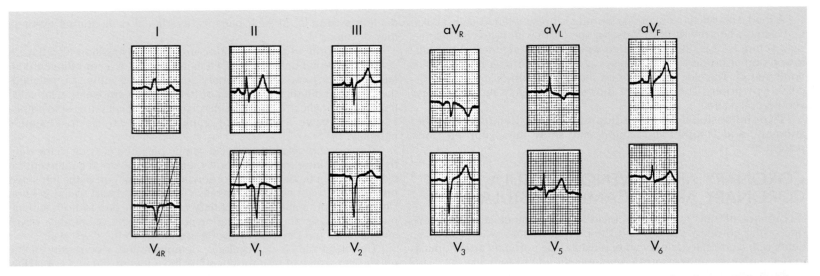

FIGURE 25.14 Corrected transposition of the great arteries. The right precordial leads (V_{4R} through V_2) show a QS pattern while there is no Q wave in V_6. This inverted pattern of septal depolarization suggests that the morphologic left ventricle is right sided and the morphologic right ventricle left sided.

REFERENCES

1. Dimich I, Steinfeld L, Park SC: Symptomatic atrial septal defect in infants. Am Heart J 85:601, 1973
2. Hunt CE, Lucas RV: Symptomatic atrial septal defect in infancy. Circulation 47:1042, 1973
3. Hislop A, Reid L: Pulmonary arterial development during childhood: Branching pattern and structure. Thorax 28:129, 1973
4. Heath D, Edwards JE: The pathology of hypertensive pulmonary vascular disease. Circulation 18:533, 1958
5. Hultgren HN, Reeve R, Cohn K et al: The ejection click of valvular pulmonary stenosis. Circulation 40:631, 1969
6. Gamboa R, Hugenholtz PG, Nadas AS: Accuracy of the phonocardiogram in assessing severity of aortic and pulmonic stenosis. Circulation 30:35, 1964
7. Vogelpoel L, Schrire V: Auscultatory and phonocardiographic assessment of pulmonary stenosis and intact ventricular septum. Circulation 22:55, 1960
8. Leatham A, Weitzman D: Auscultatory and phonographic signs of pulmonary stenosis. Br Heart J 19:303, 1957
9. Lababidi Z, Wu J-R: Percutaneous balloon pulmonary valvuloplasty. Am J Cardiol 52:650, 1983
10. Kan JS, White RI, Mitchell SE, Gardner TJ: Percutaneous balloon valvuloplasty: A new method for treating congenital pulmonic stenosis. N Engl J Med 307:540, 1982
11. Pepine CJ, Gessner IH, Feldman RL: Percutaneous balloon valvuloplasty for pulmonic valve stenosis in the adult. Am J Cardiol 50:1442, 1982
12. Oliveira Lima C, Sahn DJ, Valdes-Cruz LM et al: Non-invasive prediction of transvalvular pressure gradient in patients with pulmonary stenosis by quantitative two-dimensional echocardiographic Doppler studies. Circulation 67:866, 1983
13. Van Praagh R, Van Praagh S, Nebasar RA et al: Tetralogy of Fallot: Underdevelopment of the pulmonary infundibulum and its sequelae. Am J Cardiol 26:25, 1970
14. Lenox CC, Zuberbuhler JR: Surgical anatomy of tetralogy of Fallot. J Thorac Cardiovasc Surg 81:887, 1981
15. McMyn JK: Tetralogy of Fallot: Angiocardiographic diagnosis compared with surgical findings. Australas Radiol 13:37, 1969
16. Partridge JB, Fiddler GI: Cineangiocardiography in tetralogy of Fallot. Br Heart J 45:112, 1981
17. Bousvaros GA: The pulmonary second sound in the tetralogy of Fallot. Am Heart J 61:570, 1961
18. Tofler OB: The pulmonary component of the second heart sound in Fallot's tetralogy. Br Heart J 25:509, 1963
19. Higgins CB, Byrd BF, Farmer DW et al: Magnetic resonance imaging in patients with congenital heart disease. Circulation 70:851, 1984
20. Sabiston DC, Cornell WP, Criley JM et al: The diagnosis and surgical correction of total obstruction of the right ventricle. J Thorac Cardiovasc Surg 48:577, 1964
21. Haworth SG, Rees PG, Taylor JFN et al: Pulmonary atresia with ventricular septal defect and major aortopulmonary collateral arteries. Br Heart J 45:133, 1981
22. Vogelpoel L, Schrire V: The role of auscultation in the differentiation of Fallot's tetralogy from severe pulmonary stenosis with intact ventricular septum and right-to-left intra-atrial shunt. Circulation 11:714, 1955
23. Capelli H, Ross D, Somerville J: Aortic regurgitation in tetrad of Fallot and pulmonary atresia. Am J Cardiol 49:1979, 1982
24. Liao PK, Edwards WD, Julsrud PR, Puga FJ, Danielson GK, Feldt RH: Pulmonary blood supply in patients with pulmonary atresia and ventricular septal defect. J Am Coll Card 6:1343, 1985.
25. Hatteland K, Semb BKH: Assessment of aortic regurgitation by means of pulsed Doppler ultrasound. Ultrasound Med Biol 8:1, 1982
26. Gasul BM, Dillon RF, Vrla V et al: Ventricular septal defects: Their natural transformation into those with infundibular stenosis or into the cyanotic or noncyanotic type of tetralogy of Fallot. JAMA 164:847, 1957
27. Lynfield J, Gasul BM, Arcilla R et al: The natural history of ventricular defect in infancy and childhood. Am J Med 30:357, 1961
28. Bloomfield DK: The natural history of the ventricular septal defect in patients surviving infancy. Circulation 29:914, 1964
29. Varghese PJ, Allen JR, Rosenquist GC et al: Natural history of ventricular septal defect with right-sided aortic arch. Br Heart J 32:537, 1970
30. Ponglione G, Freedom RM, Cook D et al: Mechanism of acquired right ventricular outflow tract obstruction in patients with ventricular septal defect: An angiocardiographic study. Am J Cardiol 50:776, 1982
31. Van Praagh R, McNamara JJ: Anatomic types of ventricular septal defect with aortic insufficiency: Diagnostic and surgical considerations. Am Heart J 75:604, 1968
32. Fellows KE, Martin EC, Rosenthal A: Angiocardiography of obstructing muscle bands of the right ventricle. Am J Roentgenol 128:249, 1977
33. Lucas RV, Varco RL, Lillehei CW et al: Anomalous muscle bundle of the right ventricle. Circulation 25:443, 1962
34. Goor DA, Lillehei CW: Congenital Malformations of the Heart, pp 14–15. New York, Grune & Stratton, 1975
35. Baumstark A, Fellows KE, Rosenthal A: Combined double chambered right ventricle and discrete subaortic stenosis. Circulation 57:299, 1978
36. Van Praagh R, Corwin RD, Dahlquist EH et al: Tetralogy of Fallot with severe left ventricular outflow tract obstruction due to anomalous attachment of the mitral valve to the ventricular septum. Am J Cardiol 26:93, 1970
37. Lev M, Liberthson RR, Joseph RH et al: The pathologic anatomy of Ebstein's disease. Arch Pathol 90:334, 1970
38. Becker AE, Becker MD, Edwards JE: Pathologic spectrum of dysplasia of the tricuspid valve. Arch Pathol 91:167, 1971
39. Zuberbuhler JR, Allwork SP, Anderson RH: The spectrum of Ebstein's anomaly of the tricuspid valve. J Thorac Cardiovasc Surg 77:202, 1979
40. Perloff JK: The Clinical Recognition of Congenital Heart Disease, a, pp 244–246; b, p 248; c, p 168; d, p 597; e, pp 581–582. Philadelphia, WB Saunders, 1978
41. Crews TL, Pridie RB, Benhem R et al: Auscultatory and phonocardiographic findings in Ebstein's anomaly: Correlation of first heart sound with ultrasonic records of tricuspid valve movement. Br Heart J 34:681, 1972
42. Schiebler GL, Adams P, Anderson RC et al: Clinical study of twenty-three cases of Ebstein's anomaly of the tricuspid valve. Circulation 19:165, 1959
43. Watson H: Natural history of Ebstein's anomaly of the tricuspid valve in childhood and adolescence: An international cooperative study of 505 cases. Br Heart J 36:417, 1974

44. Smith WM, Gallagher JJ, Kerr CR et al: The electrophysiologic basis and management of symptomatic recurrent tachycardia in patients with Ebstein's anomaly of the tricuspid valve. Am J Cardiol 49:1223, 1982
45. Shiina A, Seward JB, Edwards WD et al: Two-dimensional echocardiographic spectrum of Ebstein's anomaly: Detailed anatomic assessment. J Am Coll Card 3:356, 1984
46. Shiina A, Seward JB, Tajik AJ et al: Two-dimensional echocardiographic-surgical correlation in Ebstein's anomaly: Preoperative determination of patients requiring tricuspid valve plication vs replacement. Circulation 68:534, 1983
47. Castaneda-Zuniga W, Nath HP, Moller JH et al: Left-sided anomalies in Ebstein's malformation of the tricuspid valve. Pediatr Cardiol 3:181, 1982
48. Worm AM, Ravault MC, Ethevenot G et al: Prolapsus mitral et anomalies ventriculaires gauches dans la malformation d'Ebstein de la tricuspide. Arch Mal Coeur 73:499, 1976
49. Lucas RV: Anomalous venous connections, pulmonary and systemic. In Adams FH, Emmanouilides GC (eds): Moss' Heart Disease in Infants, Children, and Adolescence, 3rd ed, p 476. Baltimore, Williams & Wilkins, 1983
50. Niwayama G: Cor triatriatum. Am Heart J 59:291, 1960
51. Pedersen A, Therkelen F: Cor triatriatum: Rare malformation of the heart, probably amenable to surgery: Report of a case with review of the literature. Am Heart J 47:676, 1954
52. Miller GAH, Ongley PA, Anderson MW et al: Cor triatriatum: Hemodynamic and angiographic diagnosis. Am Heart J 68:298, 1964
53. Ostman-Smith I, Silverman NH, Oldershaw P et al: Cor triatriatum sinistrum: Diagnostic features on cross-sectional echocardiography. Br Heart J 51:211, 1984
54. Norell MS, Lincoln C, Sutton GC: Two-dimensional echocardiographic diagnosis of cor triatriatum. J Cardiovasc Ultrason 2:369, 1983
55. Rumancik WM, Hernanz-Schulman M, Rutkowski MM et al: Magnetic resonance imaging of cor triatriatum. Ped Cardiol 9:149, 1988
56. Bisset GS, Kirks DR, Strife JL, Schwartz DC. Cor triatriatum: Diagnosis by MR imaging. AJR 149:567, 1987
57. Roberts WC: The structure of the aortic valve in clinically isolated aortic stenosis: An autopsy study of 162 patients over 15 years of age. Circulation 42:91, 1970
58. Perloff JK: Physical Examination of the Heart and Circulation, a, p 203; b, p 114. Philadelphia, WB Saunders, 1982
59. Friedman WF, Benson LN: Aortic stenosis. In Adams FH, Emmanouilides GC (eds): Moss' Heart Disease in Infants, Children, and Adolescence, 3rd ed, p 173. Baltimore, Williams & Wilkins, 1983
60. Friedman WF, Pappelbaum SJ: Indications for hemodynamic evaluation and surgery in congenital aortic stenosis. Pediatr Clin North Am 18:1207, 1971
61. Brandenburg RO, Tajik AJ, Edwards WD et al: Accuracy of 2-dimensional echocardiographic diagnosis of congenitally bicuspid valve: Echocardiographic-anatomic correlation in 115 patients. Am J Cardiol 51:1469, 1983
62. Labibidi Z, Wu J-R, Walls JT: Percutaneous balloon aortic valvuloplasty: Results in 23 patients. Am J Cardiol 53:194, 1984
63. Cyran SE, Kimball TR, Schwartz DC et al: Evaluation of balloon aortic valvuloplasty with transesophageal echocardiography. Am Heart J 115:460, 1988
64. Safian RD, Berman AD, Diver DJ et al: Balloon aortic valvuloplasty in 170 consecutive patients. N Engl J Med 319:125, 1988
65. DePace NL, Ren J-F, Iskandrian AS et al: Correlation of echocardiographic wall stress and left ventricular pressure and function in aortic stenosis. Circulation 67:854, 1983
66. Hatle L, Angelsen B, Tromsdal A: Non-invasive assessment of aortic stenosis by Doppler ultrasound. Br Heart J 43:284, 1980
67. Stamm RB, Martin RP: Quantification of pressure gradients across stenotic valves by Doppler ultrasound. J Am Coll Card 2:707, 1983
68. Berger M, Berdoff RL, Gallerstein PE et al: Evaluation of aortic stenosis by continuous wave Doppler ultrasound. J Am Coll Card 3:150, 1984
69. Feigl A, Feigl D, Lucas RV et al: Involvement of the aortic valve cusps in discrete subaortic stenosis. Pediatr Cardiol 5:185, 1984
70. Roberts WC: Valvular, subvalvular, and supravalvular aortic stenosis: Morphologic features. Cardiovasc Clin 5:97, 1973
71. Hatle L: Non-invasive assessment and differentiation of left ventricular outflow obstruction. Circulation 64:381, 1981
72. Hutchins GM: Coarctation of the aorta explained as a branch point of the ductus arteriosus. Am J Pathol 63:203, 1971
73. Perloff JK: Congenital heart disease. In Wyngaarden JB, Smith LH (eds): Cecil Textbook of Medicine, 16th ed, p 176. Philadelphia, WB Saunders, 1982
74. Cohen M, Fuster V, Steele PM et al: Coarctation of the aorta. Long-term follow-up and prediction of outcome after surgical correction. Circulation 80:840, 1989.
75. Rosenquist GC: Congenital mitral valve disease associated with coarctation of the aorta. Circulation 49:985, 1974
76. Celano V, Pieroni DR, Morera JA et al: Two-dimensional echocardiographic examination of mitral valve abnormalities associated with coarctation of the aorta. Circulation 69:924, 1984
77. Wyse RKH, Robinson PJ, Deanfield JE et al: Use of continuous wave Doppler ultrasound velocimetry to assess the severity of coarctation of the aorta by measurement of aortic flow velocities. Br Heart J 52:278, 1984
78. Hatle L, Brubakk A, Tromsdal A et al: Non-invasive assessment of pressure drop in mitral stenosis. Br Heart J 40:131, 1978
79. Veyrat C, Abitol G, Bas S et al: Quantitative assessment of valvular regurgitations using the pulsed Doppler technique: Approach to the regurgitant lesion. Ultrasound Med Biol 10:201, 1984
80. Simpson IA, Chung KJ, Glass RF et al: Cine magnetic resonance imaging for evaluation of anatomy and flow relations in infants and children with coarctation of the aorta. Circulation 78:142, 1988
81. McCormack RJ, Pickering D, Smith II: A rare type of atrial septal defect. Thorax 23:350, 1968
82. Mantini E, Grondin GM, Lillehei CW, Edwards JE: Congenital anomalies involving the coronary sinus. Circulation 33:317, 1966
83. Freedom RM, Culham JAG, Rowe RD: Left atrial to coronary sinus fenestration (partially unroofed coronary sinus). Brit Heart J 46:63, 1981
84. Carabello B, Gash A, Mayers D et al: Normal left ventricular systolic function in adults with atrial septal defect and left heart failure. Am J Cardiol 49:1868, 1982
85. Liberthson RR, Boucher CA, Fallon JT et al: Severe mitral regurgitation: A common occurrence in the aging patient with secundum atrial septal defect. Clin Cardiol 4:229, 1981
86. Sung RJ, Tamer DM, Agha AS et al: Etiology of the electrocardiographic pattern of "incomplete right bundle branch block" in atrial septal defect: An electrophysiologic study. J Pediatr 87:1182, 1975
87. Sanders SP, Yeager S, Williams RG: Measurement of systemic and pulmonary blood flow and pulmonary/systemic blood flow ratio using Doppler and 2-dimensional echocardiography. Am J Cardiol 51:952, 1983
88. McIlveen BM, Murray IPC, Giles RW et al: Clinical application of radionuclide quantitation of left to right cardiac shunts in children. Am J Cardiol 47:1273, 1981
89. Van Mill GJ, Moulaert AJ, Harinck E: Atlas of Two-Dimensional Echocardiography in Congenital Cardiac Defects, pp 53–55. Boston, Martinus Nijhoff, 1983
90. Van Mierop LHS: Pathology and pathogenesis of endocardial cushion defects. In Davila JC (ed): Second Henry Ford Hospital International Symposium on Cardiac Surgery, pp 201–207. New York, Appleton-Century-Crofts, 1977
91. Danielson GK: Correction of atrioventricular canal. In Anderson RH, Shinebourne EA (eds): Paediatric Cardiology 1977, p 470. Edinburgh, Churchill Livingstone, 1978
92. Chin AJ, Keane JF, Norwood WI et al: Repair of complete common AV canal in infancy. J Thorac Cardiovasc Surg 84:437, 1982
93. Neill CA, Ferencz C, Sabiston DC et al: The familial occurrence of hypoplastic right lung with systemic arterial supply and venous drainage "scimitar syndrome." Bull Johns Hopkins Hosp 107:1, 1960
94. Godwin JD, Tarver RD: Scimitar syndrome: Four new cases examined with CT. Radiology 159:15, 1986
95. Olson MA, Becker GJ: The scimitar syndrome: CT findings in partial anomalous pulmonary venous return. Radiology 159:25, 1986
96. Freedom RM, White RD, Pieroni DR et al: The natural history of the so-called aneurysm of the membranous ventricular septum in childhood. Circulation 49:375, 1974
97. Anderson RH, Lenox CC, Zuberbuhler JR: Mechanisms of closure of perimembranous ventricular septum in childhood. Am J Cardiol 52:341, 1983
98. Harris C, Wise J, Oakley CM: "Fixed" splitting of the second heart sound in ventricular septal defect. Br Heart J 33:428, 1971
99. Keane JF, Plauth WH, Nadas AS: Ventricular septal defect with aortic regurgitation. Circulation 56(Suppl I):1, 1977
100. Edwards JE, Burchell HB: The pathologic anatomy of deficiencies between the aortic root and the heart, including aortic sinus aneurysm. Thorax 12:125, 1957
101. Eliot RS, Woodburn RL, Edwards JE: Conditions of the ascending aorta simulating aortic valvular incompetence. Am J Cardiol 14:679, 1964
102. Chen WWC, Tai YT: Dissection of interventricular septum by aneurysm of sinus of Valsalva. Br Heart J 50:293, 1983
103. Levy MJ, Lillehei CW, Anderson RC et al: Aortico-left ventricular tunnel. Circulation 27:841, 1963
104. Gleason MM, Hardy C, Chin AJ, Pigott JD: Ruptured sinus of Valsalva aneurysm in childhood. Am Heart J 114:1235, 1987
105. Desai AG, Sharma S, Kumar A et al: Echocardiographic diagnosis of unruptured aneurysm of right sinus of Valsalva: An unusual cause of right ventricular outflow obstruction. Am Heart J 109:363, 1985
106. Peters P, Juziuk E, Gunther S. Doppler color flow mapping detection of ruptured sinus of Valsalva aneurysm. J Am Soc Echo 2:195, 1989
107. Chow LC, Dittrich HC, Dembitsky WP, Nicod PH: Accurate localization of ruptured sinus of Valsalva aneurysm by real-time two-dimensional Doppler flow imaging. Chest 94:462, 1988
108. Chia BL, Ee BK, Choo MH, Yan PC. Ruptured aneurysm of sinus of Valsalva: Recognition by Doppler color flow mapping. Am Heart J 115:686, 1988
109. Kronzon I, Winer HE, Cohen M: Non-invasive diagnosis of left coronary arteriovenous fistula communicating with the right ventricle. Am J Cardiol

49:1811, 1982
110. Calafiore PA, Raymond R, Schiavone WA, Rosenkranz ER: Precise evaluation of a complex coronary arteriovenous fistula: The utility of transesophageal color Doppler. J Am Soc Echo 2:337, 1989
111. Sanders SP, Parness IA, Colan SD. Recognition of abnormal connections of coronary arteries with the use of Doppler color flow mapping. J Am Coll Card 13:922, 1989
112. Huhta JC, Maloney JD, Ritter DG et al: Complete atrioventricular block in patients with atrioventricular discordance. Circulation 67:1374, 1983
113. Walmsley T: Transposition of the ventricles and the arterial stems. J Anat 65:528, 1931
114. Berman DA, Adicoff A: Corrected transposition of the great arteries causing complete heart block in an adult. Am J Cardiol 24:125, 1969
115. Allwork S, Bentall H, Becker A et al: Congenitally corrected transposition of the great arteries: Morphologic study of 32 cases. Am J Cardiol 38:910, 1976
116. Otero Coto E, Perez Martinez V, Palacios V et al: Ebstein's anomaly of the left-sided atrioventricular valve in AV discordance. Thorac Cardiovasc Surg 28:364, 1980
117. Engle MA, Perloff JK (eds): Congenital Heart Disease After Surgery. New York, Yorke Medical Books, 1983

SECTION 4

Section Editor
Kanu Chatterjee, MB, FRCP

Noninvasive Tests

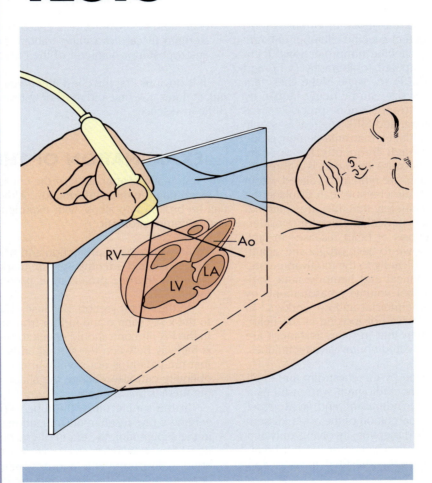

THE CHEST X-RAY FILM AND THE DIAGNOSIS OF HEART DISEASE

Melvin D. Cheitlin

WHY DO WE STILL NEED THE CHEST FILM?

The chest film is one of the oldest "noninvasive" diagnostic tests used in the diagnosis of heart disease other than physical examination. Until the advent of echocardiography, it was the most important way to evaluate the overall heart size and to detect specific chamber enlargement. With the development of more specific nonprojectional techniques such as echocardiography, computed tomography (CT), and magnetic resonance image scanning (MRI), the value of the chest film has been questioned. Specific chamber size can be better judged by the newer techniques. Ventricular hypertrophy can be precisely measured by echocardiography, CT scanning, and MRI, whereas it is only suggested in the chest film. In the chest film cardiac enlargement is due to increased chamber volume. Although frequently the specific chamber involved can be identified, because the heart is a three-dimensional structure and all the chambers are intimately related within the cardiac silhouette, enlargement of one chamber can displace the other chambers, making it appear inaccurately that they are enlarged.

What is the justification, other than historical interest, for considering the chest film of use in the diagnosis of heart disease? In fact, cardiac size by chest film has been shown to have prognostic significance in valvular disease that adds significantly to the multivariate prediction of prognosis obtained from clinical and hemodynamic variables including even the cardiac chamber volume measurements by angiocardiography in a study by Hammermeister and co-workers.[1] In addition to being the most inexpensive way of looking at the heart, there are contributions of the chest film that in many instances are unique compared with the more sophisticated noninvasive techniques:

1. Some abnormalities are best visualized by the chest film and in all likelihood might be missed if the echocardiogram were used as a screening technique. These would include aortic and great vessel aneurysms; great vessel anomalies; coarctation of the aorta; dissection of the aorta, especially type B dissection involving only the descending aorta; partial and complete absence of the left hemipericardium; pericardial cysts and perimediastinal masses; and dextrocardia with situs inversus.
2. Evaluation of pulmonary vascularity as a reflection of the physiological abnormalities of heart disease (*i.e.*, increase in pulmonary vascularity with left-to-right shunts, increase in pulmonary artery size, increase in the size of the pulmonary arterial branches compared with the sparse distal branches with pulmonary vascular disease, signs of congestive heart failure with vascular redistribution to the upper lung fields, vascular congestion, and fluid in the interstitial spaces of the lung)
3. Calcification within the heart silhouette especially if the chest film is supplemented by cardiac fluoroscopy (*i.e.*, calcification of valves, calcification of coronary arteries, calcification in left ventricular aneurysms, calcification in the walls of the heart such as the left atrium, or masses in the heart such as myxomas, calcification of the pericardium)
4. Lesions in the lung due to cardiovascular disease (*i.e.*, pulmonary arteriovenous fistulas, pulmonary emboli with pulmonary hypertension, pulmonary venous varices)
5. Other problems related to differential diagnosis in cardiovascular disease (*i.e.*, hiatal hernia, pericardial and pleural effusions, air-fluid levels in the megaesophagus, herniation of the abdominal contents into the chest, pneumomediastinum and pneumothorax)
6. Musculoskeletal abnormalities as clues to cardiovascular disease (*i.e.*, Marfan's syndrome, cervical ribs, fracture of the first rib or sternum in cardiovascular trauma, pectus excavatum and narrow anteroposterior diameter of the chest)

It is obvious that the chest film is still an important study, contributing, at times, the first and most definitive clue to the presence and type of heart disease.

EXAMINATION OF THE CHEST FILM

The systematic examination of the chest film ensures the best chance of extracting the most information. Although the systematic approach can be broken into steps, with experience these steps take little time and become automatic.

1. Identify the type of projection and whether the position is proper or slightly rotated. Identify the film marking of the right and left sides. Note whether the projection is posteroanterior (PA) or anteroposterior (AP).

    In the AP projection, because of the position of the heart closer to the x-ray source and further from the film, the heart is magnified. In the PA film one should check to see if the dorsal spinous process is halfway between the sternal ends of the two clavicles to ensure that the patient is not slightly turned to the right or left. This slight obliquity can also change the shape of the cardiac silhouette and the mediastinal shadow.

    In the supine films, the tube-to-film distance is short, and diverging x-rays result in magnification of the cardiac silhouette. Also, in the supine film, the effect of gravity on the distribution of pulmonary blood flow is lost, so the vessels to the upper lung fields appear abnormally prominent. In lordotic films the x-ray beam is no longer perpendicular to the chest and the heart, the clavicles are straight and lifted off the rib cage, and the base of the heart is narrowed.

    Attention to these details can prevent gross errors, for instance, overlooking dextrocardia and situs inversus and diagnosing displacement of the heart to the left when the patient is simply turned slightly to the left. Proper positioning allows comparison of the chest film with previous films.

    It is important to count ribs to make sure that the depth of inspiration is adequate. A film with poor inspiration can make the heart size appear to be increased and the lungs look congested, even simulating pulmonary edema. In an adult a good inspiration should bring the diaphragm to the tenth rib posteriorly or the sixth to seventh right rib anteriorly.
2. Check the exposure of the film. Underexposure or overexposure can make the pulmonary vascularity difficult to evaluate. Exposure for evaluation of pulmonary markings is adequate if the intervertebral spaces and the descending aorta behind the heart are just barely visible. If the film is overexposed, lung markings and signs of

pulmonary congestion will be lost; if it is underexposed, lung markings will be accentuated and difficult to evaluate.
3. Check for artifacts. Chest tubes, nasogastric tubes, Swan-Ganz catheters, folds of skin or clothing, protuberant nipples, absence of a breast or thoracic deformities, and electrocardiographic monitor electrodes can all cause confusing shadows which can be mistakenly interpreted. Artifacts of the development of the film due to contact of one film with another in a development tank, or electrostatic artifacts, can also be confusing.
4. Examine lung fields and mediastinum. Look for masses, calcification, and infiltrations in the lungs. Examine the position of the minor and major fissures and the position of the carina and the main stem bronchi. Identify the side of the aortic arch, whether it is left sided or right sided, the position determined by the bronchus over which it passes. Examine pulmonary vascular markings, the size of hilar vessels, the presence of calcification in the pulmonary vessels, evidence of interstitial edema (*i.e.,* Kerley's B lines, cuffing of fluid around the vessels, and the presence of pleural effusion).
5. Examine the cardiac silhouette in the PA, the lateral, and, if present, the right and left anterior oblique views. Note the overall cardiac size as measured by the cardiothoracic ratio and the position of the heart in the chest; in the PA view about a third of the heart should be to the right of the midline and two thirds to the left. Look for evidence of specific chamber enlargement and the presence of densities within the cardiac silhouette. Densities can be due to atelectasis or masses behind the heart or to calcification of valves, valve rings, or pericardium. Look for calcification in other structures (*i.e.,* the ascending aorta, the pulmonary arteries, and the aortic arch). Calcification can occur in patent ductus arteriosus, aortic aneurysms, left ventricular aneurysms, and coronary vessels.
6. Examine the skeleton and other structures.
   a. Look for air-fluid levels in the esophagus, gas in a viscus structure, or air in the mediastinum.
   b. Examine the position of the diaphragm. Normally, the diaphragm is lower on the side of the heart; therefore, usually the left diaphragm is lower than the right. If the opposite is true, this could be due to phrenic nerve paralysis, subpulmonic effusion, or subphrenic abscess.
   c. Count the ribs and look for absent ribs, cervical ribs, radiolucencies or densities in the ribs, fractures, rib notching, and changes consistent with Marfan's syndrome.
   d. Identify the stomach bubble. Examine the side of the stomach bubble as a clue to the situs of the viscera, which determine the anatomical position of the atria. Look for subdiaphragmatic densities, such as gallstones, calcification of an abdominal aneurysm, or aneurysms in subdiaphragmatic arteries, and the presence of ascites.

EVALUATION OF THE OVERALL CARDIAC SIZE

Since the heart is a three-dimensional structure, its size should be evaluated in at least two planes. At times, the heart can be displaced into the left side of the chest and give the superficial appearance of enlargement. At other times the heart can dilate anteriorly or posteriorly perpendicular to the frontal plane and therefore appear of normal size in the PA film and grossly enlarged in the lateral. The simplest way to evaluate the overall heart size is using the cardiothoracic ratio introduced by Ungerleider and Clark.[2] The measurement relates the widest diameter of the heart to the widest diameter of the thoracic rib cage measuring from the inner limits of the ribs usually at the level of the dome of the right hemidiaphragm. In normal children and adults this ratio is equal to or less than 0.5 and in infants it is up to 0.6.[3]

A second, less commonly used, measurement is a rough estimation of the cardiac volume from measurements in the frontal and sagittal films.[4] In this measurement the longest diameter (D) in the PA film, from the junction of the superior vena cava and the right atrium to the apex; the short axis (S), from the right cardiophrenic angle to the junction of the main pulmonary artery and the left atrial segments on the left heart border, and the greatest AP dimension of the heart in the lateral view (D) are measured in centimeters. The volume of the heart (V) is obtained as follows:

$$V = \frac{L \times D \times S}{\text{Body Surface Area}} \times K$$

K is a constant derived from the distance from the film to the x-ray tube and for a 6-foot chest film is 0.42. A value of 450 ml/m^2 for women and 500 ml/m^2 for men is considered normal. Above 490 ml/m^2 for women and 540 ml/m^2 for men is considered definitely enlarged.

SPECIFIC CHAMBER SIZE

Chamber size can best be estimated using the PA, left lateral, and right and left anterior oblique views. In general, chamber dilatation is necessary to influence the cardiac silhouette on the chest film. Hypertrophy of muscle can cause subtle changes in the silhouette, but enlargement is due to chamber dilatation.

In general, only four densities are distinguishable on the routine chest film: bone, air, fluid–tissue, and fat. Fluid and tissue have the same x-ray density on the chest film and cannot be separated. Since the heart is a three-dimensional structure and since the borders of the individual chambers are not separable one from the other, enlargement of one chamber can distort the cardiac silhouette in a characteristic way or can displace the heart, making it appear that the opposite border-forming part of the silhouette (*i.e.,* another chamber) is enlarged. In general, the most characteristic change in cardiac silhouette is seen when a single chamber is enlarged.[5]

The borders of the cardiac silhouette in the PA, left lateral, and right and left anterior oblique views are presented in Figures 26.1 and 26.2.

OVERALL ENLARGEMENT OF THE CARDIAC SILHOUETTE

The most common cause of enlargement of the cardiac silhouette is cardiomegaly. However, other conditions can simulate cardiomegaly: displacement of the heart into the left side of the chest, pectus excavatum, tumors applied to the left or right cardiac borders (*i.e.,* thymomas or lymphomas), pericardial cysts, and pericardial effusion.

Pericardial effusion results in enlargement of the cardiac silhouette, usually both to the right and left. The classic shape is that of a "water bottle," with a narrow neck and wide base, causing the cardiophrenic angles in the PA film to lose their acute angle and become obtuse. However, pericardial effusion filling out the lateral pouches of the pericardium and accumulating inferiorly and anteriorly can cause enlargement that exactly simulates cardiomegaly (Fig. 26.3). In general, with effusion the pulmonary vascular structures remain normal, whereas with cardiomegaly and congestive failure, they are abnormal. At times in the lateral film, a radiolucency due to the epicardial fat can be seen to be separated markedly from the retrosternal fat by the radiodense fluid, but this "epicardial fat stripe" sign is uncommon in my experience (Fig. 26.4).

SPECIFIC CHAMBER ENLARGEMENT
RIGHT ATRIUM

In the PA film, the right atrium forms the right border of the cardiac silhouette. It extends from the right cardiophrenic angle to the junction of the right atrium with the superior vena cava, where a slight indentation usually occurs (see Fig. 26.1). At times, a small part of the inferior vena cava is seen at the right cardiophrenic angle. The tricuspid valve lies over the spine, and the left border of the right atrium cannot be distinguished on the chest film. On fluoroscopy, fat in the right atrioventricular groove can be seen, and this represents the level of the tricuspid valve and the left border of the right atrium.

In right atrial enlargement the right border of the heart is displaced to the right and superiorly with the arc of the right cardiac border passing higher than normal to join the superior vena cava (Fig. 26.5). The right atrium also enlarges anteriorly and in the left anterior oblique film forms a superior shelf to the left of the cardiac silhouette. Unlike the left atrium, right atrial enlargement is rarely gigantic.

Examples of right atrial enlargement are seen classically in longstanding tricuspid insufficiency secondary to right ventricular failure, tricuspid stenosis, tricuspid atresia, and Ebstein's anomaly. Giant right atrium is a rare anomaly and can cause isolated right atrial enlargement.

RIGHT VENTRICLE

The right ventricle does not normally form a border of the cardiac silhouette in the PA film (see Fig. 26.1). In the left lateral film it forms the retrosternal border of the heart and normally fills only about one third of the retrosternal space inferiorly (see Fig. 26.2). In hypertrophy of the right ventricle, as seen in pulmonary stenosis or tetralogy of Fallot, the cardiac silhouette may not be enlarged, but in the PA film

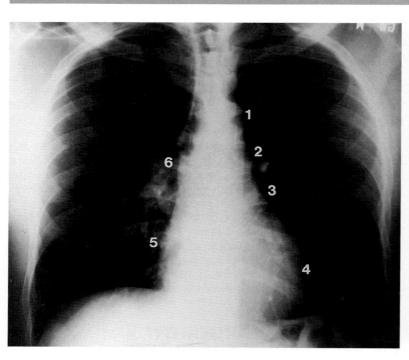

FIGURE 26.1 Posteroanterior view, normal chest roentgenogram. The borders of the cardiac silhouette are (1) aortic arch, (2) main pulmonary artery segment, (3) area of left auricular appendage, (4) left ventricle, (5) right atrial border, and (6) ascending aorta.

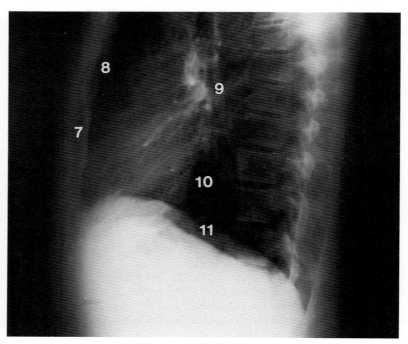

FIGURE 26.2 Left lateral view, normal chest roentgenogram. The borders of the cardiac silhouette are (7) right ventricle, (8) right ventricular outflow tract, (9) left atrium, (10) left ventricle, (11) inferior vena cava.

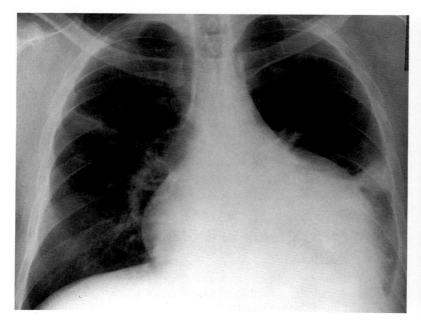

FIGURE 26.3 Posteroanterior projection of a patient with a large pericardial effusion. Note the sharp right cardiophrenic angle, normal pulmonary vascularity, and areas of atelectasis in right and left lungs.

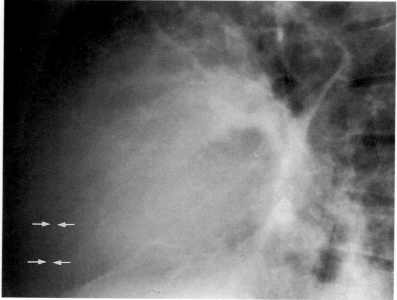

FIGURE 26.4 Left lateral projection of the same patient with pericardial effusion as in Figure 26.3. Note the radiolucent line inside the cardiac silhouette (arrows) displaced posteriorly from the retrosternal area.

the apex of the heart may be formed by the right ventricle instead of the left ventricle and classically lifts the apex of the heart off of the diaphragm (Fig. 26.6; see Fig. 26.5). In the lateral film the right ventricle fills more than one third of the retrosternal space (Fig. 26.7).

With enlargement of the right ventricular chamber, the right ventricle dilates anteriorly and to the left, eventually forming the left border of the heart, including the apex (Fig. 26.8).

Classic examples of right ventricular hypertrophy without dilatation are seen with severe pulmonary hypertension from any cause: mitral stenosis, pulmonary stenosis, pulmonary atresia (see Fig. 26.6), and tetralogy of Fallot. Right ventricular dilatation can be seen in these conditions when right ventricular failure occurs. The most common reason for right ventricular dilatation is left ventricular failure. Volume overload of the right ventricle also results in right ventricular dilatation occurring in tricuspid insufficiency, pulmonic valvular insufficiency, atrial septal defect (see Figs. 26.7 and 26.8), and anomalous pulmonary venous drainage.

LEFT ATRIUM

The left atrium is a posterior structure and normally only the tip of the left auricular appendage forms a cardiac border in the normal PA chest film. Normally the left atrium forms the superior posterior border of the cardiac silhouette in the lateral film and also in the two oblique views. The left atrium is capable of the most enormous enlargement, more than any of the other cardiac chambers. As the left atrium enlarges it dilates posteriorly, superiorly, and to the right, filling in the area under the aortic arch, the so-called aortic window, and pushing the esophagus posteriorly and usually to the right. Since the tracheal bifurcation rests on the upper posterior portion of the left atrium, left atrial enlargement pushes the left main stem bronchus posteriorly and superiorly. As the left auricle enlarges it dilates to the left and forms a convex border just under the main pulmonary artery segment. Normally, this area is concave or straight, but never convex (Figs. 26.9 and 26.10). The appendage can enlarge to an enormous extent, forming an aneurysmal mass on the left cardiac border in the PA film. Further enlargement of the body of the left atrium is to the right, resulting in a double density behind the silhouette of the right side of the heart and finally forming a bulge on the upper two thirds of the right cardiac border (see Fig. 26.9). With giant left atrium, the cardiac silhouette reaches the right thoracic wall and can form a chamber with a volume of 1000 ml to 2000 ml (Figs. 26.11 and 26.12).

Conditions resulting in left atrial enlargement are mitral valve obstruction and mitral insufficiency, as well as any reason for left ventricular failure or noncompliant left ventricle, such as arteriosclerotic heart disease and hypertrophic cardiomyopathy. When giant left atrium is seen, it is almost invariably secondary to severe mitral insufficiency.

LEFT VENTRICLE

The left ventricle normally forms the left border of the cardiac silhouette under the pulmonary outflow tract including the apex in the PA film. In the lateral film and the left anterior oblique film it forms the posteroinferior aspect of the cardiac silhouette down to and even under the left hemidiaphragm. Normally the left ventricle crosses the inferior vena cava about 1.5 cm to 2 cm above the left hemidiaphragm in the lateral film. If a line is projected vertically from the position where the inferior vena cava crosses the left ventricle in the lateral film, the posterior cardiac border formed by the left ventricle is usually no more than 2 cm posterior from this line.[6]

With left ventricular hypertrophy without dilation, there is no obvious change in the cardiac silhouette. With hypertension or aortic stenosis the left ventricle can be severely hypertrophied with left ventricular wall thickness of 2 cm and no abnormalities may be seen in the cardiac silhouette.

As left ventricular chamber enlargement occurs, the left ventricle dilates to the left, inferiorly and posteriorly. In this way the apex frequently extends under the left hemidiaphragm and the left cardiac border approaches the left thoracic wall (Fig. 26.13). In the lateral and left anterior oblique films the lower portion of the cardiac silhouette

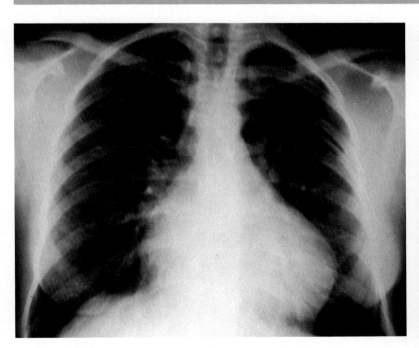

FIGURE 26.5 Posteroanterior projection of a patient with pulmonary stenosis and ventricular septal defect. Right atrial enlargement and ventricular hypertrophy are present. Note the large sweep of the right atrial border on the right from diaphragm to mediastinal shadow. Apex of the heart formed by the right ventricle is lifted off the left hemidiaphragm.

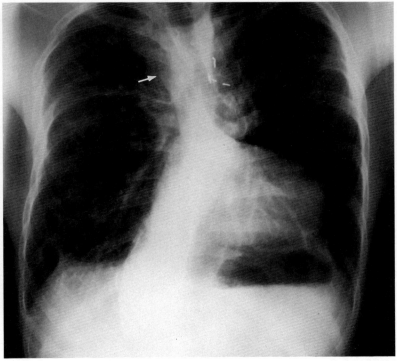

FIGURE 26.6 Posteroanterior projection of a patient with pulmonary atresia, ventricular septal defect, and a large right-to-left shunt. Postoperative bilateral Blalock-Taussig shunts (metal clips). Note the right ventricle is lifted off the diaphragm and there is absence of a main pulmonary artery segment. There is also a right-sided aortic arch (arrow).

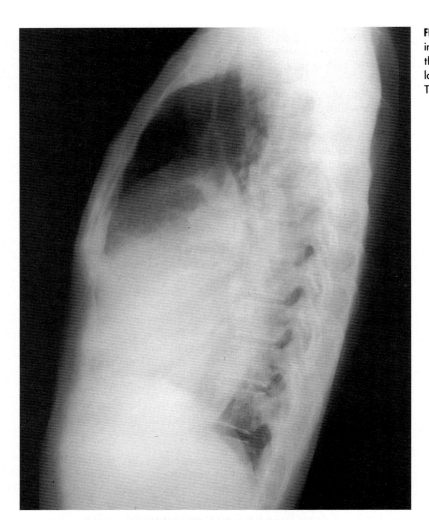

FIGURE 26.7 Left lateral projection of a patient with a large secundum interatrial septal defect and a large left-to-right shunt (pulmonary blood flow three times systemic blood flow). Note massive filling of retrosternal space by large right ventricle. Note left ventricle pushed posteriorly over the spine. There was no left ventricular enlargement.

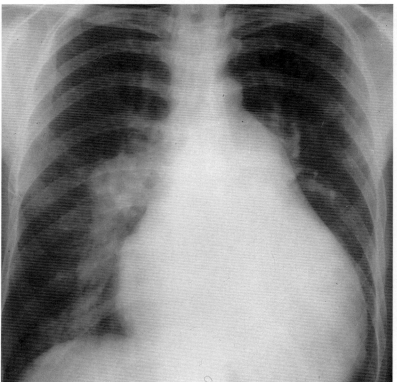

FIGURE 26.8 Posteroanterior projection of the same patient as in Figure 26.7. Note enlarged cardiac silhouette due to large right ventricle, markedly enlarged main pulmonary artery segment, and huge pulmonary arterial markings. There is no left ventricular enlargement. The right ventricle forms the apex of the heart.

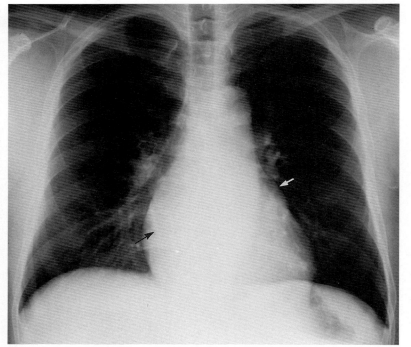

FIGURE 26.9 Posteroanterior projection a 34-year-old man with severe mitral stenosis. Note the left auricular appendage forming a convex structure (*black arrow*) under the pulmonary artery segment along the left cardiac border. Note the double density of left atrial enlargement behind the right cardiac silhouette (*white arrow*).

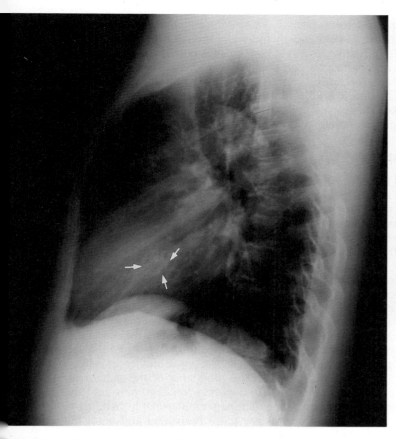

FIGURE 26.10 Left lateral projection of the same patient as in Figure 26.9. Note the large left atrium at the superoposterior aspect of the cardiac silhouette. The left atrium displaces the left main stem bronchus posteriorly. Note calcification in the mitral valve (arrows).

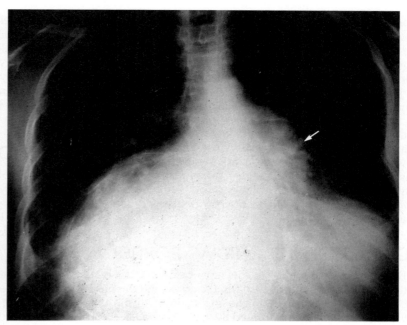

FIGURE 26.11 Posteroanterior projection of a 46-year-old woman with mitral stenosis and mitral insufficiency. Note giant left atrium with calcification of the left atrial wall and giant left atrial appendage (arrow).

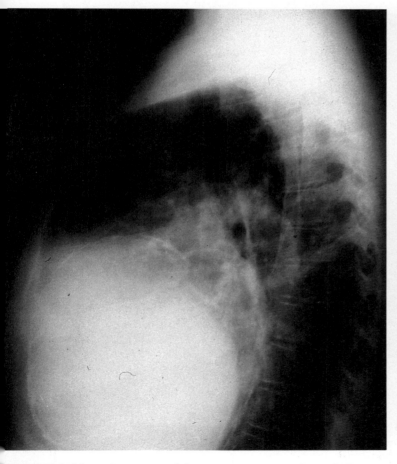

FIGURE 26.12 Left lateral projection of the same patient as in Figure 26.11. Note large calcified left atrium.

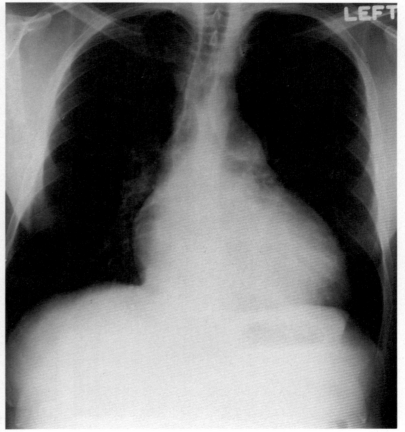

FIGURE 26.13 Posteroanterior projection of a 37-year-old patient with dilated cardiomyopathy and enlarged left ventricle, left atrium, and pulmonary artery. Note enlargement of left ventricle to the left and downward, below the diaphragm. Note large main pulmonary artery segment.

extends more posteriorly, so that in the 60° left anterior oblique film it frequently overlaps the spine posteriorly. In the left lateral film it extends more posteriorly to the inferior vena cava and crosses the inferior vena cava lower than normal and finally does not cross it at all (Fig. 26.14). Using these measurements, care must be taken to ensure a good deep inspiration or these signs are misleading.

Left ventricular hypertrophy without dilatation (concentric hypertrophy) occurs in those conditions in which left ventricular pressure is elevated, such as aortic stenosis, coarctation of the aorta, and hypertension. With failure, left ventricular dilatation occurs in these diseases as well as with coronary disease and cardiomyopathy. Volume overload lesions also result in left ventricular chamber dilatation as well as hypertrophy (eccentric hypertrophy), for instance, aortic insufficiency, mitral insufficiency, and interventricular septal defect with large left-to-right shunt.

SUPERIOR PART OF THE CARDIAC BORDER

In the PA film the three structures in the superior cardiac silhouette from right-to-left are the superior vena cava, the aorta, and the pulmonary artery. Normally, in the PA film the right border of the upper portion of the cardiac silhouette is formed by the ascending aorta. The sinuses of Valsalva are not border forming but are within the cardiac silhouette. With ascending aortic aneurysm, prominence of the right superior mediastinum may be seen (Fig. 26.15). In right ventricular failure, the superior vena cava can form the right border of the upper mediastinum. At times, the azygos vein can be seen to be dilated as a round density in this area. Occasionally, anomalous pulmonary veins can be seen in the lung, entering this area of the mediastinum.

The aorta normally arches over the left main stem bronchus and forms a left-sided aortic arch; it can be seen as a density in the upper left mediastinum, usually slightly indenting the left side of the trachea (see Fig. 26.1). Below this, on the left cardiac border the main pulmonary artery and part of the left pulmonary artery can be seen arching posteriorly and inferiorly. Normally, the main pulmonary artery is no larger than the aortic knob. On the left, superior to the aortic knob, at times it is possible to see the sweep of the left subclavian artery or, if present, a persistent left superior vena cava.

PULMONARY VASCULARITY

Because of the effect of gravity, the low pressure system of the pulmonary artery in the upright patient results in a gradient of flow from the least at the apices to the most at the bases, resulting in larger vessels to the lower lungs compared with those to the upper lung fields. Comparison of vessel size can be seen best in the PA film.

Normally, the size of the right pulmonary branches of the pulmonary artery to the lower lobes seen lateral to the cardiac silhouette does not exceed 17 mm in men and 15 mm in women. There is also a gradual decrease in size of vessels as the third, fourth, and fifth order branching occurs to the periphery of the lung where distinguishable vessels are still present. The ratio of the width of the central arteries to the segmental arteries at the lung bases varies from 3:1 to 5:1.

The pulmonary veins drain into the posterior aspect of the left atrium and gather to form four major veins, an upper and lower vein on each side. There is a difference in the branching of the pulmonary veins and pulmonary arteries with pulmonary veins coming into the cardiac silhouette lower than the pulmonary arteries exit from it. In the lower lobes the pulmonary veins are more horizontal and enter the cardiac silhouette below the pulmonary arteries. In the upper lobes the

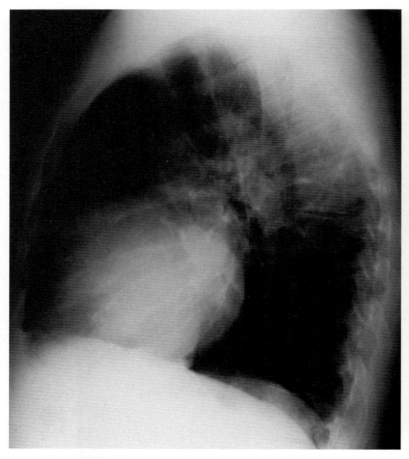

FIGURE 26.14 Left lateral projection of the same patient as in Figure 26.13. Note large left ventricle more than 2 cm posterior to the projected line of the inferior vena cava. The left ventricle crosses the inferior vena cava at the left hemidiaphragm.

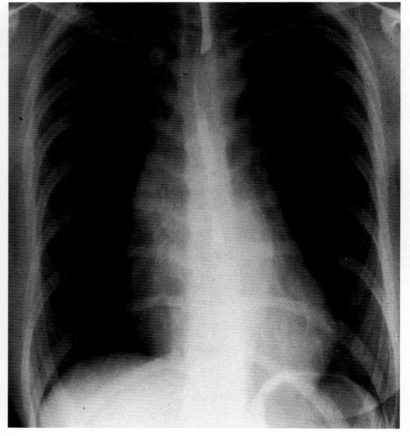

FIGURE 26.15 Posteroanterior projection of a 40-year-old man with ascending aortic aneurysm. Note prominence of the right upper mediastinal shadow and normal aortic arch.

pulmonary arteries and veins are parallel, with the pulmonary veins lateral to the arteries. In practice it is difficult, if not impossible, to distinguish one from the other.

With left-to-right shunts the pulmonary vessels, both arteries and veins, increase in size (see Figs. 26.7 and 26.8). This usually involves all the pulmonary vessels from the main pulmonary artery to the small branches all the way to the periphery of the lung fields. In this situation it is common to see pulmonary vessels well even behind the diaphragm in the PA film.

With increasing pulmonary hypertension, especially with increasing pulmonary vascular resistance, the central pulmonary arteries become large and the peripheral pulmonary vessels begin to get smaller and to disappear. With severe pulmonary vascular disease, the lateral third of the lung fields can be virtually without pulmonary vascular markings. This is termed "pruning" of pulmonary vessels seen with pulmonary hypertension. Calcification of the central, primary, and secondary pulmonary branches of the pulmonary arteries can be seen in this state (Fig. 26.16). Enormous dilatation of the main pulmonary artery and proximal pulmonary artery branches occurs in patients with congenital absence of the pulmonary valve. Prominent pulmonary artery shadow is seen in pulmonary valve stenosis (poststenotic dilatation) and in idiopathic dilatation of the pulmonary artery.

PULMONARY VASCULAR CHANGES WITH CONGESTIVE HEART FAILURE

With congestive heart failure the left atrial pressure is elevated and with it the pulmonary capillary pressure. There is increased interstitial water with increased pulmonary lymphatic drainage. This can result in the formation of "cuffing" of fluid around the small bronchi and evidence of enlargement and fuzziness of the edges of the veins. With increased interstitial water, which gravitates to the dependent areas, there is increased interstitial pressure on small vessels creating increased vascular resistance at the lung bases. There is also increased pressure on small airways, creating local hypoxia, a powerful pulmonary vasoconstrictor. This further increases pulmonary vascular resistance at the bases and results in the diversion of blood flow to the upper lungs and vascular redistribution, a sign of congestive heart failure.

Finally, the increased interstitial fluid is seen as thickening of the interlobular septa (Kerley's B lines) which are straight, thin lines, 1 cm to 2 cm long at the periphery of the lung, mostly seen in the costophrenic angles (Figs. 26.17 and 26.18). Kerley's A lines due to edema in the interstitial tissues are longer, curving lines from the hilar areas.[7] When interstitial fluid accumulates faster than it can be removed by the lymphatics, the interstitial hydrostatic pressure increases and fluid enters the alveolar spaces, resulting in the homogeneous density of alveolar pulmonary edema (see Fig. 26.17).[8] Often, early pulmonary edema is seen extending from the hilar areas in the medial one to two thirds of the lungs, the so-called bat-wing appearance. This is probably due to the pressure on the interstitial compartment of the cortex of the expanding lung during inspiration, which milks the edema fluid toward the interstitial spaces of the looser alveolar tissues of the hilus.

Pleural effusion occurs when the pleural fluid is formed, mainly from the visceral pleura, faster than it can be absorbed, primarily by the parietal pleura. This circumstance occurs when venous pressure draining the parietal pleura is elevated, that is, when systemic venous pressure is elevated owing to right ventricular failure, but most often when pulmonary venous and systemic venous pressure are both elevated as occurs in biventricular failure. Elevation of pulmonary venous pressure alone, as occurs for instance in mitral stenosis, does not result in large pleural effusions.

Several radiologic findings have been correlated to the level of pulmonary capillary wedge pressure in patients with both acute and chronic heart failure. In patients with acute myocardial infarction, radiologic findings correlate reasonably well with the severity of pulmonary venous hypertension.[9] Absence of any radiologic finding was usually associated with pulmonary capillary wedge pressure of 12 mm Hg; differential blood flow to the upper zones and hilar haze indicate pulmonary capillary wedge pressure between 12 mm Hg and 18 mm

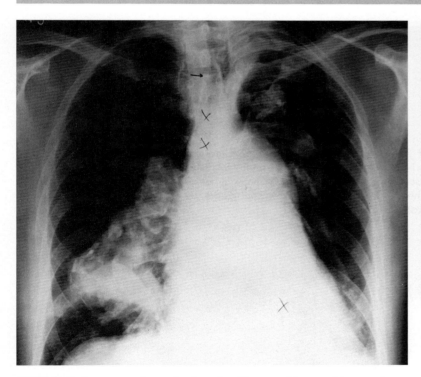

FIGURE 26.16 Posteroanterior projection of a 56-year-old man with secundum atrial septal defect and severe pulmonary hypertension. The main pulmonary artery and its primary branches are massively enlarged. There is calcification of aneurysmally enlarged secondary branches of both right and left pulmonary arteries. The peripheral lung fields are clear without pulmonary vascular markings ("pruning").

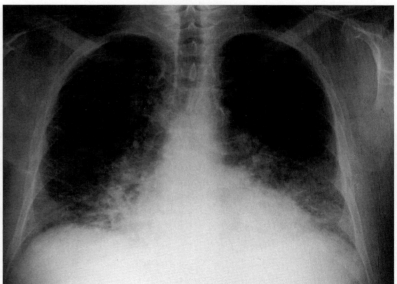

FIGURE 26.17 Posteroanterior projection of a 62-year-old patient with congestive left ventricular failure, pulmonary edema, and Kerley's B lines in lateral costophrenic angles bilaterally.

g. More severe pulmonary venous congestion (periacinar rosette formation or alveolar edema) was associated with higher pulmonary capillary wedge pressure, exceeding 20 mm Hg. It needs to be emphasized, however, that significant errors in estimating pulmonary capillary wedge pressure from the radiologic findings can occur in patients with hypoxemia and in those who receive therapy (diuretics and nitrates) before the assessment is done.

In patients with chronic congestive cardiomyopathy (ischemic and nonischemic), the usual radiologic findings of pulmonary venous congestion may not be apparent even when pulmonary capillary wedge is significantly elevated.[10] Although pulmonary venous redistribution (VR), interstitial edema (IE), alveolar edema (AE), and pleural effusion (PE) were absent in 90% of patients with pulmonary capillary wedge pressure less than 15 mm Hg, radiologic findings were also absent in many patients with significantly elevated pulmonary capillary wedge pressure. In a group of patients with pulmonary capillary wedge pressure between 15 mm Hg and 24 mm Hg, VR, IE, AE, and PE were absent in 40%, 60%, 90%, and 70% of patients, respectively. In patients with pulmonary capillary wedge pressure exceeding 25 mm Hg, VR, IE, AE, and PE were absent in 25%, 25%, 70%, and 50% of patients, respec-

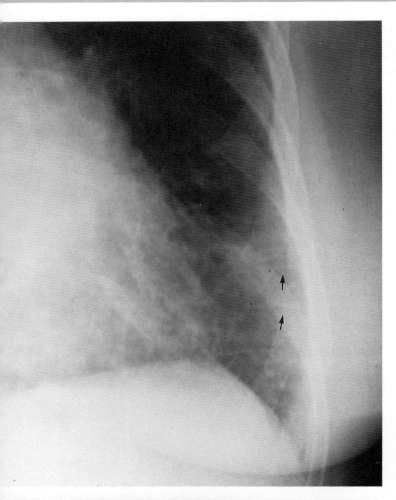

FIGURE 26.18 Detail of the left costophrenic angle in a patient with congestive heart failure. Note horizontal, thin, 1-cm to 2-cm long parallel lines of interstitial, interlobular septal edema (Kerley's B lines).

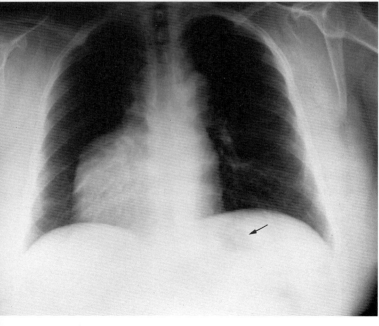

FIGURE 26.19 Posteroanterior projection. D-Loop dextrocardia in a patient with situs solitus. Note stomach bubble (*arrow*) on the left, left-sided aortic arch, and left descending aorta. Note also that the right hemidiaphragm with the right-sided heart is lower than the left hemidiaphragm. There were no additional cardiac anomalies.

tively. These findings suggest that although the presence of these radiologic signs usually indicates elevated pulmonary capillary wedge pressure, the absence does not exclude significant pulmonary venous hypertension.

POSITIONAL ABNORMALITIES OF THE HEART

The most obvious positional cardiac abnormality is dextrocardia, in which the mass of the cardiac silhouette is to the right of the midline. This can occur because of congenital rotational abnormalities, such as L-loop dextrocardia with situs inversus. Other types of dextrocardia are a D-loop dextrocardia with normal situs solitus, in which the heart has not rotated as it usually does out of the right side of the chest into the left side of the chest (Fig. 26.19); displacement of the heart to the right caused by hypoplastic anomalies of the lung, such as pulmonary sequestration; acquired loss of right lung volume such as is seen with right-sided atelectasis; and displacement of the heart by pressure into the right thorax, as is seen in left-sided tension pneumothorax. Rotational cardiac abnormalities can result in a heart that is midline, in neither the right side nor the left side of the chest.

Displacement of the heart abnormally into the left hemithorax can also be congenital, such as seen in L-loop transposition with situs inversus; caused by traction, such as seen in left-sided atelectasis; or caused by increased pressure in the right hemithorax, as is seen in right-sided tension pneumothorax.

Abnormalities of the thoracic skeleton and chest cage can also result in apparent displacement of the heart to the right, as is seen in the straight back syndrome with a narrow AP diameter of the chest, or to the left, as is seen in pectus excavatum. Thoracic skeletal abnormalities can also cause a flattening of the heart in the AP diameter, resulting in apparent cardiomegaly.

Finally, congenital absence of the left hemipericardium results movement of the cardiac silhouette abnormally into the left side of th chest and the apparent cardiomegaly. With partial absence of the le hemipericardium, only herniation of the left atrial appendage occu without cardiac displacement (Fig. 26.20).

CALCIFICATION IN THE CARDIOVASCULAR SILHOUETTE

Calcification can be seen in the plain chest film in one or more view but within the cardiac silhouette, calcification of valves and corona arteries is better detected by fluoroscopy. Since in the PA film th valves are mainly situated over the bony spine, calcification of th valves is especially difficult to detect in this projection. In the obliqu and lateral films, however, heavy calcification can frequently be eas seen. The aortic valve and the aortic ring are most frequently seen be calcified (Fig. 26.21), followed by the mitral annulus and subann lar area, whereas calcification of the tricuspid and pulmonary valves quite rare. Calcification of the mitral valve is less frequently recogniz in the lateral chest film (see Fig. 26.10) but is more easily seen c fluoroscopy.

Pericardial calcification can be massive and occurs in approx mately 50% of patients with hemodynamically significant constricti pericarditis. Calcification is most often seen in the atrioventricul groove, but frequently calcification is absent in the PA film and se only in the lateral and oblique views.

Other calcifications are as follows:

Calcification of the coronary arteries (Fig. 26.22), atherosclerot coronary artery disease, coronary artery ectasia, Kawasaki's di ease, pseudoxanthoma elasticum
Patent ductus arteriosus

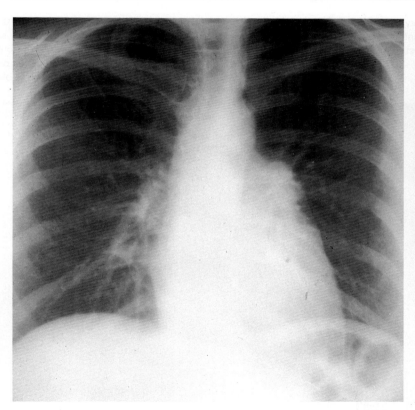

FIGURE 26.20 Posteroanterior projection. Congenital partial absence of the left hemipericardium with herniation of the left atrial appendage. Note convexity just beneath the main pulmonary artery segment along the left cardiac silhouette. The patient was asymptomatic. Major complication can be herniation of the entire heart through this restrictive defect, with strangulation of the heart and death.

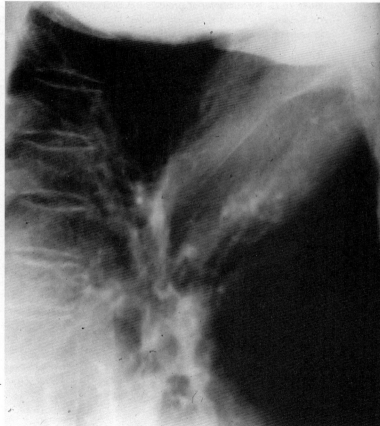

FIGURE 26.21 Left lateral projection of a patient with severe calcific aortic stenosis. Note "popcorn-like" calcification in the center of the cardiac silhouette. This is characteristic of aortic valve calcification.

Calcification of the aortic arch, which is common, and calcification of the ascending aorta, as seen in aortitis, which is not; annuloectatic disease of the aorta

Calcification in aortic aneurysms: atheromatous, syphilitic, and traumatic

Calcification in ventricular aneurysms

Calcification in tumors (*i.e.*, myxomas)

Calcification of pulmonary arteries in pulmonary hypertension (see Fig. 26.16)

Calcification of the left atrial wall with mitral stenosis (see Figs. 26.11 and 26.12), ball valve thrombus

GREAT VESSEL ABNORMALITIES

Usually the left contour of the base of the cardiac silhouette consists of the transverse aorta and arch, which loops over the left main stem bronchus, the main pulmonary artery, and the left pulmonary artery to the left of it. The arch can be right sided (see Fig. 26.6). With transposi-

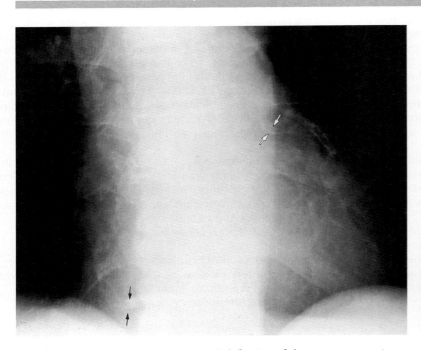

FIGURE 26.22 Posteroanterior projection. Calcification of the coronary arteries can be seen as parallel tubular calcified lines involving both left anterior descending (*white arrows*) and right coronary arteries (*black arrows*).

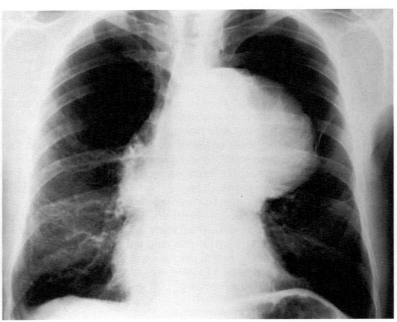

FIGURE 26.23 Posteroanterior projection. A large upper left mediastinal mass is seen adjacent to the cardiac silhouette. The aortic arch is clearly seen through the mass. The ascending aortic silhouette is also prominent. The patient had a massive aortic aneurysm arising from the superior portion of the ascending aorta and transverse aorta. It was of unknown etiology.

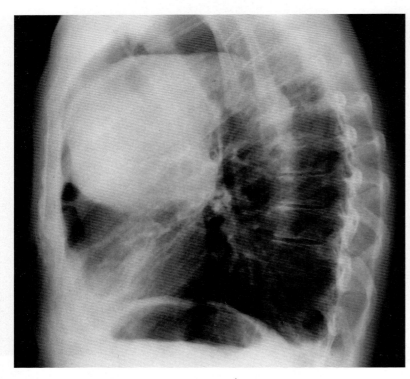

FIGURE 26.24 Left lateral projection of the same patient as in Figure 26.23. The superior mediastinal mass is associated with the upper part of the ascending aorta.

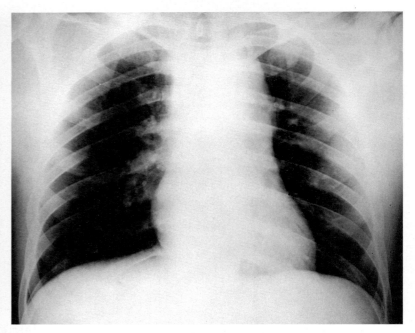

FIGURE 26.25 Posteroanterior projection of a 64-year-old hypertensive man with sudden severe back pain. Note the widened mediastinum and large aortic knob with indistinct superior border. On angiography the patient had type III dissection of the aorta.

tion of the great vessels, the two vessels are parallel and the base appears narrowed. With corrected transposition (L-transposition) of the great vessels the aortic root is abnormally to the left of the pulmonary root and the ascending aorta forms the left border of the superior cardiac silhouette.

A congenitally persistent left superior vena cava can cause a curving shadow along the left superior mediastinum. With total anomalous pulmonary venous return to the coronary sinus, the enlarged coronary sinus can be seen bulging posteriorly and to the right of the cardiac silhouette. With total anomalous pulmonary venous drainage to the left innominate vein, the vertical vein draining the common pulmonary vein passes superiorly into the left innominate vein resulting in enlargement of the left innominate vein and superior vena cava. The enlarged venous structures superior to the heart make for a characteristic "snowman" appearance.

Coarctation of the aorta can cause a notching of the descending aorta, the superior bulge being the shadow of the left subclavian artery as it rolls off the aorta near the coarctation, passing superiorly to its position over the first rib. With a barium-filled esophagus the poststenotic dilatation of the aorta beyond the coarctation can indent the esophagus just below the normal impression from the left arch, causing a reversed "3" sign. Finally, notches in the inferior rib margin from enlarged tortuous collateral intercostal arteries complete the picture.

Aneurysms of the aorta can occur from the area of the sinuses of Valsalva, where they usually do not distort the cardiac silhouette unless they are huge, to the ascending aorta, such as seen in syphilitic and poststenotic dilatation of the aorta with aortic stenosis.

Ascending aortic aneurysms can occur in tertiary syphilis or with medial necrosis with or without Marfan's disease (see Fig. 26.15). Aneurysms (Figs. 26.23 and 26.24) can involve the aortic arch itself, where they may not be seen unless they are very large, and the descending aorta, where they can be seen distorting the upper left mediastinum. These can be due to arteriosclerotic disease, aortitis, or trauma. When traumatic aneurysms occur, they are usually found just beyond the takeoff of the left subclavian artery.

Dissection of the aorta can also involve ascending aorta, arch, or descending aorta. Usually this results in a widening of the mediastinum (Fig. 26.25). Bleeding into the mediastinum can obscure the superior portion of the aortic knob, can push the trachea to the right, or, with rupture, can result in pericardial or pleural effusions.

Other abnormalities of great vessels are pulmonary venous varices, frequently related to diseases increasing pulmonary venous pressure, such as mitral stenosis, but occasionally occurring as isolated problems. These result in pulmonary nodules usually adjacent to the cardiac silhouette but sometimes out in the lung. Another pulmonary mass that is vascular is a pulmonary arteriovenous fistula. These can be single or multiple anywhere in the lung fields. They can be small or very large and obvious. Frequently the feeding vessels, arteries, and veins, and can be seen extending from the fistula toward the cardiac silhouette.

UNUSUAL DEFORMITY OF LEFT CARDIAC BORDER

Alteration of cardiac shape due to "unusual bulge" along the left border of the heart may result from a number of conditions: left atrial enlargement, left ventricular aneurysm, hypertrophic cardiomyopathy, congenital absence of the left pericardium, pericardial cysts, circumflex coronary artery to coronary sinus connection, intracardiac total anomalous venous drainage, mediastinal tumors, lymph nodes, and Ebstein's anomaly. Of these conditions, left atrial enlargement and left ventricular aneurysm are the most common in the adult.

REFERENCES

1. Hammermeister KE, Chikos PM, Fisher L et al: Relationship of cardiothoracic ratio and plain film heart volume to late survival. Circulation 59:89, 1979
2. Ungerleider HE, Clark CP: A study of the transverse diameter of the heart silhouette with prediction table based on the teleroentgenogram. Transactions of the Association of Life Insurance Medical Directors of America 25:84, 1938
3. Glover L, Baxley WA, Dodge HT: A qualitative evaluation of heart size measurements from chest roentgenograms. Circulation 47:1289, 1973
4. Amundsen P: The diagnostic value of conventional radiological examination of the heart in the adult. Acta Radiol (Suppl) 181:1–87, 1959
5. Keats TE, Enge IP: Cardiac mensuration by the cardiac volume method. Radiology 85:850, 1965
6. Hoffman RB, Rigler LG: Evaluation of left ventricular enlargement in the lateral projection of the chest. Radiology 85:93, 1965
7. Kerley PJ: Radiology in heart disease. Br Med J 2:594, 1933
8. Grainger RG: Interstitial pulmonary edema and its radiological diagnosis: A sign of pulmonary venous and capillary hypertension. Br J Radiol 31:201, 1958
9. McHugh T, Forrester JS, Adler L et al: Pulmonary vascular congestion in acute myocardial infarction: Hemodynamics as radiologic correlations. Ann Intern Med 76:29, 1972
10. Dash H, Lipton MJ, Chatterjee K et al: Estimation of pulmonary artery wedge pressure from chest radiograph in patients with chronic congestive cardiomyopathy and ischemic cardiomyopathy. Br Heart J 44:322, 1980

Electrocardiogram

Borys Surawicz

CHAPTER 27

BASIS OF THE ELECTROCARDIOGRAM

The electrocardiogram (ECG) is a record of electrical activity generated during impulse propagation in the heart. The form of the ECG recorded from the body surface depends on the properties of the generator (*i.e.,* the cardiac action potential), the spread of excitation, and the characteristics of the volume conductor. Only a general outline of these fundamental properties is presented in this chapter. A greater in-depth coverage of these subjects can be found in the appropriate handbooks and textbooks of electrophysiology.[1-4]

CARDIAC ACTION POTENTIAL

The surface ECG reflects predominantly the depolarization of the atria and the ventricles, as well as the repolarization of the ventricles. The repolarization of the atria is discernible only under special circumstances, such as complete atrioventricular dissociation or atrial infarction. The action potentials of the sinoatrial node and other parts of the specialized conducting system are not represented in the surface ECG, but the electrical activity of some of these structures, notably the bundle of His, can be identified in the local intracardiac electrograms.

The duration of the P wave and of the QRS complex is about 50 to 100 times longer than the duration of depolarization in the single cell. The atrial and ventricular depolarization complexes not only reflect the duration of the impulse propagation within these structures but provide some insight into the sequence of depolarization. In contrast, the total ventricular repolarization is only slightly longer than the duration of a single ventricular action potential. Consequently, the ST segment and the T wave, which represent the uncancelled potentials of ventricular repolarization, provide little, if any, information about the sequence of repolarization. A diagram illustrating the relation between the atrial and ventricular action potentials and the surface ECG is shown in Figure 27.1.

SPREAD OF EXCITATION

The dominant cardiac pacemaker is the sinoatrial node. Impulses originating within the sinoatrial node spread through the atria, both radially and along the interatrial tracts. The isoelectric PR segment corresponds to the conduction of the impulse through the atrioventricular node, the bundle of His, the bundle branches, and the Purkinje fibers. This interval also contains atrial repolarization, which continues throughout ventricular depolarization (see Fig. 27.1).

The order of depolarization of the ventricular myocardium is determined largely by the impulse propagation in the specialized conduction system. Normally, the more abundant left bundle branch terminals make connection with the ventricular muscle earlier than the terminals of the right bundle branch. The Purkinje network arising from bundle branches depolarizes the endocardium and conducts the impulse rapidly toward the epicardium. The paucity of Purkinje fibers at the base of the heart and in the upper septum accounts for the slow propagation of the impulse through the ventricular myocardium in these regions.

The time from the beginning to the end of ventricular depolarization corresponds to the QRS complex. The duration of the QRS complex, which is about 40 msec in newborn humans, increases with increasing ventricular mass during childhood and adolescence and reaches 80 msec to 100 msec at the completion of cardiac growth.

Depolarization of ventricular myocardium begins on the left side of the septum and spreads across the septum from left to right and anteriorly. The initial 0.02 second deflection is sometimes called "septal" although it probably contains some additional components of an early excitation wave propagating across the ventricular wall (*i.e.,* from endocardium toward epicardium). The most prominent deflection resulting from the depolarization of the free ventricular wall is directed to the left, inferiorly and posteriorly (*i.e.,* toward the apex and the mid portion of the left ventricle). The terminal portion of the QRS complex represents depolarization of the base, the upper portion of the septum, and the crista supraventricularis of the right ventricle. The activation of one or more of these structures frequently produces a separate deflection, which is directed superiorly and either posteriorly (S wave) or anteriorly (R^1). Studies of reperfused and revived hearts removed from cadavers[5] and epicardial mapping of patients during open heart surgery[6] established that early epicardial breakthrough occurs nearly simultaneously (7 msec–40 msec after the onset of QRS) at several sites (*i.e.,* anterior right ventricle near the septum, anterior left ventricle paraseptally, anterolateral left ventricle, and inferior wall of the left ventricle) (Fig. 27.2). These studies confirmed also that the basal segments of the left ventricle and the base or the pulmonary conus of the right ventricle are the sites of the latest activation (60 msec–96 msec).

PROPERTIES OF THE VOLUME CONDUCTOR

Potential differences generated during cardiac activity set up currents in the conductors surrounding the heart. The electrocardiographic theory is based on a simplified elementary model of a single fiber surrounded by a homogeneous medium. In such fibers, at rest, the positive and the negative boundaries are equal and opposite in sign for the entire extent of the conductor. This means that the polarized surface is closed and no potential is recorded (Fig. 27.3, the top tracing). When the excitation wave invades the fiber and reverses the charge across the membrane, currents flow outside the fiber, inside the fiber, and across the membrane, as indicated by the arrows in Figure 27.3, the second tracing from the top. This creates potential differences, which disappear when the double layer again becomes homogeneous in the fully activated state, as shown in the middle tracing of Figure 27.3. Subsequently a transition from activated to resting state occurs, a process of repolarization as shown in Figure 27.3, fourth and fifth tracings from top.

Each instant of depolarization or repolarization represents different stages of activity for a large number of fibers, and an electromotive force generated at each instant represents a sum of uncancelled potential differences. A potential difference between two surfaces or between two poles carrying opposite charges forms a dipole, the magnitude (moment), polarity, and direction of which can be represented by a vector. The ECG records the sequence of such instantaneous vectors attributed to an imaginary dipole that changes its magnitude and direction during impulse propagation. During activity, the recording electrode is influenced by the potential difference across the boundary, and the record of activity represented by an instantaneous vector depends on the position of the electrode within the electric field created by the dipole. Figure 27.4 shows a schematic diagram of an electric field with a central location of a dipole in an ideal homogeneous medium

dium. The solid lines represent positive and negative isopotential lines. The maximum potentials are given values of +20 and −20. They are in close proximity to the poles of the dipole, which are the source and the sink, respectively. The potentials decrease with increasing distance from the dipole. The vertical interrupted line transecting the dipole is a zero potential line. The leads to the right of this line will record positive potentials and those to the left of the line, negative potentials. No potential differences will be recorded by an electrode connecting two points on the isopotential line.

The complicated form of the thorax, the complex shape of the heart, the eccentric position of the heart within the chest, and the inhomogeneity of the electric field surrounding the heart make it practically impossible to identify accurately the sources of potentials recorded on the body surfaces.[1] In addition, it remains uncertain whether the superposition of all simultaneously generated electric fields may be regarded as the field of a single resultant dipole that may be represented by a single resultant vector.[1] An attempt to answer this question has been made by searching for mirror patterns (*i.e.*, for two electrode positions, the lead vectors of which lie in a strictly opposite direction). Although the frequent finding of only one maximum and one minimum potential on the chest wall during some portions of the QRS complex supports the single dipole concept, the cancellation usually remains incomplete and the uncancelled potentials on the torso are attributed to the proximity effects.[7] It has been suggested that the electromotive forces generated by the heart can be expressed more properly by the electric field of two or four dipoles rather than that of a single dipole.

The inability to precisely localize the source of instantaneous vectors does not detract from the applicability of physical laws governing the current flow in volume conductors to the analysis of the surface ECG. Of particular importance is the law governing the potential decline that occurs with increasing distance from the heart. It has been established that in the volume conductor with the properties of the human thorax, this potential declines approximately in proportion to the square of the distance. This means that, for practical purposes, points on the torso situated at a distance greater than two diameters of the heart are approximately "electrically" equidistant from the generator. Thus, the remoteness of the electrodes placed on the extremities is sufficient to minimize the nondipolar components of the ECG caused by the proximity effect. At the same time, it becomes understandable that the anterior precordial leads, owing to their proximity to the heart, are influenced by the local potentials generated in the structures lying directly beneath the corresponding electrodes.

Another basic concept applicable to the analysis of the body surface potentials states that at any given point the recorded potential is determined by the product of a solid angle subtended at this point by the boundary between the opposing charges, and the charge density per unit area across the boundary. This means that for any given charge

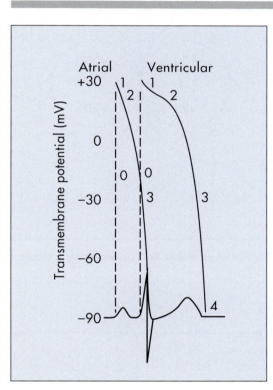

FIGURE 27.1 Diagram of atrial (A) and ventricular (V) action potential superimposed on the ECG. Dashed lines mark upstroke of action potentials. Numbers at left designate transmembrane potential in millivolts (mV). Phases of action potential are designated by numbers 0 to 4. Resting membrane potential of both fibers is approximately −90 mV. Note that the duration of the A action potential corresponds to the P wave and Ta wave which is inscribed during PQ and QRS intervals, and the duration of the V action potential corresponds to the QRS complex, ST segment, and T wave. (Surawicz B: The pathogenesis and clinical significance of primary T wave abnormalities. In Schlant RC, Hurst JW (eds): Advances in Electrocardiography. New York, Grune & Stratton, 1972)

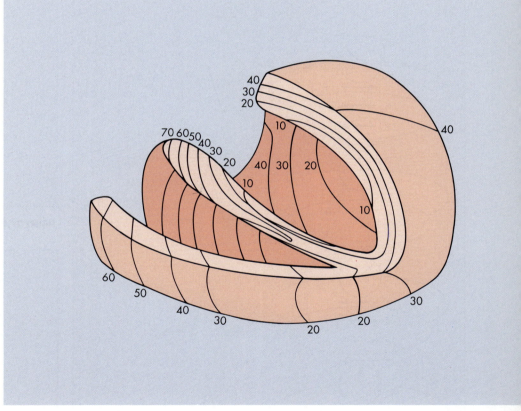

FIGURE 27.2 Pattern of excitation in the adult human heart depicted in the position it may occupy in the body. A portion of the right ventricle, septum, and left ventricle is removed, showing the open cavities. The isochrons of the 10, 20, 30, 40, 50, 60, and 70 msec are shown. Note the several sites of the epicardial breakthrough in the right ventricle (20 msec), near the apex (30 msec), and on the lateral wall of the left ventricle (40 msec). (Durrer D: Electrical aspects of human cardiac activity: A clinical-physiological approach to excitation and stimulation. Cardiovasc Res 2:1, 196

density, the deflection recorded by the electrode facing the boundary will increase with increasing surface of the boundary and, conversely, that for any given dimension of the boundary surface, the magnitude of the recorded deflection will increase with increasing charge density across the boundary. The solid angle theorem has been found useful in the analysis of potential differences caused by injury currents.[8]

The conductivity of tissues surrounding the heart influences the amplitude of the ECG deflections. Tissues with low conductivity decrease the amplitude of the ECG deflections. Low voltage is present when the lungs are hyperinflated or when the heart is insulated by a large amount of fat. Low voltage can be caused also by pericardial and pleural effusions or edema, owing to the short-circuiting action of these well-conducting fluids.

ECG LEADS

To study the electromotive forces generated during the propagation of cardiac impulses, it is necessary to attach the leading electrodes to the heart or to the body surface. When one or both electrodes are in contact with the heart, the ECG leads are called direct. When the electrodes are placed at a distance greater than two cardiac diameters from the heart, the leads are called indirect. Semidirect leads designate an arrangement in which one or both electrodes are in close proximity but not in direct contact with the heart. The leads are designated as bipolar when both electrodes face sites with similar potential variations, and as unipolar when potential variations of one electrode are negligible in comparison to those of the other. Of the 12 standard ECG leads, I, II, and III are indirect and bipolar, aV_R, aV_L, and aV_F are indirect and unipolar, and V_1 through V_6 are semidirect and unipolar.

The three standard limb leads were designed by Einthoven to represent three sides of an equilateral triangle in which the heart is positioned at the center (Fig. 27.5). The above concept sprang from an assumption that the electromotive forces of the heart could be represented by a single vector centered in this triangle. According to the law of Einthoven the magnitude of deflection in lead II equals the sum of deflections in leads I and III. Although a more accurate system of electrode placement at points equidistant from the heart has been proposed by other investigators, the use of Einthoven's leads has be-

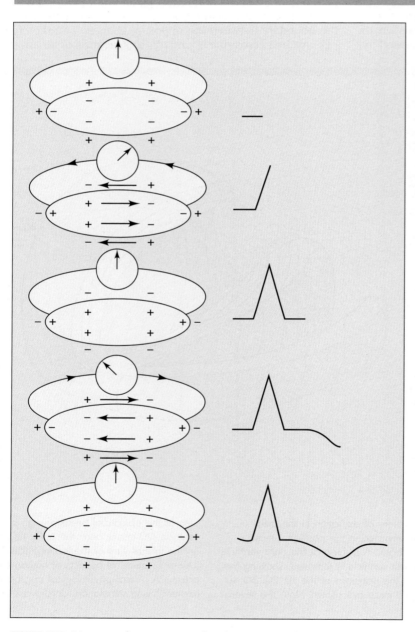

FIGURE 27.3 Diagram of resting state, depolarization, and repolarization in a single cell, the two ends of which are connected to a galvanometer. On the right are ECG deflections resulting from the polarization changes in the diagram on the left.

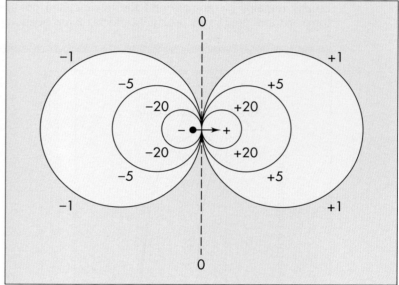

FIGURE 27.4 Diagram of an electric field generated by a dipole (−+).

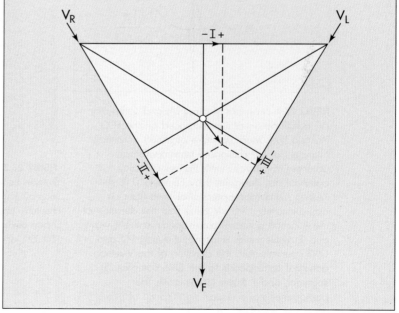

FIGURE 27.5 Diagram of Einthoven's triangle showing the projection of a vector on the axes of three standard limb leads.

come universally entrenched. The unipolar chest leads were introduced by Wilson for the purpose of diminishing the influence of the distant reference electrode. He constructed a zero potential electrode (V) by connecting the three limb electrodes through equal resistances of 5000 ohms to a central terminal. Wilson and co-workers[9] developed the system of unipolar chest leads and unipolar limb leads taken from the central terminal to the individual limb electrodes (V_R, V_L, V_F). Subsequently, Goldberger[10] disconnected the resistors placed between the limb and the central terminal and thus augmented (a) the voltage of these leads about 1.5 times (aV_R, aV_L, aV_F). The relation between the standard and unipolar augmented leads is as follows:

$$aV_R + aV_L + aV_F = 0$$

$$aV_R = \frac{-I + II}{2}$$

$$aV_L = \frac{I - III}{2}$$

$$aV_F = \frac{II + III}{2}$$

The direction of lead I is 0°; of lead II, 60°; of lead III, 120°; of lead aV_F, 90°; of lead aV_L, −30°; and of lead aV_R, −150°.

The electromotive force generated by the heart at any instant can be represented by the vector force of a single equivalent dipole situated at this point. This vector points from the negative to the positive potential (coincident with the direction of the impulse propagation), and its magnitude is proportional to the magnitude of the electromotive force. The voltage registered in a given lead corresponds to the projection of the cardiac vector on the axis of the lead (see Fig. 27.5). The maximum deflection is registered when the vector is parallel and the minimum deflection when the vector is perpendicular to the lead axis.

The maximum QRS vector is being used to define the main axis. This vector usually corresponds to the R axis. The mean QRS axis is the average of all instantaneous vectors during QRS. The general term *electrical heart axis in the frontal plane* is sometimes used in reference to the main and sometimes to the mean axis. This designation is meaningful only when one dominant deflection is present in at least one of the limb leads. When the QRS complex is biphasic in all leads, the meaning of the average QRS axis changes because the QRS loop is nearly circular. Such biphasic pattern with an indeterminate axis can be described as a sequence of two separate main axes corresponding to the initial and terminal deflections.

The normal QRS axis is about +60°, slight to moderate left axis from about +30° to 0°; slight to moderate right axis from about +90° to +120°, marked left axis about −60°, and marked right axis about +150°. An axis within the range of −60° to −90° is best designated as left superior, and one from −180° to −90° as right superior.

The semidirect precordial leads introduced by Wilson record the potential differences between the chest electrodes and the central terminal (V) electrode at locations shown in Figure 27.6.

When the electrical activity on the cardiac surface is recorded by means of a unipolar lead, the activation front approaching the electrode registers an upright deflection, but as soon as the activation front reaches the electrode, the direction changes and the electrogram records a rapid negative deflection, which is called intrinsic. This intrinsic deflection is believed to coincide with the depolarization of cells beneath the electrode. In the semidirect unipolar precordial leads, the transition from positive to negative is less abrupt than in direct leads, and this makes the intrinsic deflection less rapid and less distinct. For this reason, this deflection has been designated as intrinsicoid. The onset of intrinsicoid deflection in the precordial leads corresponds to the peak of the tall R wave or the nadir of the deep S wave. The onset of intrinsicoid deflection may be delayed if the duration of excitation wave spreading toward the recording electrode is prolonged owing to an increased ventricular wall thickness.

NORMAL ECG
P WAVE

The axis of the P wave in the frontal plane is usually about 60°. In leads I and II and in the left precordial leads, P is upright. In lead III, P is also usually upright but may be diphasic or negative. In the right precordial leads, P is usually diphasic. The initial portion of the P wave, corresponding to right atrial depolarization, is directed anteriorly, and the terminal portion, corresponding to left atrial depolarization, is directed posteriorly. Since both deflections are directed downward and to the left, they tend to fuse and form a single deflection in the frontal plane. However, careful inspection will frequently reveal a notch on the summit of normal P wave. The amplitude of normal P wave usually does not exceed 0.25 mV or 25% of the R wave. P-wave duration in adults ranges from 0.07 to 0.12 second.

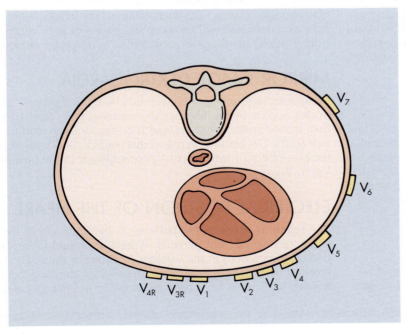

FIGURE 27.6 Cross section of the thorax illustrating the position of the unipolar precordial V leads in relation to the heart. The position of leads V_{4R} and V_{3R} on the right side of the thorax corresponds to the positions of leads V_4 and V_3 on the left side.

PR INTERVAL

The PR interval designates the interval from the beginning of the P wave to the beginning of the QRS, regardless of whether the latter begins with a Q or an R. The normal PR interval in adults ranges from 0.12 to 0.20 second, but both shorter and longer values are sometimes present in normal persons. The PR interval is shortened by increased sympathetic tone and lengthened by increased vagal tone.

QRS COMPLEX

The normal QRS duration in adults ranges from 0.07 to 0.10 second. The first downward deflection of the QRS complex is a Q wave, the second downward deflection is an S wave, and the first upright deflection is an R wave. If a second upright deflection after the S wave is present it is named R^1, and a second downward deflection after R^1, S^1. A monophasic negative deflection is designated as a QS wave. When the QRS complex is polyphasic, small letters are sometimes used to designate the low-amplitude deflections and capital letters are used for the high-amplitude deflections.

The duration of a normal Q wave is less than 0.03 second. A Q wave is seldom present in all three standard limb leads simultaneously, but may be absent in all three leads. The Q amplitude usually does not exceed 25% of the R wave in lead I but may equal or exceed the R amplitude in lead III. A slurred R wave is not considered to be an abnormal finding if the total duration of the QRS interval is not increased. The S wave may be absent in one or more of the standard leads. When present, the R/S ratio is usually greater than 1.5 in leads II and III, but in persons with left axis deviation may be less than 1 in lead III.

In the precordial leads, V_1 and V_2, R amplitude is low. Both the R amplitude and the R/S ratio increase progressively in the direction from V_1 to V_6. The transition zone at which R exceeds S is usually situated between leads V_2 and V_3 or between leads V_3 and V_4. The so-called poor R-wave progression may represent an abnormal finding signifying a decrease of the anteriorly directed forces (*e.g.,* anterior wall infarction). However, more often such pattern represents a normal variant caused by an atypical heart position or an inappropriate lead placement.

ST SEGMENT

The ST segment is the isoelectric interval interposed between the end of the QRS complex and the beginning of the T wave. The transition from the QRS to the ST segment has been designated as the RS-T junction, or the J point. The position of the J point is measured from the level of the PR segment, and the level of the ST segment is related to the level of the TP segment. The normal ST segment is usually horizontal but may be elevated or depressed by less than 0.1 mV. When the J point is shifted downward, the course of the ST segment becomes upsloping. The duration of the ST segment depends on the heart rate and parallels the rate-dependent changes of the QT interval.

T WAVE

The normal T wave is always upright in leads I and V_5 and V_6 and inverted in the lead aV_R. In leads III, aV_F, and the right precordial leads, the T wave may be upright or inverted. The normal angle between QRS complex and T-wave axis (QRS/T angle) ranges from 10° to 60°. Normally, the duration of the ascending branch of a positive T wave is longer than the descent, and the T-wave apex is reached at a point corresponding to 70% to 80% of the QT interval.[11]

QT INTERVAL

The duration of the QT interval decreases with increasing heart rate. Therefore, it is customary to correct the QT interval for the RR interval. The commonly used Bazett formula defines this value as follows: $QT = K\sqrt{RR}$. The K represents the corrected QT (*i.e.,* QTc), a value that normally averages about 0.40 in men and about 0.44 in women.[3]

U WAVE

The U wave is a broad, rounded deflection of low amplitude, appearing after the T wave and not always discernible in the limb leads. U-wave amplitude seldom exceeds 0.05 mV in the limb and 0.1 mV in the precordial leads. The normal U wave is upright in the standard limb and precordial leads. U-wave amplitude increases at slow heart rates and decreases at rapid heart rates. The U wave is inscribed during protodiastole and is attributed to potentials generated by the stretching ventricular myocardium. Other mechanisms have been also proposed.[12]

EFFECTS OF AGE, SEX, AND TRAINING

During transition from infancy to adulthood, the P, PR, and QRS intervals increase in duration. The T wave in the right precordial leads may be upright during the first few days after birth but afterward becomes inverted. During the transition to adulthood the T wave in leads V_1 to V_3 again becomes upright. The persistence of negative T wave in these leads is termed juvenile pattern. Compared with adults, the mean electrical axis in infants and young children is directed rightward. The ECG configuration in adolescents is the same as in the adults, but the QRS amplitude tends to be greater, probably due to closer proximity of the heart to the chest wall, and the J point is more frequently elevated.[13]

In aging adults, the QRS axis tends to shift progressively to the left and the T-wave amplitude tends to decrease. However, in the absence of heart disease the mean QRS axis usually does not shift to the left beyond 20°, even in the seventh to ninth decade of life.[14]

In women, the QRS duration tends to be slightly shorter than in men owing to smaller myocardial mass. Also in women, the QRS and T-wave amplitude are lower and the J point is directed more superiorly and posteriorly than in men.[15] The ST segment in women tends to be less upsloping and the QT interval is about 7% to 10% longer than in men.[15]

In athletes, the ECG tends to reflect the effects of increased vagal tone and increased ventricular mass, manifested by increased QRS duration, QRS amplitude, and J-point elevation.[16]

BODY BUILD

The QRS axis tends to be vertical in slender persons and horizontal in heavyset or obese persons. The body build needs to be taken into consideration during ECG interpretation. For instance, the presence of right axis deviation will be more suggestive of right ventricular hypertrophy (RVH) in an obese person than in a slender person.

MIRROR IMAGE DEXTROCARDIA

Dextrocardia results in a pattern in which the right and left arm electrodes appear to be intentionally reversed (*i.e.,* lead I represents its own mirror image, whereas lead II corresponds to lead III and lead III to lead II). The patterns in precordial leads V_1 and V_2 are reversed, and the placement of leads V_3 to V_6 corresponds to the positions of leads V_{3R} to V_{6R}.

ELECTRICAL POSITION OF THE HEART

The relations between the patterns in the limb and in the precordial leads vary in different persons. Wilson attributed these variable relations to differences in the variable rotations of the heart about one or more of the three separate axes: the sagittal, the longitudinal, and the transverse. Criteria have been developed for different "electrical hear

...sitions" based on the concepts of clockwise or counterclockwise ...ation about these axes. However, the presence of assumed rotations ...not well supported by the anatomical correlations and the designa...n of an electrical position has not played a major role in clinical ...actice. The two most commonly identified electrical positions are ...e vertical and the horizontal. Of these, the vertical position means ...t lead aV_L resembles V_1 to V_2 and lead aV_F resembles V_5 to V_6 ...ereas the horizontal position means that lead aV_L resembles V_5 to V_6 ...d that lead aV_F resembles V_1 to V_2. A clockwise rotation of the heart ...out its longitudinal axis is believed to cause Q-wave appearance in ...d III and S wave in lead I, while a counterclockwise rotation is ...lieved to cause Q-wave appearance in lead I and S wave in lead III. ...the precordial leads, the shift of the transition zone to the left is ...tributed to a clockwise rotation and the shift to the right is attributed ...a counterclockwise rotation of the heart.

...MPERATURE

...e effect of fever is indistinguishable from that of sympathetic stimula...n (*i.e.*, tachycardia, tall peaked P waves in leads II and III, and low T ...ves). Hypothermia causes progressive lengthening of all ECG de...ctions, but the QT interval is more sensitive to low temperature ...anges than the QRS complex and the PR interval. A rounded deflec...n resembling a P wave and designated as a J wave or Osborn wave ...ay appear after the end of the QRS complex when body temperature ...ls to less than about 32°C. The pathogenesis of this deflection has ...t been established with certainty.

VECTORCARDIOGRAPHY

...the vectors during one cardiac cycle are displayed with their origin ...a a common zero point, their ends form a vector loop beginning at ...d returning to this point. Since each of the principal ECG compo...nts, the P wave, the QRS complex, the T wave, and the U wave, starts ...om and returns to the same baseline, four separate loops can be ...corded, one for each of these four deflections. If the ST segment is ...splaced from the baseline, the QRS loop does not return to the point ...origin of the T loop and the loop remains open. Since the P, T, and U ...ops are of much lower amplitude than the QRS loop, their analysis ...quires considerable amplification.

To obtain a vectorcardiogram (VCG), two leads must be recorded ...multaneously. The modern VCG system employs a set of three or...ogonal leads, one in the right to left direction (x lead), one in the ...ead to foot direction (y lead), and one in the front to back direction (z ...ad). Sets of appropriate resistors are used to "correct" these leads ...r the varying distance of the electrodes from the heart. The leads can ...e combined to form three loops, one in the frontal plane using the x ...d y leads, one in the sagittal plane using the y and z leads, and one in ...e horizontal plane using the x and z leads. To follow the direction of ...stantaneous vectors, it is customary to interrupt the loop at 2- or ...5-msec intervals.

In addition to the enhanced accuracy of the orthogonal lead sys...m and the ability to measure accurately the direction of instanta...ous vectors at frequent intervals, the VCG displays the rotation of the ...op. This adds valuable information, not available from the inspection ...the scalar ECG. The VCG is very useful in teaching electrocardiogra...y, particularly in demonstrating how the vector loops can be used to ...rive scalar tracings. Although in principle, the scalar ECG and the ...CG have essentially the same content, in a certain number of cases, ...e VCG displays the diagnostic pattern more distinctly than the scalar ...CG.[17] In some cases, the VCG may help to clarify the diagnosis due to ...e accuracy of measured intervals and the display of the rotations of ...e QRS loop and its components. These details pertain most often to ...e analysis of the early portion of the QRS complex. The VCG has ...en most useful in clarifying the diagnosis of inferior, anteroseptal, ...d posterior myocardial infarction, as well as infarction complicated ...y bundle branch or fascicular blocks.

Notwithstanding the occasional diagnostic superiority of the VCG over the scalar ECG, the net yield of such advantages in the clinical practice is not sufficient to overcome the disadvantages of more costly equipment, a longer time needed to apply the electrodes and produce the record, and an occasional need to supplement the loops made from orthogonal leads by semidirect precordial leads. Such minor inconveniences combined with the increasing availability of technology for the assessment of wall motion abnormality and myocardial perfusion have resulted in a declining use of VCG in clinical practice.

BODY SURFACE MAPPING

Body surface mapping, facilitated by the use of a computer, provides detailed information about the distribution of QRS, ST, and T potentials on the body surfaces. Modern mapping systems analyze data at 1-msec intervals and print isopotential maps at 5-msec intervals. It has been shown that an array of 32 leads is sufficient to obtain an accurate isopotential map.[18] The clinical usefulness of body surface mapping has not been tested as widely as that of VCG. However, the relative complexity of the recording and analyzing systems, the lack of familiarity with the method of display, and the competition with other noninvasive diagnostic methods may be expected to impede the wide applicability of mapping for purposes other than analysis of cardiac arrhythmias.

CHAMBER ENLARGEMENT AND INTRAVENTRICULAR CONDUCTION DISTURBANCES
P-WAVE ABNORMALITIES

There are three distinct patterns of abnormal P waves during sinus rhythm: (1) P pulmonale, (2) right atrial enlargement, and (3) left atrial enlargement. P pulmonale is frequently present in patients with chronic lung disease, particularly in the presence of tachycardia. The pattern is most likely due to a combination of increased sympathetic stimulation and low diaphragm position. The former contributes to the increased P amplitude and the latter to the vertical P axis. The same pattern can be present during tachycardia in the absence of lung disease. Although some patients with chronic lung disease in whom this type of P-wave abnormality is present have pulmonary hypertension due to chronic cor pulmonale, there is no good overall correlation between P pulmonale and right atrial enlargement. The latter can be suspected when a tall, wide P wave is present in the limb and in the right precordial leads (Fig. 27.7), a pattern commonly present in patients with congenital heart disease, tricuspid valve disease, and pulmonary hypertension. The difference between P pulmonale and the pattern of right atrial enlargement is that the former represents an inferiorly directed P-wave vector and the latter a dominant anteriorly directed major P-wave component.

Left atrial enlargement can be suspected when a wide P wave is due to an increased duration of the terminal, posteriorly directed P-wave component. The wide separation between the anteriorly and the posteriorly directed P-wave components results in a prolonged interval between the peak of the initial upright portion and the nadir of the following inverted P-wave portion in the right precordial leads (Fig. 27.8). Such P waves are usually upright and notched in leads I, II, and V_4 to V_6 and either positive-negative or negative in the III and aV_F. Since the pattern associated with left atrial enlargement indicates an interatrial conduction disturbance rather than hypertrophy or dilation, the preferred term is *left atrial abnormality* rather than enlargement.

An additional cause of an abnormal P wave with or without displacement of the PR segment is atrial infarction. However, both the sensitivity and the specificity of P-wave abnormalities in the diagnosis of atrial infarction is low.

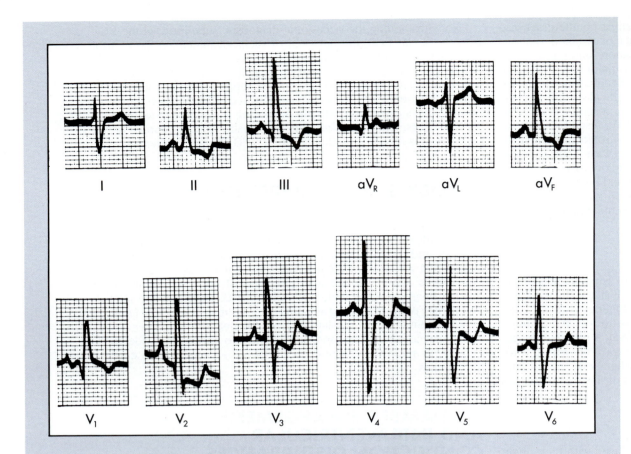

FIGURE 27.7 Typical pattern of RVH and right atrial enlargement. Note slight widening of QRS complex and Q wave in leads V_1 and V_2.

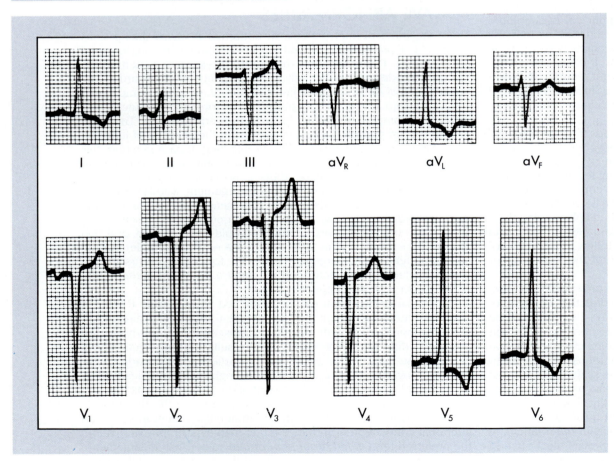

FIGURE 27.8 Typical pattern of LVH and left atrial enlargement.

LEFT VENTRICULAR HYPERTROPHY

Electrocardiographic criteria for the diagnosis of left ventricular hypertrophy (LVH) consist of increased QRS amplitude (voltage), increased QRS/T angle, intraventricular conduction delay manifested by delayed intrinsicoid deflection in the precordial leads facing the left ventricle, and occasionally left axis deviation (see Fig. 27.8). The increased voltage is attributed to one or more of the following: increased left ventricular mass, increased left ventricular surface, increased intracavitary blood volume, and closer proximity of the ventricle to the chest wall.

Deviation of the ST segment and the T wave in the direction opposite to the main QRS vector in the horizontal and frontal planes results in a widening of the QRS/T angle. The combination of increased QRS amplitude and wide QRS/T angle forms a pattern known as "left ventricular strain" (see Fig. 27.8). Although it appears inappropriate to use the word "strain" in reference to an electrical event, the term has remained popular in clinical practice.

The ST- and T-wave changes in the left ventricular strain pattern are secondary to delayed propagation of the impulse in the conducting system or hypertrophied myocardium. In theory, if the QRS area is strictly proportional to the ventricular mass and the sequence of repolarization bears the same relation to the sequence of activation as in the normal myocardium, ventricular gradient (see later) should be preserved. This occurs in uncomplicated hypertrophy, but not when the ST- and T-wave changes are due to associated myocardial ischemia, which may be present even in the absence of coronary artery disease, possibly due to a diminished number of capillaries per unit of myocardial mass in the hypertrophied myocardium.[3]

None of the numerous criteria are specific for LVH. The QRS voltage can be modified by extracardiac factors such as age, chest diameter, and body build. The QRS voltage, which tends to be greater in persons with a thin chest and a low ponderal index,[19] meets the criteria for diagnosis of LVH in about 5% of normal men.[19] Variations in precordial voltage may be due to changes in electrode position but may occur in the same person at 24-hour intervals, even independent of electrode position, perhaps due to changes in respiration and heart rate.[20]

The voltage is markedly reduced in obese persons or persons with large breasts. A significant increase in R amplitude in leads V_1 to V_5 occurs after left mastectomy, and in leads V_{3R} and V_1 after right mastectomy.[21] An erroneous diagnosis of LVH on the basis of increased voltage would be made in nearly 50% of women after mastectomy.[21] Other factors that may alter voltage in the absence of hypertrophy include myocardial ischemia, intraventricular conduction disturbance, and altered blood viscosity. A low hematocrit in anemic patients increases, and a high hematocrit in polycythemic patients decreases, QRS voltage owing to changes in blood resistivity.

The specificity of the ST and T abnormalities is even lower than that of the voltage. Also, the combination of increased voltage and wide QRS/T angle is not specific and can be due to delayed conduction in the left bundle branch system in the absence of LVH. As may be expected, the specificity and the sensitivity of the ECG criteria for LVH are related inversely to each other (*i.e.*, the stringent criteria are more specific but less sensitive and *vice versa*). In addition, the diagnostic accuracy of the LVH pattern declines in the presence of biventricular hypertrophy, myocardial infarction, and treatment with digitalis or antiarrhythmic drugs.

Perhaps the greatest diagnostic accuracy of LVH is achieved by a combined point score of Romhilt and Estes, in which increased QRS amplitude, ST-T changes, and P wave suggestive of left atrial enlargement score 3 points each, left axis deviation scores −2 points, and slight QRS widening and delayed intrinsicoid deflection score −1 point each.[22] Using this system, the LVH pattern based on the presence of more than 5 points was present in 52 of 90 patients with LVH (see Fig. 27.8) and in only 2 of 60 persons who had no LVH.[22] In patients with hypertension or valvular heart disease the echocardiographic studies confirmed that the sensitivity and specificity of the "left ventricular strain" pattern, or of the Romhilt–Estes score was better than the voltage criteria alone. However, the echocardiographic studies have underscored also the shortcomings of the ECG in the diagnosis of LVH by showing that the QRS voltage may be increased in the presence of an increased left ventricular diastolic diameter and normal thickness of the left ventricular wall[23] and that the magnitude of the maximal QRS vector in the horizontal plane cannot be used reliably to differentiate between concentric LVH and isolated left ventricular dilation.

RIGHT VENTRICULAR HYPERTROPHY

The ECG manifestations of RVH and right ventricular dilatation can be subdivided into three types: (1) typical RVH pattern with anterior and rightward displacement of the main QRS vector, (2) incomplete right bundle branch block (RBBB), and (3) posterior and rightward displacement of the main QRS axis.

The typical RVH pattern is a mirror image of the LVH pattern with right axis deviation in the frontal plane, tall R waves in the right precordial leads, deep S waves in the left precordial leads, and slight increase in the QRS duration (see Fig. 27.7). This pattern is characteristically present in patients with congenital pulmonary stenosis, tetralogy of Fallot, primary pulmonary hypertension, and other conditions in which the right ventricular mass tends to approach or exceed the left ventricular mass. The earliest portion of the QRS complex is usually unchanged because the septal activation is normal. The anterior displacement of the main QRS vector, manifested by a tall R wave in the right precordial leads, is attributed to a longer activation time of the hypertrophied right ventricular free wall.[24,25] However, the resulting lengthening of the QRS complex is usually slight, and the intrinsicoid deflection is seldom sufficiently delayed to be of diagnostic usefulness. The T waves are directed opposite to the main QRS vector and therefore are inverted in the right precordial leads and upright in the left precordial leads (see Fig. 27.7). These secondary T-wave abnormalities may be accompanied by secondary deviations of the ST segment. In some cases of severe RVH, the R wave in the right precordial leads is preceded by a Q wave (see Fig. 27.7). In such cases, the right atrium is frequently enlarged and tricuspid regurgitation is commonly present.

In adults, the suggested criteria for the diagnosis of RVH consist of R/S or R^1/S ratio in lead V_1 greater than 1.0 with R or R^1 amplitude greater than 0.5 mV and QRS duration less than 0.12 second. The sensitivity of this pattern in adults with acquired heart disease is low, and there is no strong correlation between R voltage in the right precordial leads and right ventricular pressure or weight.[26]

The incomplete RBBB causing the rSR^1 pattern in right precordial leads is attributed to the delayed activation of the hypertrophied right ventricular outflow tract. This pattern is most frequently due to factors other than RVH. However, it can signify hypertrophy, dilation, or overload of the right ventricle, perhaps most commonly in mitral valve disease with pulmonary hypertension and atrial septal defect. The prompt disappearance of this pattern observed in many cases within days after corrective surgery, suggests that the incomplete RBBB may result from slowing of intraventricular conduction due to the stretch of the peripheral conducting system in the dilated ventricle.

Posterior rightward displacement of the main QRS axis, which occurs most commonly in patients with chronic lung disease, is characterized by low QRS amplitude in limb leads, right axis deviation or $S_1S_2S_3$ pattern, and posterior, superior, and rightward deviation of the main QRS axis with deep S waves in middle and left precordial leads. Sometimes S amplitude is equal to or greater than R amplitude in all three standard limb and in all six precordial leads. The low voltage is attributed to the overinflated lungs, whereas the more vertical heart position and the abnormal R/S ratio is attributed to low diaphragm position and a higher than normal electrode position in relation to the heart. The cause of posterior and rightward displacement of the main QRS axis is not obvious but is probably related to the change in heart position within the enlarged thorax.

The best criteria for judging the severity of chronic obstructive pulmonary disease (COPD) are (1) R in V_6 less than 0.5 mV, (2) R/S in V_6 less than 1.0, and (3) increased P-wave amplitude in leads II and III.[27] Using similar criteria of low R-wave amplitude and low R/S amplitude in x lead, low voltage in x and y leads, and rightward shift of the P axis, COPD was identified correctly in 75% of patients, with only 8% false-positive cases.[28] The best indicators of deteriorating pulmonary function in patients with COPD are reported to be progressive reduction of R wave and R/S ratio in the orthogonal lead x, progressive shift of the QRS axis in the superior direction, and rightward shift of the P-wave axis.[28] In the late stages of chronic lung disease, the development of chronic cor pulmonale may cause a typical RVH pattern with tall R waves in the right precordial leads.

BIVENTRICULAR HYPERTROPHY

As the forces generated by LVH and RVH are directed opposite to each other, a partial cancellation may occur. This may sometimes obscure the established LVH pattern after the development of RVH due to pulmonary hypertension. However, the presence of concomitant LVH and RVH is frequently recognizable because of the asynchrony of ventricular depolarization and also because the precordial leads are semidirect and exaggerate the electromotive force in the proximity to the electrodes. A combined pattern of RVH and LVH is present frequently in patients with Eisenmenger's syndrome (i.e., ventricular septal defect or patent ductus arteriosus with pulmonary hypertension). In such cases, tall R waves may be present in both left and right precordial leads with tall biphasic QRS in the mid-precordial leads (Katz-Wachtel pattern). In patients with rheumatic heart disease, biventricular hypertrophy (BVH) may be suspected in the presence of tall R waves in the left precordial leads and disproportionally small S waves (i.e., less than 2 mV in V_1) or inverted T waves in the right precordial leads. Such pattern is characteristically present in patients with mitral stenosis, pulmonary hypertension, and associated mitral regurgitation or aortic valve disease. Also, right axis in the frontal plane in the presence of an LVH pattern suggests an associated right ventricular enlargement. A less reliable indicator of possible right ventricular dilation in the presence of an LVH pattern is the shift of the transition zone in the precordial leads to the left. Correlation with an echocardiogram showed that the most sensitive indicator of RVH in the presence of LVH was an R/S ratio greater than 1 in lead V_1.[29]

RIGHT BUNDLE BRANCH BLOCK

Since the initial QRS deflection is caused by depolarization transmitted to the ventricular muscle by the left bundle branch, the delay or block of the excitation wave in the right bundle branch causes no changes in the initial QRS portion.[30] As a consequence of the block in the proximal or distal right bundle branch,[31] the normal rapid activation by way of the twigs of the right bundle branch does not take place, and consequently a portion of the pulmonary outflow tract and the right ventricular base is activated predominantly by the muscle (i.e., slower than normally). This causes slowing of the terminal QRS portion, which is directed to the right and anteriorly. In the adult, the RBBB is considered as complete when QRS duration is greater than 0.12 second and incomplete when QRS duration is within the 0.09- to 0.11-second range. By comparing the complexes before and after appearance of RBBB or during RBBB alternans, it can be established that in typical RBBB cases the initial unchanged QRS portion may last 60 msec to 80 msec and that the abnormal component represents an added terminal appendage. However, in many cases the duration of the initial unchanged QRS portion is shorter because the influence of the electric forces caused by the delayed activation takes place earlier. Such pattern variations may be due to different sites of block in the right bundle branch or to different underlying basic excitation patterns. Notwithstanding such differences, some early QRS portion remains uninfluenced by the interruption of the right bundle branch in all RBBB cases. It is important to remember that the mean electrical axis in the presence of RBBB refers only to the initial narrow QRS portion. The diagnosis of RBBB is based on the presence of RSR^1 complex with a wide R^1 deflection in the right precordial leads and a wide S wave in leads I, aV_L, and left precordial leads. The T wave is directed opposite to the terminal QRS portion.

The presence of RBBB does not obscure the abnormal initial QRS force caused by transmural myocardial or preexcitation and does not interfere with the recognition of LVH based on increased voltage. However, the recognition of RVH in the presence of RBBB is more difficult. Two criteria are being used: abnormal initial rightward and anterior QRS force such as would appear in the absence of RBBB, and increased amplitude of the terminal delayed QRS portion. In the first case, this will result in a tall initial R wave, and in the second case in a tall R^1 wave in the right precordial leads.

When the QRS complex is abnormally prolonged, the presence of R^1 deflection in the right precordial leads represents a characteristic and specific marker of RBBB. However, when QRS complex is of normal duration, the significance of narrow R^1 deflection is uncertain because even in persons with a normal ECG, an exploration of the precordium using multiple chest leads frequently reveals RSR^1 complexes in some leads, above or to the right of the standard lead V_1 to V_2 positions. These R^1 deflections may represent either local depolarizations not recognizable in the QRS loop recorded with distal orthogonal leads or minor conduction delays recognizable only as a slight slowing of the terminal portion of the QRS loop. Since such R^1 deflections can be detected in many children, young adults, and persons with a thin chest, they represent a normal variant unless proven otherwise. Even a typical pattern of incomplete RBBB with a slightly prolonged QRS duration, unless known to be acquired, may be a normal variant. Also, in some cases, an anteriorly directed vector is caused by factors other than incomplete RBBB (e.g., hypertrophy of the right ventricular outflow tract, or a peri-infarction block).

Although the clinical significance of RBBB is usually determined by the presence, or absence, and the degree of associated heart disease, a QRS duration of more than 0.13 second and a QRS axis between $-45°$ and $-90°$ identify persons who most likely have associated cardiovascular abnormalities.[32]

LEFT BUNDLE BRANCH BLOCK

The intraventricular conduction disturbance resulting from left bundle branch block (LBBB) distorts the entire QRS complex. The initial deflection assumes a leftward and posterior direction and the subsequent slow transseptal activation of the left ventricle causes a wide QRS complex with a slurred middle portion. The main QRS axis is directed posteriorly in the horizontal plane; its direction in the frontal plane is variable. In a case of uncomplicated LBBB, the initial 0.02-second portion of the QRS complex is nearly always upright in leads I, II, and aV_L and left precordial leads and is either upright or inverted in III, aV_F, and right precordial leads. The QRS amplitude is usually increased and the intrinsicoid deflection delayed by more than 0.05 second. The LBBB is considered to be complete when QRS deflection is greater than 0.12 second and incomplete when QRS deflection is 0.10 to 0.11 second. The only difference between the incomplete LBBB and the LVH pattern is the direction of the initial 0.02-second QRS portion. Sometimes the LVH pattern progresses first to an incomplete and later to a complete LBBB. Sometimes Wenckebach periods within the LBBB are seen (Fig. 27.9). However, more commonly, the pattern of complete LBBB appears abruptly without evolving from an incomplete LBBB pattern.

The terminal portion of the QRS complex tends to be less wide than its middle portion. This is attributed to the probable engagement of the distal left ventricular Purkinje system after completion of the septal crossing.[33] Consistent with this explanation are the observations that in patients with LBBB who have scarred ventricular myocardium and presumed damage of the distal conducting system, the terminal QRS portion is wider and the total QRS duration longer than in persons with LBBB attributed to a block in the proximal LBBB portion alone.[34]

Because of the profoundly disturbed sequence of ventricular excitation, LBBB masks other abnormalities of the QRS complex and makes it difficult or impossible to recognize the presence or absence of transmural myocardial infarction and ventricular hypertrophy. In most cases of transmural myocardial infarction, the Q wave in the limb and precordial leads is absent because the initial "septal" depolarization is directed to the left and posteriorly. An exception to this will occur if anterior wall infarction involves both the septum and the free wall of the left ventricle. However, for unexplained reasons, low-amplitude Q waves in the anterior or "lateral" leads have been noted in a number of autopsy-proven cases of absent myocardial infarction. In the right precordial leads, a low or negative initial 0.02-second deflection may simulate an anteroseptal myocardial infarction, whereas an absent or low initial R wave in leads II, III, and aV_F may simulate an inferior myocardial infarction. The recognition of associated LVH is difficult because LBBB causes an increased QRS voltage and secondary ST- and T-wave changes that are directed opposite to the main QRS axis (i.e., in the same manner as in the presence of LVH pattern).

Although the clinical significance of LBBB depends on the underlying heart disease, in the general adult population, a newly acquired LBBB most often indicates an advanced organic heart disease. Among patients with LBBB, a superiorly oriented axis (i.e., greater than $-30°$) tends to indicate more advanced conduction diseases,[35] and many patients with such pattern have evidence of left anterior fascicular block either before the appearance or after the disappearance of LBBB.[36]

LEFT ANTERIOR FASCICULAR BLOCK (LEFT ANTERIOR HEMIBLOCK)

The ECG criteria for the diagnosis of left anterior fascicular block (LAFB) include QRS duration less than 0.12 second, direction of the main QRS axis in the frontal plane from about $-45°$ to about $-85°$, and initial QRS vector directed to the right and anteriorly (i.e., Q wave in one or more of the following leads: I, aV_L, V_6, V_7.[37] These changes reflect delayed activation of the basal anterolateral portion of the left ventricle[38] and are frequently accompanied by slurred terminal S waves in the left precordial leads. The initial R wave in leads V_1, V_2, and sometimes V_3 is low or absent probably because the onset of septal depolarization is shifted caudally. This may simulate myocardial infarction of the anterior wall. However, the initial QRS vector is directed posteriorly in the presence of myocardial infarction and anteriorly in the presence of LAFB. Therefore, these two patterns can be differentiated by recording precordial leads one or two interspaces below the standard positions of the V_1 to V_4 leads. Due to the rightward and superior course of the initial QRS deflection, LAFB may obscure the pattern of inferior myocardial infarction and simulate the pattern of anterolateral myocardial infarction. LAFB can also simulate the LVH pattern. When LAFB is combined with RBBB, the mean QRS axis representing the non-RBBB portion of the QRS complex is directed superiorly. Ventricular repolarization pattern in the presence of LAFB remains within normal limits, although the T-wave amplitude may increase in the left precordial leads.

Pathologic correlations and experimental studies suggest that the superior axis deviation is not always due to lesions in the left anterior fascicle. For instance, a similar pattern may be due to the preexcitation of the posterior fascicle believed to occur in the presence of atrioventricular cushion defect and interatrial septum primum defect. Also, superior axis deviation may be caused by other abnormalities associated with congenital heart disease and conduction through an accessory atrioventricular pathway.

Left axis deviation due to horizontal heart position may be present in obese persons, but the abnormalities of body build alone seldom cause axis deviation greater than $-30°$. In patients with chronic lung disease the QRS axis in the frontal plane may be directed superiorly, but the ECG pattern differs from the LAFB because (1) the initial Q wave is usually absent in leads I, aV_L, and V_6, (2) the S wave is usually present in all standard limb and precordial leads, and (3) R amplitude in the left precordial leads is decreased, and the mean QRS axis in the frontal plane tends to exceed $-180°$ (i.e., northwest direction).

LEFT POSTERIOR FASCICULAR BLOCK (LEFT POSTERIOR HEMIBLOCK)

Left posterior fascicular block (LPFB), attributed to a lesion in the left posterior fascicle, causes the activation to begin in the left anterior fascicle. Therefore, the initial QRS vector is directed to the left and superiorly. The subsequent QRS vector, reflecting the delayed activation of the posterior fascicle, causes rightward and inferior deviation of the main QRS axis. Thus, in the frontal plane, LPFB causes a Q wave and a tall R wave in leads III and aV_F. The mean QRS axis is greater than $+110°$.[39] The differential diagnosis of such pattern frequently includes RVH and myocardial infarction. In the presence of RBBB, the associated LPFB usually can be recognized by the presence of Q and tall R in leads III and aV_F (i.e., mean QRS axis greater than $+100°$).

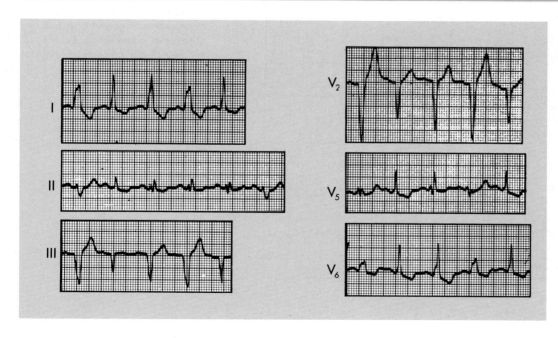

FIGURE 27.9 Second degree LBBB. Note the repetitive sequence of the LVH pattern, incomplete LBBB, and complete LBBB.

VENTRICULAR PREEXCITATION

Preexcitation of the ventricles results from the conduction of the atrial impulse through an accessory pathway that bypasses the atrioventricular node and the bundle of His. If the conduction occurs exclusively through the bypass, the ECG records a normal P wave, an absent PR segment, and a slowly inscribed delta wave, which reflects the onset of ventricular depolarization. The following QRS complex may have an abnormal morphology because the rapid impulse propagation begins at the site at which the preexcitation wave encounters the conducting system. The T wave is directed usually opposite to the delta wave. Characteristically, the morphology of the ventricular complexes varies owing to a variable degree of fusion between the impulses partly conducted through the bypass and partly through the atrioventricular node and the bundle of His.

The direction of the delta wave vector points to the approximate location of the bypass tract.[40] Conduction through a left lateral bypass tract (type A) results in a negative delta wave in lead I and left precordial leads and an upright delta wave in the right precordial leads. Conduction through a right lateral bypass tract (type B) results in an upright delta wave in leads I and left precordial leads and a negative delta wave in the right precordial leads. Other locations (i.e., anterior, posterior, and paraseptal bypass tracts) can be also deduced from the morphology of the delta wave with a fair degree of accuracy.[40] If the ECG abnormality caused by the preexcitation pattern is not correctly recognized, the pattern can be mistaken for LBBB, LVH, fascicular block, and myocardial infarction (Fig. 27.10). Conversely, the presence of preexcitation can mask the presence of other abnormalities, in particular that of myocardial infarction.

MYOCARDIAL ISCHEMIA

Manifestations of ischemia may include depression or elevation of the ST segment and U-wave inversion. T-wave changes may also occur, but they are less specific. The ST deviations are due to epicardial or endocardial injury. Figure 27.11 shows diagrammatically the effects of epicardial and endocardial injury on the ST segment in the standard limb or anterior precordial leads of the ECG. Epicardial injury may cause elevation of the ST segment and depression of the baseline, whereas subendocardial injury may cause depression of the ST segment or elevation of the baseline. The conventional ECG, recorded with alternating current coupled amplifiers, does not reveal displacement of the baseline and therefore does not differentiate between the segment displacement caused by the shift of the ST segment or shift of the baseline (i.e., systolic vs. diastolic current of injury) (see Fig. 27.11).

The ST depression in the precordial leads reflects a posteriorly directed deviation of the ST segment vector, and the ST depression in leads III and aV_F reflects a superiorly directed deviation of the ST segment vector. The ST segment depression can be due not only to subendocardial ischemia but to other causes, such as hypertrophy, conduction disturbances, digitalis, and hypokalemia.[39]

The ST elevation in precordial leads reflects an anteriorly directed deviation of the ST segment vector and, in leads III and aV_F, a superiorly directed deviation of the ST segment vector. These changes can be due not only to subepicardial or transmural ischemia but to other causes, such as hypertrophy, conduction disturbances, pericarditis, or may represent a normal variant.[39]

Acute ischemia shortens the duration of the ventricular action potential, and this shortening is expected to cause deviation of the T-wave vector toward the ischemic region. However, such T-wave abnormalities are seldom clearly recognizable in the surface ECG probably because the changes produced by ischemia are of short duration and may be obscured by other factors that affect the T wave, such as tachycardia, sympathetic stimulation, and hyperkalemia. Occasionally, a very tall upright or a very deeply inverted T wave resembling one that frequently appears within seconds or minutes after an acute experimental occlusion in the animal appears in the human ECG during the earliest phase of myocardial infarction. In such cases, the T waves are incorporated into the descending limb of the "monophasic" pattern, whereas the QT interval is usually shortened. The mechanism of occasional transient U-wave inversion during acute ischemia is unknown.

ECG IN MYOCARDIAL INFARCTION

Next to arrhythmias, the greatest usefulness of the ECG is in the diagnosis of myocardial infarction. ECG is an established standard diagnostic test for detection, localization, and estimating the approximate size of myocardial infarction. The leads facing the infarcted wall record a Q wave, and the leads facing the opposite wall record an R wave. This means that the vector of the abnormal initial QRS deflection is directed away from the infarction. The Q wave is considered abnormal when its duration is greater than 0.04 second. However, in the VCG, which more accurately measures the duration of the abnormally directed QRS forces, myocardial infarction can be diagnosed when an abnormal Q wave is greater than 0.03 second. Reliance on sheer presence or absence of a Q wave with a duration greater than 0.03 second

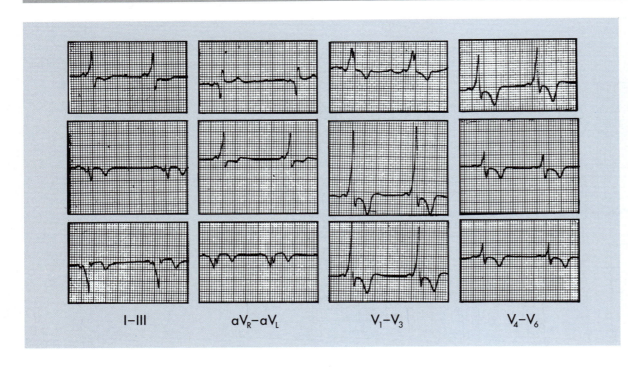

FIGURE 27.10 Typical WPW pattern simulating myocardial infarction of the inferior and posterior wall. In the absence of preexcitation, the ECG of this 37-year-old man was normal (not shown).

I–III aV_R–aV_L V_1–V_3 V_4–V_6

led to correct diagnosis of myocardial infarction in 79% of autopsy-proven cases.[41] If the infarction is nontransmural or subendocardial the QRS complex is not diagnostic of infarction. However, the characteristic morphology and the evolution of the ST segment and T-wave abnormalities are similar in the presence of both transmural and nontransmural infarction.

As a rule, the vector of the deviated ST segment is directed toward the infarction and the vector of the abnormal T wave is directed away from the infarction (Figs. 27.12 through 27.14). Thus, a large anterior wall infarction causes Q waves, ST segment elevation, and T-wave inversion in the anterior precordial leads V_1 to V_6. If the infarction is confined to the septum the corresponding QRS, ST, and T changes are present mainly in the leads facing the septum: leads V_1 and V_2 (see Fig. 27.13). If the infarction is confined to the anterior free wall or the apical region, the abnormalities are present predominantly in the mid-precordial leads, V_3 and V_4 (see Fig. 27.13). If the infarction involves the lateral wall, the abnormal QRS and T-wave vectors point to the right, resulting in a Q wave and negative T wave in lead I and aV_L and precordial leads V_5 and V_6 (see Fig. 27.14). In the presence of high anterolateral infarction, the abnormalities may be detectable only in leads aV_L and left precordial leads recorded above the normal position of V_6 and V_7. However, in these high leads, a Q wave and negative T wave may be present in the absence of infarction. In practice, myocardial infarction seldom causes a pattern in which Q waves are limited to aV_L and high precordial leads without the appearance of Q waves in the standard leads.[42] Electrocardiographic changes are of limited value for localization of "lateral wall infarctions."

Infarction of the inferior or diaphragmatic wall causes Q waves, ST segment elevation, and negative T waves in leads III, aV_F, and sometimes II, while the precordial leads show no definite abnormalities (see Fig. 27.14). Infarction of the posterior wall, or more correctly basal left lateral wall,[43] causes an increased amplitude and widening of the initial R wave (R > 0.4 second or R/S > 1 in V_1 and V_2) in the right precordial leads and increased amplitude of anteriorly directed T waves in these leads (see Fig. 27.14). In many cases, the diagnosis of posterior wall infarction is supported by the comcomitant presence of inferior or lateral infarction.

Right ventricular infarction can be diagnosed with a high degree of accuracy, based on the electrocardiographic changes; ST segment elevation or QS pattern in the right precordial leads V_{3R} or V_{4R} in the presence of inferior or inferoposterior wall myocardial infarction is strongly suggestive of involvement of the right ventricle. ST segment elevation without loss of R waves in the V_1 lead, and occasionally extending to leads V_2, V_3, and V_4, may also indicate right ventricular infarction in patients with inferior wall infarction.

In cases of typical evolution of the ECG pattern (see Figs. 27.12 and 27.13) the earliest abnormality is the deviation of the ST segment, followed by QRS abnormality and T-wave changes. However, the first appearance of T-wave abnormalities varies from minutes to hours or days after the onset of myocardial infarction. Characteristically, the T waves caused by transmural or nontransmural infarction are more symmetrical than normal. This is due to the lengthening of the interval from the apex to the end of a T wave, a pattern usually associated with moderate lengthening of the QT interval.

The term *subendocardial infarction* is used sometimes to characterize an infarction pattern resembling transient acute subendocardial ischemia but persisting for days or weeks. In such cases, QRS abnormalities are absent and the ST segment and T-wave changes are opposite in direction to those in the presence of transmural infarction (*i.e.,* in the precordial leads the ST segment is depressed and T waves are upright). Such patterns are uncommon. Frequently, the term *subendocardial infarction* is used in reference to a nontransmural infarction without Q waves and ST segment deviation (*i.e.,* anterior—subendocardial—nontransmural infarction when T waves are inverted in lead I and precordial leads, and inferior—subendocardial—nontransmural infarction when T waves are inverted in leads II, III, and aV_F).

Ventricular aneurysm may be suspected in the presence of ST segment elevation caused by myocardial infarction and persisting for longer than about a week after the onset of infarction. Multiple infarctions can be recognized if the abnormalities occur in the appropriate sets of different leads. In theory, two myocardial infarctions situated on opposing walls may be expected to normalize the ECG by cancelling the abnormal findings. However, in practice this occurs seldom. Usually both infarctions can be recognized, probably because they do not produce precise mirror image changes and also because the semi-

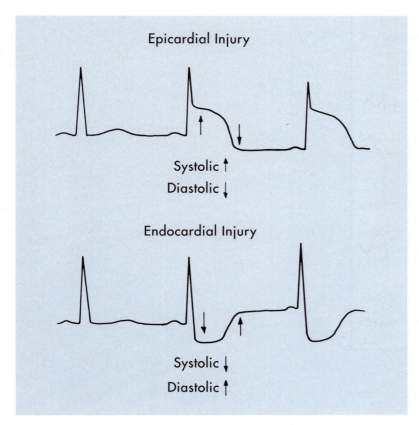

FIGURE 27.11 Diagram of the effects of epicardial and subendocardial injury on the ST segment and the baseline of the ECG. The direction of arrow signals the flow of "injury" current and not the ST segment vector. (Surawicz B, Saito S: Exercise testing for detection of myocardial ischemia in patients with abnormal electrocardiograms at rest. Am J Cardiol 41:943, 1978)

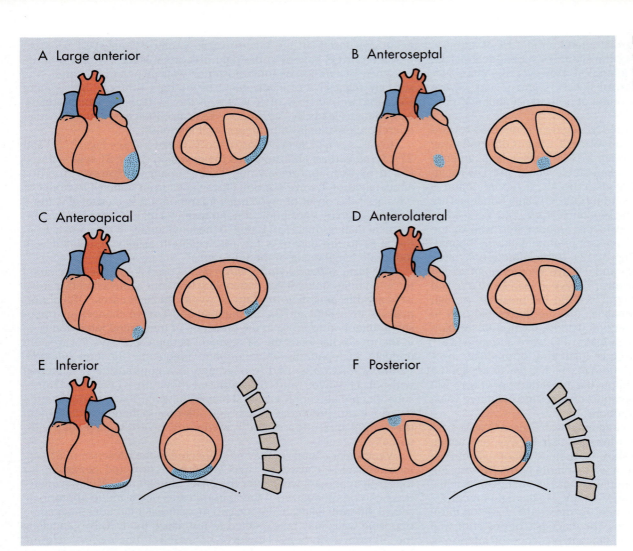

FIGURE 27.12 Diagram of the locations of the six most common sites of myocardial infarction indicated by the stippled areas.

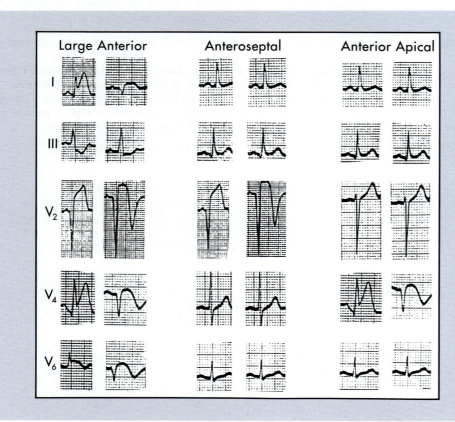

FIGURE 27.13 Each pair of leads shows the ECG patterns of the acute and the subacute stage of myocardial infarctions shown in Figure 26.12.

direct precordial leads are influenced by the proximity to the regions of the heart underlying the appropriate electrodes.

The differential diagnosis of abnormal Q waves in leads III and aV_F is difficult because Q waves in these leads may represent a normal variant in persons with horizontal heart positions. Although such noninfarction Q waves usually disappear during deep inspiration, this is not a reliable test because sometimes Q waves caused by infarction may undergo a similar change.

ABNORMAL Q WAVES AND R WAVES IN THE ABSENCE OF MYOCARDIAL INFARCTION

In the anterior precordial leads V_1 to V_4, a QS pattern in the absence of myocardial infarction is most frequently due to abnormal electrode position, atypical heart position, or superior orientation of the initial anteriorly directed QRS vector.[44] Anteroseptal infarction may be simulated by the presence of a low or isoelectric R wave in leads V_1 and V_2 (e.g., due to LBBB, LVH, LAFB, chronic lung disease, or pericardial effusion). Q waves in the anterior and lateral precordial leads are present commonly in patients with obstructive cardiomyopathy, progressive muscular dystrophy, Friedreich's ataxia, primary cardiac tumors, or metastases to the heart. The pathogenesis of these changes is similar to that in myocardial infarction, namely, replacement of muscle by scar or tumor. Also, ventricular preexcitation can simulate anterior wall infarction. Left-sided tension pneumothorax can also cause QS pattern (pseudoinfarction) in the left precordial leads.

In lead III, the sudden appearance of a Q wave may be due to an acute cor pulmonale. In patients with chronic lung disease an apparent QS pattern may occur if the initial small R wave becomes invisible owing to low voltage. The QR pattern in the ventricular premature complexes is frequently due to myocardial infarction, but the diagnostic reliability of this sign is limited, particularly in patients with inferior wall infarction. Abnormal R waves in the right precordial leads similar to those caused by posterior infarction may be due to RVH, intraventricular conduction disturbance, preexcitation, or an atypical heart position.

Transient pathologic Q waves may occur during acute ischemia (i.e., angina pectoris associated with ST segment depression or elevation) or during reperfusion. A counterpart of this finding is the disappearance of abnormal Q waves after coronary artery bypass graft operation.

CORRELATIONS WITH CORONARY ARTERY OCCLUSIONS

A pattern of anteroseptal myocardial infarction was seen in 93% of all patients with the left anterior descending coronary artery as the infarct-related artery, and a pattern of inferior myocardial infarction was seen in 53% of all patients with the right coronary artery or the left circumflex artery as the infarct-related artery. The pattern of posterior, lateral, or posterolateral infarction in the absence of changes in leads II, III, and aV_F was predictive of left circumflex artery narrowing, while the pattern of inferior infarction in the absence of associated patterns of posterior or lateral infarction was predictive of right coronary artery narrowing.[45] ECG changes fulfilled the diagnostic criteria of myocardial infarction in more than 90% of patients in whom myocardial infarction was related to the narrowing of the left anterior descending coronary artery, in about 80% of patients in whom myocardial infarction was related to the narrowing of the right coronary artery, and in only about 50% of patients in whom myocardial infarction was related to the narrowing of the left circumflex artery. Elevation of the ST segment in V_{4R} during the acute stage is reported to be predictive of proximal right coronary artery occlusion.[46]

SPECIFICITY OF ABNORMAL Q WAVE AND QRS SCORING SYSTEM

Studies of Wagner and associates established greater than 95% specificity of wide Q waves (>30 msec–40 msec) in leads I, II, aV_L, aV_F, V_3 to V_6; wide R waves (>40 msec–50 msec) in leads V_1 and V_2; and abnormal R/Q and R/S amplitude ratios in the standard 12-lead ECG for separating patients with myocardial infarction from persons with a normal ECG.[47] The QRS scoring system, based on the number of leads with abnormal Q waves and R waves, and the duration of these abnor-

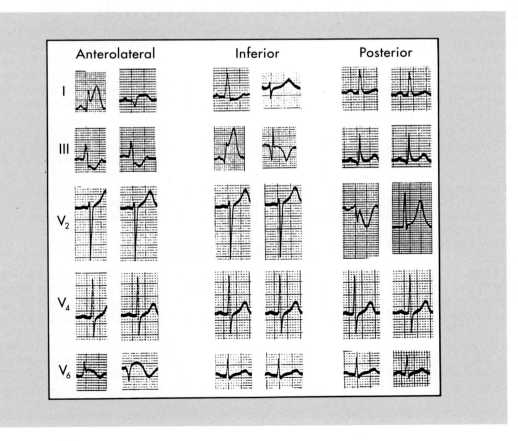

FIGURE 27.14 Each pair of leads shows the ECG patterns of the acute and the subacute stage of myocardial infarctions shown in Figure 26.12.

mal deflections were useful in the estimation of the size of uncomplicated myocardial infarction of the anterior wall[48] and uncomplicated myocardial infarction of the inferior wall.[49] The QRS scoring system is also useful in the estimation of the size of infarction of the posterolateral wall, but the QRS changes used to make this diagnosis are more subtle and diverse than in other infarction types.[50] Posterolateral myocardial infarctions are more frequently electrocardiographically silent than a single inferior or anterior infarction.[50] The QRS scores are also proportional to the severity of wall motion abnormalities and depression of global left ventricular ejection fraction.[51] The ECG is not a very sensitive indicator of apical myocardial infarction.[52] Also, Q waves are frequently absent in autopsy-proven cases of small lesions involving the lateral or posterior wall.

PERI-INFARCTION BLOCK

Studies of intramural excitation in dogs with myocardial infarction scars established evidence of slow conduction in tangential direction to the scar and the resulting late activation of the peri-infarction areas separated from the main body of myocardium by intramural fibrosis strands.[53] In the human ECG, peri-infarction block is suspected when the QRS interval is prolonged and the wide terminal QRS force is directed opposite to the initial abnormal Q wave or R wave caused by the MI. In the presence of anterior wall myocardial infarction the terminal force is directed anteriorly (anterior peri-infarction block) and in the presence of inferior myocardial infarction, inferiorly (inferior peri-infarction block).[54] The pattern of anterior peri-infarction block is similar to that of anterior myocardial infarction with LAFB. However, in the presence of LAFB the terminal QRS portion and the total QRS duration are less wide and the axis tends to be more superiorly oriented than in the presence of peri-infarction block. The pattern of inferior peri-infarction block is similar to that of inferior myocardial infarction with LPFB.

ECG IN PERICARDITIS

The ECG abnormalities produced by pericarditis[55] can be attributed to the presence of pericardial effusion, "injury" of the superficial myocardium by the presence of fluid or fibrin, and superficial myocarditis. Low ECG voltage is usually produced by the short-circuiting effect of the pericardial fluid. If voltage remains low after the removal of fluid, the decreased amplitude of deflections is probably due to the insulating effect of fibrin. The low amplitude of the ventricular complex is frequently associated with a normal amplitude of the P wave in the limb leads because of the absent effusion over the posterior surface of the atria, which is in part devoid of pericardial duplication. The variations in amplitude of the ventricular complex may be similar to the "electrical alternans" produced by an alternating configuration of the ventricular action potential or by alternating changes in intraventricular conduction. The alternans in pericarditis is due to changes in cardiac position resulting from the rotational pendular motion of the heart. Total electrical alternans involving P waves and QRS complexes, with or without ST alternans, is almost diagnostic of cardiac tamponade. The presence of ST segment alternans alone, however, may be observed in patients with evolving myocardial infarction. Electrical alternans involving only the QRS complex may be seen in severe left ventricular failure and also during or immediately after supraventricular tachycardia involving the atrioventricular bypass tract.

Injury of the superficial myocardium by the pressure of fluid or fibrin produces a "current of injury" manifested by deviation of the ST segment from the baseline and sometimes depression of the PR segment. The ST vector tends to be parallel to the lead II axis in horizontal hearts and parallel to the lead III axis in vertical hearts. The ST deviation in pericarditis is usually less pronounced than in the early stages of myocardial infarction. However, the elevation of the ST segment is recorded in more standard leads whereas the reciprocal depression of the ST segment is recorded in fewer standard leads than in myocardial infarction. The analysis of the ST vector may be helpful in the differentiation of acute pericarditis and acute myocardial infarction. In myocardial infarction, the terminal portion of the QRS complex is frequently obliterated and incorporated into the ST segment; in pericarditis the QRS complex remains unchanged, but the S wave may be pulled up by the elevated ST segment. However, such S-wave behavior can be observed in some patients with myocardial infarction and in persons without heart disease. In the acute stage of pericarditis, the amplitude and shape of the T wave is usually unchanged and the ST segment is concave; in acute myocardial infarction, the T wave is frequently obliterated and the elevated ST segment is convex.

Most patients with pericarditis have T-wave abnormalities due to superficial myocarditis (epicarditis). Characteristically, the T-wave vector is directed to the right and superiorly. In typical cases of pericarditis, the T wave becomes inverted in more standard leads but less deeply or less completely than in myocardial infarction. An incompletely inverted T wave, a diphasic T wave, or a notched T wave is a characteristic feature of the ECG pattern in pericarditis. In most cases, the QTc interval is normal, another differentiating feature from the myocardial infarction pattern. In the transitional period from acute to subacute pericarditis, different leads frequently reflect different stages of ST and T-wave abnormalities, whereas in the evolution of the infarction pattern all leads tend to reflect the same stage of abnormal repolarization. In pericarditis the elevation of the ST segment may disappear before the appearance of the T-wave abnormalities in a so-called intermediate stage during which the ECG becomes transiently normal.

The typical pattern with ST segment and T-wave changes occurs in all patients with traumatic, acute nonspecific, and purulent pericarditis, and in children. The changes appear less frequently in rheumatic, uremic, and neoplastic pericarditis and in pericarditis after myocardial infarction and cardiac surgery. The duration of ECG changes in pericarditis depends on the cause and extent of myocardial damage. They may be permanent in persistent adhesive or constrictive pericarditis, exhibiting low voltage and abnormally low, notched, or inverted T waves in many standard leads; P-wave abnormalities; and a QRS vector with an intermediate or a left axis.

ECG IN PULMONARY EMBOLISM AND ACUTE COR PULMONALE

The pattern of acute cor pulmonale described originally by McGinn and White consists of prominent S in lead I, Q in lead III, and negative T in lead III. This pattern, simulating an inferior wall myocardial infarction, occurs infrequently. More commonly, pulmonary embolism and other forms of acute cor pulmonale (e.g., acute bronchial asthma, large atelectasis) are associated with one or more of the following ECG changes: sinus tachycardia, tall P waves in leads II, III, and aV_F, transient shift of electrical axis, negative T wave in two or more right precordial leads, appearance of S waves in left precordial leads ("clockwise rotation"), complete and incomplete RBBB, and atrial arrhythmias. The other electrocardiographic changes that can be observed in pulmonary embolism are ST segment elevation in leads aV_R and V_1 to V_3; ST segment depression in leads I, II, and aV_L; left axis deviation; S_1, S_2, S_3 pattern; QS or QR in V_1 and transient low voltage.

T-WAVE ABNORMALITIES

The analysis of the T wave may be approached by relating the T-wave area to the QRS area. Wilson and co-workers pointed out that if all ventricular action potentials had the same magnitude and the same duration, the net area of the ventricular complex (QRS and T) should be zero.[56] However, in the normal heart, the mean QRS vector and the mean T vector form a narrow angle, and the area of the ventricular complex has a positive value. This indicates that in some parts of the ventricles the duration of activity must be greater than in others. They designated this difference of activity as the ventricular gradient (VG).

The main source of the VG is the nonhomogeneous duration of recovery, (*i.e.*, the difference in duration of action potentials in different parts of the ventricles).[56] The VG points from the parts of the ventricle with greater duration toward the parts with the lesser duration of activity.

The concept of VG allows one to define the primary and the secondary T-wave abnormalities according to their independence of or dependence on changes in the QRS complex.[57] A secondary T wave is a deflection that would follow a given QRS complex if ventricular recovery properties were uniform. Therefore, the area of primary T wave is equal to VG and the primary T wave describes variations of the VG as a function of time.[58]

Table 27.1 shows that primary abnormalities may be caused by uniform alteration in the shape or duration of all ventricular action potentials without a change in the sequence of repolarization, and nonuniform changes in shape or duration of the ventricular action potentials resulting in an altered sequence of repolarization. Abnormal T waves may also be caused by various combinations of primary and secondary mechanisms, as presented in Table 27.1.[57]

Certain types of primary T-wave abnormalities are labeled as functional or nonspecific. Neither of these two categories can be precisely defined. "Functional" T-wave abnormalities are usually aggravated by hyperventilation and corrected by reassurance and potassium administration.[57] "Functional" abnormalities reportedly occur more frequently in blacks and in young persons with anxiety or psychiatric disorders. Criteria for separating "functional" from "organic" T-wave abnormalities, however, should be based more on the results of clinical evaluation than on any particular ECG characteristics. The term *nonspecific* implies an abnormality of unknown cause. This term is popular among electrocardiographers but is usually unsatisfactory to the physician who receives the report. The use of the term *nonspecific abnormalities* should decline with increasing recognition of various specific causes of T-wave abnormalities.

The term *rapidly reversible primary T-wave abnormality* has been introduced to characterize a category of primary T-wave abnormality that disappears spontaneously with changes in posture or heart rate or within minutes after administration of certain drugs. Rapidly reversible T-wave abnormalities are not synonymous with "labile" T-wave abnormalities, which represent only cases of spontaneous variability. The category of rapidly reversible primary T-wave abnormalities includes most cases with functional and nonspecific T-wave abnormalities, but does not exclude T-wave abnormalities in patients with documented heart disease or with abnormalities caused by known extracardiac factors.

Primary T-wave abnormalities due to asynchronous repolarization may be associated with a prolonged or normal QTc interval. The QTc lengthening is usually attributed to some regional increase in the action potential duration. Primary T-wave abnormalities due to nonhomogeneous repolarization are frequently associated with an increased duration of the aT-eT interval. This suggests that the regional alterations of action potential duration may be due to differences in the duration of phase 3. The morphology of the abnormal T wave is usually the same in patients with and without heart disease. This similarity may lead to an erroneous diagnosis of heart disease and unnecessary diagnostic procedures in patients with benign repolarization abnormalities.

Primary T-wave abnormalities associated with myocardial infarction and pericarditis have been described in the appropriate sections. Similar T-wave abnormalities occur in patients with myocarditis or various cardiomyopathies and occasionally in association with mitral valve prolapse. The most pronounced transient and apparently functional T-wave abnormalities are due to neurogenic disorders, in particular the intracranial, usually subarachnoid, hemorrhage. This pattern is probably due to transient hypothalamic injury and has been observed after cryohypophysectomy.[57] Similar T-wave abnormalities occur occasionally in patients with adrenal or pituitary insufficiency and sometimes after truncal vagotomy.

Transient T-wave abnormalities due to extracardiac factors most frequently represent a non–steady state of repolarization accompanying rapid changes in heart rate or sympathetic tone. These changes include T-wave abnormalities associated with hyperventilation, upright position, and ingestion of large meals, as well as changes after extrasystoles and after tachycardia. Also, transient T-wave abnormalities occur during contrast injection into coronary arteries. Transient abnormalities sometimes persist for a variable period after the disappearance of LBBB and ventricular preexcitation.

Ventricular pacing frequently produces T-wave inversion in the nonpaced sinus beats. These T-wave changes occur without changes in the QRS duration. The T-wave abnormalities increase with increased duration of pacing and the amount of energy used for pacing. The site of stimulation determines the vector of the T wave. After pacing the endocardial surface of the right ventricle, abnormal T waves appear predominantly in the leads II, III, and V_3 to V_5, but after pacing the right ventricular outflow tract, the T-wave inversions occur mainly in leads V_1 and V_2.[59] The duration of the T-wave abnormalities after pacing depends on the duration of pacing. In some cases T-wave abnormalities persisted for 1 or 2 years after the termination of pacing. T-wave changes did not appear after atrial pacing or after ventricular pacing during the ventricular refractory period.[59] Thus, the T-wave abnormalities were related to the presence of abnormal depolarization in the stimulated area. It may be assumed that T-wave abnormalities are produced by lengthening of repolarization in the vicinity of the pacing electrode, but the mechanism of such lengthening is unknown. Prolonged pacing frequently produces giant T-wave inversions (1 mV or more). Giant T-wave inversions, however, can occur in other conditions: nontransmural myocardial infarction, intermittent LBBB, following Stokes-Adams attacks, intracranial lesions, markedly prolonged QT interval, and apical hypertrophic cardiomyopathy. The mechanism for the giant T-wave inversions in these conditions remains unclear.

ABNORMAL U WAVE

The amplitude of the U wave increases with increasing duration of the RR interval. The most common cause of a tall U wave in the absence of heart disease or other ECG abnormalities is bradycardia. Increased U-wave amplitude is associated also with positive inotropic interventions (*i.e.*, digitalis, isoproterenol, and hypercalcemia). Factors causing prolonged terminal repolarization at the cellular level (*i.e.*, hypokalemia, quinidinelike drugs, or thioridazine) also increase U-wave amplitude, frequently owing to fusion of T and U wave.

A negative U wave is nearly always associated with organic heart

TABLE 27.1 CLASSIFICATION OF T-WAVE ABNORMALITIES

Sequence of Depolarization	Shape and Duration of Action Potential	Sequence of Repolarization	Type of Abnormality
Abnormal	Normal	Abnormal	Secondary
Normal	Uniformly abnormal	Normal	Primary
Normal	Nonuniformly abnormal	Abnormal	Primary

disease. The three most common causes of U-wave inversion are LVH due to hypertension, hypertrophy and dilation of the left ventricle due to aortic or mitral regurgitation, and myocardial ischemia and myocardial infarction.[12]

ABNORMAL QTc DURATION

QTc may be shortened by acute ischemia, hypercalcemia, and digitalis, but the shortening is seldom greater than 20%. The QTc is lengthened by a variety of factors that prolong conduction (QRS complex) or repolarization (ST segment or T wave). The factors that cause most frequently marked (>125%) and moderate (115%–125%) QTc lengthening are listed in Tables 27.2 and 27.3.[60] Marked QTc lengthening due to increased T-wave duration is sometimes associated with increased T-wave amplitude, occasionally referred to as "giant T waves."

ELECTROLYTES AND THE ECG

High potassium (K) concentration shortens the duration of the cardiac action potential and depolarizes the membrane.[61] The earliest ECG manifestation of hyperkalemia is peaking of the T wave, which occurs when plasma K concentration (K_P) exceeds about 5.5 mEq/liter. Widening of the QRS complex is usually recognizable when K_P exceeds about 6.5 mEq/liter. The QRS lengthening is usually uniform, and the wide complex resembles a normal complex recorded at a rapid paper speed. As the K_p increases, the QRS duration increases progressively, and the widening of QRS complex correlates roughly with the severity of hyperkalemia. Occasionally, the wide QRS complex resembles the pattern of complete LBBB or LAFB.

Since atrial muscle is more sensitive to the depolarizing effect of hyperkalemia than ventricular muscle, intra-atrial conduction disturbances usually precede the intraventricular disturbances. The P wave becomes low and wide when K_p exceeds about 7.0 mEq/liter. When K_p exceeds about 8.8 mEq/liter, the P wave is usually not recognizable and the ECG pattern may be mistaken for atrial fibrillation. The pattern of advanced hyperkalemia resembles that of a dying heart. U waves in patients with hyperkalemia are either low or absent, and the PR interval is frequently prolonged. Cardiac standstill or ventricular fibrillation occurs when K_p exceeds about 10 mEq to 12 mEq/liter.

A progressive decrease in K_p results in progressive depression of the ST segment, progressive decrease in the T-wave amplitude, and progressive increase in the U-wave amplitude in the standard limb and precordial leads. As long as T and U are separated by a notch, the QT interval is unchanged; in more advanced hypokalemia the T and U waves are fused, and the QT interval cannot be accurately measured. Since the U amplitude is usually lowest in lead aV_L, this lead can be used frequently to determine the QT interval. The highest U-wave amplitude is usually in leads V_3 or V_4. The QRS complex is usually widened, but seldom by more than 0.02 second. A typical ECG pattern of hypokalemia with the depressed ST segment and U-wave amplitude exceeding T-wave amplitude in the same lead is present in about 80% of patients with K_P of less than 2.7 mEq/liter. Typically, ST-, T-, and U-wave abnormalities produced by hypokalemia can be seen more clearly at slow or normal than at fast heart rates. In the presence of tachycardia, U-wave amplitude is generally low and the U wave merges with the terminal portion of the T wave and with the P wave. In these cases, the P wave, which is superimposed on the U wave, becomes tilted. Tilting of the P wave may be the only clue to the ECG diagnosis of hypokalemia in patients with tachycardia. Hypokalemia promotes ectopic activity and contributes to lengthening of the PR interval.

Since ST and T changes caused by digitalis are similar to those produced by hypokalemia, and since quinidine-like drugs tend to increase the U-wave amplitude, the combination of digitalis and quinidine-like drugs results in a pattern that may be indistinguishable from that of hypokalemia. In the absence of hypokalemia, bradycardia may cause an increased U-wave amplitude, but, unlike hypokalemia, bradycardia is usually associated with an increased T-wave amplitude.

The duration of ventricular action potential is prolonged by hypocalcemia and shortened by hypercalcemia. As a result, low calcium concentration increases the duration of the ST segment and the QT interval, and high calcium concentration has an opposite effect. Severe hypercalcemia may also cause lengthening of the PR and QRS intervals and sometimes a second or third degree atrioventricular block.

EFFECT OF DRUGS

Many drugs produce ECG changes owing to their direct effects on the transmembrane action potential.[62] Cardiac glycosides accelerate the initial course of repolarization and shorten the ventricular action potential. This results in a typical pattern with a low or negative T wave, depressed ST segment, and shortened QTc interval. The abnormalities of ventricular repolarization produced by digitalis are frequently more pronounced at rapid than at slow rates. Consequently, during exercise-induced tachycardia ST segment abnormalities produced by digitalis may be indistinguishable from the pattern due to myocardial ischemia. Both therapeutic and toxic doses of glycosides prolong atrioventricular conduction.

Quinidine, disopyramide, procainamide, and several experimental antiarrhythmic drugs with similar action slow the velocity of ventricular depolarization and prolong the duration of ventricular action potential, causing widening of the QRS complex and lengthening of QTc interval. Therapeutic concentration of lidocaine, mexiletine, tocainide, and phenytoin cause no detectable effects on the ECG at physiologic heart rates. Phenothiazines, in particular thioridazine, cause lowering and notching of T wave and sometimes QTc lengthening. Similar changes may be produced by tricyclic antidepressant drugs, which also slow

TABLE 27.2 CAUSES OF MARKED QTc LENGTHENING* (>125%)
Congenital
Neurogenic, including organophosphorus
Severe hypothermia
Severe hypocalcemia
Fad diets
Contrast injections into coronary artery
Antiarrhythmic drugs (seldom)
Severe bradycardia, atrioventricular block, myocardial ischemia, postresuscitation, unexplained† (occasionally)
* Excluding that secondary to QRS widening.
† Probably predominantly neurogenic.

TABLE 27.3 CAUSES OF MODERATE QTc PROLONGATION* (≤125%)
Post-ischemia—transmural and nontransmural myocardial infarction
Various cardiomyopathies and after cardiac surgery or trauma
Moderate hypocalcemia
Class I antiarrhythmic agents, tranquilizers
Hypothyroidism and pituitary insufficiency (occasional)
Neurogenic or unexplained (occasionally)
* Excluding that secondary to QRS widening.

intraventricular conduction and at high concentrations cause QRS widening.

β-Adrenergic and certain calcium channel blocking drugs prolong atrioventricular conduction. Adrenaline and isoproterenol increase the heart rate, tend to shorten the QTc, and increase the T-wave and the U-wave amplitude. The effect of atropine is indistinguishable from that of the nonspecific tachycardia effect.

ECG AND ENDOCRINE AND METABOLIC DISORDERS

Hyperthyroidism usually causes sinus tachycardia, lengthening of the PR interval, and increased incidence of atrial fibrillation. Hypothyroidism causes sinus bradycardia, low-voltage QRS complexes, and lowering, or inversion, of the T wave. Changes in hypoparathyroidism and hyperparathyroidism reflect the appropriate changes in plasma calcium concentration. T-wave abnormalities and prolonged QTc occur in patients with adrenal insufficiency and hypopituitarism, probably as a result of abnormal hypothalamic activity.

The metabolic disorders usually reflect the accompanying electrolyte abnormalities. In patients with diabetes mellitus, T-wave abnormalities may be present even in the absence of hypertension, angina pectoris, or myocardial infarction. In untreated diabetic acidosis, the ECG usually reflects hyperkalemia, and the pattern of hypokalemia may appear during and after treatment. Sometimes, the ECG shows changes that cannot be explained by electrolyte abnormalities (*e.g.*, deeply inverted T waves, long QTc, and ST segment deviations).[63]

CLINICAL CONDITIONS WITH CHARACTERISTIC ECG PATTERNS

Certain diseases and clinical conditions cause characteristic ECG patterns. Experienced electrocardiographers, who are familiar with these patterns, can make sometimes useful contributions to clinical diagnosis of such conditions. Characteristic disease-specific patterns are particularly common in pediatric patients with various cyanotic and noncyanotic congenital heart diseases. In patients with suspected rheumatic fever, the presence of first and second degree atrioventricular block with atrioventricular junctional escape rhythm suggests rheumatic carditis. In patients with suspected cardiomyopathy, the presence of deep Q waves suggests septal hypertrophy. The RBBB pattern with low voltage in the right precordial leads suggests Ebstein's anomaly. Low voltage in the presence of intraventricular conduction disturbances in patients with cardiomyopathy favors the diagnosis of restrictive variety (*e.g.*, due to amyloidosis or hemochromatosis). A very high voltage is nearly pathognomonic of glycogen storage disease.

In patients with acid–base and electrolyte imbalance, the combination of hyperkalemia and hypocalcemia suggests uremia, the combination of hypokalemia with hypocalcemia suggests hypochloremic alkalosis, and the combination of hypokalemia and hypercalcemia is a common finding in patients with multiple myeloma.

ABNORMAL ECG PATTERNS IN THE ABSENCE OF HEART DISEASE

Abnormal ECG patterns occur frequently in the absence of heart disease.[64] Some of these are caused by errors in recording, such as faulty recorder (usually poor frequency response), faulty electrode placement, failure to turn the switch to proper position, excess of paste on the chest, muscle tremor, 60-cycle interference, movement of electrode (*e.g.*, on radial artery or on the apex), incorrect standardization, and incorrect mounting. However, most abnormal patterns are due to peculiarities of body build or to various physiological and pharmacologic influences.[65] The most common errors of interpretation include P-wave abnormalities that are not due to atrial enlargement, Q-wave abnormalities that are not due to myocardial infarction, and abnormal voltage that is not due to ventricular hypertrophy. Other abnormal findings in the absence of heart disease may include minor intraventricular conduction disturbances, slight lengthening of the PR interval, ventricular preexcitation, elevation or depression of the ST segment, and T-wave abnormalities that represent the effects of drugs, most frequently digitalis, electrolyte abnormalities, and various primary T-wave changes caused by nonuniform repolarization. The latter cases are sometimes attributed to neurogenic factors, or to non-steady state of ventricular repolarization, but most often remain unexplained.

REFERENCES

1. Schaefer H, Haas HG: Electrocardiography. In Hamilton WF, Dow P (eds): Handbook of Physiology, Section II, pp 323–414. Washington, DC, American Physiological Society, 1962
2. Scher AM, Spach MS: Cardiac depolarization and repolarization and the electrocardiogram. In Hamilton WF, Dow P (eds): Handbook of Physiology, Section II, p 357. Washington, DC, American Physiological Society, 1962
3. Lepeschkin E: Modern Electrocardiography: The P-Q-R-S-T-U Complex. Baltimore, Williams & Wilkins, 1951
4. Hoffman BF, Cranefield PF: The Electrophysiology of the Heart, p 824. New York, McGraw-Hill, 1971
5. Durrer D, van Dam RTh, Freud GE et al: Total excitation of the isolated human heart. Circulation 41:899, 1970
6. Wyndham CR, Meeran MK, Smith T et al: Epicardial activation of the intact human heart without conduction defect. Circulation 59:161, 1979
7. Taccardi B: Distribution of heart potentials on the thoracic surface of normal human subjects. Circ Res 12:341, 1963
8. Holland RP, Brooks H: TQ-ST segment mapping: Critical review and analysis of current concepts. Am J Cardiol 40:110, 1977
9. Wilson FN, Johnston FD, Macleod AG et al: Electrocardiograms that represent the potential variations of a single electrode. Am Heart J 9:447, 1934
10. Goldberger E: A simple, indifferent, electrocardiographic electrode of zero potential and a technique of obtaining augmented unipolar extremity leads. Am Heart J 23:483, 1942
11. Lepeschkin E, Surawicz B: The duration of the Q-U interval and its components in electrocardiograms of normal persons. Am Heart J 46:9, 1953
12. Kishida H, Cole JS, Surawicz B: Negative U wave: A highly specific but poorly understood sign of heart disease. Am J Cardiol 49:2030, 1982
13. Strong WB, Downs TD, Liebman J et al: The normal adolescent electrocardiogram. Am Heart J 83:115, 1972
14. Gorman PA, Calatayud JB, Abraham S et al: Effects of age and heart disease on the QRS axis during the seventh through the tenth decades. Am Heart J 67:39, 1964
15. Nemati M, Doyle JT, McCaughan D et al: The orthogonal electrocardiogram in normal women: Implications of sex differences in diagnostic electrocardiography. Am Heart J 95:12, 1978
16. Balady GJ, Cadigan JB, Ryan TJ: Electrocardiogram of the athlete: An analysis of 289 professional football players. Am J Cardiol 53:1339, 1984
17. Chou TC, Helm RA: Clinical Vectorcardiography. New York, Grune & Stratton, 1967
18. Green LS, Lux RL, Haws CW et al: Effect of age, sex and body habitus on QRS and ST-T potential maps of 1100 normal subjects. Circulation 71:244, 1985
19. Kilty SE, Lepeschkin E: Effect of body build on the QRS voltage of the electrocardiogram in normal men: Its significance in the diagnosis of left ventricular hypertrophy. Circulation 31:77, 1965
20. Larkin H, Hunyor SN: Precordial voltage variation in the normal electrocardiogram. J Electrocardiol 13:347, 1980
21. LaMonte CS, Frieman AH: The electrocardiogram after mastectomy. Circulation 32:746, 1965
22. Romhilt DW, Estes EH Jr: A point-score system for the ECG diagnosis of left ventricular hypertrophy. Am Heart J 75:752, 1968
23. Toshima H, Koga Y, Kimura N: Correlations between electrocardiographic, vectorcardiographic, and echocardiographic findings in patients with left ventricular overload. Am Heart J 94:547, 1977
24. Kyriacopoulos JD, Conrad LL, Cuddy TE et al: Activation of the free wall of the right ventricle in experimental right ventricular hypertrophy with and without right bundle branch block. Am Heart J 67:81, 1964
25. Durrer D: Electrical aspects of human cardiac activity: A clinical-physiological approach to excitation and stimulation. Cardiovasc Res 2:1, 1968
26. Mazzoleni A, Wolff R, Wolff L et al: Correlation between component cardiac weights and electrocardiographic patterns in 185 cases. Circulation 30:808, 1964
27. Silver HM, Calatayud JB: Evaluation of QRS criteria in patients with chronic obstructive pulmonary disease. Chest 59:153, 1971
28. Kerr A, Adicoff A, Klingeman JD et al: Computer analysis of the orthogonal electrocardiogram in pulmonary emphysema. Am J Cardiol 25:34, 1970
29. Loperfido F, Digaetano A, Santarelli P et al: The evaluation of left and right

ventricular hypertrophy in combined ventricular overload by electrocardiography: Relationship with the echocardiographic data. J Electrocardiol 15:327, 1982
30. Rosen KM, Rahimtoola SH, Sinno MZ et al: Bundle branch and ventricular activation in man: A study using catheter recordings of left and right bundle branch potentials. Circulation 43:193, 1971
31. Horowitz LN, Simson MB, Spear JF et al: The mechanisms of apparent right bundle branch block after transatrial repair of tetralogy of Fallot. Circulation 59:1241, 1979
32. Schneider JF, Thomas HE, Kreger BE et al: Newly acquired right bundle branch block. Ann Intern Med 92:37, 1980
33. Wyndham CRC, Smith T, Meeran K et al: Epicardial activation in patients with left bundle branch block. Circulation 61:696, 1980
34. Vassallo JA, Cassidy DM, Marchlinski FE et al: Endocardial activation of left bundle branch block. Circulation 69:914, 1984
35. Dhingra RC, Amat-y-Leon F, Wyndham C et al: Significance of left axis deviation in patients with chronic left bundle branch block. Am J Cardiol 42:551, 1978
36. Lichstein E, Mahapatra R, Gupta PK et al: Significance of complete left bundle branch block with left axis deviation. Am J Cardiol 44:239, 1979
37. Rosenbaum MB, Elizari MV, Lazzari JO: The Hemiblocks. Oldsmar, Fla., Tampa Tracings, 1970
38. Wyndham CR, Meeran MK, Smith T et al: Epicardial activation in human left anterior fascicular block. Am J Cardiol 44:638, 1979
39. Surawicz B, Saito S: Exercise testing for detection of myocardial ischemia in patients with abnormal electrocardiograms at rest. Am J Cardiol 41:943, 1978
40. Prystowsky EN, Miles WM, Heger JJ et al: Preexcitation syndromes: Mechanism and management. Med Clin North Am 68:831, 1984
41. Horan LG, Flowers NC, Johnson JC: Significance of the diagnostic Q wave of myocardial infarction. Circulation 43:428, 1971
42. Pearce ML, Kossowsky W, Levine R: Isolated abnormalities in high precordial leads, an infrequent sign of myocardial infarction. Am Heart J 72:442, 1966
43. Bough EW, Boden WE, Korr KS et al: Left ventricular asynergy in electrocardiographic "posterior" myocardial infarction. J Am Coll Cardiol 4:209, 1984
44. Surawicz B, Van Horne RG, Urbach JR et al: Q-S and Q-R pattern in leads V3 and V4 in absence of myocardial infarction: Electrocardiographic and vectorcardiographic study. Circulation 12:391, 1955
45. Blanke H, Cohen M, Schlueter GU et al: Electrocardiographic and coronary arteriographic correlations during acute myocardial infarction. Am J Cardiol 54:249, 1984
46. Braat SH, Brugada P, den Dulk K et al: Value of lead V_4R for recognition of the infarct coronary artery in acute inferior myocardial infarction. Am J Cardiol 53:1538, 1984
47. Wagner GS, Freye CJ, Palmeri ST et al: Evaluation of a QRS scoring system for estimating myocardial infarct size: I. Specificity and observer agreement. Circulation 65:342, 1982
48. Ideker RE, Wagner GS, Ruth WK et al: Evaluation of a QRS scoring system for estimating myocardial infarct size: II. Correlation with quantitative anatomic findings for anterior infarcts. Am J Cardiol 49:1604, 1982
49. Roark SF, Ideker RE, Wagner GS et al: Evaluation of a QRS scoring system for estimating myocardial infarct size: III. Correlation with quantitative anatomic findings for inferior infarcts. Am J Cardiol 51:382, 1983
50. Ward RM, White RD, Ideker RE et al: Evaluation of a QRS scoring system for estimating myocardial infarct size: IV. Correlation with quantitative anatomic findings for posterolateral infarcts. Am J Cardiol 53:706, 1984
51. Palmeri ST, Harrison DG, Cobb FR et al: A QRS scoring system for assessing left ventricular function after myocardial infarction. N Engl J Med 306:4, 1982
52. Rothfeld B, Fleg JL, Gottlieb SH: Insensitivity of the electrocardiogram in apical myocardial infarction. Am J Cardiol 53:715, 1984
53. Durrer D, VanLier AAW, Buller JL: Epicardial and intramural excitation in chronic myocardial infarction. Am Heart J 68:765, 1964
54. Grant RP: Peri-infarction block. Prog Cardiovasc Dis 2:237, 1959–1960
55. Surawicz B, Lasseter KC: Electrocardiogram in pericarditis. Am J Cardiol 26:471, 1970
56. Wilson FN, Rosenbaum FF, Johnston FD: Interpretation of the ventricular complex of the electrocardiogram. Adv Intern Med 2:1, 1947
57. Surawicz B: The pathogenesis and clinical significance of primary T wave abnormalities. In Schlant RC, Hurst JW (eds): Advances in Electrocardiography, p 377. New York, Grune & Stratton, 1972
58. Abildskov JA, Burgess MJ, Millar K et al: The primary T wave, a new electrocardiographic waveform. Am Heart J 81:242, 1971
59. Chatterjee K, Harris A, Davies G et al: Electrocardiographic changes subsequent to artificial ventricular depolarization. Br Heart J 31:770, 1969
60. Surawicz B, Knoebel SB: Long QT: Good, bad or indifferent? J Am Coll Cardiol 4:398, 1984
61. Surawicz B: Relationship between electrocardiogram and electrolytes. Am Heart J 73:814, 1967
62. Surawicz B, Lasseter KC: Effect of drugs on the electrocardiogram. Prog Cardiovasc Dis 13:26, 1970
63. Surawicz B, Mangiardi LM: Electrocardiogram in endocrine and metabolic disorders. Cardiovasc Clinics 8:243, 1977
64. Fisch C: The clinical electrocardiogram: A classic. Circulation 62:III-1(Suppl), 1980
65. Surawicz B: Assessing abnormal electrocardiogram in the absence of heart disease. Cardiovasc Med 2:629, 1977

Echocardiography and Doppler in Clinical Cardiology

Nelson B. Schiller • Ronald Himelman

Echocardiography is a standard diagnostic method in the clinical evaluation of cardiac disorders. Although technically demanding, the noninvasive nature of the examination and its diagnostic accuracy have made it an indispensable diagnostic tool in clinical cardiology.

The central role of echocardiography in the evaluation of heart disease makes knowledge of its applications and limitations mandatory for physicians dealing with heart disease. This chapter will survey the established applications of echocardiography while stressing its limitations.

Cardiac imaging with echocardiography generates images with both functional and anatomical information. Doppler flow detection augments echocardiographic imaging by providing information about the velocity and direction of moving red blood cells within the cardiac chambers. The complexity and wide variety of heart disease commonly encountered make echocardiography applicable to a broad array of situations.

PHYSICAL PRINCIPLES AND INSTRUMENTATION IN ECHOCARDIOGRAPHY

Echocardiography, or cardiac ultrasound, employs high-frequency sonic radiation to form images of cardiac structures or sample intravascular blood flow. High-frequency sound, well above the audible range, has the characteristic of penetrating non–air-containing structures and reflecting from interfaces formed by structures that differ from one another in acoustic impedance (tissue density × speed of sound propagation). These sonic reflections can be detected at the skin surface and can be used to construct an image (25–30 frames/second) of the interrogated object much as a petroleum engineer uses sound to construct an image of subterranean strata or a navigator uses a depth finder to locate the sea bed.

Myocardium and valve tissue have different acoustic impedances, so it is possible to image these contiguous tissues by their different reflectances. Since most of these studies are conducted without any form of contrast agent and are entirely safe and noninvasive, ultrasound provides a unique method of organ imaging.

There are three types of echocardiographic modalities in use today. These are M-mode echocardiography, two-dimensional echocardiography, and Doppler echocardiography. The more expensive instruments being manufactured at the time of this writing offer all three of these modalities combined into one package.

M-mode echocardiography was the first form of cardiac ultrasound to find wide application in cardiac diagnosis (Figs. 28.1 and 28.2).[1-3] In this technique, as in all the others, an ultrasound-generating and ultrasound-receiving transducer is placed on the anterior chest wall or other imaging windows that provide an airless pathway to the heart. Through this device a single beam of ultrasound is directed into the heart. All the structures lying along that single beam send back signals to the stationary transducer. These returning signals are recorded onto a moving strip of paper in a location determined by the distance of the reflecting object from the transducer (*i.e.*, by the transit time of ultrasound to and from the target). In addition to characteristic locations, cardiac structures have unique motion patterns that identify them; alterations in these patterns identify pathology and its severity.

A particular advantage of the M-mode method is that it allows interrogation of moving cardiac structures at sampling rates approaching 1000/sec. This rapid sampling provides images of striking time and structural resolution. Its major disadvantage is that the images are one-dimensional and, if obtained blindly, may produce unrepresentative samples of structures. An example of insufficient sampling is found when M-modes of the left ventricle are produced. Geometrically, the normal left ventricle (LV) is a truncated ellipse and the dilated LV is a sphere. Since an M-mode study only provides minor axis dimensions and no information about the LV long axis, misinformation about LV cavity volume is an almost obligatory feature of this examination.[4] Currently, isolated or stand-alone M-mode instruments are becoming rare and the standard echocardiographic examination is performed with an instrument capable of simultaneously generating two-dimensional and M-mode images. M-mode information is more reliable when obtained directly from these two-dimensional images.

Two-dimensional echocardiography is the primary ultrasound imaging method for the heart (see Fig. 28.1). A two-dimensional image should be thought of as a real-time tomograph created by rapidly sweeping an ultrasound beam back and forth across cardiac structures. Depending on the depth of the structures being imaged this modality is capable of scanning a 60-degree to 90-degree scan plane at 25 to 60 frames per second. The resolution of the image depends on how deeply into the image information is situated (the deeper, the poorer the resolution) and on the transducer carrier frequency. Higher frequencies have finer resolution but penetrate more poorly. In children, where depths are shallow and anatomical windows large, highly resolved images are usually produced because these conditions are ideal for the use of high frequencies. As electronics improve, manufacturers are offering instruments with transducers capable of imaging with frequencies of 5 MHz to 10 MHz (1 MHz = 1,000,000 cycles/sec). Up until a few years ago, the standard imaging frequency was 2.25 MHz, which was satisfactory for adults but poor for children. Now most adults can be imaged with 3.5-MHz instruments, with higher frequencies used for pediatric applications. The recent introduction of annular array technology may enable the use of frequencies as high as 5 MHz or 7 MHz in adults.[5]

There are two major types of two-dimensional echocardiographic imaging systems, mechanically driven large crystals (see Fig. 28.1) and electronically driven phased crystal arrays (32 to 64) (see Fig. 28.1).[6] The mechanical systems have enjoyed slightly better resolution but have the disadvantage of requiring bulky, motor-containing transducers, which wear out with extended use. Improvements in electronics are making the electronic phased array the predominant form of instrument. This ascendancy is accelerating with the rapid spread of Doppler ultrasound techniques. It appears to be easier for manufacturers to incorporate Doppler technology into two-dimensional instruments if the instrument is a microprocessor-driven phased array than if it is a mechanical system. In a parallel development, prototypes of annular arrays are beginning to appear that combine features of both mechanical and phased array technology.[7] It remains to be seen if the improved image quality that these devices offer will serve to divert the strong trend toward phased array systems.

Doppler echocardiography has enjoyed explosive development in the last five years. Essentially, this technique allows the indirect measurement of intracardiac flow velocities by detecting changes in the carrier frequency of reflected ultrasound returning to the transducer. When ultrasound strikes moving red cells in the heart it is not only reflected back to the transducer but, depending on the velocity of the red cells, its frequency is proportionately altered (Fig. 28.3).[8]

This velocity *difference* is oscilloscopically displayed in real time as a function of time and simultaneously converted into an audible signal. The direction of the flow relative to the detecting transducer is also indicated by displaying the spectral shift as either above or below an arbitrary baseline (Fig. 28.4). Progress in microprocessors has made the real-time generation of spectral information a major factor in the rapid proliferation of the Doppler technique. In addition to the velocity and duration of flow, the real-time spectral display provides information about the intensity of flow. The Doppler equation governing these relationships is

$$V = \frac{C}{2F_0 \times \cos\theta} Fd$$

where C = velocity of sound, F_0 = carrier frequency, θ = angle of interrogation, V = velocity, and Fd = frequency shift (Fig. 28.5).

There are two Doppler modalities required for diagnostic examinations, pulsed wave and continuous wave; these are used interactively as each has unique qualities. Pulsed-wave Doppler is able to examine a very limited region of flow and to localize flow disturbances. For example, placement of the Doppler sample volume on the atrial surface of

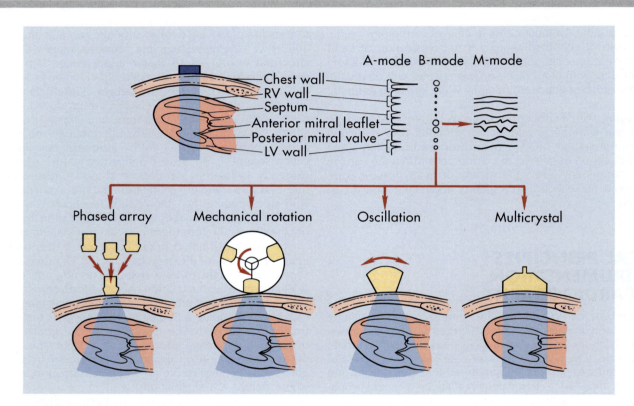

FIGURE 28.1 Instrumentation of echocardiography: M-mode and two-dimensional imaging methods. (*Top*) Long axis of the left ventricle is diagrammed showing the M-mode transducer applied to the chest wall with the ultrasound beam directed posteriorly. The stages in the production of an M-mode image are displayed to the right of the image. Each intracardiac surface or interface formed by a blood–muscle, blood–valve, or muscle–pericardium boundary gives rise to reflections that are detected by the transducer during its listening mode. The excitation of the transducer gives rise to small electrical currents that are displayed in the order they are received. If the representation of these currents is a series of spikes whose height is proportional to the strength of the signal, the display is termed an A-mode. If these spikes are modulated into dots whose size and brightness are proportional to signal strength, the display is called B-mode. Both B-mode and A-mode displays depict motion of structures in real time. However, in order to create a permanent record of the location, size, and motion of structures lying along the ultrasound beam, M-mode was developed. In M-mode, photosensitive paper is rolled or drawn across the B-mode display, creating a continuous record. (*Bottom*) Various methods of producing two-dimensional images are displayed. In these, a single beam of ultrasound is played back and forth through a sector enabling display of a cross-section of tissue in real time. In the phased array, an array of crystals with a relatively small diameter or foot print is excited. The excitation pattern allows the beam to be steered rapidly through the sector. The mechanically produced sector scans are produced by rotating three or four M-mode transducers past a window. This window is in contact with the skin surface. The motion required is supplied by a small electrical motor. In the oscillating type of mechanical two-dimensional instrument, a single M-mode type crystal is rocked back and forth to create a two-dimensional display. In the multicrystal linear array, a large line of single transducer elements is directed at a target. The result is an image of the same size as the array. The intercostal spaces are usually too large to permit the use of this type of technology for cardiac imaging. (Modified from a figure courtesy of Dr. Norman H. Silverman, Department of Pediatrics, University of California, San Francisco)

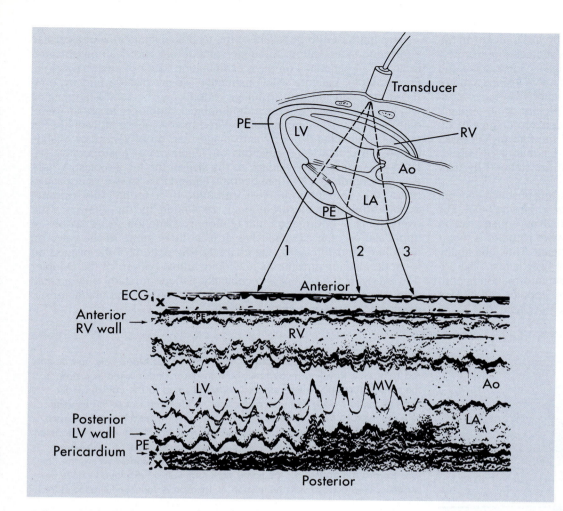

FIGURE 28.2 M-mode echocardiogram from a patient with a moderate pericardial effusion. (*Top*) Diagrammatic representation of the long axis of the heart. The transducer sits on the anterior chest wall in the precordial parasternal window and the beam is swept from apex to base. The appearance of the echogram at three beam positions on the diagram is designated by the arrows connecting the diagram to the echogram. (*Bottom*) The pericardial effusion (*PE*) is seen as an echo-free space posterior to the left ventricle. This space diminishes and finally disappears as the base of the heart is approached. (Ao, aorta; ECG, electrocardiogram; LA, left atrium; LV, left ventricle; MV, mitral valve; RV, right ventricle) (Modified from Sokolow M, McIlroy MB: Clinical Cardiology, 3rd ed. Los Altos, California, Lange Medical Publications, 1981)

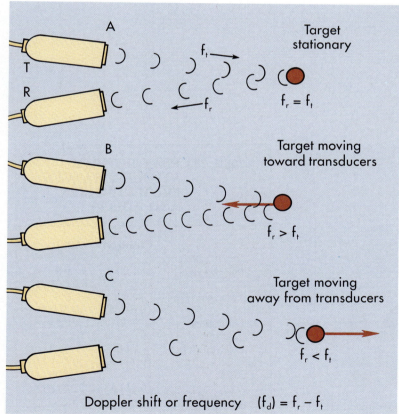

FIGURE 28.3 Pairs of transmitting and receiving transducers illustrate the Doppler effect as it occurs in relationship to targets stationary, moving toward, and moving away from the transducers. In **A**, the carrier frequency (f_t) from the transmitting transducer (T) strikes the target (e.g., a red cell) and is reflected back to the receiving transducer (R) at the reflected frequency (f_r), which is unaltered. In **B**, f_r is a higher frequency than the original transmitted frequency. An increase in frequency is typical of a target moving toward the transducer. In **C**, the carrier frequency, after being reflected from a target moving away from the transducer, is reduced. In all cases, the extent to which the carrier frequency is increased or reduced is proportional to the velocity of the target. (Modified from Feigenbaum H: Echocardiography, 4th ed. Philadelphia, Lea & Febiger, 1986)

the mitral valve can detect even trivial, clinically insignificant mitral insufficiency. Pulsed-wave Doppler has the disadvantage of accurately measuring only flow velocities in the normal range (<2 m/sec in adult patients). Rapidly moving flow, characteristic of valve lesions, cannot be measured by pulsed Doppler because rapid velocity induces aliasing. Aliasing is analogous to viewing a motion picture of an airplane propellor; as the propellor changes speed it appears to change its direction of spin because the slow frame rate of the film produces an aliased image. The relationships governing the limitations of pulsed-wave Doppler are called the *Nyquist limit* and are defined by flow theorems.[8]

Continuous-wave Doppler overcomes the aliasing problem and can be used to accurately measure high-velocity flow within the heart. For example, in critical aortic stenosis, velocities as high as 7 m/sec can be encountered. The disadvantage of continuous-wave Doppler is that it samples everything lying along the path of the beam. Thus, the ability of pulsed Doppler to precisely sample localized flow is lost. The advantage gained is that a great deal of quantitative information is contained in high-velocity jets and continuous-wave Doppler can extract that information. Normal flow velocities are given in Table 28.1.[8]

It is important to be aware of the technical limitations of a cardiac ultrasound examination. Although some information can be obtained in nearly all patients, complete examinations are not always possible. For example, patients with obstructive airway disease and hyperinflated lungs are difficult to image; often only the subcostal imaging window will allow the echocardiographic technologist to obtain useful data. A similar situation is encountered in very obese individuals. Fat conducts ultrasound poorly and images can be of very poor quality. Patients in critical care situations on ventilators or postoperative patients also present a challenge to the skill of the technologist. Whenever echocardiographic data become limited to a few views or projections, the data become less reliable. In a technically optimal echocardiogram, interpretation is facilitated by the characteristic overlapping of information that reinforces validation. For example, in mitral stenosis the examiner has at least three views of the valve on two-dimensional imaging, the characteristic pattern of the disease on M-mode imaging and the high-velocity inflow pattern of the Doppler flow study. If the patient is technically difficult to study only a small amount of this information might be available and the characteristic diagnostic certainty is compromised.

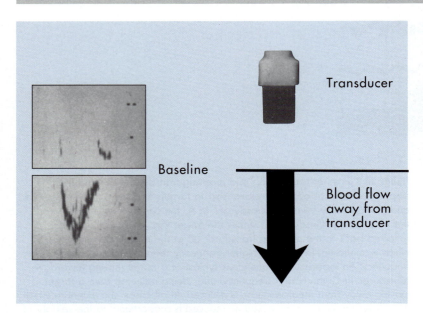

FIGURE 28.4 A typical Doppler signal from intracardiac blood flow. The moving red cells were traveling away from the transducer and resulted in a drop in the carrier frequency when reflected sound returned to the transducer. By convention, flow away from the transducer is displayed below the baseline and that toward the transducer above. Due to high-speed microprocessors this spectral information can be displayed in real time. Note that the Doppler signal portrays the entire period of flow, showing acceleration, peak flow, and deceleration. If the same event is viewed from a window where the flow runs toward the transducer the same waveform will be displayed above the baseline. (Reproduced with permission of Johnson & Johnson Ultrasound Inc.)

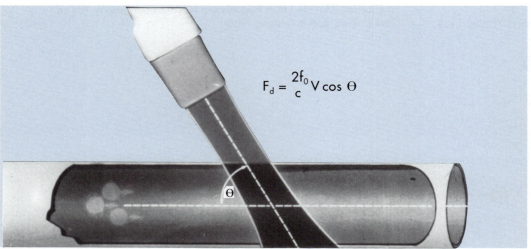

FIGURE 28.5 A diagrammatic illustration of a situation when the interrogating or insonocating beam lies at an angle to the flow of blood. Ideally, the Doppler beam should be placed parallel to blood flow. When the beam does not lie parallel it is possible to introduce a correction into the calculation of flow velocity by measuring the cosine of the angle of interrogation and introducing this value into the Doppler equation. The version of the equation in this illustration merely represents a rearrangement of the equation given in the text. (Reproduced with permission of Johnson & Johnson Ultrasound Inc.)

$$F_d = \frac{2f_0}{c} V \cos \theta$$

TABLE 28.1 PEAK DOPPLER VELOCITY RANGES FROM CHILDREN AND ADULTS

	Children	Adults
Mitral flow	1.00 (0.8–1.2)	0.9 (0.4–1.3)
Tricuspid flow	0.60 (0.5–0.8)	0.5 (0.3–0.7)
Pulmonary artery	0.90 (0.7–1.1)	0.75 (0.6–0.9)
Left ventricle	1.00 (0.7–1.2)	0.90 (0.7–1.1)
Aorta	1.5 (1.2–1.8)	1.35 (1.0–1.7)

(After Hatle L, Angelsen B: Doppler Ultrasound in Cardiology: Physical Principles and Clinical Application, 2nd ed. Philadelphia, Lea & Febiger, 1985)

ECHOCARDIOGRAPHIC EVALUATION OF THE CARDIAC CHAMBERS
EVALUATION OF THE LEFT VENTRICLE

Left ventricular (LV) evaluation is probably the single most important clinical application of echocardiography technique. Assuming that the technician performing the study and the interpreting physician have the requisite skills, a combined M-mode, two-dimensional Doppler evaluation of the LV can provide reliable information about a lengthy list of functional and anatomical parameters; principal among these is overall LV systolic function or global contractility. The concept of contractility is most commonly expressed by means of a derived parameter called *ejection fraction*. LV size or volume is another important parameter generated by an echocardiographic evaluation. Wall thickness and the motion of individual segments of the myocardium can also be reliably assessed. In fact, a reasonable perception of both diastolic and systolic behavior of the entire LV and of the behavior of local segments is usually obtained from a competently performed echocardiogram. LV masses, most commonly thrombi, are effectively identified by echocardiography and it is usually possible to differentiate thrombi from rarer neoplasms.

ASSESSMENT OF GLOBAL SYSTOLIC FUNCTION OF THE LEFT VENTRICLE

The accurate assessment of LV function requires images taken from several windows or planes. Typically, the LV is first viewed in the precordial long axis (Fig. 28.6) and short axis planes (Fig. 28.7). From these two-dimensional images, M-mode tracings are generated. Figures 28.8 and 28.9 show two-dimensional images on the left and M-

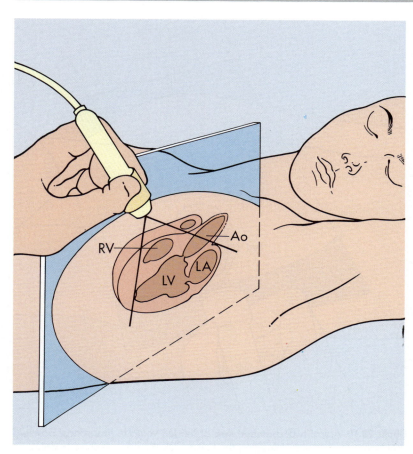

FIGURE 28.6 Long axis view of the heart. Directing the plane of the ultrasound beam from left hip to right shoulder, the heart is sectioned along its long axis. This is usually the first view obtained in a standard ultrasound cardiac examination. The left ventricular base is shown with the septum and posterior/inferior walls forming the perimeter of the chamber. (*Ao*, aorta; *LA*, left atrium; *LV*, left ventricle; *RV*, right ventricle)

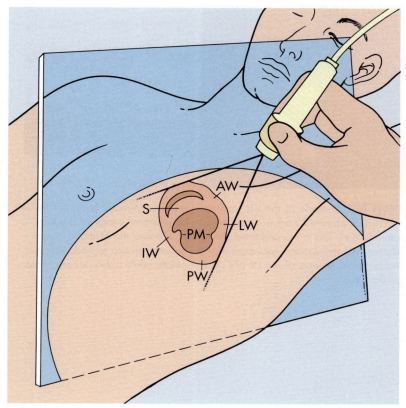

FIGURE 28.7 Short axis view of the heart. Transducer position and beam plane used for two-dimensional imaging of the heart in the short axis. In this view the plane of the cut runs through or just below the minor axis of the left ventricle. (*AW*, anteroseptal wall of the left ventricle; *IW*, inferior or diaphragmatic wall of the left ventricle; *PW*, posterior wall of the left ventricle; *S*, interventricular septum; *PM*, papillary muscles [posteromedial, right and anterolateral, left])

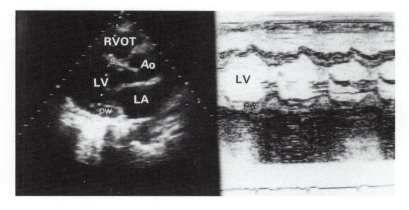

FIGURE 28.8 M-mode of the left ventricle. M-mode through the minor axis of the left ventricle (*right*) generated directly from the long axis two-dimensional view of the heart (*left*). The location of the line from which the M-mode is generated is indicated by the dotted white line running through the base of the left ventricle (*LV*) and into the posterior wall (*pw*). (*Ao*, aorta; *LA*, left atrium; *RVOT*, right ventricular outflow tract)

modes to the right. The line from which the M-mode is generated is superimposed on the two-dimensional image.[9,10] Visual integration imparted by the dynamic nature of the images contributes strongly to the information in the image and cannot be reproduced in these examples. From a technical aspect, it is essential to obtain as much of the epicardium and endocardium as possible. Failure to capture the actual boundaries of the convoluted endocardial surface is the most common source of error in LV evaluation.

All slices or tomographic planes are made so that the cavity size is maximized. In addition to precordial long and short axis views, the LV is also viewed from the apex in the two-chamber and four-chamber long axis planes and from the subcostal window. These planes are illustrated in Figures 28.10 to 28.14. Of these, M-modes, which are useful for LV function assessment, can only be derived from the subcostal plane.

The most useful M-mode indices of LV function are fractional shortening of the LV minor axis,[11] mitral septal separation,[12,13] and aortic root motion.[14–23]

Fractional shortening is simply the distance the left ventricle moves from its maximum end-diastolic dimension at the peak of the R wave to its minimum end-systolic dimension at the end of the T wave. In most situations this cavity reduction is 30% or more. Obviously the interpretation of this index and of many others depends not only on the integrity of the myocardium but on the prevailing loading conditions and inotropic environment. Figure 28.9 illustrates an M-mode tracing from an individual with a normal fractional shortening and Figure 28.15 from one with a cardiomyopathy.

A major potential source of error in the use of M-mode minor axis fractional shortening is that the sample from which this assessment of global LV function is made represents a small portion of the structure.[24]

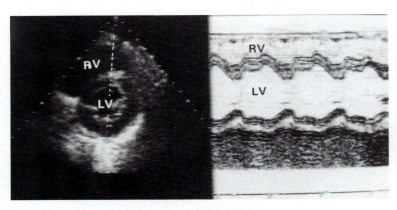

FIGURE 28.9 M-mode of the left ventricle. The same M-mode image of the left ventricle is obtained from a short axis two-dimensional image of the left ventricle (LV). This is the preferred method of directing the M-mode beam (dotted line) through the two-dimensional image to ensure reproducible M-mode measurements of the LV. (RV, right ventricle; other abbreviations same as Fig. 28.8)

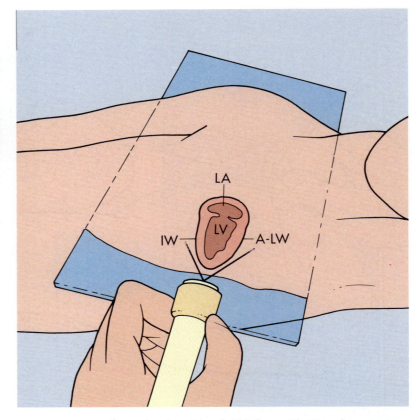

FIGURE 28.10 Apical two-chamber view of the left ventricle. Transducer position and beam plane used in imaging the heart from the apex impulse location. This view is the two-dimensional two-chamber apical view. It is similar to a right anterior oblique angiogram of the left ventricle in that the inferior wall (IW) and anterolateral walls (A-LW) are border forming.

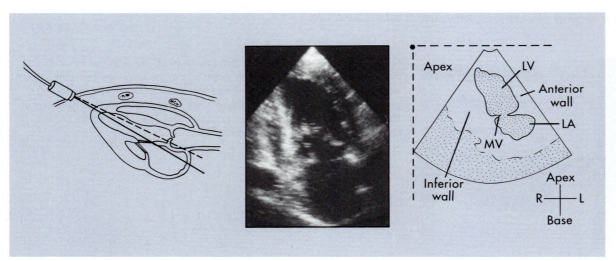

FIGURE 28.11 Apical two-chamber view of the left ventricle (LV). Diagrammatic illustration of the transducer location and beam direction used in forming the two-chamber view (left). In the center of the figure is an actual diastolic image in a patient with mild LVH and, to the right, a diagram of this image. The structure directly beneath the inferior wall is the diaphragm and beneath that the liver. (LA, left atrium; MV, mitral valve)

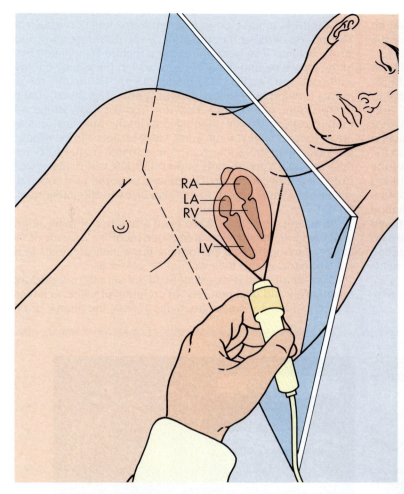

FIGURE 28.12 Apical four-chamber view. Transducer position and beam plane used to image the heart in the apical four-chamber view. The transducer is on the apex impulse location and is directed toward the right shoulder.

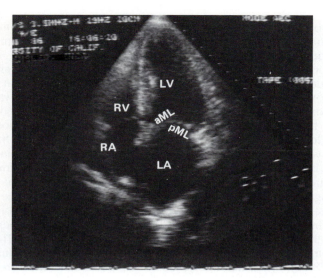

FIGURE 28.13 Apical four-chamber view. Stop-frame image of apical four-chamber view. Note that the display shows the apex at the top of the screen with the left ventricle to the viewer's right. Most laboratories choose to display the four-chamber view in this way although some reverse the ventricles and others have the apex pointing downward. (*aML*, anterior mitral leaflet; *LA*, left atrium; *LV*, left ventricle; *pML*, posterior mitral valve leaflet; *RA*, right atrium; *RV*, right ventricle)

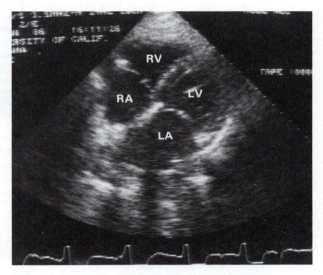

FIGURE 28.14 Subcostal four-chamber view. With the transducer in the subcostal position, a four-chamber view can be obtained. In this view, the lateral border of the LV is delimited by the mid-lateral wall as opposed to the inferolateral wall on the apical four-chamber view. The apex of the left ventricle is rarely seen in this view and the right ventricle is usually smaller than the left.

FIGURE 28.15 Cardiomyopathy. Spherical dilation and diffusely poor inward wall motion are reflected in both the two-dimensional and M-mode appearance. Compare this figure with the normal ventricle in Figure 28.9.

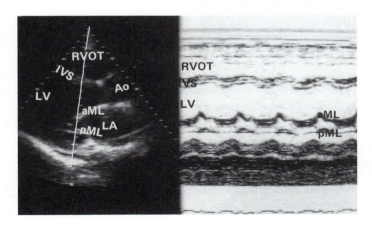

In coronary artery disease, segments remote from this site may be abnormal but this situation may not be reflected in the motion of the anterior and posterior portions of the minor axis.

E-point septal separation (EPSS) and aortic root motion are two M-mode indices that reflect global left ventricular function. In EPSS, the proximity of the most anterior opening point of the mitral valve to the most posterior systolic location of the septum is measured. Normally, the mitral valve opens to within 5 mm of the most posterior septal locus (Fig. 28.16). In most situations, when the ejection fraction of the ventricle falls, the amount of residual blood at end-systole in the cavity increases and the left ventricle dilates. At the same time, the resultant stroke volume has been reduced and the amount of blood coming across the mitral valve to replace it is also reduced. The mitral valve responds to decreased inflow by opening less. This combination of events results in the anterior excursion of the valve being decreased while the inward motion of the septum is also decreased. The two structures begin to separate in proportion to the degree of dysfunction (Fig. 28.17). In our laboratory, rather than make exact measurements of EPSS we use it as a visual or qualitative clue to the presence of LV dysfunction. For exact quantitation we prefer to use quantitative two-dimensional or Doppler methods.

A third M-mode clue to left ventricular function is also qualitative. The motion of the aortic root at the base of the heart is proportional to stroke volume. The behavior of this structure is mediated by the filling of the atrium behind the aortic root and to the kinetic energy released with each systole (Figs. 28.18 and 28.19).[17] Normally, the aortic root moves forward more than 7 mm in systole (Fig. 28.20). Caution in the interpretation of this index is advised because a low stroke volume may merely reflect altered loading conditions and not necessarily decreased contractility. If the aortic valve leaflets can be visualized simultaneously with the aortic root, it is a simple matter to derive systolic time intervals (preejection period and left ventricular ejection time) from their movement.[25,26] The degree of aortic valve opening and the shape of its motion pattern are also clues to the integrity of LV function.

In recent years there have been a number of publications dealing with computer digitization of M-mode records.[27] In view of the unavailability of computers for performing these measurements in most clinical laboratories, this area will not be covered.

Two-dimensional assessment of LV function is performed both qualitatively and quantitatively. In common practice, echocardiograms are treated like LV cineangiograms. That is, the degree of emptying is

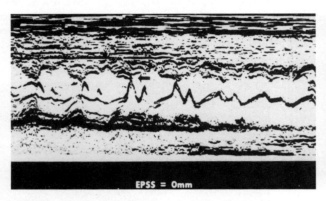

FIGURE 28.16 Determination of EPSS in a normal subject. Mitral–septal E-point separation (EPSS) is used as an M-mode index of global left ventricular function. In a normal subject, the plane of the maximum inward septal incursion and that of the maximum anterior excursion of the mitral valve are roughly the same.

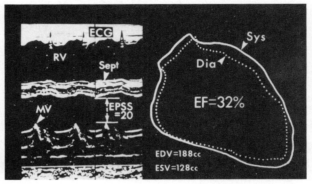

FIGURE 28.17 Marked EPSS in a patient with alcoholic cardiomyopathy. The M-mode echogram on the left and the angiogram on the right are from a patient with advanced cardiomyopathy. The EPSS is 20 mm and the ejection fraction is 32%.

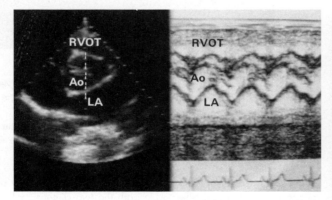

FIGURE 28.18 Normal systolic and diastolic aortic root motion in a patient with a bicuspid aortic valve. The aorta is imaged in the short axis view and on the two-dimensional image (left) appears circular. The M-mode to the right is generated from the dotted line running through the aortic root (Ao) from the right ventricular outflow tract (RVOT) anteriorly to the left atrium (LA) posteriorly. The M-mode shows that the anterior systolic motion of the root is 20 mm (scale to right of M-mode = 1 cm/division).

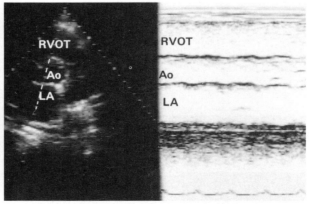

FIGURE 28.19 Depressed aortic root motion in a patient with cardiomyopathy. In comparison to Figure 28.18, note that the aortic root appears nearly motionless through the cardiac cycle. The decrease in root motion is a direct expression of the decrease in the stroke volume. If the stroke volume is depressed because of very small ventricular size, the aortic root motion will be depressed. In other words, the aortic root motion is independent of ejection fraction. Usually, of course, depressed stroke volume is associated with depressed ejection fraction. (See Figure 28.18 for abbreviations.)

judged by a visual evaluation of the contracting heart. Although it has been shown that one can reliably estimate LV ejection fraction,[28,29] we have been impressed by the occurrence of an occasional significant error when comparing visual estimation to direct quantitation.

The most accurate echocardiographic approach to the evaluation of LV contractile function by echocardiography is quantitative two-dimensional echocardiography. This statement is not meant to imply that this method is not without its problems but that it is superior to visual estimation. It remains to be seen whether Doppler techniques will surpass these techniques in accuracy.

The basic principle underlying quantitation of two-dimensional images is that a geometric model is chosen to represent the LV. Then, using values obtained by planimetry of the endocardial surfaces and linear measurements of distances between them, LV volume is calculated from an algorithm based on that model. There are numerous algorithms that have been validated (Fig. 28.21) but a comprehensive discussion of these is beyond the scope of this chapter.[30] In our laboratory we use a form of Simpson's rule to calculate ventricular volumes.[4,31] This method is relatively independent of geometry in that it reconstructs the ventricle from 20 disc-shaped slices derived from biplane two-dimensional images. The algorithm assumes that the biplane images are orthogonal to one another. This method has been validated by angiography and scintigraphy in a number of centers (Fig. 28.22)[4,31-34]. Its major shortcomings are that it underestimates angiographic volumes by approximately 25%, that tracing of endocardial surfaces can be time consuming, and that it requires a dedicated online or off-line computer system. Nonetheless, as the price of these systems falls and the quality of two-dimensional images improves, the use of quantitative methods will grow.

Figure 28.23 illustrates paired two-dimensional images from which volumes have been derived. Note that the computer has superimposed an outline on the endocardial surface. This planimetric area is used by the computer to derive volumes. Normal values for this technique are given in Table 28.2.[35]

An obvious advantage to quantitative two-dimensional LV echocardiography is that it provides volume information as well as the derived parameters, ejection fraction and stroke volume. The interpretation of a given study depends on knowledge of the clinical setting. With the development of Doppler techniques it is possible to use this information in conjunction with knowledge of valvular function. Doppler evaluation of contractile function is now under development. To date, Doppler appears to be an effective method of determining stroke volume.[36] Other indices such as acceleration of systolic aortic flow and its peak velocity appear to have promise as indices of LV function.[37,38]

As in the quantitation of two-dimensional LV echocardiograms, there are numerous proposed methods for determining the stroke volume of the left ventricle.[39-58] In our laboratory, we have used continuous-wave Doppler combined with an M-mode image of the aortic valve to generate stroke volume information.[36] All of these methods are based on the use of the flow/velocity integral and the cross-sectional area through which it is measured (Fig. 28.24). The product of the duration of flow and its mean velocity is the distance blood travels during systole. The product of this distance and the cross-sectional area through which it flows is stroke volume. The product of stroke volume and heart rate is cardiac output.

Differentiating among abnormalities of LV contractile function is difficult. If LV contraction is seen to be uniformly reduced, either by qualitative or quantitative assessment, a cardiomyopathy is implied. However, appreciation of the precise type of cardiomyopathy is usually dependent on knowledge of the clinical history or of other parameters of LV anatomy such as wall thickness. Unfortunately, our knowledge of the etiology of most cardiomyopathies remains rudimentary. Thus, our ability to differentiate among them by echocardiographic means is also primitive. Our studies show that finding segmental abnormalities favors an ischemic etiology. However, segmental variation in the degree of involvement also occurs in nonischemic cardiomyopathy.[59] The finding of depressed contractility, particularly without dilatation, should arouse suspicion of a secondary, nonmyocardial cause. For example, inappropriately rapid heart rates can be associated with decreased ejection fraction without necessarily implying myocardial disease. Certain metabolic states can also be associated with myocardial depression. Acidosis is said to cause myocardial depression. Pharmacologic agents can also temporarily depress myocardial function. Anesthetic vapors, for example, are potent myocardial depressants.[60]

LEFT VENTRICULAR SIZE, SHAPE, WALL THICKNESS, AND MASS

Left ventricular size can be assessed by the same methods used to quantitatively determine ejection fraction. In fact, some form of size determination underlies all of these methods.

M-mode determination of the LV minor axis dimension is the oldest technique for measuring LV size.[61] Although far more effective than chest roentgenography and still in widespread use today, this method can provide misleading information about global left ventricular size

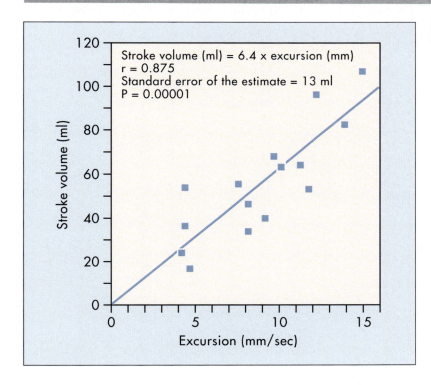

FIGURE 28.20 Quantitative relationship between aortic root excursion and angiographic stroke volume in 15 patients.

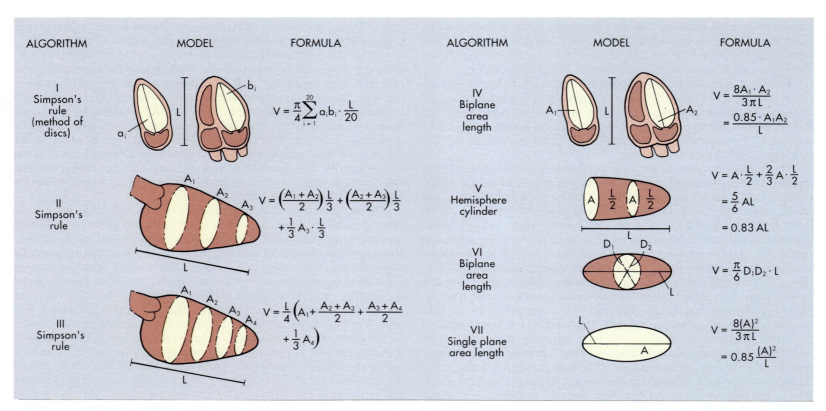

FIGURE 28.21 Algorithms for quantitative two-dimensional echocardiography. Seven algorithms used in the planimetric assessment of tomographic images of the LV. The shaded areas represent the portions of the images of ventricle that must be obtained and planimetered in order to satisfy the requirements of the various algorithms. In our laboratory, we use algorithm I (modified Simpson's rule or method of discs), IV (biplane area length), or VII (single plane area length). Wherever possible we prefer to use algorithm I. (Courtesy of Dr. Norman H. Silverman; modified from Silverman NH, Snider AR: Two-Dimensional Echocardiography in Congenital Heart Disease. Norwalk, CT, Appleton-Century-Crofts, 1982)

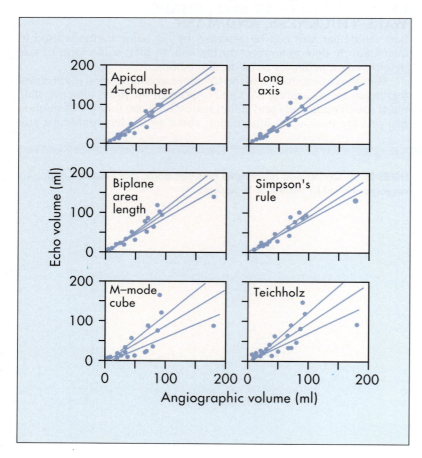

FIGURE 28.22 Relationship of angiographic LV volumes to two-dimensional and M-mode methods. Upper graphs show single-plane area–length measurements of apical four-chamber view (*top left*) and two-chamber long axis view (*top right*). Middle panels are the two biplane methods. Note that Simpson's rule is the best of all methods by a small margin. Single dimensional extrapolations from M-mode images are shown in the lower graphs and are far inferior as methods of predicting angiographic volume. This shortcoming is present despite the fact that this study was done with children with geometrically uniform ventricles. (Modified from Silverman NH, Ports TA, Snider AR et al: Determination of left ventricular volume in children—Echocardiographic and angiographic comparisons. Circulation 62:548, 1980.)

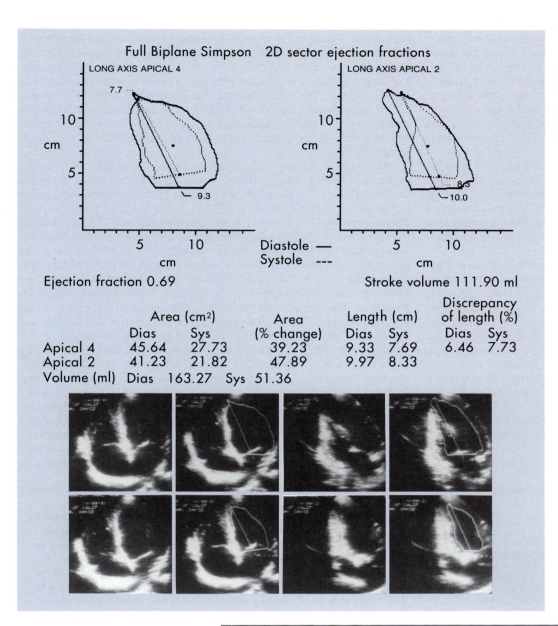

FIGURE 28.23 Quantitative two-dimensional echocardiography. A computer has been used to analyze digitized two-chamber and four-chamber apical views by a Simpson's rule algorithm. In the lower panel, two-chamber views in systole and diastole are shown on the right and four-chamber views are shown on the left both with and without their endocardial outlines superimposed.

TABLE 28.2 NORMAL VALUES FOR LEFT VENTRICULAR END-DIASTOLIC VOLUMES

Algorithm	Mean ± SD ml (Range)	Mean ± SD ml/m² (Range)
Four-Chamber Area Length		
Males	112 ± 27 (65–193)	57 ± 13 (37–94)
Females	89 ± 20 (59–136)	
Two-Chamber Area Length		
Males	130 ± 27 (73–201)	63 ± 13 (37–101)
Females	92 ± 19 (53–146)	
Simpson's Biplane Rule		
Males	111 ± 22 (62–170)	55 ± 10 (36–82)
Females	80 ± 12 (55–101)	

because it is obtained from the minor axis and gives no information about the chamber length. Nonetheless, for years it was common practice to cube the minor axis dimension as an estimation of LV volume.[33] Currently, the minor axis dimension (uncubed) and its fractional shortening are the only acceptable ways of using this information. Because of the simplicity of these linear measurements, the majority of echocardiography laboratories rely on a single minor axis LV dimension to assess LV size. Normal values for this parameter are given in Table 28.3.[62]

Two-dimensional methods of planimetry (particularly if they include all regions of the LV) provide reasonable estimation of LV size. These measurements require the use of computer-digitizing devices and knowledge of normal values (see Table 28.2). Studies presenting these values are only now appearing.[35] Additionally, as the population becomes more physically active, further modification of these normal population data may be necessary.[63-74]

As we perform more LV volume determinations in our laboratory, we have become impressed by how much additional information about LV functional status these measurements add. This situation is not surprising when one considers that volume bears a third-order relationship to dimension. Very small increments in LV diameter can introduce large increments in volume when the LV is already dilated.

The shape of the left ventricle is seldom discussed or considered. We have been impressed by the highly spherical nature of some cardiomyopathic chambers. There have also been attempts to develop a "sphericity" index which we feel will eventually aid in differentiating among types of cardiomyopathy.[59]

While generalized shape changes of the LV are seldom considered, local deformities seen in the setting of ischemic disease are commonly encountered and better appreciated.[75-80] Segmental deformity or remodeling is one of the more effective ways of identifying ischemic myocardial damage.[59] In evaluating global LV function the presence of a segmental diastolic deformity or aneurysm makes appreciation of global function more difficult. If the aneurysm is fibrous, for example, the blood within it is noncompressible (the aneurysm does not expand) and thus the deformity probably exerts little negative influence on LV performance. On the other hand, if the aneurysm is expansile, its influence on LV performance may be very important. We have, unfortunately, not yet developed methods to deal quantitatively with these shape changes.

The wall thickness of the LV has long been an informative M-mode echocardiographic measurement. Taken by itself, the linear thickness of the septum or of the posterior wall, or both, has been used as an index of LV hypertrophy (Fig. 28.25).[81] The ratio of posterior wall thickness to septal thickness has also been proposed[82-84] as an index of asymmetric hypertrophy. As in the case of LV cavitary dimension, most laboratories use the simple linear measurement of wall thickness to assess LV mass indirectly. Normal values for wall thickness obtained in this way are given in Table 28.3. With the disappearance of stand-alone M-mode echocardiographs and the availability of two-dimensional instruments, the use of wall thickness as an index of hypertrophy has been questioned. The central point of this issue is that wall thickness is being used as an indirect expression of LV mass or weight. If, for example, the weight of the left ventricle is normal, but the preload or filling volume is greatly reduced, the wall will appear to be thickened in diastole. Similarly, if the cavity is dilated the wall will appear to be thin, in spite of normal or even increased mass. For these reasons we prefer to measure left ventricular mass as an expression of left ventricular hypertrophy. There are a number of methods that have been proposed to measure LV mass from M-mode echocardiography. Unfortunately, they suffer the same theoretical limitation as the cube method of estimating LV volume from the minor axis dimension.[81] This limitation is

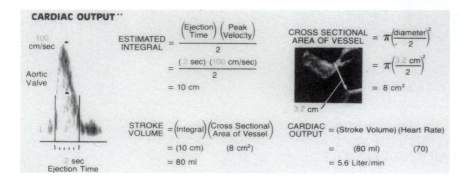

FIGURE 28.24 One of many methods for determining stroke volume by Doppler. In this method, the diameter of the left ventricular outflow tract (LVOT) is obtained from the two-dimensional long axis view on the left. From this value, the area through which blood flows is calculated. A Doppler signal from the site from which cross-sectional area was determined provides the velocity profile of systolic flow at that location. Planimetry of that signal allows determination of the mean velocity and the duration of flow. The product of the mean velocity, duration of flow, and cross-sectional area is the volume of blood flow per beat or the stroke volume. The product of the stroke volume and heart rate provides the cardiac output. (Reproduced with permission of Johnson & Johnson Ultrasound Inc.)

TABLE 28.3 LEFT ATRIAL VOLUMES OBTAINED FROM A NORMAL POPULATION

	Males		Females		Volume Index (ml/m²)	
	Mean	0.9 UCB*	Mean	0.9 UCB	Mean	0.9 UCB
Two-Chamber View Single Plane Area Length Volume (ml)						
Two-chamber view	50	82	36	57	24	41
Four-Chamber View Single Plane Area Length Volume (ml)						
Two-chamber view	41	64	34	60	21	36
Simpson's Rule Biplane Two- Plus Four-Chamber Views Volume (ml)						
Simpson's rule	41	65	32	52	21	32

* 0.9 UCB = 90% upper confidence bounds of the 95th percentile.

imposed in this case by the inability to extrapolate the volume of the myocardium from a linear dimension. This limitation is most keenly felt in attempting to deal with asymmetric hearts.[85,86] Working with more uniform hearts and in large populations where individual variations become unimportant, a number of studies have used M-mode methods and have given us valuable insight into the implications of ventricular hypertrophy, and sensitivity and specificity of electrocardiographic criteria for hypertrophy in the hypertensive population.[87]

Based on our own research and other recent work, we feel that, ultimately, LV mass should be measured directly from two-dimensional images. Our method for estimating LV mass is illustrated in Figures 28.26 to 28.29.[88] Most methods are similar in that they combine a short axis estimation of wall thickness with some estimation of ventricular length. Normal echocardiographic values for LV mass are given in Table 28.4.[89] Our preliminary observations in patients receiving aortic valve prostheses for aortic stenosis or in whom elimination of hypertension follows renal transplantation have shown rather dramatic regression of hypertrophy within the first year following therapeutic afterload reduction; in some, regression has exceeded 150 g. Others have reported similar changes following antihypertensive therapy.[90–93]

DIASTOLIC FUNCTION OF THE LEFT VENTRICLE

Almost any process that affects the systolic function of the myocardium or increases its mass affects diastolic function as well. In diastole the left ventricle should be able to accept a wide range of blood volumes without elevation of filling pressure. The healthy ventricle also has the characteristic of completing most of its filling during the initial phases of diastole. This property is particularly helpful at rapid heart rates when diastole is abbreviated.

Echocardiographic indicators of diastolic function are aortic root and mitral valve motion on M-mode, left atrial enlargement, and alterations of Doppler mitral inflow velocity patterns.

The aortic root, an intracardiac structure, sits astride the roof of the left atrium. Atrial volume changes during the cardiac cycle are reflected by the motion of the aortic root. In systole, the aortic root is propelled forward by the release of kinetic energy from the rapid ejec-

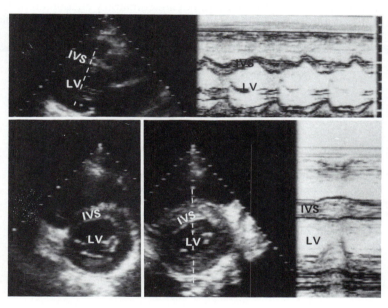

FIGURE 28.25 Left ventricular hypertrophy compared to normal. Upper half of the figure shows a long axis two-dimensional image of the LV with a dashed line indicating the plane from which the M-mode at the right was generated. Note that the walls of the LV (IVS and posterior) are thin (less than 1 cm). In the lower panel is the short axis view from the same normal patient as shown in the top panel. To the right of this short axis view is a short axis view from a patient with severe, slightly asymmetric hypertrophy. The line through this short axis view indicates the plane of the M-mode to be in the lower right. Note the obvious difference between the M-mode tracings and between the short axis views.

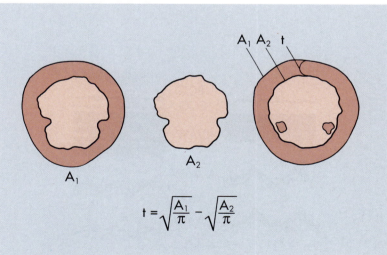

FIGURE 28.26 Wall thickness from LV short axis. By planimetry of the epicardium and endocardium in the short axis plane, mean wall thickness can be obtained as shown. This approach circumvents the obvious problems associated with estimating wall thickness at only one or two spots. Knowledge of the inner area also allows simple back calculation of the minor axis radius. (Modified from Schiller NB, Skioldebrand CG, Schiller EJ et al: Canine left ventricular mass estimation by two-dimensional echocardiography. Circulation 68:210, 1983)

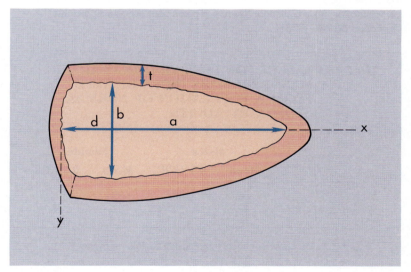

FIGURE 28.27 Dimensions from long axis LV for calculating LV mass. Using the two-chamber or four-chamber view (whichever is longer) the semimajor axis a and the truncated semiminor axis d are measured. Thickness t and minor axis radius b can be calculated from the minor axis as discussed in the legend to Figure 28.26. (Modified from Schiller NB, Skioldebrand CG, Schiller EJ et al: Canine left ventricular mass estimation by two-dimensional echocardiography. Circulation 68:210, 1983)

tion of blood and, more importantly, by the sudden expansion of the left atrium. The degree of atrial expansion is directly related to the degree of filling on the preceding beat (ventricular preload) and to the stroke volume.[94,95] In diastole, the aortic root returns posteriorly from this anterior end-systolic position. Normally, this return occurs immediately and rapidly. In fact, the posterior initial diastolic root motion is more rapid than the anterior systolic motion. Figure 28.30 shows a normal aortic root on the left and one from a patient with aortic stenosis and severe left ventricular hypertrophy (LVH) on the right. Note that in the normal example, the initial diastolic posterior motion can be easily seen to be faster. When filling is slowed and sinus rhythm present, the posterior motion during active atrial emptying becomes exaggerated and the passive filling phase blunted.[96,97] Angiographic studies have shown that normally around 50% of atrial inflow occurs during the rapid filling phase of early diastole and 30% during atrial contraction.[18] In states of decreased compliance this relationship is reversed so that the majority of filling occurs during atrial contraction.

The early diastolic filling slope of the mitral valve is also reduced in a manner similar to that seen in mitral stenosis.[98,99] This change is a less reliable indicator of decreased compliance than aortic root motion.

If a state of decreased compliance persists for an appreciable period, the left atrium will enlarge. If sinus rhythm is present and the mitral valve is normal, and if no other chamber enlargement is present, the finding of isolated atrial enlargement should suggest an abnormality of LV compliance.

Doppler demonstration of the velocity profile of LV transmitral inflow appears to be an informative method of assessing LV filling. Recent studies have demonstrated that the relationship between peak velocity and deceleration in early diastole with late diastolic velocities during atrial contraction is altered. These alterations appear to be more sensitive than the M-mode mitral filling slope (Figs. 28.31 and 28.32).[8,100] Although these Doppler parameters are dependent on heart rate, loading conditions, contractility, presence or absence of mitral regurgitation, and the patient's age,[101-104] useful information on left ventricular diastolic function can be provided in the appropriate clinical setting. For example, in a young patient with hypertension and left ventricular hypertrophy, a prominent a-wave-dominant mitral inflow pattern and a prolonged deceleration time suggest an abnormality of left ventricular diastolic relaxation.

LEFT VENTRICULAR THROMBI, TUMORS, AND MASSES

Left ventricular intracavitary thrombi are commonly encountered. The vast majority occur in the setting of recent anteroapical myocardial

$$V = \Pi \left\{ (b+t)^2 \int_0^{d+a+t} \left[1 - \frac{(x-d)^2}{(a+t)^2}\right] dx - b_2 \int_0^{d+a} \left[1 - \frac{(x-d)^2}{a^2}\right] dx \right\}$$
$$= \Pi \left\{ (b+t)^2 \left[\frac{2}{3}(a+t)+d - \frac{d^3}{3(a+t)^2}\right] - b^2 \left[\frac{2}{3}a+d - \frac{d^3}{3a^2}\right] \right\}$$

FIGURE 28.28 Formula for LV mass. The formula for LV mass derived from the method of discs and based on a model of the LV as a truncated ellipsoid is shown. Basically, the formula calculates volume from the inner and outer shells of the LV (epicardium and endocardium). The difference of these two values is the volume of the myocardium or, when multiplied by muscle density 1.05, its mass. (Modified from Schiller NB, Skioldebrand CG, Schiller EJ et al: Canine left ventricular mass estimation by two-dimensional echocardiography. Circulation 68:210, 1983)

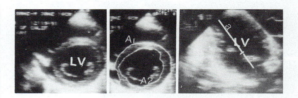

FIGURE 28.29 Computer measurement of LV mass. Although the algorithm in Figure 28.28 appears complicated, only three simple measurements are required to allow the computer to calculate LV mass. The first two measurements are of the areas subtended by the epicardium and endocardium, A1 and A2, the third of the semimajor axis a, and the fourth, the truncated semimajor axis d.

TABLE 28.4 VALUES FOR LEFT VENTRICULAR MASS AND MASS INDEX DERIVED FROM A POPULATION OF NORMAL, SEDENTARY ADULTS

	Males		Females	
	Mean	0.9 UCB*	Mean	0.9 UCB
Mass (g)	135	183	99	141
Mass index (g/m²)	71	94	62	89

* 0.9 UCB = 90% upper confidence bounds of the 95th percentile.

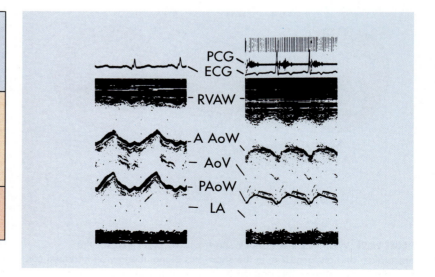

FIGURE 28.30 Decreased compliance and diastolic aortic root motion. A comparison of posterior aortic root echogram from a normal subject with one from a patient with left ventricular hypertrophy. (PCG, phonocardiogram; RVAW, right ventricular anterior wall; AAoW, anterior aortic wall; AoV, aortic valve; PAoW, posterior aortic wall; LA, left atrium) (Djalaly A et al: Diastolic aortic root motion in left ventricular hypertrophy. Chest 79:442, 1981)

infarction.[105-121] Echocardiography is highly effective in detection of thrombi and has enabled several investigators to study their formation, disappearance, and embologenic potential. Figure 28.33 demonstrates a large apical aneurysm completely filled with thrombus. In Figure 28.34, heavy trabeculations in the left ventricular apex in a patient with hypertrophic cardiomyopathy are illustrated. Differentiation of these apical structures from thrombus can present difficulties for echocardiography, and computed tomography (CT) scanning might be of help to separate these pathologic processes.[122] In one series[123] thrombi developed during serial echocardiographic evaluation in 12 of 35 patients with anterior infarction. These thrombi tended to develop on the fifth postinfarction day and were most common in older patients with more extensive infarction. The risk of embolization peaked 5 to 20 days after infarction with rapidly decreasing risk thereafter. Anticoagulation seemed to reduce the incidence of embolism and thrombus but did not seem to affect the presence of the thrombus itself. Ventricular thrombi are also encountered in congestive cardiomyopathy but are seen much less commonly than in anterior infarction. Nonthrombotic

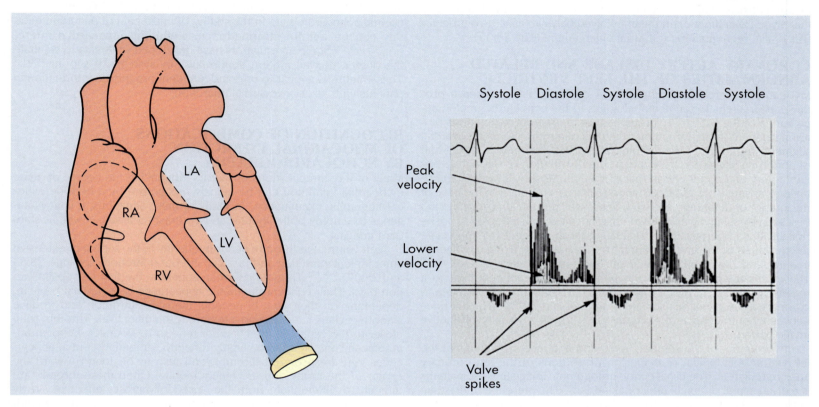

FIGURE 28.31 Normal mitral inflow Doppler tracing. The Doppler beam is directed from the apex toward the base (*left*). Mitral inflow during diastole travels toward the transducer. The Doppler frequency shift resulting from this diastolic transmitral flow is shown on the right. Note that the initial inflow signal of early diastole has the highest velocity and the late diastolic atrial inflow signal, the lowest. (Modified with permission from Hewlett Packard, Andover, MA)

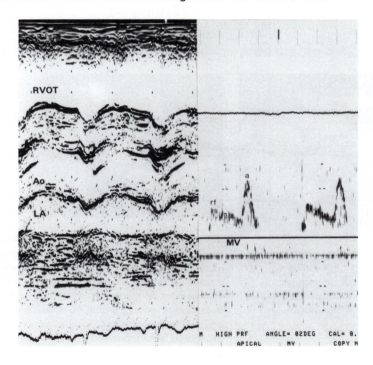

FIGURE 28.32 Decreased compliance by both aortic root motion and mitral flow. The left side of the figure is an M-mode of the aortic root showing marked slowing of the early diastolic slope and exaggeration of posterior root motion during atrial contraction. The Doppler mitral flow signal from the same patient is shown on the right. Note that the early diastolic inflow velocity is slow and the a wave velocity increased. Compare this tracing to the diagram of normal mitral flow in Figure 28.31.

masses of the left ventricle are quite rare. About 25% of the primary tumors among these masses are malignant: their approximate distribution by histologic type are 33% angiosarcoma, 20% rhabdomyomas, 10% mesotheliomas, and 11% fibrosarcomas.[124] In the pediatric population, the most common tumors are rhabdomyomata associated with tuberous sclerosis.

Other mass-like lesions of the left ventricle include endomyocardial fibrosis. This condition is most commonly encountered in the tropics and is characterized by obliteration of the apices of the LV and right ventricle (RV).[125-128] Eventually this process restricts the size of the LV cavity and leads to a severe restrictive state. The echocardiographic picture consists of apical obliteration by a partially calcified mass, normal myocardial function in the uninvolved basal areas, atrioventricular (AV) valve regurgitation, and atrial enlargement (Fig. 28.35).

CORONARY ARTERY DISEASE AND RELATED ABNORMALITIES OF THE LEFT VENTRICLE

Myocardial infarction resulting from coronary artery disease produces characteristic segmental changes in the echocardiographic appearance of the LV.[129-137] These changes range from hypokinesis of a given segment to the formation of a frank aneurysm. Some myocardial segments are much more commonly involved than others. About half of abnormal segments are found in the distribution of the right coronary artery and about half in that of the left. Most wall motion abnormalities arising from right coronary occlusion are found at the base of the inferior or diaphragmatic wall. These wall motion abnormalities are best seen by using the apical two-chamber view with a degree of posterior tilt. It is important when evaluating these segments to appreciate the thickness of the given segment, the degree of scarring, changes in texture, and how well the segment thickens with each systole.[138,139] These features give clues to the presence of old infarction or to a recent event. The abrupt demarcation of a segment typically seen in coronary disease can be ascribed as remodeling.[79,140-142] The interface between contracting and akinetic tissue forms a visually distinctive image pattern.

Involvement of the septum, apex, and anteroseptal regions of the left ventricle is typical of occlusion of portions of the left coronary artery circulation. The usual echocardiographic image in these patients is a distal septal or apical area of akinesis.[143] The presence of diastolic deformity, sharply demarcated, indicates aneurysm formation.[135,144,145] Hypokinesis, particularly without wall thinning or remodeling, suggests ischemia rather than infarction. Figures 28.36 to 28.38 illustrate the typical appearance of apical infarctions with aneurysm formation; Figure 28.39 illustrates the appearance of an anteroseptal infarction; and Figures 28.40 and 28.41 illustrate typical locations and appearance of inferior infarction.

Echocardiography is effective in detecting most areas of myocardial involvement from ischemia or infarction. In view of its reliability in this area, some laboratories have begun using it in conjunction with various forms of stress testing as a supplement to the electrocardiogram.[146-149] There have been reports that it is superior in sensitivity and specificity to scintigraphic myocardial imaging with thallium-201. Other studies, including our own, suggest that it is roughly equivalent to thallium-201 in its ability to detect areas of induced ischemia and their extent but that it falls short of scintigraphy because of its inability to provide information about the timing of reperfusion.[150-156]

The ability of echocardiography to detect segmental disease has also led to its use in acute myocardial infarction.[136,157] For example, a normal echocardiogram in the setting of chest pain of uncertain etiology can be helpful information in excluding myocardial infarction.[131,158,159] Some investigators have developed schemata to estimate the degree of wall motion abnormality by systems of scoring.[160-167] These methods appear to offer independent prognostic information in patients with acute myocardial infarction.

RECOGNITION OF COMPLICATIONS OF MYOCARDIAL INFARCTION BY ECHOCARDIOGRAPHY

Many of the complications or factors influencing the course of acute myocardial infarction can be quickly recognized by a bedside echocardiographic examination. In many of these situations, it is advantageous to employ both Doppler and contrast methods as well as standard imaging.

Left ventricular thrombi occur frequently in the setting of extensive anteroapical infarction and rarely in inferior infarction (see Figs. 28.33 and 28.37).[168-171] These masses can appear in the first few postinfarction days. Their echocardiographic appearance is somewhat protean, depending on their age. In general, the older thrombi tend to have smooth cavitary surfaces and a texture resembling liver. Thrombi lying closer to the center of the chamber tend to be younger. Echocardiographically, they tend to be highly reflective or luminescent in appearance. Very fresh or red thrombi tend also to be found toward the center of the cavity and are highly mobile. Often these thrombi are difficult to differentiate from the "pseudocontrast" effect of slowly moving cavitary blood seen within left ventricular aneurysms. Often it is possible to appreciate several layers of differing texture in larger thrombi. The more mobile and irregular the surface of the thrombus, the more likely it is to be associated with emboli. Thrombi can be difficult to differentiate from apical trabeculations, which are more pronounced in hypertrophic cardiomyopathy.

The aneurysms referred to above are also complications of myo-

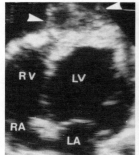
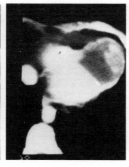

FIGURE 28.33 Apical thrombus by two-dimensional echocardiography and computed tomography. (Left) Apical four-chamber view showing large apical aneurysm filled with thrombus. (Right) The CT scan (with contrast, nongated) shows clearly that the mass is thrombus but additionally shows that the mass is partially calcified.

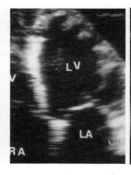

FIGURE 28.34 Apical trabeculations in hypertrophic cardiomyopathy. Heavy apical trabeculations suggested apical thrombus but an ungated computed tomography scan with contrast showed no filling defects suggestive of thrombus.

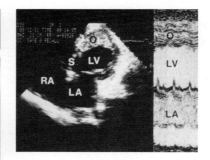

FIGURE 28.35 Endomyocardial fibrosis. Typical apical obliteration (O) by a fibrocalcific process renders the LV cavity very small. The net effect is a severe restrictive cardiomyopathy with atrial enlargement. M-mode to the right shows the characteristic echoes arising from the apical mass and the very poor mitral opening motion associated with depressed stroke volume. (Courtesy of Dr. Harry Acquatella, del Hospital Universitario de Caracas, Venezuela)

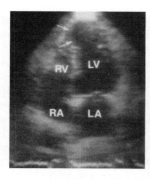

FIGURE 28.36 Apical aneurysm. Four-chamber view of a left ventricular apical aneurysm. The distribution of this lesion is typical of occlusion of the left anterior descending coronary artery.

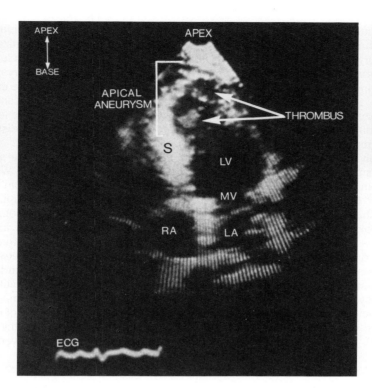

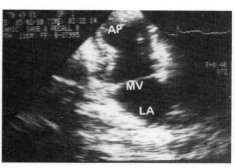

FIGURE 28.38 Apical aneurysm. This apical aneurysm (*AP*) is seen in the two-chamber view, suggesting that it is fairly extensive.

FIGURE 28.37 Apical aneurysm with thrombus. Four-chamber view with an apical aneurysm similar in appearance to Figure 28.36. This aneurysm shows intracavitary echoes consistent with thrombus. (Courtesy of Dr. Thomas A. Ports, University of California, San Francisco)

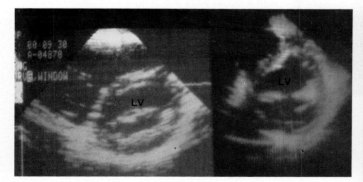

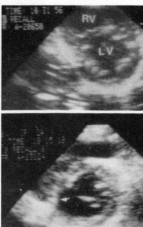

FIGURE 28.40 Inferior infarction. Normal short axis (systolic) view (*above*) and inferoposterior infarction (*below*). The arrow points to the area of segmental thinning and deformity.

FIGURE 28.39 Anteroseptal infarction. Normal short axis view (*left*) contrasted with a short axis view (*right*) in a person with an anteroseptal infarction. Note the rather striking remodeling at the anteroseptal junction.

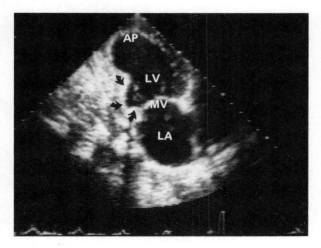

FIGURE 28.41 Inferior infarction. Two-chamber view of the LV in a patient with a moderate to large inferior myocardial infarction. Note the basal location (*arrow*) of the area of infarction and the preserved apical (*AP*) geometry.

cardial infarction.[172] Since remodeling is a feature of infarction, it is hard to define the point at which a segmental abnormality becomes an aneurysm. A simple, useful definition of aneurysm is a wall motion abnormality with the feature of *diastolic deformity*. The vast majority form at the LV apex, although an inferior basal aneurysm (Fig. 28.42) is occasionally encountered.

Pseudoaneurysms, as the name implies, resemble true aneurysms. However, these aneurysms are actually the result of frank wall rupture or cardiorrhexis. The sac of the aneurysm is composed of pericardium that contains or walls off the rupture. Since only small ruptures in the wall are compatible with survival, these aneurysms tend to have a narrow neck. True aneurysms, on the other hand, are nearly as wide at the neck as they are at their apex (Fig. 28.43).[173-175] Often echocardiography is the first modality by which these pseudoaneurysms are recognized. Unrepaired, their prognosis is poor, making their recognition much more than a matter of taxonomy.

Abrupt myocardial rupture into the pericardial sac is usually fatal and its echocardiographic recognition has little role. Slower accumulations can result in pericardial effusion and tamponade.[176] Most pericardial effusions detected by echocardiography in acute myocardial infarction are not due to wall rupture but are due to either local inflammation at the site of epicardial necrosis or post-myocardial infarction pericardial inflammation (Dressler's syndrome).[177,178] Use of anticoagulants in the presence of myocardial infarction can, of course, result in progressive fluid accumulation recognized on serial echocardiograms.

Most often, septal rupture leads to left-to-right shunt at the level of the ventricles (Fig. 28.44) and papillary muscle rupture leads to severe mitral insufficiency (Fig. 28.45). In the case of acute ventricular septal defect, Doppler and contrast studies can be diagnostic by demonstrating the appearance of bubbles on the left side after right-sided injection and by the Doppler detection of disturbed flow in and around the ventricular septal defect.[179-181]

Right ventricular infarction can be suspected by careful echocardiographic examination (Fig. 28.44). With increasing numbers of recent studies of right ventricular function in inferior infarction,[182-189] the frequency of occurrence of this complication is now appreciated as being much higher than previously thought. In fact, some studies suggest that as many as 40% of inferior infarctions are complicated by some degree of right ventricular dysfunction. However, it should be clear that there is a vast difference between depression of contractile function, which is usually subclinical and echocardiographically subtle, and severe impairment of right ventricular performance. When extensive right ventricular infarction occurs, a low output state with high mortality can occur.[190] Since patency of the foramen ovale is present in 20% to 30% of normal individuals,[191] the elevation of right-sided filling pressures accompanying severe right ventricular dysfunction can result

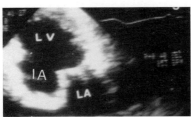
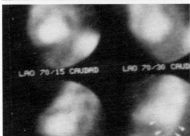

FIGURE 28.42 Inferobasal aneurysm (large). (*Upper panel*) A large inferior basal aneurysm (IA) nearly equal in size to the left atrium (LA) is seen in its usual location in the two-chamber apical view. (*Lower panel*) A blood pool scintigram of the LV showing the aneurysm in the 70٪ left anterior oblique view (LAO) (*arrows*). Contractility and uninvolved segments was excellent. (Nuclear scan courtesy of Dr. Elias H. Botvinick, University of California, San Francisco)

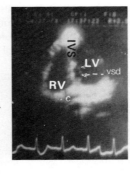

FIGURE 28.44 Ventricular septal defect and right ventricular infarction. In the setting of a recent inferior myocardial infarction this patient has developed two major complications—a ventricular septal defect (*vsd*) and a right ventricular infarction. The right ventricular infarction can be appreciated by the dilation of the right ventricle. In order to visualize the site of these abnormalities, posterior angulation of transducer is necessary. In this example, the appearance of the coronary sinus (c) in the image is proof that this posterior angulation was performed by the sonographer.

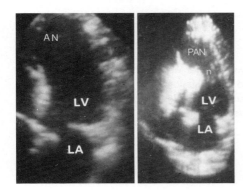

FIGURE 28.43 Aneurysm and pseudoaneurysm of the LV apex. (*Left*) An aneurysm (AN) of the LV apex is shown in the apical four-chamber view. Note that the ventricle does not narrow at the opening to the aneurysm. (*Right*) A pseudoaneurysm (PAN) identified by its connection to the LV across a narrow neck (n). (*Right*, courtesy of Dr. Ralph Clark, Pacific Medical Center, San Francisco)

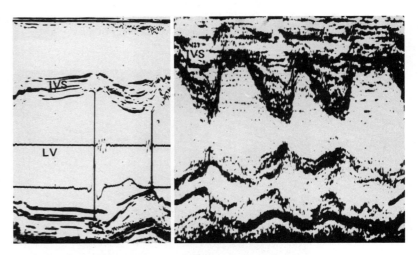

FIGURE 28.45 Mitral regurgitation complicating myocardial infarction. (*Left*) M-mode of a normal left ventricle. Note that the motion of the septum (*IVS*) and the motion of its opposing posterior wall are fairly symmetric. (*Right*) Severe mitral insufficiency arising from ischemic damage to the inferior base of the LV. This damage has undermined the support of the posteromedial papillary muscle. The resulting mitral insufficiency has exaggerated the motion of the septum. The damaged inferior wall has only poor inward motion and stands in marked contrast to the IVS.

in acute right-to-left shunting.[192] This can be easily appreciated with a simple saline echocardiographic contrast study that will demonstrate passage of microbubbles from right to left across the middle of the atrial septum.

Other two-dimensional echocardiographic findings indicative of hemodynamically significant right ventricular infarction include plethora of the inferior vena cava with blunted respiratory response (indicating elevated right atrial pressure), poor descent of the right ventricular base (indicating decreased right ventricular contractile function), and enlargement of the right ventricle relative to the left ventricle in the apical four-chamber view.[193]

RECOGNITION OF CARDIOMYOPATHIES BY ECHOCARDIOGRAPHY

There are three major types of cardiomyopathy that can be appreciated by echocardiography. The first is the dilated cardiomyopathy; the second is hypertrophic cardiomyopathy; and the third type, which is less frequently encountered and more difficult to identify by echocardiography, is the family of restrictive cardiomyopathies. Although the advanced forms of dilated cardiomyopathies are readily identified by echocardiography, the early stages are more difficult to detect. Since we seldom appreciate or encounter the early stages of this condition, this description will concentrate on the appearance of the advanced form. The most distinctive echocardiographic findings in these hearts are spherical cavitary dilation, normal or decreased wall thickness, and inward endocardial systolic motion.[194–200] On M-mode echocardiography additional features are recognized such as mitral–septal E-point separation, poor mitral valve opening, poor aortic valve opening, and poor systolic aortic root motion. In addition to the sequelae of poor ejection fraction and low stroke volume, both M-mode and two-dimensional images usually demonstrate left atrial enlargement; two-dimensional imaging also reveals four-chamber dilatation. The involvement of the right heart is important because it implies pulmonary hypertension or right ventricular failure either secondary to pulmonary pressure elevation or to involvement of the RV myocardium in the pathologic process.[201] Quantitatively, the left ventricle often exceeds 250 ml in volume while the left atrium can exceed 125 ml. The ejection fraction derived from the systolic and diastolic volume determinations can, at times, fall below 20% but is usually between 20% and 30%. In spite of the low ejection fractions, cardiac output (stroke volume × heart rate) calculations may reveal normal values. Patients with cardiomyopathy frequently have elevated heart rates, and a large end-diastolic volume may maintain adequate stroke volume. Figures 28.46 to 28.49 demonstrate some of the features of cardiomyopathy.

Doppler has been used in cardiomyopathy to measure decreased contractility. Both peak velocity and acceleration of velocity in the ascending aorta are decreased in primary myocardial dysfunction.[202]

When a cardiomyopathy is fully developed, echocardiography is a rapid and unerring method of establishing this diagnosis. Ironically, this method offers very little in establishing the etiology of dilated cardiomyopathy. Once the diagnosis is known, performing echocardiograms at frequent intervals is also relatively unrewarding unless the laboratory is equipped to make Doppler determinations of pulmonary pressure and quantitative evaluation of chamber volumes and mass. In our own laboratory, we attempted to distinguish among a group of patients with ischemic and primary cardiomyopathies using echocardiography and nuclear magnetic resonance imaging (NMR).[59] We evaluated the presence of segmental disease, remodeling of segmental abnormalities, thinning of segments, and sphericity as criteria. In patients with ischemic etiologies, segmental remodeling, thinning, and areas of

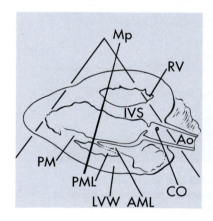
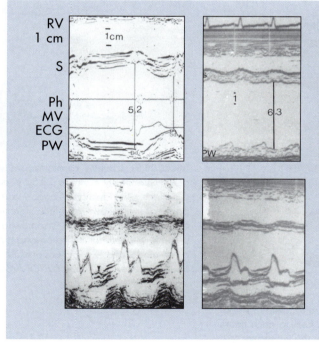

FIGURE 28.46 Cardiomyopathy compared to normal. M-mode echocardiograms illustrating some of the cardinal features of cardiomyopathy. Normal M-modes in the middle panels show the M-mode of the minor axis of the LV (upper) taken along the line (Mp) superimposed on the anatomical diagram. The panels along the right are taken from a patient with cardiomyopathy. The minor axis dimension of the normal ventricle is 5.2 cm, as compared to 6.3 cm in the patient with cardiomyopathy. The fractional shortening of the normal heart (LVEDd (5.2) − LVESd (3.4)/5.2 = 35%) is compared to that of the heart with cardiomyopathy (6.3 − 5.3/6.3 = 16%). In the lower panel, the M-mode was obtained from a level nearer to the LV base and the beam passed through the mitral valve. In the normal heart the mitral valve (MV), denoted by a small arrow, opens very near to the septum (S) while in the cardiomyopathic heart it is separated from the septum by nearly 2 cm. This separation is called mitral–septal separation, or EPSS.

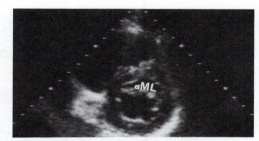
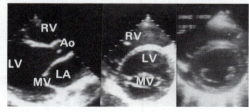

FIGURE 28.47 Cardiomyopathy compared to normal. In the upper panel, a short axis view of the left ventricle from a normal heart appears. The scale of this image is larger than the cardiomyopathic heart appearing below (each pair of dots separate 1 cm). Note the relationship between the thickness of the myocardium and that of the muscle. An exaggeration of cavitary volume and thinning of myocardial segments are typical of cardiomyopathy shown below. The left panel is a long axis view, the middle panel is a short axis view taken through the mitral valve, and the right panel is a short axis view through the papillary muscles. Note the spherical nature of the LV. (aML, anterior mitral valve leaflet)

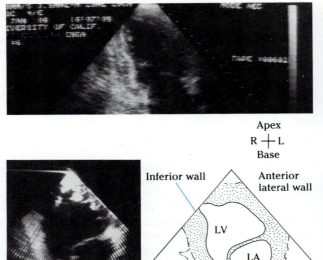

FIGURE 28.48 Cardiomyopathy compared to normal. A two-chamber apical view obtained from a normal heart is shown in the upper panel. In the lower panels, a two-chamber view from a spherically dilated cardiomyopathy heart is shown and diagrammed. Note the difference in shape between the normal and cardiomyopathy.

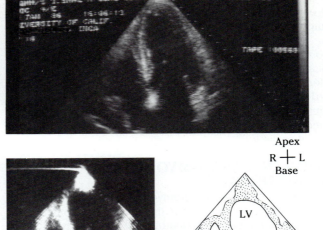

FIGURE 28.49 Cardiomyopathy compared to normal. A four-chamber view from a normal heart is shown in the upper panel. In the lower panels, a heart from a patient with cardiomyopathy is shown and diagrammed. Note that the cardiomyopathy heart is more spherical than its normal counterpart. The developing of a spherical configuration is fairly typical of cardiomyopathy.

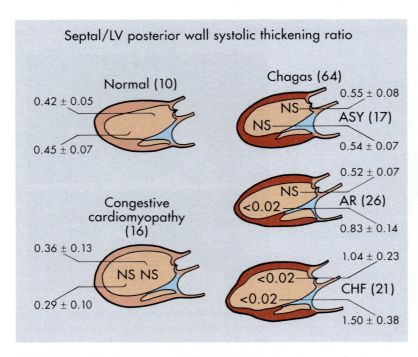

FIGURE 28.50 Diagrammatic comparison of Chagas' cardiomyopathy to non-Chagas' cardiomyopathy and normal hearts. The values next to each figure refer to the ratio of septal to posterior wall thickening at the ventricular level, indicated by the arrows. In normal hearts and non-Chagas' myopathies, the posterior wall thickening is greater than septal at all levels. In Chagas' patients, those with arrhythmias (AR) and those with congestive cardiomyopathy (CHF) show a reversal of thickening ratios in the more apical segments. In other words, relative to the septum the posteroapical segments are more scarred and less contractile. This pattern of septal scarring appears unique to Chagas' heart disease. (Modified from Acquatella H et al: M-mode and two-dimensional echocardiography in chronic Chagas' heart disease. Circulation 62:787, 1980)

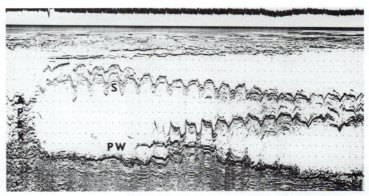

FIGURE 28.51 Chagas' cardiomyopathy. The pattern shown diagrammatically in Figure 28.50 is present on this M-mode sweep of a patient with advanced Chagas' cardiomyopathy. Note that the posterior wall shows very little sign of thickening while the septum is exaggerated. This picture is somewhat similar to that encountered in patients with inferior infarction and mitral regurgitation. (Acquatella H et al: M-mode and two-dimensional echocardiography in chronic Chagas' heart disease. Circulation 62:787, 1980)

preserved function tended to predominate. However, in some patients with no historic or angiographic evidence of ischemic disease the echocardiographic and NMR images most closely suggested a segmental or ischemic process. We believe, therefore, that the features distinguishing one process from another blend into one another and that echocardiography is not a precise method of classifying cardiomyopathies. Recent work has suggested a widening role for echocardiography in the diagnosis of cardiomyopathy by showing that it is possible to perform endocardial biopsies under echocardiographic control.[203] If greater experience in the noninvasive guidance of an invasive technique is acquired, this combination may become a standard method of refining our diagnostic and therapeutic approach to cardiomyopathies. In South American countries, the finding of a congestive or a segmental cardiomyopathy raises the possibility of Chagas' disease. In this condition, transmission of *Trypanosoma cruzi* from an insect vector eventually leads to damaging infestation of the myocardium. When the condition exists in its congestive cardiomyopathic state it is indistinguishable from any other cause of advanced myocardial disease. However, in its segmental presentation, Chagas' disease appears echocardiographically as an apical aneurysm that, unlike those most commonly seen in coronary disease, spares the interventricular septum. In a rarer segmental presentation, the inferior base can be the site of segmentally isolated thinning and scar formation (Figs. 28.50, 28.51).[204]

Hypertrophic cardiomyopathies are characterized by the presence of increased LV mass (wall thickness) without apparent etiology; in other words, the presence of LV hypertrophy (LVH) without a history of hypertension or aortic stenosis. These myopathies can be of two types, asymmetric and symmetric.[82,205–207] The echocardiogram in asymmetric septal hypertrophy (ASH) characteristically shows increased wall thickness localized or most intense in the basal septum. The patterns of distribution of this hypertrophic state are not well understood because they follow an unpredictable pattern.[208] One of the more puzzling aspects of this condition is that although it is clearly a heritable condition, the patterns of involvement differ among affected members of the same family.[209,210] In spite of its poorly understood features, the echocardiogram is the most reliable means of making the diagnosis of hypertrophic cardiomyopathy.[206,207] The usual features are selective thickening of a portion of the basal septum with sparing of the base and variable involvement of other portions of the myocardium (Fig. 28.52). In an unusual variation of ASH, the apex can become the site of the most intensive hypertrophy.[213–220] In our experience this variety is more difficult to identify by echocardiography because the apical myocardium is more difficult to image. When dynamic outflow

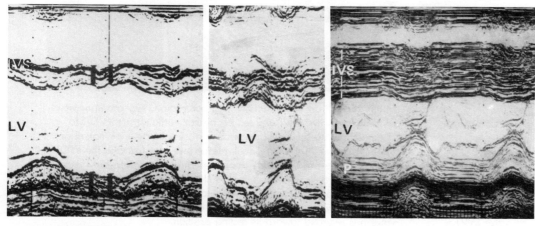

FIGURE 28.52 Symmetric and asymmetric left ventricular hypertrophy. Normal left ventricle (*left panel*) is contrasted to mild symmetric left ventricular hypertrophy (*center panel*) and marked asymmetric hypertrophy (*right panel*). Note that the a wave or presystolic ventricular filling is more exaggerated in the example of mild left ventricular hypertrophy. Exaggerated filling during the atrial phase of diastole can be a clue to decreased compliance, which may be more marked for the degree of hypertrophy.

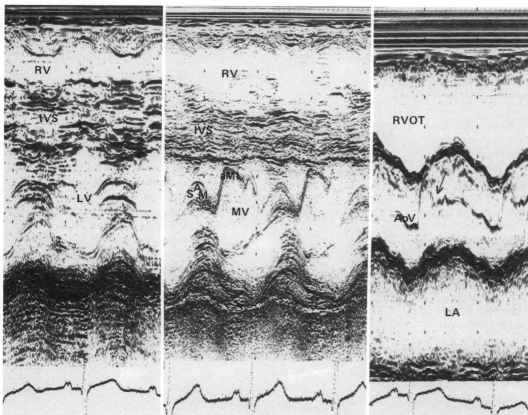

FIGURE 28.53 Hypertrophic obstructive cardiomyopathy. M-mode from a patient with resting obstruction. Left panel is from minor axis of LV and demonstrates typical asymmetric ventricular hypertrophy of the interventricular septum (IVS). Systolic anterior motion (SAM) of the mitral valve (MV) and crowded appearance of ventricle are shown in the center panel. The degree of contact between the septum and the mitral valve during systole appears minimal, suggesting that obstruction is mild. However, in the right panel, the aortic valve (AoV) demonstrates striking mid-systolic notching or closure (*arrow*), strongly suggesting that dynamic obstruction is significant.

tract obstruction accompanies ASH, the fully developed picture of obstructive hypertrophic cardiomyopathy or idiopathic hypertrophic obstructive cardiomyopathy (HOCM) is present. Echocardiographic identification of this condition is easier when the condition is fully developed (Fig. 28.53). However, when the obstruction is only provocable (Figs. 28.54 and 28.55) or slight, the task of the echocardiographer is more difficult. The features of fully-developed HOCM consist of ASH, systolic anterior motion (SAM) of the mitral valve, crowding of the LV outflow tract by the mitral apparatus and septum, partial mid-systolic closure or notching of the aortic valve, and altered diastolic compliance.[217-219,221-223] Mitral annulus calcification (MAC) also frequently accompanies HOCM. In some patients the presence of MAC may be the only clue to the potential for dynamic outflow tract obstruction. Whenever obstructive or nonobstructive HOCM is suspected it is usually desirable to perform some sort of intervention or provocation during the echocardiographic examination. If Doppler techniques are available (particularly continuous wave), simultaneous measurements of outflow tract systolic velocity with various maneuvers may not only prove diagnostic of dynamic outflow tract obstruction but provide the severity of obstruction (Figs. 28.56 and 28.57).[8] At a minimum, in laboratories having no Doppler capability, the patient should first perform a Valsalva maneuver while a clinician performs an M-mode of the mitral valve base and LV outflow tract area. The development of systolic anterior movement of the mitral valve, particularly if contact with the septum results, strongly suggests the potential for dynamic obstruction.[224] Inspection of the aortic valve at the peak of this provocation should provide secondary evidence of obstruction by demonstrating mid-systolic notching or closure (see Fig. 28.53). If a Valsalva

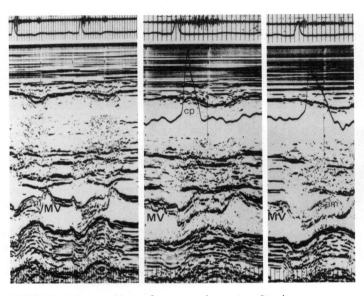

FIGURE 28.54 Provocable outflow tract obstruction. Simultaneous M-mode, phonocardiogram, and carotid pulse tracing (cp) during rest (left panel), peak amyl nitrite effect (center), and recovery (right). Note that the systolic anterior motion (sam) of the mitral valve (MV) increases markedly and lies in close apposition to the interventricular septum during the provocation. Note also that the murmur becomes more intense and the carotid pulse loses its dicrotic wave. During recovery the systolic anterior motion of the mitral valve is much less marked and only barely makes contact with the septum. It can be inferred from this study that the patient has little if any resting subaortic gradient but has easily provoked dynamic obstruction.

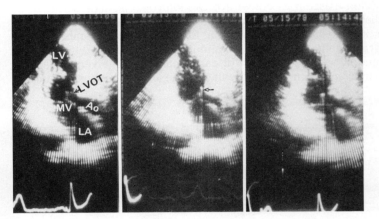

FIGURE 28.55 Provocable outflow tract obstruction. Two-chamber views of the mitral valve (MV) and left ventricular outflow tract (LVOT) to demonstrate the site and appearance of systolic anterior motion of the mitral valve. In the left panel, the patient is at rest and the LVOT is open. In the middle panel, the patient has been given amyl nitrite and the recording was made at its full effect. Note that the coapted mitral valve/chordae tip has moved into the LVOT and now abuts the septum (arrow). In the right panel, the effect has passed and the valve has returned toward its resting position.

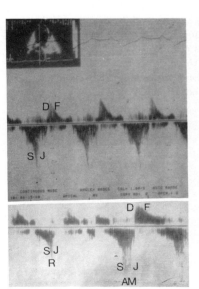

FIGURE 28.56 Doppler of dynamic subvalvular obstruction. A continuous-wave Doppler recording from the apical four-chamber view (upper left inset) records inflow across the mitral valve during diastole (DF) and outflow tract systolic jet (SJ) typical of dynamic subaortic outflow obstruction. Features of the systolic jet include transient duration, giving the velocity profile the appearance of a horse's tail. In the lower panel, the systolic jet during rest (R) has a velocity of 2.5 m/sec, suggesting a 25 mm Hg subaortic gradient. During amyl nitrite (AM) provocation, the jet increases in velocity to over 4 m/sec, consistent with a gradient of at least 65 mm Hg.

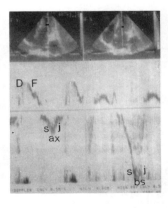

FIGURE 28.57 Dynamic subaortic outflow tract obstruction. Pulsed Doppler is used to localize the subaortic jet (sj). The location of the sample volume is shown by the black crosshatch on the line running through the four-chamber views in the upper panels. In the left upper panel, the sample volume is at the papillary muscle level, apical (ax) to the chordae, and intraventricular velocity of the subaortic jet is low. However, when the sample volume is moved basally (bs), below the contact point of the mitral valve with the septum, the subaortic jet suddenly accelerates. The high-velocity subaortic jet has the characteristic late systolic or "horse's tail" configuration, although this is partially obscured by aliasing at peak velocity.

maneuver fails to provoke changes, amyl nitrite inhalation should be applied (see Figs. 28.54 and 28.55). During this provocation, the same recordings are made. It is ideal during any intervention to have someone performing auscultation. If technical problems prevent high-quality tracings the auscultator's observations may be the only clinical data obtained. In some laboratories, a negative amyl nitrite provocation is followed by isoproterenol infusion.[225] When Doppler equipment is available, provocations are accompanied by sampling of outflow velocity recordings before and during the intervention.

Restrictive cardiomyopathies are more difficult to diagnose with echocardiography than are hypertrophic or dilated varieties. However, echocardiography may provide important diagnostic clues. The most common restrictive state is the small, stiff heart of diabetes.[226,227] However, in the vast majority of diabetics this abnormality is clinically silent. Detection is by quantitative two-dimensional echocardiography but diabetics differ only minimally from their normal counterparts. Amyloid heart disease is a condition that, although rare, is of considerable clinical importance. The prognosis is poor in those unfortunate individuals with this condition. Echocardiographically, infiltrative amyloid myocardial disease is characterized by increased LV wall thickness and peculiar glittering or scintillating appearance of the myocardium.[228-232] Superficially, amyloid disease can, in fact, resemble simple LV hypertrophy. However, in addition to the thickened, glittering myocardium, contractile function appears nearly normal or mildly depressed and the left atrium is usually enlarged. Integration of these findings with the remainder of the clinical picture (e.g., history of chronic disease, low ECG voltage, neuropathy) allows a rational decision about the final step in the diagnostic process, a gingival, rectal, or myocardial biopsy. Finally, it should be noted that not all amyloid heart disease has typical features. We have seen cases in which the echocardiogram failed to demonstrate increased left ventricular wall thickness, or in which the appearance of the myocardium made differentiation between simple LV hypertrophy and infiltrative cardiomyopathy very difficult. Endomyocardial fibrosis is a disease of North Africa and South America associated with restriction of left ventricular and right ventricular filling by obliteration of one or both cardiac apices by a thrombotic fibrocalcific process.[233] Its recognition depends on a high level of clinical suspicion and characteristic echocardiographic appearance (see Fig. 28.35). In restrictive cardiomyopathy, Doppler evaluation of mitral inflow characteristically shows an elevated early diastolic velocity, a short deceleration time, and a relatively low and abbreviated atrial flow velocity.[234]

FUNCTIONAL EVALUATION WITH STRESS TESTING

Although many patients with heart disease complain of symptoms only during exertion, cardiac investigations are usually performed at rest. Since echocardiography allows for dynamic evaluation of cardiac function during exercise, this test has rapidly become a useful diagnostic tool. Exercise two-dimensional imaging is used primarily to detect the presence and extent of coronary artery disease, whereas exercise Doppler of aortic, mitral, and tricuspid valves is used to evaluate global left ventricular systolic and diastolic function, valvular function, and pulmonary artery pressure.

EXERCISE TWO-DIMENSIONAL ECHOCARDIOGRAPHY. The goal of exercise two-dimensional echocardiography is to detect changes in left ventricular function and wall motion at rest and during peak exercise. Detection of segmental left ventricular dysfunction is useful in the diagnosis and localization of obstructive coronary artery disease. Since the normal left ventricle becomes hypercontractile during exercise, the development of reversible dyssynergy, decreased wall thickening, decreased left ventricular ejection fraction, or increased left ventricular end-systolic volume during exercise can indicate hemodynamically significant atherosclerotic coronary disease supplying the abnormal segments.

Due to improvements in echocardiographic equipment, the technical quality and popularity of this procedure has increased over the past decade.[235-239] Technically satisfactory studies can now usually be obtained in 75% to 90% of patients. Use of slow-motion bidirectional video playback units and digitized cine-loop display systems have also helped to improve offline analysis and detection of endocardial motion. Successful studies have been performed using upright treadmill, upright bicycle, supine bicycle exercise, continuous or immediate post-exercise echocardiographic monitoring, and a variety of standard echocardiographic views, including apical, parasternal, and subcostal. Due to tachypnea and tachycardia that develop at peak exercise, the heart may frequently be visible for only one or two beats at end-expiration. However, the ischemic wall motion abnormalities induced by exercise usually persist for some time after peak exercise. The apical views have also often been noted to produce a better image at peak exercise than at rest.

Advantages of exercise echocardiography relative to other diagnostic techniques include noninvasive imaging, lack of exposure to contrast agents or radiation, portability, versatility, multiple viewing planes, ability to assess wall thickening, repeatability after therapeutic interventions (such as coronary angioplasty), low expense, immediate results, and evaluation of a large number of cycles in real time throughout exercise. The widespread availability of echocardiography makes the technique accessible to small hospitals or clinics, where nuclear medicine facilities may not be available. Disadvantages of the technique include the need for a skilled operator, inability to detect all ischemic beds in multivessel coronary artery disease, and technical difficulties in muscular, obese, or emphysematous patients.

The value of exercise two-dimensional echocardiography has been validated by comparison with coronary angiography and other noninvasive techniques. Reversible areas of segmental left ventricular dyssynergy diagnosed by exercise two-dimensional imaging correlate with reversible perfusion defects identified by exercise thallium-201 perfusion scanning.[235] In addition, the sensitivity and specificity of exercise echocardiography for the diagnosis of coronary artery disease compare favorably with exercise electrocardiography, thallium-201 perfusion scanning, and radionuclide ventriculography.[237-239] Exercise echocardiography can also be helpful in predicting occurrence of adverse cardiac events after myocardial infarction.[240] The test should be considered for patients with an abnormal baseline electocardiogram, orthostatic or hyperventilation-induced electrocardiographic changes, nonspecific ST-segment and T-wave abnormalities due to drug effect, ventricular hypertrophy, or a previous nondiagnostic routine treadmill test.[237] In order to apply this diagnostic method to patients who cannot exercise, pharmacologic interventions utilizing dipyridamole, dobutamine, or adenosine infusions have been developed.

EXERCISE DOPPLER. Doppler echocardiography is widely used to assess flows and pressure gradients across heart valves. Because Doppler displays instantaneous changes in these parameters, it is an excellent technique for the study of physiologic and therapeutic interventions. Since the diameter of the aortic valve increases only minimally during exercise, integration on the continuous-wave aortic Doppler signal (flow-velocity integral) throughout exercise allows for a beat-to-beat estimation of forward left ventricular stroke volume; cardiac output can be estimated as the product of heart rate and flow velocity integral.[241-245] In addition, peak acceleration of the aortic Doppler signal correlates with left ventricular ejection fraction and has been used as an index of global left ventricular performance.[241,242] In some patients who have technically inadequate two-dimensional echocardiographic images, satisfactory aortic Doppler tracings from the ascending aorta may still be obtained from the suprasternal notch window.[243]

In young, healthy subjects, aortic flow velocity and aortic acceleration increase progressively with exercise, whereas in patients with multivessel coronary artery disease the increase in these parameters is often blunted and correlates with exaggerated increases in pulmonary artery wedge pressure.[244] However, blunted increases in peak aortic velocity and acceleration during exercise are also common in normal elderly patients or those treated with propranolol.[245,246] In children with valvar aortic stenosis, a prominent increase in peak transaortic velocity by continuous-wave Doppler during exercise suggests a critical lesion.[247]

Doppler analysis of mitral valve flow during exercise may also be helpful in evaluating patients with ischemic and valvular heart disease. Similar to aortic valve flow, a blunted increase in mean mitral flow velocity during exercise occurs in patients with stress-induced ischemia; this phenomenon may be secondary to changes in left ventricular compliance.[248] The development of mitral regurgitation by color Doppler during exercise also suggests multivessel coronary artery disease.[249] In patients with mitral stenosis, a marked and early rise in the transmitral gradient during exercise by continuous-wave Doppler echocardiography indicates hemodynamically significant stenosis.

Continuous-wave Doppler echocardiography also permits the calculation of pulmonary artery systolic pressure at rest and during exercise by evaluation of tricuspid regurgitation[250] (Fig. 28.58). Technically suboptimal right heart Doppler signals can usually be improved by the intravenous injection of agitated saline. In patients with chronic pulmonary disease, a rapid and exaggerated rise in pulmonary artery systolic pressure during exercise suggests pulmonary vascular disease.

Finally, one of the greatest advantages of exercise echocardiography is versatility. A skilled exercise technician may combine the two-dimensional imaging and the Doppler evaluations in one or more views to follow ventricular function, cardiac output, valvular gradients, and pulmonary artery systolic pressure throughout graded exercise. For example, in the presence of reversible left ventricular dyssynergy by two-dimensional echocardiography, the development of mitral regurgitation at peak exercise or the lack of increase in peak Doppler aortic flow velocity during exercise would suggest left main or multivessel coronary artery disease. Also, in the investigation of dyspnea on exertion in a 60-year-old patient with known rheumatic mitral stenosis, rapid increases in transmitral and pulmonary artery systolic pressures during exercise would indicate hemodynamically significant mitral valve disease, while reversible dyssynergy would indicate associated atherosclerotic coronary disease.

TRANSESOPHAGEAL ECHOCARDIOGRAPHY

The esophagus provides an airless posterior ultrasonic window to the heart from directly behind the left atrium. In order to circumvent the chest wall, ribs, and lungs, a miniature phased-array transducer is placed at the tip of the housing of a flexible gastroscope from which the optics have been removed.[251-253] The ultrasound beam is steerable, in that the scope can be advanced, withdrawn, or rotated within the esophagus, and the angle formed by the transducer and the esophagus can be slightly altered by manipulation of the anterior-posterior and lateral flexion controls. Commercially available transesophageal echocardiography systems provide high-resolution M-mode and two-dimensional imaging, pulsed-wave Doppler, and color-flow Doppler; newer features may include biplane imaging and continuous-wave Doppler.

Transesophageal echocardiography can be performed easily and quickly in a variety of clinical settings, including the ambulatory clinic, the operating room, and the intensive care unit. The test has an excellent safety record with no known deaths or esophageal perforations; the only major complication reported has been transient recurrent laryngeal nerve paralysis in two neurosurgical patients who were studied intraoperatively in the sitting-cervical neck flexion position.[254] Minor complications have included atrial and ventricular arrhythmias, vasovagal reactions, transient bronchospasm and hypoxemia, and minor bleeding. Relative contraindications include a history of dysphagia, prior mediastinal irradiation, esophageal pathology or surgery, coagulopathy, or active upper gastrointestinal bleeding.

Local anesthesia of the hypopharynx is achieved by having the patient gargle and swallow dilute viscous lidocaine. After the gag reflex is suppressed, the patient is placed in the left lateral recumbent position. The unlocked esophageal probe is introduced into the esophagus after endotracheal intubation and, if necessary, systemic sedation; a bite block is placed to protect both the probe and the teeth. For ambulatory studies, patients should be instructed to fast for at least 4 hours. Systemic sedation can often be avoided, but is used selectively. Intermittent suctioning of secretions is performed as needed, and vital signs and rhythm are monitored throughout the procedure. In unstable patients or those with respiratory problems, oxygen saturation is also monitored by oximeter and resuscitation equipment is kept immediately accessible.

Standard transesophageal views include the four-chamber view through the left atrium (usually obtained at about 35 to 40 cm from the incisors), short-axis views of the cardiac base through the left atrium (allows imaging of the aortic valve and surrounding structures), and short-axis view of the left ventricle (usually obtained at about 40 to 45 cm, just beyond the gastroesophageal junction). Short- and long-axis

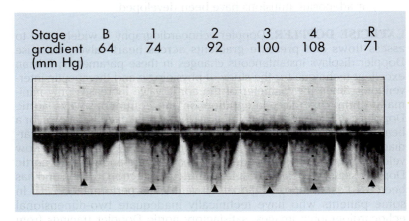

FIGURE 28.58 Representative single-beat contrast-enhanced Doppler recordings of tricuspid insufficiency at baseline (B), at the end of each stage of supine bicycle exercise (1 to 4), and at 4 minutes of recovery (R). During exercise, the width of the Doppler signal progressively decreases as heart rate increases and the maximum tricuspid insufficiency velocity increases (small black arrows). Maximum transtricuspid gradients by the modified Bernoulli equation (in mm Hg) are indicated at the top of the figure.

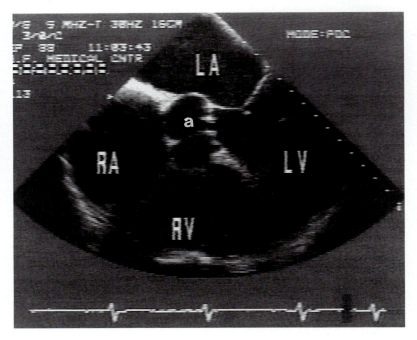

FIGURE 28.59 Standard orientation of transesophageal echocardiography. The left atrium (LA) is at the top of the screen, and the left ventricle (LV) is to the viewer's right. The aortic valve is clearly seen (a, aortic valve; RA, right atrium; RV, right ventricle)

views of the aorta can also be performed. The standard orientation (Fig. 28.59) displays the four-chamber view with the apex down and the left ventricle to the viewer's right.[255,256]

The most common indications for transesophageal echocardiography include inadequate transthoracic image, intraoperative monitoring of the left ventricle, examination for aortic pathology, left atrial thrombi and tumors, prosthetic valve regurgitation or endocarditis, and native valve disruption, vegetation, or ring abscess. Since the data obtained from transthoracic and transesophageal imaging are complementary, it is customary to perform transthoracic imaging prior to transesophageal imaging.

Transesophageal echocardiography is useful in the cardiac evaluation of patients who have technically inadequate transthoracic echocardiograms. Often such patients are obese, mechanically ventilated, or recovering from cardiothoracic surgery in the intensive care unit. For example, in a patient who develops hypotension after coronary artery bypass surgery, it may be difficult to perform precordial imaging, due to the presence of mediastinal blood and air, chest bandages, drainage tubes, positive pressure ventilation, and decreased patient mobility. However, transesophageal echocardiography can be performed at the bedside in these patients to identify cardiac tamponade, hypovolemia, or left ventricular dysfunction.[257-259]

Transesophageal echocardiography is also an important tool for the intraoperative assessment of left ventricular size, function, and wall motion in high-risk cardiac patients, including elderly patients and those with coronary artery disease or depressed left ventricular function[260-268] (Fig. 28.60). In our institution, intraoperative transesophageal monitoring has been most useful for patients undergoing coronary artery bypass or major peripheral vascular surgery. Advantages of this relatively noninvasive technique for intraoperative monitoring include rapidity of preparation, continuous evaluation, high resolution, removal from the operative field, and ease of interpretation. The short axis view of the left ventricle at the papillary muscle level provides a stable image that is convenient for long-term monitoring. Off-line digitized cine-loop display systems permit comparisons of ventricular size and segmental wall motion before and after various anesthetic and surgical procedures (i.e., induction of anesthesia, skin incision, pericardial incision, cross-clamp of the aorta, coronary artery grafting, and valve replacement) and allow for timely therapeutic interventions (i.e., administration of fluids for hypovolemia or intravenous nitroglycerine for ischemic wall motion abnormalities). Moreover, transesophageal echocardiography is more sensitive than electrocardiography for the detection of ischemia,[265] may be superior to the pulmonary artery wedge pressure as a guide to preload,[262] and readily detects intracardiac air embolism during upright neurosurgical procedures or open heart surgery.[269,270]

Transesophageal echocardiography is rapidly emerging as one of the diagnostic methods of choice for the evaluation of aortic dissection. Transesophageal imaging can be performed rapidly in the intensive care unit or emergency room to detect the extent of dissection, the site of intimal flaps, and complications such as aortic insufficiency and pericardial tamponade.[271,272] Technical factors may make it difficult to visualize pathology at the top of the aortic arch; the recent introduction of biplane instruments promises to improve access to this area. Despite this problem, the sensitivity and specificity of the technique compare favorably with those of angiography, computed tomography, and magnetic resonance imaging.

Due to the location of the transducer directly behind the left atrium, transesophageal imaging is far more powerful than transthoracic imaging for the detection of left atrial thrombus and tumor. This technique has become useful in the evaluation of patients who have emboli of unknown origin; the finding of thrombus in the body or appendage of the left atrium is an indication for long-term anticoagulation (Fig. 28.61).[273,274] By transesophageal echocardiography, patients with severe mitral stenosis often have markedly enlarged left atria, atrial fibrillation, spontaneous contrast, and a tendency to form left atrial thrombus. Since atrial thrombus can be fragmented or dislodged during catheter manipulations, we choose to refer patients with severe mitral stenosis associated with atrial thrombus for surgical therapy (open commissurotomy or valve replacement) rather than balloon valvuloplasty. For patients with atrial myxomas and other cardiac tumors, transesophageal echocardiography can be helpful in the determination of the site(s) of attachment, number, size, internal architecture, and friability (Figs. 28.62 and 28.63).[275]

The ultrasound shadowing that occurs behind mitral and aortic valve prostheses during transthoracic echocardiography often hinders adequate evaluation for prosthetic valve dysfunction (Fig. 28.64). However, transesophageal echocardiography provides a posterior approach to these structures, and thus allows for detection, localization, and semi-quantitation of prosthetic regurgitation. In patients with prosthetic mitral valves, transesophageal echocardiography with color-flow Doppler permits the differentiation between a normal "seating-puff" and pathologic regurgitation, and between valvular and perivalvular leaks[276,277] (Fig. 28.65). This technique also helps to determine the severity of mitral regurgitation; jets that occupy a large volume of the left atrium and penetrate into the left atrial appendage or pulmonary veins are usually hemodynamically severe. Note that it is our practice to administer prophylactic intravenous antibiotics to all patients with prosthetic valves (also for patients with other major indications for prophylaxis) who undergo this procedure.[278]

Transesophageal echocardiography is also useful in the evaluation of native heart valve dysfunction. In patients with endocarditis, this technique is more sensitive than transthoracic echocardiography in the detection of vegetations, ring abscesses, and fistulae[279,280] (Fig. 28.66). Precise visualization of valvular morphology and function can also enhance the preoperative assessment of mitral regurgitation. The demonstration of ruptured chordae tendineae (Fig. 28.67) or perforated valve leaflets makes mitral valve repair an excellent possibility for the cardiac surgeon, while the presence of subvalvular calcification or significant anterior mitral leaflet disease suggests that valve replacement would be more appropriate.[281-283] Furthermore, after valve repair is attempted, intraoperative transesophageal color-flow imaging provides information on the amount of residual mitral regurgitation.

Transesophageal echocardiography is valuable in the assessment

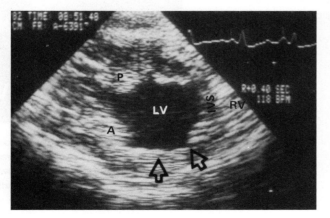

FIGURE 28.60 Intraoperative transesophageal echocardiography of the left ventricle. Short axis view of the left ventricle obtained during surgery through a transesophageal transducer. Since imaging is from behind the heart, the posterior wall and posterior medial papillary muscle (P) are at the top of the image and the anterior wall and anterolateral papillary muscle (A) are at the bottom. The arrows point to the anterior wall and its junction with the interventricular septum (IVS). During real-time examination this area was observed to have lost its normal systolic thickening, raising the possibility of intraoperative ischemia or infarction.

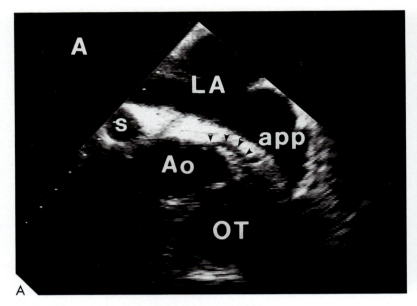
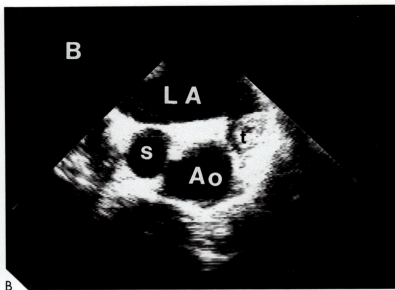

FIGURE 28.61 A. Transesophageal echocardiogram of the left atrium (LA) and left atrial appendage (app) in a normal patient. The left main coronary artery (black arrows) and its bifurcation into the left anterior descending and left circumflex coronary arteries are also noted. (Ao, aortic valve; OT, right ventricle outflow tract; s, superior vena cava) **B.** Transesophageal echocardiogram in a patient with a left atrial appendage thrombus (t).

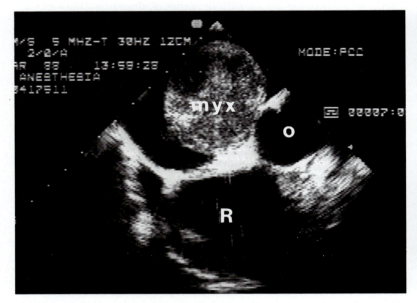
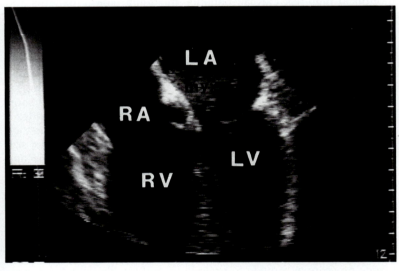

FIGURE 28.62 Intraoperative transesophageal echocardiogram demonstrating a large left atrial myxoma (myx) that is attached to the interatrial septum near the aortic valve (o). Note the multicystic internal architecture of the myxoma and the "rain-like" artifact caused by the bovie. (R, right atrium)

FIGURE 28.63 Transesophageal echocardiogram of a left atrial myxoma (myx). Compared to the pedunculated, spherical tumor in Figure 28.62, this myxoma is triangular and sessile, with a wide-based attachment to the interatrial septum. (LA, left atrium; LV, left ventricle; RA, right atrium; RV, right ventricle)

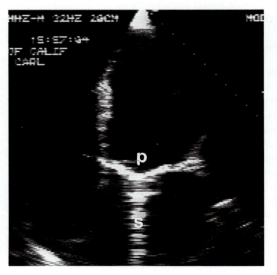

FIGURE 28.64 Apical four-chamber view of a mitral valve prosthesis (p) that causes ultrasound reverberation artifact (s) and adjacent shadowing of the left atrium; this creates difficulty in the detection of mitral regurgitation in the left atrium.

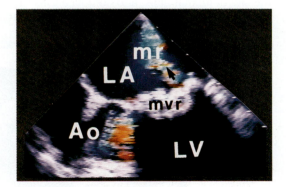

FIGURE 28.65 Transesophageal echocardiogram demonstrating paravalvular mitral regurgitation (mr, arrow) emanating from the sewing ring of a tilting-disc prosthesis (mvr). (Ao, aortic valve; LA, left atrium; LV, left ventricle)

of adults with congenital heart disease.[284,285] In atrial and ventricular septal defects, the number and location, anatomic size, and hemodynamic severity of shunts can be determined by high-resolution transesophageal imaging and color-flow Doppler (Fig. 28.68). As with mitral valve surgery, the adequacy of surgical repair of these lesions can be evaluated intraoperatively.

Finally, because of its high resolution imaging of the aortic root, transesophageal echocardiography permits identification of the proximal left and right coronary arteries in nearly all patients. Preliminary research suggests a possible role in the detection or exclusion of stenoses in the left main, proximal left anterior descending, and left circumflex coronary arteries by direct visualization of the lesion or detection of abnormal color-flow signals arising from such stenoses (see Fig. 28.61A).[286-288]

EVALUATION OF THE RIGHT VENTRICLE

Imaging the RV is an essential and highly informative portion of a comprehensive echocardiographic evaluation. Often, patients clinically suspected of having a left heart abnormality will, on echocardiographic examination, prove to have a condition affecting the right ventricle or arising in it. For example, the insidious course of primary pulmonary hypertension may lead a patient to consult a physician for progressive dyspnea. In the course of clinical evaluation, cardiomegaly on chest x-ray film may lead to echocardiography where the typical findings of cor pulmonale provide the diagnosis. In general, clinical surprises more commonly arise from right heart echocardiographic findings than from left. In patients with emphysema, echocardiography with Doppler is more sensitive in the diagnosis of cor pulmonale than the traditional clinical evaluation (physical examination, chest radiograph, and electrocardiography).[289]

ASSESSMENT OF RIGHT VENTRICULAR CONTRACTILE FUNCTION, VOLUME, AND WALL THICKNESS

The shape of the RV makes quantitation of its function and volume difficult. The LV, by contrast, has an elliptical shape and is readily modeled; its volume can be derived from relatively few dimensions. The shape of the RV has been described as a pyramid with a triangular base. However, this description fails to take into account its crescentic shape in cross-section or its outflow tract. The tomographic nature of echocardiography makes imaging this irregularly shaped organ in an encompassing plane impossible.

A number of authors have attempted to measure the size of the RV, but no method has gained wide acceptance.[290-300] In our laboratory we rely on two rather simple, qualitative approaches. The first is to inspect the standard M-mode of the RV and LV. If the RV exceeds 2.5 cm at the LV minor axis level, RV enlargement is suspected (Fig. 28.69).[301] The second is the inspection of two two-dimensional views of the chamber. The first view is the short axis through the LV minor axis. Usually, the left ventricle appears as the dominant chamber and the RV as a rather small anteriorly surrounding crescent (see Fig. 28.9). RV dilation can be strongly suspected if the RV appears to have parity to or exceed the LV in size (Fig. 28.70). Once RV dilation is suspected, particular attention is paid to the apical four-chamber view, where, in the normal heart, the LV forms the cardiac apex (see Fig. 28.13). If the RV forms or even shares the apex, RV dilation is suspected. In frank RV enlargement, the RV appears to dominate the left; in extreme cases, the LV

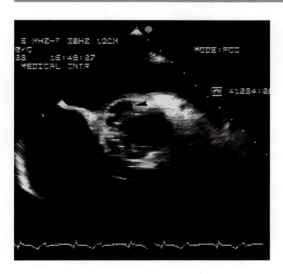

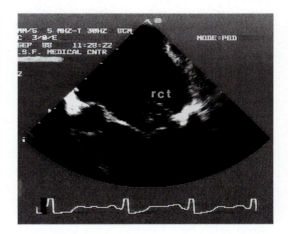

FIGURE 28.66 Transesophageal echocardiogram showing a bacterial abscess involving an aortic prosthesis. The necrotic spaces in the abscess are evident (*black arrow*) and can potentially rupture into adjacent chambers to create fistulae.

FIGURE 28.67 Transesophageal echocardiogram of a patient who has a flail posterior mitral leaflet due to ruptured chordae tendineae (*rct*). The latter is clearly visualized.

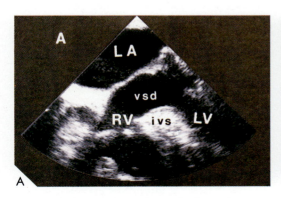
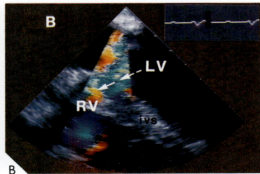
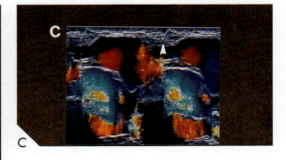

FIGURE 28.68 A. Transesophageal echocardiogram of a ventricular septal defect (*vsd*). (*ivs*, interventricular septum; *LA*, left atrium; *LV*, left ventricle; *RV*, right ventricle) **B.** Color flow demonstrates left-to-right blue flow across the defect during systole (*arrows*). **C.** Color-flow M-mode and electrocardiogram indicate that the blue flow occurs in systole, after the QRS complex (*arrow*).

appears slit-like (Fig. 28.71). Skill in performing echocardiographic examinations is required in order to avoid confusing an enlarged RV for an LV. Finally, if confusion about RV size results from the precordial short axis or apical four-chamber views, attention should be directed to the subcostal view. In our experience, this view is less likely to produce a false positive impression of RV enlargement.

RV contractile function is most commonly assessed by direct visual inspection. Since the wall of the RV is thinner, careful adjustments of instrument gain and reject settings and judicious selection of transducers may be needed to accurately detect RV inward systolic motion or wall thickening. In this application, M-mode is less useful, because most M-mode images center on the RV outflow tract region where inward motion of the wall may not be representative of the entire chamber. An M-mode taken from the subcostal view is one of the best ways of inspecting RV wall motion and of measuring RV wall thickness. Studies in which a variety of quantitative methods have been used report good correlations between these and the results of blood pool scintigraphy.[293,302] While it is always possible to identify severe RV dysfunction, difficulties may be encountered in identification of subtle degrees of RV dysfunction. Evaluation of RV wall thickness is difficult; the main difficulty lies in the numerous trabeculations and bands found in that chamber and the ambiguity they introduce into the M-mode tracing. With definition of the RV endocardium being vague, measurement of a thin structure is problematic. We consider right ventricular hypertrophy (RVH) present when the RV wall exceeds 0.5 cm in thickness.

SEGMENTAL ABNORMALITIES OF THE RIGHT VENTRICLE

The most important and common segmental RV abnormality results from right ventricular infarction. Almost all RV infarctions are seen in the setting of inferior wall myocardial infarction. Typically, the M-mode in RV infarction shows an enlarged RV.[303] Since the M-mode is taken at or near the outflow tract, the segmental RV wall motion changes appreciated on two-dimensional examination are not seen. On two-dimensional examination, the right ventricle appears dilated and portions of the anterior mid-wall and inferior RV wall may appear akinetic or even aneurysmal; a hinge point may demonstrate infarcted from normal segments (Fig. 28.72). The first clue to the presence of RV infarction may come in the short axis view where the distinctive akinesis of contiguous walls of the RV, inferior septum, and inferoposterior LV walls are seen. Inspection of the right ventricle in the apical four-chamber view will reveal not only RV dilation but may also show segmental mid-wall dyskinesis and remodeling. A clue to the hemodynamic severity of the process is provided by the degree of RV dilation and also by the degree of inferior vena caval plethora. This latter

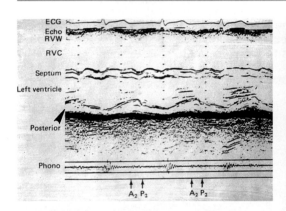

FIGURE 28.69 Right ventricular volume overload. An M-mode taken through the minor axis of the left ventricle in a patient with an atrial septal defect shows the typical appearance of right ventricular volume overload from any cause. In this example the right ventricle (RVC) is greater than 2.5 cm in diameter (~4 cm), the septum is flat (if not "paradoxical"), the left ventricle is small, and the phonocardiogram (Phono) shows a widely split second heart sound. (Posterior, posterior wall; RVW, right ventricular anterior wall)

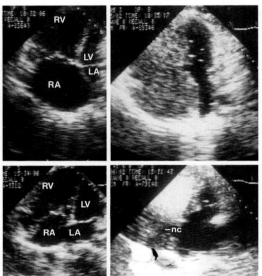

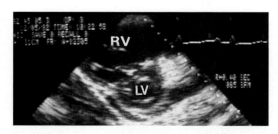

FIGURE 28.70 Right ventricular volume overload. Short axis two-dimensional view of the left (LV) and right (RV) ventricles in a patient with severe volume overload of the right ventricle. Note the relative disparity of the small LV when compared to the large RV. Note also the apparent flattening of the LV interventricular septum. This image is the counterpart of the M-mode depicted in Figure 28.69.

FIGURE 28.71 Right ventricular volume overload. Apical four-chamber views from two patients with right ventricular (RV) volume overloads of different origins. In the upper panel, the patient has end-stage primary pulmonary hypertension with associated tricuspid insufficiency. Note the large apex-forming RV, large right atrium (RA), and diminutive left ventricle (LV) and atrium (LA). Contrast is injected intravenously and results in opacification of the RA and RV. Four bubbles are seen in the LV, presumably having crossed a small patent foramen ovale. Note the bulge of the interatrial septum from right to left. Lower panels depict a superficially similar four-chamber view from a patient with a large left-to-right shunt at the level of the atrial septum. Here too the RV is apex-forming but the RV, although large, is not as large as in the example in the upper panels. Furthermore, the septum, if anything, is bulging from left to right or is in the neutral position. Contrast injection also shows a small number of contrast elements or bubbles entering the left side but, more importantly, there is a prominent negative contrast effect (nc) into the RA that not only proves the left-to-right passage of unopacified atrial blood into the contrast-filled RA but roughly outlines the size of the atrial septal defect.

structure provides information that is analogous to inspection of the jugular venous pulse but probably more reliable.[304–306] It has been our experience that when RV infarction is clinically suspected, an echocardiogram provides a rapid and reliable means of confirming this impression. The echographic study can also provide some clue to the hemodynamic importance of the process.[307–311] Chagas' disease is another process that can affect the right ventricle in a segmental fashion (see Figs. 28.50 and 28.51). In contrast to myocardial infarction, this chronic protozoan infection produces its most intense abnormality in the RV and LV apex. In half of the cases, a generalized cardiomyopathy is seen, difficult to distinguish from any other type of dilated cardiomyopathy.[204] Endocardial fibrosis (with or without eosinophilia) can also segmentally affect the apical regions of the RV. Like Chagas' disease, this condition is usually only suspected in specific geographic locations (Fig. 28.73).[126]

RIGHT VENTRICULAR MASSES

Right ventricular masses can be primary processes or metastases. For example, a mass may represent a primary, locally arising myxoma or a metastatic malignant melanoma.[312] Generally, the same masses that affect the LV can also involve the RV. Malignant processes detected by echocardiography are highly reflective of ultrasound and present a dramatic echocardiogram. It is generally impossible to differentiate one mass from another but it is often possible to deduce their origin from the clinical setting. If, however, the acoustic nature and image of a given mass fail to reveal its histology, other echocardiographic clues such as its motion pattern might. Among the wide variety of rare tumors, myxomas are probably the most common benign primary variety. Metastatic malignant tumors seem to represent one-of-a-kind situations. For example, malignant melanoma[312] and liposarcoma[88] have been encountered recently. Tumors and masses propagating along the venae cavae from distant organs are a unique feature of the right ventricle and right atrium. Hepatoma is perhaps the most common of these intracardiac masses but renal and adrenal tumors can also present in this manner. A malignant thymoma may travel down the superior vena cava and obstruct right ventricular flow. Perhaps the most important of the masses that propagate up the inferior vena cava (IVC) are thrombi arising in the lower extremities. Improved resolution of echocardiographic instruments and better training among practitioners have led to a spate of reports dealing with sightings of emboli in transit.[313–333] At times, these emboli become attached to portions of the RV and present as a localized mobile mass. Ultrasonically, these masses are not as bright as their malignant counterparts. Once these masses become impacted in the right ventricle or across the tricuspid valve, they can either go on and complete their itinerary as pulmonary emboli or the atrial portion can break off and paradoxically cross the foramen ovale.[334,335] In all cases where a right heart thrombus is identified and in most cases of pulmonary embolism we recommend that a small bolus of agitated saline be given intravenously during echocardiography. Appearance of microbubble contrast targets on the left is evidence of a patent foramen ovale and of a potential route for the paradoxical passage of thrombotic material into the systemic circulation. Regardless of which of the two routes these structures take, the echocardiographer must be aware that they have an ominous prognosis and require aggressive medical or surgical intervention.

THE RIGHT VENTRICLE IN CARDIOMYOPATHY

Primary myocardial disease isolated to the right ventricle is rarely recognized echocardiographically. However, in LV cardiomyopathy the right ventricle may or may not be abnormal. In our experience, patients in whom right ventricular involvement is as severe as left ventricular involvement have a more malignant clinical course. In some with cardiomyopathy, there inexplicably appears to be almost complete sparing of the right ventricle. In those in whom the right ventricle becomes significantly dilated and hypocontractile the echocardiogram cannot determine whether the right ventricle is involved with the same myocardial process as the left or has failed because of secondary pulmonary hypertension.

CONDITIONS ASSOCIATED WITH RIGHT VENTRICULAR DILATION

The right ventricle dilates in response to a number of situations and conditions. It is often difficult to separate these without knowledge of the clinical setting. Some of these conditions have, however, characteristics that permit echocardiographic separation. Right ventricular volume overloads without pulmonary hypertension are seen in atrial septal defect, tricuspid insufficiency, and pulmonary insufficiency. In all of these situations, the right ventricle can become enlarged, forming the cardiac apex, while the LV appears, by comparison, small (Figs. 28.71 and 28.72). Right ventricular contractile function is usually pre-

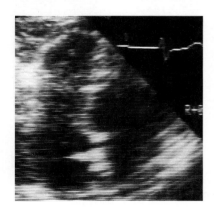
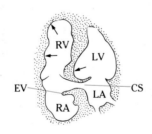

FIGURE 28.72 Right ventricular infarction. Another cause of right ventricular dilation is right ventricular infarction. This condition is distinguished from the others by a history of recent inferior wall left ventricular (*LV*) infarction. Note in this example that the RV is apex-forming. However, unlike the other cases (Fig. 28.71) of RV volume overload, real-time imaging showed dyskinesis at the arrows. Furthermore, there is remodeling or diastolic deformity of the inferior interventricular septum (*single LV arrow*). This image was taken with the proper inferior angulation to detect an abnormality in the inferior septum. Inferior angulation of the four-chamber view is documented when the coronary sinus (*cs*) and eustacian valve (*EV*) are imaged at the base of the heart. The cavity labeled *RA* probably represents the mouth of the inferior vena cava as it enters the RA.

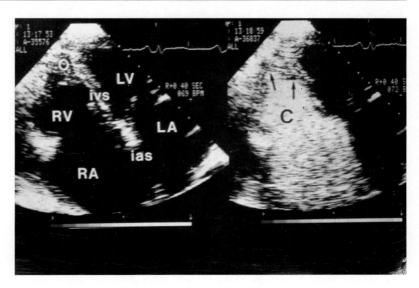

FIGURE 28.73 Endomyocardial fibrosis of the right ventricle. Another cause of segmental abnormality of the apical region of the right ventricle is endomyocardial fibrosis. In this example, the disease, often bilateral, is limited to the right ventricular apex. The characteristic apical obliteration (O) is shown and highlighted by contrast injection (*right panel*). (*ivs*, interventricular septum; *ias*, interatrial septum) (Courtesy of Dr. Harry Acquatella, Caracas, Venezuela)

served and right ventricular wall thickness remains normal. Atrial septal defect differs from valvular insufficiency in that the pulmonary artery is enlarged (Figs. 28.74 and 28.75). In our laboratory, we make a practice of evaluating the right pulmonary artery from the suprasternal window (see Fig. 28.75). The finding of a small or normal right pulmonary artery (*i.e.*, one that is smaller than the aortic arch) is rather strong evidence against a significant left-to-right shunt. Further evidence of an atrial septal defect can be obtained by performing contrast echocardiography by means of the injection of agitated saline solution into a peripheral arm vein. In atrial septal defect, a negative contrast jet[336] can be appreciated, replacing contrast-laden atrial blood with unopacified left atrial blood (Fig. 28.76). In these patients, a small amount of right-to-left shunting can also be appreciated. Imaging the defect directly is often difficult due to artifacts that occur in the echogram of the atrial septum. However, at times the defect itself can be seen. Similarly, Doppler detection of abnormal flow across the defect can also be difficult. In our hands the main value of conventional Doppler is in the evaluation of pulmonary pressure. This evaluation can be performed if

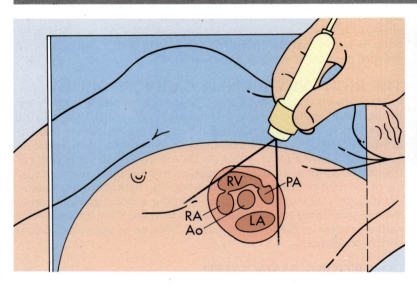
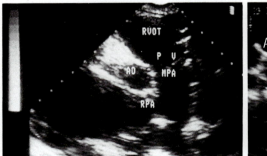
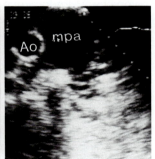

FIGURE 28.74 Main pulmonary artery dilation. Evaluation of the main pulmonary artery (*mpa*) and its branches, the right pulmonary artery (*RPA*), and the left pulmonary artery is an important echocardiographic maneuver in the evaluation of conditions associated with RV dilation. In the upper portion of the illustration, the technique for examination of the main pulmonary artery is shown. Essentially, one obtains a short axis slice through the cardiac base with slight left anterior angulation. In most patients, the pulmonic valve medial leaflet (*PV*) can be imaged in continuity with the right ventricular outflow tract (*RVOT*) and contiguous medially with the aortic root (*Ao*).

Although it is sometimes difficult to image the lateral wall of the vessel, a comparison between the diameter of the main pulmonary artery and the aortic root is the best guide to main pulmonary artery dilation. In the lower left panel is a normal study showing relative parity between the aortic root and main pulmonary artery diameters. In the lower right, a patient with an atrial septal defect shows a main pulmonary artery considerably larger than the aortic root. This window or imaging plane is also very useful for Doppler examination of pulmonary artery flow.

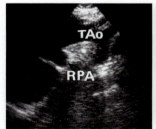
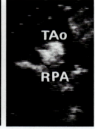
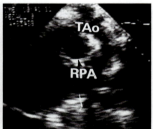
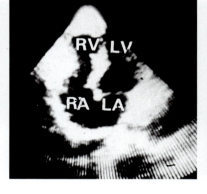
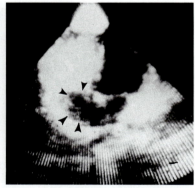

FIGURE 28.75 Right pulmonary dilation in volume overload. Imaging the aortic arch (ascending, transverse [*TAo*], and descending) from the suprasternal notch should be a standard part of every echocardiographic examination. In these three examples, the right pulmonary artery (*RPA*), when compared to the diameter of the transverse aortic arch, provides valuable information about the differential diagnosis of right ventricular enlargement. In the example on the right, the patient had a small ventricular septal defect and borderline normal right ventricular size on echocardiography. The right pulmonary artery is smaller than the transverse aortic arch and, therefore, indicative of a very small left-to-right shunt. In the middle example, a teenage girl with Ebstein's anomaly of the tricuspid valve, the large right atrium is associated with a smaller than normal right pulmonary artery, confirming the reduced pulmonary flow resulting from decreased functional volume of the right ventricle, tricuspid regurgitation, and right-to-left shunt across the atrial septum. In the example at the right, the right pulmonary artery is considerably enlarged, confirming that the atrial septal defect detected in other parts of the examination is likely to be associated with a large left-to-right shunt.

FIGURE 28.76 Demonstration of left-to-right shunt with contrast. In the four-chamber view to the left, there was only mild right ventricular (*RV*) enlargement in that the RV and left ventricle (*LV*) shared the cardiac apex. Contrast injection (*right panel*) revealed that there was a strong jet of unopacified blood passing from left to right (*arrows*). This finding led to performance of a scintigraphic shunt study, revealing a moderate-sized atrial septal defect (>2:1).

there is a small amount of tricuspid regurgitation present. In most patients with atrial septal defect and in a high percentage of the population, this functional valvular leak is present. Detection of the peak retrograde systolic velocity in the right atrium allows conversion of this parameter to pressure, using the Bernoulli equation below (Fig. 28.77).[8,306,337] Addition of an estimate of right atrium pressure yields a fairly accurate assessment of peak pulmonary systolic pressure. (Fig. 28.78).

The Bernoulli equation, of which the Toricelle portion is expressed

$$P_1 - P_2 = 4 \cdot V_m^2$$

has been modified for Doppler echocardiography by the work of Holen and Hatle. The equation states that the peak pressure gradient across a valve ($P_1 - P_2$) can be determined if the peak velocity of blood flow across the valve (V_m) is known. This equation, although simple, is revolutionary in that it allows calculation of the peak gradient in aortic, pulmonary, mitral, and tricuspid stenoses and regurgitations.

Congenital absence of the pericardium is an example of a condition associated with right ventricular enlargement, which should be separable from atrial septal defect. In this situation[338,339] the right ventricle appears to be enlarged due to rotation of the heart. The finding of a small pulmonary artery, low pulmonary pressure by Doppler, and normal contrast study should alert the echocardiographer to this condition. Severe tricuspid insufficiency and, rarely, pulmonary insufficiency produce RV enlargement. These conditions should be suspected from the clinical setting. The most common cause of severe tricuspid regurgitation is postcapillary left ventricular dysfunction, although rheumatic disease, endocarditis, and pulmonary hypertension are other commonly encountered causes. Further proof of significant tricuspid insufficiency can be obtained by pulsed-wave Doppler demonstration of a large retrograde tricuspid jet, propagating deeply into the right atrium. Systolic pulsations of the inferior vena cava and retrograde systolic incursion of right atrial saline contrast into the hepatic veins may also serve to confirm this diagnosis.[340,341] In severe primary valvular regurgitation, pulmonary pressure should remain normal unless pulmonary hypertension (primary or post-capillary) is the underlying cause. Combined volume and pressure overloads also present echocardiographic pictures that are difficult to separate from one another.

In chronic pulmonary disease, elevated pulmonary vascular resistance leads to right heart failure. This syndrome, known as cor pulmonale, presents echocardiographically as a dilated, apex-forming right ventricle. The degree of right ventricular hypertrophy is variable but is usually mild to moderate. If the patient is untreated, the inferior vena cava will be dilated and unresponsive to respiration and the pulmonary artery dilated as well. If the foramen ovale is not patent, a contrast study will rule out a right-to-left shunt. If, however, the patient is one of 20% to 30% of individuals with a probe or pencil patent foramen ovale, contrast will enter the left ventricle readily. In this circumstance, the picture will resemble an atrial septal defect. However, the absence of a negative contrast jet, atrial septal drop-out, and the presence of impaired RV function and a plethoric vena cava serve to differentiate these two entities (Fig. 28.79). Finally, the clinical history will usually provide the etiology of the condition. Most commonly, patients will have a history of chronic obstructive lung disease but such diverse entities as chronic pulmonary embolism, cystic fibrosis, bronchiectasis, connective tissue disease, adult respiratory distress syndrome, sarcoid, obesity with sleep apnea, or any chronic pulmonary infection can present an identical cardiac picture. In primary pulmo-

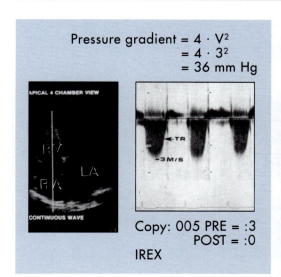

FIGURE 28.77 Calculation of gradient between right ventricle and atrium. In the presence of tricuspid insufficiency a continuous-wave Doppler can be passed from the apex to base across the tricuspid valve and the Doppler shift caused by the tricuspid insufficiency jet (TR) displayed (right). In this example, the peak velocity of the TR jet is 3 m/sec, which, by the Bernoulli equation, represents a 36 mm Hg gradient between right ventricle (RV) and right atrium (RA). If the right atrial pressure is known or can be estimated, the sum of RA pressure and the RA to RV gradient is equal to the peak pulmonary artery pressure (assuming no pulmonic stenosis). Our method for estimating right atrial pressure is shown in Figure 28.78. (Reproduced by permission of Johnson & Johnson Ultrasound Inc.)

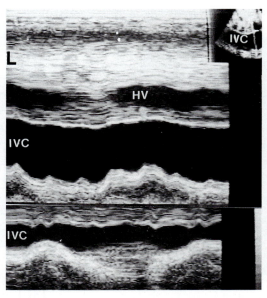

FIGURE 28.78 Inferior vena cava. The inferior vena cava (IVC) can be imaged by aligning the ultrasound beam plane parallel to the long axis of the body and placing the transducer subcostally just to the right of the midline. The resultant two-dimensional image is shown to the upper right of the image. The white line running through the image is the beam plane used to generate the M-modes of the inferior vena cava to the left. In the upper M-mode, the inferior vena cava is dilated and its collapse or narrowing in response to respiration blunted. Also, the hepatic veins (HV) are dilated. In the lower example, the inferior vena cava is of normal size and responds normally to respiration. In patients with inferior vena caval diameter greater than 20 and in whom there is poor response to respiration, the right atrial pressure is usually around 20 mm Hg or greater. In those with small inferior vena caval diameter and good respiratory response, the RA pressure is usually 0 to 5 mm Hg. Using these two inferior vena cava images as examples, the estimated RA to RV pressure gradient in Figure 28.77 would vary widely depending on which of the two inferior vena caval images was found in a patient with a 3 m/sec tricuspid regurgitation jet. For example, if a patient with a 3 m/sec jet had a normal inferior vena cava, the estimated pulmonary peak systolic pressure (RA + RA/RV gradient) would be 36 to 38 mm Hg or minimally elevated. If, on the other hand, the enlarged unresponsive inferior vena cava were encountered, the estimated peak pulmonary artery pressure could be as high as 56 mm Hg or significantly elevated.

nary hypertension, the echocardiographic findings are very similar to those in cor pulmonale. The major difference is that pulmonary hypertension is associated with more severe levels of right ventricular hypertrophy. In the earlier stages of pulmonary hypertension, the degree of hypertrophy and dilation of the right ventricle are considerably greater than the manifestations of RV failure such as vena caval plethora. Pulmonary hypertension resulting from congenital heart disease also has features that cross over with other causes of right heart dilation. In these patients, RVH is severe and findings associated with right heart failure are usually minimal. Of course, it is usually possible to detect the congenital abnormality such as a large ventricular or atrial septal defect. Isolated right ventricular dilation without findings of right heart failure, pulmonary hypertension, or hypertrophy are some of the features of arrhythmogenic right ventricular dysplasia.[342–345] In these patients, the right ventricular wall is very thin (this is also called *parchment ventricle* or *Uhl's disease*), there are often aneurysms of the RV wall, and the patients and their relatives are prone to episodes of ventricular tachycardia arising from the right ventricle. In some patients with this condition we have also noted hyperplastic moderator bands.

ECHOCARDIOGRAPHY OF THE ATRIA
THE LEFT ATRIUM

The left atrium is a roughly pillow-shaped structure that can be easily imaged from a number of echocardiographic windows and views. In fulfilling its function as a reservoir, conduit, and booster pump, the atrium commonly dilates and occasionally becomes compressed. It is also the site of rare neoplasms, most of which are benign, and occasionally gives rise to mural thrombi, some of which embolize. As a consequence of its tendency to become dilated with age, it promotes occurrence of atrial fibrillation.

ECHOCARDIOGRAPHIC ASSESSMENT OF LEFT ATRIAL VOLUME AND FUNCTION

The standard M-mode image of the left atrium (LA) represents the anterior to posterior dimension of that structure (Figs. 28.18, 28.19, 28.80, and 28.81). Because of its shape (possibly influenced by its confinement between sternum and spine), this dimension (Figs. 28.80 and 28.81) is its smallest. This dimension is also the least sensitive to enlargement but when increased is a highly specific indicator of dilation. Table 28.3 gives the range of reported normal M-mode values for this chamber. Owing to the irregular shape of the LA and the single dimension represented by the M-mode image, volume estimates require two-dimensional images, preferably obtained from two orthogonal planes. The same algorithms used for LV measurements can be used to extrapolate volume estimations from area and length measurements. We recommend the use of orthogonal biplane images obtained from the apex for computation of LA volume (Figs. 28.82 to 28.84).[346]

Use of LA volume data requires knowledge of normal population parameters. We have determined these values in normal subjects, and they are given in Table 28.4. It should be emphasized that echocardiographic values for left atrial volume may underestimate true atrial size so that the use of normal values for echocardiography is essential. By measuring the atrium during both phases of the cardiac cycle, a concept of normal atrial function can be gained.[347]

While volume changes of the LA are easy to appreciate, the actual contractility has not been studied. Atrial contractions can, however, be clearly imaged by directing the M-mode beam from the suprasternal notch toward the superior LA wall.[348] We have used these contractions to time intra-atrial conduction and to study atrioventricular dissociation.

The use of M-mode atrial dimensions to predict the success of cardioversion from atrial fibrillation to sinus rhythm has also been promoted. We, however, do not think that the M-mode single-dimensional

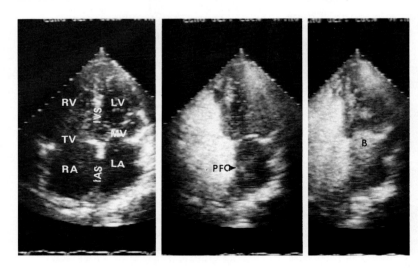

FIGURE 28.79 Pulmonary hypertension complicated by a patent foramen ovale. A 72-year-old patient with severe chronic left ventricular ischemia developed signs of pulmonary hypertension and hypoxia. Normal pulmonary function tests led to performance of a contrast echocardiogram. On the left, right atrial and ventricular (RA and RV) dilation is noted. (IAS, interatrial septum; IVS, interventricular septum; MV, mitral valve) In the middle panel, contrast has filled the right and left ventricles and the left-to-right passage of bubbles is just appearing at the arrow. (PFO, patent foramen ovale) In the right panel, this initial passage of contrast has now become a large bolus (B) of contrast seen to cross the tricuspid valve on its way into the systemic circulation. This study demonstrates that the patient's desaturation is the result of a complication of acquired pulmonary hypertension in the presence of a right-to-left shunt.

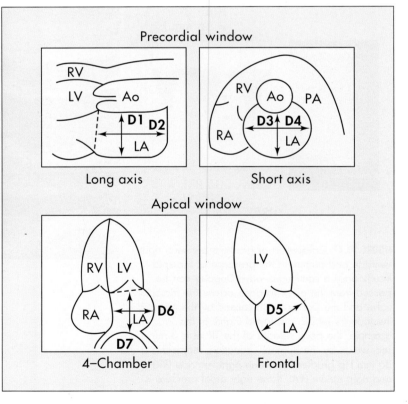

FIGURE 28.80 Standard views of the left atrium. Four commonly used windows for imaging the left atrium are diagrammed. The axes used to measure the left atrium are labeled D1 to D7. Of these, only D1 is used for both M-mode and two-dimensional imaging. The two-chamber view is called *frontal* in this diagram.

measurement of the left atrium is an adequate representation of its volume and do not favor the use of this parameter.

THE RIGHT ATRIUM

In health, the right and left atria are equal in size. The right atrium can be imaged in the precordial long and short axis views, the apical four-chamber view, and the subcostal long and short axis views. Its behavior in pathologic states is discussed in sections of this chapter dealing with the IVC, tricuspid valve, and tumors and masses of the heart.

ECHOCARDIOGRAPHY OF THE CARDIAC VALVES

While the thinness of normal valve tissues confounds most imaging methods, ultrasound, highly sensitive to the sharp difference in acoustic impedance between blood and valve tissue, easily reproduces them. The M-mode type of ultrasound examination has the advantage of high time resolution and the disadvantage of a limited scope of interrogation; it is of value in detecting the fine vibrations of a ruptured or infected valve and in recognizing the unique motion pattern of dis-

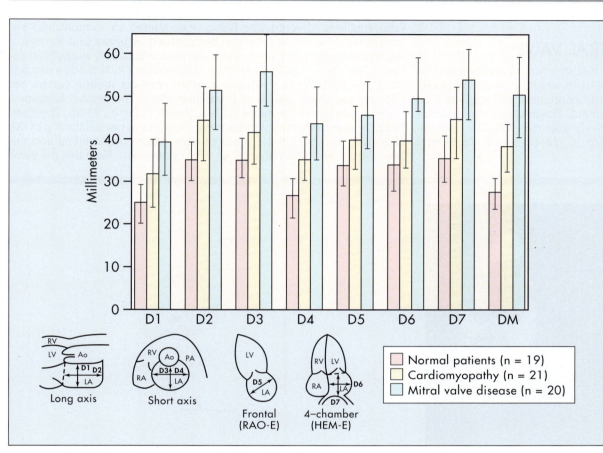

FIGURE 28.81 Left atrial dimensions in 60 patients. Using the dimensions diagrammed, the value obtained from each dimension (D1–D7) is graphed for each of three patient groups: normal, cardiomyopathy, and rheumatic mitral valve disease. Note that the D1 or M-mode dimension is the smallest of all, indicating that the anterior to posterior dimension of the LA is its smallest.

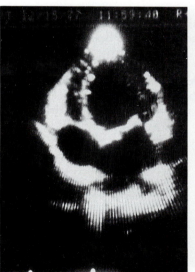 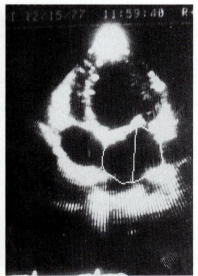 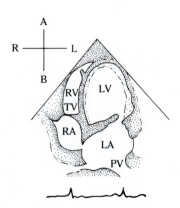

FIGURE 28.82 Planimetry of the left atrium in the four-chamber view. An end-systolic freeze-frame image is used to obtain maximum LA volume. The lines shown in the left-hand image were generated by a light-pen digitizing system that allows calculation of a single plane (area–length) volume from the outline shown or the combination of this area–length outline with that shown in Figure 28.83 to calculate atrial volume by a modified Simpson's rule or method of discs.

eases like mitral stenosis. The two-dimensional type of ultrasound examination has the advantage of showing all of a valve within a given plane and the disadvantage of low time resolution; it is of particular value in assessing the extent of a disease process such as aortic sclerosis. The Doppler type of ultrasound examination has the advantage of separating the normal from the morbid by detection and quantitation of flow patterns and the disadvantage of requiring that the sampling beam be axial to flow. The ability of Doppler to accurately quantitate aortic stenosis and pulmonary artery pressure comes close to being a revolutionary development and now stands as a major milestone in the development of noninvasive diagnostic techniques.

In this section we will examine the role and limitations of echocardiography to evaluate various abnormalities of the cardiac valves.

EVALUATION OF THE MITRAL VALVE

Historically, the mitral valve was the first structure to be identified by echocardiography.[2] The orientation of its anterior or aortic leaflet places the broad surface toward the anterior chest wall, making it an ideal target from which to reflect sound. Furthermore, the anterior leaflet is highly mobile, having a relatively large margin-to-base dimension (see Figs. 28.2, 28.11, 28.13, 28.16, 28.46, 28.47, 28.49, and 28.85).

Echocardiography can identify almost any anatomical or functional abnormality of the mitral valve. Our awareness of the omnipresence of the mitral valve prolapse syndrome is a direct result of the growing utilization of echocardiography over the past 15 years. This section will discuss the appearance of the normal mitral valve and the more commonly encountered mitral valve abnormalities.

ECHOCARDIOGRAPHY/DOPPLER OF THE NORMAL MITRAL VALVE

An adequate echocardiographic examination should consist of both an M-mode tracing and a real-time two-dimensional interrogation of the mitral valve. If Doppler is available, it is of value if mitral pathology is suspected, if quantitation of transmitral flow volume is of interest, or if abnormalities of ventricular filling (*e.g.*, altered LV compliance) are suspected. The mitral valve can be recorded by ultrasound through a variety of anatomical windows in the precordium and subxiphoid regions; we employ all of these in its examination. On M-mode examination, the normal valve exhibits a rather complex motion pattern reflecting the phasic nature of ventricular filling. The familiar M-shaped motion pattern of the mitral valve is shown in Figure 28.85. The early large opening movement of the valve (movement toward the top of the tracing is anterior) is the result of early passive rapid filling and the second reopening is the result of atrial contraction. Note that the valve

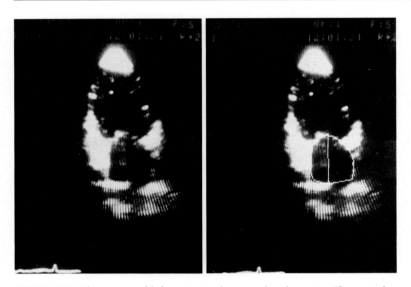

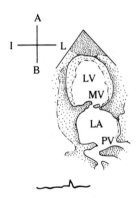

FIGURE 28.83 Planimetry of left atrium in the two-chamber view. The apical two-chamber view at end-systole is used to demonstrate the application of a computer-generated planimetric tracing from which both single and biplane atrial volumes can be generated. If possible, we prefer to combine the two- and four-chamber planimetric information to produce a biplane volume estimation.

FIGURE 28.84 Single plane volume calculation in a large left atrium. This light-pen-generated planimetric outline has been used to calculate a volume of 265 ml. As Table 28.2 shows, this is an extremely enlarged left atrium.

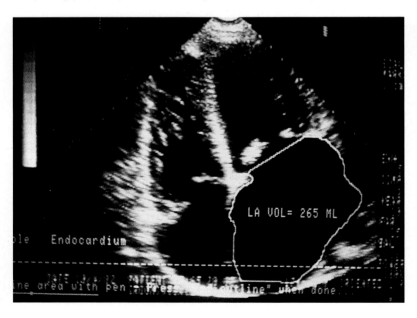

has assumed a nearly closed position during the middle of diastole, reflecting the result of deceleration of inflow as the pressure gradient between atrium and ventricle approaches parity. With atrial contraction the valve opens for a second time, completing the second peak of the letter M. Final closure is probably the combined effect of deceleration of atrial inflow[348] and isometric LV contraction. The two-dimensional appearance of the mitral valve depends somewhat on the imaging plane from which it is viewed. For example, in the short axis plane, the valve presents itself as an ovoid orifice while in the long axis it resembles clapping hands, with the anterior hand longer and more mobile than the posterior. Figures 28.46 and 28.85 are long axis views of the heart, and Figure 28.49 is a four-chamber view revealing these relationships. In general, the normal mitral valve should appear as a mobile two-leaflet structure that moves freely enough to respond to the normal flux of diastolic filling but that forms a stable coaptation plane in systole without entering the left atrium. In fact, the normally closed mitral valve descends with the cardiac base and undoubtedly makes a major contribution to left atrial filling by serving as a piston to draw blood into the atrium. Other anatomical features of the mitral apparatus appreciated on two-dimensional echocardiographic examination are the chordae, papillary muscles, and the mitral annulus. Doppler examination of the normal mitral valve reveals that the velocity pattern of blood entering the left ventricle during diastole closely resembles the M-shaped pattern of the M-mode of that structure. In other words, blood flow is most rapid during the initial phases of filling, falls to very low levels during the mid-diastolic conduit phase, and accelerates again during atrial contraction. Unlike M-mode, this inflow pattern can be sampled from more than one site. However, the apical views usually provide the most axial window from which to sample flow. The normal peak flow velocity across the mitral valve is usually just under 1 m/sec. Figure 28.86 illustrates the normal appearance of mitral inflow velocity as obtained from Doppler examination.

ECHOCARDIOGRAPHY OF MITRAL VALVE LESIONS CAUSING INFLOW OBSTRUCTION

MITRAL STENOSIS. Mitral stenosis was the first pathologic condition of the mitral valve to be identified by echocardiography.[3] In this condition, the normal, rapid biphasic motion of the valve is altered because the valve can open only partly. Anatomically, the commissural separation between the anterior and posterior or mural leaflets is diminished by partial fusion and the subvalvular apparatus altered by chordal foreshortening. These changes cause a limiting orifice that obstructs diastolic transit of blood from atrium to ventricle. Echocardiography not only can identify mitral stenosis but can also in many

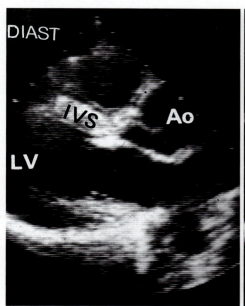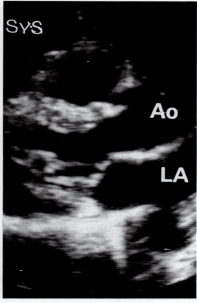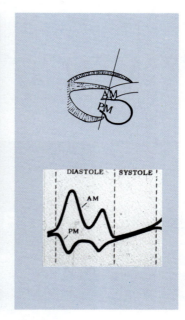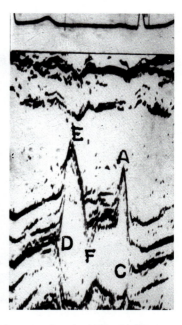

FIGURE 28.85 Normal mitral valve. The center panel diagrams the long axis plane of the left ventricle with a transecting line representing the M-mode beam path for imaging the mitral valve. For comparison, the actual two-dimensional image is shown on the left. The anterior and posterior mitral leaflets (AM and PM) are labeled. In the lower middle a schematic of the M-mode of the mitral valve is presented. Note that the valve moves in an M-shaped pattern during diastole, the anterior mitral leaflet separating from the posterior mitral leaflet. In the right panel, an M-mode tracing of the mitral valve is reproduced. The letters superimposed are the standard designations of the various waves. The initial opening motion reaches a peak at the E-point. This event is the maximal opening motion associated with rapid filling. After rapid filling is completed, temporary equalization of pressure causes the valve to move back to or near to its closed position at the F-point. The speed with which the valve travels from E to F is known as the E-F slope and can be prolonged in mitral stenosis or reduced left ventricular compliance states. The A wave is the peak opening during active or atrial filling and the C-point to closure point. The D-point is the moment just prior to opening. The C–D interval marks systole where the only movement of a normal valve is a slight anterior drift.

cases quantitate its severity accurately enough to send a patient directly to surgery without further diagnostic evaluation by catheterization. Quantitation of mitral stenosis severity can be accomplished by three direct methods and a number of indirect observations:

1. Mitral stenosis alters the appearance of the M-mode tracing of the mitral valve so that its normal early closure is delayed (Fig. 28.87). The early diastolic closure slope (so-called E–F slope) produces an easily recognized pattern and can also be quantitated to separate normal atrial inflow from obstructed flow and to differentiate among the degrees of obstruction. Although this method is the least reliable among the three[349] in our hands, a slope of less than 10 mm/sec (normal > 60) from a valve recording made during suspended respiration is strong evidence for severe mitral stenosis.

2. Mitral stenosis alters the appearance of the valve on two-dimensional echocardiography. The diastolic appearance of normal mitral valve in the long axis view shows the anterior leaflet as an extension of the posterior aortic root. In mitral stenosis, the anterior leaflet curves toward the posterior, their closest diastolic approximation occurring at their tips. Increased pressure behind the untethered belly of the anterior leaflet gives it a characteristic knee-bend appearance (Fig. 28.88). In the short axis plane, the opening of the valve can be imaged just above the tips of the papillary muscles and

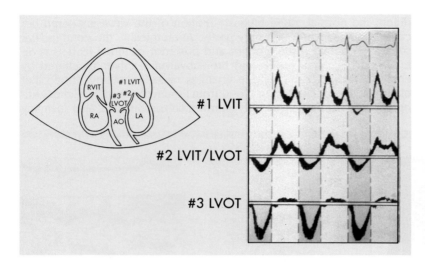

FIGURE 28.86 Normal ventricular Doppler flow patterns. With the Doppler beam directed from apex to base, a variety of Doppler flow velocity patterns can be achieved. The position of the sample volume for recording each of these patterns is shown in the diagram of an apical "five-chamber" view. Left ventricular inflow tract (#1 LVIT) records flow at the tip of the mitral valve on its left ventricular side. The M-shaped inflow pattern is nearly identical to the M-mode image of mitral leaflet motion. The initial velocity peak represents the highest velocity achieved during the passive or rapid filling phase. The lower peak velocity following represents the atrial inflow phase. Although there is similarity in the appearance of mitral M-mode motion and Doppler flow signals, there is very little predictive value of one for the other. The signal from the left ventricular outflow tract (#3 LVOT) is a systolic signal demonstrating flow away from the transducer or away from the apex. This signal represents systolic flow leaving the LV. The signal labeled #2 LVIT/LVOT is a hybrid mixture of #1 and #3 and gives inaccurate information about either. It is important to sample the Doppler flow signal axial to its flow. (Reproduced by permission, Hewlett Packard, Inc.)

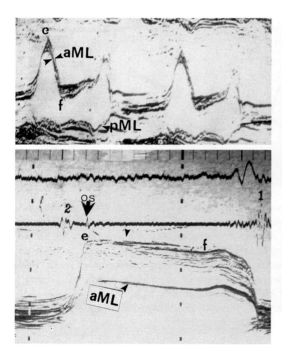

FIGURE 28.87 M-mode of mitral stenosis. The upper panel shows normal mitral valve anterior and posterior leaflets (aML and pML) and a normal E–F slope. Note that the valve thickness as demonstrated between the arrows is not increased. In the lower panel, an M-mode of a severely stenotic mitral valve shows the marked difference in its appearance from normal. Note the slow E–F slope, the thickness increase (between arrows), the second sound to opening snap interval of 0.9 sec, and the presystolic low-frequency murmur.

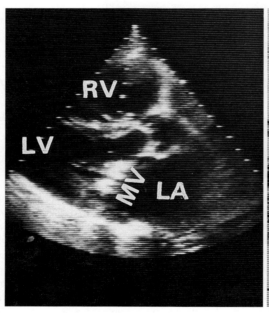

FIGURE 28.88 Mitral stenosis. The two-dimensional image on the left has been used to generate an M-mode along a line running from anterior to posterior through the tip of a heavily calcified mitral valve. The knee-bend shape characteristic of mitral stenosis is partially obscured by the heavy calcification. The M-mode to the right shows the typical pattern of mitral stenosis, as shown in Figure 28.87.

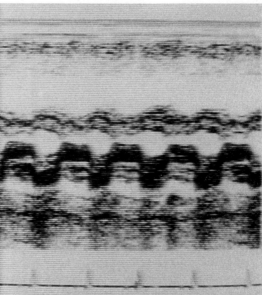

in this position its maximum diastolic opening area is measured by direct planimetry (Fig. 28.89). This method enjoys a reputation of greater reliability than the M-mode.

3. Doppler methods can measure the velocity of mitral inflow. In mitral stenosis this velocity increases from a normal value of less than 1 m/sec to 1.6 m to 2.0 m/sec. Since velocity is an expression of the pressure gradient between the ventricle and the atrium, the behavior of the transmitral pressure gradient during diastole can be quantitated directly from the Doppler velocity tracing. The most commonly used measurement for this determination is the pressure half-time.[350] Derived from hemodynamic data, the pressure half-time is an expression of how quickly the pathologic gradient between atrium and ventricle falls to one-half its initial value. In order to convert Doppler velocity into pressure gradient, the initial flow velocity is divided by 1.41 (square root of 2) because velocity bears a second-order relationship to pressure. Empirically, a pressure half-time of 220 msec has been found to indicate a valve area of 1 cm^2. In addition to valve area, the pressure half-time is influenced by flow, left atrial pressure, and compliance of left heart chambers. Erroneous results can be obtained in patients with atrial fibrillation and rapid ventricular responses or varying cycle lengths, curvilinear decay patterns, and first-degree block. In addition, in the presence of significant aortic regurgitation or cardiomyopathy, use of the pressure half-time may lead to an underestimate of the severity of mitral stenosis, due to marked increases in early diastolic left ventricular pressure and subsequent rapid fall in Doppler velocity.[351]

Of the three methods, Doppler is probably the most reliable for quantitating the severity of mitral stenosis (Fig. 28.90).

Indirect methods of identifying and assessing the severity of mitral stenosis are observing the degree of foreshortening of the chordae tendineae, assessing the extent of leaflet calcification, noting the degree of left atrial enlargement, noting the degree of LV underloading (*i.e.*, volume decrease), and studying the right heart. By noting the presence of right ventricular and atrial dilatation and of pulmonary hypertension (by Doppler of tricuspid regurgitant jet), the severity of mitral obstruction, its sequelae, and the risk of surgical intervention can be assessed. When the echocardiographic evidence is clear-cut and consonant with clinical findings, the need for catheterization is frequently obviated.

OTHER LESIONS CAUSING INFLOW OBSTRUCTION. Calcified mitral annulus is a very common echocardiographic entity usually not associated with hemodynamically important mitral insufficiency or stenosis (Fig. 28.91).[352-357] This degenerative condition is most strongly associated with age but its presence should always raise the question of hypertrophic cardiomyopathy. In renal disease it has been associated with secondary hyperparathyroidism[358] and in some series is associated with atrioventricular conduction defects. In an occasional patient the degree of calcification and the extent of subannular and leaflet infiltration become so advanced that inflow obstruction severe enough to warrant surgery develops. Doppler is the most effective

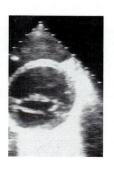
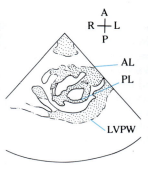
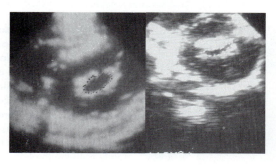

FIGURE 28.89 Mitral stenosis. Two-dimensional echocardiography has been used to estimate the severity of mitral stenosis by obtaining a short axis image through the limiting orifice. The right two panels depict the planimetric method used to outline the maximal area of the limiting orifice. The echogram at left superficially resembles those at right, but its opening is reduced by low flow. Note that while the mitral stenotic valves have central openings, the low-flow valve opens along the entire diameter of the chamber.

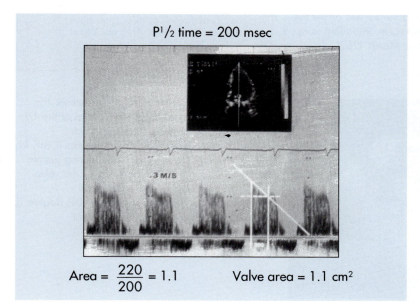

FIGURE 28.90 Doppler in mitral stenosis. The four-chamber view provides an imaging window through which the interrogating Doppler beam has been passed. In this case, continuous-wave Doppler has been used to record inflow signals across a valve suspected of being stenotic. In comparison with normal transmitral flow, which has a peak velocity no higher than 1 m/sec, the initial velocity is 3 m/sec. The standard method for estimating the severity of mitral stenosis by Doppler is to calculate the pressure half-time (P½). This is accomplished by dividing the initial velocity by 1.41 (the square root of 2) and measuring the time it takes for the initial velocity to fall to this level. In the example shown here the P½ is 200 msec. The next step is to compare the P½ to that of patients with valve areas of 1 cm^2. This value has been determined by Hatle and co-workers to be 220 msec. In this case 220/200 = 1.1 cm^2. (Reproduced with permission of Johnson & Johnson Ultrasound Inc.)

means for the identification of this rare complication of this common entity.

Congenital conditions causing mitral stenosis are very rarely encountered in an adult population. Parachute mitral valve (single papillary muscle), supravalvular mitral ring, and cor triatriatum are congenital conditions that can obstruct mitral inflow. Left atrial myxoma may cause inflow obstruction by its bulk, and mechanical trauma to the mitral valve can be associated with mitral regurgitation. When these rare tumors are encountered on two-dimensional imaging, Doppler examination can detect these complications. Carcinoid syndrome is a rare disease and in most patients involves only the right-sided valves. However, in two of 18 patients seen in our laboratory some left-sided involvement was present, presumably due to bronchial carcinoid. When bronchial carcinoid occurs alone it can result in isolated mitral stenosis.

ECHOCARDIOGRAPHY OF MITRAL VALVE ABNORMALITIES ASSOCIATED WITH MITRAL REGURGITATION

Stenotic lesions alter the diastolic motion pattern of the mitral valve and are readily identifiable by M-mode. Conversely, lesions associated with mitral insufficiency are often associated with subtle abnormalities of the valve elements and may not be recognizable. This subtlety arises because mitral motion during systole is usually minimal and a small dysfunctional area on the valve can result in significant regurgitation. Nonetheless, a large number of conditions can be recognized by anatomical imaging. In contrast to structural imaging methods, Doppler flow imaging is highly sensitive in detecting mitral regurgitation of all severities. As a measure of the importance of echocardiography to our understanding of mitral insufficiency, reference is made to a study that used echocardiography, angiography, and surgical findings to provide an assessment of the prevalence of various causes of mitral insufficiency.[359] Between 1976 and 1981, 173 patients were studied and those findings are summarized in Table 28.5. Note that mitral prolapse is now recognized as the leading cause of mitral regurgitation.

RHEUMATIC MITRAL REGURGITATION. Usually the scarring associated with the rheumatic process results in characteristic alterations in the valve's M-mode motion pattern. Even when stenosis is minimal or undetectable, the valve area is usually sufficiently reduced to alter its echographic appearance and sufficiently narrowed to separate it readily from normal. Failure of coaptation can also be seen during systole on a short axis image and its extent is proportional to the severity of regurgitation; rheumatic mitral regurgitation is the only form of insufficiency to be quantitated by failure of coaptation.[360] Figure 28.92 shows a case of rheumatic mitral regurgitation and a valve area of 4 cm^2. Since normal mitral valves have valve areas of between 6 cm^2 and 8 cm^2, this valve is anatomically stenotic. Since a measurable diastolic gradient was not present, the valve is anatomically but not hemodynamically stenotic. Note the coaptation failure on the lower panel of the figure. Doppler detection and quantitation of the severity of mitral regurgitation is the same regardless of the etiology of the incompetence. However, diastolic behavior of mitral inflow velocity will serve

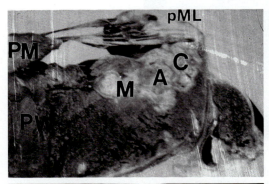
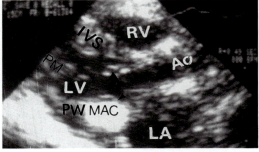

FIGURE 28.91 Mitral annular calcification. The anatomical specimen above is sectioned along the long axis of the heart. Note the infiltrative calcific process just beneath the posterior mitral valve (pML). This process is called mitral annular calcification (MAC) or subannular calcification. The latter term is probably preferable because the process actually infiltrates the posterior wall (PW) myocardium. In this case the infiltration extends nearly halfway through the basal myocardium and nearly one third of the way to the papillary muscle base (PM). In the lower panel, a long axis echocardiogram from a patient with mitral annular calcification shows that the image faithfully represents the pathologic process. Note that the calcification extends at least one third of the way from the mitral annulus to the papillary muscle base. The curved arrow designates the base of the anterior mitral valve and the tailless arrow the base of the posterior mitral valve. (Modified from Ewy GA: Consultant Journal, March 1983)

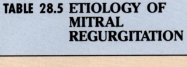

TABLE 28.5 ETIOLOGY OF MITRAL REGURGITATION

	Number of Cases	Percent of Total
Mitral prolapse	56	32.3
Rheumatic	40	23.1
Myocardial disease (dilated, 10.9%; obstructive, 6.3%)	30	17.3
Ischemic	27	15.6
Endocarditis	11	6.3
Congenital	9	5.2

(Adapted from Delaye J, Beaune J, Gayet JL et al: Current etiology of organic mitral insufficiency in adults. Arch Mal Coeur 76:1072, 1983)

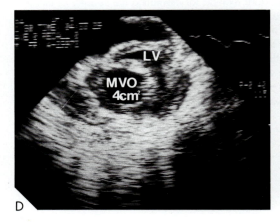
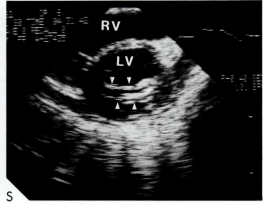

FIGURE 28.92 Rheumatic mitral regurgitation. The left panel shows a mildly stenotic mitral orifice by area. This valve presented no significant obstruction to mitral inflow and measures 4 cm^2. In the right panel, the valve is shown during systole (arrows). Note that the medial side of the valve has failed to coapt. In rheumatic mitral regurgitation, failure of coaptation of this degree is usually associated with significant mitral regurgitation.

to differentiate mixed mitral valve disease (*i.e.*, stenosis and insufficiency) from nonrheumatic varieties of "pure" mitral insufficiency. Pulsed-wave Doppler provides the most commonly employed means of detecting and assessing severity of mitral regurgitation. In this approach, the gate is set so that the area on the atrial side of the mitral valve is explored. We prefer to explore the atrial surface of the mitral valve from a variety of ultrasound windows. However, the apical approach is more likely to provide axial access to the regurgitant jet and is thus more sensitive. However, it is impossible to predict the direction of the jet and therefore all windows should be used. Careful Doppler examination with a sensitive instrument will often detect low-intensity systolic signals which we now feel represent functional regurgitation. The low intensity of these signals suggests that very few red cell targets are participating in the regurgitant stream and it is possible that this phenomenon represents the extrusion of a few red cells trapped in the infoldings of the mitral valve. In pathologic degrees of mitral regurgitation, the Doppler flow signals are of much higher intensity. Because of the high velocity of the regurgitant jet, pulsed Doppler will present an aliased signal (Fig. 28.93). As the regurgitant volume becomes larger, the strength of the signal and its apparent density on the paper increase. Mapping is a method whereby the regurgitant signal is traced from the mitral valve toward the posterior and lateral walls of the atrium. The wider the signal from the regurgitant blood flow and the deeper it penetrates, the worse the mitral regurgitation.[361] Using continuous-wave Doppler, the high-velocity jet of mitral regurgitation can be accurately measured (Fig. 28.94). However, the peak velocity of the jet provides relatively little information because it merely reflects the large gradient that normally exists between the ventricle and atrium during systole. However, in severe mitral regurgitation, left atrial pressure rises quickly and the duration of the jet is shortened and its peak velocity reduced. Doppler stroke volume methods can also be used to estimate severity of mitral regurgitation. In mitral regurgitation, the amount of blood leaving the ventricle is less than that pumped by that chamber; the difference between the two quantities represents the regurgitant volume. This difference can be calculated by measuring the stroke volume leaving the aorta by Doppler and that being pumped by the left ventricle by planimetry.[362] Although this section deals with rheumatic mitral regurgitation, Doppler is used in the same manner for all types of regurgitation. Secondary evidence of the hemodynamic importance of mitral regurgitation is gathered by noting the size of the left ventricle and left atrium. The velocity of tricuspid regurgitant jet is used to calculate the pulmonary artery pressure; pulmonary hypertension implies a more advanced degree of mitral regurgitation.

MITRAL VALVE PROLAPSE. Mitral valve prolapse was first recognized as a component of a clinical, auscultatory, and electrocardiographic syndrome in the mid 1960s when mid-to-late systolic clicks and murmurs were shown to correlate with angiographic aneurysmal protrusion of the posterior mitral leaflet. Appreciation of the prevalence and importance of this condition did not occur until independent reports in the early 1970s describing the unique and highly diagnostic echocardiographic pattern associated with this condition.[363,364] It was through echocardiography that the high prevalence of mitral prolapse in the population was appreciated. Diagnostically, this condition is best approached by the use of M-mode and two-dimensional echocardiography. Doppler is also useful to detect the late systolic pattern of the regurgitation but it is more useful to identify those individuals in whom the degree of regurgitation is more severe.

M-mode echocardiography was the only method available during our initial experience with this condition. This technique has been shown by Markiewicz[365] to have a 40% false negativity when presence of auscultatory evidence is used as a reference standard. This relatively low sensitivity might be explained in part by the work of Bon Tempo[366] and Salmon[367] and their colleagues who pointed out that chest wall deformities in mitral prolapse are very common. In fact, up to 75% of individuals with prolapse have radiographic evidence of a thoracic skeletal abnormality. These abnormalities (*e.g.*, pectus excavatum) can make M-mode evaluation (and, to a lesser extent, two-dimensional evaluation) technically difficult. Obviously, the prevalence of chest wall deformities is far more important as an indication that mitral prolapse is but a part of a generalized connective tissue/skeletal disorder rather than as a potential source for technical error in interpretation.

Ideally, any examination to detect mitral valve prolapse should combine M-mode and two-dimensional echocardiography (Figs. 28.95 to 28.98). Two-dimensional imaging allows interrogation of the entire valve and, in particular, the coaptation points of the anterior and the posterior leaflet to connote prolapse. While clear-cut displacement of the mitral valve into the left atrium poses no diagnostic problem, valves that flatten into the AV groove and no further into the atrium represent

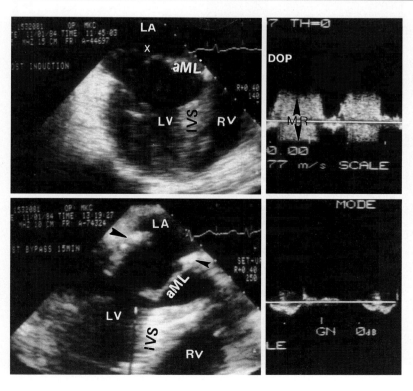

FIGURE 28.93 Pulsed Doppler detection of mitral regurgitation. Intraoperative transesophageal echocardiograms (*upper and lower right*) from a patient undergoing mitral valve replacement for mitral regurgitation (MR). Prior to valve replacement, a Doppler signal (*upper right*) was obtained from the left atrium (LA) at the site marked x. The signal obtained appeared to saturate the Doppler signal processing electronics and appeared as a dense signal on both sides of the zero line (MR and arrows). The appearance on both sides of the baseline is indicative of aliasing. Aliasing occurs when the velocity limitations imposed by the Nyquist sampling theorem on pulsed Doppler are exceeded. Postoperatively, the valve has been repaired and a Duran ring placed in the annulus (*arrows, lower panel*). Note that the valve leaflets are now contained within the LV, and the LA is much smaller. The Doppler recording to the lower right shows laminar inflow and little if any systolic signal. These findings were consistent with a successful repair.

difficult diagnostic problems. One group of investigators has proposed that since the normal human mitral annulus has a saddle-shaped configuration, with high points located anteriorly and posteriorly, leaflet displacement above the annular hinge points should be used as a criterion for mitral valve prolapse only in echocardiographic views that are oriented anteroposteriorly (*i.e.*, parasternal long-axis and apical two-chamber view, not apical four-chamber view).[368] It has been proposed that the addition of Doppler to M-mode and two-dimensional imaging will improve the specificity of diagnosis to 93%.[369] However, it appears that there is a certain amount of trivial or functional mitral regurgitation detected by Doppler in the normal population. This Doppler finding in a person with ambiguous echocardiographic findings might lead to overdiagnosis. In order for the Doppler to aid in the diagnosis of prolapse, a late systolic mitral regurgitation flow pattern should be demonstrated.

In addition to abnormal leaflet motion, mitral prolapse is also associated with leaflet thickening and deformity. Often the tips of the leaflets are most severely affected and present a club-like deformity

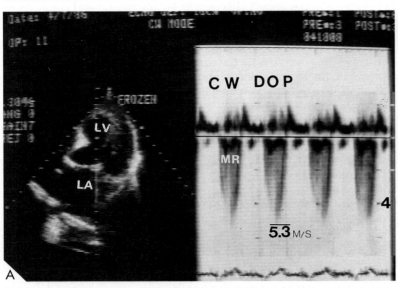
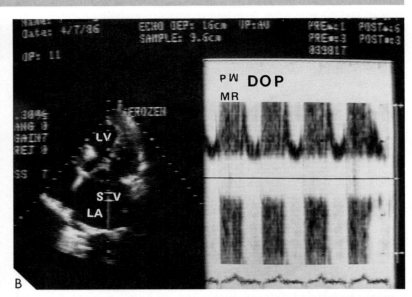
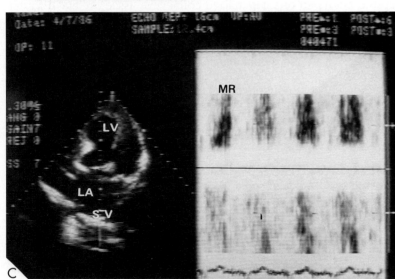
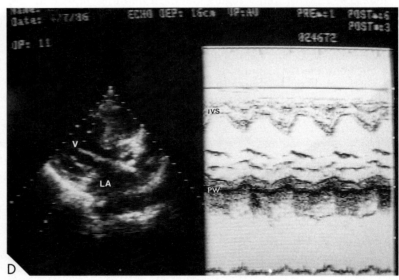

FIGURE 28.94 Doppler in mitral regurgitation. In order to determine the peak flow velocity in mitral regurgitation (MR) accurately, it is necessary to use continuous-wave Doppler (CW DOP). **A.** The four-chamber view on the left is from a patient with a large inferior wall myocardial infarction associated with significant mitral regurgitation. On the right, the continuous-wave Doppler signal was obtained from interrogation of signals reflected from structures lying along the line running through the left ventricle (LV) and left atrium (LA). The resulting signal on the spectral display to the right is a pansystolic signal reaching 5.3 m/sec peak velocity. The signal is moderately dense, suggesting mitral regurgitation of at least moderate severity. The peak velocity of the jet is merely reflective of the gradient between the ventricle and atrium and not of severity of mitral regurgitation. **B.** Pulsed-wave Doppler (PW DOP) analysis of flow in the left atrium. The sample volume (SV) is located about a third of the way toward the superior wall of the atrium. The spectral display to the right shows a saturated aliased signal in systole, indicative of disordered high-velocity flow. The density or power of the signal and the distance from the valve from which it arises suggests moderate to severe mitral regurgitation. This impression is supported by the somewhat spherical left ventricle (LV) and large left atrium (LA). **C.** The sample volume has been placed in the superior portion of the left atrium. In the spectral display to the right, a Doppler shift signal indicative of mitral regurgitation is still recorded. Mapping the signal to this portion of the atrium is supportive of moderate to severe mitral regurgitation. **D.** Long axis view of the LV with an M-mode beam directed through the tips of the mitral valve and minor axis of the LV. Note the hyperdynamic septum (IVS) in the M-mode to the right. Compare this hyperdynamic motion to the posterior wall, which is hypokinetic. This pattern, also seen in Figure 28.45, is typical of moderate to severe mitral regurgitation. Thus, in panels **A** to **D**, there is Doppler, two-dimensional, and M-mode echocardiographic evidence of significant mitral regurgitation associated with inferior wall myocardial infarction. The usual cause of this combination of wall motion abnormality and mitral regurgitation is loss of support of the base of the papillary muscle arising from extensive dysfunction of the underlying inferior wall.

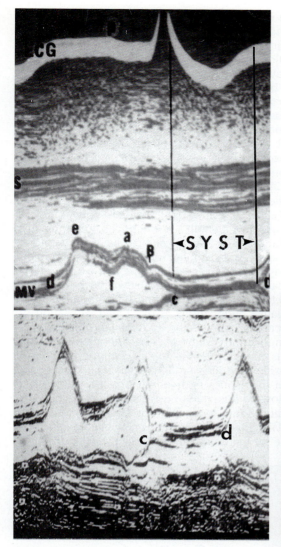

FIGURE 28.95 Mitral valve. The normal systolic (SYST) appearance of the mitral valve is seen in these two M-mode examples. In the upper tracing, the recording was made in a patient with cardiomyopathy. The B notch in diastole is supposed to indicate elevated left ventricular filling pressure. The systolic portion of the tracing is indicated and extends between the C and D points on the valve. Note that during this interval the valve migrates anteriorly without interruption. In the other example (below), the valve is recorded from a normal individual. The C–D slope has a similar smooth appearance. Compare these normal valves to those shown in Figure 28.96. For an explanation of other valve motion features, see Figures 28.85 and 28.87.

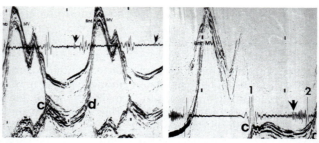 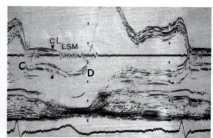

FIGURE 28.96 Mitral valve prolapse. M-mode echocardiograms and phonocardiograms from three patients with mitral prolapse. Note the posterior displacement during the course of the C–D systolic interval. Compare these three valves to the normal valves in Figure 28.95. Note that the first valve shows posterior displacement beginning in early systole and persisting throughout. In the middle and right panels, the prolapse begins roughly in mid-systole. Note also that all three valves are thickened. Finally, note that the phonocardiographic findings are not predicted by the morphologic appearance. In particular, the first valve with pansystolic prolapse has only two clicks and no murmur (arrows). The example in the middle panel has a late systolic murmur and no click, and the example in the right panel has both a click (CL) and a late systolic murmur (LSM).

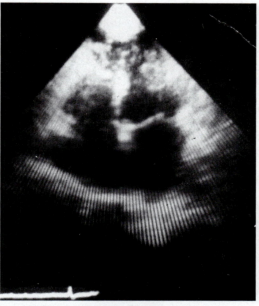 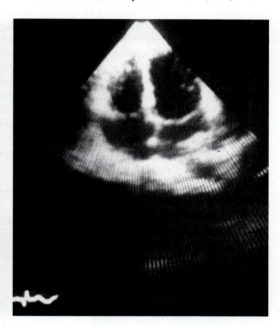

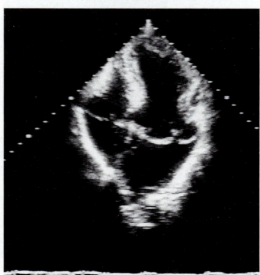 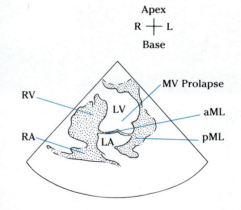

FIGURE 28.97 Mitral and tricuspid prolapse. Four-chamber view of patient with both mitral and tricuspid prolapse. Note that the posterior mitral valve leaflet (pML) is elongated. Since both the anterior and posterior leaflets (aML and pML) prolapse, the valve has a "moustache" appearance.

with a ground-glass appearance. This leaflet thickening often extends onto the inserting chordae tendineae. The more deformed the leaflet, the more likely it is that there will be an area of thickening seen along the endocardium of the septum at the point at which the hypermobile anterior leaflet abuts it. Recently it has been suggested that the more deformed the mitral valve, the more likely there is to be clinical manifestations and complications such as chest pain, arrhythmias, endocarditis, systemic emboli, and chordal rupture.[370] In extreme degrees of mitral deformity and prolapse it is often impossible to differentiate this condition from frank chordal rupture with flail mitral leaflet or from a bulky mitral vegetation.

MITRAL ENDOCARDITIS. Echocardiography has contributed to our understanding of endocarditis and has facilitated its diagnosis. In one series, Delaye and co-workers[359] (Table 28.5) found that in 6% of patients with significant mitral regurgitation, endocarditis could be implicated as a causative factor. The primary diagnostic feature of mitral or any valvular endocarditis is the vegetation. Vegetations can cause mitral insufficiency by interfering with closure of the valve or by causing disruption of leaflet or chordal continuity. Usually, patients with endocarditis and valve disruption can be identified by a constellation of findings. Prominent among these is the detection of a mass on the valve. Such masses are often assumed to represent vegetations but, on occasion, a healed vegetation, an area of myxomatous change, or a torn leaflet or chorda can mimic a true vegetation. The clinical setting can often be of considerable importance in determining the importance of an echographically detected mass lesion. On the other hand, many patients with endocarditis who are early in the course of their illness may have an entirely normal echographic examination. This lack of sensitivity for small vegetations is due to the resolution of ultrasound instruments, the signal-to-noise ratio present at the time of the examination, and the index of suspicion and skill of the operator. In an M-mode study from our laboratory, vegetations less than 5 mm in diameter escaped detection. Although two-dimensional methods might be expected to improve sensitivity to small masses, it appears as though smaller masses become confused with minor irregularities normally present or due to some other setting of preexisting valve disease. Thus, it is often impossible to distinguish the basic disease process from a vegetation. A good example of a potentially difficult diagnostic situation is an enlarged, myxomatous mitral leaflet whose chordae are ruptured. This damaged valve will appear echographically as a large, mobile, prolapsing, noncalcified mass vibrating during systole. Echocardiography cannot differentiate among these options and the clinical setting in which the patient presents is the only clue to the nature of the findings. O'Brien and Geiser[371] reviewed the literature concerning the incidence of vegetations in clinically (nonechocardiographically) proven endocarditis. Among 641 patients studied by M-mode alone, 52% had identifiable vegetations. Among 186 studied by two-dimensional echocardiography, 79% had vegetations. In other words, 21% of patients meeting clinical criteria for endocarditis will have no detectable vegetations by echocardiography. Among patients meeting the criteria for culture-negative endocarditis, 8 of 11 had vegetation on two-dimensional echocardiography. In the examination of mitral mass lesions or suspected endocarditis, M-mode echocardiography, in spite of its lower sensitivity, is extremely helpful in that disrupted portions of the mitral valve often exhibit systolic vibrations of the limited portion of the valve or vegetation that is moving freely or that has become untethered or flail. The slower frame rate of two-dimensional echocardiography usually does not permit recognition of these vibrations (Fig. 28.99). Transesophageal echocardiography has now become the most sensitive imaging mode for the detection of cardiac vegetations.[279,280]

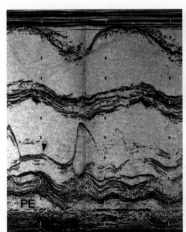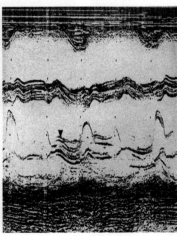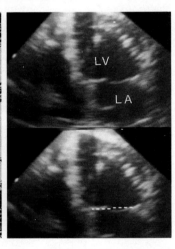

FIGURE 28.98 Mitral prolapse in pericardial effusion. M-mode (*left panel*) and two-dimensional four-chamber view (*upper right*) from a 30-year-old woman with myxedema-related pericardial effusion (*PE*). At the time of presentation, mitral prolapse (*arrow*) was noted during systole and felt to be a false positive; mitral prolapse pattern can be mimicked by increased cardiac motion associated with mitral prolapse. After treatment with thyroid hormone replacement, the effusion has resolved but the prolapse persists. In this case, the M-mode prolapse was a true positive. The two-dimensional images also demonstrated prolapse before and after treatment. In this case, however, detection of prolapse in the face of effusion is probably reliable.

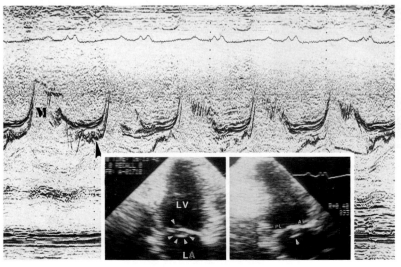

FIGURE 28.99 Mitral endocarditis. Lower insets are two-dimensional apical two-chamber views from a patient with a mitral vegetation (*arrows*) attached to both anterior and posterior mitral leaflets (*AL* and *PL*). Further evidence as to the nature of a mitral mass can be obtained from an M-mode directed through the mass. As the mitral M-mode (*M*) demonstrates, there are systolic vibrations superimposed on a pattern resembling prolapse. Systolic vibrations of the mitral valve are highly abnormal and either imply vegetation or valve disruption. With the disappearance of high-resolution stand in M-mode instruments the obtainable resolution of M-mode recordings has diminished considerably. Currently used video recordings of M-mode tracings, while inexpensive and convenient, do not offer adequate resolution to detect these fine, rapid vibrations.

EVALUATION OF THE AORTIC VALVE AND ROOT

The evaluation of the aortic valve by echocardiography has been a strength of the technique since it first gained popularity in the early 1970s. Initially, M-mode imaging reliably excluded significant aortic stenosis and sensitively detected aortic insufficiency. With the sequential development of two-dimensional imaging and Doppler flow assessment methods, these capabilities have continued to improve to the point where they now rival catheterization and angiography in the reliability and quantity of diagnostic information provided.

ECHOCARDIOGRAPHY OF THE NORMAL AORTIC VALVE AND ROOT

In current practice, M-mode echocardiography is performed in conjunction with two-dimensional imaging by targeting the M-mode beam through the aortic valve being displayed in the two-dimensional cross-sectional format. Figure 28.100 demonstrates a short axis image of the heart through which the M-mode beam has been directed to display the motion of the aortic valve and root optimally. As the figure demonstrates, the M-mode image of a normal aortic valve and root has a number of distinctive features. The aortic leaflets appear to open and close at the midpoint of the space bounded by the anterior and posterior walls of the aortic root. The opening motion of the leaflets carries them to near apposition with the aortic root where they remain until the end of systole. The net effect of these features is a "box-like" appearance of the M-mode waveform. While in their open systolic position, it is normal for the leaflets to exhibit fine vibrations. Failure to open widely or to sustain full opening usually implies a decreased stroke volume. However, a normal stroke volume and a dilated aortic root can cause open leaflets to remain at a distance from the aortic root. Also seen in low stroke volume is a tendency of the leaflets to drift shut just after achieving their maximum separation (Figs. 28.19 and 28.101). If the leaflet closes abruptly after achieving full opening, fixed subvalvular stenosis should be considered. If the leaflets close and reopen in the first third to one-half of systole, dynamic subvalvular obstruction is suspected (see Fig. 28.53). During diastole, the coapted leaflets move parallel to the aortic root. Vibrations during diastole are highly abnormal and are characteristic of rupture or disruption of the aortic valve (Fig. 28.102). Eccentricity of the opening or closure[372] is typically associated with a congenitally bicuspid or abnormal aortic valve (see Fig. 28.18).

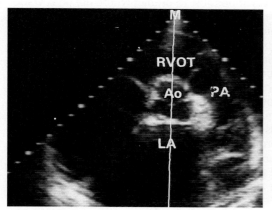
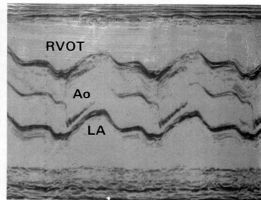

FIGURE 28.100 Normal M-mode of the aortic valve and root. On the left is a short axis two-dimensional image through the base at the level of the aortic valve. The plane of the M-mode beam (M) used to generate the M-mode to the right is shown by the solid line bisecting the aortic valve. Note that the aortic valve opens nearly to the aortic walls and, while open, has a box-like configuration. Note also the brisk anterior systolic motion of the entire aortic root and the even faster early diastolic relaxation (posterior motion). Contrast this aortic root M-mode with the one seen in Figure 28.101.

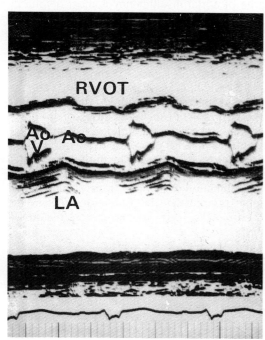

FIGURE 28.101 Aortic root in low stroke volume. M-mode of the aortic root and valve in a patient with severe cardiomyopathy. Note the loss of square wave opening motion as compared with the normal valve in Figure 28.100. Note also the poor aortic root motion.

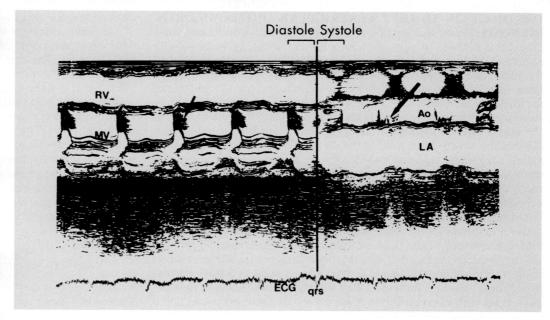

FIGURE 28.102 Bulky aortic vegetation. A bulky aortic vegetation has created a characteristic M-mode picture. On the right, the long arrow points to diastolic aortic valve/vegetation vibrations typical of bulky vegetation or of valve disruption. On the left, the short arrow points to a mass of echoes representing a prolapsing vegetation extending from the aortic valve to the upper portion of the left ventricular outflow tract. (Courtesy of Dr. Thomas Ports, University of California, San Francisco)

The motion of the aortic root is also very important and provides a considerable amount of information about global systolic and diastolic function (see Figs. 28.18 to 28.20, 28.30, 28.100, and 28.101). Normally, the aortic root moves over 7 mm anteriorly in systole and returns almost completely to its starting point immediately after the conclusion of ejection. The atrial or presystolic contribution to aortic root motion is minimal in the healthy heart. Since aortic root motion reflects the events of atrial filling and emptying, it contains a considerable amount of information. If the systolic excursion of the aortic root is decreased, a decreased stroke volume is most likely present. Note that this sign is independent of the left ventricular ejection fraction. For example, if the LV is hypovolemic but contracts normally, the aortic root motion will be decreased. Similarly, it will be decreased if the ejection fraction is severely reduced and the ventricle is increased in size. Normal or augmented systolic motion of the aortic root in the face of reduced aortic leaflet separation suggests atrial filling out of proportion to aortic flow and is typical of mitral insufficiency. If the initial diastolic posterior motion of the aortic root is slowed with augmentation of its posterior motion with atrial contraction, reduced LV compliance is suspected. (Also see the section on left ventricular function earlier in this chapter.)

Two-dimensional imaging of the normal aortic valve demonstrates a symmetric structure with uniformly thin leaflets that open equally, forming a circular orifice during most of systole. During diastole, the normal leaflets form a three-pointed star ("upside down Mercedes-Benz emblem") with a slight thickening or prominence at the central closing point formed by the aortic leaflet nodules. The aortic root has the largest diameter of the ascending aorta and is formed from the three sinuses of Valsalva; normally the root does not exceed 3.5 cm in diameter. Doppler examination of flow across a normal aortic valve results in a waveform with a peak velocity of 1 m to 1.5 m/sec. Since the aortic valve is the narrowest point in the outflow tract, velocity at the valve should be most rapid. Figure 28.24 demonstrates the normal aortic flow velocity waveform and normal flow intervals. Familiarity with Doppler evaluation of the aortic valve is important because Doppler assessment of stenotic aortic valves is one of the most successful applications of cardiac ultrasound.

PATHOLOGIC ALTERATION OF AORTIC VALVE RECOGNIZABLE BY ECHOCARDIOGRAPHY
OBSTRUCTION TO LEFT VENTRICULAR OUTFLOW/AORTIC STENOSIS.
Echocardiography in combination with continuous-wave Doppler is capable of accurate assessment of aortic stenosis. As with almost any application of echocardiography, the major limitations of the technique are dependent on the ability of the technician to obtain complete, accurate data. All three echocardiographic modalities are useful in the assessment of aortic stenosis and should be used in combination. M-mode is particularly useful in assessing the fine motion of the aortic valve. Variations in motion patterns are often useful in differentiating severe from mild aortic stenosis.[373] Typically, most aortic stenosis presents on M-mode as dense, persistent echoes replacing the normal motion patterns described above. Aortic root thickening and valve sclerosis without stenosis can mimic this pattern in that dense echoes from sclerotic areas can obscure normal leaflet motion. It is important for echocardiographers to attempt to find leaflet motion because if even one of the leaflets moves rapidly or vibrates during systole, the chances of the peak systolic gradient exceeding 50 mm Hg are significantly reduced. Other M-mode features of aortic stenosis relate to the secondary effects of the process such as left ventricular hypertrophy. Besides increased wall thickness, these include findings associated with decreased compliance such as flattened mitral filling slope, decreased early diastolic aortic root posterior motion,[96] and left atrial enlargement. Two-dimensional findings in aortic stenosis demonstrate the extent of thickening and calcification in and around the aortic root and, more importantly, the degree and pattern of leaflet motion.[374-376] If the leaflets cleanly separate, each moving in opposite directions, significant aortic stenosis is unlikely. If, however, the leaflets move together in a "doming" pattern, the possibility of significant obstruction is greater.[376] Furthermore, two-dimensional imaging can image the aorta distal to the valve, and if significant stenosis is present, poststenotic dilatation should be easily seen. Other two-dimensional findings typically present are varying degrees of left ventricular hypertrophy. In the well-compensated patient with severe aortic stenosis, a resting echocardiogram will disclose significantly increased wall thickness and normal or even hyperdynamic left ventricular function. Increased contractility seems paradoxical in the setting of chronically increased afterload. However, if wall stress is calculated while the patient is sedentary, it is usually decreased,[377] explaining the apparent increase in contractility. The degree of hypertrophy observed is, in part, a consequence of compensation for exertional states, not merely the resting state in which the patient is examined. Of course in those patients in whom hypertrophy is mild or absent while aortic stenosis is critical, a much more precarious clinical status can be inferred.

One of the most important areas for the use of Doppler echocardiography is in the assessment of aortic stenosis. With the development of continuous-wave Doppler techniques, a method for noninvasively measuring and following the pressure gradient across the aortic valve during systole became available.[378-386] Technically, it is essential to sample the jet arising across the stenotic aortic orifice from a number of sites so that the highest velocity can be recorded. Failure to perform such sampling can result in underestimation of the severity of obstruction. In our experience it is impossible to predict where the peak velocity will be found so we routinely employ the apex, suprasternal notch, and right parasternal intercostal spaces as imaging windows. In Figure 28.103, an actual spectral tracing is shown that was obtained from a right parasternal sampling site. The peak velocity of 4.3 m/sec by the simplified Bernoulli equation translates into a 74 mm Hg peak systolic gradient across the valve. It is important to note that the peak systolic gradient as measured by Doppler differs from the "peak-to-peak gradient" often used in conjunction with cardiac catheterization. The peak-to-peak gradient is derived by superimposing left ventricular and aortic pressure waveforms and is actually a nonsimultaneous estimation of gradient. In general, peak aortic velocities greater than 4.0 m/sec indicate critical aortic stenosis, whereas peak velocities less than 3.0 m/sec indicate noncritical stenosis.[387] For peak velocities between 3.0 and 4.0 m/sec, assessment of aortic valve area, left ventricular function, and the degree of aortic insufficiency is most helpful in determining the severity of the lesion (see below).

At times, relatively large peak systolic gradients can be confused with significant aortic obstruction but such confusion can be avoided in three ways. The first way is to note the rate of rise of the Doppler waveform. If the wave rises rapidly, the stenosis is more likely to be mild, but if it rises more slowly, a high gradient is likely to connote severe obstruction. The second method of avoiding confusion associated with the concept of peak gradient is by using the mean gradient across the valve. The mean gradient can be determined by planimetry, and in our experience is a more reliable predictor of hemodynamic severity, especially in milder degrees of stenosis. The third and perhaps the best method of assessing the severity of aortic stenosis is to calculate the valve area from a combination of Doppler transvalvular velocity determinations and some noninvasive determinations of cardiac output. We prefer to use the following formula[388] for the calculation of valve area:

$$\text{Valve area} = \frac{\text{Cardiac output (two-dimensional planimetry)}}{\text{HR} \times \text{Ejection time} \times \bar{V}}$$

where HR = heart rate; ejection time = jet duration; and $\bar{V}$ = mean jet velocity. Aortic valve area can also be calculated using the continuity formula; that is, based on the principle of conservation of mass, laminar blood flow volume is the product of cross-sectional area and the spatial-temporal mean flow velocity.[389] To determine aortic valve area, the continuity formula calls for measurement of the mean left ventricular outflow velocity, left ventricular outflow area, and mean aortic flow velocity. Since quantitative planimetry is not required in this method, all necessary measurements can be performed during the echocardiographic evaluation. However, the precise determination of left ventricular outflow area can be difficult in some patients. Therefore, we recommend that aortic valve area be calculated using both methods.

At the present time there is some controversy about how accurately Doppler can assess aortic stenosis in the face of significant aortic insufficiency. A recent report[390] suggests that Doppler gradients up to 40 mm Hg can result in moderate aortic insufficiency without a gradient being detected with fluid-filled catheter. Another study[391] using the continuity equation offers a rebuttal to this experience by reporting satisfactory accuracy of assessing valve area in the setting of aortic insufficiency. At the present time we are uncertain whether the controversy is merely the result of the suboptimal frequency response of fluid-filled catheters or as yet undefined factors. We therefore urge some caution in the assessment of severity of stenosis in mixed aortic stenosis and insufficiency. We also caution that subvalvular obstruction can coexist with fixed obstruction. Failure to differentiate between a subvalvular and valvular jet can result in a diagnostic error with considerable potential for patient detriment. We also caution that atrial fibrillation can introduce considerable uncertainty into these measurements.

ECHOCARDIOGRAPHIC DIFFERENTIATION AMONG THE CAUSES OF AORTIC STENOSIS

As alluded to, most aortic stenosis presenting in later life is associated with a considerable amount of thickening and calcification in and around the aortic root and valve leaflets. These degenerative changes are nonspecific and do not serve to differentiate among the possible causes of aortic stenosis. Congenitally bicuspid aortic valves are perhaps the most common precursors of progressive aortic stenosis. Before stenosis develops, these valves are recognized by eccentric opening and closure on M-mode and, more reliably, by an inability to image more than two moving leaflets and one commissure on two-dimensional echocardiographic examination (Fig. 28.104). In our experience, when the single commissure runs anterior to posterior in the short axis view, the abnormality is less likely to be artifactual than if it runs from left to right. It has also been our experience that the visualization of three commissures is no guarantee that a valve is tricuspid. In many congenitally abnormal valves, three commissures are present but one is fused. The fused commissure can be easily seen echocardiographically and the valve appears erroneously tricuspid. Clues to the true nature of these valves include apparent inequality in the size of the leaflets and eccentricity in the position of the systolic valve orifice. Patients who develop progressive stenosis of a congenitally bicuspid valve often give a lifelong history of a heart murmur. If the murmur developed late in life and if the patient had been hypertensive, then the etiology of the obstruction might be nonspecific degeneration atop a previously normal valve. How often this type of acquired stenosis might occur is very difficult to estimate. Rheumatic aortic stenosis is very difficult to separate from the more common degenerative/bicuspid types except that it is very much rarer a cause of critical aortic stenosis and is usually accompanied by significant mitral disease. In general, milder forms of rheumatic aortic valve disease seem to involve the leaflet commissures with very little, if any, involvement of the aortic ring and commissural ring attachments. Conversely, degenerative aortic disease seems to be most intense in the aortic ring, spreading centrally into the leaflets and involving the leaflet tips last.

FIXED SUBVALVULAR STENOSIS. This relatively rare congenital lesion is occasionally encountered in the adult population. The most prominent feature of the condition is narrow area of increased density best seen just proximal to the junction of the aortic root to the septum. Often the degree of narrowing is difficult to appreciate on direct inspection, and Doppler examination is indicated. The method of conducting this examination and the implications of the findings are very similar to the method of evaluating valvular aortic stenosis discussed in the preceding section.

DYNAMIC SUBVALVULAR STENOSIS OR HYPERTROPHIC OBSTRUCTIVE CARDIOMYOPATHY. This common condition is discussed under LV hypertrophy.

LESIONS ASSOCIATED WITH AORTIC REGURGITATION. Aortic regurgitation is a common lesion arising from a variety of aortic valve and root abnormalities. Many of these pathologic entities can be identified by echocardiographic imaging and the severity or degree of regurgitation assessed. First, features common to all forms of regurgitation will be discussed.

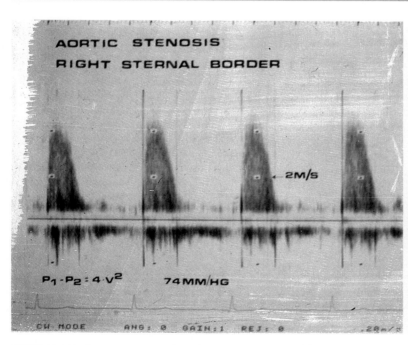

FIGURE 28.103 Continuous-wave Doppler in aortic stenosis. The peak velocity recorded by continuous-wave Doppler is 4.3 m/sec, which by the Bernoulli equation shown represents a 74 mm Hg peak pressure. (Reproduced with permission of Johnson & Johnson Ultrasound Inc.)

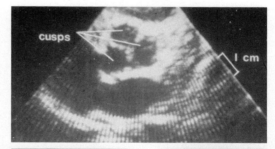
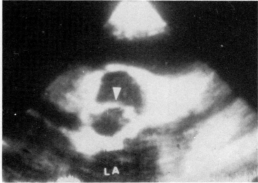

FIGURE 28.104 Bicuspid aortic valve. Short axis basal view through the aortic ring and leaflets showing the normal three-leaflet configuration (top) and an abnormal two-leaflet or cusp configuration (bottom, arrow). In the normal valve, the most anterior cusp is the right coronary cusp, the most lateral is the left, and the most medial (viewer's left) is the noncoronary cusp.

Diastolic fluttering of the anterior mitral valve leaflet was the first M-mode echocardiographic observation permitting the detection of aortic insufficiency.[392] When present, as Figure 28.105 shows, the sign is obvious. However, the reliability of this sign was uncertain until recent studies in animals[393] demonstrated that manifestation of fluttering was dependent on the leaflet or commissure from which the regurgitant jet originated rather than on the amount of regurgitation. In other words, their observations suggest that it is the direction of the regurgitant stream that determines the occurrence of mitral valve flutter. Our own experience with Doppler detection of aortic insufficiency also suggests that the regurgitant jet can propagate in a variety of directions and that when it impinges on the anterior mitral leaflet, flutter results. Ironically, with the ascendancy of digitized two-dimensional echocardiographic examinations there is a tendency to record the M-mode portion of the examination on video tape. While expensive recording paper is saved, the result is a marked decrease in the resolution of M-mode recordings and impairment of our ability to detect subtle fluttering. When aortic insufficiency is acute and severe, M-mode is of value in detecting early closure of the mitral valve.[394] This sign occurs when the patient is in precarious hemodynamic status and its occurrence usually indicates the need for pharmacologic and surgical intervention (Fig. 28.106).

There has long been considerable interest in using echocardiography to plan timely operative intervention in aortic insufficiency. One attempt to develop an echocardiographic index to suggest when surgical intervention was timely was the study[395,396] indicating that when the end-systolic dimension of the LV reached 55 mm or greater, a high likelihood of postoperative heart failure and mortality existed. The concept on which this index is based is that end-systolic volume is a sensitive angiographic indicator of LV functional status. However, since the derivation of LV volume from a single M-mode dimension is not reliable, this index may have unacceptably large variability to be a sensitive and reliable guide to operative intervention. More recently, a group[397] has reevaluated the concept that a left ventricular end-systolic

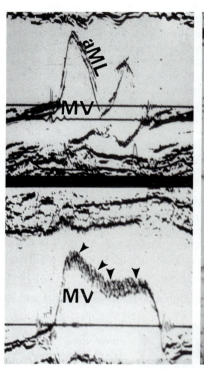
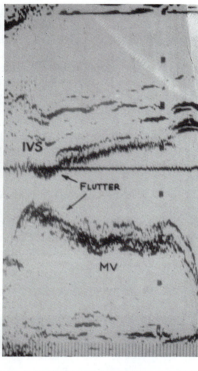

FIGURE 28.105 Mitral valve flutter in aortic insufficiency. Left panels show a normal mitral valve (MV) anterior leaflet (aML) (above) with a smooth-appearing diastolic motion pattern contrasted to a valve (below) with diastolic vibrations (arrows) of the anterior leaflet. To the right is another example of anterior leaflet flutter. Additionally, there is obvious vibratory motion of the septum (IVS). Careful inspection of the example at the left also reveals slight septal vibrations during diastole. The posterior leaflets, not well seen, can also vibrate but less prominently.

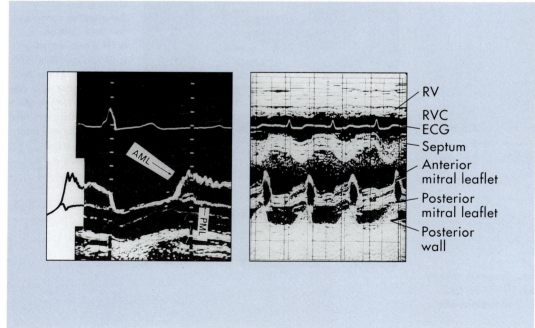

FIGURE 28.106 Severe aortic insufficiency with early closure of the mitral valve. The left panel shows a recording from a patient with marked diastolic anterior mitral leaflet (AML) and slight posterior mitral leaflet (PML) vibrations. The closure of the valve occurs on the later half of QRS. In the example to the right, no diastolic vibrations are seen, there is E-point septal separation and the valve closes well before the onset of the QRS.

dimension greater than 55 mm predicted a poor outcome of surgery. In 47 consecutive patients undergoing aortic valve replacement, 20 had a preoperative end-systolic dimension greater than 55 mm. There were no deaths in either group, symptomatic improvement was the same in both groups, and both showed similar decreases in volume and mass. The authors concluded that given newer methods of myocardial preservation, 55 mm end-systolic dimension did not seem to provide a critical index by which to judge operability. The two-dimensional assessment of aortic insufficiency severity has not been as well studied as the M-mode methods. Although it is logical to assume that the quantitative methods discussed in the first section of this chapter might provide information about the severity of the volume overload state, the degree of hypertrophy, the shape of the ventricle, and the mass to volume ratio (*i.e.,* adequacy of hypertrophic response), such studies have been scanty. Some authors claim that it is possible to visualize early closure of the mitral valve during a real-time two-dimensional examination, but the advantage of this approach is uncertain. Recently, it was reported that more significant degrees of aortic insufficiency are associated with a reversal in the curvature of the anterior leaflet of the mitral valve during diastole (Fig. 28.107).[398] However, this sign, like diastolic fluttering on M-mode, might also depend on the direction of the regurgitant jet. Presently, the broadest application of two-dimensional echocardiography seems to be in the determination of the etiology of aortic insufficiency.

Doppler echocardiography has an important role in the evaluation of the patient suspected of having aortic insufficiency. Short of direct inspection, pulsed Doppler appears to be the most sensitive method (invasive or noninvasive) for the detection of this entity.[399] In performing an examination with Doppler for aortic insufficiency, the pulsed-Doppler sample volume is placed on the ventricular side of the leaflets and their coaptation lines explored (Fig. 28.108). This maneuver is repeated from a variety of imaging windows in order to ensure that all possible jet directions will be represented and sampled. The most sensitive window is the cardiac apex but at times other windows are more informative. When a pan-diastolic jet is encountered, its penetration into the ventricle is mapped as a guide to severity.[400] In general, if a jet is found more than one-third of the way into the ventricle, the lesion is suspected of being more than mild. Recently, a more quantitative approach has been suggested by the degree of retrograde or negative flow in the descending aorta determined by measuring the reverse flow component in the descending aorta flow velocity profile.[401] Others have proposed that the stroke volume on the left side (increased) be compared to that on the right side (normal) to gain an index of regurgitant volume.[384,402] Variations on this theme have recently included the use of color-flow mapping of the regurgitant jet to provide a measurable analog of regurgitant volume.[403] Another Doppler approach to assessing the severity of aortic insufficiency has involved the use of continuous-wave Doppler to measure the velocity changes occurring across the aortic valve, between aortic root and LV, during diastole.[404] Since the velocity of retrograde flow represents the gradient between the aorta and the LV, the rate at which this velocity falls is indicative of the rate of pressure equalization across the aortic valve. In severe aortic insufficiency, pressure in the LV rises very quickly as it falls in the aorta. This phenomenon, also accounting for

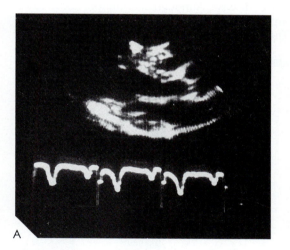
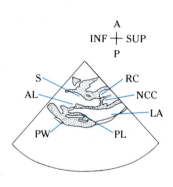
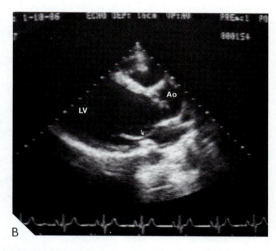

FIGURE 28.107 Anterior mitral leaflet diastolic bowing in severe aortic regurgitation. Normally, the anterior mitral leaflet (*AL*) is bowed anteriorly during diastole **A.** However, in some cases with severe aortic insufficiency (especially with posteriorly directed regurgitation jets), not only is the mitral leaflet opening motion restricted but the curvature of the leaflet is actually reversed (**B,** *arrow*). (*LA,* left atrium; *NCC,* noncoronary cusp; *PL,* posterior mitral leaflet; *PW,* posterior wall of the left ventricle; *RC,* right coronary cusp; *S,* interventricular septum)

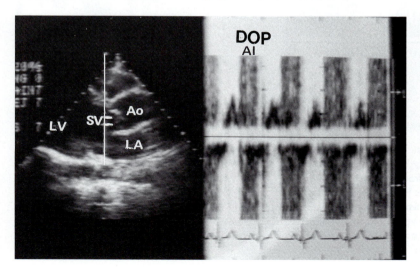

FIGURE 28.108 Pulsed-wave Doppler in aortic insufficiency. The diastolic jet of aortic insufficiency (*AI*) is directed somewhat randomly. Therefore, several windows of interrogation are used from which the Doppler jet is directed. In this patient, the Doppler sample volume (*SV*) is placed just ventral to the aortic valve (*Ao*). To the right of the two-dimensional image is the spectral display (*DOP*) from the pulsed-wave Doppler analysis performed at the site of the sample volume. The aortic insufficiency Doppler signal is seen on both sides of the baseline in diastole, indicating that the aortic insufficiency jet is high-velocity. In this case and in many others, pulsed-wave Doppler can only sample relatively normal rates of intracardiac flow before producing an aliased signal. In order to sample the high velocities encountered in aortic insufficiency, continuous-wave Doppler is employed.

early closure of the mitral valve, causes the end-diastolic velocity in the regurgitant jet to become very low or even to approach zero. The faster this velocity falls, the shorter the pressure half-time becomes.[8] This index, obtained the same way in mitral stenosis, is inversely related to regurgitant fraction and angiographic severity of aortic regurgitation. A Doppler half-time value of 400 msec separates mild from significant aortic regurgitation; a value below 200 msec indicates severe aortic regurgitation (Figs. 28.109, 28.110).[404] The Doppler half-time has also been shown to be dependent on aortic and left ventricular compliance, so that misleading half-time measurements may occasionally be recorded.[405] The Doppler signal of aortic regurgitation can be differentiated from that of mitral stenosis by the peak velocity (typically about 4 m/sec in the former and 2 m/sec in the latter); the Doppler half-time method is still useful when both valvular lesions are present.[406]

ECHOCARDIOGRAPHIC DETERMINATION OF THE ETIOLOGY OF AORTIC INSUFFICIENCY

Any process that interferes with the integrity of the aortic valve leaflets can result in aortic incompetence. The most commonly encountered abnormality associated with aortic insufficiency is chronic degeneration of the leaflets. We prefer to call this condition aortic sclerosis and usually encounter it in association with hypertension and old age. In this type of valve disease the echocardiogram demonstrates the greatest concentration of calcification or thickening at the point where the commissures meet the aortic ring. Aortic and mitral annular calcifications frequently accompany aortic sclerosis. At times, one of the leaflets may become immobile or frozen while the others move freely. When only one leaflet is immobile there is usually no significant outflow tract obstruction. The severity of aortic regurgitation in this setting is usually mild.

Aortic insufficiency in association with rheumatic mitral involvement can be readily appreciated by Doppler echocardiography. In this setting, the aortic valve leaflet edges are thickened along their entire length and the aortic ring is small and normal in appearance. While most often this type of aortic insufficiency is mild, occasionally it can be moderate or even severe.

Aortic insufficiency commonly arises in nonstenotic bicuspid aortic valves. These valves can often be recognized by two-dimensional imaging of the aorta in the precordial short axis view (see Fig. 28.104). Many of these valves are functionally bicuspid but have three leaflets. In these, two of the leaflets are fused together, leaving one commissure and two functioning leaflets. The fused commissure will often be imaged, giving the valve the appearance of a three-leaflet valve. In this situation, echocardiography detects only subtle abnormalities such as asymmetric opening motion and unequal leaflet size. Doppler examination will confirm the presence of aortic insufficiency and aid in assessment of severity.

Endocarditis of the aortic valve is probably the leading cause of acute severe aortic insufficiency. Classically, dense mobile echoes prolapsing into the LV outflow tract are diagnostic when present (Figs. 28.93 and 28.111). However, approximately 25% of clinically diagnosed endocarditis patients have no vegetations detected by echocardiography. The presence of a preexisting abnormality behaving as a nidus for infection can make vegetation detection difficult.

Aortic insufficiency can arise in association with jet lesions from subaortic stenosis. In this situation, dynamic or fixed outflow tract narrowing produces a jet of high-velocity blood, which strikes the aortic valve. The damage resulting may undermine the valve integrity and allow aortic insufficiency. Aortic insufficiency in association with mitral valve prolapse can be due to either myxomatous changes in the leaflets themselves or to aortic root disease. Although uncommon, aortic valve prolapse due to myxomatous degeneration can be seen in association with mitral prolapse. The Marfan syndrome is also associated with mi-

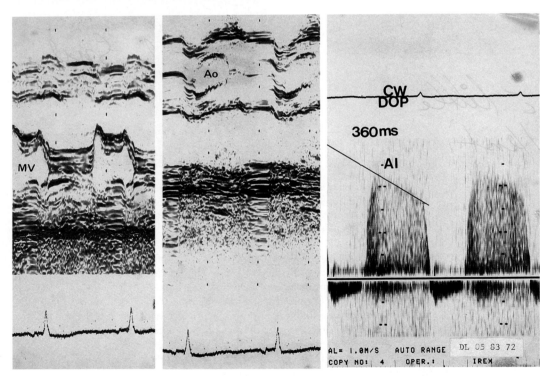

FIGURE 28.109 Continuous-wave Doppler in mild aortic insufficiency. In spite of an absence of detectable mitral valve (MV) flutter or of significant aortic valve disease, the continuous-wave (CW) Doppler display clearly demonstrates aortic insufficiency (AI). The slope of decay of the 4.5 m/sec jet is shown by the line. This line is used to find the velocity, which represents the moment when the jet represents a pressure gradient one half of the initial gradient. This moment is found by dividing the initial velocity by the square root of 2 (1.41). The time it takes from the onset of aortic insufficiency flow until this half pressure point is called the pressure half-time. In this case it is 360 msec, indicating a mild degree of regurgitation. A pressure half-time less than 250 usually indicates severe aortic insufficiency.

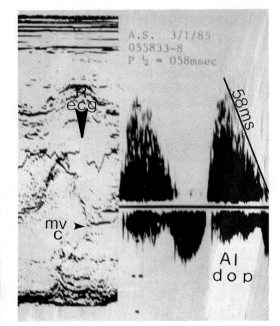

FIGURE 28.110 Continuous-wave Doppler in severe aortic insufficiency. In a patient with a large aortic vegetation the Doppler-determined pressure half-time was 58 m/sec. Note that the peak velocity is very low, suggesting that the regurgitant orifice is relatively large. In the left panel, note that the patient does not have early closure of the mitral valve. In our experience, the pressure half-time is an improved method of evaluating the severity of aortic insufficiency.

tral valve prolapse and aortic insufficiency. Although this condition appears allied with mitral valve prolapse, the appearance of the aortic valve and root are distinctly different in each.[407] In the Marfan patient, isolated dilation of the sinuses of Valsalva with sparing of the ascending aorta and a nonprolapsing aortic valve is typical but aortic valve prolapse is not seen (Fig. 28.112).

Other aortic root diseases are associated with aortic insufficiency and include proximal dissection of the aorta, hypertensive dilation, sinus of Valsalva aneurysms (with and without fistulous connection), aortoannular ectasia (Fig. 28.112), luetic aortitis, and aortic root dilation in association with ankylosing spondylitis. The echocardiographic findings in these conditions can be nonspecific and differentiation must rest on clinical or pathologic grounds. As common echocardiographic findings, dilation of the aortic root and thickening of its walls are notable. In dissection, the intimal flap can be very difficult to image but some degree of root dilation is usually present. Sinus of Valsalva aneurysms are marked by asymmetric dilation involving one of the sinuses. Often the dilated sinus will bulge in systole, facilitating detection. In the setting of a sinus of Valsalva aneurysm, a Doppler examination should be performed and both aortic insufficiency and an intracardiac communication at the site of the aneurysm sought. Rarely, aortic insufficiency can arise from a rheumatoid nodule on the valve, which produces a localized density on the leaflet.

ECHOCARDIOGRAPHY OF THE TRICUSPID VALVE

Survival in the absence of a functioning tricuspid valve is well known, and on this basis, diagnostic imaging of this structure would seem to have a lower priority than mitral imaging. However, there are numerous important conditions affecting this valve which, when recognized, yield important information about the status of the circulation. From a technical standpoint, echocardiographic and Doppler study of the tricuspid valve is somewhat more difficult than the left-sided valves. The position of this valve as the most rightward of the valves places it at or just under the sternal edge and requires that the ultrasound beam be angled sharply rightward while maintaining transducer contact with the chest wall. These constraints notwithstanding, a competent technician should successfully image this structure in the vast majority of patients.

FEATURES OF THE NORMAL TRICUSPID VALVE ECHOCARDIOGRAM

Anatomically the valve consists of anterior, septal, and posterior leaflets. The anterior leaflet is the most constant echocardiographic feature, with the septal and posterior leaflets being somewhat variable in their size and position. The echocardiographic identity of the valve leaflet being imaged is usually made by the structures of attachment. M-mode studies of the valve usually show only one of the three leaflets and their usefulness is principally timing of cardiac events or identifying systolic vibrations typical of vegetation or rupture. The motion of the anterior leaflet is similar to that of the mitral, having a large initial opening excursion followed by a secondary opening motion of less amplitude; the first motion is the result of rapid filling and the second of atrial contraction (Figs. 28.113 and 28.114). On two-dimensional imaging, the valve can be seen in long axis, precordial (Fig. 28.115), short axis, and apical four-chamber views; these projections are useful for both imaging and Doppler flow evaluation. Normally, the valve opens and closes in a manner almost identical to the mitral valve. Among the features of the normal valve is the location of the valve annulus at a more apical position than the mitral (see Figs. 28.13, 28.14, 28.49, 28.71, 28.76, 28.82, 28,84, and 28.97).

PATHOLOGIC ALTERATION OF TRICUSPID INSUFFICIENCY RECOGNIZABLE BY ECHOCARDIOGRAPHY

TRICUSPID INSUFFICIENCY AND ASSOCIATED CONDITIONS. In 1914, James Mackenzie, one of the fathers of modern cardiology, wrote, "Although actual disease of the valves is rare, incompetence of

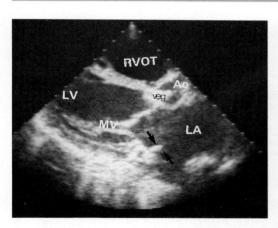

FIGURE 28.111 Aortic endocarditis. Bulky vegetation (*veg*) arising from the aortic valve. Note that the vegetation is large enough to prolapse into the left ventricular (*LV*) outflow tract. There is also a left atrial vegetation (*arrows*). Both the aortic and left atrial masses were shown to be bacterial vegetations.

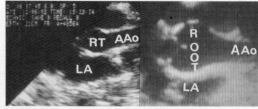
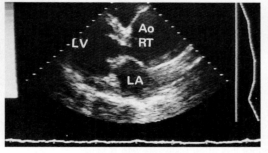

FIGURE 28.112 Aortic root enlargement. A normal aortic root (*RT*) and ascending aorta (*AAo*). Note the slight prominence of the sinuses of Valsalva. In the upper right is an aortic root and ascending aorta from a patient with the Marfan syndrome. Note the very large sinuses and the relatively normal ascending aorta. This pattern seems unique to the Marfan syndrome. In the lower panel, a greatly enlarged aortic root is also seen. Note that the pattern differs from that seen in the Marfan patient. The dilatation begins at the aortic ring and continues beyond the sinotubular junction well into the ascending aorta. We consider this pattern to represent aortoannular ectasia.

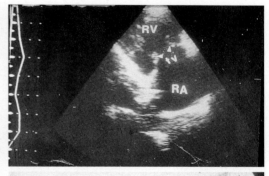
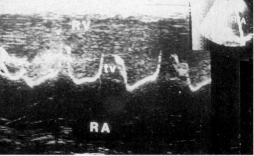

FIGURE 28.113 Normal tricuspid valve. The long axis precordial views of the tricuspid valve (*tv*) is shown above. From this view, the M-mode shown below has been generated. Note that only one leaflet (anterior or septal) is seen at a time.

the tricuspid orifice is extremely common, so common indeed, that I am inclined to look upon the valves as being barely able to close the orifice properly." The recent availability of Doppler methods has shown Dr. Mackenzie's statement to be absolutely correct in that up to 90% of normal individuals have evidence of Doppler-detected tricuspid regurgitation.[408] Obviously this "abnormality" is nothing more than a functional phenomenon but its ubiquity can be used to provide quantitative information about right heart function.

The echocardiographic findings in tricuspid insufficiency include the responsible anatomical valve abnormality (when detectable) and secondary findings. Secondary findings include right ventricular and right atrial dilation, "paradoxical" septal motion, systolic pulsations of the inferior vena cava (but not necessarily dilation), and diminished pulmonary valve opening (see Fig. 28.71). Contrast echocardiography can be performed and will demonstrate retrograde systolic filling of the vena cava and hepatic veins.[409]

The most common cause of pathologic tricuspid incompetence is right ventricular failure arising in the setting of left ventricular failure. M-mode examination of the valve reveals no characteristic findings but, in severe cases of right ventricular dilation and dysfunction, the valve leaflet tips may demonstrate poor coaptation. The Doppler findings in physiologic or pathologic tricuspid insufficiency are the same and include detection of the systolic regurgitant jet in a variety of sites. Technically, the strongest signal can be obtained by placement of the sample volume in the pulsed Doppler mode just under the coaptation point of the valve (Fig. 28.116). Depending on jet direction and the severity of the insufficiency, this jet will be detected at a variable depth into the atrium. This retrograde signal can also be detected in the hepatic veins.[410] By sampling the jet with continuous-wave Doppler from the parasternal or apical windows, its peak velocity can be measured. This determination is one of the most important parts of the Doppler examination as it provides an estimation of pulmonary artery

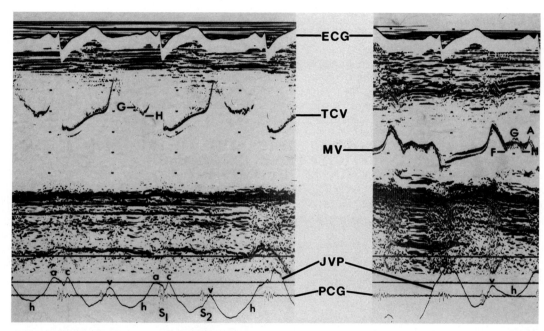

FIGURE 28.114 Normal tricuspid valve. The tricuspid M-mode (left) is compared to the mitral (right) and both are recorded simultaneously with a phonocardiogram and a jugular venous pulse tracing (JVP). In addition to the usual a, c, and v waves, a fourth positive deflection, the h wave, is seen. This wave occurs at slow heart rates in healthy individuals and its tricuspid and mitral counterparts are the f, g, and h waves, appearing between the rapid filling and atrial components of the atrioventricular valve waveform.

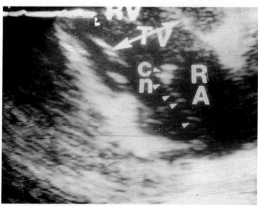

FIGURE 28.115 Normal tricuspid valve and Chiari network. The same long axis precordial view used in Figure 28.113 has been used to image the tricuspid valve (TV). Extending toward the tricuspid valve from the floor of the right atrium (RA) is a long, sinuous structure, the Chiari network. A vestige of fetal life, this structure is a net-like remnant of the baffle that directed oxygenated placental blood across the foramen ovale. The major importance of this normal structure is that it is often confused with a tumor or migrating thrombus.

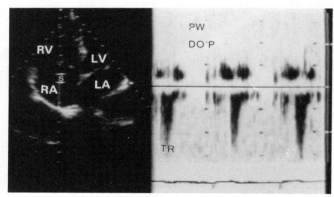

FIGURE 28.116 Doppler detection of tricuspid insufficiency. A cursor is superimposed on the apical four-chamber view on the left. The sample volume(s) is positioned just atrial to the tricuspid valve in the right atrium (RA). Pulsed-wave (PW) Doppler analysis of ultrasound at the position of the sample volume reveals that there is a 1.5 m to 2.0 m/sec retrograde systolic jet into the right atrium. This jet is consistent with normal or physiologic trivial tricuspid regurgitation (TR). A very high percentage of the normal population have at least a minor amount of tricuspid regurgitation. The importance of this observation is that it allows estimation of right ventricular pressure as described in Figure 28.77 and the surrounding text.

pressure. The peak jet across the valve, by the modified Bernoulli equation, allows calculation of the gradient between the right ventricle and right atrium (see Fig. 28.77). If right atrial pressure is known, estimation of peak right ventricular and peak pulmonary pressure (same as right ventricular peak) can be made by adding right atrial pressure to right ventricular/right atrial gradient.[411] In our laboratory we estimate this gradient by echocardiographic examination of the inferior vena cava (see Fig. 28.78). Whenever there is tricuspid regurgitation, regardless of cause, an adequately recorded signal will provide a reliable assessment of pulmonary artery pressure. Among the other causes of tricuspid insufficiency are trauma to the valve, endocarditis, rheumatic involvement, myxomatous change with prolapse, and the carcinoid syndrome. Trauma and endocarditis may appear similar echocardiographically. In both, one is likely to appreciate torn or flail portions of the valve that prolapse into the atrium during systole accompanied by systolic vibrations. In the case of a vegetation, the process may appear larger and more highly reflective. At times very large vegetations can cause a degree of inflow obstruction that can be detected by Doppler. Rheumatic involvement of the tricuspid valve is very commonly encountered in association with mitral or aortic valve disease, or both, and only rarely is of clinical importance. In most cases the degree of increased reflectance imparted by commissural scarring can be readily seen. When even minor amounts of scarring occur, there is likely to be detectable tricuspid incompetence.

Tricuspid valve prolapse occurs in up to 50% of those with mitral prolapse[412] and seems more prevalent as the patient population ages. This condition is rarely a cause for overt clinical problems and rarely occurs in isolation from mitral prolapse.

Carcinoid tumors (metastatic to liver) involve the tricuspid valve by diffuse fibrosis and shrinkage of the valve leaflets. In the more advanced cases the four-chamber apical view characteristically shows thickened, retracted tricuspid valve leaflets that are fixed in a partially open position (Fig. 28.117).[413-415] Thus, the dominant cardiac lesion identified by echocardiography and Doppler is usually severe tricuspid insufficiency with right ventricular volume overload. The acquired combination of tricuspid and pulmonary stenosis and insufficiency is nearly pathognomonic of this disorder. Carcinoid heart disease is progressive and often fatal. The development of cardiac lesions is related to chronic exposure of the right heart endocardium to high levels of circulating serotonin and other vasoactive substances.[416] Progressive hepatic dysfunction, which allows more serotonin to bypass liver enzymes and reach the right heart, may also be involved.[417]

Ebstein's anomaly of the tricuspid valve is associated with tricuspid insufficiency and a right-to-left shunt when the foramen ovale is patent. In this condition, the tricuspid valve is displaced toward the apex of the right ventricle and results in atrialization of a portion of the ventricle (Fig. 28.118). The most important feature of this condition is that the functional ventricular size, tricuspid insufficiency, and right-to-left shunting (see Figs. 28.118 and 28.119). The presence of ventricular tissue in the atrium may be detrimental in that the muscle continues to contract during systole, potentially impairing atrial filling. Echocardiography is probably the method of choice for recognition of Ebstein's anomaly in that the characteristic displacement of the tricuspid valve can be easily appreciated from the four-chamber apical view.[418] M-mode evaluation is valuable in that it can demonstrate the delayed closure of the tricuspid valve (possibly resulting from impaired atrial filling) and the simultaneous phonocardiographic occurrence of the sail sound (Fig. 28.120). Doppler flow studies in Ebstein's anomaly are also helpful in that not only is pulsed-wave Doppler a sensitive method of demonstrating tricuspid regurgitation but it can also localize the site

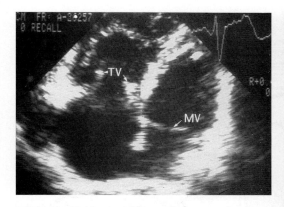

FIGURE 28.117 Carcinoid heart disease. In the most common presentation of metastatic carcinoid and associated heart disease, the patient is found to have tricuspid insufficiency/tricuspid stenosis (TI/TS). This valve condition is progressive, eventually leading to intractable heart failure and death. Note that the right ventricle is apex-forming and that the right atrium dwarfs the left. Compare the mitral (MV) and the tricuspid (TV) and note that the tricuspid is thickened. The characteristic of this stubby, thickened, and practically immobilized valve is that it has greatly limited mobility and remains partially opened during systole.

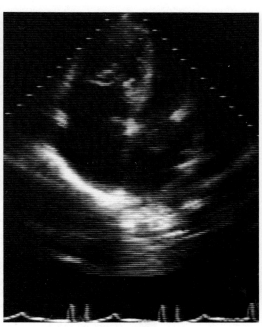

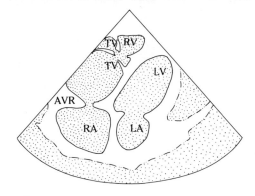

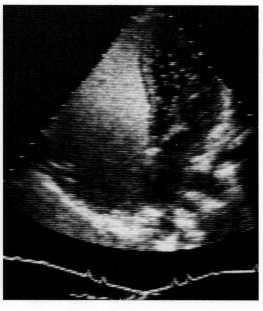

FIGURE 28.118 Ebstein's anomaly. The apically displaced tricuspid valve (TV) results in an atrialized right ventricle (RV) and a small functioning right ventricle. In the right panel, contrast has been administered and has resulted in good opacification of the right chambers. Note that several contrast targets or elements are seen in the left ventricle. This right-to-left shunt almost certainly is occurring at the atrial level.

of the abnormally placed leaflets where the abnormal flow begins. Performance of this maneuver in Ebstein's anomaly demonstrates that tricuspid regurgitation can be traced far into the body of the right ventricle, beginning at the site of displaced leaflets. The Doppler demonstration of ventricularization of tricuspid regurgitation is analogous to the demonstration at catheterization of a right ventricular intracavitary electrogram from the same location as right atrial pressures (see Fig. 28.119).

TRICUSPID STENOSIS. Tricuspid stenosis is more difficult to quantitate by echocardiography and Doppler than mitral stenosis. The diagnostic difficulties it presents arise partly from difficulties encountered in its hemodynamic evaluation and partly because it rarely occurs without at least moderate tricuspid regurgitation. The three conditions that can cause right ventricular inflow obstruction are rheumatic tricuspid stenosis, carcinoid syndrome, and prolapsing right atrial tumors. The pattern of tricuspid motion in rheumatic tricuspid stenosis resembles that seen in mitral stenosis. M-mode tracings from the precordium demonstrate a decreased E–F slope. Two-dimensional imaging from most windows shows diminished opening excursion of the leaflets and leaflet thickening. Unlike the mitral valve, it is not possible to measure the orifice diameter by two-dimensional imaging. Doppler examination demonstrates increased inflow velocity consistent with a gradient between the right atrium and ventricle. In practice, we use the same pressure half-time method employed in mitral stenosis to analyze the waveforms from the tricuspid valve. There is, however, little experimental evidence available to support this practice. It is perhaps of interest that the most frequently encountered cause of tricuspid stenosis in our laboratory is a previous tricuspid valve annuloplasty, usually performed several years prior to the onset of symptoms of right-sided inflow obstruction. The pattern of motion in tricuspid stenosis from the carcinoid syndrome is discussed under tricuspid regurgitation (see Fig. 28.117). Although carcinoid has the reputation of resulting in predominant tricuspid stenosis, insufficiency is almost always the predominant component of the hemodynamic picture.

Tumors of the right atrium can obstruct the tricuspid orifice if they become sufficiently bulky. The predominant diagnostic feature of these patients is a large mass in the right atrium or inferior vena cava which moves across the tricuspid ring during diastole. Once identified by two-dimensional echocardiography, Doppler evaluation of inflow velocity patterns can be used to confirm the degree of obstruction by estimating the gradient between ventricle and atrium. (See Echocardiography of Tumors, Masses, and Thrombi, below.)

ECHOCARDIOGRAPHY OF THE PULMONARY VALVE AND ARTERY

Diseases of the pulmonary valve are seldom encountered outside of congenital heart disease. However, like the tricuspid valve, examination of its morphology, motion, and transvalvular flow velocity patterns provides considerable information about the circulatory system. Pulmonary stenosis presents difficulties in diagnosis to the echocardiography laboratory, particularly if Doppler techniques are unavailable. These difficulties probably explain why the condition was seldom detected in our adult echocardiography laboratory population as an isolated abnormality. With the advent of Doppler techniques, mild pulmonary stenosis, while still unusual, is occasionally encountered in a patient being evaluated for a murmur. M-mode findings in pulmonary stenosis are limited to the occurrence of an exaggerated *a* wave during diastole. This *a* wave is due to a powerful right atrial contraction,

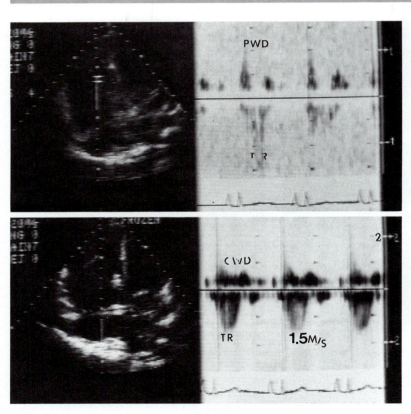

FIGURE 28.119 Doppler in Ebstein's anomaly. The pulsed-wave tracing (PWD, above right) was obtained from a sample volume just under the apically displaced tricuspid valve. Detection of a tricuspid regurgitation jet (TR) on the Doppler tracing is analogous to detection of right ventricular electrical complexes simultaneously with right atrial pressure curves. In the lower panel, a continuous-wave Doppler (CWD) has been passed along the same beam as the pulsed-wave Doppler. The tricuspid insufficiency jet peak velocity is now well recorded and, by the Bernoulli relationship, suggests peak systolic pulmonary pressure of <20 mm Hg.

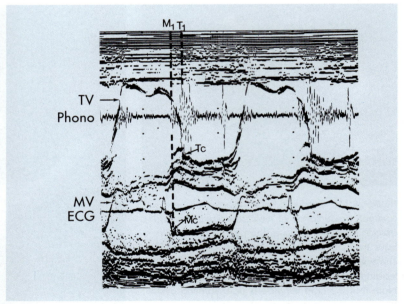

FIGURE 28.120 M-mode in Ebstein's anomaly. Compromised right ventricular volume and misplacement of contractile tissue on the wrong side of the tricuspid valve delay the closure of the tricuspid valve (TV) beyond that of the mitral valve. Although this delay is normal, in Ebstein's anomaly the delay is clearly beyond the upper limits of normal. Note that at tricuspid valve closure (T_1) the sail sound is more intense than the mitral valve closure (M_1). (MV, mitral valve; Tc, tricuspid closure; Mc, mitral closure) (Courtesy of Dr. Thomas Ports)

which, because of low diastolic pulmonary artery pressure, is able to open or at least dome the pulmonary valve. The *a* wave is most pronounced during inspiration and accounts for the disappearance of the pulmonary ejection sound at that point in the respiratory cycle. Two-dimensional findings in isolated valvular pulmonic stenosis are systolic doming of the valve, variable amounts of thickening ranging from imperceptible in the young adult to heavily calcified in the elderly, poststenotic dilation of the main pulmonary artery, decreased pulsations of the main pulmonary artery and its branches, and variable degrees of right ventricular hypertrophy. Doppler findings in pulmonic stenosis are similar to those in aortic stenosis. Continuous-wave Doppler recordings across the valve will reveal increased systolic velocity (Fig. 28.121). The peak gradient can be measured directly from this jet by the same formula used in aortic stenosis (pressure gradient = $4V^2$). If pulmonary insufficiency is detected, reversal of retrograde flow during atrial contraction can be expected. This finding is analogous to the exaggerated M-mode *a* wave. If tricuspid insufficiency is detected, the velocity of the jet will be proportional to the severity of obstruction. In this case, however, the sum of the gradient across the tricuspid valve with right atrial pressure cannot be directly translated into pulmonary systolic pressure unless the transpulmonic systolic gradient is first subtracted. This consideration becomes especially important in complex congenital heart disease where an estimation of pulmonic pressure is critical to patient management. Pulmonary insufficiency is normally present in a large percent of healthy persons (Fig. 28.122). It is a very useful finding in that end-diastolic pulmonary pressure can be estimated from the sum of right atrial pressure and the estimated end-diastolic gradient between pulmonary artery and right atrium. On rare occasions, severe pulmonary insufficiency is recognized when it occurs as the only lesion detected in the face of right ventricular volume overload.

Normal pulmonary artery flow and physiologic pulmonary insufficiency are illustrated in Figures 28.123 and 28.124. Lack of an adequate gold standard and the rarity of the lesion have hampered progress in the echocardiographic assessment of the severity of pulmonary insufficiency. Although pressure half-time measurements are not help-

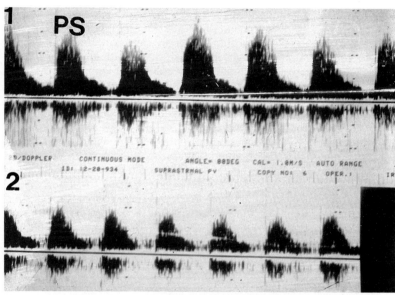

FIGURE 28.121 Pulmonary stenosis before and after pulmonary valve balloon angioplasty. (*Panel 1*) Estimated peak systolic gradient of 35 to 40 mm Hg by Doppler signal directed through the suprasternal notch. The Doppler underestimates the peak gradient because sampling of flow may not have been axial. (*Panel 2*) Decrease in peak velocity to 2 m/sec (estimated gradient = 16 mm Hg) after balloon valvuloplasty. (Tracing courtesy of Dr. Norman Silverman)

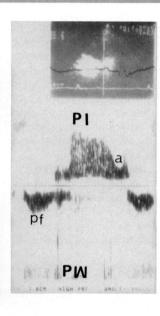

FIGURE 28.122 Pulmonary insufficiency. Pulmonary insufficiency (*PI*) is a normal finding in a high percentage of healthy individuals. Typically, the signal is recorded just central to the pulmonary valve. Note that although pulmonary insufficiency is pandiastolic, the rise in ventricular pressure caused by atrial contraction is strong enough to almost interrupt retrograde regurgitant flow. Pulmonary systolic flow (*pf*) is normal.

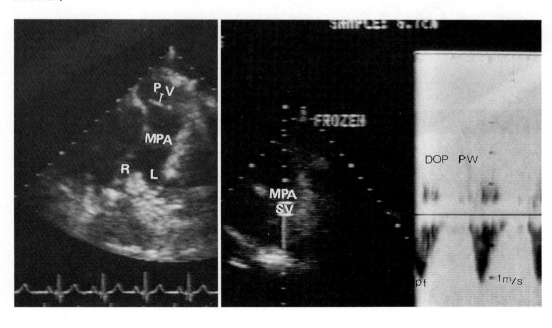

FIGURE 28.123 Normal pulmonary flow signal. The main pulmonary artery (*MPA*) and its branches are shown on the left and are normal. The pulmonary valve (*PV*) demarcates the beginning of the pulmonary artery. To the right, a Doppler cursor demonstrates the location of the sample volume (*SV*) and the site of the systolic pulmonary flow signal.

ful, we find that clinically significant pulmonary insufficiency can be identified by the intensity of the spectral Doppler signal and penetration of the pulsed-wave or color-flow jet back to the tricuspid valve in the parasternal short axis view.

COLOR-FLOW DOPPLER

Color-flow Doppler is a recent valuable advance in echocardiography that superimposes a color-coded, real-time display of blood flow velocity and direction on a two-dimensional cardiac image.[419,420] The color-flow map represents an extension of pulsed-wave Doppler technology, in that each pixel in the cardiac image is range-gated to provide selective pulsed-wave Doppler data. Commonly, about 120 sample volumes of about 0.4 mm each are placed in series along lines within the scan plane. Most systems image 90° of tissue and 30° to 45° of flow within the sector; narrowing the flow sector allows for a higher frame rate. Color frame rate is slow because each sample volume of color-flow information must be sampled at least 8 times more frequently than each unit of two-dimensional echocardiographic data. The primary colors of red, green, and blue are used singly or in combination to express direction, mean velocity, aliasing, variance, and turbulence of blood flow. According to convention, red is assigned to represent flow toward the transducer and blue to represent flow away from the transducer. In addition, color brightness is proportional to mean velocity up to the Nyquist limit. When velocity is greater than these limits, the aliasing phenomenon occurs and the opposite color is assigned. Another option, the "power mode," displays the power of the Doppler shift that is proportional to the number of red blood cells moving toward and away from the transducer. Although some systems claim to image "turbulence" in green color, there is controversy as to whether it may actually be attributable to aliasing.

In most patients, the color-flow examination of the cardiac chamber for abnormal flow signals can be performed simply by turning the color flow on and off as each standard two-dimensional echocardiographic view is imaged. Since the mean velocity of blood flow is displayed by color Doppler, aliasing of the flow signal will occur with pathologic cardiac flows, conveniently highlighting cardiac shunts, valvular stenosis, and regurgitation. Beat-to-beat flows are presented in an angiographic fashion that is familiar to most cardiologists. The major advantage provided by color-flow imaging is the immediate spatial information on cardiac flows; the major disadvantages include loss of temporal resolution and inability to measure high velocities. For accurate resolution of the timing of valve flow relative to valve motion and electrocardiography, color flow can also be overlayed on an M-mode cardiac image. Color flow can also be used in conjunction with spectral Doppler, either to align the continuous-wave cursor with stenotic or regurgitant jets or to correct for angulation. In adults, color sensitivity is optimal at relatively low frequencies (i.e., 2.5 mHz).

The appearance of color flow is influenced by numerous parameters, including loading conditions, color frame rates, pulse repetition frequency, gain settings, color map algorithms, and machine electronics.[420] In vitro studies have suggested that color jet areas are proportional to flow rates, and that jet kinetic energies are closely related to driving pressure.[421] In human subjects, reproducibility in the mapping of regurgitant color-flow jets is greater for large than for small jets and also greater for aortic than for mitral regurgitant jets; there is a minimum variability of 15%.[422-424]

Color-flow Doppler is most useful in the rapid detection and semi-quantitation of valvular regurgitation and intracardiac shunts. Although color-flow mitral, tricuspid, and pulmonary regurgitation are present in a high proportion of normal subjects of all ages, aortic regurgitation is considered to be a pathologic finding.[425] Successful grading scales of the severity of valvular regurgitation by color-flow Doppler have been developed using the depth of penetration of the jet into the receiving chamber, the area of the jet relative to that of the receiving chamber, and the width of the regurgitant jet at its origin.

Color-flow Doppler provides a near real-time flow map of the origin and direction of mitral regurgitation in the left atrium.[426] Although this information can also be obtained by interrogating the entire left atrium by pulsed-wave Doppler, this method may be tedious, technically difficult, and unreliable, especially in patients with eccentric jets. By color flow, mitral regurgitation in the apical view usually appears as a systolic flame-shaped stream of blue color flowing retrograde from the left ventricle to the left atrium (Fig. 28.125). Color-flow Doppler ap-

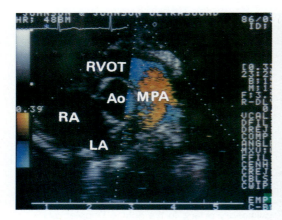

FIGURE 28.124 Doppler flow (color) mapping of the main pulmonary artery. A short axis cut through the cardiac base, similar to the left panel in Figure 28.123, demonstrates the long axis projection of the main pulmonary artery (MPA). The Doppler flow information is color-encoded so that flow in all parts of the artery can be displayed. In this systolic frame, flow should be entirely toward the transducer, or blue in color. Note that much of the color shown is red-hued, indicating flow exceeds 0.48 m/sec. Thus, the color change indicates aliasing, not reversed flow. Color-flow mapping is a promising new technique in echocardiographic imaging.

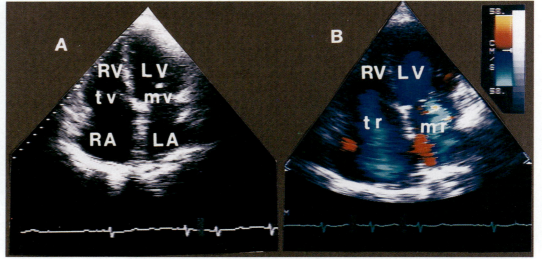

FIGURE 28.125 Color-flow Doppler of mitral regurgitation (mr) and tricuspid regurgitation (tr) in the apical view indicates streams of blue color moving from the mitral valve (mv) into the left atrium (LA) and from the tricuspid valve (tv) into the right atrium (RA), respectively. **A.** Two-dimensional imaging. **B.** Color-flow Doppler turned on. (LV, left ventricle; RV, right ventricle)

proaches ventriculography in its sensitivity to detect mitral regurgitation and its ability to grade the severity of regurgitation.[427] Although about 40% of normal subjects have mitral regurgitant color-flow jets that emanate from the posteromedial commissure, these jets are generally small in area.[425] Small jets that penetrate less than 2 cm into the left atrium generally signify mild mitral regurgitation. Large jets that fill more than half of the left atrium, extend to the posterior portion of the left atrium, or penetrate into the left atrial appendage or pulmonary veins indicate significant mitral regurgitation. In patients with very large left atria, loss of color sensitivity at maximum depths may occasionally result in the erroneous impression that mitral regurgitation is mild. The size of the jet as it forms at the valve and the convergence of the jet as it forms on the atrial (donor) side of the valve are under investigation as indicators of severity of mitral regurgitation.

Color-flow Doppler can help detect complications of bacterial endocarditis, such as perforated or flail valve leaflet, ruptured sinus of Valsalva aneurysm, and myocardial abscesses (Fig. 28.126)[428,429] In patients who develop flail mitral valve leaflet due to ruptured chordae tendineae, color flow demonstrates eccentric, turbulent mitral regurgitation jets that closely adhere to the periphery of the left atrium and move away from the damaged leaflet in a circular fashion. In flail *anterior* leaflet, mitral regurgitant jets are directed toward the posterolateral atrial wall (clockwise motion in the apical view), while in flail *posterior* leaflet, jets are directed toward the interatrial septum (counterclockwise motion) (Fig. 28.127).

Color flow is also useful to diagnose complications of acute myocardial infarction. In patients who develop new murmurs after myocardial infarction, the technique can readily distinguish interventricular shunting due to septal perforation from mitral regurgitation due to papillary muscle rupture or dysfunction.[430,431] In addition, color flow can highlight the presence of aneurysm, apical thrombus, and pseudoaneurysm.[432,433]

By color flow, aortic insufficiency appears as an abnormal mosaic of diastolic flow originating from the aortic valve and penetrating into the left ventricle (Fig. 28.128). Aortic insufficiency flow can be differentiated from mitral stenosis flow by its origin from the aortic valve in several views and its presence very early in diastole during isovolumic relaxation, before the mitral valve opens. (Figs. 28.129 and 28.130) Unlike mitral regurgitation, the maximal length and long axis area of aortic insufficiency jets do not correlate with the angiographic grade of severity.[434] However, the thickness of the aortic regurgitant jet in the long axis and area of the origin of the jet in the short axis relative to the size of the left ventricular outflow tract are better predictors of severity. The maximal mosaic pattern of diastolic flow in the left ventricle also has a fair correlation with left ventricular end-diastolic and end-systolic volumes by scintigraphy.[435] The size of the jet as it crosses the valve and the size of the convergence jet on the donor side of the valve are being investigated as further indicators of severity. Reverse flow in the descending aorta can be seen as a color reversal in the same way that pulsed-wave Doppler shows reversed diastolic flow.

Color-flow Doppler has also been applied to the detection and grading of tricuspid regurgitation (Fig. 28.131).[436,437] Tricuspid regurgitant jets can be aimed in a variety of directions, and thus should be imaged in multiple views, including apical four-chamber, right ventricular inlet, short axis parasternal through the cardiac base, and subcostal. Color-flow Doppler identifies tricuspid regurgitation with the same frequency as conventional Doppler or right ventriculography, and is more sensitive and specific than contrast two-dimensional echocardiography.[436] As with mitral regurgitation, semiquantitative grading scales are based on the depth and area of penetration of the right atrium. In addition, systolic reversal of flow in the inferior vena cava or hepatic veins indicates significant tricuspid regurgitation.

Color-flow Doppler is also useful for the assessment of prosthetic mitral valve dysfunction, especially in conjunction with transesophageal imaging. The different prostheses show specific jet patterns, which are helpful in differentiating normal from pathologic backflow.[438–441] Color flow can often distinguish paravalvular and transvalvular prosthetic mitral regurgitation and assess the severity of the leak (see Fig. 28.65). Stenotic prosthetic and native valve lesions are also readily identified and located by color Doppler[442–446]; the technique can differentiate aortic valvular, supravalvular, and various forms of subaortic stenosis. In addition, preliminary investigation suggests that the severity of stenosis may be estimated by the width of the color flow jet.

Finally, color flow is extremely helpful in the detection and assessment of congenital heart disease, especially the location, size, and number of intracardiac shunts. Advances have been made in the diagnosis of atrial septal defect, ventricular septal defect (see Fig. 28.68), coronary cameral fistulas, patent ductus arteriosus, anomalous pulmonary venous drainage, and coarctation of the aorta.[447–452] Furthermore,

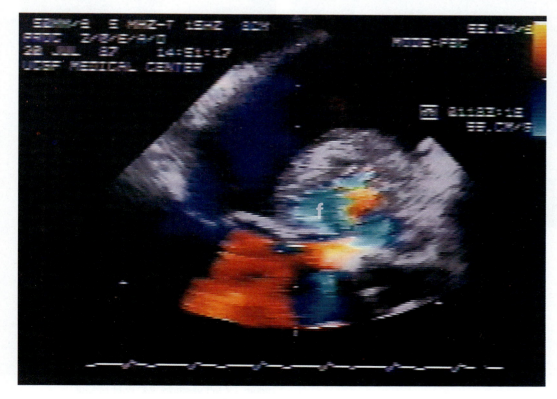

FIGURE 28.126 Transesophageal echocardiogram of an aortic abscess. Color-flow Doppler demonstrates flow (f) into the cavity of the abscess.

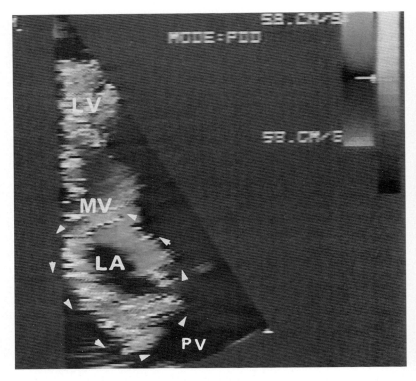

FIGURE 28.127 Apical four-chamber view showing the characteristic color-flow Doppler pattern of posterior mitral leaflet flail due to ruptured chordae tendineae. The eccentric mitral regurgitation jet moves in a counterclockwise direction (arrows) in the periphery of the left atrium (LA). (LV, left ventricle; PV, pulmonary veins)

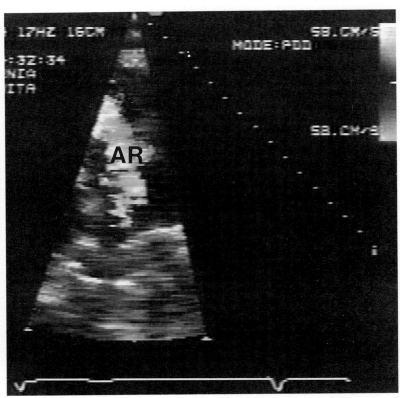

FIGURE 28.128 Apical four-chamber view with color-flow Doppler; a turbulent aortic regurgitation jet (AR) originates in the aortic valve and penetrates all the way into the apex of the left ventricle.

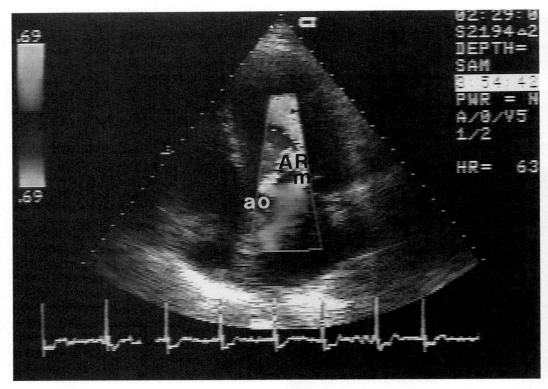

FIGURE 28.129 Apical four-chamber view with color-flow Doppler. An aaortic regurgitation jet (AR) can be seen emanating from the aortic valve (ao) and mixing with mitral inflow (m) to form a combined red jet.

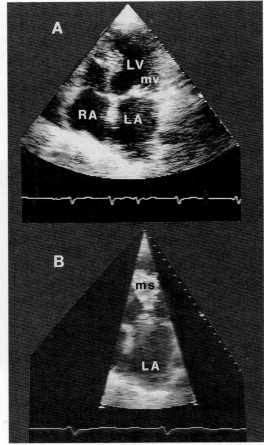

FIGURE 28.130 Apical four-chamber view in rheumatic mitral stenosis. **A.** Two-dimensional imaging shows decreased mobility and thickening of mitral valve (mv) leaflets. **B.** Color-flow Doppler indicates turbulent mitral stenosis jet (ms). (LA, left atrium; LV, left ventricle; RA, right atrium).

the diagnostic efficacy of color-flow Doppler for intracardiac shunt may be increased by the intravenous injection of contrast agents.[453,454] Intraoperative transesophageal and epicardial studies may be helpful in guiding and assessing the results of palliative surgical procedures.[455] In summary, although color flow is a semiquantitative technique, it is a major advance in cardiac imaging because it detects pathologic jets anywhere in the heart with accuracy and because it reduces the time required to perform comprehensive Doppler examinations.

ECHOCARDIOGRAPHY IN THE ACQUIRED IMMUNE DEFICIENCY SYNDROME

Although many physicians are well acquainted with the pulmonary, dermatologic, renal, neurologic, and gastrointestinal disorders associated with the acquired immune deficiency syndrome (AIDS), fewer are familiar with the cardiac disorders. With the increasing prevalence of AIDS and the widespread use of echocardiography, cardiac abnormalities are being diagnosed earlier and more frequently in the course of the disease. The major cardiac abnormalities in AIDS appear to be myocarditis, dilated cardiomyopathy, and pericarditis.[456-463] These lesions are most common in women, intravenous drug abusers, and hospitalized AIDS patients with multiple opportunistic infections and low T-helper lymphocyte counts. Isolated histologic or echocardiographic abnormalities are prevalent in AIDS, whereas symptomatic heart failure and cardiac tamponade are less common, occurring in about 5% of patients.

The most likely etiology of dilated cardiomyopathy in patients with HIV infection is infectious myocarditis. Autopsy studies in AIDS patients have demonstrated that focal nyocarditis is a common and often asymptomatic cardiac lesion. Although various cardiac pathogens have been identified, including cytomegalovirus, *Toxoplasma gondii*, *Cryptococcus neoformans*, *Candida albicans*, *Mycobacterium tuberculosis*, and *Histoplasma capsulatum*, there is no clear relationship between the presence of an opportunistic pathogen and the severity of myocarditis. Alternatively, myocardial dysfunction may be due to myocyte infection by HIV.[464] Pericardial effusions have been attributed to hypoalbuminemia, opportunistic infection in the heart or lungs, malignancy, or pericarditis. Other reports in AIDS have described primary non-Hodgkin's cardiac lymphomas,[465] disseminated Kaposi's sarcoma,[466] bacterial, fungal, and marantic endocarditis,[467-469] and severe pulmonary hypertension with cor pulmonale.[470]

Although most AIDS patients with cardiac histologic or echocardiographic abnormalities are asymptomatic, those with symptoms of congestive heart failure tend to be very ill and have an increased mortality. Despite the poor prognosis, patients with congestive heart failure often benefit symptomatically from standard medical therapy. Pericardial effusions in AIDS are usually small and benign, and only rarely cause cardiac tamponade. In the evaluation of dyspnea in AIDS, it is important to consider the cardiac as well as the pulmonary causes of this symptom. Echocardiography is recommended for hospitalized AIDS patients who have dyspnea that is out of proportion to their diagnosed pulmonary pathology or for those who have cardiac abnormalities on clinical evaluation.

ECHOCARDIOGRAPHY OF THE PERICARDIUM
DISEASES OF THE PERICARDIUM

Echocardiography is the method of choice for evaluation of most pericardial diseases. When competently performed, echocardiography detects virtually all pericardial effusions and provides clinically relevant information about their size and hemodynamic importance. The technique is less reliable in detecting and evaluating pericardial thickening and constriction but is also extremely useful in these conditions.

PERICARDIAL EFFUSION

The 1965 description of the echocardiographic diagnosis of pericardial effusion by Feigenbaum and co-workers[471] was a major stimulus to the early growth of echocardiography. In the intervening two decades, echocardiography has become the diagnostic method of choice for its identification, totally replacing more invasive procedures such as intravenous carbon dioxide during right heart fluoroscopy or blind pericardiocentesis. In addition to detection, echocardiography has a role in the assessment of the hemodynamic importance of effusions. The pericardium consists of two layers, a thick fibrous parietal layer and a thin serosal visceral layer investing the epicardium. In the normal state, there is less than 20 ml of serous fluid in the pericardial sac.[472] In pericardial effusion, the interposition of fluid between the pericardial layers results in separation of the layers to the extent that the space between can be echocardiographically resolved. In fact, as instruments with higher resolution have become available, it is not uncommon to appreciate the small separation of pericardial layers imparted by physiologic amounts of fluid. When this small separation is appre-

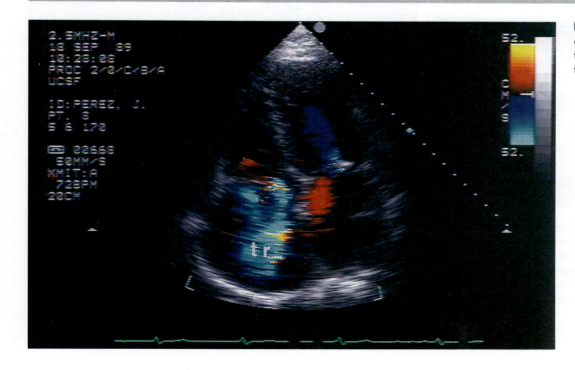

FIGURE 28.131 Severe tricuspid regurgitation (*tr*) by color-flow Doppler imaging. The blue jet emanates from two different sites on the tricuspid valve and fills most of the enlarged right atrium.

ciated, it is seen only during systole. Regardless of whether this physiologic separation is visualized, the visceral and parietal layers move in parallel to one another throughout the cardiac cycle. Appreciation of this property is important because it is altered in pericardial effusions but not in chronic pericardial inflammation without effusion. With the improvement in two-dimensional instrumentation, M-mode echocardiography has developed a subsidiary role in the evaluation of pericardial effusion. Nonetheless, its high time-resolution makes it of value in the study of pericardial motion and right ventricular dynamics. Figure 2 shows an M-mode echogram taken from a patient with disseminated testicular carcinoma, referred to our laboratory for increasing heart size. At the top of the figure is a diagrammatic representation of a long axis section of the heart cut along a line running from left hip to right shoulder. The transducer (T) sits on the anterior parasternal chest wall and the beam is swept from apex to base. The appearance of the echocardiogram at three beam positions on the diagram is designated by the arrows connecting the diagram to the echogram. Below, the pericardial effusion (PE) is seen as an echo-free space posterior to the left ventricle. This space diminishes and finally disappears as the base of the heart is approached. This distribution of pericardial effusion is due to an important anatomical relation of the pericardium to the left atrium. In this relation, the pericardium is reflected from the pulmonary veins as they enter the left atrium at its mid portion. Above this level, pericardial fluid has difficulty accumulating because the potential space available abruptly decreases. In tense pericardial effusion, the fluid migrates somewhat further behind the left atrium. For comparative purposes, Figure 28.16 shows an M-mode examination of a patient with a normal heart and pericardium. The parietal pericardium produces one of the most strongly reflective or echo-producing areas of the heart. After the second beat at the left of the figure, the gain settings of the instrument are abruptly lowered, leaving only the signals from the strongest reflector in the tracing, the pericardium. Note that the pericardium normally moves anteriorly with the epicardium. Compare this normal motion from Figure 28.132 with that of Figure 28.2. In the latter case the pericardial motion has become damped or flattened, a property typical of all freely flowing effusions. Two-dimensional echocardiography is the mainstay of the echocardiographic examination of the pericardium. The combination of its real-time format, wide-angle tomographic cuts, and multiple imaging windows affords diagnostic accuracy exceeding that available with most diagnostic tests. When its attributes of portability, safety, and repeatability are considered, its central role in effusion evaluation is easily understood. When evaluating an effusion by two-dimensional echocardiography, its presence, size, distribution, and hemodynamic importance are noted. The presence of an echo-free space between pericardial layers is the hallmark of a pericardial effusion. It is important to remember that not all pericardial spaces represent effusion. Pericardial fat is the most common source of noneffusive pericardial spaces.[473-475] This normal but highly variable tissue is most commonly seen anterior to the heart in the long axis view and in the subcostal views. The best clues to its identity as fat are its absence posteriorly, normal motion of the pericardium, low-level echoes within the space, and, perhaps most importantly, absence above the right atrium in the four-chamber view (Fig. 28.133). Of these findings, accumulation above the right atrium is, perhaps, the most important; our experience suggests that this is the first place abnormal increases in the volume of pericardial fluid are manifest. Small effusions are also reliably seen in the short axis view behind the left ventricle (Figs. 28.134, 28.135). This view is usually the only place from which normal pericardial fluid collections can be detected and is the best place from which to perform M-mode echocardiography. The use of M-mode is very important because it is the only way to appreciate the damping of the pericardium typical of a small pathologic collection of pericardial fluid. Once the effusion becomes moderate or large it is seen in every projection. If it is a simple, free-flowing effusion the damping or flattening of pericardial motion will remain a key feature. Although echocardiography is an ideal method of detection and estimation of pericardial size, it cannot quantitate effusions. Its failure in this regard arises because it is usually impossible to visualize the entire pericardial sac in any one projection and thus impossible to measure its area in that plane. It is also difficult to gain much information about the nature of the pericardial fluid; transudates, exudates, and blood are similar in appearance. Chronicity, on the other hand, is suspected if prominent strands or septations appear between the layers (Figs. 28.19 and 28.136).

Pericardial effusions come in all sizes and their hemodynamic importance is often directly proportional to their magnitude. However, very large effusions can accumulate slowly and be of only minimal hemodynamic importance and small effusions can accumulate quickly and be associated with life-threatening tamponade. A skillfully performed and interpreted echocardiogram can usually differentiate between tense, hemodynamically important effusions and benign low-pressure collections. In order to make this assessment, the size of the

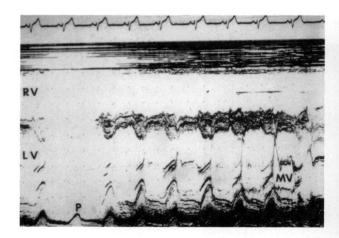

FIGURE 28.132 Normal pericardium by M-mode. M-mode echocardiogram from a normal individual demonstrating the single reflective structure that is seen posteriorly at low gain settings. This single structure (P) represents the epicardium, visceral pericardium, and parietal pericardium. Notice that at low gain this target is the only structure that can be imaged.

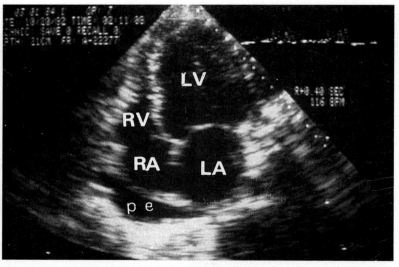

FIGURE 28.133 Pericardial effusion superior to the right atrium. Apical four-chamber view in a patient with a small pericardial effusion (pe). This effusion is seen best behind and above the right atrium. This area is the most sensitive place for detecting small effusions. In larger collections, the right atrium (RA) collapses at this point, providing a highly sensitive, minimally specific sign of cardiac tamponade.

chambers and the response of the right ventricle, right atrium, and inferior vena cava to respiration must be evaluated. Definitions of tamponade vary from hypotension caused by pericardial fluid under pressure to a less extreme state characterized by equalization of diastolic pressures. Regardless of the exact definition, pericardial tamponade has certain features that are usually present. Since the heart is generally underloaded due to impairment of filling, the chambers tend to be small. Exceptions to this finding may arise when the ventricles were enlarged prior to the accumulation of fluid. In these circumstances even slight interference with the filling of a compromised, preload-sensitive chamber may be sufficient to induce hemodynamic collapse. We have encountered tamponade in the presence of enlarged chambers due to cor pulmonale and cardiomyopathy. Tamponade is a dynamic state in which filling of the chambers is compromised. The size of the chambers is highly sensitive to respiration in that inspiration augments inflow to the volume-starved right ventricle, causing it to expand abruptly during diastole. On the other hand, expiration has the opposite effect. As inflow is decreased, pressure in the right ventricle drops and falls to or below the pressure in the pericardium. At this moment, the right ventricle and right atrium demonstrate diastolic collapse or invagination of their free walls. This phenomenon is recognized echocardiographically by a dynamic reversal of the concave outward curvature of the right ventricle (Fig. 28.137) and an indentation of the normally rounded anterosuperior right atrial wall. The M-mode also shows phasic decreases in right ventricular diameter synchronous with expiration. When the M-mode is obtained from the right ventricle, just apical to the AV groove, expiratory collapse to less than 1 cm with the patient supine is suggestive of tamponade (Figs. 28.138 and 28.139).[476-479] Because the right atrial is a thinner and more compliant structure than the right ventricle, right atrial collapse is a more sensitive

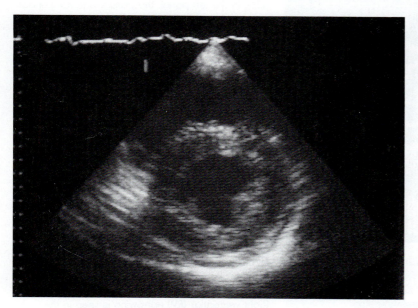
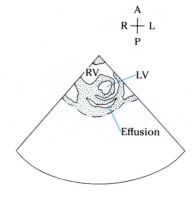

FIGURE 28.134 Small pericardial effusion. Short axis image at the level of the papillary muscles showing a small posterior collection of fluid. At times it is possible to detect physiologic accumulations of fluid behind the left atrium. In this example, the fluid could be seen in diastole and systole, suggesting a pathologic accumulation.

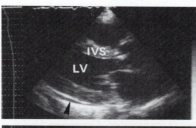
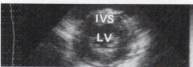
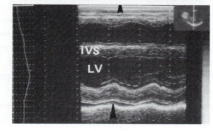

FIGURE 28.135 Small effusion. Short and long axis two-dimensional images in a patient with a small effusion (*arrowheads*). Note that the M-mode (*lower panel*) shows the posterior wall to be separated from the pericardium (*arrowhead*). All images also demonstrate considerable left ventricular hypertrophy.

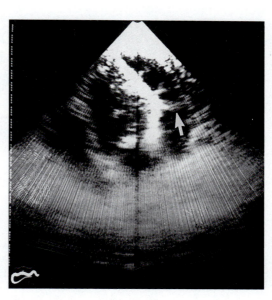

FIGURE 28.136 Stranding in chronic pericardial effusion. Two-dimensional apical four-chamber view from a patient with a chronic pericardial effusion. The transducer has been angled sharply toward the left, permitting examination of the pericardial space. Within are multiple strand-like structures (*arrow*) connecting visceral and parietal pericardium. These structures exhibited a great deal of mobility during the cardiac cycle. We consider such stranding a sign of chronicity.

but less specific sign of tamponade than right ventricular collapse (Fig. 28.140).[480,481] Similar to right ventricular collapse, the presence of this sign precedes hemodynamic evidence of tamponade and thus indicates early or incipient tamponade. While the right ventricle and right atrium collapse with expiration, the left ventricle expands. This reciprocating behavior of the ventricles is associated with the mechanism for the paradoxical pulse and arises because any increase in right ventricular volume (as in inspiration) is accompanied by a decrease in the amount of space available in the tense, fluid-filled pericardium; this extra space is contributed by the left-sided chambers, which become smaller (Fig. 28.141).

Assessment of the central venous circulation is feasible and can be reliably accomplished if a laboratory is skilled in the imaging and evaluation of the inferior vena cava (IVC). The size of the IVC and its response to respiration are the features of this structure that allow estimation of the central blood volume and the filling pressure of the right ventricle.[482–485] We define plethora of the inferior vena cava as a decrease in proximal vena caval diameter by less than 50% after deep inspiration. The vena cava can be differentiated from the descending aorta in the subcostal view by its right-sided location and lack of systolic pulsations. We have previously evaluated critically ill patients with a wide range of right atrial pressures; there is a good correlation between the change in size of the IVC after deep inspiration and right atrial pressure.[304,486] When plethora is present, the predictive value for

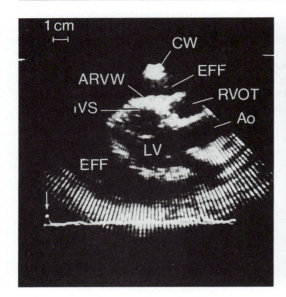
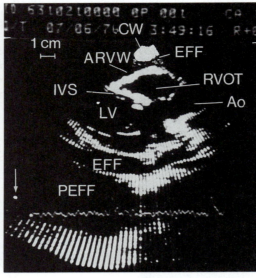

FIGURE 28.137 Tamponade. Two-dimensional long axis views from a patient with a malignant effusion (EFF). In the left panel, the patient is in tamponade and his right ventricle is compressed, leaving only the right ventricular outflow tract (RVOT) patent. In the right panel, after drainage, the right ventricle has increased considerably in size while the effusion has increased. Expansion of the scale has revealed a large left-sided pleural effusion (PEFF) posteriorly. (Schiller NB, Botvinick EH: Right ventricular compression as a sign of cardiac tamponade: An analysis of echocardiographic ventricular dimensions and their clinical implications. Circulation 56:774–779, 1977)

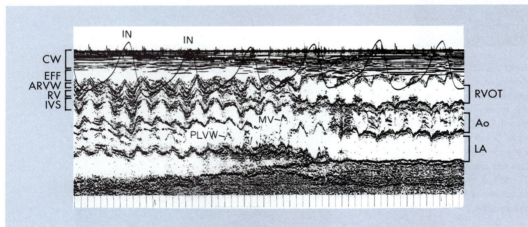

FIGURE 28.138 Tamponade. An M-mode sweep from the left ventricular cavity (left) to the aortic root (right) in a patient with cardiac tamponade. Right ventricular (RV) narrowing is seen in the minor axis. Only minimal cavitary expansion occurs with inspiration (IN), especially marked toward the right ventricular outflow tract (RVOT). (ARVW, anterior right ventricular wall; CW, chest wall; PLVW, posterior left ventricular wall) (Schiller NB, Botvinick EH: Right ventricular compression as a sign of cardiac tamponade: An analysis of echocardiographic ventricular dimensions and their clinical implications. Circulation 56:774–779, 1977)

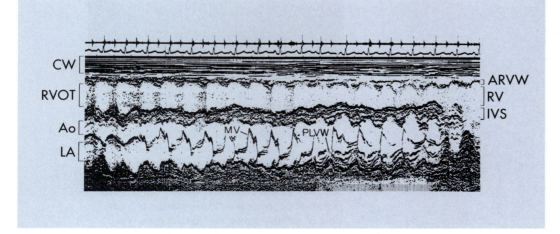

FIGURE 28.139 Tamponade. Same patient as in Figure 28.138. After pericardiotomy, the sweep, left ventricular cavity to aortic root, runs left to right. The right ventricle is decompressed and the effusion is difficult to identify. (Schiller NB, Botvinick EH: Right ventricular compression as a sign of cardiac tamponade: An analysis of echocardiographic ventricular dimensions and their clinical implications. Circulation 56:774–779, 1977)

a right atrial pressure greater than or equal to 10 mm Hg is 87%; when plethora is not present, the predictive value for a right atrial pressure less than 10 mm Hg is 82%.

In the normal patient, the development of negative intrapleural pressure with inspiration creates a pressure gradient between the abdominal IVC and the right atrium, which promotes collapse (emptying) of the IVC as blood rapidly moves into the right atrium.[27–29] In the patient who has early tamponade, elevation of pericardial pressure inhibits right ventricular filling, preventing the collapse of the IVC. Since plethora can occur when pericardial pressures exceed transdiaphragmic pressure gradients, but are still below right heart filling pressures, this sign often develops before right-sided chamber collapse and may be the last to resolve after pericardial drainage.[487] Patients with plethora have higher heart rates, lower systolic blood pressures, larger pericardial effusions, and more severe hemodynamic abnormalities than those with responsive venae cavae. As an echocardiographic marker of cardiac tamponade, plethora is far more sensitive but less specific than right-sided chamber collapse. False positives for plethora include right ventricular failure, positive pressure ventilation, and inability to inspire deeply due to decreased mentation, respiratory muscle weakness, severe breathlessness, or pleuritic chest pain. The persistence or recurrence of plethora after pericardial drainage suggests pericardial constriction, effusive-constrictive disease, or a hemodynamically significant residual effusion.

In patients recovering from cardiothoracic surgery, the added sensitivity of plethora of the IVC for the diagnosis of cardiac tamponade is especially useful. Factors contributing to the lack of sensitivity of right heart chamber collapse in cardiac surgery patients with tamponade include pericardial loculations, pulmonary hypertension, and technical problems with imaging. In these patients, it may be difficult to obtain high-quality parasternal or apical views due to the presence of mediastinal blood and air, chest bandages, drainage tubes, mechanical ventilation, and decreased patient mobility. Since right atrial or ventricular chamber inversion is often seen in only one view, this can significantly limit the usefulness of these signs. Plethora may also be absent in patients with "low-pressure" tamponade, although this entity is uncommon.[488]

Since plethora is a nonspecific marker of elevated central venous pressure, this sign should be applied in an appropriate clinical setting (i.e., presence of moderate or large pericardial effusion without right ventricular failure). However, the caval respiratory index may be most useful to exclude cardiac tamponade, since the absence of this sensitive echocardiographic sign effectively rules out a hemodynamically significant effusion that requires immediate pericardial drainage.

Other useful signs of cardiac tamponade by Doppler echocardiography include exaggerated respiratory variation in transvalvular flow velocities, isovolumic relaxation time, and reverse flow in the hepatic veins and venae cavae.[489–492] The accurate measurement of these indi-

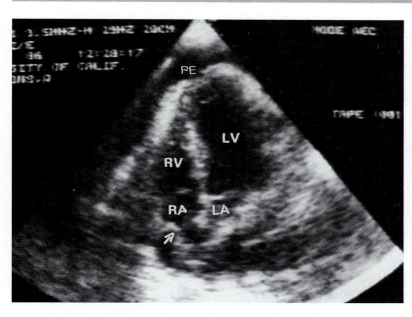

FIGURE 28.140 Tamponade. Four-chamber apical view of a patient with a large pericardial effusion (PE) well seen at the left ventricular (LV) apex. The arrow indicates the spot in the superior right atrial wall where compression is occurring. This finding is sensitive but not specific for cardiac tamponade.

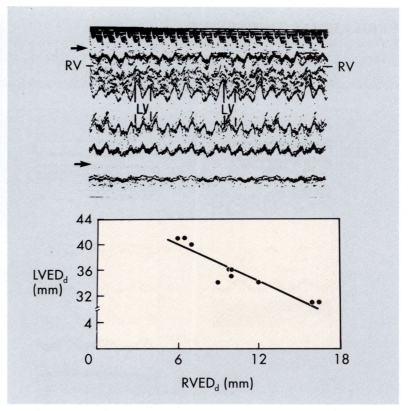

FIGURE 28.141 Tamponade. Upper panel shows M-mode through the minor axis in a patient with tamponade. During respiration, the RV fills and the LV becomes smaller; during expiration, the opposite occurs. In the graph below, RV and LV diameters are plotted against one another and demonstrate a negative correlation. This negative correlation is the result of reciprocation of the chambers within the pericardium. Since the pericardium is a rigid box, as respiration brings more blood into the RV, there is less room in the LV. Blood is pooled in the inflating lungs during inspiration. This blood plus the increased stroke volume sent to the lungs during right heart inspiratory expansion reaches the left heart during expiration. As the left heart expands, the right heart is compressed. During right heart expansion underfilling of the LV results in a drop in pulse pressure perceived as the paradoxical pulse.

ces requires that a respiratory monitor be displayed on the echocardiography screen. In patients with cardiac tamponade, the mechanism of change in these indices is probably related to respiratory variation in preload.[493] False positive results can also occur in other conditions associated with pulsus paradoxus, including acute pulmonary overload, obstructed pulmonary disease, acute left ventricular overload, and right ventricular infarction.[494] In the presence of tachycardia or arrhythmias, Doppler signals may be technically difficult to record. Furthermore, the operator must ensure that the ultrasound beam does not translocate during inspiration, causing a shift in the site or angle of interrogation.

Based on the results of the two-dimensional echocardiogram with Doppler, our initial clinical approach to patients who have moderate or large pericardial effusions is based on the presence or absence of plethora of the IVC. When this sensitive sign of a hemodynamically significant pericardial effusion is absent, we feel that there is a low probability of tamponade and generally do not recommend pericardial drainage. When plethora is present, we search for echocardiographic findings that confirm the presence of tamponade, such as right heart chamber collapse or exaggerated respiratory variation in transvalvular Doppler signals. Since plethora is not specific for tamponade, pericardial drainage is not justified without other findings. An exception to this rule is the postoperative cardiac surgical patient, where technical problems in imaging and other factors render echocardiographic confirmation of tamponade difficult. In this setting, hemodynamic data may be necessary to confirm the presence of cardiac tamponade before attempting drainage.

PERICARDIAL THICKENING

Pericardial thickening is a relatively commonly encountered echocardiographic finding, but hemodynamically important thickening or constriction is relatively rare. Diffuse or localized adhesion of the visceral and parietal layers of the pericardium is a constant feature of pericardial thickening and causes certain characteristic echocardiographic findings that facilitate its recognition. The two-dimensional recognition of pericardial thickening is somewhat difficult and is more dependent on recognition of scattered areas of adhesion interspersed with loculated areas of effusion. M-mode imaging is more sensitive to the typical motion patterns of pericardial adhesion. The cardinal feature of such adhesion is the parallel motion of the epicardium and visceral pericardium with the parietal pericardium. In other words, instead of being damped or flattened as it is in freely flowing effusion, the pericardium moves in parallel with the epicardium. Since this motion is identical to the normal behavior of the pericardium, the differentiation between normality and thickening depends on one additional feature. That feature is a separation between the visceral pericardium and epicardium, which, unlike the normal state, allows appreciation of these two distinct surfaces. This separation is present in both pericardial effusion, in which the visceral layer is flattened or damped, and pericardial thickening, in which there is parallel motion of these layers. The relatively echo-free appearance of this separating space in pericardial thickening belies the fact that it is a solid or semisolid adhesive substance pulling the pericardium inward with normal contraction. Figure 28.142 shows that the process following accumulation of pericardial fluid can pass from the free-flowing state with damped pericardium to the adhesive state to resolution. If the adhesive or thickened state fails to resolve, chronic pericardial thickening or constriction can develop.

PERICARDIAL CONSTRICTION

Pericardial thickening with constriction and pericardial thickening without constriction share several features in common but, with careful attention to the details of the echocardiographic findings, they can

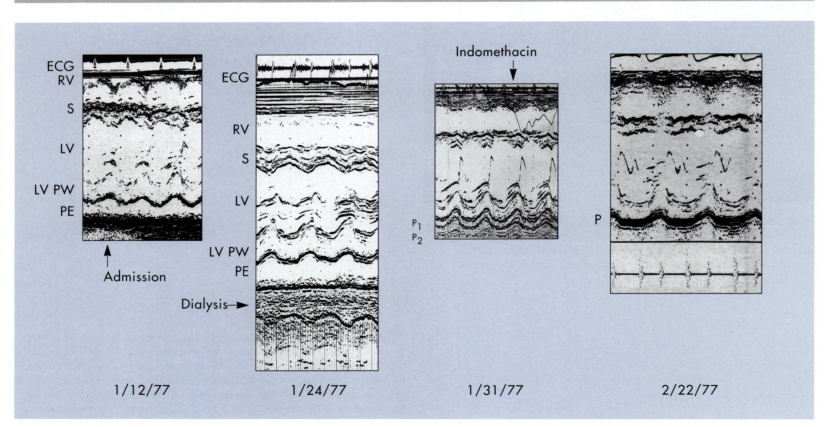

FIGURE 28.142 Pericarditis. Serial echograms from a patient with end-stage renal disease and the onset of symptoms of pericarditis. Moderate effusion was shown (*left*) and assumed secondary to uremia. The frequency of dialysis was increased, but after 12 days the effusion was larger (*left center*). Pericarditis was assumed to be inflammatory/infectious and indomethacin was administered. Seven days later (*right center*) there was resolution of effusion with evidence of pericardial thickening pattern (i.e., parallel motion of pericardial layers P_1 and P_2). Three weeks following detection of this pattern, there was no sign of pericardial space and only mild residual pericardial thickening (*right*). (Schiller NB: Echocardiography in pericardial diseases. Med Clin North Am 64:253–282, March, 1980)

often be differentiated. As with the distinction between tamponade and effusion there is a large gray zone between frank constriction and extensive pericardial thickening without hemodynamic compromise. The role of echocardiography is to interact with other clinical parameters so that patients in whom constriction is potentially present can be separated from those in whom it is unlikely; it is futile to strive for exact diagnosis where none, in fact, exists. The M-mode portion of the examination is very helpful in the evaluation of a patient suspected of constriction. As described above, the characteristic parallel motion of the epicardium and the pericardium can be positively identified by M-mode and must be present before constriction can be considered. A characteristic septal notch has also been described[495,496] in early diastole and occurs around the time of the pericardial knock. It has also been reported that the myocardium is flattened after an abbreviated rapid filling wave, that the mitral valve motion shows a diminished *a* wave, and that there is premature pulmonary valve opening.[497-499] The two-dimensional examination is the most important in identifying constriction and exhibits a number of features that are supportive of the diagnosis but not necessarily pathognomonic. Pericardial thickening can be seen by irregular reflectance of the pericardium investing various portions of the cardiac chambers. When suspected, an M-mode is passed through the area and the characteristic parallel motion of the layers is sought. In long-standing constriction, the relatively echo-free layer between the visceral and parietal pericardium can become densely fibrosed, frustrating identification by either M-mode or two-dimensional methods. In some areas it is not possible to direct the M-mode beam so that it strikes the area of interest at a 90-degree angle of incidence. In these situations the two-dimensional image must be studied in detail for evidence of adhesion of layers. The best places to look for abnormal motion of the myocardium relative to the pericardium are anterior to the right ventricular outflow tract or at the lateral apex in the four-chamber view; this finding must be sought in real time. Normal motion is characterized by the myocardium sliding or shearing along the plane of the pericardium without appearing to pull inward on the outer layers. If the myocardium appears to pull the pericardium without altering the small echo-free space separating these layers, adhesion in the area examined is suspected. When the entire pericardium is separated by a small fixed space, we call this the "halo sign" (Fig. 28.143). The finding of extensive areas of adhesion (posterior by M-mode and apical and around the right ventricular outflow tract by two-dimensional imaging) provides compelling evidence for the sort of generalized pericardial thickening needed to result in constriction. It should be noted that localized constriction is always possible albeit relatively unusual. We have seen this condition in patients who had striking loculation with intermittent areas of effusion and thickening. Usually this situation arises after cardiac surgery and is caused by postcardiotomy pericarditis.

Septal bounce is the two-dimensional counterpart of the M-mode septal notch and is often the first clue that constriction is present. This early diastolic incoordinate septal motion occurs toward the apex and is indistinguishable from the incoordinate contraction/relaxation pattern seen in left bundle branch block or paced rhythm arising from the right ventricular apex. Once the septal bounce is noted the echocardiography laboratory must exclude constriction as a possible diagnosis. If septal bounce and pericardial thickening are present the next sign that must be present in constriction is a plethoric IVC. Although this sign may not be manifest if the patient has undergone brisk diuresis or is severely dehydrated, its absence makes the diagnosis of advanced or significant constriction unlikely.

Several investigators contend that no single M-mode echocardiographic abnormality is specific for constrictive pericarditis.[500,501] For example, although rapid early diastolic filling of the ventricles, which is a physiologic hallmark of constriction, may cause premature opening of the pulmonic valve as well as abnormalities in left ventricular posterior wall and posterior aortic root motion, other conditions associated with rapid early diastolic ventricular filling, such as severe valvular regurgitation, may also demonstrate these findings.

Two-dimensional echocardiographic signs, such as early diastolic septal bounce, vena cava plethora with blunted respiratory response, and pericardial adhesion with lack of pericardial sliding, are also useful in the diagnosis of constriction and in its differentiation from hemodynamically insignificant pericardial thickening and restrictive cardiomyopathy.[502] Of these signs, plethora of the IVC and pericardial adhesion are the most sensitive for constrictive pericarditis, while diastolic septal bounce is the most specific. The complementary diagnostic value of these three echocardiographic signs reflects their dependence on disparate aspects of the physiology of constrictive pericarditis. Early diastolic septal bounce derives from transient rapid reversal of transseptal pressure gradients associated with rapid diastolic filling, plethora of the IVC reflects elevated right atrial pressures, and pericardial adhesion denotes chronic pericardial inflammation, loculation, and fibrosis. In addition, the presence of ascites and pleural effusions (Fig. 28.144) should suggest the diagnosis of pericardial constriction.

Doppler findings in pericardial constriction are related to those described for cardiac tamponade and include exaggerated respiratory variation in early mitral and tricuspid valvular flows and alterations in central venous flow patterns.[503,504] Finding constriction by echocardiography or Doppler may not always necessitate surgery. In the course of the resolution of a simple effusion, a brief constriction phase is often clinically and echographically appreciated (see Fig. 28.142).[505]

TUMORS OF THE PERICARDIUM

Localized pericardial thickening or large effusions can often represent the direct manifestation or the result of pericardial tumor.[506] It is usually impossible to separate strands and protein deposition common to all effusions from areas of tumor implantation. However, if a large tumor invades locally from the lateral chest, it is often possible to appreciate a locally dense area along the lateral border of the heart.

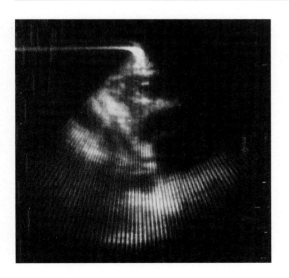 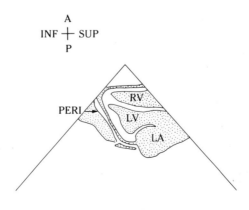

FIGURE 28.143 Subacute construction. A space separates the pericardium (*PERI*) from the RV and LV apex. This space surrounds the heart like a halo. During the cardiac cycle, this space maintains its width and the opposing layers of pericardium and myocardium do not slide across one another. Although the space has few if any reflectors within, it is clearly an adhesive, solid material. The halo sign is seen in constriction of a subacute nature.

The telling characteristic of these masses is often their seeming immobility during the cardiac cycle; as the heart abuts these masses they seem fixed in space.

ABSENCE OF THE PERICARDIUM
Complete and partial absence of the pericardium is described as being associated with enlargement of the right ventricle and paradoxical motion of the interventricular septum, findings that mimic right ventricular volume overload as seen in atrial septal defect or tricuspid insufficiency.[338,339]

PERICARDIAL CYSTS
These structures are usually suggested by the chest x-ray film. Echocardiography in the few examples we have encountered has been frustrating because the cyst lies in the lateral portion of the ultrasound beam, outside of its regions of highest resolution.[507]

ECHOCARDIOGRAPHY OF TUMORS, MASSES, AND THROMBI
Echocardiography is the method of choice for the initial evaluation of intracardiac masses, tumors, and thrombi. The first echocardiographically recognized intracardiac tumor was reported in 1959.[508] This study used M-mode, which was the established method until two-dimensional methods became available. Two-dimensional scanning has made M-mode evaluation of secondary importance in that all chambers, valves, and great vessels can be evaluated in a cross-sectional real-time format. Since most masses exhibit some degree of mobility, a real-time format offers considerable advantage in this application. Left atrial thrombi in most echocardiographic examinations are mural, immobile, poor sonic reflectors lying at a distance from the transducer and are therefore not optimally imaged. However, tumors are readily appreciated because of their size, mobility, and highly reflective nature. The most common atrial tumors are left atrial myxomata. Arising from the interatrial septum, these masses can be relatively stationary or freely prolapsing through the mitral valve. Obstruction to mitral inflow varies with their size and degree of prolapse. In Figure 28.145, a large tumor that did not prolapse is illustrated. It was of interest because it contained both cysts and bone. When studied at surgery by transesophageal echocardiography, these features were more obvious because the left atrium was very close to the intraesophageal transducer. The degree of obstruction can be assessed by Doppler. In this case, there was no increase in inflow velocity despite the large size of the mass. M-mode provides an additional clue to the degree of obstruction by noting the presence of diastolic mitral vibrations as the tumor falls through the orifice. Not all atrial tumors are benign. Figure 28.146[312,509] shows a patient in whom the tumor was at first thought to be benign but was identified as a fibrohistiocytoma which fatally recurred shortly after surgical resection. Left atrial

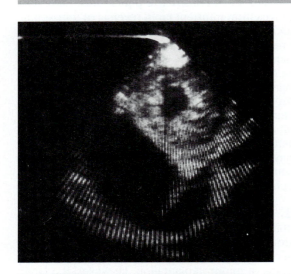
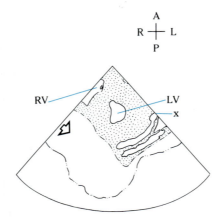

FIGURE 28.144 Pleural effusion. A large posteromedial space (open arrow) is seen behind the heart. Although superficially resembling a pericardial effusion, its sheer size, unaccompanied by any anterior collection, typifies large pleural effusion. Careful inspection reveals a small posterior pericardial effusion (x).

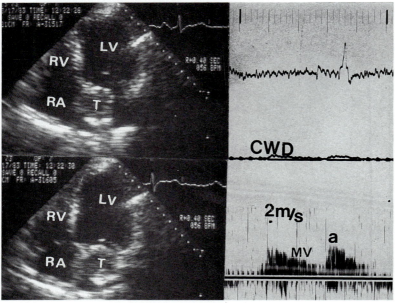

FIGURE 28.145 Left atrial myxoma. A large, partially calcified atrial myxoma (T) was found incidentally during a chest pain work-up. The tumor shows very little motion during parts of the cardiac cycle. Although the tumor appears obstructive, Doppler (right) performed with continuous wave (CWD) shows no inflow tract obstruction.

thrombi, in our experience, are very difficult to detect because of poor resolution in the distal portion of the ultrasound beam. Transesophageal imaging, on the other hand, more clearly shows these masses. Recent reports even suggest that transesophageal echocardiography can image thrombi in the atrial appendages.[510] With conventional echocardiography, there is little question that these masses are frequently overlooked.

LEFT VENTRICULAR THROMBI

Practically speaking, the recognition that left ventricular thrombi were frequent in anterior infarction is the direct result of the widespread use of echocardiography in ischemic heart disease. Because they are so common and because of their potential for embolization, this application of echocardiography is the most important when it comes to the study of intracardiac masses. The vast majority of masses arise in the setting of anteroapical infarction with aneurysm formation.[123] Inferior infarction is a rare thrombus formation site. In one series,[123] thrombi developed during serial evaluation in 12 of 35 patients (34%) with anterior infarction. On the average, the thrombi developed on the fifth postinfarction day and were more common in older patients with larger infarctions. The risk for embolization is greatest 5 to 20 days after the infarction, with rapidly decreasing incidence thereafter. Although anticoagulation does appear to reduce the incidence of systemic embolization, once thrombus is detected it does not seem to hasten its disappearance. The sensitivity of echocardiography in thrombus detection was evaluated by Visser[511] and co-workers in a series in which 51 of 67 patients had direct anatomical verification of thrombus either at surgery or postmortem. In this series the sensitivity of two-dimensional echocardiography was 92% and specificity was 88%. Myxomata of the left ventricle are extremely rare, although we have encountered two such cases.[509,512] In both cases the tumors were located at the apex, which had normal wall motion. This combination of normally moving apex and mass formation is in strong contrast to the usual setting of thrombus formation, suggesting that myxomata are not degenerated or organized thrombus. We have also encountered left ventricular masses in a patient with overwhelming staphylococcal endocarditis and have failed to detect autopsy-documented masses shown to be caused by extensive aspergillosis infection.[513]

We have encountered one hemangioma of the left ventricle, a liposarcoma,[88] and a few cases of metastatic malignant melanoma. It is important not to confuse unusual presentations of asymmetric hypertrophic cardiomyopathies (so-called Japanese or apical hypertrophic cardiomyopathy) with tumors.

It is very important that normal structures in the left ventricle not be confused with pathologic masses. Bands and trabeculations[514] are common in cardiomyopathy and particularly prominent at the apex. There is also a small muscle near the left ventricular outflow tract from which a tendon runs to the proximal interventricular septum.

RIGHT ATRIUM AND INFERIOR VENA CAVA THROMBI AND MASSES

Based on their frequency and implications, the most important right atrial masses are thrombi arising in the lower extremities that lodge in that chamber (and in the right ventricle) during their embolic migration toward the pulmonary circuit (Fig. 28.147). In the past few years (1984 and 1985) there have been 21 case reports and series dealing with these masses.[351-355,359-363,367,370] Almost all of these reports cite a high mortality in this setting.

Right atrial myxomata are less frequently encountered than left (see Fig. 28.147). At times they appear as one of bilateral atrial myxomata but most often they are solitary. Since they remain silent for longer periods than those on the left, they tend to become much larger. Once they become large enough to fill much of the inflow orifice they become symptomatic, often presenting as positional, intermittent dyspnea or syncope. As with left atrial myxomata, they are attached to the interatrial septum along the inferior margin of the foramen ovale. They are best seen in the four-chamber apical view and in the long and short axis precordial views of the right atrium. Since the right atrium can lie along the margin of the imaging plane it is important to attempt to center the right-sided structures so that these targets can reside in the most highly resolved portion of the beam plane. When encountering a right atrial mass, the most important differential diagnostic point is to determine the origin of the mass. If the mass appears attached to the interatrial septum, it is most likely a myxoma. If, however, this attachment cannot be shown, the mass may be arising from abdominal or mediastinal structures and propagating centrally within the vena cava (see Fig. 28.147). We have encountered hepatomata, renal tumors, adrenal tumors, and thymomas in the right atrium. It is essential that echocardiographers be familiar with imaging the vena cava in order that they might clearly demonstrate the nature of the right atrial tumor in question. Right atrial thrombi and tumors often extend into the right ventricle.

The real-time format of two-dimensional echocardiography allows the examiner to fix the chamber of origin in most of these cases. Tumors that arise in the right ventricle are rather unusual. We have encountered myxomata on two occasions, both of which arose in the right ventricular outflow tract. We have also encountered metastatic tumors, most commonly melanoma. Other tumors such as hemangiomata or rhabdomyoma also are seen echocardiographically. The diagnosis is often based on the clinical setting in which they are encountered. Normal right-sided structures can be confused with pathologic masses. The right ventricular AV groove near the right atrial appendage

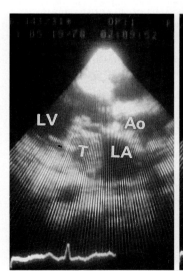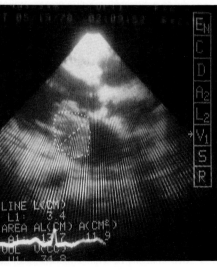

FIGURE 28.146 Mobile left atrial tumor. This was at first thought to be a left atrial myxoma. Histologically it was a fibrohistiocytoma and proved fatal despite wide atrial resection. In the right panel, a single plane area length measurement of the tumor shows a volume of 35 ml.

often appears as a dense, highly mobile region but is a normal structure. The eustachian ridge, best seen in the long axis precordial view, demarcates the entrance of the coronary sinus from the IVC and is a long projecting structure often seen in association with a vestige of fetal life, the Chiari network (see Fig. 28.115).[515] This strand-like structure attaches the eustachian valve and ridge to the inferior limb of the coronary sinus. In younger individuals it is very prominent and usually, but not always, regresses with advancing age.

Two-dimensional echocardiography utilizing high parasternal views may also be useful as a first-line test in the identification and evaluation of mediastinal masses. A disadvantage of echocardiography is that the fan-shaped field allows only a small part of the anterior mediastinum to be scanned at any one time. Thus, computed tomography, which provides anatomic sections of the entire thorax in serial planes, is useful for confirming and more completely evaluating the location and extent of mediastinal pathology.[516]

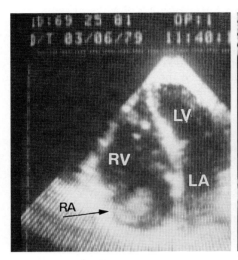
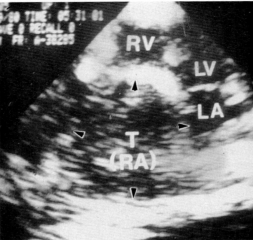
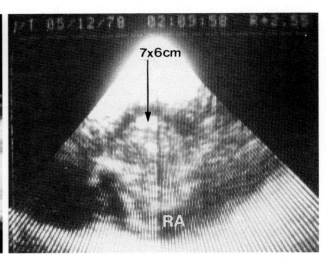

FIGURE 28.147 Right atrial masses and tumors. (*Left*) A mass protruding into the right atrium turned out to be a thrombus arising from the hepatic veins, or Budd-Chiari syndrome. Other right atrial thrombi are strongly associated with pulmonary emboli. The masses are thought to be emboli in transit, temporarily stuck to the inner architecture of the right heart. (*Middle*) A very large mass deforms and distorts not only the right atrium but the other three chambers as well. This tumor caused severe inflow obstruction as can be seen from the underloaded appearance of the rest of the chambers. This tumor was a malignant thymoma that propagated down from the superior vena cava. (*Right*) A 7 cm × 6 cm right atrial mass was asymptomatic until just prior to presentation. At this time the patient was complaining of positional syncope. The tumor was initially seen on an upper gastrointestinal series and confirmed with this echocardiogram. The patient went to surgery without catheterization.

REFERENCES

1. Hertz CH: Ultrasonic engineering in heart diagnosis. Am J Cardiol 19:6, 1967
2. Edler I: Ultrasound cardiogram in mitral valve disease. Acta Chir Scand 111:230, 1956
3. Edler I, Gustafson A: Ultrasonic cardiogram in mitral stenosis. Acta Med Scand 159:85, 1957
4. Schiller NB, Acquatella H, Ports TA et al: Left ventricular volume from paired biplane two-dimensional echocardiographs. Circulation 60:547, 1979
5. Melton HE Jr, Thurstone FS: Annular array design and logarithmic processing for ultrasonic imaging. Ultrasound Med Biol 4:1, 1978
6. Silverman NH, Snider AR: Two-Dimensional Echocardiography in Congenital Heart Disease, p 58. Norwalk, CT, Appleton-Century-Crofts, 1982
7. Collins SM, Skorton DJ: Cardiac Imaging and Image Processing, p 171. New York, McGraw-Hill, 1986
8. Hatle L, Angelsen B: Doppler Ultrasound in Cardiology: Physical Principles and Clinical Applications, 2nd ed, p 78. Philadelphia, Lea & Febiger, 1985
9. Crawford MH, Petru MA, Amon KW et al: Comparative value of 2-dimensional echocardiography and radionuclide angiography for qualitating changes in left ventricular performance during exercise limited by angina pectoris. Am J Cardiol 53:42, 1984
10. Weisse A, Jordan T: A comparison of M-mode left ventricular dimensions derived from parasternal long and short axis 2-D echocardiograms in normal and abnormal adults. J Clin Ultrasound 3:51, 1984
11. Feigenbaum H: Echocardiography, 4th ed, p 159. Philadelphia, Lea & Febiger, 1986
12. Massie BM, Schiller NB, Ratshin RA, Parmley WW: Mitral septal separation: New echocardiographic index of left ventricular function. Am J Cardiol 39:1008, 1977
13. Child JS, Krivokapick J, Perloff JK: Effect of left ventricular size on mitral E point to ventricular septal separation in assessment of cardiac performance. Am Heart J 101:797, 1981
14. Koenig W, Gehring J, Mathes P: M-mode echocardiography in the diagnosis of global and regional myocardial function in coronary heart disease: A study validated by quantitative left ventricular cineangiography. J Clin Ultrasound 3:165, 1984
15. Engle SJ, Disessa TG, Perloff J et al: Mitral valve E point to ventricular septal separation in infants and children. Am J Cardiol 52:1084, 1983
16. Djalaly A, Schiller NB, Poehlmann HW et al: Diastolic aortic root motion in left ventricular hypertrophy. Chest 79:442, 1981
17. Klauser S, Botvinick E, Schiller NB: Determination of LV stroke volume by aortic root motion: An echographic index of ventricular function (abstr). Clin Res 24:84A, 1976
18. Bryhn M: Abnormal left ventricular filling in patients with sustained myocardial relaxation: Assessment of diastolic parameters using radionuclide angiography and echocardiography. Clin Cardiol 7:639, 1984
19. O'Rourke R, Hanrath P, Henry W et al: Report of the Joint International Society and Federation of Cardiology/World Health Organization Task Force on recommendations for standardization of measurements from M-mode echocardiograms—special report (abstr). Circulation 69:854A, 1984
20. Panidis J, Ross J, Ren J et al: Comparison of independent and derived M-mode echocardiographic measurements. Am J Cardiol 54:694, 1984
21. Gardin JM, Tommaso CL, Talano JV: Echographic early systolic partial closure (notching) of the aortic valve in congestive cardiomyopathy. Am Heart J 107:135, 1984
22. Kiulzi M, Gillam L, Gentile F et al: Normal adult cross-sectional echocardiographic values: Linear dimensions and chamber areas. Echocardiography 1:403, 1984
23. Weisse A, Jordan T: A comparison of M-mode left ventricular dimensions derived from parasternal long and short axis 2-D echocardiograms in normal and abnormal adults. J Clin Ultrasound 3:51, 1984
24. Teichholz LE, Kreulen T, Herman MV, Gorlin R: Problems in echocardiographic volume determinations: Echocardiographic-angiographic correlations in the presence or absence of asynergy. Am J Cardiol 37:7, 1976
25. Vredevoe L, Creekmore S, Schiller NB: The measurement of systolic time intervals by echocardiography. J Clin Ultrasound 2:229, 1974
26. Spodick D, Doi Y, Bishop R, Hashimoto T: Systolic time intervals reconsidered—reevaluation of the preejection period: Absence of relation to heart rate. Am J Cardiol 53:1667, 1984
27. Traill TA, Gibson DG, Brown DJ: Study of left ventricular wall thickness and dimension changes using echocardiography. Br Heart J 40:162, 1978
28. Stamm RB, Carabello BA, Mayers DL, Martin RP: Two dimensional echocardiographic measurement of left ventricular ejection fraction: Prospective analysis of what constitutes an adequate determination. Am Heart J 104:136, 1982
29. Rich S, Sheikh A, Gallastegui J et al: Determination of left ventricular frac-

30. Wyatt HL, Meerbaum S, Heng MK et al: Cross-sectional echocardiography. III. Analysis of mathematic models for quantifying volume of symmetric and asymmetric left ventricles. Am Heart J 100:821, 1980
31. Silverman NH, Ports TA, Snider AR et al: Determination of left ventricular volume in children—echocardiographic and angiographic comparisons. Circulation 62:548, 1980
32. Starling MR, Crawford MH, Sorensen SG et al: Comparative accuracy of apical biplane cross-sectional echocardiography and gated equilibrium radionuclide angiography for estimating left ventricular size and performance. Circulation 63:1075, 1981
33. Wyatt HL, Haendchen RV, Meerbaum S, Corday E: Assessment of quantitative methods for 2-dimensional echocardiography. Am J Cardiol 52:396, 1983
34. Weiss JL, Eaton LW, Kallman CH, Maughan WL: Accuracy of volume determination by two-dimensional echocardiography: Defining requirements under controlled conditions in the ejecting canine left ventricle. Circulation 67:889, 1983
35. Wahr DW, Wang Y, Schiller NB: Left ventricular volumes determined by two-dimensional echocardiography in a normal adult population. J Am Coll Cardiol 1:3, 863, 1983
36. Bouchard A, Blumlein S, Schiller NB et al: New method for the measurement of stroke volume and cardiac output by M-mode/continuous wave doppler (abstr). Circulation 70:II, 1984
37. Gardin JM, Iseri LT, Elkayam U et al: Evaluation of dilated cardiomyopathy by pulsed Doppler echocardiography. Am Heart J 106:1057, 1983
38. Elkayam U, Gardin JM, Berkley R et al: The use of Doppler flow velocity measurement to assess the hemodynamic response to vasodilators in patients with heart failure. Circulation 67:377, 1983
39. Goldberg SF, Sahn DJ, Allen HD et al: Evaluation of pulmonary and systemic blood flow by two-dimensional Doppler echocardiography using fast Fourier transform spectral analysis. Am J Cardiol 50:1394, 1982
40. Nishimura RA, Callahan MJ, Schaff HV et al: Noninvasive measurement of cardiac output by continuous-wave Doppler echocardiography: Initial experience and review of the literature. Mayo Clin Proc 59:484, 1984
41. Fisher DC, Sahn DJ, Friedman MJ et al: The effect of variations on pulsed Doppler sampling site on calculation of cardiac output: An experimental study in open-chest dogs. Circulation 67:370, 1983
42. Loeppky JA, Hoekenga DE, Greene R, Luft UC: Comparison of noninvasive pulsed Doppler and Fick measurements of stroke volume in cardiac patients. Am Heart J 107:339, 1984
43. Chandraratna PA, Nanna M, McKay C et al: Determination of cardiac output by transcutaneous continuous-wave ultrasonic Doppler computer. Am J Cardiol 53:234, 1984
44. Magnin PA, Stewart JA, Myers S et al: Combined Doppler and phased-array echocardiographic estimation of cardiac output. Circulation 63:388, 1981
45. Ihlen H, Amlie JP, Dale J et al: Determination of cardiac output by Doppler echocardiography. Br Heart J 51:54, 1984
46. Schuster AH, Nanda NC: Doppler echocardiographic measurement of cardiac output: Comparison with a non-golden standard. Am J Cardiol 53:256, 1984
47. Lewis J, Kuo L, Nelson J et al: Pulsed Doppler echocardiographic determination of stroke volume and cardiac output: Clinical validation of two new methods using the apical window. Circulation 70:425, 1984
48. Nishimura R, Callahan M, Schaff H et al: Noninvasive measurement of cardiac output by continuous-wave Doppler echocardiography: Initial experience and review of the literature. Mayo Clin Proc 59:484, 1984
49. Schuster A, Nanda N: Doppler echocardiography—Part 1: Doppler cardiac output measurements perspective and comparison with other methods of cardiac output determination. Echocardiography 1:45, 1984
50. Gardin J, Dabestani A, Matin K et al: Reproducibility of Doppler aortic valve blood flow measurements: Studies on intraobserver, interobserver and day to day variability in normal subjects. Am J Cardiol 54:1092, 1984
51. Rose J, Nanna K, Rahimtoola SH et al: Transcutaneous continuous-wave Doppler computer. Am J Cardiol 54:1099, 1984
52. Barron JV, Sahn DJ, Valdes-Cruz LM et al: Clinical utility of two-dimensional Doppler echocardiographic techniques for estimating pulmonary to systemic blood flow ratios in children with L to R shunting ASD, VSD and PDA. J Am Coll Cardiol 3:169, 1984
53. Babovitz A, Buckingham T, Habermehl K et al: The effects of sampling site on the two-dimensional echo Doppler determination of cardiac output. Am Heart J 109:327, 1985
54. Zhang Y, Nitter-Hauge S, Ihlen H, Myhre E: Doppler echocardiographic measurement of cardiac output using the mitral orifice method. Br Heart J 53:130, 1985
55. Sahn D: Determination of cardiac output by echocardiographic Doppler methods: Relative accuracy of various sites for measurement. J Am Coll Cardiol 6(3):663, 1985
56. Goldberg S, Dickinson D, Wilson N: Evaluation of an elliptical area technique for calculating mitral blood flow by Doppler echocardiography. Br Heart J 54:68, 1985
57. Trompler A, Sold G, Vogt A, Kreuzer H: Noninvasive determination of stroke volume with spectral Doppler echocardiography. J Cardiol 74:322, 1985
58. Byrd BF III, Schiller NB, Botvinick EH et al: Magnetic resonance imaging and two-dimensional echocardiography in dilated cardiomyopathy (abstr). Circulation 72(III):22, 1985
59. Beaupre P, Cahalan M, Kremer P et al: Contractility depression during anesthesia: Comparison of halothane, enflurane and isoflurane by transesophageal echocardiography (abstr). Circulation 68(III):332, 1983
60. Sahn DJ, DeMaria A, Kisslo J, Weyman A: Recommendations regarding quantitation in M-mode echocardiography: Results of a survey of echocardiographic measurements. Circulation 58:1072, 1978
61. Gibson DG: Measurement of left ventricular volumes in man by echocardiography—comparison with biplane angiographs. Br Heart J 33:614, 1971
62. Schnittger I, Gordon EP, Fitzgerald PJ, Popp RL: Standardized intracardiac measurements of two-dimensional echocardiography. J Am Coll Cardiol 2:5, 1983
63. Byrd BF III, Mickelson J, Bouchard A et al: Left ventricular mechanics in distance runners. Circulation 70(II):138, 1984
64. Oakley D: Cardiac hypertrophy in athletes. Br Heart J 52:121, 1984
65. Fagard R, Aubert A, Staessen J et al: Cardiac structure and function in cyclists and runners—comparative echocardiographic study. Br Heart J 52:124, 1984
66. Shapiro LM: Physiological left ventricular hypertrophy. Br Heart J 52:130, 1984
67. Csanady M, Gruber N: Comparative echocardiographic studies in leading canoe-kayak and handball sportmen. Cor Vasa 26:32, 1984
68. Graettinger W: The cardiovascular response to chronic physical exertion and exercise training: An echocardiographic review. Am Heart J 108:1014, 1984
69. Shapiro LM, Smith RG: Effect of training on left ventricular structure and function. Br Heart J 50:534, 1983
70. Hauser A, Dressendorfer R, Vos M et al: Symmetric cardiac enlargement in highly trained endurance athletes: A two-dimensional echocardiographic study. Am Heart J 109:1038, 1985
71. Huston T, Puffer J, Rodney W, Oberman A: The athletic heart syndrome. N Engl J Med 313:24, 1985
72. Wolfe L, Martin R, Watson D et al: Chronic exercise and left ventricular structure and function in healthy human subjects. J Appl Physiol 58:409, 1985
73. Colan S, Sanders SP, MacPherson D, Borow K: Left ventricular diastolic function in elite athletes with physiologic cardiac hypertrophy. J Am Coll Cardiol 6(3):545, 1985
74. Arvan S, Varat M: Persistent ST-segment elevation and left ventricular wall abnormalities: A two-dimensional echocardiographic study. Am J Cardiol 53:1542, 1984
75. Stamm RB, Gibson RS, Bishop HL et al: Echocardiographic detection of infarction: Correlation with the extent of angiographic coronary disease. Circulation 67:233, 1983
76. Weiss JL, Bulkley BH, Hutchins GM, Mason SJ: Two dimensional echocardiographic recognition of myocardial injury in man: Comparison with post-mortem studies. Circulation 63:401, 1981
77. Wong M, Shah PM: Accuracy of two-dimensional echocardiography in detecting left ventricular aneurysm. Clin Cardiol 6:250, 1983
78. Roberts C, MacLean D, Maroko P, Kloner R: Early and late remodeling of the left ventricle after acute myocardial infarction. Am J Cardiol 54:407, 1984
79. Matsumoto M, Watanabe F, Goto A et al: Left ventricular aneurysm and the prediction of left ventricular enlargement studies by two-dimensional echocardiography: Quantitative assessment of aneurysm size in relation to clinical course. Circulation 72:280, 1985
80. Devereux RB, Reichek N: Echocardiographic determination of left ventricular mass in man. Anatomic validation of the method. Circulation 55:613, 1977
81. Abbasi AS, MacAlpin RN, Eber LM, Pearce ML: Echocardiographic diagnosis of idiopathic hypertrophic cardiomyopathy without outflow obstruction. Circulation 46:897, 1972
82. Feldman T, Borow K, Neumann A et al: Relation of electrocardiographic R-wave amplitude to changes in left ventricular chamber size and position in normal subjects. Am J Cardiol 55:1168, 1985
83. Casale P, Devereux R, Kligfield P et al: Echocardiographic detection of left ventricular hypertrophy: Development and prospective validation of improved criteria. J Am Coll Cardiol 6(3):572, 1985
84. Reichek N, Helak J, Plappert TA et al: Anatomic validation of left ventricular mass estimates from clinical two-dimensional echocardiography: Initial results. Circulation 67:348, 1983
85. Helak JW, Reichek N: Quantitation of human left ventricular mass and volume by two-dimensional echocardiography: In vitro anatomic validation. Circulation 63:1398, 1981
86. Devereux RB, Casale PN, Eiserberg RR et al: Electrocardiographic detection of left ventricular hypertrophy using echocardiographic determination of left ventricular mass as the reference standard. Comparison of standard criteria, computer diagnosis and physician interpretation. J Am Coll Cardiol 3:882, 1984
87. Godwin JD, Axel L, Adams JR et al: Computed tomography: A new method for diagnosing tumor of the heart. Circulation 63:448, 1981
88. Byrd BF III, Wahr D, Wang YS et al: Left ventricular mass and volume/mass ratio in a normal population determined by two-dimensional echocardiography. J Am Coll Cardiol 6:1021, 1985
89. Fernandez P, Kim B, Reichek N et al: The correlation of changes in systolic

blood pressure with regional anatomical regression of hypertensive left ventricular hypertrophy in patients on chronic antihypertensive therapy (more than 1 year). Curr Med Res Opin 8:720, 1984
90. Kaul U, Mohan J, Bhatia M: Effects of labetalol on left ventricular mass and function in hypertension—an assessment by serial echocardiography. Int J Cardiol 5:461, 1984
91. Dunn FG, Oigman W, Ventura HO et al: Enalapril improves systemic and renal hemodynamics and allows regression of left ventricular mass in essential hypertension. Am J Cardiol 53:105, 1984
92. Nakashima Y, Fouad F, Tarazi R: Regression of left ventricular hypertrophy from systemic hypertension by enalapril. Am J Cardiol 53:1044, 1984
93. Pratt RC, Parisi AF, Harrington JJ, Sasahara AA: The influence of left ventricular stroke volume on aortic root motion: An echocardiographic study. Circulation 53:947, 1976
94. Lalani AV, Lee SJK: Echocardiographic measurement of cardiac output using the mitral valve and aortic root echo. Circulation 54:738, 1976
95. Kramer P, Djalaly A, Poehlman H, Schiller NB: Abnormal diastolic left ventricular posterior wall motion in left ventricular hypertrophy. Am Heart J 106:5-I, 1983
96. Ambrose JA, King BD, Teicholz LE et al: Early diastolic motion of the posterior aortic root as an index of left ventricular filling. J Clin Ultrasound 11:357, 1983
97. Strunk BL, Fitzgerald JW, Lipton M et al: The posterior aortic wall echocardiogram: Its relationship to left atrial volume change. Circulation 54:744, 1976
98. Strunk BL, London EJ, Fitzgerald J et al: The assessment of mitral stenosis and prosthetic mitral valve obstruction, using the posterior aortic wall echocardiogram. Circulation 55:885, 1977
99. Miyatake K, Okamoto M, Kinoshita N et al: Augmentation of atrial contribution to left ventricular inflow with aging as assessed by intracardiac Doppler flowmetry. Am J Cardiol 53:586, 1984
100. Rokey R, Juo L, Zoghbi W et al: Determination of parameters of left ventricular diastolic filling with pulsed Doppler echocardiography: Comparison with cineangiography. Circulation 71:543, 1985
101. Nishimura RA, Abel MD, Hatle LK, Tajik AJ: Assessment of diastolic function of the heart: Background and current applications of Doppler echocardiography. Mayo Clin Proc 64:181, 1989
102. Inouye I, Massie B, Loge D et al: Abnormal left ventricular filling: An early finding in mild to moderate systemic hypertension. Am J Cardiol 53:120, 1984
103. Miller TR, Grossman WJ, Schectman KB et al: Left ventricular diastolic filling and its association with age. Am J Cardiol 58:531, 1986
104. Rokey R, Kuo LC, Zoghbi WA et al: Determination of parameters of left ventricular diastolic filling with pulsed Doppler echocardiography: Comparison with cineangiography. Circulation 71:543, 1985
105. Demaria AN, Bommer W, Neumann A et al: Left ventricular thrombi identified by cross-sectional echocardiography. Ann Intern Med 90:14, 1979
106. Asinger RW, Mikell FL, Elsperger J, Hodges M: Incidence of left ventricular thrombosis after acute transmural myocardial infarction. Serial evaluation by two dimensional echocardiography. N Engl J Med 305:297, 1981
107. Keating EC, Gross SA, Schlamowitz RA et al: Mural thrombi in myocardial infarctions. Prospective evaluation by two dimensional echocardiography. Am J Med 74:989, 1983
108. Johannessen KA, Nordrehaug JE, Von Der Lippe G: Left ventricular thrombosis and cerebrovascular accident in acute myocardial infarction. Br Heart J 51:553, 1984
109. Keren A, Billingham M, Popp R: Echocardiographic recognition and implications of ventricular hypertrophic trabeculations and aberrant bands. Circulation 70:836, 1984
110. Meltzer R, Visser C, Kan G, Roelandt J: Two-dimensional echocardiographic appearance of left ventricular thrombi with systemic emboli after myocardial infarction. Am J Cardiol 53:1511, 1984
111. Visser C, Kan G, Meltzer R et al: Embolic potential of left ventricular thrombus after myocardial infarction: A two-dimensional echocardiographic study of 119 patients. J Am Coll Cardiol 5(6):1276, 1985
112. Ezekowitz M: Acute infarction, left ventricular thrombus and systemic embolization: An approach to management. J Am Coll Cardiol 5(6):1281, 1985
113. Arvan S: Persistent intracardiac thrombi and systemic embolization despite anticoagulant therapy. Am Heart J 109:178, 1985
114. Kinney E: The significance of left ventricular thrombi in patients with coronary heart disease: A retrospective analysis of pooled data. Am Heart J 109:191, 1985
115. Singer E, Park Y: Splenic infarction following mural thrombus of the left ventricle in a patient with acute anteroseptal myocardial infarction. Cardiology Reviews & Reports 6(7):835, 1985
116. Rao A, Agatston A, Samet P: Multiple mural biventricular thrombi: Echocardiographic detection in congestive cardiomyopathy. J Clin Ultrasound 4(1):65, 1985
117. Takamoto T, Kim D, Urie P et al: Comparative recognition of left ventricular thrombi by echocardiography and cineangiography. Br Heart J 53:36, 1985
118. Lapeyre A, Steele P, Kazmier F et al: Systemic embolism in chronic left ventricular aneurysm: Incidence and the role of anticoagulation. J Am Coll Cardiol 6(3):534, 1985
119. Llorte R, Cortada X, Bradford J et al: Classification of left ventricular thrombi by their history of systemic embolization using pattern recognition of two-dimensional echocardiograms. Am Heart J 110:761, 1985
120. Keren A, Takamoto T, Harrison D, Popp R: Left ventricular apical masses: Noninvasive differentiation of rare from common ones. Am J Cardiol 56:697, 1985
121. Goldstein J, Lipton M, Schiller NB et al: Evaluation of intracardiac thrombi with contrast enhanced computer tomography and echocardiography. Am J Cardiol 49:956, 1982
122. Asinger RW, Mikell FL: Left ventricular thrombosis after myocardial infarction. Primary Cardiology 9:2, 1983
123. Vergnon JM, Vincent M, Perinetti M et al: Chemotherapy of metastic primary cardiac sarcomas. Am Heart J 110:682, 1985
124. Acquatella H, Schiller NB, Puigbo JJ et al: Value of two-dimensional echocardiography in endomyocardial disease with and without eosinophilia: A clinical and pathologic study. Circulation 67:1219, 1983
125. LeBlanc H, Collin J: Echocardiography in African endomyocardial fibrosis. Movement of the left atrial posterior wall. J Clin Ultrasound 3:13, 1984
126. Harbin A, Gerson M, O'Connell J: Simulation of acute myopericarditis by constrictive pericardial disease with endomyocardial fibrosis due to methysergide therapy. J Am Coll Cardiol 4:196, 1984
127. Silver M, Bonow RO, Deglin S et al: Acquired left ventricular endocardial constriction from massive mural calcific deposits: A newly recognized cause of impairment to left ventricular filling. Am J Cardiol 53:1468, 1984
128. Kerber RE, Abboud FM: Echocardiographic detection of regional myocardial infarction. Circulation 47:997, 1973
129. Reeder GS, Seward JB, Tajik AJ: The role of two dimensional echocardiography in coronary artery disease. Mayo Clin Proc 57:247, 1982
130. Visser CA, Durrer D: Echocardiographic determination of infarct size in acute myocardial infarction. Practical Cardiology 9:225, 1983
131. Pandian N, Skorton D, Collins S et al: Myocardial infarct size threshold for two-dimensional echocardiographic detection: Sensitivity of systolic wall thickening and endocardial motion abnormalities in small versus large infarcts. Am J Cardiol 55:551, 1985
132. Chen Y, Sherrid M, Dwyer E: Value of two-dimensional echocardiography in evaluating coronary artery disease: A randomized blind analysis. J Am Coll Cardiol 5(4):911, 1985
133. Ren J, Kotler M, Hakki A et al: Quantitation of regional left ventricular function by two-dimensional echocardiography in normals and patients with coronary artery disease. Am Heart J 110:552, 1985
134. Freeman A, Giles R, Walsh W et al: Regional left ventricular wall motion assessment: Comparison of two-dimensional echocardiography and radionuclide angiography with contrast angiography in healed myocardial infarction. Am J Cardiol 56:8, 1985
135. Matsumoto M, Watanabe F, Moto A et al: Left ventricular aneurysm and the prediction of left ventricular enlargement studies by two-dimensional echocardiography: Quantitative assessment of aneurysm size in relation to clinical course. Circulation 72:280, 1985
136. Quinones M, Roberts R: Role of two-dimensional echocardiography in acute myocardial infarction. Echocardiography 2(3):213, 1985
137. Rasmussen S, Lovelace E, Knoebel S et al: Echocardiographic detection of ischemic and infarcted myocardium. J Am Coll Cardiol 3:733, 1984
138. Franker T, Nelson A, Arthur J, Wilderson R: Altered acoustic reflectance on two-dimensional echocardiography as an early predictor of myocardial infarct size. Am J Cardiol 53:1699, 1984
139. Chandraratna P, Ulene R, Nimalasuriya A et al: Differentiation between acute and healed myocardial infarction by signal averaging and color encoding two-dimensional echocardiography. Am J Cardiol 56:381, 1985
140. Roberts C, MacLean D, Maroko R, Troner R: Early and late remodeling of the left ventricle after acute myocardial infarction. Am J Cardiol 54:401, 1984
141. Weisman H, Bush D, Mannisi J, Bulkley B: Global cardiac remodeling after acute myocardial infarction: A study in the rate mode. J Am Coll Cardiol 5(6):1355, 1985
142. Kinoshita Y, Shukuya M, Inagaki Y: Significance of a wall motion hinge point after myocardial infarction. J Cardiovasc Ultrasound 2:235, 1983
143. Nishimura R, Tajik A, Seward J: Cases from the Mayo Clinic—distinctive two-dimensional echocardiographic appearance of septal infarct secondary to isolated occlusion of first septal perforator artery. Echocardiography 1:97, 1984
144. Lapeyre A, Steele P, Kazmier F et al: Systemic embolism in chronic left ventricular aneurysm: Incidence and the role of anticoagulation. J Am Coll Cardiol 6(3):534, 1985
145. Friart A, Vandenbossche J, Hamdan B et al: Association of false tendons with left ventricular aneurysm. Am J Cardiol 55:1425, 1985
146. Maurer G, Nanda NC: Two dimensional echocardiographic evaluation of exercise induced left and right ventricular asynergy: Correlation with thallium scanning. Am J Cardiol 48:720, 1981
147. Crawford MH, Petru MA, Amon W et al: Comparative value of two dimensional echocardiography and radionuclide angiography for quantitating changes in left ventricular performance during exercise limited by angina pectoris. Am J Cardiol 53:42, 1984
148. Robertson WS, Feigenbaum H, Armstrong WF et al: Exercise echocardiography: A clinically practical addition in the evaluation of coronary artery disease. J Am Coll Cardiol 2:1085, 1983
149. Ginzton LE, Conant R, Brizendine M et al: Exercise subcostal two dimensional echocardiography: A new method of segmental wall motion analysis.

Am J Cardiol 53:805, 1984
150. Bersin R, Tubau JF, Merz R et al: Diagnostic yield of echocardiography with routine treadmill testing (abstr). Circulation 72(III):449, 1985
151. Crawford MH, Petru MA, Amon KW et al: Comparative value of 2-dimensional echocardiography and radionuclide angiography for quantitating changes in left ventricular performance during exercise limited by angina pectoris. Am J Cardiol 53:42, 1984
152. Child J: Stress echocardiography: A technique whose time has come. Echocardiography 1:107, 1984
153. Heng M, Simard M, Drake R, Udhoji V: Exercise two-dimensional echocardiography for diagnosis of coronary artery disease. Am J Cardiol 54:502, 1984
154. Berberich S, Zaer J, Plotnick G, Fisher M: A practical approach to exercise echocardiography: Immediate post exercise echocardiography. J Am Coll Cardiol 3:284, 1984
155. Glitton L, Conant R, Brizendine M et al: Exercise subcostal two-dimensional echocardiography: A new method of segmental wall motion analysis. Am J Cardiol 53:805, 1984
156. Picano E, Distante A, Masini M et al: Dipyridamole-echocardiography tests in effort angina pectoris. Am J Cardiol 56:452, 1985
157. Iskandrian A, Hakki A, Kotler M et al: Evaluation of patients with acute myocardial infarction: Which test, for whom and why? Am Heart J 109:391, 1985
158. Pandian NG, Koyanagi S, Skorton DJ et al: Relations between 2-dimensional echocardiographic wall thickening abnormalities, myocardial infarct size and coronary risk area in normal and hypertrophied myocardium in dogs. Am J Cardiol 52:1318, 1983
159. Loh I, Hubert G: Use of 2-dimensional echocardiography in the differential diagnosis of AMI in the patient presenting with chest pain. Practical Cardiology 10:185, 1984
160. Abrams DA, Starling MR, Crawford MH et al: Value of noninvasive techniques for predicting early complications in patients with clinical class II acute myocardial infarction. J Am Coll Cardiol 2:5, 1983
161. Fujii J, Sawada H, Aizawa T et al: Computer analysis of cross sectional echocardiogram for quantitative evaluation of left ventricular asynergy in myocardial infarction. Br Heart J 51:139, 1984
162. Kan G, Visser GA, Lie KI, Ferrer D: Measurement of left ventricular ejection fraction after acute myocardial infarction. Br Heart J 51:631, 1984
163. Weyman A, Franklin T, Hogan R et al: Importance of temporal heterogeneity in assessing the contraction abnormalities associated with acute myocardial ischemia. Circulation 70:102, 1984
164. Gillam L, Hogan R, Foale R et al: A comparison of quantitative echocardiographic methods for delineating infarct-induced abnormal wall motion. Circulation 70:113, 1984
165. Nishimura R, Reeder G, Miller F et al: Prognostic value of predischarge two-dimensional echocardiogram after acute myocardial infarction. Am J Cardiol 53:429, 1984
166. Freeman A, Giles R, Walsh W et al: Regional left ventricular wall motion assessment: Comparison of two-dimensional echocardiography and radionuclide angiography with contrast angiography in healed myocardial infarction. Am J Cardiol 56:8, 1985
167. Matsumoto M, Watanabe F, Moto A et al: Left ventricular aneurysm and the prediction of left ventricular enlargement studied by two-dimensional echocardiography: Quantitative assessment of aneurysm size in relation to clinical course. Circulation 72:280, 1985
168. Stratton JR: Mural thrombi of the left ventricle. Chest 83:166, 1983
169. Visser CA, Kan G, David GK et al: Two-dimensional echocardiography in the diagnosis of left ventricular thrombus: A prospective study of 67 patients with anatomic validation. Chest 83:228, 1983
170. Mongiardo R, Digaetano A, Pennestri F et al: Left ventricular thrombus evolution: Assessment by two dimensional echocardiography. G Ital Cardiol 12:308, 1982
171. Spirito P, Bellotti P, Gharela F et al: Prognostic significance and natural history of left ventricular thrombi in patients with acute anterior myocardial infarction: A two-dimensional echocardiographic study. Circulation 72:774, 1985
172. Wong M, Shah PM: Accuracy of two-dimensional echocardiography in detecting left ventricular aneurysm. Clin Cardiol 6:230, 1983
173. Knowlton A, Grauer J, Plehn J, Liebson P: Ventricular pseudoaneurysm: A rare but ominous condition. Cardiology Review 6(4):508, 1985
174. Loperfido F, Pennestri F, Mazzari M et al: Diagnosis of left ventricular pseudoaneurysm by pulsed Doppler echocardiography. Am Heart J 110:1291, 1985
175. Kaul S, Josephson MA, Tei C et al: Atypical echocardiography and angiographic presentation of a postoperative pseudoaneurysm of the LV after repair of a true aneurysm. J Am Coll Cardiol 2:780, 1983
176. Rath S, Eldar M, Shemesh Y et al: Acute cardiac rupture and tamponade: Angiographic appearance. Am J Cardiol 55:588, 1985
177. Wunderlink R: Incidence of pericardial effusions in acute myocardial infarctions. Chest 85:494, 1984
178. Kaplan K, Davison R, Parker M et al: Frequency of pericardial effusion as determined by M-mode echocardiography in acute myocardial infarction. Am J Cardiol 55:335, 1985
179. Nishimura RA, Schaff HV, Shub C et al: Papillary muscle rupture complicating acute myocardial infarction: Analysis of 17 patients. Am J Cardiol 51:373, 1983
180. Clements S, Story W, Hurst J et al: Ruptured papillary muscle, a complication of myocardial infarction: Clinical presentation, diagnosis, and treatment. Clin Cardiol 8(2):93, 1985
181. Missri JC, Spath EA, Stark S et al: Ventricular septal rupture detected by two dimensional echocardiography. J Cardiovasc Ultrasound 2:259, 1983
182. Arditti A, Lewin R, Hellman C et al: Right ventricular dysfunction in acute inferoposterior myocardial infarction. An echocardiographic and isotopic study. Chest 87:307, 1985
183. Judgutt BI, Sussex BA, Siriram CA, Rossall RE: Right ventricular infarction: Two-dimensional echocardiographic evaluation. Am Heart J 107:505, 1984
184. Panidis IP, Kotler MN, Mintz GS et al: Right ventricular function in coronary artery disease as assessed by two-dimensional echocardiography. Am Heart J 107:1187, 1984
185. Panidis JP, Ren JF, Kotler MN et al: Two-dimensional echocardiographic estimation of right ventricular ejection fraction in patients with coronary artery disease. J Am Coll Cardiol 2:911, 1984
186. Lopez-Sendon J, Garcia-Fernande Z, Coma-Canella I et al: Segmental right ventricular function after acute myocardial infarction: Two-dimensional echocardiographic study in 63 patients. Am J Cardiol 51:390, 1983
187. Kaul S, Hopkins JM, Shah PM: Chronic effects of myocardial infarction on right ventricular function: A noninvasive assessment. J Am Coll Cardiol 2:607, 1983
188. Haupt HM, Hutchins GM, Moore W: Right ventricular infarction: Role of the moderator band artery in determining infarct size. Circulation 67:1268, 1983
189. Baigrie RS, Aminul H, McLean CD et al: The spectrum of right ventricular involvement in inferior wall myocardial infarction: A clinical, hemodynamic and noninvasive study. J Am Coll Cardiol 1:396, 1983
190. Roberts N, Harrison D, Reimer K et al: Right ventricular infarction with shock but without significant left ventricular infarction: A new clinical syndrome. Am Heart J 110:1047, 1985
191. Higgins JR, Sundstrom J, Gutman J, Schiller NB: Contrast echocardiography with quantitative Valsalva maneuver to detect patent foramen ovale (abstr). Clin Res 30A:12, 1982
192. Manno BV, Bemis CE, Carver J, Mintz GS: Right ventricular infarction complicated by right to left shunt. J Am Coll Cardiol 1:554, 1983
193. Himelman RB, Goldberger JJ, Hui PY et al: Can hemodynamically significant RV infarction be identified by two-dimensional echocardiography? (abstract) J Am Coll Cardiol 13:157A, 1989
194. Corya BC, Feigenbaum H, Rasmussen S, Black MJ: Echocardiographic features of congestive cardiomyopathy compared with normal subjects and patients with coronary artery disease. Circulation 49:1153, 1974
195. Goldberg SJ, Valdes-Cruz LM, Sahn DJ, Allen HD: Two dimensional echocardiographic evaluation of dilated cardiomyopathy in children. J Am Cardiol 52:1244, 1983
196. Fortuin NJ, Pawsey CGK: The evaluation of left ventricular function by echocardiography. Am J Med 63:1, 1977
197. Tommaso CL, Talano JV: Echographic early systolic partial closure (notching) of the aortic valve in congestive cardiomyopathy. Am Heart J 107:135, 1984
198. Hayakawa M, Yokota Y, Kumaki T et al: Intracardiac flow pattern in dilated cardiomyopathy studied with pulsed Doppler echocardiography. J Cardiogr 51:317, 1983
199. Unverferth D, Magorien R, Moeschberger M et al: Factors influencing the one-year mortality of dilated cardiomyopathy. Am J Cardiol 54:147, 1984
200. Hirota Y, Shimizu G, Kaku K et al: Mechanisms of compensation and decompensation in dilated cardiomyopathy. Am J Cardiol 54:1033, 1984
201. Lambertz H: Functional tricuspid insufficiency in patients with severe heart failure: Follow-up study using echocardiography. Kardiologiia 73:159, 1984
202. Gardin JM, Iseri LT, Elkayam U et al: Evaluation of dilated cardiomyopathy by pulsed Doppler echocardiography. Am Heart J 106:1057, 1983
203. French JW, Popp RL, Pitlick TP: Cardiac localization of transvascular bioptome using 2-dimensional echocardiography. Am J Cardiol 51:219, 1983
204. Acquatella H, Schiller NB, Puigbo JJ et al: M-mode and two-dimensional echocardiography in chronic Chagas' heart disease. Circulation 62:787, 1980
205. Henry WL, Clark CE, Roberts WC et al: Difference in distribution of myocardial abnormalities in patients with obstructive and non-obstructive asymmetric septal hypertrophy (ASH): Echocardiographic and gross anatomic findings. Circulation 50:447, 1974
206. Henry WL, Clark CE, Epstein SE: Asymmetric septal hypertrophy: The unifying link in the IHSS disease spectrum: Observation regarding its pathogenesis, pathophysiology, and course. Circulation 47:827, 1973
207. Henry WL, Clark CE, Epstein SE: Asymmetric septal hypertrophy (ASH): Echocardiographic identification of the pathognomonic anatomic abnormality of IHSS. Circulation 47:225, 1973
208. Ciro E, Nichols PF, Maron BJ: Heterogeneous morphologic expression of genetically transmitted hypertrophic cardiomyopathy. Two dimensional echocardiographic analysis. Circulation 67:1227, 1983
209. Ciro E, Nicholi PF, Maron BJ: Heterogeneous morphologic expression of genetically transmitted hypertrophic cardiomyopathy. Circulation 67:6, 1983
210. Maron B, Nichols P, Pickle L et al: Patterns of inheritance in hypertrophic cardiomyopathy: Assessment by M-mode and two-dimensional echocardiography. Am J Cardiol 53:1087, 1984
211. Ballester M, Rees S, Rickards A, McDonald L: An evaluation of two-dimen-

211. sional echocardiography in the diagnosis of hypertrophic cardiomyopathy. Clin Cardiol 7:631, 1984
212. Maron B: Asymmetry in hypertrophic cardiomyopathy: The septal to free wall thickness ratio revisited. Am J Cardiol 55:835, 1985
213. Maron BJ, Bonow RO, Seshagiri TNR, Roberts WC, Epstein SE: Hypertrophic cardiomyopathy with ventricular septal hypertrophy localized to the apical region of the left ventricle (apical hypertrophic cardiomyopathy). Am J Cardiol 49:1838, 1982
214. Steingo L, Dansky R, Pocock WA, Barlow JB: Apical hypertrophic nonobstructive cardiomyopathy. Am Heart J 104:635, 1982
215. Kereiakes DJ, Anderson DJ, Crouse L, Chatterjee K: Apical hypertrophic cardiomyopathy. Am Heart J 106:855, 1983
216. Maron B, Spirito P, Chiarella F, Vecchio C: Unusual distribution of left ventricular hypertrophy in obstructive hypertrophic cardiomyopathy: Localized posterobasal free wall thickening in two patients. J Am Coll Cardiol 5(6):1474, 1985
217. Mori H, Ogawa S, Nakazawa H et al: Apical hypertrophy as a part of the morphologic spectrum of hypertrophic cardiomyopathy. J Cardiogr 14:289, 1984
218. Koga Y, Takashi H, Ifuku M et al: Hypertrophic cardiomyopathy with ventricular septal hypertrophy localized to the apical region of the left ventricle (apical ASH). J Cardiogr 14:301, 1984
219. Vacek J, Davis W, Bellinger R, McKiernan T: Apical hypertrophic cardiomyopathy in American patients. Am Heart J 108:1501, 1984
220. Koga Y, Itaya M, Takahahi H et al: Apical hypertrophy and its genetic and acquired factors. J Cardiogr 15:65, 1985
221. Martin RP, Rakowski H, French J, Popp RL: Idiopathic hypertrophic subaortic stenosis viewed by wide-angle, phased-array echocardiography. Circulation 59:1206, 1979
222. Mori H, Ogawa S, Nakazawa H et al: Apical hypertrophy as a part of the morphologic spectrum of hypertrophic cardiomyopathy. J Cardiogr 14:289, 1984
223. Sugishita Y, Iida K, Matsuda M et al: Apical hypertrophy and catecholamine. J Cardiogr 15:75, 1985
224. Spirito P, Maron B: Patterns of systolic anterior motion of the mitral valve in hypertrophic cardiomyopathy: Assessment by two-dimensional echocardiography. Am J Cardiol 54:1039, 1984
225. Baragan J, Fernandez F, Thiron JM: Dynamic auscultation and phonocardiography. In Tavel ME (ed): Dynamic Auscultation and Phonocardiography; the Contribution of Vasoactive Drugs to the Diagnosis of Heart Disease, p 115. Bowie, Maryland, The Charles Press Publishers, 1979
226. Roizen MF, Beaupre PN, Alpert RA et al: Monitoring with two-dimensional transesophageal echocardiography: Comparison of myocardial function in patients undergoing superceliac-infrarenal, or infrarenal aortic occlusion. J Cardiovasc Surg 1(2):300, 1984
227. Kereiakes DJ, Naughton JL, Brundage B, Schiller NB: The heart in diabetes. West J Med 140:4, 1984
228. Child JS, Levisman JA, Abbasi AS, MacAlpin RN: Echocardiographic manifestations of infiltrative cardiomyopathy: A report of seven cases due to amyloid. Chest 70:726, 1976
229. Siqueira-Filho AG, Cunha CL, Tajik AJ et al: M-mode and two dimensional echocardiographic features in cardiac amyloidosis. Circulation 63:188, 1981
230. Roberts WC, Waller BF: Cardiac amyloidosis causing cardiac dysfunction: Analysis of 54 necropsy patients. Am J Cardiol 52:137, 1983
231. Nicolosi GL, Pavan D, Lestuzzi C et al: Prospective identification of patients with amyloid heart disease by two dimensional echocardiography. Circulation 70:432, 1984
232. Sedlis S, Saffitz J, Schwob V, Jaffe A: Cardiac amyloidosis simulating hypertrophic cardiomyopathy. Am J Cardiol 53:969, 1984
233. Acquatella H, Schiller NB, Puigbo JJ et al: Value of two dimensional echocardiography in endomyocardial disease with and without eosinophilia. A clinical and pathologic study. Circulation 67:1219, 1983
234. Appleton CP, Hatle LK, Popp RL: Demonstration of restrictive ventricular physiology by Doppler echocardiography. J Am Coll Cardiol 11:757, 1988
235. Wann LS, Faris JV, Childress RH, Dillon JC et al: Exercise cross-sectional echocardiography in ischemic heart disease. Circulation 60:1300, 1979
236. Crawford MH, Amon KW, Vance WS: Exercise 2-dimensional echocardiography: Quantitation of left ventricular performance in patients with severe angina pectoris. Amer J Cardiol 51:1, 1983
237. Armstrong WF, O'Donnel J, Dillon JC et al: Complementary value of two-dimensional exercise echocardiography to routine treadmill exercise testing. Ann Intern Med 105:829, 1986
238. Limacher MC, Quinones MA, Poliner LR et al: Detection of coronary artery disease with exercise two-dimensional echocardiography: Description of a clinically applicable method and comparison with radionuclide ventriculography. Circulation 67:1211, 1983
239. Ryan T, Vasey CG, Presti CF, et al: Exercise echocardiography: Detection of coronary artery disease in patients with normal left ventricular wall motion at rest. J Am Coll Cardiol 11:993, 1988
240. Ryan T, Armstrong WF, O'Donnell JA et al: Risk stratification after acute myocardial infarction by means of exercise two-dimensional echocardiography. Am Heart J 114:1305, 1987
241. Harrison MR, Smith MD, Friedman BJ et al: Uses and limitations of exercise Doppler echocardiography in the diagnosis of ischemic heart disease. J Am Coll Cardiol 10:809, 1987
242. Mehta N, Boyle G, Bennett D et al: Hemodynamic response to treadmill exercise in normal volunteers: An assessment by Doppler ultrasonic measurement of ascending aortic blood velocity and acceleration. Am Heart J 116:1298, 1988
243. Mehdirad AA, Williams GA, Labovitz AJ et al: Evaluation of left ventricular function during upright exercise: correlation of exercise Doppler with postexercise two-dimensional echocardiographic results. Circulation 75:413, 1987
244. Maeda M, Yokota M, Iwase M et al: Accuracy of cardiac output measured by continuous wave Doppler echocardiography during dynamic exercise testing in the supine position in patients with coronary artery disease. J Am Coll Cardiol 13:76, 1989
245. Lazarus M, Dang TY, Gardin JM et al: Evaluation of age gender, heart rate and blood pressure changes and exercise conditioning on Doppler measured aortic blood flow, acceleration, and velocity during upright treadmill testing. Am J Cardiol 62:439, 1988
246. Harrison MR, Smith MD, Nissen SE et al: Use of exercise Doppler echocardiography to evaluate cardiac drugs: Effects of propranolol and verapamil on aortic blood flow velocity and acceleration. J Am Coll Cardiol 11:1002, 1988
247. Martin GR, Soifer SJ, Silverman NH et al: Effects of activity on ascending aortic velocity in children with valvar aortic stenosis. Am J Cardiol 59:1386, 1987
248. Mitchell GD, Brunken RC, Schwaiger M et al: Assessment of mitral flow velocity with exercise by an index of stress-induced left ventricular ischemia in coronary artery disease. Am J Cardiol 61:536, 1988
249. Zachariah ZP, Hsiung MC, Nanda NC et al: Color Doppler assessment of mitral regurgitation induced by supine exercise in patients with coronary artery disease. Am J Cardiol 59:1266, 1987
250. Himelman RB, Stulbarg MS, Kircher B et al: Noninvasive evaluation of pulmonary pressure during exercise by saline-enhanced Doppler echocardiography in chronic pulmonary disease. Circulation 79:863, 1989
251. Schluter M, Hanrath P: Transesophageal echocardiography: Potential advantages and initial clinical results. Practical Cardiology 9:149, 1983
252. Hisanaga K, Hisanaga A, Nagata K, Ichi Y: Transesophageal cross-sectional echocardiography. Am Heart J 100:605, 1980
253. Schluter M, Langenstein BA, Polster J et al: Transesophageal cross-sectional echocardiography with phased array transducer system. Technique and initial clinical results. Br Heart J 48:67, 1982
254. Schiller NB, Maurer G, Ritter SB et al: American Society of Echocardiography Committee on Special Echocardiography Procedures: Statement on Transesophageal Echocardiography. J Am Soc Echo 1990 (in press)
255. Schiller NB, Maurer G, Ritter SB et al: American Society of Echocardiography Committee on Special Procedures: Statement on Transesophageal Echocardiography. J Am Soc Echo 1989 (in press)
256. Schluter M, Hinrichs A, Their W et al: Transesophageal two-dimensional echocardiography: comparison of ultrasonic and anatomic sections. Am J Cardiol 53:1173, 1984
257. Beppu S, Nakatani S, Tanaka N et al: Transesophageal echocardiographic diagnosis of localized pericardial coagula: A special cause of cardiac tamponade (abstract). Circulation 78 (Suppl II):299, 1988
258. Chan KL: Transesophageal echocardiography in the management of intubated cardiac patients (abstract). Circulation 78 (Suppl II):299, 1988
259. Cucchiara RF, Nugent M, Seward JB et al: Air embolism in upright neurosurgical patients: Detection and localization by two-dimensional transesophageal echocardiography. Anesthesiology 60:353, 1984
260. Matsumoto M, Oka Y, Strom J et al: Application of transesophageal echocardiography to continuous intraoperative monitoring of left ventricular performance. Am J Cardiol 46:95, 1980
261. Cahalan MK, Kremer PF, Beaupre PN et al: Intraoperative myocardial ischemia detected by transesophageal 2-dimensional echocardiography. Anesthesiology 59:3, 1983
262. Beaupre PN, Cahalan MK, Kremer PF et al: Does pulmonary artery occlusion pressure adequately reflect left ventricular filling during anesthesia and surgery? Anesthesiology 59:3, 1983
263. Beaupre PN, Roizen MF, Cahalan MK et al: Hemodynamic and two-dimensional transesophageal echocardiographic analysis of an anaphylactic reaction in a human. Anesthesiology 60:482, 1984
264. Shively B, Cahalan M, Benefiel D, Schiller NB: Interoperative assessment of mitral valve regurgitation by transesophageal Doppler echocardiography (abstr). J Am Coll Cardiol 7A:228, 1986
265. Beaupre PN, Kremer PF, Cahalan MK et al: Intraoperative detection of changes in left ventricular segmental wall motion by transesophageal echocardiography (abstr). Am Heart J 107(I):1081, 1984
266. Smith JS, Cahalan MK, Benefiel DJ et al: Intraoperative detection of myocardial ischemia in high risk patients: Electrocardiography vs two-dimensional transesophageal echocardiography. Circulation 72:1015, 1985
267. Shively B, Watters T, Benefiel D et al: The intraoperative detection of myocardial infarction by transesophageal echocardiography (abstr). J Am Coll Cardiol 7A:2, 1986
268. Topol EJ, Humphrey LS, Blanck TJJ et al: Characterization of post-cardiopulmonary bypass hypotension with intraoperative transesophageal echocardiography. Anesthesiology 59:3, 1983
269. Martin RW, Colley PS: Evaluation of transesophageal Doppler detection of air embolism in dogs. Anesthesiology 58:117, 1983

270. Furuya H, Suzuki T, Okumura F et al: Detection of air embolism by transesophageal echocardiography. Anesthesiology 58:124, 1983
271. Mohr-Kahaly S, Erbel R, Rennollet H et al: Ambulatory follow-up of aortic dissection by transesophageal two-dimensional and color-coded Doppler echocardiography. Circulation 80:24, 1989
272. Borner N, Erbel R, Braun B et al: Diagnosis of aortic dissection by transesophageal echocardiography. Am J Cardiol 54:1157, 1984
273. Aschenberg W, Schlüter M, Kremer P et al: Transesophageal two-dimensional echocardiography for the detection of left atrial appendage thrombus. J Am Coll Cardiol 7:163, 1986
274. Zenker G, Erbel R, Dramer G et al: Transesophageal two-dimensional echocardiography in young patients with cerebral ischemic events. Stroke 19:345, 1988
275. Obeid AI, Marvasti M, Parker F et al: Comparison of tranthoracic and transesophageal echocardiography in diagnosis of left atrial myxoma. Am J Cardiol 63:1006, 1989
276. Taams MA, Gussenhoven EJ, Cahalan MK et al: Transesophageal Doppler color flow imaging in the detection of native and Bjork-Shiley mitral valve regurgitation. J Am Coll Cardiol 13:95, 1989
277. Lee E, Kee L, Schiler NB: Transesophageal echocardiography and color flow imaging assessment of prosthetic and native dysfunction (abstract). Circulation 78 (Suppl II):607, 1988
278. Shylman ST, Amren DP, Bisno AL et al: Prevention of bacterial endocarditis: A statement for health professionals by the Committee on Rheumatic Fever and Infective Endocarditis of the Council on Cardiovascular Disease in the Young. Circulation 70:1123A, 1984
279. Daniel WG, Schroder E, Mugge A et al: Transesophageal echocardiography in infective endocarditis. Am J Cardiac Imaging 2:78, 1988
280. Erbel R, Rohmann S, Drexel M et al: Improved diagnostic value of echocardiography in patients with infective endocarditis by transesophageal approach: A prospective study. Eur Heart J 9:43, 1968
281. Schluter M, Kremer P, Hanrath P: Transesophageal 2-D echocardiographic feature of flail mitral leaflet due to ruptured chordae tendineae. Am Heart J 108:609, 1984
282. Czer LSC, Maurer G, Bolger AF et al: Intraoperative evaluation of mitral regurgitation by Doppler color flow mapping. Circulation 76 (Suppl III):108, 1987
283. Maurer G, Czer LSC, Chaux A et al: Intraoperative Doppler color flow mapping for assessment of valve repair for mitral regurgitation. Am J Cardiol 60:333, 1987
284. Hanrath P, Schluter M, Langenstein BA et al: Detection of ostium secundum atrial septal defects by transesophageal cross-sectional echocardiography. Br Heart J 49:350, 1983
285. Oh JK, Seward JB, Khandheria BK et al: Visualization of sinus venosus defect by transesophageal echocardiography. J Am Society Echo, 1:275, 1988
286. Taams MA, Gussenhoven EJ, Cornel JH et al: Detection of left coronary artery stenosis by transesophageal echocardiography. Eur Heart J 9:1162, 1988
287. Zwicky P, Daniel WG, Mugge A et al: Imaging of coronaries by color-coded transesophageal Doppler echocardiography. Am J Cardiol 62:639, 1988
288. Yamagishi M, Miyatake K, Beppu S et al: Assessment of coronary blood flow by transesophageal two-dimensional pulsed Doppler echocardiography. Am J Cardiol 62:641, 1988
289. Himelman RB, Struve SN, Brown JK et al: Improved recognition of cor pulmonale in patients with severe chronic obstructive pulmonary disease. Am J Med 84:891, 1988
290. Cooper MJ, Teitel DF, Silverman NH, Enderlein M: Comparison of M-mode echocardiographic measurement of right ventricular wall thickness obtained by the subcostal and parasternal approach in children. Am J Cardiol 54:835, 1984
291. Silverman NH, Hudson S: Evaluation of right ventricular volume and ejection fraction in children by two-dimensional echocardiography. Pediatr Cardiol 4:197, 1983
292. Levine RA, Gibson TC, Aretz T et al: Echocardiographic measurement of right ventricular volume. Circulation 69:497, 1984
293. Starling MR, Crawford MH, Sorensen SG, O'Rourke RA: A new two-dimensional echocardiographic technique for evaluating right ventricular size and performance in patients with obstructive lung disease. Circulation 66:612, 1982
294. Hu C, Wang Y, Schiller NB: Clinical quantitative echocardiography vs. right ventricular size index in a normal adult population. Clin Res 30:12A, 1982
295. Kaul S, Tei C, Hopkins JM, Shah PM: Assessment of right ventricular function using two-dimensional echocardiography. Am Heart J 107:526, 1984
296. Levine R, Gibson T, Aretz T et al: Echocardiographic measurement of right ventricular volume. Circulation 69:497, 1984
297. Wann L, Stickels K, Bamrah V, Gross C: Digital processing of contrast echocardiograms: A new technique for measuring right ventricular ejection fraction. Am J Cardiol 53:1164, 1984
298. Panidis IP, Kotler MN, Mintz GS et al: Right ventricular function in coronary artery disease as assessed by two-dimensional echocardiography. Am Heart J 107:1187, 1984
299. Lange P, Seiffert P, Pries F et al: Value of image enhancement and injection of contrast medium for right ventricular volume determination by two-dimensional echocardiography in congenital heart disease. Am J Cardiol 55:152, 1985
300. Gibson T, Miller S, Aretz T et al: Method for estimating right ventricular volume by planes applicable to cross-sectional echocardiography: Correlation with angiographic formulas. Am J Cardiol 55:1584, 1985
301. Popp RL, Wolfe SB, Hirata T, Feigenbaum H: Estimation of right and left ventricular size by ultrasound. A study of the echoes from the interventricular septum. Am J Cardiol 24:523, 1969
302. Kimchi A, Ellrodt G, Berman D et al: Right ventricular performance in septic shock: A combined radionuclide and hemodynamic study. J Am Coll Cardiol 4:945, 1984
303. Sharpe DN, Botvinick EH, Shames DN et al: The noninvasive diagnosis of right ventricular infarction. Circulation 57:483, 1978
304. Simonson JS, Schiller NB: Sonospirometry: A new method for non-invasive estimation of mean right atrial pressure based on two-dimensional echographic measurements of the inferior vena cava during measured inspiration. J Am Coll Cardiol 11:557, 1988
305. Moreno F, Hagan A, Holmen J et al: Evaluation of size and dynamics of the inferior vena cava as an index of right-sided cardiac function. Am J Cardiol 53:579, 1985
306. Popp R, Yock P: Noninvasive intracardiac pressure measurement using Doppler ultrasound. J Am Coll Cardiol 6:757, 1985
307. Panidis IP, Kotler MN, Mintz GS et al: Right ventricular function in coronary artery disease as assessed by two-dimensional echocardiography. Am Heart J 107:1187, 1984
308. Kereiakes DJ, Ports TA, Botvinick EH et al: Right ventricular myocardial infarction with ventricular septal rupture. Am Heart J 107:1257, 1984
309. Judgutt BI, Essex BA, Sivaram CA, Rossall RE: Right ventricular infarction: Two-dimensional echocardiographic evaluation. Am Heart J 107:505, 1984
310. Cecchi F, Zuppiroli A, Favilli S et al: Echocardiographic features of right ventricular infarction. Clin Cardiol 7:405, 1984
311. Dell'Italia L, Starling M, Crawford M et al: Right ventricular infarction: Identification by hemodynamic measurements before and after volume loading and correlation with noninvasive techniques. J Am Coll Cardiol 4:931, 1984
312. Ports T, Schiller NB, Strunk B: Echocardiographic features of right ventricular tumors. Circulation 56:439, 1977
313. Felner JM, Churchwell AL, Murphy DA: Right atrial thromboemboli: Clinical, echocardiographic and pathophysiologic manifestations. J Am Coll Cardiol 4:1041, 1984
314. Rosenzweig MS, Nanda NC: Two dimensional echocardiographic detection of circulating right atrial thrombi. Am Heart J 103:435, 1982
315. Starkey IR, DeBono DP: Echocardiographic identification of right-sided cardiac intracavitary thromboembolus in massive pulmonary embolism. Circulation 66:1322, 1982
316. Van Kuyk M, Mols P, Englert M: Right atrial thrombus leading to pulmonary embolism. Br Heart J 51:462, 1984
317. Buckingham T, Williams G, Aker U, Kennedy H: Embolus to the right atrium simulating myxoma. Clin Cardiol 7:457, 1984
318. Spirito P, Bellotti P, Chiarella F et al: Right atrial thrombus detected by two-dimensional echocardiography after acute pulmonary embolism. Am J Cardiol 54:467, 1984
319. Felner J, Churchwell A, Murphy D: Right atrial thromboemboli: Clinical, echocardiographic and pathophysiologic manifestations. J Am Coll Cardiol 4:1041, 1984
320. Goldberg S, Pizzarello R, Goldman M, Padmanabhan V: Echocardiographic diagnosis of right atrial thromboembolism resulting in massive embolization. Am Heart J 108:1371, 1984
321. Lim SP, Hakim SZ, Vander Bel-Kahn JM: Two-dimensional echocardiography for detection of primary right atrial thrombus in pulmonary embolism. Am Heart J 108:1546, 1984
322. Quinn T, Plehn J, Liebson P: Echocardiographic diagnosis of mobile right atrial thrombus: Early recognition and treatment. Am Heart J 108:1548, 1984
323. Malloy P, Rippe J, Gore J et al: Transient right atrial thrombus resulting in pulmonary embolism detected by two-dimensional echocardiography. Am Heart J 108:1047, 1984
324. Percy R, Conetta D, Perryman R, Miller A: Antemortem echocardiographic identification of right atrial thromboembolus. Am Heart J 109:370, 1985
325. Nellessen U, Daniel W, Matheis G et al: Impending paradoxical embolism from atrial thrombus: Correct diagnosis by transesophageal echocardiography and prevention by surgery. J Am Coll Cardiol 5:1002, 1985
326. Cameron J, Pohlner P, Stafford E et al: Right heart thrombus: Recognition, diagnosis and management. J Am Coll Cardiol 5:1239, 1985
327. Zenker G, Gombotz H, Kandlhoffer B et al: Emergency diagnosis and treatment of a right-sided intracardiac thromboembolus in a patient with massive pulmonary embolism: An echocardiographic study. J Clin Ultrasound 4:47, 1984
328. Kinney E, Zitrin R, Kohler K et al: Sudden appearance of right atrial thrombus on two-dimensional echocardiogram: Significance and therapeutic implications. Am Heart J 110:879, 1985
329. Armstrong W, Feigenbaum H, Dillon J: Echocardiographic detection of right atrial thromboembolism. Chest 87:801, 1985
330. Busch U, Wirtzfeld A, Sebening H et al: Pulmonary and intracardiac embolectomy based on echocardiographic findings. J Clin Ultrasound 13:494, 1985
331. Kumar A, Rose JS, Reid CL et al: Echocardiographic demonstration of pulmonary embolism as it evolves through the right heart chambers. Am J

Med 79:538, 1985
332. Saner HE, Asinger RW, Daniel JA, Elsperger KJ: Two-dimensional echocardiographic detection of right-sided cardiac intracavitary thromboembolus with pulmonary embolism. J Am Coll Cardiol 4:1294, 1984
333. Nestico PF, Panidis IP, Kotler MN et al: Surgical removal of right atrial thromboembolus detected by two-dimensional echocardiography in pulmonary embolism. Am Heart J 107:1278, 1984
334. Higgins JR, Strunk BL, Schiller NB: Diagnosis of paradoxical embolism with contrast echocardiography. Am Heart J 107:375, 1984
335. Keidar S, Grenadier E, Binenboim C, Palant A: Transient right to left atrial shunt detected by contrast echocardiography in the acute stage of pulmonary embolism. J Clin Ultrasound 12:417, 1984
336. Weyman AE, Wann LS, Caldwell RL et al: Negative contrast echocardiography: A new method for detecting left to right shunts. Circulation 59:498, 1979
337. Currie P, Seward J, Chan K et al: Continuous wave Doppler determination of right ventricular pressure: A simultaneous Doppler-catheterization study in 127 patients. J Am Coll Cardiol 6:750, 1985
338. Payvandi MN, Kerber RE: Echocardiography in congenital and acquired absence of pericardium. Circulation 53:86, 1976
339. Yamamoto T, Mihata S, Tanimoto M et al: Two-dimensional echocardiography in congenital absence of the left pericardium. J Clin Ultrasound 3:69, 1984
340. Gullace G, Savoia M: Echocardiographic assessment of the inferior vena cava wall motion for studies of right heart dynamics and function. Clin Cardiol 7:393, 1984
341. Moreno F, Hagan A, Holmen J et al: Evaluation of size and dynamics of the inferior vena cava as an index of right-sided cardiac function. Am J Cardiol 53:579, 1984
342. Marcus FI, Fontaine GH, Guiraudon G et al: Right ventricular dysplasia: A report of 24 adult cases. Circulation 65:384, 1982
343. Manyari DE, Klein GJ, Gulamgusein S et al: Arrhythmogenic right ventricular dysplasia: A generalized cardiomyopathy? Circulation 68:251, 1983
344. Child J, Perloff J, Francoz R et al: Uhl's anomaly (parchment right ventricle): Clinical, echocardiographic, radionuclear, hemodynamic and angiocardiographic features in two patients. Am J Cardiol 53:635, 1984
345. Fontaine G, Frank R, Tonet J et al: Arrhythmogenic right ventricular dysplasia: A clinical model for the study of chronic ventricular tachycardia. Japan Circulation 48:515, 1984
346. Schabelman S, Schiller NB, Silverman NH, Ports TA: Left atrial estimation by two-dimensional echocardiography. Cathet Cardiovasc Diagn 7:165, 1981
347. Gutman J, Wang Y, Wahr D, Schiller NB: Normal left atrial function determined by 2-dimensional echocardiography. Am J Cardiol 51:337, 1983
348. Wang Y, Zatzkis MA, Schiller NB: Noninvasive measurement of interatrial conduction time and atrial contraction time. J Cardiovasc Ultrasound 3:3, 1984
349. Nichol PM, Gilbert BW, Kisslo JA: Two-dimensional echocardiographic assessment of mitral stenosis. Circulation 55:120, 1977
350. Hatle L, Brubakk A, Tromsdal A, Angelsen B: Noninvasive assessment of pressure drop in mitral stenosis by Doppler ultrasound. Br Heart J 40:131, 1978
351. Nakatani S, Masuyama T, Kodama K et al: Value and limitations of Doppler echocardiography in the quantification of stenotic mitral valve area: Comparison of the pressure half-time and the continuity equation methods. Circulation 77:78
352. D'Cruz I, Panetta F, Cohen H, Glick G: Submitral calcification or sclerosis in elderly patients: M-mode and two-dimensional echocardiography in "mitral annulus calcification." Am J Cardiol 44:31, 1979
353. Gabor GE, Mohr BD, Goel PC, Cohen B: Echocardiographic and clinical spectrum of mitral annular calcification. Am J Cardiol 38:363, 1976
354. Nair C, Pagano T: Mitral annular calcification: New concepts. Primary Cardiology 9:57, 1983
355. Nair CK, Aronow S, Sketch MH et al: Clinical and echocardiographic characteristics of patients with mitral annular calcification. Am J Cardiol 51:992, 1983
356. Labovitz A, Nelson J, Windhorst D et al: Frequency of mitral valve dysfunction from mitral annular calcium as detected by Doppler echocardiography. Am J Cardiol 55:133, 1985
357. Nair CK, Aronow WC, Stokke K et al: Cardiac conduction defects in patients older than 60 years with and without annular calcium. Am J Cardiol 53:169, 1984
358. Himelman RB, Helms CA, Schiller NB: Is parthormone a cardiac toxin in uremia? Int J of Cardiac Imaging 3:209, 1989
359. Delaye J, Beaune J, Gayet JL et al: Current etiology of organic mitral insufficiency in adults. Arch Mal Coeur 76:1072, 1983
360. Wann LS, Feigenbaum H, Weyman AE, Dillon JC: Cross-sectional echocardiographic detection of rheumatic mitral regurgitation. Am J Cardiol 41:1258, 1978
361. Abbasi AS, Allen MW, DeCristofaro D, Ungar I: Detection and estimation of the degree of mitral regurgitation by range-gated pulsed Doppler echocardiography. Circulation 61:143, 1980
362. Blumlein S, Bouchard A, Schiller NB et al: Quantitation of mitral regurgitation by Doppler echocardiography. Circulation 74:306, 1986
363. Dillon JC, Haisse CL, Chang S, Feigenbaum H: Use of echocardiography in patients with prolapsed mitral valve. Circulation 43:503, 1971
364. Kerber RE, Isaeff DM, Hancock EW: Echocardiographic patterns in patients with the syndrome of systolic click and late systolic murmur. N Engl J Med 284:691, 1971
365. Markiewicz W, Stoner J, London E et al: Mitral valve prolapse in one hundred presumably healthy young females. Circulation 53:464, 1976
366. Bon Tempo CP, Ronan JA Jr, De Leon AC Jr, Twigg HL: Radiographic appearance of the thorax in systolic click-late systolic murmur syndrome. Am J Cardiol 36:27, 1975
367. Salmon J, Shah PM, Heinle RA: Thoracic skeletal abnormalities in idiopathic mitral valve prolapse. Am J Cardiol 36:32, 1975
368. Levine RA, Triulzi MO, Harrigan P et al: The relationship of mitral annular shape to the diagnosis of mitral valve prolapse. Circulation 75:756, 1987
369. Abbasi AS, Decristofaro D, Anabtawi J et al: Mitral valve prolapse: Comparative values of M-mode, two-dimensional echocardiography and Doppler. J Am Coll Cardiol 2:1219, 1983
370. Nishimura RA, McGoon MD, Shub C et al: Echocardiographically documented mitral-valve prolapse. Long-term follow-up of 237 patients. N Engl J Med 313:1305, 1985
371. O'Brien JT, Geiser EA: Infective endocarditis and echocardiography. Am Heart J 108:386, 1984
372. Kececioglu-Draelos Z, Goldberg SJ: Role of M-mode echocardiography in congenital aortic stenosis. Am J Cardiol 47:1267, 1981
373. Chin ML, Bernstein RF, Child JS, Krivorapich J: Aortic valve systolic flutter as a screening test for severe aortic stenosis. Am J Cardiol 51:981, 1983
374. DeMaria AN, Bommer JW, Joye J et al: Value and limitations of cross-sectional echocardiography of the aortic valve in the diagnosis and quantification of valvular aortic stenosis. Circulation 62:304, 1980
375. Godley RW, Green D, Dillon JC et al: Reliability of two-dimensional echocardiography in assessing the severity of valvular aortic stenosis. Chest 79:657, 1981
376. Weyman AE, Feigenbaum H, Hurwitz RA et al: Cross-sectional echocardiographic assessment of the severity of aortic stenosis in children. Circulation 55:773, 1977
377. Borow KM: Adults with congenital aortic stenosis: Diagnosis and treatment. Cardiovasc Med 8:1163, 1983
378. Hatle L, Angelsen BA, Tromsdal A: Noninvasive assessment of aortic stenosis by Doppler ultrasound. Br Heart J 43:284, 1980
379. Stamm RB, Martin RP: Quantification of pressure gradients across stenotic valves by Doppler ultrasound. J Am Coll Cardiol 2:707, 1983
380. Nishimura R, Miller F, Callahan M et al: Doppler echocardiography: Theory, instrumentation, technique, and application. Mayo Clin Proc 60:321, 1985
381. Williams G, Labovitz A, Nelson J, Kennedy H: Value of multiple echocardiographic views in the evaluation of aortic stenosis in adults by continuous-wave Doppler. Am J Cardiol 55:445, 1985
382. Teirstein P, Yock P, Popp R: The accuracy of Doppler ultrasound measurement of pressure gradients across irregular, dual, and tunnel like obstructions to blood flow. Circulation 72:577, 1985
383. Krafchek J, Robertson J, Radford M et al: A reconsideration of Doppler assessed gradients in suspected aortic stenosis. Am Heart J 110:765, 1985
384. Touche T, Prasquier R, Nitenberg A et al: Assessment and follow-up of patients with aortic regurgitation by an updated Doppler echocardiographic measurement of the regurgitant fraction in the aortic arch. Circulation 72:819, 1985
385. Agatston A, Chengot M, Rao A et al: Doppler diagnosis of valvular aortic stenosis in patients over 60 years of age. Am J Cardiol 56:106, 1985
386. Nitta M, Nakamura TO, Hultgren HN et al: Progression of aortic stenosis in adult men: Detection of noninvasive methods. Chest 92:40, 1987
387. Otto CM, Pearlman AS: Doppler echocardiography in adults with symptomatic aortic stenosis: Diagnostic utility and cost-effectiveness. Arch Intern Med 148:2553, 1988
388. Warth DC, Stewart WJ, Block PC, Weyman AE: A new method to calculate aortic valve area without left heart catheterization. Circulation 70:978, 1984
389. Otto CM, Pearlman AS, Comess KA et al: Determination of the stenotic aortic valve area in adults using Doppler echocardiography. J Am Coll Cardiol 7:509, 1986
390. Krafchek J, Robertson JH, Radford M et al: A reconsideration of Doppler assessed gradients in suspected aortic stenosis. Am Heart J 110:765, 1985
391. Skjaerpe T, Hegrenaes L, Hatle L: Noninvasive estimation of valve area in patients with aortic stenosis by Doppler ultrasound and two-dimensional echocardiography. Circulation 72:810, 1985
392. Skorton DJ, Child JS, Perloff JK: Accuracy of the echocardiographic diagnosis of aortic regurgitation. Am J Med 69:377, 1980
393. Nakao S, Tanaka H, Tahara M: A regurgitant jet and echocardiographic abnormalities in aortic regurgitation: An experimental study. Circulation 67:860, 1983
394. Botvinick E, Schiller NB, Wickramasekaran R et al: Echocardiographic demonstration of early mitral valve closure in severe aortic insufficiency. Circulation 51:836, 1975
395. Henry WL, Bonow RO, Borer JS et al: Observations on the optimum time for operative intervention for aortic regurgitation. I. Evaluation of the results of aortic valve replacement in symptomatic patients. Circulation 61:471, 1980
396. Henry WL, Bonow RO, Rosing DR, Epstein SE: Observations on the optimum time for operative intervention for aortic regurgitation. II. Serial

echocardiographic evaluation of asymptomatic patients. Circulation 61:484, 1980

397. Fioretti P, Roelandt J, Bos RJ et al: Echocardiography in chronic aortic insufficiency. Is valve replacement too late when left ventricular end-systolic dimension reaches 55mm? Circulation 67:216, 1983
398. Robertson WS, Stewart J, Armstrong WF et al: Reverse doming of the anterior mitral leaflet with severe aortic regurgitation. J Am Coll Cardiol 3:431, 1984
399. Esper RJ: Detection of mild aortic regurgitation by range-gated pulsed Doppler echocardiography. Am J Cardiol 50:1037, 1982
400. Ciobanu M, Abbasi AS, Allen M et al: Pulsed Doppler echocardiography in the diagnosis and estimation of severity of aortic insufficiency. Am J Cardiol 49:339, 1982
401. Veyrat C, Lessana A, Abitbol G et al: New indexes for assessing aortic regurgitation with two-dimensional Doppler echocardiographic measurement of the regurgitant aortic valvular area. Circulation 68:998, 1983
402. Kitabatake A, Ito H, Onoue M et al: A new approach to noninvasive evaluation of aortic regurgitant fraction by two-dimensional Doppler echocardiography. Circulation 72:523, 1985
403. Bouchard A, Yock PG, Schiller NB et al: Quantitation of chronic aortic insufficiency using color Doppler flow mapping (abstr). Circulation 72(III):397, 1985
404. Teague SM, Heinsimer JA, Anderson JL et al: Quantification of aortic regurgitation utilizing continuous wave Doppler ultrasound. J Am Coll Cardiol 8:592, 1986
405. Teague SM, Marty W, Saadatmanesh V et al: The effect of mean pressure gradient, chamber compliance, and orifice size upon the Doppler halftime method. (abstract) J Am Coll Cardiol 11:204A, 1988
406. Masuyama T, Kitabatake A, Kodama K et al: Semiquantitative evaluation of aortic regurgitation by Doppler echocardiography: Effects of associated mitral stenosis. Am Heart J 117:133, 1989
407. Freed CR, Schiller NB: Echocardiographic evaluation of aortic root enlargement in mitral valve prolapse in patients with Marfan's syndrome. West J Med 126:87, 1977
408. Yock P, Popp R: Noninvasive estimation of right ventricular systolic pressure by Doppler ultrasound in patients with tricuspid regurgitation. Circulation 70:657, 1984
409. Meltzer RS, McGhie J, Roelandt J: Inferior vena cava echocardiography. J Clin Ultrasound 10:47, 1982
410. Diebold B, Touati R, Blanchard D et al: Quantitative assessment of tricuspid regurgitation using pulsed Doppler echocardiography. Br Heart J 50:443, 1983
411. Yock PG, Popp RL: Noninvasive estimation of right ventricular systolic pressure by Doppler ultrasound in patients with tricuspid regurgitation. Circulation 70:657, 1984
412. Werner J, Schiller NB, Prasquier R: Occurrence and significance of echocardiographically demonstrated tricuspid valve prolapse. Am Heart J 96:180, 1978
413. Forman MB, Myrd BF, Oates JA, Robertson RM: Two-dimensional echocardiographic features of carcinoid heart disease. Am Heart J 107:801, 1984
414. Reid CL, Chandraratna PAN, Kawanishi DT et al: Echocardiographic features of carcinoid heart disease. Am Heart J 107:801, 1984
415. Callahan JA, Wroblewski EM, Reeder GS et al: Echocardiographic features of carcinoid heart disease. Am J Cardiol 50:762, 1982
416. Lundin L, Norheim I, Landelius J et al: Carcinoid heart disease: Relationship of circulating vasoactive substances to ultrasound-detectable cardiac abnormalities. Circulation 77:264, 1988
417. Himelman RB, Schiller NB: Clinical and echocardiographic comparison of patients with the carcinoid syndrome with and without carcinoid heart disease. Am J Cardiol 63:347, 1989
418. Ports TA, Silverman NH, Schiller NB: Two-dimensional echocardiographic assessment of Ebstein's anomaly. Circulation 58:336, 1978
419. Miyatake K, Okamoto M, Kinoshita N et al: Clinical applications of a new type of real-time two-dimensional Doppler flow imaging system. Am J Cardiol 54:857, 1984
420. Sahn DJ: Instrumentation and physical factors related to visualization of stenotic and regurgitant jets by Doppler color flow mapping. J Am Coll Cardiol 12:1354, 1988
421. Simpson IA, Valdes-Cruz LM, Sahn DJ et al: Doppler color flow mapping of simulated in vitro regurgitant jets: Evaluation of the effects of orifice size and hemodynamic variables. J Am Coll Cardiol 13:1195, 1989
422. Wong M, Matsumura M, Suzuki K et al: Technical and biologic sources of variability in the mapping of aortic, mitral and tricuspid color flow jets. Am J Cardiol 60:847, 1987
423. Hoit BD, Jones M, Eidbo EE et al: Sources of variability for Doppler color flow mapping of regurgitant jets in an animal model of mitral regurgitation. J Am Coll Cardiol 13:1631, 1989
424. Smith MD, Grayburn PA, Spain MG et al: Observer variability in the quantitation of Doppler color flow jet areas for mitral and aortic regurgitation. J Am Coll Cardiol 11:579, 1988
425. Yoshida K, Yoshikawa J, Shakudo M et al: Color Doppler evaluation of valvular regurgitation in normal subjects. Circulation 78:840, 1988
426. Helmcke F, Nanda NC, Hsiung MC et al: Color Doppler assessment of mitral regurgitation using orthogonal planes. Circulation 75:175, 1987
427. Miyatake K, Izumi S, Okamoto M et al: Semiquantitative grading of severity of mitral regurgitation by real-time two-dimensional Doppler flow imaging technique. J Am Coll Cardiol 7:82, 1986
428. Miyatake K, Yamamoto K, Park YD et al: Diagnosis of mitral valve perforation by real-time two-dimensional Doppler flow imaging technique. J Am Coll Cardiol 8:1235, 1986
429. Chow LC, Dittrich HC, Dembitsky WP et al: Accurate localization of ruptured sinus of valsalva aneurysm by real-time two-dimensional Doppler flow imaging. Chest 94:462, 1988
430. Messner-Pellenc P, Leclercq F, Krebs R et al: Doppler color echocardiography in the diagnosis of 4 septal perforations complicating anterior myocardial infarction. Arch Mal Coeur 81:1243, 1988
431. Izumi S, Miyatake K, Beppu S et al: Mechanism of mitral regurgitation in patients with myocardial infarction: A study using real-time two-dimensional Doppler flow imaging and echocardiography. Circulation 76:777, 1987
432. Natello GW, Nanda NC, Zachariah ZP: Color Doppler recognition of left ventricular pseudoaneurysm. Am J Med 85:432, 1988
433. Roelandt JR, Sutherland GR, Yoshida K, Yoskikawa J: Improved diagnosis and characterization of left ventricular pseudoaneurysm by Doppler color flow imaging. J Am Coll Cardiol 12:807, 1988
434. Perry GJ, Helmcke F, Nanda NC et al: Evaluation of aortic insufficiency by Doppler color flow mapping. J Am Coll Cardiol 9:952, 1987
435. Bouchard A, Yock P, Schiller NB et al: Value of color Doppler estimation of regurgitant volume in patients with chronic aortic insufficiency. Am Heart J 117:1099, 1989
436. Suzuki Y, Kambara H, Kadota K et al: Detection and evaluation of tricuspid regurgitation using a real-time, two-dimensional, color-coded Doppler flow imaging system: Comparison with contrast two-dimensional echocardiography and right ventriculography. Am J Cardiol 57:811, 1986
437. Fisher EA, Goldman ME: Simple, rapid method for quantification of tricuspid regurgitation by two-dimensional echocardiography. Am J Cardiol 63:1375, 1989
438. Vandenberg BF, Dellsperger KC, Chandran KB et al: Detection, localization, and quantitation of bioprosthetic mitral valve regurgitation: An in vitro two-dimensional color-Doppler flow-mapping study. Circulation 78:529, 1988
439. Kapur, Fan P, Nanda NC et al: Doppler color flow mapping in the evaluation of prosthetic mitral and aortic valve function. J Am Coll Cardiol 13:1561, 1989
440. Jones M, Eidbo EE: Doppler color flow evaluation of prosthetic mitral valves: experimental epicardial studies. J Am Coll Cardiol 13:234, 1989
441. Nellessen U, Schnittger I, Appleton CP et al: Transesophageal two-dimensional echocardiography and color Doppler velocity mapping in the evaluation of cardiac valve prostheses. Circulation 78:848, 1988
442. Fan PH, Kapur KK, Nanda NC: Color-guided echocardiographic assessment of aortic valve stenosis. J Am Coll Cardiol 12:441, 1988
443. Nishimura RA, Tajik AJ, Reeder GS et al: Evaluation of hypertrophic cardiomyopathy by Doppler color flow imaging: Initial observations. Mayo Clin Proc 61:631, 1986
444. Blazer D, Kotler MN, Parry WR et al: Noninvasive evaluation of mid-left ventricular obstruction by two-dimensional and Doppler echocardiography and color flow Doppler echocardiography. Am Heart J 114:1162, 1987
445. Friedman DM, Schmer V, Rutkowski M: Two-dimensional color Doppler in discrete membranous subaortic stenosis. Am Heart J 115:686, 1988
446. Khandheria BK, Tajik AJ, Reeder GS et al: Doppler color flow imaging: A new technique for visualization and characterization of the blood flow jet in mitral stenosis. Mayo Clin Proc 61:623, 1986
447. Pollick C, Sullivan H, Cujee B et al: Doppler color-flow imaging assessment of shunt size in atrial septal defect. Circulation 78:522
448. Ludomirsky A, Huhta JC, Vick GW III et al: Color Doppler detection of multiple ventricular septal defects. Circulation 74:1317, 1986
449. Sanders SP, Parness IA, Colan SD: Recognition of abnormal connections of coronary arteries with the use of Doppler color flow mapping. J Am Coll Cardiol 15:922, 1989
450. Swensson RE, Valdes-Cruz LM, Sahn DJ et al. Real-time Doppler color flow mapping for detection of patent ductus arteriosus. J Am Coll Cardiol 8:1105, 1986
451. Vitarelli A, Sacapato A, Sanguigni V et al: Evaluation of total anomalous pulmonary venous drainage with cross-sectional colour-flow Doppler echocardiography. Eur Heart J 7:190, 1986
452. Simpson IA, Sahn DJ, Valdes-Cruz LM et al: Color Doppler flow mapping in patients with coarctation of the aorta: New observations and improved evaluation with color flow diameter and proximal acceleration as predictors of severity. Circulation 77:736, 1988
453. von Bibra H, Hartmann F, Petrik M et al: Contrast-color Doppler echocardiography. Improved right heart diagnosis following intravenous injection of Echovist. Z Kardiol 78:101, 1989
454. Becher H, Schlief R: Improved sensitivity of color Doppler by SH U 454. Am J Cardiol 64:374, 1989
455. Hagler DJ, Tajik AJ, Seward JB et al: Intraoperative two-dimensional Doppler echocardiography: Preliminary study for congenital heart disease. J Thorac Cardiovasc Surg 95:516, 1988
456. Cohen IS, Anderson DW, Virmani R et al: Congestive cardiomyopathy in association with the acquired immunodeficiency syndrome. N Eng J Med 315:628, 1986

457. Anderson DW, Virmani R, Reilly JM et al: Prevalent myocarditis at necropsy in the Acquired Immunodeficiency Syndrome. J Am Coll Cardiol 11:792, 1988
458. Baroldi G, Corallo S, Moroni M et al: Focal lymphocytic myocarditis in acquired immunodeficiency syndrome (AIDS): A correlative morphologic and clinical study in 26 consecutive fatal cases. J Am Coll Cardiol 12:463, 1988
459. Reilly JM, Cunnion RE, Anderson DW et al: Frequency of myocarditis, left ventricular dysfunction and ventricular tachycardia in the Acquired Immune Deficiency Syndrome. Am J Cardiol 62:789, 1988
460. Cammarosano C, Lewis W: Cardiac lesions in acquired immune deficiency syndrome (AIDS). J Am Coll Cardiol 5:703, 1985
461. Himelman RB, Chung WS, Chernoff DN et al: Cardiac manifestations of Human Immunodeficiency Virus Infection: A two-dimensional echocardiographic study. J Am Coll Cardiol 13:1030, 1989
462. Monsuez JJ, Kinney EL, Vittecoq D et al: Comparison among Acquired Immune Deficiency Syndrome Patients with and without clinical evidence of cardiac disease. Am J Cardiol 62:1311, 1988
463. Levy WS, Simon GL, Rios JC et al: Prevalence of cardiac abnormalities in Human Immunodeficiency Virus infection. Am J Cardiol 63:86, 1989
464. Calabrese LH, Proffitt MR, Yen-Lieberman B et al: Congestive cardiomyopathy and illness related to the Acquired Immunodeficiency Syndrome (AIDS) associated with isolation of retrovirus from myocardium. Ann Intern Med 107:691, 1987
465. Guarner J, Brynes RK, Chan WC et al: Primary non-Hodgkin's lymphoma of the heart in two patients with the acquired immunodeficiency syndrome. Lab Med 111:254, 1987
466. Silver MA, Macher AM, Reichert CM et al: Cardiac involvement by Kaposi's sarcoma in acquired immune deficiency syndrome (AIDS). Am J Cardiol 53:983, 1984
467. Henochowicz S, Mustafa M, Lawrinson WE et al: Cardiac aspergillosis in acquired immune deficiency syndrome. Am J Cardiol 5:1239, 1985
468. Laws W, Lipsick J, Cammarosano C: Cryptococcal myocarditis in acquired immune deficiency syndrome. Am J Cardiol 55:1240, 1985
469. Wilkes MS, Felix JC, Fortin AH et al: Value of necropsy in Acquired Immunodeficiency Syndrome. Lancet ii:85, 1988
470. Himelman RB, Dohrman M, Goodman P et al: Severe pulmonary hypertension and cor pulmonale in the Acquired Immunodeficiency Syndrome. Am J Cardiol 1989 (in press)
471. Feigenbaum H, Waldhausen JA, Hyde SP: Ultrasound diagnosis of pericardial effusion. JAMA 191:107, 1965
472. Horowitz MS, Schultz CS, Stinson EB et al: Sensitivity and specificity of echocardiographic diagnosis of pericardial effusion. Circulation 50:239, 1974
473. Rifkin RD, Isner JM, Carter BL, Bankoff MS: Combined posteroanterior subepicardial fat simulating the echocardiographic diagnosis of pericardial effusion. J Am Coll Cardiol 3:1333, 1984
474. Wada T, Honda M, Matsuyama S: Extra echo spaces: Ultrasonography and computerized tomography correlations. Br Heart J 47:430, 1982
475. Isner JM, Carter BL, Roberts WC, Bankoff MS: Subepicardial adipose tissue producing echocardiographic appearance of pericardial effusion. Am J Cardiol 51:565, 1983
476. Schiller NB, Botvinick EH: Right ventricular compression as a sign of cardiac tamponade. Circulation 56:774, 1977
477. Armstrong WF, Schilt BF, Helper DJ et al: Diastolic collapse of the right ventricle with tamponade: An echocardiographic study. Circulation 65:1491, 1982
478. Leimgruber PP, Klopfenstein S, Wann LS, Brooks HL: The hemodynamic derangement associated with right ventricular diastolic collapse in cardiac tamponade: An experimental echocardiographic study. Circulation 68:612, 1983
479. Williams GJ, Partridge JB: Right ventricular diastolic collapse: An echocardiographic sign of tamponade. Br Heart J 49:292, 1983
480. Gillam LD, Guyer DE, Gibson TC et al: Hydrodynamic compression of the right atrium: A new echocardiographic sign of cardiac tamponade. Circulation 68:294, 1983
481. Kronzon I, Cohen ML, Winer HE: Diastolic atrial compression: A sensitive echocardiographic sign of cardiac tamponade. J Am Coll Cardiol 2:770, 1983
482. Rein AJ, Lewis N, Forst L et al: Echocardiography of the inferior vena cava in healthy subjects and in patients with cardiac disease. Isr J Med Sci 18:581, 1982
483. Meltzer RS, McGhie J, Roelandt J: Inferior vena cava echocardiography. J Clin Ultrasound 10:47, 1982
484. Gullace G, Savoia MT: Echocardiographic assessment of the inferior vena cava wall motion for studies of right heart dynamics and function. Clin Cardiol 7:393, 1984
485. Moreno FLL, Hagan AD, Holman JR et al: Evaluation of size and dynamics of the inferior vena cava as an index of right-sided cardiac function. Am J Cardiol 53:579, 1984
486. Kircher B, Himelman RB, Schiller NB: Estimation of right atrial pressure by two-dimensional echocardiography of the respiratory behavior of the inferior vena cava. (abstract) Circulation 78 (Suppl II):550, 1988
487. Himelman RB, Kircher B, Rockey DC et al: Inferior vena cava plethora with blunted respiratory response: A sensitive echocardiographic sign of cardiac tamponade. J Am Coll Cardiol 12:1470, 1988
488. Labib SB, Udelson JE, Pandian NG: Echocardiography in low pressure cardiac tamponade. Am J Cardiol 63:1156, 1989
489. Burstow DJ, Oh JK, Bailey KR et al: Cardiac tamponade: Characteristic Doppler observations. Mayo Clin Proc 64:312, 1989
490. Leeman DE, Levine MJ, Come PC: Doppler echocardiography in cardiac tamponade: Exaggerated respiratory variation in transvalvular blood flow velocity integrals. J Am Coll Cardiol 11:572, 1988
491. Appleton CP, Hatle LK, Popp RL: Cardiac tamponade and pericardial effusion: Respiratory variation in transvalvular flow velocities studied by Doppler echocardiography. J Am Coll Cardiol 11:1020, 1988
492. Appleton CP, Hatle LK, Popp RL: Superior vena cava flow velocity patterns can diagnose cardiac tamponade in patients with pericardial effusions (abstract). J Am Coll Cardiol 9 (Suppl):118A, 1987
493. Choong CY, Herrmann HC, Weyman AE et al: Preload dependence of Doppler-derived indexes of left ventricular diastolic function in humans. J Am Coll Cardiol 10:800, 1987
494. Hoit B, Sahn DJ, Shabetai R: Doppler-detected paradoxus of mitral and tricuspid valve flows in chronic lung disease. J Am Coll Cardiol 8:706, 1986
495. Candell-Riera J, Carcia del Castillo H, Permanger-Miralda G et al: Echocardiographic features of the interventricular septum in chronic constrictive pericarditis. Circulation 57:1154, 1973
496. Gibson TC, Grossman W, McLaurin LP et al: An echocardiographic study of the interventricular system in constrictive pericarditis. Br Heart J 38:738, 1976
497. Wann LS, Weyman AE, Dillon JC, Feigenbaum H: Premature pulmonary valve opening. Circulation 55:128, 1977
498. Tei C, Child JS, Tanaka H, Shah PM: Atrial systolic notch on the interventricular septal echogram: An echocardiographic sign of constrictive pericarditis. J Am Coll Cardiol 1:970, 1983
499. Voelkel AG, Pietro DA, Folland ED et al: Echocardiographic features of constrictive pericarditis. Circulation 58:871, 1978
500. Chandraratna PAN: Uses and Limitations of Echocardiography in the Evaluation of Pericardial Disease. Echocardiography 1:55, 1984
501. Engel PJ, Fowler NO, Tei C et al: M-Mode Echocardiography in Constrictive Pericarditis. J Am Coll Cardiol 6:471, 1985
502. Himelman RB, Lee E, Schiller NB: Septal bounce, vena cava plethora, and pericardial adhesion: Informative two-dimensional echocardiographic signs in the diagnosis of pericardial constriction. J Am Soc Echo 1:333, 1988
503. Hatle LK, Appleton CP, Popp RL: Differentiation of constrictive pericarditis and restrictive cardiomyopathy by Doppler echocardiography. Circulation 79:357, 1989
504. Appleton CP, Hatle LK, Popp RL: Central venous flow velocity patterns can differentiate constrictive pericarditis from restrictive cardiomyopathy (abstract). J Am Coll Cardiol 9 (Suppl):119A, 1987
505. Sagrista-Sauleda J, Permanyer Miralc G, Candell-Riera J et al: Transient cardiac constriction: An unrecognized pattern of evolution in effusive acute idiopathic pericarditis. Am J Cardiol 59:961, 1987
506. Chandraratna PA, Aronow WS: Detection of pericardial metastases by cross-sectional echocardiography. Circulation 63:54, 1981
507. Hynes JK, Tajik AJ, Osborn MJ et al: Two dimensional echocardiographic diagnosis of pericardial cyst. Mayo Clin Proc 58:60, 1983
508. Effert S, Domanig E: The diagnosis of intra-atrial tumor and thrombi by the ultrasonic echo method. German Medical Monthly 4:1, 1959
509. Ports TA, Cogan J, Schiller NB, Rapaport E: Echocardiography of left ventricular masses. Circulation 58:528, 1978
510. Thier W, Schluter M, Krebber J et al: Cysts in left atrial myxomas identified by transesophageal cross-sectional echocardiography. Am J Cardiol 51:1793, 1983
511. Visser CA, Kan G, David GK et al: Two dimensional echocardiography in the diagnosis of left ventricular thrombus. Chest 2:228, 1983
512. Cullen JG, Korcuska K, Musser G et al: Calcified left ventricular thrombus causing repeated retinal arterial emboli. Chest 79:708, 1981
513. Peterson SP, Schiller NB, Stricker RB: Failure of two-dimensional echocardiography to detect aspergillus endocarditis. Chest 85:291, 1984
514. Keren A, Billingham ME, Popp RL: Echocardiographic recognition and implications of ventricular hypertrophic trabeculations and aberrant bands. Circulation 70:836, 1984
515. Werner JA, Cheitlin MD, Gross BW et al: Echocardiographic appearance of the Chiari network: Differentiation from right-heart pathology. Circulation 63:1104, 1981
516. Himelman RB, Abbott JA, Schiller NB: Diagnosis of mediastinal lesions by echocardiography. Echocardiography 5:219, 1988

THE SCINTIGRAPHIC EVALUATION OF THE CARDIOVASCULAR SYSTEM

Elias H. Botvinick • Michael Dae
William O'Connell
Douglas Ortendahl • Robert Hattner

The last ten years have seen a revolution in methods of cardiologic evaluation. Most prominent has been the development of noninvasive imaging techniques. Scintigraphic methods have been applied widely, impacting on the diagnosis and care of all forms of cardiac illness.[1-4] They are safe, have been adopted by the cardiologist, and have been integrated into the cardiac evaluation. However, an appreciation of the technical and physics aspects of the method[1-5] is critical if the practicing cardiologist is to employ the tool appropriately and to the best advantage of the patient.

Scintigraphy is a tracer technique. A radioactive substance, a radionuclide, physically unstable as it emits an energetic particle, is used to label a pharmaceutical or is itself administered intravenously and detected within the patient. Localization within the subject depends on the physiologic characteristics of the radiopharmaceutical. The pharmaceutical is nonallergenic, and it is given in small amounts that have no effect on the process it seeks to characterize. The label allows the body and organ pharmaceutical distribution to be determined using a radioactivity detector, generally a component of the scintillation camera. The success of cardiac scintigraphy is due to the ability of modern cameras to map accurately and computers to analyze this distribution.

▣ THE METHOD AND ITS TECHNOLOGY
THE RADIONUCLIDE

The choice of radionuclide is based on a consideration of the particle emitted; its energy level; its half-life, both physical and biological, considering both metabolism and excretion; and its labeling and localizing properties (Table 29.1). For imaging applications, gamma rays or x-rays in the energy range 70 keV to 250 keV are preferred. Lower energies are easily attenuated and have difficulty penetrating human tissue, while higher energies may be too penetrant to permit proper registration and can be accommodated only with reduced image quality. Gamma rays and x-rays are forms of electromagnetic radiation or photons. The former are the result of a nuclear interaction; the latter are due to atomic interactions. Other emissions, particularly charged particles, have reduced penetration and often deliver prohibitive radiation doses. Characteristic whole body doses for clinical tests range from 100 mrad to 300 mrad, roughly equivalent to two sets of posterior–anterior and lateral chest x-ray films, or to a flat and upright x-ray film of the abdomen. Best not performed during pregnancy and with reduced pediatric dosage, the application should be based on the overall clinical cost-to-benefit ratio. Technetium-99m, the most commonly used isotope, emits a gamma ray at 140 keV, near optimal for imaging purposes, while thallium(Tl)-201, used for cardiac perfusion studies, decays by electron capture to mercury(Hg)-201, which emits x-rays in the range of 80 keV used for imaging. ^{201}Tl has a long, 73-hour physical half-life and a significantly longer biological half-life, while the short, 6-hour physical half-life of ^{99m}Tc better suits patient evaluation and is conveniently eluted from a molybdenum-99 generator, which can be replaced weekly. While not optimal for first-pass applications, this duration does permit more prolonged imaging studies. Other imaging radionuclides, including many of those used for positron emission tomography, are short-lived and cyclotron-produced.

THE IMAGING DEVICE

Although a variety of radioisotope detectors have been used, the material of choice remains sodium iodide.[1,5] The interaction of a high-energy particle, as x-rays or gamma rays, with the sodium iodide crystal, a scintillator, causes the emission of light, which is detected and amplified by a photomultiplier tube. The magnitude of the photomultiplier signal is dependent on the amount of energy deposited in the scintillator and is proportional to the number and energy of incident photons. Relative signal strength and location of each tube determine the spatial coordinates and energy of the incident photon.

THE NONIMAGING PROBE

One early application of scintigraphy sought cardiac end-diastolic and end-systolic volumes. The simplest device for this task is the scintillation probe, which is comprised of a single sodium iodide crystal, 2 cm to 8 cm in diameter and 2 cm to 5 cm thick, viewed by a single photomultiplier tube.[1,5] To detect only radiation from the heart, the probe must be shielded within a lead cylinder with a collimator at its opening. The collimator, an adjunct of all conventional scintillation imaging devices, a lead shield penetrated by holes, provides a focusing function that permits registry of only directed photons and discourages localizing errors due to scattered radiation. Spatial resolution, limited by probe diameter, is adequate for observing the left ventricle. Modern digital electronics permit probe acquisition and display of the ventricular time versus radioactivity curve with 10-msec to 50-msec resolution, which allows beat-to-beat or averaged global volumetric and functional analysis.[6-9] While this probe system is relatively inexpensive and extremely portable, it is not an imaging detector and proper cardiac alignment might be difficult, yielding possible problems of reproducibility and accuracy, especially when evaluating ventricles with segmental abnormalities.[10]

SCINTILLATION CAMERA

Valuable information regarding regional ventricular function requires an imaging detector such as the scintillation, Anger, or gamma camera (Fig. 29.1). It consists of a larger sodium iodide crystal, at least 25 cm in diameter and 6 mm to 9 mm thick, and a bank of closely arrayed photomultiplier tubes. Sophisticated electronic circuitry senses the signal at each tube and assigns a position on the face of the crystal, localizing the point of gamma–crystal interaction. The scintillation camera analyzes a random serial sample of target radioactivity and can be set to sample regional radioactivity in brief temporal intervals. This permits the analysis and display of dynamic events. To ensure the relationship between the origin of the emitting isotope within the patient and the perceived location on the camera face, the direction of the gamma ray, constrained by means of the collimator, must be known.

CAMERA COLLIMATION

The simplest design is the pinhole collimator, which spreads emissions from a small aperture over the camera face. For small, superficial organs, such as the thyroid, this is advantageous, magnifying the image and improving its spatial resolution. However, sensitivity varies with depth, creating problems when evaluating the large, deep heart, where it has been applied to perfusion scintigraphy in adults. Pinhole and converging collimators are useful for cardiac imaging in the small pediatric patient.

The parallel hole collimator is most commonly used for cardiac applications. It constrains detected photons to travel down the length of holes that are spread uniformly over the camera face. The longer the holes and the smaller their diameter, the better will be the resultant spatial resolution. The high-resolution collimator, often used for equilibrium blood pool studies, presents the most extreme example of collimator selectivity. Yet, since this configuration rejects more photons, sensitivity is reduced, increasing the time of image acquisition. The high sensitivity is the least selective parallel hole collimator. It has advantages for use with temporally dependent studies such as first-pass blood pool and planar perfusion imaging, increasing photon acceptance and reducing imaging time. However, a price is paid in reduced spatial resolution. The optimal trade-off between resolution and sensitivity will depend on the particular application. For many cardiac applications, the low-energy, all-purpose (LEAP) collimator is used. Alternatively, the parallel slant-hole collimator can be used with intermediate sensitivity and spatial resolution.

ADAPTATIONS TO COMPENSATE FOR SCATTER

The assumption has been made that gamma rays will travel in a straight line from patient, through collimator, to detector. However, Compton scatter, due to photon interaction with free electrons in the patient or collimator, alters photon direction and reduces photon energy. Such scattered photons are projected back through the collimator to the point of scatter, not to the point of origin. The pulse height analyzer seeks to discriminate scattered photons by virtue of their reduced energy and can separate radionuclides of significantly differing emission photon energies, such as ^{201}Tl and ^{99m}Tc. However, "downscattered" energy makes it difficult to discretely identify a lower-energy emitter in the presence of a higher-energy source of relatively similar energy. Further, the relatively poor energy resolution of the scintillation camera makes it difficult to discriminate "downscattered" photons, especially when the initial energy is low and not very different from the scattered photons. Practically, ^{201}Tl would be difficult to image in the presence of ^{99m}Tc. Scatter acceptance can be reduced by choosing asymmetric energy windows.[11] In scintigraphy, the quality of photons and their proper localization may be more important than their quantity. While the latter will determine the confidence with which a particular feature may be discerned, the former affect the spatial resolution and output contrast and are determined by the properties of the collimator, the intrinsic camera resolution, and the amount of scatter rejection.

Energy resolution is further improved by correcting the measured energy for the location of the event. Detection uniformity across the field of view is also critical. Additional hardware requirements are im-

TABLE 29.1 PHYSICAL PROPERTIES OF RADIONUCLIDES COMMONLY USED IN CARDIAC EVALUATION

Radionuclide	Physical Half-Life	Principal Photon(s)
^{11}C	20.5 min	511
^{127}Cs	6.2 hr	125,411
^{129}Cs	32 hr	375,411
^{18}F	110 min	511
^{67}Ga	3.3 days	93,185,300
^{111}In	2.8 days	172,247
^{43}K	22.2 hr	373,618
^{81m}Kr	13 sec	190
^{15}O	2 min	511
^{13}N	10 min	511
^{82}Rb	75 sec	511
^{99m}Tc	6 hr	140
^{127}Xe	36 days	172,203,375
^{133}Xe	5.3 days	81
^{201}Tl	73 hr	69,083,167

Absorbed Total Body Radiation Dose for Commonly Used Radiopharmaceuticals

Radiopharmaceutical	rad/mCi
^{99m}Tc pyrophosphate	0.013
^{99m}Tc-labeled red cells	0.017
^{99m}Tc DTPA	0.016
^{99m}Tc pertechnetate	0.014
Tc-MAA	0.015
^{201}Tl	0.24
^{133}Xe	0.0009–0.0018 (single breath)
	0.0011 (5 min. rebreathing)

(Data from Freeman LM (ed): Freeman and Johnson's Clinical Radionuclide Imaging, 3rd ed. Orlando, FL, Grune & Stratton, 1984)

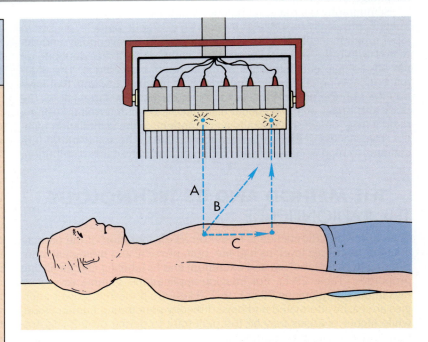

FIGURE 29.1 Scattered radiation. Shown on this schematic drawing is the path of a photon impacting on the crystal and originating in the radionuclide source (A) and two scattered photons. One photon, scattered at 45° (B), impacts on the collimator and loses energy before impacting on the crystal. Another photon undergoes Compton scatter (C), interacting with free electrons, altering photon direction. This scattered photon will impact on the crystal, projecting to the point of scatter, not to the point of origin. Such photons can only be recognized through a process of energy discrimination.

posed by cardiac first-pass studies, where peak count rates can reach 300,000 counts/sec. However, sodium iodide is not a fast material. This problem limits acquisition rates of most scintillation cameras but can be overcome in part by multicrystal cameras, used widely for first-pass blood pool studies. Newer single-crystal cameras seek to circumvent this problem by shortening the electronic pulse from the camera. However, the energy and spatial resolution are degraded.

TOMOGRAPHY
SINGLE PHOTON TOMOGRAPHIC METHODS

LIMITED ANGLE TECHNIQUES. Important information may be obscured by superimposed activity using planar imaging. This may be ameliorated in part with the acquisition of multiple projections. Spatial integration may be computerized if the relationships between projections are known, yielding tomographic images. The seven-pinhole method projects seven images of the heart onto a large-field camera face through seven holes drilled centrally into a pinhole collimator.[12] Each aperture is separated by a lead septum to prevent image overlap. The rotating slant-hole method employs a slant-hole collimator with holes tilted at 20° or 30° from the normal.[13] By rotating the collimator 60° between acquisitions, six distinct images are obtained in a given projection. In both cases, multiple projections taken at different well-defined angles with respect to the target are processed using an algebraic reconstruction technique, yielding tomographic sections at different depths. However, owing to their limited angular sampling, such reconstructions are susceptible to artifacts and do not reliably permit quantitative measurement. Although there is sufficient sampling for gross tomographic evaluation, sampling is insufficient to provide a mathematically closed solution.

SINGLE PHOTON EMISSION COMPUTED TOMOGRAPHY. Single photon emission computed tomography (SPECT) employs a camera rotating on a gantry to solve these problems.[14] Data acquired over 180° or 360° are reconstructed using standard algorithms developed for x-ray computed tomography.[15,16] One unique problem of the scintigraphic method that must be addressed is that of attenuation, producing undersampling of deep organs. Algorithms to deal with this problem are not completely satisfactory. Emission computed tomography of ^{201}Tl perfusion images applies only 180° rotation, since the posterior projections show severe attenuation of the 70-keV photons.

POSITRON EMISSION TOMOGRAPHY

Positron emission tomography (PET) is another tomographic scintigraphic modality.[16-18] The positron emitted in positron decay interacts with an electron, quickly annihilating both particles to produce two 511-keV photons, which travel at 180° to one another. By detecting each of these photons, the event is constrained to lie on the line between the two points. The reconstruction, determining the depth of origin, can then be performed using algorithms similar to those used in emission computed tomography or computed tomography, yielding highly resolved transaxial images of the target organ. PET requires completely new hardware compared to other scintigraphic studies. The high-energy 511-keV photons require a 2.5-cm crystal thickness and make the scintillation camera unsuitable for use because of its poor detection efficiency. The latter is an important issue in PET because both photons must be detected, making sensitivity proportional to the square of detection efficiency. Conversely, each of the detectors will see a large number of noncoincident events that can be automatically discounted, a kind of internal collimation. PET imaging strategy uses multiple individual detectors arranged in a ring about the patient, where components link detectors on opposite sides. This instrument provides a single cross-section or slice. If additional simultaneous sections are desired, then additional rings must be added, increasing the cost. Increased efficiency is obtained with a high-density detector such as bismuth germanate.[17] Another detection strategy employs time of flight information to improve spatial resolution.[18] Since annihilation photons are emitted simultaneously, the time to each detector could localize the event along the line. Currently fast scintillators, such as cesium fluoride, give timing resolution of 600 picoseconds and can localize the event to within 9 mm. In combination with the reconstruction algorithm, this constraint on position can lead to even better resolution. However, these faster detectors have poorer detection efficiency, and again, one must sacrifice total counts for better localizing information. It is not clear at this point which technology will prevail. PET imaging attracts special interest owing to the biologically active nature of many of the positron-emitting radionuclides. However, they are generally cyclotron-produced, their short half-life acts as both an advantage and a detriment, and they require, as shown, new expensive technology.

COMPUTERS IN CARDIAC SCINTIGRAPHY

Commercial equipment is widely available with much prepackaged software. However, the proper application and further development of these methods depend on an understanding of computer operations by physicians both generating and applying study results.

Computer applications represent a great advantage of the scintigraphic method, permitting objective, quantitative calculation of parameters measured only with difficulty by other methods or in no other way. The computer has several functions involved in the collection and storage of the study, requiring an interface to the camera and considerable mass storage. The analog data of the imaging device are easily digitized, making processing possible by microcomputers or minicomputers. The operating system provides overall control of acquisition, analysis, and display functions. Acquisition software should be adaptable, permitting the selective choice of study parameters. Analysis should be performed by programs designed to generate specific required data. Display software selects the display matrix dimension and makes the data accessible to video monitors as well as hard copy. Programs to enhance contrast and perform quantitative "washout" analysis of ^{201}Tl images should be available.[19-21]

The camera–computer interface passes the data in histogram (frame) or list mode. In histogram mode, the interface builds the digital image directly in computer memory as a two-dimensional table or histogram. As acquisition proceeds, the interface digitizes the x, y coordinates of each accepted photon and increments the corresponding pixel in the image histogram. The digital image is stored and can be displayed by letting the magnitude of data in each pixel determine its on-screen brightness. Dynamic studies can be created by beginning new images or frames at specified intervals and storing successive frames. This is the most common method of blood pool collection. In list mode, the interface passes the digitized x, y coordinates directly to memory, along with 10-msec timing marks or R wave signals. Image resolution and framing rate are deferred and are selected after acquisition from the preserved raw data. This capability is most valuable in processing gated equilibrium blood pool studies, where, in the presence of gross heart rate irregularity, the operator can choose to frame only data corresponding to a limited R-R interval. The flexibility of list mode has its price in the need for extra disk storage and added processing time.

Obviously, the capabilities of the method will depend strongly on computer capacity and versatility. For cardiac applications, the computer should have at least 80 megabytes of disk storage. The minimum memory for a cardiac acquisition and analysis station is 256 kilobytes. A large memory makes programming easier and expedites the development and implementation of new application packages by other users and vendors. Archival storage now uses magnetic tape, but in the future may employ optical disks.

The blood pool study is probably the most computer intensive and requires the greatest use of computer memory. When studies are acquired on a camera crystal 25 cm in diameter, acquisition resolution with 64 × 64 framing corresponds to a pixel size of 4 mm on a side and can adequately characterize the detail in a perfusion or blood pool scintigram. Computer memory must be at least 64 × 64 × 16 pixels large to accommodate all frames during acquisition and avoid count overflow. Analysis of ventricular counts data is facilitated and objectified by automatic edge detection methods. These work well in roughly 80% of studies and operator alteration or replacement must be easily possible.[22] A high-quality display is critically important for resolution of blood pool images and should have a raster of 256 × 256 with a broad gray scale of at least 64 shades. Since functional images are of such importance, a color display should be seriously considered. It should be capable of displaying 256 different colors simultaneously with 256 levels of brightness available for each of the primary colors, red, blue, and yellow. A joystick or trackball that permits refined cursor definition of image regions of interest is mandatory. A high-quality display also makes it possible to view two or more studies, static or dynamic cine, simultaneously, a usual feature in the evaluation of interventions or the comparison of serial studies.

MYOCARDIAL PERFUSION SCINTIGRAPHY

Myocardial perfusion scintigraphy seeks to characterize relative myocardial perfusion noninvasively.[23-25] It is among the most widely used and clinically valuable cardiac scintigraphic studies.

THE RADIONUCLIDE

Previously, potassium (K)-43 or rubidium (Rb)-81 was used.[24,25] The current methodology employs thallium-201. Each of these is an intracellular cation that is extracted rapidly following its intravenous administration, distributing intracellularly in proportion to relative myocardial perfusion.[26,27] Behaving and localizing like native body potassium, their proper intracellular localization serves also as a strong indicator of myocardial viability (Table 29.2).[3,26] Yet, these agents are not myocardial specific, but localize, according to similar kinetics, in cells of all parenchymal tissues.[23,28,29] By this mechanism, ^{201}Tl has been applied in the identification of peripheral vascular and ischemic bowel disease, and the rich thyroid perfusion permits its application in the assessment of thyroid and parathyroid disease.

This agent is a paradox of pharmaceutical chemistry; in larger doses it is an ingredient of rat poison and was the murder weapon in an Agatha Christie novel.[30] Yet, except for the small radiation dose, ^{201}Tl is entirely innocuous in the imaging dose administered. It is superior to other agents in some respects, owing to its longer half-life and the lower energy of emission; yet, it is imperfect, as the former is too long and the latter is too low for optimal image applications. Due to its rapid blood clearance, approximately 80% on the first pass, and the finite period of its intracellular localization, ^{201}Tl can be administered during a short-lived intervention and imaged shortly thereafter to reflect the distribution of perfusion at the time of administration.[28,29,31]

Except in the presence of severe obstruction, compensatory coronary arteriolar dilation or collateral perfusion permits relatively normal flow at rest through even significantly stenotic vessels. Most patients with coronary disease are asymptomatic at rest. However, as coronary flow demands increase with stress, compensation is insufficient and supply is limited. The inability to provide the full flow demands of stress represents insufficient flow reserve and is itself the pathophysiologic definition of a significant coronary stenosis. However, beds supplied by nonstenotic or minimally stenotic vessels augment regional perfusion in relation to demands (Fig. 29.2).[32] If ^{201}Tl is administered during such stress-induced regional heterogeneity, it will distribute in this heterogeneous pattern. Recognition of regions of reduced relative perfusion indicates an abnormality in the related coronary supply.

Thallium appears to gain cellular entry as does potassium, via membrane Na^+/K^+ ATPase.[33] Yet it seems relatively stable once inside. Subsequent to its localization, regional intracellular ^{201}Tl follows its gradient with the blood (Fig. 29.3).[3] Those areas with most radioactivity lose thallium most rapidly. Reappearance in the blood is followed by cellular uptake in the resting distribution. In this way, myocardial regions slowly come to equilibrium with attainment of the baseline perfusion pattern.[34,35] The regional ratio, initial radioactivity–delayed radioactivity/initial radioactivity, background and time corrected, comprises the parameter of percent washout, an established objective measure of regional perfusion (Fig. 29.4).[3,21,36] Relatively underperfused regions seen on immediate poststress imaging, which become less apparent or "fill in," are viable and indicate stress-induced regional myocardial ischemia (Fig. 29.5). If defects remain "fixed" on delayed imaging, they are, in most cases, related to irreversible infarction and scar.[35] Partial redistribution with a mixture of fixed and improving abnormalities indicates elements of both ischemia and infarction, a common clinical substrate.

THE METHOD OF DYNAMIC STRESS PERFUSION SCINTIGRAPHY

In practice, the study is performed in association with a standard stress test, generally performed on a treadmill.[37] Patients are studied in the fasting state. The stress test is conducted according to the standard method with the placement of an intravenous line to ensure accessibility during peak exercise. Symptoms, signs, blood pressure, and electrocardiogram are monitored as testing proceeds to the clinically indicated end point. The patient informs the physician of any symptoms, especially those that may limit testing, and is asked to help the physician by telling him such things as "Inject the medicine now, because I can only exercise one minute more," "Stop the test now, I can go no

---

TABLE 29.2 SCINTIGRAPHIC METHODS

For Assessment of Myocardial Viability and Functional Reversibility
1. Reversible perfusion abnormalities using ^{201}Tl or other indicator
2. Delayed redistribution on ^{201}Tl perfusion imaging
3. Normal wall motion in the presence of apparently fixed perfusion defect
4. Abnormal wall motion in the presence of apparently normal perfusion
5. Normalized or improved wall motion after nitroglycerin

For Identification of Significant Myocardium at Ischemic Risk and Poor Prognosis
1. Impressive reversible perfusion defect
2. Relatively mild perfusion defect at a low level of stress or in the presence of extensive fixed defects
3. In patients with prior infarction–perfusion defect in the distribution of a noninfarcted vessel (outside the infarct zone)
4. In the presence of ischemic heart disease—stress-induced lung uptake, "cavitary dilation," basal uptake on ^{201}Tl imaging
5. In the presence of stress-induced heart rate over 85% predicted for age—extensive washout abnormalities
6. Heterogeneity of washout in association with low achieved double product or dipyridamole infusion
7. Extensive washout in association with minor reversible perfusion defects at a low double product*
8. Preserved LVEF at rest in a patient with a history of recurrent pulmonary edema
9. Extensive stress-induced wall motion abnormalities
10. Extensive stress-induced reduction in LVEF

* Possible but not yet firmly established

further." Thirty seconds to 1 minute prior to the symptom, sign, or heart rate limited stress end point, 2 mCi of ^{201}Tl is injected through the intravenous line. A saline flush is used to clear the line as stress continues for another minute. The line is preferably placed away from joints, and the agent is administered quickly, but gently, during tension-free full arm extension to avoid back pressure and potential extravasation with infiltration or area contamination.

Full monitoring is again performed in recovery, as the scintigraphic information serves to complement the results of stress testing, not replace it. Monitoring during imaging is generally impractical. Since image data are temporally dependent, imaging is begun as soon as possible. Thus, recovery is monitored for 7 minutes to capture pertinent ST or arrhythmic abnormalities not seen during stress.[38] Imaging in multiple planar projections or using tomographic methods begins immediately on termination of monitoring, within 10 minutes of radionuclide administration, barring serious arrhythmias, hypotension, or other problems.[37,39] ST changes are not a reason to delay imaging but rather may, in fact, indicate its need. If necessary, an electrocardiogram is performed following imaging, which can confirm return to baseline. Antianginal medications can be administered following ^{201}Tl localization without influencing its distribution or test results.[3] Imaging is repeated after "redistribution," approximately four hours later.

IMAGE ACQUISITION

Both planar and tomographic methods are acceptable.[21,37,39] For the former, a state-of-the-art scintillation camera should acquire at least anterior and two left anterior oblique projections. The initial poststress projection is acquired to optimal counts, and other poststress and redistribution images are obtained to isotime at fixed intensity to permit assessment of changes in regional radioactivity over time. A LEAP collimator is most often employed as a high-resolution device adds to acquisition time. A high-sensitivity collimator decreases imaging time, permitting rapid acquisition at a small cost to resolution, and permits acquisition of additional images.[3,21,34-37] Alternatively, tomographic methods may be employed.[39,40] The multiple pinhole method, successfully used by some investigators, yields suboptimal reconstruction and is technically difficult. Currently, SPECT methods (Fig. 29.6) with an orbiting camera are optimal and can be reconstructed in cardiac long and short or off axes projections.[39,40]

IMAGE PROCESSING

Visual recognition on analog images requires gross regional perfusion differences,[4,5] while computer enhancement increases defect recognition and test sensitivity.[41,42] Computer enhancement to "correct" for background is necessary for planar image interpretation. Tomographic

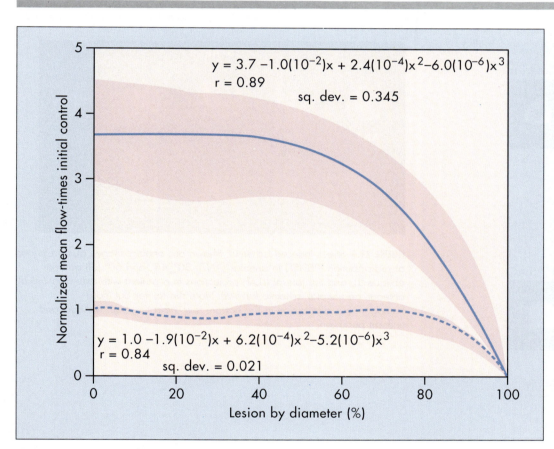

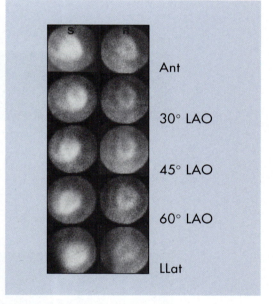

FIGURE 29.2 Coronary flow at rest and at stress. Coronary flow is measured at rest (*dotted line*) and at stress (*solid line*). Normal flow is maintained by coronary dilation at rest up to subtotal stenosis. With stress, here provided by the dilation related to intracoronary contrast infusion, flow augmentation is submaximal in relation to coronary stenosis of about 70%, defining a critical coronary lesion. Such a loss of coronary flow reserve results in regional flow heterogeneity. When ^{210}Tl is administered under such circumstances, heterogeneity of radionuclide distribution produces "cold" areas and permits regional noninvasive definition of perfusion abnormalities. (Modified from Gould KL, Lipscomb K, Hamilton GW: Physiologic basis for assessing critical coronary stenosis. Instantaneous flow response and regional distribution during coronary hyperemia as measures of coronary flow reserve. Am J Cardiol 33:87, 1974)

FIGURE 29.3 Normal planar perfusion scintigram. Shown are normal ^{210}Tl perfusion images performed at stress (*left column*) and 4 hours later with redistribution (*right column*). Images are shown in five projections: anterior, 30° left anterior oblique (LAO), 45° LAO, 60° LAO, and left lateral from above downward. Redistribution images, acquired for the same time and at the same intensity setting as poststress images, are much less intense than the poststress images, a factor related to their high washout rate. The low intensity of background supports a high level of related exercise, shifting perfusion from the soft tissues of the chest to the exercising muscles. The distribution of the radionuclide is homogeneous in the ventricles, but reduced in the less massive right ventricular and left ventricular base. The right ventricle is seen as a faint crescent-shaped uptake inferior to the left ventricle in the anterior projection and anterior to the left ventricle in the LAO projections.

images are less influenced by background and, by nature, are computer processed. However, the method is not immune to artifacts and may not be performed in large or uncooperative patients. Processing enhances image heterogeneity and makes subtle image perfusion defects more obvious (Figs. 29.7 and 29.8).[3,21,36,40,43] Yet, this may also result in reduced specificity,[42,44] and does not resolve problems related to soft tissue attenuation, most commonly the female breast,[44] probably the most common cause of false positive readings. Although tomography helps resolve this difficulty, reduced radioactivity is even seen in tomographic slices underlying the breast.[44,45]

Reduced radioactivity in the normal image relates to the ventricular base, the valve planes, membranous septum and apex, and myocardial regions with reduced mass.[27,37,44] Cardiac rotation adds to the variability (Fig. 29.9). To objectify image interpretation, circumferential profiles of the distribution of peak counts along multiple radii subtended from background subtracted poststress images have been made in populations of normal patients (Fig. 29.10).[21] Normalized to peak counts and plotted graphically in each projection, these normal values are best calculated for images rotated to a similar angulation relative to their long axis.

Similar count profiles in redistribution images, expressed in absolute counts, are compared to absolute peak radial values in each projection of the immediate poststress images. The difference in these profiles, compared to the initial radioactivity level, yields a plot of radial "washout," which appears to be an absolute perfusion indicator (Fig. 29.11).[3,21,36,40] Since the parameter depends on established myocardial/blood gradients, it is significantly affected by the achieved stress level and related double product. Washout levels below normal can be given little significance when associated with suboptimal stress.[46] An apparent perfusion defect seen best on the redistribution image has been termed *reverse redistribution*. Although originally thought to be related to widespread ischemia in other regions, the phenomenon is most frequently related to differential but normal global washout or a limited region of infarction.

Planar color functional images of regional myocardial washout have been generated that can be related to normal values.[43] Similarly, functional images of uptake, redistribution, and washout can be generated from compressed tomographic slices presented in a "bull's eye" configuration (Fig. 29.12).[40] Both methods permit a graphic, anatomical, and visual assessment of perfusion.

IMAGE INTERPRETATION

Regardless of the variety of sophisticated computer enhancement and processing methods employed, or possibly because of them, strict attention must be given to the assessment of the analog image pattern. Processed curves and images will only be as reliable as the original

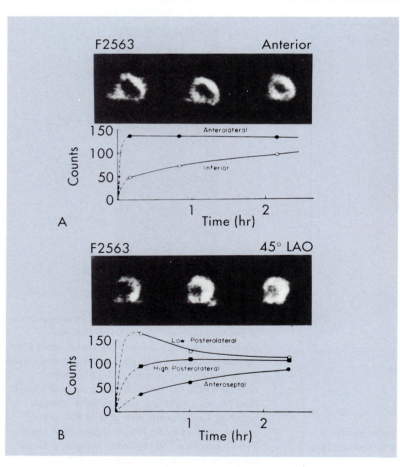

FIGURE 29.4 Myocardial washout of ^{201}Tl. Shown are perfusion images acquired serially over the course of 2 hours after stress administration of ^{201}Tl in anterior (**A**) and left anterior oblique (**B**) projections. Normal regions lose radioactivity rapidly, while visually abnormal regions show flat or upsloping curves of serial regional radioactivity. Other regions, as the high posterolateral wall in the LAO projection, may appear visually normal, yet their true relation to abnormal perfusion is exposed by the generation of an abnormal (flat) washout curve. (Reproduced with permission and modified from Campbell NP, Read EK et al: Spatial and temporal quantitation of planar thallium myocardial images. J Nucl Med 22:577, 1981)

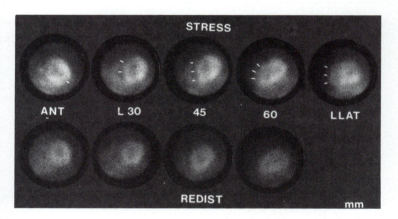

FIGURE 29.5 Stress-induced ischemia. Shown are analog images poststress and at redistribution (*REDIST*) in anterior (*ANT*), 30°, 45°, and 60° left anterior oblique (*L*), and left lateral (*LLAT*) projections in a patient with extensive apical, anterior, and septal ischemia (*arrows*). Note the fainter but more homogeneous distribution in the bottom row, indicating high washout and uniform perfusion.

data set. Without an appreciation of the baseline distribution pattern, artifacts will not be recognized. The blind acceptance of such data is fraught with danger.[41,42,44,47]

The anterior and lateral projections present as a horseshoe configuration (see Fig. 29.9). Since the left ventricle has several times the muscle mass of the right, the myocardial perfusion image is composed primarily of the left ventricular contour. The right ventricle is often only well seen in the immediate poststress image. Prominent right ventricular visualization, especially in a rest or redistribution image, often relates to the presence of right ventricular hypertrophy.[48] The identification of right ventricular perfusion defects is tenuous.

Left anterior oblique projections present as a "doughnut" configuration in horizontal hearts or as a "horseshoe" with the base oriented superiorly in vertical hearts. The septal and lateral walls have varying radioactivity depending on rotation, with the greatest intensity in walls viewed in tangent. Multiple left anterior oblique projections help visual assessment by presenting rotational progression of regional radioactivity. Both visual and circumferential profile interpretations of the perfusion scintigram are made in regions viewed in tangent. Conventional planar image evaluation permits assessment only of the walls seen in tangent. The myocardium seen *en face* is thinner, has less radioactivity, and permits the apparent imaging of the radionuclide-poor cavity. Only planar color washout images or tomographic evaluation permits assessment of the full extent of projected myocardium (see Figs. 29.11 and 29.12).[39,43]

Perfusion image interpretation requires significant experience and insight into factors related to radionuclide distribution. An evaluation of the cause of false positive perfusion images revealed that most of these occurred in females, and frequently these images revealed evidence of soft tissue breast attenuation, extending into the noncardiac soft tissues. This artifact often presents as an anterior defect, confused with pathology in the left anterior descending coronary artery distribution. Although generally fixed, some of these apparent lesions seemed reversible, but they frequently spared the apex, which was generally involved in anterior descending coronary disease.[44]

The ability to visualize the myocardium against the lung background depends on the target-to-background radioactivity ratio. This will increase with the level of exercise achieved as lower extremity perfusion increases and thoracic and subdiaphragmatic radioactivity falls. In rest or redistribution images, the target-to-background ratio is poor.

Pathologic lung uptake is related to a prolonged pulmonary transit time of any cause with increased ^{201}Tl extraction and may be seen with congestive cardiomyopathy, mitral disease, or extensive myocardial ischemia.[49-51] It must be differentiated from normal chest radioactivity seen at a low level of stress. Although nonspecific in the presence of limited but apparent perfusion abnormalities, lung uptake suggests extensive myocardium at ischemic risk.[51] It is one of three supplementary indices for image evaluation of myocardial perfusion defects in the assessment of the extent of ischemia (Fig. 29.13).[50] Another, basal uptake, reflects a general reduction of distal radioactivity in the distribution of all coronary vessels. The third, apparent cavitary dilation, is

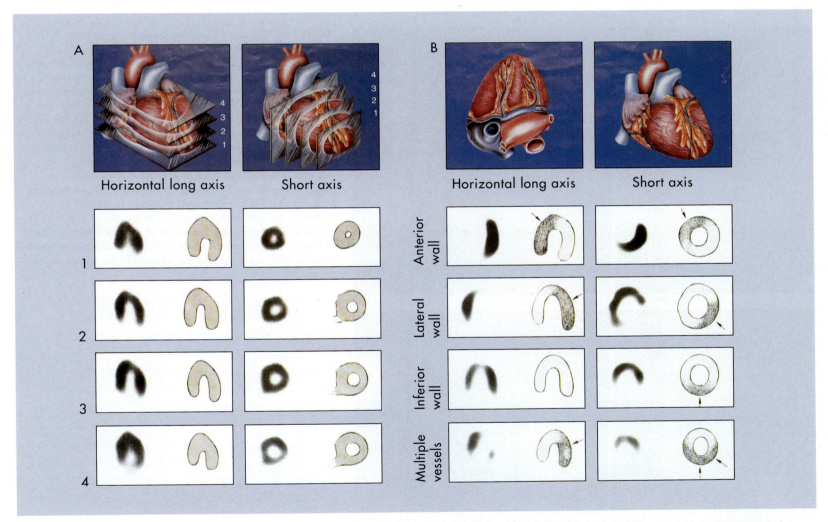

FIGURE 29.6 SPECT. **A.** Shown are long and short axes SPECT reconstruction of a normal perfusion scintigram. **B.** Here, SPECT ^{201}Tl images with a variety of perfusion abnormalities are illustrated in long and short axes. (Reproduced with permission and modified from R. VanHeertum, St. Vincent's Hospital, New York, and the General Electric Co., Milwaukee, Wisconsin)

rarely related to actual stress-induced chamber enlargement, but is probably most often due to relative underperfusion of the wall overlying the cavity.[43]

The localization of defects is broadly related to the expected distribution of coronary arteries where the septum and anterior wall relate to the left anterior descending coronary artery, the lateral wall to the circumflex, and the inferior wall to the right coronary artery (see Fig. 29.9).[26,37,44,52,73] This correlation will vary with the specific coronary distribution, collateralization, and the effects of revascularization procedures (Fig. 29.14). The absence of an apparent left ventricular cavity suggests left ventricular hypertrophy (see Fig. 29.9),[53] while reduced regional cavitary radioactivity suggests overlying scar (Fig. 29.15). Cavitary size should be assessed cautiously, owing to the ungated nature of the study. The presence of defects should be expressed as well in terms of the extent of myocardium affected, since both this parameter as well as the extent of coronary involvement are important indicators of coronary risk.[54,55] Defects must also be defined as fixed or reversible, infarcted or ischemic (Table 29.3). However, myocardial regions perfused by tight coronary lesions may not redistribute in four hours, but will show normalization on delayed imaging performed as long as 24 hours after radionuclide administration (Fig. 29.16).[56] It may be clinically important to differentiate such delayed redistribution patterns in viable myocardial regions from those of fixed scar. Functional reversibility may be expected in dysynergic myocardial segments related to normal perfusion or reversible stress-induced abnormalities post-coronary revascularization (Fig. 29.17 and Table 29.2).[57-59]

Similarly, defects seen on a rest image are generally related to infarction. Although perfusion defects are extremely sensitive indicators by which to diagnose acute infarction,[60] especially early after the event (Fig. 29.18), they are nonspecific and may relate to prior infarction or to noncoronary pathology.[53,61-64] Nevertheless, a negative study has been said to be a cost-effective measure for screening admissions to the coronary care unit.[65] Primary cardiomyopathy may present with widespread and multiple abnormalities, but may be difficult to differentiate from segmental ischemic abnormalities.[62]

The distribution of the radionuclide administered at rest need not be the same as that seen on delayed redistribution imaging.[66,67] Imaging after injection at rest, like that performed immediately poststress, reflects the relative distribution of perfusion at the time of administration. The delayed pattern rather relates to the distribution of the potassium, or viable intracellular space. Thus, if reversible ischemia exists at the time of imaging following rest injection, defects may redistribute on later image. This is a very appropriate method to assess the nature of resting symptoms and the extent of related ischemia.

ACCURACY OF DYNAMIC STRESS PERFUSION SCINTIGRAPHY

Although the method is imperfect, diagnostic accuracy of dynamic stress perfusion scintigraphy compared to coronary angiography is high.[3,21,35,37,39,68-70] Defining a significant stenosis as 50% to 70% or more area narrowing, planar methods with computer enhancement but without the application of washout techniques achieve diagnostic sensitivity in the range of 80% to 95%. Of course, when exercise is conducted to suboptimal levels, when the radionuclide is administered

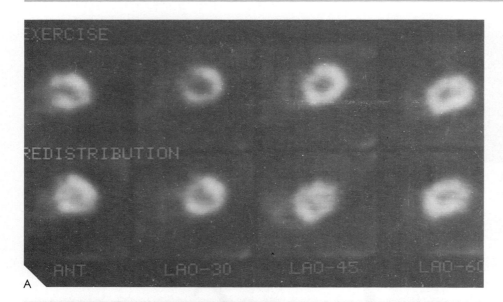
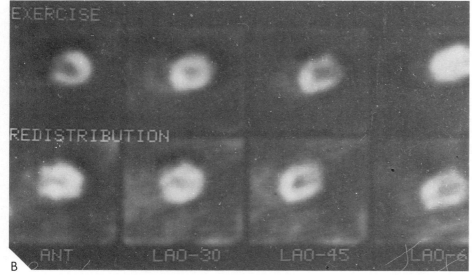

FIGURE 29.7 Planar perfusion image washout analysis. **A.** Shown are computer-enhanced images poststress (*above*) and at redistribution (*below*) in (*left to right*) anterior, 30° left anterior oblique (LAO), 45° LAO, and 60° LAO projections. The only possible abnormalities relate to subtle decreases in radioactivity at the left ventricular apex in the anterior projection and at the left ventricular base in the 30° LAO. Also, the left ventricular cavity appears somewhat larger in the poststress images. **B.** Shown above are radial counts distribution from the 12 o'clock position, progressing counterclockwise, poststress (*crosses*) and at redistribution (*dots*) in the 45° LAO projection in the same patient. Regional radioactivity and the difference between stress and redistribution radioactivity are least in the septal region at the left. Below is the radial distribution of percent washout, where the lower limit of normal varies regionally from approximately 25% to 35%. Again, washout is reduced in the septal region at the left.

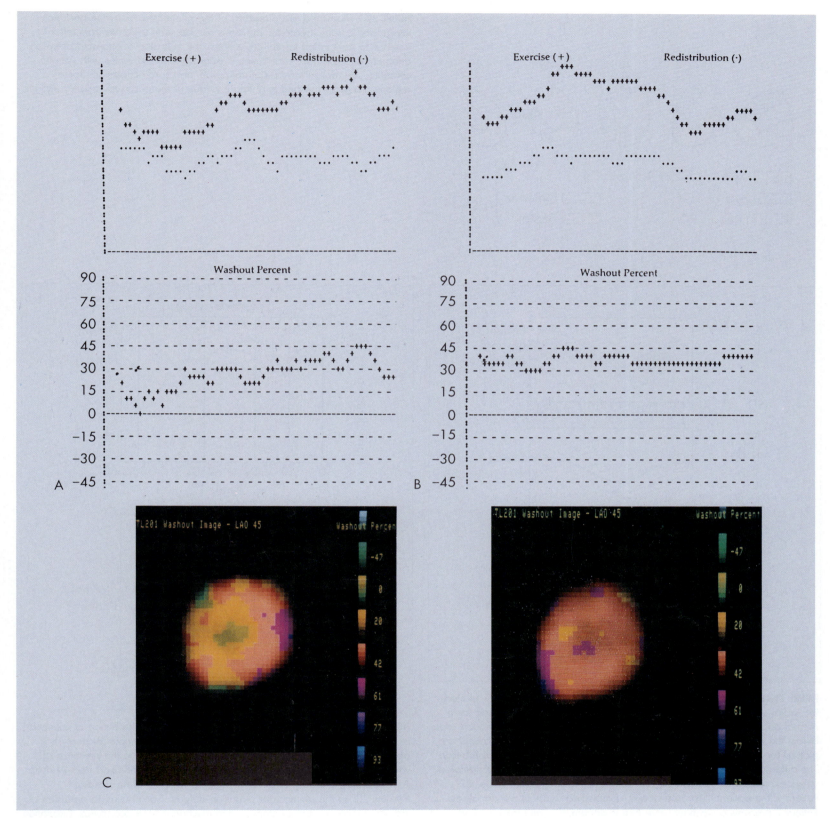

FIGURE 29.8 Planar perfusion image washout analysis. **A** and **B.** Shown according to the same format are poststress and redistribution images and radial uptake, redistribution, and washout curves in the same patient after left anterior descending (LAD) coronary angioplasty (PTCA). Images no longer reveal the suspected minor perfusion abnormalities and apparent cavitary dilation, while count and washout profiles have normalized in association with a greater achieved stress level and double percent. **C.** Shown are color washout functional images in the 45° left anterior oblique projection in the same patient before and after LAD PTCA. These functional images are color-coded for regional washout, where red-violet-blue are normal and yellow-green are abnormal. The pre-PTCA study reveals gross washout abnormalities in the region of the septum, extending over the lateral wall and the region of the cavity. Apparent cavitary dilation appears to relate, in most cases, to this relative perfusion distribution. The full distribution of washout abnormalities and their normalization postintervention are best appreciated using washout analysis and most graphically using the functional image display.

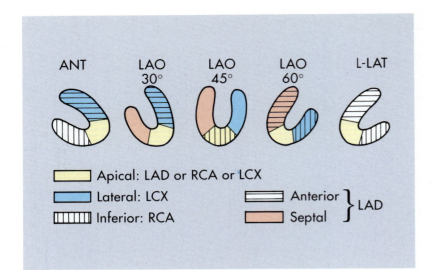

FIGURE 29.9 Illustrated are diagrams of the relationship between perfusion image and cardiac anatomy. The base can be seen to rotate from left in anterior to right in left lateral projections. The indicated relationship between anatomy and coronary distribution is approximate and varies with specific coronary size, dominance, collateralization, and cardiac rotation. Some regions are projected and may relate to any of the perfused vascular regions.

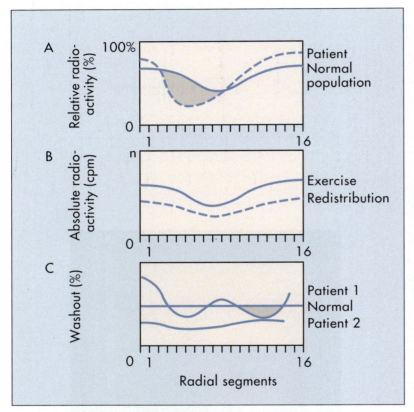

FIGURE 29.10 Radial perfusion evaluation. **A.** Relative radioactivity is plotted for radial segments around the circumference of the perfusion image for a normal population (*solid line*) and for a patient (*dotted line*). The shaded area below the normal limit subtends abnormal segments. **B.** Absolute counts are plotted for the same radial segments during exercise and with redistribution. The difference between these curves is compared to the initial stress-related value, expressed as % washout, and compared to the normal value. **C.** Patient 1, the patient illustrated above, reveals two washout abnormalities. Patient 2 presents a washout curve that is abnormal in all locations. Such balanced malperfusion may be unapparent visually, presenting as a normal pattern of relative uptake.

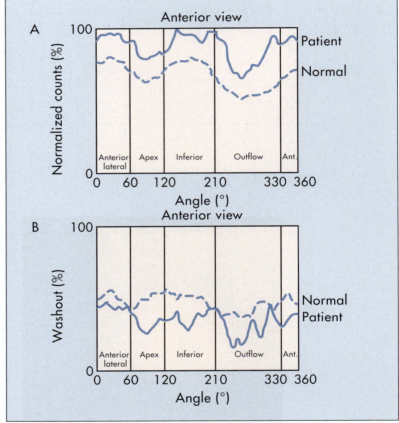

FIGURE 29.11 Advantages of washout analysis. Radial distribution of counts (**A**) in the anterior projection is normal. However, radial washout (**B**) analysis is abnormal in all segments, indicative of global ischemia in the presence of what might appear to be a normal perfusion image. (Modified from Abdulla A, Maddahi J, Garcia E et al: Slow regional washout of myocardial thallium-201 in the absence of perfusion defects. Contribution to detection of individual coronary artery stenosis and mechanisms for occurrence. Circulation 71:72, 1985)

prematurely, or when imaging is delayed, sensitivity is reduced. Similarly, the full extent of coronary involvement is less likely to be identified in the presence of collaterals.[42,71,72] This may relate to the lack of ischemia in the region of collateral supply (see Fig. 29.14). Tomographic methods appear to have added diagnostic security in image interpretation and, in some studies, have added to diagnostic sensitivity.[39,40,73] Washout methods appear to aid the more complete identification of involved coronary vessels and the full amount of myocardium at ischemic risk.[3,21,40,43,73–76] Some studies have demonstrated the ability of the method to identify almost 70% of all involved vessels.[21,77,78] Rarely, washout evaluation will identify extensive perfusion abnormalities where none are visible, apparently due to balanced ischemia.[79]

This, along with lung uptake and other indicators of widespread ischemia, has added to the ability of the method to identify patients at high coronary risk, and has helped to establish the prognostic value of the test.[51,54,77–79] Also, normal washout aids the identification of a normal study and makes coronary disease unlikely, even in the presence of induced ST depression.[80–82]

It is important to consider the difference between the pathophysiologic nature of the scintigraphic method and the anatomical nature of the angiographic technique. Although angiographic method is the "gold standard" for diagnostic assessment, interpretation of the degree and significance of coronary lesions is extremely variable.[83]

DIPYRIDAMOLE PERFUSION SCINTIGRAPHY

A large percentage of patients with known or suspected coronary disease are ill, debilitated, or even timid or anxious and cannot or should not undergo dynamic exercise stress. Nevertheless, their symptoms, when recognized, are often atypical, and the diagnosis and related risk remain in doubt. This group comprises as many as one third of all patients requiring evaluation. Compounding the problem is the fact

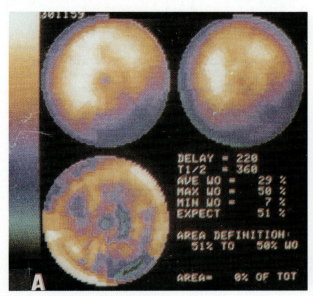
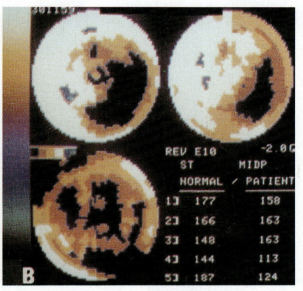

FIGURE 29.12 Tomographic display of washout. **A.** Shown is the normal "bull's eye" display of ^{201}Tl uptake in a patient with coronary disease. The "bull's eye" is formulated by placing the apical slice in the center and surrounding it with sequentially more basal, short axis slices. Regions of the left ventricular base are most peripheral and the display resembles the viewpoint of an observer at the apex looking toward the base, similar to the perspective gained viewing a rocket from its nose cone. Here, anterior regions are above, posterior, and below the lateral wall, at right, and the septum, at left. Illustrated is the "bull's eye" pattern of uptake (*upper left*), the pattern at redistribution imaging (*upper right*), and the regional washout values (*below*). Values decrease from yellow to blue. Reversible abnormalities are evident. **B.** Uptake, redistribution, and washout values in the same patient are compared to the normal control group, where values less than two standard deviations below the mean are coded black. Again, obvious uptake and washout abnormalities are evident. (Reproduced with permission from Berger HJ: Nuclear medicine's revival: New drugs and camera lead the way. Diagn Imaging 68:5, 1985)

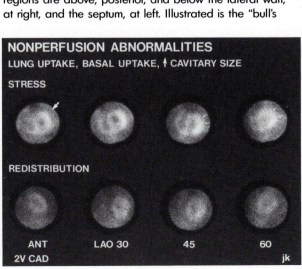

FIGURE 29.13 Example of supplementary indicators. Stress and redistribution images illustrating nonperfusion or supplementary indicators of ischemia are shown. Here, lung uptake (*arrow, upper left*), basal uptake (*arrows, upper right*), and cavitary dilatation are each evident. When seen in perfusion changes, especially in association with perfusion abnormalities, they indicate extensive myocardium at ischemic risk. (Reproduced with permission from Canhasi B, Dae M, Botvinick E et al: The interaction of "supplementary" scintigraphic indicators and stress electrocardiography in the diagnosis of multivessel coronary disease. J Am Coll Cardiol 6:581, 1985)

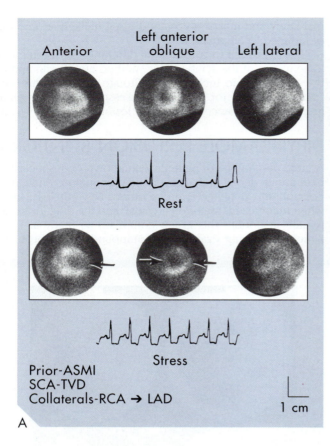
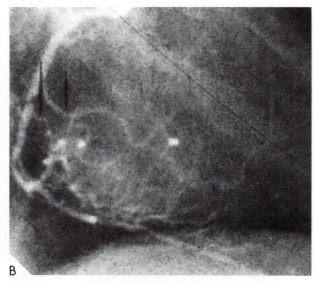

FIGURE 29.14 High-risk pattern. **A.** Shown are stress and rest ^{201}Tl perfusion images in a patient with triple-vessel disease (*TVD*) on angiography (*SCA*). A prior anteroseptal infarction (*ASMI*) is evident in the rest images. Extensive defects in the stress image indicate ischemia in the distribution of multiple vessels and extensive myocardium at risk. The inferior wall looked "normal," although the right coronary artery (*RCA*) was also stenotic. This demonstrates the relative nature of the study or relates to the fact that the RCA ischemic threshold was not reached. The RCA territory was, in fact, likely the best perfused, as the vessel served as collaterals to the left anterior descending (*LAD*) coronary artery, as shown in **B.** (Reproduced with permission from Dash H, Massie B, Botvinick E et al: The noninvasive identification of left main and three-vessel coronary artery disease by myocardial stress perfusion scintigraphy and treadmill electrocardiography. Circulation 60:276, 1979)

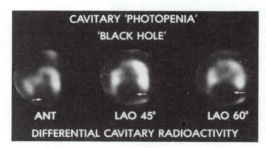

FIGURE 29.15 Cavitary photopenia. Shown in anterior (*ANT*) and 45° and 60° left anterior oblique (*LAO*) projections are perfusion scintigrams in a patient with a large apical aneurysm. Note the area of reduced radioactivity, an apparent "black hole" in the apical wall and appearing to extend into the region of the "cavity." The latter most likely relates to reduced radioactivity in the overlying myocardial wall. (Reproduced with permission from Canhasi B, Dae M, Botvinick E et al: The interaction of "supplementary" scintigraphic indicators and stress electrocardiography in the diagnosis of multivessel coronary artery disease. J Am Coll Cardiol 6:581, 1985)

TABLE 29.3 Tl-201 IMAGE INTERPRETATION*

Stress	Rest/Redistribution	Interpretation
Normal	Normal	No infarction No "ischemia"
Abnormal	Normal	Stress induced "ischemia"
Abnormal	Abnormal—less than stress	"Ischemia" and infarction
Abnormal	Abnormal—no change	Infarction without apparent "ischemia"

* General pattern for interpretation of perfusion scintigrams. Subtitles reviewed in the text provide qualification of this outline.

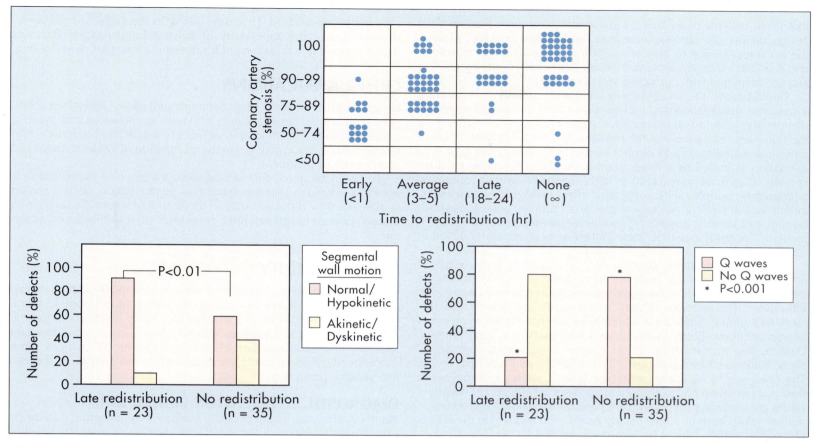

FIGURE 29.16 Delayed redistribution. Shown above is the relationship between the time to full perfusion image redistribution and the degree of coronary stenosis. The time to redistribution is directly related to the degree of narrowing. Late distributing segments, unlike those not redistributing, are viable and generally demonstrate preserved regional wall motion and no specific electrocardiographic evidence of infarction. Important clinical errors may be committed and viable segments interpreted as infarcted if delayed redistribution is not sought in select situations. (Modified from Gorman J, Berman D, Freeman M: Time to completed redistribution of Tl-201 in exercise myocardial scintigraphy: Relationship to the degree of coronary artery stenosis. Am Heart J 106:989, 1983)

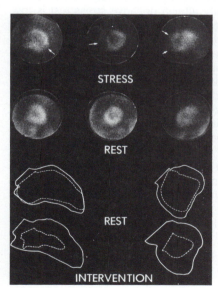

FIGURE 29.17 Functional reversibility. Large reversible abnormalities (*arrows*) are noted in the perfusion images above. Below, end-diastolic (*solid lines*) and end-systolic (*dotted lines*) outlines from the left ventriculogram of the same patient obtained at rest and postventricular ectopy indicate reversibility of wall motion abnormalities. Normal resting perfusion indicates viability and reversibility of functional abnormalities with a ventricular premature contraction (VPC), after nitroglycerin, or following successful revascularization. (Reproduced with permission from Brundage BH, Massie BM, Botvinick EH et al: Improved regional ventricular function after successful surgical revascularization. J Am Coll Cardiol 3:902, 1984)

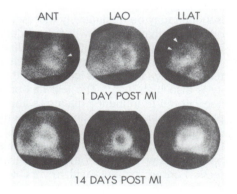

FIGURE 29.18 Serial perfusion images. Serial rest ^{201}Tl perfusion images obtained 1 day and 14 days after an acute anterior infarction demonstrate reduction of defect size. This may be due to resolution of ischemia. (Reproduced with permission from Botvinick E, Shames D: Nuclear Cardiology: Clinical Applications, p 5. Baltimore, Williams & Wilkins, 1979)

that these patients often face a significant intervention. Patients with peripheral vascular disease claudicate, and limited activities prevent the early appearance of cardiac symptoms. Yet their major morbidity and mortality relate to associated, frequently occult, coronary disease and are amplified with corrective vascular surgery.[84]

Dipyridamole inhibits circulating adenosine deaminase,[85] resulting in reduced degradation and increased levels of this potent arteriolar dilator. Administered intravenously, the agent has significant effects on the coronary resistance vessels, resulting in a three- to fivefold coronary flow augmentation in normal vessels.[86] However, this flow augmentation is limited by a fixed stenosis. Applying this differential response, Gould demonstrated a high sensitivity with a relatively unimpressive peripheral hemodynamic effect in dogs.[87] Animal experiments indicate differential augmentation of coronary perfusion in both normal and stenotic vessels,[88,89] but ischemia has rarely been documented,[90] possibly due to a "steal" effect or to an actual reduction in coronary flow.

An intravenous saline solution of 0.56 mg/kg of body weight is infused over 4 minutes, with full hemodynamic and symptomatic monitoring.[91] Ingestion of a dipyridamole slurry has also been found effective,[92] but vagaries related to the absorbed dose make this route suboptimal. Thallium is administered at the seventh minute and images acquired shortly thereafter and 4 hours later at redistribution. Uniform flow augmentation, in the absence of significant coronary lesions, leads to a homogeneous ^{201}Tl distribution and a normal image. The presence of significant coronary lesions causes heterogeneous flow augmentation and perfusion image defects (Fig. 29.19). Washout values are lower in patients who are pharmacologically stressed where normal values have not been clearly established and where the effects of the intervention cannot be clearly quantitated.[93]

The effects of the drug are generally benign, producing a mild hypotensive response and a mild increase in heart rate.[91] Side effects are generally mild and relate to vascular dilation with headache, flushing, and nausea.[91] Although ischemic indicators are uncommon, an occasional dramatic ischemic response may be seen and rare fatalities have been reported. Drug effects can be immediately reversed by the intravenous administration of aminophylline, which specifically blocks the adenosine receptors.[94] While the functional correlate of such induced ischemia may be qualitatively assessed in some cases with echocardiography,[95] that method will fail to identify the much more frequently induced malperfusion not associated with ischemia.

The diagnostic sensitivity of the imaging method approaches that related to dynamic stress imaging, in the range of 80% to 90%. Specificity is also high.[91,96-98] The test has proven extremely useful and has been noted to influence diagnosis and management in almost 80% of patients evaluated.[99] Additionally, the method, like dynamic perfusion evaluation, appears to have prognostic value.[100,101] In a group of patients studied prior to peripheral vascular surgery, perioperative coronary events were noted only in those with reversible scintigraphic defects. Further, patients with reversible perfusion abnormalities were those developing coronary events after subendocardial infarction.

While its safety in acute infarction has not yet been fully established, the method, not yet approved by the FDA, soon is likely to be made generally available for the evaluation of known or suspected coronary disease in patients who should not or cannot undergo dynamic exercise. It is already a much sought after and seemingly clinically important method. However, owing to the value of exercise-related data and the superiority of stress-related images, it is not recommended as a replacement for dynamic stress perfusion imaging.

OTHER APPLICATIONS

Maseri and co-workers have demonstrated gross reversible scintigraphic abnormalities in patients with both spontaneous and induced coronary spasm.[102] Scintigraphy appears to supplement symptoms and electrocardiographic changes in the recognition of induced spasm and its response to treatment.[103]

It should be noted that scintigraphic evidence of malperfusion is generally related to heterogeneous flow augmentation, but it is related to absolute flow reduction only in the setting of spasm. Redistribution occurs extremely quickly after resolution of spasm-induced ischemia.[102]

CLINICAL UTILITY

Thallium scintigraphy evaluates the primary pathophysiologic ischemic abnormality, insufficient myocardial perfusion. Blood pool scintigraphy and other modalities evaluate the secondary functional response. Additional ischemic responses include chest pain, a subjective and relatively insensitive measure; electrocardiographic ST changes, often a nonspecific finding; and myocardial lactate production, an insensitive invasive parameter.

DIAGNOSTIC APPLICATION (TABLE 29.4)

Many patients can be successfully evaluated for ischemic disease by exercise testing alone. A high-level stress test in the absence of pain or electrocardiographic changes may be all that is required to practically exclude the diagnosis. However, in evaluating test utility in any patient, the pre-test likelihood and Bayes theorem must be considered.[104-107] The post-test likelihood of disease is a function of test accuracy and the pre-test likelihood. The latter is a function of the patient population assessed and can be estimated.[108] Thus, if the patient is a 35-year-old man with nonanginal chest pain, representing a population with a low pre-test probability, the probability after a negative stress test is low enough to exclude coronary disease. However, if we are dealing with a 45-year-old man with atypical pain, representing a population with a 50% pre-test probability, the probability of disease after a negative stress test would still be in the range of 20%. Here, a negative perfusion scintigram reduces disease likelihood to approximately 3%, not significantly different from disease incidence in an asymptomatic population of the same age and sex (Fig. 29.20). Although it does not eliminate the diagnosis entirely, it reduces (or increases) disease likelihood to levels of diagnostic security where appropriate clinical management can be delivered.[106,107]

Scintigraphy is probably most valuable in patients presenting diagnostic difficulty (Fig. 29.21). Prominent among these are patients presenting with stress electrocardiograms that are uninterpretable for ischemia owing to the presence of bundle branch block, left ventricular hypertrophy, digitalis use, electrolyte abnormalities, or other causes for resting ST abnormalities.[37,109]

Not infrequently, patients are sent to scintigraphic study after coronary angiography. In some cases, patients are returned for noninvasive

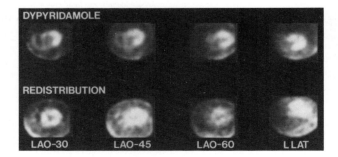

FIGURE 29.19 Abnormal dipyridamole image. The induced reversible anterior apical defect relates to left anterior descending coronary disease.

TABLE 29.4 CLINICAL APPLICATIONS OF STRESS PERFUSION OR BLOOD POOL SCINTIGRAPHY

Diagnosis of Coronary Disease
1. Where the stress test is equivocal in the presence of resting baseline electrocardiographic abnormalities
2. When the diagnosis is ambiguous and disease likelihood is indeterminant on where the stress electrocardiogram is abnormal in a patient with a low disease likelihood or the converse
3. When the stress electrocardiogram is negative at a low achieved double product*
4. To establish the pathophysiologic significance of coronary lesions of questionable significance

Evaluation of Coronary Disease Treatment
1. Localizes ischemia to specific vessels aiding the administration of revascularization procedures
2. Aids prediction of response to angioplasty or bypass surgery
3. Determines the effectiveness of collaterals
4. Determines myocardial viability, differentiating ischemia from infarction
5. Determines effectiveness of revascularization and thrombolytic therapy
6. Aids assessment of bypass graft patency

Evaluation of Coronary Disease Risk and Prognosis
1. Aids identification of main left and triple-vessel disease
2. Provides a measure of the extent of myocardium at ischemic risk, presenting an accurate independent prognostic measure
3. Assists in the selection of patients for revascularization procedures
4. Assists the evaluation and management of patients after uncomplicated infarction

* Possible but not yet firmly established.

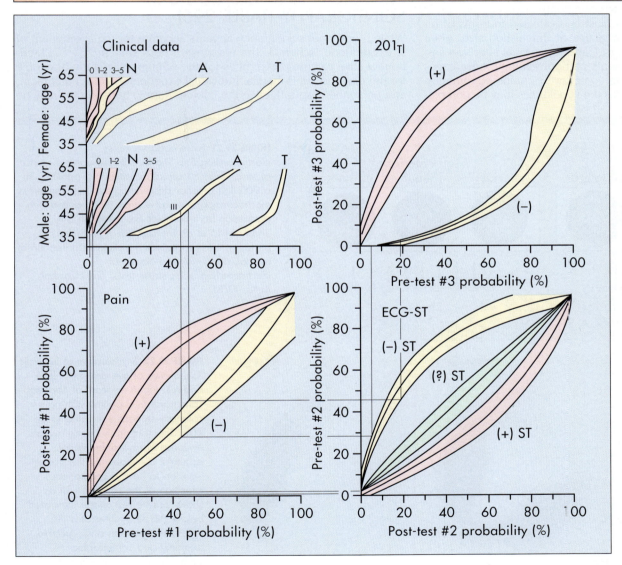

FIGURE 29.20 Diagnosis of coronary artery disease. Illustrated is the interaction of clinical data (*upper left*) and noninvasive stress-induced pain (*lower left*), ischemic electrocardiogram (*lower right*), and scintigraphic perfusion changes (*upper right*) in formulating the likelihood of coronary disease. The type of presenting pain, nonanginal (N), atypical (A), or typical angina (T), in addition to patient age and sex present an initial estimate of disease likelihood according to the data of Diamond and Forrester.[108] Thereafter, the results of noninvasive stress testing influence likelihood assessment. Charted diagrammatically are examples presenting clinical data related to low and intermediate coronary likelihood. The effects of negative noninvasive results are traced and have little impact on the patient with initial low disease likelihood. However, a patient presenting with initial, intermediate, 40% to 50% likelihood relates to a 2% to 3% likelihood of coronary disease after negative noninvasive tests. This incidence is not significantly different from a similar asymptomatic population. (Modified from Patterson RE, Eng C, Horowitz SF et al: Practical diagnosis of coronary artery disease: A Bayes' theorem nomogram to correlate clinical data with noninvasive exercise tests. Am J Cardiol 53:252, 1984)

pathophysiologic assessment when lesions are of uncertain significance or when their relation to ischemia and salvageable myocardium is questioned.

PROGNOSTIC UTILITY

Even in the clear presence of ischemic coronary disease patients are often sent for scintigraphy to determine the significance of lesions and the presence and extent of myocardium at ischemic risk (Fig. 29.22).[82,110] This measurement now more than ever appears most closely related to prognosis, an important parameter guiding management.[37,51,109,110] Further, such regions are by definition viable and present an important opportunity for aggressive treatment. Especially important is the evaluation of risk postinfarction, where both the quantitative assessment of resting ventricular function and stress-induced perfusion abnormalities have been shown to augment identification of high-risk patients.[111-113]

EVALUATION OF TREATMENT

Most valuable is the application of scintigraphic ischemic indicators to the assessment of the results of angioplasty and bypass surgery (see Figs. 29.7, 29.8, and 29.23).[51,54,112,114-118] Objective, pathophysiologic evaluation of perfusion and viability is especially important in the setting of postintervention symptoms, where a comparison baseline study is valuable. However, serial studies must be evaluated in terms of related stress level. Persistent abnormalities of diminished size, often related to a more advanced stress level, are not unusual after successful surgery. Perfusion imaging presents pathophysiologic advantages over the anatomical evaluation of graft patency by computed tomography (Fig. 29.24).[119] Yet in many cases the two studies may be complementary. Similarly, the method has been useful in determining the effects on perfusion and viability of streptokinase-induced postinfarction reperfusion.[120]

EFFECTS OF DRUGS ON STUDY INTERPRETATION

Although digitalis preparations affect membrane function, no cardiac drugs are known to interfere with the localization and dynamics of ^{201}Tl, and the method is effectively applied in patients on digitalis. Beta blockers, which reduce the achieved double product, may influence stress duration or delay the level of stress at which ischemia appears or even prevent its appearance. Most antianginal drugs affect coronary flow demands rather than the supply, which is affected by revascularization procedures. For this reason, in studies performed in patients on antianginal drugs, defects may appear unchanged but associated with higher induced stress levels. Unlike blood pool imaging, perfusion imaging may find difficulty identifying the stress level at which ischemia initially appears (Table 29.5). Although scintigraphic study while the subject is on medications is nevertheless useful for the assessment of treatment, coronary risk is best evaluated while the subject is off drugs.

PERFUSION AND BLOOD POOL SCINTIGRAPHY (TABLE 29.5)

While blood pool scintigraphy appears accurate for the assessment of stress-induced ischemia, the response is less specific.[121-123] Practitioners have varying preferences for the scintigraphic study of choice for the diagnosis of ischemia. Individual experience, skills, equipment, and personnel also influence the choice. Rarely, both studies may be

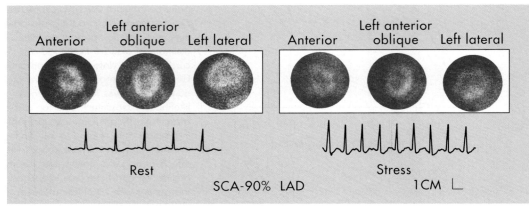

FIGURE 29.21 False negative stress electrocardiogram. Shown is scintigraphic evidence of stress-induced septal ischemia in a patient with a 90% left anterior descending stenosis. The stress electrocardiogram was normal. (Reproduced with permission from Botvinick EH, Taradash MR, Shames DM et al: Thallium-201 myocardial perfusion scintigraphy for the clinical clarification of normal, abnormal and equivocal electrocardiographic stress tests. Am J Cardiol 41:43, 1978)

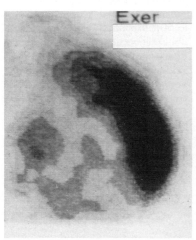
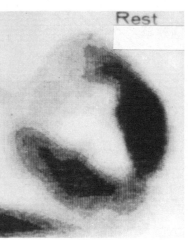
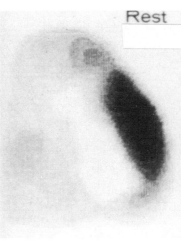

FIGURE 29.22 Myocardium at ischemic risk. Shown above are stress (*left*) and rest (*right*) myocardial perfusion scintigrams in a patient with right coronary stenosis estimated to be 40%. The scintigram clearly reveals evidence of reversible inferior ischemia. Subsequently, the patient went on to have a spontaneous infarction of the same region as shown on the rest image illustrated below. This study illustrates the difference between angiographic anatomy and scintigraphic pathophysiology while providing one form of evidence for the ability of scintigraphy to identify myocardium at ischemic risk. (Courtesy of Dr. M. Goris, Stanford University, Stanford, California)

useful. Stress blood pool evaluation is recommended when presented with a functional equivalent of angina or in evaluation of function in the setting of noncoronary heart disease.[124-126]

THE PROSPECT OF NEW IMAGING AGENTS

Radiopharmaceutical houses are now evaluating a variety of ^{99m}Tc-labeled perfusion agents.[127] Like ^{201}Tl, they distribute rapidly intracellularly in relation to relative myocardial perfusion but present the inherent imaging advantages of ^{99m}Tc. However, these agents will present a variable gastrointestinal uptake and will be relatively fixed on localization. Without the possibility of redistribution imaging, washout analysis will be lost, and the effects of stress or other interventions will have to be evaluated by serial study. Overall, improved imaging characteristics could provide a significant diagnostic advantage.

INVASIVE SCINTIGRAPHIC METHODS

There are two invasive scintigraphic methods requiring the direct intracoronary administration of a radionuclide for the evaluation of regional myocardial perfusion. Each provides complementary information to that of coronary angiography and both are most frequently employed as research tools.

"PARTICLE" EVALUATION

Myocardial perfusion scintigraphy may be performed following the intracoronary administration of radiolabeled biodegradable microspheres or macroaggregated serum albumin (MAA).[128] The latter, used for perfusion lung imaging, may be formulated in 10μ to 50μ size and labeled with ^{99m}Tc or indium-111 and employed to image individual coronary beds or the same bed serially. Each brings localization at the precapillary arteriolar level, and the lack of background radioactivity provides exquisite image resolution. Although based on coronary embolization, the technique with restricted dose and particle number has proven safe even in patients with the most severe coronary disease.

Evaluation of particle distribution at rest will underestimate lesion severity. However, particle administration after dilating intracoronary contrast produces regional heterogeneity of perfusion and particle distribution similar to the effects of dipyridamole.[129]

This method is more sensitive to the identification of small collat-

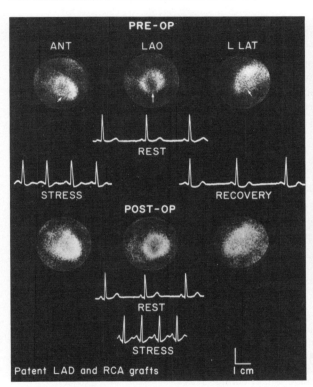

FIGURE 29.23 Effects of coronary bypass. Shown are serial perfusion studies performed before (*above*) and after (*below*) coronary artery bypass graft surgery. The induced inferior wall defect was no longer present postoperatively at a higher related double product. (Reproduced with permission from Greenberg BH, Hart R, Botvinick EH et al: Thallium-201 myocardial perfusion scintigraphy to evaluate patients after coronary bypass surgery. Am J Cardiol 42:167, 1978)

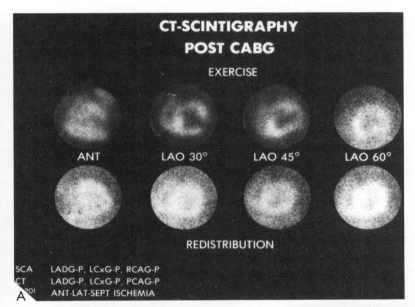

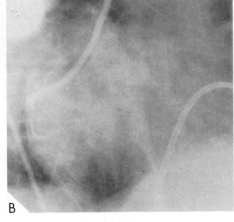 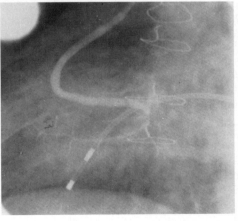

FIGURE 29.24 Computed tomography (CT) and perfusion scintigraphy. Rest CT examination of this patient with chest pain late after bypass surgery revealed flow through the left anterior descending and circumflex (*LC$_x$*) grafts, and reported them both patent. **A.** Scintigraphy reveals stress-induced ischemic changes in anterior, septal, and lateral regions (*ANT-LAT-SEPT*), the distribution of both vessels. **B.** Angiography revealed stenosis at the insertion sites of both vessels. The scintigram provides pathophysiologic information, often clarifying anatomical information. (Reproduced with permission from Englestad B, Wagner S, Herfkens R et al: Evaluation of the post coronary bypass patient by myocardial perfusion scintigraphy and computed tomography. AJR 141:507, 1983)

eral vessels than is selective angiography.[130] Most recently, serial particle injections have been applied to the evaluation of the effects of reperfusion procedures, intracoronary streptokinase infusion and angioplasty, and also to the evaluation of collateral coronary perfusion.[130,131]

INERT GAS WASHOUT

Here, an inert, freely diffusible gas, generally xenon (Xe)-133, is dissolved in saline, injected selectively as a bolus directly into a coronary artery, and followed quickly by a saline flush. Initially localized entirely in tissue, a concentration gradient is established with the blood. The rate of gas diffusion back into the blood will then depend on tissue perfusion or flow rate modified by the solubility coefficient between blood and tissue. The method presents tissue flow rates in absolute terms as milliliters per minute per 100 g.[132] For accurate results, the agent employed must be inert, not metabolized or otherwise removed from the circulation, freely diffusible, not limited by the diffusion rate in its return to the blood, and, optimally, not recirculated.

A high-sensitivity collimator with a high-sensitivity camera or probe has been successfully applied to assess rapidly changing patterns following the intracoronary administration of 20 mCi to 25 mCi of ^{133}Xe diluted in a small volume of saline. A left anterior oblique projection is used to separate coronary beds. The method utilizes the initial slope of declining radioactivity following localization, where tissue-specific flow is calculated according to the formula

$$F/W = \lambda \cdot k \cdot 100/\rho$$

where F/W is the specific flow in milliliters per minute per 100 g of tissue, λ is the blood/tissue partition coefficient, k is the slope of the washout curve, and ρ is myocardial specific gravity.

Although evaluating somewhat different parameters, such calculations have correlated well with flow measurements made by electromagnetic flow meters.[133,134] Again, owing to problems in identifying perfusion abnormalities at rest, the hyperemic effects of contrast are used to assess the presence and pathophysiologic significance of coronary lesions. The method also permits evaluation of regional native and collateral perfusion in association with pacing and a variety of drugs.

Although quantitative and independent of geometry, the method is limited. Since the partition coefficient is difficult to assess, no tracer meets the idealized method specifications; sensitivity varies with depth, and flow will be overestimated in the presence of heterogeneous flow patterns.[128]

Owing to the low energy of ^{133}Xe photon emission (81 keV), the method is relatively insensitive to perfusion in deeper tissues, and image resolution is poor. For these reasons, krypton (Kr)-81m (190 keV) has been suggested as a blood flow tracer.[135] Generated from ^{81}Rb with a 13-second half-life, the former can be perfused into the coronary and the daughter radionuclide, ^{81m}Kr, monitored to permit flow quantitation. Photon energy is nearly ideal for detection and the short half-life permits study during quick serial interventions from a single injection of the parent tracer.[135]

BLOOD POOL SCINTIGRAPHY

There are two scintigraphic methods for evaluating right and left ventricular size and function: the first-pass[136-138] and equilibrium[136,137,139] techniques. In addition to their noninvasive nature, they provide quantitative, reproducible, pathophysiologic evaluation and permit computer analysis with derivation of a variety of useful measurements. Both methods permit accurate serial volume and function measurements, as well as regional and global evaluation of ventricular function.

FIRST-PASS METHODOLOGY

This technique generates data during the first transit of a radionuclide bolus through the central circulation. Using a low radiopharmaceutical dose, only the time versus radioactivity curve can be analyzed.[8,10] With a high dose, associated images can be generated.[138,140,141] First-pass evaluation can be performed with virtually any pharmaceutical passing through the central circulation. Short-lived, rapidly excreted ^{99m}Tc diethylenetriamine pentaacetic acid (DTPA) is commonly used. However, for quantitative volume assessment or equilibrium evaluation, a long-lived blood pool marker, such as labeled red cells, should be used.[142] First-pass quantitation of ventricular size and function depends on principles of the indicator dilution technique,[143] requiring a compact bolus injection proximal to the mixing chamber and homogeneous mixing of the blood pool indicator.

A sensitive camera or probe[7,8,138,141] over the central circulation, generally in the 30° right anterior oblique projection, follows the bolus through the heart. Its arrival and departure in each chamber produce a low-frequency radioactivity peak. The sequential variations of the cardiac cycle superimpose high-frequency spikes and valleys, proportional to end-diastolic (ED) and end-systolic (ES) volumes, respectively, on the time versus radioactivity curve (Fig. 29.25). These values will yield accurate right and left ventricular ejection fractions.[136,138,140,143,144] The difference in ED and ES counts (C) is proportional to stroke volume (SV), which, divided by background-corrected EDC, yields the EF, or

$$EF = EDC - ESC/EDC - background$$

With proper choice of background, these values have been well correlated with invasive methods.[138,141,144]

The background-subtracted area under the low-frequency ventricular component of the time versus radioactivity curve is related to cardiac output and can be readily quantitated,[145] like indicator concentration, as

$$F = R/-C(t)dt$$

TABLE 29.5 COMPARISON OF PERFUSION AND BLOOD POOL SCINTIGRAPHY*

	Perfusion Imaging	Blood Pool Imaging
Images perfusion	+	−
Evaluates function	−	+
Assessment made at peak stress	+	−
Assessment averaged over last minutes of stress	−	+
Assessment made serially during stress	−	+
Multiple projections convenient	+	−
Tomography routinely possible	+	−
Cost	+	+
Technically difficult	−	+
Computer intensive	+	+
Requires most camera/computer time	−	+
Volume assessment	−	+
Test sensitivity	+	+
Test specificity	+	−
Permits objective identification of extent of myocardium at ischemic risk	+	−
Prognostic assessment	+	+
Identification of functional reversibility	+	+

* Tabulated is a comparison of perfusion and blood pool imaging. Here, + indicates an advantage in the category noted and + in both columns indicates equal capabilities in the designated category.

where F is flow or cardiac output, R is the amount of radionuclide injected in counts per minute, and the denominator is the area under the time versus radioactivity curve extrapolated to correct for recirculation. As described by Holman,[146] the total amount of radionuclide injected (R) also equals the equilibrium radionuclide concentration (Ceq) in counts per minute per millimeter times the blood volume (BV) in milliliters or

$$R = Ceq \times BV$$

and the indicator dilution equation becomes

$$F = Ceq \times BV \Big/ \int_0^x C(t)dt$$

There is no need, however, to sample this data from the total circulation. In first-pass scintigraphy, counts information is evaluated over the central circulation and over the left ventricle. The imaging device samples the same area during passage of the bolus and at equilibrium, and the fraction of the blood volume sampled need not appear in the flow equation.

In practice, measurements are made of the area under the first-pass curve and the equilibrium concentration of radionuclide is measured after a 5-minute delay. A blood sample at this time is related to the injected dose to yield the absolute blood volume in milliliters. The area under a 1-minute segment of the equilibrium curve is divided by the area under the first-pass curve to yield left ventricular (cardiac) output in volumes per minute (see Fig. 29.25). This can easily be converted to liters per minute. With the cardiac output, heart rate, and ejection fraction, the stroke volume, either right ventricular or left ventricular end-diastolic and end-systolic volumes, can be accurately calculated.[146] In addition, pulmonary transit time,[147] left ventricular ejection rate,[147] and fractional emptying measures may be generated. The dose (as low as 2 mCi) and related exposure (less than 50 mrad) permit frequent repetitive studies, and the brief acquisition time makes the study applicable, even in uncooperative patients. Nonimaging probes with high sensitivity and temporal resolution detect beat-to-beat left ventricular variations.[8,9]

To permit ventricular visualization and the assessment of ventricular shape and wall motion by first-pass techniques, a higher dose (10 mCi–20 mCi) is employed. Acquired on a high-sensitivity camera and processed on a minicomputer with high count rate acceptability,[141] the study may be displayed to reveal the anatomical features of a right-sided angiogram with subsequent levophase.[148] This flow study can be useful in the evaluation of congenital cardiac abnormalities and may demonstrate the presence and quantitate the size of central left-to-right or right-to-left shunts.[149] Subsequent temporal separation permits dynamic evaluation of ventricular wall motion, cardiac output, and ventricular volumes by the classic method noted above or employing a geometric method (Fig. 29.26).[137]

High-dose first-pass data in the temporal window of the respective ventricle can be spatially isolated and formulated using postprocessing or gated to the R wave of the electrocardiogram, yielding alternating end-diastolic and end-systolic images, or framed to provide a cyclic display of ventricular contraction. First-pass methodology requires specialized equipment for optimal performance in order to avoid statistical difficulties at low count rates. Multicrystal cameras allow count rates up to 450,000/second without significant deterioration, but their resolution is suboptimal for other techniques.

In gaining the imaging advantage, the high-dose first-pass method becomes less suitable for study repeatability. Nonetheless, such methods have been applied to the evaluation of changes in ventricular function with dynamic stress,[150-152] pharmacologic intervention,[153,154] and in a variety of clinical situations.[144,148]

It would take a count rate five times that available on first-pass analysis to reduce the statistical error to that generally obtained with equilibrium blood pool studies.[155] Nevertheless, the high-dose first-pass technique compares favorably for ejection fraction determination with equilibrium and selective ventriculographic methods,[156] with an extremely low level of intraobserver and interobserver variability.

EQUILIBRIUM METHODOLOGY

Equilibrium multiple gated blood pool scintigraphy is the most widely employed scintigraphic method for the evaluation of both right and left ventricular size and function.[157-161] Imaging is performed in synchrony with or gated to the surface electrocardiogram, at equilibrium, at least 5 minutes following intravenous administration, with complete mixing of the stable ^{99m}Tc blood pool label. At this time, each volume of blood contains the same amount of radioactivity. There are several methods to label the red cells. Although simply performed *in vivo*, greater labeling efficiency and stability are offered by the convenient modified *in vitro* method.[162] From 20 mCi to 25 mCi of ^{99m}Tc pertechnetate (O_4^-) is combined with 10 ml of the patient's blood, previously combined with stannous ions. The labeled cells are then readministered and imaged. *In vitro* labeling adds efficiency and stability, sometimes necessary in the presence of multiple medication.[163] Radionuclide stability permits repeated imaging in multiple projections without temporal constraints,

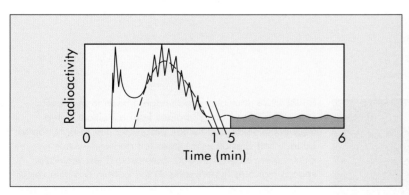

FIGURE 29.25 First-pass analysis. In this dramatic sketch of a first-pass curve, the area under the left ventricular component (*light gray*) is proportional to cardiac output. It is calibrated for volume by dividing it into the integrated area under 1 minute of the equilibrium time versus radioactivity curve (*dark gray*). Alternatively, volumes may be calculated from ventricular outlines using geometric considerations. (Modified from Botvinick EH, Glazer H, Shosa D: What is the reliability and the utility of scintigraphic methods for the assessment of ventricular function? In Rahimtoola S (ed): Controversies in Coronary Artery Disease, p 65. Philadelphia, FA Davis, 1981)

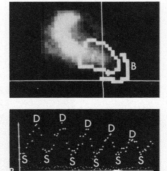

FIGURE 29.26 First-pass levophase analysis. Shown above is the levophase of a first-pass radioangiogram. A region of interest has localized the left ventricle. High-frequency analysis of the time versus radioactivity data in this region yields the curve below. Correcting for background, the peaks and valleys may be compared to calculate left ventricular ejection fraction. (Reproduced with permission from Botvinick EH, Glazer H, Shosa D: What is the reliability and the utility of scintigraphic methods for the assessment of ventricular function? In Rahimtoola S (ed): Controversies in Coronary Artery Disease, p 65. Philadelphia, FA Davis, 1981)

yet lacks the speed and temporal and spatial selectivity of first-pass methods. Resolution of anatomy and wall motion is optimized by acquisition in three projections: anterior, 70° left anterior oblique, to view the inferior wall,[164] and the "best septal" left anterior oblique projection. The latter best septal separates the two ventricles and is often obtained with a caudal tilt to reduce left atrial overlap. A high-resolution, single-crystal camera and a high-resolution or slant-hole collimator should optimally be used in adults.

Since equilibrium studies depend on image analysis of a composite sum of serial cardiac cycles, they are always computer acquired and triggered by or "gated" to the R wave. The mean length of the R-R interval is established prior to acquisition. Frame mode acquisition serially images a predetermined fraction (40 msec or less) of the mean cardiac cycle, and is best employed with regular rhythms. In each fraction, temporal interval, or frame, image data are combined to yield a summed picture over 200 to 600 cycles (Fig. 29.27). The study is terminated when each monitored frame contains sufficient data to permit the generation of images with adequate spatial resolution of chamber anatomy and to provide adequate statistical counts analysis (Figs. 29.28 and 29.29).

List mode acquisition employs an expanded computer memory to individually identify each scintillation temporally, in relation to the R wave, and spatially. Subsequently, an R-R histogram plotting beat length versus frequency can be generated and the data framed for the cycle length desired (Fig. 29.30). List mode acquisition is of particular value in the presence of a variable heart rate, or in the compilation of specific parameters referable to end-diastole, the region of the cycle most affected by heart rate variability. Again, sequential frames, regardless of the method of their derivation, can be displayed as a cyclic, endless loop movie or, alternatively, end-diastolic and end-systolic images may be extracted and viewed to evaluate wall motion.[165]

It is possible to accurately assess wall motion and calculate ejection fraction using certain classic geometric assumptions.[166] However, the great advantage of the scintigraphic method lies in the fact that counts within the ventricular region of interest are proportional to volume. Thus, in the best septal left anterior oblique projection, background-corrected ESC may be subtracted from EDC and divided by EDC to yield an ejection fraction independent of geometry (Fig. 29.31).[136,139,158,161,167] Ejection fraction, as calculated by this method, demonstrates an extremely low intraobserver and interobserver variability; however, background correction is critical.[168] Multiple gated acquisition provides a simple, reproducible, and accurate serial assessment of ventricular size and function at rest after infarction[160,169-173] and during pharmacologic interventions[174-176] or exercise,[192,122,123,168,170-183] which affect heart rate and the relative duration of systole (Fig. 29.32). Equilibrium time versus radioactivity curves can be employed as well to measure mean and peak ejection and filling rates[184,185] and a variety of other functional parameters (Fig. 29.33).[186,187] In addition, curves can be assessed serially for relative volume changes[188] or standardized for absolute volume.[189] A number of ventricular edge-detection methods are available to objectify these measurements, but all require occasional observer interventions.[190]

As for all methods, interobserver variability for the equilibrium scintigraphic calculation of right ventricular ejection fraction is greater than for left ventricular ejection fraction.[148,168] Yet, both scintigraphic methods are accurate and reproducible and have been useful for the single and serial evaluation of right ventricular ejection fraction and right ventricular wall motion in the assessment of right ventricular dis-

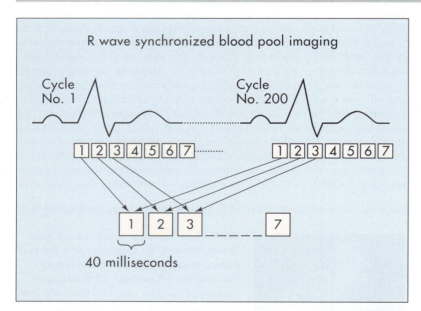

FIGURE 29.27 ECG gating of the blood pool images. With frame mode acquisition, image data representing preset fractions of the R-R interval, generally measuring 40 msec or less, are collected during each cardiac cycle. These individual frames are pooled with the same frame of subsequent beats until, after several hundred beats, summed frames (*below*) containing the sum of data representing all image intervals are displayed as an endless loop movie and analyzed for parameters of ventricular size and function. (Modified from Strauss HW, Zaret BL, Hurley PJ et al: A scintographic method for measuring left ventricular ejection fraction in man without cardiac catheterization. Am J Cardiol 28:575, 1971)

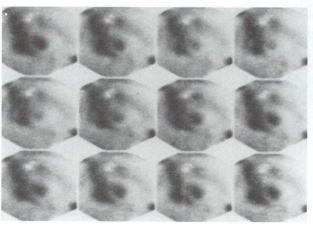
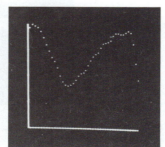

FIGURE 29.28 Multiple gated image. Shown in the "best septal" projection are 12 frames from a multiple gated equilibrium study. Contraction progresses left to right, top to bottom. End-diastole is in upper left and end-systole is immediately below it. A clear halo around left ventricular images indicates hypertrophy. At the bottom is a time versus radioactivity curve derived from left ventricular counts in this study, where peak counts are proportional to end-diastolic left ventricular volume and lowest counts are proportional to end-systolic volume. Curve count fall-off relates to irregular R-R intervals over the period of acquisition, where short cycles do not augment terminal frames. (Reproduced with permission from Green MV, Ostrow HG, Douglas MA et al: High temporal resolution ECG gated scintigraphic angiocardiography. J Nucl Med 16:95, 1975)

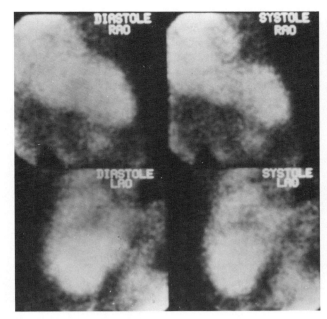
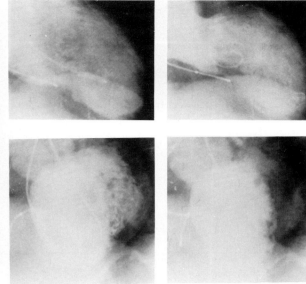

FIGURE 29.29 Blood pool/ventriculography comparison. Shown are diastolic (*left*) and systolic (*right*) frames from the rest blood pool scintigram of a patient with a left ventricular aneurysm in anterior (*above*) and "best septal" left anterior oblique projection. Similar images are shown by the same format from the selective ventriculogram in the same patient. Note both studies reveal best contraction in the posterior–lateral base in the left anterior oblique projection.

Scintigraphic anatomical information regarding regional wall motion is available and accurate and is further enhanced by functional image display. (Reproduced with permission from Botvinick EH, Glazer H, Shosa D: What is the reliability and the utility of scintigraphic methods for the assessment of ventricular function? In Rahimtoola S (ed): Controversies in Coronary Artery Disease, p 65. Philadelphia, FA Davis, 1981)

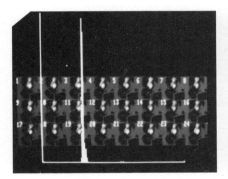
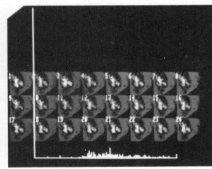

FIGURE 29.30 List mode acquisition. Shown are beat length histograms plotting R-R interval versus frequency in a patient in normal sinus rhythm (*above*) and in atrial fibrillation (*below*). Postprocessing can reconstruct dynamic blood pool images using cycles of any given R-R interval.

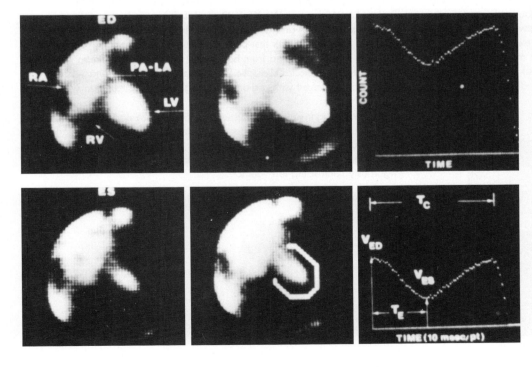

FIGURE 29.31 Equilibrium blood pool ejection fraction calculation. End-diastolic and end-systolic frames of a blood pool study are shown in the "best septal" projection (*left*). The region of the left ventricle is defined in the "best septal" projection (*middle, above*) and a background region is selected adjacent to the end-systolic left ventricle (*middle, below*). Applying this background value to the raw time versus radioactivity curve (*right, above*) generates the corrected curve (*right, below*). Since in this equilibrium method counts are proportional to volume, the curve peak is proportional to end-diastolic volume (V_{ED}), while the lowest curve value is proportional to the end-systolic volume (V_{ES}). This permits an accurate, reproducible method of ejection fraction calculation. (ED, end-diastolic frame; ES, end-systolic frame; LA, left atrium; LV, left ventricle; PA, pulmonary artery; RA, right atrium; RV, right ventricle; T_c, cycle duration; T_E, ejection time) (Reproduced with permission from Green M, Ostrow HG, Douglas MA et al: High temporal resolution ECG-gated scintigraphic angiocardiography. Circulation 56:1024, 1977)

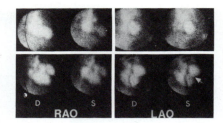

FIGURE 29.32 False left ventricular aneurysm. Above, in right anterior oblique (RAO) and left anterior oblique (LAO) projections, are end-diastolic (D) and end-systolic (S) images from the equilibrium blood pool study in a patient with a true aneurysm. Below, in the same projections and in the same format, are images from a patient with false left ventricular aneurysm. Unlike the former, the latter is not stabilized by myocardium and is actually formed by a contained myocardial rupture. The false aneurysm cavity is separated from the ventricle by a thin neck (arrow). (Reproduced with permission from Botvinick E, Shames D, Hutchinson J et al: The noninvasive diagnosis of a false left ventricular aneurysm by gated blood pool imaging. Am J Cardiol 37:1089, 1976)

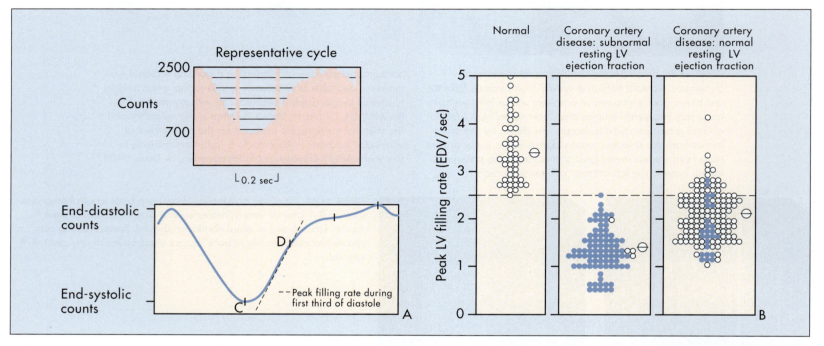

FIGURE 29.33 Evaluation and importance of diastolic filling measurements. **A.** Using first-pass data as shown here, or using equilibrium data (**B**), accurate noninvasive measurement of ventricular filling rate can be performed and applied to evaluation of a variety of problems. **B.** Bonow and co-workers found the scintigraphic peak left ventricular filling rate, expressed in end-diastolic volumes (EDV)/sec, to be lower than normal in most patients with coronary disease, studied at rest, regardless of the level of resting systolic function. While this presents the promise of noninvasive diagnosis of coronary artery disease without stress, filling rates may be nonspecific and depressed in a variety of conditions other than coronary disease. (**A**, modified from Reduto LA, Wickemyer WJ, Yang JB et al: Left ventricular diastolic performance at rest and during exercise in patients with coronary artery disease. Assessment with first-pass radionuclide angiography. Circulation 63:1228, 1981; **B**, modified from Bonow RO, Bacharach SL, Green MV et al: Impaired left ventricular diastolic filling in patients with coronary artery disease: Assessment with radionuclide angiography. Circulation 64:315, 1981)

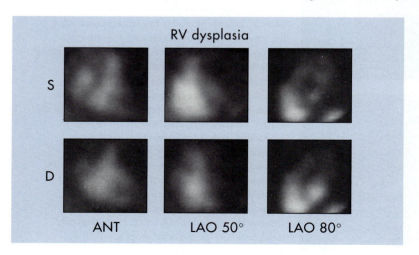

FIGURE 29.34 Right ventricular dysfunction. Shown are end-diastolic (D) and end-systolic (S) images in anterior (ANT) and 50° and 80° left anterior oblique (LAO) projections in a patient with right ventricular (RV) dysplasia. Note the large, poorly contracting right ventricle, which lifts the diminutive, vigorously contracting left ventricle.

ease (Fig. 29.34)[148,157,191,192] and in the diagnosis of right ventricular infarction.[193,194] Both calculated right ventricular and left ventricular ejection fractions correlate well with hemodynamic parameters. Serial reproducibility of functional measurements of both ventricles may be altered by changes in blood pressure and ventricular compliance,[195,196] food intake,[197] and variations in blood volume.[198]

A small, hand-guided, nonimaging probe has been developed that can perform first-pass and equilibrium studies.[9] However, in many cases problems of positioning could lead to gross inaccuracies in patients with segmental contraction abnormalities.[10] The technique has been applied to evaluate such serial changes after ergonovine administration in patients with variant angina[199] and during anesthesia administration in surgical patients with known or suspected heart disease,[200] and appears to be useful for measurement of emptying and filling phase indices. A research extension of this approach is a miniature semiconductor detector, which, when mounted as a vest on a patient, can monitor ejection fraction continuously for hours in ambulatory subjects.[201]

ABSOLUTE VOLUME CALCULATION

At equilibrium, counts are proportional to volume. Relative volumes may be converted to absolute volumes by a number of methods. The proportionality factor is related to the duration of imaging, a product of the frame duration and the number of cycles imaged, the injected dose, and the mixing volume, and is affected by the attenuation of radioactivity imaged at depth. All methods seek to normalize acquired background-corrected counts within the left ventricular region of interest for frame duration and time of acquisition, and use a blood sample to correct for the injected dose and blood volume. Links and co-workers[189] placed a radioactive marker on the left chest wall over the center of the left ventricular region of interest in the best septal left anterior oblique projection. The measured distance between the center of the left ventricle and the marker, as seen in the anterior projection, corrected for angulation, was taken as the attenuation distance of the left ventricle from the collimator face (Fig. 29.35). A number of recent studies have used phantoms or theoretical models to demonstrate the importance of attenuation and present various methods of correcting for this factor in the calculation of left ventricular volume.[202–204] Similar methods have been applied to right ventricular volume calculation. Bourguignon and co-workers[205] measured the radioactivity in a volume of the cylindrical ascending aorta and used this value to correct left ventricular counts internally and thereby derive absolute volume. Application of SPECT to the calculation of absolute ventricular volume requires extensive computer memory and software, but has obvious advantages related to spatial resolution.[206] Although some investigators have demonstrated accuracy and reproducibility for calculation of both right ventricular and left ventricular volumes in the absence of attenuation correction,[188] the physical facts make attenuation hard to ignore. Attenuation distances from 6 cm to 12 cm are common, which, when employing the attenuation coefficient of water, $\mu = 0.16/cm$, relates to an attenuation correction of roughly two to six times the measured radioactivity in the image region of interest. Practical and technical issues have led us to establish in our laboratory the relatively straightforward method of Links and co-workers.[189] The formula employed to calculate ventricular volume relates measured background-corrected left ventricular or right ventricular counts to the factors influencing its proportionality to volume:

$$\frac{\dfrac{\text{left ventricular counts*}/}{\text{time per frame} \times \text{cardiac cycles}}}{(e^{-\mu d})\dagger} \Big/ (\text{venous blood counts/cc/sec})\ddagger$$

where μ = attenuation coefficient of water and d = left ventricular depth. Practically speaking, these values are available from a combination of computer-acquired measurements and from counting a blood specimen drawn at the time of imaging. With the proper software, decay correction is automatically performed, and calculations of end-diastolic volume, end-systolic volume, stroke volume, ejection fraction, and cardiac output follow quickly. Such quantitative assessment of ventricular size and function requires careful quality control but offers important advantages in the evaluation of blood pool images. The extreme amenability of equilibrium methods to computer manipulation would then make available a variety of absolute volumetric markers related to emptying and filling phases, as well as absolute values for regional parameters of ventricular function. Additionally, computer analysis permits the generation of a variety of functional data and images that are of great potential clinical value and which, in many cases, cannot be practically obtained by other methods.[126,153,176,186,187,207–212]

Quantitation is an extremely important aspect of clinical cardiology. Whereas qualitative methods may be satisfactory for diagnostic purposes, quantitation is required for accurate serial study, the evaluation of therapeutic effects,[124,213] and prognosis.[170,171,183,184] Specifically, quantitative estimates of ventricular volumes may be quite useful for evaluating the course of illness over time,[169,182,214] the effects of exercise,[181–183] the results of pharmacologic and surgical interventions,[125,215,216] the effects of potentially cardiotoxic drugs,[36,124,213] and the functional response to conduction sequence altered by pacemakers.[217]

---

* Background-corrected end-diastolic and end-systolic counts
† Correction factor for depth and attenuation
‡ Correction for dose, blood volume, dilution

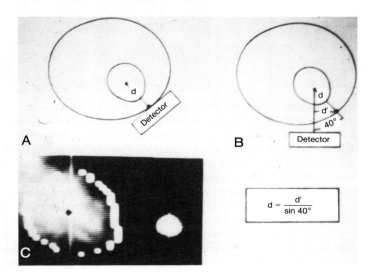

FIGURE 29.35 Attenuation correction. Shown is the mathematical basis for the measurement of an attenuation distance required to apply an attenuation correction, converting counts within the left ventricular region of interest to absolute volumes. The attenuation distance illustrated at the lower left is estimated from the measured distance from the center of the left ventricle to the chest wall marker overlying the center of the "best septal" projection, measured in the anterior projection (d'). If the "best septal" projection is the 40° left anterior oblique, the attenuation distance is given by d'/sin 40°. (Reproduced with permission and modified from Links JM, Becker LC, Schindledecker JG et al: Measurements of absolute left ventricular volume from gated blood pool studies. Circulation 65:82, 1982)

OTHER CAPABILITIES OF THE METHOD

Blood pool scintigraphy has been reported to demonstrate intracavitary masses and atrial myxomas,[218] identify the presence of ventricular hypertrophy,[219,220] differentiate pericardial effusion,[219] approximate pulmonary circuit hemodynamics from right ventricular ejection fraction,[193,194,221] and even estimate left atrial volumes.[222] Although such visual findings should be reported and such calculated measurements show promise, echocardiography appears to be the definitive and appropriately more widely used technique for the evaluation of such abnormalities. An exception in the evaluation of pericardial effusion relates to the scintigraphic ability to identify and quantitate the volume of bloody pericardial effusion, a useful aid after coronary bypass graft surgery (Fig. 29.36).[223] The scintigraphic method, however, remains the simplest and the most reproducible method for the quantitative assessment of parameters of left ventricular and right ventricular size and function after infarction, with various interventions, and during serial follow-up.[224,225]

Scintigraphic techniques afford the opportunity to quantitate left-sided or right-sided regurgitation fraction or intracardiac shunts, employing xenon washout techniques,[226] computer analysis of left-sided time versus radioactivity curves,[149,227] or the comparison of equilibrium stroke volume ratios or their equivalent (Fig. 29.37).[126,228] The latter calculation equals the left ventricular stroke volume expressed in counts divided by the counts equivalent of the right ventricular stroke volume. This regurgitant index (RI) should equal unity in normal patients, increase in the setting of left-sided regurgitant lesions and left-to-right shunts distal to the atrial level, and decrease in the setting of right-sided regurgitant lesions or right-to-left shunts. For practical purposes, the regurgitant fraction, the fraction of the total stroke volume passing retrograde through the insufficient valve, equals

$$\frac{RI - 1}{RI}$$

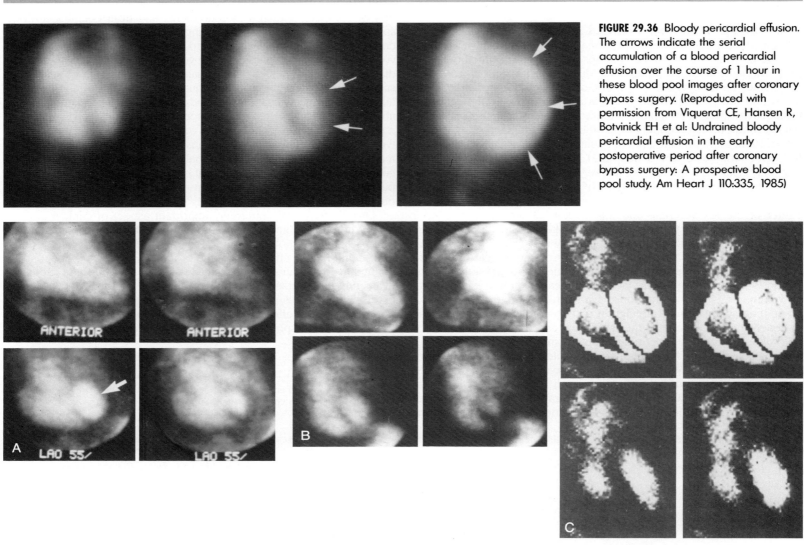

FIGURE 29.36 Bloody pericardial effusion. The arrows indicate the serial accumulation of a blood pericardial effusion over the course of 1 hour in these blood pool images after coronary bypass surgery. (Reproduced with permission from Viquerat CE, Hansen R, Botvinick EH et al: Undrained bloody pericardial effusion in the early postoperative period after coronary bypass surgery: A prospective blood pool study. Am Heart J 110:335, 1985)

FIGURE 29.37 Blood pool imaging in mitral regurgitation. **A.** Shown are end-diastolic (*left*) and end-systolic (*right*) images in the anterior (*above*) and "best septal" (*below*) projections in a patient with significant mitral regurgitation. Note the extreme intensity of the left ventricle compared to the right ventricle in diastole (*arrow*), indicative of the large left ventricular volume. This, with the dramatic left ventricular ejection compared to the right ventricular, gives visual evidence of the greater left ventricular stroke volume, indicative of a significant left-sided regurgitant lesion, which was related to a regurgitant index of 2.7 illustrated in Figure 29.45,A. **B.** Shown in the same format are the blood pool images in the same patient studied soon after mitral valve replacement. The size and relative intensity of the diastolic left ventricle are much diminished and the visual discrepancy between left ventricular and right ventricular stroke volumes is no longer present. **C.** Regurgitant index. In this initial calculation of the scintigraphic regurgitant index, the same left ventricular and right ventricular regions of interest were used in systole and diastole with efforts to exclude atrial regions. This ratio of left ventricular and right ventricular stroke volume expressed in counts relates well to the extent of valvular regurgitation but is more accurately calculated using separate end-diastolic and end-systolic regions of interest, stroke volume images, or other functional images illustrated below. (**B**, reproduced with permission from Botvinick EH, Glazer H, Shosa D: What is the reliability and the utility of scintigraphic methods for the assessment of ventricular function? In Rahimtoola S (ed): Controversies in Coronary Artery Disease, p 65. Philadelphia, FA Davis, 1981; **C**, reproduced with permission from Rigo P, Alderson PO, Robertson RM et al: Measurement of aortic and mitral regurgitation by gated cardiac blood pool scans. Circulation 60:306, 1979)

A number of investigators have reported an excellent association between scintigraphic and angiographic measurements of regurgitant fraction in patients with mitral and aortic insufficiency. While useful for assessing the major hemodynamic lesion, quantitative assessment of a regurgitant or shunt lesion by this method can only optimally be done when that lesion is strongly dominant or isolated. In the presence of mixed lesions, the scintigraphic method accurately portrays their sum. The application of mathematical assumptions and new scintigraphic methods promises to overcome difficulties related to geometry and overlap in the physiologic assessment of regurgitant lesions.[228,229]

Regional counts and their serial alterations can be compared to yield information relating to regional stroke volume, ejection fraction, and regional and global ventricular emptying and filling rates.[153,176,186] Such derived stroke volume can be compared to yield accurate, reproducible regurgitant fractions.[126,127] Additionally, parameters relating to the degree and sequence of regional ventricular or atrial emptying can be derived and displayed.

FUNCTIONAL OR PARAMETRIC IMAGING

One of the great advantages of the equilibrium scintigraphic method is its ability to generate parametric or functional images.[230] Each functional image represents the distribution of some parameter related to or derived from the time versus radioactivity curve (Fig. 29.38).

The stroke volume image is generated by a pixel-by-pixel computer subtraction of background-corrected end-systolic from end-diastolic frames. Similarly, the ejection fraction image further divides these values by regional end-diastolic counts (Fig. 29.39). In each case, regional stroke volume or ejection fraction is gray scale or color-coded for its local value.[186] These images are derived from global left ventricular end-diastolic and end-systolic frames and so are temporally dependent. That is, in the case of incoordinate contraction or conduction abnormalities, stroke volume or ejection fraction may not be accurate in image regions not sharing the systolic and diastolic timing of the global left ventricle. Regional stroke volume and ejection fraction images have been extremely useful for the assessment of changes following therapeutic interventions and after myocardial infarction[231,232] and are valuable for objectifying the response to stress or pharmacologic intervention.[153,175,176]

The phase image is a parametric image derived by fitting the time versus radioactivity curve to a cosine function of the following form on a pixel-by-pixel basis:

$$F_1(t) = A_0 + A_1 \cos(\theta_1 + W_0 t)$$

This is the first harmonic of the Fourier series, in which the frequency of the function is equal to the heart rate. For each pixel, A_1 (amplitude) is a measure of the excursion of the cosine curve approximating one-half the stroke counts. A_0 represents the mean amplitude; θ_1 is the phase angle, a measure of curve symmetry that describes the relative position of the curve peak in the acquisition interval, the R-R interval; W_0 represents a parameter that converts time to degrees as the phase angle is expressed from 0°, the onset of the R wave gating trigger, to 360°, the onset of the subsequent cycle (Fig. 29.40). Values of amplitude, A_1, and phase angle, θ_1, are extracted for each pixel and are gray scale or color-coded to provide amplitude and phase "maps" (Figs. 29.41 and 29.42). The evaluation of fitted data is employed, rather than sampling the raw data in each pixel in order to enhance sampling statistics.[187]

Unlike the stroke volume image, the amplitude image is not temporally dependent and does reflect the maximum excursion, proportional to stroke volume, regardless of where in the cardiac cycle this occurs. Although related to both systolic and diastolic curve features and influenced strongly by curve symmetry, the phase function has been related to the sequential pattern and extent of ventricular contraction and may be of value for identification of stress-induced ischemia[211] and assessment of serial function changes, as well as the extent of left ventricular aneurysm (Fig. 29.43).[209] The parameter has been applied to the assessment of the serial pattern of electrical excitation, has identified sites of ventricular impulse formation and the origin of sites of preexcitation (Fig. 29.44), has demonstrated characteristic patterns in complete bundle branch block[207,210,212] and left anterior hemiblock,[233] and has been shown to be quite accurate for the identification of the focus in patients studied during ventricular tachycardia.[207] Parametric images permit evaluation of measurements of ventricular function and structure that are not available with other methodology.

The parametric stroke volume image and the amplitude image have been employed to derive the ratio of ventricular stroke volumes or their equivalent, the regurgitant ratio. However, right atrial overlap tends to blunt the assessment of right ventricular stroke volume, falsely elevating the ratio. Using a simple correction that combines geometric considerations to correct for overlap and a regional phase evaluation to correct for incoordinate contraction, these effects can be largely eliminated (Fig. 29.45).[208]

STRESS EVALUATION

The reproducibility of blood pool measurements makes them eminently suitable for the assessment of quantitative serial changes with dynamic exercise.[158,167,168,234] These measurements have been applied to the detection of myocardial ischemia and to the evaluation of ventricular function in patients with valvular disease,[159] where it serves as a measure of valve disease severity and an indicator for surgical intervention.[235] Stress measurements have been used as well to assess the

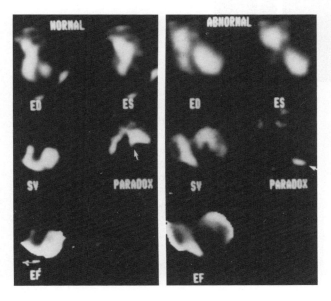

FIGURE 29.38 Functional images. Shown are end-diastolic (ED) and end-systolic (ES), stroke volume (SV), paradox, and ejection fraction (EF) images in a normal patient (left panel) and in a patient with a left ventricular aneurysm (right panel). The stroke volume image intensity codes regional, "positive" stroke volume, whereas the paradox image, made by subtracting end-diastolic from end-systolic data, reveals atrial and paradoxical ventricular segments (arrows). (Reproduced with permission from Botvinick E, Dae M, Schechtmann N: The current status of cardiovascular nuclear medicine: Selected topics. In Margulis A, Goodman C (eds): Diagnostic Radiology, p 513. St Louis, CV Mosby, 1985)

effects of chemotherapy. While the latter can probably be effectively assessed at rest,[124,216] exercise blood pool imaging appears to have diagnostic accuracy for ischemia similar to exercise perfusion scintigraphy with thallium-201 (Fig. 29.46).[123,150,178,179,236] Generally, no change or a reduced ejection fraction with stress represents a pathologic response. Yet, the response to stress varies with resting ejection fraction, age,[237] and stress end point. The complete stress evaluation should include quantitation of volumes and their alteration, since a stress-induced increase in end-systolic volume has been shown to be a sensitive indicator of the ischemic response (Fig. 29.47).[150] Similarly, filling rate may also prove sensitive to the identification of ischemia.[185,238] However, the "ischemic" response is not entirely specific and can be encountered in hypertensive patients[184,196] or in any condition with exercise-induced ventricular dysfunction. Nonetheless, the scintigraphic evaluation of the functional response to stress appears to relate to the extent of myocardium at ischemic risk, and eventual prognosis,[170,171,176,179–181] as well as to the potential for functional benefit related to invasive treatment of coronary disease.[214,225]

PITFALLS IN BLOOD POOL IMAGING

Errors in background selection are the most common type influencing blood pool results. A poor blood pool label may result in incomplete or

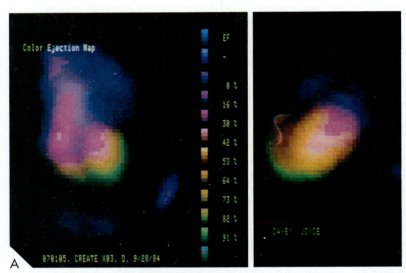

FIGURE 29.39 A. Normal ejection fraction images. Shown are color functional ejection fraction images in "best septal" (*left*) and 60° left anterior oblique projections in a normal patient. Note the yellow and green coloration, corresponding to high ejection fraction values, the "ejection shell" surrounding the ventricles. **B.** Abnormal ejection fraction image. Shown are blood pool images and derived curve (*left*) and functional ejection fraction in "best septal" (*above right*) and 70° left anterior oblique (*below right*) projections in a patient with an inferior wall contraction abnormality. Note the break in the ejection shell in the inferior wall (*arrows*) seen only in the 70° LAO projection. At the left, the automated ventricular edge fit is employed to generate the time versus radioactivity curve. The 70° LAO projection is critical for evaluating inferior wall abnormalities. The color scale at lower right codes regional ejection fraction in all functional images.

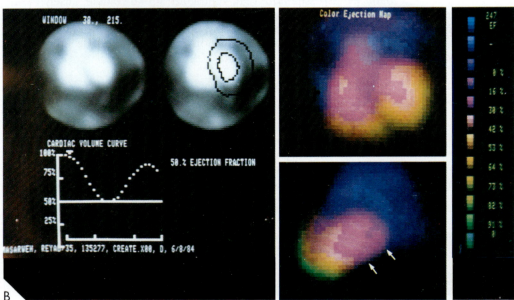

FIGURE 29.40 Cosine curve fit. Shown are the raw time versus radioactivity curve (*dots*) and first harmonic curve fit. The fitted curve peak defines the phase angle, measured from 0° to 360°, while the amplitude parallels the stroke volume and represents one-half the depth of the curve excursion. (Reproduced with permission from Frais M, Botvinick E, Shosa D et al: Phase image characterization of ventricular contraction in left and right bundle block. Am J Cardiol 50:95, 1982)

erroneous image evaluation. Omission of the priming dose, drug interference, administration through 5% dextrose in water, or label decomposition may be the cause. Errors in gating are also important and must be recognized, while soft tissue attenuation, though less common than that seen with ^{201}Tl, must still be considered. In addition to background errors, the faulty measurement of any involved parameter will lead to error in ventricular volume calculation. Most common are errors in the attenuation distance, where an underestimation will lead to a reduced volume. Particularly troublesome is the withdrawal of the blood sample from an intravenous line, where any dilution will lead to an overestimation of ventricular volume (Table 29.6).[239]

COMPARISON OF SCINTIGRAPHIC METHODS

Each scintigraphic method provides some advantages that may make it more suitable for the performance of a given task. The methodologic differences should be seriously considered to determine the most appropriate scintigraphic method (Table 29.7). Both equilibrium and first-pass methods require a computer for full analysis. In spite of their differences, both techniques are capable of providing accurate, reproducible, and quantitative data regarding both right and left ventricular size and function.[136,147,148,157,159,168] Moreover, both techniques can be employed as complementary methods in the same patient.[157–160,165,240]

OTHER LABELED CELLULAR ELEMENTS

^{111}In has been used to label both leukocytes and platelets. Although the former is a useful agent in the localization of inflammatory foci, it has found no significant cardiac application. Although labeled platelets have been applied to the identification of intravascular thrombi, reduced blood pool clearance has made its clinical use impractical.[241]

COMPARISON OF SCINTIGRAPHY WITH OTHER METHODS

In addition to scintigraphy, there are currently a number of noninvasive imaging techniques capable of assessing some aspects of left ventricular size and function. However, only echocardiography currently provides a practical noninvasive imaging method to evaluate these parameters (Table 29.8).[242] Today, echocardiography is the most widely

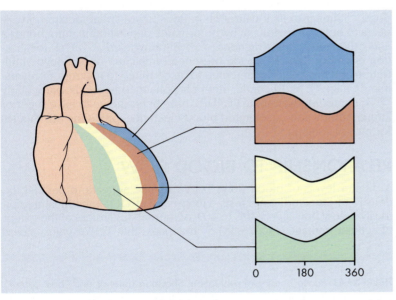

FIGURE 29.41 Phase analysis. The diagram presents a ventricle that is color-coded for increasing delay in contraction sequence, from septum to lateral wall. Resultant cosine curves fitted to the regional time versus radioactivity curves are shown below. The septum and its corresponding curve begin contraction at the R wave. The region has a phase angle of 0° and is coded green. The lateral wall and its related curve fill when the ventricle should empty. This wall would demonstrate paradoxical motion and the curve would have a phase angle of 180°. (Modified from Frais M, Botvinick E, Shosa D et al: Phase image characterization of ventricular contraction in left and right bundle branch block. Am J Cardiol 50:95, 1982)

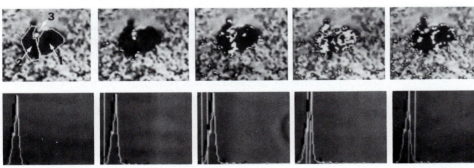

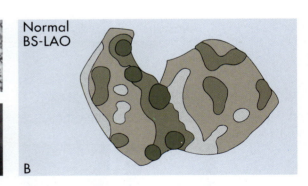

FIGURE 29.42 Normal phase analysis. **A.** Shown, above left, is the phase image in a patient with normal conduction and contraction. Early, homogeneous phase angle is evident from the dark gray shade of the left ventricle (*first arrow*) and right ventricle (*second arrow*) region of interest. The more proximal atrial regions are out of phase with the ventricles and have light gray shade and delayed phase angle in this "best septal" projection. The movement of background structures, bearing no relationship to cardiac contraction, is a random salt-and-pepper distribution of gray shades. Below are the left ventricular (*white*) and right ventricular (*black*) phase histograms generated from the respective regions above and plotting phase angle on the abscissa versus its frequency on the ordinate. Phase histograms are early, virtually superimposed and narrow based, indicating early, coordinate, and rapid onset of contraction through both ventricles. The pattern of phase progression, taken to roughly parallel the sequence of contraction, can be assessed by sequentially sampling the histograms via a set window of phase angles, vertical bars with corresponding whitening of the related pixels in the respective regions of interest. The site of earliest phase angle is seen in the proximal septum (*third arrow*), with subsequent homogeneous spread. **B.** Shown diagrammatically is the phase image of the same patient illustrated in part **A** of this figure. The site of earliest phase angle, in darkest gray, is again seen to occur in the septal region with subsequent symmetrical delay. (Reproduced with permission and modified from Botvinick E, Frais M, O'Connell W et al: Phase image evaluation of patients with ventricular pre-excitation syndrome. J Am Coll Cardiol 3:799, 1984)

employed noninvasive cardiac imaging modality, with high spatial resolution and, with newer Doppler methods,[243] the capability to assess pathophysiologic parameters. It provides excellent, largely qualitative evaluation of ventricular size and function, complementary in many ways to ventricular characterization provided by blood pool scintigraphic methods. The latter are somewhat less resolved techniques, which have as their primary advantage the ability to reproducibly, objectively, and quantitatively assess ventricular size, function, and derived parameters. Frequently, echocardiographic and scintigraphic evaluations of ventricular size and function are complementary and may both be needed. Quantitative scintigraphic or angiographic assessment early in a patient's course can be followed by qualitative echocardiography, with subsequent intermittent scintigraphic study for noninvasive confirmation of suspected functional alterations. Also, the interaction of the two tests provides strong evidence regarding the state of ventricular function, which may be all that is required in some patients.

Recently, considerable effort has been taken to employ echocardiographic methods during dynamic exercise. Analysis has not objectively demonstrated a superiority of the echocardiographic method.[244,245] While physically possible, such methodology is again qualitative and technically difficult and can only approach the indirect assessment of ischemia via its effects on ventricular function and cannot directly assess the specific effects of dynamic stress on perfusion. Although promising, the stress echocardiographic method has not yet been documented to have clinical utility compared to other methods.

Although echocardiography and scintigraphy are the most practical tools currently available for the assessment of ventricular size and function, other modalities, such as magnetic resonance imaging and cine computer tomography, loom on the horizon as alternate quantitative methods.

ACUTE MYOCARDIAL INFARCTION "INFARCT-AVID" SCINTIGRAPHY
IMAGING THE INFLAMMATORY RESPONSE

Gallium-67 citrate has long been established as an imaging agent that localizes in regions of abscess and inflammation. Recently, ^{111}In-labeled leukocytes have been introduced as a more specific marker of the inflammatory response. Although both ^{67}Ga and ^{111}In leukocytes have been applied to the visualization of vegetations in endocarditis,[246,247] this appears not to be generally useful. Over the last several years, gallium visualization of the myocardium has been reported in myocarditis and has been said to be an indicator of potential responsiveness to steroid therapy.[248]

DEVELOPMENT OF THE METHOD

While ^{67}Ga localizes in acute infarction, it requires a 1- to 2-day interval between injection and imaging for soft tissue clearance.[249] The optimal label, ^{99m}Tc, when bound to tetracycline, labeled infarction and was shown to provide a qualitative measure of infarct size. However, image evaluation could only be made after allowing 24 hours for clearance and hepatic labeling with a poor target-to-background ratio made interpretation difficult.[250] Similarly, ^{99m}Tc glucoheptonate localizes in infarction but, again, with poor resolution and distracting hepatic uptake.[251]

Shen and Jennings described calcium accumulation in myocardial cells early after the occurrence of necrosis.[252] Bonte and co-workers demonstrated the localization of ^{99m}Tc stannous pyrophosphate (TcPYP), already a common bone-imaging agent, in acute infarcts in dogs.[253] Similar to its localization in bone, myocardial localization appears to occur in regions of hydroxyapatite deposition in mitochondria and other subcellular fractions.[254,255] Intramyocardial TcPYP localization does not depend on the presence of calcium or leukocytic infiltration and has been documented to be confined to regions of irreversible damage.[256–258] Recently, other phosphate compounds, particularly ^{99m}Tc imidodiphosphonate (TcIDP), have been shown to have superior infarct affinity and accelerated blood clearance, providing advantages for infarct imaging.[259]

RELATIONSHIP TO BLOOD FLOW

At higher levels of blood flow, TcPYP uptake appears to parallel the density of myocardial necrosis. However, TcPYP uptake falls precipitously below flow levels 30% to 40% of normal, regardless of the extent of cellular damage (Fig. 29.48).[255] It appears that TcPYP gains access

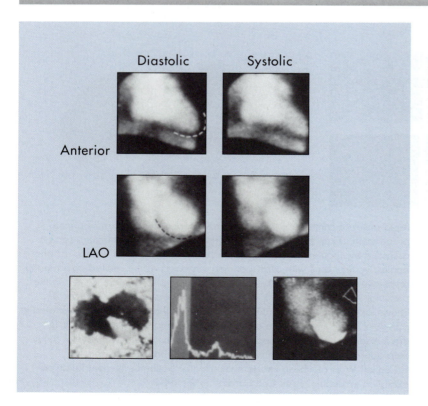

FIGURE 29.43 Phase aneurysm evaluation. Shown in anterior and "best septal" projections are diastolic (D) and systolic (S) frames of a study in a patient with large left ventricular aneurysm. The akinetic segment has been outlined. Below, the left anterior oblique (LAO) phase image and histogram are shown. Pixels corresponding to an abnormal phase angle (dark gray accentuation) are highlighted on the phase image. The related area correlates with the percent akinetic segment and can be used to estimate the extent of aneurysm involvement. (Reproduced with permission from Frais M, Botvinick E, Shosa D et al: Phase image characterization of localized and generalized left ventricular contraction abnormalities. J Am Coll Cardiol 4:987, 1984)

into acutely infarcted myocardium, in relation to a total arterial occlusion, via residual and collateral flow to the region. The "doughnut pattern" of TcPYP uptake, seen in association with proximal occlusion of the left anterior descending coronary artery in animals and humans, has been related to a poor prognosis (Fig. 29.49).[260] Some ascribe the central clear area to reduced radionuclide localization in a region of ischemic infarction. However, the origin of the pattern may relate to projectional factors.

IMAGE DYNAMICS, METHODS, AND INTERPRETATION

Postinfarction, the radionuclide depends for its localization on access to the involved area and maturation of a biochemical process. Although increased radioactivity is present in involved tissue as early as 4 to 6 hours after infarction, these cellular processes do not generally result in positive TcPYP images until at least 12 hours after the onset of

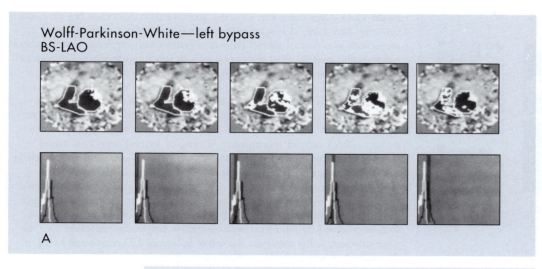

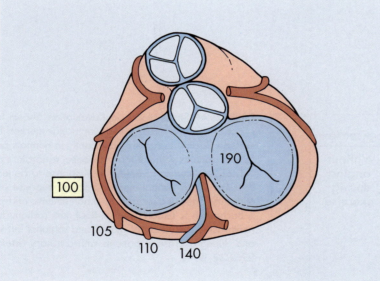

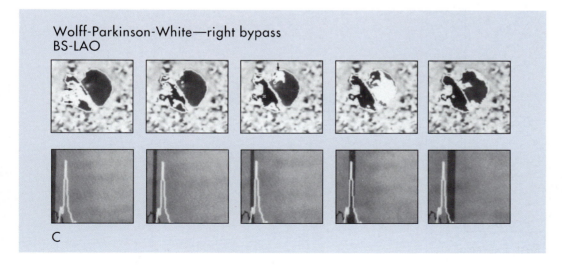

FIGURE 29.44 Phase analysis of atrioventricular connections. **A.** Shown, according to the same format as in the preceding figure, are phase images and histograms from a patient with Wolff-Parkinson-White syndrome studied during preexcitation in the "best septal" (BS-LAO) projection. Note the image site of earliest phase angle in the lateral left ventricular wall (*white arrow, above*), with parallel delay in the right ventricle phase histogram. **B.** Illustrated is the electrophysiologic map performed in the same patient as in A during preexcitation. The shortest interval of retrograde atrioventricular conduction, 100 msec, also occurred in the lateral left ventricular wall. **C.** Shown, according to the same format as shown in B, are phase images and histograms from a patient with preexcitation via a right-sided pathway. The sight of earliest phase angle appears in the lateral aspect of the right ventricle (*arrow, upper left*) with delayed phase angle in the left ventricle base (*arrow above, center panel*) and corresponding delay in the left ventricle (*white*) histogram. (Reproduced with permission and modified from Botvinick E, Frais M, O'Connell W et al: Phase image evaluation of patients with ventricular pre-excitation syndrome. J Am Coll Cardiol 3:799, 1984)

necrosis. This may relate, in part, to progressive increase in collateral supply to the infarct zone. In most patients with infarction, cardiac radioactivity is maximum at 48 to 72 hours, becomes less intense by 6 to 7 days, and is usually absent by 10 to 14 days after the event.[256-258] Reduced radionuclide avidity relates to progressive replacement of necrotic myocardium by granulation tissue and scar.

Distribution of "cardiac" radioactivity has been interpreted as localized and discrete, or diffuse (Fig. 29.50).[261] The former is specific for myocardial damage, while the latter, originally thought to be related to subendocardial infarction, is most frequently related to blood pool radioactivity.[262] Further, diagnostic security increases with the intensity of uptake, graded 1+ to 4+. "Diffuse" should not be confused with "generalized" myocardial uptake. The latter is occasionally localized to widespread subendocardial, "shell" infarction, but projected, in these ungated images, throughout the left ventricular myocardium (Fig. 29.51). Combined blood pool and infarct imaging with computer

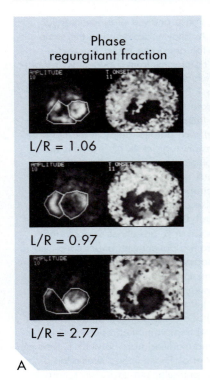
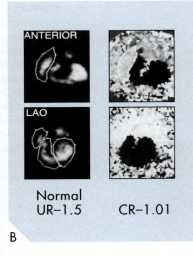

FIGURE 29.45 Atrial correction for regurgitation index. **A.** Shown are amplitude (*left*) and phase (*right*) images in the "best septal" left anterior oblique projections in a normal subject (*above*), a patient with cardiomyopathy without regurgitation (*middle*), and in the patient with mitral regurgitation illustrated in Figure 29.38. The ratio of left ventricular to right ventricular amplitude in outlined regions of interest yields a regurgitant index. While accurate and reproducible, this index tends to overestimate the amount of regurgitation owing to a blunting of the apparent right ventricular amplitude due to right atrial overlap. **B.** Shown are phase (*right*) and amplitude (*left*) images in a patient without valvular regurgitation in anterior (*above*) and "best septal" (*below*) projections. The ratio of left ventricular to right ventricular amplitude in the regions outlined in the lower amplitude image again yields an uncorrected regurgitant index. The difference between the full projected and the atrial area evident in the LAO image represents an estimate of the right ventricular region obscured by the atrium. The right ventricular amplitude is then augmented by the mean right ventricular amplitude, multiplied over the area affected. In this example, the index falls from 1.5 uncorrected to 1.0 in this patient without valvular insufficiency.

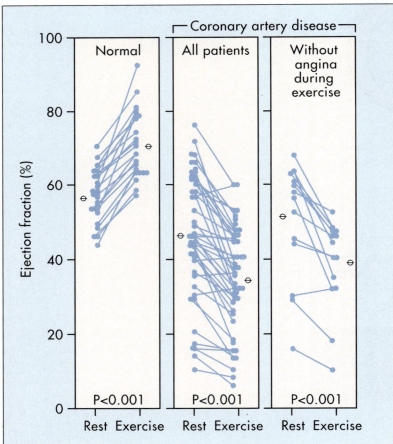

FIGURE 29.46 Stress blood pool evaluation. Shown from the initial study is the effect of dynamic stress on left ventricular ejection fraction. Left ventricular ejection fraction increases significantly in normals but shows little change or falls in patients with coronary disease, regardless of symptoms development. Subsequent studies revealed the response to be less specific and less sensitive with a normal ejection fraction response often seen in patients with coronary disease exercised to a nonischemic end-point. (Modified from Borer J, Bacharach S, Green M et al: Real time radionuclide cineangiography in the noninvasive evaluation of global and regional left ventricular function at rest and during exercise in patients with coronary artery disease. N Engl J Med 296:839, 1977)

comparison or computer subtraction of background has been suggested as a method to distinguish myocardial from cavitary radioactivity.[263] However, the interpretation of multiple projections, radiopharmaceutical choice and care in preparation, and imaging are more practical approaches. Rotating slant-hole tomography at the bedside or rotating camera ECT has recently been shown to aid diagnostic accuracy (Fig. 29.52).[264]

DIAGNOSTIC ACCURACY

Early animal studies revealed the ability of the method to detect regional transmural infarction as small as 3 g.[265] Parkey and co-workers demonstrated positive discrete uptake in all 23 patients admitted with transmural infarction.[261] Massie and co-workers revealed a direct relationship between image visualization and enzymatic infarct size.[266] They also demonstrated reduced sensitivity in subendocardial infarction, while others suggested a "diffuse" pattern of radionuclide distribution in subendocardial infarction. Soon a variety of investigators reported false-positive TcPYP scintigrams in association with valvular disease,[267] unstable angina stable angina pectoris,[268] heart failure[269] after cardiopulmonary bypass,[270] and at a time remote from past infarction.[271,272] While an occasional patient in these series revealed discrete uptake associated with a punctate area of valvular calcification, in association with unstable angina and enzyme release in relation to postinfarction pericarditis, most of these reported "false positives" were of the relatively low intensity, nonspecific "diffuse" pattern. Others, with discrete uptake, could largely be explained in reference to actual associated myocardial necrosis. Subsequent studies strongly suggested a relationship of diffuse uptake with blood pool labeling. Lyons and co-workers have reported decreased specificity of TcPYP for acute infarction due to a significant number of positive images weeks and months after the event.[271] However, a study of TcPYP scintigrams performed in 55 patients 9 days to 10 years after a documented transmural infarction revealed only two with discrete uptake. Both had extensive prior infarction and aneurysm.[272] Pathologic studies revealed evidence of ongoing necrosis in patients with remote infarction and

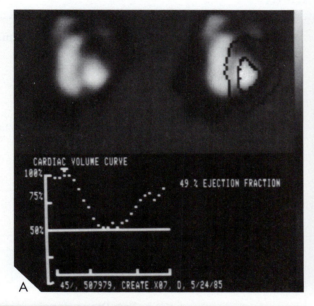

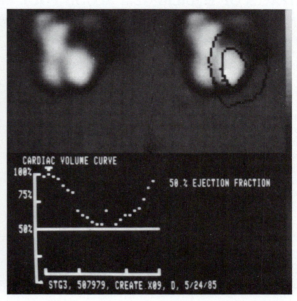

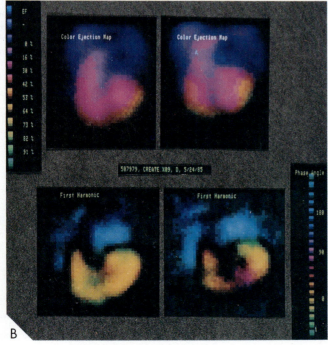

FIGURE 29.47 Functional image stress evaluation. **A.** Shown are time versus radioactivity curves generated from objectively defined left ventricular regions of interest at rest (*above*) and with stress (*below*) in a patient suspected of coronary disease. The left ventricular ejection fraction failed to augment, suggesting stress-induced ischemia. Minor curve irregularity, seen here, is related to variations in the automatic fit of the left ventricular edge. As here, they often do not significantly affect the calculation of left ventricular ejection fraction. Volume analysis revealed an abnormal stress-induced increase in end-systolic volume. Dynamic images suggested stress-induced septal hypokinesis. **B.** Color functional ejection fraction (*above*) and phase (*below*) images reveal a stress-induced fall in septal ejection fraction with a break in the yellow left ventricular ejection shell and augmentation of lateral left ventricular fraction values, and a corresponding delay in septal phase values. The phase image has been additionally intensity-coded for amplitude. The fall in septal intensity with stress represents a fall in regional stroke volume. Phase angle is color-coded, while amplitude is intensity-coded. The distribution of regions of reduced intensity (*arrows*) and shift to "hotter" colors in the stress image indicates extensive left ventricular and right ventricular involvement. Below, the color ejection fraction image codes highest ejection fraction in green and yellow. Reduced regional right ventricular ejection fraction at stress is clearly demonstrated (*arrow*).

scintigraphic myocardial uptake prior to demise in the absence of an acute coronary event.[273] Accepting the 2+ intensity classification as only equivocal, Berman and co-workers demonstrated a dramatic improvement in test specificity with only 3% false positives.[263]

Discrete uptake appears specific for acute infarction and correlates with electrocardiographic and pathologic infarct localization. Numerous studies suggest a diagnostic sensitivity to transmural infarction of 85% to 90% probably best in relation to anterior infarction.[274] However, small transmural and subendocardial infarctions are less easily resolved and the study has a sensitivity to subendocardial infarction of 60% to 70%.[266,275] Although discrete uptake is more common in transmural and dense infarction, its presence cannot itself differentiate transmural from subendocardial infarction. Further, discrete uptake may be seen as well in relation to penetrating chest trauma, tumor invasion, or other conditions related to actual myocardial necrosis and, yet, not bearing any relationship to an acute ischemic event.

"Primary" cardiac amyloidosis provides an exception to this analysis (Fig. 29.53).[276] Here, the infiltrative process is frequently associated with dense accumulation of the radiotracer. While this may relate, in part, to an associated element of necrosis, there also appears to be a relationship with the amyloid deposit itself. Images in such cases may be quite impressive and, as in all circumstances, care must be taken to relate image findings to the clinical presentation.

RELATION TO OTHER DIAGNOSTIC METHODS

While quite sensitive to the presence of acute infarction, infarct-avid scintigraphy is less sensitive than serial electrocardiographic changes, induced contraction abnormalities, serum enzyme release, and the presence of perfusion scintigraphic defects (Table 29.9). However, neither wall motion nor perfusion scintigraphic abnormalities are specific for acute infarction, and electrocardiographic changes may also be nonspecific or concealed, or mimicked by a multitude of conduc-

---

TABLE 29.6 PITFALLS OF EQUILIBRIUM BLOOD POOL IMAGING

Poor red cell label
    Stannous ions omitted
    Drug interference
    Radionuclide decomposition
    Injection in 5% dextrose in water
    ^{99}Tc administration—milking an old generator
Soft tissue attenuation
    Makes variations in right and left ventricular counts and inaccuracies in calculation of regurgitant index
Erroneous gating
    Bad beat acceptance
    Rhythm irregularity
Erroneous choice of left ventricular region of interest
Poor choice of background

Pitfalls of Equilibrium Blood Pool Volume Determination
Erroneous entry of acquisition parameters
    Time of day
    Acquisition time
    Blood sample counts
    Sample volume
Blood drawn from IV infusion—diluted specimen
Blood drawn from IV radionuclide injection site—overestimate blood counts
Error in estimate of attenuation distance
Error in delineation of left ventricular region of interest
Erroneous background correction

TABLE 29.7 RELATIVE ADVANTAGES OF BLOOD POOL IMAGING METHODS*

	First Pass		Equilibrium
	Low Dose	*High Dose*	
Technique	−	−	+
Quality control	−	−	+
Computer required	++	+	++
Acquisition time	+	+	−
Processing time	−	−	+
Radiopharmaceutical	+	+	−
Dose (radiation exposure)	+	−	−
Repeatability	++	−	+
Reproducibility	+	+	+
Image quality	−	+	++
Segmental wall motion	−	+	++
Left ventricular ejection fraction	+	+	+
Left ventricular volumes	+	+	+
Right ventricular ejection fraction	++	++	+
Functional parameters and images	−	−	+
Use with interventions	+	+	++

* Advantages of the method in the respective category are noted in increasing order from − to + to ++.

TABLE 29.8 COMPARISON OF METHODS*

	Two-Dimensional/Doppler Echocardiography	Equilibrium Blood Pool Scintigraphy
Technique	−	+
Quality control	−	+
Computer applications	−	++
Acquisition time	+	+
Processing time	++	−
Radiation exposure	++	−
Repeatability	+−	−
Reproducibility	−	+
Patient applicability	−	+
Interpretation	−	+
Image quality	+	+
Segmental wall motion	+	+
Left ventricular ejection fraction	+	++
Ventricular volumes	+	++
Functional indices	−	++
Atrial, ventricular, and intracavitary anatomy	++	−
Valvular stenosis	++	−
Valvular regurgitation	+	++

* Relative advantages of each method are shown in progressive ability from − to +− to + to ++.

tion abnormalities, drug or electrolyte effects, pericarditis, or other concomitant conditions. "Hot spot" infarct imaging maintains its specificity.

Yet, the presence of cellular damage and pathophysiologic evidence of necrosis does not itself determine clinical management. Infarction with extensive necrosis would precipitate a conservative approach. However, prolonged or recurrent episodes of chest pain with evidence of only minimal necrosis, in the setting of unstable angina and evidence of enzyme release, would encourage an aggressive approach. Acute myocardial infarction scintigraphy adds to the specificity of infarction diagnosis and provides information relating to infarct size, localization, and prognosis. The method often provides better understanding of the clinical presentation and a more rational approach to patient management. Infarct scintigraphy appears to be of greatest value for infarct diagnosis in patients where acute electrocardiographic and enzymatic findings are nonspecific or unavailable.

DIAGNOSIS OF POSTOPERATIVE INFARCTION

The diagnosis of perioperative infarction can be difficult, especially following coronary bypass graft surgery. Although the appearance of new Q waves after bypass surgery seems significant, the diagnosis may still remain in doubt. The presence of prior infarction, conduction abnormalities, nonspecific ST-T abnormalities, and pericarditis-related repolarization changes frequently make electrocardiographic findings nonspecific.[277] In this setting, even the MB-CK fraction may not be a useful clinical indicator of significant myocardial necrosis following coronary bypass surgery.[270,277,278] Several studies have demonstrated infarct scintigraphy to be a useful adjunct for the diagnosis of perioperative infarction following revascularization.[274,279] Preoperative images may be of added utility in gauging the extent of perioperative necrosis, especially in the presence of a known or potential and relatively recent preoperative event. In this case, the high specificity but limited sensitivity of the method work to clinical advantage. Patients with negative images generally bear an excellent prognosis and a benign postoperative course, regardless of associated electrocardiographic or enzymatic findings, while positive images generally relate to new contraction abnormalities and reduced ejection fraction and, occasionally, clarify the cause of new symptoms after surgery.

EVALUATION POSTCARDIOVERSION

Another important diagnostic subgroup is composed of patients in whom cardioversion or defibrillation has been carried out. Frequently comprised of patients suffering unexpected hemodynamic collapse or survivors of out-of-hospital sudden death, confirmation or exclusion of

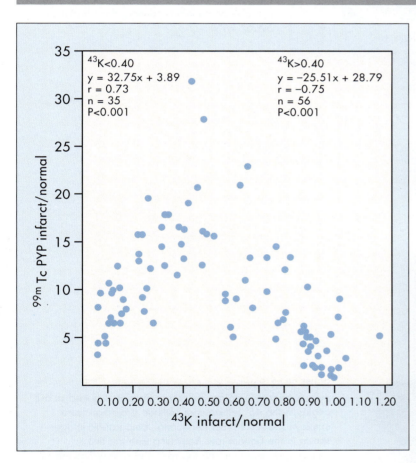

FIGURE 29.48 Relationship of ^{99m}Tc to perfusion. Shown is the relationship between ^{99m}Tc pyrophosphate (PYP) and ^{43}K infarcted and normal tissue. Although perfusion relates inversely to ^{99m}Tc pyrophosphate and apparent infarct density at high flow levels, at low flow levels, ^{99m}Tc pyrophosphate density also falls. (Modified from Zaret BL, DiCola UC, Donbedial RK et al: Dual radionuclide study of myocardial infarction. Circulation 53:422, 1976)

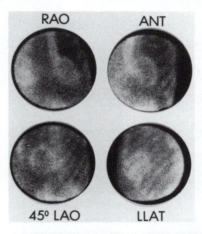

FIGURE 29.49 Doughnut configuration. Shown are ^{99m}Tc pyrophosphate images in multiple projections in a patient with a recent anterior lateral infarction. The doughnut configuration has been associated with a large infarct area and a poor prognosis, and may relate to poor central infarct perfusion. (Reproduced with permission from Botvinick E, Shames D: Nuclear Cardiology: Clinical Applications, p 5. Baltimore, Williams & Wilkins, 1979)

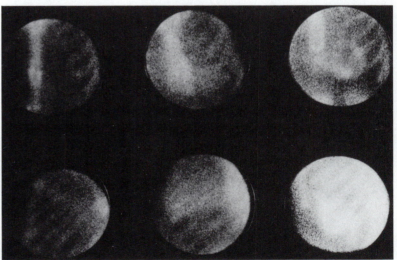

FIGURE 29.50 Patterns of ^{99m}Tc pyrophosphate uptake. Shown above, in the anterior projection, and below, in the lateral projection, are ^{99m}Tc pyrophosphate images with a normal distribution (left), diffuse radionuclide uptake (center), and discrete uptake (right). In the normal pattern, only bony structures are labeled. Discrete uptake is specific myocardial labeling. The diffuse pattern is nonspecific and likely represents blood pool activity. (Reproduced with permission from Botvinick E, Shames D: Nuclear Cardiology: Clinical Applications, p 5. Baltimore, Williams & Wilkins, 1979)

acute infarction is of considerable importance for both acute and chronic management. Yet, classification in this population may be difficult where persistent enzyme and electrocardiographic abnormalities may relate to the trauma of resuscitation or prior unrelated infarction or conduction abnormalities. Although false-positive studies have been reported with cardioversion,[279] the method appears to maintain its specificity post-coronary bypass graft surgery, even after direct electrical defibrillation,[280] and in the setting of catheter ablation of ectopic electrical foci or pathways. However, care must be taken to avoid confusion with chest wall uptake and, in turn, paddles must be placed judiciously to permit visualization of myocardial uptake.

INFARCT LOCALIZATION

The imaging method permits accurate infarct localization. While of some importance for prognostic value, this also facilitates the differentiation of current from prior infarction. With serial study, infarct imaging may permit the identification of infarct extension and its differentiation from other postinfarction pain syndromes.

A number of studies have demonstrated the relationship between right ventricular TcPYP uptake, right ventricular wall motion abnormalities, and inappropriate elevation of right-sided pressures (Fig. 29.54).[194] Such scintigraphic findings parallel pathologic findings and are seen in roughly one third of all acute inferior infarctions. TcPYP

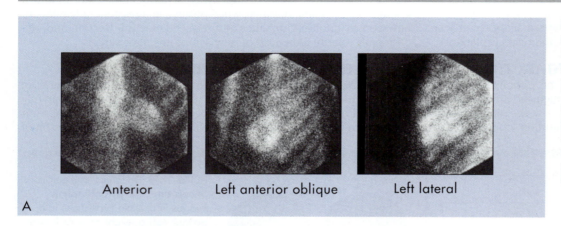

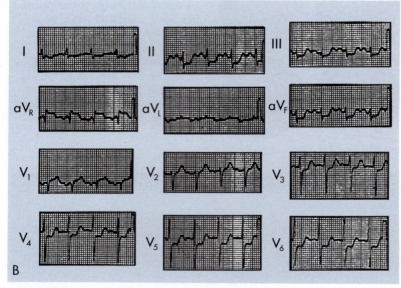

FIGURE 29.51 Extensive ^{99m}Tc pyrophosphate (TcPYP) uptake. **A.** The extensive pattern of TcPYP uptake illustrated in multiple projections is related to a poor prognosis. In surviving patients, it indicates a widespread subendocardial or shell infarction. **B.** The related electrocardiogram shows widespread ST segment depression without Q waves. (Reproduced with permission from Botvinick E, Shames D et al: Acute myocardial infarction: Clinical application of technetium 99m stannous pyrophosphate infarct scintigraphy. Circulation 59:257, 1979)

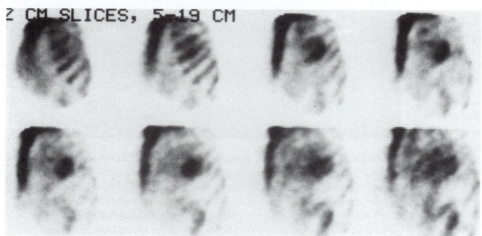

FIGURE 29.52 Rotating slant-hole tomographic ^{99m}Tc pyrophosphate imaging. Six planar images acquired at 60° angles in the 45° left anterior oblique projection were employed to reconstruct the normal tomographic images shown in the bottom row. Beginning with the first tomographic image in the top row, and proceeding left to right in this and the following row, the sternum and aspects of the ribs can be seen to come into and out of focus as slices are reconstructed from 5-cm to 19-cm depths at 2.0-cm intervals. The patient illustrated has an obvious apicolateral infarction.

imaging is the only specific direct, noninvasive method of diagnosing right ventricular infarction, which is of considerable clinical importance. To derive the full value of the method, technical errors must be avoided (Table 29.10).

PROGNOSTIC VALUE

Several reports have documented the relationship of infarct size to the development of power failure and an inverse relationship between estimates of infarct size and subsequent survival.[281] Imaging methods have been assessed for their ability to evaluate infarct size and assess methods to limit its extent and related prognosis. Although some workers have shown a correlation between CK enzyme infarct size and projected image infarct area, it is not surprising, owing to differences in their mechanisms, to note disagreement in the relationship between the amount of enzyme release and the magnitude of image infarct size.[282] TcPYP image infarct size correlated well with the weight and projected area of infarction in living dogs.[265,283,284] In patients, the infarct area correlated inversely with the stroke work index and with morbidity and mortality postinfarction (Fig. 29.55).[282] Although it was possible to differentiate infarct survivors from nonsurvivors by infarct image area, it could not be used to prognosticate subgroups among survivors, as could the size of perfusion scintigraphic abnormalities and left ventricular ejection fraction (Fig. 29.56).[115,283]

NEW AGENT

Recently, interest has focused on the ^{111}In-labeled FAB fragment of antimyosin antibody to label acute infarction.[285,286] The agent appears quite specific for acute infarction. However, it requires 24 to 48 hours for clearance of background and deposits significant radioactivity in the liver, possibly interfering with visualization of inferior infarction. Animal and patient studies thus far conducted indicate excellent diagnostic accuracy and acceptable imaging characteristics. Most enticing is the independence of agent localization from regional flow. This could make localization a more direct function of infarct density and presents an excellent prospect for accurate infarct sizing.

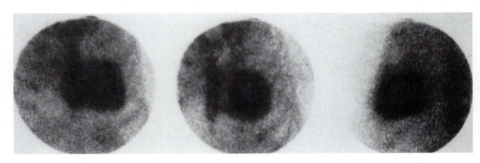

FIGURE 29.53 ^{99m}Tc pyrophosphate in amyloidosis. Shown are markedly abnormal ^{99m}Tc pyrophosphate images in (*left to right*) anterior, left anterior oblique, and left lateral projections acquired in a patient with primary amyloidosis. (Courtesy of Dr. R. Lull, Letterman Army Hospital, San Francisco, California)

TABLE 29.9 RELATIVE ACCURACY OF INFARCT DIAGNOSTIC METHODS

Sensitivity
Serial electrocardiogram changes
Wall motion abnormalities
Enzyme (CK-MB) abnormalities
Perfusion image abnormalities
Focal ^{99m}Tc pyrophosphate abnormalities

Specificity
Enzyme (CK-MB) abnormalities
Focal ^{99m}Tc pyrophosphate abnormalities
Serial electrocardiogram changes
Perfusion image abnormalities
Wall motion abnormalities

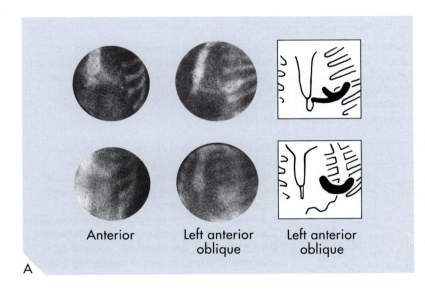
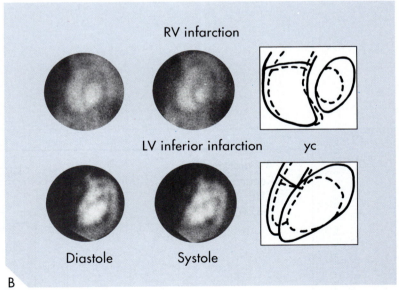

FIGURE 29.54 Right ventricular infarction. **A.** Shown are ^{99m}Tc pyrophosphate images in a patient with inferior (*below*) and **B.** added right ventricular infarction (*above*). The presence of right ventricular infarction is appreciated by the horizontal extension of radioactivity from the inferior left ventricular wall to the sternum in the left anterior oblique (*LAO*) projection. **B.** Blood pool studies in inferior infarction demonstrate related inferior contraction abnormalities, while right ventricular dysfunction is prominent in, but not specific for, right ventricular infarction. (Reproduced and modified from Sharpe DN, Botvinick E, Shames D et al: The noninvasive diagnosis of right ventricular infarction. Circulation 57:483, 1978)

SCINTIGRAPHIC EVALUATION OF HIGH-RISK CORONARY ARTERY DISEASE

A great deal of interest has been directed at the identification of coronary patients at greatest risk. This is appropriate in light of the extreme morbidity, mortality, tragedy, and suffering caused by coronary disease, as well as its cost. The importance of this effort increases along with our ability to modify that risk.

CLINICAL MEASURES OF HIGH RISK

A variety of clinical parameters, including historical factors, behavioral characteristics, and hemodynamic and anatomical variables, are known to affect the overall risk and prognosis of patients with coronary disease. Risk is certainly related to the amount of scarred myocardium.[281,287] Most important among prognostic indicators are those related to the total amount of myocardium permanently lost or at reversible ischemic risk.

THE IMPORTANCE OF ANATOMY

Early natural history studies documented the reduced survival of patients with left main and multivessel coronary disease.[54] The presence of ventricular dysfunction reduced the survival in every anatomical subgroup.

THE CONTRIBUTION AND PROBLEM OF SURGICAL STUDIES

Even if anatomy were the single determinant of coronary risk, it would be difficult to identify patients on this basis at presentation.[288] Further,

TABLE 29.10 PITFALLS OF "HOT SPOT" INFARCT-AVID SCINTIGRAPHY

Uptake in bony structures: ribs, cartilage, spine
Blood pool radioactivity
Poor label—free pertechnetate
Early imaging—prior to radionuclide localization or infarct maturation
Late imaging
Superficial uptake

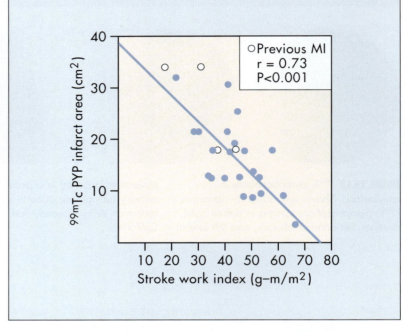

FIGURE 29.55 Function infarct size. Shown is the relationship between "hot" spot, ^{99m}Tc pyrophosphate (PYP) image infarct size and stroke work index, an index of ventricular function that correlates closely with patient prognosis. (Modified from Sharpe DN, Botvinick EH, Shames DM et al: The clinical estimation of acute myocardial infarct size with Tc-99m pyrophosphate scintigraphy. Circulation 57:307, 1978)

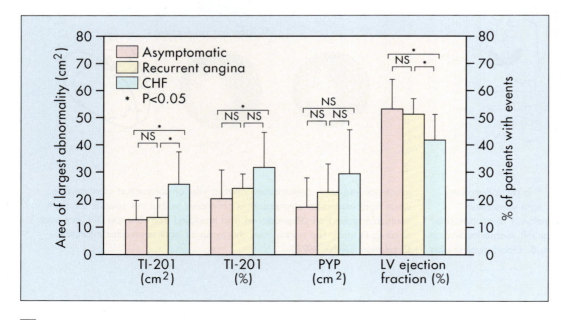

FIGURE 29.56 Scintigraphic prognosis. Perfusion defect size (Tl-201 [cm^2]) and left ventricular ejection fraction were the best discriminators of asymptomatic patients from those who suffered recurrent angina or heart failure (CHF) postinfarction. (PYP, Tc pyrophosphate image infarct size) (Modified from Perez-Gonzales J, Botvinick E, Dunn R et al: The late prognostic value of acute scintigraphic measurements of myocardial infarction size. Circulation 66:960, 1982)

the incidence of such high-risk anatomy varies widely in different coronary syndromes.[173,289] A number of controlled studies have demonstrated a limited but significant benefit of surgical intervention in the presence of triple-vessel disease, especially when related to reduced left ventricular function, and a greater benefit in the setting of left main coronary artery disease. Yet, not all patients in the groups at risk benefit from the intervention, and surgery must be performed on many patients to provide a benefit to a few.[290-292]

Further, these studies often eliminated from analysis large numbers of patients with severe ischemic symptoms,[293] employed gross clinical markers and end points, and failed to utilize established pathophysiologic indicators of ischemia or recently developed image indicators of ischemia and infarction.[49,50] They also failed to consider the difference between coronary pathophysiology and anatomy, a factor of increased importance given the documented inaccuracy and variability of the visual evaluation of coronary stenosis.

None of these studies could document either an improvement in resting left ventricular function or reduction in subsequent infarction rate. However, numerous population studies have identified those with greatest likelihood of postsurgical functional improvement, and scintigraphic studies have identified myocardial segments at greatest risk and likelihood for improvement after revascularization.[58,59,154] Would study results differ if patient populations were expanded and more selectively classified?

THE REAL CULPRIT: SALVAGEABLE MYOCARDIUM AT ISCHEMIC RISK

Since surgery and angioplasty offer nothing to infarcted, scarred segments, the full and specific component of patients at greatest risk who have the greatest possibility of benefit are those with a large or significant component of salvageable myocardium at ischemic risk.[294] This group includes postinfarction patients with preserved left ventricular ejection fraction after an episode of pulmonary edema,[295] a subgroup of those previously noted by Schuster and Bulkley to have "ischemia at a distance."[296] These and other studies suggest that the patient at greatest risk of death from coronary disease is that individual who will have extensive nonfunctioning myocardium after the next event.[51,297]

IDENTIFICATION OF MYOCARDIUM AT ISCHEMIC RISK

The extent of myocardium at ischemic risk can best be currently identified by a variety of noninvasive pathophysiologic electrocardiographic and scintigraphic markers for ischemia. Reduced exercise duration,[298] a low achieved double product,[299] the presence of stress-induced symptomatology and hypotension,[300] as well as deep ST segment depressions, particularly downsloping and early in exercise,[301] and multiple extensive perfusion abnormalities have been highly correlated with the presence of main left or triple-vessel coronary disease.[302] Although scintigraphy seems to complement electrocardiography,[51,76-78,112] Canhasi and co-workers found that many more patients with "high-risk" anatomy could be identified by the presence of lung uptake or other supplementary scintigraphic indicators.[50]

GROUPING POPULATIONS ACCORDING TO CORONARY RISK

A recent thrust in cardiology research seeks to subgroup apparently high-risk populations in an effort to identify specific individuals at risk and estimate the presence and extent of reversible ischemia.[51,109,295] Such added prognostic discrimination permits the proper diagnostic and therapeutic focus to target invasive study and aggressive treatment at those who would most likely benefit, while excluding from such consideration patients not benefiting from it.

ADVANTAGES OF SCINTIGRAPHIC EVALUATION

While able to separate patients into differing prognostic subgroups, stress tests continue to remain relatively nonspecific and insensitive, lack localizing information, and find particular difficulty in the presence of resting baseline abnormalities.[295,303] Reports document the value of both perfusion and blood pool scintigraphy in interpreting the significance of electrocardiographic changes in the setting of baseline abnormalities[37] and the importance of "reciprocal" ST depressions outside an infarct zone,[304] of ST elevations within it,[305] and of T wave normalization. Multiple perfusion scintigraphic abnormalities identified patients who became hypotensive during stress on an ischemic basis[306] better even than did extensive coronary involvement. While the relative regional sensitivity of perfusion scintigraphy varies,[72,78] visual scintigraphic patterns specific for left main or triple-vessel disease have been identified.[76] While relatively insensitive, scintigraphic and electrocardiographic findings were complementary in identifying "high-risk" coronary lesions.[76,304] Jones and co-workers demonstrated a direct relationship between the extent of decremental ejection fraction response and the extent of coronary involvement.[150] Within each coronary subgroup, however, there were wide variations, possibly related to pathophysiologic but real variation in stress response in patients with otherwise similar anatomy. Could scintigraphic variability better reflect the underlying risk than even the anatomy? The results of stress perfusion and blood pool study can be critical in determining relative coronary risk.[51,307-310]

QUANTITATIVE COMPUTER ANALYSIS

Attention to supplementary perfusion indicators and the objective, quantitative application of computer methods, including tomographic displays and "washout" analysis, promise to add to our sensitivity for the identification of extensive myocardial ischemia.[21,39,40,43,78] With this should come a further increase in our ability to assess risk and related prognosis. As important as the identification of those at greatest risk could be the elimination from consideration of those with little risk.[80,81,311]

HIGH-RISK PATIENTS POSTINFARCTION

In the setting of acute infarction, the quantitative scintigraphic assessment of resting left ventricular ejection fraction and the extent of regional akinesis have been well correlated with survival.[171,281,287,312,313] Serial measures of left ventricular ejection fraction early and late after infarction have been identified as prognostic measures.[169] Further, the effect of nitroglycerin on regional ejection fraction and the findings on perfusion scintigraphy may predict those with associated viable but ischemic and nonfunctioning myocardium after the event.[57-59,154] Brown and co-workers determined that left ventricular ejection fraction was the leading independent indicator of risk after infarction, but in the absence of infarction it was the extent and distribution of scintigraphic perfusion abnormalities.[111] However, Gibson and co-workers have shown that multiple perfusion abnormalities predicted a high complication rate in patients with inferior infarction compared to the low rate seen in patients having isolated inferior defects.[304]

"HOT SPOT" IMAGING

These agents have been shown to correlate well with pathologic measures of acute infarction size in animals and in patients.[265,314] Image infarct size related inversely to left ventricular stroke work index and directly with prognosis in patients with crescendo angina[315]; negative images related to a benign prognosis. Poor prognosis was associated with a doughnut configuration,[260] persistent image positivity,[271] and large scintigraphic abnormalities.[316,317] Infarct images were prognostic but less discriminating than the scintigraphic evaluation of function or perfusion postinfarction. This likely relates to the fact that infarct imaging cannot offer the full identification of myocardium at reversible ischemic risk (see Fig. 29.56)[112,113] including regions of prior infarction and ongoing ischemia. Differences in size of abnormalities on perfusion or blood pool and infarct images may give clues to the extent and nature of myocardium at risk and related prognosis.

PERFUSION SCINTIGRAPHY POSTINFARCTION

Wackers and co-workers have documented the extreme diagnostic sensitivity of myocardial perfusion scintigrams during the early hours to days following acute infarction.[60,61] A postmortem study by Bulkley and co-workers identified a subgroup of patients demonstrating large perfusion scintigraphic abnormalities premortem but relatively smaller areas of pathologic scar, likely owing to the prior presence of significant ischemic myocardium.[318] Recently, Becker and co-workers documented the extreme complementary prognostic value of combined scintigraphic evaluation of perfusion defect size and left ventricular ejection fraction (Fig. 29.57).[112]

Gibson and co-workers have documented the value of predischarge perfusion scintigraphy for the identification of postinfarction patients at greatest risk for future cardiac events (Fig. 29.58).[51] Most revealing was the finding that the number and extent of perfusion abnormalities were the most important predictors of a subsequent event, more predictive than stress-induced ST depression or the documented presence of multivessel coronary disease. Further, neither did the presence of multivessel disease ensure a poor prognosis, nor did its absence ensure a benign prognosis. Hung and Corbett and co-workers[170,310] have each documented a strong independent relationship between the response on stress blood pool scintigraphy and the occurrence of subsequent events in the postinfarction period.

DIPYRIDAMOLE PERFUSION SCINTIGRAPHY

Perfusion scintigraphy during infusion of dipyridamole appears able to identify coronary disease and ischemic myocardium.[91] It is most valuable in patients unable to undergo dynamic stress, a group often at greatest coronary risk. The method appears to have prognostic value in important patient subgroups.[100,101]

THE CLINICAL APPROACH TO THE HIGH-RISK PATIENT

Several recent publications have sought to integrate the results of this body of literature in the evaluation and treatment of patients with known or suspected coronary disease. Silverman and Grossman[319] mention scintigraphic evaluation of ischemia prominently in their evaluation of risk and determination of treatment of coronary patients (Fig. 29.59). DeBusk and co-workers[320] recently noted that quantitative blood pool evaluation of resting function and stress scintigraphic identification of reversible ischemia complement standard stress testing in the identification of approximately 30% of the population at high coronary risk who would not otherwise be recognized. Such analysis appreciates the relative imperfection and complementary nature of all noninvasive methods. Accepting the numerous indicators of extensive coronary disease and, more specifically, of coronary events and risk, the modern, aggressive cardiologist applies historic, physical, electrocardiographic, and scintigraphic findings to selected patients for invasive study and revascularization. Even following catheterization, proper treatment can often be designed only after the appropriate evaluation of both physiologic and anatomical assessment. Depending on the combined evaluation and the personnel and skills available, the proper course of treatment can be chosen.

A CONSIDERATION OF SCINTIGRAPHIC COST EFFECTIVENESS IN CORONARY DISEASE EVALUATION

There are a host of studies that can be performed in the evaluation of patients with known or suspected ischemic heart disease. The characteristics of the ideal imaging method can be summarized by a number of parameters related to safety, cost, and clinical effectiveness. Bell assessed clinical efficacy or utility to be of three varieties: diagnostic efficacy, confirmed by comparison with the gold standard; manage-

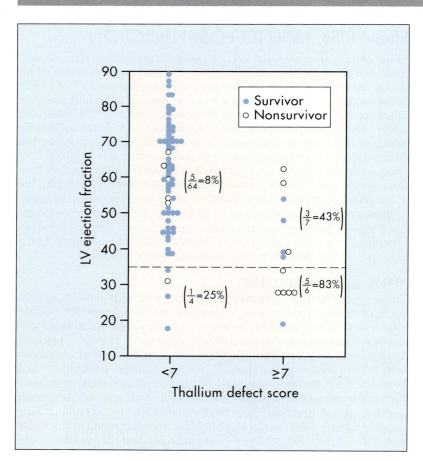

FIGURE 29.57 Prognosis postinfarction. In this study, the scintigraphic evaluation of left ventricular ejection fraction and the extent of the perfusion abnormality best subgrouped patients into risk subgroups. (Modified from Becker LC, Silverman KJ, Bulkley BH et al: Comparison of early thallium-201 scintigraphy and gated blood pool imaging for predicting mortality in patients with acute myocardial infarction. Circulation 67:1272, 1983)

ment efficacy, considering how a test influences management; and outcome efficacy, gauging the ability of the test to prognosticate the clinical outcome.[321] Scintigraphic study has been assessed from each of these perspectives.

One certain observation relates to the fact that if a test is not useful in a specific clinical situation, any advantage the test may have in other circumstances is lost. While pericardial effusion[219] and sometimes an intracavitary mass[218] can be seen on blood pool scintigraphy, or hypertrophy on perfusion scintigraphy,[62] the echocardiogram is the imaging test of choice for these abnormalities.[242,243] On the other hand, exercise echocardiography is qualitative and here scintigraphy appears to be the study of choice for the evaluation of ventricular function with stress or other intervention.[136,242,322] Cost effectiveness is clear in such situations: where the tests are of similar clinical value, the less expensive test is the clinically preferred; when the specific question clearly demands a given application, that test is to be applied. Neither do considerations related to ionizing radiation generally alter a scintigraphic preference if its advantages are otherwise apparent, since the exposure is small. Similar considerations must be made when seeking to noninvasively quantitate shunts,[149] the extent of valvular regurgitation,[278,298] or determine the location of a preexcitation pathway.[212] For these studies, there is no substitute and the choice simply relates to the clinical contribution of the data presented. Similarly, cost effectiveness of infarct-avid imaging is related to the need and ability to make the diagnosis and localize and quantitate the event without the study.[267,270,274,277,278]

Yet, cost effectiveness is often difficult to assess objectively, especially in relation to coronary disease, where the choices are numerous and varied. In considering cost effectiveness, a variety of situations and parameters must be considered. Obviously, the cost, advantages, and disadvantages of the test, the specific clinical question, and the patient population are important. Specifically, test predictive value will vary with the pretest disease likelihood, regardless of test accuracy. Any test will be somewhat less cost effective in a population with a relatively low prevalence.[323-325]

The ability of cardiac scintigraphy or any test to influence the pretest probability and come to a different post-test probability is greatest where the pretest probability is in an indeterminate range, that is, where the diagnosis is insecure.[104] Unlike the situation with populations at very low or very high levels of the scale, where test results do not strongly influence pretest probability, patients with an intermediate probability have the greatest realization of cost effectiveness.

Patterson and co-workers[106] evaluated the effects of perfusion scintigraphy on pretest probability calculated by the method of Diamond and Forrester.[108] The study illustrates test effectiveness in the diagnosis and exclusion of disease to be greatest when diagnosis is in doubt and the pretest probability is intermediate. They have also illustrated that test results in parallel (*e.g.*, an abnormal scintigram supporting an abnormal stress electrocardiogram) add a degree of diagnostic security. There is a certain potential benefit in using combined test diagnostic or predictive power. Conversely, since errors related to two tests are additive, such assessment must be carefully applied.[326]

Another study by Patterson and co-workers[105] evaluated cost effectiveness in terms of dollars and cents. Here, a theoretical population of 1000 men aged 45 was used as a model of test effectiveness for the assessment of asymptomatic coronary disease. Although costs have increased since the study publication, relative values and study conclusions still appear valid. By this analysis, were catheterization performed on patients presenting with both positive stress electrocardiogram and scintigram, rather than on all patients with a positive stress electrocardiogram alone, costs would be halved while still identifying 85% of those patients with significant coronary lesions. This excludes any benefits of eliminating the risk and discomfort of needless angiography and does not consider anatomical–pathophysiologic differences, which would add to the scintigraphic advantage.

In yet another analysis, these same investigators sought to assess coronary disease diagnosis and cost effectiveness in terms of years of life preserved in relation to four testing approaches.[105] The authors assessed costs in relation to disease prevalence as well. The lowest cost was seen in relation to the performance of angiography only if both stress test and scintigram were positive. On the other hand, when prevalence is plotted versus mortality, it is clear that this approach pays the greatest penalty for patient misdiagnosis in terms of mortality when both tests are required to be positive. Again, mortality was relatively low and stable at all prevalence rates, when angiography was done on all patients. The same data were assessed taking into account all possible factors and the cost per patient diagnosed was calculated. This parameter, most closely related to what we could call cost effectiveness, was lowest for the approach calling for angiography but only after positive scintigraphy. The difference was most significant at low disease prevalence, yet persisted to rates well over 50%. When test effectiveness was assessed in terms of survival, this approach again yielded the lowest cost per year of quality life preserved. This analysis is strictly based on diagnostic costs and fails to consider advantages related to less tangible values, which also must be factored into the cost-effectiveness equation.

This group also presented a cost-effectiveness analysis for coronary disease diagnosis in a population of 96 patients presenting with symptoms of unknown cause.[82] If stress testing, scintigraphy, and angiography were done on all patients, no patients with disease would be missed, but the cost per patient diagnosed would be high. If angiography is omitted when both stress electrocardiogram and scintigraphy are negative, or when the history is diagnostic, again no patients are missed, but the costs dramatically fall (Table 29.11). In addition to demonstrating cost effectiveness, this analysis also demonstrates the value of the scintigraphic method in excluding coronary disease. While these analyses demonstrate the interaction of tests in affecting costs, cost effectiveness must be assessed as well in terms of the diagnostic sacrifices we find acceptable. These considerations are as much ethical as clinical.

Patterson and co-workers performed a more complicated analysis in seeking to estimate the cost effectiveness of screening postinfarction patients for left main and triple-vessel disease.[74] Most cost effective was the performance of angiography on those patients with stress scintigraphic perfusion abnormalities outside the infarct zone or in those with other clinical or stress test indicators of extensive ischemia, and few patients were missed. Here, the use of all diagnostic and clinical parameters resulted in both high diagnostic and, if we recognize the poor prognosis related to the anatomy identified, outcome efficacy.

Dipyridamole perfusion scintigrams are performed in patients who cannot or should not undergo dynamic stress testing. These patients often have rest pain and, if this is ischemic in origin, it is related to severe coronary disease. Frequently, they are to undergo noncardiac surgery and are placed at significant coronary risk without any reasonable method of evaluation. Performing angiography in all of these patients is certainly ill advised, as abnormalities would be found. But could their related risk be evaluated or the anatomical information applied to properly determine the course of management?

In the initial population of 61 patients assessed with dipyridamole perfusion scintigraphy, we sought to evaluate test effects on clinical management.[99] We calculated pretest disease probability[108] and determined test influence on patient management by set criteria. These included patients with a low pretest probability and reversible image abnormalities who went on to catheterization or an aggressive medical management; patients with a high pretest probability and a benign image who were discharged or managed conservatively; and patients with an intermediate pretest probability or known coronary disease who were sent to image evaluation with ambiguous coronary anatomy and who demonstrated image findings consistent with subsequent management. The preliminary results were impressive, since dipyridamole scintigraphy influenced management in almost 80% of this initial group of patients with known or suspected coronary disease who could not undergo dynamic stress testing. Further, since scintigraphic and angiographic findings were generally consistent, such influence was apparently appropriate. The rate of such test influence is extremely high and relates to the diagnostic difficulty presented by these patients, the lack of acceptable diagnostic alternatives, and the need and willingness, more so in these patients, to let image results guide management decisions. This test then is an excellent example of high management efficacy as well as cost effectiveness. Studies have already been noted that demonstrate the potential outcome efficacy of the method.[100,101] Owing to such results and the findings of Gibson and other workers[51] documenting the value of the scintigraphic method in identifying coronary patients at greatest risk,[1-4,112,170,282,316,317] a number of recent publications indicate the importance of the role of stress scintigraphic study in the evaluation of patients with known or suspected coronary disease.[319,320]

The cost effectiveness of other diagnostic and therapeutic procedures is also of interest. In a study by Moorman and co-workers,[327] the value of 1410 rest electrocardiograms was assessed. The diagnostic yield was extremely small. Even regarding the rest electrocardiogram, the most benign test imaginable, there is still a question of cost effectiveness. Among those 775 done for screening, the electrocardiogram aided assessment in only 1% of patients, a calculated cost of $24,000 per life saved. The authors observed that much of the increased costs

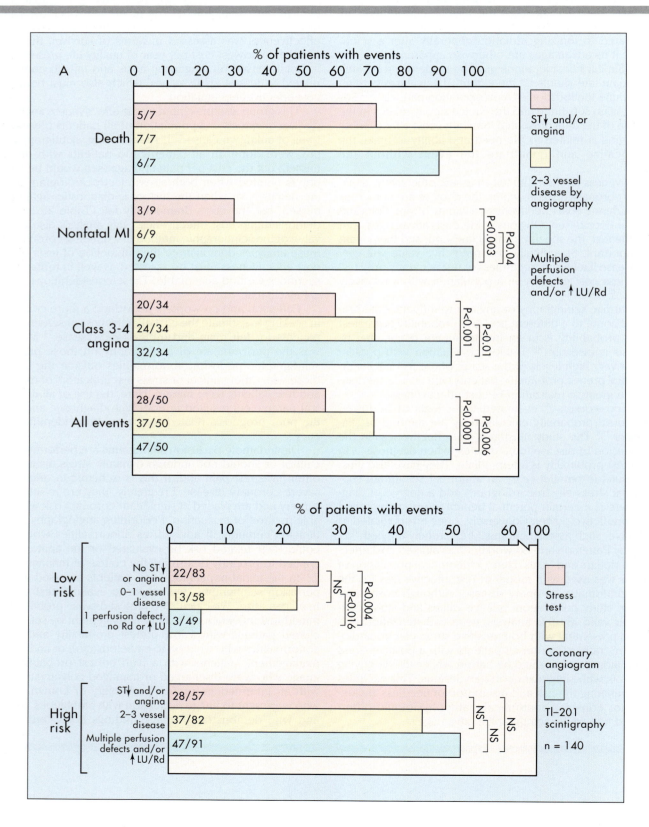

4.146

of current medical care is contributed by the widespread repeated use of individual inexpensive tests. Thus, just because a test is inexpensive, benign, and safe does not mean it is cost effective.

Evaluating coronary bypass surgery, one of the most expensive interventions, the net cost per quality-adjusted year of life gained ranges from $3800 for left main to $30,000 for single-vessel disease.[328] Again, cost effectiveness varies with the patient population as well as the anatomical and pathophysiologic nature of disease.

In this day and age, no methodology should be immune to extensive evaluation and review of cost effectiveness. The new high-tech modalities such as cine computed tomography, as well as more established methods such as echocardiography and angiography, must be evaluated as conventional scintigraphy has been. The more expensive the modality, the greater must be its demonstrated clinical advantage in order to justify its application. In the context of these new, expensive modalities, conventional scintigraphic methods must be seen as relatively inexpensive. The clinical value and expense of these tests should be evaluated in reference to the patient population and the specific clinical question being considered. Then, when the situation arises, the response will be appropriate and cost effective.

POSITRON EMISSION TOMOGRAPHY

Compared to conventional single photon scintigraphy, positron emission tomography (PET) is intrinsically tomographic and provides uniform high-efficiency event detection over an extensive field of view.[16]

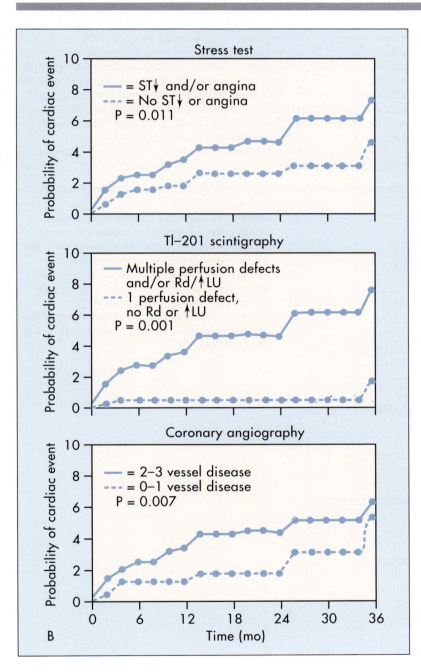

FIGURE 29.58 Prognosis of perfusion scintigraphy. **A.** Incidence of positive stress test ischemic ST depression or angina, two-or three-vessel coronary disease, or positive scintigrams—multiple perfusion defects or lung uptake (*LU*) with evidence of redistribution (*Rd*)—among patients who experienced death, nonfatal infarction (*MI*), severe angina, and all events along with the frequency of events among patients with and without these stress-induced, anatomic, or scintigraphic abnormalities. Scintigraphic findings were best both for identifying patients with highest risk of postinfarction events and separating high-risk from low-risk subgroups. Patients could not be subgrouped by any other parameter. **B.** Plotted for this same patient population is the probability, over time, of cardiac events in the presence or absence of stress test abnormalities, scintigraphic abnormalities, or multivessel coronary disease. Scintigraphy provided a significantly better separation of high-risk and low-risk subgroups than parameters noted or any others considered. (Modified from Gibson RS, Watson DD, Craddock GB et al: Prediction of cardiac events after uncomplicated myocardial infarction: A prospective study comparing predischarge exercise thallium-201 scintigraphy and coronary angiography. Circulation 68:321, 1983)

It provides high spatial resolution, inversely related to detector size and approaching 5 mm.[5,329] Resolution is independent of depth and preserved over a wide range of the solid angle of detection.[330,331] However, as detector size is reduced, sensitivity falls and instrument complexity and cost increase.[330,331] The high energy of the annihilation photon greatly reduces difficulties related to tissue attenuation so common with low-energy emitters such as ^{201}Tl. However, this high energy necessitates increased crystal thickness.[330,331] Further, technical correction for photon attenuation and characteristics of the method permit quantitation of tissue tracers.[330-332] Many positron emitters are short-lived, permitting repeated study with low radiation exposure but requiring rapid use (see Table 29.1).[16,330,331] Most important, the biologic nature of many such radionuclides, ^{11}C, ^{15}O, and ^{13}N, permits the formulation of radiopharmaceuticals, which can participate as substrates in metabolic processes.[330,333-337] This allows their application in the evaluation of myocardial metabolism. However, their generally brief half-life and mode of production make an on-site cyclotron necessary for application of many of these agents.[16,331,335]

A number of studies have demonstrated reduced regional uptake of both metabolic, ^{11}C palmitate, and perfusion markers, ^{82}Rb and ^{13}N ammonia, respectively, in myocardial infarction.[335,337,338] Positron imaging has demonstrated augmented perfusion in the hypertrophied septum of asymmetric septal hypertrophy.[339] The method has defined a specific pattern with reduced posterior wall perfusion and augmented glucose metabolism, in association with the cardiomyopathy of Duchenne's muscular dystrophy,[340] and metabolic analysis promises differentiation among other likely heterogeneous members of the currently ill-defined group of dilated cardiomyopathies.[341]

The metabolic consequences of ischemia have been imaged and applied to its diagnosis. A significant decline in the myocardial turnover rate of ^{11}C acetic acid, detected noninvasively with PET during exercise in patients with coronary disease, implies reduced activity of the citric acid cycle in ischemia.[338,342] Augmented myocardial ^{11}C palmitate uptake was noted following release of a short-duration coronary occlusion in dogs, while reduced ^{13}NH$_3$ uptake was detected distal to a coronary stenosis of even 47% following dipyridamole administration.[336] During fasting, the substrate of myocardial metabolism shifts from glucose to fatty acids. Persistent myocardial glucose utilization during fasting in regions of reduced perfusion monitored by fluorine-18 deoxyglucose (FDG) serves as the marker for ischemic myocardium and has been induced with rapid pacing (Fig. 29.60).[335,343] FDG 6-phosphate provides ample stability for imaging and is preferable to the more transient ^{11}C-labeled glucose. Visualization of such alterations with persistent image evidence of glucose metabolism in areas of apparent prior infarction appears to attest to regional tissue viability in an animal model.[343] Recently, myocardial regions of continued glucose utilization associated with abnormally perfused and contracting myocardial segments indicated viability in patient studies and served as a specific marker, superior to conventional perfusion scintigraphy, for functional improvement following revascularization.[344]

Both ^{13}NH$_3$ and ^{82}Rb distribute according to regional myocardial perfusion following their intravenous administration.[337,344-347] How-

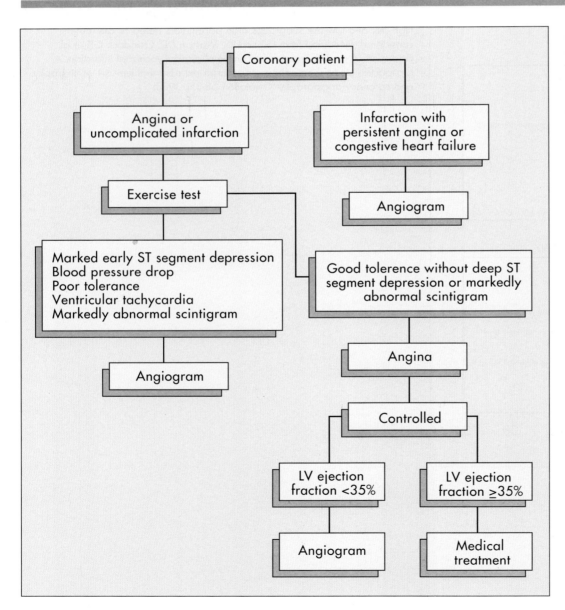

FIGURE 29.59 Coronary disease management. Shown is the relationship of scintigraphic studies with symptomatology and other test results in the determination of patient management. Left ventricular ejection fraction can be quantitatively and reproducibly calculated *only by blood pool scintigraphy*. (Modified from Silverman KJ, Grossman W: Angina pectoris: Natural history and strategies for evaluation and management. N Engl J Med 314:161, 1986)

ever, unlike most other positron emittors, ^{82}Rb is generator-produced,[347] making it potentially available as a positron perfusion agent without the need for an on-site cyclotron. Administered as a continuous infusion, its brief, 75-second half-life could permit performance of intervention evaluation in association with dipyridamole administration and baseline rest study even minutes apart. This would permit the efficient assessment of ischemia without the need for redistribution imaging, potentially increasing throughput with increased patient convenience and reduced radiation exposure compared to current methods employing ^{201}Tl.

Although gating and crude ventricular function evaluation is possible,[348] the major application of the method lies in the assessment of perfusion and metabolism. The method may provide insight into the underlying cause and earliest metabolic impairment of disease. With this comes the possibility of discriminating between currently indistinguishable conditions with individualization of therapy and of earlier disease recognition with the promise of more effective intervention. The work already done, the potential presented, and the more widespread commercial availability of perfusion and metabolically active positron imaging agents and imaging devices could make PET the next important clinical breakthrough in noninvasive cardiac imaging. Of course, the expense of method implementation and the success of current techniques make mandatory the careful evaluation of its relative diagnostic accuracy, clinical efficacy, and cost effectiveness before its conversion from its present research application to that of a widely applied clinical tool.

TABLE 29.11 ESTIMATED COST-EFFECTIVENESS OF EXERCISE TESTS TO EVALUATE PATIENTS WITH CHEST PAIN

Cost × Patients (n)	Total (Dollars)	Patients With CAD Who Would Be Missed (% of All CAD Patients)
All Tests in Every Patient		
Angiography $3000 × 96	$288,000	
Exercise tests $300 × 96	$ 28,800	
Total	$316,800	0%
Angiography Only		
Angiography $3000 × 96	$288,000	
Exercise tests $300 × None	$ 0	
Total	$288,000	0%
Avoid Angiography if Exercise Tests Are Both Negative		
Angiography $3000 × 79	$237,000	
Exercise tests $300 × 96	$ 28,800	
Total	$265,800	6%
Avoid Angiography if Exercise Tests Are Both Negative and Avoid Exercise Tests if History Reflects Typical Angina in a Patient Over 40 Years of Age		
Angiography $3000 × 82	$246,000	
Exercise tests $300 × 43	$ 12,900	
Total	$258,900	0%

(Reprinted with permission from Patterson RE, Horowitz SF, Eng C et al: Can exercise electrocardiography and thallium-201 myocardial imaging exclude the diagnosis of coronary artery disease? Am J Cardiol 49:1127, 1982)

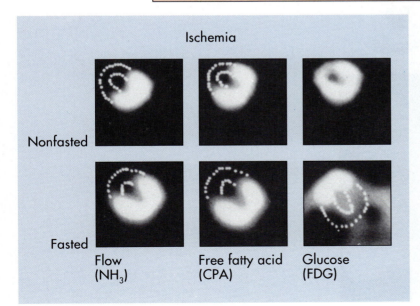

FIGURE 29.60 Metabolic PET imaging. Shown are myocardial PET images of perfusion using ^{15}N-labeled ammonia (NH$_3$), free fatty acid metabolism using ^{11}C-labeled palmitate (CPA), and glucose utilization using ^{11}F fluorodeoxglycose (FDG) acquired in fasted and nonfasted states. Fasting FDG uptake, glucose utilization in a region with reduced perfusion, indicates viable but ischemic myocardium (Reproduced with permission from Schelbert HR: The heart. In Ell PJ, Holman BL (eds): Computed Emission Tomography, p 91. Oxford, Oxford University Press, 1982)

SCINTIGRAPHIC EVALUATION OF CONGENITAL HEART DISEASE AND PEDIATRIC APPLICATIONS

Scintigraphic methods are particularly well suited to accurate, noninvasive evaluation of altered flow patterns and shunt quantitation in patients with congenital heart disease. With the growing capabilities of surgical methods, many of these patients are surviving longer and requiring evaluation for congenital disease well into adulthood.[349]

Both equilibrium blood pool and myocardial perfusion studies can be applied with clinical benefit to the pediatric age group.[124,161,191,350-353] Ventricular size and function evaluation is useful at rest and with dynamic stress in a variety of congenital lesions, both before and after surgical correction.[350,354-356] Residual structural and functional abnormalities are very common and careful, long-term follow-up is essential. It is also important to monitor age-related changes in myocardial function after appropriate interventions.[351,355-357]

In the pediatric patient, perfusion imaging has been most widely used for the noninvasive identification of the anomalous origin of coronary arteries.[351,352] Particularly, origin of the left coronary artery from the pulmonary artery produces a segmental scintigraphic abnormality on rest evaluation similar to that seen in association with extensive atheromatous involvement in adults. It is useful in the evaluation of newborns and infants presenting with an electrocardiographic pattern of infarction or unexplained deterioration in cardiac function. Perfusion abnormalities have also been induced with stress in adults with varieties of anomalous origin of the left from the right coronary artery. Evaluation of the resting pattern of ventricular perfusion and function can help differentiate segmental pathology related to large-vessel coronary disease from other causes including cardiomyopathy, myocarditis, and small-vessel embolization. Again, the pattern of ^{201}Tl uptake can suggest left or right ventricular hypertrophy and suggest the diagnosis of asymmetric septal hypertrophy.[53,62,148,157,191,192,339] In the smallest patients under a year of age, a converging or pinhole collimator should be applied to provide magnification. However, caution must be applied in analysis of such cases owing to the related field heterogeneity. While radionuclide dose should be regulated downward on a weight basis in small patients, no less than 5 mCi of ^{99m}Tc should be administered for blood pool or shunt evaluation.[358]

LEFT-TO-RIGHT SHUNT EVALUATION
FIRST-PASS METHOD

The scintigraphic study most widely applied to the evaluation of congenital disease is the first-pass evaluation of left-to-right shunts. However, while early methods aided diagnosis, they lacked reproducibility and were not reliable for quantitation.[359] The reliable scintigraphic method currently in widespread use employs the gamma variate method to analyze the pulmonary time versus radioactivity curve.[149] Clinically applied by Maltz and Treves, the method analyzes the transit of a compact radionuclide bolus, generally a variety of ^{99m}Tc, and optimally the rapidly excreted ^{99m}Tc DTPA, introduced into the central circulation.

As with first-pass methodology in general, the bolus should be ensured by injection into an external jugular vein or via a medial antecubital vein. The transit of the bolus is further monitored by imaging in the anterior projection as it courses through the heart and lungs and cardiac chambers, and into the systemic circulation. As with first-pass function analysis, a 2-minute acquisition is adequate. However, for shunt analysis, there is no need for the rapid acquisition rates required for function evaluation. Low-frequency acquisition should be performed at framing rates of two to four per second in adults and at somewhat faster rates in infants. The sequential flow study is reviewed in order to provide useful information regarding chamber orientation

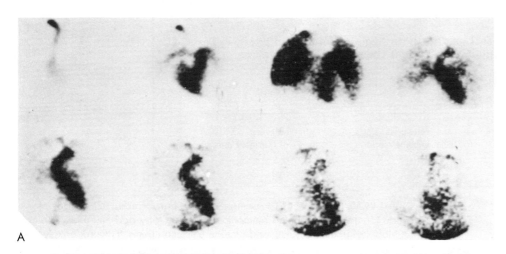

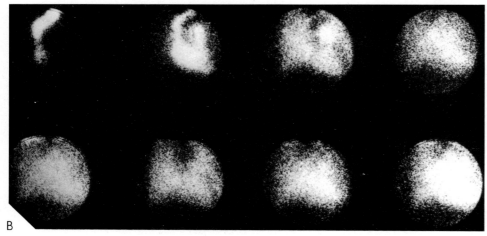

FIGURE 29.61 Radionuclide first-pass flow studies. Shown are radionuclide flow studies, progressing left to right in a patient without left-to-right shunt (A) and in a patient with left-to-right shunt (B). The absence of a levophase in the latter is consistent with a moderate to large shunt with a Qp/Qs over 1.5. (Reproduced with permission from Botvinick E, Schiller N, Shames D: The role of echocardiography and scintigraphy in the evaluation of adults with suspected left-to-right shunts. Circulation 62:1020, 1980)

and their vascular connections and even the presence and flow pattern through conduits. The absence of a good levophase is consistent with a moderate to large left-to-right shunt (Fig. 29.61). However, the levophase can be obscured as well by any condition that dilutes the bolus and is related to low flow or an enlarged right heart mixing volume. Regions of interest are drawn and time versus radioactivity curves generated over the superior vena cava to assess the quality of the bolus, and over the periphery of the right lung for actual shunt detection and quantitation. A second curve generated for the left lung may be of interest if differential shunting is suspected. Delivery of a single spike bolus, less than 3 seconds in duration, is essential to the success of the method. A fragmented bolus can give false positive results for shunt calculation. The pulmonary curve is inspected for a shoulder on the downslope, a clue to early shunt recirculation. A gamma variate, the algebraic expression describing intravascular flow and dye dilution,[360] is fit to the curve, down to the baseline. By dye dilution theory, the area under this fitted curve is proportional to pulmonary flow, Qp. The fitted curve is then subtracted from the raw data and the initial aspect of the remaining curve is again fit with a gamma variate. The area under the second fitted curve is proportional to the left-to-right shunt flow, Qsh. The difference between the two measured fitted areas is proportional to the systemic flow, Qs (Fig. 29.62). The resultant calculation of Qp/Qs is objectively performed by the computer on measured areas as

$$Qp/Qs = \frac{Qp}{Qp - Qsh}$$

Ratios less than 1.2:1 are consistent with the absence of left-to-right shunts. The Qp/Qs calculation is quantitative over a clinically significant range of 1.2:1 to 3.0:1. The gamma variate method has shown excellent agreement with shunt volume determined by oximetry. This relationship persists even in the presence of pulmonary hypertension, tricuspid regurgitation, and heart failure.[149,361] In these conditions, extensive dilution and slow flow lead to a slow downslope. However, the upslope should be proportionately slowed and the curve fit method should generally apply. Nevertheless, caution should be exercised in these cases. Since the method is predicated on the full passage of the administered radionuclide through the lungs, left-to-right shunts will be overestimated in the presence of right-to-left shunts.[362] Additionally, changes in shunt magnitude have been measured in response to oxygen therapy to assess the reactivity of the pulmonary vascular bed in patients with large shunts and pulmonary hypertension.[363]

CLINICAL APPLICATIONS. The method is most useful for quantitating known or suspected shunts in order to aid determination of its relation to symptoms and direct the clinical approach (Fig. 29.63). While anatomical information should not be disregarded, localizing the level of shunts by the scintigraphic method is difficult and depends on serial curve and image analysis. Such localization is not generally an indication for the method.[364] However, it serves as a strong complement to echocardiographic and Doppler and emerging magnetic resonance methods,[365] which frequently visualize the anatomical lesion.[242,243] A shunt caused by anomalous pulmonary venous return may be entirely missed on echocardiography.

EQUILIBRIUM APPROACH

It is possible as well, as noted above, to calculate the extent of left-to-right shunts using the stroke volume or amplitude ratio and the equilibrium blood pool approach. A good correlation (r = 0.79) has been noted between the shunt Qp/Qs ratio calculated from stroke volume ratios and oximetry.[366]

RIGHT-TO-LEFT SHUNT EVALUATION

Right-to-left shunts can be detected by inspection of the first-pass radionuclide angiogram, which reveals a premature appearance of left ventricular or aortic radioactivity (Fig. 29.64). Intravenous injections of an inert radioactive gas, such as ^{133}Xe or krypton-81m, can also be used for right-to-left shunt detection.[367] Significant systemic activity of these agents, which should be totally extracted by the lungs and exhaled in the alveolar gas, indicates shunting.

The most commonly used method is the intravenous injection of ^{99m}Tc-labeled MAA particles, similar to those used for invasive evalua-

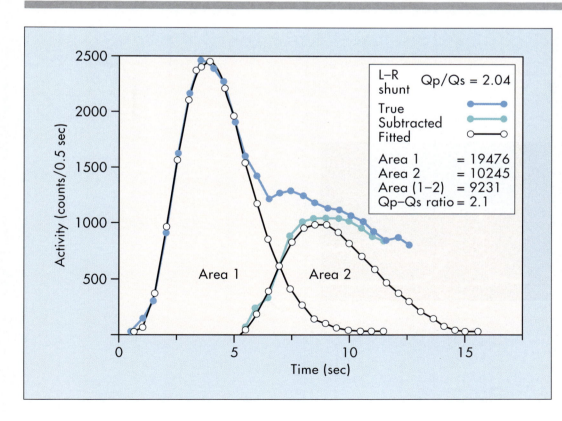

FIGURE 29.62 Left-to-right shunt calculation. Shown is a diagrammatic sketch of a time versus radioactivity curve generated from the right lung field of a patient with a left-to-right shunt, following a bolus radionuclide injection through a peripheral vein. A gamma variate function is fitted to the upslope and initial aspect of the downslope of the curve and the fitted curve is subtracted from the observed curve. A second gamma variate is fitted to the remaining curve. The ratio of fitted curve areas is used to detect the presence of left-to-right shunt, where area 1/area 2 − area 1 = Qp/Qs. The method permits accurate quantitation with Qp/Qs from 1.2 to 3:1. (Modified from Maltz DL, Treves S: Quantitative radionuclide angiocardiography: Determination of Qp:Qs in children. Circulation 47:1049, 1973)

tion of myocardial perfusion and the noninvasive assessment of pulmonary perfusion.[368] In the absence of right-to-left shunting, all of the particles are trapped in the pulmonary circulation. When right-to-left shunting occurs at any level, particles will enter the systemic circulation in proportion to the shunt flow, lodging in the capillary and precapillary beds of the systemic organs. A series of whole body images are taken to determine the percentage of right-to-left shunt as

$$\frac{\text{Whole body counts} - \text{lung counts}}{\text{Whole body counts}}$$

Such particle studies have shown a good correlation with catheterization values. In spite of the general reluctance to administer particles that will eventually lodge in the vascular network of the brain and kidneys, the method has proven quite safe. Nonetheless, caution

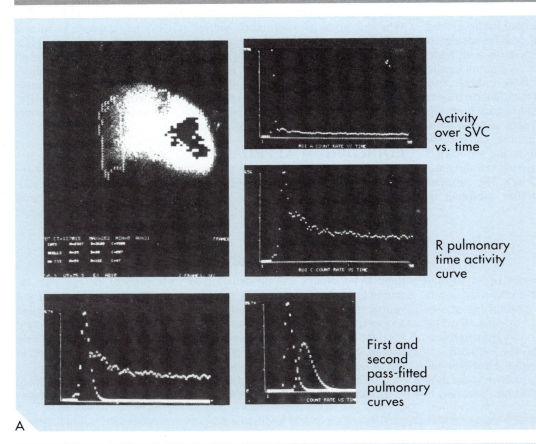

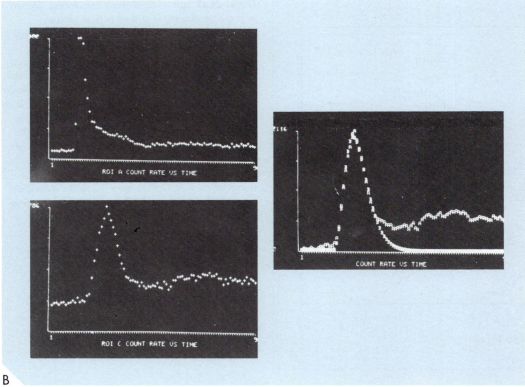

FIGURE 29.63 Atrial septal defect. **A.** Shown at upper left is the summary image marked with right (R) lung and superior vena cava (SVC) regions of interest (*upper left*), SVC and R pulmonary time versus radioactivity curves (*upper right*), and first-pass and second-pass fitted curves from the R lung region of interest (*below*) in a patient with an atrial septal defect and high Qp/Qs ratio. **B.** Shown are curves over the SVC and R lung regions of interest (*left*) in the same patient after atrial septal defect repair. The fitted lung curve reveals no significant shunt. (Reproduced with permission from Botvinick E, Schiller N, Shames D: The role of echocardiography and scintigraphy in the evaluation of adults with suspected left-to-right shunts. Circulation 62:1020, 1980)

should be applied and particle number kept low, preferably below 50,000.

THE SCINTIGRAPHIC EVALUATION OF PULMONARY THROMBOEMBOLISM

BACKGROUND

The history of perfusion lung scans is among the longest of nuclear imaging studies. It is directly traceable to Taplin's concept that biodegradable particles exceeding capillary dimensions could be deposited topographically in proportion to pulmonary perfusion.[369] If suitably labeled, these particles would render direct imaging of the pulmonary microcirculation. It soon became apparent that a normal perfusion lung scan ruled out the diagnosis of pulmonary embolism with extraordinarily high probability.

CLINICAL UTILITY

In spite of early observations, the clinical utility of perfusion lung scans remained problematic due to the lack of specificity of positive perfusion scans. Any cause of abnormal pulmonary perfusion, including primary ventilatory abnormalities, could result in a positive scan.[370-372] Many, if not the majority, of potential candidates for pulmonary embolism have parenchymal lung disease or ventilatory abnormalities. Nevertheless, lung scans were frequently useful, especially considering that the only option was contrast pulmonary angiography.

The use of concomitant ventilation imaging, made possible by the availability of an imageable radioactive gas, ^{133}Xe, and the widespread appearance of scintillation cameras simplified the diagnosis of pulmonary embolism.[373-378] It was found, as had been demonstrated experimentally, that perfusion impairment accompanied by abnormal ventilation was very rare in pulmonary embolism and, conversely, that perfusion impairment accompanied by normal ventilation was highly diagnostic of embolism.[375,379-382]

Further progress in the field followed the introduction and proliferation of ^{99m}Tc MAA. Improved spatial and contrast resolution of perfusion scans permitted the classification of perfusion defects into those representing bronchopulmonary segments and lobes typical of embolism and subsegmental and transsegmental distribution atypical of embolism. A series of studies carefully characterized ventilation/perfusion (V/Q) combinations in conjunction with a current chest x-ray film in patients with known pulmonary angiographic outcome.[380-389] Although retrospective, these studies permit classification of V/Q and chest x-ray findings into discrete probabilities predicting angiographic findings. These form the kernel of a matrix used to evaluate V/Q scans (Fig. 29.65). The retrospective approach was made necessary because a prospective study in which all patients underwent angiography, in spite of a broad spectrum of pretest probabilities, would needlessly endanger a large number of patients without emboli. Thus, these probabilities are likely overestimated for a more typical suspect patient population, and an element of clinical judgment must be reserved and applied in the image interpretation of V/Q studies.

"Matched and mismatched V/Q abnormalities" is common terminology. Matched abnormalities are improbable, whereas mismatched, ventilated but not perfused abnormalities are highly probable in pulmonary embolism. However, mismatches with nonventilated as opposed to poorly ventilated areas are probably not equivalent. Pulmonary embolism with infarction and a dense parenchymal infiltrate would show the former type of mismatch, and nonembolic abnormalities would show the latter. Other studies, similarly retrospective, have attempted to categorize embolism likelihood by the relative size of the parenchymal infiltrate compared to the perfusion defect. Another problem in interpreting V/Q scans is the presence of substantial ventilatory disease. Here, the specificity of the usual criteria used to infer embolism is impaired. This has been somewhat clarified by retrospective studies with angiographic outcome allowing a reordering of the probabilities based on a quantitative assessment of the magnitude of associated ventilatory impairment.[383,385,389]

PERFUSION IMAGING

The radiopharmaceuticals employed for perfusion evaluation are ^{99m}Tc MAA or human albumin microspheres. These particles range in size from 10μ to 50μ and occlude precapillary arterioles. About 3 mCi to 5 mCi of ^{99m}Tc tagged to 300,000 particles constitute a dose. Since there are 300,000,000 pulmonary precapillary arterioles, 0.1% of the pulmonary circulation is occluded.[390] In patients with significant pulmonary hypertension and presumably fewer precapillary arterioles, fewer particles, in the range of 100,000, are employed.[387] Images are obtained in multiple projections, assessed for number and distribution of perfusion abnormalities and to their correspondence with anatomical bronchopulmonary segments or lobes (Fig. 29.66). Symmetry of pulmonary perfusion is also noteworthy, in that a main branch partially occluding embolus will cause globally asymmetric pulmonary perfusion and, from a therapeutic standpoint, may be a critical finding.[391]

VENTILATION IMAGING

Ventilation is usually routinely carried out in association with perfusion imaging, but the choice of radiopharmaceutical and technique is not

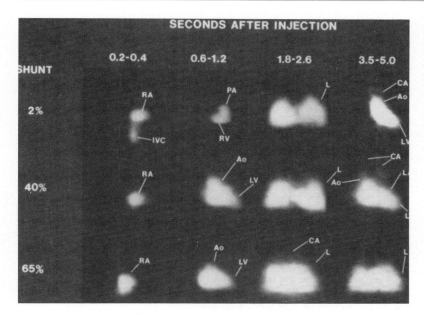

FIGURE 29.64 Scintigraphic flow studies in right-to-left shunts. The images depict tracer transit through the right heart, lung (L), and left heart in small children, ages 9 months to 3 years, with a 2% right-to-left shunt via a ventricular septal defect (top), a 40% right-to-left shunt with tetralogy of Fallot (middle), and a 65% right-to-left shunt related to transposition of the great vessels. (Ao, aorta; CA, carotid artery; IVC, inferior vena cava; LA, left atrium; PA, pulmonary artery; RA, right atrium) (Reproduced with permission from Peter C, Armstrong B, Jones R: Radionuclide quantitation of right-to-left shunts in children. Circulation 64:572, 1981)

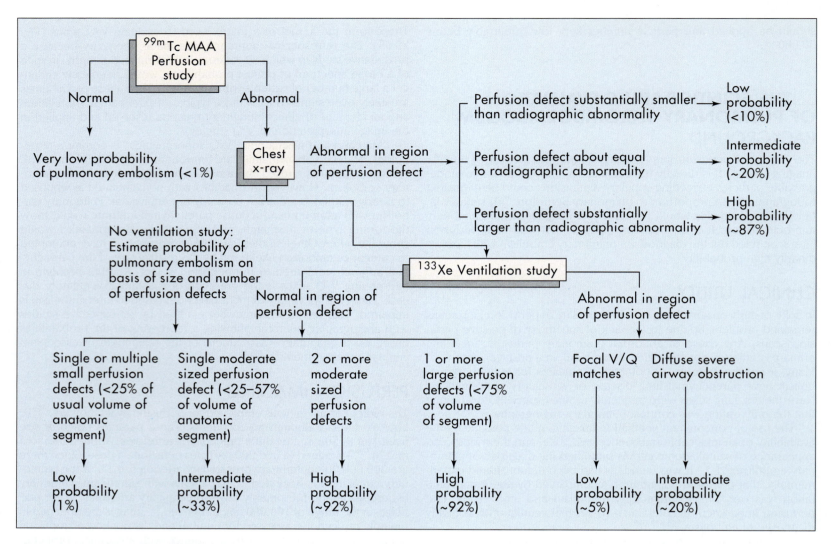

FIGURE 29.65 Embolus probability. Shown is an algorithm relating chest x-ray study and ventilation and perfusion scans to the probability of pulmonary embolus. The relationships are derived from references (adapted from a summary of available literature).

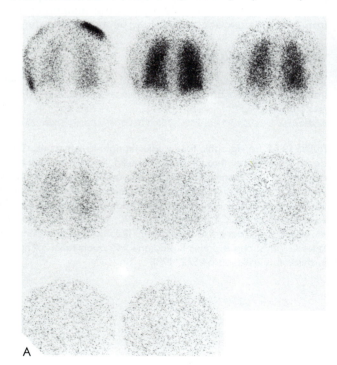

FIGURE 29.66 Normal V/Q scans. Shown are normal ^{133}Xe ventilation (**A**) and ^{99m}Tc MAA perfusion (**B**) scans in a patient with suspected pulmonary embolism. **A.** The ventilation scan is performed in the posterior projection. The single breath inhalation image (*above left*) is consistent with a poor effort. The equilibrium image, (*above center*) demonstrates homogeneous ventilation, and subsequent images acquired at 30-second intervals reveal excellent washout. **B.** Perfusion images are performed in posterior, right posterior oblique, left posterior oblique (*above, left to right*), left lateral, right lateral, and anterior (*below, left to right*) projections. Note the homogeneous distribution of radionuclide labeling. These studies are consistent with a low 1% probability of pulmonary embolus.

uniform. If one chooses to use ^{133}Xe, the ventilation scan must ordinarily be performed before the perfusion scan. Thus, the combined V/Q study costs about twice as much as an evaluation of perfusion alone. However, if the perfusion scan is normal, embolism is excluded with a probability of 0.99, and a ventilation scan is unnecessary. Because of these considerations, several methods of *post hoc* V/Q evaluation techniques have been advocated.[375,377,378,382,388]

The most readily available and acceptable ventilation study employs ^{133}Xe obtained prior to the perfusion ^{99m}Tc MAA perfusion scan. A spirometer is employed with the radioactive gas which, when exhaled, is vented to an absorbing device or to a suitable external vent to the outside atmosphere. Inhaled ^{133}Xe and oxygen are held while a posterior image is obtained, reflecting the first breath distribution. Theoretically, the first breath image distribution is a map of ventilation per unit volume. Subsequently, with the circuit closed, the patient is allowed to breathe for 3 to 5 minutes and an equilibrium distribution image is obtained. This image is theoretically a map of the total ventilated volume. The system is then vented, and a series of ambient gas dilution images is obtained consecutively for about 5 minutes. These images will reveal ventilation impairment by virtue of the topographic evaluation of retained radioactivity (Figs. 29.67 and 29.68).

A second approach to ventilation imaging is to image a relatively large 20 mCi to 30 mCi dose of ^{133}Xe during a breath-holding maneuver after the ^{99m}Tc perfusion scan is completed displaying abnormalities. The large ^{133}Xe dose dominates the image compared to the ^{99m}Tc Compton scattered photons, permitting acquisition of a relatively uncontaminated ventilation image. In this case, the projection utilized is optimized to best demonstrate the perfusion defect. Although it eliminates unnecessary ventilation studies when the perfusion study is normal, the fidelity of first breath distribution to true ventilation is poor.[377,378] Also, significant equilibration occurs during the 30 seconds of image acquisition, allowing lung parenchyma supplied by partially, but significantly, obstructed bronchioles to appear normal, resulting in false-positive findings. In a comparison study, first breath methods demonstrated a specificity of only 60% compared to washout images, a false-positive rate unacceptable to many, considering the economic justification.[377,378,388]

These problems of ^{133}Xe imaging are uniquely solved by ^{81m}Kr. The 13 second half-life daughter of ^{81}Rb can be easily obtained by a generator system in which the ^{81}Rb is absorbed to a matrix in a column. Flushing the column with oxygen washes out the ^{81m}Kr and can be directly administered to the patient by a face mask. This system is easily used, even in uncooperative, obtunded, or pediatric patients. Because of its short half-life, ^{81m}Kr represents no environmental hazard and, unlike ^{133}Xe, it does not require special venting or traps. A distinct advantage of ^{81m}Kr is that its principle photopeak energy is 191 keV, which allows uncontaminated images in the presence of ^{99m}Tc MAA, allowing ventilation evaluation after perfusion studies, thus avoiding unnecessary ventilation studies.[392-394]

^{81m}Kr images are physiologic representations of ventilation. Parenchyma with impaired ventilation appears as negative defects because the extremely short-lived ^{81m}Kr decays before reaching such regions. However, in spite of these substantial advantages, ^{81m}Kr presents two marked disadvantages. The short half-life of ^{81}Rb makes it impractical to have ^{81m}Kr continuously available. Yet, V/Q scans for pulmonary embolism are emergency studies necessarily available at all times.

Since ^{127}Xe has a principle photopeak energy of 170 keV, it can also be unambiguously imaged in the presence of ^{99m}Tc MAA, again avoiding the double costs entailed by ^{133}Xe studies.[394] However, it is not yet commercially available.

Aqueous ^{99m}Tc DTPA in an aerosolized form represents a significant competitor to ^{133}Xe for ventilation studies.[395] This was made possible by the advent of nebulizer technology, producing small (0.5-μ) uniform particles. The readily available ^{99m}Tc DTPA is injected into a disposable system and administered via a scuba-style mouthpiece for about 3 minutes. The exhaled activity is vented to a large plastic bag, allowing the undeposited particles to settle for later disposal. However, only about 3% of the activity is absorbed to bronchial surfaces, necessitating loading the nebulizer with large doses commonly approaching 50 mCi.[396] Handling of the apparatus also places an obligatory radiation exposure on the user. Although nebulized DTPA is not a gas, streaming and laminar flow may lead to a nonuniform distribution disproportionate to true ventilation. Furthermore, activity is frequently concentrated in the trachea and esophagus leading to, at minimum, distracting and, at maximum, misleading images.[396] In addition, since a time span of 3 minutes is employed to deliver the aerosol, equilibrium effects in regions of hypoventilation may be falsely represented as normal. In spite of these difficulties, many find aerosol imaging more convenient than ^{133}Xe, and high-quality investigations have shown essential equivalence in aerosol and gas images for evaluation of ventila-

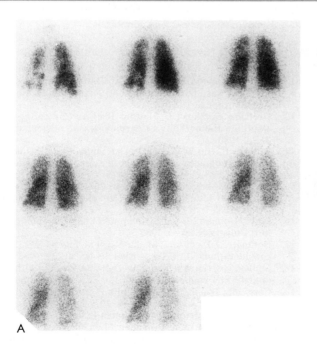

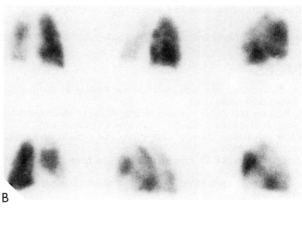

FIGURE 29.67 Nonspecific abnormal V/Q scans. Shown according to the format of the preceding figures are diffusely abnormal ^{133}Xe ventilation (**A**) and ^{99m}Tc perfusion (**B**) scans in a patient with chronic obstructive lung disease. These studies are consistent with an intermediate, approximately 20%, probability of pulmonary embolus.

tion.[396] Yet, it is necessary to do the aerosol image prior to the perfusion image, once again doubling the cost. Aerosol imaging does have cost advantages where ventilation is performed insufficiently frequently to justify maintaining continuous available ^{133}Xe in the facility. Like ^{81m}Kr and ^{127}Xe, it allows imaging in any desired projection, a specific advantage over ^{99m}Tc.

The maximum pretest probability of pulmonary embolism with a competent synthesis of all clinical, laboratory, and noninvasive roentgenographic information is only 50%. Considering the frequency of the disease in hospitalized patients, its mortality if undiagnosed, the success of treatment, and the potential danger of anticoagulating patients not needing anticoagulation, V/Q imaging has earned a strong role in evaluating patients for embolism. A thoughtful integration of V/Q scans and a current chest x-ray film logically to precise post-test probabilities of pulmonary embolism. This, in turn, permits reliable options to treat or not to treat, or to pursue further the diagnosis with pulmonary angiography, which will be required in no more than 15% of patients suspected of pulmonary embolism.[380–390,397]

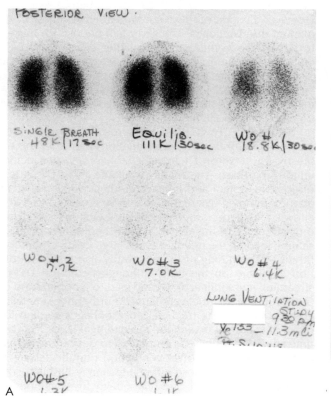 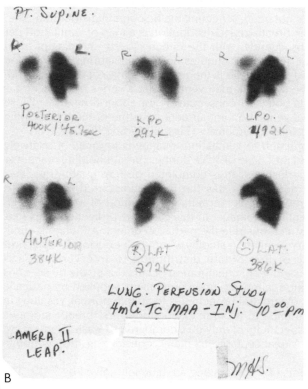

FIGURE 29.68 High-probability V/Q scans. Shown according to the same format are ^{133}Xe ventilation (**A**) and ^{99m}Tc perfusion (**B**) scans consistent with a high, over 92%, probability of pulmonary embolus. The ventilation study, as the chest x-ray film, is normal, while the perfusion scan reveals extensive segmental abnormalities.

REFERENCES

1. Freeman LM (ed): Freeman and Johnson's Clinical Radionuclide Imaging. Orlando, FL, Grune & Stratton, 1984
2. Freeman LM, Blaufox MD (eds): Cardiovascular Nuclear Medicine I–III: Seminars in Nuclear Medicine. Orlando, FL, Grune & Stratton, 1979
3. Beller G: Nuclear cardiology: Current indications and clinical usefulness. Curr Probl Cardiol 10:3, 1985
4. Cardiac Imaging Symposium I–VI. Prog Cardiovasc Dis 28:85, 1985; 29:434, 1986
5. Sorenson JA, Phelps ME (eds): Physics in Nuclear Medicine. Orlando, FL, Grune & Stratton, 1986
6. Bacharach SL, Green MV, Borer JS et al: ECG-gated scintillation probe measurement of left ventricular function. J Nucl Med 18:1176, 1977
7. Wagner HN Jr, Wake R, Nickoloff J et al: The nuclear stethoscope: A simple device for generation of left ventricular volume curves. Am J Cardiol 38:747, 1976
8. Steele PP, VanDyke D, Trow RW et al: Simple and safe bedside method for serial measurement of left ventricular ejection fraction, cardiac output and pulmonary blood volume. Br Heart J 136:122, 1974
9. Berger HJ, Davies RA, Batsford WP et al: Beat to beat left ventricular performance assessed from the equilibrium cardiac blood pool using a computerized nuclear probe. Circulation 63:133, 1981
10. Zema MJ, Restwig B, Munsey D et al: Potential pitfalls of the nuclear stethoscope. Clin Nucl Med 5:504, 1980
11. Lewellen T, Murano R, Weimen K, Graham M: The use of asymmetric energy windows. J Nucl Med 23:30, 1982
12. Vogel R, Kirsch D, LeFree M et al: Thallium-201 myocardial perfusion scintigraphy: Results of standard and multi-pinhole tomographic techniques. Am J Cardiol 43:787, 1979
13. Herfkens R, Shosa D, Hattner R et al: Clinical applications of rotating slanthole tomography to cardiovascular nuclear medicine. J Nucl Med 21:70, 1980
14. Holman B, Hill T, Wynne J et al: Single photon transaxial emission computed tomography of the heart in normal subjects and in patients with infarctions. J Nucl Med 20:736, 1979
15. Tamaki N, Mukai T, Ishii Y et al: Comparative study of thallium emission myocardial tomography with 180° and 360° data collection. J Nucl Med 23:661, 1982
16. Ell PJ, Holman BL (eds): Computed Emission Tomography. New York, Oxford University Press, 1982
17. Hoffman EJ, Ricci AR, Van der Stoe LM, Phelps ME: ECAT III—Basic design considerations. IEEE Trans Nucl Sci NS-30:729, 1983
18. Mullani NA, Gaeta J, Yerian W: Dynamic imaging with high resolution time-of flight PET camera—TOFPET I. IEEE Trans Nucl Sci NS-31:609, 1984
19. Goris ML, Daspit SG, McLaughlin P et al: Interpolative background image components. J Nucl Med 18:781, 1977
20. Ortendahl DA, Shosa DW, Kaufman L: Resolution and contrast recovery at depth in planar nuclear images. Phys Med Biol 27:257, 1982
21. Maddahi J, Garcia EV, Berman DS et al: Improved noninvasive assessment of coronary artery disease: Quantitative analysis of regional stress myocardial distribution and washout of thallium-201. Circulation 64:924, 1981
22. Goris ML, Briandet PA, Wynne J et al: A thresholding for radionuclide angiocardiography. Invest Radiol 16:115, 1981

23. Strauss HW, Harrison BS et al: Thallium 201: Noninvasive determination of regional distribution of cardiac output. J Nucl Med 18:1167, 1977
24. Zaret BL, Strauss HW, Martin ND et al: Noninvasive regional myocardial perfusion with radioactive potassium: Study of patients at exercise, rest and during angina pectoris. N Engl J Med 288:809, 1973
25. Botvinick EH, Shames DM, Gershengorn KM et al: Myocardial stress perfusion scintigraphy with rubidium-81 versus electrocardiography. Am J Cardiol 39:364, 1977
26. Nielsen AT, Morris KG, Murdock R et al: Linear relationship between the distribution of thallium-201 and blood flow in ischemic and non-ischemic myocardium during exercise. Circulation 61:797, 1980
27. Strauss HW, Harrison K, Langan JK et al: Thallium-201 for myocardial imaging. Relationship of thallium-201 to regional myocardial perfusion. Circulation 51:641, 1975
28. Beller GA, Watson DD, Pohost GM: Kinetics of thallium distribution and redistribution: Clinical applications in sequential myocardial imaging. In Strauss H, Pitt B, James AE (eds): Cardiovascular Nuclear Medicine, p 225. St Louis, CV Mosby, 1979
29. Beller GA, Watson DD, Ackell P et al: Time course of thallium-201 redistribution after transient myocardial ischemia. Circulation 61:791, 1980
30. Christie A: Ride a Pale Pony. New York, NY Pocket Books, 1982
31. Grumwald AM, Watson DD, Holzgrefe HH Jr et al: Myocardial thallium-201 kinetics in normal and ischemic myocardium. Circulation 64:610, 1981
32. Gould KL, Lipscomb K, Hamilton GW: Physiologic basis for assessing critical coronary stenosis. Instantaneous flow response and regional distribution during coronary hyperemia as measures of coronary flow reserve. Am J Cardiol 33:87, 1974
33. Britten JS, Blank M: Thallium activation of the Na^+–K^+ activated ATPase of rabbit kidney. Biochim Biophys Acta 159:160, 1968
34. Berger BB, Watson DD, Taylor GJ et al: Quantitative thallium-201 exercise scintigraphy for the detection of coronary artery disease. J Nucl Med 22:585, 1981
35. Pohost GM, Zir LM, Moore RH et al: Differentiation of transiently ischemic from infarcted myocardium by serial imaging after a single dose of thallium-201. Circulation 55:294, 1977
36. Garcia E, Maddahi J, Berman B et al: Space/time quantitation of thallium-201 myocardial scintigraphy. J Nucl Med 22:309, 1981
37. Botvinick EH, Taradash MR, Shames DM et al: Thallium-201 myocardial perfusion scintigraphy for the clinical clarification of normal, abnormal and equivocal electrocardiographic stress tests. Am J Cardiol 41:43, 1978
38. Ellestad MH: Stress Testing: Principles and Practice, 2nd ed, p 178. Philadelphia, FA Davis, 1980
39. Nohara R, Kambara H, Suzuki Y et al: Stress scintigraphy using single-photon emission computed tomography in the evaluation of coronary artery disease. Am J Cardiol 53:1250, 1984
40. Berger HJ: Nuclear medicine's revival: New drugs and cameras lead the way. Diagn Imaging 5:68, 1985
41. Massie B, Botvinick EH, Arnold S et al: Effect of contrast enhancement on the sensitivity and specificity of Tl-201 scintigraphy. Am Heart J 102:37, 1981
42. Botvinick EH, Dunn R, Hattner R et al: A consideration of factors affecting the diagnostic accuracy of thallium-201 myocardial perfusion scintigraphy in detecting coronary artery disease. Semin Nucl Med 10:157, 1980
43. Botvinick EH, O'Connell W, Hattner R et al: The color perfusion washout image provides advantages and insight. Circulation (Suppl) 72:III-424, 1985
44. Dunn R, Wolff L, Wagner S et al: The inconsistent pattern of thallium defects: A clue to the false positive perfusion scintigram. Am J Cardiol 48:224, 1981
45. VanTrain K, Maddahi J, Wong C et al: Definition of normal limits in stress Tl-201 myocardial rotational tomography. J Nucl Med 27:899, 1986
46. Kaual S, Chesler DA, Pohost GM et al: Influence of peak exercise heart rate on normal thallium-201 myocardial clearance. J Nucl Med 27:26, 1986
47. Friedman J, VanTrain K, Maddahi J et al: "Upward creep" of the heart: A frequent source of false positive reversible defection thallium-201 stress redistribution SPECT. J Nucl Med 27:899, 1986
48. Ohsuzu F, Handa S, Kondo M et al: Thallium-201 myocardial imaging to evaluate right ventricular overloading. Circulation 61:620, 1980
49. Boucher CA, Zir LM, Beller GA et al: Increased lung uptake of thallium-201 during exercise myocardial imaging: Clinical hemodynamics and angiographic implications in patients with coronary artery disease. Am J Cardiol 46:189, 1980
50. Canhasi B, Dae M, Botvinick E et al: The interaction of "supplementary" scintigraphic indicators and stress electrocardiography in the diagnosis of multivessel coronary disease. J Am Coll Cardiol 6:581, 1985
51. Gibson RS, Watson DD, Craddock GB et al: Prediction of cardiac events after uncomplicated myocardial infarction: A prospective study comparing predischarge exercise thallium-201 scintigraphy and coronary angiography. Circulation 68:321, 1983
52. Dunn RF, Freedman B, Bailey IK et al: Localization of coronary artery disease in exercise electrocardiography: Correlation with thallium-201 myocardial perfusion scanning. Am J Cardiol 48:837, 1981
53. Bulkley BH, Rouleau J, Strauss HW et al: Idiopathic hypertrophic subaortic stenosis: Detection by thallium-201 myocardial perfusion imaging. N Engl J Med 293:1113, 1979
54. Proudfit WL, Bruschke AVG, Jones FM: Natural history of obstructive coronary disease: Ten year study of 601 nonsurgical cases. Prog Cardiovasc Dis 21:53, 1978
55. Hammermeister KE, DeRouen TA, Dodge HT: Variables predictive of survival in patients with coronary disease. Circulation 59:421, 1979
56. Bateman TM, Maddahi J, Gray RJ et al: Diffuse slow washout of myocardial thallium-201: A new scintigraphic indicator of extensive coronary artery disease. J Am Coll Cardiol 4:55, 1984
57. Massie BM, Botvinick EH, Brundage BH et al: Relationship of regional myocardial perfusion to segmental wall motion: A physiologic basis for understanding the presence of reversible asynergy. Circulation 58:1154, 1978
58. Massie B, Botvinick E, Shames D et al: A physiologic basis for understanding the presence and reversibility of asynergy. Circulation 58:1154, 1978
59. Brundage BH, Massie BM, Botvinick EH et al: Improved regional ventricular function after successful surgical revascularization. J Am Coll Cardiol 3:902, 1984
60. Wackers FJT, Becker AE, Samson G et al: Location and size of acute transmural myocardial infarction estimated from thallium-201 scintiscans: A clinical pathological study. Circulation 56:778, 1977
61. Wackers FJT, Busemann-Sokole E, Samson G et al: Value and limitations of thallium-201 scintigraphy in the acute phase of myocardial infarction. N Engl J Med 295:1, 1976
62. Bulkley BH, Hutchins GM, Bailey I et al: Thallium-201 imaging and gated cardiac blood pool scans in patients with ischemic and idiopathic congestive cardiomyopathy: A clinical and pathologic study. Circulation 55:753, 1977
63. Makier PT, Lavine SJ, Denenberg BS et al: Redistribution on the thallium scan in myocardial sarcoidosis: Concise communications. J Nucl Med 22:428, 1981
64. Gaffney FA, Wohl AJ, Blomquist CQ et al: Thallium-201 myocardial perfusion studies in patients with the mitral valve prolapse syndrome. Am J Med 64:21, 1978
65. Wackers FJT, Lie KI, Liem KL et al: Potential value of thallium-201 scintigraphy as a means of selecting patients for the coronary care unit. Br Heart J 41:111, 1979
66. Brown KA, Okada RD, Boucher CA et al: Serial thallium-201 imaging at rest in patients with stable and unstable angina pectoris: Relationship of myocardial perfusion at rest to presenting clinical syndrome. Am Heart J 106:70, 1983
67. Iskandrian AS, Hakki AH, Kane SA et al: Rest and redistribution thallium-201 myocardial scintigraphy to predict improvement of left ventricular function after coronary artery bypass grafting. Am J Cardiol 51:1312, 1983
68. Rigo P, Bailey IK, Griffith LSC et al: Stress thallium-201 myocardial scintigraphy for the detection of individual coronary artery lesions in patients with and without previous myocardial infarction. Am J Cardiol 48:209, 1981
69. Ritchie JL, Zaret BL, Strauss HW et al: Myocardial imaging with thallium-201: A multicenter study in patients with angina pectoris or acute myocardial infarction. Am J Cardiol 42:345, 1978
70. Gibson RS, Beller GA: Should exercise electrocardiography be replaced by radionuclide methods? In Rahimtoola SH, Brest AN (eds): Controversies in Coronary Disease, p 1. Philadelphia, FA Davis, 1981
71. Berger BC, Watson DD, Taylor GJ et al: Assessment of the effect of coronary collaterals on regional myocardial perfusion using thallium-201 scintigraphy. Am J Cardiol 46:365, 1980
72. Massie B, Botvinick E, Brundage B: Correlation of thallium-201 scintigrams with coronary anatomy: Factors affecting region by region sensitivity. Am J Cardiol 44:616, 1979
73. Kirsch CM, Doliwa R, Buell V et al: Detection of severe coronary heart disease with thallium-201: Comparison of resting single photon emission tomography with invasive arteriography. J Nucl Med 24:761, 1983
74. Patterson RE, Horowitz SF, Eng C et al: Can noninvasive exercise test criteria identify patients with left main or three vessel coronary disease after a first myocardial infarction? Am J Cardiol 51:361, 1983
75. Rehn T, Briffith LSC, Achuff SC et al: Exercise thallium-201 myocardial imaging and left main coronary artery disease: Sensitive but not specific. Am J Cardiol 48:217, 1981
76. Dash H, Massie BM, Botvinick EH et al: The noninvasive identification of left main and three vessel coronary artery disease by myocardial stress perfusion scintigraphy and treadmill exercise electrocardiography. Circulation 60:276, 1979
77. Abdulla A, Maddahi J, Garcia E et al: Slow regional clearance of myocardial thallium 201 in the absence of perfusion defects: Contribution to detection of individual coronary stenoses and mechanism for occurrence. Circulation 71:72, 1985
78. Maddahi J, VanTrain KF, Prigent F et al: Quantitation of Tl-201 myocardial single photon emission computerized rotational tomography: Development, validation and prospective evaluation of an optimized computerized method. J Nucl Med 27:899, 1986
79. Gewirtz H, Paladino W, Sullivan M et al: Value and limitations of myocardial thallium washout rates in the noninvasive diagnosis of patients with triple vessel coronary artery disease. Am Heart J 106:686, 1983
80. Pamelia FX, Gibson RS, Watson DD et al: Prognosis with chest pain and normal thallium-201 exercise scintigrams. Am J Cardiol 55:920, 1985
81. Uhl GS, Kay TN, Hickman JR Jr et al: Computer enhanced thallium scinti-

grams in asymptomatic men with abnormal exercise tests. Am J Cardiol 48:1037, 1981

82. Patterson RE, Horowitz SF, Eng C et al: Can exercise electrocardiography and thallium-201 myocardial imaging exclude the diagnosis of coronary artery disease? Am J Cardiol 49:1127, 1982

83. Zir LM, Miller SW, Dinsmore RE et al: Interobserver variability in coronary angiography. Circulation 53:627, 1976

84. Cooperman M, Pflug B, Martin EW Jr et al: Cardiovascular risk factors in patients with peripheral vascular disease. Surgery 84:505, 1978

85. Rall TW: Central nervous system stimulants. In Gilman AB, Goodman LS, Gilman A (eds): The Pharmacologic Basis of Therapeutics, p 592. New York, Macmillan, 1984

86. Feldman RL, Nichols WW, Pepine CJ et al: Acute effect of intravenous dipyridamole on regional coronary hemodynamics and metabolism. Circulation 64:333, 1981

87. Gould KL: Noninvasive assessment of coronary stenosis by myocardial imaging during pharmacologic coronary vasodilatation: Physiologic basis and experimental vasodilation. Am J Cardiol 41:267, 1978

88. Okada RD, Leppo JA, Boucher CA et al: Myocardial kinetics of thallium-201 after dipyridamole infusion in normal canine myocardium and in myocardium distal to a stenosis. J Clin Invest 69:199, 1982

89. Beller GA, Holzgrefe HH, Watson DD: Effects of dipyridamole induced vasodilation on myocardial uptake and clearance kinetics of thallium-201. Circulation 68:1328, 1983

90. Becker LC: Conditions for vasodilator induced coronary steal in experimental myocardial ischemia. Circulation 57:1103, 1978

91. Leppo J, Boucher CA, Okada RD et al: Serial thallium-201 myocardial imaging after dipyridamole infusion: Diagnostic utility in detecting coronary stenoses and relationship to regional wall motion. Circulation 66:649, 1982

92. Jakubowski AT, Huckell VF, Cooper JA et al: Low dose oral dipyridamole produces coronary blood flow redistribution on thallium-201 myocardial imaging in patients with coronary artery disease. J Am Coll Cardiol 7:215A, 1986

93. O'Byrne GT, Maddahi J, VanTrain KF et al: Myocardial washout rate of thallium-201: Comparison between rest, dipyridamole with and without aminophylline, and exercise states. J Am Coll Cardiol 7:175A, 1986

94. Alonso S: Inhibition of coronary vasodilating action of dipyridamole and adenosine by aminophylline in the dog. Circ Res 26:743, 1970

95. Indolfi C, Giustino G, Piscione F et al: Intravenous dipyridamole in detecting coronary stenosis. Assessment by two-dimensional echocardiography and radionuclide angiography. J Am Coll Cardiol 7:212A, 1986

96. Ruddy TD, Dighero HR, Okada RD et al: Detection and localization of coronary artery disease with quantitation of dipyridamole thallium images. J Nucl Med 27:944, 1986

97. Josephson MA, Brown BG, Hecht HS et al: Noninvasive detection and localization of coronary stenosis in patients: Comparison of resting dipyridamole and exercise thallium-201 myocardial perfusion imaging. Circulation 66:649, 1982

98. Albro PC, Gould KL, Wescott RJ et al: Noninvasive assessment of coronary artery stenosis by myocardial imaging during pharmacologic coronary vasodilatation. III: Clinical trial. Am J Cardiol 42:751, 1978

99. Schechtmann N, Dae M, Lanzer P et al: The clinical impact of perfusion scintigraphy with dipyridamole. J Nucl Med 25:86, 1984

100. Boucher CA, Brewster DC, Darling RC et al: Determination of cardiac risk by dipyridamole thallium imaging before peripheral vascular surgery. N Engl J Med 312:389, 1985

101. Leppo JA, O'Brien J, Rothendler J et al: Dipyridamole thallium-201 scintigraphy in the prediction of future cardiac events after acute myocardial infarction. N Engl J Med 310:1014, 1984

102. Maseri A, Parodi O, Severi S et al: Transient transmural reduction of myocardial blood flow demonstrated by thallium-201 scintigraphy, as a cause of variant angina. Circulation 54:280, 1976

103. DiCarlo LA, Botvinick EH, Canhasi BS et al: Value of noninvasive assessment of patients with atypical chest pain in suspected coronary spasm using ergonovine infusion with thallium-201 scintigraphy. Am J Cardiol 54:744, 1984

104. Hamilton GW, Trobaugh GB, Ritchie JL et al: An analysis of clinical usefulness based on Bayes' theorem. Semin Nucl Med 8:358, 1978

105. Patterson RE, Eng C, Horowitz SF et al: Bayesian comparison of cost effectiveness of different clinical approaches to diagnose coronary artery disease. J Am Coll Cardiol 4:278, 1984

106. Patterson RE, Eng C, Horowitz SF et al: Practical diagnosis of coronary artery disease: A Bayes' theorem nomogram to correlate clinical data with noninvasive exercise tests. Am J Cardiol 53:252, 1984

107. Patterson RE, Eng C, Horowitz SF et al: Bayesian analysis of a nomogram of sequential tests for coronary disease: Indicators for exercise ECG and thallium-201 imaging. Clin Res 30:212A, 1982

108. Diamond GA, Forrester JS: Analysis of probability as an aid in the clinical diagnosis of coronary artery disease. N Engl J Med 300:1350, 1979

109. Iskandrian AS, Wasserman LA, Anderson GS et al: Merits of stress thallium-201 myocardial perfusion imaging in patients with inconclusive exercise electrocardiograms: Correlation with coronary angiograms. Am J Cardiol 46:553, 1980

110. DePace NL, Iskandrian AS, Nadell R et al: Variation in the size of jeopardized myocardium in patients with isolated left anterior descending coronary artery disease. Circulation 67:988, 1983

111. Brown KA, Boucher CA, Okada RD et al: Prognostic value of exercise thallium-201 imaging in patients presenting for evaluation of chest pain. J Am Coll Cardiol 1:994, 1983

112. Becker LC, Silverman KJ, Bulkley BH et al: Comparison of early thallium-201 scintigraphy and gated blood pool imaging for predicting mortality in patients with acute myocardial infarction. Circulation 67:1272, 1983

113. Botvinick EH, Perez-Gonzalez JF, Dunn R et al: Late prognostic value of scintigraphic parameters of acute myocardial infarction size in complicated myocardial infarction without heart failure. Am J Cardiol 53:1244, 1984

114. Gibson RS, Watson DD, Taylor GJ et al: Prospective assessment of regional myocardial perfusion before and after coronary revascularization surgery by quantitative thallium-201 scintigraphy. J Am Coll Cardiol 1:804, 1983

115. Greenberg BH, Hart R, Botvinick EH et al: Thallium-201 myocardial perfusion scintigraphy to evaluate patients after coronary bypass surgery. Am J Cardiol 42:167, 1978

116. Hirzel HO, Nuesch K, Gruentzig AR et al: Short and long term changes on myocardial perfusion after percutaneous transluminal coronary angioplasty assessed by thallium-201 exercise scintigraphy. Circulation 63:1001, 1981

117. Stuckey TD, Burwell LR, Nygaard TW et al: Value of quantitative exercise thallium-201 scintigraphy for predicting angina recurrence after percutaneous transluminal coronary angioplasty. J Am Coll Cardiol 5:531, 1985

118. DePuey EG, Roubin GS, Cloninger KG et al: Correlation of transmural coronary angioplasty parameters and quantitative thallium-201 tomography. J Nucl Med 27:900, 1986

119. Engelstad B, Wagner S, Herfkens R et al: Evaluation of the post-coronary artery bypass patient by myocardial perfusion scintigraphy and computed tomography. AJR 141:507, 1983

120. Maddahi J, Ganz W, Ninomiya K et al: Myocardial salvage by intracoronary thrombolysis in evolving acute myocardial infarction: Evaluation using intracoronary injection of thallium-201. Am Heart J 102:664, 1981

121. Osbakken MD, Okada RD, Boucher CA et al: Comparison of exercise perfusion and ventricular function imaging: An analysis of factors affecting the diagnostic accuracy of each technique. J Am Coll Cardiol 3:272, 1984

122. Berger H, Goldman L, Reduto HL et al: Global and regional left ventricular response to bicycle exercise in coronary artery disease: Assessment by quantitative radionuclide angiography. Am J Med 66:13, 1979

123. Borer JS, Bacharach SL, Green MV et al: Real time radionuclide cineangiography in the noninvasive evaluation of global and regional left ventricular function at rest and during exercise in patients with coronary artery disease. N Engl J Med 296:839, 1977

124. Alexander J, Dainiak N, Berger HF et al: Serial assessment of doxorubicin cardiotoxicity with quantitative radionuclide angiography. N Engl J Med 300:278, 1977

125. Borer JS, Rosing DR, Kent KM et al: Left ventricular function at rest and during exercise after aortic valve replacement in patients with aortic regurgitation. Am J Cardiol 44:1297, 1979

126. Rigo P, Alderson PO, Robertson RM et al: Measurement of aortic and mitral regurgitation by gated cardiac blood pool scans. Circulation 60:306, 1979

127. Williams SJ, Mousa SA, Morgan RA et al: Pharmacology of Tc-99m isonitriles: Agents with favorable characteristics for heart imaging. J Nucl Med 27:877, 1986

128. Kolibash AJ, Tetalman MR, Olsen JO et al: Intracoronary radiolabeled particulate imaging. Semin Nucl Med 10:178, 1980

129. Hamilton GW, Ritchie JL, Allen D et al: Myocardial perfusion imaging with ^{99m}Tc or ^{131m}In macroaggregated albumin: Correlation of the perfusion image with clinical, angiographic, surgical and histologic findings. Am Heart J 89:708, 1975

130. Wahr D, Ports T, Botvinick E et al: The effects of coronary angioplasty and reperfusion on myocardial flow distribution. Circulation 72:334, 1985

131. Danforth JW, Ports TA, Botvinick EH et al: Impact of sublingual nitroglycerin on the coronary collateral circulation in man. J Am Coll Cardiol 7:231A, 1986

132. Holman BL, Adams DF, Jewitt D et al: Measuring regional myocardial blood flow with ^{133}Xe and the Anger camera. Radiology 112:99, 1974

133. Klocke FJ, Bunnell IL, Green DG et al: Average coronary flow per unit weight of the left ventricle with and without coronary artery disease. Circulation 50:547, 1974

134. Cannon PJ, Schmidt DH, Weiss MB et al: The relationship between regional myocardial perfusion at rest and arteriographic lesions in patients with coronary atherosclerosis. J Clin Invest 56:1442, 1975

135. Selwyn AP, Forse G, Fox K et al: Patterns of disturbed myocardial perfusion in patients with coronary artery disease: Regional perfusion in angina pectoris. Circulation 64:83, 1981

136. Botvinick EH, Glazer H, Shosa D: What is the reliability and utility of scintigraphic methods for the assessment of ventricular function? Cardiovasc Clin 13(1):65, 1983

137. Ashburn WL, Schelbert HR, Verba JW: A review of several radionuclide angiographic approaches using the scintillation camera. Prog Cardiovasc Dis 20:267, 1978

138. Schelbert HR, Verba JW, Johnson AD et al: Nontraumatic determination of left ventricular ejection fraction by radionuclide angiocardiography. Circulation 51:902, 1975

139. Strauss HW, Zaret BL, Hurley PJ et al: A scintiphotographic method for

measuring left ventricular ejection fraction in man without cardiac catheterization. Am J Cardiol 28:575, 1971
140. Zaret BL, Strauss HW, Hurley PJ et al: A noninvasive scintigraphic method for detecting regional ventricular dysfunction in man. N Engl J Med 284:1165, 1971
141. Jengo JA, Mena I, Blaufuss A: Evaluation of left ventricular function, ejection fraction and segmental wall motion by single pass radioisotope angiography. Circulation 57:326, 1978
142. Pavel DG, Zimmer AM, Patterson VN: In vivo red blood cell labeling with ^{99m}Tc: A new approach to blood pool visualization. J Nucl Med 18:1035, 1977
143. Stewart GM: Researches on the circulation time and organs and on the influence which affect it. IV. The output of the heart. J Physiol 22:159, 1897
144. Marshall RC, Berger HJ, Cosbin JC et al: Assessment of cardiac performance by quantitative radionuclide angiography. Sequential left ventricular ejection rate and regional wall motion. Circulation 56:820, 1977
145. Harpen MD, Debulsson RL, Head B III et al: Determination of left ventricular volume from first pass kinetics of labeled red blood cells. J Nucl Med 24:98, 1983
146. Holman L: Radioisotope examination of the cardiovascular system. In Braunwald E (ed): Diseases of the Heart, p 309. Philadelphia, WB Saunders, 1980
147. Pierson RN Jr, VanDyke DC: Analysis of left ventricular function. In Pierson RN, Kriss JP, Jones RH, MacIntyre WJ (eds): New Qualitative Nuclear Cardiology. New York, John Wiley & Sons, 1975
148. Berger HJ, Matthay RA, Loke J et al: Assessment of cardiac performance with quantitative radionuclide angiocardiography: Right ventricular ejection fraction with reference to findings in chronic obstructive pulmonary disease. Am J Cardiol 41:897, 1978
149. Maltz OL, Treves S: Quantitative radionuclide angiocardiography. Determination of Qp/Qs in children. Circulation 476:1049, 1973
150. Jones RH, McEwan P, Newman GE: Accuracy of diagnosis of coronary disease by radionuclide measurement of left ventricular function during rest and exercise. Circulation 64:586, 1981
151. Bodenheimer MM, Banka VS, Fooshee CM et al: Comparison of wall motion and regional ejection fraction at rest and during isometric exercise. J Nucl Med 20:724, 1979
152. Poliner LR, Dehmer GJ, Lewis SE et al: Left ventricular performance in normal subjects: A comparison of the responses to exercise in the upright and supine positions. Circulation 62:528, 1980
153. Marshall RC, Berger HJ, Reduto LA: Assessment of cardiac performance with quantitative radionuclide angiocardiography. Effects of oral propranolol on global and regional left ventricular function in coronary artery disease. Circulation 58:808, 1978
154. Salel N, Berman D, DeNardo F et al: Radionuclide assessment of nitroglycerin influence on abnormal left ventricular segmental contraction in patients with coronary heart disease. Circulation 53:975, 1976
155. Williams DL, Hamilton GW: The effect of errors in determining left ventricular ejection fraction from radionuclide counting data. In Sorenson JA (ed): Nuclear Cardiology. Selected Computer Aspects: Symposium Proceedings, p 375. New York, Society of Nuclear Medicine, 1978
156. Burow R, Straus SH, Singleton R et al: Analysis of left ventricular function from multiple gated acquisition cardiac blood pool imaging: Comparison to contrast angiography. Circulation 56:1024, 1977
157. Maddahi J, Berman DS, Matsuoka DJ et al: A new technique for assessing right ventricular ejection fraction using multiple gated equilibrium cardiac blood pool scintigraphy. Circulation 60:581, 1979
158. Wackers FJ, Berger H, Johnston DE et al: Multiple gated cardiac blood pool imaging for left ventricular ejection fraction: Validation of the technique and assessment of variability. Am J Cardiol 43:1159, 1979
159. Borer J, Bacharach SL, Green MV: Exercise induced left ventricular dysfunction in symptomatic and asymptomatic patients with aortic regurgitation: Assessment with radionuclide cineangiography. Am J Cardiol 42:351, 1978
160. Rigo P, Murray M, Strauss HW et al: Left ventricular function in acute myocardial infarction evaluated by gated scintigraphy. Circulation 50:678, 1974
161. Dehmer GJ, Lewis SE, Hillis LD et al: Nongeometric determination of left ventricular volume from equilibrium blood pool scans. Am J Cardiol 45:293, 1980
162. Bunder RJ, Haluszcynski I, Langhammer H: In vivo/in vitro labeling of red blood cells with Tc^{99m}. Eur J Nucl Med 8:218, 1983
163. Hegge FN, Hamilton GW, Larson SM et al: Cardiac chamber imaging: A comparison of red blood cells labeled with Tc-99m in vitro and in vivo. J Nucl Med 19:129, 1978
164. Freeman M, Berman D, Stanloff H et al: Improved assessment of inferior segmental wall motion by the addition of 70-degree left anterior oblique view in multiple gated equilibrium scintigraphy. Am Heart J 101:169, 1981
165. Bacharach SL, Green MV, Borer JS: Instruments and data processing in cardiovascular nuclear medicine: Evaluation of ventricular function. Semin Nucl Med 9:257, 1979
166. Greenberg B, Drew D, Botvinick E et al: Evaluation of left ventricular volumes ejection fraction and segmental wall motion by gated radionuclide angiography. Clin Nucl Med 5:245, 1980
167. Green MV, Brody WR, Douglas MA et al: Ejection fraction by count rate from gated images. J Nucl Med 19:880, 1978
168. Okada RD, Kirshenbaum HD, Kushner FG et al: Observer variance in the qualitative evaluation of left ventricular wall motion and the quantification of left ventricular ejection fraction using rest and exercise multigated blood pool imaging. Circulation 61:128, 1980
169. Schelbert HR, Henning H, Ashburn WL et al: Serial measurements of left ventricular ejection fraction by radionuclide angiography early and late after myocardial infarction. Am J Cardiol 38:707, 1976
170. Corbett JR, Dehmer GJ, Lewis SE et al: The prognostic value of submaximal exercise testing with radionuclide ventriculography before hospital discharge in patients with recent myocardial infarction. Circulation 64:535, 1981
171. Nicod P, Corbett JR, Firth BG et al: Prognostic value of resting and submaximal exercise radionuclide ventriculography after acute myocardial infarction in high risk patients with single and multivessel disease. Am J Cardiol 52:32, 1983
172. Botvinick EH, Shames D, Hutchinson J et al: The noninvasive diagnosis of a false left ventricular aneurysm by gated blood pool imaging. Am J Cardiol 37:1089, 1976
173. Rapaport E, Remedio P: The high risk patients after recovery from myocardial infarction: Recognition and management. J Am Coll Cardiol 1:391, 1983
174. Ritchie JL, Sorensen SG, Kennedy JW et al: Radionuclide angiography: Noninvasive assessment of hemodynamic changes after administration of nitroglycerine. Am J Cardiol 43:278, 1979
175. Marshall RC, Wisenberg G, Schelbert HR et al: Effect of oral propranolol on rest, exercise and post-exercise left ventricular performance in normal subjects and patients with coronary artery disease. Circulation 63:572, 1981
176. Borer JS, Bacharach SL, Green MV et al: Effect of nitroglycerin on exercise induced abnormalities of left ventricular regional function and ejection fraction in coronary artery disease. Circulation 57:314, 1978
177. Pfisterer ME, Ricci DR, Schuler G et al: Validity of left ventricular ejection fractions measured at rest and peak exercise by equilibrium radionuclide angiography using short acquisition times. J Nucl Med 20:484, 1979
178. Gibbons RJ, Lee K, Cobb FR et al: Ejection fraction response to exercise in patients with chest pain, coronary artery disease and normal ventricular function. Circulation 66:643, 1982
179. Iskandrian AS, Hakki AH, Marsch SK et al: Prognostic implications of rest and exercise radionuclide ventriculography in patients with suspected or proven coronary heart disease. Am Heart J 110:135, 1985
180. Leong KH, Jones RH: Influence of the location of left anterior descending coronary artery stenosis on left ventricular function during exercise. Circulation 65:109, 1982
181. Bonow RO, Kent KM, Rosing DR et al: Exercise induced ischemia in mildly symptomatic patients with coronary artery disease and preserved left ventricular function: Identification of subgroups at risk of death during medical therapy. N Engl J Med 311:1339, 1984
182. Kent KM, Bonow RO, Rosing DR et al: Improved myocardial function during exercise after successful percutaneous transluminal coronary angioplasty. N Engl J Med 306:441, 1982
183. Borer J, Kent K, Bacharach SL: Sensitivity specificity and predictive accuracy of radionuclide cineangiography during exercise in patients with coronary artery disease. Circulation 60:572, 1979
184. Bonow RO, Rosing DR, Bacharach SL et al: Long-term effects of verapamil on left ventricular diastolic filling in patients with hypertrophic cardiomyopathy. Am J Cardiol 47:409, 1981
185. Bonow RO, Bacharach SL, Green MV et al: Impaired left ventricular diastolic filling in patients with coronary artery disease: Assessment with radionuclide angiography. Circulation 64:315, 1981
186. Maddox DE, Wynne J, Uren R et al: Regional ejection fraction, a quantitative radionuclide index of regional left ventricular performance. Circulation 59:1001, 1979
187. Pavel D, Sweryn S, Lam W et al: Ventricular phase analysis of radionuclide gated studies. Am J Cardiol 45:398, 1980
188. Slutsky R, Karliner J, Ricci D et al: Response of left ventricular volume to exercise in man assessed by radionuclide equilibrium angiography. Circulation 60:565, 1979
189. Links MJ, Becker LC, Shindledecker JG et al: Measurements of absolute left ventricular volume from gated blood pool studies. Circulation 65:82, 1982
190. Chang W, Henkin RE, Hals DJ et al: Methods of detection of left ventricular edges. Semin Nucl Med 10:39, 1980
191. Matthey RA, Berger HJ, Loke J et al: Right and left ventricular performance in ambulatory young patients with cystic fibrosis. Br Heart J 43:474, 1980
192. Maddahi J, Berman DS, Matsouka DT et al: Right ventricular ejection fraction during exercise in normal subjects and in coronary artery disease patients: Assessments by multi-gated equilibrium scintigraphy. Circulation 62:133, 1980
193. Rigo P, Murray M, Taylor DR et al: Right ventricular dysfunction detected by gated scintiphotography in patients with acute inferior myocardial infarction. Circulation 52:268, 1975
194. Sharpe N, Botvinick E, Shames D et al: The noninvasive diagnosis of right ventricular infarction. Circulation 57:483, 1978
195. Kolibash AJ, Leier CV, Bashore TM: Assessment of left ventricular pressure-volume relations using gated radionuclide angiography, echocardiography and micromanometer pressure recordings. Circulation 67:844, 1983
196. Wasserman AG, Katz RJ, Varghesi PJ et al: Exercise radionuclide ventriculographic responses in hypertensive patients with chest pain. N Engl J Med 311:1276, 1984

197. Brown JM, White CJ, Sobol SM et al: Increased left ventricular ejection fraction after a meal: Potential source of error in performance of radionuclide angiography. Am J Cardiol 51:1709, 1983
198. Sandler MP, Kronenberg MW, Forman MB et al: Dynamic fluctuations in blood and spleen radioactivity: Splenic contraction and relation to clinical radionuclide volume calculations. J Am Coll Cardiol 3:1205, 1984
199. Davies GJ, Chierchia S, Crea F et al: The use of a scintillation probe to investigate ischemic heart disease. J Nucl Med 22:23, 1981
200. Giles RW, Berger HJ, Barsh P et al: Left ventricular dysfunction during anesthesia induction for coronary artery surgery assessed with the computerized nuclear probe. J Nucl Med 22:17, 1981
201. Berger HJ, Hoffer PB, Steidley J et al: Serial assessments of left ventricular ejection fraction with the miniaturized Cadmium Telluride Detector Module: Potential technique for continuous monitoring of ventricular function. J Nucl Med 22:9, 1981
202. Lerman B, Lamphan R, Walton J: Count based left ventricular volume determination utilizing a left posterior oblique view for attenuation, correction. Radiology 150:831, 1984
203. Petru MA, Sorensen SG, Chandhuri TK et al: Attenuation correction of equilibrium radionuclide angiography: A noninvasive quantitation of cardiac output and ventricular volumes. Am Heart J 107:1221, 1984
204. Starling MR, Dell'Italia LI, Walsh RA et al: Accurate estimates of absolute left ventricular volumes from equilibrium radionuclide angiographic counts data using a simple geometric attenuation correction. J Am Coll Cardiol 3:789, 1984
205. Bourguignon MH, Schindledecker JG, Caret GA et al: Quantification of left ventricular volumes in gated equilibrium radioventriculography. Eur J Nucl Med 6:349, 1981
206. Bunker SR, Hartshorne MJ, Schmidt WP et al: Left ventricular volume determination from single photon emission tomography. AJR 144:295, 1985
207. Swiryn S, Pavel D, Byrom E: Sequential regional phase mapping of radionuclide gated biventriculograms in patients with ventricular tachycardia: Close correlation with electrophysiologic characteristics. Am Heart J 103:319, 1982
208. Dae MW, Botvinick EH, O'Connell W et al: Atrial corrected Fourier amplitude ratios for the scintigraphic quantitation of valvar regurgitation. J Nucl Med 25:36, 1984
209. Frais M, Botvinick E, Shosa D et al: Phase image characterization of localized and generalized left ventricular contraction abnormalities. J Am Coll Cardiol 4:987, 1984
210. Frais M, Botvinick E, Shosa D et al: Phase image characterization of ventricular contraction in left and right bundle branch block. Am J Cardiol 50:95, 1982
211. Ratib O, Heinze E, Schon H et al: Phase analysis of radionuclide ventriculograms for the detection of coronary artery disease. Am Heart J 104:1, 1982
212. Botvinick EH, Frais M, O'Connell W et al: Phase image evaluation of patients with ventricular pre-excitation syndromes. J Am Coll Cardiol 3:799, 1984
213. Colocci WS, Wynne J, Holman BL et al: Long-term therapy of heart failure with prazosin: A randomized double blind trial. Am J Cardiol 45:337, 1980
214. Nichols AB, McKusick KA, Strauss HW et al: Clinical utility of gated cardiac blood pool imaging in congestive heart failure. Am J Med 65:785, 1978
215. Kronenberg MW, Pederson RW, Harston WE et al: Left ventricular performance after coronary artery bypass surgery: Prediction of functional benefit. Ann Intern Med 99:305, 1983
216. Schwartz RG, Alexander J, McKenzie WB et al: Adherence to radionuclide angiocardiographic guidelines reduces the incidence and severity of congestive heart failure in high risk patients: The Yale doxorubicin cardiotoxicity study. J Am Coll Cardiol 7:24A, 1986
217. Nitsoh J, Seiderer M, Bull U et al: Evaluation of left ventricular performance by radionuclide ventriculography in patients with atrioventricular vs. ventricular demand pacemakers. Am Heart J 5:906, 1984
218. Pohost GM, Pastore JO, McKusick KA et al: Detection of left atrial myxoma by gated radionuclide cardiac imaging. Circulation 55:88, 1977
219. Berger HJ, Zaret BL: Radionuclide assessment of left ventricular performance. In Freeman LM (ed): Clinical Radionuclide Imaging, p 386. New York, Grune & Stratton, 1984
220. Bulkley BH, Hutchins GM, Bailey I et al: Thallium-201 imaging and gated cardiac blood pool scans in patients with ischemic and idiopathic cardiomyopathy. Circulation 55:753, 1977
221. Korr KS, Gandsman EJ, Winkler ML et al: Hemodynamic correlates of right ventricular ejection fraction measured with radionuclide angiography. Am J Cardiol 49:71, 1982
222. Bough EW, Gandsman E, Shulman R: Measurement of normal left atrial function with gated radionuclide angiography. Am J Cardiol 48:473, 1981
223. Viquerat CE, Hansen RM, Botvinick EH et al: Undrained bloody pericardial effusion in the early postoperative period after coronary bypass surgery: A prospective blood pool study. Am Heart J 110:335, 1985
224. Ramanathan KB, Bodenheimer MM, Banka VS et al: Severity of contraction abnormalities after acute myocardial infarction in man: Response to nitroglycerin. Circulation 60:1230, 1979
225. Simoons ML, Wijns W, Balakumaran K et al: The effect of intracoronary thrombolysis with streptokinase on myocardial thallium distribution and left ventricular function assessed by blood pool scintigraphy. Eur Heart J 3:433, 1982
226. Kirch D, Metz C, Steel P: Quantitation of valvular insufficiency by computerized radionuclide angiocardiography. Am J Cardiol 34:711, 1974
227. Baugh E, Gandsman E, North D et al: Gated radionuclide angiographic evaluation of valve regurgitation. Am J Cardiol 46:423, 1980
228. Sorensen SG, O'Rourke RA, Ghaudhur TK: Noninvasive quantitation of valvular regurgitation by gated equilibrium radionuclide angiography. Circulation 62:1089, 1980
229. Makler PJ Jr, McCarthy DM, Velchik MG et al: Fourier amplitude ratio: A new way to assess valvular regurgitation. J Nucl Med 24:204, 1983
230. Goris ML: Functional and parametric images. J Nucl Med 23:360, 1982
231. Wynne J, Sayres M, Moaddox DE et al: Regional left ventricular function in acute myocardial infarction: Evaluation with quantitative radionuclide ventriculography. Am J Cardiol 45:203, 1980
232. Wackers FJ, Berger HJ, Weinberg MA et al: Spontaneous changes in left ventricular function over the first 24 hours of acute myocardial infarction: Implications for evaluating early therapeutic interventions. Circulation 66:748, 1982
233. Dae M, Wen YM, Botvinick E et al: Assessment of left anterior fascicular block by scintigraphic phase analysis. J Am Coll Cardiol 3:591, 1984
234. Upton MT, Rerych SK, Newman GE et al: The reproducibility of radionuclide angiographic measurements of left ventricular function at rest and during exercise. Circulation 62:126, 1980
235. Boucher CA, Wilson RA, Kanarack DJ et al: Exercise testing in asymptomatic or minimally symptomatic aortic regurgitation. Relationship of left ventricular ejection fraction to left ventricular filling pressure during exercise. Circulation 67:1091, 1983
236. Caldwell JH, Hamilton GW, Sorensen SG et al: The detection of coronary artery disease with radionuclide techniques: A comparison of rest exercise thallium imaging and ejection fraction response. Circulation 61:610, 1980
237. Port S, Cobb FR, Coleman RE et al: Effect of age on the response of the left ventricular ejection fraction to exercise. N Engl J Med 303:1133, 1980
238. Polak JF, Kemper AJ, Bianco JA et al: Resting early peak diastolic filling rate: A sensitive index of myocardial dysfunction in patients with coronary artery disease. J Nucl Med 23:471, 1982
239. Kaul S, Boucher CA, Okada RD et al: Sources of variability in the radionuclide angiographic assessment of ejection fraction. A comparison of first pass and gated techniques. Am J Cardiol 53:823, 1984
240. Greenberg B, Drew D, Botvinick EH et al: Evaluation of left ventricular volume. Ejection fraction and segmental wall motion by gated radionuclide angiography. Clin Nucl Med 5:245, 1980
241. Ezekowitz MD, Leonard JC, Smith ED et al: Identification of left ventricular thrombi in man using indium-111 labeled autologous platelets. A preliminary report. Circulation 63:803, 1981
242. Schiller NB, Botvinick EH: Noninvasive quantitation of the left heart by echocardiography and scintigraphy. Cardiology Clinics, in press
243. Hatle L, Angelsen B: Doppler ultrasound in cardiology. In Hatle L, Angelsen B (eds): Physical Principles and Clinical Applications, p 221. Philadelphia, Lea & Febiger, 1982
244. West SR, Vasey CG, Armstrong WF et al: Comparison of continuous loop exercise echocardiography and thallium scintigraphy for detection of coronary artery disease. Circulation (Suppl) 72:III-58, 1985
245. Vasey CG, Armstrong WF, Ryan T et al: Prediction of the presence and location of coronary artery disease by digital exercise echocardiography. J Am Coll Cardiol 7:15A, 1986
246. Wiseman J, Rouleau J, Rigo P et al: Gallium-67 myocardial imaging for the detection of bacterial endocarditis. Radiology 120:135, 1976
247. Riba AL, Thakur ML, Gottschalk A et al: Imaging experimental infective endocarditis with indium-111 labeled blood cellular components. Circulation 59:336, 1979
248. O'Connell JB, Robinson JA, Henkin RE et al: Immunosuppressive therapy in patients with congestive cardiomyopathy and myocardial uptake of gallium-67. Circulation 64:780, 1981
249. Kramer RJ, Goldstein RE, Hirschfeld JW et al: Accumulation of gallium-67 in regions of acute myocardial infarction. Am J Cardiol 33:851, 1974
250. Holman BL, Lesch M, Zweiman FG et al: Detection and sizing of acute myocardial infarcts with $^{99m}Tc(SN)$ tetracycline. N Engl J Med 291:159, 1974
251. Rossman DJ, Rouleau J, Strauss HW et al: Detection and size estimation of acute myocardial infarction using ^{99m}Tc glucoheptonate. J Nucl Med 16:980, 1975
252. Shen AC, Jennings RB: Myocardial calcium and magnesium in acute ischemic injury. Am J Pathol 67:441, 1972
253. Bonte FJ, Parkey RW, Graham KD et al: A new method for radionuclide imaging of myocardial infarcts. Radiology 110:473, 1973
254. Coleman RE, Klein MS, Ahmed SA et al: Mechanisms contributing to myocardial accumulation of technetium-99m stannous pyrophosphate after coronary occlusion. Am J Cardiol 39:55, 1977
255. Zaret BL, DiCola UC, Donbedial RK et al: Dual radionuclide study of myocardial infarction. Circulation 53:422, 1976
256. Buja LM, Parkey RW, Dees JH et al: Morphologic correlates of technetium-99m stannous pyrophosphate imaging of acute myocardial infarcts in dogs. Circulation 52:596, 1975
257. Buja LM, Tofe AJ, Kulkarni PV et al: Sites and mechanisms of localization of technetium-99m phosphorous radiopharmaceuticals in acute myocardial infarcts and other tissues. J Clin Invest 60:724, 1977
258. Schelbert HR, Ingwall JS, Sybers HD et al: Uptake of infarct imaging agents in reversibly and irreversibly injured myocardium in cultured fetal mouse

259. Joseph SP, Ell PJ, Ross P: ^{99m}Tc imidodiphosphonate: A superior radiopharmaceutical for in vivo positive myocardial infarct imaging. Br Heart J 40:234, 1978
260. Rude RE, Parkey RW, Bonte FJ et al: Clinical implications of the technetium-99m stannous pyrophosphate myocardial scintigraphic "doughnut" pattern in patients with acute myocardial infarcts. Circulation 50:540, 1979
261. Parkey RW, Bonte FJ, Meyer SL et al: A new method for radionuclide imaging of acute MI in humans. Circulation 50:540, 1974
262. Prasquier R, Taradash MR, Botvinick EH et al: The specificity of the diffuse pattern of cardiac uptake in myocardial infarction imaging with technetium-99m stannous pyrophosphate. Circulation 55:61, 1977
263. Berman DS, Amsterdam DS, Hines H et al: New approach to interpretation of technetium-99m pyrophosphate scintigraphy in the detection of acute myocardial infarction. Am J Cardiol 39:341, 1977
264. Holman BL, Goldhaber SZ, Kirsch CM et al: Measurement of infarct size using single photon emission computed tomography and ^{99m}Tc-pyrophosphate: A description of the method and a comparison with patient prognosis. Am J Cardiol 50:503, 1982
265. Botvinick EH, Shames D, Lappin H et al: Noninvasive quantitation of myocardial infarction with technetium-99 pyrophosphate. Circulation 52:909, 1975
266. Massie BM, Botvinick EH, Werner JA et al: Myocardial infarction scintigraphy with technetium 99m stannous pyrophosphate: An insensitive test for nontransmural myocardial infarction. Am J Cardiol 43:186, 1979
267. Righetti A, O'Rourke RA, Schelbert N et al: Usefulness of preoperative and postoperative Tc-99m(SN) pyrophosphate scans in patients with ischemic and valvular heart disease. Am J Cardiol 39:43, 1977
268. Willerson JT, Parkey RW, Bonte FJ et al: Technetium stannous pyrophosphate myocardial scintigrams in patients with chest pain of varying etiology. Circulation 51:1046, 1975
269. Ahmed M, Dubiel JP, Logan KW et al: Limited clinical diagnostic specificity of technetium-99m stannous pyrophosphate myocardial imaging in acute myocardial infarction. Am J Cardiol 39:50, 1977
270. Klausner SC, Botvinick EH, Shames DM et al: The application of radionuclide scintigraphy to diagnose perioperative myocardial infarction following revascularization. Circulation 56:173, 1977
271. Lyons KP, Olson HG, Brown WT et al: Persistence of an abnormal pattern on ^{99m}Tc pyrophosphate myocardial scintigraphy following acute myocardial infarction. Clin Nucl Med 1:253, 1976
272. Botvinick EH, Shames DM, Sharpe DN et al: The specificity of technetium stannous pyrophosphate myocardial scintigrams in patients with prior myocardial infarction. J Nucl Med 19:1121, 1978
273. Poliner LR, Buja LM, Parkey RW et al: Clinicopathologic findings in 52 patients studied by technetium-99m stannous pyrophosphate myocardial scintigraphy. Circulation 59:257, 1979
274. Werner JA, Botvinick EH, Shames DM et al: Acute myocardial infarction: Clinical application of technetium 99m stannous pyrophosphate infarct scintigraphy. West J Med 127:464, 1977
275. Willerson JT, Parkey RW, Bonte FJ et al: Acute subendocardial infarction in patients. Circulation 51:436, 1975
276. Braun SD, Lisbona R, Novales-Diaz JA et al: Myocardial uptake of ^{99m}Tc-phosphate tracers in amyloidosis. Clin Nucl Med 6:244, 1979
277. Righetti A, Crawford MH, O'Rourke RA et al: Detection of perioperative myocardial damage after coronary artery bypass graft surgery. Circulation 5:173, 1977
278. Coleman RE, Klein MS, Roberts R et al: Improved detection of myocardial infarction with technetium-99m stannous pyrophosphate and serum MB creatine phosphokinase. Am J Cardiol 37:732, 1976
279. Pugh BR, Buja LM, Parkey RW et al: Cardioversion and "false positive" technetium-99m stannous pyrophosphate myocardial scintigrams. Circulation 54:399, 1976
280. Werner JA, Botvinick EH, Shames DM et al: Diagnosis of acute myocardial infarction following cardioversion: Accurate detection with technetium-99m pyrophosphate scintigraphy. Circulation 56:III-63, 1977
281. Page DL, Caulfield JB, Kaster JA et al: Myocardial changes associated with cardiogenic shock. N Engl J Med 285:133, 1971
282. Sharpe DN, Botvinick EH, Shames DM et al: The clinical estimation of acute myocardial infarct size with 99m technetium pyrophosphate scintigraphy. Circulation 57:307, 1978
283. Holman BL, Chishold RJ, Braunwald E: The prognostic implications of acute myocardial infarct scintigraphy with ^{99m}Tc-pyrophosphate. Circulation 57:320, 1978
284. Stokeley EM, Buja LM, Lewis SE et al: Measurement of acute myocardial infarcts in dogs with ^{99m}Tc-stannous pyrophosphate scintigrams. J Nucl Med 17:1, 1976
285. Khaw BA, Beller GA, Haber E: Experimental myocardial infarct imaging following intravenous administration of iodine-131 labeled antibody (Fab')2 fragments specific for cardiac myosin. Circulation 57:743, 1978
286. Berger H, Alderson L, Becker L et al: Multicenter trial of In-111 antimyosin for infarct-avid imaging. J Nucl Med 27:967, 1986
287. Burggraf GW, Parker JO: Prognosis in coronary artery disease: Angiographic, hemodynamic and clinical factors. Circulation 51:146, 1975
288. Block WJ Jr, Crumpacker EL, Dry TJ et al: Prognosis of angina pectoris: Observations in 6882 cases. JAMA 150:259, 1952
289. Bigger JT Jr, Heller CA, Wenger TL et al: Risk stratification after acute myocardial infarction. Am J Cardiol 42:202, 1981
290. Forrestor JS, Diamond G, Swan HJC: Classification of clinical and hemodynamic function after acute myocardial infarction. Am J Cardiol 39:137, 1977
291. Harris PJ, Lee KL, Harrell FE Jr et al: Outcome in medically treated coronary artery disease. Circulation 62:718, 1980
292. The Veterans Administration Coronary Artery Bypass Surgery Cooperative Study Group: Eleven year survival in the Veterans Administration randomized trial of coronary bypass surgery for stable angina. N Engl J Med 311:1333, 1984
293. Roberts WC, Manning MM: The coronary artery surgery study (CASS): Do the results apply to your patient? Am J Cardiol 54:440, 1984
294. Frais M, Botvinick EH, Shosa D et al: Are regions of ischemia detected on stress perfusion scintigraphy predictive of sites of subsequent myocardial infarction? Br Heart J 47:357, 1982
295. Warnowicz MA, Parker H, Cheitlin M: Prognosis of patients with acute pulmonary edema and normal ejection fraction after myocardial infarction. Circulation 67:330, 1983
296. Schuster EH, Bulkley BH: Early-post-infarction angina: Ischemia at a distance and ischemia in the infarct zone. N Engl J Med 305:1101, 1981
297. Taylor GJ, Humphries JO, Mellitis ED et al: Predictors of clinical course, coronary anatomy, and left ventricular function after recovery from acute myocardial infarction. Circulation 62:960, 1980
298. Bartel AG, Behar VS, Peter RH et al: Graded exercise stress tests in documented coronary artery disease. Circulation 49:348, 1974
299. Ellstad MH, Wan MKC: Predictive implications of stress testing. Follow-up of 2700 subjects after maximum treadmill stress testing. Circulation 51:363, 1975
300. Thompson P, Keleman M: Hypotension accompanying the onset of exertional angina. A sign of severe compromise of left ventricular ejection fraction. Circulation 52:28, 1975
301. Goldman S, Tselos S, Cohn K: Marked depth of ST segment depression during treadmill exercise testing. Indicator of severe coronary artery disease. Chest 69:729, 1975
302. Dagenais GR, Rouleau JR, Christen A et al: Survival of patients with a strongly positive exercise electrocardiogram. Circulation 65:452, 1982
303. Kattus AA: Exercise electrocardiography. In Amsterdam EA (ed): Exercise in Cardiovascular Health and Disease, p 161. New York, Yorke Medical Books, 1977
304. Gibson RS, Crampton RS, Watson DD et al: Precordial ST segment depression during acute inferior myocardial infarction: Clinical scintigraphic and angiographic correlations. Circulation 66:732, 1982
305. Haines DE, Beller G, Cooper A et al: Clinical, scintigraphic and angiographic correlates of exercise induced ST elevation, ten days after uncomplicated myocardial infarction. Circulation (Suppl)72:III-462, 1985
306. Hakki AH, Munley BM, Starvos H et al: Physiologic and anatomic determinants of abnormal blood pressure response to exercise in patients with coronary artery disease. Circulation (Suppl) 72:III-104, 1985
307. Chaitman BR, Brevers G, Dupras G et al: Diagnostic impact of thallium scintigraphy and cardiac fluoroscopy when the exercise ECG is strongly positive. Am Heart J 108:260, 1984
308. Boucher CA, Leonard M, Beller G et al: Increased lung uptake of thallium-201 during exercise myocardial imaging: Clinical, hemodynamic correlates and their relationship to coronary artery disease. Am J Cardiol 46:189, 1980
309. Weld FM, King-Lee C, Bigger JT et al: Risk stratification with low-level exercise testing 2 weeks after acute myocardial infarction. Circulation 64:306, 1981
310. Hung J, Goris M, Nash E et al: Comparative value of maximal treadmill testing, exercise thallium myocardial perfusion scintigraphy and exercise radionuclide ventriculography for distinguishing high and low risk patients soon after acute myocardial infarction. Am J Cardiol 51:361, 1983
311. Wackers FJ, Russo DJ, Russo D et al: Prognostic significance of normal quantitative planar thallium-201 stress scintigraphy in patients with chest pain. J Am Coll Cardiol 6:27, 1985
312. Dunn R, Botvinick EH, Benge W et al: The significance of nitroglycerin-induced changes in ventricular function after myocardial infarction. Am J Cardiol 49:1719, 1982
313. Misbach GA, Botvinick EH, Tyberg J et al: The functional implications of scintigraphic measures of ischemia and infarction. Am Heart J 106:996, 1983
314. Buja LM, Parkey RW, Stokely EM et al: Pathophysiology of technetium-99m stannous pyrophosphate and thallium-201 scintigraphy in acute anterior infarction in dogs. J Clin Invest 57:1508, 1976
315. Olson HG, Lyons KP, Aronow WS: The high risk angina patient: Identification by clinical features, hospital course, electrocardiography, and technetium 99m stannous pyrophosphate scintigraphy. Circulation 64:674, 1981
316. Olson H, Lyons K, Aronow W et al: Prognostic value of a persistently positive technetium-99m stannous pyrophosphate myocardial scintigram after myocardial infarction. Am J Cardiol 43:889, 1979
317. Holman LB, Chisolm RJ, Braunwald E et al: The prognostic implications of acute myocardial infarction scintigraphy with 99m technetium pyrophosphate. Circulation 57:326, 1978
318. Bulkley BH, Silverman KJ, Weisfeldt ML et al: Pathologic basis of thallium-201 scintigraphic defects in patients with fetal myocardial injury. Circulation 60:785, 1979
319. Silverman KJ, Grossman W: Angina pectoris: Natural history and strategies

320. DeBusk RF, Blomquist CG, Kouchoukos NT et al: Identification of low risk patients with acute myocardial infarction and coronary artery bypass surgery. N Engl J Med 314:151, 1986
321. Bell RS: Efficacy . . . What's that? Semin Nucl Med 8:316, 1978
322. Botvinick EH, Engelstad BL, Glazer HB et al: Blood pool scintigraphy of the heart: Current status. In Freeman LB, Wagner R (eds): Nuclear Medicine Annual. New York, Raven Press, 1982
323. Lusted LB: Introduction to Medical Decision Making. Springfield, IL, Charles C Thomas, 1968
324. Weinstein MC, Fineberg HV, Elstein AS et al: Clinical decision analysis. In Lusted LB (ed): Clinical Medicine. Philadelphia, WB Saunders, 1980
325. Weinstein MC, Stason WB: Foundations of cost effectiveness analysis for health and medical practices. N Engl J Med 296:716, 1977
326. Snedecor GW, Cochran WG: Statistical Methods, 6th ed. Ames, Iowa, Iowa State University Press, 1967
327. Moorman JR, Hlatky MA, Eddy DM et al: The yield of the routine admission electrocardiogram. Ann Intern Med 103:590, 1985
328. Weinstein MC, Stason WB: Cost-effectiveness of coronary artery bypass surgery. Circulation 66(Suppl 3):56, 1982
329. Budinger TF, Rollo FD: Physics and instrumentation. In Holman BL, Sonnenbleck EH, Lesch M (eds): Principles of Cardiovascular Nuclear Medicine, p 17. New York, Grune & Stratton, 1979
330. Goldstein RA, Mullani NA, Gould KL: Quantitative myocardial imaging with positron emittors. In Goodwin JF (ed): Progress in Cardiology, p 147. Philadelphia, Grune & Stratton, 1983
331. Phelps ME: Emission computed tomography. Semin Nucl Med 7:337, 1977
332. Henze E, Huang SC, Plummer D et al: Retrieval of quantitative information from positron emission computed tomographic images for cardiac studies with C-11 palmitate. J Nucl Med 22:21, 1981
333. Schelbert HR, Phelps ME, Hoffman EJ et al: Regional myocardial perfusion assessed with N-13 labeled ammonia and positron emission computerized axial tomography. Am J Cardiol 43:209, 1979
334. Ter-Pogossian MN, Klein MS, Markham J et al: Regional assessment of myocardial metabolic integrity in vivo by positron emission tomography with 11C labeled palmitate. Circulation 61:242, 1980
335. Marshall RC, Schelbert HR, Phelps ME et al: Evaluation of infarcted and ischemic myocardium with 18-fluoro-deoxyglucose, $^{13}NH_3$, and positron computed tomography. Am J Cardiol 47:481, 1981
336. Gould KL, Schelbert HR, Phelps ME et al: Noninvasive assessment of coronary stenoses with myocardial perfusion imaging during pharmacologic coronary vasodilatation. V. Detection of 47% diameter coronary stenosis with intravenous nitrogen-13 ammonia and emission computed transaxial tomography in intact dogs. Am J Cardiol 46:200, 1979
337. Selwyn AP, Allan RM, L'Abbate A et al: Relation between regional myocardial uptake of rubidium-82 and perfusion: Absolute reduction of cation uptake in ischemia. Am J Cardiol 50:112, 1982
338. Sobel BE, Weiss ES, Welch MJ et al: Detection of remote myocardial infarction in patients with positron emission transaxial tomography and intravenous 11C-palmitate. Circulation 55:853, 1977
339. McKenna WJ, Allan RM, Horlock P et al: Hypertrophic cardiomyopathy: Measurement of cation uptake. Am J Cardiol 47:409, 1981
340. Henze E, Perloff JK, Schelbert HR: Alterations of regional myocardial perfusion and metabolism in Duchenne's muscular dystrophy (DMD) detected by positron computed tomography (PCT). Circulation (Suppl) 64:IV-279, 1981
341. Geltman EM, Smith JL, Beecher D et al: Altered regional myocardial metabolism in congestive cardiomyopathy detected by positron tomography. Am J Med 74:773, 1983
342. Randle PJ, England PJ, Denton RM: Control of the tricarboxilic acid cycle and its interactions with glycolysis during acetate utilization in rat heart. Biochem J 117:677, 1970
343. Schelbert HR, Phelps ME, Selin C et al: Regional myocardial ischemia assessed by 18 fluoro-2-deoxyglucose and positron emission computed tomography. In Kreuzer H, Parmley WW, Rentrop P, Heiss HW (eds): Advances in Clinical Cardiology, Vol I: Quantification of Myocardial Ischemia. New York, Gehard Witzstrock, 1980
344. Tillisch J, Brunken R, Marshall R et al: Reversibility of cardiac wall motion abnormalities predicted by positron tomography. N Engl J Med 314:884, 1986
345. Schelbert HR, Wisenberg G, Phelps ME et al: Noninvasive assessment of coronary stenoses by myocardial imaging during pharmacologic vasodilation, VI: Detection of coronary artery disease in man with intravenous N-13 ammonia positron computed tomography. Am J Cardiol 49:1197, 1982
346. Marshall RC, Tillisch JH, Phelps ME et al: Identification and differentiation of resting myocardial ischemia and infarction in man with positron computed tomography, 18F-labeled fluorodeoxyglucose and N-13 ammonia. Circulation 67:766, 1983
347. Grant PM, Erdal BR, O'Brien HA: A 82Sr-82Rb isotope generator for use in nuclear medicine. J Nucl Med 16:300, 1975
348. Phelps ME, Schelbert HR, Hoffman EJ et al: Physiologic tomography of myocardial glucose metabolism, perfusion and blood pools with multiple gated acquisition. In Kreuzer H, Parmley WW, Rentrop P, Heiss HW (eds): Advances in Clinical Cardiology. New York, Gerhard Witzstrock, 1980
349. McNamara DG, Latson LA: Long term follow-up of patients with malformations for which definitive surgical repair has been available for 25 years or more. Am J Cardiol 50:560, 1982
350. Parrish MD, Graham TP Jr, Born ML et al: Radionuclide ventriculography for assessment of absolute right and left ventricular volumes in children. Circulation 66:811, 1982
351. Findley JP, Howman-Giles R, Gilday DL et al: Thallium-201 myocardial imaging in anomalous left coronary artery arising from the pulmonary artery: Applications before and after medical and surgical treatment. Am J Cardiol 42:675, 1978
352. Raifer M, Oetgen WJ, Weeks KD Jr et al: Thallium-201 scintigraphy after surgical repair of hemodynamically significant primary coronary artery anomalies. Chest 81:687, 1982
353. Rabinovitch M, Fischer KC, Treves S: Quantitative thallium-201 myocardial imaging in the assessment of right ventricular pressure in patients with congenital heart defects. Br Heart J 45:198, 1981
354. Moodie DS, Cook SA, Gill CC et al: Thallium-201 myocardial imaging in young adults with anomalous left coronary artery arising from the pulmonary artery. J Nucl Med 2:1076, 1980
355. Reduto LA, Berger HJ, Johnstone DE et al: Radionuclide assessment of right and left ventricular exercise reserve after total correction of tetralogy of Fallot. Am J Cardiol 45:1013, 1980
356. Hurwitz RA, Papanicolaou N, Treves S et al: Radionuclide angiography in evaluation of patients after surgical repair of transposition of the great arteries. Am J Cardiol 49:761, 1982
357. Robert WC (ed): Congenital Heart Disease in Adults. Cardiovasc Clinics 10/1. Philadelphia, FA Davis, 1979
358. Kereiakes JG, Feller PA, Ascoli FA et al: Pediatric radiopharmaceutical dosimetry. In Cloutier RJ, Coffey JL, Snyder WS et al (eds): Radiopharmaceutical Dosimetry Symposium, p 76. Washington, DC, US Department of Health, Education and Welfare Publication (FDA), 1976
359. Alderson PO, Jost RG, Strauss AW et al: Detection and quantitation of left-to-right cardiac shunts in children: A clinical comparison of count ratio and area ratio techniques. Circulation 51:1136, 1975
360. Cohn JD, DelGuercio LRM: Clinical applications of indicator dilution curves as gamma functions. J Lab Clin Med 69:675, 1967
361. Kuruc A, Treves S, Parker JA: Accuracy of deconvolution algorithms assessed by simulation studies. J Nucl Med 24:258, 1983
362. Parker JA, Treves S: Radionuclide detection, localization and quantitation of intracardiac shunts and shunts between the great vessels. Prog Cardiovasc Dis 20:121, 1977
363. Fujii AM, Rabinovitch M, Keane JF et al: Radionuclide angiographic assessment of pulmonary vascular reactivity in patients with left to right shunts and pulmonary hypertension. Am J Cardiol 49:356, 1982
364. Botvinick EH, Schiller NB, Shames DM: The role of echocardiography and scintigraphy in the evaluation of adults with suspected left to right shunts. Circulation 62:1020, 1980
365. Goldman MR, Pohost GM: Nuclear magnetic resonance imaging: The potential for cardiac evaluation of the pediatric patient. In Friedman WF, Higgins CB (eds): Pediatric Cardiac Imaging, p 29. Philadelphia, WB Saunders, 1984
366. Rigo P, Chevigne M: Measurement of left to right shunts by gated radionuclide angiography: Concise communication. J Nucl Med 23:1070, 1982
367. Long RTL, Braunwald E, Morrow A: Intracardiac injection of radioactive krypton. Circulation 21:1126, 1983
368. Sty JR, Starshak RJ, Miller JH: Particle body imaging in cardiopulmonary disorders. In Wagner HN (ed): Pediatric Nuclear Medicine, p 46. New York, Appleton-Century-Crofts, 1983
369. Taplin GV, McDonald NS: Radiochemistry of macroaggregated albumin and newer lung scanning agents. Semin Nucl Med 1:132, 1971
370. Greenspan RH: Does a normal isotope perfusion scan exclude pulmonary embolism? Invest Radiol 8:97, 1973
371. Poulose KP, Reba RC, Gilday DL et al: Diagnosis of pulmonary embolism: A correlative study of the clinical, scan, and angiographic findings. Br Med J 3:67, 1970
372. Shoop JD: Why do a lung scan? JAMA 229:567, 1974
373. Wagner HN, Lopez-Majano V, Langan JK et al: Radioactive xenon in the differential diagnosis of pulmonary embolism. Radiology 91:1168, 1968
374. DeNardo GL, Goodwin DA, Ravasini R et al: The ventilatory lung scan in the diagnosis of pulmonary embolism. N Engl J Med 282:1334, 1970
375. Loken MK, Westgate HD: Evaluation of pulmonary function using xenon-133 and the scintillation camera. AJR 100:835, 1967
376. Milic-Emili J: Radioactive xenon in the evaluation of regional lung function. Semin Nucl Med 1:246, 1971
377. Alderson PO, Lee H, Summer WR et al: Comparison of Xe-133 washout and single breath imaging for the detection of ventilation abnormalities. J Nucl Med 20:917, 1979
378. Alderson PO, Biello DR, Khan AR et al: Comparison of ^{133}Xe single breath and washout imaging in the scintigraphic diagnosis of pulmonary embolism. Radiology 137:481, 1980
379. McNiel BJ, Holman L, Adelstein J: The scintigraphic definition of pulmonary embolism. JAMA 227:753, 1974
380. Biello DR, Mattar AG, McKnight RC, Siegel BA: Ventilation-perfusion studies in suspected pulmonary embolism. AJR 133:1033, 1979
381. Alderson PO, Gottschalk A: Ventilation-perfusion studies for pulmonary embolism. Letter to the editor. Semin Nucl Med 9:145, 1979

382. Alderson PO, Rujanavech N, Secker-Walker RH et al: The role of ^{133}Xe ventilation studies in the scintigraphic detection of pulmonary embolism. Radiology 120:633, 1976
383. McNeil BJ: A diagnostic strategy using ventilation-perfusion studies in patients suspect for pulmonary embolism. J Nucl Med 17:613, 1976
384. McLaughlin GL, Burt RW, DePalma D et al: Effect of ventilation images on observed interpretation of lung perfusion examination. AJR 128:1037, 1977
385. McNeil BJ: Ventilation-perfusion studies and the diagnosis of pulmonary embolism: Concise communication. J Nucl Med 21:319, 1980
386. Biello DR, Mattar AG, Osei-Wusu A et al: Interpretation of indeterminate lung scintigrams. Radiology 133:189, 1979
387. Alderson PO, Biello DR, Sachariah KG, Siegel BA: Scintigraphic detection of pulmonary embolism in patients with obstructive pulmonary disease. Radiology 138:661, 1981
388. Alderson PO, Dzebolo NN, Biello DR et al: Serial lung scintigraphy: Utility in diagnosis of pulmonary embolism. Radiology 149:797, 1983
389. Carter WD, Brady TM, Keyes JW Jr et al: Relative accuracy of two diagnostic schemes for detection of pulmonary embolism by ventilation-perfusion scintigraphy. Radiology 145:447, 1982
390. Neuman RD, Sostman HD, Gottschalk A: Current status of ventilation-perfusion imaging. Semin Nucl Med 10:198, 1980
391. Caride VJ, Furi S, Slavin JD et al: The usefulness of posterior oblique views in perfusion lung imaging. Radiology 121:669, 1976
392. Fazio R, Jones J: Assessment of regional ventilation by continuous inhalation of radioactive krypton-81m. Br Med J 1:673, 1975
393. Goris ML, Daspit SG, Walter JR et al: Application of ventilation lung imaging with 81m-krypton. Radiology 122:399, 1977
394. Susskind H, Atkins HL, Goldman AG et al: Sensitivity of Kr-81m and Xe-127 in evaluating nonembolic lung disease. J Nucl Med 22:781, 1981
395. Shibel EM, Tisi GM, Moser KM: Inhalation lung scanning evaluation—radioaerosol versus radioxenon techniques. Dis Chest 56:284, 1969
396. Alderson PO, Biello DR, Gottschalk A et al: Tc99m-DTPA aerosol and radioactive gases compared to adjuncts to perfusion scintigraphy in patients with suspected pulmonary embolism. Radiology 153:515, 1984
397. Moses DC, Silver TM, Bookstein JJ: The complementary roles of chest radiography, lung scanning and selective pulmonary angiography in the diagnosis of pulmonary embolism. Circulation 49:179, 1974

NEW CARDIAC IMAGING MODALITIES

Charles B. Higgins

CHAPTER 30 VOLUME 1

The emphasis in cardiac diagnosis in recent years has been focused on noninvasive imaging techniques that provide anatomical diagnosis and physiological assessment of the severity of disease. Echocardiography and radionuclide imaging were early techniques applied for this purpose, and these have now attained a central role in cardiovascular diagnosis.

During the past few years, three new imaging modalities have been introduced: (1) magnetic resonance imaging (MRI); (2) ultrafast computed tomography (cine CT); and (3) positron emission tomography (PET). These new techniques provide the noninvasive capability for depiction of internal cardiac anatomy, myocardial tissue characterization, quantitation of blood flow, estimation and perhaps quantitation of regional myocardial perfusion, quantitation of regional myocardial contraction, and *in vivo* sampling of myocardial metabolism. Early reports have also shown the feasibility of sampling myocardial metabolism using magnetic resonance spectroscopy, in which localization is achieved by combining MRI and MR spectroscopy techniques. The current armamentarium of diagnostic techniques for cardiovascular diagnosis calls for careful consideration of the capabilities of each technique and its proper use in order to truly enhance not only the diagnosis, but also the comprehension of the pathophysiology of cardiovascular disease.

The principles and technical aspects of these new imaging modalities are described in this chapter. The early clinical experience with the use of these techniques in the evaluation of several categories of cardiac disease is also discussed.

MAGNETIC RESONANCE IMAGING

Magnetic resonance imaging (of protons) has two important attributes that make it intrinsically advantageous for imaging cardiovascular disease. The first is the natural contrast between the blood pool and the cardiovascular structures, and the second is the wide range of contrast among soft tissue, which provides the potential for myocardial tissue characterization.[1-11]

Proton magnetic resonance imaging with electrocardiographic (ECG) gating can serve as a single technique providing noninvasive evaluation of cardiovascular anatomy, physiology, and tissue characterization. Effectiveness for evaluation of anatomy and function has already been shown, while the capability for tissue characterization is not clearly established or fully developed.

PRINCIPLES AND TECHNIQUES

Magnetic resonance imaging depends on the interaction of nuclei with a strong magnetic field and the intermittently applied radiofrequency pulses to generate tomographic images of the heart. Although any atom with an odd number of protons or neutrons may be used for MRI, hydrogen is so naturally abundant and efficient (maximum number of nuclei per atomic number) that it is the most ideal nucleus for imaging. Most imaging at the current time employs hydrogen resonance and is referred to as hydrogen or proton MRI.

Localization within an imaged plane is attained by intermittent application of a magnetic field gradient. The magnetic field gradient causes hydrogen nuclei at different sites across the imaged plane to have a resonance frequency that is specific for that site and slightly different from other sites across the plane. By this means, position is encoded for MRI. The signal from any site (voxel) in the image is chiefly dependent on the concentration of hydrogen nuclei resonating at the frequency specific for that site. The signal received during the MRI process is complex. It is a multiple frequency signal dependent on the position of each signal within the varying magnetic field. The raw time domain signal undergoes Fourier transformation, which reduces the raw signal into its basic frequency components. The position of the signal depends on its specific frequency, and the amplitude of the signal depends chiefly on the concentration of mobile hydrogen nuclei at that site. Depending on the imaging technique used, the T1 (spin–lattice) and T2 (spin–spin) relaxation times also contribute to local signal intensity.

The magnetic relaxation rates or times, T1 and T2, are measures of the physiochemical interactions between hydrogen nuclei (protons) and their neighboring nuclei. These relaxation times vary among tissues and also may be markedly different for the normal compared with an abnormal component of a tissue (*i.e.*, normal vs. infarcted myocardium). The diversity of relaxation times among tissues is used to produce contrast on MR images. By varying imaging parameters contrast-dependent on hydrogen density, T1 or T2 relaxation times can be accentuated.

The spin-echo technique is sensitive to hydrogen-density T1 and T2 relaxation times and can highlight contrast between normal and abnormal tissue based on any of the three factors. Contrast based on T1 or T2 relaxation times can be accentuated by varying the imaging parameters TR (RF pulse repetition time) and TE (echo delay time). Contrast based on T1 relaxation time is accentuated with a short TR (0.5 second or gated to every heart beat) and short TE (15–30 msec). Contrast based on T2 relaxation time is accentuated with a longer TR (2.0 seconds or gated to every other heart beat) and longer TE (60–120 msec). The intensity of one region (voxel) in an MR image increases with increasing hydrogen density, decreasing T1 time, and increasing T2 time. The gradient-echo technique is also sensitive to T1 and T2 relaxation times. Contrast based on T1 and T2 times can be accentuated by varying TR and TE, but in a manner different than for the spin-echo technique.[1]

An important feature of MRI of the cardiovascular system is that no contrast media are needed to mark the blood pool.[1,4,12–14] The MR process is sensitive to blood flow and can be used to measure blood flow velocity. Moreover, a very practical result of this flow sensitivity for cardiac imaging is that it causes high contrast between the blood pool (no signal) and the myocardial walls when using the spin echo technique.

MRI TECHNIQUES FOR EVALUATION OF THE HEART

The techniques used in MRI of the heart depend on the primary goal of the procedure. When the evaluation of anatomical abnormalities is paramount, the use of the ECG-gated spin-echo technique provides static images with high signal-to-noise ratios. When the primary goal is to assess cardiac contractile function, cine MRI is important.[1] This technique uses narrow flip angles (<90°) and gradient-refocused echoes. Because the TR and TE values are 20 to 30 msec and 10 to 15 msec, respectively, the cardiac cycle can be divided into more or less than 30 time frames. By lacing these together in a cinematic format, tomograms of the beating heart are obtained.

The imaging plane used for a specific study also depends on the information desired. When purely anatomical information is sought, imaging in a transverse, coronal, or sagittal plane is desirable. However, when measurements of cardiac dimensions, such as diameter of the ventricle and ventricular wall thickness or derivation of functional parameters are required, imaging in the plane perpendicular to the cardiac long axis (short axis plane) is indicated. These cardiac axis planes are oblique to the long axis of the body. The most useful plane, referred to as the short-axis plane, is perpendicular to the long axis of the left ventricle. The long axis of the left ventricle is a plane that transects the middle of the aortic valve and the apex of the left ventricle. Achieving such short-axis images generally requires a two-step angulation of the slice-selective gradient relative to the orthogonal axis of the body and, consequently, usually increases the total imaging time.

The blood pool has a unique signal on both spin-echo and gradient-refocused images. The blood pool on the ECG-gated spin-echo images generally is a signal void, which provides high contrast between blood and the myocardial wall (Fig. 30.1 and 30.2). On the other hand, the blood pool produces a very bright signal when the gradient-refocused technique is used (Fig. 30.3). This also causes high contrast between the blood pool and the myocardial wall. Abnormal flow patterns cause intraluminal bright signal in the signal void on the spin-echo images and, alternately, a focal signal void within high-intensity blood pool on the gradient-refocused images.

IMAGING PLANES

Imaging can be done in any plane desired. The plane is specified prior to imaging, and the tomograms are produced in the specified plane. As opposed to some techniques, such as computed tomography, the images obtained in the sagittal and coronal planes are directly acquired rather than reconstructed planes; there is no loss of spatial resolution in these planes in comparison to the transverse plane. Most MRI studies of the heart have been done in the transverse plane, with supplemental studies obtained in the coronal and sagittal planes in some instances. However, it should be noted that three planes are orthogonal to the body as a reference structure, but produce oblique sections of the heart, since the heart is oriented in the thorax at approximately a 45° angle to the sagittal plane. Consequently, images parallel (long axis plane) or perpendicular (short axis) to the long axis of the heart are sometimes needed. Preliminary images, usually in the transverse or coronal plane, are done in order to calculate the angle of the slice-selective gradient needed for acquiring short or long axis images (see Fig. 30.1). In addition, rotation of the patient can be done to acquire sections approximating the left anterior and right anterior oblique views (see Fig. 30.2).

TISSUE CHARACTERIZATION

The range of contrast among soft tissues provided by MRI is enormous in comparison to roentgenography and other imaging techniques. Harnessing and quantitating these capabilities should provide some

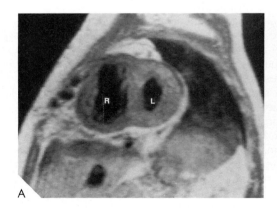
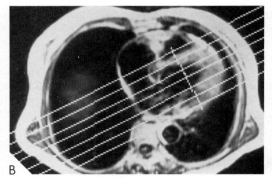
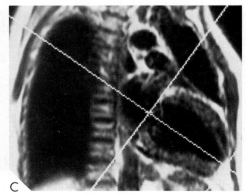

FIGURE 30.1 A. ECG-gated MR image acquired using the spin-echo technique in a short axis plane. There is increased thickness of the free wall of the right ventricle, indicating right ventricular hypertrophy. (L, left ventricle; R, right ventricle) **B.** Images are done initially in the transverse plane in order to define the plane parallel to the long axis of the left ventricle. **C.** Using the long axis images, planes are assigned perpendicular to it.

degree of pathology-specific tissue characterization. At this early stage in the development and understanding of MRI, the parameters used for tissue characterization are relatively primitive and incompletely validated. There are at least seven parameters that can be used for tissue characterization on MRI: (1) longitudinal relaxation time (T1), (2) transverse relaxation time (T2), (3) spin density, (4) molecular self-diffusion, (5) proton chemical shift, (6) magnetic susceptibility changes and differences; and (7) blood flow[15] or blood content of a tissue. The influence of the last factor on the intensity of the image is profound, but poorly understood at the current time.

Until now, magnetic relaxation times have been used to characterize pathologic processes. These times are only roughly approximated by MRI. Initial studies on excised myocardial tissue using MR spectrometers[16] and *ex situ* hearts employing small bore imagers[17] indicated that T1 and T2 relaxation times were prolonged in the acutely injured myocardium. Subsequently, ECG-gated MRI in animals[2] and humans[10] has revealed significant alterations of myocardial T2 relaxation times in acute infarcts, fully evolved infarcts replaced by scar,[9] and cardiac transplant rejection.[18]

Relaxation times are calculated from MR images by constructing regions of interest over the myocardium. These are average relaxation times for the tissue contained within the region of interest. Calculation of the relaxation times is done using the double spin-echo formula:

$$I = N(H)f(v) \exp(-TE/T2) \times [1 - \exp(-TR/T1)]$$

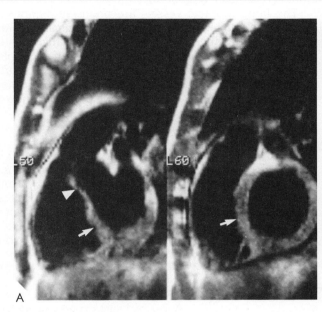
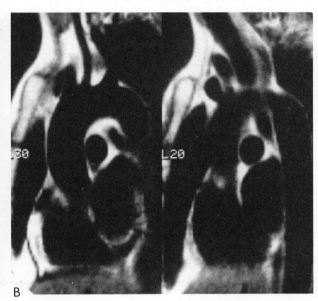

FIGURE 30.2 Gated images with the patient rotated into a position equivalent to the left anterior oblique view. **A.** Tomograms through the ventricles (*left*) show the perimembranous (*arrowhead*) and muscular (*arrow*) portions of the ventricular septum. **B.** Tomograms through the aorta show the entire aortic arch and arch vessels and descending aorta. (Didien D, Higgins CB: Identification and localization of ventricular septal defects by gated magnetic resonance imaging. Am J Cardiol 57:1363, 1986)

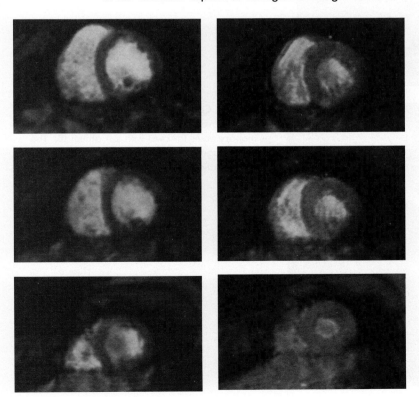

FIGURE 30.3 MR images acquired using the gradient-echo technique in a short axis plane. Images correspond to end diastole (*left*) and end systole (*right*). Images are acquired at basal, mid, and apical levels of the left ventricle. Note the thickening of the left ventricular wall from diastole to systole.

To use this formula the intensity values of a region must be measured from at least two intensity images of an anatomical level. For estimating T1 it requires two images obtained with different TR values. For estimating T2 it requires two images with different TE values. On ECG-gated images the TR is equivalent to the RR interval of the ECG. In order to measure T1, images must be obtained gated to every heart beat and then repeated with gating to every other heart beat. On the other hand, two sets of images with two TE values are generally obtained during a single-gated acquisition. Most *in vivo* studies have used only the MR intensity measurement and calculated T2 relaxation time to characterize abnormal from normal myocardium. Differential myocardial tissue characterization is at an inchoate stage, and much work remains to be done in this area.

DEMONSTRATION OF CARDIAC ANATOMY ON MR IMAGES

The natural contrast between blood and the cardiac wall is evident in Figure 30.1. Because of the unique signal from the blood pool, both sides of the ventricular septum are well seen, as are the left and right ventricular walls. With such resolution, wall thickness and chamber dimensions may be easily measured. The trabeculations of the right ventricle and the papillary muscles of the left ventricle are usually demonstrated on transverse or short axis images through the middle of the ventricles (see Fig. 30.1). On the other hand, the cardiac valves are so thin and mobile that they are not always visualized. The valve leaflets and cusps are visualized in motion on cine MRI.[1] The direct visualization of the myocardium is attained by MRI in a manner superior to that which has previously been possible with any imaging modality.

The normal pericardium is composed of fibrous tissue that produces low signal intensity owing to its relatively low water content (see Fig. 30.1). The normal pericardium frequently is only visualized anterior to the right ventricle and apex as a thin dark line sandwiched between myocardium or epicardial fat and pericardial fat. Proximal portions of the coronary arteries may be seen on MR images without using contrast medium because of the high contrast between moving intraluminal blood and the surrounding epicardial fat (Fig. 30.4). The larger coronary veins are frequently discernible, and the coronary sinus almost always is visualized on transverse MR images.

The transaxial images have been the most useful ones for depicting normal intracardiac anatomy as well as for identifying pathologic structures. Complete evaluation of the left ventricle by MRI is achieved by also obtaining images in the sagittal and coronal planes. The sagittal plane demonstrates the thickness of the anteroseptal and posterior walls of the left ventricle. The coronal plane will demonstrate various regions of the ventricular septum and lateral and diaphragmatic walls of the left ventricle (Fig. 30.5).

The large thoracic vessels are precisely demonstrated on MR images. The relationship of the aorta and pulmonary arteries to each other, as well as their connection to the ventricles, is unequivocally defined. Imaging in the sagittal plane or a plane equivalent to the left anterior oblique demonstrates most of the thoracic aorta on a single image (see Figs. 30.1 and 30.2). The connection of the venae cavae and pulmonary veins to the right and left atria are shown by MRI.

ANATOMICAL DIAGNOSIS

The advantages of MRI in comparison to other cardiac imaging techniques are the clear delineation of the endocardial and epicardial margins of the cardiac walls; the discrimination of the internal cardiac structures including normal trabecular structures as well as intraluminal tumors and thrombi; and direct visualization of the pericardium, intrapericardial fluid, and paracardiac masses. Considerable attention has been directed toward the use of MRI for the evaluation of ischemic

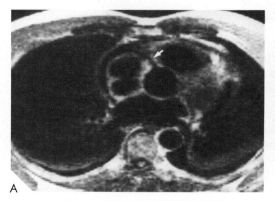
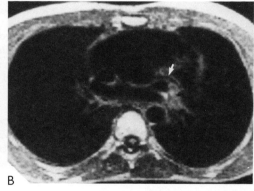

FIGURE 30.4 MR images at the base of the aorta. **A.** Proximal right coronary artery (*arrow*). **B.** Left coronary artery (*arrow*).

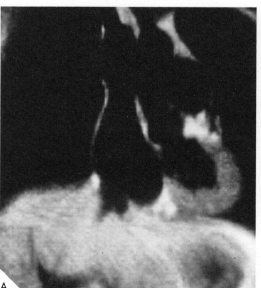
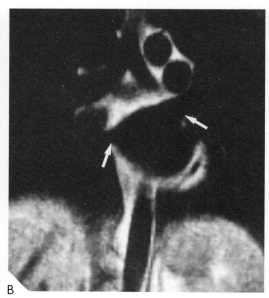

FIGURE 30.5 Coronal MR images show the junction of venae cavae with right atrium (**A**) and pulmonary veins (*arrows*) with left atrium (**B**). The coronal image also provides direct imaging of the diaphragmatic wall of the left ventricle.

heart disease, and its role in this disease is evolving. The clinical indications for MRI that are established at the current time include evaluation of diseases afflicting the myocardial walls; pericardial disease; cardiac and paracardiac masses; and some aspects of congenital heart disease. MRI may be the most effective technique for definitive diagnosis of abnormalities of the thoracic aorta, such as aneurysm and dissection, and some abnormalities of the central pulmonary arteries, such as chronic thromboembolic disease.

ISCHEMIC HEART DISEASE

For the evaluation of ischemic heart disease MRI is indicated for showing the extent of myocardial loss after an acute myocardial infarction and complications of infarctions, such as ventricular aneurysms and mural thrombus. Studies in animals[2,16,18] and in humans[10] have revealed that acute infarctions are readily visualized on MR images as regions of increased signal intensity. In regard to the differential signal intensities and relaxation times between normal and infarcted myocardium, it should be remembered that signal intensity on spin-echo images increases with increase in hydrogen (spin) density, shortening of T1, and lengthening of T2. Acutely infarcted myocardium is edematous, and this state is associated with an increase in hydrogen density and prolongation of T1 and T2 relaxation times.[2,10,17] The contrast between normal and infarcted myocardium is increased on the second echo (TE = 56–60 msec) image compared with the first echo (TE = 28–30 msec) image; the second echo image accentuates the T2 difference between the normal and edematous myocardium (Fig. 30.6).

Regions of old myocardial infarction can be discerned due to the clear demonstration of wall thinning on MR images (Figs. 30.7–30.9). The transition between normal myocardial wall thickness and wall thinning is well defined; this enables a confident estimation of the extent of the left ventricle involved by the prior infarction.[3,11]

In some patients with remote infarctions, the residual myocardial wall had sufficient thickness that measurements of signal intensity were possible.[11] In these instances, signal intensity of the infarcted region was decreased compared with normal myocardium. In contradistinction to acute infarctions, the T2 relaxation times were prolonged relative to normal myocardium in these patients. The current notion on the relationship between histology and relaxation times in acute and chronic myocardial infarctions is summarized in Table 30.1.

Complications of myocardial infarctions have been clearly demonstrated on MR images.[3] Gated MR images displayed regions of extreme wall thinning and bulging of segments of the left ventricle in patients with aneurysms (see Figs. 30.8 and 30.9); such MR findings have cor-

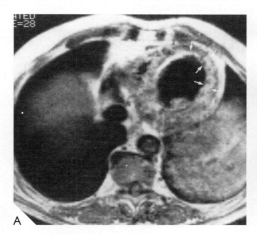

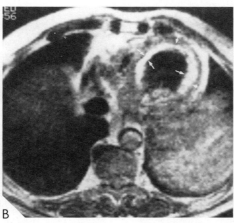

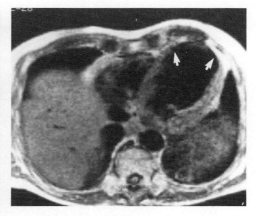

FIGURE 30.6 Transverse images through the apical portion of the left ventricle in a patient with acute infarction. **A.** First echo (TE = 28 msec) image. **B.** Second echo (TE = 56 msec) image. The increased intensity of the infarcted myocardium (*small arrows*) is more evident on the second echo image owing to the substantial decline in signal of the surrounding normal myocardium with the longer TE time. (McNamara MT, Higgins CB, Schechtmann N et al: Detection and characterization of acute myocardial infarctions in man using gated magnetic resonance imaging. Circulation 71:717, 1985, by permission of the American Heart Association)

FIGURE 30.7 Gated transverse image through the middle of the left ventricle of a patient with a chronic anteroseptal myocardial infarction. MR image shows thinning of the anterior portion of the septum and the anterior segment (*arrows*).

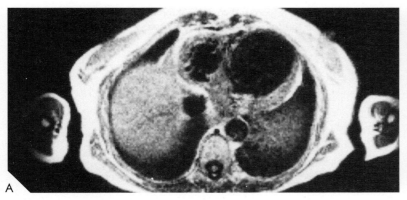

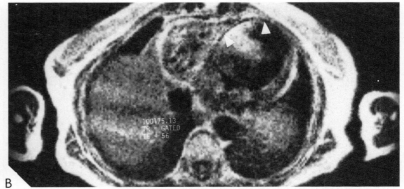

FIGURE 30.8 First (**A**) and second (**B**) images of the left ventricle from a patient with an old anteroseptal myocardial infarction. There is anteroseptal wall thinning. Note on the second echo image there is a rim of very low signal (*arrowheads*) on this more T2-weighted image, consistent with the shorter relaxation time of fibrous scar compared with muscle. The strong signal from stagnant blood adjacent to the infarct is also evident on the second echo image. (Higgins CB, Lanzer P, Stark D et al: Nuclear magnetic resonance imaging in chronic ischemic heart disease in man. Circulation 69:523, 1984, by permission of the American Heart Association)

related with left ventriculography or echocardiography.[3] The MR tomogram can provide visualization of the ostium of the aneurysm; a small ostium compared with the diameter of the aneurysm suggests a false aneurysm (see Fig. 30.9). Mural thrombi have also been shown projecting into the signal void within the left ventricular chamber (see Fig. 30.9).

Important questions regarding the potential use of MRI are how early after coronary occlusion can MRI detect myocardial ischemic injury and whether it can accurately quantitate infarct size. Initial canine studies have indicated that MRI can identify and depict increase in signal intensity of jeopardized myocardium within 3 hours after coronary occlusion.[18] Significant increases in intensity and T2 relaxation time have been measured in the infarct region compared with the normal myocardium by 3 hours after occlusion.

New paramagnetic contrast media have been used to outline the region at jeopardy after acute coronary occlusion in animals.[19] Contrast media have also been used to distinguish between occlusive and reperfused myocardial infarctions.[20]

CARDIOMYOPATHIES

Since MRI provides sharp delineation of the left ventricular wall, it is an excellent technique for evaluating the presence and severity of cardiomyopathies. Magnetic resonance imaging has provided accurate definition of the extent, location, and severity of left ventricular hypertrophy in hypertrophic cardiomyopathy (Fig. 30.10).[21] Hypertrophy exists only in the outflow septum in many patients. In others the entire septum is hypertrophied, and in still others, hypertrophy may extend from the septum into the free wall or apex. MRI has been particularly useful in defining the variant forms of this disease. Regions of ischemic myocardial injury due to hypertrophy out of proportion to the blood supply of the region have also been shown by MRI (Fig. 30.11).

The patterns of distribution of hypertrophic cardiomyopathy shown by MRI have correlated well with two-dimensional echocardiography.[21] Often the resolution of MRI is superior to echocardiography, and, in particular, it more clearly discriminates the endocardial and epicardial borders of the left ventricular wall. Moreover, the larger field of view of MRI may be useful in depicting the overall extent of hypertrophy. MRI has been an effective method for measuring left ventricular mass in animals[22] and humans.[23] The accuracy of the technique for measuring mass has been shown in animals.[22]

MRI demonstrates the dilatation of the cardiac chambers characteristic of congestive cardiomyopathy (Fig. 30.12). This technique has shown that ischemic cardiomyopathy can usually be recognized by the presence of disproportionate wall thinning in one or more regions of the left ventricle. Idiopathic cardiomyopathy is usually characterized by normal wall thickness or mild generalized wall thinning. Cine MRI

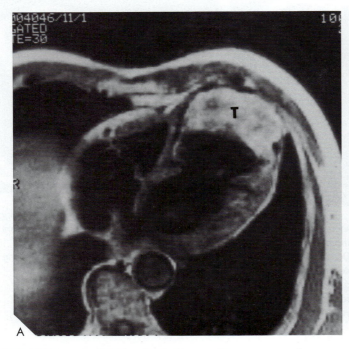
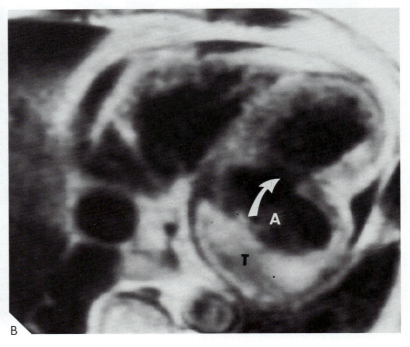

FIGURE 30.9 A. ECG-gated spin-echo images acquired in transverse plane demonstrate complications of myocardial infarctions. True aneurysm involves the anteroapical region and contains mural thrombus (*T*). **B.** False aneurysm (A) involves posterior region and contains thrombus (*T*). True aneurysm has a wide ostium while the false aneurysm has a narrow ostium (*curved arrow*).

TABLE 30.1 RELATIONSHIP BETWEEN HISTOLOGY AND RELAXATION TIMES IN ACUTE AND CHRONIC MYOCARDIAL INFARCTION

	Acute Infarction	Chronic Infarction
Signal intensity (compared with normal myocardium)	Increased	Decreased
T2 relaxation time	Increased	Decreased
Pathology	Edema	Fibrosis

has been used to quantitate left ventricular volumes, ejection fraction, and mass. The cine MRI measurements show a considerable increase in left ventricular mass, but a reduced ratio of left ventricular mass to end-diastolic volume.[23]

Measurement of relaxation times in groups of patients with hypertrophic and congestive cardiomyopathies has shown no significant difference in relaxation times compared with normal subjects. Tissue characterization by relaxation times is considered crude at present. It may become more specific as additional quantitative parameters of magnetic resonance are further developed for imaging.

PERICARDIAL DISEASE

The normal pericardium is only 1 mm to 2 mm in thickness, and the visceral and parietal layers are closely applied to each other. The normal pericardium in some regions, especially near the diaphragm, can measure up to 4 mm. A measurement greater than 5 mm on MRI is considered pericardial thickening. The normal pericardium is composed primarily of fibrous tissue, which produces little MRI signal. Both pericardial and subepicardial fat produce an area of high MRI signal intensity at the external margin of the heart; consequently, there is high contrast between the pericardium and adjacent fat (Fig. 30.13). The pericardial line is recognized as a thin lucent line surrounding portions of the circumference of the heart, where it is highlighted by adjacent fat. In most normal patients the pericardium is visualized only over the right anterior aspect of the heart. Since pure fluid also produces little or no MRI signal, this lucent line is usually composed of normal pericardial fluid as well as the two layers of pericardium.

Increase in thickness of the dark rim around the myocardium has

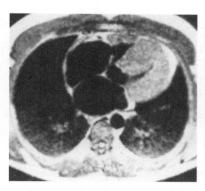 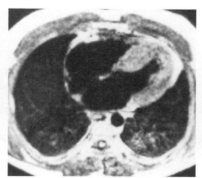 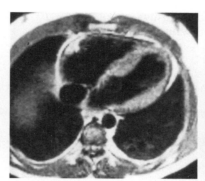 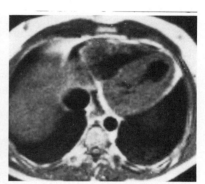

FIGURE 30.10 Series of transverse images extending from the base (*left*) to the apex (*right*) of the left ventricle in a patient with hypertrophic cardiomyopathy. In the left ventricular outflow region there is severe hypertrophy of the septal and lateral walls. In the middle of the left ventricle the hypertrophy involves only the septal region. (Higgins CB, Byrd BF III, Stark D et al: Magnetic resonance imaging of hypertrophic cardiomyopathy. Am J Cardiol 55:1121, 1985)

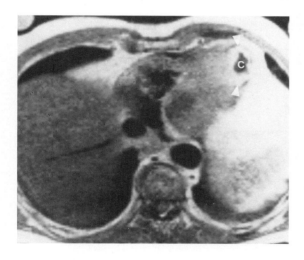

FIGURE 30.11 Transverse image through the apical level of the left ventricle in a patient with a variant form of hypertrophic cardiomyopathy. The left ventricular chamber at the apex is almost completely obliterated by extreme hypertrophy. Note the high signal intensity of the anterior myocardial region due to acute subendocardial infarction (*arrowheads*). The high intensity region has a subendocardial location around the small residual cavity (c) near the apex.

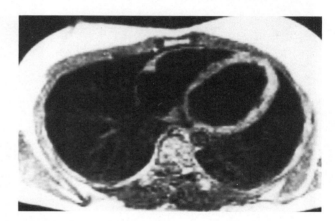

FIGURE 30.12 Transverse MR image of a patient with congestive cardiomyopathy shows dilation of the right and left ventricular chambers.

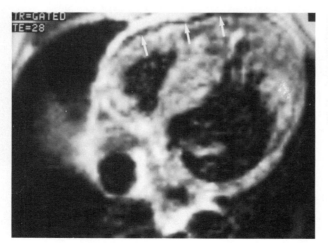

FIGURE 30.13 Transverse image shows the low intensity pericardium (*arrows*) between the pericardial and subepicardial fat layers over the anterior surface of the heart. Note also the posterior wall thinning in this patient with a previous myocardial infarction.

been observed in the presence of thickened pericardium in patients with constrictive pericarditis (Fig. 30.14).[29] The low signal intensity of the thickened pericardium suggests that it is composed mostly of fibrous tissue, as would be expected in chronic constrictive pericarditis. Gated MRI has defined a number of pericardial abnormalities, including pericardial effusions, tumors, cysts, and several inflammatory pericardial processes. In some patients with uremic pericarditis the MR images demonstrated pericardial effusion and abundant inflammatory exudate on the pericardium. In contradistinction to the normal pericardium, the inflamed pericardium produced strong MRI signal intensity, as did adhesions between the visceral and parietal pericardium (Fig. 30.15). Moreover, the signal intensity of the pericardium under such circumstances is greater on the image with a longer delay time, which is consistent with a long T2 relaxation time observed with other edematous tissues.

Most pericardial effusions have low signal on spin-echo images (see Fig. 30.15, A). On T1-weighted spin-echo images, bloody effusions are represented by high signal intensity (see Fig. 30.15, B). MRI can usually demonstrate pericardial hematomas.

PARACARDIAC MASSES

The attributes of MRI useful in evaluating mass lesions are the clear delineations of the cardiac walls and cardiac chambers; the direct and definitive visualization of the pericardium; spatial separation of the various chambers and various regions of each chamber (e.g., septal from the lateral wall); and the large field of view that shows the cardiac chambers in relation to other mediastinal and pulmonary structures.

It can unequivocally distinguish between paracardiac and intracardiac masses (Figs. 30.16–30.19). It also can determine the extent of mass lesions of the thorax and whether mediastinal, lung, and pericardial tumors extend into the heart (see Fig. 30.16). MRI can determine the presence and volume of pericardial effusions encountered in association with malignant cardiac and paracardiac tumors. Finally, it can be used to establish the presence of pericardial involvement by tumor as the etiology of recurrent pericardial effusions.

INTRACARDIAC MASSES

Magnetic resonance imaging displays the mass within the signal void of the cardiac chambers. The absence of signal from blood in motion within the chambers provides contrast for visualizing the mass (see Figs. 30.17 and 30.19). MRI should be used for assessing the possibility of direct extension or metastasis of tumors to the heart (see Fig. 30.19). An intracavitary tumor on MRI must be differentiated from thrombi, normal structures, and intracavitary signal generated from stasis of blood flow in a chamber. The signal associated with stasis of flow increases dramatically on images using the second spin echo (TE

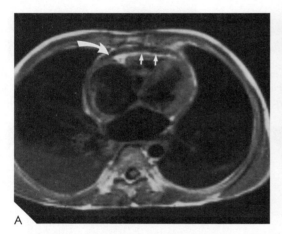
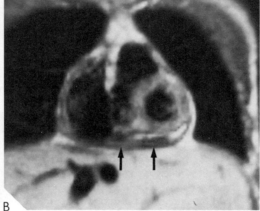

FIGURE 30.14 Transverse (**A**) and coronal (**B**) MR images of a patient with constrictive pericarditis. The thickened pericardium is visible as a low signal intensity line (*curved arrow*) between the high intensity regions produced by pericardial and epicardial fat (*small arrows*). There are pleural effusions bilaterally. Note the thick pericardium along the diaphragmatic surface of the heart.

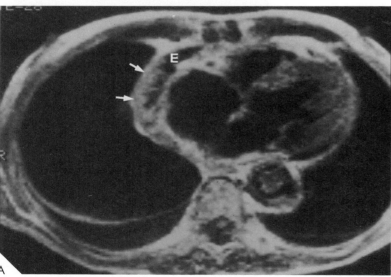
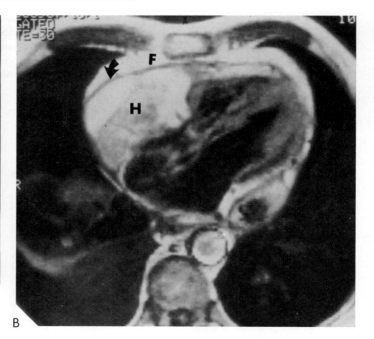

FIGURE 30.15 ECG-gated spin-echo images of two patients with inflammatory effusion and pericardial hematoma. **A.** The thickened parietal (*arrows*) and visceral pericardium have high signal intensity, consistent with inflammatory pericardial thickening caused by uremic pericarditis. The nonhemorrhagic effusion (*E*) causes low intensity. **B.** The pericardial hematoma (*H*) produces high signal intensity on this T1-weighted image. The hematoma has signal intensity equivalent to the fat (*F*) on the surface of the parietal pericardium (*curved arrow*).

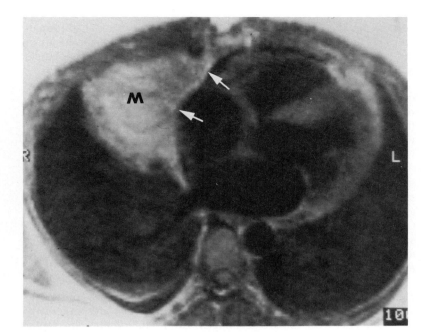

FIGURE 30.16 ECG-gated spin-echo image in transverse plane shows a mass (M) abutting the pericardium. The pericardial line separates the mass from the cardiac structures. Visualization of the pericardial line (arrows) suggests that the pericardium has not been invaded by tumor.

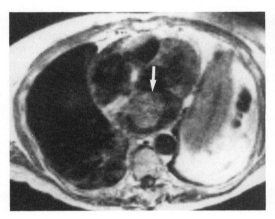

FIGURE 30.17 Transverse MR image displays an atrial myxoma (arrow). The solid tissue in the left hemithorax is liver and subdiaphragmatic fat occupying this position due to eventration of the left hemidiaphragm.

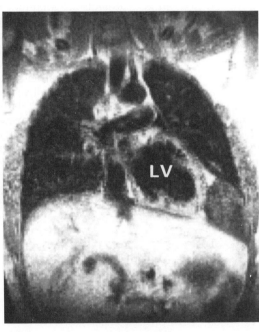

FIGURE 30.18 Coronal MR image shows pericardial cyst adjacent to the left ventricle (LV). Simple cyst with low protein content produces low MR signal intensity.

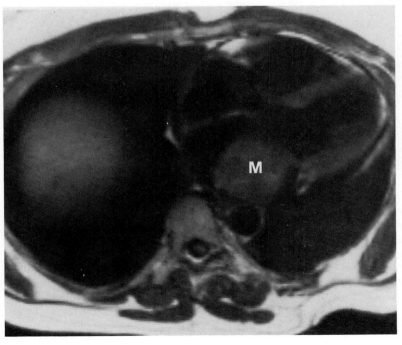

FIGURE 30.19 ECG-gated spin-echo image shows a mass (M) attached to the wall of the left atrium diagnosed as metastatic giant cell tumor of the pelvis.

= 56–60 msec) compared with those produced by the first spin echo (TE = 28–30 msec). Moreover, the signal from blood stasis varies or appears only at certain phases of the cardiac cycle; signal within the ventricles usually occurs in late diastole, and signal within the atrium usually appears in systole.[12] Consequently, it is possible to distinguish between blood stasis and tumors by observing images acquired at different phases of the cardiac cycle.

Intramural masses produce an increase in thickness of the involved cardiac wall and a contour abnormality of the involved region. Since the cardiac walls are well delineated on MR images, this technique is effective for the evaluation of such lesions. Experience is too limited at this time with the MRI evaluation of cardiac tumors to indicate whether there are consistent differences in intensity between the tumor and normal myocardium.

PERICARDIAL MASSES

Pericardial cysts and tumors have been clearly defined by MRI. Indeed, the pericardial origin of such masses and whether the masses are cystic or solid are usually better defined by MRI than any other imaging modality. Since MRI defines the low-signal intensity pericardial layer, it can show the presence of the usually high intensity masses in relationship to the outside or inside of the pericardium (see Figs. 30.16 and 30.18). MRI has been useful for distinguishing between pericardial masses and atypical pericardial effusions, as depicted by two-dimensional echocardiography. One such enigmatic effusion has been pericardial hematoma causing compression of cardiac chambers (see Fig. 30.19).

CONGENITAL HEART DISEASE

Internal cardiac anatomy is well defined without the use of contrast media or ionizing radiation. The latter is an important consideration in children, since angiography is associated with a high radiation dose. The tomographic imaging format facilitates definition of congenital lesions at the various levels, such as is needed for unraveling the components of complex anomalies involving great vessel orientation, type of bulboventricular loop, and visceroatrial situs. When considered in relation to the effectiveness and current reliance on echocardiography in congenital heart disease, the major indications for MRI are thoracic aortic anomalies (Figs. 30.20 and 30.21); pulmonary arterial abnormalities (Fig. 30.22), especially pulmonary atresia; complex anomalies of the ventricles, especially single ventricle; and postoperative conduits and anastomoses (*i.e.*, Rastelli and Fontan procedures).

Analysis of complex cardiac relationships is facilitated by a series of transverse images encompassing the base of the heart to the superior aspect of the liver. This series defines the type of ventricular loop, the relationship of the atria to the ventricles, the relationship of atria to visceral situs, and the atrial connections of the systemic and pulmonary veins.

Positional abnormalities of the great vessels are clearly demonstrated on transaxial images. These include anterior and rightward position of the aorta with d-transposition of the great vessels, anterior and leftward position of the aorta with l-transposition of the great vessels (see Figs. 30.20 and 30.22), and side-by-side position of the great vessels with double-outlet right ventricle and the single large vessel, indicative of truncus arteriosus. Coarctation of the aorta is also well evaluated on the sagittal or oblique sagittal images (see Fig. 30.21).

MRI has consistently demonstrated ventricular septal defects (see Fig. 30.22).[24,25] These include defects of both the inflow (posterior) and outflow (anterior) portions of the septum, which are particularly well delineated on transverse images. Even small ventricular septal defects are identified on transverse images as abrupt truncation of the septum compared with the usual appearance in which the septum is seen to smoothly taper from the muscular into the membranous portion. Delineation of common ventricle with a rudimentary septum and single ventricle with a hypoplastic inverted right ventricular outflow chamber has been documented on transverse images and has been particularly well shown on coronal images (see Fig. 30.22).

Atrial septal defects have been consistently demonstrated on transverse MR images. In the secundum type, the cranial portion of the atrial septum is clearly visible, as is the residual septum adjacent to the defect (Fig. 30.23). In contrast to this appearance, in some normal patients there is poor signal intensity of the septum adjacent to the central portion of the septum where signal dropout is occasionally observed (region of the fossa ovalis). The caudal portion of the atrial septum is absent, and the inflow ventricular septum is truncated on transverse images in primum atrial septal defect.[24]

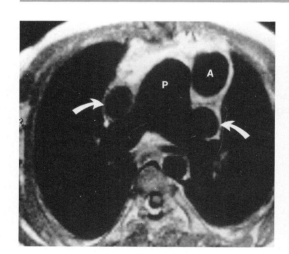

FIGURE 30.20 Transverse MR image at level of great vessels in patient with l-transposition. The aorta (A) is positioned anteriorly and to the left of the pulmonary artery (P). Note bilateral superior venae cavae (*curved arrows*). (Fisher MR, Lipton MJ, Higgins CB: Magnetic resonance imaging in congenital heart disease. Semin Roentgenol 20:272, 1985)

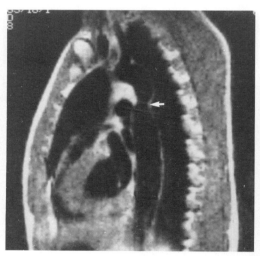

FIGURE 30.21 MR image in a position equivalent to the left anterior oblique view shows discrete coarctation of the aorta (*arrow*). Image also displays left ventricular hypertrophy. (Fisher MR, Lipton MJ, Higgins CB: Magnetic resonance imaging and computed tomography in congenital heart disease. Semin Roentgenol 20:272, 1985)

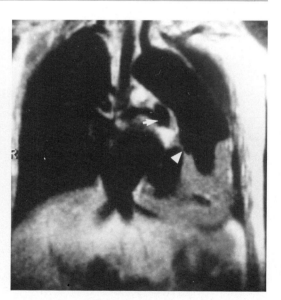

FIGURE 30.22 Coronal MR image of a patient with single ventricle and l-transposition of great vessels and pulmonary atresia. Note the bulboventricular foramen (*arrowhead*) connecting the infundibular chamber to the dominant ventricular chamber. The central pulmonary artery is demonstrated (*arrow*). (Higgins CB: Overview of MR of the heart—1986. AJR 146:907, 1986)

Complete absence of the atrial septum is demonstrable in patients with a common atrium. Associated abnormalities, such as severe right ventricular hypertrophy secondary to Eisenmenger's syndrome, may be observed with MRI. In the complete type of atrioventricular canal defect, the large atrial septal defect and common atrioventricular valve have been completely defined on transverse MR images. Additionally, in patients with atrial septal defects it is possible to assess the pattern of drainage of the pulmonary veins, which may be anomalous.

It is too early in the clinical use of MRI for the evaluation of congenital heart disease to be able to predict the eventual role of this modality compared with angiography. However, even at this early time it defines intracardiac, great vessel, and visceral situs at least as well as, and in some instances more definitively than, angiography.

Patients with congenital heart disease are evaluated initially with two-dimensional echocardiography, and in many congenital lesions MR is the secondary diagnostic technique. However, MR provides images in which the anatomy is displayed with the precision of angiography. Consequently, the evaluation of congenital heart disease, in many instances, is less costly, safer, and at least as effective when echocardiography is followed by MRI. In anomalies of the aortic arch, such as coarctation, MRI can be considered the procedure of choice. MRI frequently is the most useful study for the demonstration of pulmonary arterial abnormalities and for the identification of the presence and size of central pulmonary arteries in patients with pulmonary atresia.[26] Likewise, MRI can be used to evaluate the status of the pulmonary arteries after central shunt operations have been performed.

Finally, the accuracy of MRI has been compared with that of angiography for the evaluation of complex ventricular anomalies (Diethelm and associates, unpublished data). In a group of 17 patients with such complex ventricular anomalies, along with anomalies of the great vessels, the evaluation of all lesions was accomplished more completely with MRI than with angiography. There was agreement between the two techniques in about 90% of the instances in which the possible lesion was evaluated by both studies.

ABNORMALITIES OF THE GREAT VESSELS

THORACIC AORTIC DISSECTION. The initial experience with MRI for the evaluation of aortic dissection has demonstrated accuracy in diagnosis and determination of the extent of the dissection (Fig. 30.24). Definitive diagnosis of dissection requires demonstration of the intimal flap; the sensitivity and specificity of MRI for the diagnosis of aortic dissection exceed 90%.[27] The technique also determined in each instance whether the flap extended into the ascending aorta and was thus effective in differentiating type A (involvement of ascending aorta) and type B (involvement of the descending aorta only) dissections. The transverse plane has been found to be the most reliable one for demonstration of the intimal flap.

MRI can frequently distinguish the true and false channels. Since slow flow or thrombus occurs in the false channel, MR images frequently show moderate to high signal intensity of blood in this channel. If there is brisk flow in both channels, then a complete flow void is observed on both sides of the intimal flap. The dissection has been observed extending into branches of the aortic arch and through the entire extent of the aorta into the iliac arteries. The origin of visceral vessels from the true or false channels can be defined by MRI.

THORACIC ANEURYSM. MRI has defined atherosclerotic and traumatic (false) aneurysms of the thoracic aorta. The depiction of the aneurysms on both transverse and sagittal images provides more precise anatomical information than aortography. MRI shows the outer wall of the aneurysm (true size), the size of the aneurysmal lumen, the aneurysmal wall thickness, and the thrombus engrafted on the aneurysmal wall. It is also likely that MRI can demonstrate perivascular hemorrhage and transudation.

PULMONARY ARTERIES. MRI has been used to demonstrate several abnormalities of the pulmonary arteries. Dilatation of the central pulmonary arteries and abnormal intraluminal signal consistent with slow flow has been shown in pulmonary arterial hypertension.[14] The presence, location, and severity of intraluminal thrombus have been depicted by MRI in pulmonary hypertension caused by chronic thromboembolic disease (Fig. 30.25).[28] MRI is an alternative to angiography in patients with pulmonary hypertension when there is the need to exclude pulmonary thromboembolism. The slow flow accompanying pulmonary hypertension can cause substantial intraluminal signal on MR images. Thrombus can usually be distinguished from slow blood flow by acquiring images at multiple phases of the cardiac cycle (see Fig. 30.25). The thrombus is unchanged on images at the various phases of the cardiac cycle, while the signal from slow blood flow varies during the cardiac cycle. Obstruction and stenosis of the central pulmonary arteries due to extrinsic masses or mediastinal fibrosis can also been demonstrated by MRI.

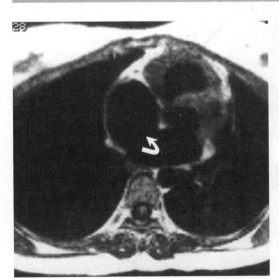

FIGURE 30.23 Transverse image of a patient with a secundum atrial septal defect and pulmonary arterial hypertension. Transverse images show the defect in the secundum septum (curved arrow). Note the increase in thickness of the walls of the right ventricle.

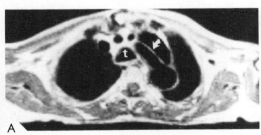

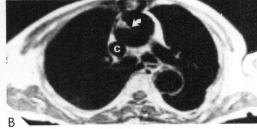

FIGURE 30.24 Aortic dissection. MR images through the ascending aorta (**A**) and aortic arch (**B**) show the intimal flap in the aortic lumen (curved arrow). (c, superior vena cava; t, trachea) (Amparo EG, Higgins CB, Hricak H et al: Aortic dissection: Magnetic resonance imaging. Radiology 155:399, 1985)

ASSESSMENT OF FUNCTION

Functional evaluation of the cardiovascular system is now practical with cine MRI.[1] Several reports have indicated the capability of multiphasic or cine MRI for the evaluation of abnormal blood flow patterns,[1,6] left ventricular and right ventricular dimensions and stroke volumes,[30] left ventricular mass,[22,23] and regional myocardial function.[30]

By achieving a temporal resolution of more than 30 frames per cardiac cycle, cine MRI successfully captures end-diastole and end-systole, such that end-diastolic and end-systolic volumes, stroke volume, and ejection fraction can be calculated accurately.[1,30] Good correlation has been found between left ventricular volumes measured from cine MR images with similar volumes measured by two-dimensional echocardiography.[30] The volumes measured from cine MRI in general are smaller than those that have been traditionally accepted from angiographic measurements. The advantages of MRI for such measurements are that this technique is a truly three-dimensional imaging technique when tomographic images are acquired, encompassing the entire chamber being assessed. However, angiographic measurements depend on geometric assumptions of varying validity, which is influenced by the shape of the chamber.

Measurement of left ventricular mass with MRI has correlated closely with postmortem measurements in animals.[22] Accurate measurement of a left ventricular mass is important because changes in the mass may be the most effective way to monitor the response to therapy in diseases causing left ventricular hypertrophy. Sequential measurements of a mass could be used effectively to monitor the myocardial response to aortic valve replacement or pharmacologic treatment of hypertension.

Functional evaluation in ischemic heart disease is achieved with MRI by monitoring wall thickening during the cardiac cycle. One study in normal persons and patients with prior myocardial infarction demonstrated that MRI readily distinguished the site of previous myocardial injury by a diminution or absence of wall thickening during systole.[30]

IDENTIFICATION AND QUANTITATION OF VALVULAR REGURGITATION

The blood pool usually has a homogeneous high signal intensity throughout most of the cardiac cycle on cine MRI. An exception to this is a diminution in signal intensity that occurs near the opening tricuspid and mitral valves during early diastole. There may also be a momentary signal loss behind the tricuspid and mitral valves during their rapid closure. Regurgitation through either the atrioventricular or semilunar valves is associated with a high-velocity jet that causes a signal void within the otherwise high signal intensity chamber (Fig. 30.26). The appearance of this signal void emanating from the insufficient valve can be used to identify the presence of valvular regurgitation.[1,30] In aortic regurgitation, the signal void is in continuity with the closed aortic valve (see Fig. 30.26), whereas in mitral regurgitation it is in continuity with the closed mitral valve.

Quantitation of the severity of valvular regurgitation can be accomplished by measuring the right and left ventricular stroke volumes and then using these measurements to calculate the regurgitant fraction or regurgitant volume with standard formulas.[1,30] This is accomplished by measuring the blood pool region on all images encompassing the two ventricles at end-diastole and end-systole; the difference between the volumes at these phases is the stroke volume. In the normal subject, the stroke volume should be equal for the two ventricles. However, the stroke volume of the left ventricle exceeds that of the right ventricle by a value equivalent to the regurgitant volume in patients with aortic or mitral regurgitation. With this technique, patients with moderate and severe regurgitation can be distinguished from normal persons and patients with mild regurgitation, as shown by independent imaging techniques.[30] Quantitation of regurgitation can also be done by various measurements of the dimension of the signal void (Fig. 30.27). This has been accomplished by measuring the entire volume of the signal void as it appears on multiple tomographic images encompassing the recipient chamber. Another technique is to measure the length of the regurgitant jet and the width of the base of the regurgitant jet at the point

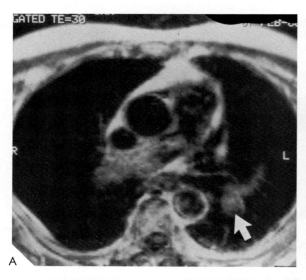
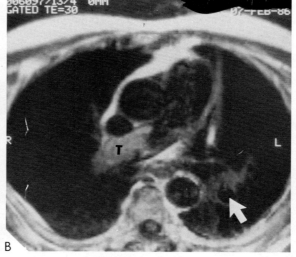

FIGURE 30.25 Pulmonary embolism in patient with pulmonary arterial hypertension. ECG-gated images during diastole (**A**) and systole (**B**). Image at late diastole shows signal in right and descending branch of left pulmonary artery, while the image in systole shows clearing of signal in descending branch of left pulmonary artery (arrow), indicating slow blood flow at this site. Persistence of signal at all phases of the cardiac cycle indicates thrombus (T) in the right pulmonary artery.

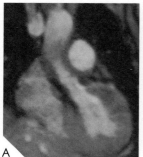
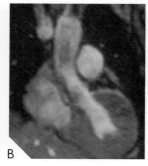
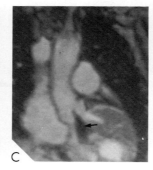
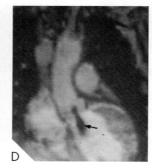

FIGURE 30.26 Cine MRI (gradient refocused technique) in the coronal plane in aortic regurgitation. Images acquired in systole (A and B) and diastole (C and D). Note the signal void (arrow) emanating from the closed aortic valve.

where it emanates from the insufficient valve. The severity of aortic regurgitation is quantitated by measuring the size of the signal void during diastole at each of the tomographic levels beneath the aortic valve and extending to the apex of the left ventricle.

Mitral regurgitation has been quantitated by monitoring the signal intensity within the left atrium during the systolic phase of the cardiac cycle.[1,30] In normal persons there is a moderate increase in signal intensity within the left atrium during systole. However, in patients with mitral regurgitation there is a distinct decline in signal intensity within the left atrium during this phase. The magnitude of the decrease in signal intensity in the left atrium seems to bear an approximate relationship to the severity of mitral regurgitation.[30] In a pilot study, this parameter distinguished patients with moderate and severe mitral regurgitation from those with mild regurgitation.[30]

The early studies with cine MRI for the estimation of the severity of regurgitation are encouraging but need to be evaluated further in a large group of patients with both normal and abnormal chamber sizes and ventricular function. The high-velocity flow pattern associated with valvular stenosis also produces a signal void in the vessel or chamber distal to the stenosis.

Sophisticated measurements of myocardial function can also be achieved with MRI.[30] Wall stress of the left ventricle can be estimated by using the combination of automated digital blood pressure measurements referenced to the carotid pulse tracing and the recording of cine MR images. With this technique, the end-systolic and peak-systolic wall stress can be calculated. As expected, these measurements are markedly elevated in patients with congestive (dilated) cardiomyopathy in comparison with normal persons.[30] This technique may prove useful for assessing the effectiveness of various pharmacologic therapies in patients with congestive cardiomyopathies and other types of dilated cardiac diseases.

COMPUTED TOMOGRAPHY

Computed tomography until recently had had little influence on the clinical diagnosis of heart disease in the United States. Some experience at a few centers in Europe and Japan have shown that ECG-gated and even ECG-nongated CT can be useful for the assessment of a number of cardiac and pericardial diseases.[31,32] Precise depiction of internal cardiac anatomy and quantitation of cardiac dimension with CT has generally required ECG gating. The acquisition of gated CT images has been difficult and has not achieved widespread acceptance for clinical diagnosis of heart disease. Although considerable information has been gained in ischemic heart disease in humans and in experimental animals using standard CT scanners,[33] CT has not been considered competitive with other noninvasive techniques, such as echocardiography and cardiac scintigraphy.

The previously nihilistic approach to CT of the heart must be reconsidered, since it has been shown that CT scans of the heart can be produced at exposure times of 50 msec or less.[34] The inherent advantages of CT for cardiac diagnosis now become very relevant. These advantages include high spatial resolution, but even more importantly for the evaluation of regional myocardial disease, distinct and unequivocal spatial separation of the various walls of the left ventricle on the CT scans.

Contrast-enhanced CT scans define both the inner and outer margins of the left ventricular walls and, consequently, this technique is effective for assessing abnormalities of the myocardial walls,[31] for quantitating regional wall thickness[35,36] and left ventricular mass,[37] for measuring ventricular volumes,[38] and for evaluating wall thickening dynamics.[35,36] When transverse scans are obtained at multiple levels from the base to apex of the heart, CT serves as a three-dimensional imaging technique and thus can provide quantitation of left ventricular mass[37] and myocardial infarctions. Computed tomography also clearly depicts the pericardium and is useful for the definitive diagnosis of pericardial thickening and other pericardial abnormalities.[31]

PRINCIPLES AND TECHNIQUES

The influence of cardiac motion and, to a lesser extent, respiratory motion, significantly degrades image quality because of the long scan time of standard CT in relation to the cardiac cycle. Finally, the ability to image only one slice at a time is a major drawback for cardiac purposes. A further disadvantage of CT imaging when used to assess cardiac function is the necessity for using contrast media. Standard ionic contrast media can have important effects on cardiac performance and regional blood flow.

The approach to CT scanning of the heart usually requires modification of standard CT techniques used for investigating other parts of the body. For some purposes, such as the evaluation of pericardial disease and patency of coronary arterial bypass grafts, standard CT techniques are usually adequate. Assessment of cardiac function and

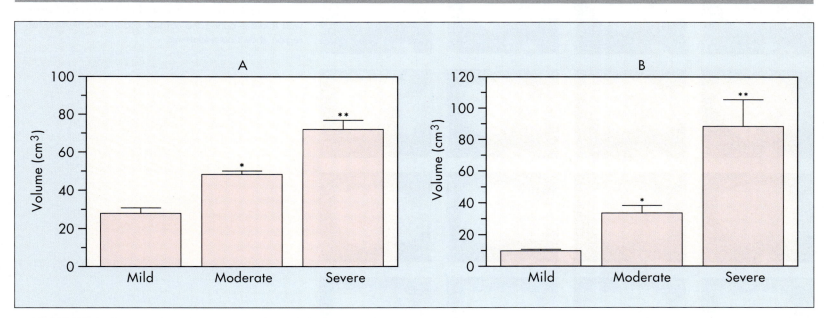

FIGURE 30.27 Block diagram shows the average volume of the signal void in relation to the severity of regurgitation as graded by angiography and/or echocardiography. **A.** Aortic regurgitation. **B.** Mitral regurgitation.

precise definition of intracardiac anatomy necessitates either ECG gating of standard CT scanners or, preferably, the use of a millisecond scanner.

GATED CT SCANNING

Gated CT scanning is one method of overcoming the problem of cardiac motion and is critical in obtaining quantitative dimensional data and ejection fractions. It can also be used to measure the extent of wall thickening during the cardiac cycle.

Gated CT scanning is more complicated than standard CT scanning. To obtain a reconstructed image of a stationary object by standard CT, a nearly full complement of angular radiographic data must be obtained over the scanning cycle from 0° to 360° without significant gaps in the angular data set. Multiple scans are required to obtain the necessary angular data to reconstruct a gated image of the heart.

Two gating techniques have been used: retrospective and prospective gating. With retrospective gating, the CT scan data and the ECG are simultaneously recorded, but the ECG signal does not guide the acquisition in any manner. Subsequently, the image is reconstructed from data obtained within a selected time window (biologic window), bracketing the desired portion of the ECG signal, such as the QRS complex at end-diastole.

The prospective gating system allows preselection of a fraction of the RR interval to be monitored. The biologic window width sets the fraction of the cardiac cycle to be represented by each image. Prospective gating ensures the even distribution of R waves throughout the scanning cycle in the minimal number of scans. This is accomplished by launching the x-ray tube at the appropriate time relative to the R wave on the ECG input, such that one of the following R waves falls in the largest gap in the already acquired angular x-ray data. In most studies, the width of the biologic window has generally been set at 10% of the RR interval. With the heart rate at 100 beats per minute, each frame represents 60 msec. With the biologic window set at 10% of the RR interval, approximately eight scanner rotations are required to obtain a full complement of gated angular radiographic data, requiring approximately 45 seconds of breath holding.

FAST CT SCANNER

The introduction of electronic scanning methods such as those used in the fast CT scanner provide the capability for complete cardiac imaging in real-time without the need for ECG gating.[34] The exposure time of each scan is 50 msec. A series of scans obtained during the same cardiac cycle in a patient with left ventricular hypertrophy is shown in Figure 30.28.

The fast CT scanner is not limited by inertia associated with moving mechanical parts, but rather uses a focused electron beam that is swept at the speed of light across four cadmium tungstate target arcs in succession (see Fig. 30.27). Each of four targets generates a fan beam of photons that passes from beneath the patient to a bank of photon detectors arranged in a semicircle above the patient. The cine CT scanner can be operated in three different modes. The cine mode is used to assess global and regional myocardial function. The scans are obtained in an exposure of 33 msec to 50 msec and at a rate of 17 to 24 scans per second. The triggered mode is used for flow analysis and employs a series of 20 successive scans in which each of the 50-msec exposures is triggered (ECG triggered) at a specific phase of the cardiac cycle of successive heart beats. From such a series of scans, time–density curves can be constructed for specific regions of interest in the cardiac chamber or regions of the myocardium in order to provide an estimate of transit time, perfusion, or blood flow. The third mode is the volume mode, in which eight scans are obtained by using all four target areas. These eight transverse scans (1-cm thickness) can usually encompass the entire left ventricular chamber and thus provide an estimate of the left ventricular volumes and myocardial mass.

CAPABILITIES OF CINE CT

Cine CT provides transverse tomograms of the heart without image degradation associated with normal cardiac motion (see Fig. 30.28). The tomographic format attains distinct spatial separation of most left ventricular segments. An exception is the diaphragmatic segment of the left ventricle, which is oriented parallel to the transverse plane and consequently is not adequately evaluated by the single plane for direct

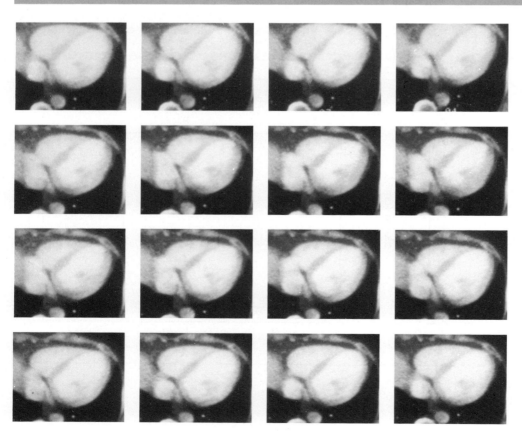

FIGURE 30.28 Series of fast CT scans during a single cardiac cycle in a patient with a prior anteroseptal myocardial infarction. Note the wall thinning in the anterior region of the left ventricle. Although the lateral wall thickens during the cardiac cycle, the anteroseptal region shows no thickening.

imaging provided by CT scanners. Both the endocardial and epicardial borders are delineated on contrast-enhanced CT. Consequently, wall thickening dynamics, as well as wall motion, can be measured during the cardiac cycle with the high temporal resolution afforded by cine CT. Studies have revealed that cine CT can be used to measure left ventricular mass[37] and have shown the variability of myocardial wall motion at multiple levels through the left ventricle.[39]

CARDIAC OUTPUT AND MYOCARDIAL BLOOD FLOW

Cardiac output has been estimated by constructing CT attenuation versus time curves from regions of interest placed in the thoracic aorta or the left ventricular chamber using a series of cine CT scans. This technique has correlated well with thermodilution measurements of cardiac output over a range of outputs induced by pharmacologic interventions.[40]

It seems to be theoretically possible to quantitate regional myocardial perfusion and even blood flow using such attenuation time curves from regions of interest placed in the ventricular myocardium. With this technique CT scans are gated to the same phase of the cardiac cycle of 20 to 40 consecutive or alternate heart beats in order to construct attentuation-time curves during the wash-in and wash-out phases of contrast opacification of the myocardium (Fig. 30.29). Since images are gated to the same phase of the cardiac cycle, the region of interest does not vary across the myocardial wall and phasic differences in coronary blood flow are vitiated. An initial study involving the measurement of myocardial blood flow by parameters derived from the CT attenuation time curve has shown good correlation with radionuclide microsphere measurements of myocardial blood flow.[41]

Thus, considerable physiological information can be derived from cine CT studies. In essence, it combines in one study the information contained in radionuclide gated blood pool imaging and thallium perfusion imaging. Cine CT is currently the only imaging modality that achieves evaluation of myocardial wall contraction and perfusion in spatially identical regions of the left ventricle. Such cine CT studies have been acquired at rest and during supine exercise.

CLINICAL APPLICATIONS

Various congenital and acquired disorders have been effectively examined by CT. The use of CT for cardiovascular diagnosis of several groups of abnormalities is described here. The use of cine CT for the clinical evaluation of heart disease has only been underway for a few years. Consequently, the role of this technique is unclear at present, but the initial experience in using cine CT for the evaluation of regional myocardial contraction and the patency of coronary artery bypass grafts has been encouraging.

ISCHEMIC HEART DISEASE

Quantitation of regional myocardial wall thickening dynamics is effective for evaluating regional myocardial contractile function in ischemic situations. Gated CT scans in an animal model of regional ischemia have identified the region of ischemia by demonstrating the loss of wall thickening during the cardiac cycle.[35]

A number of patients with documented coronary artery disease have now been evaluated by the fast CT scanner in order to define the capability of the technique for demonstrating regional contraction abnormalities.[42] These patients had prior myocardial infarctions documented by ECG and elevations in enzyme levels. Regional wall thickening and inward motion were assessed by fast CT in order to detect regional contraction abnormalities. The presence and site of regional contraction abnormalities defined by fast CT correlated with wall motion abnormalities demonstrated on left ventriculography and critical coronary stenoses shown by coronary arteriography. The correlation between fast CT and ventriculography for detecting regional contraction abnormalities was 91%.

Considerable information regarding the site, size, and complications of myocardial infarctions has been shown by standard CT and cine CT. These transverse CT scans have displayed the extent of wall thinning of the anterior and posterior regions of the left ventricle in patients with previous infarctions.[31] Computed tomography has also defined the presence and differentiated between true and false aneurysm of the left ventricle. It has clearly demonstrated the differentiating features of false aneurysm; namely, the small ostium between the left

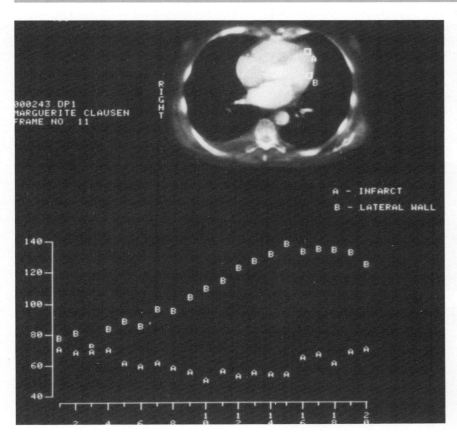

FIGURE 30.29 Regions of interest placed on various regions of the left ventricular myocardium are used to generate density (CT attenuation number) versus time curves from the sequential CT scan acquired during passage of contrast media. In this patient with a previous anterior infarct, the curve for this region (**A**) shows no rise in density during passage of the contrast through the myocardium. A normal curve is shown for the lateral wall (**B**).

ventricular cavity and the aneurysm, the usual posterior site, and the usual large size projecting well beyond the left ventricular contour.

Computed tomography has also been found to be equally as accurate as two-dimensional echocardiography for identifying left ventricular mural thrombus.[32] Indeed, comparative studies have shown greater accuracy of CT compared with two-dimensional echocardiography in the demonstration of thrombus in the left atrium. The technique has shown better capability for demonstrating thrombus situated on the lateral atrial wall and in the appendage.

EVALUATION OF CORONARY ARTERY BYPASS GRAFTS

Standard CT (nongated) as well as cine CT has accurately demonstrated patency of coronary artery bypass grafts. A multicenter prospective study using cine CT has shown a greater than 90% accuracy of CT for this purpose; patient validation of CT findings was done with coronary angiography.[43] The accuracy of CT has been better for grafts to the left anterior descending and right coronary artery than for grafts to the circumflex septum. The optimal CT scan level is free of metallic clips and is situated at approximately the level of the pulmonary artery bifurcation. The site of the bypass graft on contrast-enhanced CT scans can be related to a clock viewed from the feet looking upward. The grafts to the right coronary artery are situated between 9 and 11 o'clock. The grafts to the left anterior descending artery are situated at 12 to 2 o'clock, while the graft to the circumflex system is located at 2 to 4 o'clock. Diagnostic confidence is enhanced by visualizing the grafts at two adjacent anatomical levels and by showing contrast enhancement of the graft coincident with aortic opacification. Dynamic CT scanning (multiple segmental CT scans at the same level) demonstrates opacification and washout of contrast from the grafts. Sequential CT scans during the opacification and clearance of contrast media from the grafts can be used to generate radiographic attenuation versus time curves for regions of interest over the grafts and thus at least roughly assess the adequacy of blood flow in the graft.

PERICARDIAL ABNORMALITIES

Established noninvasive techniques (notably echocardiography) have proved valuable in reliably detecting pericardial effusions. However, CT is emerging as perhaps a more sensitive method for identifying constrictive pericarditis, effusive-constrictive pericarditis, pericardial cyst, and tumors and mediastinal mass lesions adjacent to the pericardium.[44] Localized or generalized pericardial fluid can also be identified and quantitated by CT. Since the whole chest is readily scanned by CT, associated abnormalities elsewhere in the mediastinum and lungs can be detected during the same procedure. Pericardial constriction can be reliably diagnosed when symptoms and signs of elevated diastolic pressure are present and CT demonstrates thickened pericardium (Fig. 30.30). Normally, the pericardium is represented as a thin line only 1 mm to 2 mm in thickness; it is always less than 4 mm in the normal person. The diagnosis of constriction by CT is aided by scanning after the administration of contrast medium. The ventricles are usually seen as compressed, tubular-shaped cavities, and the atrioventricular groove is narrowed. Calcification of the pericardium is an important suggestive sign, although it is not essential for the diagnosis of constriction.

ABNORMALITIES INVOLVING THE GREAT VESSELS AND VENOUS STRUCTURES

Computed tomography serves as an effective method for defining vascular mediastinal masses, aortic aneurysms, and aortic dissections.[28,45] With thoracic aortic aneurysm, the transverse scans display a markedly dilated ascending aorta and depict areas of calcification along its outer margin (Fig. 30.31). The presence of peripheral calcification favors a true aneurysm as opposed to a dissecting aneurysm. This can be seen before the infusion of contrast medium, which confirms (by its uniform enhancement) that the mass is indeed vascular.

True aortic aneurysms can be distinguished from classic aortic dissection. The findings of this condition have been described in detail previously.[28,46] Dissecting aneurysms can also be diagnosed by CT. False and true lumens may opacify differentially. Unequivocal diagnosis of dissection on CT scan requires the visualization of the intimal flap. Aortic arch anomalies have been clearly displayed by CT.[45]

ASSESSMENT OF FUNCTION

The fast CT scanners have the capability for the evaluation of cardiac function. The exposure time of 50 msec attained by cine CT is adequate for quantitating many aspects of cardiac function. The three-dimensional nature of the technique permits precise measurement of chamber volume, which has now been verified by several investigations. Right and left ventricular volumes can be assessed with equivalent accuracy. While right ventricular end-diastolic and end-systolic volumes are larger than left ventricular volumes, stroke volumes of the two ventricles measured by cine CT are nearly equal for the two ventricles in normal subjects. A disparity in stroke volumes is caused by volume overload lesions, such as shunts and valvular regurgitation. The precision demonstrated by cine CT for measuring volumes of the right as well as the left ventricle and the demonstration of equivalent stroke volumes of the two ventricles indicate that this technique should be reliable for quantitating volume overload lesions.

Because sequential images can be acquired during a single heart beat, cine CT is ideal for monitoring the effect of interventions on the right and left ventricles. Cine CT performed at peak effort during supine bicycle exercise has been used to identify the abnormal response ex-

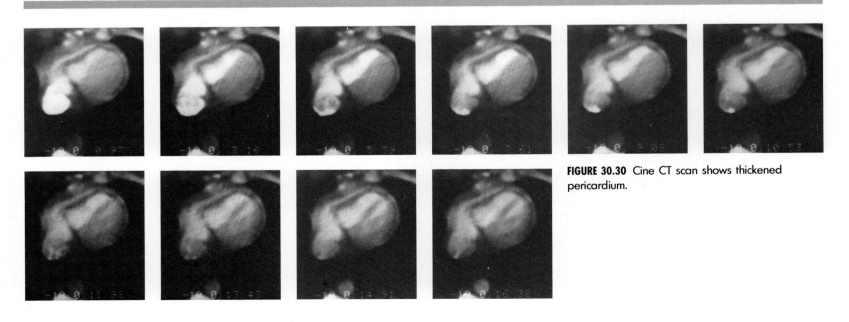

FIGURE 30.30 Cine CT scan shows thickened pericardium.

pected for patients with hemodynamically significant coronary arterial stenoses.[38] The abnormal response is characterized by a less than 5% increase in ejection fraction or the elicitation of a regional wall motion abnormality between the rest and exercise study. Cine CT has also been effective for the detection of abnormal right ventricular function. It has depicted structural and functional abnormalities in a subset of patients with ventricular arrhythmias originating from a right ventricular focus (Abbott J: unpublished data).

Functional abnormalities at rest and during bicycle exercise in patients with chronic lung disease have been detected using cine CT. Cine CT performed at rest in patients with severe pulmonary arterial hypertension shows dilated right-sided chambers and inferior vena cava, indicative of tricuspid regurgitation and loss or reversal of the normal curvature of the ventricular septum. Tomographic images of normal subjects show that the septal curvature is convex toward the right ventricle during systole. Because of the frequently associated tricuspid regurgitation, the ejection fraction and stroke volume may not be reduced even in the presence of severe pulmonary arterial hypertension and right ventricular heart failure. The volume of tricuspid regurgitation is the difference between right ventricular and left ventricular stroke volume. Thus, the left ventricular stroke volume is equivalent to the effective (forward) right ventricular stroke volume. The level of exercise achieved by many patients with severe lung disease (and presumably pulmonary arterial hypertension) is submaximal, but most patients display an abnormal response. The abnormal response consists of an increase in right ventricular end-diastolic volume; a less than 5% increase of ejection fraction of the left or both ventricles; and an increase in the right ventricular regurgitant volume. The ability to obtain a cine CT study during a single heart beat makes this technique effective for the evaluation of ventricular function during peak exercise and other transient interventions.

Fast (cine) CT has also been proposed as a method for measuring regional myocardial perfusion at rest and in comparison to interventions that increase myocardial blood flow, such as exercise and vasodilators.[41] Perfusion is estimated by monitoring density values of the myocardium over time on CT scans exposed sequentially during peak opacification and washout of contrast media from regional myocardium. The goal is to simulate the rest–exercise thallium perfusion study, but with a substantially greater degree of spatial resolution and separation of myocardial regions.

POSITRON EMISSION TOMOGRAPHY

Positron emission tomography (PET) has the capability for the evaluation of regional myocardial blood flow and regional myocardial metabolism. The transverse tomograms provide distinct spatial separation between various regions of the left ventricle, so that the distribution of myocardial blood flow and the uptake of metabolic markers can be assigned to the various myocardial regions. Experience with this technique in recent years suggests that it may provide the capability to predict the response of the myocardium to therapeutic interventions.[47,48] By monitoring changes in metabolic patterns or substrate uptake, it may also prove capable of monitoring early response to therapy.

ASSESSMENT OF REGIONAL MYOCARDIAL BLOOD FLOW

Since the various regions of the left ventricle are unequivocally separated from each other on the transverse tomographic images, PET scans using perfusion markers can be used to detect and localize coronary artery disease. Two perfusion markers have been used extensively with PET. The metabolic rates and tissue kinetics of nitrogen-13 ammonia ($^{13}NH_3$)[49,50] and rubidium-82[51] are now well understood.

Gould and co-workers[49] used $^{13}NH_3$ to assess regional myocardial blood flow at rest and in a hyperemic state induced by the powerful vasodilator dipyridamole. This technique has shown regional reduction of the positron emitter in the presence of stenoses, reducing luminal diameter by 40% to 50%.

Assessment of regional blood flow with rubidium-82 PET scans has shown segmental defects in coronary patients during mental exercise[52] and has shown segmental defects in the absence of ischemic symptoms or ECG changes.[51] These observations document the occurrence of "silent ischemia."

MYOCARDIAL METABOLISM

The most unique and innovative feature of PET is its capability to measure regional myocardial substrate uptake and metabolic kinetics in a noninvasive and nonperturbing fashion. The "proviso" in assessing myocardial metabolism is that, in general, the natural metabolic moieties are not monitored by PET but rather by injected positron-labeled analogs of the natural metabolites. PET has demonstrated the capability to (1) measure regional myocardial uptake of exogenous glucose and free fatty acid[53–59]; (2) quantitate free fatty acid metabolism in the myocardium under various physiologic states[56,57]; (3) define the preferential myocardial energy source (fatty acid versus glucose) under various physiologic states[47,48,55–58]; and (4) evaluate myocardial chemical receptor sites.

PET employing $^{13}NH_3$ and fluorine-18 fluorodeoxyglucose (^{18}FDG) has been used to evaluate simultaneously regional myocardial perfusion and glucose uptake, respectively, in an effort to distinguish regions with a perfusion defect, but containing viable myocardium from irreversibly infarcted myocardium. Tillisch and colleagues have used these two positron traces to define residual myocardial viability after acute myocardial infarction and to predict reversal of regional wall motion

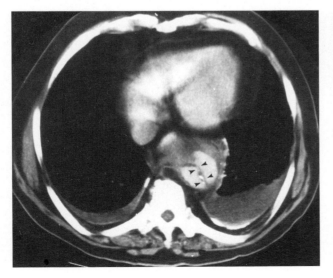

FIGURE 30.31 CT scan of thoracic aorta dissection identifies the intimal flap (arrow). There is a hematoma surrounding the aorta and a left pleural effusion. (White RD, Lipton MJ, Higgins CB et al: Noninvasive evaluation of suspected thoracic aortic disease by contrast enhanced computed tomography. Am J Cardiol 57:282, 1986)

abnormalities in response to revascularization surgery.[47] Preservation of myocardial uptake of [18]FDG in association with decreased uptake of [13]NH$_3$ correlated with ischemia without infarction. Nonviable myocardium (infarction) was defined as a concordant decrease in uptake of [18]FDG and [13]NH$_3$ (Fig. 30.32), whereas ischemic, but viable, myocardium caused a discordant pattern characterized by decrease in [13]NH$_3$ uptake and a normal or increased uptake of [18]FDG in the same myocardial region (Fig. 30.33).

The discordant distribution (mismatch) of the two tracers achieved an 85% accuracy in predicting improvement in contraction after revascularization.[47] On the other hand, a concordant decrease predicted nonsalvageable infarcted myocardium with a 92% accuracy. The study demonstrates the capability of this modality to accurately predict response to therapy in ischemic heart disease.

This mismatch in [18]FDG and [13]NH$_3$ has also been observed in patients with exercise-induced ECG abnormalities or persistent angina after myocardial infarction.[58] Moreover, those patients displaying this mismatch after recent myocardial infarction had a higher frequency of recurrent chest pain or transient ECG abnormalities than did patients with completed myocardial infarction.[58] Consequently, this mismatch pattern may identify patients who will benefit from angioplasty or surgical revascularization after acute myocardial infarction.

PET employing the positron emitter carbon-11 palmitic acid has identified the consequences of myocardial ischemia and infarction on myocardial free fatty acid metabolism.[53,55-58] These studies revealed that exogenous ^{11}C-labeled palmitic acid can enter two metabolic pools within the myocardium: namely a rapidly metabolized pool in which the fatty acid is immediately oxidized to carbon dioxide or a storage pool of triglycerides. During myocardial ischemia, myocardial uptake of ^{11}C-labeled palmitic acid and its distribution into the two pools are altered. The free fatty acid pathway most vulnerable to ischemia is β-oxidation, and consequently the amount of ^{11}C-labeled palmitic acid entering this pathway is decreased initially.

Prediction of a successful salvage of myocardium after thromboly-

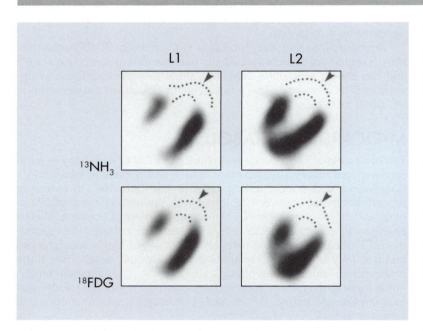

FIGURE 30.32 The positron emission tomogram at two levels through the left ventricle showing the myocardial distribution of nitrogen-13 ammonia ([13]NH$_3$), a perfusion marker, and fluorine-18 fluorodeoxyglucose ([18]FDG), a marker of glucose uptake. In this patient with a prior anterior wall infarct there are matched perfusion and metabolic defects. (Courtesy of Dr. Heinrich Schelbert)

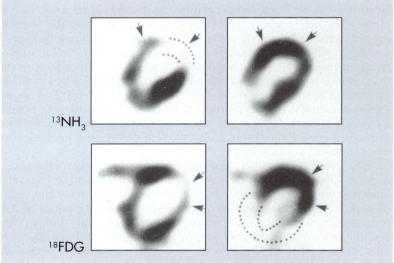

FIGURE 30.33 Mismatched pattern in another patient with prior infarct shows a perfusion ([13]NH$_3$) defect, but persistent glucose ([18]FDG) uptake in the anterior wall. (Courtesy of Dr. Heinrich Schelbert)

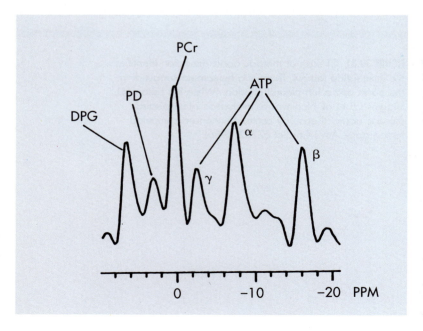

FIGURE 30.34 Phosphorus-31 magnetic resonance spectrum from a normal subject. The important spectral peaks are phosphocreatine (PCr), the three for adenosine triphosphate (ATP), phosphodiester (PD), and 2,3-diphosphoglycerate (DPG).

sis with streptokinase has been achieved by PET imaging of ^{11}C-labeled palmitic acid uptake in the jeopardized myocardium.[59] Successful thrombolysis was associated with resumption of uptake of ^{11}C-labeled palmitic acid in the jeopardized region.

MAGNETIC RESONANCE SPECTROSCOPY

MR spectroscopy has provided a new research tool for the evaluation of myocardial metabolism. It can be used to investigate the link between myocardial function and metabolism, assess the early response of the myocardium to various therapeutic and pharmacologic interventions, establish myocardial viability, and assess beneficial or detrimental effects of reperfusion on the ischemically injured myocardium.

MR spectroscopy operates on the same principle as MRI in that the nuclei of some atoms (those with an odd number of nuclear particles) resonate when radiofrequency energy is applied at a frequency specific for a particular atom. After this energy is applied, each nuclei resonates at a characteristic frequency so that the presence of a particular atom within a chemical compound or tissue can be identified by the MR process. In distinction to imaging, which is usually only sensitive to the presence of a certain atom within a compound, MR spectroscopy can provide a map of the various sites where an atom exists within a compound. MR spectroscopy depicts the very slight differences in resonant frequencies of the same nuclei when it exists in different compounds. The slight variation in resonant frequencies of the same nuclei in various compounds is called *chemical shift,* and the graphic display of the various frequencies is the MR spectrum of the nuclei. An example of this is the MR spectrum of phosphorus-31 (^{31}P), where the multiple spectral peaks represent ^{31}P in the compounds: inorganic phosphate, creatine phosphate, adenosine triphosphate, and so on (Fig. 30.34). The MR spectra are displayed in a convention whereby the position of the peak in the spectrum (horizontal axis) indicates the specific compound (*i.e.,* creatine phosphate) while the height of the peak (vertical axis) and an area under the peak indicate the relative concentration of the compound.

At the current time MR spectroscopy is for the most part a research technique, although clinical uses have been proposed. The nuclei for which MR spectroscopy seems the most intriguing for diagnostic purposes are hydrogen-1, carbon-13, and phosphorus-31. Hydrogen-1 (proton) spectroscopy has been used to detect lactate in ischemic tissue[60] and lipid accumulation in ischemically injured tissue.[61] Metabolism of energy substrates in the myocardium has been approached using carbon-13; the technique has the potential for monitoring the use of fat and glucose by the myocardium and the manner in which ischemia influences their use. At this time most attention has been devoted to ^{31}P MR spectroscopy as a method for studying high energy phosphate stores in various myocardial disease states and alterations of high energy phosphate stores in response to therapeutic interventions.[62,63]

Phosphorus-31 spectroscopy in experimental preparations has been used to evaluate the influence of potentially toxic agents on the myocardium, such as doxorubicin[64] and ethanol.[62] Some experiments also indicate the potential of using MR spectroscopy to evaluate the effects of pharmacologic therapy on myocardial metabolism. For instance, calcium channel blockers have been found to enhance recovery of both function and high energy phosphate stores of the ischemically injured myocardium.[65]

The possibility of reperfusion of the ischemically injured myocardium in humans using streptokinase and other thrombolytic agents has aroused intense interest in pathophysiology of the reperfused myocardium. Specifically, it is important to determine myocardial viability in a region that has been reperfused. ^{31}P MR spectroscopy may be a method for accomplishing this. Recent studies of regional myocardial ischemia in an animal model have compared the pattern of alteration in the ^{31}P MR spectroscopy of the myocardium that has been irreversibly injured and then reperfused with the ^{31}P spectroscopic pattern of the reversibly injured reperfused myocardium.[63,66]

^{31}P spectroscopy of the myocardium has now been accomplished in humans in several laboratories around the world. Abnormal spectra have been observed in patients with myocardial disease.[67] However, the sensitivity, specificity, and, indeed, the clinical use of ^{31}P MR spectroscopy have yet to be established.

CONCLUSIONS

The newer imaging techniques provide the capability for definitive diagnosis and comprehensive evaluation of cardiac anatomy and function. Because these techniques provide three-dimensional information, they can attain a high level of quantitative accuracy and reproducibility. Some of these techniques extend the diagnostic evaluation beyond anatomy and function by sequentially sampling myocardial metabolism.

It is likely that the role of new cardiac imaging modalities in the evaluation of cardiac disease will change rapidly in the next few years. Unlike imaging techniques introduced at earlier periods, the development of these techniques will be importantly influenced by the growing cost-containment concern now extant in most countries.

REFERENCES

1. Sechtem U, Pflugfelder PW, White RD et al: Cine MRI: Potential for the evaluation of cardiovascular function. Am J Radiol 148:239, 1987
2. Wesbey G, Higgins CB, Lanzer P et al: Imaging and characterization of acute myocardial infarctions in vivo using gated nuclear magnetic resonance. Circulation 69:125, 1984
3. Higgins CB, Lanzer P, Stark D et al: Nuclear magnetic resonance imaging in chronic ischemic heart disease in man. Circulation 69:523, 1984
4. Kaufman L, Crooks L, Sheldon P et al: The potential impact of nuclear magnetic resonance imaging on cardiovascular diagnosis. Circulation 67:251, 1983
5. Lanzer P, Lorenz V, Schiller NB et al: Cardiac imaging using gated nuclear magnetic resonance. Radiology 150:121, 1984
6. Fisher MR, von Schulthess GK, Higgins CB: Quantitation of regional left ventricular wall thickness using rotated gated magnetic resonance imaging. Am J Radiol 145:27, 1985
7. Dinsmore RE, Wismer GL, Levine RA et al: Magnetic resonance imaging of the heart: Positioning and gradient angle selection for optimal imaging planes. Am J Radiol 143:1135, 1984
8. Go RT, MacIntyre WJ, Yeung HN et al: Volume and planar gated cardiac magnetic resonance imaging: A correlative study with thallium 201 SPECT and cadaver sections. Radiology 150:129, 1984
9. Fletcher BD, Jacobstein MD, Nelson AD et al: Gated magnetic resonance imaging of congenital cardiac malformations. Radiology 150:1378, 1984
10. McNamara MT, Higgins CB, Schechtmann N et al: Detection and characterization of acute myocardial infarctions in man using gated magnetic resonance imaging. Circulation 71:717, 1985
11. McNamara MT, Higgins CB: Magnetic resonance imaging and characterization of chronic myocardial infarction. Am J Radiol 146:315, 1986
12. von Schulthess GK, Fisher MR, Crooks LE et al: The nature of intracardiac signal on gated NMR images in normals and patients with abnormal left ventricular function. Radiology 156:125, 1985
13. Bradley WG Jr, Waluch V, Lai KS et al: The appearance of rapidly flowing blood on magnetic resonance images. Ann Intern Med 103:317, 1985
14. von Schulthess GD, Fisher MR, Higgins CB: Detection of abnormal pulmonary flow pattern by magnetic resonance imaging in pulmonary arterial hypertension. Ann Intern Med 103:317, 1985
15. Feinberg DA, Crooks LE, Hoenninger J et al: Pulsatile blood velocity in human arteries displayed by magnetic resonance imaging. Radiology 153:177, 1984
16. Williams ES, Kaplan JI, Thatcher F et al: Prolongation of proton spin lattice relaxation time in regionally ischemic tissue from dog hearts. J Nucl Med 21:449, 1980
17. Tscholakoff D, Aherne T, Yee ES et al: *In vivo* evaluation of cardiac allograft rejection in dogs using magnetic resonance imaging. Radiology 157:697, 1985
18. Tscholakoff D, McNamara MT, Derugin N et al: Early detection of myocardial ischemic injury by MRI. Radiology 159:667, 1986
19. Brown JJ, Higgins CB: Myocardial contrast agents for magnetic resonance imaging. Am J Radiol 151:239, 1988
20. Saeed M, Wagner S, Wendland MF et al: Occlusive and reperfused myocardial infarcts: differentiation with Mn DPDP-enhanced MR imaging. Radiology 172:59, 1989
21. Higgins CB, Byrd BF III, Stark D et al: Magnetic resonance imaging of hypertrophic cardiomyopathy. Am J Cardiol 55:1121, 1985
22. Caputo GR, Sechtem U, Tscholakoff D et al: Measurement of myocardial in-

23. Buser PT, Auffermann W, Holt WW et al: Noninvasive evaluation of the global left ventricular function using cine MR imaging. J Am Coll Cardiol 13:1294, 1989
24. Jacobstein MD, Fletcher BD, Goldstein S et al: Evaluation of atrioventricular septal defect by magnetic resonance imaging. Am J Cardiol 55:1158, 1985
25. Higgins CB, Byrd BF III, Farmer D et al: Magnetic resonance imaging in patients with congenital heart disease. Circulation 70:851, 1984
26. Sommerhoff BK, Sechtem UP, Higgins CB: Evaluation of pulmonary blood supply by nuclear magnetic resonance imaging in patients with pulmonary atresia. J Am Col Cardiol 11(1):166, 1988
27. Kersting-Sommerhoff BA, Higgins CB, White RD et al: Aortic dissection: Sensitivity and specificity of MR imaging. Radiology 3(166):651, 1988
28. White RC, Dooms GC, Higgins CB: Advances in imaging thoracic aortic disease. Invest Radiol 21:761, 1986
29. Soulen RL, Stark DD, Higgins CB: Magnetic resonance imaging of constrictive pericardial heart disease. Am J Cardiol 55:480, 1985
30. Higgins CB, Holt W, Pflugfelder P, Sechtem U: Functional evaluation of the heart with magnetic resonance imaging. Magn Reson Med 6:121, 1988
31. Lackner K, Thurn P: Computed tomography of the heart: ECG gated and continuous scans. Radiology 140:413, 1981
32. Tomada H, Hoshai M, Fururja H et al: Evaluation of intracardiac thrombus with computed tomography. Am J Cardiol 51:843, 1983
33. Higgins CB, Carlssen E, Lipton MJ (eds): CT of the Heart and Great Vessels, pp 167–168. Mount Kisco, NY, Futura Publishing, 1983
34. Lipton MJ, Higgins CB, Farmer D et al: Cardiac imaging with a high-speed cine-CT scanner: Preliminary results. Radiology 152:579, 1984
35. Mattrey RF, Higgins CB: Detection of regional myocardium dysfunction during ischemia with computerized tomography. Documentation and basis. Invest Radiol 17:329, 1982
36. Farmer DW, Lipton MJ, Higgins CB et al: *In vivo* assessment of left ventricular wall and chamber dynamics during transient myocardial ischemia using cine CT. Am J Cardiol 55:560, 1985
37. Feiring AJ, Rumberger JA, Reiter SJ et al: Determination of left ventricular mass in dogs with rapid-acquisition cardiac computed tomographic scanning. Circulation 72(6):1355, 1985
38. Caputo GR, Lipton MJ: Evaluation of regional left ventricular function using cine CT. In Pohost GM, Higgins CB, Morganroth J et al (eds): New Concepts in Cardiac Imaging, Year Book Medical Publishers, Chicago, 1988
39. Rumberger JA, Fiering AJ, Skorton DJ et al: Sectional and segmental variability of left ventricular function: experimental and clinical studies using ultrafast computed tomography. J Am Coll Cardiol 12:415, 1988
40. Garrett J, Lanzer P, Higgins CB et al: Quantitation of cardiac output by cine CT. Am J Cardiol 56:657, 1985
41. Gould RG, Lipton MJ, McNamara MT et al: Measurement of regional myocardial flow in dogs using ultrafast CT. Invest Radiol 23(5):348, 1988
42. Lipton MJ, Farmer DW, Killebrew E et al: Evaluation of regional myocardial function with fast CT in patients with prior myocardial infiltration. Radiology 157:735, 1985
43. Sanford W, Brundage B, McMillan R et al: Sensitivity and specificity of assessing coronary bypass graft patency with ultrafast computed tomography: Results of a multicenter study. J Am Coll Cardiol 12:1, 1988
44. Moncada R, Baker M, Salinas M et al: Diagnostic role of computed tomography in pericardial heart disease. Am Heart J 103:263, 1982
45. McLaughlin MJ, Weisbrod G, Wise DJ et al: Computed tomography in congenital anomalies of the aortic arch and great vessels. Radiology 138:399, 1981
46. Goodwin JD, Herfkens RJ, Skioldebrand CB et al: Evaluation of dissections and aneurysms of the thoracic aorta by conventional and dynamic CT scanning. Radiology 136:125, 1980
47. Tillisch J, Marshall R, Schelbert H et al: Reversibility of wall motion abnormalities: Preoperative determination using positron tomography [18]fluorodeoxyglucose and [13]NH$_3$ (abstr). Circulation 68:III-387, 1983
48. Marshall RC: Identification and differentiation of resting myocardial ischemia and infarction in man with positron computed tomography, ^{18}F-labelled fluorodeoxyglucose and N-13 ammonia. Circulation 64:766, 1983
49. Gould KL, Schebert HR, Phelps ME et al: Noninvasive assessment of coronary stenoses with myocardial perfusion imaging during pharmacologic coronary vasodilation: V. Detection of 47 percent diameter coronary stenosis with intravenous nitrogen-13 ammonia and emission-computed tomography in intact dogs. Am J Cardiol 43:200, 1979
50. Schelbert HR, Wisenberg G, Phelps ME et al: Noninvasive assessment of coronary stenosis by myocardial imaging during pharmacologic coronary vasodilation: VI. Detection of coronary artery disease in human beings with intravenous N-13 ammonia and positron computed tomography. Am J Cardiol 49:1197, 1982
51. Selwyn AP, Allan RM, L'Abbate A et al: Relation between regional myocardial uptake of rubidium 82 and perfusion: Absolute reduction of cation uptake in ischemia. Am J Cardiol 50:112, 1982
52. Deanfield J, Sheam M, Wilson R et al: Mental stress and ischemia in patients with coronary disease (abstr). Circulation 58:III–258, 1983
53. Schelbert HR, Henze E, Schon HR et al: C-11 palmitate for the noninvasive evaluation of regional myocardial fatty acid metabolism with positron computed tomography: III. In vivo demonstration of the effects of substrate availability on myocardial metabolism. Am Heart J 105:492, 1983
54. Henze E, Schelbert HR, Barrio JR et al: Myocardial uptake and clearance of C-11 palmitic acid in man: Effects of substrate availability and cardiac work. J Nucl Med 23:P12, 1982
55. Schelbert HR, Henze E, Keen R et al: C-11 palmitate for noninvasive evaluation of regional myocardial fatty acid metabolism with positron computed tomography: IV. In vivo evaluation of acute, experimentally induced myocardial ischemia in dogs. Am Heart J 106:736, 1983
56. Schon HR, Schelbert HR, Robinson G et al: C-11 labelled palmitic acid for the noninvasive evaluation of regional myocardial fatty acid metabolism with positron computed tomography: I. Kinetics of C-11 palmitic acid in normal myocardium. Am Heart J 103:532, 1982
57. Schon HR, Schelbert HR, Najafi A et al: C-11 labelled palmitic acid for the noninvasive evaluation of regional myocardial fatty acid metabolism with positron computed tomography: II. Kinetics of C-11 palmitic acid in acutely ischemic myocardium. Am Heart J 103:548, 1982
58. Schelbert HR, Buxton D: Insights into coronary artery disease gained from metabolic imaging. Circulation 78:496, 1988
59. Ludbrook PA, Geltman EM, Tiefenbrunn AJ et al: Restoration of regional myocardial metabolism by coronary thrombolysis in patients (abstr). Circulation 68:III–325, 1983
60. Richards T, Terrier F, Sievers R et al: Lactate accumulation in ischemic and anoxic isolated rat hearts measured by H-1 spectroscopy. Invest Radiol 22:638, 1987
61. Richards T, Tscholakoff D, Higgins CB: Proton NMR spectroscopy in canine myocardial infarction. Magn Reson Med 4(6):555, 1987
62. Wu S, White R, Wikman-Coffelt J et al: The preventative effect of verapamil on ethanol-induced cardiac depression: P-^{31} NMR and high pressure liquid chromotographic studies of hamsters. Circulation 75(5):1058, 1987
63. Wendland MF, White RD, Derugin N et al: Characterization of high-energy phosphate compounds during reperfusion of the irreversibly injured myocardium using ^{31}P MRS. Magn Reson Med 7:172, 1988
64. Ng TC, Dougherty JP, Evanchko WT et al: Detection of antineoplastic agent induced cardiotoxicity by ^{31}P NMR of perfused rat hearts. Biochem Biophys Res Commun 110:339, 1983
65. Buser PT, Wikman-Coffelt J, Wu S: Post-ischemic recovery of mechanical performance and energy metabolism in the presence of left ventricular hypertrophy. A ^{31}P MRS study. Circ Res 1990 (in press)
66. Holt WH, Wendland M, Derugin N et al: Effect of repetitive brief episodes of cardiac ischemia on ^{31}P MRS in the cat. Circulation 76(Suppl IV):246, 1987
67. Auffermann W, Chew W, Tavares NJ et al: Characterization of phosphorus metabolism in dilated cardiomyopathy: A gated, localized P-31 MR spectroscopy study in humans (abstr). Radiology 169(p):345, 1988

# EXERCISE STRESS TESTING: PRINCIPLES AND CLINICAL APPLICATION

Myrvin H. Ellestad • Robert J. Stuart

The material in this chapter is presented as an introduction to exercise testing. It is hoped that it will provide a framework on which to build a comprehensive knowledge of exercise physiology and exercise testing.

Exercise testing has become established as one of the most widely used tests in clinical cardiology. We hope the reader will appreciate that an evaluation by the methods presented here should provide more than a positive or negative diagnosis. The competent physician will often be able to estimate the severity of the disability, the percent of probability of significant coronary narrowing, and the prognosis. As with any test, all of the known clinical information must be synthesized to interpret the findings in a meaningful way.

HISTORY

Although William Cubitt, a British civil engineer who designed the first treadmill, had no interest in cardiac patients, his elongated "stepping wheel" may have been a precursor of our present technique. "Treading the wheel" became a common method of punishment in the early 19th century in British prisons, but it was outlawed after only a few years because it was considered inhumane and unhealthy.[1] Now thousands of patients pay good money for the same treatment under the guise of testing their heart. Edward Smith in 1846 began to use a similar device to study exercise performance and measure respiratory rate, stroke volume, heart rate, and oxygen utilization.[2] Thus, the stage was set for modern efforts to better understand exercise in both normal subjects and those with coronary heart disease.

Modern exercise testing probably dates from the empirical discovery that ST depression reflects myocardial ischemia. Einthoven may have recognized this in 1908, when he published a postexercise tracing showing ST segment depression, but he failed to comment on these specific changes. In 1918, Blousfield[3] correlated ST segment depression with angina, and in 1928, Feil and Siegel deliberately exercised patients to bring on angina and ST segment changes.[4] They suggested that the ST segment depression was due to a decreased blood flow to the heart and published electrocardiographic tracings before and after the ischemic event.

In 1929, Master started exercise testing with his steps, but counted the pulse and recorded the blood pressure to evaluate cardiac function.[5] Twelve years later, he reported the use of the electrocardiogram and thereafter popularized the use of the "step test" for the diagnosis of coronary heart disease.

From then on, many cardiac physiologists, including Katz, Brouha, Wood, and Hellerstein,[6] expanded our knowledge of the mechanisms of the changes occurring during exercise in patients with ischemia. About 1959, Hellerstein began to use the treadmill to evaluate the work capacity of postinfarction patients in preparation for their return to their usual employment. These "work classification" clinics were sponsored by the American Heart Association and evolved into our present cardiac rehabilitation programs. They helped establish the safety of exercise testing in patients with known myocardial ischemia.

About 1956, Bruce[7] began his extensive studies in exercise physiology and popularized the protocol that has become standard in the United States. Since that time, correlation of exercise data with coronary angiograms and with epidemiologic data has allowed us to better characterize our findings and has helped establish the method as an indispensable part of patient evaluation in ischemic heart disease.

PHYSIOLOGY OF EXERCISE AND MYOCARDIAL PERFUSION

SYSTEMIC CHANGES WITH EXERCISE

Exercise can be broadly characterized as dynamic when the motion is rhythmic and repetitive, and isometric where sustained muscle contraction occurs. Because the latter has much less effect on the heart, we will concentrate on dynamic or isotonic exercise in this discussion.

As exercise is initiated, vagal tone declines rapidly, resulting in an increase in the heart rate, venous return, stroke volume, and cardiac output. The increase in cardiac output is almost linear with the increase in oxygen uptake by the respiratory apparatus. The changes in heart rate, cardiac output, and stroke volume are facilitated by sympathetic stimuli, both neurogenic and humoral. If exercise is maintained at a submaximal level, the patient is said to be at a "steady state," in which the intake of oxygen and the increased needs of the metabolic processes are in balance. If this is sustained for an extended time, the subject eventually gets into a "drift phase," in which the elimination of heat by sweating and the water lost through breathing result in a drop in central blood volume and cause changes in heart rate, stroke volume, and arterial pressure (Fig. 31.1).[8]

MYOCARDIAL PERFUSION

In the peripheral circulation, the metabolic demands of exercising muscles can be increased several times more than the increase in blood flow because of the ability to increase oxygen extraction. In the heart at basal state (heart rate about 60–70 beats per minute), the oxygen extraction is very near maximal capacity. This requires that increased cardiac work be associated with an almost linear increase in myocardial perfusion. Thus, an increase in systemic oxygen uptake is usually linear with an increase in myocardial blood flow, unless other physiological events also add work to the heart, such as an increase in blood pressure or peripheral resistance. This is the reason why the so-called double product (heart rate times systolic blood pressure) is such an excellent index of myocardial blood flow and myocardial work.

CORONARY RESISTANCE

The driving force for perfusing the heart is primarily the diastolic pressure minus the resistance in the heart itself. This is because the compressive forces of systolic contraction inhibit flow to the middle and inner layers of the myocardium. Thus, most of the myocardial perfusion occurs during diastole, and this flow is regulated by the precapillary sphincters. They respond almost exclusively to the metabolic demands of the heart, probably mediated by local pH changes, bradykinins, and other substances still incompletely understood.

INTRAMYOCARDIAL TENSION

As the tension or pressure generated during systole by cardiac contraction increases, the need for oxygen responds accordingly. The tension is a function not only of pressure but of wall thickness and the radius of the ventricular cavity. As the radius increases, myocardial tension also increases. These forces are important during diastole because the blood has to overcome the increased stiffness often associated with myocardial hypertrophy and a dilated left ventricular cavity.

SYSTOLIC AND DIASTOLIC INTERVALS

Because the time during diastole is about two thirds of the cardiac cycle at heart rates of about 70, there is adequate time to nourish the heart effectively. As the heart rate increases with exercise, however, the systolic time decreases only slightly, but the diastolic time progressively shortens, so that at a heart rate of 180, diastole comprises only about 20% of the cardiac cycle. Thus, the time available to perfuse the muscle is so attenuated that there is a marked reduction in flow and, thus, a limit to the performance. This reduction in diastolic time may be the reason the heart rate has a maximum level for each age-group.

DETERMINANTS OF MYOCARDIAL OXYGEN CONSUMPTION

The three major determinants of myocardial oxygen utilization are heart rate, myocardial contractility, and wall stress. Wall stress equals volume times chamber pressure/wall thickness. Shortening, activation, and basal metabolic requirements are minor determinants. The total requirements of the heart can be accurately assessed only when all of these are known.[9] The percent increase of each factor with exercise is illustrated in Figure 31.2. It becomes obvious that if one can reduce the heart rate and contractility, a major reduction in demand will occur. On the other hand, exercise increases both heart rate and catecholamine concentration, and this provides the greatest stimulus to an increase in myocardial oxygen consumption.

TRANSMURAL DISTRIBUTION OF BLOOD FLOW

There is no evidence to demonstrate that there are variations in transmural blood flow among animal species, so data in dogs can be presumed to pertain to man.[9] In dogs, the endocardial one third of the heart receives more blood than the middle or subepicardial areas, because wall stress in this area increases myocardial oxygen demands. It is ironic that this area is the most vulnerable in ischemic heart disease.

NEUROGENIC CONTROL

Until a few years ago, it was believed that coronary flow in normal subjects was always mediated primarily by metabolic demands of the myocardium. It is now known that epicardial arteries may be constricted in apparently normal segments of the coronary arteries or in areas where a plaque has already partly reduced flow.[10] These reflexes can be mediated by aortic blood pressure, emotion, cold, altered pH, and probably other factors. Thus, there are times when vasomotion of the coronary circulation reduces flow below that required by the metabolic demands of the myocardium, even in the absence of coronary obstructive lesions.

PHYSIOLOGICAL MECHANISMS IN MYOCARDIAL ISCHEMIA

As the myocardial oxygen demand rises owing to exercise or other causes, the subendocardium, being the most metabolically active and also the most vulnerable from an anatomical standpoint, is the first area to be affected. As the subendocardial cells become starved because of an inadequate oxygen supply, they probably take in excess calcium and lose some of their ability to relax. This stiffness in the inner layers of the myocardium reduces ventricular compliance, which causes the filling pressure to rise. This increase in filling pressure may further suppress diastolic blood flow, thus aggravating the ischemic process. This is the concept of the subendocardial clamp (Fig. 31.3). However, hemodynamic causes, such as increase in left ventricular afterload and ventricular interaction, may also contribute to increased left ventricular diastolic pressure during myocardial ischemia.

As the ischemic process progresses, there is a leak in potassium from subendocardial cells causing a current flow toward the epicar-

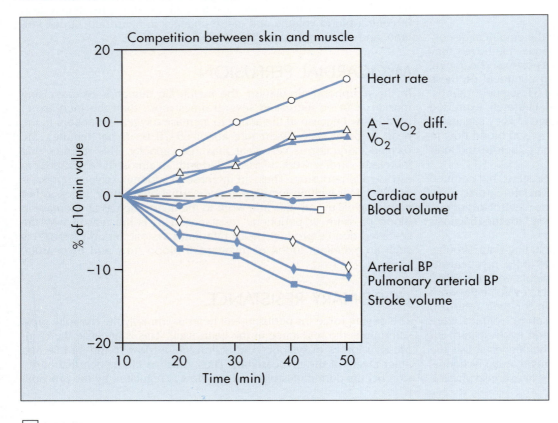

FIGURE 31.1 The trends in physiological measurements with time during a 50-minute run in man. Note the decrease in blood volume caused by sweating, which caused a drop in stroke volume and an increase in heart rate, so that the cardiac output remains stable. (Modified from Nadel ET: Problems with Temperature Regulation During Exercise. New York, Academic Press, 1977)

dium and usually toward the precordial monitoring electrodes. This diastolic current of injury displaces the baseline upward. When ventricular depolarization occurs with the QRS complex, all the cardiac cells are depolarized, and at this point (onset of the ST segment) the galvanometer records no current and returns the deflection to the null point, or zero, which is below the baseline previously deflected upward during diastole by the potassium current (Fig. 31.4). After the T wave is inscribed, the diastolic potassium current again deflects the baseline during the QT interval to its position above the zero line. If the process involves enough of the muscle, contraction of the ischemic area will decrease or cease, allowing an outward bulge during systole.

This may result in a drop in cardiac output and blood pressure or may be associated with anginal pain, which occurs in about 20% to 30% of subjects with ischemic myocardium.

INDICATIONS FOR EXERCISE TESTING
CORONARY ARTERY DISEASE

Since the days of the Master "2-step" test, the exercise test has been used to discover or confirm the presence of coronary narrowing. It remains one of the most practical and commonly used tests in cardiol-

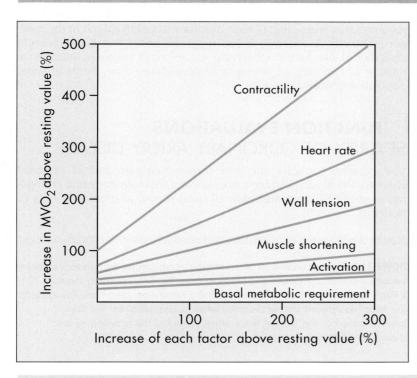

FIGURE 31.2 The changes in various factors contributing to myocardial oxygen requirements during exercise in percent. (Modified from Marcus ML: The Coronary Circulation in Health and Disease. New York, McGraw-Hill, 1983)

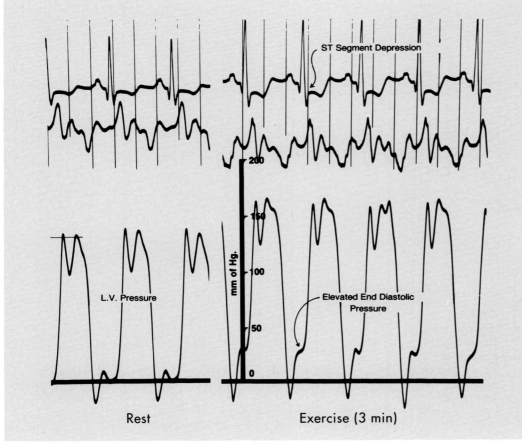

FIGURE 31.3 The left ventricular (L.V.) end-diastolic pressure rises as ischemia increases with exercise, causing subendocardial ischemia and ST segment depression.

ogy. Because these patients so commonly have no resting physical findings or symptoms, a dynamic test is essential.

ETIOLOGY OF CHEST PAIN

Observing a person during exercise and being able to assess his or her heart rate, rhythm, blood pressure response, and electrocardiographic changes provide information obtained in no other way. If pain is induced by exercise, observing the patient's response and asking questions provide important insights.

CARDIAC ARRHYTHMIAS

The ability to observe the onset or termination of arrhythmias with exercise adds diagnostic value of considerable importance. When these are correlated with symptoms, the clinical significance becomes more obvious.

DETECTION OF LABILE HYPERTENSION

It is now known that a hypertensive response to exercise may be the first indicator that the patient is destined to have significant clinical hypertension in the future.

PROGNOSIS

Even when the anatomy of the coronary tree has been studied, the prognosis of the subsequent outcome of the patient can be predicted more accurately after exercise testing. Predictions can also be made from the exercise test alone in patients with coronary artery disease prior to, as well as after, a myocardial infarction. Recent work has also demonstrated that the outcome of some patients undergoing coronary bypass surgery can be predicted prior to surgery by exercise testing. Postangioplasty exercise testing can also help predict those who will have restenosis.

PREVENTIVE MEDICINE

In asymptomatic well subjects, the exercise response, when combined with risk factor analysis, can be used to identify patients needing preventive medicine and life-style change. It is also useful in evaluation of patients undergoing coronary rehabilitation in an effort to prevent a recurrence or worsening of their coronary disability. Much of the present emphasis on exercise is based on the belief that it can prevent disability in the future. Observing the exercise response may be as reliable as coronary angiography in predicting future events in some population groups.[11]

FUNCTION EVALUATIONS
SEVERITY OF CORONARY ARTERY DISEASE

The exercise capacity, the time of onset of pain and ST segment changes, the blood pressure response, and the magnitude and configuration of the ST response, have all been shown to predict severity of ischemia.

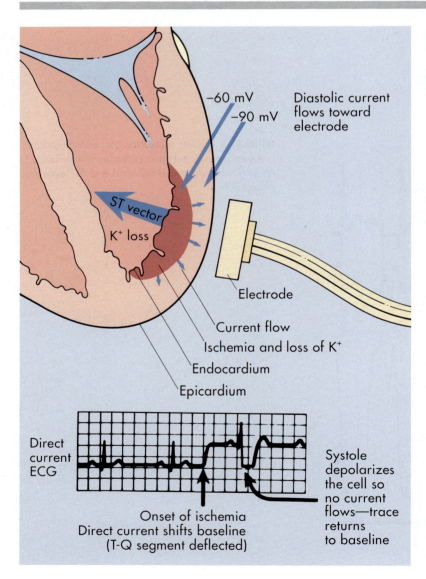

FIGURE 31.4 The mechanism of ST segment depression as the subendocardium becomes ischemic. The loss of potassium from the cells causes a diastolic current flow toward the epicardium and the monitoring electrode. This deflects the baseline upward during diastole, which is unmasked by the total depolarization at the time of the R wave, returning the baseline to zero during the ST interval.

MYOCARDIAL CONTRACTILITY

In patients with previous myocardial infarction, myocardiopathies, or vascular disorders, the performance of the patient during exercise allows one to decide on methods of management. Observing function will supplement the data collected during the history and give insight into the contractile state of the heart.

EVALUATING THERAPEUTIC INTERVENTIONS

When drugs are given to reduce ischemia or to control arrhythmias or hypertension, the most efficient way to determine the efficacy is to do an exercise test. The same can be said for any intervention from the prescribing of exercise to the evaluation of the results of coronary angioplasty, coronary bypass surgery, or valve replacement.

RESEARCH

Each year new applications of exercise testing are reported in research papers. The evaluation of various treatments and drugs and the study of mechanisms of ischemia, substrate utilization, and other physiological adaptive mechanisms are all facilitated by the use of exercise testing, not to mention the search for new exercise findings that will have predictive or diagnostic power in the understanding of circulatory disorders.

CONTRAINDICATIONS

The safety of exercise has been discussed at length, and there is still considerable disagreement. With the American public pursuing fitness by the millions, it seems trite but obvious that it is much safer to exercise in a good stress laboratory than in a health spa or a park or by hiking in the high mountains.

The most important aspect of safety in the stress laboratory is the experience and knowledge of those performing the test. Needless to say, they should be familiar with the rudiments of exercise physiology, as well as fully qualified to perform resuscitation, if needed. Knowledge of the risks and careful observation of patients during the test will circumvent all but the rare catastrophe in the stress laboratory.

ABSOLUTE

It is generally agreed that stress testing should not be done on the following:

- Patients with an acute myocardial infarction
- Patients suffering from acute myocarditis or pericarditis
- Patients exhibiting signs of unstable progressive angina, including the patient who has recent onset of long periods of angina at rest
- Patients with rapid ventricular or atrial arrhythmias
- Patients with second or third degree heart block and patients with known severe left main coronary artery disease
- Acutely ill patients such as those with infections, hyperthyroidism, or severe anemia
- Patients with locomotion problems

Over the years, exercise was believed to be dangerous in certain conditions, which led to these conditions being included in a list of absolute contraindications to exercise testing. In some of these, such as unstable angina, experience led to this conclusion, while in others, common sense seemed to justify such a statement. Every so often, one of the absolutes is moved to the relative contraindications list. In the past few years, this was the case for both aortic stenosis and congestive heart failure; it may soon pertain to left main coronary artery disease and various types of heart block. Thus, the above list comprises a current consensus but may be changed as new knowledge is accumulated.

RELATIVE
AORTIC STENOSIS

If the signs and symptoms suggest a severe process, such as a very long systolic murmur, a low or narrow pulse pressure, or a history of syncope or anginal pain, stress testing should be avoided. In those with moderate disease, however, a diagnosis usually easily made clinically, it is safe to proceed with the test, especially if the patient is fairly young or in the pediatric age range. Exercise testing may be helpful to determine whether patients with valvular heart diseases (aortic stenosis, aortic regurgitation, mitral stenosis or regurgitation) are truly asymptomatic.

SUSPECTED LEFT MAIN CORONARY ARTERY DISEASE OR LEFT MAIN EQUIVALENT

If very severe ischemia is suspected from the history or if resting ST segment depression is marked, stress testing should be done with extreme caution. Early termination of exercise, liberal use of nitroglycerin, and careful monitoring of blood pressure are essential.

SEVERE HYPERTENSION

When malignant hypertension or very severe fixed blood pressure elevation of 240/130 is present, caution is necessary. In younger patients without obvious end-organ disease, however, one can proceed to test most hypertensive patients.

OBSTRUCTIVE CARDIOMYOPATHY (IDIOPATHIC HYPERTROPHIC SUBAORTIC STENOSIS)

Sudden severe arrhythmias have occurred with exercise, especially during recovery, and are not necessarily related to the presence or degree of outflow obstruction. Thus, patients with this syndrome should be exercised only if other strong indications exist.

CONGESTIVE HEART FAILURE

Patients with compensated failure may be tested with caution, but when overt failure is present, exercise is definitely detrimental, although these patients have been tested in a few research projects.[12]

WHEN TO TERMINATE EXERCISE

Careful observations and continued communication with the patient will usually alert the experienced physician when to terminate exercise. The following list provides the common reasons:

- Patient request
- Maximum capacity obviously reached
- Progression of anginal chest pain
- Ataxia, vertigo, pallor, cyanosis
- Serious arrhythmias, multifocal premature ventricular contractions, sustained tachycardia heart block, ventricular tachycardia, or ventricular fibrillation
- Drop in systolic blood pressure below control

Deep ST depression or submaximal target heart rates need not be cause to terminate exercise. Excessive increase in blood pressure also should not be regarded as an indication for termination of exercise, as this usually indicates excellent left ventricular function. A drop in blood pressure is, of course, an immediate cause for termination.

EQUIPMENT AND DRUGS

Adequate monitoring equipment, a defibrillator, and appropriate emergency supplies and drugs are essential. A supply of drugs and the function of the emergency equipment must be checked at frequent intervals.

RISKS AND LEGAL IMPLICATIONS

It would appear that exercise testing is becoming safer. Sheffield and co-workers recently reported on 9000 tests done on patients in the lipid research clinics without a death.[13] Scherer and Kaltenbach reported on over 1 million persons undergoing exercise tests, 750,000 of whom had coronary disease.[14] The test done mostly on a bicycle resulted in 17 deaths (2 per 100,000) in the coronary patients, but there was no mortality in over 300,000 "sports persons." These figures are better than those reported by Rochimis, in 1971, who found 1 death per 10,000 using primarily treadmill stress testing. Recent legal decisions emphasized the importance of following established guidelines as listed here and of having a published procedure to be followed for routine testing and for the management of emergencies. The courts favor the plaintiff in the absence of these safeguards.

BAYESIAN ANALYSIS: SENSITIVITY AND SPECIFICITY

Although it is common knowledge that stress testing and most other tests are imperfect, the factors that influence the degree of imperfection are often obscure. The concept of Bayesian analysis helps us understand some of these discrepancies. Bayes's theorem is a mathematical rule that relates past experiences to our present observations to predict the reliability of the final result, or the "post-test probability" of uncertainty.

Information content pertains to how much we know about the presence or absence of disease before the test and its effect on the reliability of the diagnosis of the test. In Figure 31.5, the pretest information (10%) is added to the test information (50%), leaving us with 40% of the information still unknown. If the pretest information content were greater (e.g., 40%) and the test information were the same, then the post-test uncertainty would be only 10%.

Diamond and colleagues[15] and others have proposed that the pretest information content, or pretest probability, can be predicted from the patient's symptoms. Typical angina, for example, almost ensures the presence of coronary artery disease (nearly 90%), so a test that increases the probability by 50% would only increase the post-test probability to 95%. On the other hand, Diamond's group found nonanginal chest pain to be associated with an intermediate pretest probability of about 35%; thus, when exercise-induced ST segment depression increased the probability 50%, it added much more information and, thus, made a greater contribution to the diagnosis. It is known, of course, that the symptoms are only one of the determinants of coronary disease probability; some of the others are sex, age, family history, and smoking. Figure 31.6 illustrates this concept on the significance of the magnitude of ST segment depression as related to the pretest probability. The greater the magnitude of ST segment depression, the more post-test certainty of coronary disease or the least post-test uncertainty.[16] Once the post-test probability of a test is determined, another test confirming the diagnosis (such as a thallium stress test) will increase the probability of disease and reduce the uncertainty. On the other hand, if the second test suggests disease is absent (a negative thallium test), the post-test probability will decrease significantly.

Because the prevalence of coronary artery disease is very low in certain population groups, such as young asymptomatic men or women, an abnormal response (such as ST segment depression) has little likelihood of indicating disease. Thus, in this setting, most of the abnormal responders are likely to be "false-positive." The Bayesian

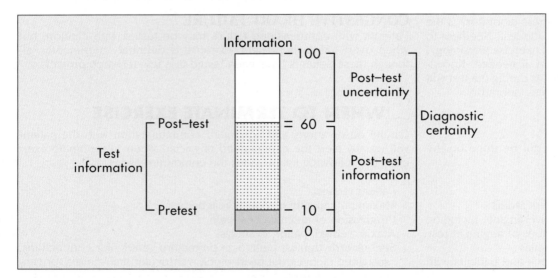

FIGURE 31.5 The information content. The pretest information (shaded area), 10% in this example, is added to the information gained from the test (stippled area), leaving the post-test information or post-test probability at 60%. Thus, the post-test uncertainty is still 40%. Factors improving the post-test certainty or probability are greater pretest probabilities, associated with higher disease prevalence or more information content in the test itself. (Modified from Diamond GA, Hirsch M, Forrester JS et al: Application of information theory to clinical diagnostic testing. Circulation 63(4):915, 1981)

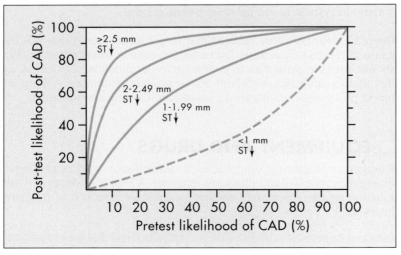

FIGURE 31.6 Family of ST segment depression curves and the likelihood of coronary artery disease (CAD), depending on the pretest probability of disease. (Modified from Epstein SE: Implications of probability analysis on the strategy used for noninvasive detection of coronary artery disease. Am J Cardiol 46:491, 1980)

theorem thus explains why stress testing, when used as a diagnostic tool, is more useful in populations with an intermediate prevalence of disease.

PROBLEMS WITH THE USE OF THE BAYESIAN THEOREM IN CLINICAL MEDICINE

The prevalence of disease in the population, to which each individual subject belongs, is modified by many factors. The Framingham risk factors, for instance, are important. Patients referred to a hospital for a coronary angiogram will have a very high prevalence and those who go to a cardiac center for exercise testing and who have been screened by other physicians will have a prevalence that is only moderately less than those having an angiogram. The prevalence of ST segment depression in two groups of patients, according to age and sex, is illustrated in Table 31.1. The difference in the prevalence of ST segment depression on patients referred for evaluation of coronary artery disease (Memorial Hospital, Long Beach) and in asymptomatic volunteers (Long Beach Heart Association) is striking.

Finally, a number of exercise findings, besides ST segment depression, are used as discriminators, such as chest pain, heart rate, blood pressure, and exercise duration, to name a few. The information content of the various combinations of these variables in conjunction with ST segment depression is yet to be defined. To further compound the uncertainty, Marcus[9] has demonstrated that the physiological significance of angiographically measured disease correlates very poorly with the degree of stenosis. Thus, all our statistical data based on the concept that a stenosis of greater than 70% causes ischemia and one less than this does not, need reevaluation.

Because much of the analysis of exercise testing has been done by comparing ST segment depression with coronary angiographic anatomy, the terms *sensitivity* and *specificity* are commonly used. Sensitivity describes how often one can identify subjects with significant coronary narrowing (usually obstructions from 50%–75% or more).

$$\text{Sensitivity} = \frac{\text{true-positives}}{\text{true-positives plus false-negatives}}$$

Specificity describes how often subjects with normal coronary arteries (usually those with obstruction less than 50%) are identified.

$$\text{Specificity} = \frac{\text{true-negatives}}{\text{true-negatives plus false-negatives}}$$

These values are also markedly affected by the prevalence of disease in the population. When a test is very sensitive (*i.e.*, when it identifies a very high percentage of the diseased patients) it is likely to reduce the specificity. It will label some of those without disease improperly. These subjects can then be called false-positives. Increasing the specificity likewise usually reduces the sensitivity, resulting in more false-negatives.

Predictive value of an abnormal test

$$= \frac{\text{true-positives}}{\text{true-positives plus false-positives}}$$

In a population with low prevalence, the predictive value of an abnormal test will be low because a greater number of those with abnormal tests will be false-positives. In populations with a very high prevalence of disease, the predictive value of a negative test will be low because a significant number of subjects with a negative test will, in reality, have disease.

VARIABLES USED FOR DIAGNOSIS AND PROGNOSIS OF ISCHEMIA

The three types of events commonly used for evaluating an ischemic response are electrocardiographic, hemodynamic, and symptomatic.

ELECTROCARDIOGRAPHIC RESPONSES

NORMAL RESPONSE TO EXERCISE. It has been shown by Blomqvist[17] and others that a moderate amount of J point and ST segment depression is common in a normal subject (Fig. 31.7). Thus, an awareness of this is important in the interpretation of abnormal ST changes.

ABNORMAL ST SEGMENT DEPRESSION. ST segment depression in the lateral precordial leads has long been the hallmark of exercise-induced ischemia. Most experts use an ST segment depression of approximately 0.1 millivolts (1 mm) if the ST is inscribed as horizontal or downsloping. When the ST is upsloping, a 1.5-mm depression at 80 msec from the J point is usually required.

ST VARIABLES

CONFIGURATION OF THE ST RESPONSE. UPSLOPING RESPONSE. Until about 10 years ago, an ST response that was upsloping was believed to be normal, in spite of the magnitude of depression. Epidemiologic studies[18] demonstrated that subjects with this configuration had the same prevalence of cardiac events during follow-up as those with horizontal ST response. When correlated with coronary angiography,[19] upsloping response is reported to have a slightly lower specificity than horizontal depression, but should still be regarded as a useful marker for ischemia in most subjects.

HORIZONTAL AND DOWNSLOPING ST RESPONSE. Horizontal and downsloping patterns are not only predictive of coronary events in a follow-up study (Fig. 31.8), but also have a reasonable sensitivity and specificity when evaluated by coronary angiography. A downsloping pattern appears to predict a higher prevalence of subsequent coronary events than the horizontal pattern (Fig. 31.9). When horizontal ST segment depression evolves into a downsloping pattern during recovery, it indicates an increased probability of subsequent coronary problems.

ST SEGMENT ELEVATION. When patients have had a previous infarction and Q waves by electrocardiography, elevation of the ST segment with exercise is commonly due to an aneurysmal scar. If the patient has never had an infarction, ST segment elevation may be associated with severe ischemia, especially proximal left anterior descending disease. It is believed that ST segment elevation represents transmural ischemia, while ST segment depression is generated by subendocardial tissue only. Ischemia can be predicted from ST segment

TABLE 31.1 PERCENTAGE OF POSITIVE MAXIMUM TREADMILL STRESS TESTS

	Female		Male	
Age	MHLB	LBHA	MHLB	LBHA
21–30	0	0	2.5	1.2
31–40	10.1	2.1	11.7	4.3
41–50	19.9	2.0	29.5	11.4
51–60	29.1	7.4	48.0	26.9
Over 60	43.3	12.1	58.2	29.3
Mean	23.3	4.6	34.3	13.5

(*MHLB*, Memorial Hospital, Long Beach; *LBHA*, Long Beach, California Heart Association)

elevation, either in the left anterior precordial leads or in lead V_1. Coronary spasm can also produce ST segment elevation during exercise, but it is very unusual. Most patients with vasospastic angina, who have ST changes, have ST segment depression. When this occurs, it usually indicates both vasospasm and fixed coronary atherosclerotic stenosis.

ST INTEGRAL AND SLOPE. As on-line computers become more and more common, the use of the ST integral and slope may play a larger role in patient evaluation. These measurements, first proposed by Sheffield,[20] have been used as another way of quantitating the magnitude of the ST segment depression. Although there has been limited enthusiasm in the early years of their introduction, more interest has been generated recently. It was recently reported that an abnormal integral of 16 microvolt seconds (mVμ) or greater identified a threefold increase in risk of coronary death over a 6- to 8-year follow-up. Thus, the use of this measurement in a large multicenter trial, MRFIT (Multiple Risk Factor Intervention Trial), may encourage others to study its predictive power. The ST integral is the area subtended by the depressed ST segment and the horizontal line through the P-Q junction (Fig. 31.10).

MAGNITUDE OF ST DEPRESSION. The magnitude of ST depression contains some of the same data available in the integral. A good deal has been written about the "markedly positive exercise electrocardiogram." Some claim it is a reliable marker for severe coronary disease,

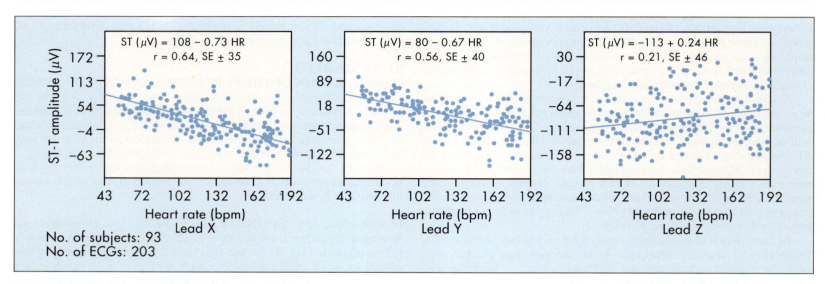

FIGURE 31.7 Variations in ST segment depression in normal subjects as the heart rate increases. (Modified from Blomqvist CG: Heart disease and dynamic exercise testing. In Willerson JT, Sanders CA (eds): Clinical Cardiology. New York, Grune & Stratton, 1977)

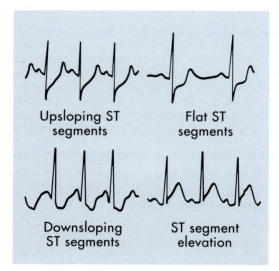

FIGURE 31.8 Family of ST segment changes seen with ischemia.

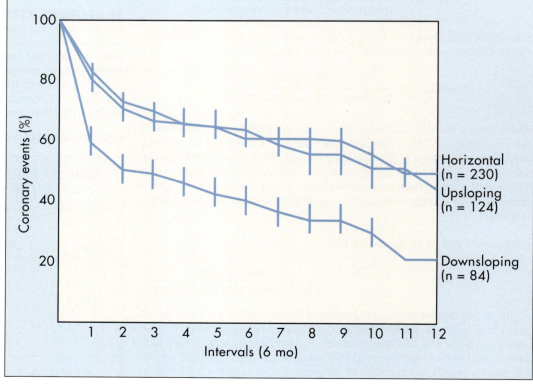

FIGURE 31.9 Prevalence of coronary events per year in subjects with upsloping, horizontal, and downsloping ST segment depression. Note more serious implications in those with downsloping STs.

while others feel it has little importance. The important issue has to do with the work load necessary to induce major magnitudes of ST segment depression. If it comes on at a low work load, it will usually identify severe ischemia (usually multivessel coronary disease and a poor prognosis). If it occurs at a high work load, it may be associated with mild to moderate pathology and has few of the ominous implications ascribed to the former.

NON-ST VARIABLES

R-wave amplitude increases with exercise in some patients with severe ischemia and helps identify this process.[21] It is a rather nonspecific change, however, and a decrease in R-wave amplitude, which is a normal phenomenon, occurs in a fairly high number of patients with significant disease. This is particularly true if they are able to exercise to a high heart rate.

If the septal Q wave increases with exercise, this provides strong evidence against the presence of ischemia, particularly in the left anterior descending coronary artery.[22] Patients with nonspecific cardiomyopathies often have ST depression and increasing septal Q waves with exercise. Unfortunately, less than 50% of the usual population tested have resting septal Q waves. If the septal Q waves are present at rest and reduced during exercise, this provides very good evidence of ischemia due to narrowing of the left anterior descending coronary artery.

It has long been known that the QT interval becomes prolonged with ischemia or infarction; however, patients with a rapid heart rate have electrocardiograms that make it difficult to measure because of the overlapping of the P wave. Evidence is now available that the interval from the Q to the peak of the T wave provides the same data and is usually easier to measure. Vasilomanolakis and associates were able to correctly diagnose half of the false-negative responders with this measurement.[23]

If exercise causes the QRS to widen, either moderately or to the point that bundle branch block can be diagnosed, the probability of ischemia is markedly increased. This is probably a weaker predictor for ischemia than ST segment depression, but in appropriate age-groups this is still important.

NONELECTROCARDIOGRAPHIC PARAMETERS
SYMPTOMS

In many diseases, the patient is not evaluated until symptoms appear. Unfortunately, more than 50% of patients with coronary artery disease have as their first symptom a myocardial infarction or death. Therefore, symptoms are not the only important determinant of disease. However, in most doctors' practices, the prevalence of coronary heart disease in their patients without symptoms is quite low, as compared with those with typical angina, who, when in the appropriate age and sex category, have a prevalence of coronary artery disease of about 90%.

CHEST PAIN

A history of exertional chest pain is important in the diagnosis of coronary artery disease. When this occurs during the exercise test, it has special significance, even though it occurs in only about 30% of patients with significant coronary narrowing. Follow-up studies have demonstrated that those who have this finding, combined with ST depression, have a much higher incidence of subsequent cardiac events.[24] Weiner and colleagues found a predictive accuracy during exercise testing even in the absence of ST depression.[25]

AGE AND SEX

Age and sex are well-known discriminators and need little amplification. Coronary artery disease would be a very unlikely cause of chest pain in a 17-year-old girl; instead, a search should be made for mitral valve prolapse or some noncardiac cause for the pain.

CONVENTIONAL RISK FACTORS

Smoking, hypertension, high cholesterol, diabetes, and a family history for coronary heart disease should alert the physician to an increased prevalence, and, thus, a greater likelihood, of disease. Excellent tables from the Framingham study have been published to illustrate the effect of these findings.[26]

HEMODYNAMIC RESPONSE
EXERCISE BLOOD PRESSURE RESPONSE

Failure to increase the blood pressure or a drop in the early stages is strong evidence in support of poor ventricular function when no other recognizable cause is obvious. This drop in blood pressure early on in the exercise test should be distinguished from the normal drop occurring in all subjects when reaching maximum capacity and persisting, in spite of the onset of anaerobic metabolism. A very early drop in pressure is predictive of left main vessel or three-vessel disease in over 50% of those demonstrating this finding.

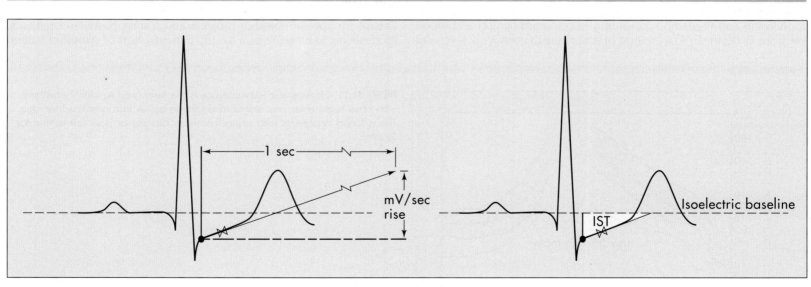

FIGURE 31.10 ST integral. The area subtended by the ST segment depression and the projected baseline constitutes the integral.

RECOVERY BLOOD PRESSURE

Amon and co-workers reported that the persistence of an elevated blood pressure for the first 2 to 3 minutes of recovery may indicate ischemia.[27] This finding may be useful in some patients, but further studies will be required to confirm the validity of this concept.

HEART RATE RESPONSE

The failure to accelerate the heart rate normally or to reach a significant percentage of the expected predicted maximum identifiers reduced left ventricular function, often due to coronary artery disease. Because of this, it is important to know the predicted heart rate for each age-group and what heart rate response is appropriate for whatever protocol the examiner uses. A slower than normal rate for a given submaximal work load has been termed *chronotropic incompetence* (Fig. 31.11). This has been found to be a predictor of subsequent coronary events in a 5-year follow-up.

ENDURANCE

A short exercise time or low maximum aerobic capacity is a useful indicator of poor function. Subjects who are very sedentary, however, may respond this way without cardiovascular disease, but usually can be identified from the history or their appearance. Bruce has found this to be an excellent predictor of subsequent cardiac events,[28] and his conclusions were recently confirmed in the Coronary Artery Surgical Study (CASS) study.[29]

COMBINING MULTIPLE VARIABLES

Figure 31.12 provides a logic tree that can be used as a guide to the use of the various variables in decision making. As mentioned in the beginning, our instinctive understanding of patients tends to provide us with ways to use the information based on these various types of steps. Mechanical or conceptual ways of organizing this information into a final diagnostic score have been designed and are now undergoing validations. A multivariable analysis program that has an accuracy of over 90% in the test patients has been developed. The prospective use of this methodology is now under study.

EXERCISE TEST PROTOCOLS
REQUIREMENTS

Exercise test protocols should be structured to provide (1) activity that can be performed by sedentary as well as athletic subjects; (2) a variable work load so that the energy expenditure of patients can be compared over time and with others; (3) continuous electrocardiographic monitoring and repeated recording of electrocardiograph and blood pressure as desired; (4) a method of estimating at each work level, but short enough to allow patients to reach their peak work load without becoming exhausted; and (5) a sufficient body of information so that the response of patients and normal subjects can be categorized.

SINGLE LOAD TESTS

The Master test, performed as a subject walks over a small set of steps at a prescribed rate and speed, was very popular prior to the advent of treadmill testing. The heart rate and blood pressure were not recorded, and the electrocardiograms were taken after exercise was discontinued. The postexercise electrocardiogram was examined for ST segment depression, and no effort was made to quantify the exercise tolerance, blood pressure, or heart rate responses.

INTERMITTENT TESTS

Mixing short periods of exercise and rest with progressive increases in the magnitude of work performed is an excellent approach, yet very few laboratories do this because it takes longer to complete.

CONTINUOUS TESTING
BICYCLE

The use of the bicycle is preferred in Europe, probably because of the cost and because more Europeans bicycle regularly and, thus, are able to perform this type of exercise well. It has the advantage of less torso and arm movement, so that electrocardiograms and blood pressure measurements are easier. On the other hand, horizontal or supine bicycle testing rarely result in a work response close to maximum, and patients with coronary artery disease may develop pulmonary edema when using this approach.

TREADMILL

The treadmill has been the preferred approach in the United States in the past 10 to 15 years. Walking or running on a grade makes it easy to estimate body work and compare it to others, and it probably represents the most physiologic approach. The subject's maximum oxygen consumption is usually somewhat greater when tested on a treadmill than when tested on a bicycle, probably because more muscles are used. Popular exercise protocols are listed below and in Tables 31.2 through 31.4.

WORK LOAD

Except for special research projects and testing postinfarct patients, there seems to be no reason to stop patients short of symptom-limited

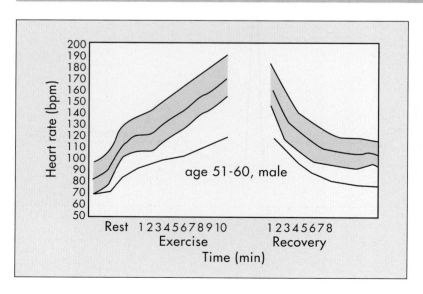

FIGURE 31.11 *Chronotropic incompetence* is the term used to identify patients who have heart rates one standard deviation below that predicted for age. This is found in patients with severe coronary disease or poor left ventricular function.

maximal exercise. The predicted maximal heart rate is used as a guide, but patients should be encouraged to exercise as long as they can. There is no evidence that stopping at 85% or 90% of predicted maximum heart rate is safer than going to the maximum. There is probably little to be recommended between the popular treadmill protocols used in the United States. The Bruce protocol has become the most commonly used, and because of this it enjoys the widest familiarity. Figure 31.13 depicts the oxygen requirements of the Bruce protocol, as compared with some others from a study by Pollock.[30]

CLIMBING STAIRS

Besides the single-stage Master test, a continuous step climbing test requiring the use of the arm muscles (as on a ladder) has been used by Kaltenbach.[31] There is some advantage in including the arms, but it precludes blood pressure measurements and, thus, reduces safety somewhat.

ARM ERGOMETRY

When claudication or orthopaedic problems preclude walking, arm testing can be an excellent substitute. It is usually done with a standard electrically braked bicycle adapted for use by the arms. It is especially useful in men who have strong arms, and in this setting the work achieved may be about 80% of that expected by the legs.

ISOMETRIC EXERCISE

Isometric exercise is usually accomplished with a hand grip dynamometer at about one third to one half of maximum grip strength and sustained pressure for as long as possible. The increase in heart work is

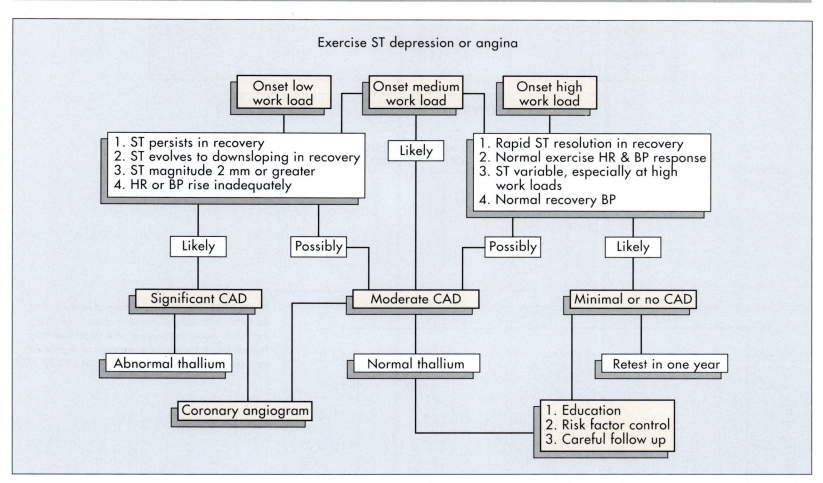

FIGURE 31.12 Logic tree. By applying the above information in a logical format, as depicted, one can decide whether or not to proceed to angiography. Note that in many cases we do not believe an angiogram is necessary in coronary patients.

TABLE 31.2 ELLESTAD PROTOCOL

Stage	Speed (mph)	Grade (%)	Duration (min)	METs (units)	Total Time Elapsed (min)
1	1.7	10	3	4	3
2	3.0	10	2	6–7	5
3	4.0	10	2	8–9	7
4	5.0	10	3	10–12	10
5	5.0	15	2	13–15	12
6	6.0	15	3	16–20	15

TABLE 31.3 NAUGHTON PROTOCOL

Stage	2.0 mph Grade (%)	3.0 mph Grade (%)	3.4 mph Grade (%)	Duration (min)	METs (units)	Total Time Elapsed (min)
1				2	1.0	2
2	0.0			2	2.0	4
3	3.5	0.0		2	3.0	6
4	7.0	2.5	2.0	2	4.0	8
5	10.5	5.0	4.0	2	5.0	10
6	14.0	7.5	6.0	2	6.0	12
7	17.5	10.0	8.0	2	7.0	14
8		12.5	10.0	2	8.0	16
9		15.0	12.0	2	9.0	18
10		17.5	14.0	2	10.0	20
11		20.0	16.0	2	11.0	22
12		22.5	18.0	2	12.0	24
13		25.0	20.0	2	13.0	26
14		27.5	22.0	2	14.0	28
15		30.0	24.0	2	15.0	30
16		32.5	26.0	2	16.0	32

TABLE 31.4 McHENRY PROTOCOL

Stage	Speed (mph)	Grade (%)	Duration (min)	Total Time Elapsed (min)
1	2.0	3	3	3
2	3.3	6	3	6
3	3.3	9	3	9
4	3.3	12	3	12
5	3.3	15	3	15
6	3.3	18	3	18
7	3.3	21	3	21

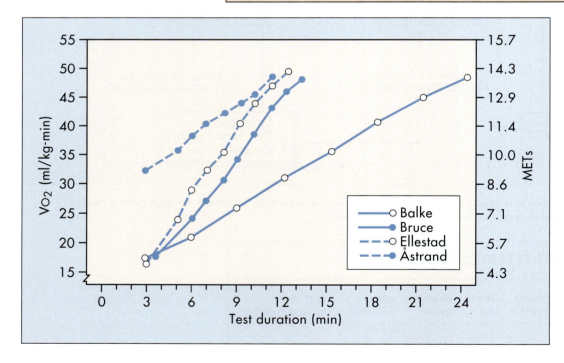

FIGURE 31.13 The oxygen uptake of various protocols according to minutes of exercise. (MET, metabolic equivalent system unit) (Modified from Pollock ML: A comparative analysis of 4 protocols for maximal exercise testing. Am Heart J 93:39, 1976)

due to the rise in systolic blood pressure, as well as some increase in heart rate. In attempting to initiate ischemia in coronary patients, this method may be about one half as effective as dynamic exercise.

EMOTIONAL STRESS TESTING

All poker players know that the heart rate can be increased by excitement as well as by fear and anger. The latter two emotions are usually induced by questions that threaten a patient and are often associated with a rise in blood pressure and may produce ischemia in subjects with severe coronary disease. Most of the reports using this method are research oriented, but it may be useful in special situations.[32] It may also initiate coronary spasms.

DRUGS

Catecholamines and other drugs are occasionally used to initiate ischemia or to accentuate it during exercise. Dipyridamole may, when infused intravenously, cause ischemia by initiating a "coronary steal."[33] That is, it may result in an increase in blood flow to the areas of myocardium perfused by normal coronary arteries and, thus, divert blood away from the areas where coronary stenosis limits flow.

ATRIAL PACING

Increasing the heart rate with atrial pacing has been popular in the catheterization laboratory and has had limited use in the coronary care unit. Although it may produce ischemia, the stroke volume decreases as the heart rate increases, so that the myocardial work is less for any given heart rate than it would be in the case of dynamic exercise. Its convenience when testing subjects in special settings recommends it as a useful modality.

PROCEDURE FOR TREADMILL TESTING

After becoming familiar with the patient's history and general physical findings, the testing physician should review a resting electrocardiogram. This tracing is often taken with the Mason–Likar modified lead placement, so that the same leads can be used (Fig. 31.14) during exercise testing. This test should be thoroughly explained to the patient, and a signed consent should be obtained. A demonstration of treadmill walking and the method of getting on and off the belt should follow.

The monitoring leads and the blood pressure should be recorded supine, standing, and after hyperventilation prior to the test.

The first stage of exercise should be slow enough so that the patient can become familiar with walking on the belt. During this time, conversation during the test and advice on walking technique and body position will reassure the patient and provide confidence during the warm-up period (Fig. 31.15). Following the warm-up stage, the work load is increased by increasing either belt speed or the grade of the treadmill or both. Electrocardiographic strips and blood pressure should be recorded at each work level, and some believe at each minute. Continuing conversation with the patient, asking about symptoms and providing reassurance, is essential during the test, as well as observing the electrocardiographic monitor for arrhythmias and ST changes and the general condition of the patient. When it is deemed time to terminate exercise (see under reasons for termination), the patient is warned; the treadmill is turned off or slowed, depending on the protocol; and the subject is helped to a chair or preferably a broad bench or low bed. During this time, the electrocardiogram should be continuously recorded to detect changes that may occur immediately after exercise. The blood pressure should be recorded as soon as practical either in the sitting or recumbent position, depending on the preferences of the attending physician. Intermittent recording of the

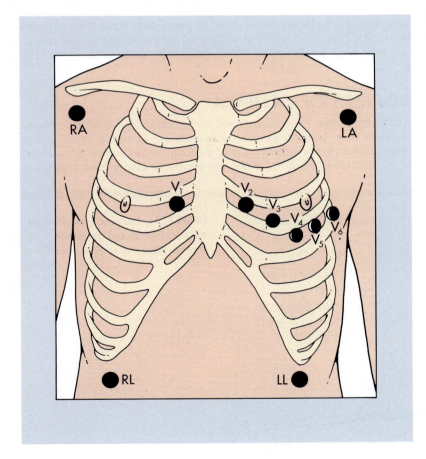

FIGURE 31.14 Lead positions commonly used in exercise testing as modified by Mason and Likar.

electrocardiogram and blood pressure should be taken during recovery. In those who have myocardial ischemia, the recumbent position may accentuate the ischemic process because cardiac inflow is accentuated in this position and may cause ST segment depression to be more pronounced. Recovery is usually monitored for a period until the patient is deemed stable, usually 6 to 10 minutes.

REASONS FOR TEST TERMINATION

The reasons for terminating the test are the same as for terminating any exercise test:

    Patient request
    Maximum capacity obviously reached
    Progression of anginal chest pain
    Ataxia, vertigo, pallor, cyanosis
    Serious arrhythmias, multifocal premature ventricular contractions, sustained tachycardia, heart block, ventricular tachycardia, or ventricular fibrillation
    Drop in systolic blood pressure below control

FINAL REPORT

The records of the test and report should be organized in a way that presents a summary of the work load used, the heart rate and blood pressure response, the patient's symptoms, and labeled copies of the electrocardiographic strips at each level of work and during recovery. A summary of the findings with an impression should also be included.

A number of excellent commercially designed monitoring devices are now on the market that make testing more efficient and that facilitate a complete and accurate final record. Most of these use computers to help analyze and organize the data and are a significant step forward in technology.

EXERCISE TESTING AFTER MYOCARDIAL INFARCTION

Studies have indicated not only that most myocardial infarctions are unexpected, but that they initiate a chain of events that often lead to further problems. Death after recovery from a myocardial infarction is often sudden and is most likely to occur in the ensuing 6 months.[34] Because of increased recurrent infarction and sudden death in some patients, strategies to identify patients at high risk and those who might need special attention have been developed.

Exercise testing has been proposed and generally accepted as the most practical way to identify patients in this category. Initially, it was believed that exercise-induced ST segment depression was the most reliable predictor of subsequent coronary events. Theroux and associates[35] reported that post-myocardial infarction patients with 1 mm or greater ST segment depression within 2 to 3 weeks of their infarction had a mortality rate of 27%, while those with a normal ST response had only a 2% mortality rate. A similar predictive power was reported by Sami and others. More recently, however, Williams and Deckers and co-workers[36] have questioned the value of ST segment depression and claim exercise duration has more predictive capacity. The latter authors, reporting from Europe, use a more strenuous protocol than is popular in the United States and may also be testing a somewhat different population. The predictive value reported by Deckers' duration, blood pressure, and heart rate is depicted in Figure 31.16.

SAFETY AND PATIENT SELECTION

It is generally agreed that only those with uncomplicated infarction should have early testing. Those with hypotension, heart failure, serious arrhythmias, and continued or prolonged pain should not be tested within the first few weeks.

Serious complications from this type of testing are almost as common when tests are done on the above high-risk subjects. Prudent low-level testing in the younger patient population with an uncomplicated myocardial infarction has been reported to be safe and useful.

PROTOCOL

Because the testing end point and time from the infarction have varied a good deal, it is difficult to be arbitrary as to the work load. Some investigators have used a high-level symptom-limited test at 3 weeks without reporting problems. Because most asymptomatic patients are now being discharged much earlier (average of 10 days), it is recommended that a limited protocol terminating exercise from 3 to 5 METs and at a heart rate of 120 to 130 beats per minute be used. It has been suggested that coronary angiography should be performed in patients who manifest ischemia at this level of exercise prior to their hospital discharge. This is especially true if the patients have had a subendocardial infarction, in whom the likelihood of a second event is known to be high in the ensuing year.

MARKERS OF ISCHEMIA

Although angina, exercise-induced arrhythmias, and a drop in blood pressure have been correlated with ongoing ischemia, there is less agreement as to the significance of these findings than the occurrence of ST depression. Further work will probably clarify how aggressive

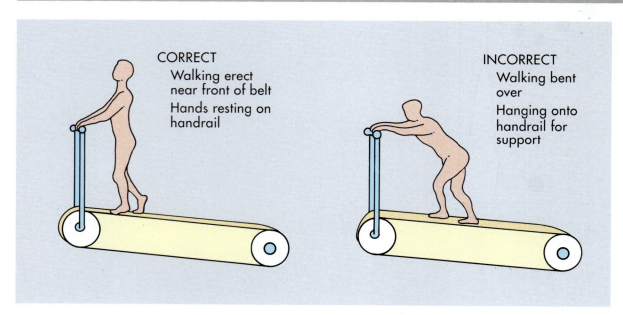

FIGURE 31.15 The proper position on the treadmill should be demonstrated. Note the vertical stance.

one should be based on these events. It may turn out after more experience that angioplasty might be indicated in some cases and bypass surgery would be more appropriate in others.

ISOTOPE TECHNIQUES

Because thallium imaging can be an aid in localizing the obstructed vessel, in some cases it can also be used in the post-myocardial infarction patient as an aid to stratification. Reports are now available indicating that both thallium scintigraphic images and exercise gated blood pool imaging provide predictive information.[37]

CLINICAL APPLICATION

Figure 31.17 provides a logic tree that might be used as a guide when managing patients after a myocardial infarction. Because it is well known that poor ventricular function places patients in a high risk for subsequent events, some of these patients should probably have coronary angiography in the early post-myocardial infarction period. Evidence of this, either from clinical events, such as severe heart failure or hypotension, or after isotopic ventricular function studies have been done, will help determine the most prudent course of action.

EXERCISE TESTING AFTER SURGERY AND ANGIOPLASTY

Exercise testing after bypass surgery and coronary angioplasty has proven to be of definite clinical value.

Ryan and colleagues[38] recently reported that when exercise testing is used prior to surgery, those with a short exercise time have been shown to do better with surgery than if they are treated medically. When surgery or angioplasty results in reversion of preoperative ST segment depression to normal after surgery, one can predict with considerable likelihood that the ischemia has been improved. A significant depression does not always predict graft closure, but seems to suggest that less than ideal results have been obtained, particularly after angioplasty. Although patients with improved perfusion usually increase their exercise tolerance, the same thing can be said for a fair number of patients who have all of their grafts closed. This may be due to the fact that angina is often abolished after bypass surgery, even when there are no patent grafts. Thus, the reason for stopping the exercise test preoperatively may be eliminated postoperatively, even though myocardial perfusion does not seem to be improved.

Improved perfusion is suggested by elimination of ST segment depression or a delay in ST segment depression, so that it occurs at a higher double product (heart rate times blood pressure). In some patients, ST segment depression can occur postoperatively, even in the presence of functioning coronary artery bypass grafts.

When a postoperative patient has been without ST depression or pain for a time and then these changes return during an exercise test, it is a reliable indicator of progressive ischemia due to either graft closure or progression of disease in the native circulation.

Recent reports indicate that exercise testing performed 2 days after angioplasty in asymptomatic patients is a reliable predictor of restenosis.[39] This would imply that reclosure, when it occurs, begins to take place very early.

Serial exercise testing after coronary artery bypass or angioplasty has proved to be one of the most useful tools in the determination of the ultimate progress of coronary atherosclerosis.

STRESS TESTING IN WOMEN

Until about 10 years after menopause, the prevalence of coronary artery disease in women is very low, yet exercise-induced ST segment depression is quite common. Wu and co-workers found that ST segment depression in females under age 45 exceeded that found in men by five times.[40] Yet, as they grow older and coronary artery disease becomes more common, the prevalence of ST segment depression with exercise decreases. Various studies have demonstrated a very high false-positive ST response in women undergoing coronary angiograms. Why does a woman have exercise-induced ST segment depression often associated with anginal-like chest pain and still have a normal coronary angiogram? It may be that as exercise increases the

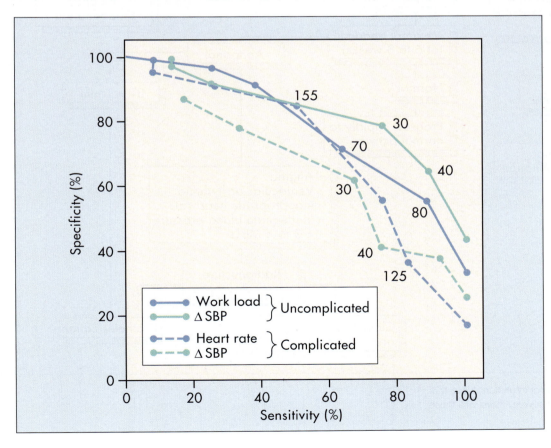

FIGURE 31.16 Exercise findings predictive of mortality after myocardial infarction. Note that in uncomplicated infarction, maximal workload and systolic blood pressure (SBP) are useful, and in the more severe cases, maximal achieved heart rate is useful as well as blood pressure. (Modified from figure courtesy of Dr. J. W. Deckers)

myocardial oxygen demands, the cardiac muscle actually becomes ischemic. This could be due to a disturbance in the regulators controlling myocardial perfusion. The ability of the microvasculature to dilate and reduce resistance to flow with exercise has been shown to be inadequate and has been called "reduced vasodilator reserve."[9] Are there abnormal humoral vasoconstrictors circulating in the blood of women? There is some evidence that estrogen may be one. Other agents, still poorly understood, may also be present.

It is apparent, however, that ST segment depression in women under 55 to 60 may not be due to epicardial coronary narrowing. Because so-called false-positive ST segment depression is very common in women, other exercise variables must be taken into consideration to reach a proper diagnosis. These include short exercise time, sudden drop in blood pressure early in the exercise protocol, and ST evolution to a downsloping pattern during recovery. Causes of false-positive ST segment depression also include mitral valve prolapse, reduced serum potassium, and chronic hyperventilation. It is of interest that exercise-induced angina is a much weaker predictor of coronary artery disease in women than in men.[41]

Radioisotope scintigraphy is helpful, but also has a higher false-positive rate in women than it does in men.[42]

ANGINA AND NORMAL CORONARY ARTERIES

In many cardiac centers, 10% or more of the patients studied for classic angina turn out to have normal or near normal coronary arteries. Although many are tested with ergonovine, few develop high-grade localized narrowing. Many patients with this syndrome have effort angina, exercise-induced ST segment depression, and relief of pain by nitroglycerin, and in some patients, myocardial lactate production has been observed during atrial pacing. It appears that myocardial ischemia develops in the face of normal coronary arteries. Likoff and associates labeled these patients as having "syndrome X" as early as 1966.[43] Recently, Marcus[9] has demonstrated that the capacity of the intramyocardial coronary circulation to dilate adequately to provide appropriate perfusion is impaired in some of these patients, suggesting "inadequate" or "reduced vasodilator reserve." Although the patients

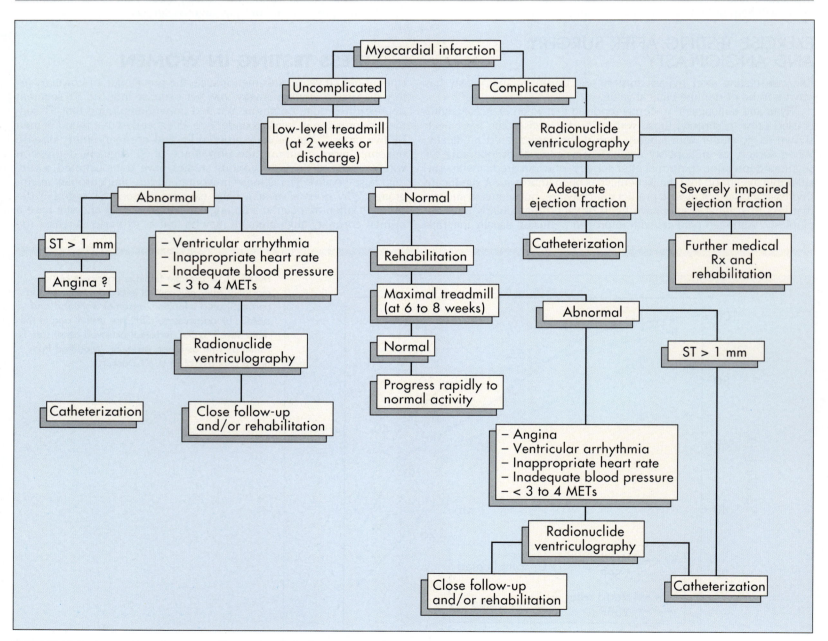

FIGURE 31.17 Logic tree of management after myocardial infarction. Note that among the uncomplicated mild patients and the most severe, there are those who may not need angiography.

with this syndrome may have multiple causes, it is now suspected that many have myocardial ischemia. This is especially true if they have exercise-induced ST segment depression.

Even in patients who have never had chest pain but have ST segment depression and normal coronary vessels, there is evidence to indicate that exercise-induced ST segment depression is associated with myocardial pathology. Erikssen and co-workers followed 36 men with this syndrome for 7 years and found that 22% developed myocardial disease, classified as cardiomyopathy, and half of them had an abnormal ejection fraction with an exercise gated radionuclide ventriculogram.[44]

Although some patients with this syndrome have a myocardial cause for their symptoms, one should not ignore the possibility of esophageal disease. It is often so similar to angina that it almost defies differentiation.[45] Exercise-induced pain is common in esophageal dysfunction, and Harrison and associates recently demonstrated gastroesophageal reflux during exercise in patients with this syndrome.[46] This was present especially when the exercise followed eating. Testing these patients in the fasting state will not usually induce gastroesophageal reflux and therefore may not initiate chest pain. Occasionally, esophageal motility studies are necessary to make this diagnosis.

ISCHEMIA IN ASYMPTOMATIC SUBJECTS

A report by Gordon and Kannel that the first sign of coronary heart disease in men is a myocardial infarction or death in 55% of those studied in the Framingham study emphasizes that the absence of symptoms is not universally predictive of a benign course.[47] The prevalence of asymptomatic, significant coronary heart disease is still unknown, but may well be as high as 20% in men over age 50.

The reasons ischemia is not associated with recognizable anginal pain are complex and still poorly understood. Some may have inadequate or impaired pain perception and others may have an "anginal equivalent," such as indigestion, breathlessness, and severe fatigue. Performing a Holter monitor in patients with clinical angina reveals that over 80% of ischemic episodes identified by ST segment depression are "silent." Although there has been considerable criticism of routine testing in asymptomatic subjects,[48,49] there is considerable evidence to justify exercise testing in those with multiple risk factors who might belong to a group who have a high prevalence of disease.

Exercise testing is commonly performed for the evaluation of arrhythmia or as a screening test as part of an executive physical. If electrocardiographic evidence of myocardial ischemia is observed, true-positives should be differentiated from false-positive results. Some findings usually associated with true-positive stress testing are listed in Table 31.5. Clinical findings suggest a significant possibility of a false-positive test, especially if the ST segment depression occurs at high work loads. Testing can be repeated at intervals, usually 6 months or so, and if there is no change, further investigation such as coronary angiography is not required. If changes occur at a lower level of exercise, one might try repeating the test after a full dose of β-blockade. If the ST segment depression is abolished, it provides strong evidence to support the absence of significant disease. Some patients with normal coronaries, however, will have a reduction in ST segment depression, but some residual changes will persist. Thus, the exercise test does not always give a conclusive result for the diagnosis of coronary artery disease. Isotope imaging or angiography may be required, depending on the clinical circumstances.

In some subjects, ST segment depression may indicate important changes in left ventricular function, even when the coronary arteries are normal. Thus, abnormal ST segment depression must be correlated with the total clinical picture when deciding on patient management. When ischemia appears on subsequent testing at lower work loads in asymptomatic patients with known coronary artery disease, it may be an indication to intervene more aggressively. Myocardial infarction is not always heralded by the appearance of symptoms.

METABOLIC AND DRUG EFFECT IN THE EXERCISE TEST

Although hypothyroidism and hypokalemia will cause exercise-induced ST segment depression, the most vexing problems in this category are the changes associated with various drugs.

DIGITALIS

Digitalis remains the agent most likely to cause exercise-induced ST segment depression in patients with normal coronary arteries. Because this substance is a vasoconstrictor, a reduction in left ventricular subendocardial blood flow may be the mechanism of action. If this were so, it would explain the increased likelihood that older subjects will have ST segment depression with digitalis. Estrogens may produce the same effect and, thus, explain the high prevalence of exercise-induced ST segment depression in young premenopausal females. After menopause, ST segment depression in normal females becomes less common and one can suspect that its reliability as a marker for coronary heart disease will increase to close to that found in men.

ANTIANGINAL AGENTS

It has long been believed that nitroglycerin, β-blockers, and now probably calcium blockers will normalize ST segment depression and mask ischemia during stress testing. Although this may be true in some cases, it has been reported that when a progressive work load is used, these agents only delay ischemia and will rarely ever cause a false-negative test if exercise is continued to the patient's maximum capacity.[50]

ANTIHYPERTENSIVE AGENTS

Most drugs that reduce resting blood pressure will also cause a reduction in peak exercise blood pressure. Stress testing in hypertensive patients is often useful to titrate the therapeutic effect of the agent being prescribed. It would be desirable to give enough drug to reduce exercise-induced, as well as resting, blood pressure. Drugs that reduce peripheral resistance, such as the vasodilators, angiotensin-converting enzyme inhibitors, diuretics, and α-blockers, usually result in a lower exercise pressure and may favor an improved exercise tolerance. Propranolol and other β-blockers, however, increase peripheral resistance and usually reduce exercise tolerance as well as heart rate. Careful attention to the period immediately after exercise is necessary when testing patients on antihypertensive medications. There may be a sudden drop in pressure requiring a period of recumbency until the auto-

TABLE 31.5 FINDINGS ASSOCIATED WITH TRUE-POSITIVE STRESS TESTING

Short exercise time
Less than normal increase in heart rate or blood pressure during the test
Early onset of ST segment depression with progression during exercise
Evolution to downsloping ST pattern during recovery
Persistence of systolic hypertension during the first 2 or 3 minutes of recovery
Marked increase in R-wave amplitude
Reduction in amplitude of the septal Q, if present
Prolongation in Q peak–peak T interval with exercise
Widening of the QRS with exercise
High post-test probability on multivariate analysis (MVA) or likelihood ratio
Abnormal cardiokymogram (CKG) (part of our routine exercise test)
Confirmation with radionuclide stress testing

nomic system readjusts and allows for resumption of normal redistribution of blood flow.

The final drug needing consideration is alcohol. More than two drinks will reduce myocardial contractile strength and, thus, exercise capacity. This effect is more marked if there is an underlying process causing myocardial dysfunction; thus, while alcohol will probably not effect the ST segment response, it will confuse the issue as to the exercise capacity. It should, therefore, be avoided prior to exercise testing, as should the ingestion of tranquilizers and stimulants.

EXERCISE TESTING IN REHABILITATION AND SPORTS MEDICINE

Exercise testing was applied to problems related to work capacity and to exercise capacity in sportsmen long before it was used as a diagnostic aid in coronary artery disease. The ability to observe a subject performing exercise and to take appropriate measurements while the exercise load and the environment are altered usually tells a good deal more about the patient's function than by observing him at rest.

Testing patients prior to starting an exercise program after coronary bypass surgery, or after a myocardial infarction, provides guidelines that can be used to regulate exercise at work and at play. The *target heart rate*, a level of work that increases the heart rate to a point that will improve conditioning but still be less than that necessary to bring on ischemia or produce arrhythmias, is the backbone of the exercise prescription. After this has been determined, the patient may exercise for several weeks or months until his status allows for an adjustment, depending on the degree of improvement. Once it appears that he has improved his work capacity, a second test can give objective evidence of this improvement and provide guidelines for future activity.

With the popularization of exercise as a means to fitness, controversy has arisen as to the need for exercise testing prior to embarking on a strenuous exercise program. If the subject is 45 years of age or older, or if he has several risk factors that increase his probability of coronary disease, a test prior to starting a program is prudent, although it has been pointed out that it will not be abnormal in all those who will eventually have a coronary event while training.

When testing athletes, ST- and T-wave changes are quite common in normals, as are episodes of first and second degree heart block, as well as left ventricular hypertrophy.

The erroneous idea that marathon running will prevent the progression of coronary artery disease has finally been disproven by the reports of numerous deaths in long distance runners, including the well-known author James Fixx. The life-style and diets associated with endurance training may have more protective impact than exercise itself. Regular exercise may, however, give some protection from coronary artery disease and may retard its evolution.[51] It would appear that a moderate program of exercise three or four times a week for ½ to 1 hour will provide all the health benefits that are worthwhile. There is no evidence that a much more vigorous program will add to the benefits, and in older subjects the probability of injuries increases dramatically. Exercise testing remains an excellent way to monitor progress and aerobic capacity and can serve as a guideline to improvement during a conditioning program. The reduction in heart rate and often blood pressure at any given work load will provide the sportsman with an objective measure of his improved ability to use oxygen and perform work.

COMPUTERS IN STRESS TESTING

Although the average physician is still unfamiliar with the intricacies of computer technology, our lives are already being influenced in many ways by these technologic advances. Because computers are well suited to the measurement and the calculations necessary in the analysis of exercise tests, we are likely to see a rapid proliferation of this technology. The advantages of computer processing of the electrocardiogram are considerable.

STORAGE OF DATA

The large volume of electrocardiographic and other data recorded during an exercise test can be easily stored, and the important elements can be accessed at will.

NOISE REDUCTION

Electrical noise, which causes difficulty in interpreting tracings, is a common problem. This is often generated at the electrode–skin interface and can be reduced by proper skin preparation. It is also due to respiration, muscle contraction, and electrical interference. Signal averaging after analog-to-digital conversion can largely eliminate most of these problems.

INTEROBSERVER AGREEMENT AND ACCURACY OF MEASUREMENTS

The lack of agreement between several observers in the measurement of ST segment depression and the failure of experts to agree with themselves on repeat examination of tracings are well known. Crow and Campbell tested a commercially available system (Quinton) and found the measurement of ST segment depression to be accurate within ±0.1 mm 79% of the time on repeat analysis.[52] Heart rate and ST slope were also highly repeatable measurements. This type of consistency is far in excess of that possible by visual analysis.

SIGNAL PROCESSING

The analog signal (the familiar electrocardiogram) is really a time voltage record that can be easily converted to a series of numbers. This is called "analog-to-digital" (A–D) conversion. The speed of sampling of the voltage change determines how accurately the wave can be reproduced and measured. Speeds of 200 to 500 samples per second are commonly used. This sequence of numbers (representing voltage changes) is then stored and can be used for the many measurements necessary.

A program that can recognize an electrocardiographic complex is fairly easy to construct. Different approaches have been used, using different fiduciary points to identify the complex. The peak of the R wave has been the most popular point because of its short time duration and high voltage. Other points can then be identified as being within a predictable time interval from the original point. ST measurements are often done at 60 msec or 80 msec after the R wave. Other methods such as the measurement of the *slew rate* (the rapidity of voltage change) have also been used. Methods to separate normal from abnormal complexes are also used, sometimes based on variations in timing or the width of the QRS complex for premature ventricular contractions. Abnormal beats must be excluded when measurements of ST segment depression, heart rate, and other parameters are made to ensure accuracy.

USEFUL MEASUREMENTS NOT EASILY DONE VISUALLY

Not only is it possible to measure ST segment depression more accurately, but the ST slope and the ST integral (area subtended by the ST segment depression) can be easily and accurately measured and recorded. The slope and integral (see Fig. 31.10) have been reported to be useful adjuncts in the analysis of exercise tracings, but it still remains to be determined if they are superior to ST segment displacement. Other measurements such as R-wave amplitude and QT interval can also be done.

CALCULATIONS

It has been popular to calculate an estimate of oxygen uptake, percentage of predicted heart rate, maximum double product, and the percentage of estimated aerobic capacity as part of the test report. These can be more easily done by the computer than manually. A number of treadmill scores have been used that are helpful in estimating the severity of ischemia. A computer-generated multivariant analysis can be used to calculate the post-test probability of coronary disease using several clinical and exercise variables. This improves the discriminatory power of exercise testing considerably. Similar approaches have been reported by Diamond and Forrester[53] and are commercially available. It is likely that this type of analysis will become commonplace in the near future and will provide a more useful concept of disease probability.

PRINTOUT OF THE RECORD

With the newer printers available, the final report of a stress test can be generated in detail. This final record can be more complete, with illustrations of appropriate ST changes, and graphs of blood pressure and heart rate change can be obtained, if desired. The machine can easily produce an abbreviated report or a detailed one from the information stored in the computer during the test.

COMMENT

It can be appreciated from the preceding information that the advantage of a computer system in the exercise laboratory is considerable. Simoons has reported that the sensitivity of electrocardiographic analysis can be improved from 10% to 40% with only a small loss of specificity (3%–10%).[54] This is primarily due to an increased accuracy of measurements. It is important to recognize that the implementation of insufficiently tested computer programs may introduce errors difficult to recognize by those unfamiliar with computer technology. Careful overreading of the output will be mandatory because even in the most sophisticated systems, errors will be present. Eventually standards for computer systems should be developed and adopted by professional organizations as guidelines for those attempting to evaluate the commercial products being placed on the market.

The information presented in this chapter will provide the reader with an overview of the "state of the art." For additional detail, more comprehensive monographs are available.[41,55]

REFERENCES

1. Fletcher GF, Cantwell JD: Historical Aspects of Exercise and Coronary Heart Disease, 2nd ed. Springfield, IL, Charles C Thomas, 1979
2. Chapman CB, Smith E: 1818–1874: Physiologist, human ecologist reformer. J Hist Med 22:1, 1967
3. Blousfield G: Angina pectoris: Changes in electrocardiogram during paroxysm. Lancet 2:457, 1918
4. Feil H, Siegel M: Electrocardiographic changes during attacks of angina pectoris. Am J Sci 175:225, 1928
5. Master AM, Oppenheimer EJ: A simple exercise tolerance test for circulatory efficiency with standard tables for normal individuals. Am J Med Sci 177:223, 1929
6. Hellerstein HK, Newman B, Goldston E et al: Results of an integrative method of occupational evaluation of persons with heart disease. J Lab Clin Med 38:821, 1951
7. Bruce RA: Evaluation of functional capacity and exercise tolerance of cardiac patients. Mod Concepts Cardiovasc Dis 25:321, 1956
8. Nadel ET: Problems with Temperature Regulation During Exercise. New York, Academic Press, 1977
9. Marcus ML: The Coronary Circulation in Health and Disease. New York, McGraw-Hill, 1983
10. Maseri A, Miami R, Chierchia S et al: Coronary artery spasm as a cause of acute myocardial ischemia in man. Chest 68:625, 1975
11. Ellestad MH, Wan MKC: Predictive implications of stress testing: Following up of 2700 subjects after maximum treadmill stress testing. Circulation 51:363, 1975
12. Franciosa JA: Exercise testing in chronic congestive heart failure. Am J Cardiol 53:1447, 1984
13. Sheffield LT, Haskell W, Heiss G et al: Safety of exercise testing volunteer subjects: The Lipid Research Clinics' prevalence study experience. J Cardiac Rehab 2(5):395, 1982
14. Scherer D, Kaltenbach M: Frequency of life-threatening complications associated with stress testing. Dtsch Med Wochenschr 104:1161, 1979
15. Diamond GA, Hirsch M, Forrester JS et al: Application of information theory to clinical diagnostic testing. Circulation 63(4):915, 1981
16. Epstein SE: Implications of probability analysis on the strategy used for noninvasive detection of coronary artery disease. Am J Cardiol 46:491, 1980
17. Blomqvist CG: Heart disease and dynamic exercise testing. In Willerson JT, Sanders CA (eds): Clinical Cardiology. New York, Grune & Stratton, 1977
18. Stuart RJ, Ellestad MH: Upsloping ST segments in exercise testing: Six year follow-up of 438 patients and correlation with 248 angiograms. Am J Cardiol 37:19, 1976
19. Goldschlager N, Selzer A, Cohn K: Treadmill stress tests as indicators of presence and severity of coronary artery disease. Ann Intern Med 85:277, 1976
20. Sheffield LT, Holt JH, Lester FM et al: On-line analysis of the exercise electrocardiogram. Circulation 40:935, 1969
21. Bonoris P, Greenberg P, Christison G et al: Evaluation of R wave amplitude changes versus ST segment depression in stress testing. Circulation 57:904, 1978
22. Morales-Ballejo H, Greenberg PS, Ellestad MH: The septal Q wave in exercise testing. Am J Cardiol 48:247, 1981
23. Vasilomanolakis E, Damian A, Mahan G et al: Treadmill stress testing in geriatric patients (abstr). J Am Coll Cardiol 3(2):520, 1984
24. Cole JP, Ellestad MH: Significance of chest pain during treadmill exercise: Correlation with coronary events. Am J Cardiol 41:277, 1978
25. Weiner DA, McCabe C, Hueter DC et al: The predictive value of anginal chest pain as an indicator of coronary disease during exercise testing. Am Heart J 96(4):458, 1978
26. McGee R, Gordon T: The results of the Framingham Study applied to 4 other U.S.-based studies of cardiovascular disease. The Framingham Study (76-1083), sec 31. Washington, U.S. Government Printing Office, 1976
27. Amon KW, Crawford MH, Petra MA et al: Value of post exercise systolic blood pressure in diagnosing coronary disease (abstr). Circulation II (6B):36, 1983
28. Hossack KF, Bruce RA, Fisher L et al: Prognostic value of risk factors and exercise testing in men with atypical chest pain. Int J Cardiol 3:37, 1983
29. Weiner DA, Ryan TJ, McCabe CH et al: Prognostic importance of a clinical profile and exercise test in medically treated patients with coronary artery disease. J Am Coll Cardiol 3(3):772, 1984
30. Pollock ML: A comparative analysis of 4 protocols for maximal exercise testing. Am Heart J 93:39, 1976
31. Kaltenbach M: Exercise Testing of Cardiac Patients. Baltimore, Williams & Wilkins, 1976
32. McNeil MS: Continuous monitoring during stress interviews in coronary patients: Scope of ambulatory monitoring in ischemic heart disease. Seattle, Washington, Medical Communications and Services Administration, 1977
33. Slany J, Mosslacher H, Kronik G et al: Einfluss von dipyridamole aug das ventrikulogramm bei koronarer herzkrankheit. Z Kardiol 66:389, 1977
34. Moss AJ, DeCamilla J, Davis H et al: The early posthospital phase of myocardial infarction: Prognostic stratification. Circulation 54:58, 1976
35. Theroux P, Waters DD, Halphen C et al: Prognostic value of exercise testing soon after myocardial infarction. N Engl J Med 301:342, 1979
36. Deckers JW, Fioretti MD, deFeyler PC et al: Bayesian analysis of exercise test after myocardial infarction (abstr). J Am Coll Cardiol 5(2):503, 1985
37. Gibson RS, Taylor GJ, Watson DD et al: Predicting the extent and location of coronary artery disease during the early post infarction period by quantitative thallium-201 scintigraphy. Am J Cardiol 50:1271, 1982
38. Ryan TJ et al: The role of exercise in the randomized cohort of CASS (abstr). Circulation II-70:78, 1984
39. Marco J, Fajadet J, Fournial G et al: Two years and more follow-up after successful percutaneous transluminal coronary angioplasty (abstr). Eur Heart J 5(Suppl 1):76, 1984
40. Wu SC, Secchi MB, Radice M et al: Sex differences in the prevalence of ischemic heart disease and in the response to a stress test in a working population. Eur Heart J 2:461, 1981
41. Ellestad MH: Stress Testing: Principles and Practices, 2nd ed. Philadelphia, FA Davis, 1980
42. Greenberg PS, Bible M, Ellestad MH: Prospective application of the multivariate approach to enhance the accuracy of the treadmill stress test. J Electrocardiol 15(2), 1982
43. Likoff W, Segal BL, Kasparian H: Paradox of normal coronary arteriograms in patients considered to have unmistakable coronary heart disease. N Engl J Med 276:1063, 1966
44. Erikssen J, Dale J, Rootwelt K et al: False suspicion of heart disease: A 7 year

follow-up study of 36 apparently healthy middle-aged men. Circulation 68(3):490, 1983
45. Tibbling L: Angina-like chest pain in patients with dysfunction. Acta Med Scand (Suppl)644:56, 1981
46. Harrison MR, Lehman GA, Faris JV: Gastroesophageal reflux occurring during treadmill exercise testing. (in press)
47. Gordon T, Kannel WB: Premature mortality from coronary artery disease. JAMA 215(10):1617, 1971
48. Epstein SE, Kent KM, Goldstein RE et al: Strategy for evaluation and surgical treatment of the asymptomatic or mildly symptomatic patient with coronary artery disease. Am J Cardiol 43:1015, 1979
49. Selzer A, Cohn K: Asymptomatic coronary artery disease and coronary bypass surgery. Am J Cardiol 39:614, 1977
50. Marcomichelakis J, Donaldson R, Green J et al: Exercise testing after beta-blockade: Improved specificity and predictive value in detecting coronary heart disease. Br Heart J 43:252, 1980
51. Paffenbarger PS, Hale WE: Work activity and coronary heart mortality. N Engl J Med 292:545, 1975
52. Crow SR, Campbell S: Accurate automatic measurement of ST segment response in the exercise electrocardiogram. Comput Biomed Res 11:243, 1978
53. Diamond GA, Forrester JS: Analysis of probability as an aid in the clinical diagnosis of coronary artery disease. N Engl J Med 300:1350, 1979
54. Simoons ML: Optimal measurements for detection of coronary artery disease by exercise electrocardiography. Comput Biomed Res 10:483, 1977
55. Chung E: Exercise Electrocardiography: Practical Approach. Baltimore, Williams & Wilkins, 1980

Exercise Evaluation of Cardiorespiratory Function

Karl T. Weber • Joseph S. Janicki

The heart and lungs, together with hemoglobin, represent the body's respiratory gas transport system, which links the metabolizing tissues to the atmosphere for the purpose of obtaining O_2 and eliminating CO_2. Together, the heart and lungs form a metabolic unit, termed the *cardiopulmonary unit*, whose purpose is to provide the movement of air and blood into and out of the thorax in a manner commensurate with the metabolic requirements of the tissues.[1]

When a person is at rest, the O_2 and CO_2 transport function of the cardiopulmonary unit is modest: 3.5 ml of O_2 per minute is consumed per kilogram of body weight, while 75% to 80% of the O_2 utilized is converted to CO_2. During muscular work, O_2 consumption ($\dot{V}O_2$) and CO_2 production ($\dot{V}CO_2$) increase, placing the metabolic function of the unit under an increased demand to bring O_2 to and remove CO_2 from the tissues. The increased gas transport requirements that accompany exercise mandate that the functional integrity of the unit be intact and its integrated behavior be precise. A disease that affects the cardiocirculatory system, respiratory system, or both jeopardizes the ability of the cardiopulmonary unit to support O_2 and CO_2 transport, a condition that may either be evident when the patient is at rest or become apparent only during physical activity.

The purpose of this chapter is to review the noninvasive monitoring of respiratory gas exchange and air flow during the physiologic stress of isotonic exercise, which we call cardiopulmonary exercise testing (CPX); to identify how noninvasive CPX can be used clinically to elicit an abnormality of the cardiopulmonary unit in such conditions as chronic cardiac failure, valvular heart disease, and pulmonary hypertension; and to identify the cause of exertional dyspnea in patients with heart or lung disease.

CARDIOPULMONARY EXERCISE TESTING

Exercise is a physiologic stress that can be used clinically to evaluate the respiratory gas transport function of the heart and lungs. Subtle or latent abnormalities that exist in the cardiocirculatory and respiratory systems become manifest during the increased metabolic requirements attendant on muscular work, and the severity of clinically overt disease can also be assessed. The advent of rapidly responding O_2 and CO_2 analyzers, together with air flow–sensing devices, makes the noninvasive evaluation of the body's gas transport and exchange system a practical reality for the clinical laboratory or office practice. The continuous monitoring of $\dot{V}O_2$, $\dot{V}CO_2$, minute ventilation ($\dot{V}E$), respiratory rate, and tidal volume at rest and during exercise can be performed simply and on a breath-by-breath basis. More cumbersome methods of gas collection and analysis used in the past are no longer necessary.

A variety of exercise tests can be used together with the analysis of respiratory gas exchange and air flow to address a particular clinical disorder of the cardiopulmonary unit. The choice of test and the parameters measured depend primarily on the nature of the clinical problem and the patient and secondarily on the individual preferences of the physician.

NONINVASIVE CPX TESTING

Various types of isotonic exercise can be used to evaluate disorders of the cardiopulmonary unit.[2]

CPX is not a diagnostic test. It does not identify the underlying mechanism that is responsible for an abnormal response. For this purpose, complementary procedures and tests of cardiocirculatory and respiratory function are required. For example, echocardiographic imaging of the heart may identify a thickened pericardium or stenosed mitral valve that is responsible for the impaired aerobic capacity of a particular patient. Moreover, it should be noted that whenever possible, imaging techniques should be used to identify abnormalities in valve function, myocardial wall motion, or myocardial perfusion that appear only during exercise. Invasive monitoring procedures of intracardiac, intravascular, and pleural pressures and arterial blood gases may need to be used during exercise to identify the abnormalities that impair effort tolerance. We consider these various procedures to represent invasive forms of CPX. They are reviewed later in this chapter.

Walking is the most common form of daily exercise, and it does not involve a specialized skill as does bicycling or swimming. If a patient can walk into the physician's office and walk the corridors of the hospital, he can walk on the treadmill at 1 mile per hour, zero grade. Physicians and patients alike frequently consider treadmill exercise to be an athletic activity. Given that most treadmills are programmable, each patient and his exercise capacity can be accommodated without the test's becoming an "athletic event."

We have chosen a protocol of gradual, progressive treadmill exercise to evaluate cardiorespiratory function in the wide range of patients commonly seen in our hospital-based practice.[3] The protocol uses 2-minute stages of exercise and is given in Table 32.1. We prefer this test for most of our patients because walking not only represents a nonspecialized skill, but it is also easily negotiable, acceptable, reproducible, and reliable while working a large muscle mass to stress the cardiopulmonary unit adequately. With the monitoring of $\dot{V}_{O_2}$, $\dot{V}_{CO_2}$, $\dot{V}_E$, and end-tidal O_2 and CO_2 on a breath-by-breath basis, we are able to determine the anaerobic threshold and the maximal O_2 uptake ($\dot{V}_{O_2}$ max) of a patient during a single treadmill exercise test. The first two stages of exercise represent very low workloads. They can be viewed as a warm-up for most patients. However, for patients with advanced cardiac failure or pulmonary hypertension, walking the corridor amounts to nearly maximal exercise. Therefore, in order to keep the test uniform for all patients and to draw comparisons between normal and abnormal responses, we use this common protocol for each patient.

MAXIMAL O_2 UPTAKE

Maximal O_2 uptake ($\dot{V}_{O_2}$ max), also termed *aerobic capacity*, is defined as $\dot{V}_{O_2}$ remaining invariant (<1 ml/min/kg) for 30 seconds or more despite an increment in workload. We prefer to have an invariant $\dot{V}_{O_2}$ for at least two full stages of exercise whenever possible. Patients must be supervised during the test to ensure that they cross their anaerobic threshold and achieve their $\dot{V}_{O_2}$ max. Figure 32.1 depicts the $\dot{V}_{O_2}$ max determination from the breath-by-breath gas exchange data obtained in a patient with cardiovascular disease. The $\dot{V}_{O_2}$ max associated with treadmill exercise provides the largest aerobic capacity of any standard exercise test because it involves the largest muscle mass (*vis-à-vis* leg or arm ergometry).

$\dot{V}_{O_2}$ max is a function of the maximal cardiac output the heart can generate (*i.e.*, the *cardiac reserve*) and the maximal amount of O_2 the tissues can extract. We have divided the aerobic capacity observed during CPX with incremental treadmill exercise into four classes, each of which represents a given degree of functional impairment (Table 32.2).[4] This four-class breakdown was chosen to avoid any confusion with the New York Heart Association's classification, which is frequently used to derive similar information from historical data obtained through patient interview.

Our classification is the following: (1) *Class A* indicates that little or no impairment in aerobic capacity is present when $\dot{V}_{O_2}$ max exceeds 20 ml/minute/kg. For age- and sex-corrected $\dot{V}_{O_2}$ max in the normal adult population commonly seen in practice, $\dot{V}_{O_2}$ max is above this level;[5] (2) *class B* indicates that a mild to moderate impairment is present when $\dot{V}_{O_2}$ max ranges between 16 ml/minute/kg and 20 ml/minute/kg; (3) in *class C*, a moderate to severe impairment exists when $\dot{V}_{O_2}$ max falls to between 10 ml/minute/kg and 16 ml/minute/kg; and (4) *class D* represents a severe impairment with $\dot{V}_{O_2}$ max ranging between 6 ml/minute/kg to 10 ml/minute/kg. A very severe impairment in aerobic capacity is present in class E patients, who are markedly symptomatic and anaerobic at rest with a $\dot{V}_{O_2}$ below 6 ml/minute/kg.[6] We do not recommend exercising these patients.

We do not recommend substituting the duration of symptom-free treadmill exercise for the $\dot{V}_{O_2}$ max determination, because treadmill time is far less precise in characterizing aerobic capacity.[2] Moreover, treadmill time suffers from not having an objective, quantitative end point to predict aerobic capacity. Individual differences in gait and body weight create variations in the level of work performed for equivalent stages of treadmill exercise. Finally, symptom-limited exercise time is clouded by patient and physician bias. The maximum heart rate attained with exercise is also not as reliable a measure of $\dot{V}_{O_2}$ max because of individual variations in the exercise response.[7]

$\dot{V}_{O_2}$ *max is a function of the maximal cardiac output and the maximal level of O_2 extraction by the tissues.* The relationship between systemic O_2 extraction, or the ratio of the arteriovenous O_2 difference and the arterial O_2 content, and normalized aerobic capacity for each functional class is given in Figure 32.2. The data represented were obtained in 76 patients with myocardial disease (*i.e.*, ischemic heart disease and dilated cardiomyopathy). It is apparent that although there are differences in the resting arteriovenous O_2 difference from class to class, there is a progressive rise in O_2 extraction during incremental exercise.[4,8,9] At 80% of aerobic capacity, systemic O_2 extraction exceeds 70%. A number of laboratories have reported that O_2 extraction within the exercising limb itself may exceed 80%, particularly when systemic blood flow is impaired.[9-11] Hence, tissue O_2 extraction is not the impediment to tissue O_2 availability. What therefore determines aerobic capacity is the cardiac output response to isotonic exercise, or the cardiac reserve.

The relationship between cardiac output and normalized aerobic capacity for the four functional classes is given in Figure 32.3, where it can be seen that the maximum cardiac output differs for each class. These differences in cardiac output are statistically significant. Thus, the measurement of respiratory gas exchange at the mouth and the determination of $\dot{V}_{O_2}$ max is a noninvasive method to assess cardiac reserve. The relationship between maximum exercise cardiac output and $\dot{V}_{O_2}$ max is depicted in Figure 32.4 for a 70-kg adult of average body surface area (1.75 m^2).

Irrespective of the etiologic basis of their heart disease, class A patients generate a cardiac output in excess of 8 liters/minute/m^2. Patients in classes B and C are able to raise cardiac output during exercise to a value between 6 liters and 8 liters/minute/m^3 and between 4 liters and 6 liters/minute/m^2, respectively. Class D patients never generate more than 4 liters/minute/m^2 of systemic blood flow.

The impairment in exercise cardiac output depends on the nature of the underlying disease. For example, myocardial failure secondary to previous myocardial infarction or dilated cardiomyopathy is responsible in some patients, and chronic mitral valvular incompetence and elevated pulmonary vascular resistance with right heart failure might be at fault in others. Those conditions that compromise myocardial contractility directly are considered to represent examples of chronic *cardiac* (or *myocardial*) *failure*, and diseases extrinsic to the myocardium, such as valvular heart disease, are considered to represent examples of *circulatory failure*.[12] Examples of conditions that lead to cardiac and circulatory failure are given in Table 32.3.

The etiologic basis of the disease cannot be determined from the $\dot{V}_{O_2}$ max determination. For this purpose, ancillary studies including invasive hemodynamic monitoring during exercise are required. These issues are addressed elsewhere in this chapter.

TABLE 32.1 TREADMILL PROTOCOL FOR THE DETERMINATION OF AEROBIC CAPACITY AND ANAEROBIC THRESHOLD IN PATIENTS WITH CARDIOVASCULAR OR RESPIRATORY DISEASE OF DIVERSE ETIOLOGY AND SEVERITY

Stage*	Speed (mph)	Grade (%)
1	1.0	0
2	1.5	0
3	2.0	3.5
4	2.0	7.0
5	2.0	10.5
6	3.0	7.5
7	3.0	10.0
8	3.0	12.5
9	3.0	15.0
10	3.4	14.0
11	3.4	16.0
12	3.4	18.0
13	3.4	20.0
14	3.4	22.0

* 2-minute stages

It should be noted here that a number of laboratories have reported that there is no relationship between resting indices of left ventricular function and $\dot{V}O_2$ max.[13–18] For example, resting cardiac output, left ventricular filling pressure, and the ejection fraction do not correlate with $\dot{V}O_2$ max and therefore do not predict cardiac reserve. The same can be said of the poor correlation that exists between estimates of heart size (*i.e.*, the radiographic measurement of cardiac–thoracic ratio or echocardiographic end-diastolic left ventricular internal dimension) and cardiac reserve.[19] Hence, it is necessary to stress the heart to determine its pumping reserve. The physiologic stress of exercise is an excellent means to obtain this information and also provides objective data on patients' functional capacity and the severity of their disease.

The reproducibility of the $\dot{V}O_2$ max determination for treadmill exercise in patients with cardiovascular disease is shown in the left panel of Figure 32.5. The values were obtained days to weeks apart. We have

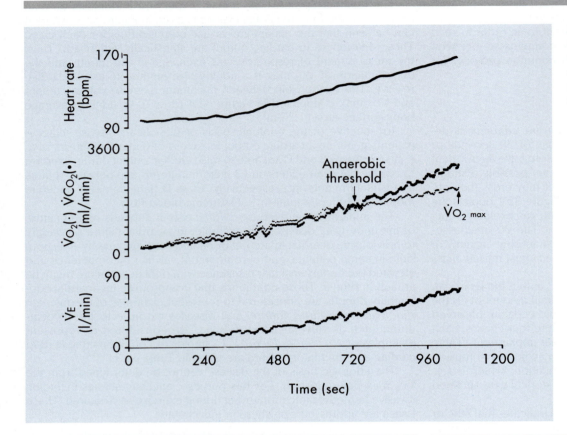

FIGURE 32.1 The breath-by-breath response of respiratory gas exchange to incremental treadmill exercise in a 98 kg, 28-year-old man. Note the onset of anaerobic metabolism at a $\dot{V}O_2$ of 15 ml/minute/kg and an invariant $\dot{V}O_2$ for two consecutive stages of exercise (i.e., $\dot{V}O_2$ max of 22 ml/minute/kg).

TABLE 32.2 FUNCTIONAL IMPAIRMENT IN AEROBIC CAPACITY AND ANAEROBIC THRESHOLD AS MEASURED DURING INCREMENTAL TREADMILL CPX

Class	Severity	$\dot{V}O_2$ max (ml/minute/kg)	Anaerobic Threshold (ml/minute/kg)
A	Mild to none	>20	>14
B	Mild to moderate	16–20	11–14
C	Moderate to severe	10–16	8–11
D	Severe	6–10	5–8
E	Very severe	<6	<4

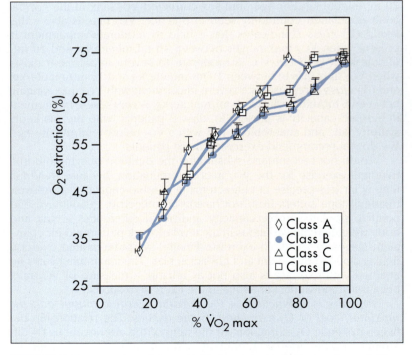

FIGURE 32.2 The response of systemic O_2 extraction to incremental treadmill exercise for each exercise class. (Modified from Weber KT, Janicki JS: Cardiopulmonary exercise testing for evaluation of chronic cardiac failure. Am J Cardiol 55:22A, 1985)

had the opportunity to follow the exercise response of a number of patients over a period of several months. These patients had agreed to participate in a controlled clinical trial in which they received placebo instead of the drug under evaluation in a double-blind study over a period of 12 weeks.[20] Our findings again indicate the reproducibility of the aerobic capacity determination and underscore the fact that serial exercise testing does not introduce a training response.

Patients generally adapt very rapidly to the treadmill protocol, particularly with the low level of work involved in stages 1 and 2. The major learning portion of the procedure is focused on familiarizing the patient with the fact that he is not expected to run, that he should find a comfortable gait that does not require his walking too quickly at low levels of exercise, and that he must not lean on the handrails of the treadmill to support his weight. This learning curve is necessitated in part by the preconceived notion of what a treadmill exercise test represents or the fact that the patient has previously been exercised with the Bruce protocol. Once he has been familiarized with the test procedure, the $\dot{V}O_2$ max determination is reproducible. This familiarization process should not be confused with the exercise training response, which is a distinct physiologic process that evolves over many weeks of regular exercise.

ANAEROBIC THRESHOLD

When working muscle does not receive an adequate amount of O_2 relative to its aerobic requirements, it uses less efficient, anaerobic pathways to derive its energy. As a result, lactate is produced and subsequently enters the vascular compartment. Lactate is buffered by bicarbonate. This leads to an additional, nonmetabolic source of $\dot{V}CO_2$ and a chemical stimulus to respiration. The fall in hydrogen ion concentration as bicarbonate is consumed also stimulates ventilation. The carotid bodies mediate the ventilatory response through these chemical stimuli. Once anaerobiosis occurs, $\dot{V}E$ rises in a manner that is

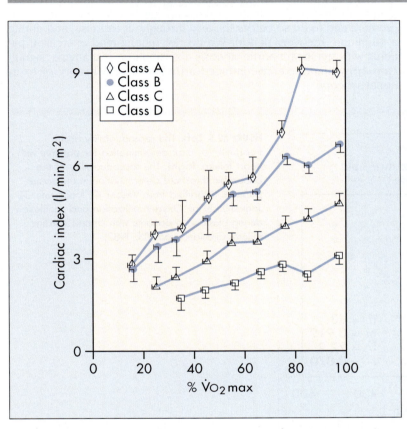

FIGURE 32.3 The interrelationship between normalized $\dot{V}O_2$ and cardiac output for each functional class. (Modified from Weber KT, Janicki JS: Cardiopulmonary exercise testing for evaluation of chronic cardiac failure. Am J Cardiol 55:22A, 1985)

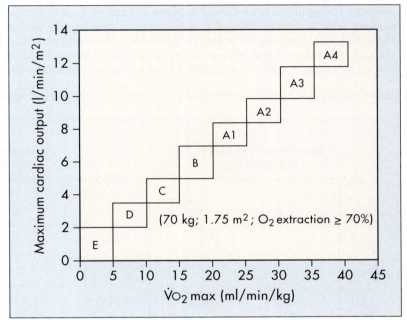

FIGURE 32.4 The relationship between the maximum cardiac output attained during incremental treadmill exercise and the maximum O_2 uptake. The letters refer to the functional classes (see text). Class A has been broken down into four subcategories: A_1, A_2, A_3, and A_4. (Modified from Weber KT, Janicki, JS: Cardio-pulmonary exercise testing: Physiologic principles and clinical applications. Philadelphia, WB Saunders, 1986)

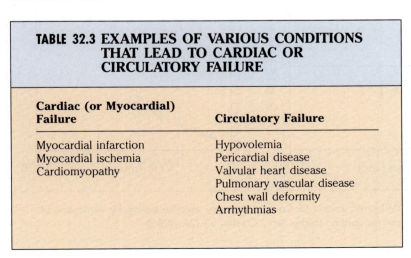

TABLE 32.3 EXAMPLES OF VARIOUS CONDITIONS THAT LEAD TO CARDIAC OR CIRCULATORY FAILURE

Cardiac (or Myocardial) Failure	Circulatory Failure
Myocardial infarction	Hypovolemia
Myocardial ischemia	Pericardial disease
Cardiomyopathy	Valvular heart disease
	Pulmonary vascular disease
	Chest wall deformity
	Arrhythmias

disproportionate to $\dot{V}O_2$. The corresponding level of work or $\dot{V}O_2$ at which anaerobiosis occurs has been termed the *anaerobic threshold*.[21]

The anaerobic threshold determination is generally defined according to five criteria, including the disproportionate rise (relative to $\dot{V}O_2$) in $\dot{V}CO_2$, R (or the ratio $\dot{V}CO_2/\dot{V}O_2$), $\dot{V}E$ and the ventilatory equivalent for O_2 or $\dot{V}E/\dot{V}O_2$, and the disproportionate rise in end-tidal O_2 relative to end-tidal CO_2. These criteria can best be applied to breath-by-breath respiratory gas exchange data obtained during incremental exercise. Figure 32.1 depicts the anaerobic threshold determination based on the disproportionate rise in $\dot{V}CO_2$ that can be observed directly during the exercise test. Figure 32.6 depicts other relations for determining anaerobic threshold that are obtained after the test. In our laboratory, we make no attempt to define the absolute time or absolute workload at which anaerobiosis occurs. Rather, we identify the stage of exercise and its corresponding level of work as being the anaerobic threshold.

The onset of anaerobic metabolism by these noninvasive criteria has also been validated by monitoring the response in mixed venous lactate concentration in the pulmonary artery.[4,8] A lactate concentration over 12 mg/dl has been chosen to represent lactate production by working skeletal muscle. This value is more than 2 standard deviations above the normal resting value for our laboratory. The studies of Donald and co-workers[22] and Wilson and co-workers,[9] in which femoral venous lactate was measured during bicycle exercise in patients with cardiovascular disease, indicate that the rise in lactate is the result of lactate production by the working limb and a function of the impairment in O_2 delivery.

The relationship between mixed venous lactate concentration and the normalized aerobic capacity in treadmill exercise for the four functional classes is given in Figure 32.7. It is apparent from these data that the onset of anaerobiosis occurs at different workloads for each class. For classes A to D, the range of $\dot{V}O_2$ at which lactate production occurs (the anaerobic threshold) is quite distinct (see Table 32.2) at above 14 ml, 11 ml to 14 ml, 8 ml to 11 ml, and 5 ml to 8 ml/minute/kg, respectively. Hence, the noninvasive determination of anaerobic threshold is yet another predictor of the impairment in systemic blood flow that can be obtained from measurements of respiratory gas exchange and used to grade the severity of cardiac and circulatory failure (see Table 32.2). Finally, like $\dot{V}O_2$ max, the anaerobic threshold determination has been found to be reproducible when measured days or weeks apart (see Fig. 32.5, right panel).[4]

In addition to monitoring respiratory gases and air flow, we recommend monitoring the electrocardiogram, heart rate, and cuff blood pressure and to do so before the test, throughout exercise, and during a 10-minute recovery period. We do not recommend exercising patients with significant aortic stenosis, exertional or rest angina, significant arrhythmia, exercise-induced arrhythmia, or a history of exertional syncope.

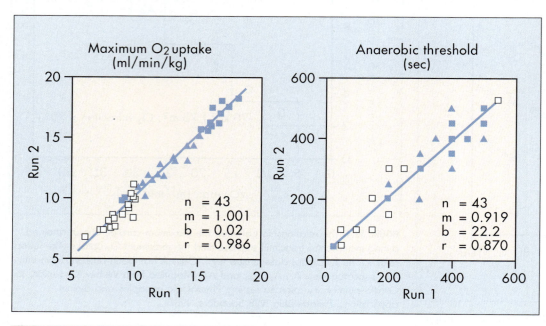

FIGURE 32.5 Left. The reproducibility of the treadmill $\dot{V}O_2$ max determination for patients with heart failure. **Right.** The reproducibility of the anaerobic threshold determination in the same patients. (Modified from Weber KT, Kinasewiz GT, Janicki JS et al: Oxygen utilization and ventilation during exercise in patients with chronic cardiac failure. Circulation 65:1213, 1982)

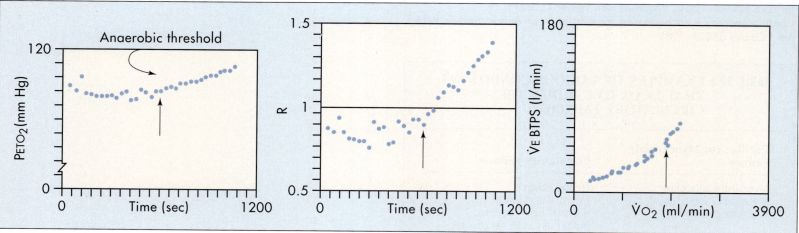

FIGURE 32.6 Relations used to identify the anaerobic threshold from (*arrows*) the respiratory gas exchange response. (PET, end-tidal pressure; R, ratio of $\dot{V}CO_2$ to $\dot{V}O_2$; BTPS, body temperature, pressure, saturated). (Modified from Weber KT, Janicki JS: Cardiopulmonary exercise testing for evaluation of chronic cardiac failure. Am J Cardiol 55:22A, 1985)

The normal heart rate and blood pressure responses to our treadmill exercise protocol are given in Table 32.4, and the heart rate–$\dot{V}O_2$ relation is shown for each of the four functional classes in Figure 32.8. The slope of the relation between heart rate and $\dot{V}O_2$ is not statistically different between classes. What distinguishes the classes is the maximum heart rate they achieve. Given that class D patients reach their $\dot{V}O_2$ max at less than 10 ml/minute/kg, their maximum heart rate does not generally exceed 120 beats per minute respectively. The usual maximum heart rates for classes C, B, and A are 130, 145, and 160 beats per minute. These findings imply that although there is a withdrawal of vagal tone and activation of the adrenergic nervous system during exercise, the dominant influence on the heart rate response to exercise is the afferent signals that arise from the exercising muscles. It is known that various muscle groups evoke different heart rate responses.[23] For example, arm exercise is always associated with a faster heart rate than exercise performed by the lower extremity for comparable workload. The expected heart rate–$\dot{V}O_2$ relation for treadmill or any exercise modality allows one to identify an inappropriate tachycardia or bradycardia with exercise.[24] Specialized studies to evaluate the nature of this disturbance can be pursued.

Given the maximum cardiac output and heart rate responses to exercise in classes A to D, it should be apparent that the maximum stroke volume response to exercise is quite different for each class. Class D patients are unable to increase their resting stroke volume during any level of treadmill exercise (Fig. 32.9). Accordingly, their modest cardiac output response (<4 liters/minute/m²) is mediated

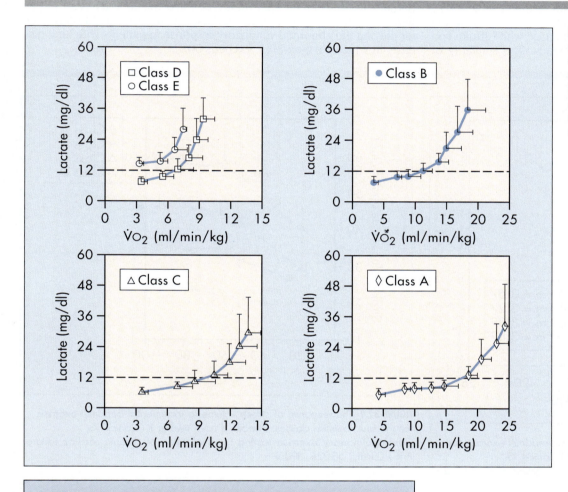

FIGURE 32.7 The response of mixed venous lactate concentration is given as a function of $\dot{V}O_2$ for each exercise class. A mixed venous lactate concentration of 12 mg/dl is identified by the broken horizontal line. (Modified from Weber KT, Janicki JS: Lactate production during maximal and submaximal exercise in patients with chronic cardiac failure. J Am Coll Cardiol 6:717, 1985)

TABLE 32.4 NORMAL RESPONSE IN HEART RATE AND BLOOD PRESSURE TO INCREMENTAL TREADMILL EXERCISE PROTOCOL

Stage	Heart Rate (beats per minute)	Systolic/Diastolic Pressure (mm Hg)
Standing	86 ± 13	130 ± 8/92 ± 11
1	96 ± 15	140 ± 13/96 ± 8
2	98 ± 14	141 ± 12/93 ± 8
3	104 ± 13	145 ± 13/91 ± 7
4	110 ± 13	150 ± 13/87 ± 8
5	118 ± 14	155 ± 13/92 ± 11
6	126 ± 13	159 ± 21/87 ± 8
7	135 ± 15	168 ± 19/88 ± 9
8	144 ± 15	166 ± 19/91 ± 11
9	155 ± 14	169 ± 25/88 ± 10
10	162 ± 15	179 ± 21/86 ± 14

solely by the increase in heart rate. In class C patients, there is a reserve in stroke volume, albeit of modest proportion (an average increase of 27%). Class B and A patients come closer to the expected normal response: stroke volume is increased 45% and 50% respectively above its resting value during the transition from standing rest to low and moderate levels of exercise (<60% $\dot{V}O_2$ max); thereafter, the increase in stroke volume is modest.

VENTILATION

The measurement of air flow and its integral to obtain tidal volume can be used to monitor the ventilatory response to exercise. The normal *ventilatory response* to incremental treadmill exercise consists of an increase in tidal volume and respiratory rate at light to moderate workloads.[2] At higher loads, the elevation in respiratory rate may become dominant with little or no change in tidal volume (Table 32.5). This latter response is somewhat similar to that of the heart, in which heart rate increases throughout incremental exercise while stroke volume rises predominantly during lighter workloads. The similarity of these responses underscores the close coupling that exists within the cardiopulmonary unit.

In patients with pulmonary venous hypertension and pulmonary congestion, a pattern of rapid shallow breathing characterizes the ventilatory response to exercise. We have observed this response in class C and D patients with chronic cardiac and circulatory failure.[4]

Another point of interest concerning the ventilatory response to upright exercise is the ratio of the $\dot{V}E$ max achieved with exercise to the maximum voluntary ventilation (MVV) determined during routine pulmonary function testing. Unless there is coexistent lung disease, most patients with cardiovascular disease rarely exceed 50% of their MVV in developing their exercise ventilatory response.[4] The same can be said of the ratio of maximum exercise tidal volume to vital capacity. Thus, the ventilatory reserve, represented by MVV and vital capacity, is only partially utilized during light, moderate, and maximal exercise in patients with heart disease. This ventilatory pattern forms the basis for identifying the abnormal ventilatory response in patients with lung disease, in which $\dot{V}E$ max/MVV exceeds 50%.

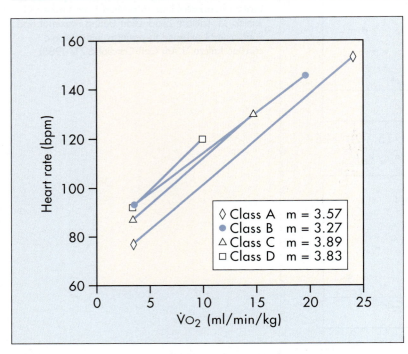

FIGURE 32.8 The response of heart rate to incremental treadmill exercise for the four functional classes. (Modified from Weber KT, Janicki JS: Pathophysiologic responses to exercise in patients with chronic cardiac failure. Heart Failure 1:131, 1985)

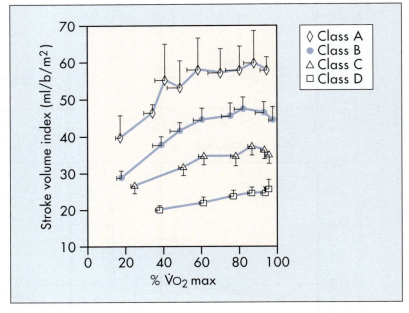

FIGURE 32.9 The response of stroke volume to incremental treadmill exercise for the four exercise classes. (Modified from Weber KT, Janicki JS: Cardiopulmonary exercise testing for evaluation of chronic cardiac failure. Am J Cardiol 55:22A, 1985)

TABLE 32.5 NORMAL RESPONSE IN VENTILATION TO INCREMENTAL TREADMILL EXERCISE

Stage	Minute Ventilation (liters/minute)	$\dot{V}E$/MVV (%)	Tidal Volume (ml)	Forced Vital Capacity (%)	Respiratory Rate (breaths per minute)
1	18 ± 6.1	12 ± 3.7	1153 ± 417	25 ± 7.6	17 ± 4.0
2	20 ± 5.3	14 ± 3.4	1162 ± 450	26 ± 8.2	19 ± 3.5
3	24 ± 7.2	17 ± 3.7	1270 ± 368	29 ± 6.5	20 ± 3.9
4	29 ± 8.5	20 ± 4.9	1388 ± 394	31 ± 6.2	22 ± 3.6
5	33 ± 9.3	23 ± 5.8	1468 ± 405	33 ± 6.9	24 ± 2.8
6	40 ± 12.2	27 ± 6.9	1628 ± 456	36 ± 6.9	25 ± 3.9
7	46 ± 13.7	31 ± 7.8	1776 ± 502	40 ± 7.6	27 ± 5.8
8	52 ± 17.3	35 ± 9.1	1921 ± 502	42 ± 9.8	28 ± 6.6
9	61 ± 18.9	41 ± 8.9	2153 ± 681	47 ± 9.4	29 ± 7.2
10	72 ± 25.0	46 ± 12.6	2216 ± 700	48 ± 9.7	33 ± 10.2

ARTERIAL O_2 SATURATION

Ear oximetry is an indirect, noninvasive method of monitoring arterial O_2 saturation that can be used as part of CPX. This is a particularly useful screening procedure in cases in which O_2 desaturation might be anticipated (*e.g.*, congenital heart disease with right-to-left shunt, restrictive or obstructive lung disease, or pulmonary embolic disease). Normal subjects and patients with chronic cardiac failure do not experience a fall in O_2 saturation during exercise.[25,26] The ear oximeter, however, may give erroneous information from the hyperpigmented skin of some black patients or when the earlobe is pierced. In cases in which O_2 desaturation is suspected or evident from ear oximetry, arterial O_2 saturation should be measured directly in arterial blood, which can be sampled directly from an indwelling catheter placed in the radial artery.

INVASIVE CPX TESTING

In patients with cardiopulmonary disease, it may be necessary to use invasive hemodynamic monitoring to define better the nature and severity of the underlying disorder. The information that can be gathered from such an approach is described below.

The advent of the flexible triple-lumen flotation catheter has simplified the process of hemodynamic monitoring during exercise. The catheter can be inserted at the bedside in the exercise laboratory without fluoroscopic imaging and left in place during exercise, whether it be on the treadmill or on the cycle ergometer. Importantly, an overnight hospital stay is not required.

In brief, the triple-lumen flotation catheter with thermistor is inserted through an antecubital vein and advanced into the terminal portion of the pulmonary circulation to obtain pulsatile pulmonary artery and occlusive wedge pressures. In reaching the smaller arteries of the pulmonary circulation, there is minimal catheter whip present during exercise unless exercise cardiac output is high. Right atrial pressure monitoring is obtained through the proximal part of the catheter. Determination of O_2 saturation of mixed venous blood, subsequent determination of cardiac output by Fick principle, and determination of lactate concentration can be obtained at each stage of exercise or whenever desired from the distal port of the catheter. Cardiac output is obtained using thermodilution during each stage to indicate the direction of the flow response. We, however, rely on the Fick cardiac output determinations for making our final determination of the hemodynamic response to exercise. Advances in fiberoptic technology now make it possible also to monitor mixed venous O_2 saturation on a continuous basis with the flotation catheter.[27] This technique simplifies the need to obtain multiple blood samples during exercise for the Fick cardiac output determination.

A catheter inserted into the radial or brachial artery of the same arm permits direct monitoring of arterial pressure and sampling of arterial blood for its O_2 tension and saturation and CO_2 tension.

PULMONARY CAPILLARY WEDGE PRESSURE

In normal subjects or patients with minimal cardiovascular disease, a progressive rise in cardiac output accompanies incremental treadmill work. For every 100 ml/minute/m^2 increase in $\dot{V}O_2$ there is a 600 ml/minute/m^2 rise in cardiac output. The maximal cardiac output response to exercise was considered earlier in this chapter. Generally speaking, and irrespective of its etiologic basis, the elevation in systemic flow with chronic cardiac failure is accomplished with a minimal elevation in left ventricular filling pressures that rarely exceeds 18 mm Hg (Fig. 32.10).[4,8] In patients with chronic cardiac failure of mild, moderate, or marked severity, the elevation in exercise cardiac output is accomplished with a greater elevation in left ventricular filling pressure. In class B, the resting wedge pressure may be only slightly elevated; with upright exercise, wedge pressure exceeds 20 mm Hg at aerobic capacity. In classes C and D, the resting wedge pressure is elevated to a greater degree and with exercise can frequently exceed 30 mm Hg. In these patients, however, clinically overt pulmonary congestion may not occur during or after the exercise test and marked exertional dyspnea may be absent; fatigue is a more frequent complaint.

In patients with valvular heart disease and chronic aortic or mitral regurgitation, the rise in wedge pressure can be more dramatic than that observed with chronic cardiac failure (see Fig. 32.10). In general, however, the same generalizations noted for chronic cardiac failure hold true for class A patients, in whom the elevation in wedge pressure is the least of the four classes. In the case of pulmonary vascular disease, wedge pressure rarely exceeds 18 mm Hg in any functional class. Patients with systemic hypertension may have diastolic dysfunction of the left ventricle that leads to a marked increase in wedge pressure during exercise. With a marked elevation in exercise arterial pressure, as occurs in patients with systemic hypertension, mitral regurgitation may appear.

SYSTEMIC VASCULAR RESISTANCE

Systolic and mean arterial pressure are increased during upright exercise (see Table 32.4); however, because of the vasodilatation that occurs in working skeletal muscle, arterial diastolic pressure remains

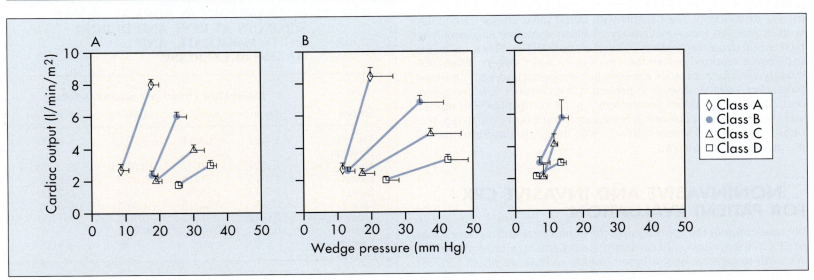

FIGURE 32.10 The exercise ventricular function curve for the left heart, comparing cardiac output and wedge pressures. **A.** Function curves for patients with chronic cardiac failure. **B.** Curves for patients with chronic mitral or aortic regurgitation. **C.** Curves for patients with pulmonary vascular disease. Because patients with pulmonary hypertension are not seen until late in the course of their disease, there are no class A patients represented in part **C**.

essentially invariant. Resting systemic vascular resistance, which normally averages 1200 dynes/second/cm^{-5}, falls by 50% during maximal isotonic treadmill exercise.[8] The autoregulation of the large muscle mass involved with walking accommodates a greater proportion of systemic blood flow. Other circulatory beds, such as the splanchnic and cutaneous circulations, that are less metabolically active vasoconstrict, permitting enhanced O_2 delivery to working muscle while preserving mean arterial pressure. Table 32.6 details the reapportionment of systemic blood flow that occurs among the various organs during mild, moderate, and heavy isotonic exercise, including the rise in skeletal muscle blood flow. An abnormal fall in vascular resistance or cardiac output during exercise may account for exertional hypotension. On the other hand, inadequate vasodilation secondary to medial hypertrophy within the arterioles of skeletal muscle results in exertional hypertension. In patients with established systemic hypertension, in whom resting systemic resistance may be abnormally elevated and vasodilatory capacity may be impaired, there can be a dramatic rise in systolic arterial pressure as well as an elevation in arterial diastolic pressure with upright exercise.

PULMONARY VASCULAR RESISTANCE

Because of the low impedance characteristics of the pulmonary circulation, which are normally 10% of the systemic vascular resistance, pulmonary artery systolic, mean, and diastolic pressures rise only minimally with exercise. It is only at higher workloads, when $\dot{V}O_2$ max exceeds 30 ml/minute/kg and cardiac output averages 15 liters/minute or more, that pulmonary artery systolic pressure may approach 50 mm Hg. Pulmonary vascular resistance, like systemic vascular resistance, falls by 50% during incremental isotonic exercise. However, once again, pulmonary resistance is only 60 dynes/second/cm^{-5}, or 10% that in the systemic circulation, at maximal exercise.

The normal relationship between the gradient in pressure across the lung and cardiac output is shown in Figure 32.11 against isopleths of constant pulmonary vascular resistance. This relationship is important in the evaluation of pulmonary vascular disease that may or may not accompany other disorders that produce pulmonary venous hypertension or intrinsic pulmonary vascular disease. We have found that the occlusive wedge pressure is the appropriate downstream pressure to use in calculating this gradient despite the existence of a critical closing pressure in the pulmonary circulation.[28]

In patients with an elevated left ventricular filling pressure secondary to ischemic or myopathic heart disease, pulmonary vascular resistance at rest and during exercise generally falls between 200 dynes/second/cm^{-5} and 400 dynes/second/cm^{-5}. With mitral valve disease, in which there is more longstanding pulmonary venous hypertension, pulmonary resistance can be elevated beyond that seen with left ventricular dysfunction. For patients with mitral valve disease commonly seen in practice today, pulmonary vascular resistance is generally as high as 600 dynes/second/cm^{-5}, but it is rarely higher. This is unlike the experience reported before the era of open heart surgery. When pulmonary vascular resistance exceeds 600 dynes/second/cm^{-5}, intrinsic pulmonary vascular disease is present.[29] We consider 600 dynes/second/cm^{-5} to 1000 dynes/second/cm^{-5} to be compatible with moderately severe vascular disease. A resistance in excess of 1000 dynes/second/cm^{-5} connotes severe disease within the arteries and arterioles of the pulmonary circulation.

☐ NONINVASIVE AND INVASIVE CPX FOR PATIENT EVALUATION

We now consider the application of the noninvasive and invasive forms of CPX in the evaluation of cardiocirculatory and pulmonary disorders. We wish to provide only a broad outline of how we select CPX for general categories of patients that are commonly seen in the clinical exercise laboratory. Based on this information, the choice of therapy can also be obtained. For a more detailed discussion of our experience, the interested reader is referred elsewhere.[2] Based on this information, the choice of therapy can also be obtained.

HEART DISEASE

Patients with documented evidence of myocardial or valvular heart disease or those with chronotropic dysfunction (e.g., sick sinus syndrome, atrioventricular block, inappropriate sinus tachycardia, or atrial fibrillation) should have a noninvasive CPX test using incremental treadmill exercise to determine their aerobic capacity and anaerobic threshold. This indicates the severity of their disease, their cardiac reserve, and their functional capacity, which can now be objectively monitored over time or as it relates to a particular therapeutic intervention.

Resting pulmonary function studies need to be obtained beforehand in patients with heart disease who also have a history or clinical evidence of lung disease. This information aids in excluding ventilatory dysfunction and identifies the ventilatory reserves. Should there be evidence of obstructive or restrictive lung disease or a reduced diffusing capacity (suggesting a perfusion defect), it is wise to add ear oximetry to the test to exclude exercise-induced arterial O_2 desaturation.

After the aerobic capacity and anaerobic threshold of an individual with heart disease have been determined and a ventilatory component to effort intolerance in patients with coexistent heart and lung disease has been excluded, the following approach is recommended regarding any additional exercise studies:

1. In patients with *dilated cardiomyopathy*, there is no need for additional testing because one can predict cardiac reserve, severity of cardiac failure, and functional capacity. These patients can be followed by noninvasive CPX to assess the course of their disease or its response to therapy.
2. In patients with *ischemic heart disease* who are in functional class B, C, or D, one may wish to recommend invasive CPX with hemodynamic monitoring to understand why the cardiac reserve is reduced (e.g., onset of mitral regurgitation vs. a noncompliant ventricle), to guide therapy, and to identify why there may be a disparity between the clinical evaluation and CPX.
3. In *mitral* or *aortic valvular incompetence* there may exist a disparity between cardiac catheterization findings obtained at rest in the supine position to indicate the severity of disease and the heart's response to exercise. Here invasive CPX with hemodynamic moni-

TABLE 32.6 O_2 TRANSPORT IN NORMAL HUMAN SUBJECTS AT REST AND DURING LIGHT, MODERATE, AND MAXIMUM EXERCISE

	Blood Flow (liters per minute/% total)			
Organ	Resting	Light	Moderate	Maximum
Viscera Skeleton	1.4/24	1.1/11	0.60/3	0.30/1
Muscle	1.2/21	4.50/47	12.50/71	22.00/88
Kidneys	1.1/19	0.90/10	0.60/3	0.25/1
Brain	0.7/13	0.75/8	0.75/4	0.75/3
Skin	0.5/8	1.50/15	1.90/12	0.60/2
Other organs	0.6/10	0.40/4	0.40/3	0.10/1
Heart	0.3/3	0.35/4	0.75/4	1.00/4
Overall	5.8	9.50	17.50	25.00

(Adapted from Wade OL, Bishop JM: Cardiac Output and Regional Blood Flow. Philadelphia, FA Davis, 1962; and Falls HB (ed): Exercise Physiology. New York, Academic Press, 1968)

toring can provide invaluable information relevant to the issues of cardiac reserve, left ventricular dysfunction (both diastolic and systolic), and the patient's candidacy for valve replacement. For example, a patient who still has a considerable cardiac reserve (class B) and aerobic capacity that cannot be assessed from resting hemodynamic data may not be a candidate for surgery, whereas class C and D patients have a considerable impairment in aerobic capacity and should have valve replacement. Moreover, the relation of the pressure gradient to cardiac output across the pulmonary circulation identifies an abnormal pulmonary vascular resistance that influences the decision on remedial surgery and aids in predicting the postoperative rate of recovery (*i.e.*, the higher the vascular resistance, the slower the recovery).

4. In patients with suspected or occult *pericardial* disease, the heightened venous return of exercise can aid in eliciting the constrictive element of the pericardium. Monitoring the response in right atrial and wedge pressures during exercise enables identification of the presence of pericardial disease and its severity in compromising the cardiac output response to exercise.
5. In patients with *chronotropic dysfunction* at rest and during noninvasive CPX, there is no need for invasive studies. Functional capacity can be monitored in response to various therapeutic interventions (*e.g.*, pacemaker, hydralazine, β-blockade) that are dictated by the nature of the underlying disease and the abnormality in cardiac rhythm and rate.

VASCULAR DISEASE
SYSTEMIC HYPERTENSION
In patients with systemic hypertension, the noninvasive incremental treadmill test is recommended with noninvasive monitoring of arterial blood pressure. If the patient's $\dot{V}O_2$ max is compatible with class B, C, or D, a repeat test with pulmonary artery catheter is recommended to assess the degree of left ventricular diastolic dysfunction. In class B, C, or D patients it does not appear wise to use β-adrenergic blockade because their cardiac output response to exercise is suboptimal. On the other hand, it is unlikely that the cardiac output response is impaired in class A patients. If the patient has a normal aerobic capacity (*i.e.*, class A), but the arterial systolic or diastolic pressure response to exercise is markedly abnormal, the test should be repeated with an arterial catheter for the direct recording of arterial pressure. This information serves as an important baseline for monitoring the response in ambulatory blood pressure to antihypertensive therapy, as well as for the correlating the noninvasive cuff technique in follow-up tests.

ATHEROSCLEROTIC DISEASE
Normotensive patients with atherosclerotic cardiovascular disease of the lower extremity may experience claudication during treadmill exercise and therefore fail to attain their anaerobic threshold and $\dot{V}O_2$ max. There is little reason to recommend an invasive study. The noninvasive test permits an objective assessment of the severity of occlusive disease. The efficacy of various medical and surgical therapies for vascular disease can be serially evaluated with noninvasive CPX, and the level of $\dot{V}O_2$ can be identified at the onset of limiting leg pain. In cases in which the anaerobic threshold can be determined before the appearance of claudication and the patient's functional class is C or D, an improvement in cardiac output and large-vessel limb blood flow with vasodilators or inotropic agents may enhance limb blood flow and improve exercise capacity.

PULMONARY VASCULAR DISEASE
Patients with pulmonary vascular disease (intrinsic vascular disease or thromboembolic disease) and pulmonary hypertension should have an invasive incremental test after noninvasive CPX testing with ear oximetry has been obtained. After assessment of the aerobic capacity of these patients and determination of whether they have arterial O_2 desaturation, the invasive test can be completed more efficiently and intelligently. An arterial line should be inserted for the invasive test to document the fall in arterial O_2 tension and for subsequent repeat testing with supplemental O_2. We recommend the invasive test in these patients, even if they are class A, for the following reasons

1. It is often difficult to predict the severity of the pulmonary hypertension on clinical grounds.
2. Serial noninvasive measurements of pulmonary artery pressure cannot be obtained as is true for the systemic circulation, and the exercise response can be invaluable for subsequent evaluation.
3. Early treatment of pulmonary hypertension with vasodilators may

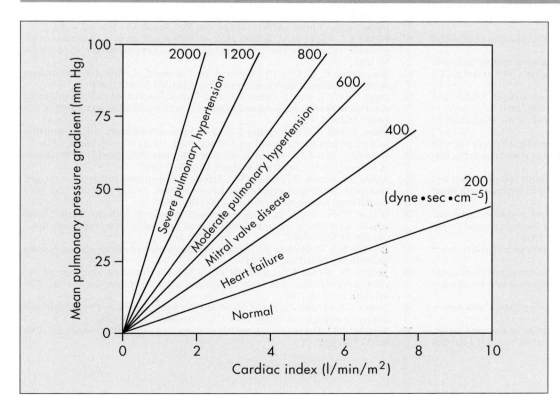

FIGURE 32.11 The interrelationship between the pressure gradient across the lung and cardiac output, plotted against a background of isopleths of constant pulmonary vascular resistance. The normal range of resistance and the ranges observed for various cardiopulmonary disorders are given.

be effective in retarding the development of right heart failure. The choice of vasodilator that is most effective and the dosage that can be safely administered without systemic hypotension can be assessed by bedside hemodynamic monitoring after the exercise test. The baseline pressure–flow relation of the diseased pulmonary circulation (at least three points are required) obtained at rest and two levels of exercise can be compared with that following drug intervention if one of the vasodilators appears to be effective in reducing resting mean pulmonary artery pressure and pulmonary vascular resistance.

4. The response in pulmonary artery pressure and vascular resistance to supplemental O_2 can also be assessed, and physical activity at home can be restricted to those levels of work that are not associated with marked right ventricular pressure overload.

LUNG DISEASE

Patients with restrictive or obstructive lung disease are rarely able to cross their anaerobic threshold and attain their $\dot{V}O_2$ max before becoming dyspneic. Pulmonary function studies should be obtained prior to noninvasive CPX in order to identify the ventilatory reserves (i.e., the vital capacity and MVV) so that exercise tidal volume and $\dot{V}E$ can be examined in relation to these reserves. Generally speaking, these patients use more than 50% of these reserves during exercise when they become dyspneic. Ear oximetry should be included with the noninvasive test to examine for arterial hypoxemia that appears during exercise. If there is no evidence of cor pulmonale in these patients, there is little need to proceed to the invasive exercise test, except with an arterial line to quantify directly the severity of arterial O_2 desaturation. The arterial line can be left in place and the exercise test repeated with supplemental inspired O_2.

EXERTIONAL DYSPNEA

The following clues aid in identifying whether exertional dyspnea is secondary to ventilatory dysfunction: (1) the appearance of arterial hypoxemia, (2) maximum $\dot{V}E$ on exercise that is more than 50% of MVV, and (3) a patient who is unable to reach aerobic capacity when symptomatic dyspnea prohibits further exercise. This is also true in patients with coexistent heart and lung disease when the ventilatory impairment is dominant and is consistent with the limited ventilatory effort that can be voluntarily sustained before the appearance of fatigue or the sensation of breathlessness in normal subjects.[30] When heart or circulatory disease is dominant, patients are able to cross their anaerobic threshold and attain their aerobic capacity. These patients do not develop arterial hypoxemia and do not use more than 50% of their ventilatory reserves.

DISABILITY, WORK CAPACITY, AND REHABILITATION

The noninvasive CPX test permits a determination of aerobic capacity and identifies aerobic and anaerobic levels of work. This information should prove invaluable in objectively assessing disability and work capacity and writing an individualized exercise prescription. These results can also be followed over time to assess the results of exercise training. It needs to be emphasized, however, that all the potentials of CPX described above have not been systematically tested, and their practical values in clinical practice need to be determined by further studies. Nevertheless, CPX based on sound physiological principles provides useful information regarding the pathophysiologic conditions in patients with various cardiovascular disorders and should be regarded as a valuable and clinically relevant investigation in the assessment of these patients.

REFERENCES

1. Weber KT, Janicki JS, Shroff SG et al: The cardiopulmonary unit: The body's gas transport system. Clin Chest Med 4:101, 1983
2. Weber KT, Janicki JS (eds): Cardio-Pulmonary Exercise Testing: Physiologic Principles and Clinical Applications. Philadelphia, WB Saunders, 1986
3. Weber KT, Janicki JS, Likoff MJ: Exercise testing in the evaluation of cardiopulmonary disease: A cardiologist's point of view. Clin Chest Med 5:173, 1984
4. Weber KT, Kinasewiz GT, Janicki JS et al: Oxygen utilization and ventilation during exercise in patients with chronic cardiac failure. Circulation 65:1213, 1982
5. Astrand PO: Quantification of exercise capability and evaluation of physical capacity in man. Prog Cardiovasc Dis 19:51, 1976
6. Weber KT, Janicki JS: Lactate production during maximal and submaximal exercise in patients with chronic cardiac failure. J Am Coll Cardiol 6:717, 1985
7. Davies CTM: Limitations to the prediction of maximum oxygen intake from cardiac frequency measurements. J Appl Physiol 24:700, 1968
8. Weber KT, Janicki JS: Cardiopulmonary exercise testing for evaluation of chronic cardiac failure. Am J Cardiol 55:22A, 1985
9. Wilson JR, Martin JL, Schwartz D et al: Exercise intolerance in patients with chronic heart failure: Role of impaired nutritive flow to skeletal muscle. Circulation 69:1079, 1984
10. Wilson JR, Martin JL, Ferraro N et al: Effect of hydralazine on perfusion and metabolism in the leg during upright bicycle exercise in patients with heart failure. Circulation 68:425, 1983
11. Kugler J, Maskin C, Fishman WH et al: Regional and systemic metabolic effects of angiotensin-converting enzyme inhibition during exercise in patients with severe heart failure. Circulation 66:1256, 1982
12. Katz LN, Feinberg H, Shaffer AB: Hemodynamic aspects of congestive heart failure. Circulation 21:95, 1960
13. Gelberg HJ, Rubin SA, Ports TA et al: Detection of left ventricular functional reserve by supine exercise hemodynamics in patients with severe, chronic heart failure. Am J Cardiol 44:1062, 1979
14. Benje W, Litchfield RL, Marcus ML: Exercise capacity in patients with severe left ventricular dysfunction. Circulation 61:955, 1980
15. Franciosa JS, Park M, Levine B: Lack of correlation between exercise capacity and indices of left ventricular performance in heart failure. Am J Cardiol 47:33, 1981
16. Engler R, Ray R, Higgins C et al: Clinical assessment and follow-up of functional capacity in patients with chronic congestive cardiomyopathy. Am J Cardiol 49:1832, 1982
17. Higginbotham MD, Morris KG, Conn EH et al: Determinants of variable exercise performance among patients with severe left ventricular dysfunction. Am J Cardiol 51:51, 1983
18. Szlachcic J, Massie BM, Kramer BL et al: Correlates and prognostic implication of exercise capacity in chronic congestive heart failure. Am J Cardiol 55:1037, 1985
19. Weber KT, Wilson JR, Janicki JS et al: Exercise testing in the evaluation of the patient with chronic cardiac failure. Am Rev Respir Dis 192:S60, 1984
20. Weber KT, Andrews V, Janicki JS et al: Pirbuterol, an oral beta-adrenergic receptor agonist, in the treatment of chronic cardiac failure. Circulation 66:1262, 1982
21. Wasserman K, McIlroy M: Detecting the threshold of anaerobic metabolism in cardiac patients during exercise. Am J Cardiol 14:844, 1964
22. Donald KW, Glostor J, Harris EA et al: The production of lactic acid during exercise in normal subjects and in patients with rheumatic heart disease. Am Heart J 62:494, 1961
23. Vokac Z, Bell H, BautzoHolter E et al: Oxygen uptake/heart rate relationship in leg and arm exercise, sitting and standing. J Appl Physiol 39:54, 1975
24. Weber KT, Likoff MJ, McCarthy D: Low dose beta blockade in the treatment of chronic cardiac failure. Am Heart J 104:877, 1982
25. Rubin SA, Brown HV, Swan HJC: Arterial oxygenation and arterial oxygen transport in chronic myocardial failure at rest, during exercise and after hydralazine treatment. Circulation 66:143, 1982
26. Wilson JR, Ferraro N: Exercise intolerance in patients with chronic left heart failure: Relation to oxygen transport and ventilatory abnormalities. Am J Cardiol 51:1358, 1983
27. Divertie MB, McMichan JC: Continuous monitoring of mixed venous oxygen saturation. Chest 85:423, 1984
28. Janicki JS, Weber KT, Likoff MJ et al: The pressure-flow response of the pulmonary circulation in heart failure and pulmonary vascular disease. Circulation 72:1270, 1985
29. Weber KT, Janicki JS, Shroff SG et al: The right ventricle: Physiologic and pathophysiologic considerations. Crit Care Med 11:323, 1983
30. Shephard RJ: The maximum sustained voluntary ventilation in exercise. Clin Sci 32:167, 1967

NONINVASIVE EVALUATION OF PERIPHERAL VASCULAR DISEASE

D. E. Strandness, Jr

Although noninvasive tests for evaluating the peripheral circulation have been available since the 1960s, it was several years before they were accepted by the medical profession.[1] Most physicians, particularly surgeons, felt comfortable with the findings of the history, physical examination, and arteriography. Prior to the introduction of ultrasonic duplex scanning in 1974, nearly all tests of the peripheral circulation were indirect, that is, they generated physiologic data for a limb segment but were unable to interrogate directly the specific vascular segments.[2] These devices were largely plethysmographic and detected volume changes that could be used to measure limb pressures and flow and record the periodic changes in limb and digit volume associated with each heartbeat.[1] From a clinical standpoint, the measurements that finally were determined to be of clinical use were the measurement of limb segmental and ankle systolic blood pressures and the estimation of volume pulsations. The value of the ankle systolic blood pressure is increased when measured both at rest and after exercise.[3,4] The measurement of limb blood flow, while theoretically attractive, has not found a useful place in diagnostic medicine. Limb blood flow is maintained at normal levels even with extensive chronic arterial disease. The most important change to take place was the introduction of continuous-wave Doppler methods in the 1960s. The development of the pulsed Doppler system was rapidly followed by its union with imaging methods in the 1970s.[2,5,6] In this chapter techniques in current use are reviewed.

EVALUATION OF THE EXTREMITIES

The diseases that affect the large- and medium-sized arteries mainly include atherosclerosis and thromboangiitis obliterans. Because thromboangiitis obliterans is uncommon, atherosclerosis is considered the major vascular disease in the western world. It is a segmental disease of branch points and bifurcations, and it produces problems by one of two mechanisms: (1) a reduction in pressure and flow and (2) emboli from ulcerated plaques. A reduction in flow is the most common cause of symptoms in the lower limbs. In contrast, it is believed that emboli are the most common basis for cerebral ischemic events.

The simplest method of establishing the presence of arterial obstruction is to measure the pressure beyond the area of involvement. Hemodynamically significant lesions will produce a pressure drop that is directly related to the higher resistance of the collateral circulation and other associated stenoses or occlusions that exist in the adjacent segments.[7]

However, there are circumstances in which the lesions are not occlusive and estimation of hemodynamic significance may be more difficult. If this is the case it may be necessary to study the lesions under conditions of stress that may bring out the functional abnormality, that is, a drop in pressure secondary to the increased flow demand.[3]

BASIC SCREENING TESTS

For patients who present with symptoms or are considered to be at high risk for peripheral arterial disease the basic study is simply to measure the ankle systolic blood pressure (by Doppler) and relate it to arm systolic blood pressure, arriving at the ankle/arm index (AAI).[8] If this index is greater than or equal to 1.0, the result is considered normal. If it is below 0.95, the patient's condition is definitely abnormal, with the value depending on the level and, most importantly, on the extent of the occlusive disease. For example, with only one segment involved at the popliteal artery or higher, the AAI is usually greater than 0.50. With more than one level of stenosis or occlusion, it is below 0.50. The absolute level of ankle systolic blood pressure is important as a rough index of perfusion. Rest pain and/or ulceration rarely occur with a pressure greater than 40 mm Hg. Below that level the flow is marginal and the patient should be so warned.

If the ankle systolic blood pressure is normal and the clinical picture, particularly for claudication, is suspicious, the patient should have the ankle systolic pressures measured after treadmill exercise.[3] Normal subjects at a modest workload (2 mph on a 12% grade) will not experience a decrease in their pressures. This is in contrast to patients with atherosclerosis and significant lesions, in whom the pressure falls, often to unrecordable levels, and requires several minutes to return to the pre-exercise level.[4] This testing approach is adequate for baseline tests, and the results can serve as markers for further evaluation.

With the availability of continuous-wave Doppler studies and an experienced observer, it is possible to perform a quick screening of the common and superficial femoral, popliteal, and tibial arteries to estimate the probable level(s) of occlusion and/or stenosis. In some cases this screening can permit a reasonable estimate of where the disease is and how it might be treated.[5,6,9,10] Continuous-wave Doppler screening is inexpensive, available, and applicable to nearly all patients, and it serves as a baseline for longitudinal follow-ups and monitoring of the status of the disease (Table 33.1). The time this watchful approach changes is when the patient is considered a candidate for a direct procedure to improve flow. Then it is vital to know not only where the disease is but also its hemodynamic significance. The standard method of making this determination has been arteriography.

ROLE OF ARTERIOGRAPHY

In recent years arteriography has undergone several improvements, including the development of catheters for insertion into the arterial system, the implementation of digital computer methods, and the development of a hypo-osmolar contrast material that is less painful and perhaps less toxic. However, it still represents only a two-dimensional display of three-dimensional lesions.[11] In the past arteriography has been used to demonstrate the location and extent of disease with an attempt (based on dimensions of stenosis) to predict the hemodynamic significance of apparent lesions. It is generally agreed that for peripheral arteries, a reduction of 50% or greater in the diameter of an arterial segment is sufficient to produce an abnormal pressure gradient and a reduction in flow even under resting flow conditions.[7] However, it is also known that lesser degrees of narrowing may become hemodynamically significant if there is an increase in flow across a stenosis of less than 50% diameter. Because of its invasive nature and the availability of sensitive noninvasive test, arteriography is not required to make a clinical diagnosis. Its use should be limited to those patients in whom an interventional therapeutic method is intended.[12] This intervention is nearly always based on the patient's presentation and an estimate of the severity of the problem. For example, nearly all patients with advanced ischemia presenting with rest pain and/or limited area of tissue loss will be candidates for intervention if the anatomical distribution of the disease is suitable. On the other hand, patients who present with intermittent claudication will be evaluated only if the problem limits the patient's life-style or interferes with gainful employment. The only exception to this relates to those patients with iliac stenoses and moderately severe claudication who may be candidates for transluminal angioplasty, which is a simple, direct approach that can now be done with a minimum of risk, a much lower cost, and the prospects for good, long-term success.

ULTRASONIC DUPLEX SCANNING

With the routine use of the indirect tests, the following questions can be quickly and accurately answered: Is disease present? Is it functionally mild or severe? Does it involve a single or multiple segments? Are further tests such as duplex scanning required?

In practice, arterial disease can be ruled out if the following findings are noted:

1. An AAI of 1.0 or greater.
2. Triphasic velocity tracing recorded from all peripheral arteries—from the femoral to the tibial arteries at the ankle.
3. No fall in ankle systolic pressure after a workload sufficient to bring out this problem. In my experience, a 5-minute walk on a treadmill set for 2 mph on a 12% grade is sufficient to bring this out.

In most cases, the clinical presentation is sufficient to determine the functional status of the circulation to the limb. However, there are useful clues from the noninvasive test results that signify advanced disease:

1. An AAI less than 50% (0.50) or an absolute ankle systolic blood pressure of less than 50 mm Hg.
2. The absence of arterial velocity signals from the tibial and peroneal artery at the level of the ankle.
3. A walking time on the treadmill of less than 1 minute with a greater than 20-minute period required for the pressure to return to baseline.

Whether the disease involves single or multiple arterial segments is certainly an important question because single segment disease, such as in the iliac or superficial femoral artery, is rarely associated with the occurrence of ischemic symptoms at rest or disabling claudication. On the other hand, multisegment disease is more prone to lead to limb loss and is more difficult to approach therapeutically.[13] It is multisegment disease that taxes the talents of the vascular surgeon and interventional radiologist. The following data provide useful clues:

1. An AAI less than 0.50.
2. An absolute pressure below 40 mm Hg.
3. Unrecordable ankle systolic blood pressures.
4. The absence of detectable flow from the tibial arteries.
5. No recordable pressure from the toes or a level below 20 mm Hg.

Combinations of these findings present a dismal prognosis *unless* more blood can be brought to the limb by either surgery or angioplasty. It is also in this group of patients where the most accurate information regarding the exact location of disease is essential in planning therapy.

If the clinical presentation combined with appropriate test results suggest that intervention will be required, ultrasonic duplex scanning can be performed.[14,15] This modality combines B-mode ultrasound with a pulsed Doppler study. Although the major use of this procedure is to study the carotid bulb, several innovations in technology have made it practical to use ultrasonic duplex scanning to evaluate the peripheral arteries. These include the following:

1. A variety of transmitting frequencies (2.5–10 MHz). For deeply placed arteries, such as the aorta, it may be necessary to go as low as 2.5 MHz to obtain a satisfactory image of the vessels and to characterize the flow.
2. Fast Fourier Transform spectral analysis to provide comprehensive information on the data in the spectra of velocities that are recorded.
3. Computer-based algorithms that simplify the study procedure, data acquisition, and analysis.

The data needed to institute therapy are precise localization of the disease and an objective estimate of hemodynamic severity. The finding of an occlusion is nearly certain evidence that its correction will result in a significant increase in both pressure and flow either to the distal limb or to the next system of collaterals.

For less than occlusive lesions, not only their localization but also an estimate of hemodynamic severity become the key issues in managing the disease. Although this represents an oversimplification, the following disease patterns will in general demand certain therapeutic approaches:

1. Single-segment occlusions (aortoiliac, femoropopliteal). Direct arterial surgery with some form of bypass graft will be required.
2. Single-segment, high-grade stenoses (aortoiliac, femoropopliteal). Angioplasty is clearly the treatment of choice for the proximal dis-

TABLE 33.1 DIAGNOSTIC CRITERIA BY INDIRECT TESTING FOR OCCLUSIVE ARTERIAL LESIONS*

Finding	Systolic Pressure (Ankle)	Velocity Waveform	Exercise Test
Normal	AAI > 1.0†	Triphasic	<20% fall in ankle pressure
Occlusion	AAI > 0.95	Monophasic	>20% fall in ankle pressure
Stenosis (>50%)	AAI < 0.95	↑Systolic velocity in stenosis ↑↓Systolic velocity distal to stenosis Monophasic waveform	>20% fall in ankle pressure
Stenosis (<50%)	AAI > 0.95	Minimal velocity change in stenosis Normal distal to stenosis Triphasic waveform	Variable; with stenosis approaching 50%, test results may be abnormal.

* These are lesions in or proximal to the popliteal artery.
† AAI, ankle/arm index.

ease. Bypass surgery is probably best for femoropopliteal disease because of the high rate of restenosis that occurs after angioplasty in this group.
3. Multisegment disease
   a. Aortoiliac and femoropopliteal. Correction of the proximal disease alone is sufficient to relieve rest pain and heal open lesions but will not restore walking distance to normal.
   b. Femoropopliteal and tibial-peroneal involvement. This pattern of disease will usually require some form of distal bypass from the femoral to lower limb vessels, often at the level of the ankle.

DIAGNOSTIC CRITERIA

The most accurate method at the moment for predicting normalcy is the finding of a triphasic velocity waveform throughout all segments of the arterial system, from the level of the abdominal aorta to the tibial arteries at the ankle. These three phases represent, in order, the forward flow with systole, the reverse flow in early diastole, and a second forward flow component in late diastole (Fig. 33.1). A loss of the second and third phase, resulting in a monophasic waveform, is diagnostic of arterial narrowing and/or occlusion. In previous years, it was thought that once the reverse flow component was lost it was never recovered beyond sites of narrowing. It is now known that this may not necessarily be the case. For example, the finding of a triphasic waveform at the level of the femoral artery does not conclusively rule out disease in the proximal iliac arteries.

One other aspect of the velocity pattern that may be of diagnostic importance is the amount of spectral broadening that is present. In a laminar flow system, the red blood cells generally move at similar velocities except near the wall where the velocity gradients are steep, which results in a very narrow band of frequencies with a clear window beneath the systolic peak.

Whenever the speed and direction of the red blood cells randomly change in regions of turbulent flow, the systolic window will begin to fill in and is referred to as spectral broadening. Although spectral broadening cannot be quantitated, it is a useful diagnostic feature when seen.

When disease develops it does so in stages, some of which are clinically relevant. In our studies with ultrasonic duplex scanning and arteriography, my colleagues and I have chosen to use the following categories (Fig. 33.2)[13,14].

1. One to 19% (wall roughening). For minimal wall disease in this category, these lesions are not clinically significant except for the rare situation in which emboli may arise from areas of ulceration. Since there is initially no narrowing of the artery, one would not expect an increase in the peak systolic velocity. The only change would be some alteration in the velocity profile with disturbances manifested by spectral broadening.
2. Twenty to 49% stenosis. These lesions, while not hemodynamically significant, can lead to an increase in the peak systolic velocity in the narrowed segment. There are basically four features of the waveform that are relevant:
   a. An increase in peak velocity of greater than 30% from the adjacent proximal segment
   b. Spectral broadening
   c. Preservation of reverse flow
   d. No post-stenotic turbulence
3. Fifty to 99% stenosis. A stenosis of this magnitude will produce both a drop in pressure and a reduction in flow to the limb. These are clinically important lesions characterized by the following criteria:
   a. An increase in peak systolic velocity of greater than 100% from the prestenotic segments
   b. Spectral broadening
   c. Loss of reverse flow
   d. The appearance of post-stenotic turbulence
4. Total occlusion. In this setting, no flow is detected from an observed segment.

At this point, it is important to comment on the role of the imaging as distinguished from the use of the pulsed Doppler velocity data that have just been reviewed. Plaques, calcification, and, in some cases, narrowing can be seen, but the resolution is not sufficient to make an estimate of the degree of narrowing. In addition, it is difficult if not impossible to estimate the stenotic dimensions of a three-dimensional plaque from a two-dimensional view. Until three-dimensional imaging along with methods of estimating boundaries is developed, we must

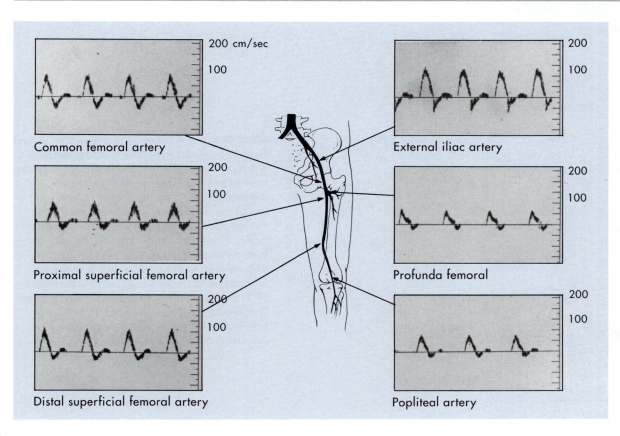

FIGURE 33.1 The velocity waveforms recorded from the sites shown were done using an ultrasonic duplex scanner. The spectral display was analyzed using the Fast Fourier Transform approach. The waveforms are quite uniform in their shape and phasic qualities with the three components shown and include the prominent forward flow component with systole, the reverse flow component in early diastole, and the second forward low component noted in late diastole. The clear window beneath the systolic peak is typical of the patterns seen when the flow is laminar. (Reproduced and modified from Jager KA, Ricketts HJ, Strandness DE Jr. Duplex scanning for the evaluation of lower limb arterial disease. In Bernstein EF [ed]: Noninvasive Diagnostic Techniques in Vascular Disease, p 619. St. Louis, CV Mosby, 1985)

depend on velocity indices as estimators of the degree of narrowing (Fig. 33.3).

ACCURACY

Validation of duplex scanning has gone through several phases. There are only two alternative methods against which such scanning can be compared: arteriography and direct intra-arterial pressure measurements.[11] The latter are generally done only across the aortoiliac segment.

During our initial duplex studies, we carried out two projects: comparison of duplex scanning with arteriography and comparison of the readings of one radiologist with another when each read the same films.[13] As is shown in Table 33.2, these comparisons provided some interesting surprises. The most notable finding was how often two radiologists might differ when reading the same film. In this study, calipers were used to measure and classify the degree of stenosis.

The data can be expressed in four ways as related to arteriography: sensitivity, specificity, and positive and negative predictive value.[14] The first two, sensitivity and specificity, refer to the global accuracy, either in detecting the presence of disease or ruling it out. This is adequate information for epidemiologic studies, but more information is needed when applying therapy, particularly interventional methods. When the data are used for specific treatment purposes, precise localization and estimates of hemodynamic significance become of paramount importance. It is at this point when positive and negative predictive values for each vascular segment become extremely important (Table 33.3).

APPLICATION TO PRACTICE

It is clear that duplex scanning represents an emerging technology that will require more time to evaluate at several centers. Nonetheless, given the present data, there are conclusions that do appear warranted:

1. The method is not needed to establish the diagnosis.
2. The severity of the illness still depends on the patient's presentation and findings on physical examination.
3. It is currently not a replacement for arteriography, which has to be done prior to intervention.
4. It can provide useful data for patients who could be scheduled for angioplasty without waiting for the definitive arteriographic study.
5. It is the best method for evaluating long-term results of both angioplasty and direct arterial surgery, particularly in situ and in reversed saphenous vein grafts.

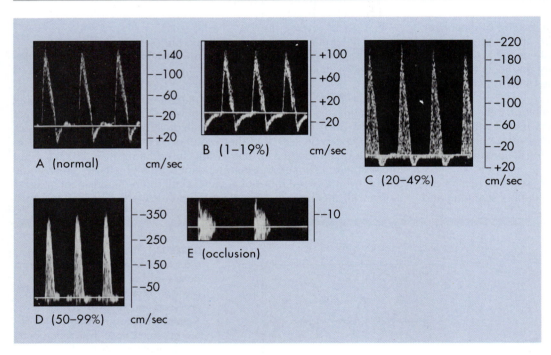

FIGURE 33.2 The patterns seen in the study of peripheral arterial patterns and reviewed in the text are illustrated. The major differences seen between the non-flow- and flow-reducing lesions (C and D) are with the loss of reverse flow and the dramatic increase in peak systolic velocity in the high-grade lesions. When the sample volume of the pulsed Doppler is placed just proximal to a total occlusion, a biphasic "thumping" sound is heard.

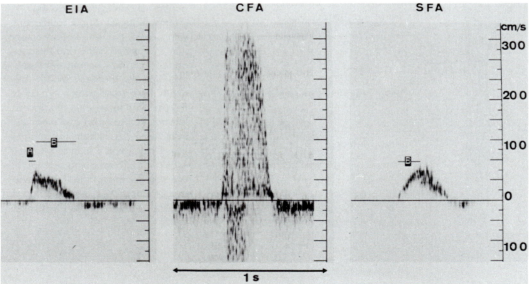

FIGURE 33.3 The waveforms just proximal to, in, and distal to a greater than 50% diameter reducing lesion are shown. The major changes relate to the marked increase in velocity in the narrowed segment (greater than three times normal) with loss of the reverse flow component and the marked spectral broadening. The waveforms just proximal and distal to the involved segment are normal in most respects. (EIA, external iliac artery; CFA, common femoral artery; SFA, superficial femoral artery) (Jager KA, Ricketts HJ, Strandness DE Jr. Duplex scanning for the evaluation of lower limb arterial disease. In Bernstein EF [ed]: Noninvasive Diagnostic Techniques in Vascular Disease, p 619. St. Louis, CV Mosby, 1985)

EVALUATION OF THE RENAL ARTERIES

The renal arteries are of greatest interest because of the association of hypertension with high-grade renal artery stenoses. The problem with the diagnostic approaches to these arteries is that short of highly selective arteriography, none of the noninvasive tests designed to uncover these lesions has been successful. Although the prevalence of hypertension is high in the United States the percentage of patients with an underlying cause due to renal artery stenosis is relatively low. In this setting the test used must have a very high specificity, that is, it must be able to distinguish the normal patient with a high degree of accuracy. False-positive tests will often lead the patient to an invasive test such as arteriography, which should be avoided if at all possible.

ROLE OF ARTERIOGRAPHY

Arteriography has remained the definitive test for the diagnosis of renal artery stenosis. There was an attempt to replace it with intravenous digital subtraction methods, but the resolution was not good enough and the dye load required to obtain adequate films was too great. The intra-arterial digital method appears to be a satisfactory compromise, but even it has some shortcomings. The best images and information are still obtained by the selective injection approach with both anteroposterior and oblique views of the renal artery ostia.

ULTRASONIC DUPLEX SCANNING

With the availability of low-frequency scanheads (2–3 MHz), it is now possible to reach the posterior aspect of the abdomen and evaluate the renal arteries. Although the imaging component of these systems has improved, it is not possible to use the ultrasonic image to make the diagnosis of renal artery atherosclerosis or estimate its significance. It is necessary to depend on the velocity changes that occur along the length of the vessel and relate them to those recorded from the adjacent aorta.

The ultrasound anatomy used to find the renal arteries is not difficult. One must first identify the left renal vein, which crosses the aorta anterior to and directly over the renal arteries. In the course of our studies my colleagues and I tested several approaches but finally determined the following criteria to make the diagnosis of renal artery stenosis:

1. The normal peak systolic velocities in the aorta and the renal arteries are in the range of 100 cm/sec (SD ± 20 cm/sec).
2. The blood flow pattern to the kidney is dominated by the low resistance nature of the organ. Like the brain and the liver there is a very high mean flow component that is characterized by a high end-diastolic flow. This is in contrast to the flow to the aorta, which should always have a reverse flow component in early diastole (Fig. 33.4).
3. Because it appears that the renin–angiotensin system is not activated until the renal artery is narrowed by more than 60%, this is the degree of narrowing that must be detected.
4. Of all the algorithms tested, the one that seems most suitable for clinical purposes is the ratio of the peak systolic velocity in the renal artery to that in the aorta (RAR ratio). When the RAR ratio exceeds 3.5, a high-grade stenosis is suggested (Fig. 33.5).
5. If the length of the kidney as measured from the flank is less than 9 cm, total occlusion of the renal artery is likely.

In the latest evaluation of these parameters, we were able to validate duplex scanning against arteriography in 58 cases.[16] From this study, we assessed the role of duplex scanning as a screening test. The method has a sensitivity of 84% and a specificity of 97%, with an overall accuracy of 93% (Fig. 33.6).

TABLE 33.2 COMPARISON OF READINGS: ULTRASONIC DUPLEX SCANNING VS. ARTERIOGRAPHY AND TWO RADIOLOGISTS READING THE SAME FILMS

Category*	Duplex vs. Arteriography	Radiologist 1 vs. Radiologist 2
Normal	81%	68%
1–19%	83%	58%
20–49%	83%	57%
50–99%	60%	70%
Occlusion	94%	100%

* Arteriography estimated by caliper measurements of single plane arteriogram.

TABLE 33.3 PREDICTIVE VALUE OF DUPLEX SCANNING COMPARED WITH ARTERIOGRAMS FOR SPECIFIC VASCULAR SEGMENTS

Artery	N	Sensitivity	Specificity	Positive Predictive Value	Negative Predictive Value
Iliac	70	81%	91%	77%	96%
Profunda femoris	47	67%	83%	57%	88%
Superficial femoral	121	84%	94%	92%	87%
Popliteal	37	75%	96%	86%	93%
All	394	81%	94%	83%	93%

The standard criteria for screening should be the guidelines for ordering this test and include the following:

1. Any young person with severe hypertension.
2. Any patient with the acute onset of hypertension for no apparent cause.
3. The finding of an upper abdominal or flank bruit in a patient with hypertension.
4. Any patient with malignant hypertension.

EVALUATION OF THE MESENTERIC ARTERIES

Although atherosclerotic involvement of the aorta is common, the development of disease in the celiac and superior mesenteric arteries is much less common. This is also reflected in the rarity of the syndrome of chronic mesenteric angina, which is characterized by the development of abdominal cramps and diarrhea after ingesting a meal. These problems become progressively more serious over time, leading to the small meal syndrome and severe weight loss.

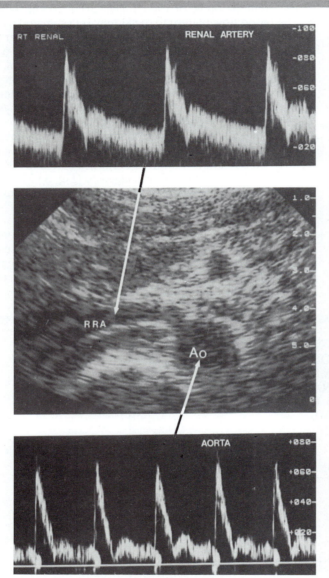

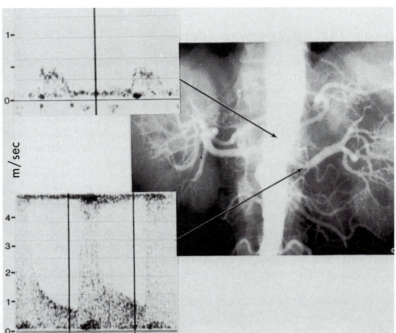

FIGURE 33.5 In the case shown the left renal artery has a very high peak systolic velocity detected in the proximal renal artery that exceeds 500 cm/sec. When compared with the adjacent aorta with a peak velocity of 50 cm/sec, the RAR ratio (see text) is greater than 10. (Taylor DC, Kettler MD, Moneta GL et al: Duplex ultrasound scanning in the diagnosis of renal artery stenosis: A prospective evaluation. J Vasc Surg 7:363, 1988)

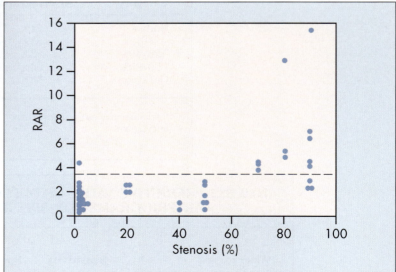

FIGURE 33.6 The relationship between the RAR ratio and the degree of narrowing as determined by arteriography is shown. See text for details. (Modified from Taylor DC, Kettler MD, Moneta GL et al: Duplex scanning in the diagnosis of renal artery stenosis: A prospective evaluation. J Vasc Surg 7:363, 1988)

For this entity to occur both the celiac and superior mesenteric arteries must be involved. It will not develop with involvement of either artery alone because of the excellent collateral circulation that exists in the area.

ROLE OF ARTERIOGRAPHY

Until recently, lateral aortography to show the origins of both the celiac and superior mesenteric arteries was necessary to confirm the diagnosis.

ULTRASONIC DUPLEX SCANNING

As these arteries are readily accessible to ultrasound, it is only natural to use ultrasonic duplex scanning to study these patients. To date we have verified the diagnosis in 5 patients, who were subsequently treated by either surgery or angioplasty.[17] In each case there have been very tight stenoses of these vessels, which made the diagnosis very easy to make. Unless we can demonstrate these changes we will not proceed with arteriography. The results in a normal subject before and after a meal are shown in Figure 33.7. The findings in a patient with high-grade stenoses in both the celiac and superior mesenteric arteries are shown in Figure 33.8.

One false-positive result occurred in a young woman who had sustained an abdominal injury. After the injury she began to develop what appeared to be the small meal syndrome and weight loss. By duplex scanning she was found to have peak systolic velocities of greater that 350 cm/sec in the proximal superior mesenteric artery. Her celiac artery was normal. Because we had no other explanation for her symptoms, we proceeded with arteriography. The test did not reveal any anatomical abnormality in the suspicious area, and we have no explanation for the finding. Anyone in whom the diagnosis of celiac and superior mesenteric artery disease is suspected should have the duplex scan performed to confirm the diagnosis.

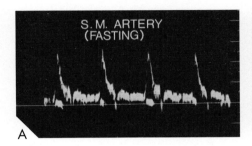
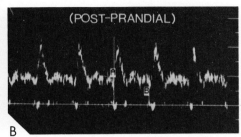

FIGURE 33.7 A. The velocity pattern recorded in the superior mesenteric artery under fasting conditions is much the same as that seen in any peripheral artery. **B.** However, after eating the resistance to flow decreases and the end-diastolic flow increases. (Nicholls SC, Kohler TR, Martin RL et al: Use of hemodynamic parameters in the diagnosis of mesenteric insufficiency. J Vasc Surg 3:507, 1986)

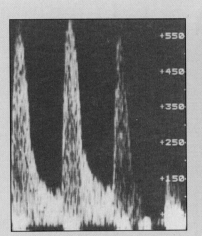
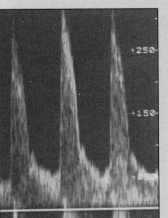

FIGURE 33.8 In the case shown the peak velocities are several times greater than those noted normally. When arteriography was done a 50% stenosis of the celiac artery and a 90% stenosis of the superior mesenteric artery were found.

REFERENCES

1. Strandness, DE Jr: Peripheral vascular disease: Diagnosis and objective evaluation using a mercury strain gauge. Ann Surg (Suppl) 161:1, 1965
2. Barber FE, Baker DW, Strandness DE Jr: Duplex Scanner II. For simultaneous imaging of artery tissues and flow. Ultrasonic Symp Proc IEEE No. 74, CHO89615V, 1974
3. Carter SA: Response of ankle systolic pressure to leg exercise in mild or questionable arterial disease. N Engl J Med 287:578, 1972
4. Strandness DE Jr: Abnormal exercise response after successful reconstructive arterial surgery. Surgery 59:325, 1966
5. Strandness DE Jr, McCutcheon EP, Rushmer RF: Application of a transcutaneous Doppler flowmeter in evaluation of occlusive arterial disease. Surg Gynecol Obstet 122:1039, 1967
6. Strandness DE Jr, Schultz RD, Sumner DS et al: Ultrasonic flow detection: A useful technique in the evaluation of peripheral vascular disease. Am J Surg 113:311, 1967
7. May AG, Van de Berg L, DeWeese JA et al: Critical arterial stenosis. Surgery 54:250, 1963
8. Carter SA, Lezak JD: Digital systolic pressures in lower limbs in arterial disease. Circulation 43:905, 1971
9. Gosling RG, Dunbar G, King DH et al: The quantitative analysis of occlusive arterial disease by a noninvasive ultrasonic technique. Angiology 22:52, 1971
10. Sumner DS, Strandness DE Jr: The relationship between calf blood flow and ankle blood pressure in patients with intermittent claudication. Surgery 65:763, 1969
11. Slot HB, Strijbosch L, Greep JM: Interobserver variability in single plane arteriography. Surgery 90:497, 1981
12. Thiele BL, Bandyk DF, Zierler RE: A systematic approach to the assessment of aortoiliac disease. Arch Surg 118:477, 1983
13. Sumner DS, Strandness DE Jr: Aortoiliac reconstruction in patients with combined iliac and superficial femoral obstruction. Surgery 82:785, 1977
14. Jager KA, Phillips DJ, Martin RL: Noninvasive mapping of lower limb arterial lesions. Ultrasound Med Biol 11:515, 1985
15. Kohler TR, Nance DR, Cramer MM et al: Duplex scanning for diagnosis of aortoiliac and femoropopliteal disease. Circulation 5:1074, 1987
16. Taylor DC, Kettler MD, Moneta GL et al: Duplex ultrasound in the diagnosis of renal artery stenosis: A prospective evaluation. J Vasc Surg 7:363, 1988
17. Nicholls AC, Kohler TR, Martin RL et al: Use of hemodynamic parameters in the diagnosis of mesenteric insufficiency. J Vasc Surg 3:507, 1986

SECTION 5

Section Editor
Kanu Chatterjee, MB, FRCP

Invasive Tests

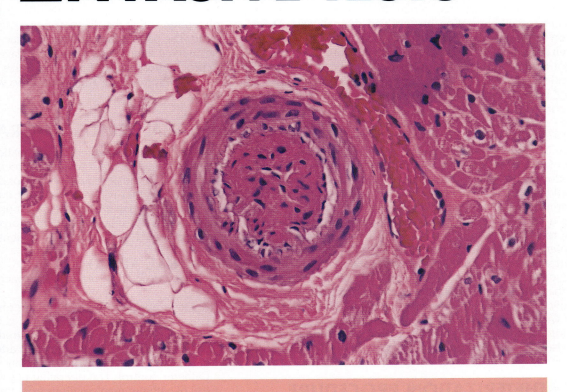

CARDIAC CATHETERIZATION
Blase A. Carabello

Human cardiac catheterization began in 1929 when Werner Forssmann, searching for a method to deliver medications rapidly, introduced a catheter into his own right atrium from an antecubital vein.[1] Since then cardiac catheterization has evolved dramatically. At first, catheterization was primarily a scientific tool used to gain insight into normal as well as pathologic physiology.[2-4] In the 1950s it evolved into a clinical tool as the primary method of establishing the severity of congenital and valvular heart disease. The advent of coronary arteriography in 1959[5] placed cardiac catheterization in a preeminent position to diagnose coronary artery disease, the full impact of which would be realized when coronary artery bypass surgery became commonplace in the early 1970s. Throughout the next decade catheterization underwent a series of technological refinements, which together with increased skill of operators led to increasing safety and diagnostic yield of the procedure. Currently, cardiac catheterization still remains the diagnostic gold standard for most cardiac lesions. Further, with the advent of percutaneous transluminal angioplasty, the catheter began evolving into a therapeutic modality, the full potential for which has still not been realized.

This chapter will acquaint the reader with the fundamentals of cardiac catheterization. It will discuss the principles of the procedure, basic hemodynamics, assessment of cardiac function, and indications and risks of the procedure. It is not the intent of this chapter to teach the reader how to perform cardiac catheterization. Rather, the chapter will focus on what information can be gained from the procedure on a lesion by lesion basis. The specific topic of coronary arteriography will be covered elsewhere in this volume.

THE CATHETERIZATION PROCEDURE
PATIENT PREPARATION

It is essential that the patient and the physician or team performing the cardiac catheterization meet to discuss the procedure prior to the actual catheterization. As the emphasis on shortening hospital stays increases, it may become general practice for patients to be admitted to the hospital on the day of the procedure. In such cases, it will be necessary for the operator to meet with the patient prior to hospital admission. During the precatheterization interview, the operator assesses what diagnostic questions need to be addressed at catheterization so that he can plan a procedure that will answer these questions. After he makes this assessment it will be possible for the physician to advise the patient about the nature of the procedure and its length, discomforts, and risks. The more the patient knows about the procedure, the more comfortable he will be with it, enhancing the ease with which the catheterization can be performed.

Two misconceptions regarding cardiac catheterization seem to be prevalent. The first concerns the route by which the procedure will be performed. Since cardiac catheterization has become commonplace, many patients are acquainted with persons who have previously had a cardiac catheterization. They may know of a friend who has had the procedure performed from the femoral approach and are surprised, confused, or upset to find that their procedure will be performed from the brachial approach or *vice versa*. It is helpful for the referring physician to advise the patient prior to his meeting with the operator that the approach chosen will be the one felt to be the best for the patient but that this decision will not be made until the operator has had a chance to interview and examine the patient. A second common misconception is that the diagnostic cardiac catheterization will be therapeutic. The patient may confuse cardiac catheterization with coronary transluminal angioplasty or he may have misunderstood the intent of the procedure. It is helpful to emphasize to the patient that the cardiac catheterization will be only diagnostic with no expectant therapeutic benefit.

BRACHIAL VERSUS FEMORAL APPROACH

A question frequently asked by both patients and physicians is which is better, the brachial approach with direct surgical exposure of the brachial vessels or the percutaneous femoral approach. The answer is that the procedure that will yield the best data at the lowest risk and discomfort to the patient should be employed. Both approaches have their inherent advantages and limitations and these should be considered with regard to the particular patient being catheterized.

BRACHIAL APPROACH
The advantages of the brachial approach are

1. Relative absence of brachial atherosclerosis. Atherosclerotic involvement of the brachial vessels is rare compared to that of the femoral and iliac vessels. It is extremely unusual to be unable to pass a catheter from the brachial artery into the central aorta because of atherosclerotic obstruction.
2. Catheter control. The operating physician generally has more control of catheter manipulations from the brachial approach than from the femoral approach.
3. Hemostasis. Since the brachial approach requires direct surgical isolation of the brachial artery and arteriotomy for catheter insertion, bleeding is controlled by arteriotomy repair instead of indirect arterial compression through the soft tissues. Patients with clotting disorders, particularly those with abnormal platelet function (*e.g.*, uremia), are best catheterized from the brachial approach. Hemostasis is generally also easier to obtain from the brachial approach in patients with aortic insufficiency, where the presence of a wide pulse pressure tends to dislodge the hemostatic plug in the femoral artery, and in obesity, where direct compression of the artery is difficult. Finally, since hemostasis is gained by direct closure of the arteriotomy, patients need not remain supine for several hours following the procedure, allowing for rapid mobilization after the catheterization is completed.

Disadvantages of the brachial approach include the following:

1. A cutdown must be performed for exposure of the artery.
2. Smaller brachial than femoral arteries, particularly in women, may lead to spasm of the artery during catheter passage, resulting in difficult manipulation, and subsequent arterial complications.
3. Difficulty may be encountered in negotiating the catheter around the shoulder into the ascending aorta, particularly in elderly or hypertensive patients in whom the great vessels tend to be tortuous.

FEMORAL APPROACH

Advantages to the percutaneous femoral approach are

1. The artery is entered percutaneously by the Seldinger technique and does not require a cutdown. Hemostasis is obtained by indirect compression of the artery and no arterial repair is required.
2. Arterial size. The femoral artery is larger than the brachial artery and thus catheter-induced femoral arterial spasm is quite rare. The femoral approach is particularly facilitatory in women and children, where the brachial artery tends to be small.

Disadvantages of the femoral approach include the following:

1. Atherosclerotic obstruction of the femoral or iliac arteries may prevent catheter passage into the descending aorta.
2. The need for prolonged bed rest (24 hr) to allow the hemostatic plug to form after the catheterization procedure increases hospital stay and patient discomfort. However, the recent introduction of small-bore (No. 5 French) catheters requires less bed rest for satisfactory hemostasis following the procedure and allows for more rapid mobilization.
3. Reliance on indirect compression of the artery for hemostasis may not be adequate in cases of extreme obesity or when the patient has a hemostatic defect.

TRANSSEPTAL APPROACH

In transseptal catheterization a catheter is introduced percutaneously into the right femoral vein and advanced to the right atrium or superior vena cava. A stiff hollow trocar with a needle tip is advanced through the catheter until the tip of the needle lies just inside of the catheter. The catheter and needle are then maneuvered into the fossa ovalis where the needle is advanced outside of the catheter and used to puncture the atrial septum. Catheter and needle are then advanced into the left atrium where the needle-tipped trocar is removed. From there the catheter can be advanced into the left ventricle. Transseptal technique is employed to

1. Enter the left ventricle antegrade when retrograde catheterization is made difficult by the presence of aortic stenosis or a prosthetic valve;
2. Obtain a direct left atrial pressure recording if doubt exists about the veracity of the pulmonary capillary wedge pressure, especially in cases of mitral stenosis where the gradient between left atrium and left ventricle is a key parameter to be derived from the procedure; or
3. Avoid catheter entrapment as a cause of a false gradient in cases of idiopathic hypertrophic subaortic stenosis.

RIGHT HEART CATHETERIZATION

During right heart catheterization a catheter is passed from the superior vena cava or inferior vena cava into the right atrium, right ventricle, pulmonary artery, and pulmonary capillary wedge positions. Pressures and oxygen saturations are obtained at each position. A right heart catheterization is also performed when it is necessary to measure cardiac output.

Right heart catheterization may be performed with a flow-directed balloon flotation catheter such as the Swan-Ganz catheter, or with a stiffer woven Dacron Cournand or Goodale-Lubin catheter. The Swan-Ganz catheter is a soft catheter with little potential for cardiac perforation. When fitted with a thermistor, the catheter may be used to obtain cardiac output by the thermodilution technique. However, in cases of extreme dilatation of the right atrium or right ventricle, or both, such as might occur in tricuspid regurgitation, it may be difficult to negotiate a balloon catheter into the pulmonary artery and pulmonary capillary wedge position. In this case, selection of a stiffer catheter offers the operator better catheter control, facilitating catheter passage.

There is debate as to whether a right heart catheterization needs to be performed in every cardiac catheterization. In common practice, in the catheterization of patients with coronary artery disease where pre-catheterization evaluation has indicated the absence of heart failure and the presence of good left ventricular function, only a left heart catheterization is performed. However, right heart catheterization should be performed whenever information regarding cardiac filling pressures and cardiac output will add to the overall picture of a patient with coronary artery disease. In cases of intracardiac shunts, valvular heart disease, and cardiomyopathy, a right heart catheterization is always performed.

LEFT HEART CATHETERIZATION

Left heart catheterization is performed to obtain aortic and left ventricular pressures, to perform left ventriculography and aortography when indicated, and to obtain coronary arteriograms. The left heart catheterization is begun by passing a ventriculographic catheter (pigtail, NIH, Eppendorf, Sones) into the aorta, where central aortic pressure is recorded. The catheter is then passed to the left ventricle, where left ventricular pressure is recorded and left ventricular end-diastolic pressure is recorded on high gain. If a right heart catheterization has been performed, simultaneous pulmonary capillary wedge pressure (or left atrial pressure) and left ventricular pressure are recorded as shown in Figure 34.1. If cardiac output is to be calculated during the procedure, it should be done during the recording of the pressure tracings so that they can be matched temporally for calculation of vascular resistance. After recording the left ventricular pressure, left ventriculography is usually performed. Following the left ventriculogram, a "pullback" pressure from left ventricle to central aorta is performed to rule out an aortic valve pressure gradient. At this time the ventriculographic catheter is exchanged for a coronary arteriographic catheter (i.e., Judkins, Amplatz, or Sones type). Following satisfactory completion of the coronary arteriograms, the catheters are removed and hemostasis is gained by femoral artery compression or brachial artery repair.

☐ DETERMINING CARDIAC OUTPUT

Although an endocrinologic function of the heart has been recently described, the heart's major function is to pump blood. The amount of blood that the heart pumps per unit of time is the cardiac output, and one would expect that there would be an accepted accurate way of calculating this simple parameter. Unfortunately, all methods of cardiac output calculation have significant limitations. The Fick method, the dye indicator method, the thermodilution method, and the angiographic method are those currently used for determining the cardiac output.

FICK METHOD

The determination of the cardiac output by the Fick method is described by the formula[6]

$$\text{Cardiac output (CO)} = \frac{O_2 \text{ consumption}}{(A\text{-}V\ O_2\Delta)}$$

where $A\text{-}V\ O_2\Delta$ = arterial–venous oxygen difference. The concept is clarified by rearranging the terms such that O_2 consumption = CO $\times$ $A\text{-}V\ O_2\Delta$. Thus, all the oxygen consumed by the body is accounted for by that which is delivered to the tissues by the heart (cardiac output) and extracted from the delivered blood ($A\text{-}V\ O_2\Delta$). By calculating oxygen consumption and A–V O_2 difference one can calculate cardiac output.

Oxygen consumption is determined by collecting the entire volume of the patient's expired air in a collection bag over a known period of time. The oxygen content in the expired air is subtracted from the oxygen content in the atmosphere and multiplied by the volume of air in the bag. Thus, one calculates how much oxygen the patient's body removed from the atmosphere and was consumed during the time of collection.

Arterial–venous oxygen difference is calculated by subtracting the oxygen content of a well-mixed venous sample (such as taken from the pulmonary artery) from the oxygen content of a blood sample taken from the systemic circulation (peripheral artery, central aorta, or left ventricle). Oxygen content is equal to the patient's hemoglobin times the carrying capacity of oxygen per gram of hemoglobin (hb) times the percent saturation (sat) of oxygen (determined by oximetry) for that sample. Arterial–venous oxygen difference is then calculated as

$$\text{A--V } O_2\Delta \text{ (ml } O_2) = \text{hb (g/dl)} \times 1.36 \text{ ml } O_2/\text{g hb}$$
$$\times \text{ (\% sat artery} - \text{\% sat mixed venous sample)} \times 10$$

The cardiac output determined by the Fick method is only as accurate as the determination of the oxygen consumption and the A–V $O_2\Delta$. Determination of the A–V $O_2\Delta$ relies on well-standardized determinations of the patient's hemoglobin and oxygen saturation and this portion of the cardiac output determination is usually accurate. However, accurate determination of oxygen consumption is dependent on fastidious collection of the patient's expired air. Any leakage of expired air into the atmosphere (via a ruptured tympanic membrane or improper seal around the mouthpiece, and so on) will result in a falsely low oxygen consumption and a falsely low cardiac output. In order to circumvent the tedious and sometimes inaccurate calculation of oxygen consumption, the normal resting oxygen consumption of 125 ml/min/m^2 has been assumed as a standard oxygen consumption. However, a recent study has shown a wide variation in normal oxygen consumption (126 ± 26 ml/min/m^2).[7] In the case of an A–V $O_2\Delta$ of 40 ml/liter, this variation in oxygen consumption would result in the cardiac index varying from 2.5 liters/min/m^2 to 3.8 liters/min/m^2, a potential 53% difference. Thus, substituting an assumed oxygen consumption for a measured one is unlikely to improve the accuracy of the cardiac output determination. Measurement of the A–V $O_2\Delta$ alone produces a good estimation of the adequacy of a patient's cardiac output without actually calculating it. If the A–V $O_2\Delta$ is normal, the implication is that the cardiac output is adequate to meet tissue oxygen demand. On the other hand, if A–V $O_2\Delta$ is increased, it implies that the tissues are forced to increase the extraction of oxygen from the hemoglobin delivered, indicating that cardiac output is inadequate regardless of whether its calculated numerical value is within the "normal" range. The Fick determination is most accurate when cardiac output is normal or reduced. At high cardiac output when A–V $O_2\Delta$ is a small number, slight changes in A–V $O_2\Delta$ produce large changes in cardiac output, reducing accuracy of the method.

INDICATOR DILUTION METHOD

The volume of a chamber of fluid could be measured by injecting a known quantity of an indicator and then measuring the concentration of the indicator once it was totally mixed in the fluid. The formula for the volume (V) would be V = I/C, where I = the amount of indicator injected in milligrams, and C = the concentration of the indicator in milligrams per liter. The milligrams cancel out, leaving the result in liters of fluid. To convert this principle to flow, the indicator is mixed in a moving fluid as a bolus and its concentration is measured over time downstream.[8] The longer it takes the bolus of indicator to pass a given point, the slower the rate of flow. Flow calculated by the indicator technique uses the formula

$$Q = \frac{I}{\int_0^\infty c(t)dt}$$

where Q = blood flow, I = the amount of indicator injected and $\int_0^\infty c(t)dt$ = integral of the area under the concentration–time curve as shown in Figure 34.2. Indocyanine green is the indicator most widely used currently. In practical use, a bolus of a known quantity of indocyanine green is injected into the pulmonary artery where it is completely mixed in the circulation. Blood is withdrawn from the arterial tree and passed through a densitometer, which records the concentration of indocyanine green. Since the concentration of the indicator

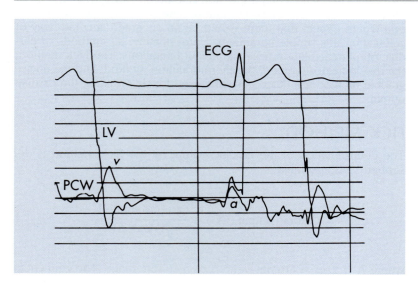

FIGURE 34.1 Normal left ventricular and pulmonary capillary wedge pressure tracings, recorded simultaneously. The v wave is recorded slightly later than it physiologically occurred because of the normal delay in pressure wave transmission (a, a wave; EKG, electrocardiogram; LV, left ventricular pressure tracings; PCW, pulmonary capillary wedge pressure tracing; v, v wave)

is identical everywhere in the arterial tree because of complete mixing, blood from any major artery can be sampled. The amount of indicator injected divided by its concentration represents the entire volume of the vasculature from the point of injection to the point of sampling. The higher the concentration produced by a known quantity injected, the less volume must be present, and the longer the time over which the bolus passes the densitometer, the slower that volume must be moving. Thus, a large concentration–time curve indicates a lower cardiac output for any given amount of indicator injected. As shown in Figure 34.3, concentration rises and then falls and then rises again as it is recirculated. In order to calculate cardiac output, one plots the linear decay of the time–concentration curve and extrapolates it to zero as shown in Figure 34.3. In most catheterization laboratories, the concentration–time plot is done with the assistance of a small computer. In patients with a low cardiac output, intercardiac shunts, or valvular regurgitation, recirculation may occur before the extrapolation of the down-slope can be made accurately. In such cases the indicator dye dilution technique cannot precisely calculate cardiac output.

THERMODILUTION METHOD

The thermodilution technique is a widely employed special modification of the dye indicator technique. It can be used during cardiac catheterization as well as in the intensive care unit setting. Typically, a Swan-Ganz catheter is fitted with a distal thermistor. A known quantity of saline of known temperature is injected proximally.[9] A microcomputer calculates the cardiac output using the formula

$$CO = \frac{V_I(T_B - T_I)}{\int_0^\infty \Delta T_B(t)dt}$$

where V_I = volume of the injectate, T_B = temperature of the blood, T_I = temperature of the injectate, and $\int_0^\infty \Delta T_B(t)dt$ = the area under the temperature–time curve in °C times seconds. The basic principle involved is that in low flow states the indicator becomes warmer than in high flow states and thus the area of the curve is larger. The thermodilution technique has an advantage over the dye indicator technique because it does not require an arterial puncture for sampling and it does not require blood withdrawal. Accurate cardiac output determination using the thermodilution technique requires that the injectate not be allowed to warm up prior to injection and that an exact amount of injectate be delivered. The thermodilution technique is inaccurate in low cardiac output states and when tricuspid regurgitation is present.

ANGIOGRAPHIC CARDIAC OUTPUT

Since cardiac output is equal to the stroke volume times the heart rate, one can calculate cardiac output using ventriculography. End-diastolic volume (EDV) and end-systolic volume (ESV) are calculated as discussed below. Cardiac output is calculated as (EDV − ESV) × heart rate.

CALCULATION OF SYSTEMIC AND PULMONARY RESISTANCE

Ohm's Law as it applies to the heart is

$$P = Q \times R$$

where P = pressure, Q = blood flow, and R = resistance. Total systemic or total pulmonary resistance cannot be measured directly, but rather is calculated as pressure divided by flow, R = P/Q. Most of the

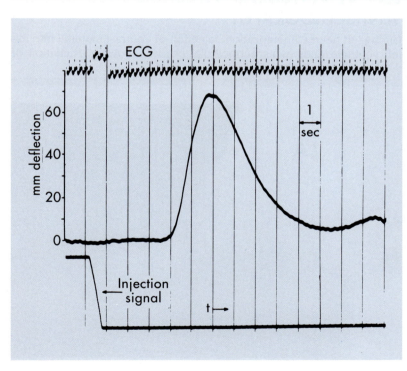

FIGURE 34.2 A dye dilution curve recorded after injection of indocyanine green. The larger the area under the curve, the smaller is the cardiac output for any given amount of dye indicator injected. (ECG, electrocardiogram; t, time) (Reproduced by permission from Milnor WR: The heart as a pump. In Mountcastle VB (ed): Medical Physiology, 14th ed. St. Louis, CV Mosby, 1980)

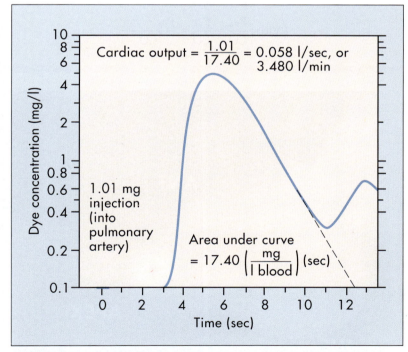

FIGURE 34.3 Calculation of cardiac output using the indicator dilution method. The dashed line indicates extrapolation of the down-slope of the concentration–time curve at the point of recirculation. (Modified from Milnor WR: The heart as a pump. In Mountcastle VB (ed): Medical Physiology, 14th ed. St. Louis, CV Mosby, 1980)

resistance to flow is offered by the blood vessels. Poiseuille, in 1842, devised a series of empiric formulas describing flow through rigid glass tubes. He derived the formula

$$Q = \frac{\pi(P_i - P_o)r^4}{8nl}$$

where Q = the volume of flow, $P_i - P_o$ = inflow pressure minus outflow pressure, r = radius of the tube, l = length of the tube, and n = viscosity of the fluid. Since $R = \frac{P_i - P_o}{Q}$, $R = \frac{8nl}{\pi r^4}$. This equation emphasized that the radius of the vessel is the key determinant of resistance since resistance varies inversely with the *fourth* power of the radius.

PULMONARY VASCULAR RESISTANCE

The heart may be viewed as two pumps (right and left ventricles) operating in series. The right ventricle must generate enough pressure to move blood through the resistance offered by the pulmonary artery as well as the resistance produced by the filling of the left ventricle (left ventricular filling pressure or left atrial pressure). In most clinical applications, it is the specific resistance offered by the pulmonary vasculature (pulmonary vascular resistance) that is useful in patient care. For example, by being able to calculate the pulmonary vascular resistance, the effect of a given medication in changing this resistance could be evaluated. In calculating pulmonary vascular resistance, the resistance offered by the left ventricle–left atrium complex must be subtracted from the total pulmonary resistance. The formula for pulmonary vascular resistance (PVR) is

$$PVR = \frac{P_{PA}}{CO} - \frac{P_{LA}}{CO} = \frac{P_{PA} - P_{LA}}{CO}$$

where P_{PA} = mean pulmonary artery pressure and P_{LA} = mean left atrial (or pulmonary capillary wedge) pressure. Resistance is expressed either in simple units (Woods units) or is converted to metric resistance units using the following formula:

$$R = \frac{\Delta P}{Q} \frac{(mm\ Hg) \times 1332\ dynes/cm^2/mm\ Hg}{liters/min \times 1000\ ml/liter \div 60\ sec}$$

$$= \frac{\Delta P}{Q} \times 80,\ expressed\ as\ dynes - sec - cm^{-5}$$

SYSTEMIC VASCULAR RESISTANCE

The left ventricular pump, in order to propel the blood to the next pump (right ventricle), must overcome the resistance offered by the systemic vasculature and the resistance offered by the filling of the right ventricle (right ventricular filling pressure or right atrial pressure). Thus, systemic vascular resistance is calculated as

$$\frac{\overline{A_oP} - \overline{RAP}}{CO}$$

where $\overline{A_oP}$ = mean arterial pressure and $\overline{RAP}$ = mean right atrial pressure. Evaluation of systemic vascular resistance is helpful in assessing the success of vasodilator therapy for heart failure or hypertension.

LEFT VENTRICULOGRAPHY, AUGMENTATION VENTRICULOGRAPHY, AORTOGRAPHY, AND CALCULATION OF LEFT VENTRICULAR VOLUMES AND MASS

VENTRICULOGRAPHY

During left heart catheterization, injection of contrast material into the left ventricle outlines its endocardial border, allowing evaluation of

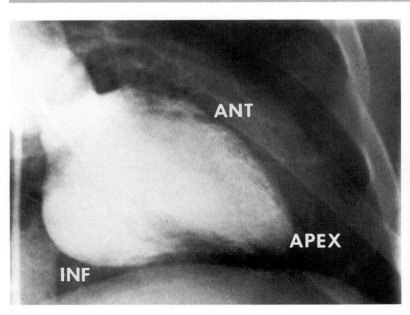

FIGURE 34.4 A 30° right anterior oblique (RAO) projection of the end-diastolic frame of a left ventriculogram. Anterior (*ANT*), apical (*APEX*), and inferior (*INF*) segments of the left ventricle are demonstrated in this view.

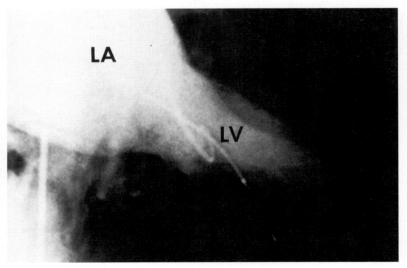

FIGURE 34.5 The right anterior oblique projection of the end-systolic frame of a left ventriculogram from a patient with severe mitral regurgitation demonstrates an enlarged, densely opacified left atrium (*LA*). (*LV,* left ventricle)

regional and global cardiac motion. Single plane left ventriculography is usually performed in 30° right anterior oblique projection. As shown in Figure 34.4, anterior, apical, and inferior regions of the left ventricle are seen in this view. Mitral regurgitation, if present, is best evaluated in the right anterior oblique position (Fig. 34.5). When biplane left ventriculography is performed, the 60° left anterior oblique projection is filmed simultaneously with the 30° right anterior oblique view. As shown in Figure 34.6, this allows for the additional evaluation of the left ventricular posterior wall and septum.

LEFT VENTRICULAR VOLUMES AND MASS

The left ventricle has the shape of a prolate ellipse. The formula for volume of a prolate ellipse is $V = 4/3\pi \times L/2 \times M/2 \times N/2$, where L is the long axis of the ellipse, and M and N are the two minor axes of the ellipse. As shown in Figure 34.7, in single plane ventriculography, M and N are considered to be equal and are expressed as the minor axis or diameter of the heart, D. Thus $V = 4/3\pi \times L/2(D/2)^2$. The minor axis of the heart (D) is equal to $4A/\pi L$, where A = area planimetered around the endocardial edge of the chamber. Substituting $4A/\pi L$ for D derives the formula

$$V = \frac{4}{3}\pi \cdot \frac{L}{2}\left(\frac{4A}{\pi L}/2\right)^2$$

which is simplified to the formula $V = 0.85A^2/L$.[10] Since the angiographic equipment (image intensifier, projector, and so on) magnifies the real image of the heart, this magnification correction factor must be calculated and applied to each axis. The magnification correction factor is derived by positioning a grid of known size at the level of the patient's heart and then obtaining the x-ray image of the grid. The correction factor (CF) is

$$CF = \sqrt{\frac{\text{known actual area}}{\text{planimetered area}}}$$

When biplane cineangiography is used to obtain the ventriculogram, the following formula is used to calculate volumes:

$$V = \frac{8}{3}\pi \frac{A_{RAO} \cdot A_{LAO}}{L\ min} \cdot CF_{RAO} \cdot CF_{LAO} \cdot CF_{min}$$

where A_{RAO} = planimetered area in the RAO projection, A_{LAO} = area from the LAO projection, L min = long axis from the view with the shorter long axis (usually the LAO), and CF = angiographic correction factor.[11]

A high correlation exists between angiographically calculated volumes and actual volumes obtained from ventricular casts. However, angiographic volumes usually overestimate true volumes (after correction for magnification). A number of regression equations derived by plotting known volume against calculated volume have been developed to correct this overestimation.[12-14]

As can be seen in Figure 34.7, myocardial thickness can often be assessed during left ventriculography. It is measured as the distance from the air–soft tissue border (epicardial border) to the soft tissue–contrast border (endocardial border) in diastole along the mid anterior wall. This measurement is multiplied by the angiographic correction factor. By knowing the thickness, the volume of the chamber can be subtracted from the volume of the myocardium to obtain left ventricular mass using the following formula:

$$Mass = \left[\left(\frac{4}{3}\pi \cdot \frac{L + 2h}{2}\left(\frac{m + 2h}{2}\right)^2\right) - V\right]1.05$$

where L = ventricular long axis, m = minor axis, h = wall thickness, and v = ventricular volume.[15]

AUGMENTATION VENTRICULOGRAPHY

Dyssynergy frequently accompanies coronary artery disease. A frequent question of important clinical significance is whether contractile

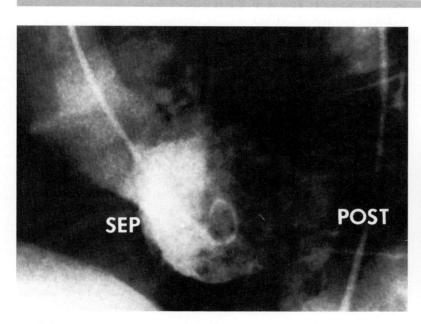

FIGURE 34.6 The end-systolic frame from a 60° left anterior oblique (LAO) projection of a left ventriculogram demonstrates the septal (SEP) and posterior (POST) segments of the left ventricle.

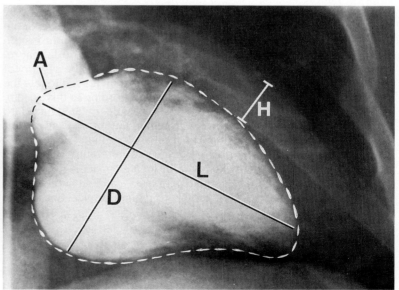

FIGURE 34.7 An RAO projection of an end-diastolic frame from a left ventriculogram. The minor axis (D, substituted for axes M and N) and the long axis (L) from the aortic valve to the apex are diagrammed. The area used to calculate left ventricular volume (A) is shown in dashed lines. Left ventricular wall thickness is measured along the anterior border of the heart (H).

function of a dyssynergic ventricular segment will improve if the segment is revascularized. Although one cannot usually expect an improvement in ventricular function after bypass grafting or angioplasty, several studies indicate that contractile function occasionally increases in hypokinetic or akinetic segments after revascularization.[16-18] The question about which segments will improve and therefore benefit from revascularization can be addressed using augmentation ventriculography. The premise of augmentation ventriculography is that scar tissue and nonviable areas of the ventricle cannot be made to contract under any circumstances, whereas noncontractile but potentially viable segments can be induced to contract with the augmentation maneuver. The two commonly used methods of augmentation are administration of nitroglycerin and induction of a premature ventricular contraction.

Administration of sublingual nitroglycerin reduces ventricular volume and systolic pressure, the key determinants of ventricular afterload. Nitroglycerin may also improve myocardial perfusion. Thus, nitroglycerin probably produces augmentation of ventricular shortening by reducing afterload or potentially by reducing ischemia, thereby increasing contractile function. Substantiation for the use of nitroglycerin for augmentation was provided by Helfant and co-workers, who found a good correlation between segments that augmented with nitroglycerin preoperatively and those that improved following bypass surgery.[19]

During augmentation ventriculography with a premature ventricular contraction, catheter manipulation is used to cause the extrasystolic beat. The post-premature beat is augmented by post extrasystolic potentiation. The augmentation in ventricular contractility that occurs in a post-premature beat is probably due to increased calcium release or decreased calcium uptake as well as the Frank-Starling principle. Cohn and associates demonstrated that patients with a low ejection fraction who augmented their ejection fraction by more than 0.1 ejection fraction units had a significantly better prognosis at surgery.[20] Thus, augmentation ventriculography may be a useful adjunct in helping to make the decision of whether a bypass graft (or transluminal angioplasty) is likely to improve contractile function of a given ventricular segment.

AORTOGRAPHY

Aortography is employed during cardiac catheterization to evaluate suspected aortic insufficiency, to identify the false lumen in aortic dissection, or to reveal the presence of a patent ductus arteriosus. It may also be used to identify the ostia of coronary artery bypass grafts or the site of a coarctation of the aorta. In the evaluation of aortic insufficiency, the relative amount of contrast injected into the aorta that returns to the left ventricle in diastole is used to evaluate the severity of the lesion. Conventionally, a qualitative rating system is used to rate the amount of regurgitation on a 1+ to 4+ scale. According to this system, 1+ indicates that only a trace amount of dye has regurgitated back into the ventricle; 2+ indicates that enough regurgitation has occurred to fully opacify the left ventricle but to a lesser extent than the aorta; 3+ indicates equal opacification of the aorta and left ventricle; and 4+ indicates severe aortic regurgitation with greater opacification of the left ventricle than the aorta. Generally, grades 3+ and 4+ indicate that the aortic insufficiency is severe enough to require surgical correction.

EVALUATION OF CARDIAC FUNCTION

The amount of cardiac dysfunction produced by a given cardiac lesion is a key determinant of prognosis. Thus, during cardiac catheterization it is not adequate merely to identify and evaluate the severity of a lesion, but it is also necessary to evaluate the amount of cardiac dysfunction caused by the lesion since this information will be used to evaluate prognosis and the likely response to surgery. The following is a summary of the various indices of contractile and pump function currently used to make this assessment.

INDICES OF CONTRACTILE FUNCTION
EJECTION FRACTION

Contractile function is defined as the force-generating capacity of the myocardium at a given preload. Currently, the most commonly employed index of contractile function is the ejection fraction. Conceptually, ejection fraction is the percentage of the diastolic volume of the ventricle expelled during systole. Ejection fraction is described by the formula

$$\frac{EDV - ESV}{EDV}$$

where EDV = end-diastolic volume and ESV = end-systolic volume. Ejection fraction has gained popularity because it has accurately predicted surgical outcome[21,22] and because it is easy to obtain both invasively and noninvasively. At catheterization left ventricular ejection fraction is obtained by calculating volumes of the left ventricle at end-diastole and end-systole using the formula described above.

Ejection fraction is particularly useful in describing the contractile performance of patients with coronary disease and cardiomyopathy.[21,22] Unfortunately, ejection fraction is affected not only by contractile state but also by preload and afterload.[23,24] In patients with valvular or congenital heart disease where preload and afterload may be greatly altered by the lesion present, ejection fraction may either seriously overestimate or underestimate contractile function. In mitral regurgitation, for instance, preload is greatly increased by the volume overload of the lesion itself. Afterload may be normal or reduced.[25] These loading conditions increase ejection fraction, and thus ejection fraction may be normal even when significant contractile dysfunction exists.[26] In aortic stenosis, on the other hand, increased afterload may be present, which reduces ejection fraction even though contractile function may be relatively normal.[27]

MEAN VELOCITY OF CIRCUMFERENTIAL FIBER SHORTENING

Mean velocity of circumferential fiber shortening (VcF) describes the rate and extent of shortening. It is the shortening fraction divided by ejection time and is described by the formula

$$VcF = \frac{EDD - ESD}{EDD \times ET}$$

where EDD = end-diastolic minor axis, ESD = end-systolic minor axis, and ET = ejection time. VcF has the advantage over ejection fraction of being relatively insensitive to changes in preload.[28] However, VcF is still sensitive to changes in afterload, and thus may also fail to describe contractile function accurately if the cardiac lesion has altered afterload significantly.

AFTERLOAD CORRECTED EJECTION PHASE INDICES

By plotting ejection fraction or VcF against afterload, one can correct them for the afterload present, thus factoring out afterload to yield a better descriptor of contractile function. Many studies have demonstrated a strong inverse linear correlation between afterload and ejection fraction or VcF as shown in Figure 34.8.[27] The ventricle of a patient whose ejection performance and afterload fall downward and to the left of this normal relationship demonstrates less shortening for any given load, suggesting impaired contractile function. One falling above and to the right of the relationship shows enhanced shortening for any given load, suggesting increased inotropic state.

END-SYSTOLIC INDICES OF VENTRICULAR FUNCTION

Because ejection phase indices are altered by loading conditions, an interest has developed in using the more load-independent end-systolic indices to examine contractile function. The cornerstone of the end-systolic indices of ventricular function rests on the fact that end-systolic volume is independent of preload, as shown in Figure 34.9.[29] Since end-systolic volume is preload independent, it is not surprising that the end-systolic volume index has been shown to be useful in predicting outcome in diseases such as valvular regurgitation where preload is increased.[30] Although end-systolic volume is not affected by changes in preload, it varies nearly linearly with afterload, as shown in Figure 34.10.[29,31] By altering load, one can develop this relationship, the slope of which is an indicator of contractile function. As shown in Figure 34.11, the slope of the end-systolic afterload–end-systolic volume relationship steepened when isoproterenol, a positive inotropic stimulus, was infused into the bath supporting an isolated canine ventricle. The steepening of the slope occurs because the ventricle now contracts to a smaller volume against the same load, indicating increased inotropic state. Figure 34.12 demonstrates a similar relationship obtained from two different loading conditions in humans in the catheterization laboratory.[32] In this example, patients with cardiomyopathy had a flatter slope than normal subjects properly indicating the reduced inotropic state in congestive cardiomyopathy.

In deriving the end-systolic relationship, afterload must be quantified. Afterload has usually been expressed as end-systolic pressure or end-systolic wall stress. End-systolic stress has an advantage over end-systolic pressure as an expression of afterload because it accounts for the radius and thickness over which the pressure is distributed. Stress is described by the Laplace relationship

$$\text{Stress} = \frac{P \cdot r}{2h}$$

where P = pressure, r = ventricular radius, and h = wall thickness. This relationship calculates that a pressure of 100 mm Hg in a ventricle with

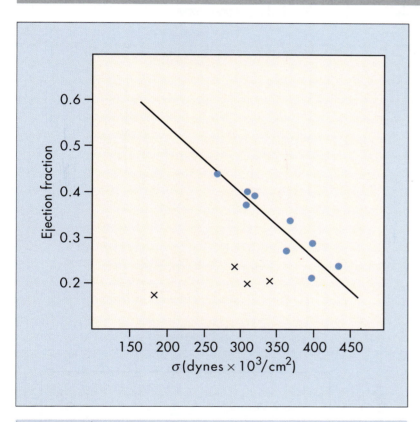

FIGURE 34.8 Ejection fraction and wall stress (σ) are plotted in patients with severe aortic stenosis. The linear inverse correlation between ejection fraction and wall stress in patients with a good surgical outcome (*solid circles*) suggests that the existing reduction in ejection performance was due to the presence of increased afterload. On the other hand, patients with a poor surgical outcome (×) had lower ejection performance for any given afterload, suggesting an intrinsic contractile deficit.

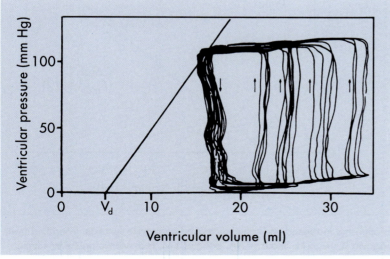

FIGURE 34.9 Pressure–volume loops from an isolated beating canine left ventricle. End-systolic volume is constant despite large variations in end-diastolic volume. Thus, end-systolic volume is shown to be independent of preload. (Suga H, Sagawa K, Shoukas AA: Load independence of the instantaneous pressure–volume ratio of the canine left ventricle and effects of epinephrine and heart rate on the ratio. Circ Res 32:314, 1973. Reproduced by permission of the American Heart Association, Inc.)

a 2-cm end-systolic radius and a 1-cm end-systolic thickness would represent twice the afterload (expressed as stress) as the same pressure in a ventricle with a 2-cm radius and a 2-cm end-systolic thickness. Mirsky and others have refined this relationship as it relates to the prolate ellipsoid of the human left ventricle.[33] Mirsky's formula for wall stress is

$$\text{Stress} = \frac{P \cdot b}{h}\left(1 - \frac{h}{2b} - \frac{b^2}{2a^2}\right) \times 1332 \text{ dynes/cm}^2/\text{mm Hg}$$

where P = pressure, b = ventricular semi–minor axis $\left(\frac{D + h}{2}\right)$ and a = semi–major axis $\left(\frac{L + h}{2}\right)$.

Thus, in developing the end-systolic relationship, end-systolic stress can be substituted for end-systolic pressure. Stress is usually used in place of pressure in conditions where eccentric or concentric left ventricular hypertrophy causes systolic pressure to be a poor estimator of afterload.

Currently, derivation of the slope of the end-systolic afterload–volume relationship is probably the most reliable load-independent method for evaluating acute changes in contractile function. However, in the catheterization laboratory the need to perform ventriculography at several different loading conditions to establish the end-systolic afterload–end-systolic volume relationship is cumbersome, and in ill patients potentially dangerous. The advent of digital subtraction angiography, which may permit ventriculography using small quantities of contrast, should facilitate obtaining the relationship.

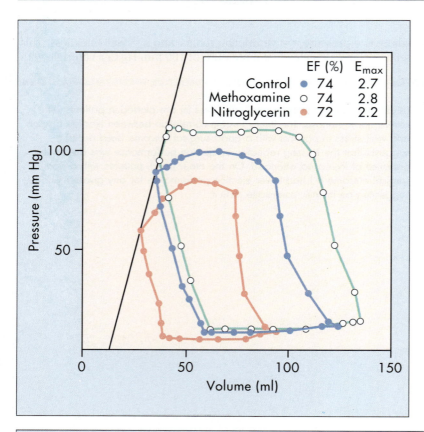

FIGURE 34.10 Pressure and volume were plotted at different afterloads (pressure). End-systolic volume increased linearly with end-systolic pressure. The slope of the line described by this relationship is an indicator of contractile function. (Modified from Nivatpumin T, Katz S, Scheuer J: Peak left ventricular systolic pressure/end-systolic volume ratio: Sensitive detector of left ventricular disease. Am J Cardiol 43:969, 1979)

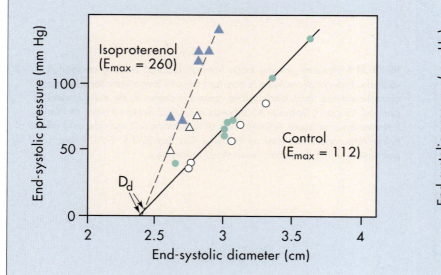 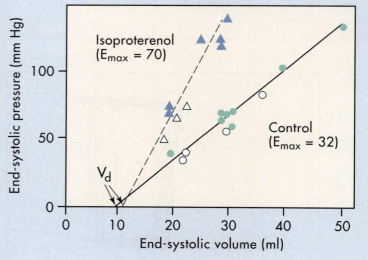

FIGURE 34.11 Pressure–volume relationship of an isolated contracting canine ventricle is shown at different inotropic states. During isoproterenol infusion (*dashed line*) the slope of the pressure–volume or pressure–diameter relationship increased, indicating increased contractile function. (Modified from Sagawa K, Suga H, Shoukas AA, Bakalar KM: End-systolic pressure/volume ratio: A new index of ventricular contractility. Am J Cardiol 40:748, 1977)

A potential limitation of the end-systolic relationship exists in eccentric hypertrophy states. When eccentric hypertrophy such as occurs in volume overload develops, it increases end-systolic volume. Thus, in eccentric hypertrophy states, end-systolic volume could be increased either because sarcomeres have failed to shorten properly against the load (reduced inotropic state) or end-systolic volume could be increased because of the addition of normally contracting sarcomeres in series (eccentric hypertrophy). In the latter case, the increase in end-systolic volume will reduce the slope of the stress–volume relationship even though inotropic state is not impaired. Ways to correct for this situation are currently under investigation.

Other limitations of the end-systolic afterload–volume relationship have recently been defined. The relationship is not entirely linear and the degree of nonlinearity may vary with inotropic state. The relationship appears to become concave at higher inotropic states and may become convex at severely reduced inotropic states.[34] Thus, the search for applicable, accurate clinical measures of contractile function will continue. Other measures currently under investigation include recruitable stroke work[35] and end-systolic stiffness.[36]

INDICES OF PUMP FUNCTION

Indices of pump function describe the heart's ability to deliver cardiac output. Although changes in contractile function may be mirrored by changes in pump function, these two types of indicators of cardiac performance can be quite discordant. For instance, in acute mitral regurgitation the contractile function of the muscle of the left ventricle is normal or supernormal secondary to sympathetic stimulation. However, regurgitation of a substantial part of the left ventricular output into the left atrium may reduce cardiac output substantially below normal.[37] In this example, an index of contractile function may indicate normal muscle function, yet pump function is reduced. On the other hand, in a case of dilated cardiomyopathy, where the end-diastolic volume has increased to 400 ml and the ejection fraction is 20%, the stroke volume would be 80 ml. The index of contractile performance (ejection fraction) is extremely reduced, yet the indicator of pump function—the stroke volume—is normal. In this example, cardiac dilatation has allowed pump function to remain adequate, at least at rest, while contractile function is severely compromised.

STROKE WORK INDEX

Stroke work is the area under the pressure–volume curve as shown in Figure 34.13. Work = F × d, where F = force and d = distance. Pressure = F/A, where F = force and A = area over which the force is applied. Thus, P × A = F. By multiplying both sides of the equation by distance (d), one obtains the formula P × A × d = F × d (work). An area multiplied by another dimension (in this case, distance) yields a volume. Thus, stroke work equals pressure times volume. While stroke work could be derived by planimetering the area under the pressure–volume curve, it is more conventionally calculated as stroke volume × developed left ventricular pressure:

$$SW = SV(LVSP - LVEDP) \times 0.0136 \text{ g-m/mm Hg}$$

where SW = stroke work, SV = stroke volume, LVSP = left ventricular peak systolic pressure, and LVEDP = left ventricular end-diastolic pressure. Stroke work index is obtained by dividing by body surface area.

CARDIAC FUNCTION CURVES

By plotting an index of pump performance such as cardiac output or stroke work index against a parameter of filling such as left ventricular end-diastolic pressure or end-diastolic volume, one can assess pump performance in relation to cardiac filling. The rationale behind developing this relationship is that not only must the heart produce an adequate cardiac output or stroke work, it must do it at a filling pressure or

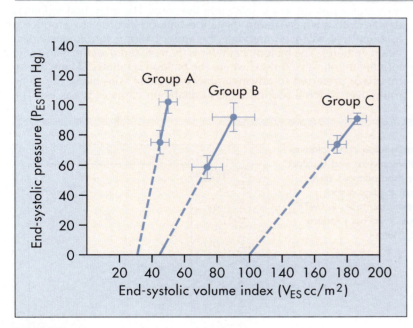

FIGURE 34.12 The end-systolic pressure–end-systolic volume index relationship for patients with normal ejection fraction (Group A), moderate reductions in ejection fraction (0.41–0.59, Group B), and more severe left ventricular dysfunction (ejection fraction < 0.4, Group C). The slope of the pressure–volume relationship is less in the two groups with left ventricular dysfunction, indicating reduced shortening for any given afterload. (Modified from Grossman W, Braunwald E, Mann T et al: Contractile state of the left ventricle in man as evaluated from end-systolic pressure-volume relations. Circulation 56:845, 1977)

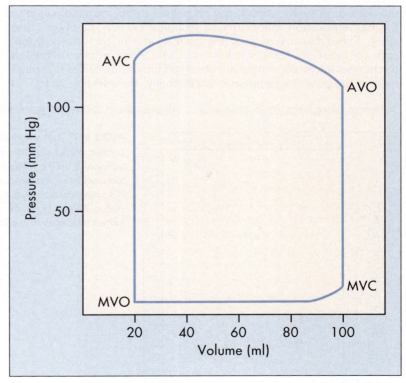

FIGURE 34.13 The area under this pressure–volume loop is the stroke work done by the ventricle during the beat. (MVO, mitral valve opening; MVC, mitral valve closure; AVO, aortic valve opening; AVC, aortic valve closure)

filling volume at which the patient does not experience symptoms of congestive failure. A plot of cardiac output against left ventricular end-diastolic pressure is shown in Figure 34.14. Note that although a normal cardiac output is maintained, a high left ventricular end-diastolic pressure of 25 mm Hg is required to produce this normal output, indicating cardiac dysfunction. At lower end-diastolic pressures, the cardiac output is subnormal. The relationship between cardiac output and filling pressure examines overall cardiac function but does not give insight into inotropic state. Left ventricular end-diastolic pressure could be high because preload is high (suggesting reliance on increased preload) or because cardiac compliance is low. In a noncompliant heart such as is seen in valvular aortic stenosis, a high filling pressure might actually be coincident with subnormal preload (reduced fiber stretch).[38] A low cardiac output could be due to reduced inotropic state, reduced preload, or increased afterload. Thus, a curve such as displayed in Figure 34.14 is useful in describing whether cardiac function is improving or worsening for a given patient, but the mechanisms responsible cannot be dissected. In Figure 34.15, stroke work index is plotted against end-diastolic volume. Since stroke work index incorporates afterload (expressed as pressure) into its expression, and end-diastolic volume more nearly represents preload than end-diastolic pressure, this curve is more indicative of contractile state than the one shown in Figure 34.14. However, in cases of volume or pressure overload where either eccentric or concentric left ventricular hypertrophy is present, the ventricular function curve again does not allow one to ascertain whether changes in contractile state, afterload, or preload have resulted in any abnormalities present. Eccentric hypertrophy will cause an increase in end-diastolic volume independent of changes in preload, making end-diastolic volume a poor indicator of preload. Concentric hypertrophy, as noted above, makes pressure an inadequate indicator of load on a given muscle fiber. Thus, the stroke work index–end-diastolic volume curve cannot adequately account for changes in preload or afterload under these circumstances.

PUMP FUNCTION DURING EXERCISE

If a patient referred for evaluation of symptoms of congestive heart failure has normal cardiac pump function and filling pressure at rest, a hemodynamic explanation for the patient's symptoms has not been uncovered. In such cases, it may be helpful to exercise the patient in the catheterization laboratory to examine cardiac function under stress. Either dynamic or isometric exercise may be preformed. During dynamic exercise, changes in left ventricular filling pressure in relation to changes in cardiac output are observed for abnormalities that might explain the patient's symptoms. Additionally, the exercise factor can be calculated. The exercise factor is the relationship between the increase in cardiac output and the increase in oxygen consumption that occur during exercise. In normal subjects the cardiac output increases approximately 600 ml/min for every 100 ml/min increase in oxygen consumption.[39] By measuring oxygen consumption during rest and exercise and by measuring cardiac output during rest and exercise, one can calculate this exercise factor. Failure of the cardiac output to increase adequately in relationship to oxygen consumption indicates impaired cardiac function under stress.

Isometric exercise is usually performed by hand grip. It produces an increase in afterload by causing an increase in aortic pressure as well as an increase in cardiac output usually produced by an increase in heart rate. By measuring left ventricular filling pressure (PCW), cardiac output, and aortic pressure during isometric exercise, one can plot stroke work against filling pressure at rest and with exercise. Examples of normal and abnormal relationships obtained in this fashion are demonstrated in Figure 34.16.

ADVANCEMENT OF THE CATHETER AS A DIAGNOSTIC AND THERAPEUTIC TOOL

In addition to its use in routine diagnostic cardiac catheterization, the catheter has assumed an increasingly diverse role as a diagnostic and therapeutic tool. Additional uses are listed in Table 34.1.

Most recently, following the reports of successful balloon valvuloplasty in children,[48,49] there has been an explosion of reports of successful balloon valvuloplasty for aortic and mitral stenosis in adults. Discussed briefly below, a more detailed description is presented in Chapter 85.

MITRAL VALVULOPLASTY

As depicted in Figure 34.17, mitral valvuloplasty is performed following percutaneous transseptal catheterization. After standard transseptal catheterization, a guide wire is advanced across the interatrial septum and then across the mitral valve with the aid of a flow-directed balloon catheter. The wire is further advanced into the aortic outflow tract and across the aortic valve into the aorta. The interatrial septum is dilated with a small 10-mm dilatation balloon in order to produce a foramen that will accommodate the larger balloon valvuloplasty dilatation catheter. The balloon catheter is then passed over the guide wire into the mitral valve orifice, where the balloon is inflated. Many operators have preferred to advance a second guide wire along the same route over which a second balloon dilatation catheter is passed. The

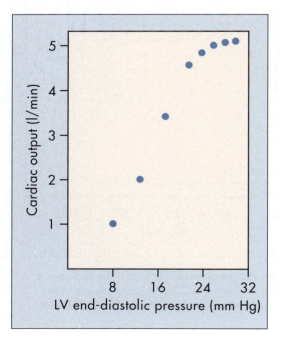

FIGURE 34.14 Left ventricular function curve plotting cardiac output against left ventricular end-diastolic pressure (LVEDP). A higher than normal LVEDP is required to maintain normal cardiac output, indicating cardiac dysfunction. Increases in LVEDP above 22 mm Hg in this case did not produce further increases in cardiac output.

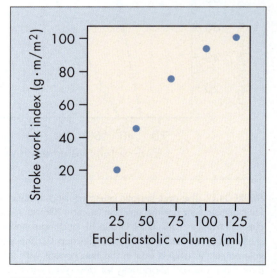

FIGURE 34.15 Ventricular function curve plotting stroke work index against end-diastolic volume.

two balloons are then inflated simultaneously in the mitral valve orifice. Clinical and postmortem studies suggest that mitral valvuloplasty causes increased mitral valve leaflet mobility by separation of the leaflets along the natural planes of the commissures.[50,51] Thus, mitral valvuloplasty done percutaneously produces similar mechanical effects to that which occurs in surgical commissurotomy. Both invasive and noninvasive studies indicate this procedure results in a greater than twofold increase in mitral valve area.[50-52] The development or worsening of mitral regurgitation following balloon valvuloplasty is usually mild. In a representative study of balloon mitral valvuloplasty, left atrial pressure fell from 27 ± 2 mm Hg to 14 ± 1 mm Hg. At the same time, cardiac output increased from 3.9 ± 0.2 liters/min to 4.6 ± 0.2 liters/min.[52]

Complications from this procedure include mild worsening of mitral regurgitation, perforation of the left ventricle by the dilating balloon with subsequent tamponade, new atrial septal defect, and transient or complete heart block. Thromboembolic complications can also occur. However, as with most new procedures, the incidence of complications will probably decrease as further investigation improves catheterization techniques.

From this early experience, it appears that percutaneous mitral valvuloplasty might be as effective as surgical commissurotomy in the relief of mitral stenosis. Long-term follow-up studies will of course be necessary to judge the procedure's ultimate benefits and risks.

AORTIC VALVULOPLASTY

As shown in Figure 34.18, aortic valvuloplasty is performed by percutaneous retrograde catheterization of the left ventricle. A standard end-hole catheter is negotiated across the stenotic valve through which a guide wire is passed and the catheter is then removed. The valvuloplasty catheter is inserted over the guide wire through a large femoral sheath into the aortic valve orifice. The balloon is then inflated to perform the valvular dilation. During inflation there is usually enough flow around the balloon to maintain a modest but adequate peripheral blood pressure of 50 mm Hg to 60 mm Hg.

Pathologic studies suggest that unlike mitral valvuloplasty, aortic valvuloplasty produces dilatation by stretching of the valve leaflets or by fracturing of the calcium nodules in the aortic valve.[53] Because the calcium is endothelialized, its embolic potential is small. Indeed, the risk of thromboembolic disease following aortic valvuloplasty is probably less than 1%. Even in the cases of reported thromboembolism, the embolus is probably due to the atheromatous material scraped from the aorta rather than particles embolized from the valve itself.

The results of aortic valvuloplasty have been less encouraging than those from mitral valvuloplasty. The average orifice area has increased from approximately 0.5 cm² to 0.9 cm², with a reduction in aortic valve gradient of approximately 50%.[53-55] In patients with reduced ejection fraction prior to the procedure, there have been some improvements in ejection performance. The incidence of recurrence in aortic stenosis following valvuloplasty is not certain but may be as high as 50% in 6 months.

The mortality associated with this procedure is approximately 2%. Complications include vascular trauma at the site of catheter insertion, ventricular perforation and tamponade, myocardial infarction, and cerebrovascular accident.

Aortic valvuloplasty in its current stage of development appears to be primarily a palliative procedure suitable for those patients who cannot tolerate surgical aortic valve replacement.

INDICATIONS, TIMING, AND EXPECTATIONS OF CARDIAC CATHETERIZATION

The two general broad indications for cardiac catheterization are (1) to establish a specific cardiac diagnosis and (2) to perform a complete cardiac evaluation prior to cardiac surgery. In many cases it may be necessary to establish a diagnosis even when surgery is not contemplated. For instance, in the patient with atypical chest pain who has a nondiagnostic exercise test, it is important for the patient and his physician to know whether or not he has heart disease, which in turn will be useful in prescribing a rational therapeutic plan for the patient. In the patient whose history, physical examination, and noninvasive data suggest that cardiac surgery may be indicated, the catheterization can further establish cardiac anatomy and physiology to help assess whether surgery will be beneficial and, in some cases, what type of surgery is required. The following is a summary of the data provided by cardiac catheterization for cardiac lesions encountered in the adult patient.

VALVULAR DISEASE
AORTIC STENOSIS

The natural history of aortic stenosis is well known. When patients develop angina, syncope, or symptoms of congestive heart failure, life span is substantially shortened unless the mechanical obstruction to aortic outflow is relieved.[56] Thus, the onset of symptoms together with

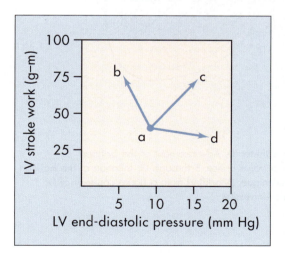

FIGURE 34.16 Changes in left ventricular stroke work and end-diastolic pressure following hand-grip exercise. The response a–b is normal, suggesting that contractile function has increased during hand-grip exercise because stroke work has increased despite a fall in preload suggested by the fall in end-diastolic pressure. The abnormal response a–c demonstrates the ability to increase the stroke work by using preload reserve, indicating a contractile deficit forced the patient to rely on increasing preload rather than contractile reserve to produce the increase in stroke work. The response a–d indicates severe left ventricular dysfunction. In this case the increased afterload produced a fall in stroke work index that could not be overcome by maximum use of preload reserve and any additional contractile reserve. (Modified from Lorell BH, Grossman W: Dynamic and isometric exercise during cardiac catheterization. In Grossman W (ed): Cardiac Catheterization and Angiography, 3rd ed. Philadelphia, Lea & Febiger, 1986)

TABLE 34.1 NEWER USES FOR THE CARDIAC CATHETER

Electrophysiologic testing and stimulation
Ablation of preexcitation pathways, and arrhythmogenic foci[40,41]
Cardiac biopsy[42]
Coronary angioplasty[43]
Coronary thrombolysis[44]
Valvuloplasty[45]
Septostomy[46]
Pulmonary embolectomy[47]

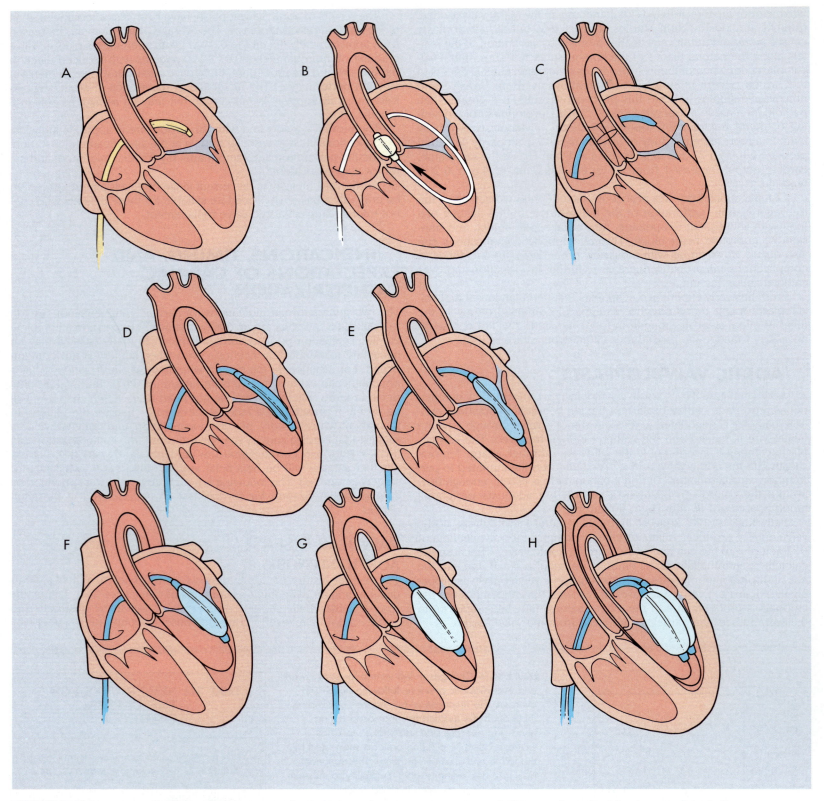

FIGURE 34.17 The sequence of events occurring in a mitral valvuloplasty. **A.** Transseptal interatrial puncture. **B.** Advancement of a flow-directed balloon-tipped catheter and guide wire across the septum through the mitral valve into the aortic outflow tract and aortic arch. **C.** Insertion of the small interatrial septal dilating catheter. **D.** Advancement of the balloon valvuloplasty into the mitral valve orifice. **E** through **G.** Inflation of the balloon. **H.** The double balloon technique. (Modified from a figure courtesy of Dr. J. Patrick Kleaveland, Temple University)

a physical examination and noninvasive studies that are concordant with the diagnosis of significant aortic stenosis are indications for cardiac catheterization prior to aortic valve replacement. During the cardiac catheterization, accurate determination of the pressure gradient across the aortic valve (Fig. 34.19) together with a simultaneous determination of cardiac output is performed so that the aortic valve area can be calculated by the Gorlin formula:[57]

$$AVA = \frac{CO/SEP \cdot HR}{K44.3\sqrt{G}}$$

where CO = cardiac output, SEP = systolic ejection period, HR = heart rate, and G = mean valvular pressure gradient. Valve areas of less than 0.7 cm^2 indicate critical aortic stenosis requiring aortic valve replacement. It should be noted that discrepancies between actual valve areas and those calculated by the Gorlin formula have been emphasized recently.[58,59] These discrepancies relate primarily to the constant in the equation. They are important clinically in that they can cause misjudgment about the severity of aortic stenosis in low output states where a severely reduced aortic valve area is calculated, but only mild aortic stenosis is actually present.

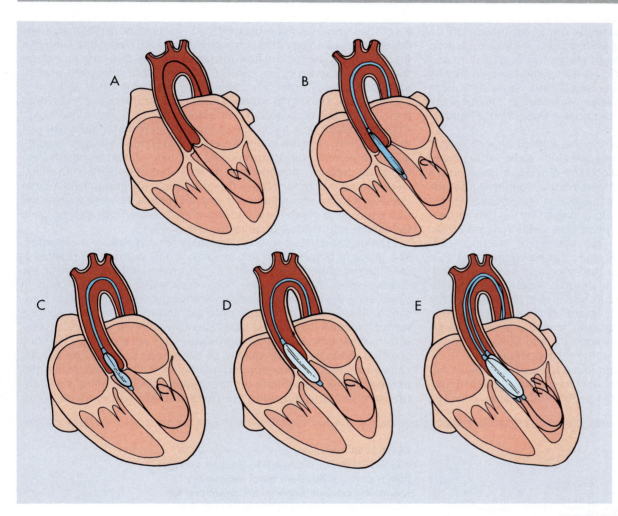

FIGURE 34.18 Aortic valvuloplasty. **A.** The guide wire has been placed in the left ventricle via retrograde aortic valve catheterization. **B.** Advancement of the balloon valvuloplasty catheter over the wire into the aortic valve. **C** and **D.** Inflation of the balloon. **E.** The double-valve technique in aortic valvuloplasty. (Modified from a figure courtesy of Dr. J. Patrick Kleaveland, Temple University)

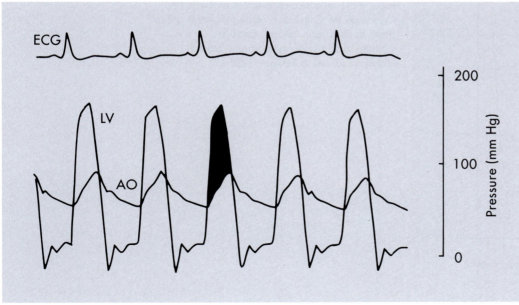

FIGURE 34.19 Pressure tracings from a patient with severe aortic stenosis are shown. The gradient between left ventricle (*LV*) and aorta (*AO*) is shown in black. (*EKG*, electrocardiogram) (Hershman MV, Cohn PF, Gorlin R: Resistance to blood flow by stenotic valves. In Grossman W (ed): Cardiac Catheterization and Angiography, 2nd ed. Philadelphia, Lea & Febiger, 1980)

Since there is significant discordance between the presence and absence of angina and the presence and absence of coronary artery disease, coronary arteriography should generally be performed in patients with aortic stenosis. In patients with hemodynamic evidence of congestive heart failure at the time of cardiac catheterization, ventriculography need not be performed since ventricular performance data can be obtained noninvasively. Furthermore, most patients with aortic stenosis who have a reduced preoperative ejection fraction have improvement in ejection performance postoperatively. Thus, a subnormal ejection fraction usually does not indicate a poor outcome of surgery.[27]

AORTIC REGURGITATION

The proper timing of aortic valve replacement for aortic regurgitation, and thus the need for cardiac catheterization, is controversial.[60] In general, I would recommend cardiac catheterization for patients who have developed even mild symptoms of congestive heart failure and who have evidence of early left ventricular dysfunction as indicated by noninvasive techniques that show an enlarged end-systolic dimension or volume. During cardiac catheterization intracardiac pressures are obtained. Cardiac output should be performed using the thermodilution or Fick techniques.

Aortography is performed to examine the amount of aortic regurgitation qualitatively. The amount of regurgitation can be further quantified by calculating regurgitant fraction. The difference between angiographic end-diastolic volume and end-systolic volume equals the angiographic stroke volume, which is the total stroke volume ejected from the left ventricle. The cardiac output derived by the Fick or thermodilution methods divided by the heart rate yields forward stroke volume "seen" by the periphery. The regurgitant fraction (ASV − FSV)/ASV, where ASV = angiographic stroke volume and FSV = forward stroke volume, quantitates the amount of volume regurgitated back into the left ventricle during diastole. Regurgitant fractions of <40% indicate that the aortic regurgitation is mild to moderate, not usually requiring aortic valve replacement. A regurgitant fraction > 60% indicates severe aortic regurgitation requiring aortic valve replacement. Regurgitant fractions between 40% and 60% represent a middle ground of moderately severe aortic regurgitation.

End-systolic volume index has been found to be prognostic of outcome in this disease and should be obtained from the ventriculogram.[30] Increasing end-systolic volume probably indicates increased left ventricular dysfunction. In the past decade improvements in surgical technique have permitted patients to have a good response to aortic valve replacement in spite of relatively poorer ventricular function. Thus, the "cut-off" for end-systolic volume index consistent with good surgical results has increased from 60 cc/m^2 [30] to approximately 100 cc/m^2.[61,62]

MITRAL STENOSIS

Patients with late New York Heart Association Class II or more severe symptoms due to mitral stenosis are candidates for surgery when the mitral valve area is <1.2 cm^2. Since the development of pulmonary hypertension increases operative mortality rate, timing of surgery should be prior to the onset of severe pulmonary hypertension. However, if surgery has been delayed until pulmonary hypertension has developed, pulmonary artery pressure usually falls following surgery if the patient can be successfully managed through the early perioperative period. Whether or not cardiac catheterization is required prior to mitral valve replacement or mitral valve repair for mitral stenosis is controversial. Modern two-dimensional echocardiographic techniques permit accurate visualization and assessment of mitral valve area.[63] Current Doppler flow techniques permit an accurate estimation of pulmonary artery pressure in the presence of even mild tricuspid regurgitation. In general, most cardiologists feel that cardiac catheterization including coronary arteriography is indicated in patients with mitral stenosis in the coronary artery disease–prone age group. Evidence of coexistent mitral regurgitation on physical examination or a suspicion of the presence of other cardiac abnormalities also indicates the need for cardiac catheterization prior to surgery.

During catheterization the pulmonary artery pressure is recorded. The gradient between the left atrium and left ventricle in diastole is carefully measured (Fig. 34.20) at the time of measurement of the cardiac output. Although some controversy exists about the validity of substituting the pulmonary capillary wedge pressure for left atrial pressure in this disease, a carefully obtained and oximetrically confirmed wedge pressure is recorded simultaneously with left ventricular pressure in most laboratories to approximate left atrial pressure.[64] If any question exists as to the validity of the wedge pressure, transseptal catheterization can be performed to obtain left atrial pressure in order to measure the transmitral pressure gradient directly. Mitral valve orifice area is calculated using the Gorlin formula as described above

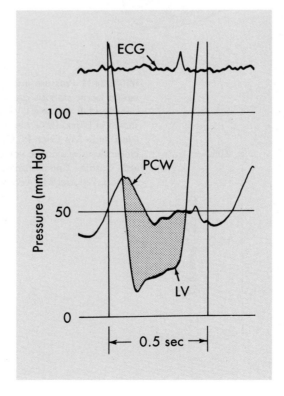

FIGURE 34.20 Pulmonary capillary wedge (PCW) and left ventricular diastolic (LV) pressure tracings from a patient with severe mitral stenosis are shown. The gradient between left atrium and left ventricle in diastole is depicted by the stippled area. (ECG, electrocardiogram) (Carabello BA, Grossman W: Calculation of stenotic valve orifice area. In Grossman W (ed): Cardiac Catheterization and Angiography, 3rd ed. Philadelphia, Lea & Febiger, 1986)

under Aortic Stenosis. In mitral stenosis the diastolic filling period is substituted for the systolic ejection period and the empiric constant of 0.85 instead of 1.0 is used. Left ventriculography should be performed to detect mitral regurgitation, which might be present, since the presence of mitral regurgitation may alter the surgical choice of whether to repair or replace the mitral valve. Coronary arteriography is usually performed in the coronary-prone age group. Since mitral stenosis can cause underestimation of the severity of coexistent aortic regurgitation, aortography should be performed in most cases of mitral stenosis where physical examination and noninvasive studies have demonstrated the presence of aortic insufficiency.[65]

MITRAL REGURGITATION

In mitral regurgitation, the presence of reduced or normal afterload and increased preload causes ejection phase indices of contractile function to overestimate left ventricular performance. By the time patients become even mildly symptomatic from chronic mitral regurgitation, significant left ventricular dysfunction may be present.[26] If valve replacement or repair is delayed further, there is likely to be substantial persistent postoperative fall in left ventricular performance. Thus, cardiac catheterization is indicated prior to surgery in chronic mitral regurgitation when patients first become symptomatic. During cardiac catheterization, pulmonary artery pressure and pulmonary capillary wedge pressure are obtained. An enlarged v wave (2 to 3 times the mean wedge pressure) in the pulmonary capillary wedge pressure tracing helps to confirm that severe mitral regurgitation is present. However, the correlation of the size of the v wave with the amount of mitral regurgitation is inconsistent and cannot be relied upon to indicate severity of the lesion. Left ventriculography gives a qualitative estimation of the amount of mitral regurgitation present using the same grading scale as described under aortography for aortic regurgitation. Regurgitant fraction can be calculated as it is for aortic regurgitation to help quantify the severity of the lesion. End-systolic volume index and the ratio of end-systolic stress to end-systolic volume index have been useful in assessing outcome for mitral valve replacement and can be obtained during cardiac catheterization.[26,30,61] Recent reports indicate that mitral valve repair offers a distinct advantage over mitral valve replacement by helping to preserve left ventricular performance postoperatively.[66] Thus, development of techniques at catheterization to help the surgeon decide whether repair is possible or whether replacement will be necessary may become an important part of catheterization for this lesion.

TRICUSPID REGURGITATION

Cardiac catheterization is limited in ability to assess the severity of tricuspid regurgitation. A catheter crossing the tricuspid valve to perform right ventriculography in order to estimate tricuspid regurgitation causes tricuspid incompetence by itself. Thus, right ventricular angiography has not been used extensively to estimate the amount of tricuspid regurgitation. Simultaneous recordings of the right atrial and right ventricular pressure tracings can demonstrate the amount of "ventricularization" of the right atrial pressure tracing. A giant v wave in the right atrial pressure tracing indicates that severe tricuspid regurgitation is present but does not help to quantify severity of the lesion.

MYOCARDIAL AND PERICARDIAL DISEASE
DILATED CONGESTIVE CARDIOMYOPATHY

Catheterization in dilated congestive cardiomyopathy is usually performed in younger patients with the disease to ensure that no other correctable lesion is present. Current noninvasive techniques are usually adequate to rule out concealed aortic or mitral regurgitation that could present as dilated cardiomyopathy. However, with the increasing use of cardiac transplantation to treat end-stage cardiomyopathy, catheterization is usually performed in order to be certain that transplantation is indicated. During cardiac catheterization, pulmonary artery pressure must be obtained to ensure that severe pulmonary artery hypertension does not exist since it can preclude cardiac transplantation. If severe pulmonary hypertension is present but reversible with vasodilators, it increases the likelihood that the patient could undergo a successful cardiac transplantation. The potential for mitral and aortic valve gradients is assessed and ventriculography is performed. Once it is clear that no other cardiac lesion exists, acute interventions with vasodilator therapy to assess its effect on cardiac output and filling pressures may be useful in directing the patient's medical management.

IDIOPATHIC HYPERTROPHIC SUBAORTIC STENOSIS

The diagnosis of idiopathic hypertrophic subaortic stenosis (IHSS) is primarily made echocardiographically. Unlike valvular aortic stenosis where the amount of obstruction determines the outcome of the disease, outcome in IHSS is not related directly to the gradient.[67] Only when medical therapy has failed to control symptoms is myomectomy indicated. Thus, cardiac catheterization is reserved for those patients in whom either a poor echocardiographic window prohibits noninvasive detection of IHSS or those who have failed medical therapy. During cardiac catheterization, the gradient between the left ventricle and the aorta is recorded at rest and during maneuvers known to increase the gradient. Recording of the gradient during the Valsalva maneuver, during amyl nitrite inhalation, and following a premature ventricular contraction is performed. Following a premature ventricular contraction in IHSS one expects a fall in the aortic pulse pressure because of the increased obstruction that occurs after post-extrasystolic potentiation (Brockenbrough's sign). The aortic pressure trace is recorded and examined for the presence of the typical "spike and dome" pattern. As in aortic stenosis, there is no concordance between the presence of chest pain and the presence of coronary disease; thus, coronary arteriography is usually performed. Left ventriculography is usually indicated. If left ventriculography demonstrates severe coexistent mitral regurgitation, mitral valve replacement instead of myomectomy may be indicated to ablate the outflow gradient.

CONSTRICTIVE PERICARDITIS AND RESTRICTIVE CARDIOMYOPATHY

The presence of biventricular failure with right-sided failure out of proportion to left-sided failure together with noninvasive studies that show good systolic ventricular function but no regurgitant valvular lesions suggests the presence of restrictive cardiomyopathy or constrictive pericarditis. Since constrictive pericarditis is a treatable disease, such patients are candidates for cardiac catheterization and surgery. During cardiac catheterization, one tries to establish the hallmark of constrictive pericarditis, the equalization of all diastolic pressures. Right ventricular and left ventricular diastolic pressure tracings are recorded simultaneously. In constrictive pericarditis, left and right ventricular diastolic pressure tracings are superimposable and show a characteristic dip and plateau. The right atrial pressure tracing typically shows a steep y descent in constrictive pericarditis. Unfortunately, if the restriction present in restrictive cardiomyopathy affects the right and left ventricles to a similar degree, it may mimic constrictive pericarditis. At the end of the catheterization it may be impossible for the operator to say with certainty which lesion is present. In such cases ventricular biopsy or a limited thoracotomy to examine the pericardium is generally indicated.

CONGENITAL HEART DISEASE IN THE ADULT
ATRIAL SEPTAL DEFECT

Because an atrial septal defect (ASD) with a greater than 2-to-1 left-to-right shunt may lead to the development of pulmonary hypertension or to the worsening of the shunt as left ventricular compliance is reduced with age, correction of large ASDs is currently recommended even in asymptomatic patients. Whether catheterization is indicated in patients with ASD is controversial. Noninvasive techniques can generally establish that an ASD is present and can determine with relative accuracy the size of the shunt. If there is suspicion of an ostium primum ASD, catheterization should be performed to assess the mitral valve and the amount of mitral regurgitation, which is usually present. When catheterization is performed for ASD, it is usually performed from the femoral vein approach, which facilitates crossing the atrial septal defect so that left atrial pressure and pulmonary vein oxygen saturations can be measured directly. During catheterization, left and right atrial pressures should be obtained. Oxygen saturations are obtained from the superior vena cava, the inferior vena cava, the right atrium, the right ventricle, pulmonary artery, pulmonary veins, and aorta. A step-up in oxygen saturation at the level of the right atrium indicates the presence of the left-to-right shunt. The ratio of pulmonic flow to systemic flow is calculated using the formula

$$\frac{PV\ sat - [(3\ SVC\ sat + IVC\ sat)/4]}{PV\ sat - PA\ sat}$$

where SVC = superior vena cava, IVC = inferior vena cava, PV = pulmonary vein, and PA = pulmonary artery.[68] If a pulmonary vein saturation is not obtained because of failure to cross the defect, aortic saturation is substituted for pulmonary vein saturation. Pulmonary artery pressure is also obtained and, if elevated, the ratio of pulmonary vascular resistance to systemic vascular resistance is calculated. If this ratio is greater than 0.7, it is likely that severe pulmonary vascular changes have occurred and correction of the ASD will not yield clinical improvement.

VENTRICULAR SEPTAL DEFECT

Usually, a large ventricular septal defect (VSD) is detected and corrected in childhood because of the loud murmur present. Failure to correct VSDs in childhood often leads to severe pulmonary hypertension by adulthood. During catheterization of a patient with a suspected VSD, pressures and oxygen saturations are obtained as in ASD. An oxygen saturation step-up at the level of the right ventricle confirms the presence of the VSD and the quantification of the left-to-right shunt is performed as with an ASD. Left ventriculography in the left anterior oblique view demonstrates radiographic contrast crossing the VSD.

PATENT DUCTUS ARTERIOSUS

As with ASD and VSD, the noninvasive suggestion that a patent ductus arteriosus (PDA) is present is an indication for cardiac catheterization to assess the magnitude of the shunt. A left-to-right shunt of a magnitude greater than 2 to 1 should be surgically corrected. During cardiac catheterization, pressures and oximetry are performed. An oxygen saturation "step-up" in the left pulmonary artery confirms the presence of a PDA. Aortography performed in a steep left anterior oblique position will demonstrate the presence of a PDA. Frequently during a right heart catheterization, the catheter will inadvertently enter the PDA and cross into the aorta, confirming the presence of the shunt.

COARCTATION OF THE AORTA

When hypertension together with the absence of peripheral pulses suggests that coarctation of the aorta is present, cardiac catheterization prior to correction of the coarctation is indicated. During cardiac catheterization the gradient across the coarctation is measured. Angiographic demonstration of the coarctation is provided by aortography.

RISKS AND CONTRAINDICATIONS

The risks of cardiac catheterization include death, myocardial infarction, stroke, perforation of the great vessels, dye reactions, vagal reactions, arrhythmias, and local arterial complications. A recent report from the Registry of the Society for Cardiac Angiography found an incidence of death of 0.14% out of 53,581 cases.[69] The reported incidence of myocardial infarction ranges from 0.07% to 2.6%. Cerebral vascular complications occurred in 0.2% of the patients in the cooperative study. However, these figures represent the statistics from a large pool of patients with varying degrees of risk. The risks in any particular patient depend on the experience of the operator and the severity of the disease process involved. Thus, patients with severe aortic stenosis and heart failure are at much higher risk than the patient who is ultimately found to have a normal cardiovascular system.

Local complications of catheter insertion have been estimated by the Registry report at 0.56%. From the brachial approach, local arterial thrombus is the major complication. This problem can usually be corrected by Fogerty catheterization and repair of the vessel. From the femoral approach, distal thrombosis or embolism, false aneurysm, and hematoma are the major problems encountered. The incidence of perforation of the heart or great vessels was reported in the Registry study to be 0.8%. However, 30 of the 100 perforations reported were secondary to transseptal catheterization. The next most frequent site of perforation is the right heart during right heart catheterization. Right heart perforation is extremely unusual when a Swan-Ganz catheter is used. However, in situations requiring the stiffer Cournand-type catheter the incidence of perforation is increased.

The only total contraindication to the procedure is refusal of the patient to undergo it. However, severe congestive heart failure, fever, coagulopathy, digitalis intoxication, electrolyte abnormalities, and renal dysfunction are relative contraindications to the procedure. If it is possible to reverse or lessen these contraindications, it should be done prior to catheterization.

REFERENCES

1. Forssmann W: Die Sondierung des rechten Herzens. Klin Wochenschr 8:2085, 1929
2. Cournand AF, Ranges HS: Catheterization of the right auricle in man. Proc Soc Exp Biol Med 46:462, 1941
3. Richards DW: Cardiac output by the catheterization technique in various clinical conditions. Fed Proc 4:215, 1945
4. Dexter L, Haynes FW, Burwell CS et al: Studies of congenital heart disease. II. The pressure and oxygen content of blood in the right auricle, right ventricle, and pulmonary artery in control patients, with observations on the oxygen saturation and source of pulmonary "capillary" blood. J Clin Invest 26:554, 1947
5. Sones FM Jr, Shirey EK, Proudfit WL, Westcott RN: Cine coronary arteriography. Circulation 20:773, 1959
6. Fick A: Über die Messung des Blutquantums in den Herzventrikeln, p 16. Sitz der Physik-Med ges Wurtzberg, 1870
7. Dehmer GJ, Firth BG, Hillis LD: Oxygen consumption in adult patients during cardiac catheterization. Clin Cardiol 5:436, 1982
8. Guyton AC, Jones CE, Coleman TG: Circulatory Physiology: Cardiac Output and Its Regulation, 2nd ed, pp 4–80. Philadelphia, WB Saunders, 1973
9. Forrester JS, Ganz W, Diamond G et al: Thermodilution cardiac output determination with a single flow-directed catheter. Am Heart J 83:306, 1972
10. Sandler H, Dodge HT: The use of single plane angiocardiograms for the calculation of left ventricular volume in man. Am Heart J 75:325, 1968
11. Dodge HT, Sandler H, Ballew DW, Lord JD Jr: The use of biplane angiocardiography for the measurement of left ventricular volume in man. Am Heart J 60:762, 1960
12. Wynne J, Green LH, Mann T et al: Estimation of left ventricular volumes in man from biplane cineangiograms filmed in oblique projections. Am J Cardiol 41:726, 1978
13. Graham TP Jr, Jarmakani JM, Canent RV Jr, Morrow MN: Left heart volume estimation in infancy and childhood. Reevaluation of methodology and normal values. Circulation 43:895, 1971
14. Kennedy JW, Baxley WA, Figley MM et al: Quantitative angiocardiography. I. The normal left ventricle in man. Circulation 34:272, 1966
15. Rackley CE, Dodge HT, Coble YD Jr, Hay RE: A method for determining left ventricular mass in man. Circulation 29:666, 1964
16. Kleinman LH, Hill RC, Chitwood WR Jr et al: Regional myocardial dimensions following coronary artery bypass grafting in patients. Relationship of functional deterioration to graft occlusion. J Thorac Cardiovasc Surg 77:13, 1979
17. Sesto M, Schwarz F: Regional myocardial function at rest and after rapid ventricular pacing in patients after myocardial revascularization by coronary bypass graft or collateral vessels. Am J Cardiol 43:920, 1979
18. Wolf NM, Kreulen TH, Bove AA et al: Left ventricular function following coronary bypass surgery. Circulation 58:63, 1978
19. Helfant RH, Pine R, Meister SG et al: Nitroglycerin to unmask reversible asynergy. Correlation with post coronary bypass ventriculography. Circulation 50:108, 1974
20. Cohn PF, Gorlin R, Herman MV et al: Relation between contractile reserve and prognosis in patients with coronary artery disease and a depressed

ejection fraction. Circulation 51:414, 1975
21. Cohn PF, Gorlin R, Cohn LH, Collins JJ: Left ventricular ejection fraction as a prognostic guide in surgical treatment of coronary and valvular heart disease. Am J Cardiol 34:136, 1974
22. Singh R, Green W, McGuire LB: Left ventricular ejection fraction and results of cardiac surgery. Cardiology 59:342, 1974
23. Mahler F, Ross J Jr, O'Rourke RA: Effects of changes in preload, afterload and inotropic state on ejection and isovolumic phase measures of contractility in the conscious dog. Am J Cardiol 35:626, 1975
24. Quinones MA, Gaasch WH, Alexander JK: Influence of acute changes in preload, afterload, contractile state and heart rate on ejection and isovolumic indices of myocardial contractility in man. Circulation 53:293, 1976
25. Wisenbaugh T, Spann JF, Carabello BA: Differences in myocardial performance and load between patients with similar amounts of chronic aortic versus chronic mitral regurgitation. J Am Coll Cardiol 3:916, 1984
26. Carabello BA, Nolan SP, McGuire LB: Assessment of preoperative left ventricular function in patients with mitral regurgitation: Value of the end-systolic wall stress–end-systolic volume ratio. Circulation 64:1212, 1981
27. Carabello BA, Green LH, Grossman W et al: Hemodynamic determinants of prognosis of aortic valve replacement in critical aortic stenosis and advanced congestive heart failure. Circulation 62:42, 1980
28. Nixon JV, Murray RG, Leonard PD et al: Effect of large variations in preload on left ventricular performance characteristics in normal subjects. Circulation 65:698, 1982
29. Suga H, Sagawa K, Shoukas AA: Load independence of the instantaneous pressure-volume ratio of the canine left ventricle and effect of epinephrine and heart rate on the ratio. Circ Res 32:314, 1973
30. Borow KM, Green LH, Mann T et al: End-systolic volume as a predictor of postoperative left ventricular performance in volume overload from valvular regurgitation. Am J Med 68:655, 1980
31. Weber KT, Janicki JS, Hefner LL: Left ventricular force-length relations of isovolumic and ejecting contractions. Am J Physiol 231:333, 1976
32. Grossman W, Braunwald E, Mann T et al: Contractile state of the left ventricle in man as evaluated from end-systolic pressure-volume relations. Circulation 56:845, 1977
33. Mirsky I: Left ventricular stress in the intact human heart. Biophys J 9:189, 1969
34. Kass DA, Beyar R, Lankford E, Heard M, Maughan WL, Sagawa K: Influence of contractile state on curvilinearity of in situ end-systolic pressure–volume relations. Circulation 79:167, 1989
35. Glower DD, Spratt JA, Snow ND et al: Linearity of the Frank-Starling relationship in the intact heart: The concept of preload recruitable stroke work. Circulation 71:994, 1985
36. Mirsky I, Tajimi T, Peterson KL: The development of the entire end-systolic pressure–volume and ejection fraction–afterload relations: A new concept of systolic myocardial stiffness. Circulation 76:343, 1987
37. Carabello BA, Grossman W: Effect of acute and chronic mitral regurgitation of left ventricular mechanics and contractile muscle function. In Duran C, Angell WW, Johnson AD, Oury JH (eds): Recent Progress in Mitral Valve Disease, pp 181–190. London, Butterworths, 1984
38. Gaasch WH, Battle WE, Oboler AA et al: Left ventricular stress and compliance in man: With special reference to normalized ventricular function curves. Circulation 45:746, 1972
39. Dexter L, Whittenberger JL, Haynes FW et al: Effects of exercise on circulatory dynamics of normal individuals. J Appl Physiol 3:439, 1951
40. Scheinman MM, Evans-Bell T: Catheter ablation of the atrioventricular junction: A report of the percutaneous mapping and ablation registry. Circulation 70:1024, 1984
41. Hartzler GO: Electrode catheter ablation of refractory focal ventricular tachycardia. J Am Coll Cardiol 2:1107, 1983
42. Mason JW: Technique for right and left ventricular endomyocardial biopsy. Am J Cardiol 41:887, 1978
43. Simpson JB, Baim DS, Robert EW, Harrison DC: A new catheter system for coronary angioplasty. Am J Cardiol 49:1216, 1982
44. Reduto LA, Smalling RW, Freund GC, Gould KL: Intracoronary infusion of streptokinase in patients with acute myocardial infarction: Effects of reperfusion on left ventricular performance. Am J Cardiol 48:403, 1981
45. McKay RG, Safian RD, Lock JE et al: Balloon dilatation of calcific aortic stenosis in elderly patients: Postmortem, intraoperative, and percutaneous valvuloplasty studies. Circulation 74:119, 1986
46. Rashkind WJ: Transcatheter treatment of congenital heart disease. Circulation 67:711, 1983
47. Scoggins WG, Greenfield LJ: Transvenous pulmonary embolectomy for acute massive pulmonary embolism. Chest 71:213, 1977
48. Lock JE, Castaneda-Zuniga WR, Buhrman BP, Bass JL: Balloon dilation angioplasty of hypoplastic and stenotic pulmonary arteries. Circulation 67:962, 1983
49. Kan JS, White RI Jr, Mitchell SE, Gardner TJ: Percutaneous balloon valvuloplasty: A new method for treating congenital pulmonary valve stenosis. N Engl J Med 307:540, 1982
50. McKay RG, Lock JE, Safian RD et al: Balloon dilatation of mitral stenosis in adult patients: Postmortem and percutaneous mitral valvuloplasty studies. J Am Coll Cardiol 9:723, 1987
51. Reid CL, McKay CR, Chandraratna PAN et al: Mechanisms of increase in mitral valve area and influence of anatomic features in double-balloon, catheter balloon valvuloplasty in adults with rheumatic mitral stenosis: A Doppler and two-dimensional echocardiographic study. Circulation 76:628, 1987
52. Palacios I, Block PC, Brandi S et al: Percutaneous balloon valvotomy for patients with severe mitral stenosis. Circulation 75:778, 1987
53. McKay RG, Safian RD, Lock JE et al: Balloon dilatation of calcific aortic stenosis in elderly patients: Postmortem, intraoperative, and percutaneous valvuloplasty studies. Circulation 74:119, 1986
54. Cribier A, Savin T, Berland J et al: Percutaneous transluminal balloon valvuloplasty of adult aortic stenosis: Report of 92 cases. J Am Coll Cardiol 9:381, 1987
55. Isner JM, Salem DN, Desnoyers MR et al: Treatment of calcific aortic stenosis by balloon valvuloplasty. Am J Cardiol 59:313, 1987
56. Rapaport E: Natural history of aortic and mitral valve disease. Am J Cardiol 35:221, 1975
57. Gorlin R, Gorlin G: Hydraulic formula for calculation of area of stenotic mitral valve, other cardiac values and central circulatory shunts. Am Heart J 41:1, 1951
58. Cannon SR, Richards KL, Crawford M: Hydraulic estimation of stenotic orifice area: A correction of the Gorlin formula. Circulation 71:1170, 1985
59. Carabello BA: Advances in hemodynamic assessment of stenotic cardiac valves. J Am Coll Cardiol 10:912, 1987
60. Bonow RO, Picone AL, McIntosh CL et al: Survival and functional results after valve replacement for aortic regurgitation from 1976 to 1983: Impact of preoperative left ventricular function. Circulation 72:1244, 1985
61. Carabello BA, Williams H, Gash AK: Hemodynamic predictors of outcome in patients undergoing valve replacement. Circulation 74:1309, 1986
62. Carabello BA, Usher BW, Hendrix GH, Assey ME, Crawford FA, Leman RB: Predictors of outcome in patients with aortic regurgitation and left ventricular dysfunction: A change in the measuring stick. J Am Coll Cardiol 10:991, 1987
63. Martin RP, Rakowski H, Kleiman JH: Reliability and reproducibility of two dimensional echocardiographic measurement of the stenotic mitral valve orifice area. Am J Cardiol 43:560, 1979
64. Alpert JS: The lessons of history as reflected in the pulmonary capillary wedge pressure (Editorial). J Am Coll Cardiol 13:830, 1989
65. Gash AK, Carabello BA, Kent RL: Left ventricular performance in patients with coexistent mitral stenosis and aortic insufficiency. J Am Coll Cardiol 3:703, 1984
66. Goldman ME, Mora F, Fuster V et al: Is mitral valvuloplasty superior to mitral valve replacement for preservation of left ventricular function. J Am Coll Cardiol 7:160A, 1986
67. Frank S, Braunwald E: Idiopathic hypertrophic subaortic stenosis. Clinical analysis of 126 patients with emphasis on natural history. Circulation 37:759, 1968
68. Flamm MD, Cohn KE, Hancock EW: Measurement of systemic cardiac output at rest and exercise in patients with atrial septal defect. Am J Cardiol 23:258, 1969
69. Kennedy JW: Complications associated with cardiac catheterization and angiography. Cathet Cardiovasc Diagn 8:5, 1982

GENERAL REFERENCES

Grossman W (ed): Cardiac Catheterization and Angiography, 3rd ed. Philadelphia, Lea & Febiger, 1986

Kennedy RH, Kennedy MA, Frye RL et al: Cardiac-catheterization and cardiac-surgical facilities: Use, trends, and future requirements. N Engl J Med 307:986, 1982

Rahimtoola S: The need for cardiac catheterization and angiography in valvular heart disease is not disproven. Ann Intern Med 97:433, 1982

CORONARY ARTERIOGRAPHY INCLUDING QUANTITATIVE ESTIMATION OF CORONARY ARTERY STENOSIS

*George T. Kondos • Jeffrey G. Shanes
Bruce H. Brundage*

Coronary arteriography continues to be the cornerstone by which clinicians make diagnostic and therapeutic decisions regarding patients with coronary artery disease, coronary vasospasm, and congenital coronary anomalies. It is therefore imperative that cardiologists become familiar with coronary anatomy and its variations so as to make appropriate clinical decisions. With the advent of better radiographic imaging techniques, catheter improvements, coronary angioplasty, and thrombolytic techniques, coronary arteriography has become a safe and commonplace procedure. The ultimate goal of coronary arteriography is the complete visualization of the coronary anatomy including assessment of coronary artery collaterals, the type of coronary pathology, and the presence of coronary anomalies. Without assessing each of these important factors an incomplete study eventuates.

NORMAL CORONARY ANATOMY

DEFINITION OF SEGMENTS

For the purposes of description, the left anterior descending, left circumflex, and right coronary arteries are subdivided into segments. The names given to the branches and the definition of the segments are highly variable. For uniformity, we have chosen to use the Coronary Artery Surgery Study (CASS) system for defining coronary segments and names of branches (Fig. 35.1).[1]

RIGHT CORONARY ARTERY

The ostium of the right coronary artery is generally located in the right half of the right aortic sinus; the ostium may originate near the aortic valve or near the sinotubular ridge.

The proximal portion of the right coronary artery extends from the origin of the vessel to a point halfway to the take-off of the acute marginal branch. After the initial take-off, the right coronary artery travels within the right atrioventricular sulcus. The proximal segment is best seen in a 60° left anterior oblique (LAO) projection (Fig. 35.2); in this projection the first branch of the right coronary artery is the conus branch, which encircles the right ventricular outflow tract. The conus branch is directed superiorly and anteriorly; in 40% of patients the conus branch will have a separate orifice a few millimeters anterior to the orifice of the right coronary artery. Selective cannulation of this vessel may lead to the erroneous conclusion that the right coronary artery is totally occluded or that a left dominant system exists (Fig. 35.3). Selective cannulation of the conus branch is considered when a right posterior descending is not visualized via left-to-right collaterals or a posterior descending artery does not arise from the left circumflex vessel. The next branch of the right coronary artery is the sinus node artery. In 60% of patients the sinus node artery arises from the proximal right coronary artery, 38% from the circumflex, and 2% from both right

coronary artery and circumflex vessels. The sinus node artery is directed opposite the conus branch running posteriorly toward the spine and superiorly. In the right anterior oblique (RAO) projection the conus branch is directed anteriorly and the sinus node artery is directed posteriorly (Fig. 35.4). In the LAO projection the sinus node artery is easily recognizable by its constant division into two distinct rami. The ramus directed anteriorly encircles the superior vena cava and supplies the sinus node. The ramus directed posteriorly supplies the superior and posterior walls of the left atrium. In a small percentage of patients the sinus node artery may have a separate orifice in the right aortic sinus. Because the orifice is usually small, inadvertent cannulation is uncommon. The last vessels arising from the distal portion of the

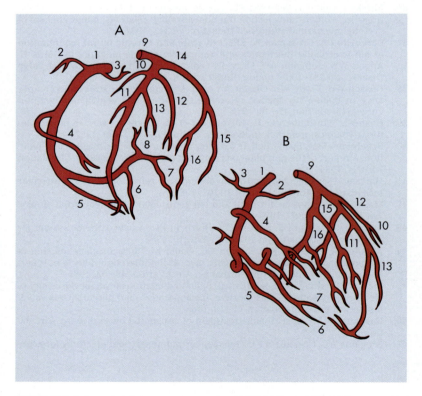

FIGURE 35.1 Left and right coronary arteries in (**A**) LAO and (**B**) RAO views. (*1*, right coronary artery; *2*, conus branch; *3*, sinus node artery; *4*, right ventricular branch; *5*, acute marginal; *6*, right posterior descending; *7*, right posterolateral branch; *8*, AV nodal artery; *9*, left main; *10*, left anterior descending; *11*, first septal; *12*, first diagonal; *13*, second diagonal; *14*, left circumflex; *15*, obtuse marginal; *16*, left posterolateral)

proximal right coronary artery are a variable number of right ventricular branches directed anteriorly, which encircle and supply the right ventricular free wall. These vessels are best visualized in the RAO projection.

The mid right coronary artery extends from the end of the proximal right coronary artery to the take-off of the acute marginal branch, which marks the termination of the right coronary artery. The mid right coronary artery continues to travel in the right atrioventricular sulcus and is best seen in the LAO view. The branches of the mid right coronary artery include a variable number of right ventricular branches encircling the right ventricle. The terminal branch of the mid right coronary artery is the acute marginal branch, which supplies the acute margin of the right ventricle. This margin or border is formed by the anterior and inferior walls of the right ventricle. Occasionally a right atrial artery may arise opposite the acute marginal branch, which runs posteriorly supplying the right atrium. These vessels are best seen in the RAO projection.

The distal right coronary artery begins just beyond the acute marginal branch and ends with, and includes, the take-off of the posterior descending artery. The posterolateral segment begins after the take-off of the posterior descending artery, continuing in the right atrioventricular groove, terminating with the take-off of the last right posterolateral branch. Both of these segments of the right coronary artery are foreshortened in the standard oblique projections. As a result of this, inadequate visualization of coronary stenosis may occur. To avoid this problem, steep cranial angulation in either the RAO or LAO projections with deep inspiration to avoid diaphragmatic or hepatic interposition is done. In the LAO view, the distal right coronary artery appears in an inverted U shape (Fig. 35.5). From the first segment of the inverted U arises the posterior descending artery, directed caudally and toward

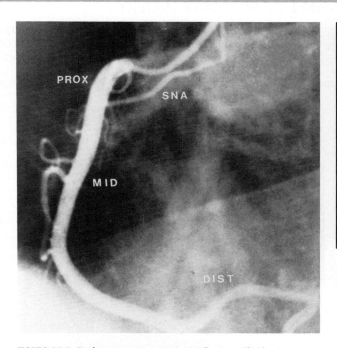

FIGURE 35.2 Right coronary artery, LAO view. (*SNA*, sinus node artery; *PROX*, proximal; *MID*, middle; *DIST*, distal)

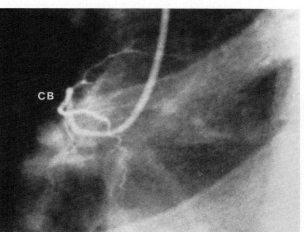

FIGURE 35.3 LAO view, selective cannulation of the conus branch (*CB*).

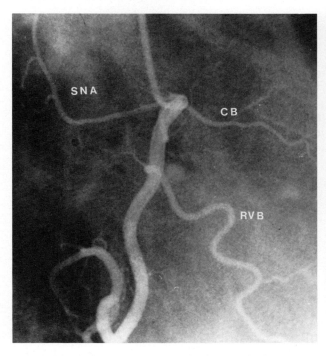

FIGURE 35.4 Right coronary artery, RAO view. (*SNA*, sinus node artery; *CB*, conus branch; *RVB*, right ventricular branch)

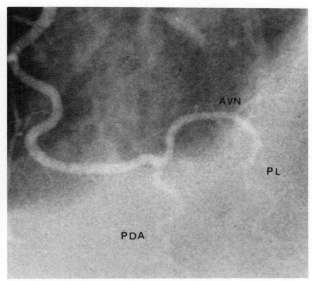

FIGURE 35.5 Right coronary artery, LAO cranial view. (*AVN*, AV nodal artery; *PDA*, posterior descending artery; *PL*, right posterolateral artery)

the apex. At the top of the inverted U is the origin of the AV nodal artery, which is directed cephalad and in opposite direction to the left ventricular branches. Where the inverted U is located is termed the *crux of the heart*, implying the center point of the heart where both atria and ventricles meet. As the right coronary artery continues beyond the AV nodal artery, one or several posterolateral branches may arise, which supply the posterior walls of the left ventricle. Occasionally confusion may arise in distinguishing the posterior descending artery and posterolateral branches. In the RAO view, small septal perforators extend cephalad throughout the course of the posterior descending artery. These branches are not seen from the posterolateral branches. Also, posterolateral branches arise distal to the AV nodal artery, whereas the posterior descending artery arises proximal to the AV nodal artery.

Considerable variability exists as to the anatomy of the posterior descending and posterolateral vessels. This variability may be dependent on a relationship that exists between the left and right coronary systems. In general, this relationship exists between the left anterior descending and the posterior descending from the right coronary artery. The larger the left anterior descending, the smaller the posterior descending vessel. A similar relationship exists between the posterolateral branches from the right coronary artery and those arising from the circumflex.

Occasionally two posterior descending vessels may run together in the posterior interventricular sulcus. Another variation occurring in approximately 3% of cases is the circum-marginal posterior descending (Fig. 35.6).[2] The circum-marginal arises from the right coronary artery before the acute margin of the heart. Its course crosses the acute margin. The circum-marginal ends in the posterior interventricular sulcus as the only posterior descending vessel or can be seen complementing another posterior descending artery with a more standard course. Occasionally a nondominant right coronary artery will be seen. In this instance the right coronary artery is a small vessel that bifurcates early, supplying the right atrium and right ventricle (Fig. 35.7). It is important to recognize a nondominant right circulation to avoid mistaking this for an obstructed right coronary artery.

LEFT CORONARY ARTERY

The origin of the ostium of the left main coronary artery is extremely variable. It generally arises from the middle of the left coronary sinus. The left main coronary artery generally travels to the left and slightly

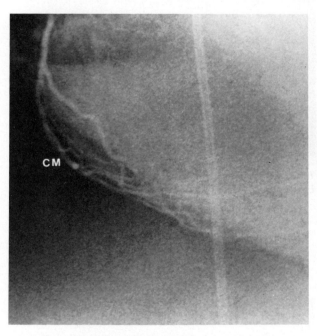

FIGURE 35.6 Right coronary artery, RAO view. (CM, circum-marginal)

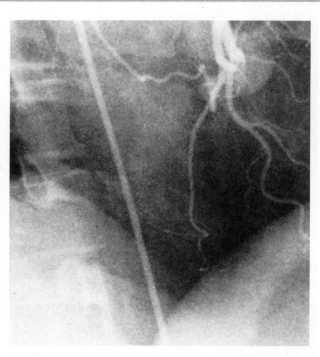

FIGURE 35.7 Nondominant right coronary artery, RAO view. The two branches supply the right ventricle and right atrium.

FIGURE 35.8 Shallow RAO view visualizing the proximal and mid left main coronary artery (LM).

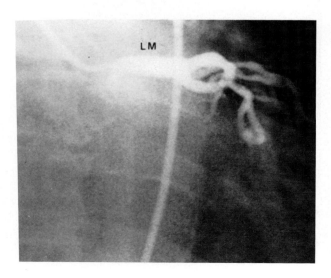

posterior, and has a variable length from 1 mm to 25 mm. In 2% of cases the left main coronary artery is nonexistent and separate orifices exist for the left anterior descending and circumflex vessels. Importantly, this variation must be realized at the time of angiography to avoid misinterpreting it as a total occlusion of either major left vessel. In 12% of patients an extremely short left main coronary exists. It is important to realize this condition because selective opacification generally occurs of either the left anterior descending or circumflex. In addition, the left main coronary artery may not be adequately visualized. Under these conditions, selective cannulation of these vessels must be done in addition to a pullback or cusp injection to visualize the left main.

The entire left main is best seen in the shallow RAO projection such that the left main is just positioned off the spine (Fig. 35.8). However, the RAO projection generally will not visualize the bifurcation of the left main. Usually the left main travels in a horizontal or cephalad direction so that a shallow LAO with caudal angulation helps define the bifurcation; in other instances a shallow LAO with steep cranial angulation is most useful. Because of overlap that may occur between the left anterior descending, circumflex, and intermediate vessels at their origin it is important that these other views are considered.

The left main generally terminates into two branches, the left anterior descending, which continues anteriorly in its course in the anterior interventricular sulcus, and the circumflex, which travels posteriorly in the left atrioventricular sulcus. Occasionally the left main terminates in a trifurcation, giving off an intermediate vessel that is directed laterally. The trifurcation is best visualized in either the LAO or RAO caudal views.

The course of the entire left anterior descending and its branches is relatively uniform. The left anterior descending may be divided into three segments: proximal, middle, and distal.

The proximal left anterior descending extends from the origin of the left anterior descending to the origin of the first septal perforator. The middle segment extends from the first septal perforator to the take-off of the second diagonal. The distal segment extends from the second diagonal to the termination of the vessel.

In general, complete opacification of the proximal left anterior descending may be difficult because of overlap between the circumflex and intermediate vessels in the standard LAO and RAO projections (Figs. 35.9 and 35.10). The overlap may be averted with either of the following projections: LAO with steep cranial angulation; RAO with steep caudal angulation; LAO with caudal angulation; or a straight left lateral with slight caudal angulation.

Along the entire course of the left anterior descending two or more diagonal vessels may originate that supply the anterolateral wall of the left ventricle. In the LAO view the diagonal vessels are directed downward and to the right; in contrast, the left anterior descending is directed straight downward. The origins of the diagonal vessels will be best seen in an LAO projection with steep cranial angulation. In the RAO projection the general direction of the left anterior descending and diagonal branches may be quite similar and difficulty in distinguishing them may occur. In the shallow RAO view the diagonals are seen to course over the anterolateral surface of the heart, whereas the left anterior descending is seen to travel inside the border of the heart. Another feature that is helpful in distinguishing the left anterior descending is its lack of lateral motion during systole compared to the diagonal and obtuse marginal vessels of the circumflex, which move toward one another during systole.

A variable number, usually from one to six, of septal vessels may originate from the left anterior descending. The most proximal septal perforator may vary considerably in size and caliber and on occasion is as large as a major diagonal branch. Since in the standard LAO projection the left anterior descending and septal perforators course in the same direction, the LAO cranial view is a helpful differentiator. In this projection the septal vessels course downward and to the left, as opposed to the left anterior descending, which follows a straight down-

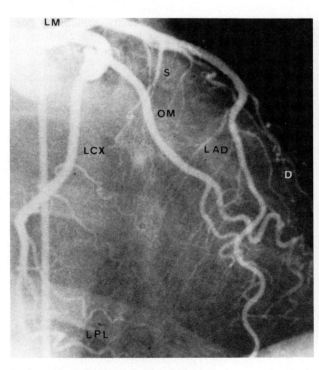

FIGURE 35.9 Left coronary artery, shallow RAO view. (*LM*, left main; *LCX*, left circumflex; *OM*, obtuse marginal; *LPL*, left posterolateral; *LAD*, left anterior descending; *S*, septal; *D*, diagonal). In the shallow RAO projection the left anterior descending artery travels within the border of the heart while the two diagonal arteries course over the anterolateral aspect of the heart.

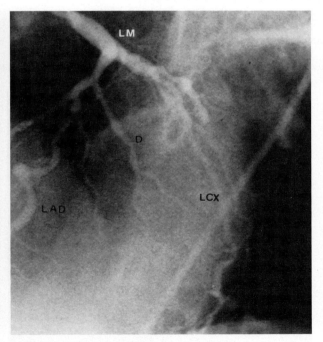

FIGURE 35.10 Left coronary artery, LAO view. (*LM*, left main; *LAD*, left anterior descending; *D*, diagonal; *LCX*, left circumflex)

ward course. In the shallow RAO, the septal vessels are seen at 90° angles to the left anterior descending.

An interesting variant of the left anterior descending coronary artery is a dual left anterior descending system (Fig. 35.11).[3] It is important that this anatomical variant be identified because of the important surgical implications. A dual left anterior descending system is present in less than 1% of angiographic studies. In this circumstance the left anterior descending bifurcates into short and long left anterior descendings. The short left anterior descending generally supplies the anterior interventricular septum traveling in the anterior interventricular groove and terminating before the apex. The long left anterior descending has a variable course, traveling for a short time in the anterior interventricular sulcus and then on the epicardial surface of the left ventricle, reentering the anterior interventricular sulcus near its distal third. The long left anterior descending may also travel entirely intramyocardially deep in the interventricular septum. Alternatively, the long left anterior descending may travel on the anterior wall of the right ventricle. If this anatomical variant is not recognized, the wrong left anterior descending may be bypassed. In addition, this variant may help explain the presence of an akinetic basal septum with good anterolateral wall motion or, conversely, the presence of normal anterior interventricular septal motion with abnormal anterior left ventricular wall motion.

Immediately after the circumflex arises from the left main it angulates in a posterior direction and is directed into the left atrioventricular sulcus. The circumflex may be arbitrarily divided into three segments to simplify description: proximal, distal, and atrial ventricular. The proximal segment of the circumflex extends from the origin of the circumflex vessel to and including the origin of the first obtuse marginal vessel. After the branching of the first obtuse marginal vessel, the entire circumflex vessel is divided in half as it courses in the AV sulcus. The first half is referred to as the distal circumflex and the remaining portion, the atrial ventricular segment. In 40% of patients a sinus node artery may arise from the circumflex. The sinus node artery may best be seen in a shallow RAO projection where it is directed posteriorly and superiorly toward the superior vena cava.

As the circumflex reaches the obtuse margin of the heart, defined as the border of the inferior and lateral walls of the left ventricle, three obtuse marginal branches arise that run parallel to the diagonal and intermediate vessels. The first obtuse marginal or anterolateral marginal arises from the proximal circumflex and supplies the lateral wall of the left ventricle superior to the obtuse margin of the heart. The second obtuse marginal is generally the largest of the obtuse marginal branches. It arises from the distal circumflex and supplies the obtuse margin of the heart. The third obtuse marginal or posterolateral marginal branch arises from the distal circumflex and courses toward the lateral wall of the left ventricle inferior to the obtuse margin of the heart. The anatomy of the three obtuse marginal branches is best appreciated in a shallow RAO projection.

A great deal of variation in anatomy exists with respect to the obtuse marginal branches. Often a very large single obtuse marginal may arise from the circumflex and run in the distribution of the obtuse margin of the left ventricle and supply areas of the heart supplied by the first and second obtuse marginal branches by sending secondary branches that course inferiorly and superiorly. On occasion, the obtuse marginal vessel may functionally represent the termination of the circumflex vessel.

After the obtuse marginal branches are given off, the circumflex usually continues in the left atrioventricular sulcus and gives off at least one posterior left ventricular branch. In the case of a left dominant coronary system, the posterior descending and AV nodal artery also arise from the circumflex.

As with the distal and posterolateral segments of the right coronary artery, the distal and atrial ventricular segments of the circumflex are best seen in an LAO cranial projection. Frequently a left atrial branch or left atrial circumflex artery arises from the distal circumflex, continuing in the AV groove and finally coursing to the left atrium. This vessel may supply most of the left atrial wall.

CORONARY ARTERY DOMINANCE

The left ventricle receives the majority of its blood supply from the left coronary system. Coronary anatomy has traditionally been divided into three general types of circulations: right dominant, left dominant, and co-dominant or balanced. Coronary dominance does not refer to the amount of myocardium supplied by the coronary arteries; rather, it refers to which coronary system, the left coronary artery or the right

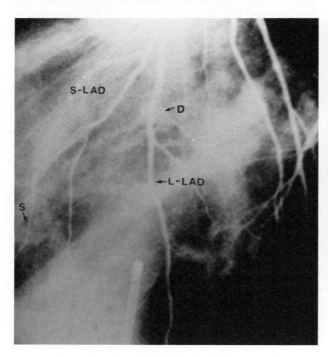

FIGURE 35.11 Dual left anterior descending, LAO view. (*L-LAD*, long left anterior descending; *S-LAD*, short left anterior descending; *S*, septal artery; *D*, diagonal artery)

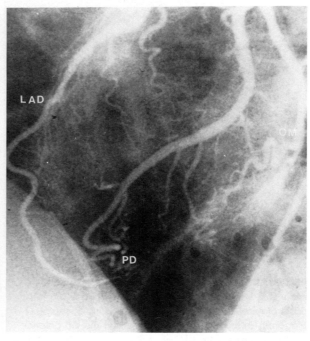

FIGURE 35.12 Left dominant circulation, LAO view. (*LAD*, left anterior descending; *PD*, left posterior descending)

coronary artery, supplies most of the posterior wall of the left ventricle. If the right coronary artery terminates before giving off a posterior descending branch, a left dominant system is present (Fig. 35.12). If the terminal branch of the right coronary artery is the posterior descending with at least one posterolateral branch, a right dominant system is present. If the terminal branch of the right coronary is the posterior descending only, a codominant or balanced circulation is present. A right dominant system is present in 84% of people, a left dominant in 12%, and the remaining 4% have a balanced circulation.

CORONARY ARTERY COLLATERALS

Intricate coronary arterial communications exist, anastomosing all of the major coronary arteries. The development of flow in these connecting channels is dependent on the presence of acquired stenosis of the coronary vasculature, namely, the development of coronary atherosclerotic obstructive disease. As the degree and duration of obstructive disease increase, angiographically visible collaterals develop. In the normal heart, collaterals are generally not visualized angiographically. However, their significance in patients with obstructive coronary disease is important. Collaterals may preserve myocardial function. In general, collaterals, if supplied by a nondiseased vessel, are capable of providing adequate resting coronary blood flow. Ischemia may occur during conditions that need increased myocardial blood flow. There is no formal classification system of coronary collaterals. In general, two types of collateral pathways exist. Intercoronary collaterals supply communications between the major coronary arteries, and intracoronary collaterals are communications that exist between the same coronary arteries. Typical routes of collateral circulation in cases of left anterior descending, circumflex, and right coronary artery occlusions are illustrated in Figures 35.13 to 35.15.

The absence of coronary collaterals coupled with the absence of major coronary arteries without regional wall motion abnormality signifies to the angiographer that the major artery has not been visualized due to selective cannulation or the presence of anomalous origin. Furthermore, the presence of collaterals to an area of myocardium supplied by what appears to be a relatively normal-appearing vessel should encourage the angiographer to search for angiographically hidden obstructive disease. The absence of collaterals to an area subtended by an occluded coronary artery may signify recent occlusion.

To better visualize collateral vessels the angiographer must continue to record on cine images for a longer period of time than usual in the first LAO and RAO projections of the left and right coronary arteries. Visualization of the collaterals is important because they may provide the only means of assessment of an occluded vessel. Occasionally, in cases of left anterior descending obstruction, the left anterior descending may be supplied by collaterals from the conus artery. Because this branch arises from a separate orifice in 40% to 50% of patients, the left anterior descending may not be visualized if only the right coronary is injected. The angiographer must then selectively inject the conus branch. Coronary collaterals may be better visualized after the injection of 300 µg of intracoronary nitroglycerin. Examples of collateral circulation are demonstrated in Figures 35.16 to 35.18.

CORONARY ANGIOGRAPHIC TECHNIQUES

Key to successful coronary arteriography involves optimal patient preparation. The more prepared and comfortable the patient is, the

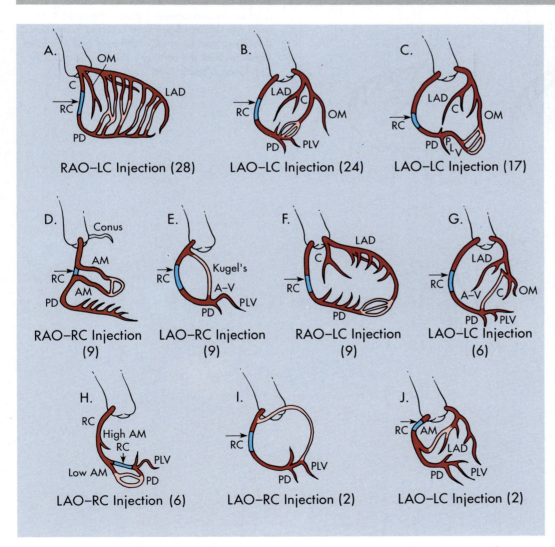

FIGURE 35.13 Right coronary obstruction, collateral supply. (LC, left coronary; RC, right coronary). The numbers in parentheses indicate the number of times the collateral pathway occurred in this series. (Modified from Levin DC: Pathways and functional significance of the coronary collateral circulation. Circulation 50:831, 1974)

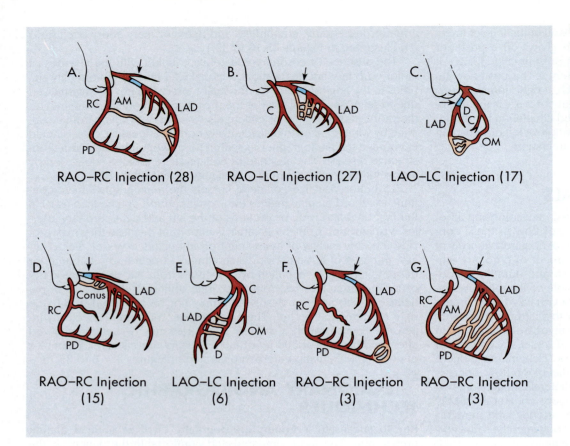

FIGURE 35.14 Left anterior descending obstruction, collateral supply. (*LC*, left coronary artery; *RC*, right coronary artery). The numbers in parentheses indicate the number of times the collateral pathway occurred in this series. (Modified from Levin DC: Pathways and functional significance of the coronary collateral circulation. Circulation 50:834, 1974)

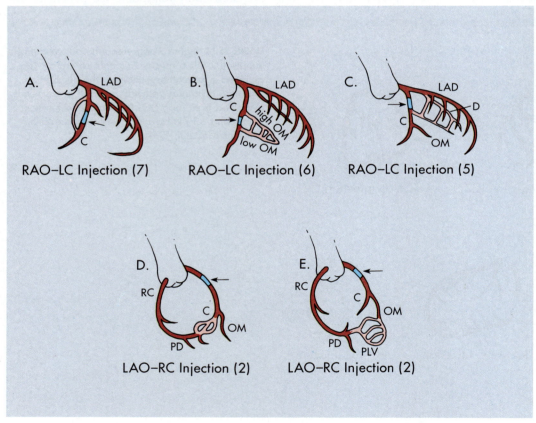

FIGURE 35.15 Left circumflex obstruction, collateral supply. (*LC*, left coronary; *RC*, right coronary) The numbers in parentheses indicate the number of times the collateral pathway occurred in the series. (Modified from Levin DC: Pathways and functional significance of the coronary collateral circulation. Circulation 50:835, 1974)

easier the procedure becomes. The angiographer or a member of the catheterization team must evaluate the patient prior to the cardiac catheterization to determine the need for the procedure and the questions to be addressed. In addition, the procedure, along with the potential complications and risks, is explained. A careful history may uncover a prior anaphylactoid reaction to contrast material. The physical examination may be helpful in deciding the optimal approach (*i.e.*, via femoral, brachial, or axillary artery). For example, the brachial approach may be preferred in patients with severe peripheral vascular disease or in extremely obese individuals.

The patient is instructed to take medications and small amounts of liquids for the 8 hours prior to the procedure. Appropriate sedation is administered prior to arrival at the catheterization laboratory. The authors recommend diazepam, 10 mg PO, and diphenhydramine, 50 mg PO, prior to the procedure. Meperidine, 50 mg IM, is an alternative regimen.

PERCUTANEOUS FEMORAL APPROACH

The angiographer must be familiar with the anatomy of the inguinal area (Fig. 35.19). The inguinal ligament extending from the anterior superior iliac spine to the pubic symphysis is palpated. The femoral artery is palpated as it courses under the inguinal ligament. The femoral artery is entered approximately two fingerbreadths below the inguinal crease. With a 25-gauge needle the skin and subcutaneous tissue are infiltrated with lidocaine anesthesia. Intermittent aspiration during lidocaine administration is important to avoid intravascular injection of

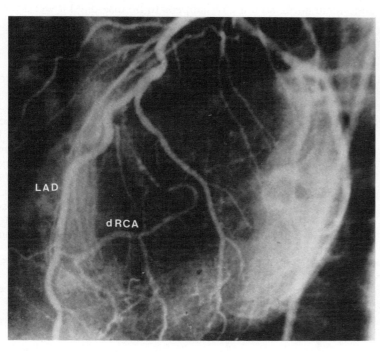

FIGURE 35.16 Left coronary artery injection. LAO view demonstrating the distal right coronary (*dRCA*) filling by collaterals from the left anterior descending (*LAD*).

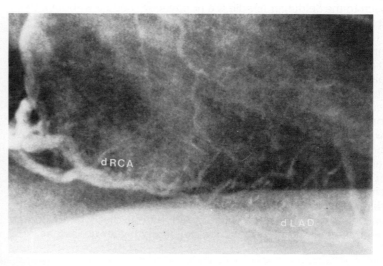

FIGURE 35.17 Right coronary artery injection. RAO view demonstrating the distal left anterior descending (*dLAD*) filling from collaterals from the distal right coronary artery (*dRCA*).

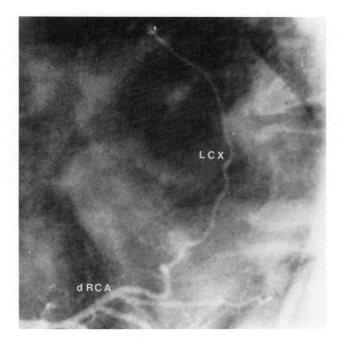

FIGURE 35.18 Right coronary artery injection. LAO view demonstrating the left circumflex (*LCX*) filling from collaterals from the distal right coronary artery (*dRCA*).

the anesthetic agent. After infiltration, a small stab wound is made over the femoral artery, and the area is enlarged with a small straight Kelly clamp. While palpating the femoral artery with the left hand, the Seldinger needle is advanced at a 30° to 45° angle with respect to the horizontal plane of the patient. Steeper angulation may make passage of the guidewire difficult, and lesser angulation may result in entrance of the femoral artery above the inguinal ligament with the subsequent inability to maintain hemostasis after the catheters are removed. When the angiographer feels the artery has been entered, the stylet is removed. The free flow of blood from the needle signals the artery has been entered. If both sides of the artery have been entered and the needle hits the periosteum of the pelvic bone, the stylet should be removed and local anesthesia given after initial aspiration. The patient will sense a pressure-like sensation with the administration of lidocaine anesthesia. The Seldinger needle is continuously pulled back while watching for a free flow of blood from the needle. An alternative approach to the Seldinger needle is a hollow-core needle without a stylet that allows one to puncture one side of the artery.

Once free flow of blood is established, a 0.035 J-tipped movable or nonmovable core guidewire (Fig. 35.20) is inserted through the needle and advanced to the level of the diaphragm. If difficulty is encountered in passing the guidewire the angiographer determines the cause of the difficulty by fluoroscopic examination. If the guidewire is seen not to advance beyond the tip of the needle, subintimal or extravascular position of the needle is likely. The guidewire is removed and free backflow is reestablished. If backflow is not seen, the needle is repositioned. If the original needle puncture was made too low in the inguinal area, the superficial femoral artery may be entered rather than the common femoral artery. If the superficial femoral is small, it may be occluded by the guidewire or catheter or the guidewire may enter preferentially one of the superficial femoral branches rather than the main body of the vessel. In either case, the needle is removed and another attempt at entering the femoral artery higher up is done.

Once the wire is above the level of the diaphragm, the needle is removed while constant pressure is applied over the artery to prevent the formation of a hematoma. The guidewire is then wiped with a saline-soaked gauze to remove any clots that may have formed. A No. 8 French dilator is placed over the guidewire with a twisting motion and the subcutaneous tissue and femoral artery are dilated. The dilator is removed, the guidewire is wiped to remove any clots, and the appropriate angiographic catheter is inserted over the wire and placed in the descending aorta. Some angiographers prefer to use one of the various sheaths with a hemostatic valve to facilitate catheter exchanges instead of repeatedly exchanging over a guidewire.

Once the catheter is in position, the guidewire is removed and wiped. The catheter is aspirated to remove any clot that may have formed and is then vigorously flushed. After the catheter has been flushed, 3,000 units of heparin is given and the catheter is advanced around the aortic arch. All catheter flushing should be done in the abdominal aorta, so if a clot happens to be dislodged it will travel to the lower extremities rather than to the central nervous system.

LEFT CORONARY ARTERY CANNULATION

The cannulation of the left coronary artery with a Judkins preformed catheter is generally easily accomplished. The left Judkins catheter is available in four sizes (3.5–6) (Fig. 35.21). The numbers refer to the length of the secondary curve in centimeters (Fig. 35.22). The catheter is advanced retrograde into the aortic root on profile. Once the left coronary is cannulated the operator notes the distal catheter tip pressure waveform to avoid damping or ventricularization. Either of these phenomena—damping, a fall in systolic pressure, or ventricularization, a decrease in the diastolic pressure—may signal that either a proximal high-grade stenosis with subsequent wedging of the catheter is present or the tip of the catheter is against the wall of the coronary artery. Injection of contrast in the presence of damping or ventricularization

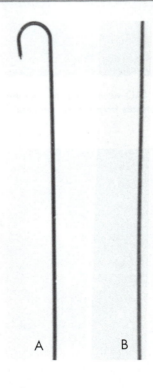

FIGURE 35.20 Guidewires used in coronary arteriography. **(A)** 0.035 J-tipped movable core wire; **(B)** 0.035 straight movable core wire.

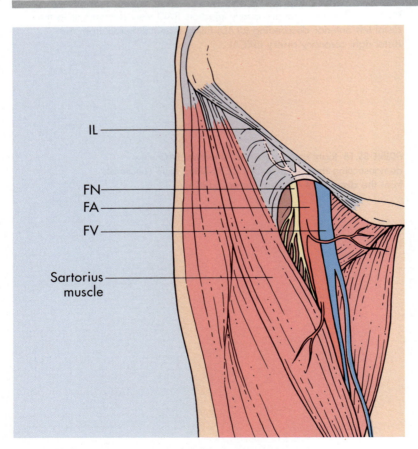

FIGURE 35.19 Anatomy of the right inguinal area. (*FN*, femoral nerve; *FA*, femoral artery; *FV*, femoral vein; *IL*, inguinal ligament)

may lead to dissection of the coronary artery. The operator must either reposition the catheter, make small injections of contrast into the left sinus of Valsalva to detect any proximal high-grade obstructions, or use small intracoronary injections with immediate removal of the catheter.

In patients with dilated aortic roots or superior take-offs of the left coronary artery, a number 5-cm or 6-cm Judkins catheter is usually employed. Conversely, in patients with small aortic roots a 3.5-cm catheter is preferred. Upon entering the left coronary ostium, the tip of the left Judkins catheter should be in the horizontal position. If the catheter tip is pointing in an upward direction a larger secondary curve is used. Conversely, if the tip of the catheter is pointing downward the catheter is too large and a Judkins catheter with a smaller secondary curve is used. If a 4.0 Judkins catheter is still too large the operator may advance the catheter into the left sinus of Valsalva in an attempt to decrease the primary curve. After the catheter has been held in this position for 15 seconds it is slowly withdrawn until the left coronary ostium is engaged. Care is necessary doing this procedure to avoid dissection of the left main coronary artery.

In patients with a short left main coronary artery, superior take-offs of the left main, or separate origins of the left anterior descending and left circumflex arteries, the Amplatz type of catheters may be useful. These catheters are available in four sizes, each with a larger curve (I–IV) (Fig. 35.23). Another advantage of the Amplatz catheter is its responsiveness to rotation, which is clearly better than the conventional Judkins catheter.

The Amplatz catheter is advanced on profile across the aortic root and retrograde into the ascending aorta. The tip of the catheter will pass the left ostium and generally lodge in the left sinus of Valsalva. With continued advancement of the catheter, the tip will move superiorly and engage the ostium of the left coronary artery. Once the ostium is engaged, slight withdrawal of the catheter will allow for better engagement of the coronary ostium. Further advancement of the Amplatz catheter will generally disengage the tip from the coronary ostium.

RIGHT CORONARY ARTERY CANNULATION

The cannulation of the right coronary artery requires more catheter manipulation than cannulation of the left coronary. The Judkins right coronary catheter is available in four sizes (3–6), which reflect the distance in centimeters from the primary curve to the halfway point of the secondary curve (Fig. 35.24).

The right coronary catheter is advanced to the ascending aorta to a position of approximately 4 cm above the aortic valve. The catheter is rotated in a clockwise manner. The catheter is then moved inferiorly approximately 2 cm to 3 cm into the right sinus of Valsalva. As rotation is continued slowly in a clockwise direction, the catheter will usually engage the right coronary ostium. Alternatively, the catheter may be placed at the level of the aortic valve. The catheter is rotated in a clockwise manner and pulled back to allow the clockwise torque to be imparted to the catheter. Once the right coronary orifice has been engaged, the catheter tip pressure waveform is checked to detect damping and a small test injection is done to verify the correct catheter position.

The most common error in right coronary artery cannulation is overtorquing of the catheter. The catheter must be slowly rotated by the operator to allow the catheter to position itself. Occasionally selective cannulation of the conus branch occurs because of a separate orifice. If this happens the catheter is removed and selective cannula-

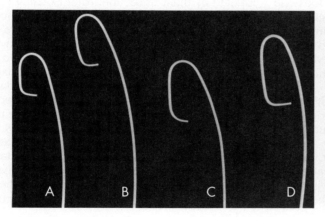

FIGURE 35.21 Left Judkin's coronary catheters: **(A)** 3.5L; **(B)** 4.0L; **(C)** 5.0L; **(D)** 6.0L.

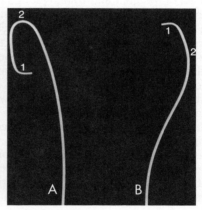

FIGURE 35.22 Judkin's coronary catheters: **(A)** 4.0L; **(B)** 4.0R. (1, primary curve; 2, secondary curve)

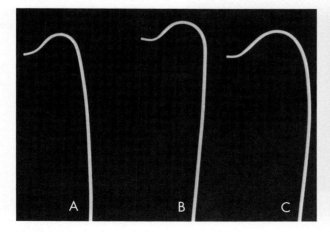

FIGURE 35.23 Amplatz catheters: **(A)** AL I; **(B)** AL II; **(C)** AL III.

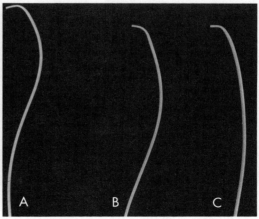

FIGURE 35.24 Right Judkins coronary catheters: **(A)** 3.5R; **(B)** 4.0R; **(C)** 5.0R.

tion of the right coronary is done. The conus branch may also branch superiorly from the proximal right coronary artery. In this case the right coronary catheter may also selectively seek this vessel. If this occurs the catheter is removed and selective recannulation of the right coronary artery is attempted. If this fails a larger right coronary catheter is used that allows the tip of the catheter to point more inferiorly, thus avoiding selective cannulation of the conus branch. High-grade proximal right coronary stenosis may cause damping of the pressure no matter how the catheter is manipulated. In this case, small injections of contrast are done with immediate removal of the catheter from the ostium with each injection.

BYPASS GRAFT AND INTERNAL MAMMARY ARTERY CANNULATION

Numerous catheters have been used for visualization of coronary bypass grafts. The angiographer must be familiar with the surgeon's graft placement. In addition, the operative report should be reviewed prior to the coronary angiogram.

In general, the graft to the right coronary artery is attached to the aorta approximately 2 cm above the native right coronary orifice. The grafts to the left anterior descending and diagonal branches are attached to the aorta slightly superior and to the left of the native right coronary artery or right coronary graft. The aortic origins of grafts to the circumflex system are generally superior and to the left of anterior descending grafts.

Each of these grafts may be cannulated with either a Judkins right coronary catheter or right bypass graft catheter. The left anterior descending and circumflex grafts may also be entered with a left bypass graft catheter (Fig. 35.25).

Right coronary grafts are cannulated by advancing the catheter to a level slightly above the level of the graft and rotating it in a clockwise direction similar to the technique described for the native right coronary artery. Cannulation of left anterior descending and circumflex coronary artery grafts is similar. The catheter is advanced to the appropriate level above the graft and rotated clockwise until beyond the midportion of the ascending aorta. The catheter is then advanced and the appropriate graft entered.

Internal mammary artery cannulation is accomplished with an internal mammary artery catheter. This catheter resembles the right coronary artery catheter with the exception of a tighter primary curve (less than 90°) and a longer tip (1.5 cm–2.0 cm) (Fig. 35.26).

The origin of the internal mammary is from the anterior, inferior surface of the subclavian artery. To cannulate this vessel, the catheter is advanced to the origin of the left subclavian. The catheter tip is slowly rotated anteriorly until the left internal mammary is cannulated. If difficulty is encountered in entering the left subclavian artery, a 0.35 straight movable-core guidewire may be inserted into the catheter and advanced into the subclavian artery. The catheter may then be successfully advanced over the wire into the main body of the subclavian. The catheter is further manipulated until the left internal mammary is cannulated.

Cannulation of the right internal mammary is more difficult. The internal mammary catheter is advanced into the aortic arch. The catheter is then rotated counterclockwise and advanced. With this maneuver, the catheter tip will point superiorly and preferentially enter the innominate artery and subclavian artery rather than the ascending aorta. Once in the subclavian, the catheter is manipulated anteriorly and inferiorly by rotation until the internal mammary is cannulated.

Prior to injecting the internal mammary artery the distal pressure is noted. Injection of contrast when the pressure is damped may result in dissection of the vessel. If the subclavian artery is dilated, an internal mammary catheter with a longer tip may be required.

The injection of the internal mammary will cause the patient to experience an unpleasant burning feeling in the anterior chest. This results from branches of the internal mammary artery that supply muscles of the chest wall. The pain may be alleviated by the use of nonionic contrast agents or the dilution of ionic contrast material, 1:1, with 1% lidocaine.

THE BRACHIAL APPROACH

The angiographer must become familiar with the anatomy of the left and right antecubital fossae prior to attempting the brachial approach (Fig. 35.27). The brachial artery is palpated at the level of the median epicondyle or approximately 2 to 3 fingerbreadths above the elbow crease. A horizontal incision is made over the artery, and the artery is isolated by blunt dissection. After isolating the artery, umbilical tapes are placed proximally and distally and used for traction. A small transverse arteriotomy is made with iris scissors, a No. 11 blade, or an 18-gauge needle, and 5000 units of heparin is introduced distally to prevent thrombosis from distal stasis. A No. 7 or 8 French, 80-cm Sones catheter is introduced into the brachial artery and passed with fluoroscopic guidance to the ascending aorta (Fig. 35.28). Occasionally spasm occurs on insertion of the catheter into the brachial artery. Spasm may cause extreme discomfort to the patient as well as making catheter advancement difficult. If this occurs, the catheter is removed and reintroduced after the patient has relaxed. Care is taken not to force the catheter into the ascending aorta. Not uncommonly the catheter follows one of the branches of the brachial or subclavian arteries. Whenever resistance is met, the catheter is withdrawn, slightly rotated, and readvanced. If difficulty is encountered in entering the

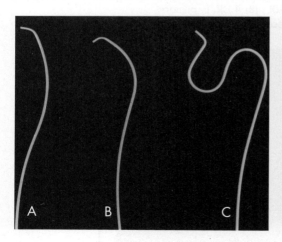

FIGURE 35.25 Saphenous vein bypass catheters: (A) right saphenous vein graft catheter; (B) left saphenous vein graft catheter; (C) Fromm graft catheter.

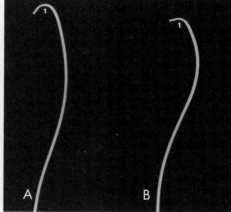

FIGURE 35.26 Comparison of (A) internal mammary artery catheter and (B) right coronary artery catheter. Note the tighter primary curve (1) of the internal mammary catheter compared to the right coronary catheter.

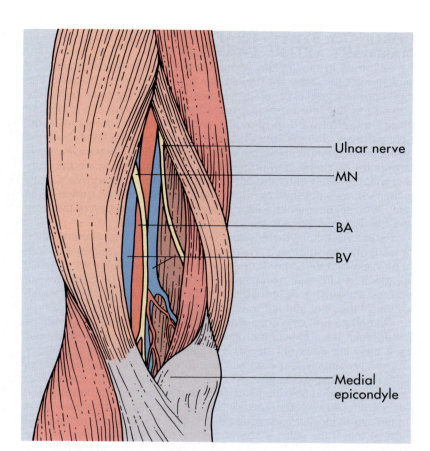

FIGURE 35.27 Anatomy of the right antecubital fossa. (*BV*, brachial vein; *BA*, brachial artery; *MN*, median nerve). On occasion the vein may lie on top of the artery. Careful dissection is required to separate the vessels.

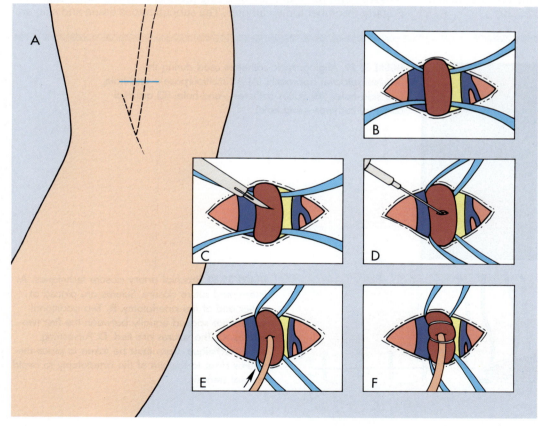

FIGURE 35.28 Brachial cutdown technique. **A.** A transverse incision is made in the skin overlying the brachial artery. **B.** The brachial artery is isolated by two umbilical tapes placed proximally and distally. **C.** A transverse incision is made in the artery. **D.** Heparin, 5000 units, is delivered distally. **E.** Insertion of Sones catheter through the arteriotomy. **F.** Rubber band in place over the proximal portion of the brachial artery to aid in hemostasis.

ascending aorta, a 0.35 J-tipped guidewire is inserted into the Sones catheter and advanced to the ascending aorta. This is especially helpful in large tortuous subclavian vessels where the catheter preferentially travels down the descending aorta.

LEFT CORONARY ARTERY CANNULATION

The Sones catheter is advanced with the imaging system in a 45° LAO projection. In this projection, the left and right sinuses of Valsalva are on the left and right of the fluoroscopic image screen, respectively. The noncoronary cusp is posterior in location. The catheter is advanced to the left sinus of Valsalva and a small loop is formed so the tip points superiorly; by continually advancing the catheter, the tip moves up the aortic wall until the left ostium is selectively engaged. When a high take-off of the left ostium is encountered, a large loop may be formed by continually moving the catheter tip superiorly. In this instance selective engagement may be difficult and arteriography is done with the catheter holes adjacent to the coronary ostium.

RIGHT CORONARY ARTERY CANNULATION

The Sones catheter is advanced to the right sinus of Valsalva and a small loop is formed. The tip of the Sones catheter is slowly moved superiorly until the orifice of the right coronary is engaged. Alternatively, the Sones catheter may be advanced into the left sinus of Valsalva where a small loop is formed. The catheter is slowly turned in a counterclockwise direction sweeping the anterior aortic wall until the right coronary ostium is engaged. Care must be taken in cannulation of the right coronary with the Sones catheter—at times the catheter may deeply penetrate the right coronary lumen.

Numerous other catheters, including right and left Amplatz catheters, the A2 multipurpose catheter, or Judkins catheters, may also be used via the brachial approach with success (Fig. 35.29).

CORONARY BYPASS GRAFT AND INTERNAL MAMMARY ARTERY CANNULATION

As described in the Judkins approach, the proximal anastomoses of saphenous vein grafts are predictably positioned in most cases. The right coronary graft is generally the most anterior. The next graft more leftward is the left anterior descending. All subsequent grafts are placed more leftward, posteriorly, and superiorly. To cannulate the right coronary graft the Sones catheter is advanced to a level above the orifice of the graft. With further advancement, the catheter will usually engage the lip of the graft orifice. Then with slight retraction the catheter will selectively enter the orifice. Cannulation of left coronary grafts is similarly accomplished by advancing the catheter to the orifice of the graft. With slight counterclockwise rotation and retraction of the catheter, the left graft orifices are selectively cannulated.

Catheterization of the left internal mammary is best accomplished by a left brachial approach. Therefore, if a left internal mammary needs to be visualized the entire procedure may be done via the left brachial approach. An internal mammary artery catheter may be used and positioned similarly as described under the Judkins approach for visualization of the right and left internal mammary arteries.

On completion of coronary arteriography, the catheter is removed and forceful back bleeding proximally and distally is allowed. If brisk back bleeding does not occur, a Fogarty thrombectomy catheter is inserted proximally and distally. Once forceful back bleeding is seen, 3000 units of heparin is given via the arteriotomy distally and arterial clamps are placed proximal and distal to the brachial arteriotomy. The artery is closed with 6.0 Tevdek via a pursestring or transverse interrupted suture closure technique (Fig. 35.30). An adequate radial pulse must be felt. If the pulse is absent the brachial arteriotomy sutures are removed and forceful back bleeding produced by repeat passage of a Fogarty thrombectomy catheter. The subcutaneous tissue and skin are

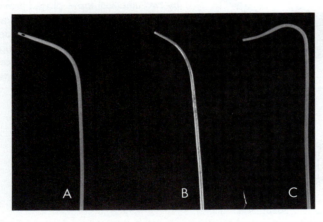

FIGURE 35.29 Angiographic catheters used during the brachial cutdown approach: **(A)** A2 multipurpose—end-hole, two side-holes; **(B)** Sones catheter—end-hole; **(C)** brachial coronary catheter—end-hole.

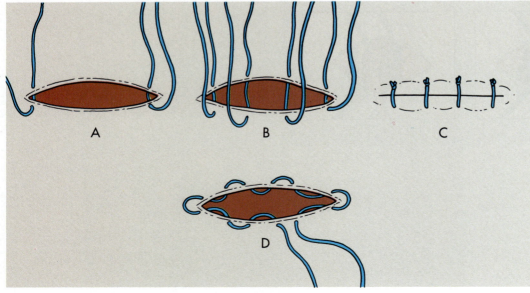

FIGURE 35.30 Brachial artery closure techniques. **A.** Interrupted suture closure. Sutures are placed at either end of the arteriotomy. **B.** Two additional sutures are spaced equally between the first two sutures. **C.** The sutures are tied. **D.** Pursestring suture technique. Care must be taken to place the sutures close to the site of the arteriotomy to avoid arterial stenosis.

then approximated with 3.0 silk, using an interrupted mattress suturing technique.

PERCUTANEOUS BRACHIAL APPROACH

An alternative to the brachial cutdown approach is the percutaneous brachial approach.[4] The brachial artery is palpated slightly above the elbow crease. The skin and subcutaneous tissue are infiltrated with 1% lidocaine anesthesia. The skin above the brachial artery is punctured with a No. 11 blade. A hollow Cook needle is advanced at a 70° angle with the skin surface. When free flow of blood is encountered a .035 guidewire is advanced through the needle into the brachial artery. The needle is removed with continual pressure to the puncture site to prevent hematoma formation. A No. 7 or 8 French sheath is inserted over the wire. The No. 7 French sheath should be used in females or patients with small brachial arteries. The Sones catheter is advanced through the sheath. Once in the brachial artery 4000 units of heparin is given. The catheters used and their manipulation are identical to the cutdown technique. When the procedure is finished the catheter and sheath are removed and adequate hemostasis is obtained by enough pressure over the brachial artery while allowing the radial pulse to be faintly felt.

PERCUTANEOUS TRANSAXILLARY APPROACH

Rarely difficulty may be encountered with both the percutaneous femoral approach and the brachial approach because of advanced vascular disease or unusual tortuosity of the vessels. In those circumstances, the percutaneous left or right transaxillary is an alternative approach.[5] The same catheters used for femoral artery cannulation may be used with the transaxillary approach.

The patient is placed in the supine position with the appropriate hand behind the neck. The elbow is flexed and the arm supinated and abducted. The axillary artery is palpated with the index and middle fingers. The axillary artery is punctured approximately 4 cm proximal to the deltopectoral groove. Once free backflow of blood is established, a guidewire is inserted via the needle. The subcutaneous tissues are dilated with an arterial dilator and catheter exchanges are accomplished over the guidewire. The insertion of a sheath facilitates catheter exchanges.

Upon completion of the examination the catheter is removed and the area over the puncture site is compressed until adequate hemostasis is achieved. Good radial and ulnar pulses after the procedure indicate reestablishment of adequate circulation.

The major hazards of the transaxillary approach include neurologic and vascular injury. Damage to the brachial plexus from needle trauma during lidocaine infiltration may occur. In addition, hematoma formation may compress the brachial plexus and produce motor or sensory symptoms and signs in the upper extremity.

EVALUATION OF CORONARY ARTERY SPASM

It is important for the angiographer to consider coronary vasospasm or variant angina as a possible etiology for a patient's chest pain syndrome.[6-8] This is especially true if a typical history of coronary vasospasm is elicited. The authors recommend that patients with a significant chest pain history suggestive of coronary vasospasm with normal or insignificant coronary artery disease undergo provocative ergonovine testing. Reportedly patients with ectatic coronary arteries without significant obstructive disease may have severe coronary vasospasm induced by ergonovine testing.[9] Review of the videotape is important prior to ergonovine testing to rule out any significant obstructive coronary disease.

After routine arteriography is completed the patient is given incremental doses of ergonovine at 3-minute intervals (0.05 mg, 0.1 mg, 0.15 mg, 0.2 mg). Aortic pressure is measured before each injection. Two minutes after administration, a 12-lead electrocardiogram is obtained and aortic pressure is measured. If there are no significant changes the next dose is given. Generally, a total dose of 0.4 mg of ergonovine is given; occasionally, an additional 0.3 mg may be given if no significant increase in heart rate or elevation of mean systolic arterial pressure is observed. In patients with a strong likelihood of coronary vasospasm, an initial dose of 0.025 mg of ergonovine may be prudent.

After the last dose of ergonovine is given, if the patient has not developed electrocardiographic changes or chest pain, coronary arteriography in multiple views is done. Because the Judkins technique requires a catheter exchange to visualize both coronary arteries, the angiographer determines which coronary is most likely to have spasm present by prior electrocardiographic changes. Alternatively, the brachial approach may be used or an A2 multipurpose catheter is used via the percutaneous femoral approach, which obviates catheter exchanges. If the angiographer notes electrocardiographic changes or the patient develops the typical chest pain syndrome, further doses of ergonovine are not given until the coronary arteries are visualized.

In instances of ergonovine-induced coronary vasospasm the angiographer is prepared to give intracoronary doses of 300 μg of nitroglycerin along with nifedipine, 10 mg sublingually. These doses are repeated until the coronary vasospasm is relieved, which must be documented arteriographically.

The authors recommend that nitrate and calcium channel blocker preparations be stopped at least 24 to 48 hours prior to ergonovine administration. Furthermore, if ergonovine is given to patients on nitrates or calcium channel blockers it is difficult to interpret negative results. The authors recommend that ergonovine only be administered in the cardiac catheterization laboratory where direct intracoronary instillation of nitroglycerin is possible (Figs. 35.31 and 35.32). Hyperventilation with or without infusion of sodium bicarbonate can also induce coronary artery spasm, but the technique is seldom used and an ergonovine-provocative test is preferable.

RADIOGRAPHIC EVALUATION OF CORONARY ANATOMY

To quantitate the degree of coronary artery stenosis accurately the vessel must be visualized in several profiles. Foreshortening, or visualizing the vessel on end, along with vessel overlap, must be avoided. When selective coronary arteriography was first developed, x-ray systems were only capable of rotating the table or x-ray tube in a transverse plane perpendicular to the long axis of the body. As a result of this, the images obtained were not always perpendicular to the coronary arteries. With the advent of modern radiographic equipment the x-ray tube and image intensifier may be rotated in the sagittal plane. Because of this, the coronaries are visualized with x-ray beams directed perpendicularly to them, thus minimizing foreshortening. With the various degrees of rotation and angulation, vessel overlap is also avoided.

Much confusion exists in today's literature regarding radiographic projections. Most cardiovascular angiographers define the projection by the position of the image intensifier rather than the direction the x-ray beam is traveling. The degree of angulation in the transverse plane is measured from the midline whereas the degree of angulation in the sagittal plane is measured from the vertical. For example, if the image intensifier is located on the patient's left side, 30° from the midline, this is a 30° LAO projection. If the image intensifier were moved toward the patient's feet approximately 20° from the vertical, this is considered a 20° caudal projection (Fig. 35.32).

Multiple views must be obtained in the cardiovascular laboratory. The authors routinely use the following views: left coronary artery, 10° to 20° LAO, 60° LAO, left lateral/10° caudal, 45° LAO/20° cranial, 10° RAO, 60° RAO/20° caudal; right coronary artery, 30° LAO, 30° RAO.

Not every patient may tolerate all of the contrast injections. The

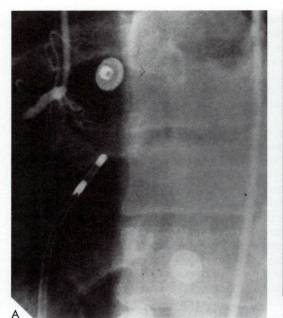
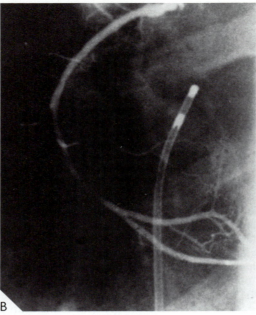

FIGURE 35.31 A. Right coronary after administration of 0.15 mg of ergonovine. **B.** Spasm was relieved after 300 μg of intracoronary nitroglycerin was given. No significant obstructive disease is seen.

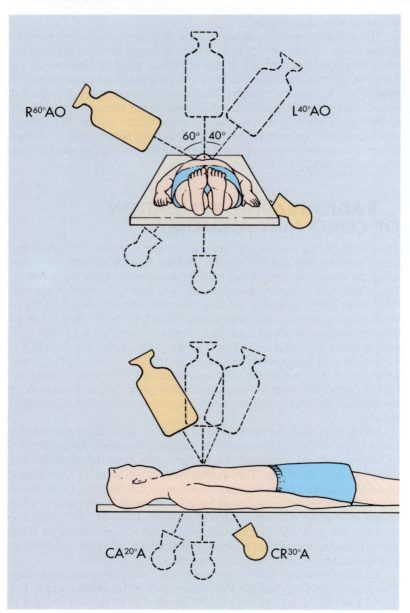

FIGURE 35.32 Cardiovascular nomenclature. **A.** The image intensifier has been rotated in a transverse plane around the long axis of the body. **B.** The image intensifier has been rotated in the sagittal plane. ($R^{60°}AO$, 60° right anterior oblique projection; $L^{40°}AO$, 40° left anterior oblique projection; $CR^{30°}A$, 30° cranial angulation; $CA^{20°}A$, 30° caudal angulation) (Modified from Paulin S: Terminology for radiographic projections in cardiac angiography. Cathet Cardiovasc Diagn 7:341, 1981)

angiographer must decide, after a few test injections, which projections will be most helpful. Table 35.1 lists useful radiographic projections.

ANALYSIS OF THE CORONARY ARTERIOGRAM

Prerequisite to correct interpretation of the coronary arteriogram is the presence of an excellent x-ray imaging system, a good projector to view the 35-mm cine film, and an experienced angiographer. Any weakness in this linkage leads to misinterpretation and a nondiagnostic study.

The angiographer must obtain the required views, which eliminate vessel overlap and foreshortening. Presently with x-ray systems this is accomplished easily because of the ease with which the image intensifier is readily angulated in either the sagittal or transverse planes. Each coronary artery is visualized in at least two views, preferably orthogonal to one another.

SYSTEMATIC APPROACH TO THE IDENTIFICATION OF VESSELS

The coronary arteriogram is analyzed in a systematic fashion. Each angiographer develops a plan for interpreting the arteriogram. A cursory review of the film is definitely inadequate. Each coronary segment must be examined closely. All areas of the myocardium are supplied by coronary arteries; if the supply to a region of myocardium is not identified, occlusion or anomalous origin of the coronary artery must be suspected.

The left main coronary artery is best seen in a shallow RAO projection. If the vessel is not seen well in this view or questions exist as to the presence of left main stenosis, other views are obtained. The distal left main is well seen in the 20° to 30° cranial projection, because modern equipment provides adequate penetration of the overlying spine. When the left main travels in a horizontal or cephalad direction, a 45° LAO/20° caudal projection is used to evaluate the distal left main bifurcation. When an intermediate vessel is present, the trifurcation can also be well visualized. Patients with a left main that travels in an inferiorly directed position are imaged with the 45° LAO/20° cranial view, which will elongate the left main and provide good visualization of the distal bifurcation. Severe left main obstruction is demonstrated with ostial injections. Occasionally total occlusion of the left main coronary artery is encountered. It is important for the angiographer to be aware of this unusual situation. If repeated attempts at cannulation of the left main are unsuccessful or if only a stump of the left anterior descending is visualized, the angiographer must proceed with injection of the right coronary artery to look for any collateralization to the left coronary system. Usually extensive collateral formation is evident (Fig. 35.33).[10,11]

TABLE 35.1 RADIOGRAPHIC PROJECTIONS OF THE CORONARY ARTERIES

Coronary Artery	Radiographic Projections	Comments
Left Main	10° RAO	Generally the best view for the left main
	45° LAO/20° cranial	Evaluation of the left main bifurcation with an inferior orientation
	45° LAO/20° cranial	Horizontal left main, distal left main, and distal left main bifurcation
	20°–30°/cranial	Distal left main evaluation
Left Anterior Descending	30° LAO	Evaluation of proximal and mid left anterior descending
	30° RAO	Evaluation of proximal and mid left anterior descending
	45° LAO/30° caudal	Evaluation of proximal left anterior descending with a horizontal orientation
	45° LAO/20° cranial	Evaluation of proximal and mid left anterior descending and origins of diagonals
	Left lateral/10° caudal	Evaluation of proximal, mid, and distal portions of the left anterior descending
	30° RAO/20° caudal	Evaluation of mid, distal left anterior descending
Left Circumflex	45° LAO/20° cranial	Evaluation of proximal circumflex
	40° LAO	Evaluation of mid circumflex
	30°–40° RAO	Evaluation of the obtuse marginal vessels
	45° LA/20° cranial	Evaluation of obtuse marginal vessels
	10°–20° RAO/20° caudal	Evaluation of proximal and mid circumflex
	45° LAO/20° cranial	Evaluation of the bifurcation of the right coronary artery and posterior descending branches
	45° RAO/20° cranial	Evaluation of posterior descending and posterolateral branches
Right Coronary	30° RAO	Evaluation of the mid right coronary artery posterior descending and posterolateral branches
	30° LAO	Evaluation of proximal right coronary artery

Evaluation of the left anterior descending and left circumflex coronary arteries depends on the angle subtended by the two vessels. When the angle formed by these vessels is less than 30°, considerable overlap exists in the RAO projection. The standard 60° LAO and 45° LAO/20° cranial projections are helpful or a 45° RAO/20° caudal projection will display the proximal left anterior descending and circumflex vessels.[12-15] Occasionally the 45° RAO/20° caudal projection is not helpful and a 45° RAO/20° cranial is used. In a horizontal heart, the proximal left anterior descending and circumflex vessels may be best evaluated with an LAO/caudal projection (Fig. 35.34).[16,17] A much underutilized view is the left lateral projection with 10° to 15° caudal angulation. In this view, the proximal, mid, and distal portions of the left anterior descending are well visualized (Fig. 35.35). In some cases the RAO/cranial projection will best identify the mid portion of the left anterior descending. Significant image degradation may occur with the sagittal projections because the x-ray is attenuated by the liver and spleen.

The origins of the diagonal vessels are best visualized in the LAO/cranial projection. In the RAO projection, errors occur in some cases. Because of a totally occluded left anterior descending, a diagonal vessel or a large septal perforator may resemble the occluded vessel.

The proximal left circumflex coronary artery may be obscured by the left main, left anterior descending, or intermediate coronary arteries in the standard RAO projection (Fig. 35.36). The RAO/caudal projection helps to increase the angle between the left anterior descending and the circumflex. The proximal circumflex may also be visualized in the left lateral or in the 45° LAO/30° cranial projection. Because of foreshortening, the LAO projection is not optimal for visualization of the obtuse marginal branches. The standard RAO projections along with the RAO/caudal projection best profile these vessels.

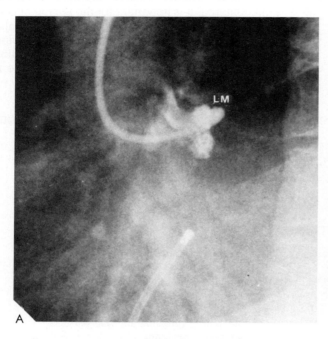
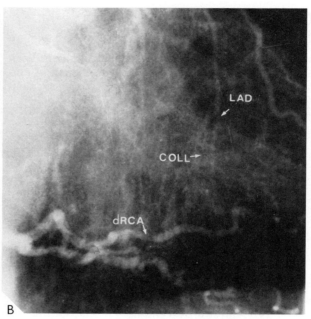

FIGURE 35.33 A. Total occlusion of the distal left main (*LM*) coronary artery, LAO projection. **B.** Right coronary artery injection showing collaterals to the left system. (*dRCA*, distal right coronary artery; *COLL*, collaterals; *LAD*, left anterior descending)

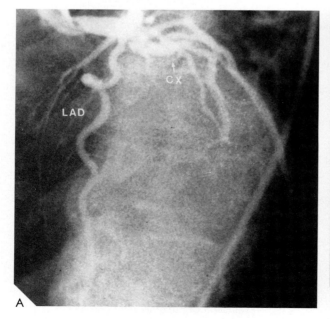
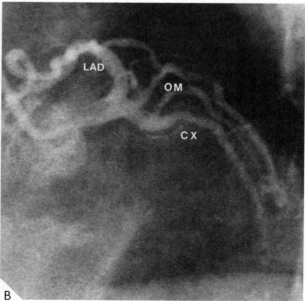

FIGURE 35.34 Left coronary artery. **A.** LAO view. **B.** LAO caudal view. The origins of the left anterior descending (*LAD*), left circumflex (*CX*), and obtuse marginals (*OM*) are clearly seen in the caudal view without overlap.

Adequate views of the right coronary artery may be difficult to obtain. The LAO view demonstrates the proximal and conduit portions of the right coronary artery well. However, in the LAO view the posterior descending and posterior lateral vessels tend to be foreshortened and overlap. The RAO view eliminates the foreshortening and depicts the mid right coronary, posterior descending, and posterior lateral branches well. Occasionally the bifurcation of the distal right coronary artery and take-off of the posterior descending are hard to visualize. In this case, cranial angulation to either the RAO or LAO views is helpful (Fig. 35.37).[18]

EVALUATION OF CORONARY ARTERY STENOSIS

The degree of coronary artery stenosis is subjectively assessed by the experienced angiographer. The degree of diameter reduction is compared to the apparently normal adjacent segments. This assessment is generally accurate in mild or severe stenosis; however, considerable interobserver variability exists in assessing lesions in between the range of mild to severe. This topic is further discussed in the section on Quantitative Coronary Arteriography, below.

Hemodynamically significant stenoses are usually in the range of

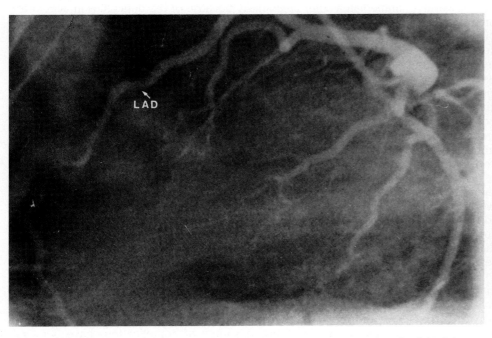

FIGURE 35.35 Left lateral projection with 10° caudal angulation. The entire length of the left anterior descending (LAD) artery is visualized.

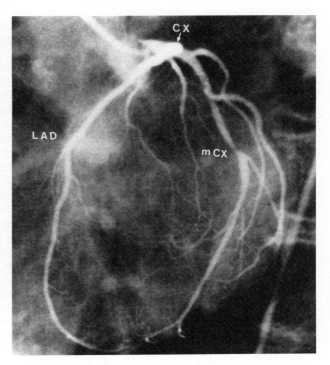

FIGURE 35.36 Left coronary artery, LAO projection. The proximal circumflex (CX) is obscured by overlap from the proximal left anterior descending (LAD). A lesion is seen in the mid circumflex (mCX).

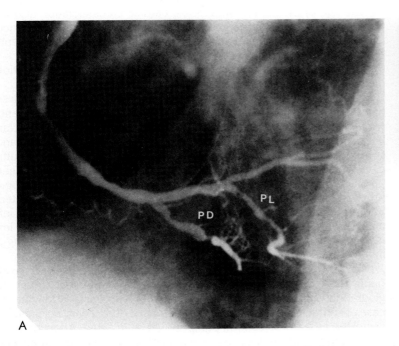

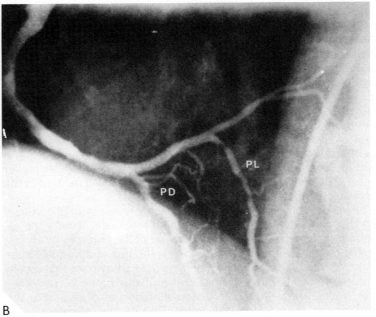

FIGURE 35.37 A. Right coronary artery, LAO projection. **B.** Right coronary artery, LAO/cranial projection. With cranial angulation, foreshortening is eliminated; the distal vessels are better visualized. (PD, posterior descending; PL, right posterolateral)

70% diameter reduction, which correlates with a 90% reduction in cross-sectional area. Quantitative coronary arteriography and indirect measurement of blood flow are being done with increasing frequency because of the recognition that coronary angiographic assessment of anatomy does not always accurately predict the physiology produced by the stenosis.

QUANTITATIVE CORONARY ANGIOGRAPHY

Clinicians accept the coronary angiogram as the court of last resort and ultimate truth in the evaluation of coronary artery disease. However, there is increasing awareness that the coronary arteriogram may often underestimate and in some instances even overestimate the severity of coronary arterial stenosis.[19] These inaccuracies are further compounded by the rather large interobserver and intraobserver interpretive variability that is demonstrated whenever comparative analysis is made.[20] Comparison of readers skilled in coronary arteriographic interpretation demonstrates a 20% to 40% interobserver variability and a 7% to 10% intraobserver variability.[21] Because of these observations there have been major efforts made over the past ten years to develop more objective means of evaluating the severity of coronary artery disease by coronary angiography. Initially, studies were performed using optical magnification and calipers to measure the percent reduction in the coronary arterial diameter produced by atherosclerotic disease.[22,23] However, a recent report by White and co-workers comparing this measurement with the reactive hyperemic response of coronary flow to transient arterial occlusion in the operating room demonstrated a very poor correlation.[24] This study emphasizes the difficulties encountered in interpreting coronary arteriograms and extrapolating the changes in anatomy to physiologic effects.

Brown and associates developed a computerized quantitative technique for measuring coronary arterial stenosis, and the validity of this method has been confirmed by several other research groups.[25-27] This method analyzes two orthogonal cine views of a coronary lesion and requires manual tracing of the optically magnified arterial border. Corrections are made for pin-cushion distortion, and magnification is determined by using the coronary catheter tip as a scaling device. The computer program assumes an elliptical lumen and calculates the absolute and percentage reduction in diameter and cross-sectional area of the vessel. Comparison of the intraoperative coronary reactive hyperemic response with the minimal cross-sectional area determined by this method has correlated well.[26] This is the first validation in humans that a quantitative anatomical method of evaluating coronary artery stenosis accurately predicts the physiologic effects of the disease.

Selzer and Blankenhorn and associates have emphasized the need for an objective method of determining the edge of the arterial lumen in order to make quantitative angiography totally operator independent.[28] They and others have developed objective computer methods for determining coronary vessel edge.[29-31] After several years of development and improvement, reasonably accurate and precise determinations of vessel edge can be made. Variation in the measurement of percent arterial narrowing of less than 3% has been achieved.[32] The advent of decreasing computer costs and increasing computer power makes it likely that quantitative methods of analysis will be used in the clinical angiographic laboratory.

The major problem with any morphometric assessment of coronary artery disease is defining a normal arterial reference. Usually the assumption is made that the greatest diameter of the coronary artery just proximal or distal to an area of stenosis is the true and normal lumen diameter. Pathologic studies have demonstrated, however, that usually the blood vessel is diffusely diseased and this frame of reference causes frequent arteriographic underestimation of disease. For this reason, several investigators have advocated the measurement of the smallest cross-sectional area of a stenosis as the best indicator of severity of disease.[25,26]

Video densitometry is another approach to quantitating the severity of coronary artery disease. This technique is performed by digitizing a single frame of a technically excellent coronary angiogram. Computer algorithms are employed to define changes in contrast density from one edge of the vessel to the other. Scanning the entire lesion in this manner produces a profile of brightness values from which the background contribution is subtracted and a net cross-sectional absorption profile is obtained. Integration of this function gives a measure of the cross-sectional area.[14] The correlation between morphometric measurements of coronary artery stenosis and densitometric methods is good. A recent report indicates that video densitometry may be superior to morphometric methods analyzing residual coronary stenosis immediately after angioplasty because of the difficulties in accurately determining vessel edge.

Significant progress in the analysis of coronary arteriograms has been made over the past decade. Clinicians recognize there are serious pitfalls in "eyeballing" the coronary angiogram. Because of the diffuse nature of coronary artery disease, even the employment of quantitative methods may significantly underestimate the severity of coronary obstructions if the regions proximal and distal to the area of greatest stenosis are used to calculate percent stenosis. The best quantitative method is a biplane orthogonal evaluation of a lesion and the use of computer edge-detection algorithms to determine the minimal cross-sectional area.

COMPLICATIONS OF CORONARY ARTERIOGRAPHY

MAJOR COMPLICATIONS

DEATH, MYOCARDIAL INFARCTION, AND CEREBROVASCULAR COMPLICATIONS

Prior to undergoing any invasive procedure, the benefits accrued should outweigh the risks of the procedure. Four studies in the literature address the issue of complications (Table 35.2)[33-36] resulting from cardiac catheterizations. A variety of complications have been reported involving cardiac catheterization. Table 35.2 lists some of these complications.

Overall, certain conclusions may be drawn from the various studies. The more advanced the coronary atherosclerotic disease, the higher the complication rate. In patients with significant left main coronary artery disease, the mortality rates ranged from 0.76% to 0.86%.[33,34]

The age of the patient undergoing cardiac catheterization also influences the complication rates. If the incidence of death is examined it varies from 1.75% of patients less than 1 year old to 0.25% of patients older than 60 years.[33]

The major complications associated with cardiac catheterization include death, acute myocardial infarction, and stroke.

Death can be prevented if high-risk patients are identified. These high-risk patients include (1) infants less than 1 year old; (2) patients with advanced coronary atherosclerotic disease, especially significant left main coronary artery disease; (3) left ventricular dysfunction; and (4) other severe noncardiac medical conditions such as renal insufficiency or severe peripheral or carotid vascular disease. Hemodynamic parameters must be monitored in these patients and pharmacologic pretreatment given to optimize abnormal hemodynamic parameters prior to catheterization. In patients suspected of having significant left main disease, the angiographer must be careful in cannulating the left main ostium, watching the catheter pressure waveform, and using a limited number of projections.

Factors leading to death may also predispose the patient to developing acute myocardial infarction. To avoid this complication the angiographer must medically pretreat patients with unstable angina. In cases of refractory angina that occur before or during cardiac catheterization an intra-aortic balloon pump should be inserted. Adequate heparinization has also helped to prevent myocardial infarction during cardiac catheterization. It has been the authors' practice not to reverse systemic anticoagulation for the brachial or femoral approaches. In patients with allergies to fish or insulin-dependent diabetics, protamine should not be given. If protamine is given the patient should be carefully watched for the development of an anaphylactoid reaction.[37]

The development of central nervous system complications may best be avoided by observing good angiographic techniques. Guidewires must be wiped carefully and catheters aspirated and flushed after guidewire removal.

In patients with advanced cerebrovascular disease the angiographer must avoid entering any of the arch vessels. Likewise, in patients with abdominal or thoracic aneurysms, catheter exchanges must be made above the aneurysm to avoid plaque embolization. Also in patients with suspected left ventricular thrombus, care must be used when advancing the catheter into the left ventricle to avoid dislodging the thrombus. Systemic heparinization has helped to lessen some of these complications; however, the best way to avoid these central nervous system complications is by good catheter technique and speed with which the procedure is done.

MINOR COMPLICATIONS
ARTERIAL INJURY

In earlier studies of cardiac catheterization the rates of arterial complications range from 3.6% to 6% of cases. In Kennedy's study the vascular complication rate was much lower, occurring in approximately 0.57% of patients.[34,35]

The major vascular complications vary depending on the route of arterial entry. Thrombosis and trauma to the artery are more common with the brachial approach, especially in laboratories where this approach is done infrequently. The vascular complications include vascular dissection, which may involve the femoral, aortic, subclavian, or coronary arteries. To avoid this complication, careful technique with respect to guidewire and catheter advancement should be used. Catheters and guidewires must never be forced. If difficulty is encountered with respect to advancement, free backflow of blood must be established before catheter and guidewire manipulation is continued. Dissection of the coronary arteries is a rare complication of coronary arteriography. This generally results from vigorous catheter manipulation or injection of contrast when the catheter is wedged against the arterial wall. Dissection more commonly occurs in the right coronary artery and it occurs more commonly in patients with normal coronary arteries. This complication may result in myocardial infarction. Surgical intervention is usually indicated when coronary dissection occurs.

Thrombosis is best prevented with good catheterization technique. When employing the brachial approach, distal systemic anticoagulation is mandatory, along with routine Fogarty catheter use prior to arterial repair. If the radial pulse is not felt after repair of the artery, the sutures must be removed and the vessel explored.

When using the percutaneous femoral approach, similar vascular complications may occur. In addition, hemorrhage and pseudoaneurysm formation may occur. Hemorrhage generally occurs as a result of early ambulation. It is the authors' practice to delay ambulation for at least 6 hours after catheterization. In patients who are heavy or in whom difficulty in maintaining hemostasis was encountered, ambulation is allowed after 12 hours of bed rest. The development of a pseudoaneurysm that is a hematoma communicating with a ruptured artery generally results from poor compression of the femoral artery. In this case the patient will complain of pain and local swelling in the leg. This complication may not be manifest at times until several weeks after the angiographic procedure. Peripheral vascular surgical intervention is always required because of the high incidence of rupture.

The development of arteriovenous fistulas following cardiac catheterization has also been reported. This generally results when the vein and artery are overlying one another, with the subsequent catheter entrance going through both vessels. Surgical repair is mandatory when a continuous murmur is heard over this area.

When peripheral pulses are not palpated after cardiac catheterization surgical exploration is mandatory to avoid ischemic complications and loss of limb. Occasionally if the pulses are weaker after catheterization, systemic heparinization with careful patient monitoring for a short period of time may be done. If improvement is not evident within hours, arterial exploration to remove the thrombus or to repair an intimal flap must be done. Thrombosis of the femoral artery requires surgical exploration with subsequent removal of the clot.

LOCAL NEUROLOGIC COMPLICATIONS

Local neurologic complications may result from either the brachial or femoral approaches. These complications result from damage to the median or femoral nerve during anesthetic administration from the needle. Other median nerve complications may result during the cutdown or during suturing of the arteriotomy.

Occasionally the development of a large hematoma may compress the brachial or femoral nerve, resulting in neurologic symptomatology.

In general, insignificant injury to the median nerve results in a sensation of numbness, tingling, and slight weakness of the hand. These symptoms generally resolve in approximately two weeks. Alternatively, if the patient is complaining of significant hand pain and weakness, exploration of the area must be done.

ELECTROPHYSIOLOGIC DISTURBANCES

Numerous cardiac arrhythmias may occur during the course of catheterization. These may include ventricular fibrillation, ventricular tachycardia, asystole, or bradydysrhythmias. The incidence of ventricular fibrillation varies between 0.56% to 1.28% of cases.[33-36]

Major arrhythmias resulting from coronary arteriography result from inadvertent entry of the catheter into the left ventricle or after injection of the coronary arteries. In the latter instance, the coronary arteries are generally normal. Injection of the right coronary artery more commonly produces this problem. To avoid ventricular fibrilla-

TABLE 35.2 COMPLICATIONS OF CARDIAC CATHETERIZATION

Investigator	Years Study Conducted	Number of Patients	Complications* (%)	
Braunwald[36]	1966–1968	12,367	Death	(0.44)
			MI	(0.4)
			VF	(0.7)
			Arterial	(1.4)
			CNS	(0.5)
Adams et al[33]	1970–1971	46,904	Death	(0.45)
			MI	(0.61)
			VF	(1.28)
			Arterial	(1.62)
			CNS	(0.23)
Davis et al[34]	1975–1976	7,515	Death	(0.2)
			MI	(0.25)
			VF	—
			Arterial	(0.74)
			CNS	—
Kennedy et al[35]	1978–1979	53,581	Death	(0.14)
			MI	(0.07)
			VF	(0.56)
			Arterial	(0.57)
			CNS	(0.07)

* MI, myocardial infarction; VF, ventricular fibrillation; CNS, central nervous system.

tion in these instances, smaller injections of contrast material and disengagement of the catheter between injections are done. If ventricular fibrillation persists, prompt defibrillation and resuscitative measures are indicated. With the development of asystole or bradycardia, a standby ventricular pacemaker is used. It is the authors' practice during arteriography not to leave the pacing catheter in the right ventricle. If one of the rhythm disturbances necessitating pacing ensues, the pacemaker is advanced to the right ventricle and left in position until the procedure is terminated.

In general, three factors are important when trying to minimize complications. It is clear from numerous studies that the greater the catheterization laboratory volume (*i.e.*, greater than 200 cases/2 years), the lower the complication rate. In Kennedy and co-workers' study the risk of complications was eight-fold higher in catheterization laboratories where less than 200 procedures/2 years were performed.[34] In addition to case load, constant monitoring of catheterization technique and the speed with which the procedure is done will help to reduce the complication rate significantly. Finally, despite attention to all of the above details, complications will occur. Complications occur in the population with advanced atherosclerotic disease or advanced age. In these circumstances, prompt recognition of the complication is mandatory, with appropriate actions taken.

ERRORS IN INTERPRETATION OF THE CORONARY ARTERIOGRAM

Numerous factors either related to the angiographic technique or to the patient may result in erroneous interpretation of the angiogram.

INCOMPLETE STUDY. An incomplete study occurs when an inadequate number of projections have been taken. There are no standard numbers or even standard projections in coronary arteriography. The number and type of projection must be sufficient to define the entire

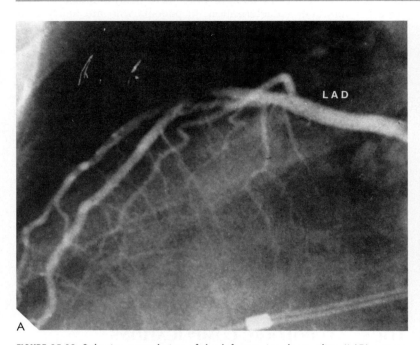

FIGURE 35.38 Selective cannulation of the left anterior descending (*LAD*) artery. The circumflex vessel is not visualized.

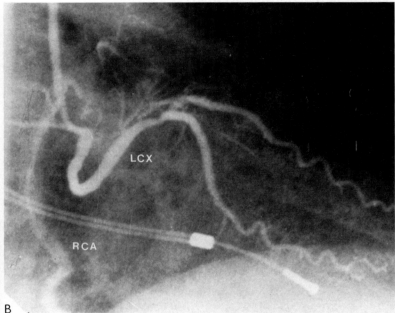

FIGURE 35.39 Anomalous origin of the left circumflex from the right aortic sinus. The right coronary artery is faintly visualized. (*CX*, circumflex; *RCA*, right coronary artery)

FIGURE 35.40 Anomalous origin of a nondominant right coronary artery (*RCA*) from the noncoronary sinus.

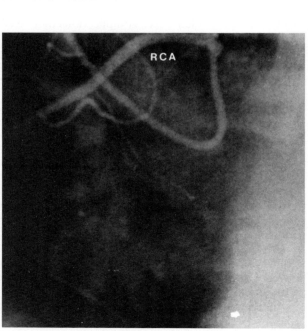

coronary arterial tree. Furthermore, the study should be tailored to the patient's individual needs.

POOR CONTRAST INJECTION. Poor injections of contrast into the arterial tree result in the layering of the contrast material and overall poor opacification of the vessel. This results in the appearance of luminal narrowing when the vessel may be normal. In addition, critical branches may not be visualized. The force and amount of contrast injected should be enough to opacify the entire vessel by ensuring good mixing of the contrast agent and blood.

SELECTIVE CANNULATION OF CORONARY VESSELS. Selective cannulation may lead to the inappropriate conclusion of total occlusion of the unopacified vessel (Fig. 35.38). In some instances of selective injection (*i.e.*, the injection of the conus branch), ventricular fibrillation may occur. In areas where no regional wall motion abnormality exists, if there is absence of collaterals to the area or no visible major coronary artery is present, selective cannulation must be considered.

Occasionally, selective injections may be indicated to visualize collateral blood supply or in cases of a short or absent left main coronary artery.

INADEQUATE X-RAY PENETRATION OR PROJECTIONS. Poor x-ray penetration occurs especially with the newer sagittal projections and when the liver is penetrated. In addition, when the patient does not breathe properly to move the diaphragm down, especially in the RAO projections, poor visualization of the coronaries may ensue, making interpretations impossible or erroneous. To avoid these problems, proper breathing instructions are given, along with appropriate x-ray settings in heavy patients.

CATHETER-INDUCED CORONARY SPASM. Coronary spasm related to the arteriographic catheter may lead to the false conclusions of significant atherosclerotic disease. The angiographer should be alerted to the possibility of coronary spasm when (1) damping of the catheter waveform occurs; (2) backflow of contrast into the appropriate aortic

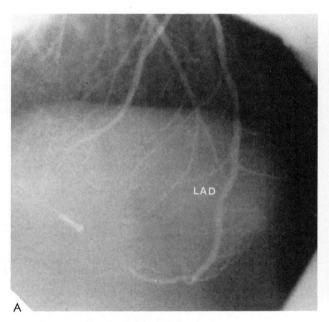
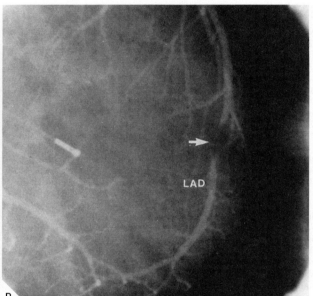

FIGURE 35.41 Myocardial bridging. **A.** Normal-appearing left anterior descending (*LAD*) artery. **B.** During systole, apparent narrowing of the left anterior descending is indicated by arrow.

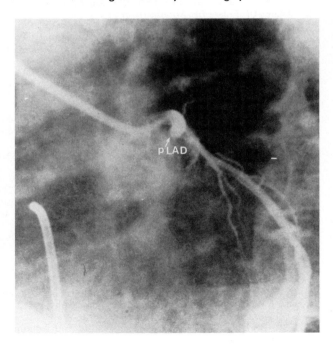

FIGURE 35.42 Left coronary artery, LAO projection demonstrating total occlusion of the proximal left anterior descending (*pLAD*) artery.

sinus is not visible with each injection; or (3) there is absence of chest pain during ergonovine administration. Catheter spasm may occur with any coronary vessel, more commonly with the right coronary artery. When coronary spasm is noted, 300 µg of intracoronary nitroglycerin should be given and arteriography repeated. Occasionally, if spasm continues to occur, cusp injections are done to rule out significant proximal obstructive coronary disease.

CONGENITAL CORONARY ANOMALIES. The presence of congenital coronary anomalies, when unsuspected, may lead to erroneous conclusions of total occlusions. The same maxims pertain in this situation as with selective cannulation of coronary vessels. When the angiographer suspects the presence of coronary anomalies, the use of a right coronary catheter or an A2 multipurpose catheter may make cannulation of these vessels easier. Occasionally, review of the ventriculogram or an aortic root injection may help to nonselectively identify the origin of these vessels, thereby allowing subsequent selective opacification of these vessels (Figs. 35.39 and 35.40).[37-40]

MYOCARDIAL BRIDGES. The epicardial coronary arteries may on occasion course intramyocardially. If this occurs, the result may be bridged by ventricular muscle. In this instance, during systole an area of obstruction may be seen (Fig. 35.41). The key to recognition of myocardial bridging is the absence of the stenosis during diastole.[41,42] Myocardial bridging uncommonly may be associated with ischemic episodes. In general, it is an inconsequential phenomenon, especially when unassociated with a significant clinical counterpart.

TOTAL OCCLUSION OF A CORONARY ARTERY. One of the most difficult problems to identify is total "flush" occlusion of a coronary artery at its origin. This may be mistaken for selective cannulation. On occasion, large septal perforators or diagonal vessels may be mistaken for the left anterior descending coronary artery. To avoid misinterpretation, the angiographer must be familiar with the typical course of the vessel in the various radiographic projections. In addition, the careful search for collateral vessels in the presence of a total proximal occlusion may be helpful (Fig. 35.42).

REFERENCES

1. The Principal Investigators of CASS and Their Associates: The National Heart, Lung and Blood Institute Coronary Artery Surgery Study (CASS). Circulation 63 (Suppl I):I-1, 1981
2. McAlpine WA: Heart and Coronary Arteries, p 203. New York, Springer-Verlag, 1975
3. Spindola-Franco H, Groser R, Solomon N: Dual left anterior descending coronary artery: Angiographic description of important variants and surgical implications. Am Heart J 105:445, 1983
4. Fergusson DJG, Kamada RO: Percutaneous entry of the brachial artery for left heart catheterization using a sheath: Further experience. Cathet Cardiovasc Diagn 12:209, 1986
5. Valeix B, Labrunie P, Jahjah F et al: Selective coronary arteriography by percutaneous transaxillary approach. Cathet Cardiovasc Diagn 10:403, 1984
6. Maseri A, Severi S, De Res M et al: Variant angina: One aspect of a continuous spectrum of vasospastic myocardial ischemia. Am J Cardiol 42:1019, 1978
7. Heupler FA, Proudfit WL, Razqui M et al: Erogonovine maleate provocative test for coronary arterial spasm. Am J Cardiol 41:631, 1978
8. Heupler FA: Syndrome of symptomatic coronary arterial spasm with nearly normal coronary arteriograms. Am J Cardiol 45:873, 1980
9. Bove AA, Vliestra RE: Spasm in ectastic coronary arteries. Mayo Clin Proc 60:822, 1985
10. Crosby JK, Mellons HA, Burwell L: Total occlusion of the left coronary: Incidence and management. J Thorac Cardiovasc Surg 77:389, 1979
11. Goldberg S, Grossman W, Markis JE et al: Total occlusion of the left main coronary artery: A clinical hemodynamic and angiographic profile. Am J Med 64:3, 1978
12. Bunnell IL, Greene DG, Tandon RN et al: The half-axial projection: A new look at the proximal left coronary artery. Circulation 68:1151, 1973
13. Green CE, Elliot LP, Rogers WJ et al: The importance of angled right anterior oblique views in improving visualization of the coronary arteries. Part I: Caudocranial view. Diagnostic Radiology 142:631, 1982
14. Elliot LP, Green CE, Rogers WJ et al: The importance of angled right anterior oblique views in improving visualization of the coronary arteries. Part II: Craniocaudal view. Diagnostic Radiology 142:637, 1982
15. Grover M, Slutsky R, Higgins C et al: Terminology and anatomy of angulated coronary arteriography. Clin Cardiol 7:37, 1984
16. Elliot LP, Bream PR, Soto B et al: Significance of the caudal left anterior oblique view in analyzing the left main coronary artery and its branches. Diagnostic Radiology 139:39, 1981
17. Arani DT, Bunnel IL, Greene DG et al: Lordotic right posterior oblique projection of the left coronary artery. Circulation 52:504, 1975
18. Miller RA, Felix WG, Warkentin DL et al: Angulated views in coronary anteriography. AJR 134:407, 1980
19. Staiger J, Dieckmann H, Adler CP et al: Post mortem angiographic and pathologic-anatomic findings in coronary artery disease: A comparative study using planimetry. Cardiovasc Intervent Radiol 3:139, 1980
20. Zir LM, Miller SW, Dinsmore RE et al: Interobserver variability in coronary angiography. Circulation 53:627, 1976
21. DeRouen TA, Murray JA, Owen W: Variability in the analysis of coronary arteriograms. Circulation 55:324, 1977
22. Gensini GG, Kelly AE, DaCosta BCB et al: Quantitative angiography: The measurement of coronary vasomobility in the intact animal and man. Chest 60:522, 1971
23. Feldman RL, Pepine CJ, Curry RC et al: Quantitative coronary arteriography using 105-mm photospot angiography and an optical magnifying device. Cathet Cardiovasc Diagn 5:195, 1979
24. White CW, Creighton BW, Doty DB et al: Does visual interpretation of the coronary arteriogram predict the physiologic significance of a coronary stenosis? N Engl J Med 310:819, 1984
25. Brown BG, Bolson E, Frimer M et al: Quantitative coronary arteriography: Estimation of dimensions, hemodynamic resistance, and atheroma mass of coronary artery lesions using the arteriogram and digital computation. Circulation 55:329, 1977
26. Harrison DG, White CW, Hiratzka CF et al: The value of lesion cross-sectional area determined by quantitative coronary angiography and assessing the physiologic significance of a proximal left anterior descending coronary artery stenosis. Circulation 69:1011, 1984
27. Gould KL, Kelley KO, Bolson EL et al: Experimental validation of quantitative coronary arteriography for determining pressure-flow characteristics of coronary stenosis. Circulation 66:930, 1982
28. Selzer RH, Blankenhorn DH, Crawford DW et al: Computer analyses of cardiovascular imaging. In Proceedings of the Caltext/JPL Conference on Image Processing Technology, Data Sources and Software for Commercial and Scientific Applications, p 1. Pasadena, 1976
29. Ledbetter DC, Selzer RH, Gordon RN et al: Computer quantitation of coronary angiograms. In Miller HA, Smitch EV, Harrison DC (eds): Noninvasive Cardiovascular Measurements. Society of Photo-Optical Instrumentation 167:17, 1978
30. Reiber JH, Serruys PW, Kooijman CJ et al: Assessment of short-, medium-, and long-term variations in arterial dimensions for computer-assisted quantitation of coronary angiograms. Circulation 71:280, 1985
31. Aldermane E, Berte LE, Harrison DC et al: Quantitation of coronary artery dimensions using digital image processing. In Brodey WR (ed): Digital Radioarteriography. Society of Photo-Optical Instrumentation 314:273, 1982
32. Serruys PW, Reiber JHC, Wijns W et al: Assessment of percutaneous transluminal coronary angioplasty by quantitative coronary angiography: Diameter vs. densitometric area measurements. Am J Cardiol 54:482, 1984
33. Adams DF, Fraser DB, Abrams HL et al: The complications of coronary arteriography. Circulation 48:609, 1973
34. Davis K, Kennedy WJ, Kemp HG et al: Complications of coronary arteriography from the collaborative study of coronary artery surgery (CASS). Circulation 59:1105, 1979
35. Kennedy WJ, Baxley WA, Bunnell IL et al: Mortality related to cardiac catheterization and angiography. Cathet Cardiovasc Diagn 8:323, 1982
36. Braunwald E: Deaths related to cardiac catheterization. Am Heart J 38–39:III-17, 1968
37. Stewart WJ, McSweeney SM: Increased risk of severe protamine reactions in NPH insulin-dependent diabetics undergoing cardiac catheterization. Circulation 70:788, 1984
38. Roberts WC: Major anomalies of coronary arterial origin seen in adulthood. Am Heart J 111:941, 1986
39. Liberthson RR, Dinsmore RE: Aberrant coronary artery origin from the aorta: Diagnosis and clinical significance. Circulation 50:774, 1974
40. Blake HA, Manion WC: Coronary artery anomalies. Circulation 30:927, 1964
41. Blook CM, Lowman RM: Myocardial bridges in coronary angiography. Am Heart J 654:1985, 1963
42. Geiringer E: The mural coronary artery. Am Heart J 50:359, 1950

GENERAL REFERENCES

Gensini GG: Coronary Arteriography, p 163. Mount Kisko, NY, Futura, 1975
Grossman W: Cardiac Catheterization and Angiography, p 173. Philadelphia, Lea & Febiger, 1986
King SB, Douglas JS: Coronary Arteriography and Angioplasty. New York, McGraw-Hill, 1985

Cardiac Digital Angiography

Neal Eigler ▪ James S. Forrester

CHAPTER 36 · VOLUME 1

Although film-based ventriculography and coronary angiography are standards against which noninvasive diagnostic tests are assessed and are often the basis for therapeutic decisions, they have four important limitations: (1) Chemical processing delays review of the definitive image until it is generally too late to repeat an inconclusive study, which frequently results in the acquisition of more views than are actually needed for diagnosis. (2) There is redundancy in the information content of the 150 to 200 images of a typical cineangiographic run, resulting in unnecessary radiation exposure to the patient and angiographer. (3) Subjective image interpretation is neither accurate nor reproducible. (4) The images may contain hidden diagnostic information that is not readily extracted by visual inspection.

Since the early 1980s, the development of cardiac digital angiography has been based on the premise that a digital format would hasten image processing and display, allow more flexible image acquisition protocols, and facilitate the extraction of quantitative parameters from images, improving diagnostic accuracy and reducing subjective variability. In this chapter the focus is on the established and potential advantages as well as the limitations of digital angiography for the quantitative assessment of cardiac function and coronary anatomy.

TECHNICAL CONSIDERATIONS

Digital angiographic systems acquire, store, retrieve, and process radiographic images in an electronic format used by digital computers. A digital angiographic system for cardiac evaluation must accommodate the special requirements of ventricular and coronary angiographic imaging created by cardiac and respiratory motion as well as the small size of objects to be evaluated diagnostically (*e.g.*, coronary stenoses). A detailed discussion of the technology supporting digital angiography is beyond the scope of the chapter, and the reader is referred to previous comprehensive reviews.[1,2]

Figure 36.1 is a simplified schematic diagram of a typical cardiac digital system consisting of (1) a cine x-ray generator/x-ray tube capable of continuous fluoroscopy or production of pulsed x-rays of 60 kVp to 120 kVp at 1 mA to 1000 mA for 1 msec to 8 msec at rates up to 30 pulses per second; (2) an image receptor system comprising a cesium iodide image intensifier tube, coupling optical lenses, and a low noise, linear, progressive scan video camera[3]; (3) an analog-to-digital (A/D) converter, or image digitizer, that changes the video signal into a series of digital numbers; (4) an image processor, which is a highly specialized computer for accepting digital images and performing mathematical operations on one or several images simultaneously; (5) digital storage devices, such as digital disks for temporary storage at transfer rates of up to 30 frames per second or magnetic tapes for long-term storage at slow transfer rates (1 frame per second); (6) display devices, such as a video monitor, videotape recorder, or multiformat camera; and (7) a host computer for controlling the previously listed devices and communicating with the operator. During image acquisition, the host computer must synchronize the x-ray generator pulses with the television camera, A/D converter, image processor, and image storage devices. The same computer controls the recall of images from storage to the image processor for postacquisition processing and subsequent display.

Images are created and transmitted as follows: X-rays striking the input phosphor of the image intensifier are converted into a two-dimensional visible light image on the output phosphor. The light image is focused onto the video camera pickup tube, where it is scanned by an electron beam from top to bottom as a stack of parallel horizontal lines or rasters and thus converted into an electronic video signal. Most video systems use 525 lines per image, although newer systems are capable of higher spatial resolution at 1023 lines per image. Digitization converts the video signal into a two-dimensional matrix of rectangular picture elements (pixels), each with unique coordinates corresponding to a position in the image. Most commonly, digital images are composed of matrices of 256^2, 512^2, or, with high-resolution systems, 1024^2 pixels. Each pixel is assigned to its own address within the image processor memory and given a discrete integer value proportional to its brightness (gray level). For example, in many systems, the pixel values range from 0 = black to 255 = white; thus, there are 256 gray levels. A new video picture is generated 30 times each second. Therefore, to acquire images at maximal frame rates, a typical system must be capable of digitizing, storing, and processing information at a rate of $512^2 \times 30 = 7.86 \times 10^6$ pixels per second. Following acquisition, digital image processing techniques are used to enhance image contrast; to quantify cardiac function, coronary stenosis, and myocardial perfusion; and to display complex information in clinically useful formats.

The major and most vexing limitation of cardiac digital angiographic systems available today is cumbersome image archiving and retrieval. Commercially available digital disks can temporarily store enough images for one or two complete patient examinations. Although large numbers of images can be conveniently transferred for long-term storage in analog form on videotape or disk, image quality is seriously degraded by the technical limitations of these media. Newer systems allow simultaneous acquisition of digital and standard cine film images. Selected digital images may be saved for subsequent processing and quantification while cine film provides a high-resolution durable long-term record. A satisfactory method for archiving and retrieving digital information with the storage capacity, speed, and reliability required for practical daily use remains an elusive goal that will have to be resolved before digital angiography can totally replace film in the cardiac catheterization laboratory.

CONTRAST ENHANCEMENT

Image contrast differences can be enhanced by alteration of the gray scale, temporal subtraction, and digital spatial filtering.[1,4] A window can be created that looks at only a portion of the gray scale where all pixel values below the window will be changed to black and all values above the window will become white. Additionally, the level of the center of the window on the gray scale can be changed or the gray scale itself can be transformed from a linear function of pixel intensity by any mathematical function (*e.g.*, a logarithmic function).

Two temporal image subtraction methods have been applied to increase contrast. Mask-mode subtraction creates an image of iodine-containing vessels by subtracting preinjection images (the mask) from those containing contrast material. This requires that the heart be in the same position for both the mask and the angiographic image, because nonalignment causes misregistration artifacts in the subtracted image. It is possible largely to eliminate these artifacts by either prospectively gating image acquisitions to the electrocardiogram or retrospectively subtracting masks that correspond to the same portion of the cardiac cycle.[5,6] Additionally, patient immobility, and thus rigorous breath holding, is required. Although these images are often spectacular (Fig. 36.2) because of the uniform background and high contrast, they may, even under ideal circumstances be misregistered because of respiratory motion and beat-to-beat changes in heart rate, cardiac chamber volume, and contractility. Reregistration algorithms have been developed, but they are time consuming and may create additional artifacts.

The second form of subtraction is time interval difference subtraction. Sets of frames separated by only a few frame times are subtracted, resulting in images of the difference in contrast levels between each frame pair. Both forms of temporal subtraction were widely applied in early investigations of digital coronary angiography; however, motion misregistration artifacts often make these images difficult to subjectively interpret or to apply automated quantification techniques.

Image contrast can also be enhanced by digital spatial filtration. Each raw image can be considered to contain true information plus artifacts that degrade the image but that may be removed by spatial filtration. One major artifact is image unsharpness or blur due to focal spot unsharpness and light diffusion in the input phosphor of the image intensifier tube. Focal spot unsharpness occurs because x-rays emanate from a spatially extended source on the anode instead of from a

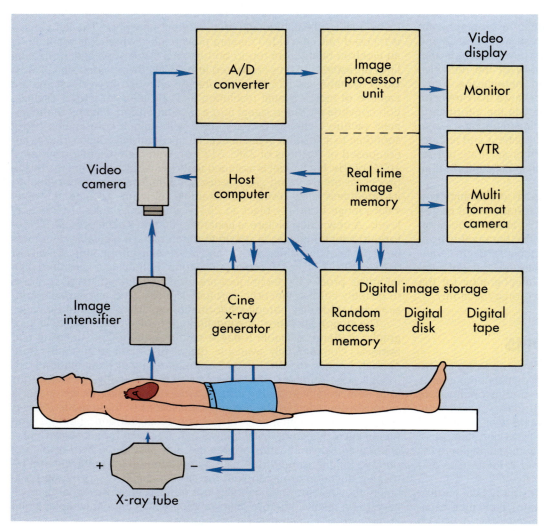

FIGURE 36.1 Schematic diagram of a typical cardiac digital angiography system.

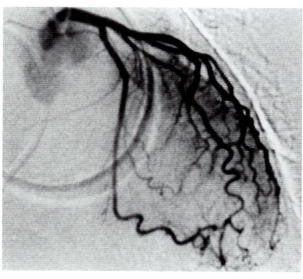

FIGURE 36.2 ECG-gated masked-mode digital subtraction coronary angiogram. Although this image is of diagnostic quality with high contrast and low noise and much of the underlying background structure has been removed, misregistration artifacts are present and may contribute to errors in stenosis quantification.

single point source. Thus objects do not cast single sharp shadows. Typical values for the width of these sources of blur are about 0.3 mm. The system blur can be measured and removed from the image by a process called deconvolution in which every pixel is modified according to the values of surrounding pixels. An advantage of this technique is that there are no misregistration artifacts due to motion. The filtered image has sharper, more distinct vessel edge borders that make their perception and quantification easier. Such edge-enhancing filters are now commercially available and are capable of performing at video acquisition rates (real time).

A primary source of contrast loss is due to scattered x-rays and to light and electron scattering within the image intensifier tube, known as veiling glare. Scatter is spatially variant within the image and may typically account for 30% to 50% of pixel brightness, thus reducing image contrast. Digital filters have been developed to remove scatter;[7-9] however, at present, these techniques require a calibration object to be present in the image, are slow, and must be performed offline. Both spatial filter techniques can be used to improve image quality (spatial and contrast resolution), which may enhance the clinical utility of these images.

In the future, another form of subtraction that makes use of the differential absorption characteristics of iodine for x-rays according to their energy (energy subtraction) may play an important role. With this technique, the iodine-containing vessels are alternately pulsed only a few milliseconds apart with nearly monochromatic x-ray beams at different energies just above and below the K-edge of iodine (33 keV) to take advantage of the large difference in x-ray absorption. If x-rays can be pulsed in very quick succession (*i.e.*, within 4 msec to 6 msec), minimal appreciable motion will occur and therefore perfectly registered subtraction can be performed with maximal contrast enhancement and complete elimination of background structures. This technique requires extremely sophisticated x-ray generating and image-acquisitions equipment including a linear accelerator to provide an intense synchrotron radiation source. These devices are only in the early stages of development but appear to hold promise because preliminary studies suggest that diagnostic quality coronary angiograms can be obtained following less invasive intravenous contrast injections.[1,10-12]

IMAGE QUALITY

Reliable computer quantification of stenosis requires high-quality images. Image quality is determined by the imaging systems spatial resolution, contrast resolution, and system noise and is limited by permissible radiation dose to the patient and x-ray tube loading. Development of automated quantification programs requires strict attentions to these aspects.[13,14]

The spatial resolution inherent in a digital image is particularly important. One advantage of conventional cine angiography is that the tiny grains of photographic film resolve objects smaller than the ideal limits of the x-ray imaging chain (four to five line pairs per millimeter using a 15-cm image intensifier). In contrast, the individual pixels of a typical digital image are roughly two times larger (1.9 line pairs per millimeter for a 512 × 512-pixel matrix) and thus introduce a potential source of inaccuracy. There are three lines of evidence to suggest that this inherent difference in spatial resolution is not a limiting problem. First, the effective spatial resolution of a cine film image in the clinical setting is no more than two line pairs per millimeter because motion unsharpness, quantum mottle, scatter, glare, and x-ray focal spot blurring degrade the image.[13,14] Second, a 512 × 512-pixel matrix can detect angiographic contrast medium–containing vessels with a cross-sectional area of 0.3 mm^2, the expected size of a "critical" coronary stenosis where flow is reduced under resting conditions.[15-17] Third, we and others have shown that the subjective interpretation of percent diameter coronary stenosis using a 512 × 512-pixel digital format correlates closely with the same interpretations from 35-mm cine film.[18,19] Accurate vessel edge detection is equally dependent on high-contrast resolution, an area in which digital angiography excels. Tobis and co-workers have demonstrated that the mask-mode subtraction 512 × 512-pixel format yields values for coronary stenosis similar to those obtained by direct caliper measurement from cine film.[20] This suggests that, although the spatial resolution for 512 × 512-pixel digital images may not be optimum, the enhanced contrast detectability may provide diagnostic perceptibility equal to that of film.

System noise is the major reason for loss of image detail. The major source of this noise is x-ray quantum mottle, the statistical fluctuation in the number of x-ray photons striking the image intensifier. Quantum noise produces random error in the perception and measurement of arterial diameter. This error is greatest for small-diameter vessels because of their lower radiographic contrast. Quantum mottle can be reduced by increasing the x-ray dose for each frame because noise is proportional to $1/(dose)^{1/2}$. The problems encountered in increasing radiation dose are patient safety and excessive tube loading. ECG-gated image acquisition protocols may reduce the number of images obtain from standard 30 frames per second by a factor of 10. This permits a 10-fold increase in dose per frame and thus a 68% reduction in quantum noise. Whether slow acquisition frame rates will miss stenoses that are only demonstrated by the rapid cardiac rotation during systole remains to be determined. A second significant noise source, background clutter, also known as patient structure noise, is caused by overlying anatomy, including bones and soft tissue. This type of noise can be largely removed by mask-mode subtraction.

DIGITAL ANGIOCARDIOGRAPHY AND QUANTITATIVE MEASUREMENTS OF MYOCARDIAL FUNCTION

Digitized ventricular images can be processed to quantify ejection fraction, chamber volumes, and segmental wall motion by two independent analytic techniques. The first technique (geometric) uses manual or automatic edge detection to delineate physical dimensions to which established formulas (*e.g.*, area × length equations) are then applied. The second approach (densitometric) uses videodensitometry to estimate iodine concentration, which can be calibrated to determine blood volume.

Vas and colleagues[21] first demonstrated that intravenous digital angiography could accurately quantify left ventricular volume and ejection fraction in animals and humans using standard geometric formulas developed by Sandler and Dodge.[22] Subsequently, chamber volume, cardiac output, left ventricular wall thickness, and left ventricular mass measurements by digital left ventriculography have been validated in animal studies.[23-25] Using a geometric approach, multiple investigators have reported excellent correlations between intravenous or direct-injection digital left ventriculography with standard cine left ventriculography in human subjects for the calculation of ejection fraction and end-systolic and end-diastolic volumes.[26-34] Mask-mode subtracted intravenous digital ventriculography underestimates ventricular volume by 2% to 7%; however, this does not occur following direct left ventricular injection. These differences are probably due to errors introduced by suboptimal ventricular opacification and difficulty in estimating the location of the mitral valve plane following intravenous contrast injection. These differences are minor, correctable, and not likely to be of clinical significance.

The most popular geometric algorithms measure left ventricular volume by assuming that the chamber is an ellipsoid. This assumption breaks down, however, when segmental contraction abnormalities alter the basic shape of the ventricle. Densitometric assessment of relative left ventricular volume is independent of geometric assumptions and provides accurate estimates of ejection fraction.[35-37] Densitometric measurements of absolute chamber volume are somewhat less accurate than geometric measurements because of uncorrected error caused by x-ray scatter, image receptor veiling glare, and beam-hardening artifacts.[38-41]

Diagnostic quality digital left ventriculograms can be routinely obtained in 90% to 95% of patients following a 30-ml to 50-ml peripheral or central venous contrast medium injection with fluoroscopic doses of x-ray without ventricular ectopy. Alternatively a 5-ml to 10-ml direct left ventricular injection yields good ventricular opacification with minimal hemodynamic derangement.

Both geometric and densitometric techniques have been applied to quantify right ventricular function. Lange and associates reported that right ventricular volumes determined geometrically from biplane digital angiograms were concordant with a similar cineangiographic method in 25 children.[42] The digital technique required only one third the dose of contrast material and 60% less x-ray dose and produced 60% fewer ventricular ectopic beats than conventional angiography. Detrano and co-workers used a videodensitometric method and found a high correlation between right ventricular ejection fraction and first-pass radionuclide imaging.[43]

Because the ventricular image obtained by venous injection of contrast material is substantially superior to technetium-99m blood pool imaging, digital ventriculography has been used to assess left ventricular function in response to stress in patients with suspected coronary artery disease. Goldberg and colleagues studied intravenous digital ventriculography during supine bicycle exercise.[44] Acceptable images were obtained in 29 of 31 patients, and exercise ejection fraction correlated closely with radionuclide ventriculography. Nevertheless, the procedure has not found wide acceptance because digital subtraction imaging requires breath holding, which is difficult during and immediately after strenuous exercise.

To circumvent this problem, other investigators have performed digital ventriculography in conjunction with rapid atrial pacing. Tobis and colleagues showed that the response of ejection fraction to pacing has a sensitivity of 93% and a specificity of 83% for the detection of stenoses of more than 70% diameter narrowing in patients with suspected coronary artery disease.[45] Johnson and co-workers demonstrated that the development of new regional wall motion abnormalities accurately predicted the presence of coronary stenosis in 89% of patients referred for coronary angiography.[46] In comparison, a fall in left ventricular ejection fraction during exercise as determined by intravenous digital subtraction angiography is also a sensitive way (greater than 90%) to detect coronary disease in patients without infarction and to detect multivessel disease in patients with previous myocardial infarction; however, the specificity was much lower (less than 72%), indicating a high false-positive rate.[47,48] The development of a new regional wall motion abnormality in response to exercise was only moderately sensitive and specific for the detection of coronary artery disease in these same groups of patients. These results suggest that pacing or stress digital ventriculography will remain a secondary tool for evaluating the severity of disease, because it as yet offers no clear advantages over noninvasive methods already in widespread use.

An important contribution of digital ventriculographic analysis is its potential to resolve the high variability among angiographers in the subjective assessment of regional wall motion.[49-51] The magnitude of this problem is substantial: we found disagreement between three independent observers in 60% of myocardial regions analyzed, and 53% of the disagreements were major (two or more grades on a 0-5 scale).[28] Furthermore, we have found that angiographers systematically modify their interpretation of wall motion to make it consistent with coronary anatomy when this information is provided.[52] In 56% of cases, angiographers' interpretations overestimated regional dysfunction when they knew that the coronary artery supplying the regions was narrowed or underestimated dysfunction when they knew that the vessels were normal. Automated analysis of regional function eliminates this subjective bias.

Mancini and co-workers compared mask-mode intravenous digital subtraction angiography with direct left ventricular injection using an automated geometric regional wall motion algorithm in 45 patients with suspected coronary artery disease.[53] Percentage of shortening was measured along seven radii at 45° angles originating from the centroid of the end-diastolic left ventricular cavity tracing. "Normal" shortening for each ray was defined as the mean ± 1.5 standard deviations of fractional shortening observed in segments subjectively evaluated as normal by three observers. Overall agreement between techniques was 87%, with identical categorization for 274 of the 315 radii examined. Interobserver and intraobserver variability for shortening measurements were ±5.3% and ±8.8%, respectively. Using the same analysis, digital ventriculograms performed following rapid atrial pacing correctly differentiated a small number of patients for the presence or absence of coronary artery disease. There is as yet no evidence that computer quantification of regional wall motion is more accurate than subjective evaluation; however, these early results suggest that reproducibility is improved.

Automatic quantification of regional wall motion creates two new problems. First, there is no agreed reference system for superimposing the end-diastolic and end-systolic silhouettes. Second, conventional descriptors of wall motion, such as dyskinesis, akinesis, and hypokinesis, have no widely accepted method of measurement and no established range of normal and abnormal excursion.[54-57]

To address these problems, we studied 767 direct-injection left ventriculograms in patients referred for the diagnosis of coronary artery disease.[58] Following subjective analysis, 442 (57%) were interpreted as having normal wall motion in all segments and 83 of these ventriculograms were associated with normal coronary angiograms. Fractional shortening was determined for each of 100 rays extending from the end-diastolic centroid to the cavity perimeter. Four different orientations of the end-systolic and end-diastolic silhouettes were examined: (1) no correction (i.e., fixed external reference), (2) correction for rotation by alignment of the two long axes, (3) correction for translation by superimposition of the two area centroids, and (4) correction for rotation and translation.

For "normal" ventricles, the values for systolic shortening were similar for all four orientations, but the variance of the uncorrected algorithm was 53% lower than in the other three reference systems, which suggests that this reference system is the most reproducible. This finding is consistent with the prior work of Sheehan and co-workers.[56] This uncorrected reference system also most closely corresponds to the traditional external reference employed in visual assessment and thus represents a quantification of subjective judgment. Therefore, we chose this model to develop our normal and abnormal categories.

The "normal" range was established for each of the 100 rays by modeling the distribution of fractional shortening of each ray from the normal ventriculograms as a β-distribution and determining the 90% confidence intervals. Similar distribution modeling was performed for rays in regions labeled as hypokinetic, akinetic, or dyskinetic. No significant differences in fractional shortening were seen between regions designated akinetic and dyskinetic, and enormous overlap was observed between hypokinetic and normal regions. This overlap is the result of the inherently high variability of subjective interpretation. Therefore, subjective analysis of regional wall motion is unreliable and impractical because normal shortening varies widely from segment to segment.

The advantages of this system of automated regional wall motion analysis are that it was derived from a large clinical experience; it is highly reproducible for the categorization of segments as normal, equivocal, or abnormal; and it takes into account regional variations in segment shortening. Figure 36.3 is an example of our automated analysis program for digital left ventriculography.

Densitometric methods have also been applied to quantify regional left ventricular ejection fraction before and after rapid atrial pacing.[59,60] Preliminary studies indicate that densitometry is simpler, faster, more reproducible, and more sensitive and specific for detecting coronary artery disease than geometric measurements of area or radial ejection changes. The other advantages of regional densitometric measurements are (1) it is independent of ventricular geometry and thus allows a three-dimensional assessment of the left ventricle from a single projection and (2) precise detection of either the end-diastolic or end-systolic cavity borders are not required.

Digital ventriculography thus has several advantages in comparison with conventional film-based angiography. Analysis of both global and regional ventricular performance is quick, simple, and highly reproducible. In practice, intravenous contrast injection is less invasive, produces no ventricular ectopy, and yields a homogeneously opacified ventricular image that is beneficial for densitometric analysis; conversely, direct left ventricular injection reduces the contrast dose to less than one third of that needed for cineangiography and allows serial assessment of ventricular function during cardiac catheterization.

Densitometric quantification of the severity of valvular regurgitation is another area where digital angiography may be advantageous. Aortic regurgitant fraction can be measured following aortic root injection as the difference in areas under simultaneous time-density curves acquired over the aortic root and the left ventricle. Animal validation studies have shown excellent correlations between densitometric quantification and direct flowmeter measurements.[61] The theoretical advantages of densitometry are that it is independent of geometric assumptions and may be less influenced by mitral regurgitation than the standard comparison of angiographic and Fick or thermodilution-determined cardiac output.

Researchers from Kiel, West Germany, and the Cleveland Clinic have examined the application of digital angiography following intravenous or arterial contrast medium injection in pediatric and adult patients with congenital heart disease.[62,63] These studies show that adequate visualization of the size, shape, and relationship of cardiac chambers and great vessels can be achieved, and intracardiac shunts can be measured by densitometric quantification for the full spectrum of congenital heart disease, including suspected left-to-right shunts (atrial septal defect, ventricular septal defect, patent ductus arteriosus), cyanotic heart disease (tetralogy of Fallot, transposition, truncus, tricuspid atresia, total anomalous pulmonary venous return, single ventricle), and aortic coarctation. Furthermore, digital angiographic findings were judged to be sufficiently diagnostic to exclude totally or eliminate part of a cardiac catheterization procedure in over 90% of patients studied. The effectiveness of surgical repair can often be confirmed by central venous contrast injection during the immediate postoperative period. Selective injection digital angiography may be helpful during cardiac catheterization in identifying poorly opacified structures, reducing contrast dose, or minimizing the hemodynamic effects of large bolus contrast injection. For these indications, digital angiography appears to be an acceptable alternative to film-based angiography, with the inherent advantages of being less invasive and requiring smaller doses of contrast material and radiation exposure. As such, many diagnostic procedures in the pediatric age group may now be performed on an outpatient basis. The eventual role of digital angiography in the diagnosis of congenital heart disease remains uncertain, however, because advances in nonradiographic imaging technologies such as color Doppler echocardiography may permit noninvasive visualization and quantification of these abnormalities.

CORONARY ANGIOGRAPHY

The initial results that showed excellent coronary opacification following aortic root contrast injection in animals have not been obtained in human subjects. In general, images of only fair quality are obtained. Contrast filling of the coronary arteries by aortic root injection is limited by the injectate volume that can be delivered during the diastolic coronary filling period. Very little of the injectate delivered during systole passes into the coronary circulation; therefore, aortic root injections need to be electrocardiographically triggered during two to three diastoles. Additionally, at least one coronary ostia is obscured by the

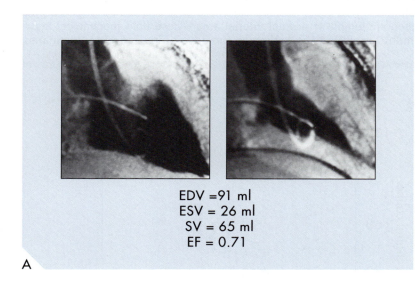

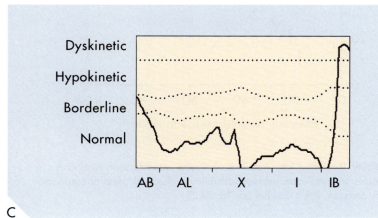

FIGURE 36.3 Automated global and regional wall motion analysis. **A.** End-diastolic and end-systolic frames of a digital left ventriculogram obtained in the 30° right anterior oblique projection following direct injection of 10 ml of radiographic contrast medium. After tracing the silhouettes with a light pen, the computer calculates end-diastolic volume (*EDV*), end-systolic volume (*ESV*), stroke volume (*SV*), and ejection fraction (*EF*). **B.** The two silhouettes are superimposed to demonstrate the extent of regional shortening. **C.** Regional shortening of each of 100 rays (*dark line*) originating from the end-diastolic centroid. The x axis is the position of each ray with respect to five cardiac segments. The y axis is the percentage of regional shortening. For each ray, the limits for normal and abnormal shortening (*dotted lines*) were determined by β-distribution modeling of 767 angiograms.

opacified aortic root, leaving a sometimes crucial coronary segment unvisualized. Digital aortic root injection may serve a minor role in delineating the origin of a coronary artery or documenting bypass graft patency when selective cannulation is difficult; however, similar information is often obtained following intravenous injection, albeit with a lower sensitivity (95% vs. 75%).[64-67] We believe, however, that digital aortic root injection is unlikely to challenge selective coronary angiography as the primary diagnostic procedure for the evaluation of coronary artery disease. Nevertheless, digital angiography has an important role in coronary angiography.

A major weakness of conventional coronary angiography is that subjective interpretation of coronary stenosis severity is inaccurate. Whereas several investigators have compared coronary stenoses measured from the coronary angiogram with direct postmortem studies and have reported that "angiographers routinely and significantly underestimate the severity of stenoses,"[68,69] others have reported that the frequency of overestimation and underestimation are approximately the same.[70,71] Two morphologic features explain these findings: (1) atherosclerosis is often diffuse, thus the diameter of the 'normal' coronary segment is underestimated, and (2) stenoses are frequently eccentric or polymorphous and, in the extreme case, may have a slit-like lumen.[72-74]

Subjective stenosis evaluation is further complicated because interpretations between observers, and even for the same observer, are not reproducible. Bjork and co-workers reported complete agreement between four observers in only 37% of coronary angiographic interpretations, and in 40% of the observations the variability was greater than 20%.[75] This lack of agreement in the subjective interpretation of coronary angiograms has been confirmed repeatedly.[76-79] For example, in the Coronary Artery Surgery Study (CASS), interobserver disagreement between normal and more than 50% diameter narrowing occurred in 15% of the coronary arteries studied.[79] Intraobserver reproducibility may be improved by the use of broad categories[80]; however, Galbraith and co-workers found an 18% misclassification rate using the broadest possible categories (greater or less than 50% diameter stenosis).[70] These data substantiate the need for a less subjective, more reproducible technique for quantifying coronary stenosis severity.

These limitations seem ideally suited to resolution by automated computer processing. A detailed discussion of the methods and limitations in quantifying coronary anatomy from coronary angiography can be found in several recent reviews.[81-83]

Early attempts to objectively assess coronary anatomy employed mechanical or electromechanical calipers to measure the percentage of vessel diameter narrowing from cine-film images.[72,80,84] Similarly, digital calipers using movable cursor points can be conveniently applied directly to digital images. Digital caliper measurement markedly and significantly improves intraobserver and interobserver reproducibility (Fig. 36.4).[18,85,86] For subjective analysis, variability is largest for stenoses of moderate severity; with digital calipers, both intraobserver and interobserver variability were narrow and uniformly distributed without relation to the severity of stenosis.[18]

Although the percentage of diameter measurements are currently the standard for determining severity of coronary artery disease, they are limited by three problems: (1) lack of an objective criteria for choosing the "normal" coronary diameter, especially when diffuse atherosclerosis or post-stenotic dilatation is present; (2) poor definition of vessel boundaries resulting from x-ray/optical system noise; and (3) inaccurate analysis of asymmetrical lesions in single-plane projections. Even if these problems were resolved, fundamental objections to using a relative measurement like the percentage of stenosis still remain. These measurements are poor predictors of the physiologic importance of coronary stenoses with regard to resting flow or coronary vasodilatory reserve, and, in practice, they are of only limited use for predicting the development of unstable ischemic syndromes and mortality.[87-91] A crucial issue, therefore, is to determine which morphologic feature(s) of coronary stenosis best reflects its functional significance.

Fluid mechanical principles have been applied to develop the relationship between pressure gradient, flow, and vascular resistance under ideal circumstances.[92,93] These studies show that the hemodynamic significance of a stenosis is primarily affected by the minimal stenotic cross-sectional area as its influence is squared compared with stenotic length or normal arterial area. These fluid mechanical arguments provided the rationale for developing more sophisticated

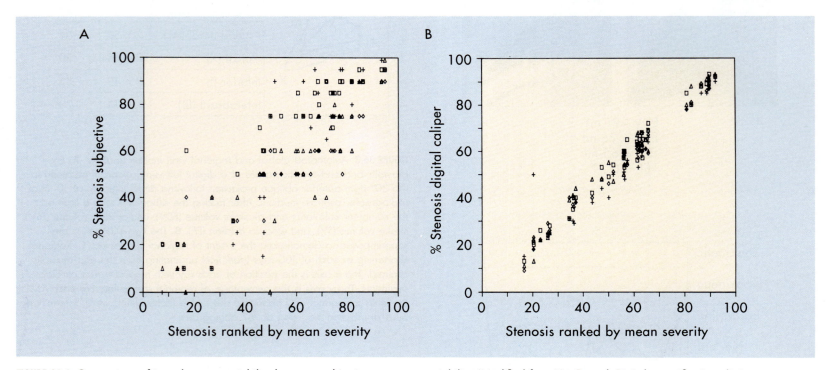

FIGURE 36.4 Comparison of interobserver variability between subjective reading (A) and digital caliper measurement of the percentage diameter stenosis (B). Thirty-six stenoses were evaluated by four angiographers using both methods. Digital caliper measurement significantly reduced interobserver variability. (Modified from Vas R et al: Digital quantification eliminates intraobserver and interobserver variability in the evaluation of coronary artery stenosis. Am J Cardiol 56:718, 1985)

methods to quantify the three-dimensional attributes of coronary stenoses.

Brown and colleagues developed quantitative coronary angiography (QCA), a technique for three-dimensional reconstruction of selected coronary arteries from biplane angiograms.[94] Single-frame images from orthogonal projections during the same portion of the cardiac cycle are selected and magnified five times, and the coronary edges are manually traced with a device that digitized the coordinates. Coronary dimensions are corrected for magnification by measuring the projected size of a known object such as a catheter and for radially symmetrical image intensifier pincushion distortion. The minimal cross-sectional area is calculated by assuming the minimal diameters in the two tracings are the major and minor axes of an ellipse. Values for minimal stenotic area, ellipticity, atheroma mass, and segmental resistance are derived from the elliptical reconstruction. Although phantom and injected postmortem sections suggest that this method is highly accurate and reproducible to within 0.10 mm to 0.15 mm, concern has been expressed that system blur, motion, scatter, complex plaque geometry, and contrast dilution make this degree of accuracy overly optimistic for clinical application.[95,96] Furthermore there are errors associated with subjective edge tracing, with the assumption that minimal diameter in each view occurs at the same point, that the calibration object has the same magnification as the stenosis, and with reconstructing eccentric stenoses from two arbitrary orthogonal projections.[97,98]

Nevertheless, QCA clearly represents a significant improvement over previous methods. Although QCA has not achieved clinical acceptance because it is too cumbersome and time consuming for routine use (20 minutes per stenosis), it has been extensively used as a clinical research tool. McMahon an co-workers found that QCA differentiated patients with rest angina from non–Q wave infarction (minimal stenotic area 0.63 ± 0.19 mm^2 vs. 0.35 ± 0.11 mm^2) and suggested that small increases in lesion severity may precipitate myocardial infarction.[17] Harrison and colleagues measured coronary flow reserve by epicardial Doppler flow probe during cardiac surgery in 23 patients with isolated stenosis of the proximal left anterior descending artery and found that minimal stenotic area predicted flow reserve while relative measurements such as percent diameter or percent area narrowing did not.[99] Gould and colleagues found a good correlation between QCA predicted and measured trans-stenotic pressure gradients over the full range of coronary flow rates in dogs.[100] Using sophisticated fluid mechanical modeling, this group has been able to integrate multiple QCA parameters including minimal stenotic cross-sectional area, normal artery cross-sectional area, and stenosis length to accurately predict coronary flow reserve for ideal stenoses.[101] Despite these data, the use of coronary dimensions to predict individual patient flow dynamics is limited by the complex nature of coronary atherosclerosis, which include asymmetric morphology, changes in severity during the cardiac cycle, multiple serial stenoses, diffuse atherosclerosis, multivessel disease, coronary collaterals, and so on.

Although automatic edge detection would eliminate subjective bias, there is no widely agreed upon algorithm for finding the true vessel edges from noisy/blurred images. In the absence of these artifacts, the edges of an artery can be very precisely defined as both the first and second derivative of the contrast density profile are maximum at the edge (Fig. 36.5). In practice, however, there are systematic errors, with the first derivative underestimating and the second derivative overestimating the true vessel diameter. One method to minimize these errors uses an empirically weighted average of the maximum first and second derivative edges.[102]

A second method for locating the edges of an artery is to find the best match between the blurred edge of the angiographic image and a mathematical model that is calibrated to represent the actual blurring characteristics of the imaging system.[13,103] This process is called cross-correlation. Its primary advantage over the differentiation-based methods is that it is less sensitive to noise.

Both of these automatic edge detection methods have a precision of 0.15 mm; however, neither is capable of accurately measuring cross-sectional area of asymmetrical or eccentric stenoses. An additional limitation is that vessels with diameters smaller than about twice the blur size will be overestimated. This means that the smallest stenosis that can be accurately quantified by edge detection is approximately 0.6 mm in diameter, which corresponds to an 80% stenosis in a 3-mm artery.[15]

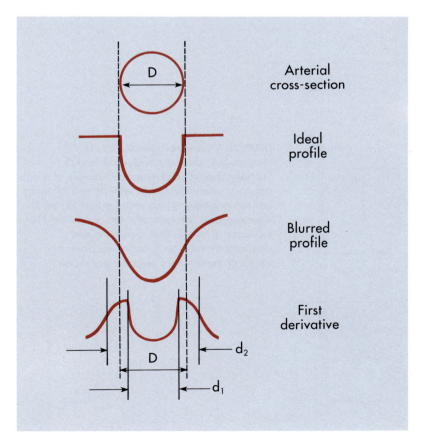

FIGURE 36.5 Schematic representation of how image unsharpness makes edges ambiguous in the density profile of a coronary artery. The true artery diameter is underestimated by the distance between the locations of the peak first derivative (d_1) and underestimated by the peak second derivative (d_2).

These limitations of edge detection may be overcome by using videodensitometry to determine the cross-sectional area from a single view.[104] This concept is illustrated in Figure 36.6, which shows that integrating the contrast density under the densitometric profile is directly proportional to the cross-sectional area of the artery irrespective of the shape of the lumen. The densitometric approach is also much less sensitive to quantum noise and image blur. Unlike edge detection, however, the densitometric approach depends on the assumption that contrast material completely displaces blood in the artery. In addition, to achieve a linear relationship between contrast material thickness and image brightness it is necessary to correct for scatter and veiling glare.

Automatic edge detection and densitometric integration techniques have now been validated extensively in x-ray phantoms and with *in vitro* histopathologic correlations. In animal models with artificial coronary stenoses, edge detection techniques appear to have less variability. On the other hand, densitometric techniques have been shown to be more accurate for assessing eccentric stenoses. Studies in humans have had promising results showing good correlations with epicardial echo coronary imaging and coronary flow reserve before and after interventions such as balloon angioplasty.[16,105-118] Figure 36.7 is a clinical example of our current coronary analysis algorithm that generates geometric and densitometric coronary indices.

In the past several years there has been evolving evidence from pathologic and angioscopic studies that atherosclerotic plaque disruption (fissuring, ulceration, or hemorrhage, with or without thrombosis) is present in an overwhelming percentage of patients presenting with sudden death, myocardial infarction, or unstable angina.[119-122] Qualitative angiographic features of plaque disruption, including a "complicated" angiographic appearance characterized by irregular luminal borders and filling defects, have been described for unstable angina and Q wave and non–Q wave acute myocardial infarction, however, the sensitivity of these subjective findings has been low.[123-126] As yet, only one study has tried to detect and quantify atherosclerotic plaque surface irregularities by developing a numerical index of ulceration that appears to segregate patients according to their clinical syndromes.[91] Patients with unstable angina or acute myocardial infarction had objective evidence of plaque ulceration, whereas patients with stable angina did not. In the same study, the percentage of stenosis and the absolute minimum cross-sectional area did not distinguish between patients with stable versus unstable ischemic syndromes. This appears to be an important area in which computer quantification of plaque morphology may prove useful, particularly if surface morphology abnormalities can predict a high-risk subset of patients with stable symptoms.

Despite the proliferation of experience using quantitative coronary angiography, no single method has achieved the status of a "standard," and each has recognized technical limitations. There is clearly,

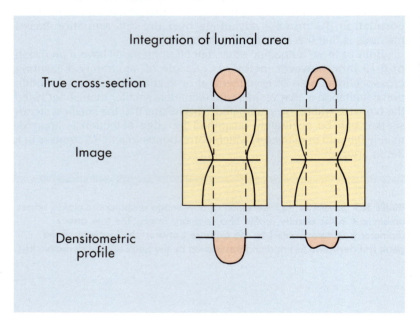

FIGURE 36.6 Densitometric coronary stenosis analysis. Although two stenoses may have different cross-sectional areas owing to lesion eccentricity, they may appear similar in planar coronary images. Integration of the densitometric profile across each stenosis yields a correct approximation of the cross-sectional area.

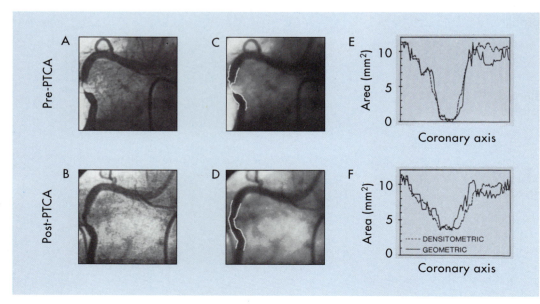

FIGURE 36.7 Combined geometric and densitometric coronary analysis. **A** and **D**. Spatially filtered edge-enhanced images of a right coronary artery are shown prior to and following balloon angioplasty. The vessel edges (**B** and **E**) were detected automatically with a matched filter technique. **C** and **F**. Both geometric and densitometric cross-sectional areas along the length of the coronary segment are shown

however, mounting evidence that quantitative coronary angiography improves accuracy, reduces variability among observers, and may provide important information about the hemodynamic properties of coronary stenoses, thus warranting expanded and widespread investigational and clinical use. The eventual role of quantitative coronary angiography will thus depend on how this kind of information impacts on clinical decision making and prognosis.

MYOCARDIAL PERFUSION IMAGING

Digital image processing can extract information not readily available from subjective image interpretation. Figure 36.8 illustrates that the transit of contrast material through the coronary arteries and into the myocardial microcirculation can be visualized and quantified by digital angiography using videodensitometry to construct regional myocardial time-density curves. These curves resemble indicator dilution curves and may be analyzed to estimate regional perfusion. Several methods for analyzing these curves have been developed, all of which are based on the principle that the time required for contrast material to transit the coronary circulation is inversely proportional to regional flow and directly proportional to its distribution volume. Transit time parameters can be derived from either the appearance or washout phases of the regional contrast dilution curve.

Vogel and colleagues have developed the contrast medium appearance picture (CMAP), which is a parametric image that displays the time (in cardiac cycles) following injection required to produce an empirically determined level of pixel brightness over the myocardium. Good correlations have been achieved between the percentage of caliper-measured stenosis, the coronary sinus thermodilution blood flow measurements, and the transstenotic pressure gradients before and after coronary angioplasty. A limitation of this technique is that it significantly underestimates coronary flow reserve as measured by the ratio of regional appearance time at rest to that following hyperemia induced by either ionic contrast material, intravenous dipyridamole, or intracoronary papaverine.[127-129] This method has been modified by using the ratios of peak myocardial densities to account for relative changes in distribution volume between rest and hyperemic states. This approach gives coronary flow reserve that compare favorably with direct flowmeter measurements.[130,131] Another appearance phase index, time to peak concentration, has also been demonstrated to correlate with hyperemic/rest flow ratios and with absolute regional flow.[132,133] Color displays of regional myocardial coronary flow reserve are now available.[131] These methods are now being used in clinical investigation to determine the functional significance of coronary artery disease and the effects of interventional therapies.[16,134] One obvious limitation of using appearance time to assess flow is that the measurement is exquisitely sensitive to injection rate and volume and thus requires preset coronary power injection.

An appealing alternative approach is the quantification of myocardial contrast washout. The critical assumption with this technique is that a given myocardial region behaves as a single, well-mixed compartment, which can be modeled by a declining monoexponential decay function whose time constant or washout half-time is inversely proportional to flow. Strong linear relationships have been documented between washout parameters and electromagnetic coronary flow and thermodilution great cardiac vein flow in animal models, and these indices appear to differentiate normal from both infarcted myocardium and viable myocardium supplied by severely stenotic vessels.[135-137] Other investigators, however, have demonstrated that these measurements may be highly variable.[133] The major drawbacks of this approach are that the monoexponential function may be an inadequate model for contrast washout, especially because the washout phase occurs while flow is rapidly changing following the hyperemic effects of contrast media, and that many patients cannot hold their breath for the 15 to 20 seconds required to obtain adequate washout-phase data. As in all planar projection imaging techniques, myocardial contrast perfusion imaging requires multiple projections to minimize overlap of different vascular territories and is incapable of separating endocardial and epicardial perfusion bed difference.

Another approach quantifies coronary flow reserve as the ratio of

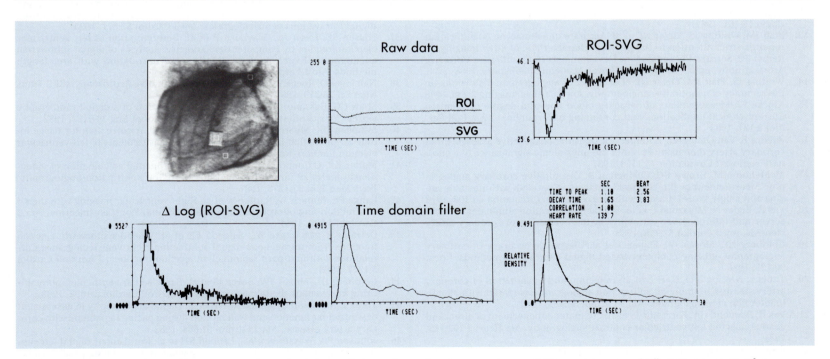

FIGURE 36.8 Generation of time-density curves. The upper left panel shows the placement of three regions of interest: one over the coronary ostium to define the time of injection, one over a lead blocker to determine the background level due to x-ray scatter and image receptor veiling glare (SVG), and one over the region of interest (ROI) that is to be measured in the myocardium. The raw image intensities of SVG and ROI are plotted as a function of time in the upper center panel. The next two panels illustrate processing for correction of background and logarithmic transformation to obtain a curve that is proportional to the amount of contrast material in the myocardium. The curve is then smoothed and analyzed to determine the time to peak and the exponential washout decay half-time.

the areas under time-density curves obtained directly over epicardial coronary arteries following subselective coronary injections of the same amount of contrast material before and after a hyperemic stimulus.[133] Although this has the advantage of being less affected by the overlap of projection imaging, the unfulfilled assumption of complete mixing of contrast material with blood in the proximal coronary tree and the requirement for subselective coronary injections are limiting factors. As with all of the densitometric methods described, strict attention to system calibration and correction of important sources of densitometric nonlinearities such as scatter and veiling glare are critical.[14,132]

At this time, therefore, the role of digital angiography in the assessment of regional myocardial perfusion appears promising. Despite its theoretical and practical limitations, digital coronary perfusion imaging may ultimately provide a convenient means for assessing both the rate and distribution of blood flow through coronary stenoses and coronary bypass grafts and the patient's status following interventions such as coronary angioplasty.

REFERENCES

1. Kruger RA, Riederer SJ: Basic Concepts of Digital Subtraction Angiography. Boston, GK Hall, 1984
2. Heintzen PH, Brennecke R (eds): Digital Imaging in Cardiovascular Radiology: International Symposium Kiel. Stuttgart, Georg Thieme Verlag, 1983
3. Holmes DR, Bove AA, Wondrow MA et al: Video x-ray progressive scanning: New technique for decreasing x-ray exposure without decreasing image quality during cardiac catheterization. Mayo Clin Proc 61:321, 1986
4. Hardin CW, Kruger RA, Anderson FL et al: Real time digital angiocardiography using a temporal high-pass filter. Radiology 151:517, 1984
5. Brennecke R, Hahne JH, Modenhauer K et al: Improved digital real-time processing and storage techniques with applications to intravenous contrast angiography. IEEE Proc Comp Cardiol 78:191, 1978
6. Bogren HG, Seibert JA, Hines HH et al: The beneficial effects of short pulse width acquisition and ECG-gating in digital angiocardiography. Invest Radiol 19:284, 1984
7. Seibert JA, Nalcioglu O, Roeck WW: Characterization of the veiling glare point spread function in x-ray image intensified fluoroscopy. Med Phys 11:172, 1984
8. Seibert JA, Nalcioglu O, Roeck WW: Deconvolution technique for the improvement of contrast of image intensifiers. Society of Photo-optical Instrumentation Engineers 314:310, 1981
9. Shaw CG, Ergun DL, Myerowitz PD et al: A technique of scatter and glare correction for videodensitometric studies in digital subtraction videoangiography. Rad Phys 142:209, 1982
10. Thompson AC, Zeman HD, Otis JN et al: Transvenous coronary angiography in dogs using synchrotron radiation. Int J Cardiac Imaging 2:53, 1986
11. Rubenstein ER, Hofstadter R, Zeman HD et al: Transvenous coronary angiography in humans using synchrotron radiation. Proc Natl Acad Sci USA 83:9724, 1986
12. Rubenstein E: Synchrotron radiation for angiography. Ann Rev Biophys Chem 16:161, 1987
13. Pfaff JM, Whiting JS, Eigler NE et al: Accurate densitometric quantification requires strict attention to the physical characteristic of x-ray imaging. In Reiber JC, Serruys PW (eds): New Developments in Quantitative Coronary Arteriography, pp 22–33. Boston: Kluwer Academic Publishers, 1988
14. Whiting JS, Pfaff JM, Eigler NL et al: Effect of angiographic distortions on the accuracy of quantitative angiography. Am J Cardiac Imaging 2:239, 1988
15. Klocke FJ: Measurements of coronary blood flow and degree of stenosis: Current clinical implications and continuing uncertainties. J Am Coll Cardiol 1:131, 1983
16. Zijlstra F, Van Ommeren J, Reiber JH: Does the quantitative assessment of coronary artery dimensions predict the physiologic significance of a coronary stenosis? Circulation 75:1154, 1987
17. McMahon MM, Brown BG, Cukingnan R: Quantitative coronary angiography: Measurement of the "critical" stenosis in patients with unstable angina and single-vessel disease without collaterals. Circulation 60:106, 1979
18. Vas R, Eigler N, Miyazono C et al: Digital quantification eliminates intraobserver and interobserver variability in the evaluation of coronary artery stenosis. Am J Cardiol 57:718, 1985
19. Goldberg HL, Moses JW, Fisher J et al: Diagnostic accuracy of coronary angiography utilizing computer-based digital subtraction methods. Chest 90:793, 1986
20. Tobis J, Nalcioglu O, Iseri L et al: Detection and quantitation of coronary artery stenosis from digital subtraction angiograms compared with 35-millimeter film cineangiograms. Am J Cardiol 54:489, 1984
21. Vas R, Diamond GA, Forrester JS et al: Computer enhancement of direct and venous-injected left ventricular contrast angiography. Am Heart J 102:719, 1981
22. Sandler H, Dodge HT: The use of single plane angiocardiograms for the calculation of left ventricular volumes in man. Am Heart J 75:325, 1968
23. Carey PH, Slutsky RA, Ashburn WI et al: Validation of cardiac output estimates by digital video subtraction angiography in dogs: Correlation with thermodilution values. Radiology 143:623, 1982
24. Higgins CB, Norris SL, Gerber KH et al: Quantitation of left ventricular dimensions and function by digital video subtraction angiography. Radiology 144:461, 1982
25. Radtke W, Bursch JH, Brennecke R et al: Assessment of left ventricular muscle volume by digital angiocardiography. Invest Radiol 18:149, 1983
26. Sasayama S, Nonogi H, Kawai C et al: Automated method for left ventricular volume measurement by cineventriculography with minimal doses of contrast medium. Am J Cardiol 48:746, 1981
27. Kronenberg MW, Price RR, Smith CW et al: Evaluation of left ventricular performance using digital subtraction angiography. Am J Cardiol 51:837, 1983
28. Vas R, Diamond GA, Forrester JS et al: Computer-enhanced digital angiography: Correlation of clinical assessment of left ventricular ejection fraction and regional wall motion. Am Heart J 104:732, 1982
29. Engels PHC, Ludwig JW, Verhoeven LAJ: Left ventricle evaluation by digital video subtraction angiocardiography. Radiology 144:471, 1982
30. Tobis J, Nacioglu O, Johnston WD et al: Left ventricular imaging with digital subtraction angiography using intravenous contrast injection and fluoroscopic exposure levels. Am Heart J 104:20, 1982
31. Goldberg HL, Borer JS, Moses JW et al: Digital subtraction intravenous left ventricular angiography: Comparison with conventional intraventricular angiography. J Am Coll Cardiol 1:858, 1983
32. Greenbaum RA, Evans TR: Investigation of left ventricular function by digital subtraction angiography. Br Heart J 51:163, 1984
33. Norris SL, Slutsky RA, Mancini GBJ et al: Comparison of digital intravenous ventriculography with conventional direct left ventriculography for quantitation of left ventricular volumes and ejection fractions. Am J Cardiol 51:1399, 1983
34. Felix R, Eichstadt H, Kempter H et al: A comparison of conventional contrast ventriculography and digital subtraction ventriculography. Clin Cardiol 6:265, 1983
35. Detrano R, MacIntyre WJ, Salcedo EE et al: Videodensitometric ejection fractions from intravenous digital subtraction left ventriculograms: Correlations with conventional direct contrast and radionuclide ventriculography. Radiology 155:19, 1985
36. Tobis J, Nacioglu O, Seibert A et al: Comparison of videodensitometry and area-length methods for computing left ventricular ejection fraction from digital intravenous ventriculograms. Am J Cardiol 52:871, 1983
37. Nissen SE, Elion JL, Grayburn P et al: Determination of left ventricular ejection fraction by computer densitometric analysis of digital subtraction angiography: Experimental validation and correlation with area-length methods. Am J Cardiol 59:675, 1987
38. Nalcioglu O, Roeck W, Pearce JG et al: Quantitative fluoroscopy. IEEE Trans Nucl Sci 28:219, 1981
39. Shaw CG, Bassano DA, Grossman ZD: Calibration of a digital radiography system for quantitative studies. Proc Soc Photoopt Eng 347:122, 1982
40. Swanson DK, Myerowitz PO, Van Lysel M et al: A correction for tissue iodine accumulation in videodensitometric measurements of left ventricular ejection fraction. Radiology 37:1437, 1983
41. Maher KP, O'Connor MK, Malone JF: Experimental examination of videodensitometry of large opacifications in digital subtraction angiography. Phys Med Biol 32:1273, 1987
42. Lange PE, Budach W, Radtke W et al: Right ventricular imaging with digital subtraction angiography using intraventricular contrast injection. Am J Cardiol 54:839, 1984
43. Detrano R, MacIntyre WJ, Salcedo EE et al: Videodensitometric ejection fractions from intravenous digital subtraction right ventriculograms: Correlations with first-pass radionuclide ejection fractions. J Am Coll Cardiol 5:1377, 1985
44. Goldberg HL, Moses JW, Borer JS et al: Exercise left ventriculography utilizing intravenous digital angiography. J Am Coll Cardiol 2:1092, 1983
45. Tobis J, Nalcioglu O, Johnston WD et al: Digital angiography in assessment of ventricular function and wall motion during pacing in patients with coronary artery disease. Am J Cardiol 51:668, 1983
46. Johnson RA, Wasserman AG, Leoboff RH et al: Intravenous digital left ventriculography at rest and with atrial pacing as a screening procedure for coronary artery disease. J Am Coll Cardiol 2:905, 1983
47. Detrano R, Simpfendorfer C, Day K et al: Comparison of stress digital ventriculography, stress thallium scintigraphy and digital fluoroscopy in the diagnosis of coronary artery disease in subjects without prior myocardial infarction. Am J Cardiol 56:434, 1985
48. Bellamy GR, Yiannikas J, Detrano R et al: Detection of multivessel disease after myocardial infarction using intravenous stress digital subtraction angiography. Radiology 161:685, 1986
49. Tzivoni D, Diamond GA, Pichler M et al: Analysis of regional ischemic left

ventricular dysfunction by quantitative cineangiography. Circulation 60:1278, 1979
50. Chaitman BR, DeMots H, Briston JD et al: Objective and subjective analysis of left ventricular angiograms. Circulation 52:420, 1975
51. Kussmaul WG, Kleaveland JP, Seevi GR: Sources of subjective variability in the assessment of left ventricular regional wall motion from contrast ventriculogram. Am J Cardiol 60:153, 1987
52. Diamond GA, Vas R, Forrester JS et al: The influence of bias on the subjective interpretation of cardiac angiograms. Am Heart J 107:69, 1984
53. Mancini GBJ, Norris SL, Peterson KL: Quantitative assessment of segmental wall motion abnormalities at rest and after atrial pacing using digital intravenous ventriculography. J Am Coll Cardiol 2:70, 1983
54. Gelberg HJ, Brundage BH, Glanz S et al: Quantitative left ventricular wall motion analysis: A comparison of area, chord, and radial methods. Circulation 59:991, 1979
55. Fujita M, Sasayama S, Kawai C et al: Automatic processing of cineventriculograms for analysis of regional myocardial function. Circulation 63:1065, 1981
56. Sheehan FH, Stewart DK, Dodge HT et al: Variability in the measurement of regional left ventricular wall motion from contrast angiograms. Circulation 68:550, 1983
57. Nissen SE, Booth D, Waters J: Evaluation of contractile pattern by intravenous digital subtraction left ventriculography: Comparison with cineangiography and assessment of intraobserver variability. Am J Cardiol 52:1293, 1983
58. Vas R, Diamond GA, Hu ZX et al: Quantitative analysis of left ventricular regional wall motion. In Sigwart U, Heintzen PH (eds): Ventricular Wall Motion: International Symposium Lausanne. Stuttgart, Georg Thieme Verlag, 1984
59. Chappuis FC, Widmann T, Buth B et al: Quantitative assessment of regional left ventricular function by densitometric analysis of digital-subtraction ventriculograms: Correlation with myocardial systolic shortening in dogs. Circulation 77:457, 1988
60. Chappuis FP, Widmann TF, Nicod P et al: Densitometric regional ejection fraction: A new three-dimensional index of regional left ventricular function—comparison with geometric methods. J Am Coll Cardiol 11:72, 1988
61. Grayburn PA, Nissen SE, Elion JL et al: Quantitation of aortic regurgitation by computer analysis of digital subtraction angiography. J Am Coll Cardiol 10:1122, 1987
62. Brogren HG, Bursch JH: Digital angiography in the diagnosis of congenital heart disease. Cardiovasc Intervent Radiol 7:180, 1984
63. Buonocore E, Pavlicek W, Modic MT et al: Anatomic and functional imaging of coronary heart disease with digital subtraction angiography. Radiology 147:647, 1983
64. Steffenino G, Meier B, Boop P et al: Non-selective intra-arterial digital subtraction angiography for the assessment of coronary artery bypass grafts. Int J Cardiac Imaging 1:209, 1987
65. Myerowitz PD, Turnipseed WD, Swanson DK et al: Digital subtraction angiography as a method for screening for coronary artery disease during peripheral vascular angiography. Surgery 92:1042, 1982
66. Myerowitz PD, Turnipseed W, Shaw CG et al: Computerized fluoroscopy: New technique for the non-invasive evaluation of the aorta, coronary artery bypass grafts, and left ventricular function. J Thorac Cardiovasc Surg 83:65, 1982
67. Lupon-Roses J, Montana J, Domingo E et al: Venous digital angio-radiography: An accurate and useful technique for assessing coronary bypass graft patency. Eur Heart J 7:979, 1986
68. Blankenhorn DH, Curry PJ: The accuracy of arteriography and ultrasound imaging for atherosclerosis measurement: A review. Arch Pathol Lab Med 106:483, 1982
69. Arnett EN, Isner JM, Redwood CR et al: Coronary artery narrowing in coronary heart disease: Comparison of cineangiographic and necropsy findings. Ann Intern Med 91:350, 1979
70. Galbraith JE, Murphy ML, DeSoyza N: Coronary angiogram interpretation: Interobserver variability. JAMA 240:2053, 1981
71. Hutchins GM, Bulkley BH, Ridolfi RL et al: Correlation of coronary arteriograms and left ventriculograms with post mortem studies. Circulation 56:32, 1977
72. Isner JM, Kishel J, Kent KM: Accuracy of angiographic determination of left main coronary arterial narrowing. Circulation 63:1056, 1981
73. Roberts WC, Jones AA: Quantitation of coronary arterial narrowing at necropsy in sudden coronary death. Am J Cardiol 44:39, 1979
74. Vlodaver Z, Frech R, Van Tassel RA et al: Correlation of the antemortem coronary arteriogram and the postmortem specimen. Circulation 48:162, 1973
75. Bjork L, Spindola-Franco H, Van Houten FX et al: Comparison of observer performance with 16 mm cinefluorography and 70 mm camera fluorography in coronary arteriography. Am J Cardiol 36:474, 1975
76. Zir LM, Miller SW, Dinsmore RE et al: Interobserver variability in coronary angiography. Circulation 53:627, 1976
77. Detre KM, Wright E, Murphy ML et al: Observer agreement in evaluating coronary angiograms. Circulation 52:979, 1975
78. DeRouen TA, Murray JA, Owen W: Variability in the analysis of coronary arteriograms. Circulation 55:324, 1977
79. Fisher LD, Judkins MP, Lesperance J et al: Reproducibility of coronary arteriographic reading in the Coronary Artery Surgery Study (CASS). Cathet Cardiovasc Diagn 8:565, 1982
80. Trask N, Califf RM, Conley MJ et al: Accuracy and interobserver variability of coronary cineangiography: A comparison with postmortem evaluation. J Am Coll Cardiol 3:1145, 1984
81. Pfaff JM, Eigler N, Whiting J et al: Quantitative coronary angiography. In Wasserman AG, Ross A (eds): Digital Angiography. Futura Publishing, 1988
82. Brown BG, Bolson EL, Dodge HT: Quantitative computer techniques for analyzing coronary arteriograms. Prog Cardiovasc Dis 28:403, 1986
83. Reiber JHC, Kooijman CJ, Slager CJ et al: Computer assisted analysis of the severity of obstructions from coronary cineangiograms: A methodological review. Automedica 5:219, 1984
84. Scoblionko DP, Brown BG, Mitten S et al: A new digital electronic caliper measurement of coronary arterial stenosis: Comparison with visual estimates and computer-assisted measurements. Am J Cardiol 53:689, 1984
85. Simons MA, Bastian BV, Bray BE et al: Comparison of observer and videodensitometric measurement of simulated coronary artery stenosis. Invest Radiol 22:562, 1987
86. Schweiger MJ, Stanek E, Iwakoshi K et al: Comparison of visual estimate with digital caliper measurement of coronary artery stenosis. Cathet Cardiovasc Diagn 13:239, 1987
87. White CW, Wright CB, Doty DB et al: Does visual interpretation of the coronary arteriogram predict the physiologic importance of a coronary stenosis? N Engl J Med 310:819, 1984
88. Friesinger GC, Page II, Ross RS: Prognostic significance of coronary arteriography. Trans Assoc Am Physicians 83:78, 1970
89. CASS principal investigators and their associates: Myocardial infarction and mortality in the Coronary Artery Surgery Study randomized trial. N Engl J Med 310:750, 1984
90. Califf RM, Tomabechi Y, Lee KL et al: Outcome of one-vessel coronary artery disease. Circulation 67:283, 1983
91. Wilson RF, Holida MD, White CW: Quantitative angiographic morphology of coronary stenoses leading to myocardial infarction or unstable angina. Circulation 73:286, 1986
92. Gould KL: Pressure-flow characteristics of coronary stenoses in unsedated dogs at rest and during coronary vasodilatation. Circ Res 43:242, 1978
93. Gould KL, Kelley KO: Physiological significance of coronary flow velocity and changing stenosis geometry during coronary vasodilatation in awake dogs. Circ Res 50:695, 1982
94. Brown BG, Boson E, Frimer M et al: Quantitative coronary angiography: Estimation of dimensions, hemodynamic resistance, and atheroma mass of coronary artery lesions using the arteriogram and digital computation. Circulation 55:329, 1977
95. Gensini GG, Lelly AE, DaCosta BCB et al: Quantitative angiography: The measurement of coronary vasomobility in the intact animal and man. Chest 60:522, 1971
96. Crawford DW, Beckenbach ES, Blankenhorn DH et al: Grading of coronary atherosclerosis: Comparison of a modified IAP visual grading method and a new quantitative angiographic technique. Atherosclerosis 19:231, 1974
97. Spears JR, Sandor T, Balm DS et al: The minimum error in estimating coronary luminal cross sectional area from cineangiographic diameter measurements. Cathet Cardiovasc Diagn 9:119, 1983
98. Gottwik MG, Siebes M, Bahawar H et al: Quantitative angiographic assessment of coronary stenosis: Problems and pitfalls. Z Kardiol 72:111, 1983
99. Harrison DG, White CW, Hiratza LF et al: The value of lesion cross-sectional area determined by quantitative coronary angiography in assessing the physiologic significance of proximal left anterior descending coronary arterial stenosis. Circulation 69:1111, 1984
100. Gould KL, Kelley KO, Bolson EL: Experimental validation of quantitative coronary arteriography for determining pressure-flow characteristics of coronary stenosis. Circulation 66:930, 1982
101. Kirkeeide RL, Gould KL, Parsel L: Assessment of coronary stenoses by myocardial perfusion imaging during pharmacologic coronary vasodilatation: VII. Validation of coronary flow reserve as a single integrated functional measure of stenosis severity reflecting all its geometric dimensions. J Am Coll Cardiol 7:103, 1986
102. Reiber JHC, Cornelis JK, Cornelis JS et al: Coronary artery dimensions from cineangiograms: Methodology and validation of a computer assisted analysis procedure. IEEE Medical Imaging 3:131, 1984
103. Fujita H, Doi K, Fencil LE et al: Image feature analysis and computer-aided diagnosis in digital radiography: II. Computerized determination of vessel sizes in digital subtraction angiography. Med Phys 14:549, 1987
104. Kruger RA: Estimation of the diameter of and iodine concentration within blood vessels using digital radiography devices. Med Phys 8:652, 1981
105. Nichols AB, Christopher FO, Gabrieli BA et al: Quantification of relative coronary arterial stenosis by videodensitometric analysis of coronary arteriograms. Circulation 69:512, 1984
106. Serruys PW, Reiber JHC, Wijns W et al: Assessment of percutaneous transluminal coronary angioplasty by quantitative coronary angiography: Diameter versus densitometric area measurements. Am J Cardiol 54:482, 1984
107. Johnson RA, Wasserman AG, Katz RJ et al: Correlation of coronary stenosis and contrast density decay curves by on-line subtracted digital fluoroscopy. J Am Coll Cardiol 3:588, 1984

108. Wiesel J, Grunwald AM, Tobiasz C et al: Quantitation of absolute area of a coronary stenosis: Experimental validation with a preparation in vivo. Circulation 74:1099, 1986
109. Shea S, Sciacca RR, Esser P et al: Progression of coronary atherosclerotic disease assessed by cinevideodensitometry: Relation to clinical risk factors. J Am Coll Cardiol 8:1325, 1986
110. Mancini BGJ, Simon SB, BcGillem MJ et al: Automated quantitative coronary arteriography: Morphologic and physiologic validation *in vivo* of a rapid digital angiographic method. Circulation 75:452, 1987
111. Tobis J, Nalcioglu O, Johnston WD et al: Videodensitometric determination of minimum coronary artery luminal diameter before and after angioplasty. Am J Cardiol 59:38, 1987
112. Sanz ML, Mancini GBJ, LeFree MT et al: Variability of quantitative digital subtraction coronary angiography before and after percutaneous transluminal coronary angioplasty. Am J Cardiol 60:55, 1987
113. Klein LW, Agarwal JB, Rosenberg MC et al: Assessment of coronary artery stenoses by digital subtraction angiography: A pathoanatomic validation. Am Heart J 113:1011, 1987
114. Skelton TN, Kisslo KB, Mikat EM et al: Accuracy of digital angiography for quantitation of normal coronary luminal segments in excised, perfused hearts. Am J Cardiol 59:1261, 1987
115. Johnson MR, McPherson DD, Fleagle SR et al: Videodensitometric analysis of human coronary stenoses: Validation in vivo by intraoperative high-frequency epicardial echocardiography. Circulation 77:328, 1988
116. Rosenberg MC, Klein LW, Agarwal JB et al: Quantification of absolute luminal diameter by computer-analyzed digital subtraction angiography: An assessment in human coronary arteries. Circulation 77:484, 1988
117. Serruys PW, Luijten HE, Beatt KJ et al: Incidence of restenosis after successful coronary angioplasty: A time-related phenomenon: A quantitative angiographic study in 342 consecutive patients at 1, 2, 3, and 4 months. Circulation 77:361, 1988
118. Ellis S, Sanders W, Goulet C et al: Optimal detection of the progression of coronary artery disease: Comparison of methods suitable for risk factor intervention trials. Circulation 74:1235, 1986
119. Chapman I: Morphogenesis of occluding coronary artery thrombosis. Arch Pathol 80:256, 1965
120. Falk E: Unstable angina with fatal outcome: Dynamic coronary thrombosis leading to infarction and/or sudden death. Circulation 71:699, 1985
121. Sherman CT, Litvack F, Grundfest W et al: Coronary angioscopy in patients with unstable angina pectoris. N Engl J Med 315:913, 1986
122. Brown BG, Gallery CA, Badger RS et al: Incomplete lysis of thrombus in the moderate underlying atherosclerotic lesion during intracoronary infusion of streptokinase for acute myocardial infarction: Quantitative angiographic observation. Circulation 73:653, 1986
123. Levin DC, Fallon JT: Significance of the angiographic morphology of localized coronary stenosis: Histopathologic correlations. Circulation 66:316, 1982
124. Ambrose JA, Winters SL, Stern A et al: Angiographic morphology and the pathogenesis of unstable angina pectoris. J Am Coll Cardiol 5:609, 1985
125. Ambrose JA, Winters SL, Arora RR et al: Coronary angiographic morphology in myocardial infarction: A link between the pathogenesis of unstable angina and myocardial infarction. J Am Coll Cardiol 6:1233, 1985
126. Ambrose JA, Hjemdahl-Monsen CE, Borrico S et al: Angiographic demonstration of a common link between unstable angina pectoris and non-Q wave acute myocardial infarction. Am J Cardiol 61:244, 1988
127. Vogel RA, LeFree M, Bates ER et al: Application of digital techniques to selective coronary arteriography: Use of myocardial contrast appearance time to measure coronary flow reserve. Am Heart J 107:153, 1984
128. Vogel RA, Bates ER, O'Neill WW et al: Coronary flow reserve measured during cardiac catheterization. Arch Intern Med 144:1773, 1984
129. O'Neill WW, Walton JA, Bates ER et al: Criteria for successful coronary angioplasty as assessed by alteration in coronary vasodilatory reserve. J Am Coll Cardiol 3:1382, 1984
130. Hodgson JMcB, Legrand V, Bates ER et al: Validation in dogs of a rapid digital angiographic technique to measure relative coronary blood flow during routine cardiac catheterization. Am J Cardiol 55:188, 1985
131. Cumsa JT, Toggart EJ, Folts JD et al: Digital subtraction angiographic imaging of coronary flow reserve. Circulation 75:461, 1987
132. Whiting JS, Drury JK, Pfaff JM et al: Digital angiographic measurement of radiographic contrast material kinetics for estimation of myocardial perfusion. Circulation 73:789, 1986
133. Nissen SE, Elion JL, Booth DC et al: Value and limitations of computer analysis of digital subtraction angiography in the assessment of coronary flow reserve. Circulation 73:562, 1986
134. Hodgson JMcB, Riley RS, Most AS et al: Assessment of coronary flow reserve using digital angiography before and after successful percutaneous transluminal coronary angioplasty. Am J Cardiol 60:61, 1987
135. Ikeda H, Yoshinori K, Fumihiko U et al: Quantitative evaluation of regional myocardial blood flow by videodensitometric analysis of digital subtraction coronary arteriography in humans. J Am Coll Cardiol 8:809, 1986
136. Takeda T, Matsuda M, Akatsuka T et al: Digital subtraction angiography: Image-sequence analysis for regional myocardial perfusion dynamics. J Cardiol 16:1, 1986
137. Takeda T, Matsuda M, Akatsuka T et al: Clinical validity of washout time constant images obtained by digital subtraction angiography. J Cardiol 16:841, 1986

Assessment of Ventricular Diastolic Function

Derek G. Gibson

It is no longer necessary to plead the case that diastolic abnormalities are a clinically significant cause of impaired cardiac function. Over the past 10 years, there has been increasing interest in this phase of the cardiac cycle. Such activity may have led to the impression that concern with diastolic function of the ventricles is a recent phenomenon. However, this is far from the case. In 1904, a literature of nearly 200 references was reviewed in detail by Ebstein, who wrote an account that can still be read with great interest, showing that many current ideas on diastolic function had already been considered in detail by the end of the nineteenth century.[1] If there has been any discontinuity in thought, it has been among cardiologists who have interpreted impaired left ventricular performance almost exclusively in terms of disturbed systolic function over the past 20 years. This trend has now been reversed, and in the present review, an account is given of methods of assessing normal diastolic function in humans and of abnormalities that may occur in disease. It is concerned to a great extent with the function of the left rather than the right ventricle, because the latter has received much less attention in the literature. The field is an active one, involving complementary use of invasive and noninvasive methods. As in any rapidly developing subject, general agreement does not exist on important questions of definition, technique, and interpretation, nor has the clinical significance of many departures from normality yet been established.

PHASES OF DIASTOLE

The terminology used for describing the phases of diastole is based on that elaborated by Wiggers from his observations of pressure pulses and valve motion.[2] The onset of *protodiastole* is taken as that of the rapid fall in aortic pressure during late ejection, and its end as aortic valve closure. *Isovolumic relaxation* is the interval between aortic valve closure and mitral opening. The filling period itself can be divided into three phases, that of *rapid early diastolic filling*, a mid-diastolic period of *diastasis,* and finally *atrial systole*. This division is used as the basis for the present discussion, and although there are difficulties in its implementation in individual patients, it has nevertheless proved useful in practice.

There is little more to say about protodiastole than was said by Wiggers 60 years ago. The timing of the onset of relaxation in the myocardium itself is still uncertain. There is no information even as to whether it is normally synchronous in different parts of the ventricle, though the complex fiber structure and stress distribution across the ventricular wall during systole and dependence of the onset and rate of relaxation on systolic loading conditions suggest that this may well not be the case.[3] By implication, diastole follows immediately after end-systole, which itself remains a poorly defined landmark in the cardiac cycle. From the clinical point of view, therefore, this earliest phase is not considered, and diastole is taken as starting with aortic valve closure.

ISOVOLUMIC RELAXATION
DEFINITION AND MEASUREMENT

Isovolumic relaxation represents the time interval from aortic valve closure until mitral valve opening. Aortic valve closure can be defined in a number of ways. The most direct is the timing of apposition of the valve cusps on an M-mode echocardiogram. This coincides with A_2, the initial high-frequency vibration of the aortic component of the second heart sound. It is essential that the phonocardiogram is recorded from the left sternal edge and not the apex, where A_2 is delayed. The timing of aortic valve closure can be defined invasively from that of the dicrotic notch on the pressure pulse recorded with a micromanometer just above the valve. Valve closure can also be recognized angiographically, but such estimates are likely to be limited by the frame rate. Mitral valve opening is usually taken as the time of cusp separation on M-mode echocardiography from a record taken at a level showing the cusps themselves.[4] The onset of rapid anterior motion of the anterior cusp (D' point) follows mitral valve opening and is an unreproducible landmark. The start of filling can be taken as the timing of first appearance of unopacified dye within the left ventricular cavity on a contrast left ventriculogram. Mitral opening bears no fixed relation to the "O" point of the apexcardiogram, or to the time of cross-over of atrial and ventricular pressure.[5] Practical problems in the definition of mitral valve opening remain. The M-mode echogram samples only one region of the valve, so the possibility of earlier opening in some other region exists. In addition, the valve cusps bulge into the left ventricle before actually separating, effectively increasing left ventricular volume. The period from A_2 to mitral valve opening need not be isovolumic in patients with aortic or mitral regurgitation or a ventricular septal defect. Aortic valve closure may not be recognizable in patients with severe aortic valve disease. The interval from pulmonary valve closure to tricuspid opening cannot be used to define a corresponding period on the right side of the heart. In contrast to the left side of the heart, pressure in the pulmonary artery is delayed with respect to that in the right ventricle in late ejection. It is the former that determines the timing of P_2, which may thus occur at a time when right ventricular pressure has fallen to atrial levels, a phenomenon termed "hang-out."[6] Hang-out results from the low impedance of the pulmonary vascular bed and is lost in severe pulmonary hypertension.

DURATION

In normal adults, the duration of isovolumic relaxation is remarkably uniform, being in the range of 60 ± 10 msec (mean ± 1 SD) with significantly lower values in children.[4] In normal subjects, there is a weak negative correlation with heart rate.[4] In left ventricular disease, two processes can be identified. The first is a nonspecific lengthening so that it may be 100 msec or more in coronary artery disease, hypertrophy,[7] or in diabetics with microvascular disease.[8] Occasionally this prolongation may be very striking (Fig. 37.1, *A*). The second process is shortening due to raised left ventricular filling pressure[8] up to as low as 10 msec when end-diastolic pressure is around 30 mm Hg, or even becomes negative when end-diastolic pressure is higher (Fig. 37.1, *B*). This abbreviation counteracts prolongation by left ventricular disease (Fig. 37.2), and in individual patients the result is a balance between the two. Aortic diastolic pressure has less effect, probably because pressure is dropping rapidly at the time of aortic closure. In normal subjects, isovolumic relaxation time is unchanged during isometric or dynamic exercise, but in patients with left ventricular hypertrophy or coronary artery disease, it is shortened by both types. Isovolumic relax-

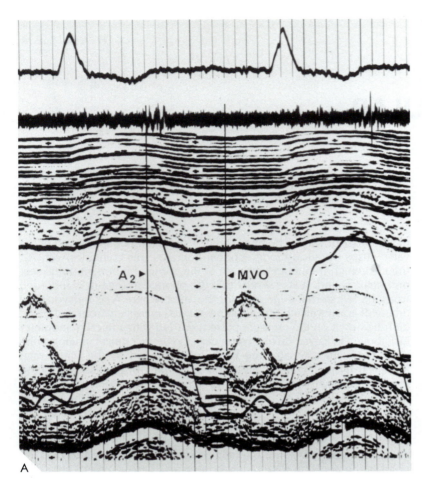

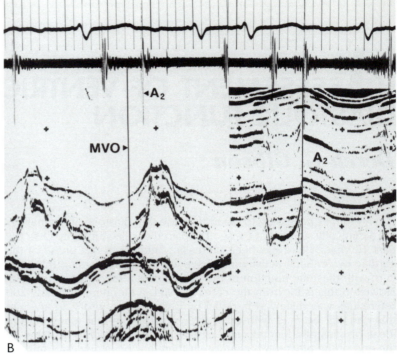

FIGURE 37.1 Measurement of isovolumic relaxation from simultaneous M-mode echo and phonocardiogram. **A.** Prolongation of isovolumic relaxation time to 240 msec in a patient with coronary artery disease. Note that a considerable increase in left ventricular dimension has occurred before mitral valve opening. **B.** (*Left*) Mitral echogram from a patient with severe left ventricular disease and aortic Starr-Edwards prosthesis. Mitral valve opening (MVO) precedes aortic valve closure (A_2) by 60 msec. (*Right*) Echogram of prosthesis confirms that A_2 coincides with the ball impinging on the ring at the end of ejection. Time marker: 40 msec.

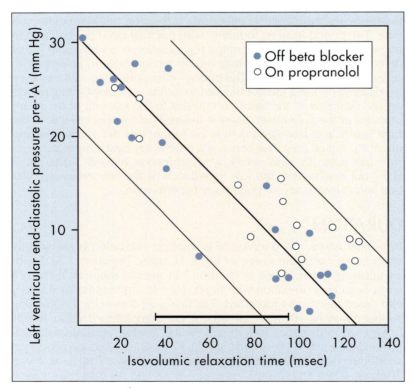

FIGURE 37.2 Relation between isovolumic relaxation time and left ventricular end-diastolic pressure in patients with coronary artery disease. Horizontal bar represents 95% confidence limits of normal. (Modified from Mattheos M, Shapiro E, Oldershaw PJ et al: Non-invasive assessment of changes in left ventricular relaxation by combined phono-, echo-, and mechanography. Br Heart J 47:253, 1982)

ation time is lengthened by nitrate administration when end-diastolic pressure is high[7] and shortened by verapamil or nifedipine in patients with hypertrophic cardiomyopathy when it is prolonged in the control state.[9,10] The ratio of Q–MVC to A_2–E point is inversely proportional to left atrial pressure, where Q represents the Q wave of the ECG, MVC represents mitral closure, and the E point represents the timing of maximum opening of the mitral echogram.[11] The interval of A_2–E point closely approximates isovolumic relaxation time and shows the same sensitivity to left atrial pressure,[12] while Q–MVC considered in isolation is independent of it. The overall sensitivity of the ratio to left ventricular filling pressure is thus likely to depend on inclusion of isovolumic relaxation time.

VENTRICULAR PRESSURE CHANGES

Peak rate of fall of pressure during isovolumic relaxation can be derived by simple differentiation of the output of a micromanometer pressure record. The maximum rate of fall of left ventricular pressure, i.e. peak negative dP/dt, is influenced by systolic events and peak systolic pressure.[13] It falls in pacing-induced ischemia,[14] in chronic coronary artery disease,[15] and in hypertrophic cardiomyopathy,[15] but not in left ventricular hypertrophy due to hypertension or aortic stenosis.[15,16] A second approach has been to assume that the rate of fall of left ventricular pressure is exponential from the time of peak negative dP/dt to mitral valve opening, allowing the time constant (T) of pressure decay to be calculated.[17] Although there is no theoretical basis for exponential pressure decline within the left ventricle, the correlation between predicted and observed values is close in normal subjects (Fig. 37.3). Use of T has advantages over use of peak negative dP/dt, because in experimental animals it is independent of peak systolic pressure, stroke volume, heart rate, and peak systolic shortening rate.[18] In humans, T increases with advancing age[15] and shortens with tachycardia due to atrial pacing or exercise.[19,20] Deviations from normal have been reported in patients with left ventricular disease, although results from different series can be compared only when the exact method of derivation is taken into account. In the earliest determinations, a simple plot of ln P against time (t) was used, ln P here being the natural logarithm of ventricular pressure and this relation assumes that the arbitrary zero, usually atmospheric pressure, used for setting up the catheter system is identical to the pressure in the unstressed ventricle. Although this approach is adequate for an open chest preparation, it does not take into account the possibility that in intact humans baseline shift might have occurred or that some additional extracavitary pressure is present, arising, for example, from the pericardium. This additional pressure (P_b) is not usually known. An alternative method of calculation was thus proposed by Murgo and Craig. If the time course of pressure fall is exponential, then P is given by:

$$P = P_0 e^{-t/T} + P_b$$

where P_0 = pressure at time zero. It follows that it is ln $(P - P_b)$ rather than ln P that is a linear function of t. Thus,

$$dP/dt = -1/T(P - P_b)$$

that is, a graph of $-dP/dt$ against measured pressure has a slope of 1/T. It is thus unnecessary to know P_b in order to derive T, but only to calculate the intercept. The relation is linear only if the fall in pressure is exponential, providing a method by which the original assumption can be checked. Although such plots are nearly linear in normal subjects, with very high correlation coefficients, consistent departures are seen, with the slope increasing as pressure falls.[21] More marked deviations are seen in patients with hypertrophic cardiomyopathy and to a lesser extent in those with secondary left ventricular hypertrophy.[19]

The magnitude of P_b itself can be estimated by allowing the zero pressure as well as T to vary when calculating the exponential best fit. This theoretic zero pressure is termed the *asymptote*. Calculated values for T differ strikingly using these two methods; thus Thompson and colleagues noted the average time constant to be 31 ± 9 msec (mean ± 1 SD) in normal subjects using the simple semilogarithmic method and 55 ± 12 msec when the asymptote is varied.[22] The mean value of the asymptote itself was notable, being −25 ± 9 mm Hg in normal subjects. Any physical significance this may have remains to be determined. T is prolonged in patients with coronary artery disease, and pacing-induced ischemia is associated with a reduction in the asymptote toward zero. Regardless of the method of calculation used,

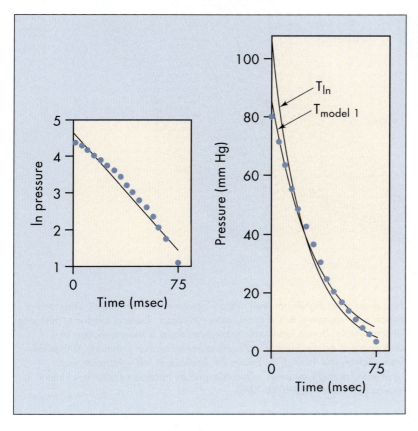

FIGURE 37.3 Estimation of time constant of relaxation in a patient with coronary artery disease, without angina. (*Left*) Simple semilogarithmic plot of ln pressure against time after peak dP/dt. Although correlation coefficient is −0.98, deviations from linear relation are not random, but slope becomes steeper as pressure falls. (*Right*) Measured pressures (dots) compared with those predicted from simple semilogarithmic plot (T_{ln}), and from a single exponential with variable asymptote ($T_{model\ 1}$). (Modified from Thompson DS, Waldron CB, Coltart DJ et al: Estimation of time constant of left ventricular relaxation. Br Heart J 49:250, 1983)

T is consistently prolonged in hypertrophic cardiomyopathy and secondary left ventricular hypertrophy.[16,23] Such an increase might reflect a uniform change in relaxation rate but could also be the result of an increased spread of values of relaxation rates in different regions of the myocardium. Rousseau and associates suggested that the fall was biexponential in a large majority of cases with coronary artery disease, with selective prolongation of T derived from the first 40 msec.[24] However, a biexponential curve was also noted in nearly half the normal controls, and values in both were prolonged to a similar extent by nifedipine. In addition, an apparently biexponential course of pressure fall can be converted to a monoexponential one simply by shifting the asymptote.[25]

REGIONAL WALL MOTION

The most comprehensive methods of observing regional left ventricular wall motion during isovolumic relaxation are those based on contrast angiography. Because it is necessary to distinguish slow from incoordinate or asynchronous motion, the wall must be shown throughout the cardiac cycle rather than only at end-diastole and end-systole. Figure 37.4 demonstrates one way in which this can be done.[26] Left ventricular wall motion is displayed as an array of plots of displacement against time, taken in a standardized order around the cavity outline. The display from a normal subject is shown in Figure 37.4, *A*. Uniform inward motion, shown as upward displacement, is apparent around the cavity outline throughout ejection. However, during the period of isovolumic relaxation, endocardial position changes little. After mitral valve opening, there is rapid and synchronous outward motion. This should be contrasted with a display from a patient with coronary artery disease (Fig. 37.4, *B*). In the anterior part of the cavity, there is uniform inward motion, while hypokinesis can be seen inferiorly. During isovolumic relaxation, there is early outward motion of endocardium in the anterior region associated with abnormal inward motion inferiorly. This results in a striking change in cavity shape. Such asynchronous wall motion is very common during isovolumic relaxation in patients with coronary artery disease. The primary abnormality appears to be in the segment showing delayed inward motion, which is to be found in the territory of the affected coronary artery in patients with single-vessel disease. Asynchronous relaxation may thus be the cause of the increase in T of pressure fall. Plots of regional wall thickness based on the same principle have demonstrated that these abnormalities of endocardial position are due to corresponding disturbances of wall dynamics rather than to overall motion of the heart in space.[27] Analysis of a large series of cases has shown that with triple vessel involvement of the coronary arteries, these changes are not randomly distributed around the left ventricular cavity outline, but that inward motion during isovolumic relaxation is much more common along the inferior wall of the ventricle, while outward motion is almost confined to the mid-portion of the free wall,[28] where it is frequently referred to as *segmental early relaxation phenomenon* (SERP).[29]

A related series of abnormalities can be detected by M-mode echocardiography.[30] Normally, mitral valve opening corresponds to peak thickness of the posterior wall of the left ventricle and minimum transverse cavity dimension. In many patients with coronary artery disease, a striking increase in cavity dimension before mitral valve opening can be seen, again reflecting a change in cavity shape (see Fig. 37.1, *A*). This is the result of asynchronous relaxation, the region of the ventricle studied by M-mode echocardiography being similar to that in the upper part of the display in Figure 37.3, *B*. It is thus not the site of the primary abnormality but is a normal region whose behavior has been affected by a disturbance elsewhere in the ventricle.

CLINICAL SIGNIFICANCE OF ABNORMALITIES

Although many abnormalities can be recognized during isovolumic relaxation, it is still not clear whether these should be regarded as

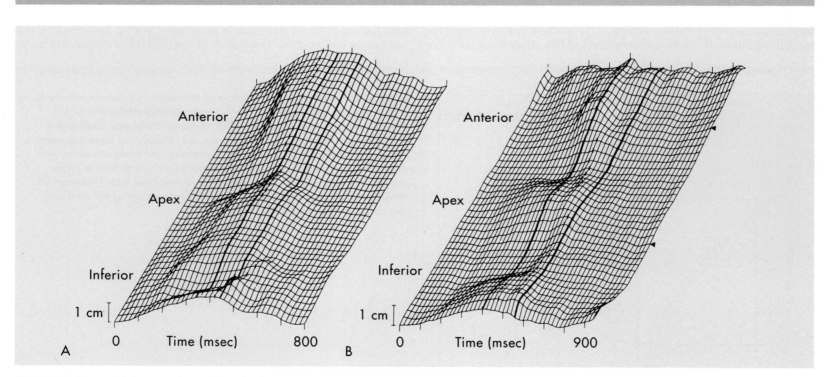

FIGURE 37.4 Regional left ventricular wall motion during isovolumic relaxation derived from a contrast angiogram. Plots represent regional endocardial motion from around the circumference of the right anterior oblique (*RAO*) projection. Inward movement is shown by upward displacement. The site around the cavity from which plot is derived is shown on the left of the display. Diagonal lines correspond to the timing of each cine frame; those corresponding to minimum cavity area and mitral opening are accentuated. **A.** Normal subject. Inward motion is synchronous around the cavity outline, and there is no significant wall motion between minimum cavity area and mitral valve opening. **B.** Coronary artery disease. There is inferior hypokinesis during systole. During isovolumic relaxation, there is inward motion of endocardium on the inferior wall and outward motion anteriorly. (Modified from Gibson DG, Prewitt TA, Brown DJ: Analysis of left ventricular wall movement during isovolumic relaxation and its relation to coronary artery disease. Br Heart J 38:1010, 1976)

potential pathogenic mechanisms or simply as markers of disease. Abbreviation of isovolumic relaxation time provides the basis for noninvasive methods of detecting high left ventricular filling pressure, at the same time stressing the importance of considering loading conditions when interpreting these measurements. Shortening of an abnormally prolonged isovolumic relaxation time by a drug or other maneuver does not necessarily imply improved relaxation, but may merely indicate an increase in filling pressure. Lack of coordinate wall motion during isovolumic relaxation leads to practical problems in defining the timing of end-systole. The start of diastole is spread over a period of up to 100 msec at a time when cavity shape may be changing rapidly. Analysis of regional wall motion based on apparent motion between two frames leads to ambiguity in approximately half of patients with coronary artery disease, the apparent pattern of wall motion displayed depending critically on the exact timing during isovolumic relaxation of the frame identified as end-systolic (Fig. 37.5).[31] Finally, in both left ventricular hypertrophy and coronary artery disease, abnormalities of isovolumic relaxation are associated with a reduction in peak filling rate during early diastole. It has been suggested that prolonged isovolumic relaxation may contribute to impaired myocardial perfusion in hypertrophic cardiomyopathy; however, such a mechanism remains conjecture.

RAPID VENTRICULAR FILLING
LEFT VENTRICULAR FILLING TIME

Opening of the mitral valve marks the start of filling, which continues until the start of the succeeding ventricular systole. The total time during which the mitral valve is open during diastole thus represents the time available for ventricular filling. It can be measured relatively simply using M-mode echocardiography, both at rest and on exercise, and beat-to-beat changes can be documented in atrial fibrillation. At rest, ventricular filling time is significantly longer than the time available for ejection, being 400 msec to 500 msec at a heart rate of 60 beats per minute.[32] However, as heart rate rises, there is a disproportionate reduction in filling time, which drops to 150 msec to 200 msec at a rate of 120 beats per minute and to 100 msec or less when the rate is above 160 beats per minute, considerably less than that available for ejection which is approximately 150 msec at this rate. If stroke volume is assumed to be around 100 ml, then the mean ventricular filling rate on exercise is approximately 1 liter per second. These considerations give some idea of the effectiveness of the physiologic mechanisms underlying normal rapid filling in humans.

NORMAL LEFT VENTRICULAR FILLING
VOLUME CHANGES

The first direct measurements of ventricular volume changes during diastole in man were made using contrast angiography, with the cavity area being estimated on successive frames. The results of Hammermeister and Warbasse confirmed the presence in humans of the pattern of left ventricular filling known from animal experiments.[33] An example of a left ventricular filling curve from a normal subject is given in Figure 37.6. Peak rate of inflow into the normal left ventricle occurs early in diastole and reaches a value of approximately 500 ml/second to 700 ml/second. The corresponding values for normalized filling rate obtained by nuclear angiography are in the range of 3.1 to 3.3 sec^{-1}.[36-38] There is a considerable increase in peak filling rate on exercise, whether measured by contrast[34] or nuclear angiography. From the nuclear time-activity curve, peak filling occurs 130 msec to 170 msec after minimum counts.[35] The corresponding interval determined angiographically from mitral valve opening to peak filling rate is approximately 60 msec.[36] The difference probably reflects the difficulty in determining the exact time of start of filling from a time-activity curve, that of minimum counts probably occurring some time during the period of isovolumic relaxation.[37] The normal value of *filling fraction*, the proportion of the stroke volume to enter the ventricle during the first third of diastole, is 47 ± 15% at rest.[38]

LEFT VENTRICULAR DIMENSION AND WALL THICKNESS CHANGES

The pattern of left ventricular dimension and wall thickness changes during filling can be assessed by digitizing a directed M-mode record.[30] Such information is similar to measurements of dimension or segment length made by implanted ultrasonic crystals in experimental animals. Rates of change of transverse dimension do not directly reflect those of volume (see Fig. 37.6).[39] In normal subjects, the two are related in a semiquantitative way, both demonstrating a phase of rapid early diastolic increase after mitral valve opening followed by a period of diastasis. However, comparison of the two curves shows that the peak rate of increase in transverse dimension characteristically precedes that of volume by 20 msec to 40 msec, reflecting an early diastolic change in cavity shape toward a more circular configuration. Dimension changes elsewhere in the ventricle must thus be delayed with respect to those of volume. The timing of the end of rapid volume and of dimension increase, however, are indistinguishable. The extent of volume increase during left atrial systole is consistently underestimated from transverse dimension and frequently undetectable on an M-mode echocardiogram. Major discrepancies may occur between the extent and timing of volume and dimension changes in disease. Dimension may alter during isovolumic periods; in coronary artery disease, for example, the greater part of transverse dimension increase may occur before mitral valve opening, with a corresponding reduction in local movement during filling. Asynchronous wall motion may be accentuated with abnormal filling, as in mitral valve disease, even in the absence of significant left ventricular involvement. Finally, the relation between peak rate of dimension increase and volume increase depends directly on left ventricular cavity size. At constant filling rate, peak rate of dimension increase is inversely proportional to the square of simultaneous dimension. Subject to these limitations, M-mode echocardiography has proved a valuable tool in studying disturbances of left ventricular filling. Peak rate of dimension increase from digitized records in normal subjects is 15 ± 3 cm per second. Peak rate of dimension increase occurs 80 msec to 120 msec after mitral valve opening, and the rate of increase has returned to 20% of its peak value by 160

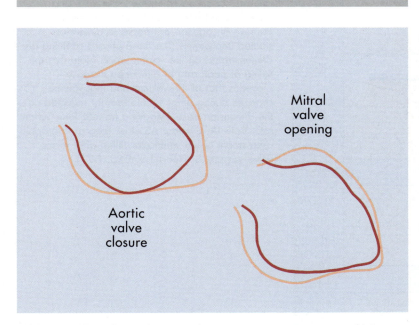

FIGURE 37.5 Effect of asynchronous relaxation on apparent pattern of left ventricular wall motion shown by two-frame display. Both panels are derived from the same beat of the angiogram of a patient with coronary artery disease. On the left, end-systole has been taken as coinciding with aortic valve closure, and on the right with mitral valve opening. Note the striking difference in the apparent pattern of regional wall motion.

± 40 msec. This latter interval defines the early diastolic period of rapid dimension increase.

The earliest method by which left ventricular wall thickness was measured *in vivo* in humans was with angiography, as the distance between the epicardial border of the heart shadow and the outer edge of the ventricular cavity opacified by dye. It is possible to demonstrate reciprocal relations between dimension and wall thickness changes.[27] After mitral valve opening, there is a rapid fall in free wall thickness as dimension increases during the period of early diastolic left ventricular filling. A more satisfactory means of studying these relations is to use M-mode echocardiography, which allows them to be extended to the interventricular septum.[30] The rate of thinning of the posterior wall at the level of the chordae during early diastole is high, 10.7 ± 1.7 cm per second, considerably higher than the rate of increase in thickness during ejection, 4.6 ± 1.2 cm per second. This rapid thinning period is coterminous with that of the rapid dimension increase and has a mean duration of 100 ± 20 msec. Rapid thinning is not shown by the septum, while in the posterior wall, its rate varies with position, being maximum at mid-cavity level.

PRESSURE CHANGES

Extrapolation of the exponential pressure decline during isovolumic relaxation suggests that significant tension may still be present at the time of mitral valve opening and persist during early filling. This phenomenon has been termed *incomplete relaxation*.[18] In open-chest dogs, no such effect could be detected beyond a period of three times T after the timing of peak minimum dP/dt. At rapid heart rates, passive ventricular stiffness was increased at intervals less than this. Incomplete relaxation has not been definitely identified in normal humans, but it may be responsible for maintaining ventricular pressure early during the filling period and possibly causing a small increase in wall stiffness at this time. Related to incomplete relaxation is the idea of *diastolic tone*, which refers to sustained tension developed by myofibrils, rather than the simple termination of the relaxation process. There is no evidence to suggest that any such effect can be recognized under normal circumstances, but it may be induced by prolonged ischemia and thus be related to the contracture that occasionally occurred after cardiopulmonary bypass operations when ischemic arrest of the heart was used.

Peak left ventricular filling rate is correlated with atrioventricular pressure difference, both at rest and on exercise. Both pressures continue to fall after mitral valve opening in normal subjects during the early part of the filling period, that in the left ventricle reaching a minimum value 140 ± 50 msec after mitral valve opening as determined angiographically, and 55 ± 60 msec after the time at which peak filling rate occurs. This period of falling left ventricular pressure thus includes the greater part of rapid filling, including all that of accelerating flow, and accounts for 30% to 50% of the total stroke volume at rest. When heart rate is rapid and filling time short, this percentage is even higher. The cause of this delay in minimum left ventricular pressure has not been established but is likely to involve the interaction of a number of factors including the termination of relaxation, dynamic flow, and possibly the dissipation of potential energy within the myocardium generated during the previous systole.

The possible presence of ventricular pressures negative to atmospheric early in diastole is referred to as *ventricular suction*.[40,41] Its demonstration in intact humans presents problems owing to difficulty in defining the zero for pressure measurement, particularly because there is evidence to suggest that normal tissue pressure is negative to atmospheric. Recent suggestive evidence for the presence of ventricular suction comes from the demonstration of subatmospheric pressure early in diastole in the left ventricle in patients in whom normal rapid ventricular filling was prevented by mitral stenosis.[42] These were not seen in normal subjects.

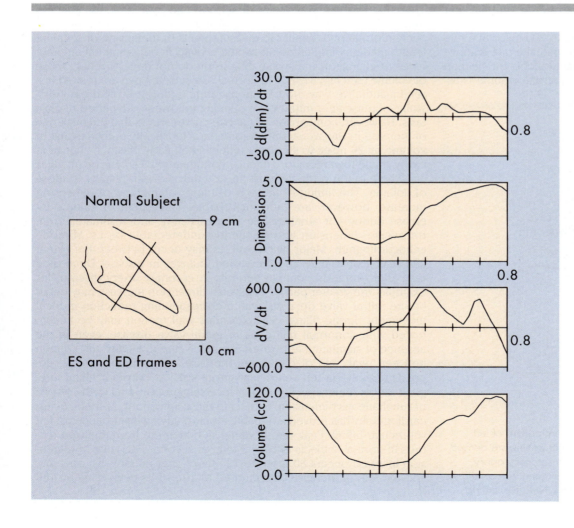

FIGURE 37.6 Volume and dimension changes during filling in a normal subject. Changes in cavity volume, calculated from right anterior oblique projection (*bottom trace*), include the rate of change of volume [d(vol)/dt], transverse dimension, rate of change of dimension [d(dim)/dt], and superimposed end-diastolic and end-systolic frames with position of transverse dimension studied (*top panel*). The three phases of filling are demonstrated on the volume trace. Note that the timing of peak rate of dimension increase precedes that of the volume and that volume changes during atrial systole are not reflected on the dimension trace. (Modified from St John Sutton MG, Traill TA, Ghafour AS et al: Echocardiographic assessment of left ventricular filling after mitral valve surgery. Br Heart J 39:1283, 1977)

ABNORMAL LEFT VENTRICULAR FILLING

MITRAL STENOSIS

Rapid left ventricular filling is very abnormal in mitral stenosis. Peak filling rate, determined angiographically, is reduced to values of 390 ± 110 msec,[33,43] and the pattern of filling is modified, with loss of differentiation into the early diastolic rapid filling period and mid-diastolic period of diastasis. This abnormal filling pattern is also reflected in disturbed transmitral flow, assessed by Doppler echocardiography.[44] This method shows that peak velocity is increased along with the diastolic pressure gradient and is maintained throughout the filling period rather than falling normally during mid-diastole. M-mode echocardiography shows a reduction in the peak rate of dimension increase and prolongation or complete loss of the early rapid filling period.[30] The low rate of increase in cavity volume has been demonstrated angiographically to be accompanied by incoordinate rather than slow regional outward wall motion. In one third of cases, the cavity appears to oscillate with 2 mm or more of inward wall motion during filling in one part of the cavity associated with accelerated outward movement elsewhere.[43] These findings suggest some independence of regional wall motion from transmitral flow.

HYPERTROPHIC CARDIOMYOPATHY

Indirect evidence for an abnormal pattern of left ventricular filling in hypertrophic cardiomyopathy came from the observation of a slow y descent on the left atrial pressure pulse and a reduced diastolic closure rate on the mitral echogram. However, both these measurements have a multifactorial basis, and neither is now considered to give a valid estimate of filling rate. A reduced left ventricular filling rate was seen in a small number of cases studied angiographically.[45] In a larger series,[46] however, the mean value of filling rate was normal at 770 ± 260 ml per second, but scatter was increased. In eight out of twenty patients, the rapid filling phase was abnormally prolonged. There was negative correlation between peak filling rate and isovolumic relaxation time, so that if isovolumic relaxation time was prolonged, filling rate was low. Clinically, patients whose exercise tolerance was limited by chest pain had significantly lower filling rates than those in whom the limiting symptom was breathlessness. Similar observations have been made more recently by nuclear angiography.[47]

Diastolic abnormalities can also be demonstrated by M-mode echocardiography. The rate of transverse dimension increase and posterior wall thinning are reduced in approximately half.[30] Mitral valve opening is delayed with respect to minimum cavity dimension, and isovolumic relaxation is prolonged unless severe left ventricular outflow tract obstruction is present. These changes are reversed by verapamil administration.[9] Regional abnormalities of ventricular function have been studied angiographically, and slow filling has been shown to be on the basis of incoordinate rather than uniformly slow outward motion.[48] The mechanism underlying these diastolic changes is not clear. It is possible that they are due to incomplete relaxation, but because pressure decay is frequently not exponential, T cannot be calculated. Alternatively, these abnormalities may reflect loss of normal fiber architecture, either locally or generally throughout the ventricle with fiber disarray.

Diastolic abnormalities have also been demonstrated in patients with secondary left ventricular hypertrophy due to a variety of causes, including aortic stenosis and systemic hypertension. On M-mode echocardiography, it is possible to demonstrate prolongation of the interval from A_2 to mitral valve opening and reduction in peak rate of dimension increase in over 50% of cases.[4,49] These abnormalities are distributed unimodally, with a median value and distribution indistinguishable from those seen in hypertrophic cardiomyopathy. More recently, similar disturbances of filling have been documented by radionuclide angiography.[50] Both techniques have clearly demonstrated that diastolic abnormalities can occur in the absence of any detectable depression of systolic function. During exercise, patients with left ventricular hypertrophy show further abnormalities of diastolic time intervals. Left ventricular filling time does not show its normal shortening with tachycardia, and at a heart rate of 160 beats per minute, it is approximately double the normal value. This increase is accommodated in part by a striking reduction in isovolumic relaxation time and in part by shortening of QA_2.[32]

CORONARY ARTERY DISEASE

A reduced rate of early diastolic filling is frequently seen in patients with coronary artery disease. Values for peak filling rate obtained using contrast angiography are in the range of 340 ml to 600 ml per second, though there is considerable scatter depending on the population studied.[54-56] Early diastolic filling rates, normalized to end-diastolic volume, are also reduced to the range of 1.34 sec^{-1} to 4.07 sec^{-1}, measured either by contrast or by radionuclide angiography.[20,34,35] As with mitral stenosis, the pattern of inflow is modified, with prolongation of the early diastolic filling period and loss of the normal period of diastasis. Filling fraction is reduced,[38] and the time interval from minimum counts to that of peak inflow rate is increased, particularly in patients in whom the ejection fraction is low.[36] The overall specificities and sensitivities of these indices of ventricular filling are too low to allow them to be used as reliable noninvasive markers of significant coronary artery disease in individual patients. In patients with coronary artery disease, peak diastolic filling rate increases significantly with exercise, although the differences with respect to normal persist.[34]

The mechanism of these diastolic abnormalities is not clear. The most consistent clinical association has been with ejection fraction. When the ejection fraction is normal, the filling rate ranges from 2.1 sec^{-1} to 2.4 sec^{-1}, while values of only half this are seen when the ejection fraction is depressed and particularly when end-systolic volume is increased. The number and site of coronary arteries involved, the presence of Q waves on the electrocardiogram, and β-blocker therapy all seem to be without influence. However, as in hypertrophic cardiomyopathy, events occurring during isovolumic relaxation can also affect peak filling rate. The time constant of relaxation as measured from the left ventricular pressure pulse is prolonged[19,20] and is correlated inversely with filling rate at rest and with atrial pacing.[19] In addition, the extent of change in cavity shape during isovolumic relaxation[35] is increased in patients in whom filling is slow. Thus, asynchronous relaxation seems to be a significant factor in the pathogenesis of the reduced rate of ventricular filling in coronary artery disease. Even when the filling rate is within normal limits, incoordinate wall motion after mitral valve opening has been demonstrated by radionuclide[51] and contrast angiography,[35] and as in mitral stenosis oscillations of the ventricle can be demonstrated in approximately one third of cases.

MECHANISMS AND CLINICAL SIGNIFICANCE

The physical basis of rapid filling remains uncertain, although it is a period of considerable functional significance in the cardiac cycle, accounting for at least half the stroke volume at rest and more on exercise. The consistent finding of falling pressure and increasing volume seems to exclude a purely passive basis, and a variety of mechanisms have been proposed to explain it. These depend on the idea that energy stored from the previous systole is coupled to the circulation early in diastole, as a result of the action of restoring forces. These forces are proportional to the degree of deformation of the left ventricular cavity from its end-diastolic configuration. There is still no agreement as to whether they have a single anatomical basis, possible mechanisms having been identified at the levels of the myofibril, the single cell, and the isolated heart.[52] All cause the sarcomere length to return toward its resting length in the absence of hydrostatic gradient when contraction has ceased. The presence of such forces might also be expected to interact with the relaxation process itself, owing to its load dependence.[3] If the storage of such forces were related to myocardial fiber structure, then a basis for the consistent patterns of wall motion seen in humans during rapid filling would be provided.

Because the major part of the stroke volume enters the left ventricle during the period of rapid filling, its impairment in left ventricular disease is likely to be of considerable clinical significance, particularly during exercise, when filling time is limited. A promising group of patients to study is those with isolated disturbances of diastolic function (*e.g.*, particularly left ventricular hypertrophy). In such patients, systolic function is frequently normal, but exercise tolerance is reduced, with clinical evidence of "heart failure." Treatment with diuretics and vasodilators has proved unsatisfactory or even dangerous,[53] while improvement follows administration of negative inotropic agents such as slow channel or β-adrenergic blocking agents.

PASSIVE VENTRICULAR FILLING

Study of the passive properties of the left ventricle has evolved into a subject of considerable complexity that has, as yet, contributed disappointingly little to the understanding and treatment of disease. Nevertheless, this body of information is worthy of review, if only to give some idea of the complexity of diastolic function in humans, and to guard against simplistic interpretations of the effects of drugs or disease.

VENTRICULAR CHAMBER STIFFNESS

The period of passive filling of the ventricle can be said to start when pressure and volume increase together toward the end of rapid filling and to last until the start of atrial systole. Even when heart rate is slow, only 10% to 20% of the total stroke volume enters the ventricle during this phase, and the proportion is even smaller during exercise. If pressure and volume do increase together, it is possible to plot one against the other and so obtain a pressure–volume curve. The *stiffness* of the ventricle is defined as the slope of this curve and expressed as the ratio dP/dV, where dP and dV are small increments of pressure and volume, respectively, so that the ratio represents the pressure increase brought about by unit increase in volume expressed in millimeters of mercury per milliliter (Fig. 37.7). The reciprocal of stiffness, dV/dP, is referred to as *compliance* or *distensibility*. This definition implies that if two ventricles are similar in all respects except that their volumes differ, then their relative stiffnesses measured in terms of dP/dV will be inversely proportional to volume. This effect can be allowed for by considering not an absolute increment in volume but a relative one, dV/V,

i.e., volume change per unit volume, and defining *volume elasticity* as V · dP/dV or rate of change of pressure with relative volume changes. The reciprocal of this quantity, 1/V · dV/dP, is referred to as *specific compliance*, and represents compliance normalized to unit volume.

The left ventricular pressure–volume curve is not linear, but becomes steeper as filling proceeds, with a corresponding increase in slope corresponding to dP/dV. This increase is such that there is an approximately linear relation between cavity pressure and dP/dV, whose slope is the *stiffness constant*. A linear relation between pressure and stiffness implies an exponential relation between pressure and volume of the form

$$P = Ke^{av} + b$$

where a corresponds to the stiffness constant and b and k are empirical constants. It follows from these considerations that simple measurements of stiffness vary considerably through diastole, so that it is necessary to specify either the pressure at which they were made or the time in the cardiac cycle, for example, at end-diastole, to avoid ambiguity. In normal subjects, end-diastolic stiffness is in the range 0.15 mm Hg to 0.4 mm Hg per milliliter, but it is several times greater in patients with hypertrophic or congestive cardiomyopathy.[54,55] The stiffness constant itself is not a direct measure of cavity stiffness. Its units are not those of stiffness, but ml^{-1} or reciprocal volume, so it expresses the dependence of stiffness on cavity pressure. A ventricle in which pressure and volume were linearly related throughout passive filling (*i.e.*, one that obeyed Hooke's law) would have a stiffness constant of zero, regardless of the steepness of the slope of the pressure–volume relation itself. Values of the stiffness constant have been reported by several authors. Diamond and Forrester found values of 0.005 ml^{-1} in normal subjects, 0.011 ml^{-1} in chronic coronary artery disease, and 0.045 ml^{-1} after acute myocardial infarction.[54,55] Mirsky reported 0.027 ml^{-1} in normal subjects, 0.038 ml^{-1} in those with hypertrophic cardiomyopathy, and 0.016 ml^{-1} in those with dilated cardiomyopathy.[56] There is considerable variation in the stiffness constant among normal individuals, and it is little different from that in patients with severe left ventricular disease. In addition, the derivation of the stiffness constant itself depends on pressure–volume relation's being exponential. There is no theoretical reason why this should be the case. In practice, deviations are frequently seen, particularly at the extremes of pressure, and values at diastolic pressures lower than 5 mm Hg are usually disregarded.

Possible relations between cavity stiffness and end-diastolic pressure are summarized in Figure 37.7. *AB* represents a normal pressure–volume curve, and the point *b* the end-diastolic values. If the properties

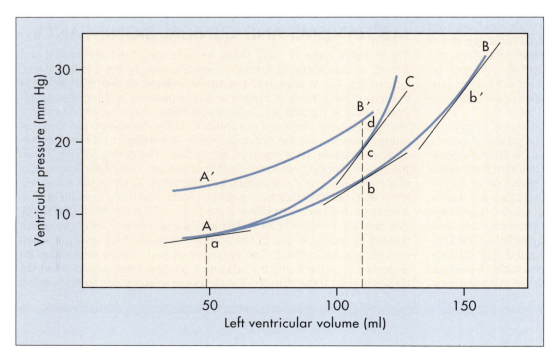

FIGURE 37.7 Passive left ventricular filling. Normal pressure–volume curve is represented by *AB*, and that from a ventricle with increased stiffness constant by *AC*. *A'B'* represents the effect of upward displacement of *AB*. The slopes of the pressure–volume curves (i.e., stiffness values) are shown as tangents at *a*, *b*, *b'*, and *c*.

of the ventricle remain unchanged, but end-diastolic volume enlarges to the point corresponding to b' by increasing venous return, there will be a rise in end-diastolic pressure and in stiffness (corresponding to the slope of the curve at b') but not in the stiffness constant. Alternatively, if the pressure–volume characteristics of the ventricle change to those of the curve AC, then end-diastolic pressure will rise although volume remains constant. The increase in end-diastolic stiffness at point c is identical to that seen at point b', although the stiffness constant of the curve itself has now increased. Finally, if there is upward displacement of the whole pressure–volume curve as a whole as shown by $A'B'$, then end-diastolic pressure will rise to point d, at constant end-diastolic volume, although the stiffness constant and end-diastolic stiffness both remain unchanged. It follows from these considerations that no predictions about the pressure–volume curve of the ventricle or its stiffness can be made from simple measurements of end-diastolic pressure and volume.

The apparent stiffness of a ventricle is affected by the velocity with which it fills, owing to viscous and inertial effects. Viscous forces are proportional to rate of stretching of myocardium and cause measured stiffness to be greater than in the static situation. Indirect evidence for their presence in humans was reported by Gaasch and associates, who noted the pressure–volume curve deviated from an exponential early in diastole and during atrial contraction both in normal subjects and patients with hypertrophic or dilated cardiomyopathy.[57] The maximum deviation between observed and expected values came during atrial systole and ranged from 0.9 mm Hg to 4.8 mm Hg. Although these results are suggestive, they are not conclusive, because the evidence for viscous forces depends simply on deviation of the observed curve from the theoretic exponential. Inertial forces result from outward acceleration of the wall and lead to a reduction in cavity stiffness. The maximum acceleration seen in humans is on the order of 0.25 g, suggesting that such forces are small and unlikely to cause pressure changes of more than 1 mm Hg.

VARIATION IN PRESSURE–VOLUME RELATIONS

A much more fundamental objection to the idea that the left ventricle in intact humans consistently behaves as a simple elastic structure has come from the observation of acute shifts in the pressure-volume curve by pharmacologic or other interventions. Angiotensin administration shifts the whole pressure–volume curve upwards, and nitroprusside has the reverse effect.[58] The changes are large, being on the order of 5 mm Hg to 20 mm Hg at an identical ventricular volume. There is no associated change in mean ventricular filling rate, T, or pleural pressure. Similar shifts have been observed with isometric handgrip,[59] and during pacing-induced angina,[60] which increase ventricular pressure at any given volume, and with propranolol,[61] nifedipine,[62] or nitrates, which have the reverse effect. The mechanism underlying these changes remains uncertain. In acute angina, a true change in ventricular diastolic properties may well occur. The elevation of diastolic pressure has been related to prolongation of the time constant of relaxation and also to a striking increase in the asymptote, which approaches zero.[19] Such an analysis clearly depends on the assumption of monoexponential pressure decay in a ventricle likely to be the seat of regional abnormalities of relaxation during angina.

EFFECTS OF PERICARDIAL RESTRAINT

One possible mechanism underlying shifts in the pressure–volume relation is interference with ventricular filling by the pericardium. Ventricular diastolic pressure measured relative to some external reference such as mid-chest or atmosphere may increase because of a rise in pericardial pressure, with the pressure difference across the myocardium remaining unchanged.[63,64] If it is assumed that the pericardium restricts ventricular filling in intact humans, then a drug or maneuver that increases cardiac volume, such as angiotensin or isometric handgrip, might be expected to cause an increase in pericardial pressure, and a reduction in cardiac volume would have the reverse effect. There is much evidence in the dog to support this hypothesis, where volume expansion caused a marked upward shift of the left ventricular pressure-dimension curve only when the pericardium was intact.[63,64] The exact nature of this restriction to ventricular filling is complex. In part, it is due to simple elevation of the hydrostatic pressure within the pericardial space. This is particularly likely to occur if there is a pericardial effusion, and the measurement of such pressures is straightforward with a standard catheter system. A second mechanism of restraint is by direct pressure of the pericardium or other extracardiac structures on the epicardium of the ventricle. This need not be associated with an increase in simple hydrostatic pressure in the pericardial space and might be caused, for example, by surrounding the heart with a net. Both these mechanisms restrict ventricular filling by exerting a pressure (*i.e.*, a force per unit area) on the epicardial surfaces, and it is the sum of these forces, *surface pressure*, that must be measured.[64] This cannot be done with a simple fluid-filled catheter in the pericardial space, but a satisfactory method is to introduce a small balloon with a volume of 1 ml to 2 ml, and measure the pressure inside it. In humans, the evidence for pericardial involvement is not so clear. When left ventricular pressure–volume relations were displaced upward during pacing-induced angina, there was no corresponding change in right ventricular pressure, which would have been the case if pericardial pressure had increased.[60] In postoperative patients, surface pressure can be measured by solid-state transducers directed toward the epicardium, which are left in place at the time of surgery. Up to a 10% change in transverse left ventricular dimension measured by echocardiography, caused by isometric handgrip or nitroglycerin administration, was not associated with measurable change in pericardial pressure.[65] Nevertheless, the role of the pericardium should always be considered in the analysis of diastolic events. Normal pericardial pressure is low, but it varies during the cardiac cycle. Pericardial disease leads to the classic disturbances of pericardial constriction and tamponade. Direct measurement of pericardial pressure after open heart surgery has demonstrated that elevated values may persist, leading to a corresponding increase in ventricular filling pressures.[66] A similar increase can be postulated when ventricular dilatation occurs owing to disease, particularly when there is an associated pericardial effusion. Such an elevated pericardial pressure must cause a corresponding increase in the filling pressure of both ventricles. An isolated change in left ventricular diastolic pressure cannot be due to the effects of the pericardium alone. In addition, the effects of the pericardium are likely to be greater toward the end of diastole, causing an increased slope in the pressure–volume relation rather than simple upward displacement.[63] It is of interest that elevated left ventricular end-diastolic pressure due to pericardial effusion or constriction occurring clinically differs from that due to left ventricular disease in that it seldom causes pulmonary congestion or edema.

ALTERATION IN RIGHT VENTRICULAR VOLUME

Changes in right ventricular cavity size and pressure may also modify left ventricular diastolic properties. In dogs, an increase in right ventricular volume is associated with upward displacement of the left ventricular pressure volume curve. In humans, there is substantial evidence to support this interaction, which may presumably be mediated through either the interventricular septum or the pericardium. Distortion of the left ventricular cavity by right ventricular enlargement can readily be demonstrated by two-dimensional echocardiography, and acute shifts of the septum follow volume loading in humans. The possibility that changes in right ventricular function might underlie acute shifts in the left ventricular pressure-volume relation was also supported by a comparison of the effects of nitroglycerin and amyl nitrite.[67] Both drugs caused a substantial reduction in aortic pressure. Only nitroglycerin caused a reduction in right ventricular end-diastolic pressure, which was associated with downward displacement of the left ventricular pressure–volume curve. Both right ventricular end-diastolic pressure and the left ventricular pressure–volume curve were unchanged after amyl nitrite. However, it seems unlikely that unloading was responsible for the effects of nifedipine in patients with hypertrophic cardiomyopathy, because both it and nitroprusside cause a reduction in end-diastolic pressure, but nitroprusside causes a fall and nifedipine causes an increase in end-diastolic volume.[68]

CORONARY PERFUSION PRESSURE

Changes in coronary artery perfusion pressure represent a third mechanism by which ventricular pressure–volume relations might be altered. Experimentally, a significant effect of perfusion pressure on ventricular diastolic properties has been reported only at pressures below 80 mm Hg. Those within the physiologic range have been without effect.[69] The significance of coronary perfusion pressure in humans as a determinant of left ventricular diastolic properties remains unsubstantiated.

CAVITY SHAPE

A final mechanism by which left ventricular pressure–volume relations could potentially be altered is by a change in cavity shape. If cavity shape is allowed to vary, then volume can increase as the ventricle assumes a more spherical configuration without any distention of the myocardium. Such a volume increase might thus be associated with a smaller pressure increase than an identical one with which cavity shape remained constant. Changes in cavity shape are a prominent feature of the normal cardiac cycle but are frequently lost in disease, particularly when the ejection fraction is low.

LEFT VENTRICULAR STRESS–STRAIN RELATIONS

An alternative approach to the study of the passive diastolic properties of the left ventricle may be taken by investigating stress–strain relations of the wall rather than the stiffness of the cavity. A *stress* is a force per unit area, and it has direction as well as magnitude. If the force is perpendicular to the cross section, it is described as a *normal stress;* if it is parallel, it is described as a *shear stress*. Stresses need not be uniformly distributed, and there is much evidence to suggest that in the left ventricular wall they are not. Such nonuniformity may be due to the structure of the myocardium, the shape of the cavity, or variation with position across the wall.

DERIVATION OF WALL STRESS

Left ventricular wall stress is commonly calculated using Laplace's law:

$$p = t(1/r + 1/R)$$

where p is cavity pressure, t is wall tension, and r and R are the principal radii of curvature. This formulation makes a number of significant assumptions. The myocardium is assumed to be *linearly elastic* (*i.e.,* to obey Hooke's law) and to be *isotropic* and *homogeneous* (*i.e.,* its properties are uniform with respect to direction and position). It is treated as being in equilibrium, so that dynamic components are not considered. Wall stress is assumed to be constant across the wall, which is unlikely to be the case if the wall's thickness is greater than one tenth that of the radius of curvature. A number of formulations based on these assumptions have been proposed, a widely used one for a thin-walled ellipsoid being that of Falsetti[70]:

$$\sigma = \frac{Pb}{h} \cdot \frac{(2a^2 - b^2)}{2a^2 + bh}$$

where a and b are endocardial major and minor axes, respectively, P is cavity pressure, and h is wall thickness. Estimates of left ventricular wall stress based on Laplace's law have been widely used to derive stress–strain relations. A *strain* is a proportional deformation, defined as increase in length divided by unstressed length, and so is dimensionless. As with the relation between pressure and volume, the stress–strain curve of the normal left ventricle is nonlinear, so that at any point *elastic stiffness* (E) can be defined as the slope of the curve ($d\sigma/d\epsilon$). Experimentally, the curve has been shown to approximate an exponential form, because stiffness increases with strain. In order to construct such curves, it is necessary to measure left ventricular cavity size, wall thickness, or left ventricular mass and cavity pressure throughout diastole. Standard analysis of right anterior oblique (RAO) angiograms allows minor and major axes to be measured, along with free wall thickness. Pressure is measured with a micromanometer during the angiogram. An alternative approach has been to use a simultaneous M-mode echocardiogram recorded at a paper speed of 100 msec per second and a high-fidelity pressure.[71] Such estimates of wall stress are obviously approximations. The simple Laplace formulation cannot take into account regional variations in geometry such as the reversal of curvature frequently seen on the inferior wall of the heart or the complex fiber structure of the myocardium. It is inadequate to describe any disease pattern that is regional in its involvement. Alternative methods for calculating wall stress have been described. These include a true thick-walled model that allows for variation in stress across the wall.[72] Although the mathematics of this model are more complex, calculated average stresses are still of the same order as those from the simpler Laplace equation, with significant differences occurring only at the apex. A second approach is to use the finite element method, which is particularly suitable for structures of complex shape and composition. In this method, the whole structure is broken down into smaller elements of simpler geometry.[73] The elements can be reconstructed to form the required shape and material properties to the desired degree of complexity.

A number of approaches have been used to analyze left ventricular stress–strain relations. That most commonly used has been to assume an exponential relation between the two of the form

$$d\sigma/d\epsilon = k\sigma + c$$

where σ is stress, ϵ is strain, k is the elastic constant, and c is an empirical constant. This implies that, as for the pressure–volume relation, left ventricular wall stiffness is a function of strain. It is thus possible to define an *elastic constant* which is dimensionless, that expresses this dependence of E on strain. Normal values are in the range of 10 to 20,[54,55] although exact comparison between reported series is not always possible owing to differences in the method by which they are derived. High values of the elastic constant are seen when the left ventricular cavity is dilated and the ejection fraction is reduced as in dilated cardiomyopathy or severe coronary artery disease. By contrast, in left ventricular hypertrophy, whether it is due to aortic stenosis or hypertrophic cardiomyopathy, values overlap the normal range.[54,55,74] Corresponding values of E at end-diastole are 10 kN to 20 kN per square meter (100 to 200 g/cm²) in normal subjects. Values are considerably increased with cavity dilatation and low ejection fraction,[55,74] but they are normal or only slightly raised with hypertrophy. Apart from limitations inherent in the wall stress calculations, these estimates are open to a number of criticisms. They do not take into account the possible effects of pericardial pressure, right ventricular abnormalities, or coronary perfusion. They make the fundamental assumption that throughout diastole, volume increase occurs by simple stretching of myocardium along its long axis. This is questionable. During systole, minor axis shortening is 30% to 40% of end-diastolic length, very much greater than the 10% shortening of normally loaded sarcomeres. The difference seems to result from thickening of myocardial fibers and their oblique arrangement. The same conditions must apply in reverse during diastole, indicating that cavity dimensions increase significantly more than the myocardial fibers themselves are stretched. Thus stress–strain relations as measured in the intact heart need bear no clear relation to the material properties of the myocardial fibers themselves.

DYNAMIC FACTORS

Dynamic factors may also affect stress–strain relations. Viscosity leads to an increase in wall stiffness when the cavity is being distended rapidly. *In vitro* evidence suggests that it becomes significant in papillary muscles at rates of distention of more than 1 sec^{-1} and more pronounced as fiber length increases.[75] The simplest assumption is that its main determinant is the rate of increase of strain (*strain rate*). In instrumented dogs, departures from the theoretic exponential stress–strain relation have indeed been detected that are greater at times of rapid filling[76] and approximately proportional to strain rate, so that values for the constant of viscosity can be calculated. A similar approach in humans has yielded a value of 0.3 ± 0.1 N/sec/m^2 for the constant in patients in whom left ventricular function was normal, with similar values in those with aortic valve disease.[77] However, in these studies, other factors were not considered, including the length dependence of viscosity and the possibility of an effect on stress–strain relations during early diastole by incomplete relaxation.[78] It is thus doubtful whether all departures from the theoretic exponential can uniquely be ascribed to viscosity, particularly when the effects of loading by the pericardium and the right ventricle have not been excluded. In patients with mitral stenosis, in whom filling is much slower than normal, similar departures from the exponential relation are seen in early diastole,[71] raising the possibility that some different mechanism is involved.

Stress–strain relations may alter over a period that is long in comparison with a cardiac cycle. *Creep* is time-dependent lengthening of a material held at constant stress. When it is released, it does not return to its initial length. A related process is *stress relaxation,* which describes a reduction in stress in a material when strain is held constant. These two are described as *plastic properties*. The possibility arises that they, or some related effect, may be the basis of chronic enlargement of the left ventricular cavity such as occurs with chronic volume overload. There is no clear evidence for their involvement in humans, in whom cavity dilatation is due not to stretching of sarcomeres, but rather to realignment of muscle fibers.[79]

CLINICAL SIGNIFICANCE OF ABNORMALITIES OF PASSIVE FILLING

Variation in diastolic pressure–volume relation with drugs or other interventions has considerable clinical significance. It means that measurements of left ventricular end-diastolic pressure cannot be used to assess left ventricular volume or sarcomere length during acute interventions or taken as identical with preload as a basis for constructing Starling curves. This variability is of considerable therapeutic importance and may well be the basis of the favorable effects of nitrates or slow channel blocking agents in patients with cavity dilatation or left ventricular hypertrophy and even of the paradoxical effects of β-blockers in those with congestive cardiomyopathy.[80] The genesis of a raised end-diastolic pressure, commonly used as clinical evidence of left ventricular disease can be seen as very complex, with no clear relation to any single aspect of systolic or diastolic function. The variable relation between end-diastolic pressure and volume implies that if ventricular diastolic properties are to be studied, the possible effects of the pericardium and right ventricle must be taken into account. It is often implied that there is a direct relation between the passive properties of the left ventricle and peak filling rate such that when compliance is reduced, filling is slow. The basis for this supposition is not clear. Peak filling rate occurs before the ventricle has begun to show passive properties, excluding a direct physical relation between the two. The possibility of a biologic correlation exists, but in order for it to be confirmed, the time in the cardiac cycle or the pressure at which measurements of compliance are made must be specified, and these figures must be correlated with peak filling rate determined by some validated method. No such study has been reported. Whether filling rate alters ventricular stiffness in any clinically significant way as the result of viscosity remains uncertain; increased filling rate in early diastole may cause the pressure to rise a few millimeters of mercury, but there is little evidence to suggest any clinically significant effect on end-diastolic or left atrial pressure. Efforts to correlate stiffness indices with objective myocardial abnormalities have not proved successful. In left ventricular hypertrophy, cavity stiffness is increased but elastic modulus is normal. The most obvious disturbances of these indices are seen in congestive cardiomyopathy or coronary artery disease with cavity dilatation. Although it seems possible that the underlying abnormality is myocardial fibrosis, direct evidence for any but the most tenuous relation is lacking.[81] Finally, passive ventricular filling occurs only when heart rate is slow. It is unlikely, therefore, that abnormalities of this period of the cardiac cycle has any significant effect on exercise tolerance when the heart rate is rapid and the filling time is short.

ATRIAL SYSTOLE
VENTRICULAR FILLING

The effects of atrial systole are apparent from examination of the left ventricular volume trace recorded by contrast or radionuclide angiography. In normal subjects, in whom heart rate is slow enough for a well-developed period of diastasis to be present, atrial systole accounts for approximately 20% of the stroke volume. The rate of ventricular filling also increases to around 200 ml per second or approximately one third to one half of that during the early diastolic rapid filling phase.[33] The effects of atrial systole cannot be clearly identified on the volume trace when heart rate is rapid, because filling is rapid throughout diastole. The contribution of atrial systole to stroke volume is increased in patients with left ventricular disease to approximately 30% of stroke volume, although the absolute volumes are not increased. The increase in cavity volume during atrial systole is not accommodated by uniform outward wall motion but mainly by upward motion of the mitral valve ring. The functional significance of the resulting contribution to stroke volume is apparent with the clinical deterioration that may occur when patients with left ventricular disease develop atrial fibrillation.

PRESSURE CHANGES

Atrial contraction is associated with an increase in left ventricular pressure that is on the order of 2 mm Hg to 5 mm Hg in normal subjects but that may be considerably increased in patients with left ventricular disease. The ratio of pressure to volume increase can be used as a measure of left ventricular stiffness at this stage of the cardiac cycle.[82] A larger pressure increment per unit volume change was particularly characteristic of patients with cardiographic evidence of left ventricular hypertrophy.

CONCLUSION

Major abnormalities of diastolic ventricular function are common in patients with heart disease of all types, including the two most common: hypertrophy and ischemia. They cause limitation of exercise tolerance and pulmonary congestion and can occur in patients in whom systolic function is normal. It is thus clear that the traditional analysis of left ventricular disease in terms of preload, afterload, and contractility is no longer adequate and that if ideas such as "heart failure" or "decompensation" are to be used at all, they must take into account diastolic as well as systolic abnormalities. Further investigation of the events of diastole, particularly those occurring during relaxation and rapid filling, is likely to prove rewarding, not only in gaining an increased understanding of this fascinating aspect of cardiac function at rest and particularly during exercise, but also in laying the basis for the development of new approaches to the treatment of patients with heart disease.

REFERENCES

1. Ebstein E: Die diastole des Herzens. Erg der Physiol 3:130, 1904
2. Wiggers CJ: Studies on the duration of the consecutive phases of the cardiac cycle. I: The duration of the consecutive phases of the cardiac cycle and criteria for their precise determination. Am J Physiol 56:415, 1921
3. Brutsaert DL, Housmans PR, Goethals MA: Dual control of relaxation: Its role in the ventricular function in the mammalian heart. Circ Res 47:637, 1980
4. Chen W, Gibson DG: Relation of isovolumic relaxation to left ventricular wall movement in man. Br Heart J 42:51, 1979
5. Tsakiris AG, Gordon DA, Padiyar R et al: Relation of mitral valve opening and closure to left atrial and ventricular pressures in the intact dog. Am J Physiol 234:H146, 1978
6. Curtiss EI, Matthews RG, Shaver JA: Mechanism of normal splitting of the second heart sound. Circulation 51:157, 1975
7. Mattheos M, Shapiro E, Oldershaw PJ et al: Non-invasive assessment of changes in left ventricular relaxation by combined phono-, echo-, and mechanography. Br Heart J 47:253, 1982
8. Shapiro LM: Echocardiographic features of impaired ventricular function in diabetes. Br Heart J 47:439, 1982
9. Hanrath P, Mathey D, Kremer P et al: Effect of verapamil on left ventricular isovolumic relaxation time and regional left ventricular filling in hypertrophic cardiomyopathy. Am J Cardiol 45:1258, 1980
10. Lorell BH, Paulus W, Grossman W et al: Modification of abnormal left ventricular diastolic properties by nifedipine in patients with hypertrophic cardiomyopathy. Circulation 65:499, 1982
11. Askenazi J, Koenigsberg DI, Ribner HS et al: Prospective study comparing different echocardiographic measurements of pulmonary capillary wedge pressure in patients with organic heart disease other than mitral stenosis. J Am Coll Cardiol 2:919, 1983
12. Gamble WH, Salerni R, Shaver JA: The noninvasive assessment of pulmonary capillary wedge pressure in mitral regurgitation. Am Heart J 107:950, 1984
13. Cohn PF, Liedtke AJ, Serur J et al: Maximal rate of pressure fall (peak negative dP/dt) during ventricular relaxation. Cardiovasc Res 6:263, 1972
14. McLaurin LP, Rolett EL, Grossman W: Impaired left ventricular relaxation during pacing-induced ischemia. Am J Cardiol 32:751, 1973
15. Hirota Y: A clinical study of left ventricular relaxation. Circulation 62:756, 1980
16. Eichhorn P, Grimm J, Koch R et al: Left ventricular relaxation in patients with left ventricular hypertrophy secondary to aortic valve disease. Circulation 65:1395, 1982
17. Weiss JL, Fredericksen JW, Weisfeldt ML: Hemodynamic determinants of the time-course of fall in canine left ventricular pressure. J Clin Invest 58:751, 1976
18. Weisfeldt ML, Weiss JL, Frederiksen JT et al: Quantification of incomplete left ventricular relaxation: Relationship to the time constant for isovolumic pressure fall. Eur Heart J 1:A119, 1980
19. Carroll JD, Hess OM, Hirzel HO et al: Exercise-induced ischemia: The influence of altered relaxation on early diastolic pressures. Circulation 67:521, 1983
20. Fioretti P, Brower RW, Meester GT et al: Interaction of left ventricular relaxation and filling during early diastole in human subjects. Am J Cardiol 46:197, 1980
21. Raff GL, Glantz SA: Volume loading slows left ventricular isovolumic relaxation rate. Circ Res 48:813, 1981
22. Thompson DS, Waldron CB, Coltart DJ et al: Estimation of time constant of left ventricular relaxation. Br Heart J 49:250, 1983
23. Thompson DS, Wilmshurst P, Juul SM et al: Pressure-derived indices of left ventricular isovolumic relaxation in patients with hypertrophic cardiomyopathy. Br Heart J 49:259, 1983
24. Rousseau MF, Veiter C, Detry J-M et al: Impaired early left ventricular relaxation in coronary artery disease: Effects of intracoronary nifedipine. Circulation 62:764, 1980
25. Thompson DS, Waldron CB, Juul SM et al: Analysis of left ventricular pressure during isovolumic relaxation in coronary artery disease. Circulation 65:690, 1982
26. Gibson DG, Prewitt TA, Brown DJ: Analysis of left ventricular wall movement during isovolumic relaxation and its relation to coronary artery disease. Br Heart J 38:1010, 1976
27. Gibson DG, Traill TA, Brown DJ: Changes in left ventricular free wall thickness in patients with ischaemic heart disease. Br Heart J 39:1312, 1977
28. Greenbaum RA, Gibson DG: Regional non-uniformity of left ventricular wall movement in man. Br Heart J 45:29, 1981
29. Gaasch WH, Blaustein AS, Bing OHL: Asynchronous (segmental early) relaxation of the left ventricle. J Am Coll Cardiol 5:891, 1985
30. Upton MT, Gibson DG: The study of left ventricular function from digitized echocardiograms. Prog Cardiovasc Dis 20:359, 1978
31. Gibson DG, Marier DL: Limitations of the two frame method in displaying left ventricular wall motion. Br Heart J 44:555, 1980
32. Oldershaw PJ, Dawkins KD, Ward DE et al: Effect of exercise on left ventricular filling in left ventricular hypertrophy. Br Heart J 49:568, 1983
33. Hammermeister KE, Warbasse JR: The rate of change of left ventricular volume in man. II: Diastolic events in health and disease. Circulation 49:739, 1974
34. Carroll JD, Hess OM, Hirzel HD et al: Dynamics of left ventricular filling at rest and during exercise. Circulation 68:59, 1983
35. Hui WKK, Gibson DG: Mechanisms of reduced left ventricular filling rate in coronary artery disease. Br Heart J 50:362, 1983
36. Bonow RO, Bacharach SL, Green MV et al: Impaired left ventricular diastolic filling in patients with coronary artery disease: Assessment with radionuclide angiography. Circulation 64:315, 1981
37. Iskandrian AS, Hakki AH, DePace NL et al: Evaluation of left ventricular function by radionuclide angiography during exercise in normal subjects and in patients with chronic coronary artery disease. J Am Coll Cardiol 1:1518, 1983
38. Reduto LA, Wickemeyer WJ, Young JB et al: Left ventricular diastolic performance at rest and during exercise in patients with coronary artery disease: Assessment with first pass radionuclide angiography. Circulation 63:1228, 1981
39. St. John Sutton MG, Traill TA, Ghafour AS et al: Echocardiographic assessment of left ventricular filling after mitral valve surgery. Br Heart J 39:1283, 1977
40. Brecher GA: Critical review of recent work on ventricular diastolic suction. Circ Res 6:554, 1958
41. Katz LN: The role played by the ventricular relaxation process in filling the ventricle. Am J Physiol 95:542, 1930
42. Sabbah HN, Anbe DT, Stein PD: Negative intraventricular diastolic pressure in patients with mitral stenosis: Evidence of left ventricular diastolic suction. Am J Cardiol 45:562, 1980
43. Hui WKK, Lee PK, Chow JSF et al: Analysis of regional left ventricular wall motion during diastole in mitral stenosis. Br Heart J 50:231, 1983
44. Hatle L, Brubakk A, Tromsdal A et al: Noninvasive assessment of pressure drop in mitral stenosis by Doppler ultrasound. Br Heart J 40:131, 1978
45. Holt JH, Frank M, Dodge HT: Ventricular ejection and filling rates in idiopathic hypertrophic subaortic stenosis (abstr). Circulation [Suppl III] 40:108, 1969
46. Sanderson JE, Gibson DG, Brown DJ et al: Left ventricular filling in hypertrophic cardiomyopathy: An angiographic study. Br Heart J 39:661, 1977
47. Bonow RO, Leon MB, Rosing DR et al: Effects of verapamil and propranolol on left ventricular systolic function and diastolic filling in patients with coronary artery disease: Radionuclide angiographic studies at rest and during exercise. Circulation 65:1337, 1982
48. Gibson DG, Sanderson JE, Traill TA et al: Regional left ventricular wall movement in hypertrophic cardiomyopathy. Br Heart J 40:1327, 1978
49. Gibson DG, Traill TA, Hall RJC et al: Echocardiographic features of secondary left ventricular hypertrophy. Br Heart J 41:54, 1979
50. Fouad FM, Slominski MJ, Tarazi RC: Left ventricular diastolic function in hypertension: Relation to left ventricular mass and systolic function. J Am Coll Cardiol 3:1500, 1984
51. Yamagishi T, Ozaki T, Kumada T et al: Asynchronous left ventricular diastolic filling in patients with isolated disease of the left anterior descending coronary artery: Assessment with radionuclide ventriculography. Circulation 69:933, 1984
52. Winegrad S, Weisberg A, McClennan G: Are restoring forces important to relaxation? Eur Heart J 1[Suppl]:A59, 1980
53. Topol EJ, Traill TA, Fortuin NJ: Hypertensive hypertrophic cardiomyopathy of the elderly. N Engl J Med 312:277, 1985
54. Diamond G, Forrester JS: Effect of coronary artery disease and acute myocardial infarction on left ventricular compliance in man. Circulation 45:11, 1972
55. Fester A, Samet P: Passive elasticity of the human left ventricle. The "parallel elastic element." Circulation 50:609, 1974
56. Mirsky I: Assessment of passive elastic stiffness ot cardiac muscle: Mathematical concepts, physiologic and clinical considerations, direction of future research. Prog Cardiovasc Dis 18:277, 1976
57. Gaasch WH, Cole JS, Quinones MA et al: Dynamic determinants of left ventricular pressure–volume relations in man. Circulation 51:317, 1975
58. Alderman EL, Glantz SA: Acute hemodynamic interventions shift the diastolic pressure-volume curve in man. Circulation 54:662, 1976
59. Flessas AP, Connelly GP, Handa S et al: Effects of isometric exercise on the end-diastolic pressure, volumes, and function of the left ventricle in man. Circulation 53:839, 1976
60. Mann T, Goldberg S, Mudge GH Jr et al: Factors contributing to altered left ventricular diastolic properties during angina pectoris. Circulation 59:14, 1979
61. Coltart DJ, Alderman EL, Robison SC et al: Effect of propranolol on left ventricular function, segmental wall motion, and diastolic pressure-volume relation in man. Br Heart J 37:357, 1975
62. Ludbrook PA, Teifenbrunn AJ, Reed FR et al: Acute hemodynamic responses to sublingual nifedipine: Dependence on left ventricular function. Circulation 65:489, 1982
63. Tyberg JV, Misbach GA, Galnyz SA et al: A mechanism for shifts in the diastolic, left ventricular, pressure-volume curve: The role of the pericardium. Eur J Cardiol 7[Suppl]:163, 1978
64. Smiseth OA, Frais MA, Kingma I et al: Assessment of pericardial constraint in dogs. Circulation 71:158, 1985
65. Oldershaw PJ, Shapiro E, Mattheos M et al: Independence of changes in left ventricular diastolic properties of pericardial pressure. Br Heart J 48:125, 1982
66. St. John Sutton MG, Gibson DG: Measurement of postoperative pericardial

pressure in man. Br Heart J 39:1, 1977
67. Ludbrook PA, Byrne JD, MacKnight RC: Influence of right ventricular hemodynamics on left ventricular diastolic pressure-volume relations in man. Circulation 59:21, 1979
68. Paulus WJ, Lorell BH, Craig WE et al: Comparison of the effects of nitroprusside and nifedipine on diastolic properties in patients with hypertrophic cardiomyopathy: Altered left ventricular loading or improved muscle inactivation. J Am Coll Cardiol 2:879, 1983
69. Olsen CO, Attarian DE, Jones RN et al: The coronary pressure-flow determinants of left ventricular compliance in dogs. Circulation 49:856, 1981
70. Falsetti HL, Mates RE, Greene DG et al: Left ventricular wall stress calculated from one-plane cineangiography: An approach to force-velocity analysis in man. Circ Res 26:71, 1970
71. Gibson DG, Brown DJ: Relation between diastolic left ventricular wall stress and strain in man. Br Heart J 36:1066, 1974
72. Mirsky I: Left ventricular stresses in the intact human heart. Biophys J 9:189, 1969
73. Yin RCP: Ventricular wall stress. Circ Res 49:829, 1981
74. Mirsky I, Parmley WW: Assessment of passive elastic stiffness for isolated heart muscle and the intact heart. Circ Res 33:233, 1973
75. Noble MIM: The diastolic viscous properties of cat papillary muscle. Circ Res 40:288, 1977
76. Rankin JS, Arentzian CE, McHale PA: Viscoelastic properties of the diastolic left ventricle in the conscious dog. Circ Res 41:37, 1977
77. Hess OM, Grimm J, Krayenbuehl HP: Diastolic simple elastic and viscoelastic properties of the left ventricle in man. Circulation 59:1178, 1979
78. Pouleur H, Karliner JS, LeWinter M et al: Diastolic viscous properties of the left ventricle. Circ Res 45:410, 1979
79. Linzbach AJ: Heart failure from the point of view of quantitative anatomy. Am J Cardiol 5:370, 1960
80. Vedin A, Wikstrand J, Wilhelmsson C et al: Left ventricular function and beta blockade in chronic ischaemic heart failure. Br Heart J 44:101, 1980
81. Hess OM, Ritter M, Schneider J et al: Diastolic stiffness and myocardial structure in aortic valve disease before and after valve replacement. Circulation 69:855, 1984
82. Grossman W, Stefadouros MA, McLaurin LP et al: Quantitative assessment of left ventricular diastolic stiffness in man. Circulation 47:567, 1973

GENERAL REFERENCES

Glantz SA, Parmley WW: Factors which affect the diastolic pressure-volume curve. Circ Res 42:171-180, 1978
Grossman W, McLaurin LP: Diastolic properties of the left ventricle. Ann Intern Med 84:316, 1976
Traill TA, Gibson DG: Left ventricular relaxation and filling: Study by echocardiography. In Yu PN, Goodwin JF (eds): Progress in Cardiology. Philadelphia, Lea & Febiger, 1979
Yellin EL, Sonnenblick EH, Frater RWM: Dynamic determinants of left ventricular filling: An overview. In Baan J, Arntzenius AC, Yellin EL: Cardiac Dynamics, p. 145. The Hague, Martinus Nijhoff, 1980

CARDIAC BIOPSY

Margaret E. Billingham • Henry D. Tazelaar

CHAPTER 38 VOLUME 1

Before 1962, the only type of diagnostic biopsy of the myocardium described was transthoracic needle biopsy, and this was rarely performed. Since then, the percutaneous transvenous catheter bioptome has become available which has greatly aided our ability to examine the myocardial pathology. This technique has for the first time allowed documentation of the earliest morphologic changes of cardiac disease in the living patient. In addition, it is now possible to follow the evolution of the disease and to document changes following treatment. The endomyocardial biopsy is now recognized as a relatively safe procedure that, if intelligently interpreted, may be of considerable use in the diagnosis, management, and prognosis of patients with cardiac disease. The purpose of this chapter is to describe the technique of endomyocardial biopsy, the methods of handling a biopsy specimen, and the pitfalls of biopsy diagnosis and to survey the diagnoses attainable by endomyocardial biopsy. The practical use of the cardiac biopsy by the clinician is emphasized.

ENDOMYOCARDIAL BIOPTOMES

There have been a number of catheter bioptomes designed or modified for the performance of endomyocardial biopsies. This section deals with only those instruments that are the most frequently used bioptomes in the United States.

THE KONNO-SAKAKIBARA BIOPTOME

The Konno-Sakakibara bioptome,[1] the first endomyocardial bioptome, was developed in 1962. It is approximately 100 cm long with the diameter of a No. 8 French or No. 9 French sheath. This bioptome has two elliptical cutting spoons that measure either 2.5 mm (8 French) or 3.5 mm (9 French) in diameter and produce a relatively large specimen of 3 mm to 4 mm in maximum dimension. The bioptome may be introduced from the neck, leg, or arm and usually requires a vascular cutdown because it is wide. A clinical disadvantage is that it is not flexible and is, therefore, somewhat more difficult to manipulate than either of the two bioptomes described below.

THE CAVES-STANFORD BIOPTOME

The Caves-Stanford bioptome was originally developed by Caves and associates[2] in 1972 and was modified by Mason[3] in 1978. This bioptome is one of the two most frequently used bioptomes in the United States. It was originally designed for a transjugular approach to the right ventricle and is therefore shorter than the Konno-Sakakibara bioptome (about 50 cm in length). It has the outer diameter of a No. 9 French sheath and two cuplike cutting tools, one of which is 2.5 mm in diameter and the other of which is 1.5 mm in diameter. This bioptome produces tissue specimens of 2 mm to 3 mm in diameter. The instrument is flexible and is easy to maneuver. A longer version of this bioptome has been designed for left ventricular biopsies and for the femoral approach to the right ventricle.

THE CORDIS BIOPTOME

The Cordis bioptome is the second most commonly used instrument in the United States. The cutting end is modified from the Olympus Bronchoscope biopsy forceps and in 1974 was known as the King's bioptome. The Cordis bioptome is available in two sizes: a shorter version for a transjugular approach and a longer version for left ventricular biopsy or a femoral approach to the right ventricle. This bioptome is disposable; however, it can be cleaned and reused safely in the same patient. The disadvantage of this bioptome is that it uses a No. 7 French sheath, resulting in biopsy specimens that are much smaller (1–2 mm) than those obtained with either the Konno-Sakikibara or Caves-Stanford bioptome (Fig. 38.1).

TECHNIQUE OF ENDOMYOCARDIAL BIOPSY

The three bioptomes described above have established endomyocardial biopsy as a diagnostic procedure that can be performed with safety in a cardiac catheterization laboratory on an outpatient basis. The detailed procedure for endomyocardial biopsy has been described by Mason[3] and Weiss.[4] It is recommended that the procedure be performed in the cardiac catheterization laboratory with the availability of fluoroscopy. Before the procedure, a complete history should be obtained and a physical examination should be performed. Blood should be obtained for prothrombin time, activated partial thromboplastin time (APTT), and a platelet count in order to exclude patients with a significant bleeding diathesis. Weiss[4] recommends that a prothrombin time or APTT that is prolonged beyond 50% of control or a platelet count of less than 75,000 should exclude a patient from biopsy. Other reasons for exclusion are the presence of a pneumothorax or the inability to cooperate properly with breath holding. For a percutaneous transjugular biopsy, the skin overlying the right internal jugular vein, between the two heads of the sternocleidomastoid muscle and 3 cm above the superior border of the clavicle, is prepared and draped for a sterile procedure. This area is then infiltrated with a local anesthetic of 2% lidocaine (Xylocaine) using a 25-gauge needle. A 22-gauge, 1.5-inch needle is then attached to the syringe and Xylocaine is infiltrated deeply. Care must be taken not to enter the carotid artery. A puncture site is made with a scalpel and hemostat in the usual matter for percutaneous catheterization. A 1.5-inch, 21-gauge probing needle is then directed at an angle of 30° to 45° caudal from the vertical and 10° to 20° toward the right shoulder and advanced with syringe suction until blood is drawn back from the internal jugular vein. The syringe is removed and the needle left in place as a marker. An 18-gauge, thin-walled needle is introduced into the vein alongside the probing needle, and suction is applied while the needle is advanced. Once the needle is placed in the internal jugular vein, a standard Seldinger technique is used to advance a No. 9 French sheath into the vein. The sheath should be equipped with a one-way check valve to prevent an embolism or backflow of blood and with a side arm for flushing. This type of sheath is made by Cordis and has greatly simplified and improved the safety of the technique because it allows the operator to flush the sheath with heparin saline (25,000 units in 500 ml of normal saline) between biopsies during the procedure to prevent thrombus formation. The operator then inserts the bioptome into the sheath and directs it to the lower third of the right atrium with the tip pointed toward the lateral right atrial wall. The bioptome is rotated so that the tip lies medially and is advanced across the tricuspid valve. The tip is kept pointed toward the septum and advanced slowly toward the apex. The right ventricular positioning is verified by the occurrence of premature ventricular beats, the sensation of ventricular myocardial contraction transmitted to the operator's hand, and a fluoroscopic image of the catheter position. When the correct position for the biopsy is reached, the bioptome is withdrawn 1 cm and the bioptome jaws are opened and gently repositioned against the septum. The operator then briskly closes the jaws of the bioptome and removes the specimen with a gentle tug. This procedure is repeated until an adequate amount of tissue is obtained. The patient is asked to hold his breath as the bioptome is withdrawn from the sheath. The sample is removed from the bioptome directly into the fixative with a needle, with care taken not to damage the sample. At the conclusion of the procedure, the thorax is examined fluoroscopically for evidence of pericardial effusion, pleural effusion, or pneumothorax. The patient is then placed in a sitting position to lower venous pressure, and pressure is applied to the area above and below the puncture site for at least 10 minutes. The puncture site is then covered with a Band-Aid.

The bioptome can also be inserted through a femoral vein or brachial artery. A longer bioptome is required, and the long-sheath technique is preferred. For left ventricular biopsy, the technique is similar to that outlined above, but the bioptome is passed retrograde through the aortic valve, usually through the brachial artery.

SAFETY AND COMPLICATIONS

There has been one death to date from the use of the endomyocardial bioptome.[5] At Stanford University, where more than 8000 right ventricular endomyocardial biopsy procedures have been performed, there have been no deaths and the morbidity has been below 0.3%, which is lower than that from liver or renal biopsies. Endomyocardial biopsy is, therefore, a relatively safe procedure.

Complications from endomyocardial biopsy have included the formation of a hematoma at the site of percutaneous insertion, the occurrence of a small apical pneumothorax, and a case of Horner's syndrome and right recurrent laryngeal nerve paralysis most likely due to local anesthesia at the site of skin insertion. Although ventricular ectopic beats are usually induced during cardiac biopsy, sustained ventricular tachyarrhythmias have not been reported. There have been

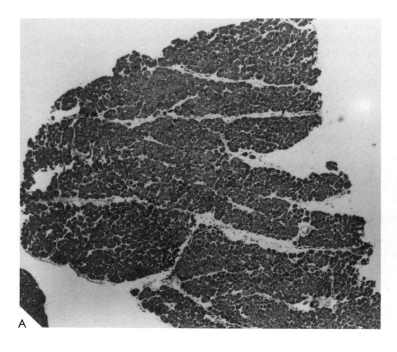
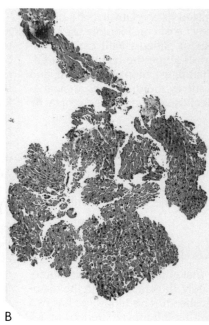

FIGURE 38.1 Comparison of the size of endomyocardial biopsy specimens obtained with the 9 French catheter sheath (**A**) versus a 7 French catheter sheath (**B**). These pieces are of the average size obtained by each bioptome, and they have been photographed at the same low-power magnification. Note that there is two to three times as much myocardium sampled by the larger bioptome.

reports, however, of the induction of atrial fibrillation in a small number of patients, which in some cases has required cardioversion. The most serious complication of the endomyocardial biopsy has been cardiac perforation with tamponade, which has occurred primarily in patients without prior chest surgery. (After cardiac transplantation, for example, the pericardial cavity, if present at all, usually has too many adhesions to make this a significant problem.) In the Stanford series, cardiac tamponade has occurred in fewer than 0.2% of cases, and surgical drainage has been required in only a few of these cases. Because the biopsy is done under fluoroscopic monitoring, cardiac tamponade is usually dealt with immediately by pericardiocentesis. In the case of left ventricular biopsies, there have been several reports of cerebral embolism and for this reason most patients undergoing left ventricular endomyocardial biopsy are given heparin.

RIGHT VERSUS LEFT VENTRICULAR BIOPSY

In general it is agreed that most cardiac disorders that are diffuse in nature such as acute allograft rejection, hemochromatosis, amyloidosis, and dilated cardiomyopathy can be evaluated from a right-sided septal endomyocardial biopsy, and this is the most widely used method because it is the most convenient. Obviously, if there is some particular disorder involving solely the left ventricle (e.g., endocardial fibroelastosis in infants), it is preferable to perform the biopsy on the left side. Other processes that may preferentially involve the left ventricle (e.g., radiation toxicity due to the location of the port of delivery) require that the biopsy be done on the left. Although the risk of complication is essentially the same on the left as on the right side, the consequences of complications on the left are more serious. The relative ease of right ventricular endomyocardial biopsy and the fact that it can be performed on an outpatient basis make it preferable in most circumstances.

INFANTS AND CHILDREN

The myocardial biopsy technique described above can be performed in infants as young as 3 months as well as in older children. The bioptomes used are smaller versions of the adult type. As a consequence of this, the pieces of myocardium obtained are usually much smaller and, therefore, sampling error is greater unless many pieces are taken. In infants and very young children it is necessary to administer general anesthesia when taking an endomyocardial biopsy to prevent sudden movements or crying, which might result in air emboli. For this reason, the risk from biopsy is greater in children. Many children who are being treated with antineoplastic anthracyclines require endomyocardial biopsy for assessment of cardiotoxicity, and the biopsy has been used successfully in this population. There are also more children receiving cardiac allografts. At Stanford it has been possible to monitor acute rejection in these children by biopsy without undue complications. If the biopsy follows cardiac catheterization, the patient is usually already anesthetized. It has been suggested by those with the greatest experience that biplane fluoroscopic facilities contribute to the safety of performing endomyocardial biopsies in infants.

SAMPLING ERROR

One of the most important considerations in using endomyocardial biopsy for the diagnosis of cardiac disease is adequate sampling. This is the responsibility of the cardiologist or surgeon performing the procedure. For most diagnostic analyses, it is mandatory to have at least three pieces of tissue from different areas of the interventricular septum. In some cases (e.g., to rule out the presence of myocarditis or acute rejection), it is preferable to have more than three pieces. It has been shown that in diffuse but multifocal diseases such as acute cardiac rejection there is a false-negative rate of 5% if three pieces of tissue are obtained; and this false-negative rate is reduced to 2% if there are four pieces of tissue.[6] To ensure that different areas of myocardium are sampled, it is important that the operator move the bioptome up and down the interventricular septum whenever possible. Otherwise, the bioptome is often guided back to the same location by the configuration of the ventricular trabeculae. This can result in the biopsy of a previous biopsy site. It should also be noted that if a bioptome that produces smaller samples is used (e.g., the Cordis bioptome), extra pieces should be taken to compensate for the smaller size.

TISSUE HANDLING AND PROCESSING

For optimal results with endomyocardial biopsy, the tissue should be handled very carefully to minimize artifacts. The myocardial fragments should be picked off the bioptome jaws with a needle point rather than forceps, which may cause unnecessary handling artifacts (Fig. 38.2). Although biopsies may be divided into two fragments by the single stroke of a sharp blade, this is to be avoided because it may cause crushing or shearing artifacts. If additional pieces are needed for special studies, it is preferable to obtain another piece directly from the heart.

For light microscopy the biopsy fragment should be transferred immediately to 10% phosphate buffered formalin or another standard fixative, sent to the pathology department, and processed in the usual way. If the biopsy floats in formalin it is most likely that adipose tissue from the subepicardial area has been sampled, and an extra piece of myocardium should be obtained to replace it. It is recommended that all endomyocardial biopsies be stained with hematoxylin and eosin and with a connective tissue stain. Appropriate special stains should be used for individually suspected diseases, for example, a Congo red stain for amyloidosis or an iron stain for hemochromatosis. The paraffin-embedded biopsy specimens should be cut in levels to avoid missing diagnostic changes at deeper levels in the block. The biopsy should also be sectioned at $0.4\ \mu m$ to $0.6\ \mu m$ because thicker sections appear to be more cellular than they really are. Contraction bands (Fig. 38.3) occur as a normal consequence of the endomyocardial biopsy procedure, so it is recommended that the biopsies be fixed in solutions that are at room temperature. Ice-cold solutions appear to accentuate the contraction artifact.

For electron microscopy, the endomyocardial biopsy tissue should be fixed immediately in a buffered 2.5% glutaraldehyde and 2% paraformaldehyde solution and embedded in epon for thin sectioning in the usual way. Thick sections ($0.5\ \mu m$ to $1\ \mu m$) stained with toluidine blue provide excellent diagnostic information, and at least five to ten blocks should be screened carefully for each diagnostic endomyocardial biopsy. Selected thin sections can then be examined ultrastructurally.

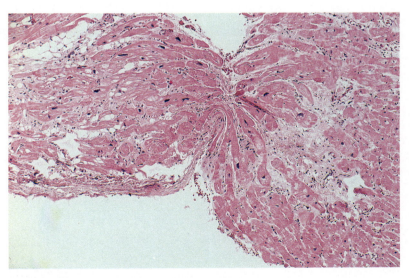

FIGURE 38.2 Endomyocardial biopsy artifact induced by forceps. This type of artifact is avoidable through proper handling.

Endomyocardial biopsies can be easily "snap frozen" in liquid nitrogen or isopentane (2-methylbutane) and dry ice for immunohistochemistry, immunofluorescence, or other studies requiring frozen tissue. It is recommended that these tissue pieces be preserved in freezing mixture within a small Beem capsule to prevent drying. The tissue thus prepared and labeled can be stored indefinitely at −70°C and still retain its immunogenicity. We have successfully used tissue stored in this manner for up to 7 years.

It is strongly recommended that before a biopsy procedure is begun, the type of fixative and the amount of tissue required be discussed with the pathologist who will be examining the tissue. If this is not done, the biopsy may become valueless because the appropriate test cannot be performed. For example, with endomyocardial biopsy for the purpose of assessing cardiotoxicity due to anthracycline drugs, all the tissue should be fixed in a glutaraldehyde for electron microscopy. Anthracycline cardiotoxicity cannot generally be assessed by light microscopy.

With the advent of microtechniques and new technology, the endomyocardial biopsy can be used for scanning electron microscopy, elemental studies, x-ray diffraction, elemental diffraction analysis by x-ray (EDAX), and morphometrics. For each of these types of studies the collection and quantity of tissue and fixative must be discussed with the responsible technician.

INTERPRETATION

It must be reemphasized that sufficient numbers of pieces of myocardium should be examined to avoid a sampling error, and a minimum of three pieces is required in most instances. The tissue should be well prepared and as artifact free as possible. It is not uncommon to find fragments of blood clot, old thrombus, or adipose tissue from the subepicardial layer. If epicardial mesothelial cells are attached to the adipose tissue, perforation of the ventricle has occurred. If only adipose tissue is seen, the ventricle has not necessarily been perforated. The subepicardial adipose tissue, however, is generally not useful for diagnosis and may be misleading if the patient has had recent cardiac surgery. It is also important that endomyocardial biopsy interpretation be done by a pathologist who has had some experience in biopsy pathology or who has taken a course to acquire this knowledge. There are many small diagnostic points in the examination of endomyocardial biopsies that are not readily appreciated by a general pathologist. Ultrastructural interpretation particularly relies heavily on the pathologist's experience and the availability of control human heart biopsies for comparison. It must be understood by the clinician that in many cases the biopsy may not provide a definitive diagnosis. Nevertheless, useful information may be obtained from the biopsy: the suspected disease may not be present or the findings may substantiate a clinical diagnosis by showing features that are consistent with, but not necessarily diagnostic of, the disease in question. For example, the clinical presentation of congestive cardiomyopathy can be mimicked by such diseases as acute myocarditis. If myocarditis is not present on the biopsy and the somewhat nonspecific findings of congestive cardiomyopathy (see below) are, the pathologist should be able to comment that the biopsy shows features consistent with the latter diagnosis assuming there is no coronary or valvular disease. Repeat endomyocardial biopsies following treatment of some disease entities such as myocarditis or acute cardiac rejection may help to determine whether the treatment has been effective and whether it should be continued or altered. In a Stanford series of 450 cardiac biopsies in nontransplant patients, a definite diagnosis, exclusion of a clinical diagnosis, or supporting evidence of a diagnosis has been made in 60% of cases.[7] In only 13% was a new and previous unsuspected diagnosis made. These figures are similar to those published in a report by Olsen on a series of 81 biopsies in which confirmation or exclusion of a clinical diagnosis was made in 65% of cases.[8]

PROBLEMS AND PITFALLS

The most annoying artifact of the biopsy procedure is the occurrence of myocardial contraction bands (see Fig. 38.3). Because this is a common problem, contraction bands should not be interpreted as indicating myocytic ischemia as they may in an autopsy sample. It is also important that myocytic nuclear morphology be well described because this is meaningful in a biopsy that undergoes rapid fixation, whereas it is not as important in autopsy tissue in which autolysis has taken place. Another pitfall of biopsy interpretation is that of the diagnosis of edema, which should not be made in the absence of other findings. The reason for this is that even with careful handling myocytic separation can easily occur. The diagnosis of small vessel thrombosis is sometimes inadvertently made based on biopsy specimens. However, this appearance may be due to a biopsy artifact caused by the telescoping of the small vessels into themselves, creating in effect an "intussusception" that in cross section resembles an organized thrombus (Fig. 38.4). In patients who are having serial biopsies, one of the most annoying problems is that of performing a biopsy on a previous biopsy site. Although this would seem to be unlikely, the configuration of the trabeculae within the ventricle often guides the bioptome to the same spot as before. Every effort should be made by the operator to manipulate the bioptome so as to avoid going back to the same place. Biopsy sites are usually readily identifiable by having a crater-like shape at the endocardial surface and being composed of an admixture of granulation tissue and fibrin. An older fibrotic biopsy site is covered by a thickened endocardium, is frequently associated with myocytic disarray at the junction with normal myocardium, and contains residual inflammatory cells including hemosiderin-laden macrophages.

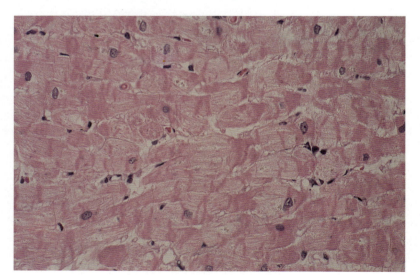

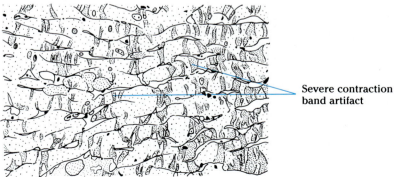

FIGURE 38.3 Endomyocardial biopsy with severe contraction band artifact. The contraction bands are formed by the clumping of sarcomeres. This type of artifact may be minimized by using room temperature (not cold) fixatives.

INDICATIONS

The clinical indications for endomyocardial biopsy are multiple and may somewhat arbitrarily be grouped by the principal mode of presentation of the disease in question (Table 38.1). The following discussion focuses primarily on the clinically relevant points of endomyocardial biopsy diagnosis.

CARDIAC TRANSPLANTATION

The least controversial use of the endomyocardial biopsy, and the most common one, is in cases of heart and combined heart–lung transplants. Initially the biopsy is useful for pretransplant confirmation of the suspected disease, because occasionally a patient with an apparent end-stage dilated cardiomyopathy actually has sarcoidosis (Fig. 38.5). In this case a steroid trial is recommended before transplantation. If amyloidosis (Fig. 38.6) were found, transplantation would in most cases be precluded.

Once cardiac transplantation has been performed, the use of endomyocardial biopsy for the diagnosis and management of acute cardiac rejection has proved to be reliable and of great practical importance.[9-11] Once again, it is important to have at least four pieces of tissue in order to rule out the presence of acute rejection. This group of patients requires many biopsies, particularly in the first 3 months following cardiac transplantation, when they are most likely to reject their grafts. At most centers biopsies are performed every 5 to 7 days for the first 4 to 6 weeks. Many patients have had more than 30 endomyocardial biopsy procedures. At Stanford, 39 biopsies have been performed in one heart without any adverse sequelae.

The histologic features of acute cardiac rejection may be graded as follows.

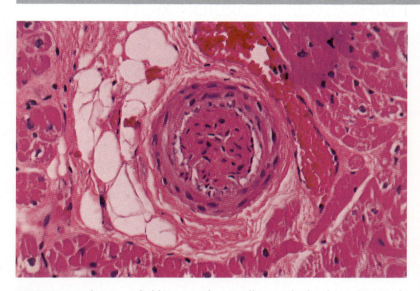

FIGURE 38.4 Endomyocardial biopsy with a small arteriole that has telescoped into itself, simulating a small thrombus. This type of artifact is unavoidable.

TABLE 38.1 INDICATIONS FOR ENDOMYOCARDIAL BIOPSY

Pretransplant evaluation and post-transplant monitoring of cardiac allograft recipients
Patients presenting with heart failure
  Anthracycline-induced cardiotoxicity
  Idiopathic dilated cardiomyopathy
  Myocarditis: idiopathic, infectious, or drug-induced
  Specific heart muscle disease (see Table 38.6)
Patients presenting with arrhythmias
  Myocarditis: idiopathic, infectious, or drug-induced
  Right ventricular dysplasia
  Infiltrations by hematologic malignancies
  Ischemic disease
  Sarcoidosis
Patients presenting with restrictive disease
  Radiation effect
  Amyloidosis
  Fibroelastosis
  Restrictive cardiomyopathy (endomyocardial fibrosis and Löffler's disease)

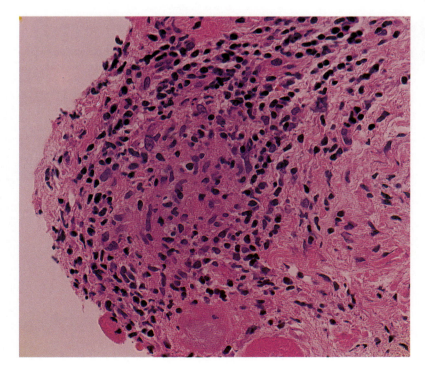

FIGURE 38.5 Endomyocardial biopsy showing the presence of a discrete noncaseating granuloma. Special stains for the presence of organisms were negative in this case; therefore, this biopsy is consistent with the diagnosis of cardiac sarcoidosis.

1. *Mild acute rejection* (Fig. 38.7) is characterized by the presence of a scant perivascular or interstitial lymphocytic infiltrate. The lymphocytes or immunoblasts are of T-cell origin and are pyroninophilic (the cytoplasm stains with methyl green pyronine indicating a high ribonucleic acid [RNA] content). An endocardial infiltrate of similar-appearing lymphocytes is also usually present.
2. *Moderate acute rejection* (Fig. 38.8) is characterized by spreading of the perivascular infiltrate into the interstitium. The infiltrate is usually present in several, if not all, of the pieces of tissue. In addition, focal myocytic damage and necrosis are usually present.
3. *Severe acute rejection* (Fig. 38.9) is characterized by the presence of a mixed (neutrophils and lymphocytes) interstitial inflammatory infiltrate as well as interstitial hemorrhage. There are usually large numbers of necrotic myocytes as well as vascular necrosis. If the patient is being treated with cyclosporine, the mixed infiltrate often includes eosinophils.

Following treatment, a new biopsy may be interpreted as signifying "ongoing rejection" if the degree of cellular infiltration and necrosis are the same as or worse than the previous biopsy; "resolving acute rejection" if it appears to be improving and there is evidence of early scar-tissue formation associated with proliferating fibroblasts; or "resolved acute rejection" if there is no evidence of an inflammatory infiltrate and perhaps only a residual scar.

In addition to the presence of rejection as described above, approximately 10% of patients treated with cyclosporine-A–based immunosuppression may also have an endocardial accumulation of lymphocytes (Fig. 38.10), which does not require treatment for acute rejection. The lymphocytes are primarily T-cells and can be present with or without rejection in the same biopsy and may outlast a treated and resolved rejection episode on subsequent biopsies. The phenomenon is referred to as the *Quilty effect*, a term derived from the surname of the first patient in which it was recognized. It has not been associated with the development of malignant lymphoma or any other adverse sequelae.

In this immunosuppressed group of patients the presence of eosinophils in any of the biopsies should alert the clinician to check *Toxoplasma gondii* titers if organisms have not been identified on the biopsy. Eosinophils may also be seen with cytomegalovirus infection involving the myocardium.

ANTHRACYCLINE CARDIOTOXICITY

Doxorubicin (Adriamycin) and its anthracycline analogues, either by themselves or in combination, are some of the most useful cancer chemotherapeutic agents available. Unfortunately, some patients develop irreversible heart failure as a toxic side-effect, with an incidence that increases after a cumulative dose of 550 mg per square meter. For

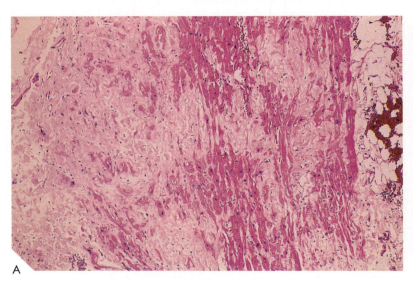
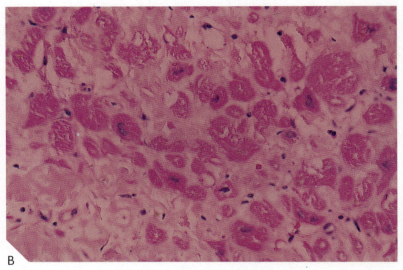

FIGURE 38.6 A. Endomyocardial biopsy showing replacement of much of the myocardium by amyloid in a patient with multiple myeloma. **B.** The higher power photomicrograph with the myocytes cut in cross section demonstrates the characteristic perimyocytic pattern frequently found in cardiac amyloidosis.

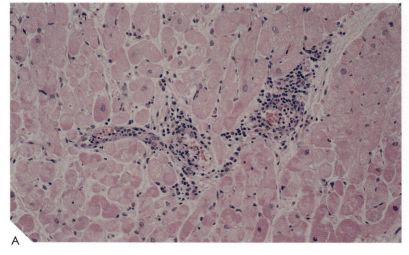
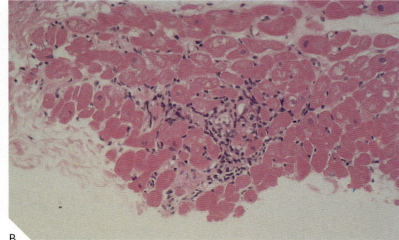

FIGURE 38.7 Mild acute cardiac allograft rejection characterized by either **(A)** a sparse perivascular infiltrate or **(B)** a sparse interstitial infiltrate.

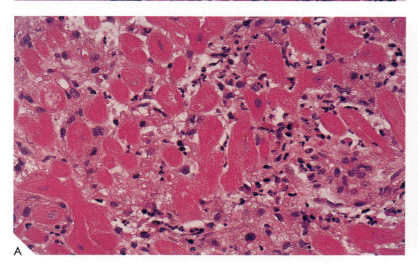

FIGURE 38.8 Endomyocardial biopsy from a cardiac transplant recipient shows a marked interstitial lymphocytic infiltrate characteristic of moderate acute rejection.

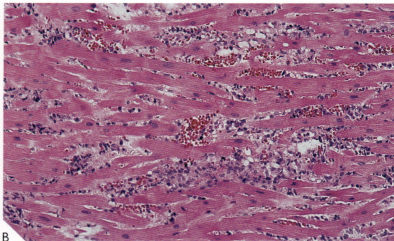

FIGURE 38.9 A. Severe acute cardiac allograft rejection showing the presence of an interstitial inflammatory infiltrate composed of lymphocytes and neutrophils with myocyte damage. **B.** Other areas of the biopsy show the presence of interstitial hemorrhage.

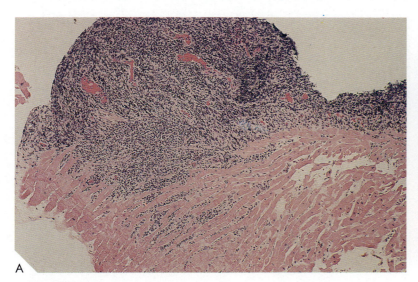
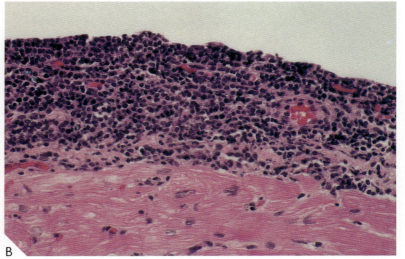

FIGURE 38.10 A. Endomyocardial biopsy from a cardiac transplant recipient on cyclosporine-A-based immunosuppression showing the presence of an endocardial infiltrate. This appearance is known as the Quilty effect. Occasionally there is subendocardial involvement as seen in this case. **B.** The higher power shows the cells to be round, regular lymphocytes set in a vascular stroma.

this reason, many clinicians use this dose as an arbitrary cutoff for the drug, although it has demonstrated good tumoricidal activity. Some patients go into heart failure at a lower cumulative dose (*e.g.*, 180 mg to 300 mg/m^2) if they have certain risk factors. The use of the endomyocardial biopsy in this group of patients, however, has allowed the development of a clinically useful toxicity grading scheme (Table 38.2).[12-14] The morphologic grading, usually used in combination with right heart catheterization, accurately reflects the cardiac damage present at the time of biopsy. Furthermore, it enables prediction at low cumulative doses which patients will develop heart failure if more drug is given because there is a linear relationship between the toxicity grade and the drug dose. In patients who do not have toxic cardiac effects and in whom it is important to give more anthracycline drug, it has been possible to deliver over 1000 mg per square meter without the development of heart failure if they are followed carefully by endomyocardial biopsy.

The morphologic changes due to anthracyclines can be focal or widespread and are best appreciated by electron microscopic examination. Light microscopic examination has proved unreliable in this setting. The lesions in human myocardium are of two main types. In the first, myocytes may show partial or total myofibrillar loss with only peripheral Z-band remnants remaining (Fig. 38.11). The second type of myocytic injury caused by anthracycline drugs is sarcotubular dilatation (Fig. 38.12), which may progress to sarcotubular coalescence. Eventually the myocyte may look entirely vacuolated. The mitochondria may remain unaffected in these damaged cells. The two types of myocyte damage may occur in the same cell or in separate cells, and there appears to be no predictive value to the type of damage that appears first. For this reason both types of abnormality are counted equally in the grading system. Interstitial fibrosis does occur with anthracycline-induced cardiotoxicity; however, this is not included in the grading system because it is a nonspecific change and may be due to other factors (*e.g.*, irradiation). The changes described have been seen in all the anthracycline analogues that have been produced so far, although damage may occur at different cumulative doses depending on the particular drug. The changes described may also be seen in end-stage cardiomyopathy of the dilated type; however, the assumption is made that patients in these cases do not have cardiomyopathy before the onset of treatment, and a baseline biopsy is obtained at some institutions to confirm this. Moreover, the heart failure due to Adriamycin also develops much more rapidly and without the extreme dilatation and cardiomegaly that occurs in end-stage congestive cardiomyopathy. The fact that these two entities are different is borne out by recent studies that have shown that there are definite morphometric changes that can be used to separate them.[15]

Risk factors for the development of Adriamycin cardiotoxicity include cardiac irradiation[16] either before or following anthracycline treatment, the presence of hypertension, advanced age, and very young age. In practice it is necessary to biopsy only those patients who have risk factors or who must have more than 500 mg per square meter of anthracycline. To date endomyocardial biopsy is the only method that shows evidence of cardiac damage at low doses. Hemodynamic and other functional tests reflect cardiotoxicity only when there has already been enough damage to result in heart failure; they are not predictive. Therefore, endomyocardial biopsy grading provides a useful method for arriving at rational dose optimization.

TABLE 38.2 MORPHOLOGIC GRADING SYSTEM FOR ANTHRACYCLINE CARDIOTOXICITY

Grade	Morphology
0	Normal myocardial ultrastructure
1	Isolated myocytes affected by distended sarcotubular system or early myofibrillar loss; damage to fewer than 5% of all cells in ten plastic embedded blocks of tissue
1.5	Changes similar to those in grade 1 but with damage to 6%–15% of all cells in ten plastic embedded blocks of tissue
2.0	Clusters of myocytes affected by myofibrillar loss or vacuolization, with damage to 16%–25% of all cells in ten plastic embedded blocks of tissue
2.5	Many myocytes, 26%–35% of all cells in ten plastic embedded blocks, affected by vacuolization or myofibrillar loss. Only one more dose of anthracycline should be given without further evaluation
3.0	Severe and diffuse myocytic damage (more than 35% of all cells in ten plastic embedded blocks) affected by vacuolization or myofibrillar loss. No more anthracycline should be given

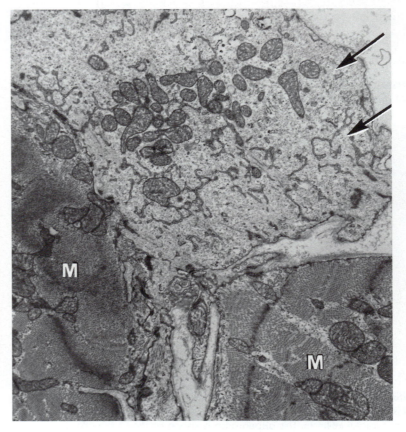

FIGURE 38.11 Electron micrograph showing an anthracycline-damaged myocyte with total myofibrillar loss and Z-band remnants (*arrows*) compared with adjacent unaffected myocytes, M. Note the smaller but intact mitochondria in the damaged cell. (Lead citrate stain, original magnification ×4400) (Billingham ME: Endomyocardial changes in anthracycline-treated patients with and without irradiation. Front Radiat Ther Oncol 13:72, 1979; reproduced by permission of S Karger AG, Basel)

IDIOPATHIC DILATED CARDIOMYOPATHY

There are many conditions that can result in a dilated heart with a reduced ejection fraction. The endomyocardial biopsy is useful in both confirming congestive heart failure due to cardiomyopathy and diagnosing other conditions that may simulate end-stage dilated cardiomyopathy. Before the endomyocardial biopsy is done, however, it is necessary to exclude coronary artery disease or valvular heart disease as possible causes for the heart failure[17] because they may cause pathologic changes similar to those seen in idiopathic dilated cardiomyopathy. Only if these are absent are the morphologic changes in the biopsy useful in confirming that end-stage dilated cardiomyopathy is present. Although there is some debate as to the value of the biopsy, at Stanford biopsies done for end-stage dilated cardiomyopathy are examined routinely by electron microscopy. Many of the pathologic features of idiopathic dilated cardiomyopathy, such as the presence of large, bizarre-shaped nuclei with low form factors and myofibrillar loss, correlate with the degree of the ventricular dilatation, and these can be appreciated only at the ultrastructural level. On light microscopy, however, fibrosis, large hyperchromatic bizarre-shaped myocyte nuclei, and myocytic hypertrophy can be appreciated and confirm the presence of a dilated cardiomyopathy (Figs. 38.13, 38.14, and 38.15) if ischemic,

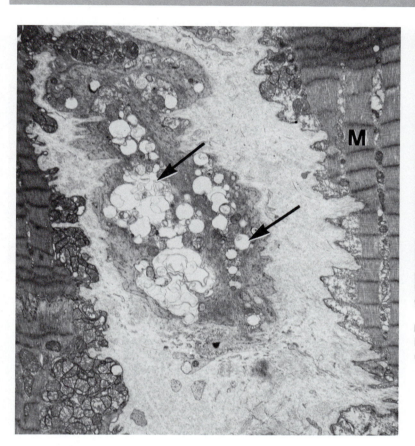

FIGURE 38.12 Electron micrograph demonstrating vacuolization of the sarcotubular system in an anthracycline-damaged mycoyte (*arrows*) compared with an adjacent unaffected mycoyte, M. (Lead citrate stain, original magnification ×2300) (Billingham ME: Endomyocardial changes in anthracycline-treated patients with and without irradiation. Front Radiat Ther Oncol 13:72, 1979; reproduced by permission of S Karger AG, Basel)

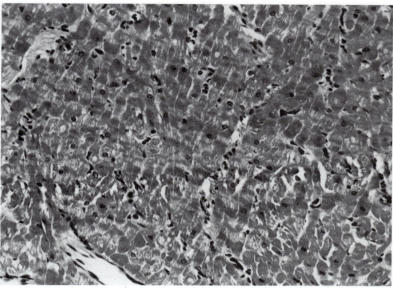

FIGURE 38.13 Normal myocardial morphology as seen in an endomyocardial biopsy. Note the regularity of the nuclei and the width of myocytes. (Hematoxylin and eosin, original magnification ×200)

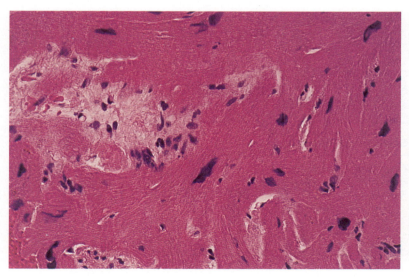

FIGURE 38.14 Endomyocardial biopsy from a patient with idiopathic dilated cardiomyopathy showing the bizarre nuclear shapes characteristic of this entity. For comparison see Figure 38.13 of normal myocardium, taken at the same magnification. (Hematoxylin and eosin, original magnification ×200)

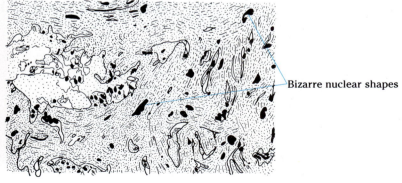

hypertensive, and valvular disease are not present.[18] It has been shown that patients with end-stage dilated cardiomyopathy may also have mononuclear inflammatory cell infiltrates within the interstitium; however, at the present time we do not think these represent an active myocarditis (which might be treated with immunosuppression).[19]

HYPERTROPHIC CARDIOMYOPATHY

There is some debate about the usefulness of endomyocardial biopsy in the setting of idiopathic hypertrophic subaortic stenosis (hypertrophic cardiomyopathy).[20-23] It has been shown that the characteristic myocytic disarray is frequently confined to the inner third of the septum,[24] an area out of reach of the 3-mm piece of tissue obtained at endomyocardial biopsy. It is also clear that myocytic disarray is nonspecific and can be seen in many biopsies from patients in whom there is no other clinical evidence of hypertrophic cardiomyopathy. If myocytic disarray is seen on the biopsy it may be prudent to examine the patient more carefully to rule out the presence of hypertrophic cardiomyopathy; however, if a biopsy is done in a patient with hypertrophic cardiomyopathy, it should be done to rule out other possibly coexisting disease and not primarily to make the diagnosis of hypertrophic cardiomyopathy.

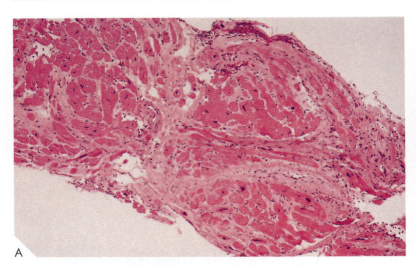

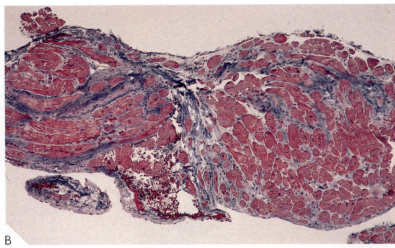

FIGURE 38.15 Endomyocardial biopsy from an 18-year-old, demonstrating characteristic features of idiopathic dilated cardiomyopathy. **A.** There is moderate myocyte hypertrophy associated with interstitial fibrosis. This is highlighted on the trichrome stain (**B**), where the collagen stains blue. Note the characteristic pericellular pattern of interstitial fibrosis. (**A**, hematoxylin and eosin; **B**, Masson's trichrome)

FIGURE 38.16 Endomyocardial biopsy from a 50-year-old man showing the features of idiopathic myocarditis. There is a marked, predominantly lymphocytic, interstitial inflammatory cell infiltrate with evidence of myocyte damage.

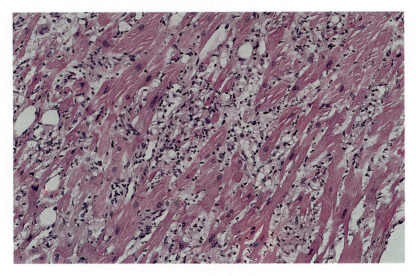

TABLE 38.3 DIAGNOSTIC CATEGORIES OF IDIOPATHIC MYOCARDITIS SUGGESTED BY THE DALLAS MYOCARDITIS PANEL

First Biopsy	Subsequent Biopsies
Active myocarditis with myocytic necrosis (with or without fibrosis)	Ongoing (persistent myocarditis)
Borderline myocarditis (biopsy results not diagnostic; suggest rebiopsy)	Resolving (healing myocarditis)
No evidence of myocarditis	Resolved (healed myocarditis; this group may have some of the features of dilated cardiomyopathy)

MYOCARDITIS

The endomyocardial biopsy can be very useful in making the diagnosis of idiopathic (viral?) myocarditis[25,26] as well as myocarditis secondary to bacteria, fungi, protozoa, rickettsia, readily recognizable viruses (*e.g.*, cytomegalovirus), and drugs. The diagnosis of myocarditis requires adequate sampling and the presence of an inflammatory infiltrate associated with myocytic necrosis (Fig. 38.16).[27] The diagnostic categories suggested by the Dallas Myocarditis Panel are shown in Table 38.3.[27] Whenever the diagnosis of idiopathic myocarditis is considered on biopsy, secondary causes must be ruled out first. Particularly important in this regard is to rule out drug-related myocarditis. A detailed drug history should be obtained because many drugs can cause a toxic or hypersensitivity-related myocarditis (Table 38.4).[30,31]

The type of infiltrate in myocytic necrosis should be carefully examined to rule out ischemia (Fig. 38.17), drug-related myocarditis, or hematologic malignancies infiltrating the heart. There are many pitfalls in the diagnosis of acute myocarditis by endomyocardial biopsy[28,29] and guidelines for ensuring that these pitfalls are kept to a minimum are outlined in Table 38.5.

Because of the potentially adverse effects of immunosuppressive treatment and the nonspecific nature of the presenting symptoms in most cases, a confirmatory biopsy should be performed before treatment is instituted. It must be emphasized, however, that although anecdotal reports continue of contributions of immunosuppressive therapy to the recovery of patients with idiopathic myocarditis (Figs. 38.16 and 38.18),[26,32] a prospective randomized trial studying this issue has not yet been performed.

TABLE 38.4 DRUGS ASSOCIATED WITH MYOCARDITIS

Toxic Myocarditis*			Hypersensitivity Myocarditis†		
Anthracyclines	Catecholamines	Histamine-like drugs	Sulfonamides	Tetracyclines	Methyldopa
Amphetamines	Paraquat	Lithium compounds	Izoniazid	Phenylbutazone	Cocaine
Antihypertensives	Cyclophosphamide	Phenothiazines	Penicillin	Thiazide diuretics	Streptomycin
Barbiturates	Fluorouracil	Theophylline		Horse serum	

* Dose-related lesions of different ages with necrotizing vasculitis.
† Non–dose-related lesions of same age with eosinophilic infiltrate.

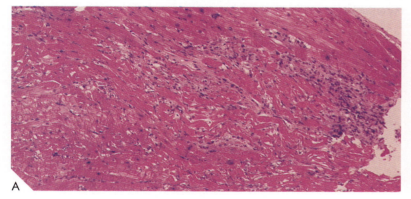

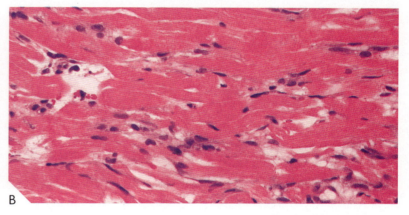

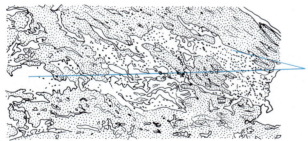

Granulation tissue

FIGURE 38.17 A. Low power photomicrograph of an endomyocardial biopsy from a 61-year-old woman shows features of an organizing infarct. There is early granulation tissue at the edge of the infarct. **B.** The higher power shows that the myocytes in the center of the infarct have lost their nuclei and cross striations; these features are characteristic of ischemic damage.

TABLE 38.5 GUIDELINES FOR THE BIOPSY DIAGNOSIS OF MYOCARDITIS

Perform the biopsy *early* in the course of the disease.
In order to reduce sampling error, at least three pieces (processed at three levels) should be obtained.
Take a careful drug history.
Take a careful history to rule out secondary causes of myocarditis.

SPECIFIC HEART MUSCLE DISEASE

Endomyocardial biopsy is very useful in making the diagnosis of many specific heart muscle diseases, such as those listed in Table 38.6. Probably the most common diagnosis made by biopsy in this group is that of amyloid heart disease. Because amyloidosis is partly focal and does not always stain with the usual light microscopic stains, it is recommended that one piece of the biopsy be studied by electron microscopy if the light microscopic stains are negative and the clinical suspicion that the disease is present is high. In some clinical situations it is difficult to distinguish between constrictive and restrictive heart disease (see below). Rather than have a patient subjected to open heart surgery for pericardial biopsy, an endomyocardial biopsy is frequently diagnostic of amyloidosis. However, it is important to remember that normal biopsy results do not exclude the diagnosis. The biopsy samples only a small portion of heart, and if clinical suspicion is high for any of the specific heart muscle diseases, a repeat biopsy may be warranted.

PATIENTS PRESENTING WITH ARRHYTHMIAS

Endomyocardial biopsy is useful in patients presenting with arrhythmias, because some potentially treatable underlying causes of arrhythmias such as myocarditis or sarcoidosis may be identified. A list of conditions presenting with arrhythmias that may be diagnosable by endomyocardial biopsy and that we have identified is given in Table 38.1. Right ventricular dysplasia is a somewhat nonspecific diagnosis morphologically[33]; however, a biopsy may show the characteristic features and aid in ruling out other causes for the arrhythmias (Fig. 38.19).

PATIENTS PRESENTING WITH RESTRICTIVE OR CONSTRICTIVE MYOCARDIAL DISEASE

In some patients, hemodynamic and electrophysiologic studies are unable to distinguish restrictive from constrictive disease, and the endomyocardial biopsy may be useful in making this distinction. Frequently, amyloidosis may be found in an endomyocardial biopsy, which would account for restrictive hemodynamics. With respect to radiation effect, it may not be clear whether previous irradiation to the unscreened heart has caused enough interstitial fibrosis to cause restrictive physiology or whether some other process is responsible. An endomyocardial biopsy may be able to shed light on this problem. Endomyocardial fibrosis also causes a restrictive pattern physiologically and sometimes this diagnosis can be made by biopsy; however, a focally thickened endomyocardium is nonspecific and not pathologically diagnostic of restrictive disease. Fibroelastosis, on the other hand, particularly in infants, is an easily made diagnosis on endomyocardial biopsy although the biopsy specimen in this instance may need to be taken from the left ventricle. Many of these conditions can be ruled out by biopsy and thus save the patient from open chest surgery or pericardial biopsy for presumed constriction.

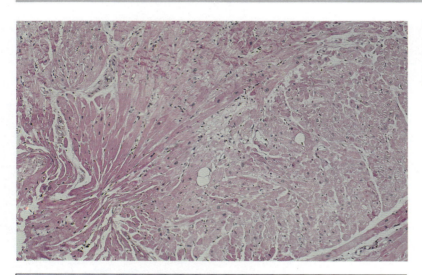

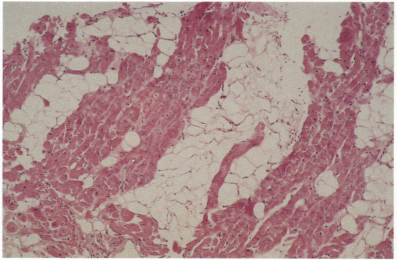

FIGURE 38.18 This endomyocardial biopsy from the patient in Figure 38.16 2 weeks after the initiation of immunosuppressive therapy shows the features of a resolving myocarditis. The inflammatory infiltrate is significantly reduced, and there is a mild increase in interstitial connective tissue and focal myocyte hypertrophy.

TABLE 38.6 SPECIFIC HEART MUSCLE DISEASES FOR WHICH ENDOMYOCARDIAL BIOPSY IS USEFUL

Inflammatory—bacterial, viral, rickettsial, fungal, protozoal, Whipple's disease
Metabolic—amyloidosis, hemochromatosis, oxalosis, storage diseases (*e.g.*, Fabry's)
Endocrine—hypo- and hyperthyroidism, pheochromocytoma, carcinoid syndrome
Neuromuscular—progressive muscular dystrophy, Friedreich's ataxia
Rheumatic—rheumatic heart disease, rheumatoid heart disease
Toxic—radiation effect, anthracycline drugs, others (see Table 38.5)
Hematologic infiltrates—leukemia, lymphoma

FIGURE 38.19 Endomyocardial biopsy shows features consistent with right ventricular dysplasia. There is abundant adipose tissue not confined to either the subendocardial or the subepicardial zone admixed with relatively little intervening myocardium and areas of fibrosis.

REFERENCES

1. Sakakibara S, Konno S: Endomyocardial biopsy. Jpn Heart J 3:537, 1962
2. Caves PK, Schulz WP, Dong E Jr et al: A new instrument for transvenous cardiac biopsy. Am J Cardiol 33:264, 1974
3. Mason JW: Techniques for right and left endomyocardial biopsy. Am J Cardiol 41:887, 1978
4. Weiss MB: Right ventricular biopsy. In Fenoglio JJ (ed): Endomyocardial Biopsy: Techniques and Applications, p. 8. Boca Raton, CRC Press, 1983
5. Hess ML: Personal communication, 1986
6. Spiegelhalter DJ, Stovin PGI: An analysis of repeated biopsies following cardiac transplantation. Stat Med 2:33, 1983
7. Billingham ME: Some recent advances in cardiac pathology. Hum Pathol 10:367, 1979
8. Olsen EGJ: Diagnostic value of the endomyocardial bioptome. Lancet 1:658, 1974
9. Billingham ME: Endomyocardial biopsy detection of acute rejection in cardiac allograft recipients. Heart Vessels 1(Suppl):86, 1985
10. Gokel JM, Reichart B, Struck E: Human cardiac transplantation—evaluation of morphological changes in serial endomyocardial biopsies. Pathol Res Pract 178:354, 1985
11. Pomerance A, Stovin PGI: Heart transplant pathology: The British experience. J Clin Pathol 38:146, 1985
12. Billingham ME, Bristow MR: Evaluation of anthracycline cardiotoxicity: Predictive ability and functional correlation of endomyocardial biopsy. Cancer Treat Symposia 3:71, 1984
13. Billingham ME, Mason J, Bristow M et al: Anthracycline cardiomyopathy monitored by morphologic changes. Cancer Treat Rep 62:865, 1978
14. Legha SS, Benjamin RS, MacKay B et al: Reduction of doxorubicin cardiotoxicity by prolonged continuous intravenous infusion. Ann Intern Med 6:133, 1982
15. Rowan RA, Masek MA, Billingham ME: Anthracycline cardiotoxicity and dilated cardiomyopathy: Morphometric distinctions. J Am Coll Cardiol 7:121A, 1986
16. Billingham ME, Bristow MR, Glastein E et al: Adriamycin cardiotoxicity: Endomyocardial biopsy evidence of enhancement by irradiation. Am J Surg Pathol 1:17, 1979
17. World Health Organization/International Society and Federation of Cardiology. Report of the task force on the definition and classification of cardiomyopathies. Br Heart J 44:672, 1980
18. Roberts WC, Ferrans VJ: Pathologic anatomy of the cardiomyopathies: Idiopathic dilated and hypertrophic types, infiltrative types and endomyocardial disease with and without eosinophilia. Hum Pathol 6:287, 1975
19. Tazelaar HD, Billingham ME: Leucocytic infiltrates in idiopathic dilated cardiomyopathy: A source of confusion with active myocarditis. Am J Surg Pathol 10:405, 1986
20. Alexander CS, Gobel FL: Diagnosis of idiopathic hypertrophic subaortic stenosis by right ventricular septal biopsy. Am J Cardiol 34:142, 1974
21. Olsen EGJ, Spry CJF: Endomyocardial fibrosis and eosinophilic heart disease. Prog Cardiol 8:281, 1979
22. Ferrans VJ, Roberts WC: Myocardial biopsy: A useful diagnostic procedure or only a research tool? Am J Cardiol 41:965, 1978
23. Tazelaar HD, Billingham ME: The surgical pathology of hypertrophic cardiomyopathy. Arch Pathol Lab Med (in press)
24. Maron BJ, Roberts WC: Quantitative analysis of cardiac muscle cell disorganization in the ventricular septum of patients with hypertrophic cardiomyopathy. Circulation 59:689, 1979
25. Kereiakes DJ, Parmley WW: Myocarditis and cardiomyopathy. Am Heart J 108:1318, 1984
26. Dec GW Jr, Palacios IF, Fallon JT et al: Active myocarditis in the spectrum of acute dilated cardiomyopathies. Clinical features, histologic correlates and clinical outcome. N Engl J Med 312:885, 1985
27. Aretz HT, Billingham ME, Edwards WE et al: Myocarditis—a histologic definition and working classification. Am J Cardiovasc Pathol 1:5, 1986
28. Edwards WD: Current problems in establishing quantitative histopathologic criteria for the diagnosis of lymphocytic myocarditis by endomyocardial biopsy. Heart Vessels 1(Suppl):138, 1985
29. Billingham ME: The diagnostic criteria of myocarditis by endomyocardial biopsy. Heart Vessels 1(Suppl):130, 1985
30. Billingham ME: Morphologic changes in drug-induced heart disease. In Bristow MR: Drug-Induced Heart Disease, p 127. Amsterdam, Elsevier-North-Holland Biomedical Press, 1980
31. Fenoglio JJ: The effects of drugs on the cardiovascular system. In Silver MD (ed): Cardiovascular Pathology, p 1085. New York, Churchill Livingstone, 1983
32. Mason JW, Billingham ME, Ricci DR: Treatment of acute inflammatory myocarditis assisted by endomyocardial biopsy. Am J Cardiol 45:1037, 1980
33. Marcus FI, Fontaine GH, Guiraudon G et al: Right ventricular dysplasia: a report of 24 adult cases. Circulation 65:384, 1982

GENERAL REFERENCES

Fenoglio JJ Jr (ed): Endomyocardial Biopsy: Techniques and Applications. Boca Raton, CRC Press, 1982

Fowles RE, Mason JW: Role of cardiac biopsy in the diagnosis and management of cardiac disease. Prog Cardiovasc Dis 27:153, 1984

Przybojewski JZ: Endomyocardial biopsy: A review of the literature. Cathet Cardiovasc Diag 11:287, 1986

Robinson JA, O'Connell JB: Myocarditis: Precursor of Cardiomyopathy. Lexington, MA, Collamore Press, 1983

Sekiguchi M, Olsen EGJ, Goodwin JF (eds): Myocarditis and related disorders. Proceedings of the International Symposium on Cardiomyopathy and Myocarditis. Heart Vessels 1(Suppl):11-320, 1985

Ursell PC, Fenoglio JJ: Spectrum of cardiac disease diagnosed by endomyocardial biopsy. In Sommers SC, Rosen PP (eds): Pathology Annual, p 197. Norwalk, CT, Appleton-Century-Crofts, 1984

BEDSIDE HEMODYNAMIC MONITORING

Kanu Chatterjee

Hemodynamic monitoring is the application of the principles of right heart catheterization at the bedside and the knowledge of central and peripheral hemodynamics thus derived permits diagnosis of the various pathologic conditions that alter cardiac function.[1-4] The nature and severity of cardiac failure can be assessed by hemodynamic monitoring. Prompt evaluation of results of therapy can be made. Assessment of prognosis is also possible in certain cardiac patients. Thus, bedside hemodynamic monitoring has emerged as an integral part of critical care in recent years.

HEMODYNAMIC MONITORING

The hemodynamic variables that provide useful information about the etiologic diagnosis and management of altered cardiac performance in critically ill patients are heart rate and rhythm; arterial pressure; right atrial, pulmonary arterial, and pulmonary capillary wedge pressures; and cardiac output. From the directly determined hemodynamic parameters, a number of additional hemodynamic indices can be derived that are helpful in assessment of the etiology and severity of cardiac failure as well as the appropriate selection of therapy. For normal values of determined and derived hemodynamic parameters, see Table 39.1.

HEART RATE AND RHYTHM

The electrocardiographic monitor with an automatic rate meter is most frequently used to determine the instantaneous changes in heart rate. Movement artifacts, however, can trigger the heart rate meter and display an inaccurately high heart rate. An increased amplitude of T or P waves may also trigger the meter and indicate a heart rate higher than the actual heart rate. On the other hand, if the amplitude of the QRS complex is too low to trigger the counter, the displayed heart rate may be lower than the actual heart rate.

The heart rate may be accurately measured from an electrocardiographic printout. When the electrocardiogram is recorded at a 25 mm/sec paper speed, the time interval between the two darker vertical lines is 0.2 seconds, and between the two smaller vertical lines it is 0.04 seconds. Heart rate can be determined by dividing 60 seconds by the time interval between two consecutive QRS complexes.

The nature and frequency of dysrhythmias are frequently monitored on-line with the use of automated computerized arrhythmia detection devices.

ARTERIAL PRESSURE

Monitoring the arterial pressure either directly or indirectly provides useful information about cardiovascular dynamics and is an important component of hemodynamic monitoring. Indirect measurement of arterial pressure by the cuff method is rapid and fairly accurate; however, continuous monitoring of arterial pressure by this technique is not feasible. Furthermore, in patients with low cardiac output and stroke volume, Korotkoff sounds may be inaudible and in such patients indirect measurement of arterial pressure by the cuff method should be avoided. Direct determination of arterial pressure by inserting an arterial cannula allows accurate measurement of systolic and diastolic pressures and is used increasingly in the critical care and postsurgical units. Accurate arterial pressure monitoring is critically important during the therapy of "low output state" and cardiogenic shock. In patients with severe peripheral vasoconstriction, a significant disparity can exist between central and peripheral arterial pressures. In such patients, femoral or brachial artery cannulation is preferable to radial artery cannulation.

RIGHT HEART PRESSURES, CATHETER DESIGNS, AND CATHETER PLACEMENT

In medical or surgical intensive care units, pressures on the right side of the heart are measured almost exclusively with the use of balloon-tipped flotation catheters. The flow-directed pulmonary artery catheters were introduced into clinical practice in 1970[1] and the initial catheters were No. 5 French size containing two lumens; one lumen was used to inflate a 1 ml latex balloon positioned just proximal to the tip of the catheter and the second lumen, terminating at the tip, was used for monitoring pulmonary artery pressure and for obtaining blood

TABLE 39.1 NORMAL VALUES OF DETERMINED AND DERIVED HEMODYNAMIC PARAMETERS

Parameter	Normal Value
Arterial pressure (mm Hg)	
Systolic	100–140
Diastolic	60–90
Mean	70–105
Mean pulmonary artery wedge pressure (mm Hg)	<15
Mean pulmonary artery pressure (mm Hg)	<18
Mean right atrial pressure (mm Hg)	<8
Cardiac index (liter/min/m^2) = Cardiac output/body surface area	2.8–4.2
Stroke volume index (ml/m^2) = Cardiac index/heart rate	30–70
Left ventricular stroke work index (g-m/m^2) = [stroke volume index × (mean arterial systolic pressure − mean pulmonary artery wedge pressure)] × 0.0136	40–65
Right ventricular stroke work index (g-m/m^2) = [stroke volume index × (mean pulmonary artery pressure − mean right atrial pressure) × 0.0136]	8–12
Systemic vascular resistance (dynes/sec/cm^{-5}) = (mean arterial pressure − mean right atrial pressure/cardiac output) × 80	900–1400
Pulmonary vascular resistance (dynes/sec/cm^{-5}) = [(mean pulmonary artery pressure − mean pulmonary artery wedge pressure)/cardiac output] × 80	150–250

samples from the pulmonary artery. Balloon flotation catheters, however, have undergone several modifications and new features have been incorporated. Presently, a quadruple-lumen No. 7 French catheter is most frequently employed.[2] Two lumens serve to transmit pressure signals and aspiration of blood samples from the pulmonary artery and the right atrium, respectively. One lumen is used for balloon inflation and the remaining lumen carries cables for a thermistor located approximately 4.5 cm proximal to the tip. The four-lumen catheter thus allows (1) monitoring of pulmonary artery pressure (distal lumen, balloon deflated); (2) monitoring of pulmonary artery wedge pressure (balloon inflated); (3) monitoring of right atrial pressure; (4) determination of cardiac output by thermodilution technique; and (5) aspiration of blood samples from the pulmonary artery and right atrium.

Multipurpose electrode catheters incorporate atrial and ventricular electrodes, which can be used for recording intra-atrial and intraventricular electrograms and which facilitate diagnosis of complex arrhythmias. Intra-cardiac electrograms provide signals of considerably larger amplitude than those produced by surface electrograms. Therefore, intraventricular electrograms monitored by multipurpose electrode catheters can be used to trigger QRS sensing devices, such as intra-aortic balloon counterpulsation, when the QRS amplitudes recorded by the surface electrograms fall below the threshold values. Atrial and ventricular electrodes can be employed for temporary atrial and ventricular pacing respectively, and atrioventricular sequential pacing can also be achieved in the absence of atrioventricular conduction by simultaneous use of atrial and ventricular electrodes. When multipurpose electrode catheters are used for transvenous temporary pacing, the pacing threshold is usually much higher than when conventional pacing electrode catheters are used, because adequate endocardial contact with these electrodes is rarely achieved. Lack of endocardial contact is observed more frequently in patients with considerable right atrial and right ventricular enlargement. Loss of electrode contact with the endocardium and failure of pacing may also occur when the balloon is inflated to record pulmonary artery wedge pressure or when the intracardiac catheter position changes with the movement of the patient. Thus, the use of multipurpose electrode catheters should be avoided if consistent and prolonged transvenous pacing is desired. In patients with markedly dilated right heart chambers, reliable pacing is rarely achieved with the use of multipurpose electrode catheters. In the presence of a normal-sized heart, reliable atrial and ventricular pacing are expected in approximately 70% to 90% of patients respectively.[3] Recently, right ventricular port multipurpose balloon flotation catheters have been introduced, and in these catheters an additional right ventricular lumen has been incorporated. This lumen can be used either for monitoring right ventricular pressure or for introducing a thin flexible electrode into the right ventricle for right ventricular pacing. Reliable ventricular pacing with the use of the right ventricular port catheter is expected in the vast majority of patients, irrespective of heart size.[4]

Newer catheters also incorporate a fifth lumen containing fiberoptic bundles to measure mixed venous oxygen saturation. When oxygen consumption remains constant, arterial–mixed venous oxygen content varies inversely to cardiac output, and mixed venous oxygen saturation is higher with higher cardiac output. Thus, monitoring of changes in mixed venous oxygen saturation provides information about changes in cardiac output.

In the newer catheters, an additional lumen designed to terminate in the right atrium and to be used for fluid infusions is frequently incorporated. This not only provides an additional central line, but also eliminates the necessity to interrupt intravenous therapy during cardiac output determinations, when the proximal right atrial lumen is used for intravenous infusions.

The insertion of balloon flotation catheters should be undertaken under strictly sterile conditions, and the appropriate preparation of the skin is extremely important to minimize the risk of sepsis. Access to the right side of the heart can be achieved by a number of venous routes. The choice of veins depends not only on the operator's preference and experience, but also on the indications and anticipated duration of hemodynamic monitoring. The antecubital veins are usually chosen in patients with coagulopathies and who are on anticoagulant therapy or in patients who have received thrombolytic therapy (e.g., streptokinase for acute myocardial infarction). Another common peripheral vein used for pulmonary artery catheterization is the external jugular vein. It may often be cannulated percutaneously and a J guide wire can be employed to navigate the junction of the external jugular vein with the central venous system.[5] Manipulation of the catheter, however, is more difficult and the incidence of venous thrombosis is higher when peripheral veins are used.

The internal jugular or subclavian veins (central veins) are preferable when prolonged hemodynamic monitoring (more than 24 hours) is anticipated. The disadvantages of the internal jugular approach include puncture of the common carotid artery and, rarely, the trachea. It is also difficult to maintain sterile conditions for prolonged periods of time. Subclavian venous access should not be attempted in patients with bleeding disorders or in those who have received anticoagulation or thrombolytic therapy, because direct pressure cannot be applied to the puncture site to control bleeding.

Elderly patients with tortuous major arterial vessels are at a higher risk of arterial laceration, so the subclavian approach in these patients should be attempted with caution. The femoral vein is infrequently used for the placement of flotation catheters for hemodynamic monitoring. Because of the risk of deep vein thrombosis and subsequent pulmonary emboli, this approach should be avoided if possible. It is also difficult to maintain sterility of the insertion site, and the incidence of sepsis appears to be higher.

Balloon-tipped flow-directed catheters can be placed into the pulmonary artery, in most instances, without the use of fluoroscopy. In patients with markedly dilated right heart chambers or with severe chronic pulmonary hypertension, fluoroscopy aids in the prompt placement of the flotation catheters. The location of the catheter tip is identified by recognizing the pressure tracings characteristic of different intracardiac chambers (Fig. 39.1). Intrathoracic location of the catheter can be appreciated by observing the changes in the pressure tracing during respiration. If the patient is breathing spontaneously, this is characterized by a sudden decrease in pressure during the inspiratory phase of respiration. With increased intrathoracic pressure, such as during coughing or during positive pressure ventilation, the pressure tracing demonstrates an increase along with an increase in intra-aortic pressure. As the catheter is advanced with the balloon inflated, it traverses the tricuspid valve, and the right ventricular pressure tracing becomes visible. The right ventricular pressure tracing is characterized by a sharp upstroke, a peak pressure significantly higher than that seen in the right atrial tracing, and sharp downstroke without the presence of a dicrotic notch. As the catheter is advanced further, it traverses the pulmonary valve, and a change in the pressure tracing characteristic of pulmonary artery pressure is recognized. The pressure tracing in the pulmonary artery demonstrates a dicrotic notch on the downstroke of the wave form. The pulmonary artery end-diastolic pressure is usually higher than the right ventricular end-diastolic pressure. If the dicrotic notch is not obvious, the end-systolic pressure in the pulmonary artery can be estimated by determining the pressure at the end of the T wave of the QRST complex in the simultaneously recorded electrocardiogram. The end-systolic pressure in the pulmonary artery is higher than the end-diastolic pressure. In the right ventricle, however, the end-systolic pressure is lower than the end-diastolic pressure. Once the pulmonary artery pressure tracing is recognized, the catheter tip should be advanced slowly with the balloon inflated until the character of the pressure tracing again changes and the wedge pressure tracing is visible. The wedge pressure tracing shows a low-amplitude phasic wave form similar to the right atrial pressure tracing. The wedge position of the catheter tip can be verified by demonstrating a higher oxygen tension in the blood sample drawn from this position (balloon inflated) than that in the sample drawn when the catheter tip is in the pulmonary artery (balloon deflated). Before the catheter is secured in the correct position, the difference between the pulmonary artery end-diastolic pressure and the pulmonary capillary wedge pressure should be noted.

In the absence of any significant difference, pulmonary artery end-diastolic pressure can be substituted for the wedge pressure, and further manipulation of the catheter to obtain wedge pressure can be avoided. At the end of the procedure, a chest radiograph should always be taken to ascertain the location of the catheter tip.

CENTRAL VENOUS PRESSURE

Central venous pressure[6-15] and right atrial pressure are equal to right ventricular diastolic pressure in the absence of tricuspid valve obstruction and represent right ventricular filling pressure. Until the advent of balloon flotation pulmonary artery catheters, central venous pressure was used to assess the status of intravascular volume and to estimate right and left ventricular filling pressures. Although in the presence of normal right and left ventricular function and in the absence of any cardiopulmonary disease a reasonable correlation exists between central venous, right atrial, and pulmonary artery wedge pressures,[6] with altered right or left ventricular function such correlations are no longer observed. The correlation between central venous pressure and pulmonary capillary wedge pressure in patients with coronary artery disease is reasonably good in the presence of normal left ventricular ejection fraction (>0.5) and in the absence of left ventricular dyssynergia.[7] A poor correlation is found in patients with ejection fractions below 40% and with left ventricular dyssynergia.[7] Central venous pressure has been shown to correlate poorly with left atrial or pulmonary capillary wedge pressure in patients with valvular heart disease,[8,9] coronary artery disease,[7,10] or pulmonary hypertension.[11] Even in the absence of cardiopulmonary disease, the correlation between the central venous pressure (right atrial pressure) and pulmonary capillary wedge pressure is only modest.[12] A poor correlation between right atrial pressure and pulmonary artery wedge pressure is found in patients with acute myocardial infarction,[13] partly owing to the preponderance of coexisting right ventricular failure resulting from either right ventricular infarction or left ventricular failure. Thus, monitoring of both right atrial and pulmonary capillary wedge pressures is preferable to assess right and left ventricular dysfunction and their causes.

PULMONARY ARTERY WEDGE PRESSURE

Pulmonary artery pressure is identical to right ventricular pressure during systole in the absence of right ventricular outflow obstruction. Pulmonary artery end-diastolic pressure is similar to pulmonary artery wedge pressure in the absence of elevated pulmonary vascular resistance. Pulmonary artery wedge pressure reflects fairly accurately left atrial pressure. By balloon inflation, which occludes a pulmonary artery branch, or by wedging a catheter into a small branch of a pulmonary artery, one abolishes the pressure differential between the pulmonary artery branches distal to the tip of the catheter and the pulmonary capillaries and veins and the left atrium, and flow across the vascular segments is absent. Interruption of forward flow in this manner allows a fairly accurate measurement of pulmonary venous and left atrial pressures from a proximal source (pulmonary artery branches distal to balloon occlusion). In experimental animal studies, it has been demonstrated that when a cardiac catheter is wedged into a small branch of the pulmonary artery until the vessel is occluded, the distal opening of the catheter establishes a free communication with the pulmonary capillaries and veins.[16] The phasic variations in the wedge pressure tracing obtained this way are similar to those of left atrial pressure tracings.[17] Pulmonary artery occluded pressure obtained with the use of a balloon flotation catheter is virtually identical to that obtained by wedging a standard catheter.[18] During left ventricular diastole and in the absence of mitral valve obstruction, left atrial and left ventricular diastolic pressures correlate fairly closely, except in certain conditions (described below). Thus, by determining the pulmonary artery occluded or pulmonary artery wedge pressure, an estimate of left ventricular diastolic pressure can be obtained.

At end-diastole, pressures in the pulmonary artery, left atrium, and left ventricle are virtually identical in the absence of certain cardiovascular disorders.[19-21] An excellent correlation between pulmonary artery wedge pressure and left atrial pressure has been demonstrated in patients with coronary artery disease and valvular heart disease.[22-24] The differences between mean pulmonary artery wedge and left atrial pressure usually do not exceed ±2 mm Hg.[22] However, at higher levels of pulmonary artery wedge pressure (exceeding 25 mm Hg), the discrepancy tends to increase.[25] The wider discrepancies between pulmonary artery wedge and left atrial pressures at higher levels of pressure are likely to be related to differences in the compliance of pulmonary veins and the left atrium.

Mechanical ventilation and positive end-expiratory pressure (PEEP) produce variable differences between pulmonary artery wedge and left atrial pressure. Increasing levels of PEEP increase right atrial, pulmonary arterial, pulmonary arterial wedge, and pleural pressures.[26-36] Although in general pulmonary artery wedge pressure tends to increase with PEEP, decreases and no change have been re-

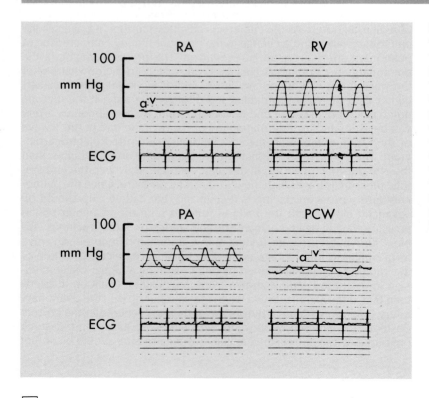

FIGURE 39.1 Right atrial (RA) pressure tracing shows a low-amplitude phasic wave form with a and v waves. As the catheter traverses the tricuspid valve, the right ventricular (RV) pressure tracing becomes visible. The right ventricular pressure tracing is characterized by a sharp upstroke, a peak pressure higher than the right atrial pressure, and a sharp downstroke without a dicrotic notch. With further advancement of the catheter, the pulmonary artery (PA) pressure wave form is shown by the presence of the dicrotic notch. The end-diastolic pulmonary artery pressure is higher than the right ventricular end-diastolic pressure. The catheter is then advanced with the balloon inflated until the character of the pressure tracing again changes and the wedge (PCW) pressure tracing is visible. The pulmonary artery wedge pressure tracing also shows a low-amplitude phasic wave form similar to that of the right atrial pressure tracing. (Chatterjee K: Bedside hemodynamic monitoring. In Bolooki H (ed): Clinical Applications of Intra-aortic Balloon Pump, p 197. Mt Kisco, NY, Futura Publishing, 1977)

ported.[28,30] A number of factors such as catheter position, lung compliance, level of PEEP, type of ventilation, and the initial level of left atrial pressure contribute to these discrepancies. With PEEP below 10 cm H_2O, the differences between pulmonary artery wedge and left atrial pressures are minimal; the disparity increases when the level of PEEP exceeds 10 cm H_2O.[27,36] The catheter position in the thorax and its relation to left atrium are also important for the adequate reflection of left atrial pressure to pulmonary artery wedge pressure. The assessment of left atrial pressure by measuring pulmonary artery wedge pressure depends on the presence of fluid (blood)-filled vascular segments between the catheter tip and left atrium. Whether the intervening vascular segments (capillaries and veins) are relatively empty or remain fluid filled depends on a number of factors: pulmonary artery pressure, alveolar pressure, left atrial pressure, and the hydrostatic relation of the vessels to the left atrium.[37] When alveolar pressure exceeds both pulmonary arterial and pulmonary venous pressures, as in zone 1 of West's model (top of the lung),[38] pulmonary microvasculature is compressed and the fluid-filled system ceases to exist. Airway pressure is then transmitted to the collapsible portion of the pulmonary vasculature. The center of the lung is in zone 2, where alveolar pressure is greater than the pulmonary venous pressure but less than the pulmonary artery pressure, and pulmonary microvasculature may be only partially collapsed. The bottom of the lung is in zone 3, because pulmonary arterial and pulmonary venous pressures are greater than alveolar pressure. In this zone, pulmonary vasculature remains "fluid filled" without being compressed. Pulmonary artery wedge pressure reflects left atrial pressure accurately when zone 3 conditions are fulfilled. In the supine position, most of the lung is found in zone 3. However, alveolar pressure might exceed pulmonary venous pressure under conditions of high alveolar pressure (PEEP) or when the catheter tip is above the level of the left atrium. In these circumstances, considerable discrepancy between pulmonary artery wedge and left atrial pressure is expected. When the left atrial and pulmonary venous pressures are significantly higher than the alveolar pressure, pulmonary vasculature between the catheter tip and the left atrium may not be compressed, even with the addition of PEEP. Thus, in patients with pulmonary venous hypertension, measured pulmonary artery wedge pressure is likely to reflect accurate left atrial pressure. In the presence of normal pulmonary artery or pulmonary venous pressure, accurate assessment of left atrial pressure by measuring pulmonary artery wedge pressure is not possible when significant PEEP is applied. Variable effects of PEEP on lung compliance produce changes in extramural and transmural pressure. During routine clinical practice, left atrial pressure can be approximated by subtracting the magnitude of PEEP applied from the pulmonary artery wedge pressure determined at end-expiration. Marked fluctuations in pulmonary artery wedge pressure, along with respiratory fluctuations, are common in patients with chronic pulmonary disease, and the accurate measurement of pulmonary artery wedge pressure is often difficult in such patients. Furthermore, pulmonary artery wedge pressure may not reflect left atrial or left ventricular diastolic pressure owing to alterations in alveolar and intrathoracic pressures. Increased alveolar pressure due to airway obstruction might compress the vascular segments and interrupt the static column of blood distal to the tip of the catheter. On the other hand, increased pulmonary venous pressure due to increased intrathoracic pressure may prevent collapse of the pulmonary vasculature. An increase in intrathoracic pressure is accompanied by a rise in pressure in the intrathoracic blood vessels. Thus, elevated pulmonary artery wedge pressure, observed in some patients with chronic pulmonary disease,[39,40] may be a reflection of increased intrathoracic pressure rather than an indication of left ventricular failure. Despite these limitations, a correlation between pulmonary artery wedge pressure and left atrial and left ventricular end-diastolic pressures exists in the majority of patients with chronic pulmonary disease.[39,40] The magnitude of change in pulmonary artery wedge pressure also correlates to the magnitude of change in esophageal pressures during respiratory fluctuation.[40,41] When mean pulmonary artery wedge pressure (atmospheric) was compared to the effective pulmonary artery wedge pressure (atmospheric pulmonary artery wedge pressure–esophageal pressure), the difference was 0.5 ± 1.6 mm Hg in all patients with intrathoracic pressure changes of less than 20 mm Hg.[41] With intrathoracic pressure above 20 mm Hg, mean pulmonary artery wedge pressure may be considerably higher than the effective pulmonary artery wedge pressure. During marked respiratory fluctuations in patients with severe chronic pulmonary disease or with Cheyne-Stokes respiration, accurate determination of pulmonary artery wedge pressure is difficult. In clinical practice, the mean pressure at end-expiration during several respiratory cycles is determined to approximate the left ventricular diastolic pressure.

PULMONARY ARTERY END-DIASTOLIC PRESSURE

Pulmonary artery end-diastolic pressure is frequently used to reflect pulmonary artery wedge pressure and hence left ventricular filling pressure. Pulmonary artery end-diastolic pressure correlates fairly closely with mean pulmonary artery wedge pressure in normal subjects and in patients with acute myocardial infarction or left ventricular failure.[19,42-44] Pulmonary artery end-diastolic pressure is usually 1 mm Hg to 2 mm Hg higher than the mean pulmonary artery wedge and left atrial pressures. In patients with left ventricular dysfunction, particularly in the presence of decreased left ventricular compliance, left ventricular end-diastolic pressure is usually higher than pulmonary artery end-diastolic pressure.[19,21,42,45] Directional changes in pulmonary artery end-diastolic pressure, pulmonary artery wedge pressure, and left ventricular end-diastolic pressure are usually concordant and a correlation may exist between the changes in these pressures in normal subjects as well as in patients with left ventricular dysfunction.

In certain clinical conditions, a significant disparity between pulmonary artery end-diastolic and pulmonary artery wedge pressures is observed, and pulmonary artery end-diastolic pressure cannot be used to reflect pulmonary artery wedge or left ventricular filling pressure. Pulmonary artery diastolic pressure is considerably higher than the pulmonary artery wedge pressure in patients with precapillary pulmonary arterial hypertension. Increased pulmonary vascular resistance, irrespective of its etiology, is associated with higher pulmonary artery diastolic pressure. If pulmonary artery end-diastolic pressure exceeds pulmonary artery wedge pressure by 4 mm Hg to 5 mm Hg, increased pulmonary vascular resistance should be suspected.[46] The difference between the pulmonary artery diastolic pressure and the pulmonary artery wedge pressure also reflects the magnitude of increase in pulmonary vascular resistance.[46,47] Pulmonary vascular resistance is elevated in patients with precapillary pulmonary arterial hypertension such as (1) primary pulmonary hypertension; (2) thromboembolic pulmonary hypertension; (3) acute and chronic cor pulmonale; (4) some cases of increased pulmonary flow, as in left-to-right shunt; (5) Eisenmenger's syndrome; (6) hypoxia; (7) some cases of chronically elevated pulmonary venous pressure (valvular heart disease, chronic left ventricular failure); and (8) pulmonary venous obstruction.

Changes in pulmonary artery diastolic pressure may not reflect changes in left atrial pressure in patients undergoing open heart surgery.[48] The reasons for discrepancies, however, remain unclear. In the presence of excessive tachycardia, pulmonary artery diastolic pressure is higher than the pulmonary artery wedge pressure, because the time for adequate runoff is curtailed. Increasing disparity between pulmonary artery diastolic and left ventricular diastolic pressures has been noted with increasing heart rate.[21]

At the time of placement of flotation catheters, the difference between pulmonary artery end-diastolic pressure and pulmonary artery wedge pressure should be noted. In the absence of significant difference (less than 4 mm Hg), pulmonary artery diastolic pressure can be monitored instead of pulmonary artery wedge pressure to estimate left ventricular filling pressure.

PULMONARY ARTERY WEDGE PRESSURE— A REFLECTION OF LEFT VENTRICULAR FILLING PRESSURE

Filling pressure of the left ventricle is its transmural pressure, which is the difference between the distending pressure at end-diastole (left ventricular end-diastolic pressure) and the extramural pressures resisting its filling. Intrapericardial and intrapleural pressures and lung compliance contribute to the resistance of extramural pressures to left ventricular diastolic filling. With normal intrapericardial and intrapleural pressure (usually zero or negative pressure), left ventricular end-diastolic pressure reflects left ventricular filling pressure. Elevated intrapericardial or intrapleural pressures are associated with passive elevation of pressures of intracardiac chambers, including the left ventricle. However, transmural pressures may not change concurrently. Because pulmonary artery wedge pressure increases parallel to left ventricular diastolic pressure, it cannot be used to estimate left ventricular filling pressure in these circumstances.

Pulmonary artery wedge pressure may not reflect left ventricular filling pressure in other clinical situations in which intrapericardial or intrapleural pressures are not elevated. In patients with hemodynamically significant mitral valve obstruction, pulmonary artery wedge pressure is higher than left ventricular diastolic pressure and, therefore, does not reflect left ventricular filling pressure. Also, in some patients with severe mitral regurgitation, a discrepancy between pulmonary artery wedge and left ventricular end-diastolic pressure is observed. In the presence of a hypertrophied, relatively noncompliant left ventricle, as in patients with aortic stenosis, systemic hypertension, or hypertrophic cardiomyopathy, left ventricular end-diastolic pressure may be considerably higher than pulmonary artery wedge pressure. In some patients with acute myocardial infarction, atrial systole may be associated with a marked increase in left ventricular end-diastolic pressure, which may be considerably higher than pulmonary artery wedge pressure.[42] A difference of 5 mm Hg or more between left ventricular end-diastolic and pulmonary artery wedge pressures can be observed when large left ventricular a waves are present. Left atrial contraction can cause a significant increase in left ventricular end-diastolic pressure without a proportional increase in left atrial and pulmonary artery wedge pressures. In the presence of large a waves, the pre-a left ventricular diastolic pressure correlates better with pulmonary artery wedge pressure.

Lack of correlation between the changes in pulmonary artery wedge pressure and left ventricular diastolic volume, determined by radioisotope angiograms, has been observed in the immediate postoperative period in patients undergoing coronary artery bypass surgery. Discordant changes between pulmonary artery wedge pressure and left ventricular volume were reported in many instances.[49] The precise mechanisms for such divergent changes have not been clarified. These observations suggest that in certain clinical circumstances, pulmonary artery wedge pressure does not reflect changes in left ventricular filling pressure or its diastolic volume. In most patients, however, estimation of pulmonary artery wedge pressure provides an approximation of left ventricular filling pressure. Furthermore, monitoring of pulmonary artery wedge pressure is necessary to determine the risk of developing pulmonary edema in critically ill patients.

CARDIAC OUTPUT

The thermodilution technique is employed almost exclusively for measurement of cardiac output in intensive care units. The thermodilution principle for determination of cardiac output was introduced as early as 1954,[50] and the reliability of the technique has been confirmed in animal studies.[51] The technique is based on the indicator–dilution principle, whereby a solution having a known temperature is injected into the bloodstream and the resulting temperature change is recorded downstream. Balloon flotation catheters, which incorporate thermistors, allow determination of cardiac output. A bolus of cold dextrose or saline solution or a fluid at room temperature is injected into the right atrium through the proximal lumen of the catheter; the resulting temperature change is detected by the thermistor in the catheter tip in the pulmonary artery and is recorded as a temperature–time curve. The principle for calculating the cardiac output is based on the fact that the heat gained by the injectate after it is mixed with blood equals the heat lost by the blood.

Comparison of thermodilution cardiac output with cardiac output determined simultaneously by the dye-dilution technique showed close agreement of the two methods (96%).[52] The reproducibility of cardiac output measurements was 4.1% with thermodilution and 5.4% with the dye-dilution technique. The variability of cardiac output measurements with a flow-directed catheter with a single thermistor has also been determined, and it was usually 2% or less.[53] In vitro experimental thermodilution flow measurements using the single-thermistor catheter were validated by comparing thermodilution flow with the actual flow measured in a continuous flow rate. Thermodilution flow was accurate to within 2.2% of actual flow.[53]

Potential sources of error, however, exist in determining cardiac output by the thermodilution technique. Infusion of an inaccurate volume of the injectate introduces considerable error; with less volume of the injectate, the measured cardiac output is erroneously high, and with greater volume of the injectate it is erroneously low. If the proximal lumen of the catheter is not located in the right atrium, the mixing of the injectate with blood may be inadequate and the measured cardiac output may be falsely high or low. In patients with severe tricuspid regurgitation, potential exists for inaccurate measurements of cardiac output resulting from nonuniform mixing of the injectate. The thermistor remaining in contact with the wall of the pulmonary artery may introduce error in determining cardiac output by the thermodilution technique. When the catheters migrate to the wedge position or fall back to the right ventricle, measured cardiac output is inaccurate owing to inadequate mixing. With proper and detailed attention to the procedures, however, determination of cardiac output by the thermodilution technique is accurate and reproducible in the majority of patients.

CLINICAL APPLICATIONS

In intensive care units, measurements of right heart pressures and cardiac output by bedside hemodynamic monitoring aid in the diagnosis and management of various pathophysiologic conditions associated with altered cardiac performance (Table 39.2). Furthermore, determination of hemodynamic indices provides information regarding prognosis in some critically ill cardiac patients.

HYPOVOLEMIC SHOCK

Reduction of systemic output in hypovolemic shock results from decreased effective intravascular and intracardiac volumes due to hemorrhage, fluid loss to the extravascular space, or decreased venous return to the heart due to abnormalities of the peripheral circulation. The characteristic hemodynamic abnormalities of hypovolemic shock are decreased right atrial and pulmonary artery wedge pressures in addition to hypotension and decreased cardiac output. Reflex tachycardia is frequently observed. In the absence of preexisting cardiopulmonary disease, pulmonary artery pressure decreases or remains within the normal range.

PREDOMINANT LEFT VENTRICULAR FAILURE

In left ventricular failure with and without clinical features of shock, pulmonary artery wedge pressure is elevated and is higher than the right atrial pressure, which may be normal or increased depending on the presence or absence of associated right ventricular failure. Cardiac output, stroke volume, and stroke work decrease, and the magnitudes of reduction are proportional to the severity of pump failure. Arterial pressure falls in patients with severe heart failure and cardiogenic shock. Pulmonary artery pressure tends to increase along with increased pulmonary venous pressure, and in some patients, pulmonary vascular resistance increases. This hemodynamic profile is seen in both acute and chronic left ventricular failure, irrespective of the primary etiology.

PULMONARY CONGESTION WITH NORMAL CARDIAC OUTPUT

In some patients with symptoms and signs of pulmonary venous congestion (e.g., dyspnea and pulmonary edema), cardiac output may remain in the normal range although pulmonary artery wedge pressure may be elevated. This hemodynamic profile is observed in some patients with acute myocardial infarction and in patients with hypertrophied noncompliant left ventricle (e.g., hypertrophic cardiomyopathy, aortic stenosis, hypertensive heart disease). The diagnosis of this subset is important, because therapy in these patients is different from that in other patients who also have low cardiac output.

PREDOMINANT LEFT VENTRICULAR FAILURE

Predominant right ventricular failure can also be associated with low systemic output. Acute and chronic right ventricular failure produce qualitatively similar hemodynamic abnormalities. Acute right ventricular failure can result from right ventricular infarction, acute severe tricuspid regurgitation (bacterial endocarditis, trauma) and acute massive pulmonary embolism. In the adult population, chronic predominant right ventricular failure is most commonly seen in patients with severe pulmonary arterial hypertension. The relatively common causes of chronic pulmonary hypertension include obstructive pulmonary disease, secondary pulmonary hypertension (thromboembolism, systemic lupus erythematosus, scleroderma), and Eisenmenger's syndrome. Severe mitral valve obstruction due to mitral valve stenosis or left atrial myxoma can be associated with marked pulmonary arterial hypertension and right ventricular failure. Chronic right ventricular failure may also be caused by primary tricuspid regurgitation (bacterial endocarditis), Ebstein's anomaly, hypoplastic right ventricle (Uhl's syndrome), atrial septal defect, left ventricular–right atrial shunt, and occasionally infiltrative disease primarily involving the right ventricle.

The hemodynamic abnormalities in predominant right ventricular failure are disproportionate elevation of right atrial pressure in relation to pulmonary artery wedge pressure and hemodynamic evidence of depressed right ventricular systolic function (decreased right ventricular stroke work). The etiology of predominant right ventricular failure can also be suspected from the associated hemodynamic abnormalities. Precapillary pulmonary hypertension is associated not only with elevated pulmonary artery pressure, but also with pulmonary artery diastolic pressure significantly higher than the mean pulmonary artery

TABLE 39.2 HEMODYNAMIC DIFFERENTIAL DIAGNOSIS OF CONDITIONS ASSOCIATED WITH LOW CARDIAC OUTPUT OR PULMONARY EDEMA, FREQUENTLY SEEN IN CORONARY CARE UNITS

Hemodynamic Status	RAP	PAWP	PADP	PADP–PAWP	RAP = PAWP	Disproportionate Elevation of RAP	CO	PVR	SVR
Hypovolemic shock	Low	Low	Normal	Normal	Absent	Absent	Low	Normal	Normal or high
Predominant left ventricular failure with or without shock	Normal or high	High	High	Normal	Absent	Absent	Low	Normal or high	Usually high
Primary right ventricular failure	High	Normal or high	Normal or high	Normal or increased	Depends on etiology—usually present in RV infarct	Present	Low	Normal or elevated	Usually normal
Secondary right ventricular failure	High	Normal or high	High	Increased	Usually absent	Present	Low	High	Normal or high
Cardiac tamponade	High	High	High	Normal	Present	Present	Low	Normal	High or normal
Acute, severe mitral regurgitation	Usually high, maybe normal	High peaked v wave	High	Usually normal	Absent	Absent	Low	Normal or high	High or normal
Acute ventricular septal defect	Usually high	High	High	Usually normal	Absent	Usually absent	Low	Normal or high	High or normal
Septic shock	Usually low	Usually low or maybe high	Normal or high	Normal or increased	Absent	Absent	High or normal	Normal or high	Low or normal
Adult respiratory distress syndrome	Normal or high	Normal	Normal or high	Usually increased	Absent	Maybe present	Depends on etiology	High or normal	Depends on etiology

(RAP, right atrial pressure; PAWP, pulmonary artery wedge pressure; PADP, pulmonary artery diastolic pressure; PADP–PAWP, pulmonary artery diastolic and wedge pressure gradient; RAP = PAWP, equalization of diastolic pressures; CO, cardiac output; PVR, pulmonary vascular resistance; SVR, systemic vascular resistance; RV, right ventricle; LV, left ventricle)

wedge pressure, and the calculated pulmonary vascular resistance is markedly elevated. In contrast, in patients with right ventricular infarction or primary tricuspid regurgitation, pulmonary artery pressure and pulmonary vascular resistance are only modestly elevated or may even be normal. Usually no significant difference is observed between pulmonary artery end-diastolic pressure and pulmonary artery wedge pressure. Severe tricuspid regurgitation can be suspected from the accentuated v wave (regurgitant wave) and occasionally ventricularization of the right atrial pressure wave. In some patients with severe right ventricular infarction, the pulmonary artery pressure wave form is distorted and is difficult to recognize (Fig. 39.2). The pulmonary artery pressure wave forms may appear similar to right atrial pressure wave forms, probably related to marked loss of right ventricular contractility.[54]

In right ventricular infarction, right ventricular and pulmonary artery systolic pressures do not increase proportionately to the increase in right atrial pressure. The ratio of right atrial pressure to pulmonary artery wedge pressure is usually greater than 0.65 to 1 and not infrequently equal to or greater than 1 to 1.[55-61] The square root configuration of the right ventricular diastolic pressure wave form, similar to that seen in constrictive pericarditis, can be seen in some patients with right ventricular infarction.[58] These hemodynamic abnormalities, however, have relatively low sensitivity. In the presence of relatively low right atrial and pulmonary artery wedge pressures, these expected hemodynamic abnormalities may not be apparent and volume loading may sometimes be necessary to identify predominant right ventricular failure.[57,60]

EQUALIZATION OF RIGHT ATRIAL AND PULMONARY ARTERY WEDGE PRESSURES

When equal right atrial and pulmonary artery wedge pressures are observed, a number of clinical conditions should be considered in the differential diagnosis. Similar right atrial and pulmonary artery wedge pressures suggest equalization of right and left ventricular end-diastolic pressures, the hemodynamic abnormality that is frequently seen in cardiac tamponade and constrictive pericarditis. Similar hemodynamic changes can also result from severe predominant right ventricular failure associated with right ventricular and right atrial dilatation. In patients with right ventricular infarction, severe tricuspid regurgitation, and acute right ventricular failure secondary to massive pulmonary embolism, right atrial and pulmonary artery wedge pressures can be identical (Fig. 39.3).[62,63] In predominant right ventricular failure, as in right ventricular infarction, equalization of diastolic pressures probably results from an increased intrapericardial pressure due to marked dilatation of the right heart chambers within the confinement of the pericardium.[64] The differentiation between cardiac tamponade and severe right ventricular failure associated with right ventricular dilatation cannot be made based on hemodynamic abnormalities. Echocardiography is particularly useful for confirming the diagnosis of cardiac tamponade or right ventricular failure. Pericardial fluid, decreased ventricular volumes, and right ventricular compression are detected in cardiac tamponade. In right ventricular failure, on the other hand, a dilated, poorly contracting right ventricle can be visualized by echocardiography.

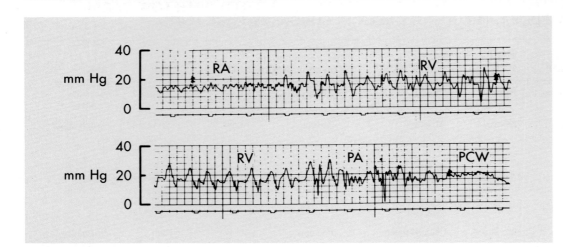

FIGURE 39.2 Hemodynamic abnormalities in acute right ventricular infarct are characterized by a disproportionate elevation of right atrial (RA) pressure in relation to pulmonary capillary wedge (PCW) pressure. RAP may be equal to PCWP, and the pulmonary artery pressure wave form may be distorted. (Chatterjee K: Bedside hemodynamic monitoring. In Bolooki H (ed): Clinical Applications of Intra-aortic Balloon Pump, p 197. Mt Kisco, NY, Futura Publishing, 1977)

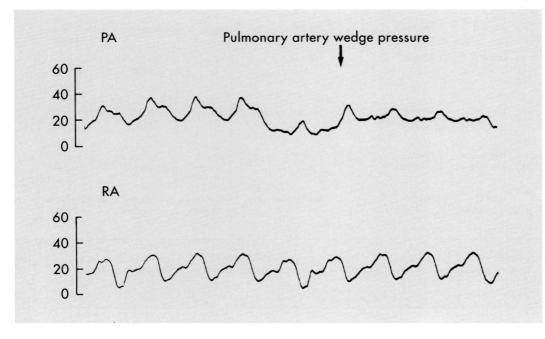

FIGURE 39.3 Simultaneous recording of pulmonary artery, pulmonary artery wedge, and right atrial pressures in a patient with severe tricuspid regurgitation. Mean pulmonary artery wedge and right atrial pressures were equal. Severe tricuspid regurgitation was evident from the "ventricularization" of right atrial pressure morphology.

MITRAL REGURGITATION

Both papillary muscle infarct and ventricular septal rupture are relatively uncommon but catastrophic complications of acute myocardial infarction. The sudden appearance of a pansystolic murmur associated with severe pump failure may herald the onset of either of these complications. The diagnosis of these complications can be established at the bedside by hemodynamic monitoring.[65] In patients with acute severe mitral regurgitation, irrespective of its cause, a giant v wave (regurgitant wave) is frequently present in the pulmonary artery wedge pressure tracing (Fig. 39.4). The onset and peak of the regurgitant v wave tend to occur earlier than those of the normal v wave without mitral regurgitation, and the regurgitant v wave frequently incorporates the c wave in the pulmonary artery wedge pressure tracing. A separate c wave may not be discernible in severe acute mitral regurgitation. However, a giant v wave (height of the v wave exceeding the mean pulmonary artery wedge pressure by 10 mm Hg or more) can occur in the absence of mitral regurgitation.[66] In patients with mitral stenosis, aortic stenosis, and aortic regurgitation with prosthetic mitral valve and congestive heart failure associated with coronary artery disease, large v waves have been observed in the absence of mitral regurgitation.[66] Furthermore, in patients with congenital ventricular septal defect and ventricular septal rupture following acute myocardial infarction, a giant v wave identical in morphology to that seen in severe mitral regurgitation can be identified in the pulmonary artery wedge pressure tracing.[66]

In some patients with angiographically documented severe mitral regurgitation, a large v wave in the pulmonary artery wedge pressure tracing may be absent.[66,67] The predictive value of the finding of a large v wave in diagnosing severe mitral regurgitation was 64% in patients with chronic mitral regurgitation.[66] The reflected v wave in the pulmonary artery pressure tracing usually indicates severe and relatively acute mitral regurgitation. The pulmonary artery v waves due to mitral regurgitation occur in early diastole, after the dicrotic notch, and are associated with large v waves in the pulmonary artery wedge pressure tracings. In patients with pulmonary artery v waves, early closure of the pulmonary valves preceding the aortic valve closure can occur.[68] Retrograde flow in the pulmonary artery can also be detected, associated with large pulmonary artery v waves.[68]

VENTRICULAR SEPTAL DEFECT

Hemodynamic diagnosis of ventricular septal defect with a relatively large left-to-right shunt depends on the detection of higher oxygen saturation in the right ventricular and pulmonary artery blood samples as compared with that in the right atrial blood sample (Fig. 39.5). In patients with acute myocardial infarction, the ventricular septal defect is usually large, and there is a considerable step-up in oxygen saturation in the pulmonary artery over the oxygen saturation in the right atrial blood sample. In the presence of severe mitral regurgitation with large v waves, a higher oxygen saturation can be found in blood sam-

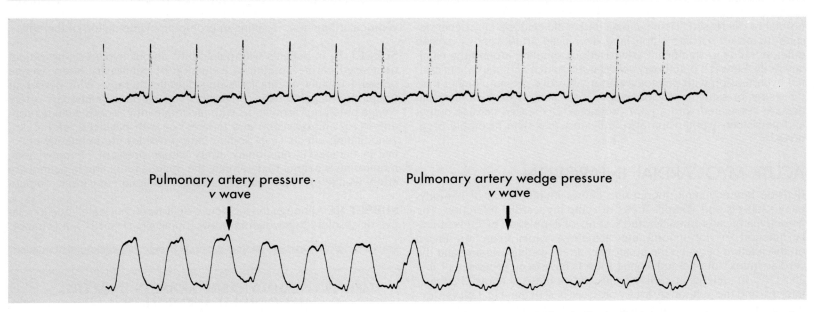

FIGURE 39.4 A giant peaked v wave in the pulmonary artery wedge pressure tracing (after balloon inflation) and a reflected v wave in the pulmonary artery pressure tracing (before balloon inflation) suggest acute severe mitral regurgitation.

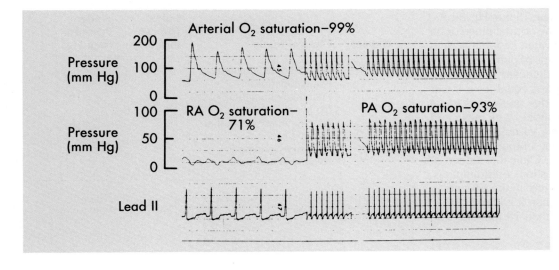

FIGURE 39.5 Simultaneous determinations of right atrial (RA), pulmonary arterial (PA), and systemic arterial (ART) oxygen saturation allow determination of the presence and the magnitude of left-to-right shunt. Higher pulmonary artery O_2 saturation compared with right atrial O_2 saturation indicates left-to-right shunt. (Chatterjee K: Bedside hemodynamic monitoring. In Bolooki H (ed): Clinical Applications of Intra-aortic Balloon Pump, p 197. Mt Kisco, NY, Futura Publishing, 1977)

ples drawn from the distal pulmonary artery branches. Thus, in the diagnosis of ventricular septal defect, when blood samples are taken for the determination of oxygen saturation, it is necessary to ensure that the tip of the catheter is in the main pulmonary artery and not in the distal pulmonary artery branches.

NONCARDIOGENIC PULMONARY EDEMA

The diagnosis of noncardiogenic pulmonary edema and adult respiratory distress syndrome can frequently be established by bedside hemodynamic monitoring. The adult respiratory distress syndrome is associated with radiologic evidence of bilateral pulmonary infiltrates consistent with edema and also hypoxemia ($Po_2/Fio_2 < 160$). However, normal pulmonary artery wedge pressure distinguishes noncardiogenic pulmonary edema from cardiogenic pulmonary edema. Increased difference between pulmonary artery diastolic and pulmonary artery wedge pressures and increased pulmonary venous–arterial admixture, in addition to normal pulmonary artery wedge pressure, are frequent in respiratory failure due to primary pulmonary causes.

SEPTIC SHOCK

The hemodynamic responses in patients with bacterial shock are variable.[69] Septic shock is usually associated with marked hypotension, but cardiac output may be increased, normal, or decreased. During the early stage of shock, especially due to gram-negative sepsis, systemic vascular resistance is lower than normal and cardiac output is increased. Right atrial and pulmonary artery wedge pressures may be normal or decreased. Tissue anoxia and lactic acidosis may occur despite increased cardiac output and decreased arteriovenous oxygen difference due to significant arteriovenous shunting around the capillary beds. Elevated pulmonary vascular resistance and pulmonary arterial hypertension with pulmonary artery diastolic pressure higher than the wedge pressure may be observed. These hemodynamic abnormalities are associated with a poor prognosis. Decreased cardiac output and persistent hypotension also indicate a less than favorable prognosis.[69,70]

ACUTE MYOCARDIAL INFARCTION

Bedside hemodynamic monitoring allows identification of hemodynamic subsets and complications of acute myocardial infarction. The hemodynamic abnormalities and severity of depression of left ventricular function are not uniform after acute myocardial infarction. Based on the relation between the pulmonary artery wedge pressure and the cardiac index, four hemodynamic subsets have been proposed (Table 39.3).[71,72] In patients in *subset I*, the cardiac index is above 2.2 liters/min/m^2 and the pulmonary artery pressure is ≤18 mm Hg. Left ventricular stroke work index, arterial pressure, and systemic vascular resistance are usually normal. Clinical evidence of pulmonary congestion or hypoperfusion is absent in the majority of patients. In *subset II*, the cardiac index is adequate (above 2.2 liters/min/m^2), but the pulmonary artery wedge pressure is elevated and is higher than 18 mm Hg. Stroke work index and arterial pressure may remain in the normal range or be only slightly decreased. Normal or modestly elevated systemic vascular resistance is also observed. Signs and symptoms of pulmonary congestion without evidence of hypoperfusion are detected in these patients. In patients in *subset III*, the cardiac index is equal to or lower than 2.2 liters/min/m^2, and pulmonary artery wedge pressure is equal to or less than 18 mm Hg, along with decreased stroke work index and decreased arterial pressure. Changes in systemic vascular resistance depend on the magnitude of reduction of cardiac output and arterial pressure, and not infrequently it remains normal. Clinical evidence of hypoperfusion, rather than of pulmonary congestion, predominates. Depression of left ventricular function is more severe in the patients in *subset IV*; the cardiac index is equal to or less than 2.2 liters/min/m^2 and pulmonary artery wedge pressure is higher than 18 mm Hg. The stroke work index is decreased, and in the absence of marked hypotension, systemic vascular resistance is elevated. When arterial pressure is also low, systemic vascular resistance remains normal. Clinical signs and symptoms of both hypoperfusion and pulmonary congestion are present in the majority of patients. Clinical manifestations of cardiogenic shock may accompany severe depression of left ventricular function.

Besides these broad subsets, hemodynamic monitoring permits diagnosis of special complications of acute myocardial infarction: predominant right ventricular infarct, mitral regurgitation, and ventricular septal rupture. The hemodynamic differentiation of these complications already has been outlined.

HEMODYNAMIC MONITORING DURING THERAPEUTIC INTERVENTION

In patients with acute myocardial infarction, hemodynamic monitoring not only permits identification of hemodynamic subsets, but also helps to provide a rational therapeutic approach.

SUBSET I. In patients with uncomplicated myocardial infarction with normal hemodynamics, no specific therapy is necessary aside from close observation for development of complications. Some patients in this subset may have tachycardia and arterial hypertension and may develop postinfarction angina requiring therapy with β-adrenergic blocking agents or calcium channel blocking agents. In some patients with initially compensated left ventricular function, pump failure may supervene owing to reinfarction or extension of the infarct. Hemodynamic monitoring may be useful to detect early deterioration of left ventricular function, resulting in prompt implementation of therapy.

SUBSET II. In patients with pulmonary venous hypertension without decreased cardiac output, a reduction of pulmonary artery wedge pressure usually occurs following diuretic therapy. With persistent symptoms of pulmonary congestion and elevated pulmonary artery wedge pressure, vasodilators with predominantly venous dilating properties (*e.g.*, nitroglycerin and nitrates) or with balanced arterial and venodilating effects (*e.g.*, sodium nitroprusside) are frequently effective in decreasing pulmonary artery wedge pressure. Hemodynamic monitoring is helpful to determine the optimal reduction in pulmonary artery wedge pressure without causing a reduction in cardiac output.

SUBSET III. Although the incidence of "low output state" due to relative or absolute hypovolemia is low (approximately 15%), it is impor-

TABLE 39.3 HEMODYNAMIC SUBSETS IN ACUTE MYOCARDIAL INFARCTION

Subset	Clinical Signs	Cardiac Index (liters/min/m^2)	Pulmonary Artery Wedge Pressure (mm Hg)
I	No pulmonary congestion No hypoperfusion	>2.2	≤18
II	Pulmonary congestion No hypoperfusion	>2.2	>18
III	No pulmonary congestion Hypoperfusion	≤2.2	≤18
IV	Pulmonary congestion Hypoperfusion	≤2.2	>18

Forrester JS, Diamond G, Chatterjee K et al: Hemodynamic therapy of myocardial infarction. N Engl J Med 295:1356, 1404, 1976. Reprinted by permission.

tant to identify these patients, because their hemodynamic derangement can usually be rectified by volume repletion. During fluid infusion, monitoring of pulmonary artery wedge pressure helps to determine the optimal filling pressure. In most patients with recent myocardial infarction with relatively normal left ventricular size, optimal filling pressure, in terms of stroke output, is 14 mm Hg to 18 mm Hg.[73] Further increase in pulmonary artery wedge pressure enhances the risk of pulmonary edema. In some patients who initially appear hypovolemic, increasing pulmonary artery wedge pressure with administration of intravenous fluids does not result in a significant increase in cardiac output. In such patients, concomitant left ventricular pump failure exists, and therapy for pump failure is indicated while optimal filling pressures are maintained.

SUBSET IV. Hemodynamic monitoring is required to determine the severity of left ventricular failure and hemodynamic derangement so that appropriate therapy can be chosen in individual patients. Acute pump failure is generally treated initially with parenteral vasodilators, inotropic agents, vasopressors, or intra-aortic balloon counterpulsation, depending on the severity of pump failure. The most commonly used vasodilators are sodium nitroprusside, phentolamine, and nitroglycerin. The expected hemodynamic effects of sodium nitroprusside and phentolamine are an increase in cardiac output and a decrease in pulmonary artery wedge and right atrial pressures.[74] Phentolamine tends to increase heart rate, which does not change or decrease with sodium nitroprusside. The principal hemodynamic effects of nitroglycerin and nitrates are a decrease in right atrial and pulmonary artery wedge pressures with only a modest increase or no change in cardiac output.[74] Arterial pressure may decrease, however, with any of these vasodilator agents. It is apparent that the determination of initial hemodynamics is helpful for selection of a vasodilator in a patient with pump failure. If cardiac output is only slightly decreased but the pulmonary artery wedge pressure is elevated, any of these vasodilator agents is likely to correct the hemodynamic abnormalities and to improve left ventricular function. In patients with significantly decreased cardiac output and elevated pulmonary artery wedge pressure without marked hypotension (systolic blood pressure above 90 mm Hg), sodium nitroprusside or phentolamine produces better hemodynamic responses. During vasodilator therapy, hypotension is a potential undesirable hemodynamic response. Hypotension tends to occur when the increase in cardiac output is not proportional to the decrease in systemic vascular resistance. Furthermore, cardiac output may not increase, or may even decrease, if pulmonary artery wedge pressure decreases to a very low level during vasodilator therapy.[74] Hemodynamic monitoring, therefore, is required not only for the selection of vasodilators, but also to optimize the hemodynamic response and to avoid complications such as hypotension. The guidelines for intravenous vasodilator therapy in acute pump failure are outlined in Table 39.4.[75] In patients with hypotension (systolic blood pressure below 90 mm Hg) or in whom vasodilator therapy fails to produce adequate beneficial hemodynamic effects, inotropic and vasopressor therapy and intra-aortic balloon counterpulsation are frequently required. During combined inotropic and vasodilator therapy, hemodynamic responses are monitored to adjust the doses of inotropic and vasodilator agents.

RIGHT VENTRICULAR INFARCT

Hemodynamic monitoring is necessary during management of the low output state resulting from right ventricular failure in patients with predominant right ventricular infarct. Systemic output tends to increase following intravenous administration of fluids, presumably from the increase of left ventricular preload.[76] Changes in right atrial and pulmonary artery wedge pressures and cardiac output need to be determined during intravenous fluid therapy. Excessive increase in right atrial pressure usually reflects marked dilatation of the right ventricle. Marked right ventricular dilatation may compromise left ventricular filling owing to a further increase in intrapericardial pressure, which is usually elevated in right ventricular infarct.[64] The optimal right atrial pressure that is associated with a maximum increase in cardiac output needs to be determined in individual patients by hemodynamic monitoring during intravenous fluid therapy. Vasodilator drugs (sodium nitroprusside) and inotropic agents (dobutamine) increase cardiac output in patients with predominant right ventricular failure, presumably by increasing right ventricular stroke output, which increases left ventricuar preload. However, concomitant reduction in right ventricular preload as manifested by a reduction in right atrial pressure during vasodilator or inotropic therapy may curtail the magnitude of increase in cardiac output. Hemodynamic monitoring is required to determine the optimal right atrial pressure during vasodilator or inotropic therapy and during concomitant administration of intravenous fluid.

MITRAL REGURGITATION AND VENTRICULAR SEPTAL DEFECT

Hemodynamic monitoring aids not only in the diagnosis of mitral regurgitation and ventricular septal rupture, but also in the assessment of response to therapy. Beneficial hemodynamic and clinical effects of vasodilator therapy have been documented in patients with severe mitral regurgitation.[74] Forward stroke volume and cardiac output increase and regurgitant fraction decreases. Decreased regurgitant volume is associated with decreased v-wave magnitude and mean pulmonary artery wedge pressure (Fig. 39.6). Changes in regurgitant v waves indirectly reflect changes in regurgitant volume. Thus, monitoring changes in pulmonary artery wedge pressure and cardiac output is helpful in assessing the response to vasodilator therapy. Vasodilator therapy appears to be more effective in the presence of elevated systemic vascular resistance. When marked hypotension is associated with decreased cardiac output and systemic vascular resistance is normal or minimally elevated, vasodilator therapy may not be effective. Combined inotropic and vasodilator therapy with or without intra-aortic balloon counterpulsation may be required, and hemodynamic monitoring is helpful to assess therapeutic response.

In patients with ventricular septal rupture, cardiac output determined by the thermodilution technique reflects pulmonary flow, and the precise estimation of the magnitude of left-to-right shunt is not possible. However, a rough assessment of the severity of left-to-right shunt can be made at the bedside by determining the ratio of the pulmonary to systemic flow (QP/QS). The larger the magnitude of the

---

TABLE 39.4 GUIDELINES FOR INTRAVENOUS VASODILATOR THERAPY FOR ACUTE PUMP FAILURE

1. Determine initial hemodynamics for selection of vasodilator.
2. Start therapy with low initial dose (nitroprusside 15 μg/min, phentolamine 0.1 mg/min, nitroglycerin 10 μg/min).
3. Gradually increase infusion rate every 5 to 15 minutes.
4. Monitor changes in blood pressure, heart rate, left ventricular filling pressure, cardiac output, and systemic vascular resistance.
5. If cardiac output increases with a decrease in systemic vascular resistance and left ventricular filling pressure and little change in blood pressure, maintain same infusion rate.
6. If blood pressure decreases without change in cardiac output or left ventricular filling pressure, discontinue vasodilator or add inotropic agent.
7. Monitor thiocyanate level during prolonged nitroprusside infusion.
8. Substitute nonparenteral vasodilator when chronic therapy is indicated.

Massie BM, Chatterjee K: Vasodilator therapy for pump failure. Med Clin North Am 63:32, 1979.

left-to-right shunt, the higher is the ratio of QP/QS. The QP/QS ratio can be estimated by determining the arterial, pulmonary arterial, and right atrial oxygen saturations (QP/QS = [arterial − right atrial/(arterial−pulmonary atrial)] × %O$_2$ saturation). Determination of QP/QS is helpful to evaluate the results of therapy in these patients. This is particularly relevant when vasodilator therapy is employed. The magnitude of left-to-right shunt in ventricular septal defect is related to the size of the defect and the ratio of the pulmonary and systemic vascular resistances. When the size of the defect is large, as in most patients with postinfarction ventricular septal rupture, the magnitude of left-to-right shunt is largely determined by the ratio of pulmonary to systemic vascular resistance, because the defect itself offers little resistance to left-to-right shunt. Some vasodilator drugs (*e.g.*, sodium nitroprusside, nitroglycerin, and nitrates) can potentially decrease pulmonary vascular resistance more than the systemic vascular resistance and enhance the left-to-right shunt reflected in increased QP/QS. Increased right atrial oxygen saturation and lower pulmonary artery oxygen saturation indicate increased systemic output and decreased left-to-right shunt.

CRITICALLY ILL PATIENTS WITHOUT ACUTE MYOCARDIAL INFARCTION

The knowledge of hemodynamic status is helpful for the management of critically ill patients with multiple organ system disease. Prediction

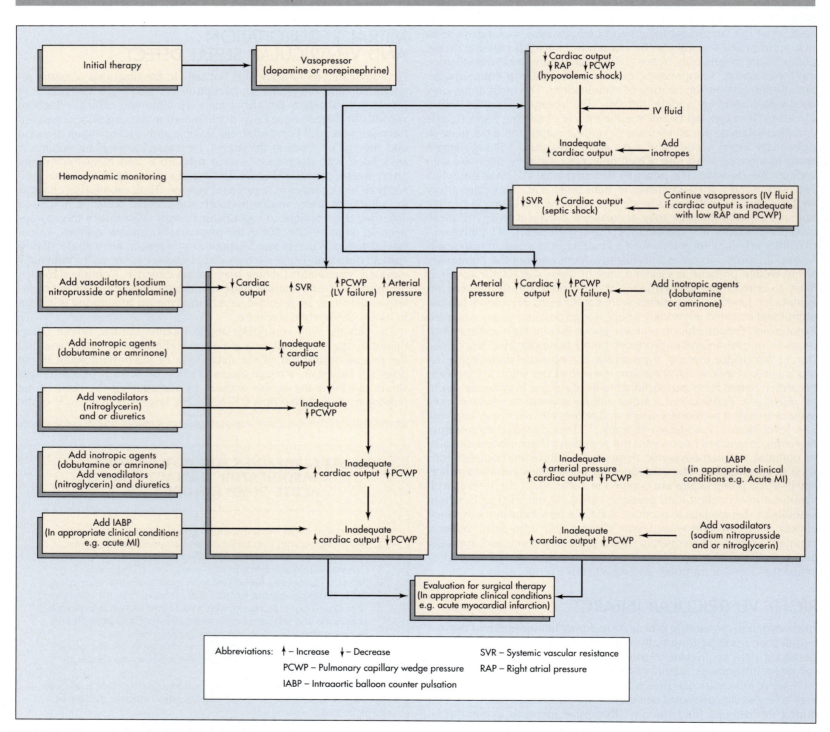

FIGURE 39.6 Stepwise therapeutic approach for hypotension in critically ill patients, based on hemodynamic changes. (↑, increase; ↓, decrease; *CO*, cardiac output; *SV*, systemic vascular resistance; *PCWP*, pulmonary capillary pressure; *AP*, arterial pressure; *RAP*, right atrial pressure; *IABP*, intra-aortic balloon counter-pulsation)

of hemodynamic status by physical examination and by chest roentgenographic findings is frequently in error in patients with hypotension, respiratory failure, congestive heart failure, sepsis, pulmonary edema, or renal failure.[77] These severely ill patients are often difficult to examine. They have altered mental status or require mechanical ventilation. These factors interfere with optimal physical examination. The percentage of accurate clinically useful predictions for right atrial, pulmonary artery wedge, and pulmonary artery pressures and cardiac index in these patients varied between 42% and 44%.[77] Furthermore, the information obtained by hemodynamic monitoring prompted a change in therapy in approximately 50% of these patients. Although the presence of a left ventricular S_3 gallop indicated elevated left ventricular end-diastolic pressure in patients with chronic congestive heart failure, the accurate assessment of the magnitude of elevation of left ventricular diastolic or pulmonary artery wedge pressure is not possible by physical examination. Similarly, the radiologic findings of pulmonary venous hypertension are frequently absent in patients with chronic left ventricular failure with markedly elevated pulmonary artery wedge pressure.[78]

Although alveolar edema is highly specific for elevated pulmonary capillary wedge pressure (25 mm Hg or higher), it occurs in only approximately 30% of patients with markedly elevated pulmonary venous pressure. The sensitivity of other radiologic "fluid abnormalities" such as venous redistribution, interstitial edema, and pleural effusion in the diagnosis of elevated pulmonary artery wedge pressure appears to be low in patients with chronic left ventricular failure.[78]

Management of hypotension in critically ill patients is also aided by hemodynamic monitoring, because it provides information regarding the mechanism of hypotension (Fig. 39.7). Hypotension may result from low cardiac output, particularly when the compensatory increase in systemic vascular resistance is inadequate (arterial pressure = cardiac output × systemic vascular resistance). Hypotension may also be caused by disproportionately low systemic vascular resistance, despite normal or even increased cardiac output, as observed in some patients with sepsis. Hemodynamic monitoring is helpful to adjust vasopressor therapy to correct hypotension in these patients. If hypotension is primarily due to low cardiac output, it is necessary to determine its cause: hypovolemia or predominant right or left ventricular failure.

When patients with chronic left ventricular failure become hemodynamically unstable, parenteral vasodilator and inotropic therapy are often required, and the assessment of the hemodynamic status allows selection and dosage adjustment. During vasodilator therapy, knowledge of the level of pulmonary artery wedge pressure is particularly informative, because marked reduction of pulmonary artery wedge pressure may be associated with decreased cardiac output.

PROGNOSTIC INDICES

Measurements of cardiac index, pulmonary artery wedge pressure, and other indices of left ventricular function allow assessment of prognosis of patients with acute myocardial infarction. In patients with normal cardiac index (>2.2 liters/min/m^2) and pulmonary artery wedge pressure of 18 mm Hg or less, the immediate prognosis is excellent and the hospital mortality in this group was found to be only 3%. Mortality increases to approximately 10% when pulmonary artery wedge pressure exceeds 18 mm Hg and to 50% when pulmonary artery wedge pressure is high (>18 mm Hg) and cardiac index is low (>2.2 liters/min/m^2).[71,72] In patients with clinical features of shock, a low stroke work index (≤20[g/m]^2), low cardiac index (≤2.0 liters/min/m^2), and elevated pulmonary artery wedge pressure (≥15 mm Hg) are associated with a hospital mortality rate of approximately 96%.[79] Determination of cardiac output, pulmonary artery wedge pressure, and stroke work index by hemodynamic monitoring coupled with clinical examination can potentially identify the high-risk subsets of acute myocardial infarction.

Measurement of systemic hemodynamics and cardiac output also provides prognostic information about patients with chronic heart failure due to dilated cardiomyopathy. In patients with either ischemic or nonischemic dilated cardiomyopathy, markedly elevated pulmonary artery wedge pressure (exceeding 25 mm Hg) was associated with a higher 1-year mortality rate than in those patients with lower pulmonary artery wedge pressure.[80,81] Decreased cardiac index (2.2 liters/min/m^2 or less) and stroke work (45 g-m/m^2 or less) and significantly elevated systemic vascular resistance (more than 1800 dynes/sec/cm^{-5}) were also found to be associated with a worse prognosis.[80] It is

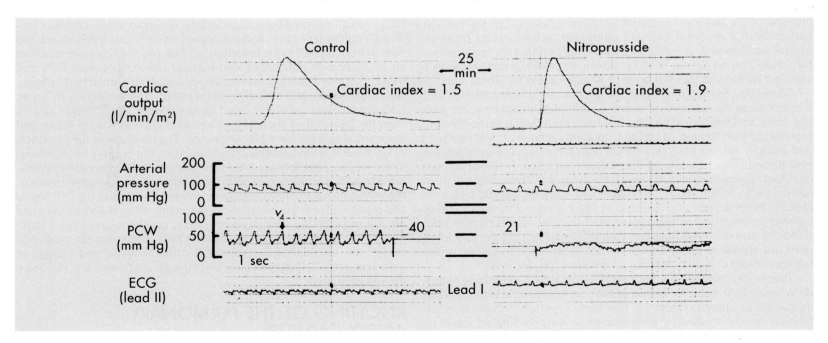

FIGURE 39.7 Evaluation of response to sodium nitroprusside by hemodynamic monitoring in acute mitral regurgitation complicating myocardial infarction. During nitroprusside infusion, cardiac index (CI) increased and the pulmonary artery wedge pressure (PCW) and the magnitude of the peak v wave decreased, indicating reduction in the severity of mitral regurgitation. (Chatterjee K: Bedside hemodynamic monitoring. In Bolooki H (ed): Clinical Applications of Intra-aortic Balloon Pump, p 197. Mt Kisco, NY, Futura Publishing, 1977)

apparent that the more severe the hemodynamic derangement, the worse the outcome, and measurement of hemodynamics is helpful to assess the prognosis of such patients.

COMPLICATIONS

The most common complications of pulmonary catheterization are *atrial and ventricular arrhythmias*. In addition to premature atrial contractions, atrial fibrillation and atrial flutter with varying atrioventricular block can be precipitated during manipulation of the catheter in the right heart. Ventricular arrhythmias include premature ventricular contractions, nonsustained and sustained ventricular tachycardia, and rarely ventricular fibrillation. The incidence of ventricular ectopy has varied from 1% to 68%.[82] Similarly, a wide variability in the frequency of ventricular tachycardia (1% to 53%) has been reported during pulmonary artery catheterization.[83,84] Ventricular arrhythmias are most prone to occur in critically ill patients during emergency bedside catheterization. Shock, hypoxemia, acidosis, hypokalemia, hypocalcemia, myocardial ischemia, and infarction all increase the risk of ventricular arrhythmia. It has been suggested that prophylactic lidocaine can decrease the incidence of ventricular tachycardia during the insertion of flotation catheters.[83] However, the pulmonary artery catheter must be withdrawn from the right ventricle if sustained ventricular tachycardia occurs during catheterization.

The development of *new right bundle branch block*, presumably due to mechanical irritation of the right bundle branch by the balloon-tipped catheter, has been observed in 3% to 6% of patients.[82] New left anterior or posterior fascicular block, in addition to right bundle branch block, has also been reported during catheterization,[85] and it has been assumed to be a result of direct trauma to the bundle of His. In patients with preexisting left bundle branch block, development of a right bundle branch block may be associated with complete atrioventricular block and ventricular standstill.[86] This complication is usually transient, and normal atrioventricular conduction returns within a few hours in almost all patients. Although insertion of a temporary right ventricular pacing electrode prior to the placement of balloon catheter prevents ventricular asystole, such a practice is rarely required if catheter manipulation in the right ventricle is avoided. *Balloon rupture* may be encountered during prolonged hemodynamic monitoring. Balloon rupture is diagnosed by the loss of resistance during deflation and inflation of the balloon; occasionally blood leaks through the balloon lumen. With a ruptured balloon, pulmonary artery wedge pressure cannot be obtained. A ruptured balloon may contribute to thrombus formation around the tip of the catheter; therefore, a catheter with a ruptured balloon should not be kept *in situ* for any length of time.

Thrombus formation around the pulmonary artery catheter and thrombosis of the subclavian, external, and internal jugular veins, axillary veins, and superior vena cava have occurred during hemodynamic monitoring with the use of balloon flotation catheters.[82] Venographic and autopsy studies have reported a high incidence (66%) of jugular vein thrombosis at the site of the catheter insertion; however, no patient had clinical evidence of venous thrombosis.[87] Thrombus can form fairly rapidly, within 60 to 130 minutes of catheter insertion, despite heparin pretreatment and flushing of the catheter. Pulmonary artery catheterization also has been associated with increased platelet consumption and decreased platelet counts[88]; however, this complication does not appear to be clinically relevant. With the introduction of the heparin-bound catheter, thrombus formation has declined.[89]

Pulmonary infarction is a potential complication of bedside hemodynamic monitoring with the use of balloon flotation catheters, and an incidence of approximately 7% has been reported.[90] Pulmonary infarction may be caused by embolization of thrombi formed inside or around the catheter or by migration of the catheter to the wedge position. Endothelial injury of the pulmonary artery by the catheter may initiate thrombus formation, and subsequent embolization may produce pulmonary infarction. The incidence of pulmonary infarction can be reduced by the use of continuous heparinized flush solution through the pulmonary artery catheter.

PULMONARY ARTERY PERFORATION

Pulmonary artery perforation, although rare, is a potentially fatal complication of pulmonary artery catheterization. The reported incidence is approximately 0.2%,[91] and it manifests clinically by the sudden onset of hemoptysis, which may range from blood-tinged sputum to massive hemorrhage. Radiologic changes include pulmonary infiltrates in the area of the catheter tip or even hemothorax. Diagnosis can be confirmed by injection of radiographic contrast media through the pulmonary artery catheter, which localizes the site of rupture. Pulmonary artery rupture tends to occur most frequently in patients with severe pulmonary hypertension and in surgical patients. The precise mechanism for pulmonary artery perforation by the balloon flotation catheters remains unknown. Migration of the catheter tip to the distal pulmonary artery branches appears to be a common occurrence before pulmonary artery perforation. Overdistention of the balloon or eccentric balloon inflation while the tip of the catheter is in the smaller peripheral pulmonary artery branches may cause pulmonary artery perforation. The catheter should be withdrawn from the site of the injury to prevent further bleeding. Injection of clotted blood through the pulmonary artery catheter may occasionally prevent further bleeding.[92] However, emergency thoracotomy with resection of the involved pulmonary segment may be required. The risk of pulmonary artery rupture can be minimized if the migration of the catheter to the smaller pulmonary artery branches is prevented. After the initial passage of the catheter, balloon inflation should be done slowly and with a small volume of air. Smaller inflation volume than recommended (1.5 ml for a No. 7 French) to obtain wedge pressure indicates migration of the catheter to small pulmonary artery branches; the catheter should be pulled back to a position in which full or nearly full recommended inflation volume is required to record pulmonary artery wedge pressure. This ensures that the catheter tip is in the central, larger pulmonary artery branches. The balloon should not be inflated with fluid, which may cause pulmonary artery rupture.

ENDOCARDIAL LESIONS

Endocardial lesions of the right atrium, tricuspid valve, chordae tendineae, pulmonary valve, and pulmonary arteries have been associated with pulmonary artery catheterization. Autopsy studies have reported an incidence of right-sided endocardial lesions between 53% and 61%.[87,93] Endocardial lesions consisted of subendocardial hemorrhage, sterile thrombus, and infective endocarditis. The incidence of septic endocarditis was relatively low (approximately 7%).[93] Septic emboli from the bacterial endocarditis of tricuspid and pulmonary valves and myocardial abscess have been reported. The mechanism for formation of right-sided endocardial lesions is unclear, but is likely to be related to the endocardial damage from flow-directed pulmonary artery catheterization. The incidence of septicemia during hemodynamic monitoring with balloon flotation catheters is between 2% and 8%.[94,95] Sepsis and septic endocarditis occur more frequently when flotation catheters are left in place for long periods of time, usually longer than 3 days. Repeated manipulations of the catheter also predispose the patient to septicemia. Avoidance of prolonged catheterization and change of catheters every 3 days, with insertion through a different site, minimize the risk of sepsis.

KNOTTING OF THE PULMONARY ARTERY CATHETER

Knotting of the pulmonary artery catheter within the vascular space or around the cardiac structures is an infrequent complication of pulmonary artery catheterization with the use of flow-directed catheters. Kinking and looping due to insertion of excessive lengths of catheter predispose the catheter to knotting.

Other complications of pulmonary artery catheterization are similar to those that occur during placement of central venous lines. These complications include bleeding; hematoma; pain and swelling; inflammation; infection at the site of catheter insertion; thrombophlebitis; arterial puncture; pneumothorax, hemothorax, or hydrothorax; air embolism; and thoracic duct and brachial nerve injury. Bernard-Horner syndrome, pneumoperitoneum, hematuria, catheter tip in the wall of the internal carotid artery, and fracture of a flotation catheter have been reported as complications of pulmonary artery catheterization;[96] however, these complications are extremely rare. Arterial cannulation may also be associated with complications, which include infection and thrombosis. The rate of sepsis is about 4% and tends to occur more frequently with surgical cutdowns and when the catheter is left in place for prolonged periods of time. The incidence of thrombotic complications may be as high as 38%,[97] but the affected vessels almost always recanalize. Vascular insufficiency associated with skin or finger necrosis occurs very rarely. Percutaneous insertion of the catheter rather than surgical cutdown, change of the infusion apparatus every 48 to 72 hours, and removal of the catheters every 3 to 4 days minimize the risk of thrombosis and infection following arterial cannulation.

REFERENCES

1. Swan HJC, Ganz W, Forrester J et al: Catheterization of the heart in man with the use of a flow-directed balloon tipped catheter. N Engl J Med 283:447, 1970
2. Forrester JS, Ganz W, Diamond G et al: Thermodilution cardiac output determination with a single flow directed catheter for cardiac monitoring. Am Heart J 83:306, 1972
3. Chatterjee K, Swan HJC, Ganz W et al: Use of balloon-tipped flotation electrode catheter for cardiac monitoring. Am J Cardiol 36:56, 1975
4. Chatterjee K: Bedside hemodynamic monitoring. In Bolooki H (ed): Clinical Applications of Intra-aortic Balloon Pump, p 197. Mt Kisco, NY, Futura Publishing, 1977
5. Blitt C: Central venous catheterization via the external jugular vein: A technique employing the "J" wire. JAMA 229:817, 1974
6. Civetta JM, Gabel JC: Flow directed pulmonary artery catheterization in surgical patients: Indications and modifications of techniques. Am Surg 176:753, 1972
7. Mangano DT: Monitoring pulmonary arterial pressure in coronary artery disease. Anesthesiology 53:364, 1980
8. Sarin CL, Yalav E, Clement AJ et al: The necessity for measurement of left atrial pressure after cardiac surgery. Thorax 25:185, 1970
9. Bell H, Stubbs D, Pugh D: Reliability of central venous pressure as an indicator of left atrial pressure: A study in patients with mitral valve disease. Chest 59:169, 1971
10. Byrick RJ, Nobel WH: Influence of elevated pulmonary vascular resistance on the relationship between central venous pressure and pulmonary artery occluded pressure following cardiopulmonary bypass. Can Anaesth Soc J 25:106, 1978
11. Del Guercio LRM, Cohn JD: Monitoring: Methods and significance. Surg Clin North Am 56:977, 1976
12. Toussaint GP, Burgess JH, Hampson LG: Central venous pressure and pulmonary wedge pressure in critical surgical illness. Arch Surg 109:265, 1974
13. Forrester JS, Diamond G, McHugh TJ et al: Filling pressures in the right and left sides of the heart in acute myocardial infarction. N Engl J Med 285:190, 1971
14. Civetta JM, Gabel JC, Larer MB: Disparate ventricular function in surgical patients. Surg Forum 22:136, 1971
15. Delaurentis DA, Hayes M, Matsumoto T et al: Does central venous pressure accurately reflect hemodynamic and fluid volume patterns in the critical surgical patient? Am J Surg 126:415, 1973
16. Hellems HK, Haynes FW, Dexter L et al: Pulmonary capillary pressure in animals estimated by venous and arterial catheterization. Am J Physiol 155:98, 1948
17. Lagerlof M, Werko L: Studies on the circulation of blood in man. Scand J Clin Lab Invest 1:147, 1949
18. Batson GA, Chandra Sekhar KP, Payas Y et al: Measurement of pulmonary wedge pressure by the flow directed Swan-Ganz catheter. Cardiovasc Res 6:748, 1972
19. Falicor RE, Resnekov L: Relationship of the pulmonary artery end diastolic pressure to the left ventricular end-diastolic and mean filling pressures in patients with and without left ventricular dysfunction. Circulation 42:65, 1970
20. Jenkins BS, Bradley RD, Branthwaite MA: Evaluation of pulmonary arterial end-diastolic pressure as an indirect estimate of left atrial mean pressure. Circulation 42:75, 1970
21. Bouchard RJ, Gault JH, Ross J: Evaluation of pulmonary arterial end-diastolic pressure as an estimate of left ventricular end-diastolic pressure in patients with normal and abnormal left ventricular performance. Circulation 44:1072, 1971
22. Lappas D, Leu WA, Gabel JC et al: Indirect measurements of left atrial pressure in surgical patients—pulmonary capillary wedge and pulmonary artery diastolic pressures compared with left atrial pressure. Anesthesiology 38:394, 1973
23. Epps RG, Adler RH: Left atrial and pulmonary capillary pressures in mitral stenosis. Br Heart J 15:298, 1953
24. Fitzpatrick GF, Hampson LG, Burgess JH: Bedside determination of left atrial pressure. Can Med Assoc J 106:1293, 1972
25. Watson A, Kendall ME: Comparison of pulmonary wedge and left atrial pressure in man. Am Heart J 86:159, 1973
26. Hobelmann CF, Smith DE, Virgilio RW et al: Left atrial and pulmonary artery wedge pressure difference with positive end-expiratory pressure. Surg Forum 25:232, 1974
27. Lozman J, Powers SR, Older T et al: Correlation of pulmonary wedge and left atrial pressures. Arch Surg 109:270, 1974
28. Ovist J, Pontoppidan H, Wilson RS et al: Hemodynamic response to mechanical ventilation with PEEP: The effect of hypovolemia. Anesthesiology 42:45, 1975
29. Hobelmann CF, Smith DE, Virgilio RW et al: Hemodynamic alterations with positive end-expiratory pressure: The contribution of the pulmonary vasculature. J Trauma 15:951, 1975
30. Downs JB, Douglas ME, Sanfelippo PM et al: Ventilatory pattern, intrapleural pressure and cardiac output. Anesth Analg 56:88, 1977
31. Scharf SM, Caldiri P, Ingram RH: Cardiovascular effects of increasing airway pressure in the dog. Am J Physiol 232:H35, 1977
32. Zapol WM, Snider MT: Pulmonary hypertension in severe acute respiratory failure. N Engl J Med 296:476, 1977
33. Roy R, Powers SR, Fenstel PJ et al: Pulmonary wedge catheterization during positive end-expiratory pressure ventilation in the dog. Anesthesiology 46:385, 1977
34. Manny J, Patten MT, Leibman PR et al: The association of lung distention, PEEP and biventricular failure. Am Surg 189:15, 1978
35. Cassidy SS, Robertson CH, Pierce AK et al: Cardiovascular effects of positive end-expiratory pressures in dogs. J Appl Physiol 44:743, 1978
36. Jadin F, Farcot JC, Boisante L et al: Influence of positive end-expiratory pressure on left ventricular performance. N Engl J Med 304:387, 1981
37. Neville JF, Askanazi J, Mon RL et al: Determinants of pulmonary artery wedge pressure. Surg Forum 26:206, 1975
38. West JB, Dollery CT, Naimark A: Distribution of blood flow in isolated lung: Relation to vascular and alveolar pressure. J Appl Physiol 19:713, 1964
39. Lockhart A, Tzareva M, Nader FL et al: Elevated pulmonary artery wedge pressure at rest and during exercise in chronic bronchitis: Fact or fancy. Clin Sci 37:503, 1969
40. Rice DL, Awe RJ, Gaasch WH et al: Wedge pressure measurements in obstructive pulmonary disease. Chest 66:628, 1974
41. Rao BS, Chon KE, Eldridge FL et al: Left ventricular failure secondary to chronic pulmonary disease. Am J Med 45:229, 1968
42. Rahimtoola SH, Leb HS, Ehsami A et al: Relationship of pulmonary artery to left ventricular diastolic pressures in acute myocardial infarction. Circulation 46:290, 1972
43. Rackley CE, Russell RO Jr, Mantle JS: Clinical considerations of hemodynamic measurements and left ventricular function in myocardial infarction. In Rackle CE (ed): Hemodynamic Monitoring in a Coronary Intensive Care Unit, p 173. Mount Kisco, NY, Futura Publishing, 1976
44. Scheinman M, Evans TG, Weiss A et al: Relationship between pulmonary artery end-diastolic pressure and left ventricular filling pressure in patients in shock. Circulation 47:317, 1973
45. Fisher ML, DeFelice CE, Parisi AF: Assessing left ventricular filling pressure with flow direction (Swan-Ganz) catheters. Chest 68:542, 1975
46. Gabriel S: The difference between pulmonary artery diastolic pressure and the pulmonary wedge pressure in chronic lung disease. Acta Med Scand 190:555, 1971
47. Jonsson B, Sanai S: The reliability of diastolic pressure measurement in the pulmonary artery as an index of mean left atrial pressure. Cardiologia 54:329, 1969
48. Subramanian VA, Hai MA, Sherman MM et al: Filling pressure of the heart following open heart surgery. Surg Forum 26:236, 1975
49. Hansen R, Viquerat C, Mathasy M et al: Pulmonary artery wedge pressure and left ventricular preload do not correlate immediately postcoronary artery bypass graft surgery. Clin Res 33:8A, 1985

50. Fegler G: Measurement of cardiac output in anesthetized animals by a thermodilution method. J Exp Physiol 39:153, 1954
51. Rapaport E, Ketterer SG: The measurement of cardiac output by the thermodilution method. Clin Res 6:214, 1958
52. Ganz W, Donoso R, Marcus HS et al: A new technique for measurement of cardiac output by thermodilution in man. Am J Cardiol 27:392, 1971
53. Forrester JS, Ganz W, Diamond G et al: Thermodilution cardiac output determination with a single flow directed catheter. Am Heart J 83:306, 1972
54. Kulbertus HE, Rigo P, Legrand V: Right ventricular infarction: Pathophysiology, diagnosis, clinical course and treatment. Mod Concepts Cardiovasc Dis 54:1, 1985
55. Cohn JN, Guiha NH, Broder MI et al: Right ventricular infarction: Clinical and hemodynamic features. Am J Cardiol 33:209, 1974
56. Lorell B, Leinbach RC, Pohost GM et al: Right ventricular infarction: Clinical diagnosis and differentiation from cardiac tamponade and pericardial constriction. Am J Cardiol 43:465, 1979
57. Lopez-Sendow J, Coma-Canella J, Gamallo C: Sensitivity and specificity of hemodynamic criteria in the diagnosis of acute right ventricular infarction. Circulation 64:515, 1981
58. Lloyd EA, Gersh BJ, Kennelly BM: Hemodynamic spectrum of dominant right ventricular infarction in 19 patients. Am J Cardiol 48:1016, 1982
59. Rackley CE, Russel RO: Right ventricular function in acute myocardial infarction. Am J Cardiol 33:927, 1974
60. Lopez-Sendow J, Coma-Canella I, Vinuelas-Adamez J: Volume loading in patients with ischemic right ventricular dysfunction. Am Heart J 2:329, 1981
61. Sharpe DN, Botvinick EH, Shames DM et al: The noninvasive diagnosis of right ventricular infarction. Circulation 57:483, 1978
62. Chatterjee K: Bedside hemodynamic monitoring in the cardiac care unit. In Schroeder JS, Bresl AN (eds): Invasive Cardiology, p 253. Philadelphia, FA Davis, 1985
63. Higgins JR, VanReet RE, Gregory JD et al: Equalization of diastolic pressures in severe tricuspid regurgitation: Ventricular diastolic interdependence. J Am Coll Cardiol 5:448, 1985
64. Goldstein JA, Vlahakes GJ, Verrier ED et al: The role of right ventricular systolic dysfunction and elevated intrapericardial pressure in the genesis of low output in experimental right ventricular infarction. Circulation 65:513, 1982
65. Meister SG, Helfant RH: Rapid bedside differentiation of ruptured intraventricular septum from acute mitral insufficiency. N Engl J Med 287:1024, 1972
66. Fuchs RM, Henser RR, Yin FCP et al: Limitations of pulmonary wedge V waves in diagnosing mitral regurgitation. Am J Cardiol 49:849, 1982
67. Braunwald E, Awe WC: The syndrome of mitral regurgitation with normal left atrial pressure. Circulation 27:29, 1963
68. Grose R, Strain J, Cohen MV: Pulmonary artery 'V' waves in mitral regurgitation: Clinical and experimental observations. Circulation 69:214, 1984
69. Weil MH, Nishijima H: Cardiac output in bacterial shock. Am J Med 64:920, 1978
70. Sibbald WJ, Paterson AM, Holliday RL et al: Pulmonary hypertension in sepsis. Chest 73:583, 1978
71. Forrester JS, Diamond G, Chatterjee K et al: Hemodynamic therapy of myocardial infarction (first of two parts). N Engl J Med 295:1356, 1976
72. Forrester JS, Diamond G, Chatterjee K et al: Hemodynamic therapy of myocardial infarction (second of two parts). N Engl J Med 295:1404, 1976
73. Crexells C, Chatterjee K, Forrester JS et al: Optimal level of left heart filling pressures in acute myocardial infarction. N Engl J Med 289:1263, 1973
74. Chatterjee K, Parmley WW: The role of vasodilator therapy in heart failure. Prog Cardiovasc Dis 19:301, 1977
75. Massie BM, Chatterjee K: Medical therapy for pump failure complicating acute myocardial infarction. In Scheinman MS (ed): Cardiac Emergency, p 29. Philadelphia, WB Saunders, 1984
76. Goldstein JA, Vlahakes GJ, Verrier ED et al: Volume loading improves low cardiac output in experimental right ventricular infarction. J Am Coll Cardiol 2:270, 1983
77. Connors AF Jr, McCaffree DR, Gray BA: Evaluation of right heart catheterization in the critically ill patients without acute myocardial infarction. N Engl J Med 308:263, 1983
78. Dash H, Lipton MJ, Chatterjee K et al: Estimation of pulmonary artery wedge pressure from chest radiography in patients with chronic congestive cardiomyopathy and ischemic cardiomyopathy. Br Heart J 44:322, 1980
79. Weber KT, Janicki JS, Russell RO et al: Identification of high risk subsets of acute myocardial infarction: Derived from the Myocardial Infarction Research Units Cooperative Study Data Bank. Am J Cardiol 41:197, 1978
80. Franciosa JA, Wilen M, Ziesche S et al: Survival in men with severe chronic left ventricular failure due to either coronary artery disease or idiopathic dilated cardiomyopathy. Am J Cardiol 51:831, 1983
81. Unverferth DV, Magorien RD, Moschberger ML et al: Factors influencing the one-year mortality of dilated cardiomyopathy. Am J Cardiol 54:147, 1984
82. Sprung CL: Complications of pulmonary artery catheterization. In Sprung CL (ed): The Pulmonary Artery Catheter, Methodology and Clinical Applications, p 73. Baltimore, University Park Press, 1983
83. Shaw TJI: The Swan-Ganz pulmonary artery catheter. Anesthesia 34:495, 1979
84. Sprung CL, Pozen RG, Rozanski JJ et al: Advanced ventricular arrhythmias during bedside pulmonary artery catheterization. Am J Med 72:203, 1982
85. Castellanos A, Ramirez AV, Mayorga-Cortes A et al: Left fascicular blocks during right heart catheterization using the Swan-Ganz catheter. Circulation 64:1271, 1981
86. Abernathy WS: Complete heart block caused by the Swan-Ganz catheter. Chest 65:349, 1974
87. Chastre J, Cornud F, Bouchama A et al: Thrombosis as a complication of pulmonary-artery catheterization via the internal jugular vein. N Engl J Med 306:278, 1982
88. Kim YL, Richman KA, Marshall BE: Thrombocytopenia associated with Swan-Ganz catheterization in patients. Anesthesiology 55:261, 1980
89. Hoar PF, Wilson RM, Mangano DT et al: Heparin bonding reduces thrombogenicity of pulmonary artery catheters. N Engl J Med 305:993, 1981
90. Foote GA, Schabel SI, Hodges M: Pulmonary complications of the flow directed balloon tipped catheter. N Engl J Med 290:927, 1974
91. McDaniel DD, Stone JG, Faltas AN et al: Catheter induced pulmonary artery hemorrhage. J Thorac Cardiovasc Surg 82:1, 1981
92. Rubin SA, Puckate RP: Pulmonary artery bronchial fistuli: A new complication of Swan-Ganz catheterization. Chest 75:515, 1979
93. Rowley KM, Clubb S, Walker-Smith GJ et al: Right sided infective endocarditis as a consequence of flow directed pulmonary artery catheterization. A clinico-pathological study of 55 autopsied patients. N Engl J Med 311:1152, 1984
94. Elliot CG, Zimmerman GA, Clemmer TP: Complications of pulmonary catheterization in the care of critically ill patients. Chest 76:647, 1979
95. Sise MJ, Hollingsworth P, Brimm JE et al: Complications of the flow directed pulmonary artery catheter. A prospective analysis of 219 patients. Crit Care Med 9:315, 1981
96. Teich SA, Halprin SL, Tay S: Horner's syndrome secondary to Swan-Ganz catheterization. Am J Med 78:168, 1985
97. Goldenheim PD, Kazemi H: Cardiopulmonary monitoring of critically ill patients. N Engl J Med 311:776, 1984

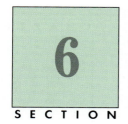

SECTION 6

Section Editor
Melvin M. Scheinman, MD

Electrophysiology

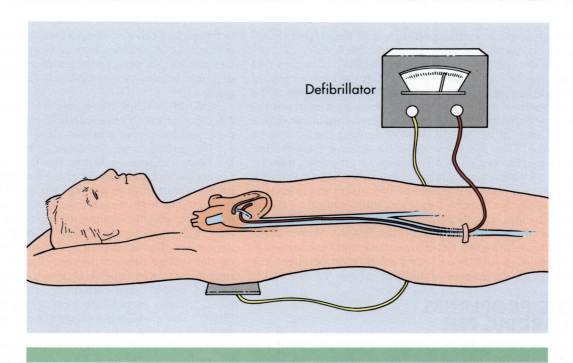

Mechanisms of Cardiac Arrhythmias

Richard J. Kovacs • John C. Bailey
Douglas P. Zipes

Abnormalities of the cardiac rhythm present one of the most common clinical problems in cardiology. Observations at the bedside and deductive analysis of the surface electrocardiogram (ECG) have provided insights into the mechanisms of arrhythmias, but the introduction of the microelectrode has provided a tool for the systematic study of the basic electric properties of the cardiac cell. An understanding of the characteristics of the transmembrane action potential has allowed for a greater understanding of the mechanisms underlying the genesis of clinical arrhythmias. This chapter reviews the fundamental electric properties of the cardiac cell and correlates these properties with the basic mechanisms for arrhythmogenesis. Using data acquired from the cellular laboratory, a scheme is presented categorizing arrhythmias as those caused by abnormal impulse formation, those caused by abnormal impulse conduction, and those involving both abnormal impulse formation and abnormal conduction. This classification of arrhythmogenesis has proven useful in understanding cellular and clinical mechanisms for arrhythmias as well as providing information pertinent to a rational approach to the treatment of disorders of cardiac rhythm.

ELECTRIC PROPERTIES OF THE CARDIAC CELL

The cardiac cell membrane, or sarcolemma, creates a barrier that is semipermeable to several ionic species. This property allows for unequal distribution of the ionic species between the inside and outside of the cardiac cell (Table 40.1). Unequal distribution of the ions produces electrochemical gradients across the cell membrane, the magnitude of which can be predicted by the Nernst equation:

$$E = \frac{RT}{ZF} \ln \frac{C_o}{C_i}$$

where E is the equilibrium potential for a given ionic species, R is the gas constant, T is the absolute temperature, Z is the valency of the ion, F is the Faraday constant, ln is the natural logarithm, and C_o and C_i are the extracellular and intracellular ion concentrations, respectively.

Maintenance of the large differences in sodium and potassium concentrations across the sarcolemma is made possible by an energy-dependent Na/K pump. The Na/K pump requires adenosine triphosphate (ATP) for energy and is membrane bound. The pump is capable of transporting three Na ions out of the cell for every two K ions moved into the cell. Therefore, the pump tends to move a net positive charge from the interior of the cell, and hence is termed *electrogenic*.[1] The cardiac glycosides (such as digitalis and ouabain) are specific inhibitors of the Na/K pump.

Intracellular calcium is largely bound or sequestered by intracellular proteins and organelles, especially the sarcoplasmic reticulum. Small changes in transsarcolemmal calcium flux may thus have a large effect on free intracellular calcium concentrations. Although the calcium gradient across the sarcolemma contributes little to resting membrane potential, levels of intracellular calcium may affect the movement of other ionic species across the membrane. For example, potassium conductance may be increased by an increase in intracellular calcium. Calcium exchanges for sodium across the sarcolemma and depends on the maintenance of the sodium gradient by the Na/K pump.

Chloride is felt to move passively across the sarcolemma, although the intracellular Cl concentration may be somewhat higher than that predicted by passive diffusion alone.

The sarcolemmal membrane at rest provides a high resistance to the flow of current across it. The flow of ions across the membrane occurs through ion-specific channels. These channels are presumably protein-containing structures that provide a low-resistance conduit through the high-resistance phospholipid bilayer. Ion movement through a specific channel is controlled by a system of gates (Fig. 40.1).[2] The opening and closing of the gates are both voltage and time dependent. The number of ions conducted across a channel depends on the voltage required to open the gate and the time that the gate remains activated (open). Channels, however, do not necessarily behave as simple linear conductors. Potassium conductance, for example, decreases as depolarization occurs despite a larger chemical gradient.[3] The potassium channels are said to show inward-going rectification, that is, they pass inward-going currents more easily than outward-going currents. The basis for this property is not known, but it allows for a smaller loss of intracellular potassium with depolarization than would be expected if such inward-going rectification did not exist.

Insertion of a glass microelectrode into a cardiac cell allows for the measurement of the transmembrane potential changes produced when ions flow across the membrane.[4] The electrode measures intracellular potential referenced to an electrode external to the cell. Although some cardiac cells display spontaneous activity (discussed below), other cells remain quiescent until stimulated. When a cell is stimulated, the change in transmembrane voltage with respect to time is called an action potential. The relationship of the cellular action potential to the surface ECG is shown in Figure 40.2.

TABLE 40.1 CARDIAC INTRACELLULAR AND EXTRACELLULAR IONIC CONCENTRATIONS

Ionic Species	Intracellular Concentration	Extracellular Concentration
Na^+	5–10 mmol	145 mmol
K^+	150 mmol	4 mmol
Ca^{2+}	0.1 μmol	2–4 mmol
Cl^-	5 mmol	120 mmol

IONIC BASIS FOR THE CARDIAC ACTION POTENTIAL

When a sufficiently strong stimulus is applied to a cell from atrial or ventricular myocardium or the His-Purkinje system, voltage-dependent activation of the sodium channel occurs, and sodium moves down its electrochemical gradient producing depolarization of the cell. This rapid phase of depolarization is referred to as phase 0. The stimulus needs to be sufficiently strong to raise membrane potential to about −70 mV in order for the sodium channels to be activated. In general, larger stimuli fail to produce a greater depolarization, and conversely smaller stimuli fail to produce any activation at all; hence the action potential is an "all-or-none" phenomenon. Figure 40.3 demonstrates the transmembrane ion fluxes during the cardiac action potential.

Following phase 0, the membrane rapidly repolarizes (phase 1) due to several factors: (1) inactivation of the inward sodium current, (2) activation of transient outward potassium current, and (3) possibly some inward movement of chloride. Phase 1 repolarization does not return the membrane to its resting potential but is terminated by the plateau phase of the action potential.

Phase 2 or the plateau phase represents the sum of several currents, producing a net balance in inward and outward movement. Outward potassium current is markedly decreased due to the inward-going rectification that this current exhibits, and few potassium ions cross the membrane. In addition, electrogenic Na/K exchange occurs through the Na/K pump, and a small amount of chloride may continue to enter the cell. These net outward currents are balanced by the slow inward current carried primarily by calcium. Although sodium channels are to a large extent inactivated at the level of membrane potential present in phase 2, recent work has described a tetrodotoxin-sensitive sodium current that flows during phase 2. Tetrodotoxin, derived from the puffer fish, specifically blocks sodium but not calcium channels. This inward sodium current, or window current, that is blocked by administration of tetrodotoxin also contributes to the plateau.[5] Depending on the cell type and other factors such as stimulation rate, the plateau phase of the action potential may last for several hundred milliseconds.

During phase 3 of the action potential, rapid repolarization of the cell occurs due to inactivation of the slow inward calcium current and by net outward potassium movement. Phase 3 repolarization returns the membrane to its resting membrane potential.

Phase 4 of the action potential represents electric quiescence in normal atrial and ventricular muscle. Spontaneous diastolic depolariza-

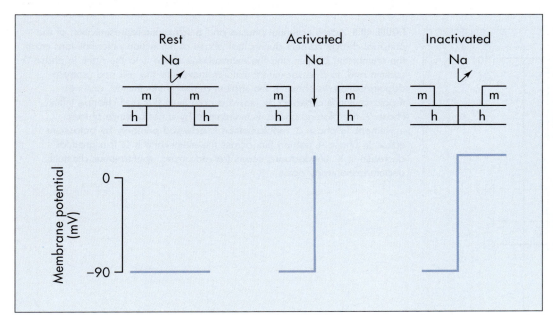

FIGURE 40.1 A schematic diagram illustrating the gated channel mechanism controlling sodium influx across the sarcolemmal membrane. The m gate faces the extracellular space, and the h gate faces the intracellular space. The membrane potential corresponding to the state of the channel is illustrated below the schematic of the channel. In the left panel the membrane is at the resting membrane potential. The inactivation (or h) gate is open, but the m gate is closed and the channel is impermeable to sodium. In the center panel the membrane has been stimulated to threshold and the m gate opens, allowing depolarization of the membrane. Inactivation through closure of the h gate lags behind, but by the right panel it is completed. A similar gating mechanism is proposed to control the calcium channel as well.

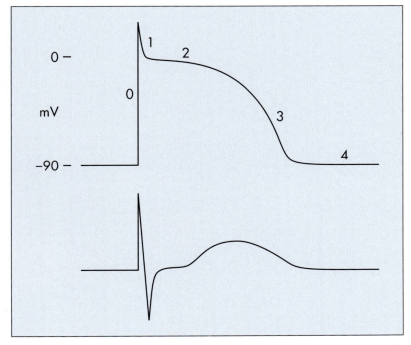

FIGURE 40.2 A correlation of the transmembrane action potential of a cardiac cell with the surface ECG. In the top panel the phases of the action potential are labeled 0–4. In the bottom panel, cardiac activity as detected by the surface ECG is compared to the timing of the cellular events. During phase 0, the cell depolarizes rapidly (1–2 msec), the sum of the depolarizing currents being reflected in the QRS complex of the surface tracing. Owing to the larger mass of the entire heart as compared with the single cell, the QRS complex is significantly wider than the upstroke of the single cell (usually about 80 msec). In phase 2, or the plateau phase, no net current flows. During phase 3, the T wave of the surface tracing is inscribed, and the end of the T wave reflects the return of the cell to its resting potential.

tion does occur in several cell types during phase 4 and is discussed subsequently.

Action potentials arising from resting membrane potentials from −80 mV to −95 mV are typically seen in atrial and ventricular muscle and in the His-Purkinje system. These action potentials display a rapid upstroke of phase 0 and the maximal upstroke velocity (V_{max}) is on the order of 200 V to 1000 V per second. These action potentials are called fast responses, and they rapidly propagate. A second type of action potential, called a slow response, can be seen in normal sinoatrial (SA) and atrioventricular (AV) nodal cells as well as in other cell types under specific laboratory conditions or disease states. Depolarization of the membrane under these conditions is due to an inward flow of calcium ions[6] (and, to a lesser extent, sodium).

Several factors distinguish slow-response action potentials from fast-response action potentials. Slow responses take off from a much lower membrane potential, usually from −40 mV to −70 mV. The V_{max} of these action potentials is on the order of 1 V to 10 V per second. These action potentials propagate more slowly than fast responses. Activation of the slow channel typically occurs at a transmembrane potential of −30 mV to −40 mV, and both activation and inactivation of this channel occur much more slowly than in the fast-channel response (one to two orders of magnitude more slowly). In addition, recovery of the channel from inactivation is slow, requiring additional time after the action potential returns to its maximum diastolic potential before the channels can again be activated and another action potential can occur. These characteristics contribute to the slow conduction and prolonged refractoriness present in tissues displaying slow response activity. Fast and slow responses may also be distinguished by the use of specific channel blockers. As mentioned above, tetrodotoxin specifically blocks sodium but not calcium channels. Antiarrhythmic agents such as lidocaine, quinidine, procainamide, and disopyramide also block the fast channel, although they also affect other membrane currents. A variety of new agents have been introduced that specifically block slow channels. These include D-600, verapamil, nifedipine, and diltiazem.

The types of action potentials seen in specific regions of the heart and the characteristics of the specific cell type are summarized in Figure 40.4. The cellular properties of these tissue types account for certain clinical electrocardiographic phenomena. Conduction velocity through the SA and AV nodes is quite slow because of the low resting potentials, high currents required to excite the cells, and low V_{max}. Although conduction time out of the SA node is not reflected on the surface ECG, slow propagation through the AV node is principally responsible for the PR interval, which on the surface ECG normally

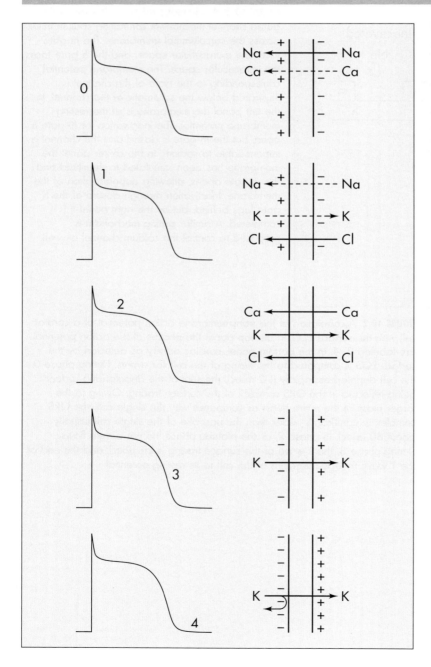

FIGURE 40.3 Action potential phases and a schematic representation of the principal charge carriers during that phase of the action potential. Ions cross the membrane bilayer, and the extracellular space is to the right. In phase 0, sodium and, to a lesser extent, calcium move into the cell and produce depolarization. In phase 1, the sodium current is inactivated, and net repolarization is achieved by outward potassium flux and chloride influx. Phase 2, the plateau phase, is maintained by a net balance of ionic movement. In phase 3, repolarization is achieved primarily by potassium efflux. In phase 4, net ion flux across the membrane is 0. If a gradual decrease in K^+ conductance occurs (curved arrow), spontaneous diastolic depolarization may occur.

ranges up to 200 msec. Transmission of an impulse through the His-Purkinje system, on the other hand, is quite rapid. Ventricular muscle exhibits relatively rapid conduction, and despite the great bulk of the ventricular tissue, ECG depolarization (QRS complex) occurs in less than 100 msec.

EXCITABILITY AND REFRACTORINESS

Although some cardiac cells display spontaneous action potentials, most cardiac fibers require a stimulus sufficient to move the membrane potential to threshold potential in order to produce an all-or-none depolarization. If the cell is capable of producing an action potential, it is said to be excitable. The cardiac cell is not uniformly excitable throughout the cardiac cycle. Periods during which an action potential cannot be elicited despite suprathreshold stimuli are termed *refractory periods*. The phases of excitability of a typical Purkinje cell are illustrated in Figure 40.5. In general, when phase 4 potential is steady and maximal, a constant amount of depolarizing current is required to elicit an action potential. If stimuli reach the cell late in phase 3, they may require larger amounts of current to stimulate the cell, and in addition the action potentials elicited exhibit slow upstrokes and low amplitude, making them less likely to propagate. During other periods of phase 3 it is possible to stimulate the cell with less current than is necessary during phase 4; these periods are defined as the period of supernormal excitability.

The refractory period of a typical cardiac cell is, in general, related to the duration of the action potential. The action potential duration, and hence refractoriness, is related to the frequency of stimulation. Rapid stimulation rates result in short-duration action potentials and abbreviated refractoriness, and slow stimulation rates result in prolonged refractoriness. Cycle length–dependent changes in action potential duration and refractoriness may become manifest within a single cycle; thus it is not necessary to maintain the cycle length alteration for a period of time in order to observe clinically relevant alterations in refractoriness. This observation forms the basis for Ashman's phenomenon, in which a sudden prolongation of cycle length prolongs the refractory period of the subsequent impulse, and a second impulse arriving sufficiently early may find refractory tissue, producing slow conduction through that area. This is manifested on the ECG as aberrant conduction of the QRS complex. Refractoriness is not determined only by stimulation frequency, however, but may also be affected by the external ionic environment, neural influences, drugs, and pathologic states such as ischemia or hypoxia.

CELL-TO-CELL COMMUNICATION

Although each cardiac cell functions as a single unit, the heart beats as a functional syncytium. The mechanism by which communication between cardiac cells occurs is not completely understood. Cell-to-cell coupling contributes to both normal and abnormal conduction patterns, which are discussed below. Adjacent cells share specialized structures known as intercalated discs. These structures provide mechanical adhesion among the cells but in addition contain gap junctions, structures in which the opposing cell membranes are closely approximated. These gap junctions probably provide low ohmic resistance connections between the cells as well as allow for the intercellular movement of ions and small molecules.[7] The way in which this movement is controlled is not known.

In addition to its active properties, such as excitability and spontaneous automaticity, the cell membrane also has passive electric properties. The cell membrane resists current flow and also functions as a capacitor (is capable of storing a charge). This membrane capacitance must be overcome by any stimulus applied to the cell in order to depolarize the membrane. It is also important to realize that heart cells do not exist in isolation from one another electrically. The physical proximity of the cells allows for current spread among cells along the paths of lowest resistance. The path of current spread in three dimensions is difficult to predict. The simplest experimental models can approximate

Tissue		Type of response	Take off potential (mV)	Conduction velocity (m/sec)	$\dot{V}_{max}$ (V/sec)	Duration (msec)
Sinoatrial node	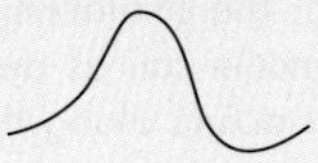	Slow	−60	< 0.05	1–2	100–300
Atrium	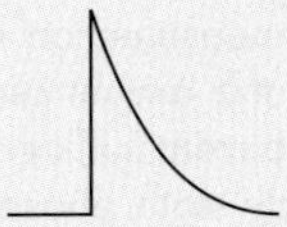	Fast	−90	~1	100–200	100–300
Atrioventricular node	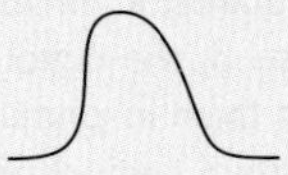	Slow	−60	< 0.05	5	100–300
His-Purkinje	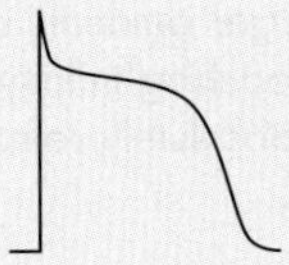	Fast	−95	3	500–1000	300–500
Ventricle	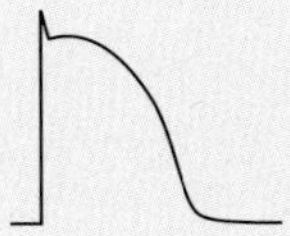	Fast	−90	1	100–500	100–200

FIGURE 40.4 A comparison of action potential characteristics in different regions of the heart. The morphology of the action potential in a given region is shown in the second column. Note that slow response action potentials in the sinoatrial node and atrioventricular node are associated with the low take off potential seen in these regions. These slow response action potentials conduct slowly as opposed to the impulses in atrium, ventricle, or His-Purkinje fibers. (Take off potential is the level of membrane potential from which the action potential arises; V_{max}, the first derivative of the cardiac cell upstroke with respect to time, or dV/dt.)

cells placed end to end as an electric cable.[8] Because resistance across gap junctions is lower than the transmembrane resistance, current tends to flow down the cable. The cable is not, however, perfectly insulated, and current is able to leak across the membrane. Current injection at one end of the cable does not produce a uniform change in voltage all along the cable. Mathematical predictions can be made under the assumption that current flows along a cable, and predictions may be tested in Purkinje fibers (which most closely approximate a cable), but cardiac muscle presents a much more complicated three-dimensional structure. Such interactions among the cells of a matrix are of considerable importance. Local interactions allow a cell to influence many neighboring cells. For example, a depolarized cell can produce slight depolarization in neighboring cells because of local current spread, and electrotonus from the leading edge of a wave of depolarization may depolarize cells ahead of the wavefront. Such electrotonic interactions can influence both automaticity and conduction, as is seen below.

EFFECTS OF THE AUTONOMIC NERVOUS SYSTEM ON CELLULAR ELECTROPHYSIOLOGY

The autonomic nervous system is a major regulator of cardiac electric function at the cell level as well as an influence on the heart as a whole. The adrenergic nervous system may influence the heart through local release of norepinephrine from nerve endings or through circulating catecholamines. Adrenergic stimuli tend to increase automaticity and conduction velocity and may alter cellular refractoriness as well. In addition, β-adrenergic stimulation is capable of inducing slow-response action potentials in depolarized cells. Stimulation of the β-receptor results in an increase in intracellular cyclic adenosine monophosphate (cyclic AMP) levels. Increase in cyclic AMP may, in turn, be responsible for phosphorylation of a membrane protein that allows increased calcium influx through the slow channel.[9]

The vagus nerve exerts influence on both atrial and ventricular tissue by local release of its neurotransmitter, acetylcholine, from the parasympathetic nerve terminals. Parasympathetic stimuli produce direct effects on automaticity and conduction, tending to slow the rate of spontaneous discharge and to slow conduction speed, especially in the AV node. These effects are mediated by acetylcholine-induced alterations in potassium conductance.[10] The vagus produces direct effects on the action potential duration and refractoriness of atrial cells (shortening the action potential duration). In ventricular myocardium, vagal stimulation produces no direct effects *in vitro*, but may prolong ventricular refractoriness in man.[11] In His-Purkinje tissue, acetylcholine can affect automaticity and conduction.[12] Interactions between the limbs of the autonomic nervous system are important in governing cardiac electrophysiology as well, as exemplified by vagal antagonism of the effects of β-adrenergic stimulation.[13,14]

NORMAL AUTOMATICITY

Specific cells of the heart are capable of producing action potentials spontaneously. These cells are said to possess the property of automaticity. Cells displaying automaticity are located in the sinus node, parts of the atrium, the His-Purkinje system, and possibly the AV node. The hallmark of all automatic cells is the presence of spontaneous diastolic depolarization. A microelectrode recording of an automatic cell reveals a slow decrease in membrane potential during phase 4 of the action potential (Fig. 40.6).

Although the ionic basis for diastolic depolarization is still a focus of debate, the slow, spontaneous depolarization during phase 4 must be explained by a net shift in balance of inward- and outward-going currents toward a depolarizing current. This is due to shift in the balance of net outward-going potassium current and net inward-going sodium current.

Pacemaker currents, at least in Purkinje fibers, have been felt to be due to a gradual time-dependent decrease in potassium conductance (less potassium leaves the cell), allowing an increase in sodium influx and a gradual decrease in membrane potential toward threshold.[14,15] An alternative explanation has been proposed: a separate pacemaker current carried by inward-going sodium increases with time, while the net outward potassium current remains constant.[16] This argument has not been resolved.

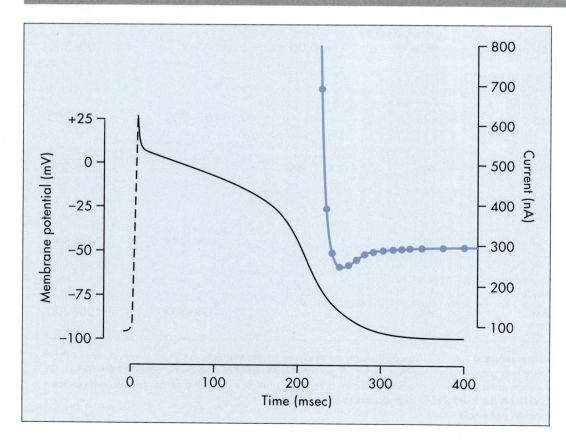

FIGURE 40.5 The excitability of a normal canine cardiac Purkinje cell as determined by current injection at points along the action potential. The amount of current required to elicit a second action potential is measured on the right-hand axis. Each point along the current curve represents the injection of current sufficient to excite the cell. During steady-state phase 4, a constant amount of current is required to produce an action potential. Late in phase 3, the amount of current required is actually less than in phase 4, which is defined as the supernormal period of excitability. Early in phase 3, larger amounts of current are required, eventually reaching infinity. At this point the cell is said to be absolutely refractory.

The spontaneous rate of cardiac pacemakers is under extrinsic control by the autonomic nervous system. Application of acetylcholine or vagal stimulation produces hyperpolarization of sinus nodal cells and decreases the slope of phase 4. This is presumed to be due to an increase in membrane potassium conductance by acetylcholine. Sympathetic stimulation produces an increase in phase 4 slope and an increase in the spontaneous rate of discharge of the sinus node. The increase in spontaneous rate appears to be due to an increase in calcium as well as potassium currents. In fibers with more negative membrane potentials, such as Purkinje fibers, the effects on calcium influx may be less important, because the calcium channel is largely inactivated at the more negative potentials.

Several factors determine which potential or latent cardiac pacemaker becomes manifest as the controlling pacemaker of the entire heart. The first factor is the relative rates of discharge of the potential pacemakers. It is clear that faster pacemakers tend to dominate because other latent pacemakers may be reached by the depolarization wavefront before phase 4 depolarization would allow them to reach threshold.

A second factor determining pacemaker hierarchy is overdrive suppression of automaticity.[17] Overdrive suppression of a latent pacemaker is achieved by driving the pacemaker cell faster than its intrinsic rate. With each depolarization, sodium enters the cell. Na/K pump activity is enhanced by the increased intracellular sodium activity. As discussed above, the Na/K pump is electrogenic, moving relatively more sodium out of the cell than potassium into the cell. This net hyperpolarizing current suppresses spontaneous depolarization. When the period of overdrive is terminated, there is still a lag time before the decrease occurs in the intracellular sodium concentration, as well as in the Na/K pump current, allowing the intrinsic rate to resume. This process occurs gradually and thus explains the warm up period observed in the latent pacemaker after overdrive stimulation ceases.

The final factor contributing to the determination of pacemaker latency is the interaction of pacemaker cells with nonautomatic cells. As mentioned previously, electrotonic interactions can occur between cells. Suppression of spontaneous depolarization and hence automaticity can occur through interactions of pacemaker cells with cells having more negative resting membrane potentials. This mechanism has been proposed to explain the suppression of AV nodal automaticity by surrounding atrial tissue. Conversely, elimination of such electrotonic interactions could result in suppressed pacemakers' becoming manifest.

ABNORMAL AUTOMATIC MECHANISMS

In addition to the normal mechanism for automaticity discussed above, impulses may be formed by abnormal mechanisms. Abnormal impulse generation forms one of the two major mechanisms of arrhythmogenesis, the other being abnormal impulse conduction. Furthermore, these two mechanisms may operate simultaneously, and we discuss below certain situations in which both abnormal impulse formation and abnormal conduction play a role in arrhythmogenesis.

Abnormal impulses may be generated in two major ways, either *de novo* or as the consequence of a preceding impulse. Impulses that arise without dependence on the previous impulse are defined as automatic. Abnormal automatic impulses have been observed in dog Purkinje fibers following myocardial infarction,[18] in myocardium damaged by catecholamines,[19] in some atrial tissue,[20] and in tissue removed for abnormal human ventricle at surgery.[21] Impulses that depend on a previous impulse for their generation are said to be triggered and arise by a different mechanism. These mechanisms are discussed below.

Abnormal automaticity may become manifest in cardiac cells when transmembrane potential has been reduced to about −50 mV.[22] This abnormal automaticity, in contrast to normal SA and AV nodal automaticity, which occurs at about the same level of membrane potential, is termed *abnormal* because these cells normally have resting membrane potentials in excess of −50 mV, usually closer to −90 mV. Action potentials generated by this mechanism are of the slow response type because at the low membrane potentials the fast sodium channels are inactivated. Slow channel blockers are capable of blocking the activity in these preparations. The mechanism of automaticity at low levels of membrane potential may be different in different tissue preparations, but in at least some experiments a deactivation of an outward-going potassium current (normally functioning as a repolarizing current) produces the depolarization necessary to reach threshold.[23]

The low level of membrane potential associated with abnormal automatic foci may determine two clinically relevant characteristics of such activity. First, abnormal automatic foci may not be sensitive to overdrive suppression because the sodium current is inactivated (and Na/K pump activity reduced) at this level of membrane potential.[21] Second, areas surrounding a focus of abnormal automaticity may also be partially depolarized. Conduction of impulses into such a depolarized area is depressed (see discussion of conduction below); as a result, the abnormal focus may be protected from other pacemakers (see also the discussion of parasystole).

AFTERDEPOLARIZATIONS AND TRIGGERED ACTIVITY

Triggered activity, as defined above, is dependent on an initiating depolarization. Triggered activity may be of two types, depending on the temporal relationship of the triggered activity to the initiating impulse. The triggered depolarization may occur before full repolarization has been achieved, in which case it is termed an *early afterdepolarization* (EAD) (Fig. 40.7), or it may occur after full repolarization has been achieved, in which case it is termed a *delayed afterdepolarization* (DAD) (Fig. 40.8). Triggered activity may arise in fibers with either high or low resting membrane potentials and has been observed in a wide variety of cardiac tissues including atrial and ventricular myocardium, the His-Purkinje system, fibers taken from mitral and tricuspid valves, and cells from the coronary sinus.[24]

EADs occur during the repolarization phase of action potentials in cells with high resting membrane potentials. EADs may occur singly or as multiple transient depolarizations occurring during the plateau phase. Occasionally sustained rhythmic activity may ensue, or the membrane potential may "hang up" for an extended period of time at a potential less negative than the resting potential of the cell. Some

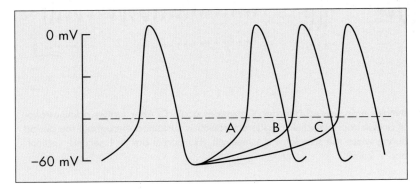

FIGURE 40.6 Transmembrane action potentials from a cell exhibiting spontaneous diastolic depolarization. The action potentials are typical of those seen in pacemaker areas of the SA node. The dashed line defines the threshold potential at which an action potential is generated. If the slope of phase 4 is decreased from B to C (as might occur with vagal stimulation or the application of acetylcholine), the time required to reach threshold is increased, and the rate of discharge slows. An increase in the slope of phase 4 depolarization (as might occur with sympathetic stimulation or the application of norepinephrine) from B to A results in take off potential being reached sooner and an increase in rate of discharge.

EADs may elicit a second action potential before complete repolarization of the cell. These second action potentials are of the slow response type.[25] The ability of EADs to provoke second upstrokes has sparked interest in EADs as potential causes of clinical arrhythmias. Various factors have been shown to promote the production of EADs. These include hypoxia,[26] hypercarbia,[27] catecholamine excess,[28] physical injury or stretch of the fiber,[29] and drugs that prolong action potential duration.[30] Because these factors play a clinically important role in myocardial ischemia or infarction, dilation of a cardiac chamber, and antiarrhythmic drug therapy, EADs have been suggested as a basis for clinically relevant arrhythmias. Although EADs have been demonstrated in diseased human myocardium removed at surgery,[21] their clinical importance has not been proven.

DADs are transient depolarizations occurring after complete repolarization of the cell membrane and are dependent on the previous activity for expression. DADs may fail to reach threshold potential (in which case the membrane potential returns to its resting value) or reach threshold and elicit an action potential. In some cases the triggered activity becomes sustained (see Fig. 40.8). DADs have been described in multiple types of cardiac tissue. DADs may occur in cells with either high or low levels of resting membrane potential, confounding determination of the primary charge carrier across the membrane. In fact, more than one mechanism for DADs may be present. In some preparations DADs arise from low membrane potential and are suppressed by slow channel blocking agents,[31] suggesting that calcium is the charge carrier. In other preparations, DADs may arise from membrane potentials at which the calcium channel would be inactivated. Although the carrier of the inward current is as yet undefined, there is evidence to suggest that the current is at least partly carried by sodium ions.[32] Despite the fact that DADs may be a heterogeneous group of depolarizations, there is some evidence that large increases in intracellular calcium may be a common feature.[33] Increases in intracellular calcium may produce oscillations in release of calcium and other ions from the sarcoplasmic reticulum. The phasic release of calcium may influence the permeability of the sarcolemma to other ions.

DADs may be induced by toxic concentrations of digitalis and by exposure to catecholamines but also may be present in the absence of either of these agents. Digitalis inhibits the Na/K pump, producing an increase in intracellular sodium. The accumulated sodium is exchanged for calcium by the Na/Ca exchange mechanism, which in turn leads to an elevated level of intracellular calcium.[34] Catecholamines directly increase calcium flux across the cell membrane by increasing the slow inward current.[35]

The production of triggered activity in a preparation displaying DADs may be influenced by the rate of stimulation. Increasing the rate of stimulation, even for one cycle, may result in a previously subthreshold DAD's reaching threshold and causing triggered activity. Triggered activity may also display overdrive acceleration.[36] A train of

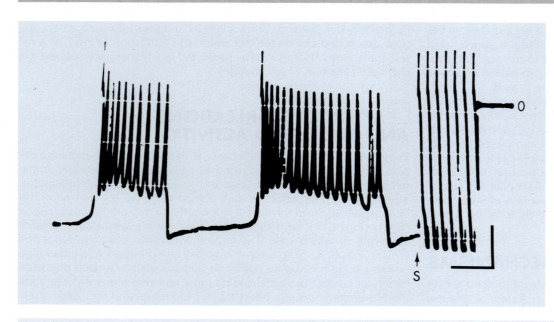

FIGURE 40.7 Early afterdepolarizations (EADs) produced spontaneously in a canine cardiac Purkinje fiber in the presence of a lowered concentration of extracellular potassium. Note that there is spontaneous phase 4 depolarization. The initial upstroke of the two action potentials on the left is followed by several depolarizations before the membrane returns to its maximum diastolic potential. At point S the cell is stimulated electrically and normal action potentials are produced. (Horizontal calibration bar = 5 seconds; vertical bar = 25 mV.)

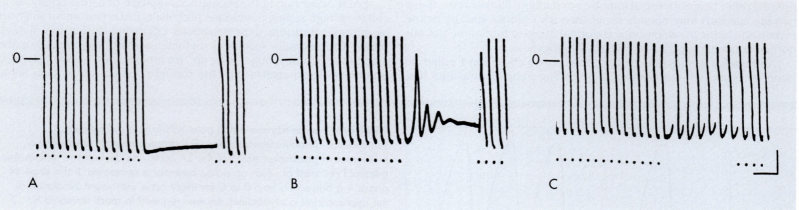

FIGURE 40.8 Delayed afterdepolarizations (DADs) and triggered activity in a canine Purkinje fiber intoxicated with digitalis. Transmembrane potentials are recorded, and marks in the lower trace record the stimulus train. **A.** Prior to digitalis administration, cessation of the stimulus train results in electric quiescence. **B.** Acetylstrophanthidin is applied, and at the termination of the stimulus train several afterdepolarizations occur. **C.** After further administration of acetylstrophanthidinin, triggered activity is sustained throughout the period during which the stimulator is turned off. (Horizontal bar = 1 second; vertical bar = 25 mV.)

paced impulses faster than the triggered rate may result in an increase in the rate of triggered responses after the pacing train is stopped.

Termination of triggered activity may occur through several mechanisms. Activity due to catecholamine excess or digitalis excess may terminate spontaneously despite continued exposure to the agent. One mechanism by which triggered activity may be terminated may be an increase in sodium pump activity stimulated by the increased intracellular sodium concentration. Intracellular sodium concentration rises because of the increase in sodium influx during the rapid triggered activity. The net outward current produced by enhanced sodium pump activity may slow the rate of triggered activity or if of sufficient magnitude may terminate it. Clearly digitalis-induced triggered activity does not terminate by this mechanism, because the Na/K pump is inhibited, so other mechanisms are probably capable of terminating triggered activity. An alternate way by which activity could be terminated is by accumulation of intracellular sodium or calcium. If sufficient sodium or calcium accumulates, the electrochemical gradient for the ion may decrease, resulting in a loss of action potential amplitude and ultimately a cessation of activity. Triggered activity may be terminated by a single premature stimulus or by overdrive pacing, making it difficult to distinguish from reentrant activity. Whether a period of overdrive pacing results in acceleration of the rate or termination of the triggered rhythm depends on the particular preparation, the level of membrane potential, and the rate and duration of the stimulation train.

Although triggered activity has been described in numerous preparations, its correlation with clinical arrhythmias has been difficult. Accelerated junctional rhythms, as well as some atrial tachycardias and ventricular rhythms, have been suggested as being compatible with triggered activity.[37]

ABNORMAL CONDUCTION

Early in the twentieth century it was recognized that reentry of a wave of excitation into a previously excited area could reactivate that area.[38] It was also recognized that such a reentrant impulse could continue to circulate and perpetuate an arrhythmia. In normally functioning myocardium, the activation wavefront rapidly depolarizes each cell, and at the completion of depolarization the cell is absolutely refractory. If all cells in a circuit are simultaneously refractory, the propagating wavefront is extinguished. Reentry may occur only if conduction of the cardiac impulse is altered in such a way that a reentering impulse can reach tissue that has recovered excitability. Expressed mathematically, the wavelength of the reentrant impulse must be shorter than the length of the circuit it must traverse. The wavelength of the impulse is directly related to the conduction velocity as well as the refractory period of the tissue. Whether reentry occurs in a given circuit depends on the critical relationship of pathway length, refractoriness, and conduction velocity. Reentry is favored by slowing conduction velocity or shortening the refractory period. Conversely, reentrant arrhythmias may be terminated by altering either refractoriness or conduction velocity to upset the critical relationship. Multiple factors, including the ionic environment of the cell, the presence of ischemia or hypoxia, heart rate, neural influences, and drugs may combine to determine the refractoriness of a given cell (see the discussion of action potential duration above). Conduction velocity also depends on multiple factors, including the magnitude and velocity of sodium influx during phase 0, excitability, the efficiency of cell-to-cell coupling, the geometry of the tissue through which conduction occurs, electrotonic interactions, drug effects, and effects of the autonomic nervous system.

The magnitude of sodium influx during phase 0 is determined by the number of sodium channels opening with stimulation and the electrochemical gradient for sodium across the cell membrane. At membrane potentials greater than -70 mV the fraction of sodium channels available to conduct is large enough that conduction velocity depends mainly on the excitability of the tissue. Thus, the closer the membrane is to threshold potential, the less current is required to raise the potential to threshold and propagate the impulse. At membrane potentials less negative than -70 mV, inactivation of the sodium channel becomes an important factor, and action potential amplitude and V_{max} become important determinants of the ability to conduct an impulse (Fig. 40.9). Premature stimulation of the heart may thus provide a substrate for reentry when premature impulses reach relatively refractory tissue. Partial inactivation of the sodium channel at the less negative membrane potentials leads to slow propagation of that impulse and, if the other criteria for reentry are met, may result in a reentrant arrhythmia. Generalized depolarization of the cell membrane also produces slowing of conduction but does not require a premature impulse, because partial inactivation of the sodium channel occurs at the low resting potentials of such a cell (Fig. 40.10).

Reentrant excitation occurring in macroscopic circuitous pathways has been demonstrated in several systems (Fig. 40.11).[39] Such circuits may consist of loops of Purkinje fibers, muscle surrounding an area of infarction or fibrosis, and accessory atrioventricular pathways. Such a circuit must contain a segment in which unidirectional block occurs, as well as the geometry necessary to meet the criteria for impulse wavelength mentioned above. An impulse circulating around the loop will continue to circulate unless it encounters refractory tissue ahead of the depolarization wavefront. Alterations in conduction velocity around the loop may permit the wavefront to encounter refractory tissue. If conduction velocity around the loop is increased, the impulse may reenter an area before refractoriness has dissipated. If conduction velocity slows, impulses from other foci may penetrate the loop and depolarize tissue ahead of the reentrant wavefront, making the tissue inexcitable.

Reentrant extrasystoles often exhibit a fixed coupling interval to the basic stimulus rate if the stimulus rate remains constant. However, alterations in stimulus rate may alter the coupling interval. Generally, increases in the stimulus rate lead to further slowing in the circuit or even to complete block.[40] Premature stimuli may serve either to initiate or to terminate reentry in a loop through effects on conduction velocity. Premature stimuli entering the loop may traverse a depressed segment more slowly than impulses arriving at a slower rate and may render that segment refractory, extinguishing the reentrant impulse. Conversely, a premature impulse entering the circuit where reentry was not present may conduct slowly and initiate reentry if the other criteria for reentry were met.

Gross anatomical loops are not required for reentry of a cardiac impulse. Reentry can occur in the SA and AV nodes, where anatomically distinct loops do not occur. Presumably reentry can occur through functional longitudinal dissociation of pathways within these structures. This type of mechanism has been demonstrated in unbranched sheets of muscle or unbranched Purkinje fibers (see Fig. 40.11). If functionally different pathways occur in such a preparation, it is possible for an impulse to be slowly conducted in one direction and to return in the opposite direction through the other pathway. The characteristics of such reentry are analogous to reentry in a gross circuit and may be regarded as a form of microscopic reentry.[41]

True reflection (return of the impulse through its original path) has been described in a situation that involves the delayed activation of a segment distal to a region of inexcitability.[42] Activation of the distal segment occurs via the electrotonic spread of current across the inexcitable region. If the inexcitable segment is shorter than the length constant for the decay of current across the inexcitable gap, current reaches the distal cells. If current strength is sufficient, the distal cells may be depolarized to threshold and an action potential generated in the distal segment. Conduction occurs with a great deal of delay. The action potential generated in the distal segment may not only propagate anterogradely, but may also cause retrograde current flow across the inexcitable segment. If retrograde current flow is of sufficient intensity and reaches the proximal segment after refractoriness has dis-

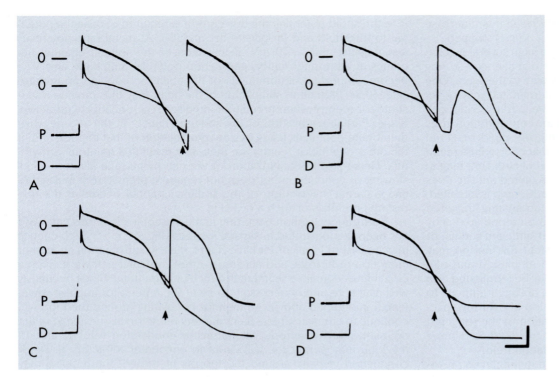

FIGURE 40.9 Conduction delay produced by premature stimulation. Two cells, one proximal (*P*) and one distal (*D*) are recorded simultaneously. Arrows mark the point at which the second stimulus occurs. **A.** The second stimulus conducts with very little delay to the distal cell. **B.** A more closely coupled premature stimulus conducts with significant delay to the distal cell. **C.** With a slightly more premature impulse, conduction is blocked and only a slight prolongation of the action potential of the distal cell is seen, a consequence of electrotonic spread of current from the proximal impulse. **D.** The premature stimulus occurs too early to capture the proximal cell, and no effects are observed distally. (Calibration vertical bar = 25 mV; horizontal bar = 50 msec.)

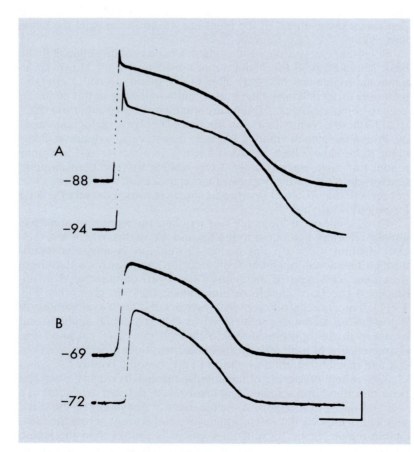

FIGURE 40.10 Conduction delay due to generalized depolarization. Two cells are recorded simultaneously along the same Purkinje fiber. The impulse travels from the proximal cell (*top action potential*) to the distal cell (*bottom action potential*). The conduction time is reflected in the distance between the upstrokes of the two cells. **A.** With normal resting potentials (−94 mV and −88 mV), conduction is rapid. **B.** Resting membrane potential is reduced by raising extracellular potassium. Note the marked increase in conduction time between the cells. (Vertical bar = 25 mV; horizontal bar = 50 msec.)

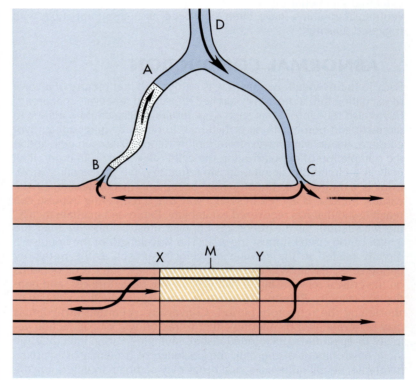

FIGURE 40.11 Reentry as described in the model of Schmitt and Erlanger in 1928. The top panel depicts reentry through a branched Purkinje fiber at its junction with the myocardium. Unidirectional block is produced in the stippled segment. The impulse originating at (*D*) conducts normally from (*D*) to (*C*) and depolarizes the distal myocardium. The impulse is able to reenter at point (*B*) and conduct retrograde through the area of unidirectional block and complete the circuit. In the bottom panel, reentry is achieved without a gross anatomic loop in two pathways that exhibit functional longitudinal dissociation. Unidirectional block occurs in the hatched area of pathway (*A*). Impulse conduction occurs normally in pathway (*B*). The distal segment of pathway (*A*) is excited by the impulse from (*B*), and the impulse propagates retrograde from point (*Y*) to point (*X*) and reenters the proximal segment of pathway (*A*). (Modified from Schmitt FO, Erlanger J: Directional differences in the conduction of the impulse through heart muscle and their possible relation to extrasystolic and fibrillatory contractions. Am J Physiol 87:326, 1928)

sipated, an action potential may be propagated retrogradely through the proximal segment (Fig. 40.12).

Reentry may occur without anatomic obstacles. The substrate necessary for this type of reentry is a tissue in which cells of differing refractoriness lie in close proximity. This situation has been investigated in rabbit atrial muscle.[43] In that model, an impulse conducts in fibers with short refractory periods but blocks in the fibers with longer refractory periods. The slowly conducting impulse traverses a circle of 6 mm to 8 mm, returning to the initial point of propagation after refractoriness has dissipated. Impulses moving toward the center of the circle keep the central cells in a steady state of refractoriness, and the central cells show only local electrotonic responses. This type of reentry has been called a "leading circle" (Fig. 40.13).

Reentry is postulated as the mechanism for a wide variety of clinical arrhythmias including both supraventricular and ventricular tachycardias. Although in the laboratory it has been possible to measure carefully the sequence of depolarization around a reentrant loop, such a task presents a formidable clinical problem. Tachycardias involving reentry through an accessory AV bypass tract have been the clinical prototype of reentrant arrhythmias, and knowledge of basic reentry phenomena has enabled a rational approach to the diagnosis and treatment of these arrhythmias. The application of our knowledge of reentry to other arrhythmias has been more difficult, primarily because of the limited resolution of clinical electrophysiologic techniques.

ABNORMAL AUTOMATICITY AND CONDUCTION

Parasystole is the prototype of a disorder combining both abnormal automatic discharge of a focus and abnormal conduction. Depressed conduction into the automatic focus serves to protect the focus from depolarization by other pacemakers. The clinical result is an independent ectopic pacemaker capable of becoming the dominant rhythm if its discharge coincides with a period of excitability. Block surrounding the focus may not be unidirectional, and depressed conduction may produce exit block from the focus as well. Parasystolic foci are probably not perfectly isolated from the influence of surrounding pacemakers, and electrotonic interactions across the region of depressed conduction may still produce enough current flow to modulate the abnormal pacemaker.[44] Whether this modulating influence alters the clinical characteristics of rhythms presumed to be parasystolic has yet to be proven.

Deceleration-dependent aberrancy, or phase 4 aberrancy, in which bundle branch block appears during periods of relative slowing of the

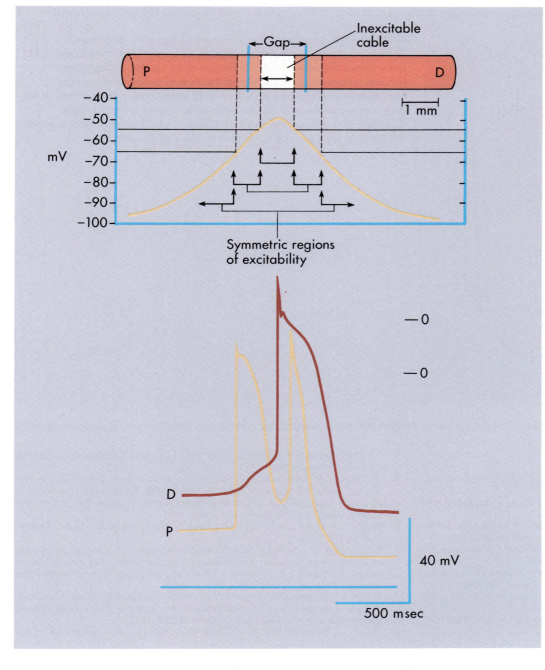

FIGURE 40.12 Reentry by the mechanism of reflection is illustrated. In the top panel, a segment of Purkinje fiber is displayed, the central section of which has been depolarized, producing an inexcitable gap. The level of membrane potential is shown in the graph below the corresponding segment of fiber. Impulse transmission across the gap does not occur, but electrotonic spread of current occurs slowly across the gap. If it is of sufficient amplitude, this current may excite the distal segment. In the lower panel, the proximal segment, (P), is stimulated, and electronic current spreads slowly across the gap, depolarizing the distal segment, (D), to threshold. The delay across the gap is sufficient to allow the distal segment to reexcite the proximal segment (the second upstroke in the proximal recording). The impulse is said to reenter by means of reflection. (Modified from Antzelevich C, Moe GK: Electrotonically-mediated delayed conduction and reentry in relation to "slow responses" in mammalian ventricular conducting tissue. Circ Res 49:1129, 1981)

dominant supraventricular rhythm, is the second example of a conduction abnormality produced by combined abnormal automaticity and abnormal conduction. The exact electrophysiologic mechanism for deceleration-dependent aberrancy is unknown, but spontaneous depolarization of the specialized intraventricular conducting system has been suggested. It is proposed that depolarization of the affected bundle branch to about −70 mV or −60 mV by phase 4 depolarization produces responses to stimuli that exhibit depressed V_{max} and low amplitude of phase 0, propagate slowly, and are easily extinguished.[45] Normal pacemaker cells within the His-Purkinje system have a take off potential of about −70 mV, and action potentials from this level propagate normally. Therefore, it has been postulated that the cells responsible for deceleration-dependent aberrancy must also be somewhat depolarized, with a shift of the threshold potential to less negative potentials, and at least some experimental models of deceleration-dependent aberrancy support this.[46] Thus, the manifestation of deceleration-dependent aberrancy has been postulated to require a combination of phase 4 depolarization of the specialized conduction system as well as a generalized depolarization, with a shift of the threshold potential to a less negative potential, and a spontaneous change from a positive slope of phase 4 to a slope approaching zero. Recent data raise the possibility that other mechanisms may be responsible for deceleration-dependent aberrancy as well. Jalife and associates have demonstrated time-dependent variations in excitability in depressed cardiac Purkinje fibers.[47] In their experiments, conduction delay or block occurred if pacing rates were more rapid or slower than an optimal intermediate pacing rate. Phase 4 depolarization did not contribute to conduction delays at slow pacing rates. Rather, conduction was facilitated in the presence of phase 4 depolarization. They postulated that both acceleration- and deceleration-dependent intraventricular conduction delays might be due to this mechanism. Similarly, Gilmour and associates demonstrated overdrive and underdrive suppression of conduction in depressed cardiac Purkinje fibers, also temporally related to changes in diastolic excitability.[48] However, neither of these two studies accounts for the frequently observed ventricular escape complexes, probably arising from the affected bundle branch, seen in clinical instances of deceleration-dependent bundle branch block. The presence of ventricular escape complexes strongly implies that phase 4 depolarization is operative, at least in some way, in this conduction disturbance.

CONCLUSIONS

Cardiac arrhythmias present a myriad of clinical manifestations. The study of the basic electric activity of the heart has provided a model of arrhythmogenesis based on the findings of abnormal automaticity and abnormal conduction. The use of microelectrode techniques has been central to the basic understanding of these mechanisms.

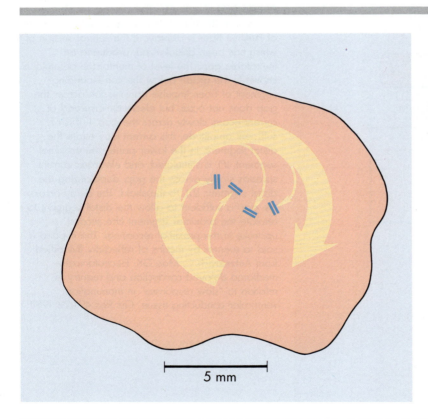

FIGURE 40.13 A schematic diagram of reentry by the leading circle mechanism. The outline traces the borders of a sample of atrial tissue. Bold arrow shows the path of slow conduction of an impulse through areas of variable refractoriness. The center of the circle is depolarized by impulses from multiple points on the circle that block (*double bars*), in the center of the circle. Circus movement is thus achieved without an anatomic obstacle. (Modified from Allessie MA, Bonke F, Schopman F: Circus movement in rabbit atrial muscle as a mechanism of tachycardia. Circ Res 41:9, 1977)

REFERENCES

1. Thomas RC: Electrogenic sodium pump in nerve and muscle cells. Physiol Rev 52:563, 1972
2. Hodgkin AL: The ionic basis of electrical activity in nerve and muscle. Biol Rev 26:339, 1951
3. Noble D, Tsein RW: The kinetics and rectifier properties of the slow potassium current in cardiac Purkinje fibers. J Physiol (Lond) 195:185, 1968
4. Draper MH, Weidmann S: Cardiac resting and action potentials recorded with an intracellular electrode. J Physiol 115:74, 1951
5. Coraboeuf E, Deroubaix E, Coulombe A: Effect of tetrodotoxin on action potentials of the conducting system in the dog. Am J Physiol 236:H561, 1979
6. Reuter H: Divalent cations as charge carriers in excitable membranes. Prog Biophys 26:1, 1973
7. Lowenstein WR, Kanno V, Socolar SJ: The cell to cell channel. Fed Proc 37:2645, 1978
8. Jack JJB, Noble D, Tsien RW: Electric Current Flow in Excitable Cells. Oxford, Clarendon Press, 1975
9. Watanabe AM, Lindemann JP, Jones LR et al: Biochemical mechanisms mediating neural control of the heart. In Abboud FM, Fozzard HA, Gilmore JP et al (eds): Disturbances in the Neurogenic Control of the Circulation. Bethesda, American Physiological Society, 1981
10. Hutter OF: Mode of action of autonomic transmitters on the heart. Br Med Bull 13:176, 1957
11. Prystowsky EN, Jackman WM, Rinkenberger RL et al: Effect of autonomic blockade on ventricular refractoriness and atrioventricular conduction in humans: Evidence supporting a direct cholinergic action on ventricular muscle refractoriness. Circ Res 49:511, 1981
12. Bailey JC, Greenspan K, Elizari MV et al: Effects of acetylcholine on automaticity and conduction in the proximal portion of the His-Purkinje specialized conduction system of the dog. Circ Res 30:210, 1972
13. Bailey JC, Watanabe AM, Besch HR Jr et al: Acetylcholine antagonism of the

14. Takahashi N, Zipes DP: Vagal modulation of adrenergic effects on canine sinus and atrioventricular nodes. Am J Physiol 13:H775, 1983
15. Vassalle M: Analysis of cardiac pacemaker potential using a "voltage clamp" technique. Am J Physiol 208:770, 1965
16. Carmeliet E, Sailawa T: Shortening of the action potential and reduction of pacemaker activity by lidocaine, quinidine, and procainamide in sheep cardiac Purkinje fibers. An effect on Na or K currents? Circ Res 50:257, 1982
17. Vassalle M: Electrogenic suppression of automaticity in sheep and dog Purkinje fibers. Circ Res 27:361, 1970
18. Friedman PL, Stewart JR, Wit AL: Spontaneous and induced cardiac arrhythmias in subendocardial Purkinje fibers surviving extensive myocardial infarction in dogs. Circ Res 22:612, 1973
19. Gilmour RF Jr, Zipes DP: Electrophysiologic characteristics of rodent myocardium damaged by adrenaline. Cardiovasc Res 14:582, 1980
20. Ten Eick RE, Singer DH: Electrophysiological properties of diseased human atrium. I. Low diastolic potential and altered cellular response to potassium. Circ Res 44:545, 1979
21. Gilmour RF Jr, Heger JJ, Prystowsky EN et al: Cellular electrophysiological abnormalities of diseased human ventricular myocardium. Am J Cardiol 51:137, 1983
22. Surawicz B, Imanishi S: Automatic activity in depolarized guinea pig ventricular myocardium: Characteristics and mechanisms. Circ Res 39:751, 1976
23. Carmeliet E: The slow inward current, non-voltage clamp studies. In Zipes DP, Bailey JC, Elharrar V (eds): The Slow Inward Current and Cardiac Arrhythmias. The Hague, Martinus Nijhoff, 1980
24. Zipes DP: A defense of triggered automaticity (symposium). In Harrison DC (ed): Cardiac Arrhythmias: A Decade of Progress. Boston, GK Hall, 1981
25. Cranefield PF: Action potentials, afterpotentials, and arrhythmias. Circ Res 41:415, 1977
26. Trautwein W, Gottstein V, Dudel J: Der aktionsstrom der myokardfaser in sauerstoffmanel. Pflugers Arch 260:40, 1954
27. Coraboef E, Boistel J: L'action des taux eleves de gaz carbonique sur le tissu cardiaque etudiee a l'aide de microelectrodes intracellulaires. Compt Rend Soc Biol (Paris) 147:654, 1953
28. Brooks CM, Hoffman PF, Suckling EE et al: Excitability of the Heart. New York, Grune and Stratton, 1955
29. Wit AL, Cranefield PF, Gadsby DC: Triggered activity. In Zipes DP, Bailey JC, Elharrar V (eds): The Slow Inward Current and Cardiac Arrhythmias. The Hague, Martinus Nijhoff, 1980
30. Dangman KH, Hoffman BF: In vivo and in vitro antiarrhythmic and arrhythmogenic effects of N-acetyl procainamide. J Pharmacol Exp Ther 217:851, 1981
31. Wit AL, Fenoglio JJ, Hordof AJ et al: Ultrastructure and transmembrane potentials of cardiac muscle in the human anterior mitral valve leaflet. Circulation 59:1284, 1979
32. Kass RS, Tsien RW, Weingart R: Ionic basis of transient inward current induced by strophanthidin in cardiac Purkinje fibers. J Physiol 281:209, 1978
33. Wit AL: Cardiac arrhythmias: Electrophysiologic mechanisms. In Reisen HJ, Horowitz LN (eds): Mechanism and Treatment of Cardiac Arrhythmias: Relevance of Basic Studies to Clinical Management. Baltimore, Urban and Schwarzenberg, 1985
34. Ferrier GR: Digitalis arrhythmis: Role of oscillatory afterpotentials. Prog Cardiovasc Dis 19:459, 1977
35. Nathan D, Beeler GW: Electrophysiologic correlates of the inotropic effects of isoproterenol in canine myocardium. J Mol Cell Cardiol 7:1, 1975
36. Vassalle M, Commins M, Castro C et al: The relationship between overdrive suppression and overdrive excitation in ventricular pacemakers in dogs. Circ Res 38:367, 1976
37. Rosen MR, Fisch C, Hoffman BF et al: Can accelerated atrioventricular junctional escape rhythms be explained by delayed afterdepolarizations? Am J Cardiol 45:1272, 1980
38. Mines GR: On circulating excitations in heart muscle and their possible relations to tachycardia and fibrillation. Trans Roy Soc Can 8:43, 1914
39. Wit AL, Cranefield PF: Reentrant excitation as a cause of cardiac arrhythmias. Am J Physiol 235:H1, 1978
40. Cranefield PF, Wit AL, Hoffman BF: Genesis of cardiac arrhythmias. Circulation 47:190, 1973
41. Wit AL, Hoffman BF, Cranefield PF: Slow conduction and reentry in the ventricular conducting system. I. Return extrasystoles in canine Purkinje fibers. Circ Res 30:1, 1972
42. Antzelevich C, Jalife J, Moe GK: Characteristics of reflection as a mechanism of reentrant arrhythmias and its relationship to parasystole. Circulation 61:182, 1980
43. Allessie MA, Bonke FM, Schopman FJG: Circus movement in rabbit atrial muscle as a mechanism of tachycardia. III. The "leading circle" concept: A new model of circus movement in cardiac tissue without the involvement of an anatomical obstacle. Circ Res 41:9, 1977
44. Antzelevich C, Moe GK, Jalife J: Electrotonic modulation of pacemaker activity. Further biological and mathematical observations in the behavior of modulated parasystole. Circulation 66:1225, 1982
45. Singer DH, Lazarra R, Hoffman BF: Interrelationships between automaticity and conduction in Purkinje fibers. Circ Res 21:537, 1967
46. El-Sherif N, Scherlag BJ, Lazarra R et al: Pathophysiology of tachycardia and bradycardia dependent block in the canine proximal His-Purkinje system after acute myocardial ischemia. Am J Cardiol 33:529, 1979
47. Jalife J, Antzelevitch C, Lamanna V et al: Rate-dependent changes in excitability of depressed cardiac Purkinje fibers as a mechanism of intermittent bundle branch block. Circulation 67:912, 1983
48. Gilmour RF, Salata J, Zipes DP: Rate related suppression and facilitation of conduction in isolated canine cardiac Purkinje fibers. Circ Res 57:35, 1985

PHARMACODYNAMICS OF ANTIARRHYTHMIC DRUGS

Peter Danilo, Jr • Michael R. Rosen

This chapter consists of two sections. In the first section we review briefly the mechanisms for arrhythmias that are presented in detail elsewhere in these volumes and then consider how representative antiarrhythmic drugs act to modify these electrophysiologic mechanisms. In the second section, we discuss both the cellular electrophysiologic effects and the indirect actions of individual antiarrhythmic drugs to provide a basis for the discussion of their clinical use, which is presented in another chapter. The reader should note that before reading this chapter it is essential to review the principles of normal and abnormal cardiac electrophysiology discussed elsewhere in these volumes because this provides the descriptions of cellular electrophysiologic phenomena and the definitions of a number of terms used in this chapter. In addition, the description of toxicity of antiarrhythmic drugs is provided elsewhere in these volumes.

MECHANISMS RESPONSIBLE FOR ARRHYTHMIAS AND MODIFICATION BY ANTIARRHYTHMIC DRUGS

There are two major categories used to describe the mechanisms responsible for cardiac arrhythmias: abnormalities of impulse conduction and abnormalities of impulse initiation.[1,2]

ABNORMALITIES OF IMPULSE CONDUCTION

In the normal heart, impulse initiation by the sinus node is followed by ordered activation of the atria and ventricles. However, in the presence of disease or anatomical abnormalities (such as atrioventricular bypass tracts), abnormal conduction and reentry may occur. A model of unidirectional conduction block with retrograde conduction is summarized in Figure 41.1, A. The primary requisites for reentry here are unidirectional conduction block and a pathway through which the retrogradely propagating impulse can travel at a velocity sufficiently low to permit refractoriness to terminate in the tissue into which it is propagating. In this model, the conditions of timing, conduction velocity, and termination of refractoriness must be met or reentry will not occur.[3-6]

To start our consideration of how drugs might affect reentry, we must recognize that at different sites in any reentrant circuit there may be different transmembrane potential characteristics. Some of these are depicted in the reentrant pathway (modeled in Fig. 41.1, A).

Two mechanisms whereby reentry might be abolished in this model are reviewed in Figures 41.1, B and 41.1, C. In Figure 41.1, B, the action of the drug has been to improve antegrade propagation, removing unidirectional block and restoring a normal activation pattern. It is uncertain whether any antiarrhythmic drugs act in this way clinically, although in cellular electrophysiologic studies phenytoin[7] and lidocaine[8] have been shown to exert such an effect.

Another means whereby a drug might improve antegrade propagation is if depressed conduction occurs because phase 4 depolarization has reduced the activation voltage for the action potential (Fig. 41.2). Here, a drug that decreases the slope of phase 4 depolarization, thereby hyperpolarizing the membrane, might improve conduction even if the drug itself depresses conduction. Such an effect has been demonstrated for procainamide.[9]

Another means for terminating reentry is through depression of conduction and the induction of bidirectional conduction block (see Fig. 41.1, C). The site at which bidirectional conduction block is induced by a drug varies depending on the mechanism of action of that drug. For example, quinidine depresses the rapid inward current in fibers having the fast response[10,11] as well as the depressed fast-response action potential.[12] As a result, it would be anticipated to depress conduction at both sites (a) and (b) in Figure 41.1, C. In addition to slowing conduction, quinidine also prolongs repolarization and refractoriness.[13] This provides another means for inducing bidirectional block (see Fig. 41.1, C), because throughout much of the potentially reentrant circuit it increases the interval during which cardiac fibers are protected from the propagation of premature beats. In contrast to these effects of quinidine are those of verapamil. This and other slow channel blockers depress slow inward current carried by Ca^{2+} and to a lesser extent Na^+ through the so-called slow channel. If this slow-response action potential is an important component of a reentrant circuit (as in Fig. 41.1, A) then verapamil, if it could gain access to the site of slow conduction, would be expected to terminate reentry through its action at this site. Unlike quinidine, it would have little or no effect on normal action potentials at other sites in the circuit.

Thus far, we have outlined how the direct effects of individual antiarrhythmic drugs can modify conduction in one type of reentrant circuit. Moreover, we have shown that drugs having different mechanisms of action can act at different sites in the circuit. For quinidine, the actions of importance in Figure 41.1 involve (1) depression of the fast inward sodium current, leading to slowed conduction in normal and depressed fibers having the fast response action potential; and (2) attenuation of repolarizing K^+ currents in the same fibers, prolonging action potential duration and refractoriness. For verapamil, the action of importance is depression of slow inward current in still other fibers in the same reentrant circuit.

It must be stressed that these direct actions of drugs on tissues in the reentrant loop are only one means whereby reentry may be suppressed in this model. Another possibility is considered in Figure 41.3. Here, we see that a drug-induced change in heart rate alone may have an antiarrhythmic action. Figure 41.3, A demonstrates that at a given heart rate, some fibers in the reentrant circuit, although not firing spontaneously, manifest phase 4 depolarization (a); there is very slow conduction through the depressed segment (cross-hatched area), and reentry (b). In Figure 41.3, B a drug has slowed sinus rate considerably. Depending on any additional effect of the drug on phase 4 depolarization, two different effects on conduction may be seen. If phase 4 is unchanged (and only sinus rate is slowed), the membrane may be depolarized further at the time of action potential initiation, and conduction velocity may slow or be blocked. If, alternatively, the slope of phase 4 is decreased by the drug, then subsequent action potentials will occur at higher levels of membrane potential, and conduction velocity may increase. In both examples, sinus slowing is associated with changes in the determinants of conduction velocity, which in turn can result in suppression of reentry. In addition, the slowing of sinus rate tends to be accompanied by a prolongation of repolarization and refractoriness. This, too, modifies the propagation of premature depolarizations.

Another possibility is explored in Figure 41.3, C. Here sinus rate increases, resulting in the acceleration of repolarization (*b*). However, the effect of the increase in stimulation rate may also be to overdrive-suppress those fibers having phase 4 depolarization. As a result, action potentials may be initiated at higher levels of membrane potential than previously and may propagate more rapidly (*a*). Again, the critical timing requirement for reentry may not be met, and the arrhythmia may terminate.

Still another means whereby a drug may modify conduction through the reentrant circuits depicted in Figures 41.1 and 41.3 is via indirect actions exerted through the autonomic nervous system or β- and α-adrenergic and muscarinic receptors. The sympathetic nervous system, through its β-adrenergic component, tends to hyperpolarize ventricular and Purkinje fibers, to increase slow inward current, to accelerate repolarization, and to increase the slope of phase 4 depolar-

ization. Any of these actions of β-adrenergic catecholamines may contribute to the conduction characteristics of a reentrant loop. By inducing β-adrenergic blockade or by reducing efferent sympathetic activity (as with a drug like phenytoin) we might expect some change in membrane potential and the slope of phase 4 depolarization (and attendant changes in conduction), a suppression of slow responses and their contribution to reentry, and alterations in repolarization and refractoriness. Interventions that enhance vagal function also tend to counteract β-adrenergic mechanisms, whereas vagolytic actions tend to enhance sympathetic effects.

Summarizing our analysis of this model of reentry, we have attempted to show that drugs may act in at least three different ways to modify conduction through the circuit: by exerting a direct effect on the electrophysiologic properties of cells in the reentrant loop, by di-

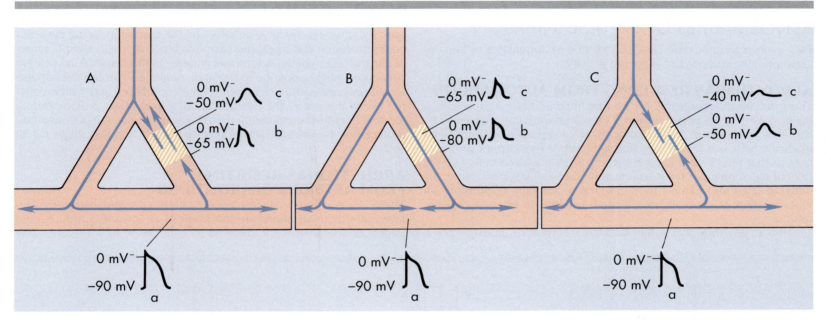

FIGURE 41.1 Mechanisms whereby an antiarrhythmic drug might suppress a reentrant rhythm. This model for reentry was initially described by Schmitt and Erlanger.[3] **A.** Antegrade conduction block of an impulse in the shaded area. Propagation proceeds through the remainder of the conducting system, reenters the depressed segment and propagates slowly through it until it reaches the interface with normal tissue. If refractoriness at the site has terminated, the impulse can reenter the proximal conducting system. The following assumptions have been made for the sake of this figure: The electrophysiologic properties and action potentials of much of the conducting system are normal, as exemplified by action potential (*a*). There is slow conduction secondary to slow-response action potentials in the depressed segment indicated as (*c*). At intermediary sites there are depressed fast-response action potentials (*b*). **B.** Results that might occur if a drug hyperpolarized the depressed tissues at sites (*b*) and (*c*). Antegrade conduction resumes and reentry no longer occurs. **C.** Results that might occur if a drug further depressed the already abnormal tissues at sites (*b*) and (*c*). This would induce bidirectional block in the depressed segment of the conducting system and, again, the reentrant rhythm would be suppressed. (Modified from Reiser HJ, Horowitz LN (eds): Mechanisms and Treatment of Cardiac Arrhythmias. Urban and Schwarzenberg, Baltimore-Munich, 1985)

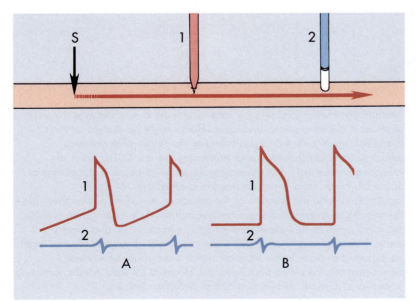

FIGURE 41.2 An unbranched Purkinje fiber bundle is depicted that is stimulated at one end (s), and is impaled with a microelectrode in the center (1). A bipolar recording electrode is placed at the other end (2). The pathway of activation is from (s) to (2). **A.** Marked phase 4 depolarization. The conduction time from the microelectrode site to the electrogram site can be estimated by observing the relationship of the upstroke of the action potential (1) and the electrogram (2). **B.** Through the action of a drug, the slope of phase 4 depolarization has decreased, the action potential is initiated at a higher level of membrane potential, and propagation is more rapid. (Modified from Reiser HJ, Horowitz LN (eds): Mechanisms and Treatment of Cardiac Arrhythmias, Urban & Schwarzenberg, Baltimore-Munich, 1985)

rectly or indirectly modifying heart rate, and by exerting actions mediated via the autonomic nervous system or its cardiac receptors. We again emphasize the fact that this approach and model are very simplistic. We state this in large part because the model presented in Figures 41.1 and 41.2 is an example of only one type of reentry. Reentry can result from anatomical abnormalities (such as bypass tracts) or pathologic changes (such as infarction and scarring) in the heart. It can occur as a result of slow conduction secondary to the slow response or the depressed fast response (as shown in Fig. 41.1 and Fig. 41.3),[14,15] as a result of complete conduction block associated with electrotonic current flow inducing reexcitation or reflection,[14] or as a functional abnormality as well as an anatomical or pathologic abnormality.[16] In each of these situations the ability of a drug to modify ionic currents directly, to modify cardiac rate, and to modify autonomic input can critically alter abnormal conduction and suppress reentry.

ABNORMALITIES OF IMPULSE INITIATION

Two major categories are used to describe abnormalities of impulse initiation: automaticity and triggered activity.

ARRHYTHMIAS RESULTING FROM AUTOMATICITY

The mechanism responsible for normal Purkinje fiber automaticity is the so-called i_f pacemaker current. This is an inward current carried by Na^+ that is activated on the completion of repolarization and then gradually increases in intensity during phase 4. This current is in contrast to that responsible for automaticity in depolarized cells (≤ -70 mV) of the ventricular myocardium and conducting system. Here, the outward i_x current carried by K^+, which is normally responsible for repolarization, is gradually deactivated, resulting in phase 4 depolarization.

Hence, any drug that suppresses the i_f current or increases the i_x current should be able to modify automaticity. It should be understood that by depressing the i_f current, not only might an ectopic pacemaker resulting from this current be suppressed, but the normal sinus node pacemaker mechanism to which this same current contributes also might be suppressed.

Another mechanism for suppressing some automatic arrhythmias is to increase the rate of impulse initiation by the sinus node pacemaker. This can induce overdrive suppression of the ectopic pacemaker. For this to occur, two conditions must be met. Not only must there be an increase in the rate of the sinus pacemaker, but the propagating cardiac impulse then must have access to the site of ectopic impulse initiation. In other words, there must be little or no entry block protecting this ectopic automatic pacemaker such that it can be excited by the impulse propagating from the region of the sinus node.

Another means for suppressing automatic activity would be to modify the ability of the ectopic impulse to propagate from its site of initiation to the rest of the heart. This could occur in two ways: First, even if a drug did *not* have an effect on the current inducing the automatic rhythm, it still might increase exit block by depressing conduction in the region of the ectopic pacemaker. In this instance the ectopic pacemaker might continue to fire at an unaltered rate but the impulse would propagate into a region of conduction block and hence could not excite the rest of the heart. Second, a drug might prolong refractoriness in tissues surrounding the ectopic pacemaker. In this situation propagation beyond the site of increased refractoriness might fail as well.

ARRHYTHMIAS RESULTING FROM AFTERDEPOLARIZATIONS

There are two types of afterdepolarizations: delayed and early. Delayed afterdepolarizations are the result of an inward current carried largely by sodium ion but triggered by an increase in intracellular cal-

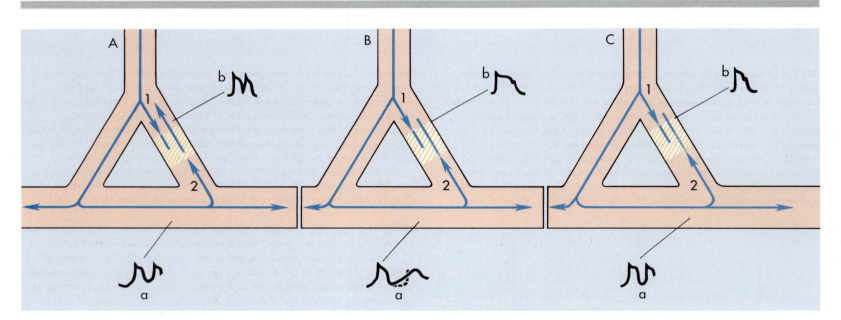

FIGURE 41.3 The modification of reentry by changing heart rate. **A.** The same reentrant model as demonstrated in Figure 41.1. Again there is a depressed segment in the cross-hatched area with antegrade conduction block and slow retrograde propagation. An action potential at a normal site in this instance has phase 4 depolarization (a), but this fiber is not firing automatically; it is being driven by the basic sinus rhythm of the heart. In (b), an action potential in the proximal conducting system demonstrates that the reentrant impulse arrives after the termination of refractoriness and propagates further in the conducting system. **B.** Cardiac rate has slowed. The broken trace at (a) shows the effect of a drug that not only slows rate but also decreases the slope of phase 4 depolarization. The result is that propagation proceeds more rapidly. The slowing of rate also prolongs repolarization and refractoriness at site (b). As a result the reentrant impulse now arrives before termination of the effective refractory period and there is failure of retrograde propagation. Alternatively, if with the slowing of rate in (a) there is no change in the slope of phase 4 depolarization, conduction velocity might be slowed further or conduction might even fail, again changing the relationship between refractoriness and conduction and terminating reentry. **C.** The result of increasing cardiac rate and decreasing the slope of phase 4 depolarization at site (a). Again there is an acceleration in conduction. At site (b) repolarization and the duration of the refractory period have shortened, but if the velocity of propagation has increased sufficiently the retrograde impulse still might arrive at (b) before termination of refractoriness, and reentry will cease. It must be emphasized that these are simplified models of what might be expected to occur in this situation, rather than actual experimental demonstrations. (Modified from Reiser HJ, Horowitz LN (eds): Mechanisms and Treatment of Cardiac Arrhythmias, Urban & Schwarzenberg, Baltimore-Munich, 1985)

cium ion.[17–19] Any drug that increases outward or repolarizing current would be expected to decrease the magnitude of the delayed afterdepolarization, as would any event that decreases inward current carried by sodium ion. Moreover, any intervention that decreases the intracellular concentration of calcium (the triggering event for the afterdepolarization) would be expected to be antiarrhythmic as well.

Less is known about the ionic mechanisms responsible for early afterdepolarizations, although these arise in situations where either repolarizing current (i_x) is diminished or inward current (i_{si}) is increased.[20–24] It should be apparent that any event that increases repolarizing current or decreases inward current should be antiarrhythmic. Hence, interventions that increase i_x or suppress i_{si} might be anticipated as effective in suppressing early afterdepolarizations.

One important property shared by delayed and early afterdepolarizations is that both require preceding action potentials for their induction and both have particular cardiac rate requirements for the initiation and propagation of arrhythmias. That is, early afterdepolarizations tend to become larger in amplitude and to induce arrhythmias as cardiac rate slows, and the reverse is true of delayed afterdepolarizations.

Given these factors, any event that changes cardiac rate such that the afterdepolarizations diminish in magnitude is antiarrhythmic. In addition, as for automatic rhythms, any event that either increases exit block around the site of ectopic impulse initiation or prolongs repolarization and refractoriness is antiarrhythmic.

ADDITIONAL FACTORS MODIFYING ANTIARRHYTHMIC DRUG ACTIONS

Thus far we have considered the means whereby antiarrhythmic drugs might be expected to modify cardiac arrhythmias. The points to be stressed again are that there are particular ionic mechanisms that antiarrhythmic drugs can modify, which in turn result in an antiarrhythmic action. Drugs may exert their effects on these ionic currents either by a direct interaction with the cell membrane and its ionic channels or indirectly through interactions with the modifiers of ionic currents and channels such as catecholamines and acetylcholine. Moreover, the interactions of any drug with the sinus node pacemaker to change heart rate also could induce important antiarrhythmic effects.

There are other factors to consider, as well, before we proceed to a consideration of individual antiarrhythmic drugs. These relate to the following: in any situation in which an antiarrhythmic drug is administered, the effects it exerts ultimately depend on its gaining access to a specific site on or in the membrane.[25–27] Based on its actions at the site, it then can interfere with an ionic current or currents. This phenomenon has been studied most completely with respect to drugs that modify fast channel function, and these are used as the major example here.

To consider the accessibility of any drug to the fast channel, it is convenient to use the model proposed by Hille for nerve (Fig. 41.4). As shown here, the fast channel is considered as a transmembrane pore whose ability to admit and transfer ions is limited by a so-called selectivity filter. This may be a functional or anatomical barrier that appears to have a diameter of <6Å and whose selectivity is largely for Na^+ (although some studies suggest it is permeable to H^+ as well).[28] On the internal side of the membrane are two "gates," m and h, initially described by Hodgkin and Huxley.[29] When the cell is in the resting state, the m gate is closed and h is open. In this situation, ions are not admitted through the channel. When stimulation occurs, the m gate opens and Na^+ (and perhaps H^+) passes through the channel into the cell. It is this sequence that is responsible for the occurrence of the rapid, phase 0 upstroke of the action potential. After the m gate opens, the h gate begins to close. As it does so, the rapid inward Na^+ diminishes, and with the h gate closed, the channel is effectively inactivated. A state of inactivation of fast channels also may be attained by depolarizing fibers to approximately −60 mV. Consequently, the m gates close and the h gates open, again returning the fiber to the resting state.

There are a number of experiments that suggest that the site of action of local anesthetic antiarrhythmic drugs is between the selectivity filter and the m and h gates.[25,30,31] It is important to recognize, however, that because of the locus of the "receptor," local anesthetic antiarrhythmic drugs cannot be thought of simplistically as molecules that merely approach a channel from its external surface and "plug" it from the outside. This is in sharp contrast to agents such as tetrodotoxin that have binding sites superficial to the selectivity filter. For tetrodotoxin, channel blockade is thought to occur as a result of occlusion of the selectivity filter by its guanidium group.[32]

Let us consider first how a local anesthetic molecule gains access

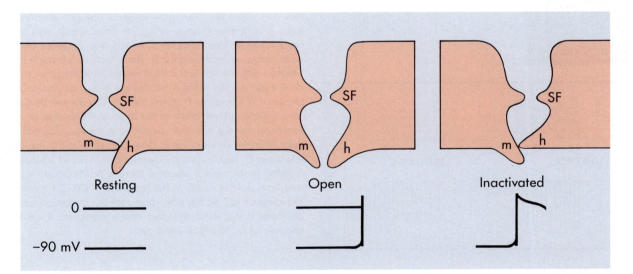

FIGURE 41.4 This is a diagram of a fast sodium channel of a cardiac cell. Three channel states are depicted: resting, open, and inactivated. Within the channel there is a so-called selectivity filter (SF) as well as the m and h gates. The lower panels under each representation of the channel state depict the concurrent transmembrane potential. With the heart in the resting state and all channels closed, one might record a resting potential of only approximately −90 mV in the Purkinje system. In the open state, sodium ion is permitted to enter the channel as the m gate opens, and there is the inscription of phase 0 of the action potential. In the inactivated state the h gate has closed, and the initial repolarization of the action potential is seen. (Modified from Hondeghem LM, Katzung BG: Time and voltage-dependent interactions of antiarrhythmic drugs with cardiac sodium channels. Biochim Biophys Acta 472:373, 1977)

to its receptor site. This depends on the ability of the molecule to pass *through the membrane* (and not through the fast channel) to the receptor. The membrane is a lipoprotein structure, and it has been clearly demonstrated that lipophilic molecules pass through this structure far more readily than do hydrophilic molecules.[25-27] Another important variable is molecular weight, with large molecules again dissociating far more slowly from the fast channel receptor site than small molecules.[33-35]

Experimental evidence supporting the view that differences in lipid solubility and ionization of local anesthetic–type drugs play an important role in their antiarrhythmic actions is presented by using three drugs as examples (Fig. 41.5). These are benzocaine, which is un-ionized and highly lipid soluble, lidocaine, which at physiologic pH exists in both the ionized and un-ionized forms, and QX-314, a permanently ionized derivative of lidocaine that is highly hydrophilic. If each of these agents is equilibrated with cardiac fibers at a physiologic pH, the following occurs: Benzocaine binds readily to the cell membrane, reaching a steady-state effect in less than 10 minutes, and its ability to block the channel is minimally influenced by stimulation rate (Fig. 41.5, *A*). In contrast, therapeutic concentrations of lidocaine, which is partially ionized at physiologic pH, exerts a slight "tonic" blocking effect (*i.e.*, block of the fast channel at slow stimulation rates) within 20 to 30 minutes but as stimulation rate is increased, its extent of fast channel block is augmented (referred to as a frequency or "use"-dependent effect) (Fig. 41.5, *B*).[36,37] Finally, QX-314 requires about an hour to attain a steady-state effect. Moreover, its tonic blocking action is minimal but it has a marked frequency-dependent effect (Fig. 41.5, *C*).

Studies of cardiac muscle and of nerve have suggested that for tonic block to occur, the drug gains access to the channel simply by passing through the lipid membrane to the receptor site. This explains the ready access of benzocaine and of the un-ionized fraction of lidocaine to the receptor permitting the reduction of fast Na^+ entry. Because the passage of un-ionized molecules is little influenced by stimulation rate, the magnitude of block of the fast channel and of maximum uptake velocity ($\dot{V}_{max}$) does not change with stimulation rate.

In contrast, the permanently charged QX-314 requires a long time to exert its effect, presumably reflecting the relative inability of such ionized molecules to pass through a lipid barrier. Whereas such transit requires a long time in cardiac muscle, in nerve it has been possible to demonstrate an effect of QX-314 only after it has been iontophoresed into the cytoplasm.[30] Once the ionized molecule has reached the cytoplasm (*i.e.*, the aqueous phase), it is capable of gaining access to the receptor site only through the channel itself. This requires that an open pathway be present; that is, the *m* and *h* gates must be open to permit passage of the molecule. The more rapid the heart rate, the more frequently channel openings occur and the more drug gains access to the receptor. This, then, is the basis for the ability of ionized molecules to exert a use-dependent effect in the fast channel and to reduce $\dot{V}_{max}$ (and conduction velocity) more markedly at rapid stimulation rates. If a molecule like lidocaine, present in both ionized and un-ionized forms at physiologic pH, is placed in a milieu where there is an increase in the ionized fraction (such as a reduced pH), then its depressant effects on $\dot{V}_{max}$ will increase secondary to prolongation of the recovery time constant from use-dependent block.[38] Hence, the situation of ischemia and acidosis augments the frequency-dependent (and channel blocking) effect of lidocaine.[39]

Thus far we have seen how lipid solubility and molecular charge

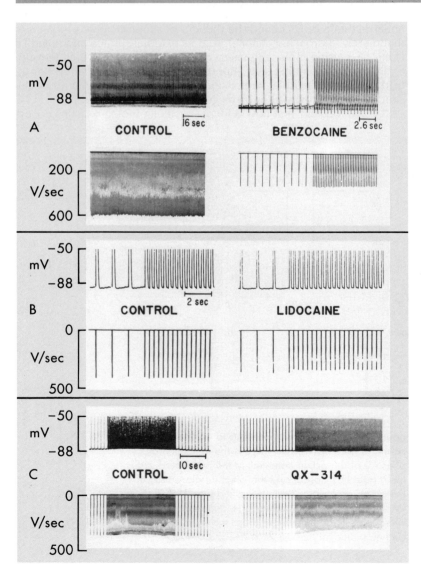

FIGURE 41.5 Effects of benzocaine, lidocaine, and QX-314 on electrophysiologic properties of canine Purkinje fibers. On the lower traces are the differentiated $\dot{V}_{max}$ of phase 0, expressed as a downward deflection. Records were made using a peak-hold unit. **A.** The effects of benzocaine, a highly lipid-soluble local anesthetic that does not show use-dependent properties. The membrane potentials at which the action potentials are initiated are shown on the upper traces of all panels. On the left is a control record at a drive cycle length of 800 msec. On the right are the results of superfusion with benzocaine, 132 µg/ml, for 10 minutes. At a basic cycle length of 1300 msec, there has been a marked reduction of $\dot{V}_{max}$ as compared with control. However, when the drive cycle length is abruptly shortened to 300 msec, there is no further change in $\dot{V}_{max}$. In other words, no use-dependent effect of benzocaine is demonstrable; its effects are consistent and equivalent over a wide range of cycle lengths. **B.** The effects of lidocaine in a comparable situation. On the left is a control record indicating that at slow and at fast drive cycle lengths there is no change in $\dot{V}_{max}$ of phase 0. On the right in the presence of lidocaine, 8 µg/ml, there is a reduction of $\dot{V}_{max}$ at the slow drive rate, indicating tonic block of the channel. When the drive rate is abruptly increased there is a further decrease in the $\dot{V}_{max}$, demonstrable within one beat after the onset of rapid drive. This reflects the use-dependent effect of lidocaine. **C.** Results with the permanently ionized lidocaine derivative, QX-314, 5 µg/ml. In the control situation, there is no change in $\dot{V}_{max}$ on changing drive rate from slow to rapid. In the presence of QX-314 there is only minimal reduction of $\dot{V}_{max}$ at the slow drive rate but a marked use-dependent decrease in $\dot{V}_{max}$ when the drive rate is increased. (Experiments in **B** and **C** courtesy of Dr. Yoshiyuki Morikawa)

play a role in determining the access of local anesthetic antiarrhythmics to their receptor sites. As mentioned above, another important determinant is molecular weight. This is a major determinant of the duration of binding of the molecule to its receptor.[33-35] To illustrate, studies of the time constant of recovery from frequency-dependent block (*i.e.*, the time required for $\dot{V}_{max}$ to return to its tonic level following cessation of rapid drive) have demonstrated that drugs having low molecular weights "unbind" much more rapidly than those having high molecular weights (Fig. 41.6). For example, mexiletine, whose molecular weight is 179, has a time constant for recovery from channel blockade of about 0.5 second, whereas flecainide, with molecular weight of 408, has a recovery time constant of 15.5 seconds. Drugs like mexiletine and lidocaine (molecular weight = 234), which have rapid time constants, may dissociate so rapidly from the channel during diastole that at the time of onset of the next action potential there is little residual block of the channels (although at high drug concentrations or very fast stimulation rates the magnitude of block will increase).[33-35] In contrast, for drugs of high molecular weight a large number of channels remain inactivated at the end of diastole, such that the subsequent action potential adds its fast channel blocking effects to an already extensive residuum of channels blocked.[33,35,39]

Hence, we can see that for the fast sodium channel, the equilibration of drugs with their binding sites is determined by several important factors, including lipid solubility, ionization, and molecular weight. Factors that influence either the state of the molecule, such as pH, or the extent of activation or inactivation of the fast channel, such as membrane potential, can further modify the access of drugs. For example, local anesthetics such as lidocaine can more prominently depress V_{max} in situations in which membrane potential is low and channels are partially inactivated.[40,41] Similar but less extensive information is available concerning the binding of calcium channel blocking drugs, for which frequency dependence also is of importance.

The effects of drugs on the fast channel are thus viewed as reflecting shifts in equilibrium between blocked channels (which are nonconducting) and unblocked channels (which conduct). Moreover, these shifts appear to be voltage dependent. Several hypotheses have been formulated to describe the binding of drugs to the fast channel. One, the modulated receptor hypothesis,[37] is based on the observation that fast Na^+ channels in the cell membrane may be present in resting, activated, and inactivated states (Fig. 41.7). It postulates that shifts in the equilibrium between blocked and unblocked channels are the result of a receptor that has *variable* affinity and a modified inactivation (*h*) gate in the channels complexed with drug. The association and dissociation rate constants differ for the resting, activated, and inactivated states as well as for individual drugs, and these determine the affinity of the drug for the receptor or channel site.

A second point of view is presented by the guarded receptor hypothesis.[42] This proposed that the channel receptor to which the drug binds is a *constant* affinity receptor. The channel gates (*m* and *h*) regulate access to the receptor. When both gates are open, the receptor is accessible to drug; when gates are closed not only drug access is limited, but so is the ability of a drug to leave the vicinity of the receptor.

The key factor to be understood in reviewing the actions of antiarrhythmic drugs is that they cannot be conceived of simply as molecules that plug channels. Rather, they bear many similarities to ligands to specific receptors. Their access is controlled by molecular size, ionization, and lipid solubility. It is further limited by the state of the channel (which, in effect, modulates drug access to the receptor). Finally, changes in the environment such as acidosis or membrane depolarization can modify drug ionization and channel state, respectively, and further influence drug action. Although these considerations may appear at first glance far afield for the consideration of drug actions in the clinic, they may go a long way toward explaining much of the variability that is seen in antiarrhythmic drug actions both among patients and within one patient over a period of time.

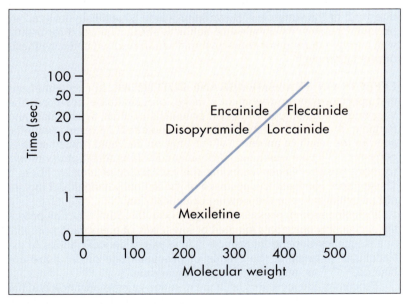

FIGURE 41.6 Relationship between the log of the time constant of recovery from frequency dependent block and the molecular weight of a series of antiarrhythmic drugs. Correlation coefficient for this line equalled 0.94. (Modified from Reiser HJ, Horowitz LN (eds): Mechanisms and Treatment of Cardiac Arrhythmias. Urban & Schwarzenberg, Baltimore-Munich, 1985)

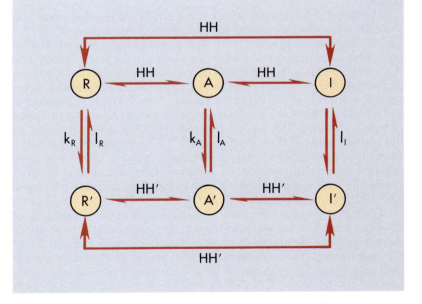

FIGURE 41.7 The modulated receptor hypothesis used to describe antiarrhythmic drug action. (R), (A), and (I) represent the resting, activated (or open), and inactivated states of the membrane referred to in Figure 41.4. (R), (A), and (I) are unoccupied by drug, whereas (R'), (A'), and (I') represent channels occupied by drug. The channels can move between the (R), (A), and (I) and (R'), (A'), and (I') stages via Hodgkin-Huxley (*HH*) kinetics. The constants (*k*) and (*l*) are respectively the association and dissociation rate constants for interactions of drug with the sodium channels in each state. The constants are characteristic for each drug and for each channel state. (Modified from Hondeghem L, Katzung B: Test of a model of antiarrhythmic drug action. Effects of quinidine and lidocaine on myocardial conduction. Circulation 61:1217, 1980)

MECHANISMS OF ACTION OF ANTIARRHYTHMIC DRUGS
DRUGS THAT DEPRESS THE FAST INWARD CURRENT AND PROLONG REPOLARIZATION

QUINIDINE

Quinidine, an optical isomer of quinine, was originally prepared by Pasteur for the therapy of malaria in 1853.[43] Although reports as many as 200 years earlier had suggested that cinchona bark derivatives might modify the rapid or irregular pulse, it was not until 1918 that the effects of cinchonine, quinine, and quinidine were recognized as effective in the treatment of atrial fibrillation.[44]

EFFECTS ON TRANSMEMBRANE POTENTIAL. Quinidine exerts its effects on atrial, ventricular, and Purkinje fiber transmembrane potentials. In concentrations that do not alter the resting membrane potential, the drug decreases the upstroke velocity of phase 0 of the action potential.[10,11,37,40,45,46] This results from its ability to decrease the conductance of sodium through the fast channel. This action of quinidine is frequency dependent, with depression of $\dot{V}_{max}$ being greater at high than at slow drive rates.[37,46,47] The magnitude of the reduction of $\dot{V}_{max}$ induced by quinidine is enhanced when pH is reduced from the neutral to the acid range, an effect that results from an increase in the proportion of the drug molecules existing in the charged form.[47,48] Increasing extracellular potassium also enhances the reduction in $\dot{V}_{max}$ induced by quinidine as a result of the decrease in membrane potential as described by the Nernst equilibrium, relating membrane potential to extracellular potassium.[49,50] As indicated above, when membrane potential is reduced there is slower dissociation of local anesthetics such as quinidine from receptor sites because a larger number of the sodium channels are in the inactivated state.[36]

In addition to its depressant action on $\dot{V}_{max}$, quinidine also displaces the threshold potential for the initiation of the action potential to more positive values, resulting in a reduction of excitability.[51] As a result, a greater stimulus intensity is needed to initiate the action potential.

Quinidine prolongs the voltage-time course of repolarization and the effective refractory period of atrial and ventricular fibers[11,13,37,40,45] as well as Purkinje fibers.[10,48,52,53] The prolongation of repolarization has a frequency-dependent component, being more prominent at slow drive rates.[50] This is the result of a decrease in potassium conductance of the membrane, which reduces the net outward current that is responsible for repolarization of the cardiac fiber.[13] The prolongation of the effective refractory period, however, is greater than that of action potential duration. This occurs because quinidine delays recovery of the sodium channel from inactivation[10,36,37,40] such that repolarization must move the membrane potential to more negative values than were required prior to drug exposure. A minor effect of quinidine is to decrease the slow inward current, which in turn may decrease the amplitude of the action potential plateau.[54]

Quinidine also has a profound depressant effect on automaticity of cardiac fibers. The normal pacemaker mechanism that is responsible for automaticity of Purkinje fibers (*i.e.*, the i_f pacemaker current),[10] and the mechanism that is responsible for impulse initiation in normal sinoatrial node fibers (incorporating both i_f and i_x)[45] both are suppressed by quinidine. This decrease in the slope of phase 4 in itself would be sufficient to decrease automatic rate, but the suppression of automaticity is enhanced further by the fact that quinidine displaces threshold potential to more positive voltages.

Quinidine has dual effects on delayed afterdepolarizations. It depresses digitalis-induced delayed afterdepolarizations in the Purkinje system, probably by decreasing the slow inward calcium current as well as the transient inward current (t_i) carried by sodium that is the primary current responsible for the afterdepolarizations.[55] In contrast, quinidine increases the amplitude of delayed afterdepolarizations in atrial fibers exposed to norepinephrine.[56] This is based on the quinidine-induced increase in action potential duration, which is thought to enhance calcium influx into the cell.[54]

There are no data available concerning suppression of early afterdepolarizations by quinidine. In contrast, under certain circumstances, quinidine actually can induce early afterdepolarizations.* This is seen most readily in situations in which the extracellular potassium concentration is reduced, decreasing K^+ conductance of the membrane and prolonging the duration of the action potential.

EFFECTS ON THE HEART AND CIRCULATION. Quinidine can induce profound hypotension indirectly by blocking α-adrenergic receptors[57,58] and directly through a vasodilator effect.[59] As a result of both of these effects, quinidine given intravenously decreases the systemic vascular resistance.

Quinidine has a direct negative inotropic effect on ventricular muscle[54,60] that can result in an elevated left ventricular end-diastolic pressure. Such an effect is seen especially when the drug is given intravenously.[62] Following oral administration there usually is little effect on left ventricular performance.[62,63] In addition, quinidine has a major parasympatholytic effect.[64] Because of this effect and because of the α-adrenergic blocking effects of quinidine (which reflexly increase heart rate), quinidine may increase the ventricular rate in patients who have atrial fibrillation.

The actions of quinidine on cardiac rhythm result from both its direct and its indirect effects. Quinidine can increase sinus rate and enhance atrioventricular conduction indirectly through its vagolytic effects.[64] Ventricular activation and recovery are depressed by its direct effects, resulting in an increase in QRS duration and the QT interval. The quinidine-induced increase in QRS duration is used to monitor the therapeutic effect. Increases in duration of approximately 40% to 50% above predrug values indicate impending toxicity, and quinidine administration should be terminated.[61,65]

PROCAINAMIDE

In 1936, Mautz demonstrated that procaine increased the stimulation threshold of the ventricle.[66] Because procaine is rapidly hydrolyzed by plasma esterases, its duration of action is short. The need for a drug with a longer duration of antiarrhythmic action resulted in the synthesis of procainamide.[67]

EFFECTS ON TRANSMEMBRANE POTENTIAL. In concentrations that approximate the therapeutic range, procainamide decreases the $\dot{V}_{max}$ and the amplitude of action potentials in atrial, ventricular, and Purkinje fibers. Such concentrations have no effect on resting potential and are the result of an effect of the drug on the rapid inward sodium current.[10,68-70] Like quinidine, procainamide shifts threshold potential to more positive values, reducing the excitability of cardiac fibers.[71] These effects on both the upstroke of the action potential and threshold potential result in the slowing of conduction.

Procainamide depresses the $\dot{V}_{max}$ of both the normal action potential and action potentials initiated at low levels of membrane potential in a frequency-dependent fashion.[72] At elevated concentrations of extracellular potassium, the effects of procainamide on $\dot{V}_{max}$ are enhanced,[49,50,68] as described above for quinidine.[69]

Procainamide increases both the duration of repolarization and the effective refractory period of atrial, ventricular, and Purkinje fibers.[10,68,70] The increase in the effective refractory period is greater than that of the action potential duration. This is consistent with a delayed removal of inactivation of the sodium channel, requiring that the membrane attain higher levels of potential than occurred prior to drug administration before the fast inward current can be induced. The prolongation of repolarization and refractoriness is more prominent at anatomical sites in the conducting system that have relatively short

---

* B. Hoffman, personal communication

action potential durations.[69] As a result, the drug tends to increase the homogeneity of repolarization in the ventricular conducting system.

Normal automaticity of Purkinje fibers is attenuated by procainamide through a reduction in the slope of phase 4 depolarization.[10,68,69] In addition, procainamide shifts threshold potential in a positive direction, tending to suppress automatic rhythms.[71] Triggered activity induced by delayed afterdepolarizations in digitalis-toxic Purkinje fibers is suppressed by procainamide, as are the afterdepolarizations themselves.[73] In contrast, studies of atria from diseased human hearts having abnormal automaticity at low levels of membrane potential show no pacemaker suppression by procainamide.[74]

EFFECTS ON THE HEART AND CIRCULATION. Procainamide administered as a rapid intravenous injection may induce hypotension and reduce myocardial contractility.[75–77] Vasodilation probably occurs as a result of ganglionic blockade.[78] Although procainamide has anticholinergic properties, they are not nearly as marked as those of quinidine or disopyramide. Its parasympatholytic effects are minimal and usually are not a major problem during clinical use.

The effects of procainamide on cardiac electric activity are similar to those of quinidine. Therapeutic plasma levels of procainamide may increase sinus rate slightly as a result of an anticholinergic action but, unlike quinidine, procainamide does not have the α-blocking properties of quinidine that can result in reflex increases in rate.[78] Individuals with existing sinus node dysfunction may show a decrease in sinus rate due to procainamide.[79] Atrioventricular conduction usually is not altered by therapeutic levels of procainamide, although there have been reports of slight depression of conduction.[79–81] Ventricular activation and recovery are prolonged by procainamide.[82,83]

DISOPYRAMIDE

Disopyramide was synthesized in 1954 and has been used extensively outside the United States since that date. Approval for U.S. use was given in 1978.

EFFECTS ON TRANSMEMBRANE POTENTIAL. Like quinidine and procainamide, concentrations of disopyramide that have no effect on the resting potential of atrial, ventricular, and Purkinje fibers decrease the amplitude and $\dot{V}_{max}$ of the action potential.[84–87] The effect on $\dot{V}_{max}$ is enhanced as extracellular potassium concentration is increased and membrane potential decreases.[87,88] As a result, Purkinje fibers having depressed fast-response action potentials show more depression of the action potential than fibers having normal fast responses. The antiarrhythmic effects of disopyramide appear to be frequency dependent, increasing in magnitude at rapid drive rates.[89]

Disopyramide induces equivalent increases in action potential duration and the effective refractory period of atrial, ventricular, and Purkinje fibers.[84–87] This effect differs somewhat from those of quinidine and procainamide, which tend to prolong refractoriness more than the duration of repolarization. Like procainamide, disopyramide tends to prolong repolarization and refractoriness less in regions where these are initially long.[90] Hence, it increases homogeneity of repolarization in the ventricular conducting system.

Disopyramide decreases the automaticity of normal Purkinje fibers by decreasing the slope of phase 4 depolarization.[87] Its actions on early and delayed afterdepolarizations have not as yet been reported. Disopyramide has no effect on slow-response action potentials in canine Purkinje fibers.[87]

EFFECTS ON THE HEART AND CIRCULATION. Disopyramide has important anticholinergic effects.[91] It appears to have little effect on impulse initiation in the normal sinus node, although its direct depressant effects can often be seen when there is preexisting sinus node disease.[92] Similarly, in normal hearts, disopyramide exerts little effect on the electrocardiographic PR interval,[93] probably because the anticholinergic actions counteract the direct effects of the drug. Its depressant effects on conduction in the ventricle result in prolongation of the QRS complex, and its prolongation of repolarization is reflected by prolongation of the QT interval.[93,94]

Disopyramide has clinically important hemodynamic effects. It exerts negative chronotropic effects, which are more pronounced in failing than in normal hearts.[95] There are reports of its induction of congestive heart failure as well.[96,97] In addition to these direct effects on cardiac contractility, disopyramide can cause arteriolar constriction[98] through direct actions on vascular smooth muscle.[99]

DRUGS THAT DEPRESS THE FAST INWARD CURRENT AND ACCELERATE REPOLARIZATION

Lidocaine, tocainide, mexiletine, phenytoin, aprindine, and ethmozin all depress the fast inward current but, in contrast to the above agents, they accelerate repolarization.

LIDOCAINE

Lidocaine was synthesized in 1946[100] and was first used by Southworth and associates to prevent ventricular tachyarrhythmias.[63] In concentrations that have no effect on the resting membrane potential, lidocaine induces a small decrease in $\dot{V}_{max}$ of normal cardiac cells.[99–101] This effect is far less than that induced by quinidine, procainamide, or disopyramide and does not significantly modify conduction.

EFFECTS ON TRANSMEMBRANE POTENTIAL. Lidocaine's actions on $\dot{V}_{max}$ are dependent on the rate of action potential initiation.[37,102] It is thought that lidocaine associates with the sodium channel when it is in the inactivated and open states and dissociates from it most rapidly when it is in the resting state. The effect of lidocaine on $\dot{V}_{max}$ is greatly augmented by a decreased membrane potential such as may occur as a result of increasing the extracellular potassium concentration.[103,104] Decreasing the pH also enhances the depressant action of lidocaine on $\dot{V}_{max}$, because a greater amount of the molecule exists in its ionized and active form at an acid pH.[38,48]

Because the effects of lidocaine are more prominent in fibers having lower than normal membrane potentials, its most significant action is on the depressed fast response.[40,104,105] It decreases $\dot{V}_{max}$ and conduction far more markedly in ischemic or depressed regions of the heart than in normal regions. Lidocaine has little effect on the threshold potential.

The duration of the action potential of normal Purkinje fibers is decreased by lidocaine.[106,107] A greater degree of shortening occurs in those fibers that initially have the longest duration.[108] The acceleration of repolarization appears to result from a decrease in inward sodium current during the plateau through those sodium channels remaining open at this time.[53,109] In normal Purkinje fibers, lidocaine shortens the refractory period to a lesser extent than the duration of the action potential.[106,107] In contrast, there is little effect of therapeutic concentrations of lidocaine on the effective refractory period of normal ventricular or atrial muscle.[106,110]

In partially depolarized ventricular muscle having depressed fast-response action potentials, lidocaine may prolong the effective refractory period.[111] In this situation, because the effect of the drug on action potential duration is not marked, refractoriness may outlast complete repolarization. A larger fraction of sodium channels remain inactivated in partially depolarized than in normal fibers. Lidocaine dissociates far less readily from inactivated than from resting channels, and this provides a basis for the greater prolongation of refractoriness in diseased or depolarized tissues.[37,45]

Therapeutic concentrations of lidocaine have no effect on sinus node automaticity but decrease the slope of phase 4 depolarization of normal Purkinje fibers, resulting in a slowing of automatic rate.[107,110] In this same concentration range, lidocaine has little or no effect on pacemaker activity in depolarized Purkinje fibers showing so-called abnormal automaticity or in depolarized ventricular muscle fibers.[112,113]

Lidocaine can hyperpolarize partially depolarized fibers, presumably by decreasing the background sodium current.[114] In this fashion, it can terminate automatic rhythms occurring at low membrane potentials simply by hyperpolarizing the membrane. Similarly, although lidocaine has no effect on early afterdepolarizations, it may hyperpolarize or accelerate repolarization in fibers demonstrating early afterdepolarizations, terminating the associated arrhythmia.[4] Delayed afterdepolarizations induced by digitalis or by infarction also are suppressed by lidocaine.[115]

EFFECTS ON THE HEART AND CIRCULATION. Lidocaine has little effect on the electrocardiogram. Except in cases in which there is preexisting sinus node disease, lidocaine has no significant effect on sinus rate.[110,116,117] Similarly, neither the PR interval[118] nor the QRS duration[119] is affected by therapeutic concentrations of lidocaine. Lidocaine has little effect on cardiac contractility except in individuals in whom ventricular function is abnormal.[120] The peripheral circulation is unaffected by lidocaine.

TOCAINIDE

The antiarrhythmic drug tocainide is structurally similar to lidocaine and its actions on the transmembrane potential are essentially identical to those of lidocaine. Tocainide slightly decreases $\dot{V}_{max}$ and the amplitude of normal action potentials in a frequency-dependent manner. In therapeutic concentrations, however, these effects are minimal. When extracellular potassium is elevated, these effects of tocainide are augmented; conversely, when extracellular potassium is decreased, these effects are attenuated.[121,122]

EFFECTS ON TRANSMEMBRANE POTENTIAL. Although the effects of tocainide on abnormal action potentials have not been studied directly, it is expected that its actions are similar to those of lidocaine (i.e., tocainide will significantly decrease $\dot{V}_{max}$ of already depressed fast-response action potentials while exerting little effect on slow responses). In normal Purkinje fibers, tocainide decreases both the duration of the action potential and the effective refractory period. It also depresses normal automaticity occurring at high levels of membrane potential.[121]

EFFECTS ON THE HEART AND CIRCULATION. Tocainide has little effect on the normal electrocardiogram or on cardiac contractility of normal or diseased hearts. However, clinical experience suggests that tocainide may precipitate or worsen congestive heart failure in some patients with severely depressed left ventricular function. Sinus rate is not altered by tocainide in therapeutic doses, nor does it change refractoriness of atrial and ventricular myocardium or of the atrioventricular conducting system.[123,124] The duration of the QRS complex is not changed by tocainide, although the QT interval may decrease slightly.[125,126]

Although tocainide exerts no significant effect on sinus rate in patients with normal sinus nodes, asystole has been reported when it was administered concurrently with β-adrenergic blocking agents to patients with sinus node dysfunction.[128] No adverse effects of tocainide on atrioventricular conduction have been noted, even in patients with preexisting conduction disturbances.[123] Tocainide has little effect on hemodynamics in normal individuals, although in patients with cardiac disease, aortic and pulmonary arterial pressure and systemic vascular resistance may increase.[123,127]

MEXILETINE

Mexiletine, another analogue of lidocaine, was first used as an antiarrhythmic drug in Europe in 1969. In concentrations that have no effect on the resting potential of atrial, ventricular, and Purkinje fibers, mexiletine decreases $\dot{V}_{max}$ and action potential amplitude.[129-132] These effects are associated with a depression of conduction velocity and of membrane responsiveness. These effects of mexiletine, like those of lidocaine, are the result of a similar blockade of fast inward sodium channels. This occurs in a frequency-dependent fashion. However, because mexiletine has a rapid dissociation constant from the fast channel (see above), its frequency-dependent actions are best seen at fast drive rates and high drug concentrations.

EFFECTS ON TRANSMEMBRANE POTENTIAL. Mexiletine has little effect on the voltage-time course of repolarization of atrial myocardium,[130] but in Purkinje fibers it does decrease action potential duration and the effective refractory period (the latter less than the former).[133] It decreases automaticity of normal Purkinje fibers, but it does so less as a result of its action on phase 4 than as a result of shifting threshold potential to more positive values.[131,132] Digitalis-induced delayed afterdepolarizations and abnormal automaticity at low levels of membrane potential both are suppressed by mexiletine.[131]

EFFECTS ON THE HEART AND CIRCULATION. Mexiletine has little effect on the normal electrocardiogram. Sinus rate, PR interval, and QRS duration are usually unchanged by mexiletine.[134,135] However, the preexistence of disorders of impulse initiation or conduction can result in atrioventricular block[135] or in severe sinus bradycardia.

Mexiletine can decrease cardiac contractility and systemic arterial pressure in individuals with prior myocardial infarction,[136-138] although the changes induced are small and usually are of little clinical importance.

PHENYTOIN

Although phenytoin (structurally related to the barbiturates) was first introduced for use as an anticonvulsant in 1938,[139] it was not until 1958 that it was used in the treatment of cardiac arrhythmias.[140]

EFFECTS ON TRANSMEMBRANE POTENTIAL. The actions of phenytoin on the cardiac transmembrane potential are complex and depend in large part on the concentration of the drug and the extracellular potassium concentration as well as the level of resting potential when the drug is administered.

At normal potassium concentrations and low drug concentrations, phenytoin has no effect on $\dot{V}_{max}$ of phase 0 or the amplitude of the action potential.[141,142] Some reports have shown increases in action potential amplitude and $\dot{V}_{max}$ of atrial fibers.[142,143] However, action potential amplitude, $\dot{V}_{max}$, and membrane responsiveness usually are depressed by higher concentrations of phenytoin.[141,143,144]

Increasing the extracellular potassium concentration can significantly augment the depressant effect of phenytoin on $\dot{V}_{max}$.[144] However, if resting potential and maximum upstroke velocity are depressed by a variety of experimental manipulations, phenytoin may increase both of these variables[144,145] and presumably improve impulse conduction. Studies of slow-response action potentials suggest that phenytoin does decrease the slow inward current carried by calcium, although not with the same magnitude of effect as that seen with calcium blockers such as verapamil.[144]

Therapeutic concentrations of phenytoin accelerate repolarization and shorten the effective refractory periods of Purkinje fibers, the latter decreasing less than the former.[144,146] Phenytoin has no effect on the duration or refractoriness of atrial fibers, however.[147] Phenytoin decreases the slope of phase 4 depolarization of Purkinje fibers having normal or partially depolarized maximum diastolic potentials.[144,146,148] Delayed afterdepolarizations occurring in Purkinje fibers as a result of digitalis toxicity are suppressed by phenytoin as well.[144]

EFFECTS ON THE HEART AND CIRCULATION. Phenytoin decreases sympathetic discharge in cardiac efferent sympathetic fibers, resulting in reduced sympathetic traffic to the heart.[149,150] Thus, the effects of phenytoin on the electrocardiogram result from both indirect and direct actions. Sinus rate is usually unaffected by phenytoin but is most likely to decrease in individuals with sinus node disease.[147,151]

Atrial conduction and P wave duration are not changed by phenytoin.[152] Clinically relevant concentrations of phenytoin may have no effect on or may accelerate atrioventricular conduction,[153-155] the latter effect being most pronounced in cases of digitalis intoxication.[153] Phenytoin has no significant effect on QRS duration.[153-156]

Phenytoin can induce significant hypotension[157,158] and pronounced negative inotropic effects.[158-169] These effects are most likely to occur when phenytoin is administered rapidly as an intravenous injection. These effects result not only from the drug itself but also from the diluent, propylene glycol and alcohol.[161]

APRINDINE
Aprindine, developed in Europe, is a local anesthetic compound that has been used in the United States primarily as an investigational drug.

EFFECTS ON TRANSMEMBRANE POTENTIAL. In therapeutic concentrations, aprindine decreases action potential amplitude and $\dot{V}_{max}$ of phase 0 of atrial, ventricular, and Purkinje fibers.[131,132] There appears to be a frequency-dependent component of these effects of aprindine. It also depresses membrane responsiveness. These actions are associated with a decrease in conduction velocity. The drug has no apparent effect on the slow-response action potential.[164]

Aprindine decreases Purkinje fiber action potential duration and reduces plateau height.[162,163] It shortens the effective refractory period as well, but to a lesser extent than action potential duration in atrial and ventricular myocardium and in Purkinje fibers.[162,163] It has been suggested that the decrease in action potential duration results from a decrease in inward sodium current during the plateau, because aprindine does not increase potassium efflux from myocardial fibers.[162,163]

Aprindine reduces the slope of phase 4 depolarization, decreasing automaticity of Purkinje fibers having normal levels of membrane potential.[162,166] It apparently induces no change in threshold potential. Aprindine also reduces the spontaneous rate of fibers having low levels of membrane potential as a result of potassium-free superfusates, hypoxia, digitalis, or stretch.[163,166] Digitalis-induced delayed afterdepolarizations in canine Purkinje fibers also are suppressed by aprindine.[164]

Aprindine has little or no interaction with the autonomic nervous system.[107,168] Nonetheless, it does alter impulse initiation and conduction and has some negative inotropic actions which can be important in patients with poor cardiac function.

EFFECTS ON THE HEART AND CIRCULATION. Clinically effective concentrations of aprindine have little effect on sinus rate in normal individuals.[169,170] Intra-atrial and atrioventricular conduction are depressed by aprindine,[169,170] and the QRS complex is prolonged. Aprindine given orally can slightly decrease blood pressure,[171] and it has direct negative inotropic effects in normal individuals.[172] The extent of these effects in the presence of heart disease is not yet known.[173]

ETHMOZIN
Ethmozin is a phenothiazine derivative developed in Russia for use as an antiarrhythmic drug.[173,174] It currently is undergoing clinical testing in the United States.

EFFECTS ON TRANSMEMBRANE POTENTIAL. Ethmozin's electrophysiologic effects have been studied mostly in canine Purkinje fibers, in which it reduced $\dot{V}_{max}$ of phase 0 and action potential amplitude.[175,176] It has no effect on the slow-response action potential.[177] Although its actions on the effective refractory period have not been studied using cellular electrophysiologic techniques, ethmozin does decrease the duration of Purkinje fiber action potentials[175,176] and presumably shortens the effective refractory period as well.

Unlike most of the other antiarrhythmic drugs discussed thus far, ethmozin does not affect the slope of phase 4 depolarization of Purkinje fibers.[175] Although it may decrease spontaneous rate by shifting threshold potential to more positive values, it only slightly depresses normal automaticity in the Purkinje system.[175,176] In contrast, it markedly reduces the slope of phase 4 depolarization and automaticity in Purkinje fibers having abnormal automaticity induced either by barium chloride or by experimental myocardial infarction.[177] It decreases the amplitude of delayed afterdepolarizations of Purkinje fibers in the digitalis-toxic[74] or infarcted canine heart.[177]

EFFECTS ON THE HEART AND CIRCULATION. Although ethmozin is a phenothiazine derivative, it has only minimal central nervous system effects.[178,179] Ethmozin administered orally to humans slows atrioventricular conduction and increases QRS duration; the QT interval is not changed.[179-181] Available data suggest that oral ethmozin has little effect on blood pressure.

DRUGS THAT DEPRESS THE FAST INWARD CURRENT AND HAVE LITTLE OR NO EFFECT ON REPOLARIZATION
ENCAINIDE
EFFECTS ON TRANSMEMBRANE POTENTIAL. Encainide, a compound structurally similar to procainamide, decreases the $\dot{V}_{max}$ of phase 0 and conduction velocity[182,183] in concentrations that have little or no effect on the resting potential. These concentrations also depress membrane responsiveness in Purkinje and myocardial cells.[183] The actions of encainide are frequency dependent. As a relatively large molecule, it associates slowly with the channel and tends to dissociate slowly as well. As a result of its slow dissociation, its depressant effects on $\dot{V}_{max}$ are profound. Encainide accelerates repolarization of the Purkinje fibers' action potential and has a lesser effect on the effective refractory period.[182,183] Encainide has no significant effect on the duration of the ventricular muscle action potential. The change in refractoriness is less than that in repolarization.

Encainide reduces the slope of phase 4 depolarization, decreasing automaticity of Purkinje fibers having normal or partially depolarized membrane potentials.[182] It has no effect on slow-response action potentials,[183] and its actions on delayed and early afterdepolarizations and triggered activity have not as yet been reported. Two metabolites of encainide have been isolated and their cellular electrophysiologic effects studied: these are o-demethylated encainide (MJ-9444) and 3-methoxy-4-hydroxy encainide (MJ-14030). Both derivatives appear to have more potent cellular electrophysiologic effects than the parent compound.[183] In Purkinje fibers, both derivatives reduce $\dot{V}_{max}$ and the duration of the action potential. Neither metabolite alters automaticity arising in normally polarized or partially depolarized Purkinje fibers.[183]

EFFECTS ON THE HEART AND CIRCULATION. Encainide has no effect on sinus rate or atrioventricular conduction when administered intravenously.[184-186] Ventricular depolarization and repolarization are prolonged, however.[184-186] When administered orally for longer than 72 hours, encainide depresses conduction through the atrioventricular node and within the His-Purkinje system.[187] The difference in the magnitude of effects of encainide by the parenteral and oral routes is consistent with the formation, probably in the liver, of active metabolites when encainide is given orally. Clinically relevant doses of encainide have no significant effect on systemic blood pressure[186] or the systolic ejection fraction.[188]

FLECAINIDE
Flecainide, a benzimide derivative, is an antiarrhythmic agent with local anesthetic properties. It became available for clinical trials in 1975.

EFFECTS ON TRANSMEMBRANE POTENTIAL. Flecainide decreases $\dot{V}_{max}$ and action potential amplitude without affecting maximum diastolic potential in atrial and ventricular muscle[188,189] or in Purkinje fibers.[190] These effects are frequency dependent and are augmented by increases in extracellular potassium concentration.[191] Available data indicate that flecainide may slightly increase action potential duration in ventricular muscle but decrease it in Purkinje fibers.[189,190] It has minimal effects on slow-response action potentials induced by isoproterenol in K^+-depolarized ventricular muscle.[189] Automaticity of the rabbit sinoatrial node and of Purkinje fibers is decreased by flecainide.[190]

EFFECTS ON THE HEART AND CIRCULATION. Flecainide depresses conduction in atrial myocardium and the atrioventricular node[192-194] and increases refractoriness in atrial, atrioventricular nodal, and ventricular tissues.[192-196] The former effect is probably related to the depressant action of flecainide on $\dot{V}_{max}$. The effects of flecainide on the atrioventricular node appear to be the result of a prolongation in both AH and HV intervals, although HV conduction is depressed to a greater extent.[192,194,195] In patients with preexisting Wenckebach periodicity or 2° atrioventricular block, flecainide may induce complete heart block.[195] As a result of the atrioventricular nodal effects of flecainide, the PR interval may be prolonged as much as 17% to 27% above control values.[197] The QRS duration is increased by flecainide,[197] presumably through the drug's effect on phase 0 depolarization (i.e., $\dot{V}_{max}$). The QT interval may be unchanged or slightly prolonged by flecainide,[197] an action consistent with the minimal effects of this agent on action potential duration. Ventricular refractoriness is prolonged by flecainide by up to 10% above control values.[192,194-196]

Flecainide has been reported to have no effect on impulse initiation by the normal sinus node[198,199] or to decrease[195,200] or increase[201] it slightly. In patients with preexisting sinus node dysfunction, although sinus rate was not significantly altered by flecainide, the corrected sinus node recovery time was increased markedly.[194]

Flecainide exerts negative inotropic effects in isolated ventricular muscle preparations and in the intact heart.[202] In patients with coronary artery disease,[202,203] flecainide increases right atrial and pulmonary artery pressure. Systemic vascular resistance is increased slightly. Cardiac index, stroke volume index, stroke work index, and left ventricular ejection fraction are decreased by flecainide.

DRUGS WHOSE MAJOR EFFECT IS ON REPOLARIZATION

The drugs described above share a marked frequency-dependent effect on the upstroke of the action potential and on conduction. Some, like quinidine, disopyramide, and procainamide, tend to prolong repolarization whereas others such as lidocaine and related drugs tend to accelerate repolarization and still others like encainide and flecainide have little effect on repolarization. In this section we deal with drugs that exert a major effect on repolarization: bretylium and amiodarone.

BRETYLIUM

Bretylium is a drug whose primary effect initially was thought to be related to an interaction with the sympathetic nervous system. It is taken up by and concentrated in adrenergic nerve terminals, resulting in a release of norepinephrine and a brief sympathomimetic effect. Following this initial effect, subsequent norepinephrine release is inhibited. The result is that the drug blocks the response to sympathetic nerve stimulation but does not block the response to catecholamines of the end organ.[204,205] Although it was initially used as an antihypertensive drug and then withdrawn,[206] it was found in 1966 to elevate the ventricular fibrillation threshold in animals.[207] Subsequently, it has proven to be of limited use in treating arrhythmias and ventricular fibrillation in patients.

EFFECTS ON TRANSMEMBRANE POTENTIAL. Most of the initial electrophysiologic effects of bretylium described in isolated tissue studies appear to result from norepinephrine release from nerve fibers,[208-211] which may increase resting potential and $\dot{V}_{max}$ and accelerate conduction in atrial and Purkinje fibers. Concentrations greater then 20 mg/ml decrease the action potential amplitude, overshoot V_{max}, and depress conduction and membrane responsiveness as well.[208,211] However, it is unlikely that such concentrations are consistent with those obtained in clinical situations.

The major effect of bretylium (in concentrations that do not depress $\dot{V}_{max}$) is to increase the duration of the action potential and the effective refractory period in atrial, ventricular, and Purkinje fibers.[208-210,212] This occurs in hearts having normal catecholamine quantities as well as in those depleted of catecholamines. Bretylium tends to prolong the action potential and the effective refractory period to the greatest extent in areas where they are short and in this way it decreases inhomogeneities of repolarization and refractoriness. It is this action of bretylium on repolarization that is thought to be the major basis for its antiarrhythmic effects. Bretylium has no effect on the slope of phase 4 depolarization and automaticity as a result of its direct actions, although by releasing catecholamines it may transiently increase automaticity.[208,209]

EFFECTS ON THE HEART AND CIRCULATION. Bretylium exerts biphasic effects on impulse initiation and conduction. After an intravenous dose, sinus rate first increases as endogenous catecholamines are released and then may decrease as sympathetic tone decreases.[213,214] The atrial effective refractory period increases, presumably as a result of an increase in action potential duration.[213,215] Bretylium has little effect on atrioventricular conduction in humans, although atrioventricular nodal refractoriness may decrease.[214] When administered to dogs, bretylium's anti-adrenergic effect results in an increase in atrioventricular conduction time. In contrast, neither the HV interval nor the duration of the QRS complex is altered by bretylium. Bretylium does, however, increase the ventricular fibrillation threshold by a mechanism not yet fully elucidated.[207,208,216]

Because bretylium blocks the effects of sympathetic nerves on peripheral arterioles it may induce some degree of hypotension.[206,217] Although there is no evidence that it has direct effects on myocardial contractility, the catecholamine release that occurs may transiently increase contractility.

AMIODARONE

Amiodarone is an iodine-containing benzofuran derivative that initially was introduced as a coronary vasodilator and antianginal drug. Subsequently, it was found to have antiarrhythmic actions. It is used as an antiarrhythmic and an antianginal agent in Europe and South America and, to a limited extent, in the United States.

EFFECTS ON TRANSMEMBRANE POTENTIAL. One of the major difficulties in studying amiodarone is that its effects appear to develop over a long period of time when the drug is given chronically by the oral route. As a result it is sometimes difficult to relate amiodarone's effects on isolated tissues acutely superfused with this compound to its mechanism of action. Nonetheless, it appears that atrial, ventricular, and Purkinje fibers show reduction of action potential amplitude and $\dot{V}_{max}$ with this drug as well as depression of membrane responsiveness. These all are associated with slowing of conduction. Initially, this mechanism of action of amiodarone was not thought to be important,[218] but more recent studies have shown that the drug has a prominent frequency-dependent action, which is presumably important to its antiarrhythmic efficacy.

The frequency-dependent effect is due mainly to binding of the drug with sodium channels that are in the inactivated state.[219] This effect, which has been demonstrated following acute or chronic administration of amiodarone, is dependent on the frequency of stimulation, being greater at greater rates of stimulation.[220] Recovery from this effect is a voltage-dependent phenomenon; thus, amiodarone slows impulse conduction more in depolarized tissue. The result of this action of amiodarone is that it would further depress $\dot{V}_{max}$ of cells whose action potential duration was longer. In addition, depolarized cells (as a result of infarction, for example) are more sensitive to amiodarone. The precise mechanism for the antiarrhythmic effect of amiodarone remains to be determined.

Perhaps more important to the antiarrhythmic efficacy of amiodarone is the marked prolongation of action potential duration and the effective refractory period in the presence of amiodarone. It is of interest that when superfused over isolated tissues, amiodarone's effects on repolarization are not seen; only those on the action potential upstroke are apparent.[218] In contrast, when amiodarone is administered chronically to animals, subsequent study of the ventricular transmembrane potentials reveals marked prolongation of repolarization.[221]

Amiodarone has little or no effect on phase 4 depolarization and automaticity of Purkinje fibers.[221] It has been stated to decrease the slope of phase 4 depolarization of sinus node pacemaker cells in isolated rabbit atria, however, and to slow their spontaneous rate of firing.

EFFECTS ON THE HEART AND CIRCULATION. Amiodarone exerts important effects on the heart through both direct and indirect mechanisms. The indirect effects are mediated primarily through the autonomic nervous system. Amiodarone is a noncompetitive antagonist of cardiac adrenergic stimulation.[222-224] Decreases in sinus rate associated with intravenous amiodarone administration are due to both an antiadrenergic action and direct suppression of phase 4 depolarization in sinus node cells.[225] The diluent for amiodarone (ethanol + polysorbate) causes transient tachycardia.[226] Conduction through the atrioventricular node is depressed so that the PR interval is prolonged.[227-229] Similarly, impulse conduction through the His-Purkinje system is slowed, especially when there is preexisting bundle branch block.[230-232] Refractoriness is prolonged throughout the heart by amiodarone.[230-233]

Hemodynamic effects of amiodarone result from a direct relaxation of vascular smooth muscle. Intravenous injection of amiodarone decreases peripheral resistance, decreasing afterload. This effect, in conjunction with the negative chronotropic effect of amiodarone, can result in a decrease in cardiac work and also myocardial oxygen consumption.[223,234,235] These effects may explain the antianginal action of amiodarone. Rapid intravenous injections of amiodarone may result in severe hypotension, marked negative inotropic effects, and increased left ventricular and diastolic pressure. Despite these occasionally severe hemodynamic effects of parenteral amiodarone, when the drug is administered orally on a chronic basis, few important hemodynamic side effects are observed.

DRUGS THAT MODIFY THE SLOW INWARD CURRENT: VERAPAMIL

In the past few years, increasing attention has been given to drugs that modify the slow inward current carried by calcium. To a very great extent such drugs do not affect the rapid upstroke of phase 0 carried by sodium ion but rather modify the current carried by calcium that contributes to the plateau phase of the normal action potential. Although antiarrhythmic capabilities have been described for diltiazem, we use verapamil, which has been studied more extensively, as an example here.

Verapamil was initially introduced as a coronary vasodilator.[236] It was thought to act as a β-adrenergic blocking agent,[237,238] although this has been shown not to be the case.

EFFECTS ON TRANSMEMBRANE POTENTIAL. In concentrations that have no significant effect on the resting membrane potential, the $\dot{V}_{max}$ of phase 0, or the amplitude of the action potential of fibers having the fast response, verapamil markedly depresses the slow inward current and, as a result, the plateau.[239-241] This action is largely the function of the L-isomer; the D-isomer has some local anesthetic actions.[242] Because it depresses the slow inward current, verapamil has major effects on the upstroke and action potential amplitude of cells in the sinus and atrioventricular nodes.[240,241] These effects result in slowing of sinus rate and depression of sinoatrial and atrioventricular nodal conduction.[240,243] The action of verapamil on slow responses is such that concentrations of the drug that are too low to affect the normal action potential markedly depress the slow response.[244,245] This action can be reversed in part by elevating the extracellular calcium concentration.[241] The basis for verapamil's suppression of the slow response is the reduction of the slow channel conductance of both calcium and sodium ions.[244,245]

In addition, verapamil prolongs the time for recovery from inactivation of the slow channel and, as a result, markedly prolongs the effective refractory period of fibers having the slow response.[245] Refractoriness may be prolonged to a far greater extent than the duration of the action potential.

Verapamil decreases the automatic firing rate of normal Purkinje fibers by depressing the slope of phase 4 depolarization.[239] It also depresses automaticity in fibers having low levels of membrane potential, whether resulting from disease or from experimental reductions in membrane potential.[241,243,246] Verapamil also suppresses triggered activity resulting from digitalis-induced delayed afterdepolarizations[247] and those induced in potassium-free superfusates or by catecholamines.[115,248]

EFFECTS ON THE HEART AND CIRCULATION. Because of the hypotensive effects of intravenous verapamil, sinus rate may reflexly increase.[249] This effect is reduced in patients on chronic verapamil therapy because of the direct depression of sinus node automaticity. In patients with sick sinus syndrome, verapamil may cause a profound bradycardia.[249]

Verapamil does not significantly decrease the rapid, inward sodium current ($\dot{V}_{max}$) and therefore has no important effect on impulse conduction in working myocardial cells or in the ventricular specialized conduction system. Thus, although the AH interval is prolonged by verapamil,[250-252] the HV interval is unchanged. The net result is an increase in the PR interval.

Atrioventricular nodal functional and effective refractory periods are prolonged by verapamil in the orthograde more than the retrograde direction.[253,254] It is this action of verapamil that probably underlies its effectiveness in abolishing reentrant atrioventricular nodal tachyarrhythmias.

The hemodynamic effects of verapamil are due to its calcium blocking properties as well as to reflex changes resulting from the resultant vasodilation. Verapamil decreases cardiac contractility and relaxes vascular smooth muscle.[251-257] Parenterally administered verapamil can cause modest decreases in systemic blood pressure; however, the reflex increase in heart rate is less pronounced than with other calcium entry blocking agents such as nifedipine. It may increase ejection fraction and cardiac index[249] in some patients. The expected decrease in blood pressure following chronic administration may be compensated for by the reflex increase in sympathetic tone.[258]

β-ADRENERGIC BLOCKING DRUGS: PROPRANOLOL

An increasing number of β-adrenergic blocking drugs are becoming available in the United States today. However, the major drug in use still is propranolol, which is the subject of this presentation. It is important to stress that the actions of the β-adrenergic blocking drugs we are referring to are specifically related to their interaction with the β-receptor. Among the β-blockers are some drugs with partial agonist activity, such as acebutolol, practolol, and pindolol.

EFFECTS ON TRANSMEMBRANE POTENTIAL. The concentrations of propranolol that induce β-blockade have no direct membrane effects. They do not affect the resting membrane potential, amplitude, or $\dot{V}_{max}$ of atrial, Purkinje, or ventricular muscle fibers.[259] Nonetheless, one should be aware that at high concentrations (equal to or greater than 10 μg/ml to 20 μg/ml) propranolol depresses $\dot{V}_{max}$ of the action potential, its amplitude, membrane responsiveness, and conduction velocity in Purkinje, ventricular, and atrial fibers.[259-261] These actions are the result of depression of the fast inward (Na^+) current. Propranolol accelerates repolarization and the effective refractory period as well. Such acceleration is greatest where the duration of the action potential is longest. The reduction of refractoriness is not as great as that of action potential duration.[259]

Propranolol alone in high concentrations can decrease the slope of phase 4 depolarization and suppress automaticity.[259,261] In addition it depresses delayed afterdepolarizations induced by digitalis.[262,263] It is to be stressed that all of these latter actions are the result of the direct effect of propranolol on the heart at concentrations exceeding those required for β-blockade.[264]

EFFECTS ON THE HEART AND CIRCULATION. Propranolol exerts most of its clinically relevant effects by blocking β-adrenergic receptors and the effects of sympathetic activation. To a large extent, therefore, the effects of propranolol ultimately depend on the level of preexisting sympathetic tone. When this tone is high, propranolol exerts relatively greater effects than when sympathetic activity is low.[265]

Sinus rate is slowed by propranolol, more so in the presence of sick sinus syndrome than in normal individuals. These negative chronotropic effects on the diseased sinus node may be the result of a direct effect[265] as well as β-blockade. As a result of its antiadrenergic effects, propranolol can depress atrioventricular conduction when this has been enhanced by a high sympathetic tone; the PR interval thus is increased. Under normal resting conditions, however, the PR interval may be unchanged. Conduction through the His-Purkinje system of normal individuals is not affected by propranolol.[264] Further, there is no effect of propranolol on impulse conduction through ventricular myocardium, so the QRS duration is unchanged.[264]

The magnitude of the effects of propranolol on hemodynamic variables depends on the level of sympathetic tone and is thus due to its β-blocking properties rather than its direct actions. In normal therapeutic doses, propranolol decreases heart rate and contractility and thus cardiac output is decreased. Because of the decrease in contractility and cardiac output, peripheral resistance may reflexly increase. All of these effects of propranolol on hemodynamics are more pronounced during exercise. However, the negative inotropic effects of propranolol can reduce the oxygen demand of the heart, an action that may be desirable in some patients. Another possible result of the negative inotropic effects of propranolol is the precipitation of cardiac failure, especially (but not only) in individuals who are dependent on a high sympathetic tone for the maintenance of cardiac output.

REFERENCES

1. Wit AL, Rosen MR, Hoffman BF: Electrophysiology and pharmacology of cardiac arrhythmias. II. Relationship of normal and abnormal electrical activity of cardiac fibers to the genesis of arrhythmias. A. Automaticity. Am Heart J 88:515, 1974
2. Wit AL, Rosen MR, Hoffman BF: Electrophysiology and pharmacology of cardiac arrhythmias. II. Relationship of normal and abnormal electrical activity of cardiac fibers to the genesis of arrhythmias. B. Reentry. Am Heart J 88:664, 1974
3. Schmitt FO, Erlanger J: Directional differences in the conduction of the impulse through heart muscle and their possible relation to extrasystolic and fibrillary contractions. Am J Physiol 87:326, 1967
4. Moe GK: Evidence for reentry as a mechanism for cardiac arrhythmias. Rev Physiol Biochem Pharmacol 72:56, 1975
5. Wit AL, Hoffman BF, Cranefield PF: Slow conduction and re-entry in the ventricular conducting system. Circ Res 30:1, 1972
6. Wit AL, Cranefield PF: Reentrant excitation as a cause of cardiac arrhythmias. Am J Physiol 235:H1, 1978
7. Bigger JT, Strauss HC, Basset AL et al: Electrophysiological effects of diphenylhydantoin on canine Purkinje fibers. Circ Res 22:221, 1968
8. Weld FM, Bigger JT Jr: The effect of lidocaine on diastolic transmembrane current determining pacemaker depolarization in cardiac Purkinje fibers. Circ Res 38:203, 1976
9. Singer DH, Strauss HC, Hoffman BF: Biphasic effects of procainamide on cardiac conduction. Bull NY Acad Med 43:1194, 1967
10. Hoffman BF: The action of quinidine and procainamide on single fibers of dog ventricle and specialized conducting system. Ann Acad Bras Cienc 29:365, 1958
11. Vaughan Williams EM, Szekeres L: A comparison of tests of antifibrillatory action. Br J Pharmacol 17:424, 1961
12. Hondeghem LM: Effects of lidocaine, phenytoin and quinidine on ischemic canine myocardium. J Electrocardiol 9:203, 1976
13. Vaughan Williams EM: The mode of action of quinidine on isolated rabbit atria interpreted from intracellular potential electrodes. Br J Pharmacol 13:276, 1958
14. Cranefield PF: The Conduction of the Cardiac Impulse: The Slow Response and Cardiac Arrhythmias. Mt Kisco, NY, Futura Publishing, 1975
15. El-Sherif N, Scherlag BJ, Lazzara R et al: Reentrant ventricular arrhythmias in the late myocardial infarction period. Circulation 56:395, 1977
16. Janse MJ, van Capelle F, Morsink H et al: Flow of 'injury' current and patterns of excitation during early ventricular arrhythmias in acute regional myocardial ischemia in isolated porcine and canine hearts. Circ Res 47:151, 1980
17. Kass RS, Tsien RW, Weingart R: Ionic basis of transient inward currents induced by strophanthidin in cardiac Purkinje fibers. J Physiol (Lond) 281:209, 1978
18. Tsien RW, Carpenter DO: Ionic mechanisms of pacemaker activity in cardiac Purkinje fibers. Fed Proc 37:2127, 1978
19. Lederer WJ, Tsien RW: Transient inward current underlying arrhythmogenic effects of cardiotonic steroids in Purkinje fibers. J Physiol 263:73, 1976
20. Hoffman BF, Cranefield PF: Electrophysiology of the heart. New York, McGraw-Hill, 1960
21. Schmidt RF: Versuche mit Acontin zum Problem der spontanen Erregungsbildun in Herzen. Pflugers Arch 271:526, 1960
22. Dangman KH, Hoffman BF: Effects of N-acetylprocainamide on cardiac Purkinje fibers. Pharmacologist 20:150, 1978
23. Strauss HC, Bigger JT, Hoffman BF: Electrophysiological and beta-receptor blocking effects of MJ 1999 on dog and rabbit cardiac tissue. Circ Res 26:661, 1970
24. Brown BS: Early afterdepolarizations induced by batrachotoxin: Possible involvement of a sodium current. Fed Proc 42:1692, 1983
25. Hille B: Local anesthetics: Hydrophilic and hydrophobic pathways for the drug-receptor reaction. J Gen Physiol 69:497, 1977
26. Narahashi T, Frazier DT, Yamada M: The site of action and active forms of local anesthetics. I. Theory and pH experiments with tertiary compounds. J Pharmacol Exp Ther 171:32, 1970
27. Frazier DT, Narahashi T, Yamada M: The site of action and active forms of local anesthetics. Experiments with quaternary compounds. J Pharmacol Exp Ther 171:45, 1970
28. Schwarz W, Palade PT, Hille B: Local anesthetics: Effect of pH on use-dependent block of Na^+-channels in frog muscle. Biophys J 20:343, 1977
29. Hodgkin AL, Huxley AF: A quantitative description of membrane current and its application to conduction and excitation in nerve. J Physiol (London) 117:500, 1952
30. Strichartz GR: The inhibition of sodium currents in myelimated nerve by quaternary derivative of lidocaine. J Gen Physiol 62:37, 1973
31. Hille B: Local anesthetic action on inactivation of the Na channel in nerve and skeletal muscle: Possible mechanisms for antiarrhythmic agents. In Morad M (ed): Biophysical Aspects of Cardiac Muscle, p 55. New York, Academic Press, 1978
32. Armstrong CM: Sodium channels and gating currents. Physiol Rev 61:644, 1981
33. Campbell DT: Importance of physico-chemical properties in determining the kinetics of the effects of class I antiarrhythmic drugs on maximum rate of depolarization in guinea-pig ventricle. Br J Pharmacol 80:33, 1983
34. Courtney KR: Fast frequency-dependent block of action potential upstroke in rabbit atrium by small local anesthetics. Life Sci 24:1581, 1979
35. Courtney KR: Interval-dependent effects of small antiarrhythmic drugs on excitability of guinea-pig myocardium. J Mol Cell Cardiol 12:1273, 1980
36. Hondeghem L, Katzung B: Time and voltage-dependent interactions of antiarrhythmic drugs with cardiac sodium channels. Biochim Biophys Acta 472:373, 1977
37. Hondeghem L, Katzung B: Test of a model of antiarrhythmic drug action. Effects of quinidine and lidocaine on myocardial conduction. Circulation 61:1217, 1980
38. Grant AO, Strauss LJ, Wallace AG et al: The influence of pH on the electrophysiological effects of lidocaine in guinea pig ventricle myocardium. Circ Res 47:542, 1980
39. Vaughan Williams EM: The classification of antiarrhythmic drugs reviewed after a decade. In Reiser HJ, Horowitz LN (eds): Mechanisms and Treatment of Cardiac Arrhythmias: Relevance of Basic Studies to Clinical Management, p 153. Baltimore, Urban and Schwarzenberg, 1985
40. Chen C-M, Gettes LM, Katzung BG: Effects of lidocaine and quinidine on steady-state characteristics and recovery kinetics of (dv/dt) max in guinea pig ventricular myocardium. Circ Res 37:20, 1975
41. Singh BN, Vaughan Williams EM: Effect of altering potassium concentration on the action of lidocaine and diphenylhydantoin on rabbit atrial and ventricular muscle. Circ Res 29:286, 1971
42. Starmer CF, Grant AO, Strauss HC: Mechanisms of use-dependent block of sodium channels in excitable membranes by local anesthetics. Biophys J

43. Moe GK, Abildskov JA: Antiarrhythmic Drugs. In Goodman LS, Gilman A (eds): The Pharmacological Basis of Therapeutics, p 709. New York, Macmillan, 1970
44. Frey W: Weitere Erfahrungen mit Chiniden bei absoluter Herzunregelmassigkeit. Wien Klin Wochenschr 55:849, 1918
45. West TC, Amory DW: Single fiber recording of the effect of quinidine at atrial pacemaker sites in the isolated right atrium of the rabbit. J Pharmacol Exp Ther 130:183, 1960
46. Johnson EA, McKinnon MG: The differential effect of quinidine and pyrilamine on the myocardial action potential at different rates of stimulation. J Pharmacol Exp Ther 120:460, 1957
47. Grant AO, Trantham JL, Brown KK et al: pH-Dependent effects of quinidine on the kinetics of dv/dt_{max} in guinea pig ventricular myocardium. Circ Res 50:210, 1982
48. Nattel S, Elharrar V, Zipes D et al: pH-dependent electrophysiological effects of quinidine and lidocaine on canine cardiac Purkinje fibers. Circ Res 48:55, 1981
49. Dreifus LS, Azevedo IH, Watanabe Y: Electrolyte and anti-arrhythmic drug action. Am Heart J 88:95, 1974
50. Watanabe Y, Dreifus L, Likoff W: Electrophysiological antagonism and synergism of potassium and antiarrhythmic agents. Am J Cardiol 12:702, 1963
51. Hoffman BF, Rosen MR, Wit AL: Electrophysiology and pharmacology of cardiac arrhythmias. VII. Cardiac effect of quinidine and procainamide. Am Heart J 90:117, 1974
52. Mirro MJ, Watanabe AM, Bailey JC: Electrophysiologic effects of the optical isomers of disopyramide and quinidine in the dog. Dependence on stereochemistry. Circ Res 48:867, 1981
53. Colatsky T: Mechanisms of action of lidocaine and quinidine on action potential duration in rabbit cardiac Purkinje fibers: An effect on steady-state sodium currents? Circ Res 50:17, 1982
54. Nawrath H: Action potential, membrane currents and force of contraction in mammalian heart muscle fibers treated with quinidine. J Pharmacol Exp Ther 216:176, 1981
55. Henning B, Vereecke J, Carmeliet E et al: Block transient inward current by TTX and local anesthetic. Circulation (Suppl) II:356, 1982
56. Henning B, Wit AL: Multiple mechanisms of antiarrhythmic drug action on delayed afterdepolarizations in canine coronary sinus. Am J Cardiol 49:913, 1982
57. Roberts J, Stadter RP, Cairoli V et al: Relationship between adrenergic activity and cardiac action on quinidine. Circ Res 11:758, 1962
58. Schmid PG, Nelson LD, Mark AL et al: Inhibition of adrenergic vasoconstriction by quinidine. J Pharmacol Exp Ther 188:124, 1974
59. Lu G: The mechanism of the vasomotor action of quinidine. J Pharmacol Exp Ther 103:441, 1951
60. Parmley WW, Braunwald E: Comparative myocardial depressant and antirrhythmic properties of d-propranolol, dl propranolol and quinidine. J Pharmacol Exp Ther 158:11, 1967
61. Bigger JR Jr: Management of arrhythmias. In Braunwald E (ed): Heart Disease: A Textbook of Cardiovascular Medicine, p 691. Philadelphia, WB Saunders 1980
62. Ferrer IM, Harvey RM, Wrko L et al: Some effects of quinidine sulfate on the heart and circulation in man. Am Heart J 36:816, 1948
63. Markiewicz W, Winkle RA, Binetti G et al: Normal myocardial contractile state in the presence of quinidine. Circulation 53:106, 1948
64. Mirro MJ, Manalan AS, Bailey JC et al: Anticholinergic effect of disopyramide and quinidine on guinea pig myocardium: Mediation by direct muscarinic receptor blockade. Circ Res 47:855, 1980
65. Heissenbuttel RH, Bigger JT Jr: The effect of oral quinidine on intraventricular conduction in man: Correlation of plasma quinidine with changes in QRS duration. Am Heart J 80:453, 1970
66. Mautz FR: The reduction of cardiac irritability by the epicardial and systemic administration of drugs as a protection in cardiac surgery. J Thorac Surg 5:612, 1936
67. Mark LC, Kayden HJ, Steele JM et al: The physiological disposition and cardiac effects of procaine amide. J Pharmacol Exp Ther 102:5, 1951
68. Rosen MR, Gelband H, Hoffman BF: Canine electrocardiographic and cardiac electrophysiologic changes induced by procainamide. Circulation 46:528, 1972
69. Rosen M, Gelband H, Merker C et al: Effects of procaine amide on the electrophysiological properties of the canine ventricular conducting system. J Pharmacol Exp Ther 185:438, 1973
70. Sada H, Kojima M, Ban T: Effect of procainamide on transmembrane action potential in guinea pig papillary muscle as affected by external potassium concentration. Naunyn Schmiedebergs Arch Pharmacol 309:179, 1979
71. Arnsdorf MF, Bigger JT Jr: The effect of procaineamide on components of excitability in long mammalian cardiac Purkinje fibers. Circ Res 38:115, 1976
72. Ehring G, Hondeghem LM: Antiarrhythmic structure-activity relationships in a series of lidocaine procainamide derivatives. Proc West Pharmacol Soc 24:221, 1981
73. Hewett K, Gessman L, Rosen MR: Effects of procainamide, quinidine and ethmozin on delayed afterdepolarizations. Eur J Pharmacol 96:21, 1983
74. Hordof A, Edie R, Malm J, Rosen M: Effects of procainamide and verapamil on electrophysiologic properties of human atrial tissues. Pediatr Res 9:267, 1975
75. Giardina EGV, Heissenbuttel RH, Bigger JT Jr: Intermittent intravenous procainamide to treat ventricular arrhythmias. Correlation of plasma concentration with effect on arrhythmias, electrocardiogram and blood pressure. Ann Intern Med 78:183, 1973
76. Bigger JT Jr, Giardina EGV: The pharmacology and clinical uses of lidocaine and procainamide. Medical College of Virginia Quarterly 9:65, 1973
77. Bigger JT Jr, Heissenbuttel RH: The use of procaine amide and lidocaine in the treatment of cardiac arrhythmias. Prog Cardiovasc Dis 11:515, 1969
78. Schmid PG, Nelson LD, Heistad DD et al: Vascular effects of procaineamide in the dog. Predominance of the inhibitory effect on ganglionic transmission. Circ Res 35:948, 1974
79. Wyse DG, McAnulty JH, Stadius M et al: Electrophysiologic effects of procainamide in patients with normal and prolonged sinoatrial conduction times. Am J Cardiol 41:386, 1978
80. Scheinman MM, Weiss AN, Shafton E et al: Electrophysiologic effects of procaine amide on patients with intraventricular conduction delay. Circulation 49:522, 1974
81. Josephson ME, Carcacta AR, Riccuiti MA et al: Electrophysiologic properties of procainamide in man. Am J Cardiol 33:596, 1974
82. Arnsdorf MF: The effect of antiarrhythmic drugs on triggered sustained rhythmic activity in cardiac Purkinje fibers. J Pharmacol Exp Ther 201:689, 1977
83. Giardina EGV, Bigger JT Jr: Procaine amide reentrant ventricular arrhythmias: Lengthening R-V intervals of coupled ventricular premature depolarizations as an insight into the mechanism of action of procaine amide. Circulation 48:959, 1973
84. Mirro MJ, Watanabe AM, Bailey JC: Electrophysiological effects of disopyramide and quinidine on guinea pig atria and canine cardiac Purkinje fibers. Circ Res 46:660, 1980
85. Sekija A, Vaughan Williams EM: A comparison of the antifibrillatory actions and effects on intracellular cardiac potentials of pronetholol, disopyramide, quinidine. Br J Pharmacol 21:473, 1963
86. Kus T, Sasyniuk BI: Electrophysiological actions of disopyramide phosphate on canine ventricular muscle and Purkinje fibers. Circ Res 37:844, 1975
87. Danilo P Jr, Hordof AJ, Rosen MR: Effect of disopyramide on electrophysiologic properties of canine cardiac Purkinje fibers. J Pharmacol Exp Ther 201:701, 1977
88. Kus T, Sasyniuk BI: The electrophysiological effects of disopyramide phosphate on canine ventricular muscle and Purkinje fibers in normal and low potassium. Can J Physiol Pharmacol 56:139, 1978
89. Vassallo JA, Cassidy DM, Frame LH et al: Prevention of ventricular tachycardia induction: Frequency-dependent effects of type I drugs. Circulation 68(III):381, 1983
90. Sasyniuk BI, Kus T: Effects of disopyramide phosphate (DP) on membrane responsiveness, conduction and refractoriness in infarcted canine ventricle. Fed Proc 35:235, 1976
91. Mokler CM, Van Arman CG: Pharmacology of new antiarrhythmic agent alpha-disopropylamino alpha-phenyl-alpha-(2-pyridyl)-butyramide (SC-7031). J Pharmacol Exp Ther 136:114, 1962
92. LaBarre A, Strauss HC, Scheinman MM et al: Electrophysiologic effects of disopyramide phosphate on sinus node function in patients with sinus node dysfunction. Circulation 59:226, 1979
93. Josephson ME, Carcacta AR, Lau SH et al: Electrophysiological evaluation of disopyramide in man. Am Heart J 86:771, 1973
94. Befeler B, Castellanos A, Wells DE et al: Electrophysiologic effects of the antiarrhythmic agent disopyramide phosphate. Am J Cardiol 35:282, 1975
95. Marrott PK, Ruttley MST, Winterbottam JT et al: A study of the acute electrophysiologic and cardiovascular action of disopyramide in man. Eur J Cardiol 4:303, 1976
96. Podrid PJ, Schoeneberger A, Lown B: Congestive heart failure caused by oral disopyramide. N Engl J Med 302:614, 1980
97. Lawrie TDV: Comparison of newer anti-arrhythmic agents. Am Heart J 100(2):990, 1980
98. Kotter V, Linderer T, Schroder R: Effects of disopyramide on systemic and coronary hemodynamics and myocardial metabolism in patients with coronary artery disease: Comparison with lidocaine. Am J Cardiol 46:469, 1980
99. Walsh RA, Horwitz LD: Adverse hemodynamic effects of intravenous disopyramide compared with quinidine in conscious dogs. Circulation 60:1053, 1979
100. Lofgren N: Studies on local anesthetics. Xylocaine, A New Synthetic Drug. Stockholom, Ivar Haeggstroms, 1948
101. Southworth JL, McKusick VA, Pierce EC et al: Ventricular fibrillation precipitated by cardiac catheterization. JAMA 143:717, 1950
102. Gintant G, Hoffman BF, Naylor RE: The influence of molecular form on the interactions of local anesthetic-type antiarrhythmic agents with canine cardiac Na^+ channel. Circ Res 52:735, 1983
103. Obayaski H, Hayakawa H, Mandel WJ: Interrelationships between external potassium concentration and lidocaine: Effects on the canine Purkinje fibers. Am Heart J 89:221, 1975
104. Brennan FJ, Cranefield PF, Wit AL: Effects of lidocaine on slow response and depressed fast response action potentials of canine cardiac Purkinje fibers. J Pharmacol Exp Ther 204:312, 1978
105. Lazzara R, Hope RR, El-Sherif N et al: Effects of lidocaine on hypoxia and

ischemic cardiac cells. Am J Cardiol 41:872, 1978
106. Davis LD, Temte JV: Electrophysiological actions of lidocaine on canine ventricular muscle and Purkinje fibers. Circ Res 24:639, 1969
107. Bigger JT Jr, Mandel WT: Effect of lidocaine on transmembrane potentials of ventricular muscle and Purkinje fibers. J Clin Invest 49:63, 1970
108. Wittig J, Harrison LA, Wallace AG: Electrophysiological effects of lidocaine on distal Purkinje fibers of the canine heart. Am Heart J 86:69, 1973
109. Carmeliet E, Saikawa T: Shortening of the action potential and reduction of pacemaker activity by lidocaine, quinidine and procainamide in sheep cardiac Purkinje fibers: An effect on Na or K currents? Circ Res 50:257, 1982
110. Mandel WJ, Bigger JT Jr: Electrophysiologic effects of lidocaine on isolated canine and rabbit atrial tissues. J Pharmacol Exp Ther 178:81, 1971
111. Gettes LS, Reuter H: Slow recovery from inactivation of inward currents in mammalian myocardial fibers. J Physiol (Lond) 240:703, 1974
112. Imanishi S, McAllister RG Jr, Surawicz B: The effects of verapamil and lidocaine on the automatic depolarizations in guinea-pig ventricular myocardium. J Pharmacol Exp Ther 207:294, 1978
113. Arita M, Nagamoto Y, Saikawa T: Automaticity and time dependent conduction disturbance produced in canine ventricular myocardium. Jpn Circ J 40:1408, 1976
114. Gadsby DC, Cranefield PF: Two levels of resting potential in cardiac Purkinje fibers. J Gen Physiol 70:725, 1977
115. Rosen MR, Danilo P: Effects of tetrodotoxin, lidocaine, verapamil and AHR-2666 on ouabain-induced delayed afterdepolarizations in canine Purkinje fibers. Circ Res 46:117, 1980
116. Cheng TO, Wadhwa N: Sinus standstill following intravenous lidocaine administration. JAMA 223:790, 1973
117. Lippestad CT, Forgang K: Production of sinus arrest by lignocaine. Br Med J 1:537, 1971
118. Rosen KM, Lau SH, Weiss MB et al: The effect of lidocaine on atrioventricular and intraventricular conduction in man. Am J Cardiol 25:1, 1970
119. Frieden J: Antiarrhythmic drugs. VI. Lidocaine as an antiarrhythmic agent. Am Heart J 70:713, 1965
120. Grossman JI, Cooper JA, Frieden J: Cardiovascular effects of infusion of lidocaine in patients with heart disease. Am J Cardiol 24:191, 1969
121. Moore EM, Spear JF, Horowitz LN et al: Electrophysiologic properties of a new anti-arrhythmic drug-tocainide. Am J Cardiol 41:703, 1978
122. Oshita S, Sada H, Kojima M et al: Effects of tocainide and lidocaine on the transmembrane action potentials as related to external potassium and calcium concentrations in guinea pig papillary muscles. Naunyn Schmeidebergs Arch Pharmacol 314:62, 1980
123. Anderson JF, Mason JW, Winkle RA et al: Clinical electrophysiologic effects of tocainide. Circulation 57:685, 1978
124. McDevitt DG, Nies AS, Wilkinson GR et al: Antiarrhythmic effects of lidocaine congener, tocainide, 2-amino-2′, 6′-propionoxylidine, in man. Clin Pharmacol Ther 19:396, 1976
125. Coltart DJ, Berndt TB, Kernoff R et al: Antiarrhythmic and circulatory effects of astra W36075, a new lidocaine like agent. Am J Cardiol 34:35, 1974
126. Nyquist O, Forssell G, Nordlander R et al: Hemodynamic and antiarrhythmic effects of tocainide in patients with heart disease. Circulation 57:787, 1980
127. Winkle RA, Anderson JL, Peters F et al: The hemodynamic effects of intravenous tocainide in patients with heart disease. Circulation 57:787, 1978
128. Ikram H: Hemodynamic and electrophysiologic interactions between antiarrhythmic drugs and beta blockers, with special reference to tocainide. Am Heart J 100:1076, 1980
129. Singh BN, Vaughan Williams EM: Investigations of the mode of action of a new antidysrhythmic drug (KO1173). Br J Pharmacol 44:1, 1972
130. Yamaguchi I, Singh B, Mandel W: Electrophysiological actions of mexiletine on isolated rabbit atria and canine ventricular muscle and Purkinje fiber. Cardiovasc Res 13:288, 1979
131. Weld FM, Bigger JT Jr, Swistel D et al: Electrophysiological effects of mexiletine (Ko 1173) bovine cardiac Purkinje fibers. J Pharmacol Exp Ther 210:222, 1979
132. Iwamura N, Shimizu T, Toyoshima H et al: Electrophysiological actions of a new antiarrhythmic agent on isolated preparations of the canine Purkinje fiber and ventricular muscle. Cardiology 61:329, 1976
133. Vaughan Williams EM: Mexiletine in isolated tissue models. Postgrad Med J 53:(Suppl I)30, 1977
134. McComish M, Robinson C, Kitson D et al: Clinical electrophysiological effects of mexiletine. Postgrad Med J 53(Suppl I):85, 1977
135. Roos JC, Paalman DCA, Dunning AJ: Electrophysiological effects of mexiletine in man. Postgrad Med J 53(Suppl I):92, 1977
136. Saunamaki KI: Haemodynamic effects of a new antiarrhythmic agent, mexiletine (Ko 1173) in ischemic heart disease. Cardiovasc Res 9:788, 1975
137. Pozenel H: Hemodynamic studies on mexiletine, a new antiarrhythmic agent. Postgrad Med J 53(Suppl I):78, 1977
138. Shaw TRD: The effect of mexiletine on left ventricular ejection: A comparison with lidocaine and propranolol. Postgrad Med J 53(Suppl I):69, 1977
139. Merrit HH, Putnam TJ: Sodium diphenylhydantoin in treatment of convulsive disorders. J Am Med Assoc III:1068, 1938
140. Leonard WA: The use of diphenylhydantoin (Dilantin) sodium in the treatment of ventricular tachycardia. Arch Intern Med 101:714, 1958
141. Singh BN, Vaughan Williams EM: Effect of altering potassium concentrations on the action potentials of lidocaine and diphenylhydantoin on rabbit atrial and ventricular muscle. Circ Res 29:286, 1971
142. Jensen RA, Katzung BG: Electrophysiological actions of diphenylhydantoin on rabbit atria. Circ Res 26:17, 1970
143. Katzung BG, Jensen RA: Depressant action of diphenylhydantoin on electrical and mechanical properties of isolated rabbit and dog atria: Dependence on sodium and potassium. Am Heart J 80:80, 1970
144. Rosen MR, Danilo P Jr, Alonso MB et al: Effects of therapeutic concentrations of diphenylhydantoin on transmembrane potentials of normal and depressed Purkinje fibers. J Pharmacol Exp Ther 197:594, 1974
145. Bassett AL, Bigger JT Jr, Hoffman BF: 'Protective' action of diphenylhydantoin on canine Purkinje fibers during hypoxia. J Pharmacol Exp Ther 173:336, 1970
146. Bigger JT, Strauss HC, Bassett AL et al: Electrophysiological effects of diphenylhydantoin on canine Purkinje fibers. Circ Res 22:221, 1968
147. Strauss HC, Bigger JT Jr, Bassett AL et al: Actions of diphenylhydantoin on the electrical properties of isolated rabbit and canine atria. Circ Res 23:463, 1968
148. Bigger JT Jr, Weinberg DI, Kovalik ATW et al: Effects of diphenylhydantoin on excitability and automaticity of canine heart. Circ Res 26:1, 1970
149. Gillis RA, McClellan JR, Sauer TS et al: Depression of cardiac sympathetic nerve activity by diphenylhydantoin. J Pharmacol Exp Ther 179:599, 1971
150. Evans DE, Gillis RA: Effect of diphenylhydantoin and lidocaine on cardiac arrhythmias induced by hypothalamic stimulation. J Pharmacol Exp Ther 191:506, 1974
151. Unger AH, Sklaroff HJ: Fatalities following intravenous use of sodium diphenylhydantoin for cardiac arrhythmias. Report of two cases. JAMA 200:335, 1967
152. Russell JM, Harvey SC: Effects of diphenylhydantoin on canine atria and A-V conducting system. Arch Int Pharmacodyn Ther 182:219, 1969
153. Helfant RH, Scherlag BJ, Damato AN: The electrophysiological properties of diphenylhydantoin sodium as compared to procaine amide in the normal and digitalis-intoxicated heart. Circulation 36:108, 1967
154. Bigger JT Jr, Schmidt DH, Kutt H: Relationship between the plasma level of diphenylhydantoin sodium and its cardiac antiarrhythmic effects. Circulation 38:363, 1968
155. Damato AN, Berkowitz WD, Patton RD et al: The effects of diphenylhydantoin on atrioventricular and intraventricular conduction in man. Am Heart J 79:51, 1970
156. Dhatt MS, Gomes JAC, Reddy CP et al: Effects of phenytoin on refractoriness and conduction in the human heart. J Cardiol Pharmacol 1:3, 1979
157. Harris AS, Kokernot RH: Effects of diphenylhydantoin (Dilantin sodium) and phenobarbital sodium upon ectopic ventricular tachycardia in acute myocardial infarction. Am J Physiol 163:505, 1950
158. Mixter CG III, Moran JM, Austen WG: Cardiac and peripheral vascular effects of diphenylhydantoin sodium. Am J Cardiol 17:332, 1966
159. Lieberson AD, Schumacher RR, Childress RH et al: Effect of diphenylhydantoin on left ventricular function in patients with heart disease. Circulation 36:692, 1967
160. Puri PS: The effect of diphenylhydantoin sodium (Dilantin) on myocardial contractility and hemodynamics. Am Heart J 82:62, 1971
161. Louis S, Kutt H, McDowell F: The cardiocirculatory changes caused by intravenous Dilantin and its solvent. Am Heart J 74:523, 1967
162. Verdonck F, Vereecke J, Vleugels A: Electrophysiological effects of aprindine on isolated heart preparations. Eur J Pharmacol 26:338, 1974
163. Steinberg MI, Greenspan K: Intracellular electrophysiological alterations in canine cardiac conducting tissue induced by aprindine and lidocaine. Cardiovasc Res 10:236, 1976
164. Elharrar V, Bailey JC, Lathrop DA et al: Effects of aprindine on slow channel action potentials and transient depolarizations in canine Purkinje fibers. J Pharmacol Exp Ther 205:410, 1978
165. Gilmour RF Jr, Chikhaev VN, Jurevichus JA et al: Effect of aprindine on transmembrane currents and contractile force in frog atria. J Pharmacol Exp Ther 217:390, 1981
166. Carmeliet E, Verdonck F: Effects of aprindine and lidocaine on transmembrane potentials and radioactive K efflux in different cardiac tissues. Acta Cardiol [Suppl] (Brux) 18:73, 1974
167. Georges A, Hosslet A, Duvernay G: Pharmacological evaluation of aprindine (AC 1802). A new antiarrhythmic agent. Acta Cardiol (Brux) 28:166, 1973
168. Elharrar V, Foster PR, Zipes DP: Effects of aprindine HCl on cardiac tissues. J Pharmacol Exp Ther 195:201, 1975
169. Seipel L, Both A, Breithardt G et al: Action of antiarrhythmic drugs on His bundle electrogram and sinus node function. Acta Cardiol [Suppl] (Brux) 18:251, 1974
170. Breithardt G, Gleichmann V, Seipel L et al: Long term oral anti-arrhythmic therapy by antiarrhythmic drugs. Acta Cardiol [Suppl] (Brux) 18:341, 1974
171. Rousseau MF, Brasseur LA, Detry JM: Hemodynamic effects of aprindine during upright exercise in normal subjects. Acta Cardiol [Suppl] (Brux) 18:195, 1974
172. Piessens J, Willems J, Kesteloot H et al: Effects of aprindine on left ventricular contractility in man. Acta Cardiol [Suppl] (Brux) 18:203, 1971
173. Remme WJ, Verdouw PD: Cardiovascular effects of aprindine, a new antiarrhythmic drug. Eur J Cardiol 314:307, 1975
174. Kaverina NV, Senova ZP: Ethmozin—a new preparation for treating cardiac rhythm disorders. Proc First US–USSR Sym on Sudden Death, Yalta, Oct 3–5, 1977. US Dept of HEW, PHS, NTH, DHEW Publ No 78:1470, 1978

175. Danilo P Jr, Langan WB, Rosen MR et al: Effects of the phenothiazine analog EN 313 on ventricular arrhythmias in dogs. Eur J Pharmacol 45:127, 1977
176. Ruffy R, Rozenshtraukh LV, Elharrar V et al: Electrophysiological effects of ethmozine on canine myocardium. Cardiovasc Res 13:354, 1979
177. Dangman KH, Hoffman BF: Effects of ethmozin on automatic and triggered impulse initiation in canine cardiac Purkinje fibers. J Pharmacol Exp Ther 227:578, 1983
178. Morganroth J, Pearlman AS, Dunkman WB et al: Ethmozine: A new antiarrhythmic agent developed in the USSR. Efficacy and tolerance. Am Heart J 98:621, 1979
179. Podrid PJ, Lyakishev A, Lown B et al: Ethmozine, a new antiarrhythmic drug for suppressing ventricular premature complexes. Circulation 61:450, 1980
180. Morganroth J, Michelson EL, Klitchen JG et al: Ethmozin: Electrophysiologic effects in man. Circulation 64:263, 1981
181. Singh SN, DiBianco R, Fletcher RD et al: Ethmozin shown effective in reducing chronic high frequency: Results of a prospective controlled trial. Am J Cardiol 49:1015, 1982
182. Gibson JK, Somani P, Bassett AL: Electrophysiologic effects of encainide (MJ9067) on canine Purkinje fibers. Eur J Pharmacol 52:161, 1978
183. Elharrar V, Zipes DP: Effects of encainide and metabolites (MJ14030 and MJ9444) on canine cardiac Purkinje and ventricular fibers. J Pharmacol Exp Ther 220:440, 1982
184. Sami M, Mason JW, Oh G et al: Canine electrophysiology of encainide, a new antiarrhythmic drug. Am J Cardiol 43:1149, 1979
185. Sami M, Mason JW, Peters F et al: Clinical electrophysiologic effects of encainide, a newly developed antiarrhythmic agent. Am J Cardiol 44:526, 1979
186. Jackman WM, Zipes DP, Naccarelli GV et al: Electrophysiology of oral encainide. Am J Cardiol 49:1270, 1982
187. Roden DM, Reele SB, Higgins SB et al: Total suppression of ventricular arrhythmias by encainide: Pharmacokinetic and electrocardiographic characteristics. N Engl J Med 302:877, 1980
188. Barchard U, Borsten M: Effect of flecainide on action potentials and alternating current-induced arrhythmias in mammalian myocardium. J Cardiovasc Pharmacol 4:205, 1982
189. Schulze JJ, Knops J: Effects of flecainide on contractile force and electrophysiological parameters in cardiac muscle. Arzneim Forsch 32:1025, 1982
190. Kvam DC, Banitt EH, Schmid JR: Antiarrhythmic and electrophysiologic action of flecainide in animal models. Am J Cardiol 53:22B, 1984
191. Cambell CJ, Vaughan-Williams EM: Characterization of a new oral antiarrhythmic drug, flecainide (R-818). Eur J Pharmacol 73:333, 1981
192. Olsson SB, Edvardsson N: Clinical electrophysiologic study of antiarrhythmic properties of flecainide. Am Heart J 102:864, 1981
193. Muhiddin KA, Hellestrand KJ, Nathan A et al: The electrophysiological effects of flecainide acetate (R-818) on the cardiac conduction system. Br J Clin Pharmacol 13:286, 1981
194. Vik-mo H, Ohm OJ, Lund-Johnson P: Electrophysiologic effects of flecainide acetate in patients with sinus node dysfunction. Am J Cardiol 50:1090, 1982
195. Hellestrand KJ, Bextan RS, Nathan AW et al: Acute electrophysiologic effects of flecainide acetate on cardiac conduction and refractoriness in man. Br Heart J 48:140, 1982
196. Hellestrand KJ, Nathan AW, Bextan RS et al: Cardiac electrophysiologic effects of flecainide acetate for paroxysmal re-entrant junctional tachycardias. Am J Cardiol 51:770, 1983
197. Estes NAM, Garon H, Ruskin JN: Electrophysiologic properties of flecainide acetate. Am J Cardiol 53:26B, 1984
198. Abitbol H, Colipno JE, Abote C et al: Use of flecainide acetate in the treatment of premature ventricular contraction. Am Heart J 105:227, 1983
199. Somani R: Antiarrhythmic effects of flecainide. Clin Pharm Ther 27:464, 1980
200. Anderson JF, Stewart JR, Perry BA et al: Oral flecainide acetate for the treatment of ventricular arrhythmias. N Engl J Med 305:473, 1981
201. Hellestrand KJ, Nathan AW, Bexton PS, Comm AJ: Electrophysiologic effects of flecainide acetate on sinus node function, anomalous atrioventricular connections, and pacemaker thresholds. Am J Cardiol 53:30b, 1984
202. Josephson MA, Ikeda N, Singh BN: Effects of flecainide on ventricular function: Clinical experimental correlations. Am J Cardiol 53:95B, 1984
203. Legrand V, Vandromoal M, Collignon P et al: Hemodynamic effects of a new antiarrhythmic agent, flecainide (R-818), in coronary heart disease. Am J Cardiol 51:422, 1983
204. Boura ALA, Green AF: The actions of bretylium: Adrenergic neurone blocking and other effects. Br J Pharmacol 14:536, 1959
205. Boura ALA, Green AF: Adrenergic neurone blocking agents. Ann Rev Pharmacol 5:183, 1965
206. Heissebuttel RH, Bigger JT Jr: Bretylium tosylate: A newly available antiarrhythmic drug for ventricular arrhythmias. Ann Intern Med 91:229, 1979
207. Bacaner MG: Bretylium tosylate for suppression of induced ventricular fibrillation. Am J Cardiol 17:528, 1966
208. Bigger JT Jr, Jaffe CA: The effect of bretylium tosylate on the electrophysiological properties of ventricular muscle and Purkinje fibers. Am J Cardiol 27:82, 1971
209. Wit AL, Steiner C, Damato AN: Electrophysiologic effects of bretylium tosylate on single fibers of the canine specialized conducting system and ventricle. J Pharmacol Exp Ther 173:344, 1970
210. Namm DH, Wang CM, El-Sayad S et al: Effect of bretylium on rat cardiac muscle: The electrophysiologic effects and its uptake and binding in normal and immunosympathectomized rat hearts. J Pharmacol Exp Ther 193:194, 1975
211. Papp JG, Vaughan Williams EM: The effect of bretylium on intracellular cardiac action potentials in relation to its antiarrhythmic and local anesthetic activity. Br J Pharmacol 37:380, 1969
212. Cardinal R, Sasyniuk BI: Electrophysiological effects of bretylium tosylate on subendocardial Purkinje fibers from infarcted canine hearts. J Pharmacol Exp Ther 204:159, 1978
213. Glassman RD, Wit AL: Electrophysiological effect of bretylium tosylate. In Bretylium Tosylate: Current Scientific and Clinical Experience. Amsterdam Excerpta Medica, 1979
214. Touboul P, Porte J, Huerta F et al: Etude des proprietes electrophysiologiques du tosylate de bretylium chez l'homme. Arch Mal Coeur 69:503, 1976
215. Waxman MB, Wallace AG: Electrophysiologic effects of bretylium tosylate on the heart. J Pharmacol Exp Ther 183:264, 1972
216. Allen JD, Pantridge JF, Shanks RG: Effects of lignocaine, propranolol and bretylium on ventricular fibrillation threshold. Am J Cardiol 28:555, 1971
217. Sanna G, Arcidiacono R: Chemical ventricular defibrillation of the human heart with bretylium tosylate. Am J Cardiol 32:982, 1973
218. Singh BN, Vaughan Williams EM: The effects of amiodarone, a new antianginal drug, on cardiac muscle. Br J Pharmacol 39:657, 1970
219. Mason JW, Hondeghem LM, Katzung BG: Amiodarone blocks inactivated cardiac sodium channels. Pflug Arch 396:79, 1983
220. Mason JW, Hondegham LM, Katzung BG: Block of inactivated sodium channels and of depolarization-induced automaticity in guinea-pig papillary muscle by amiodarone. Circ Res 55:277, 1984
221. Rosenbaum MB, Chiale PA, Halpern MS et al: Clinical efficacy of amiodarone as an antiarrhythmic agent. Am J Cardiol 38:934, 1976
222. Charlier R, Deltour G, Baudine A et al: Pharmacology of amiodarone, an antianginal drug with a new biological profile. Arzneimittelforsch 11:1408, 1968
223. Charlier R: Cardiac actions in the dog of a new antagonist of adrenergic excitation which does not produce competitive blockade of adrenoceptors. Br J Pharmacol 39:668, 1970
224. Bacq ZM, Blakeley AGH, Summers RJ: The effects of amiodarone, an alpha and beta receptor antagonist, on adrenergic transmission in the cat spleen. Biochem Pharmacol 25:1195, 1976
225. Goupil N, Lenfant J: The effects of amiodarone on the sinus node activity of the rabbit heart. Eur J Pharmacol 39:23, 1976
226. Sicart M, Besse P, Choussat A et al: Action hemodynamique de l'amiodarone intraveineuse chez l'homme. Arch Mal Coeur 70:219, 1977
227. Touboul P, Huerta F, Porte J et al: Bases electrophysiologiques de l'action antiarrhythmnique de l'amiodarone chez l'homme. Arch Mal Coeur 69:845, 1976
228. Cabasson J, Puech P, Mellet JM et al: Analyse des effets electrophysiologiques de l'amiodarone par l'enregistrement simultane des potentiels d'action monophasiques et du faisceau de His. Arch Mal Coeur 69:691, 1976
229. Coulte R, Fontaine G, Franks R: Etude electrocardiologique des effets de l'amiodarone sur la conduction introcardiaque chez l'homme. Ann Cardiol Angiol (Paris) 18:543, 1977
230. Rosenbaum MB, Chiale PA, Ryba D et al: Control of tachyarrhythmias associated with Wolff-Parkinson-White syndrome by amiodarone hydrochloride. Am J Cardiol 34:215, 1974
231. Wellens HJJ, Lie KI, Bar FW et al: Effect of amiodarone in the Wolff-Parkinson-White syndrome. Am J Cardiol 38:189, 1976
232. Rowland E, Krikler DM: Electrophysiological assessment of amiodarone in treatment of resistant supraventricular arrhythmias. Br Heart J 44:82, 1980
233. Rasmussen V, Berning J: Effect of amiodarone in the Wolff-Parkinson-White syndrome. Acta Med Scand 205:31, 1979
234. Petta JM, Zaccheo VJ: Comparative profile of L3428 and other antianginal agents on cardiac hemodynamics. J Pharmacol Exp Ther 176:328, 1971
235. Cote P, Bourassa MG, Delaye J et al: Effects of amiodarone on cardiac and coronary hemodynamics and on myocardial metabolism in patients with coronary artery disease. Circulation 59:1165, 1979
236. Haas H, Hartfelder G: Alpha-Isopropyl-alpha(N-methyl-N-homoveratryl-alpha-amino propyl)-3-4-dimethoxyphyenyl acetonstrol, eine Substanz mit Coronasgefass-Eigenschaften. Arzneimittelforsch 11:1408, 1968
237. Nayler WG, McInnes I, Swann JP et al: Some effects of iproveratril (isoptin) on the cardiovascular system. J Pharmacol Exp Ther 161:247, 1968
238. Fleckenstein A, Doring HJ, Kammermaier H: Einfluss von beta-receptor Entblocker und verwandten Substanzen auf Erregung, Kontraktion und Energiestoffwechsel des Myokordifasers. Klin Wochenschr 46:343, 1968
239. Rosen MR, Ilvento JP, Gelband H et al: Effects of verapamil on electrophysiologic properties of canine Purkinje fibers. J Pharmacol Exp Ther 189:414, 1974
240. Wit AL, Cranefield P: Effect of verapamil on the sinoatrial and atrioventricular nodes of the rabbit and the mechanism by which it arrests reentrant atrioventricular nodal tachycardia. Circ Res 35:413, 1974
241. Cranefield PF, Aronson RS, Wit AL: Effect of verapamil on the normal action potential and on a calcium-dependent slow response of canine Purkinje fibers. Circ Res 34:204, 1974
242. Bayer R, Kalusche D, Kaufmann R et al: Inotropic and electrophysiological actions of verapamil and D600 in mammalian myocardium. III. Effects of the

243. Danilo P Jr, Hordof AJ, Reder RF et al: Effects of verapamil on electrophysiologic properties of blood superfused cardiac Purkinje fibers. J Pharmacol Exp Ther 213:222, 1980
244. Kohlhardt M, Bauer B, Krause H et al: Differentiation of the transmembrane Na + Ca channels in mammalian cardiac fibers by the use of specific inhibitors. Pflugers Arch 335:309, 1972
245. Kohlhardt M, Muich Z: Studies on the inhibitory effect of verapamil on the slow inward current in mammalian-ventricular myocardium. M Mol Cell Cardiol 10:1037, 1978
246. Gettes LS, Saito T: Effect of antiarrhythmic drugs on the slow inward current system. In Zipes DP, Bailey JC, Elharrar V (eds): The Slow Inward Current and Cardiac Arrhythmias, p 455. The Hague, Martinus Nijhoff, 1980
247. Wit AL, Wiggins JR, Cranefield PF: Some effects of electrical stimulation on impulse initiation in cardiac fibers: Its relevance for the determination of the mechanism of clinical cardiac arrhythmias. In Wellens HHJ, Lie KI, Janse M (eds): The Conduction System of the Heart: Structure, Function and Clinical Implications, p 163. Philadelphia, Lea and Febiger, 1976
248. Wit AL, Cranefield PF: Triggered and automatic activity in the canine coronary sinus. Circ Res 41:435, 1977
249. Angus JA, Richmond DR, Dhumma-Upakorn LB et al: Cardiovascular action of verapamil in the dog with particular reference to myocardial contractility + atrioventricular conduction. Cardiovasc Res 10:623, 1976
250. Neuss H, Schlepper M: Der Einfluss von Verapamil auf die atrioventrikulare Uberleitung, Lokalisation des Wirkungsortes mit His Bundel Elektrogrammen. Verh Dtsch Ges Herz Kreislaufforsch 37:433, 1971
251. Kriklr DM, Spurrell RAJ: Verapamil in the treatment of paroxysmal supraventricular tachycardia. Postgrad Med J 50:447, 1974
252. Huisiani MH, Klvasnicka J, Ryden L et al: Action of verapamil on sinus node, atrioventricular and intraventricular conduction. Br Heart J 35:734, 1973
253. Wellens HJJ, Tan SL, Bar FWH et al: Effect of verapamil studied by programmed electrical stimulation of the heart in patients with paroxysmal reentrant SVT. Br Heart J 39:1058, 1977
254. Roy PR, Spurrell RAJ, Sowton E: The effect of verapamil on the cardiac conduction system in man. Postgrad Med J 50:270, 1974
255. Nayler WG, Szeto J: Effect of verapamil on contractility, oxygen utilization and calcium exchange ability to mammalian heart muscle. Cardiovasc Res 6:120, 1972
256. Smith HJ, Goldstein RA, Griffith JM et al: Regional contractility: Selective depression of ischemic myocardium by verapamil. Circulation 54:629, 1976
257. Haeusler G: Differential effect of verapamil on excitation conduction coupling in smooth muscle and on excitation secretion coupling in adrenergic terminals. J Pharmacol Exp Ther 180:672, 1972
258. Baky SH, Kirsten EB: Verapamil. In Goldberg ME (ed): Pharmacological and Biochemical Properties of Drug Substances. Washington, American Pharmaceutical Association, Academy of Pharmaceutical Science, 1981
259. Davis LD, Temte JV: Effects of propranolol on the transmembrane potentials of ventricular muscle and Purkinje fibers in the dog. Circ Res 22:661, 1968
260. Pitt WA, Cox AR: The effect of the beta-adrenergic antagonist propranolol on rabbit atrial cells with the use of the ultramicroelectrode technique. Am Heart J 76:242, 1968
261. Papp JG, Vaughan Williams SM: A comparison of the antiarrhythmic action of 1C1 50172 and (−) propranolol and their effects on intracellular cardiac action potentials and other features of cardiac function. Br J Pharmacol 36:391, 1969
262. Koerpel BJ, Davis LD: Effects of lidocaine, propranolol and sotalol on ouabain-induced changes in transmembrane potential of canine Purkinje fibers. Circ Res 30:681, 1972
263. Hewett K, Rosen MR: Beta adrenergic modulation of delayed afterdepolarizations. Am J Cardiol 49:913, 1982
264. Wit AL, Hoffman BF, Rosen MR: Electrophysiology and pharmacology of cardiac arrhythmias. IX. Cardiac electrophysiologic effects of beta adrenergic receptor stimulation and blockade. Part C. Am Heart J 90:795, 1975
265. Gibson D, Sowton E: The use of beta-adrenergic receptor blocking drugs in dysrhythmias. Prog Cardiovasc Dis 12:16, 1969

Certain of the studies referred to were supported by USPHS-NHLBI grants HL-28958, HL-28223, and 5-KO4-HL-00853.

Use of Antiarrhythmic Drugs: General Principles

Kelley P. Anderson • Roger A. Freedman
Jay W. Mason

Despite substantial progress in the understanding of mechanisms of antiarrhythmic drugs, it is not yet possible to select a drug on the basis of known actions on known mechanisms of specific arrhythmias. Currently, therefore, antiarrhythmic drug therapy is largely empiric, and several drug trials are often necessary before an effective agent can be identified. A systematic approach to arrhythmia management is needed to distinguish efficiently and unequivocally effective and ineffective drugs. In advance of therapy, the clinician should define (1) the goals of therapy (*e.g.*, reduction of palpitations, elimination of syncope, prevention of sudden death); (2) the target arrhythmia (*e.g.*, atrial premature beats, ventricular premature beats, ventricular tachycardia induced by programmed stimulation); (3) the method to be used to evaluate medications (*e.g.*, patient's symptoms, ambulatory electrocardiographic monitoring, electrophysiologic testing); and (4) the criteria to be used to define drug success (*e.g.*, 80% reduction in ventricular premature beats, failure to induce supraventricular tachycardia). A drug is usually considered a failure when it does not adequately suppress or prevent the target arrhythmia despite plasma concentrations or doses well within the therapeutic range or when it causes unacceptable adverse reactions.

PHARMACOKINETICS OF ANTIARRHYTHMIC DRUGS

The effects of an antiarrhythmic drug are assumed to be related to its concentration at the effector site. This concentration cannot be directly measured, but for most antiarrhythmic agents the concentration at the effector site is related to the plasma concentration, which often can be measured. Both plasma and effector site concentrations are governed by the pharmacokinetics of a particular drug in an individual patient. This topic is covered in detail elsewhere in this volume, but a few pertinent aspects will be discussed here. The basic determinants of the plasma concentration of a given drug are its bioavailability, volume of distribution, and clearance.

BIOAVAILABILITY

Bioavailability is the fraction of unchanged drug reaching the systemic circulation. Some antiarrhythmic drugs are given intravenously, which achieves maximum bioavailability. Oral administration reduces the bioavailability of antiarrhythmic medications primarily by incomplete intestinal absorption or by liver extraction from the splanchnic circulation. Bretylium is an example of an antiarrhythmic drug that cannot practically be used orally because of limited and erratic intestinal absorption. Lidocaine, on the other hand, is well absorbed but is subject to extensive first-pass liver metabolism, which produces metabolites with central nervous system toxicity but little antiarrhythmic activity.[1] Bioavailability may be affected by disease. The absorption of several antiarrhythmic drugs is unpredictable and erratic in acute myocardial infarction, perhaps because of changing splanchnic blood flow or because of alterations in intestinal motility caused by narcotics.[2] Hepatic extraction can be reduced by liver disease, causing increased bioavailability. Importantly, small changes in bioavailability of drugs with low bioavailability can result in large changes in the amount of drug reaching the circulation. For instance, if the amount of drug extracted changes from 95% to 90%, the amount of drug entering the circulation will double.

VOLUME OF DISTRIBUTION

The volume of distribution (V) is a proportionality constant that relates the amount of drug in the body (A) with the plasma or blood concentration (C): $V = A/C$. It is the volume of plasma or blood that it would take to dissolve the amount of drug in the body to give the measured concentration. It is called an apparent volume because it does not describe an actual space. Nevertheless, it is a useful concept because it can be used to estimate the amount of drug needed to obtain a certain plasma concentration. Some disease states may alter the volume of distribution, causing changes in the plasma concentration.[2] Acute myocardial infarction and congestive heart failure reduce the volume of distribution for lidocaine and may cause unexpected elevation of the plasma levels.[3]

CLEARANCE

Clearance (Cl) relates the rate of elimination (E) and the plasma (or blood) concentration (C): $Cl = E/C$. Clearance indicates the rate at which plasma is cleared of drug and is usually expressed in milliliters per minute. For most antiarrhythmic drugs, the rate of elimination is directly proportional to the concentration, so that the clearance is constant over the range of plasma concentrations. Drugs such as phenytoin exhibit saturable elimination, so that the rate of elimination is concentration dependent.

The elimination of most antiarrhythmic drugs occurs by renal excretion or by hepatic biotransformation. Renal disease, hepatic disease, or disorders causing decreased perfusion of these organs may markedly increase plasma drug concentrations. Other drugs may also affect elimination; for example, propranolol and cimetidine reduce hepatic flow and increase lidocaine levels.

HALF-LIFE

In a one-compartment model, drug disposition is assumed to be instantaneous into a single, homogeneous compartment with a size equal to the volume of distribution. A constant fraction of drug is assumed to be eliminated per unit time, so-called first-order kinetics. The half-life ($t_{1/2}$) is the time required to remove one half of the amount of drug in the body and is an expression of the relation between the volume of distribution (Vd) and clearance (Cl):

$$t_{1/2} = 0.693(Vd/Cl)$$

Elimination of drugs with first-order kinetics follows an exponential curve. The constant 0.693 is obtained from the natural logarithm of one-half. It can be seen from the above equation that the half-life alone cannot completely describe drug disposition. For instance, in congestive heart failure the volume of distribution and clearance of lidocaine decrease by similar proportions, so the half-life remains unchanged. However, the infusion rate needed to maintain a therapeutic concentration depends on the clearance and must be reduced in order to avoid toxic levels.[3,4] The half-life of a drug is very useful for estimating the time it will take to reach steady-state conditions after initiating therapy or after changing the dose. Assuming a constant dose and frequency of administration, this time interval is approximately four times the half-life.

MODELS OF DRUG DISPOSITION

The one-compartment model mentioned above does not adequately explain the behavior of all drugs. Instead of one homogeneous compartment in which drug distribution occurs rapidly relative to drug elimination, a two-compartment model assumes the presence of a central compartment and a peripheral compartment. Drug absorption and elimination occur via the central compartment, and elimination follows first-order kinetics. Instead of instantaneous distribution as occurs in the one-compartment model, drug passes slowly from the central compartment into the peripheral compartment along an exponential curve characteristic for that drug. Drug molecules must pass back into the central compartment before elimination can occur. Two half-lives describe this process: the distribution or α-half-life describes movement from the central to the peripheral compartment, and the elimination or β-half-life reflects drug clearance.

The pharmacokinetic behavior of some drugs cannot be modeled using just one or two compartments. A drug may distribute differently in each of several organs and tissues. Multicompartment models are needed for such drugs. Furthermore, distribution between compartments and elimination from compartments are not necessarily exponential, so that more complicated mathematical descriptions are necessary.

PLASMA CONCENTRATION

The increasing sophistication of models of drug distribution has not eliminated the need for determining plasma concentrations of antiarrhythmic drugs. The reason for this is that most antiarrhythmic medications have relatively small therapeutic to toxic ranges, and many patients with heart disease have abnormalities in absorption, distribution, and elimination that may have unpredictable effects on the pharmacokinetic behavior of a drug. Moreover, several factors may alter the relation between the effects of antiarrhythmic drugs and the measured plasma concentration.

PROTEIN BINDING

Clinical laboratories measure total plasma concentrations, that is, drug bound to plasma proteins plus free (unbound) drug, whereas only free drug concentration is in equilibrium with the concentration at the cellular effector site. Usually, the total plasma level parallels the concentration of free drug; however, this may not be the case when (1) the extent of protein binding varies from patient to patient (e.g., quinidine); (2) the extent of protein binding changes in certain disease states (e.g., lidocaine in acute myocardial infarction); (3) the proportion of protein-bound drug changes with drug concentration (e.g., disopyramide); and (4) the degree of protein binding is high, so that small changes in binding cause large changes in the unbound drug (e.g., phenytoin).

DOSING HISTORY

The plasma concentration must be interpreted in light of the patient's dosing history. Plasma drug levels should be measured after steady-state concentrations are reached, just before the next regularly scheduled dose so that the minimum (trough) levels are measured. Plasma levels may also be useful at times of suspected drug toxicity or at the time of arrhythmia recurrence.

METABOLITES

The presence of metabolites may confound the relation between plasma concentration and drug effects. Metabolites may have no effects, effects (cardiac or noncardiac) similar to those of the parent drug, or different effects. Also, metabolite accumulation may vary between patients. Unmeasured active metabolites can cause toxic effects despite "therapeutic" levels of the parent compound. Active metabolites may have different kinetics than the parent compound and result in therapeutic or toxic effects after the plasma level of the parent compound has diminished.

INTERACTIONS OF ANTIARRHYTHMIC DRUGS

Antiarrhythmic drugs interact in important ways with other medications. Pharmacokinetic interactions refer to those that alter the concentration of the antiarrhythmic drug at the active site but do not alter the relationship between effect of the drug and its concentration. Pharmacokinetic interactions may be caused by changes in absorption, distribution, metabolism, or clearance. Interactions in which the response of an antiarrhythmic drug is changed without altering its concentration are termed *pharmacodynamic*. Pharmacodynamic interactions may involve inhibition (antagonism) or augmentation (summation or potentiation). An antiarrhythmic medication may have numerous effects, each of which could be affected differently by another drug. Some drug interactions involve both pharmacokinetic and pharmacodynamic processes. Many of the known interactions that occur with antiarrhythmic drugs are listed in Table 42.1.

PHARMACOKINETIC INTERACTIONS

ABSORPTION

The absorption of antiarrhythmic drugs may be altered by changes in intestinal motility, pH, and intestinal flora or by the formation of insoluble complexes.[5] Antacids and cholestyramine decrease the absorption of digitalis by forming insoluble complexes. Sodium bicarbonate will increase the un-ionized portion of weak bases such as quinidine, procainamide, and disopyramide and cause increased gastric absorption. Other antacids cause increased gastric motility, which may cause more rapid absorption of these weak bases that are absorbed primarily in the small intestine. A fraction of digoxin is metabolized by intestinal bacteria. Antibiotic therapy may increase the amount of digoxin absorbed.[5]

DISTRIBUTION

Several antiarrhythmic drugs are highly bound to serum proteins or nonreceptor tissues. Phenylbutazone may displace digitoxin from protein binding sites and increase its concentration at effector sites.[5] Quinidine may increase digoxin levels in part by displacing it from nonreceptor binding sites.[6] Disease states may affect the amount of protein available for binding or result in the production of substances that compete for binding sites.

METABOLISM

Reduction of hepatic blood flow by drugs or other factors may reduce metabolism of drugs such as propranolol and lidocaine. The addition of drugs such as isoniazid, chloramphenicol, dicumarol, and cimetidine increases the concentration of phenytoin by competing for metabolic enzymes. Phenothiazines and oral contraceptive agents may decrease the metabolism of imipramine. Drugs such as phenobarbital, phenytoin, and rifampin may increase the metabolic activity of certain enzyme systems that will reduce concentrations of antiarrhythmic agents such as disopyramide, quinidine, and imipramine.[5]

EXCRETION

The concentrations of digoxin, disopyramide, and procainamide may be increased by agents that decrease renal blood flow. Quinidine, verapamil, and spironolactone reduce digoxin clearance by interfering with active tubular secretion. Medications that increase the pH of the urine, for example, diuretics (furosemide, thiazides, and acetazolamide), may increase reabsorption of weak bases such as quinidine, procainamide, disopyramide, and mexiletine.[5]

PHARMACODYNAMIC INTERACTIONS

INHIBITION

Inhibition of a drug response may occur as a result of competition by an agonist and an antagonist for an active site. An obvious example is inhibition of catecholamines by β-adrenergic blocking agents. Quinidine and disopyramide block muscarinic receptors, which facilitates atrioventricular node conduction and causes some of the unpleasant side effects associated with these medications.[7] Pyridostigmine, which impairs acetylcholinesterase, increases the concentration of acetylcholine competing for the muscarinic receptors and inhibits the anticholinergic effects of these antiarrhythmic agents.[8] Digoxin increases vagus nerve activity, which increases the concentration of acetylcholine available to compete with muscarinic blockers. This interaction is frequently used to counteract the tendency for quinidine and disopyramide to increase the ventricular rate response during treatment of atrial tachyarrhythmias. Verapamil interferes with calcium ion transport across cell membranes. The administration of calcium salts can be used to inhibit the hypotensive effects of verapamil.[9,10] Interestingly, calcium administration does not reduce the electrophysiologic effects of verapamil and may actually enhance them.[9,11]

An important theory postulates a common receptor site for antiarrhythmic drugs with sodium channel blocking activity.[12] This raises the possibility of competitive interactions at this site. For instance, bupivacaine is a local anesthetic with sodium channel blocking activity that

TABLE 42.1 ANTIARRHYTHMIC DRUG INTERACTION

Antiarrhythmic Drug	Interacting Drug	Type of Interaction*	Effect†	Mechanism
Bretylium	Digitalis	A	↑ Digitalis toxicity	↑ Catecholamines
	Norepinephrine	A	↑ Norepinephrine effect	?↑ Sensitivity
	Phenylephrine	A	↑ Phenylephrine effect	?↑ Sensitivity
	Quinidine	A	↓ Antiarrhythmic effect	?
	Tricyclic antidepressants	I	↓ Vasodilation	↓ Neuronal uptake
	Vasodilators	A	↑ Vasodilation	Additive
Disopyramide	Digoxin	I	↓ Vagolytic effect	
	Myocardial depressants	A	↓ Contractility	Additive
	Pyridostigmine	I	↓ Anticholinergic effect	↓ Muscarinic blockade
	Phenytoin	C	↓ Concentration	↑ Metabolism
	Rifampin	C		↑ Metabolism
	Tocainide	A	↑ Antiarrhythmic effect	↑ Sodium channel block
	Verapamil	A	Sinus arrest	?
Lidocaine	Cimetidine	C	↑ Concentration	↓ Hepatic flow or uptake
	Metoprolol	C	↑ Concentration	↓ Hepatic flow or uptake
	Propranolol	C	↑ Concentration	↓ Hepatic flow or uptake
	Smoking	C	↓ Unbound concentration	↑ Protein binding
Magnesium sulfate	Aminoglycosides	A	↑ Neuromuscular effects	?
	Calcium chloride	I	↓ Neuromuscular effects	?
Phenytoin	Alcohol	C	↓ Concentration	↑ Metabolism
	Aspirin	C	↑ Concentration	↓ Protein binding
	Cimetidine	C	↑ Concentration	↓ Clearance
	Oral contraceptives	C	↑ Concentration	?
	Phenobarbital	C	↓ Concentration	↑ Metabolism
Procainamide	Alcohol	C	↓ Concentration	↑ Hepatic clearance
	Aminoglycosides	A	↑ Neuromuscular effects	?
	Cimetidine	C	↑ Concentration	↓ Renal clearance
Quinidine	Amiodarone	A	↑ Proarrhythmic effect	?↑ QT
	Digoxin	C	↑ Digoxin concentration	↓ Renal clearance and tissue binding of digoxin
	Dieuretics	C	↑ Concentration	↓ Renal clearance
	Phenobarbital	C	↓ Concentration	↑ Metabolism
	Phenytoin	C	↓ Concentration	↑ Metabolism
	Skeletal muscle relaxant	A	↑ Neuromuscular effect	?
	Warfarin	?	↑ Anticoagulation	?

* A, augmentation; I, inhibition, C, change in concentration.

† Refers to effect on antiarrhythmic drug unless otherwise stated.

(Compiled from references cited in the text and data from Griffin JP, D'Arcy PF: A Manual of Adverse Drug Interactions. Bristol, Wright, 1984)

causes serious arrhythmias and myocardial dysfunction when excessive amounts reach the systemic circulation. Bupivacaine's high affinity for sodium channels and its slow dissociation rate may be partly responsible for its toxicity. Lidocaine, which dissociates rapidly from the sodium channel permitting recovery at normal heart rates, competes for sodium channels and has been shown to reduce the sodium channel blocking actions of bupivacaine *in vitro*.[13] This is presumably the mechanism by which lidocaine exerts a therapeutic effect on ventricular arrhythmias caused by toxic doses of propafenone, an investigational sodium channel blocking drug.[14] Certain antiarrhythmic drugs with sodium channel blocking properties resembling those of bupivacaine (*e.g.*, amiodarone),[15] may also be subject to competitive inhibition. Although further investigations will be needed to assess the efficacy and safety of this approach, this concept may prove useful for treating some toxic reactions of antiarrhythmic therapy. Also, in theory, the empiric combination of certain antiarrhythmic drugs should result in *reduced* antiarrhythmic action.

Other inhibitory interactions involve noncompetitive or unknown mechanisms. Prostigmine and other tricyclic antidepressants block neuronal uptake of bretylium and reduce its hypotensive effects.[16] Phenytoin and lidocaine sometimes eliminate digitalis-toxic arrhythmias.

AUGMENTATION

Most augmentation interactions that involve antiarrhythmic drugs are undesirable. Antiarrhythmic agents cause vasodilation (quinidine, procainamide, verapamil), reduce contractility (disopyramide, procainamide, verapamil), and block reflex sympathetic activity (β-adrenergic blockers, bretylium). Combinations of these medications or concomitant use of cardiovascular drugs with similar properties can result in serious hypotension or myocardial dysfunction, especially in patients with limited cardiovascular reserve. Most antiarrhythmic drugs affect sinus node automaticity and atrioventricular conduction. Drug combinations may enhance these effects, causing sinus arrest or heart block. Primarily at risk are patients with preexisting sinus node dysfunction or conduction disturbances. Augmentation of proarrhythmic effects have been reported.[17-19]

Relatively little information exists concerning augmentation of antiarrhythmic effect by combinations of antiarrhythmic drugs. A few investigations have addressed the usefulness of drug combinations in patients undergoing electrophysiologic study for ventricular arrhythmias. Ross and co-workers retrospectively examined the benefit of administering two antiarrhythmic agents for preventing arrhythmia induction in patients with ventricular tachycardia.[20] The individual drugs were ineffective. Lidocaine in combination with quinidine was effective in 3% of the trials and with procainamide in 5% and was not effective with encainide. Similarly, another group reported little additional benefit with the combination of mexiletine and disopyramide.[21] However, Greenspan and associates reported that the combination of mexiletine with quinidine or procainamide prevented arrhythmia induction in 8 of 23 patients with ventricular tachycardia.[22] In another study, intravenous procainamide was added to quinidine or disopyramide at electrophysiologic study in patients with ventricular tachycardia. Ventricular tachycardia remained inducible in all patients and could be induced using a less vigorous stimulation protocol in most patients.[23]

Somewhat better results have been obtained in patients treated for ventricular ectopic activity. Duff and colleagues found the combination of mexiletine and quinidine to be very effective in patients with ventricular ectopic activity who did not respond to either agent alone.[24] Furthermore, this combination permitted lower doses of each drug, resulting in fewer adverse reactions. Similar observations have been made using the combination of procainamide and quinidine.[25]

In general, we believe the concomitant administration of drugs with similar properties (*e.g.*, quinidine plus disopyramide or procainamide, flecainide plus encainide) should be performed cautiously because of increased risk of adverse reactions, unpredictable interactions, and lack of evidence of benefit.

COMPLICATIONS OF ANTIARRHYTHMIC DRUGS

Antiarrhythmic drugs are associated with a wide variety of adverse reactions. The most important reactions are peripheral vasodilation, decreased contractility, depression of normal automaticity, conduction disturbances, and proarrhythmic effects.

HEMODYNAMIC COMPLICATIONS
VASCULAR RESISTANCE

Quinidine, procainamide, phenytoin, verapamil, bretylium, and amiodarone decrease peripheral vascular resistance. This effect is usually enhanced during rapid intravenous administration except in the case of bretylium, which may cause hypertension initially. Disopyramide and tocainide cause vasoconstriction,[26] but this rarely results in serious consequences.

CONTRACTILITY

Disopyramide and verapamil have prominent negative inotropic activity. β-Adrenergic blocking agents may reduce left ventricular function in patients dependent on sympathetic activity for support of a failing heart. In addition, these agents and bretylium may impair reflex sympathetic activity. Quinidine, procainamide, and phenytoin mildly depress contractility, but these effects are not apparent at usual doses. However, with high doses and in patients with severe left ventricular dysfunction, any of the antiarrhythmic drugs may cause significant hemodynamic embarrassment. Amiodarone also exerts negative inotropic effects, but concomitant peripheral vasodilatation prevents deterioration of left ventricular pump function.

ARRHYTHMIC COMPLICATIONS
NORMAL AUTOMATICITY

Almost all antiarrhythmic agents depress sinus node or subsidiary pacemaker automaticity (Fig. 42.1). Other drug-related effects such as anticholinergic activity or vasodilation and reflex stimulation may inhibit the direct effect. Serious bradyarrhythmias are rarely a problem, but patients with sinus node dysfunction should be observed carefully during the initiation of antiarrhythmic therapy, and antiarrhythmic agents should be prime suspects in patients who develop abnormalities of sinus node function.

CONDUCTION

Several antiarrhythmic medications alter conduction. Digoxin and verapamil slow conduction in the atrioventricular node but have little impact on atrial and ventricular tissue, although they may facilitate conduction through an accessory atrioventricular connection. Flecainide, encainide, and amiodarone profoundly depress conduction in atrial, nodal, and ventricular tissue. Quinidine, procainamide, and disopyramide also reduce conduction in most cardiac tissues, although simultaneous anticholinergic effects mask the change in atrioventricular node conduction. Lidocaine and tocainide have little effect on conduction at normal heart rates but at rapid heart rates slow conduction in ventricular tissue. Other sodium channel blockers also exhibit rate-dependent effects on conduction. Although there is a potential for precipitating complete heart block with many antiarrhythmic drugs, in practice this rarely occurs at the usual doses even in patients with preexisting conduction disturbances. Nevertheless, patients with evidence of conduction abnormalities should receive gradual dose increments and close observation.

PROARRHYTHMIC EFFECTS

All antiarrhythmic drugs have a potential for precipitating or exacerbating serious ventricular tachyarrhythmias and are responsible for a small but significant fraction of patients who die suddenly.[27] Several types of proarrhythmic responses have been described. A fourfold increase in the frequency of ventricular premature beats or a tenfold increase in repetitive forms without the development of sustained arrhythmias was reported in 5% of drug trials for treatment of ventricular arrhythmias.[28] This complication may be seen with any antiarrhythmic drug but does not contraindicate the use of another antiarrhythmic drug in the same class or subclass.[28]

Another form of arrhythmia exacerbation is an increased frequency of recurrent, sustained ventricular tachycardia. The arrhythmia is similar in morphology to the ventricular tachycardia present before therapy, although the rate is often slower. It is sometimes difficult to distinguish this proarrhythmic effect from drug ineffectiveness and spontaneous recurrence of the arrhythmia. If the arrhythmia does not terminate spontaneously it should be treated with nonpharmacologic means, either direct-current shock or ventricular pacing. It is usually easily controlled and does not contraindicate the use of a similar antiarrhythmic agent, although careful observation is warranted in a patient with this complication.

Sustained ventricular tachyarrhythmias may be provoked in patients without a previous history of such rhythms. This complication occurs in about 6% of drug trials in patients treated for ventricular arrhythmias. These arrhythmias are usually polymorphic and have been reported to complicate therapy with nearly every antiarrhythmic drug.[28]

The drug conversion of nonsustained to sustained ventricular tachycardia during drug testing using programmed electrical stimulation is another type of proarrhythmic effect. A series of patients with this complication developed sustained ventricular tachyarrhythmias, although only nonsustained ventricular tachycardia was inducible before drugs were given.[29] The sustained arrhythmias induced during drug therapy were morphologically similar to the induced nonsustained rhythms and were easily terminated with countershock or rapid pacing. The culprit drugs in this series included amiodarone, disopyramide, encainide, and quinidine.

Torsade de pointes is a form of polymorphic ventricular tachycardia associated with a long QT interval with features and response to therapy that may distinguish it from other arrhythmias.[17,30] It occurs primarily as a complication of therapy with quinidine, disopyramide, or procainamide but is also seen with other drugs, including those that do not normally prolong the QT interval.[17,30] It is associated with other conditions such as hypokalemia and hypomagnesemia. No risk factors reliably identify susceptible patients, although preexisting QT interval prolongation is often present.[31] This reaction usually occurs in the first week after initiation of therapy,[30,31] and plasma drug levels are usually within the usual therapeutic range. Torsade de pointes may also occur spontaneously after several years of therapy, although a precipitating factor can be identified in some cases such as an increased dose, the addition of another antiarrhythmic medication, or the development of hypokalemia or hypomagnesemia. The arrhythmia is usually preceded by a long QT interval, usually greater than 0.59 second.[17,30] The arrhythmia often begins with short bursts of polymorphic ventricular tachycardia followed by longer runs of torsade de pointes, which may terminate spontaneously or degenerate into ventricular fibrillation (Fig. 42.2). Direct-current shock is usually only transiently effective, and other antiarrhythmic drugs are rarely helpful and may exacerbate the condition. The treatment of choice is atrial or ventricular pacing at 90 to 150 beats per minute, which almost always dramatically inhibits the arrhythmia. Magnesium sulfate has been successfully used,[32] although it is not certain if it has usefulness beyond correction of magnesium deficiency. Isoproterenol has also been reported to be effective in some cases,[17] but therapy with this drug should only be attempted if emergency pacing is unavailable.

A more refractory drug-induced ventricular tachyarrhythmia has been encountered during therapy with encainide,[33] flecainide,[34] amiodarone,[35] pirmenol, and propafenone.[36] The configurations of the arrhythmia include ventricular flutter, polymorphic ventricular tachycardia, and monomorphic ventricular tachycardia, which may resemble the patient's clinical arrhythmia. The arrhythmia is often preceded by marked QRS widening, which may be rate dependent and abrupt in onset. We have observed this proarrhythmic effect during exercise testing and rapid atrial pacing in patients in whom these methods previously did not provoke arrhythmias (Fig. 42.3). It is often accompanied by marked hypotension and cardiogenic shock even with rates of ventricular tachycardia that were well tolerated before treatment. This tachyarrhythmia is remarkably resistant to direct-current shock. It may terminate transiently or fail to respond at all. Rapid pacing is rarely useful for termination or inhibition, and pharmacologic therapy is rarely fruitful, although a response to magnesium sulfate has been noted.[33] Resuscitative efforts must often be carried out for several hours until the drug concentration diminishes. Although plasma concentrations are often in the "therapeutic" range, this reaction appears to be dose related and is probably a toxic effect resulting in both the arrhythmia and myocardial dysfunction. This complication is usually seen in patients treated for recurrent, sustained ventricular tachyarrhythmias. It occurs less frequently in patients treated for ventricular ectopic activity and is rarely seen in healthy subjects without ventricular arrhythmias receiving the drugs in research protocols.[33]

INDIVIDUAL ANTIARRHYTHMIC DRUGS

Approved medications (Table 42.2) will be discussed here. The mechanisms of antiarrhythmic drugs and characteristics of new antiarrhythmic agents are discussed elsewhere in this volume.

SODIUM CHANNEL BLOCKING DRUGS
DISOPYRAMIDE
Disopyramide is available in the United States in the oral form only and is approved for the treatment of ventricular arrhythmias. It is also effective for atrial arrhythmias, arrhythmias using accessory atrioventricular connections, and atrioventricular nodal reentrant tachycar-

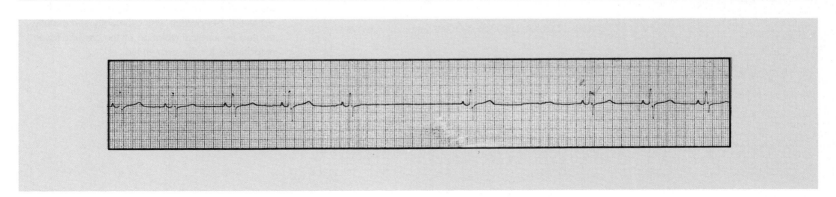

FIGURE 42.1 Sinus pauses (type II second-degree sinoatrial block) developed in this patient treated with procainamide. This rhythm disturbance disappeared after discontinuation of the procainamide.

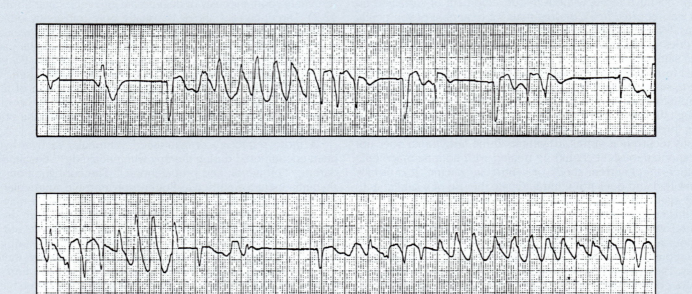

FIGURE 42.2 Rhythm strip obtained from a woman treated with procainamide for a four-beat run of wide QRS complex tachycardia that occurred during an exercise treadmill test. The top recording of polymorphic ventricular tachycardia was recorded after the patient complained of a syncopal episode that occurred approximately 1 year after the initiation of therapy. The patient was treated with intravenous procainamide and developed longer runs of polymorphic ventricular tachycardia that deteriorated into ventricular fibrillation. Numerous other antiarrhythmic drugs were administered without improving the arrhythmia. Finally, ventricular pacing was initiated, which completely suppressed the arrhythmia. After discontinuation of all antiarrhythmic drugs, programmed stimulation was performed, which failed to induce a ventricular arrhythmia. The patient was discharged on no medications and has had no further recurrences.

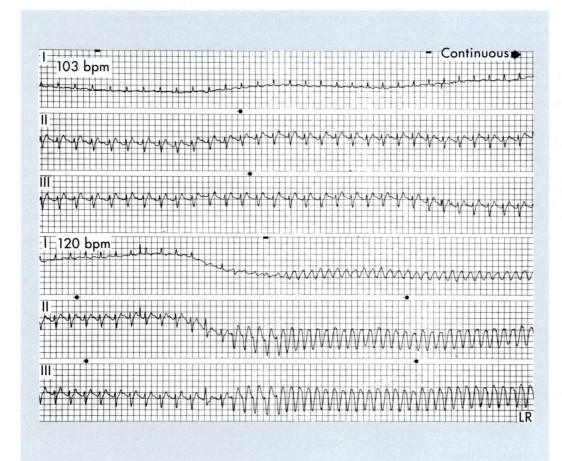

FIGURE 42.3 This tracing was obtained from a patient treated with flecainide, 200 mg twice a day, for recurrent ventricular tachycardia that had not responded to several antiarrhythmic agents, including amiodarone. The patient had moderate left ventricular dysfunction. In the lower panel obtained during exercise, sinus tachycardia developed into ventricular tachycardia that caused marked hypotension in this patient. The patient's clinical ventricular tachycardia had a different morphology and did not result in immediate hypotension. Although the arrhythmia could be terminated with direct-current cardioversion, sinus tachycardia was followed in several seconds by resumption of the above arrhythmia. Lidocaine and ventricular pacing failed to suppress the arrhythmia. After several hours of cardiopulmonary resuscitation, sustained sinus rhythm was finally achieved. The patient was eventually successfully treated by surgical ablation of the cardiac tissue responsible for the arrhythmia.

dias.[37,38] When the drug is used against atrial arrhythmias, concurrent therapy with digoxin may be warranted to inhibit disopyramide's vagolytic effects. Disopyramide does not appear to affect digoxin concentration.[39] Disopyramide has been shown to exacerbate sinus node dysfunction and should be used cautiously in patients with this disorder.[37] In addition, the combination of disopyramide and verapamil has been shown to have a strong depressant action on sinus node function.[40] Disopyramide depresses conduction and can cause complete heart block in patients with severe conduction system disease,[41] but the data suggest this occurs rarely and that it may be safely administered to patients with first- and second-degree type I atrioventricular block and bundle branch block.[37] Disopyramide may cause polymorphic ventricular tachycardia and ventricular fibrillation associated with QT interval prolongation. This effect may occur with plasma concentrations in the therapeutic range and often occurs within the first 10 days of treatment.[37]

Disopyramide has a prominent negative inotropic effect and a peripheral vasoconstrictive effect.[42] It should be used cautiously in patients with mild ventricular dysfunction and should be avoided in patients with severe myocardial dysfunction. On the other hand, the negative inotropic effects may be useful for treating arrhythmias in patients with hypertrophic obstructive cardiomyopathy in whom disopyramide has been shown to have a beneficial hemodynamic effect.[43]

Other than the hemodynamic effects, the side effects associated with disopyramide are largely related to its anticholinergic actions and include partial or complete urinary obstruction, especially in patients with prostatism; dry mouth; blurred vision; headaches; and abdominal distress. The use of pyridostigmine, an anticholinesterase inhibitor, has been proposed to relieve some of these side effects.[8]

The usual daily dosage is 400 mg to 800 mg in three or four divided doses. Therapy may be initiated by a loading dose of 200 mg to 300 mg. The therapeutic level is 2 μg to 5 μg/ml, and the half-life is 7.3 hours (range of 4 to 10 hours).[39] The fraction of protein-bound drug is 40% to 70% in the therapeutic range and is inversely proportional to the plasma concentration. Protein binding is primarily to α_1-acid glycoprotein, which may fluctuate substantially during disease. The fraction of disopyramide bound to protein may increase 30% during the first week after myocardial infarction and remain higher than control levels for several weeks.[44] Fluctuations in the unbound fraction can result in changes in antiarrhythmic and toxic effects without alterations in dose or plasma level. The mono-N-dealkylated metabolite of disopyramide does not have significant antiarrhythmic activity and does not normally accumulate, although it may have greater anticholinergic effects than the parent compound.[39] Excretion is principally renal so that the dose should be adjusted in patients with renal failure.

LIDOCAINE

Lidocaine is approved for parenteral treatment of ventricular arrhythmias. Oral use is precluded by first-pass hepatic degradation. Lidocaine is effective against ventricular tachyarrhythmias associated with acute myocardial infarction and may be used prophylactically in this circumstance. It is rarely effective in patients with chronic, recurrent ventricular arrhythmias and is not believed to be useful for treatment of atrial arrhythmias. Lidocaine may be used to slow conduction in accessory atrioventricular connections but has been reported to increase the ventricular rate during atrial fibrillation in patients with Wolff-Parkinson-White syndrome.[45] Lidocaine has been successfully used for treatment of atrial and ventricular arrhythmias associated with digitalis toxicity.[46]

Lidocaine has fewer proarrhythmic effects than other antiarrhythmic medications. It may rarely alter sinus node function, depress escape rhythms, and cause His-Purkinje system block.[47] It has minimal hemodynamic effects in normal doses, but excessive doses have resulted in circulatory collapse and asystole. Other adverse effects include dose-related signs of central nervous system toxicity, including tremors, tinnitus, slurred speech, dizziness, paresthesias, delirium, hallucinations, and seizures.

The intravenous loading dose is 1 mg to 2 mg/kg administered slowly, which is sometimes followed by a second bolus of half the initial dose 15 to 30 minutes later. The usual maintenance rate is 1 mg to 4 mg/min. The intramuscular dose is 300 mg to 400 mg (4 mg to 5 mg/kg), which results in therapeutic serum levels in about 15 minutes and lasts for about 90 minutes.[48,49] The therapeutic range of plasma concentrations is 2 μg to 6 μg/ml. Lidocaine is roughly 50% protein bound, largely to α_1-acid glycoprotein, an acute-phase reactant that increases after myocardial infarction among other disease states.[50] The unbound concentration of constant dose lidocaine changes little after myocardial infarction despite increased binding and total plasma concentration. The elimination half-life is 1 to 2 hours in normal subjects, and clearance is by hepatic metabolism. Smaller boluses and infusion rates should be used in patients with heart failure or hepatic disease or in older patients because of reduced volumes of distribution and hepatic clearance. Propranolol, metoprolol, and cimetidine have been shown to increase lidocaine concentrations by decreased hepatic blood flow or uptake.[51,52] Plasma concentrations also may increase during prolonged infusions (greater than 24 hours).[53] Monoethylgly-

TABLE 42.2 DOSES AND PHARMACOKINETIC PROPERTIES OF ANTIARRHYTHMIC DRUGS

Drug	Route	Usual Dose Load	Usual Dose Maintenance	Therapeutic Level (mg/ml)	Half-life (hours)	Major Elimination Route	Percent Protein Bound
Bretylium	IV	5–10 mg/kg	1–4 mg/min	0.7–1.5	13.6	Renal	<1
Disopyramide	Oral	200–300 mg	400–800 mg/day	2–4	7.3	Renal	40–70*
Lidocaine	IV	1–2 mg/kg	2–4 mg/min	2–6	1–2	Hepatic	40–80
	IM	4–5 mg/kg					
Magnesium sulfate	IV	1–3 g	15–50 mg/min	2–4			
Phenytoin	IV	10–14 mg/kg		10–18	22	Hepatic	90
	Oral	1 g	200–400 mg/day				
Procainamide	IV	10–14 mg/kg	1–6 mg/min	4–10	3–4	Hepatic	15–20
	Oral		1–4 g/day				
Quinidine	IV	6–10 mg/kg					
	Oral	600–1000 mg	1000–2000 mg/day	2–4	6	Hepatic	60–90

*Concentration dependent.

cinexylidide is an active metabolite that may accumulate significantly during lidocaine administration.[54]

PHENYTOIN

Phenytoin is not approved for use as an antiarrhythmic agent but has been shown to be effective in the treatment of children with ventricular arrhythmias[55] and of atrial and ventricular tachyarrhythmias caused by digitalis excess.[56,57] Because of its effects on cardiac sympathetic activity,[58] it has been used for patients with the idiopathic long QT interval syndrome.[59] It does not appear to be effective for supraventricular arrhythmias in general[60] and is of limited use for ventricular arrhythmias due to chronic coronary artery disease.[58,61] Because of its greater ease of use, lidocaine should be the drug of first choice for digitalis-associated arrhythmias that require treatment. Phenytoin appears to have few proarrhythmic effects. It has minimal hemodynamic effects in usual doses, but severe transient hypotension may occur with excessive rates of intravenous administration. Common adverse reactions involve dose-related central nervous system effects such as nystagmus, ataxia, delirium, and coma and features such as nausea and abdominal pain. Long-term use may cause bizarre side effects such as hyperglycemia, pseudolymphoma, drug-induced systemic lupus erythematosus, megaloblastic anemia, and gingival hyperplasia.

The intravenous dose is 10 mg to 14 mg/kg administered slowly (less than 50 mg/min). An oral loading dose of 1000 mg followed by 200 mg to 400 mg/day as a single dose is standard. The pharmacokinetics are nonlinear so that small changes in dose may result in large changes in plasma concentration. Ninety percent of the drug is protein bound. The therapeutic range is 10 μg to 18 μg/ml, and the half-life in this range is 22 hours but increases with higher doses.[4] Metabolism is hepatic and may be altered by numerous medications.

PROCAINAMIDE

Procainamide is approved for the treatment of atrial and ventricular arrhythmias and is useful for both chronic and emergent therapy of a wide spectrum of arrhythmias except those caused by sodium channel blocking agents. It is the second drug of choice after lidocaine for ventricular ectopic activity in the acute phase of myocardial infarction. Sinus node function is minimally affected normally but may be markedly affected in patients with sinus node dysfunction (see Fig. 42.1).[62] Procainamide has a direct depressant action on atrioventricular conduction, which may be partially offset by its vagolytic effect, although this anticholinergic effect is much less than that of quinidine or disopyramide.[7] It may be used for arrhythmias associated with accessory atrioventricular connections because it increases the effective refractory period of accessory pathways. It is the drug of choice for the emergent treatment of atrial tachyarrhythmias causing rapid ventricular rates due to conduction over accessory pathways and for wide complex tachycardias of uncertain etiology not caused by drugs.

Procainamide, like quinidine and disopyramide, may cause fatal ventricular tachyarrhythmias even in patients treated for atrial arrhythmias who have normal cardiac function (see Fig. 42.2). Complete heart block is possible in patients with severe His-Purkinje system disease but is rarely a problem in most patients with chronic bundle branch block. In patients with atrial tachyarrhythmias, procainamide may result in salvos of aberrantly conducted beats owing to aberration that are sometimes misdiagnosed as ventricular tachycardia. The evidence regarding the effect of procainamide on hemodynamic variables is conflicting.[42] It is reasonable to conclude that it produces a negative inotropic effect that is mild at the usual doses but that may become pronounced at high doses. Hypotension is often observed during intravenous administration. Noncardiac side effects of procainamide include gastrointestinal symptoms, central nervous system symptoms, fever, agranulocytosis, and rash. An important adverse reaction that often limits chronic use of procainamide is the systemic lupus erythematosus–like syndrome, which may be manifested by malaise, arthritis, arthralgia, or serositis. Positive responses to antinuclear antibody tests develop in 60% of patients, although the lupus-like syndrome occurs in approximately 15% of patients.[63] The likelihood of developing this complication increases with larger doses and with the duration of therapy. Patients who acetylate the compound slowly are more likely to develop this syndrome.

The intravenous loading dose is 10 mg to 14 mg/kg or 1000 mg administered slowly (less than 50 mg/min) or intermittently, preferably with continuous blood pressure monitoring and frequent electrocardiographic recordings to assess changes in QRS complex duration. Hypotension should be managed by discontinuing the infusion and by administering normal saline. The infusion can be reinitiated after the blood pressure returns to normal. QRS complex widening (greater than 25%) suggests a toxic effect. The usual maintenance infusion rate is 1 mg to 6 mg/min. Intramuscular administration is possible but offers few advantages over the oral route. The usual target plasma concentration is 4 μg to 10 μg/ml. The short half-life, 3 to 4 hours, requires frequent oral doses; 250 to 1000 mg every 4 hours. Sustained-release forms allow every 6 hours dosing (500 to 1500 mg). We have encountered patients in whom the sustained-release forms appeared to result in very high peak concentrations, causing myocardial depression and death in one case and seizures in another. Peak plasma levels should be obtained if this phenomenon is suspected. Also, patients should be warned that the drug vehicle will be excreted apparently intact (little change in color and texture). Procainamide is 15% to 20% protein bound and 50% to 70% excreted unchanged in the urine.[4,44] The rate of hepatic metabolism shows a bimodal distribution in the population with patients being either fast or slow acetylators.[4] Procainamide is metabolized in the liver to n-acetylprocainamide (NAPA), which has different electrophysiologic effects from the parent compound, and patients who respond to procainamide do not necessarily respond to NAPA.[4,64,65] The routine monitoring of NAPA concentrations has little role in the management of patients receiving procainamide,[4] but it should be performed in patients with renal failure.

QUINIDINE

Quinidine is approved for the treatment of supraventricular and ventricular arrhythmias. Its antiarrhythmic spectrum is similar to that of procainamide. Quinidine may be used safely in patients with sinus node dysfunction,[66] although sinus slowing has been reported.[67] It is useful for the prevention of arrhythmias associated with accessory atrioventricular connections. Because of its vagolytic effects, it should be combined with digoxin for treatment of atrial arrhythmias in the absence of Wolff-Parkinson-White syndrome. Quinidine should not be used to treat arrhythmias caused by drugs. It also should be avoided in patients with the idiopathic long QT interval syndrome and in patients with a history of drug-induced torsade de pointes.

Polymorphic ventricular tachycardia (torsade de pointes) and ventricular fibrillation complicate quinidine therapy of atrial or ventricular arrhythmias in 1% of patients.[31,67] Patients who develop this complication are usually receiving digoxin and often have prolonged QT intervals before therapy.[31] Whether these factors alter the propensity for torsade de pointes is uncertain. In most cases this drug-induced arrhythmia occurs within the first week, but it may occur after several years of quinidine therapy. Patients must be closely observed during the first week of quinidine administration, and if they are not hospitalized, arrangements should be made for rapid access to medical services. The QT interval should be monitored. QT interval prolongation is an expected effect of quinidine; however, further precautions are needed in patients with preexisting QT interval prolongation or in patients who develop marked QT interval prolongation after therapy.

As with procainamide and disopyramide, there is a small risk of complete heart block in patients with severe conduction disturbances. Also, quinidine-induced aberrant conduction may mimic ventricular arrhythmias. Quinidine may exert a minor negative inotropic effect[42] but does not usually exacerbate congestive heart failure.[67] In fact, its peripheral vasodilating effects could exert a beneficial hemodynamic effect in some patients with myocardial dysfunction. Quinidine causes vasodilating effects both directly and by α-adrenergic receptor blockade.[42,68] Its vagolytic effects are mediated by blockade of muscarinic receptors.[7] Side effects occur frequently with quinidine. Various degrees of diarrhea are common and can sometimes be managed with an antacid containing aluminum hydroxide. Numerous other gastrointestinal, central nervous system, allergic, and hematologic reactions occur.[67] A number of important drug interactions are seen with quinidine. Quinidine may cause significant elevations in serum digoxin levels so that the dose of digoxin should be lowered or its effects monitored. This interaction is discussed in more detail elsewhere in this volume. Phenytoin and phenobarbital may increase hepatic metabolism of quinidine and increase its clearance. The intravenous administration of verapamil to patients receiving quinidine orally may cause severe hypotension.[69] The combination of quinidine and mexiletine has been reported to be effective against ventricular arrhythmias unresponsive to either agent alone and to permit lower doses of each.[24]

The intravenous dose of quinidine gluconate is 6 mg to 10 mg/kg administered slowly (less than 30 mg/min). Blood pressure and QRS duration should be monitored. Hypotension usually responds to discontinuation of the infusion and saline administration.[70] The oral loading dose is 600 mg to 1000 mg. The sulfate preparation is used for oral loading because of its more rapid absorption. The usual oral maintenance dosage is 200 mg to 500 mg of quinidine sulfate every 6 hours or one to two tablets of quinidine gluconate (324 mg to 648 mg) every 8 hours. The slower absorption of the sustained-release gluconate preparation permits greater dosing intervals. Polygalacturonate and slow-release sulfate forms are also available. Therapeutic levels are 2 μg to 4 μg/kg, and the half-life is about 6 hours. Protein binding is 60% to 90% but varies between patients. It is important to follow dose-related effects since plasma levels alone may not precisely reflect free drug concentration. Metabolism is primarily hepatic, but 10% to 20% is excreted in the urine.

β-ADRENERGIC BLOCKING DRUGS

β-Adrenergic blocking agents are useful for a wide spectrum of supraventricular and ventricular arrhythmias, although not all agents are approved for arrhythmia treatment. A variety of agents are available differing in β-receptor subtype selectivity, intrinsic sympathetic activity, sodium channel blocking properties, and pharmacokinetics. The impact of these characteristics on antiarrhythmic therapy has not been completely elucidated. Both β_1- and β_2-receptor subtypes are present in the human heart, but the electrophysiologic roles of each have not been well delineated. An additional benefit of β-adrenergic blocking agents could be the prevention of hypokalemia caused by sympathetic activity mediated by β_2-receptors.[71]

β-Blocking drugs are most effective for arrhythmias dependent on sympathetic stimulation such as those associated with exercise, pheochromocytoma, thyrotoxicosis, and some forms of general anesthesia. β-Blockers can be used to reduce the ventricular response rate to atrial tachyarrhythmias but are rarely effective for converting or preventing atrial fibrillation or flutter or other arrhythmias originating in the atria. By slowing conduction through the atrioventricular node, β-blockers are variably effective for terminating and preventing reentrant tachycardias that use this structure.[72-75] β-Blocking agents have no consistent effect on accessory pathway refractory periods.[74,75]

β-Adrenergic blockers are moderately effective against chronic ventricular ectopic activity[76-78] and recurrent, sustained ventricular tachycardia.[79] They are especially useful against exercise-induced ventricular arrhythmias.[76,77] β-Adrenergic blocking agents have been demonstrated to reduce the incidence of ventricular fibrillation and sudden death after myocardial infarction, although ventricular ectopic activity is not dramatically reduced.[80,81] It is uncertain whether this effect is primarily due to antiarrhythmic, anti-ischemic, or other properties of β-adrenergic antagonists.[76,80] β-Adrenergic blocking therapy also plays an important role in the therapy of patients with the congenital long QT interval syndrome.[59]

β-Adrenergic receptor blocking drugs typically cause sinus bradycardia and depress atrioventricular nodal conduction, but these effects are rarely clinically significant except in patients with preexisting sinus or atrioventricular node dysfunction. Proarrhythmic reactions occur with β-blockers but are infrequent and rarely, if ever, cause the type of malignant arrhythmias seen with sodium channel blockers.

CALCIUM CHANNEL BLOCKING DRUGS
VERAPAMIL

Intravenous verapamil is approved for the termination of paroxysmal supraventricular tachycardia and for rapid, temporary control of the ventricular rate in atrial fibrillation or flutter. Oral verapamil is not approved in the United States as an antiarrhythmic drug but certainly has a role for this purpose. Verapamil is most useful for the termination and prevention of arrhythmias in which the atrioventricular node is part of the reentrant circuit, such as atrioventricular nodal reentry and circus movement tachycardias involving accessory pathways and the atrioventricular node. It is also very useful for controlling the ventricular response rate to atrial tachyarrhythmias that are conducted over the atrioventricular node. Verapamil often provides effective control of ventricular rate in atrial fibrillation with or without digitalis. Furthermore, verapamil may be more effective than digoxin alone in preventing an excessive increase in ventricular rate during exercise in patients with atrial fibrillation.[82] Verapamil rarely prevents atrial tachyarrhythmias (*i.e.*, arrhythmias originating in the atria). Theoretically, however, atrial arrhythmias caused by calcium currents could respond to this medication.[83] Verapamil may be effective against ventricular tachycardia,[84] particularly exercise-induced sustained ventricular tachycardia[85] and ventricular tachycardia with features suggestive of triggered automaticity.[86]

Verapamil may cause sinus bradycardia or various degrees of atrioventricular nodal block, although these effects can be offset to a variable extent by reflex sympathetic activity caused by hypotension. Verapamil may accelerate the ventricular rate to atrial fibrillation in patients with Wolff-Parkinson-White syndrome[87] and should be avoided in this circumstance.

Verapamil may cause an accelerated junctional escape rhythm that may be manifest as "regularization" of the ventricular rate in patients with atrial fibrillation[88] but may also occur during therapy for other arrhythmias.[89] Curiously, this arrhythmia is less often seen in patients receiving verapamil for nonarrhythmic reasons.[89] Verapamil has a negative inotropic effect and causes peripheral vasodilation so that profound hypotension may occur, especially in patients with left ventricular dysfunction or hypovolemia or in combination with drugs having similar effects. Calcium administration may reverse or prevent these complications without affecting the antiarrhythmic effects of verapamil.[9,10] Other frequent side effects are constipation and headaches.

The usual intravenous dose is 5 mg to 10 mg administered slowly (5 mg/min). Additional boluses to 25 mg may be necessary, but since the electrophysiologic effects may be delayed, a 10- to 15-minute interval between boluses is advised. A method of determining a maintenance infusion rate has been designed,[90] or the infusion can be increased from 0.0025 mg/kg/min as needed. The usual oral dosage is 80 mg to 120 mg every 6 to 8 hours. The half-life is 4 to 8 hours but may increase with chronic oral dosing in patients with chronic atrial fibrillation, allowing less frequent dosing.[91] Ninety percent of verapamil is protein bound, and metabolism is primarily hepatic. Norverapamil is produced, but the clinical significance of this active metabolite is unknown. Verapamil causes a reduction in digoxin clearance, so digoxin doses should be lowered when this drug is used with verapamil. The combination of verapamil with other negative inotropic agents or vasodilators should be undertaken very cautiously.

MISCELLANEOUS DRUGS

BRETYLIUM

Bretylium tosylate was originally introduced as an antihypertensive agent but was subsequently noted to have prominent antifibrillatory effects in ventricular muscle.[92] Because the oral route results in erratic absorption, only the parenteral form is approved for use. It is primarily used for the emergency treatment of ventricular tachycardia or ventricular fibrillation that is refractory or recurs despite direct-current shock and lidocaine. Bretylium is not clearly superior to lidocaine against ventricular fibrillation or prophylactically during acute myocardial infarction.[93] It has limited activity against ventricular ectopic activity or chronic, recurrent ventricular tachycardia[93,94] and is believed to be ineffective against atrial arrhythmias. Bretylium does not appear to alter sinus node function or affect atrioventricular conduction 60 to 90 minutes after administration.[93]

The antiarrhythmic effects of bretylium may occur within 5 minutes of infusion or be delayed by several hours.[95] Bretylium initially causes release of norepinephrine, resulting in a transient increase in heart rate and blood pressure. During this early period there is a potential for myocardial ischemia[93] and arrhythmia exacerbation,[96] which may be facilitated by digitalis.[97] Later, it blocks release of norepinephrine from adrenergic nerve terminals, which causes mild bradycardia and hypotension by peripheral vasodilation. Bretylium appears to have a minor positive inotropic effect, but the clinical significance of this is uncertain.[42] The drug may cause hemodynamic deterioration in patients with compromised ventricular function who are dependent on sympathetic stimulation for inotropic support. On the other hand, the unloading effects of bretylium could conceivably improve cardiac function in some patients.

Nausea and vomiting may be precipitated by excessively rapid infusion of bretylium. The major side effect is orthostatic hypotension, which sometimes confines the patient to a supine position. Mild hypotension may be ameliorated by fluid administration. Because catecholamine sensitivity may occur, pressor agents must be administered cautiously. Tricyclic antidepressants have been reported to prevent orthostatic hypotension in patients receiving bretylium (e.g., protryptyline, 5 mg to 10 mg every 6 to 8 hours)[12] but have also been shown to alter its antifibrillatory effects.[98]

The usual loading dose for emergent therapy is 5 mg to 10 mg/kg administered rapidly intravenously. This may be repeated, but there is little experience with doses greater than 40 mg/kg. For hemodynamically stable arrhythmias, the same loading dose can be diluted and administered over 10 to 30 minutes to prevent nausea and vomiting. The maintenance infusion rate is 1 mg to 4 mg/min. Since perfusion of intramuscular injection sites may be erratic, and repeated injections painful, the intravenous route is usually preferred. The therapeutic range is unknown, ranging from 0.07 μg to 5 μg/ml,[99,100] but plasma concentration measurements are not yet widely available. The mean plasma elimination half-life is 13.5 hours, so the antiarrhythmic and side effects may persist for days after discontinuation of bretylium. Excretion is primarily renal; therefore, maintenance dosage should be reduced in patients with renal insufficiency.

We use bretylium for the emergent management of patients who are experiencing repeated bouts of ventricular fibrillation or rapid ventricular tachycardia not caused by drugs who have not responded to lidocaine. We would discourage its use in patients with well-tolerated ventricular tachycardia since bretylium may cause rapid hemodynamic embarrassment in this situation when other agents and maneuvers may be safer and more effective.

DIGITALIS

Cardiac glycosides are considered in detail elsewhere. A few aspects related to their antiarrhythmic and arrhythmogenic properties are discussed here. Digoxin and digitoxin are the most commonly used forms of digitalis and are approved for the treatment both of atrial fibrillation or atrial flutter in the absence of ventricular preexcitation and of paroxysmal supraventricular tachycardia. Digitalis reduces the ventricular response rate to atrial fibrillation and atrial flutter. Conversion of atrial fibrillation to sinus rhythm is often noted after administration of digitalis,[101] but it is unclear if this is caused by digitalis. There is greater uncertainty regarding the value of digitalis in preventing atrial fibrillation or flutter. In some cases, especially when the arrhythmia appears to be vagally induced, digitalis may increase the frequency of attacks[102] and has been used to promote chronic atrial fibrillation.[103] Digitalis is useful for the termination and prevention of reentrant arrhythmias using the atrioventricular node but should be used cautiously if at all in adult patients with the Wolff-Parkinson-White syndrome and paroxysmal atrial fibrillation.[104] A digitalis preparation has been reported to reduce the frequency of ventricular premature beats,[105,106] but it is not widely used for this purpose.

Digitalis toxicity may cause almost any rhythm disturbance, but some are more common than others. There appear to be little published data to support the contention of several texts that ventricular premature beats are the most frequent arrhythmia produced by digitalis.[107-109] In a small, controlled study of digitalis toxicity, the only arrhythmias found to be significantly more frequent in the digitalis-toxic patients were ventricular tachycardia, junctional rhythm, and atrial tachycardia with block.[109] Excessive bradycardia or atrioventricular block may occur in some patients, particularly those with abnormal sinus or atrioventricular node function.

The plasma concentration of digitalis preparations may increase with the concomitant administration of other drugs such as quinidine, verapamil, and amiodarone.[107,110] Hypokalemia and hypomagnesemia may lower the threshold for digitalis-associated arrhythmias. Therefore, potassium and magnesium concentrations should be monitored in patients receiving digitalis and diuretics. Direct-current cardioversion should be avoided in patients with digitalis toxicity but appears safe in patients receiving digitalis without evidence of toxicity or electrolyte disturbances.[107,111,112] The benefits of digitalis in patients with congestive heart failure and sinus rhythm have been questioned,[113] and digitalis may unfavorably affect prognosis after myocardial infarction.[114,115] Given the arrhythmogenic potential of digitalis drugs, we believe it should be prescribed only when the indications for its use are clear, and it should be discontinued if the benefits are equivocal.

MAGNESIUM

Magnesium sulfate is not approved for treatment of arrhythmias but has been effective in terminating refractory ventricular arrhythmias. Magnesium deficiency may cause polymorphic ventricular tachycardia or ventricular fibrillation, and it may reduce the threshold for digitalis-associated arrhythmias.[116-119] Magnesium sulfate has been successfully used to treat (1) arrhythmias associated with magnesium deficiency,[116-118] (2) digitalis-toxic arrhythmias with normal serum magnesium levels,[114] (3) drug-induced torsade de pointes with normal serum magnesium levels,[32,120] and (4) refractory ventricular tachyarrhythmias associated with encainide.[33] In most of these cases the arrhythmias were refractory to several conventional antiarrhythmic agents. However, cellular magnesium may be reduced despite normal serum magnesium concentration, so that it is not clear if magnesium sulfate therapy is useful for treating arrhythmias in the absence of abnormal cellular magnesium content.

Magnesium sulfate may be administered orally, intramuscularly, or intravenously. The latter is the preferred route for rapid effect. One gram of magnesium sulfate should be administered intravenously slowly (over 3 to 5 minutes) and repeated up to three times, until the desired effect is achieved or toxicity results. A continuous intravenous infusion may be used (1 g to 3 g/hr). Excessively rapid administration may cause hypotension, and excessive doses may cause respiratory arrest or asystole. Serum levels should not exceed 4 mEq/liter. Loss of deep tendon reflexes is an early sign of toxicity. Calcium chloride may reverse the neuromuscular effects of magnesium toxicity, but its effects on the cardiac actions are not well described.

ARRHYTHMIAS REQUIRING ANTIARRHYTHMIC DRUG THERAPY

The decision to treat a patient with arrhythmias involves an assessment of the severity of symptoms and the risk of morbidity and mortality associated with the arrhythmias. This must be balanced against the risk, time, and expense of therapy and procedures used to evaluate drug efficacy. The needs and concerns of the patient, in addition to his or her age, life-style, co-morbidity, and resources are individual factors that must also be weighed.

VENTRICULAR PREMATURE BEATS

Ventricular premature beats (VPBs) are treated either to reduce the risk of sudden death or to alleviate symptoms. A wide variety of symptoms are associated with VPBs, including lightheadedness, palpitations, chest pain, anxiety, dyspnea, abdominal discomfort, fatigue, and lethargy. In our experience, these symptoms are highly idiosyncratic and do not correlate well with VPB frequency or cardiac function. Nevertheless, the symptoms improve with drugs that eradicate the arrhythmia but not with placebos or ineffective drugs and the symptoms return on withdrawal of the medications. Some patients who initially deny symptoms claim to feel much better once on medications that control VPBs. The risk of arrhythmic death associated with VPBs depends on the type and severity of underlying cardiac disease and on the frequency and complexity of the VPBs. VPBs are common in the general population and appear to be a benign abnormality in healthy subjects.[121] Even patients with frequent and repetitive forms who have normal cardiac function have a good prognosis.[122]

VPBs have prognostic implications in patients with ischemic heart disease. VPB frequency determined by 24-hour ambulatory electrocardiographic monitoring before hospital discharge following acute myocardial infarction is an independent risk factor for subsequent death; the higher the frequency (up to 30 VPBs per hour) the greater the mortality.[123,124] The impact of VPB frequency on mortality is less than that of measures of cardiac function, but the risk of death is magnified when frequent VPBs occur in the presence of left ventricular dysfunction.[124] The presence of repetitive ventricular beats in a predischarge 24-hour recording also contributes independently to the risk of mortality.[125]

The importance of VPBs has not been as carefully scrutinized in patients with rarer forms of myocardial disease. Patients with idiopathic dilated cardiomyopathy are at increased risk for sudden death and have a high prevalence of frequent and complex VPBs. However, the results of studies assessing the clinical significance of ventricular ectopic activity in this population are contradictory.[126,127] Short runs of asymptomatic ventricular tachycardia have been shown to predict sudden death or cardiac arrest in patients with hypertrophic cardiomyopathy, while other characteristics of ventricular arrhythmias are not predictive.[128]

In general, patients with extensive myocardial disease are prone to sudden, presumably arrhythmic, death. With few exceptions, the risk of sudden death correlates better with the severity of cardiac dysfunction than with the frequency or complexity of VPBs. It has long been hypothesized that VPBs presage fatal ventricular arrhythmias. Accumulating evidence supports this theory, although the support is not overwhelming. It has also been assumed that eradication of VPBs will prevent arrhythmic death. There is little solid evidence to support this idea. Nevertheless, the standard of practice is to suppress frequent or complex VPBs, especially in patients with ventricular dysfunction.

There are no universally accepted criteria for "frequent" or "complex" VPBs. A widely used grading system introduced by Lown and co-workers has been aptly criticized.[123] What constitutes effective suppression is also in dispute. Many clinicians aim for "significant" suppression, that is, a level of VPB reduction that is unlikely to be due to chance. Because of the enormous spontaneous variation in VPB frequency, long-term ambulatory monitoring has become the standard method of gauging the effectiveness of therapy against VPBs. If 24-hour recordings are used, an antiarrhythmic drug must reduce the patient's VPB frequency by at least 80% in order for it to be considered effective by most authorities.[129,130] This value is based on the spontaneous variability observed in 24-hour recordings obtained within days of each other. However, one study suggests that even greater deviations in VPB frequencies are observed in 24-hour recordings obtained several months apart.[131]

When treating VPBs the clinician must be aware of the so-called "riding the downslope to glory" phenomenon. It is intuitively obvious that a patient with VPBs is most likely to present during a period when his VPB frequency and complexity are greatest, because this is the time when symptoms are most likely to be present or when an "irregular" heart beat is most likely to be detected. An electrocardiographic recording obtained during some other period will probably reflect the patient's usual VPB frequency (regression to the mean). Drug therapy directed against VPBs initiated during the period of most frequent VPBs may appear successful because of the spontaneous decrease of the patient's VPB frequency.

It is rarely possible to predict in advance which antiarrhythmic agent will effectively reduce VPBs. After excluding drugs that are contraindicated, it is prudent to initiate therapy with the least dangerous agents (*e.g.*, β-adrenergic blocking agent, mexiletine, or tocainide). Unfortunately, these agents are effective in only a minority of patients so drugs such as quinidine, disopyramide, or procainamide can be tried but the potential for serious proarrhythmic effects may impel hospitalization. If these are ineffective, the addition of mexiletine or tocainide may improve VPB suppression. Some clinicians may prefer to use the newly approved drug flecainide as a first-line agent because of its effectiveness against VPBs. These recommendations must be considered tentative pending the results of ongoing and future studies.

REFERENCES

1. Burney RG, DiFazio CA, Peach MJ et al: Anti-arrhythmic effects of lidocaine metabolites. Am Heart J 88:765, 1974
2. Prescott LF: Pharmacokinetic abnormalities in myocardial infarction. In Sandoe E, Julian DG, Bell JW (eds): Management of Ventricular Tachycardia—Role of Mexiletine, pp 465–471. New York, Excerpta Medica, 1978
3. Thompson PD, Melmon KL, Richardson JA et al: Lidocaine pharmacokinetics in advanced heart failure, liver, disease, and renal failure in humans. Ann Intern Med 78:499, 1973
4. Winkle RA: Class I and III drugs. In Winkle RA (ed): Antiarrhythmic Therapy. Menlo-Park, CA, Addison-Wesley, 1983
5. Bigger JT, Giardina ELV: Drug interactions in antiarrhythmic therapy. In Lucchesi BR, Dingell JV, Schwartz RP (eds): Clinical Pharmacology of Antiarrhythmic Therapy. New York, Raven Press, 1984
6. Kim DH, Akera T, Brody TM: Interactions between quinidine and cardiac glycosides involving mutual binding sites in the guinea pig. J Pharmacol Exp Ther 218:108, 1981
7. Mirro MJ, Manalan AS, Bailey JC et al: Anticholinergic effects of disopyramide and quinidine on guinea pig myocardium. Circ Res 47:855, 1980
8. Teichman S, Fisher JD, Matos JA et al: Disopyramide: Byridostigmine: Report of a beneficial drug interaction. J Cardiovasc Pharmacol 7:108, 1985
9. Hariman RJ, Mangiardi LM, McAllister RG Jr et al: Reversal of the cardiovascular effects of verapamil by calcium and sodium: Differences between electrophysiologic and hemodynamic responses. Circulation 59:797, 1979
10. Weiss AT, Lewis BS, Halon DA et al: The use of calcium with verapamil in the management of supraventricular tachyarrhythmias. Int J Cardiol 4:275, 1983
11. Bristow MR, Daniels JR, Kernoff RS et al: Effect of D600, practolol, and alterations in magnesium on ionized calcium concentration: Response relationships in the intact dog heart. Circ Res 41:574, 1977
12. Hondeghem LM, Katzung BG: Mechanism of action of antiarrhythmic drugs. In Sperelakis N (ed): Physiology and Pathophysiology of the Heart. Boston, Martinus Nijhoff, 1984
13. Clarkson CW, Hondeghem LM: Evidence for a specific receptor site for lidocaine, quinidine and bupivacaine associated with cardiac sodium chan-

14. Stevens CS, McGovern B, Garan H et al: Aggravation of electrically provoked ventricular tachycardia during treatment with propafenone. Am Heart J 110:24, 1985
15. Mason JW, Hondeghem LM, Katzung BG: Block of inactivated sodium channel and of depolarization-induced automaticity in guinea pig papillary muscle by amiodarone. Circ Res 44:277, 1984
16. Woosley RL, Reele ST, Roden DM et al: Pharmacologic reversal of hypotensive effect complicating antiarrhythmic therapy with bretylium. Clin Pharm Ther 32:313, 1982
17. Keren A, Tzivoni D, Gavish D et al: Etiology, warning signs and therapy of torsade de pointes. Circulation 64:1167, 1981
18. Tatini R, Steinbrunn W, Kappenberger L et al: Dangerous interaction between amiodarone and quinidine. Lancet 1:1327, 1982
19. Derrida JP, Ollagnier J, Benaim R et al: Amiodarone et propranolol: Une association dangereuse? Nouv Presse Med 8:1429, 1979
20. Ross DL, Sze DY, Keefe DL et al: Antiarrhythmic drug combinations in the treatment of ventricular tachycardia: Efficacy and electrophysiologic effects. Circulation 66:1205, 1982
21. Breithardt G, Seipel L, Abendroth RR: Comparison of the antiarrhythmic efficacy of disopyramide and mexiletine against stimulus-induced ventricular tachycardia. J Cardiovasc Pharm 3:1026, 1981
22. Greenspan AM, Spielman SR, Webb CR et al: Efficacy of combination therapy with mexiletine and a type IA agent for inducible ventricular tachyarrhythmias secondary to coronary artery disease. Am J Cardiol 56:277, 1985
23. Duffy CE, Swiryn S, Bauernfeind RA et al: Inducible sustained ventricular tachycardia refractory to individual class I drugs: Effect of adding a second class I drug. Am Heart J 106:450, 1983
24. Duff HF, Roden D, Primm RK et al: Mexiletine in the treatment of resistant ventricular arrhythmia: Enhancement of efficacy and reduction of dose-related side effects by combination with quinidine. Circulation 67:1124, 1983
25. Kim SG, Seiden SW, Matos JA et al: Combination of procainamide and quinidine for better tolerance and additive effects for ventricular arrhythmias. Am J Cardiol 56:84, 1985
26. Winkle RA, Anderson JL, Peters F et al: The hemodynamic effects of intravenous tocainide in patients with heart disease. Circulation 57:787, 1978
27. Ruskin JN, McGovern B, Garan H et al: Antiarrhythmic drugs: A possible cause of out-of-hospital cardiac arrest. N Engl J Med 309:1302, 1983
28. Velebit V, Podrid P, Lown B et al: Aggravation and provocation of ventricular arrhythmias by antiarrhythmic drugs: Circulation 65:886, 1982
29. Rinkenberger RL, Prystowsky EN, Jackman WM et al: Drug conversion of nonsustained ventricular tachycardia to sustained ventricular tachycardia during serial electrophysiologic studies: Identification of drugs that exacerbate tachycardia and potential mechanisms. Am Heart J 103:177, 1982
30. Kay GN, Plumb VJ, Arciniegas JG et al: Torsade de pointes: The long-short initiating sequence and other clinical features: Observations in 32 patients. J Am Coll Cardiol 2:806, 1983
31. Bauman JL, Bauernfeind RA, Hoff JV et al: Torsade de pointes due to quinidine: Observations in 31 patients. Am Heart J 107:425, 1984
32. Tzivoni D, Keren A, Cohen AM et al: Magnesium therapy for torsade de pointes. Am J Cardiol 53:528, 1984
33. Winkle RA, Mason JW, Griffin JC et al: Malignant ventricular tachyarrhythmias associated with the use of encainide. Am Heart J 102:857, 1981
34. Hohnloser S, Zeiher A, Hust MH et al: Flecainide-induced aggravation of ventricular tachycardia. Clin Cardiol 6:130, 1983
35. Fogoros RN, Anderson KP, Winkle RA et al: Amiodarone: Clinical efficacy and toxicity in 96 patients with recurrent, drug-refractory arrhythmias. Circulation 68:88, 1983
36. Connolly SJ, Kates RE, Lebsack CS et al: Clinical efficacy and electrophysiology of oral propafenone for ventricular tachycardia. Am J Cardiol 52:1208, 1983
37. Morady F, Scheinmen MM, Desai J: Disopyramide. Ann Intern Med 96:337, 1982
38. Brugada P, Wellens HJJ: Effects of intravenous and oral disopyramide on paroxysmal atrioventricular nodal tachycardia. Am J Cardiol 53:88, 1984
39. Karim A, Nissen C, Azarnoff DL: Clinical pharmacokinetics of disopyramide. J Pharmacokin Biopharm 10:465, 1982
40. Lee JT, Kates RE, Winkle RA et al: Post-tachycardia cardiac standstill: A disopyramide-verapamil interaction in dogs (abstr). J Am Coll Cardiol 1:700, 1983
41. Bergfeldt L, Rosenqvist M, Vallin H et al: Disopyramide induced second and third degree atrioventricular block in patients with bifascicular block: An acute stress test to predict atrioventricular block. Br Heart J 53:328, 1985
42. Block PJ, Winkle RA: Hemodynamic effects of antiarrhythmic drugs. Am J Cardiol 52:14C, 1983
43. Pollick C: Muscular subaortic stenosis: Hemodynamic and clinical improvement after disopyramide. N Engl J Med 307:997, 1982
44. David BM, Ilett KF, Whitford EG et al: Prolonged variability in plasma protein binding of disopyramide after acute myocardial infarction. Br J Pharmacol 15:435, 1983
45. Akhtar M, Gilbert CJ, Shenasa M: Effect of lidocaine on atrioventricular response via the accessory pathway in patients with Wolff-Parkinson-White syndrome. Circulation 63:435, 1981
46. Castellanos A, Ferreiro J, Pefkaros K et al: Effects of lignocaine on bidirectional tachycardia and on digitalis-induced atrial tachycardia with block. Br Heart J 48:27, 1982
47. Edvardson N, Holmberg S, Talwar KK et al: Electrophysiological effects of lidocaine in acute myocardial infarction with bifascicular block or complete A-V block. Cardiology 70:333, 1983
48. Lie KI, Liem KL, Louridtz WJ et al: Efficacy of lidocaine preventing primary ventricular fibrillation within one hour after a 300 mg intramuscular injection: A double-blind randomized study of 300 hospitalized patients with acute myocardial infarction. Am J Cardiol 42:486, 1978
49. Koster RW, Dunning AF: Intramuscular lidocaine for prevention of lethal arrhythmias in the prehospitalization phase of acute myocardial infarction. N Engl J Med 313:1105, 1985
50. Routledge PA, Shand DG, Barchowsky A et al: Relationship between alpha$_1$-acid glycoprotein and lidocaine disposition in myocardial infarction. Clin Pharm Ther 30:154, 1981
51. Knapp AB, Maguire W, Keren F et al: The cimetidine–lidocaine interaction. Ann Intern Med 98:174, 1983
52. Conrad KA, Byers JM, Finley PR et al: Lidocaine elimination: Effects of metoprolol and of propranolol. Clin Pharm Ther 33:133, 1983
53. Bauer JA, Brown T, Bibaldi M et al: Influence of long-term infusions on lidocaine kinetics. Clin Pharmacol Ther 31:433, 1982
54. Drayer DE, Lorenzo B, Werns S et al: Plasma levels, protein binding and elimination data of lidocaine and active metabolites in cardiac patients of various ages. Clin Pharmacol Ther 34:14, 1983
55. Garson A Jr: Evaluation and treatment of chronic ventricular dysrhythmias in the young. Cardiovasc Rev Rep 2:1164, 1981
56. Damato AN: Diphenylhydantoin: Pharmacological and clinical use. Prog Cardiovasc Dis 12:1, 1969
57. Atkinson AJ, Davison R: Diphenylhydantoin as an antiarrhythmic drug. Annu Rev Med 25:99, 1974
58. Gillis RA, McClellan JR, Sauer TS et al: Depression of cardiac sympathetic nerve activity by diphenylhydantoin. J Pharmacol Exp Ther 179:599, 1971
59. Moss AF, Schwartz PJ: Delayed repolarization (QT or QTU prolongation) and malignant ventricular arrhythmias. Mod Concept Cardiovasc Dis 51:85, 1982
60. Wit AL, Rosen MR, Hoffman BF: Electrophysiology and pharmacology of cardiac arrhythmias: VIII. Cardiac effects of diphenylhydantoin. Am Heart J 90:397, 1975
61. Peter T, Ross D, Duffield A et al: Effect on survival after myocardial infarction of long-term treatment with phenytoin. Br Heart J 40:1356, 1978
62. Goldberg D, Reiffel JA, Davis JC et al: Electrophysiologic effects of procainamide on sinus function in patients with and without sinus node disease. Am Heart J 103:75, 1982
63. Giardina EGV: Procainamide: Clinical pharmacology and efficacy against ventricular arrhythmias. Ann NY Acad Sci 432:177, 1984
64. Jaillon P, Winkle RA: Electrophysiologic comparative study of procainamide and n-acetylprocainamide in anesthetized dogs: Concentration-response relationships. Circulation 60:1385, 1979
65. Jaillon P, Rubenson D, Peters F et al: Electrophysiologic effects of n-acetylprocainamide in human beings. Am J Cardiol 47:1134, 1981
66. Vera Z, Awan NA, Mason DT: Assessment of oral quinidine effects on sinus node function in sick sinus syndrome patients. Am Heart J 103:80, 1982
67. Cohen IS, Jick H, Cohen SI: Adverse reactions to quinidine in hospitalized patients: Findings based on data from the Boston collaborative drug surveillance program. Prog Cardiovasc Dis 20:151, 1977
68. Motulsky HJ, Maisel AS, Snavely MD et al: Quinidine is a competitive antagonist at alpha$_1$ and alpha$_2$-adrenergic receptors. Circ Res 55:376, 1984
69. Maisel AS, Motulsky HJ, Insel PA: Hypotension after quinidine plus verapamil. N Engl J Med 312:167, 1985
70. Swerdlow CD, Yu JO, Jacobson E et al: Safety and efficacy of intravenous quinidine. Am J Med 75:36, 1983
71. Brown MJ, Brown DC, Murphy MB: Hypokalemia from beta$_2$ receptor stimulation by circulating epinephrine. N Engl J Med 309:1414, 1983
72. Wu D, Denes P, Dhingra R et al: The effects of propranolol on induction of A-V nodal reentrant paroxysmal tachycardia. Circulation 50:665, 1974
73. Chang M, Sung RF, Tai T et al: Nadolol and supraventricular tachycardia: An electrophysiologic study. J Am Coll Cardiol 2:894, 1983
74. Denes P, Cummings JM, Simpson R et al: Effects of propranolol on anomalous pathway refractoriness and circus movement tachycardias in patients with preexcitation. Am J Cardiol 41:1061, 1978
75. Kou H, Yeh S, Lin F et al: Effects of acebutolol on paroxysmal atrioventricular reentrant tachycardia in patients with manifest or concealed accessory pathways. Chest 83:92, 1983
76. Roden DM, Wang T, Woosley RL: Antiarrhythmic effects of beta-blocking drugs. In Lucchesi BR, Dingell JV, Schwarz RP Jr: Clinical Pharmacology of Antiarrhythmic Therapy, pp 95–103. New York, Raven Press, 1984
77. Pratt CM, Yepsen SC, Bloom MGK et al: Evaluation of metoprolol in suppressing complex ventricular arrhythmias. Am J Cardiol 52:73, 1983
78. Podrid PJ, Lown B: Pindolol for ventricular arrhythmia. Am Heart J 104:491, 1982
79. Mason JW, Swerdlow CD, Winkle RA et al: Ventricular tachyarrhythmia induction for drug selection: Experience with 311 patients. In Lucchesi BR, Dingell JV, Schwarz RP Jr (eds): Clinical Pharmacology of Antiarrhythmic Therapy, pp 229–239. New York, Raven Press, 1984

80. Hjalmarson A: Beta-blocker effectiveness post infarction: An antiarrhythmic or anti-ischemic effect. Ann NY Acad Sci 427:101, 1984
81. Herlitz J, Edvardsson N, Holmberg S et al: Göteborg metoprolol trial: Effects on arrhythmias. Am J Cardiol 53:27D, 1984
82. Klein HO, Kaplinsky E: Verapamil and digoxin: Their respective effects on atrial fibrillation and their interaction. Am J Cardiol 50:894, 1982
83. Wyndham CRC, Arnsdorf MR, Levitsky S et al: Successful surgical excision of focal paroxysmal atrial tachycardia. Circulation 62:1365, 1980
84. Mason JW, Swerdlow CD, Mitchell LB: Efficacy of verapamil in chronic, recurrent ventricular tachycardia. Am J Cardiol 51:1614, 1983
85. Wu D, Kou H, Hung J: Exercise-triggered paroxysmal ventricular tachycardia. Ann Intern Med 95:410, 1981
86. Sung RJ, Shapiro WA, Shen EN et al: Effects of verapamil on ventricular tachycardias possibly caused by reentry, automaticity and triggered activity. J Clin Invest 72:350, 1983
87. Gulamhusein S, Ko P, Carruthers SG et al: Acceleration of the ventricular response in the Wolff-Parkinson-White syndrome after verapamil. Circulation 65:348, 1982
88. Neusee H: Control of ventricular rate in atrial fibrillation: Role of verapamil. In Kulbertus HE, Olsson SB, Schlepper M: Atrial Fibrillation. Mölndal, Sweden, AB Hässle, 1982
89. Schwartz JB, Jeang M, Raizner AE et al: Accelerated junctional rhythms during oral verapamil therapy. Am Heart J 107:440, 1984
90. Reiter MJ, Shand DG, Aanonsen LM et al: Pharmacokinetics of verapamil: Experience with a sustained infusion regimen. Am J Cardiol 50:716, 1982
91. Kates RF, Keefe DLD, Schwartz J et al: Verapamil disposition in chronic atrial fibrillation. Clin Pharmacol Ther 30:44, 1981
92. Bacaner MB: Bretylium tosylate for suppression of induced ventricular fibrillation. Am J Cardiol 17:528, 1966
93. Anderson JL: Bretylium: An update on pharmacokinetic studies and clinical uses. In Rapaport E: Cardiology Update 1983, p 24. New York, Elsevier Biomedical, 1983
94. Bauernfeind RA, Hoff JV, Swiryn S et al: Electrophysiologic testing of bretylium tosylate in sustained ventricular tachycardia. Am Heart J 105:973, 1983
95. Bacaner MB: Treatment of ventricular fibrillation and other acute arrhythmias with bretylium tosylate. Am J Cardiol 21:530, 1968
96. Anderson JL, Popat KD: Paradoxical ventricular tachycardia and fibrillation after intravenous bretylium therapy. Arch Intern Med 141:801, 1981
97. Gillis RA, Clancy MM, Anderson RJ: Deleterious effects of bretylium in cats with digitalis induced ventricular tachycardia. Circulation 57:974, 1973
98. Kopia GA, Hess TA, Lucchesi BR: Role of the sympathetic nervous system in bretylium's antifibrillatory action (abstr). Fed Proc 41:1737, 1982
99. Anderson JL, Patterson E, Wagner JG et al: Clinical pharmacokinetics of intravenous and oral bretylium tosylate in survivors of ventricular tachycardia or fibrillation: Clinical application of a new assay for bretylium. J Cardiovasc Pharm 3:485, 1981
100. Noneman JW, Batenhorst RL, Jones MR et al: Treatment of refractory ventricular arrhythmias: High dose parenteral and oral bretylium tosylate. Chest 4:517, 1982
101. Weiner P, Bassan MM, Jarchovsky J et al: Clinical course of acute atrial fibrillation treated with rapid digitalization. Am Heart J 105:223, 1983
102. Coumel P, Leclercq J-F, Attuel P: Paroxysmal atrial fibrillation. In Kulbertus HE, Olsson SB, Schlepper M (eds): Atrial Fibrillation. Mölndal, Sweden, AB Hässle, 1982
103. DeSilva RA, in discussion section of Campbell RWF: Drug prophylaxis of atrial fibrillation. In Kulbertus HE, Olsson SB, Schlepper M (eds): Atrial Fibrillation, p 284. Mölndal, Sweden, AB Hässle, 1982
104. Sellers TD Jr, Bashore TM, Gallagher JJ: Digitalis in the pre-excitation syndrome: Analysis during atrial fibrillation. Circulation 56:260, 1977
105. Lown B, Graboys TB, Podrid PJ et al: Effect of a digitalis drug on ventricular premature beats. N Engl J Med 296:301, 1977
106. Podrid P, Lown B, Zielonka J et al: Effects of acetyl-strophanthidin on left ventricular function and ventricular arrhythmias. Am Heart J 107:882, 1984
107. Smith TW, Antman EM, Friedman PL et al: Digitalis glycosides: Mechanisms and manifestations of toxicity. Prog Cardiovasc Dis 26 (I):413; (II):495; (III):21, 1984
108. Beller GA, Smith TW, Abelmann WH et al: Digitalis intoxication: A prospective clinical study with serum level correlations. N Engl J Med 284:989, 1971
109. Bernabei R, Perna GP, Carosella L et al: Digoxin serum concentration measurement in patients with suspected digitalis-induced arrhythmias. J Cardiovasc Pharm 2:319, 1980
110. Fenster PE, White NW, Hanson CD: Pharmacokinetic evaluation of the digoxin-amiodarone interaction. J Am Coll Cardiol 5:108, 1985
111. Ditchey RV, Karliner JS: Safety of electrical cardioversion in patients without digitalis toxicity. Ann Intern Med 95:676, 1981
112. Mann DL, Maisel AS, Atwood JE et al: Absence of cardioversion-induced ventricular arrhythmias in patients with therapeutic digoxin levels. J Am Coll Cardiol 5:882, 1985
113. Fleg JL, Lakatta EG: How useful is digitalis in patients with congestive heart failure and sinus rhythm? Int J Cardiol 6:295, 1984
114. Moss AJ, Davis HT, Conard DL et al: Digitalis-associated cardiac mortality after myocardial infarction. Circulation 64:1150, 1981
115. Bigger JT Jr, Fleiss JL, Rolnitzky LM et al: Effect of digitalis on survival after acute myocardial infarction. Am J Cardiol 55:623, 1985
116. Iseri LT, Freed J, Bures AR: Magnesium deficiency and cardiac disorders. Am J Med 58:837, 1975
117. Levine SR, Crowley TJ, Hai HA: Hypomagnesemia and ventricular tachycardia. Chest 81:244, 1982
118. Ramee SR, White CJ, Svinarich JT et al: Torsade de pointes and magnesium deficiency. Am Heart J 109:164, 1985
119. Cohen L, Kitzes R: Magnesium sulfate and digitalis-toxic arrhythmias. JAMA 249:2808, 1983
120. Iseri LT, Chung P, Tobis J: Magnesium therapy for intractable ventricular tachyarrhythmias in normomagnesemic patients. West J Med 138:823, 1983
121. Moss AJ: Clinical significance of ventricular arrhythmias in patients with and without coronary artery disease. Prog Cardiovasc Dis 23:33, 1980
122. Kennedy HL, Whitlock JA, Sprague MK et al: Long-term follow-up of asymptomatic healthy subjects with frequent and complex ventricular ectopy. N Engl J Med 312:193, 1985
123. Bigger JT, Weld FM: Analysis of prognostic significance of ventricular arrhythmias after myocardial infarction: Shortcomings of Lown grading system. Br Heart J 45:717, 1981
124. Multicenter Postinfarction Research Group: Risk stratification and survival after myocardial infarction. N Engl J Med 309:331, 1983
125. Bigger JT Jr, Fleiss JL, Kleiger R et al: The relationships among ventricular arrhythmias, left ventricular dysfunction, and mortality in the 2 years after myocardial infarction. Circulation 69:250, 1984
126. Von Olshausen K, Schafer A, Mekmel HC et al: Ventricular arrhythmias in idiopathic dilated cardiomyopathy. Br Heart J 51:195, 1984
127. Meinertz T, Hofmann T, Kasper W et al: Significance of ventricular arrhythmias in idiopathic dilated cardiomyopathy. Am J Cardiol 53:902, 1984
128. Anderson KP: Sudden death in patients with hypertrophic cardiomyopathy. Cardiovasc Rev Rep 5:363, 1984
129. Morganroth J, Michelson EL, Horowitz LN et al: Limitations of routine long-term electrocardiographic monitoring to assess ventricular ectopic frequency. Circulation 58:408, 1978
130. Thomas LJ Jr, Miller JP: Long-term ambulatory ECG recording in the determination of antidysrhythmic drug efficacy. In Lucchesi BR, Dingell JV, Schwarz RP Jr: Clinical Pharmacology of Antiarrhythmic Therapy, p 249. New York, Raven Press, 1984
131. Pratt CM, Delclos G, Wierman AM et al: The changing base line of complex ventricular arrhythmias. N Engl J Med 313:1444, 1985

Clinical Use of Newer Antiarrhythmic Drugs

Samuel Levy

In the past decade, our therapeutic armamentarium has been enriched by a number of new antiarrhythmic agents. These new agents provide an alternative therapy to conventional antiarrhythmic agents, which are, in a significant number of patients, ineffective or associated with intolerable side effects. Most of the newer antiarrhythmic agents are now available for clinical use in Europe and for clinical or investigational use in the United States. The large number of new antiarrhythmic agents cannot be covered in a single chapter, and the discussion here is restricted to selected antiarrhythmic drugs that it is believed will be of practical importance for the clinician. The extensive use of some of these agents, as reflected by the abundant literature, will help to define their electrophysiologic properties, clinical efficacy, dosage, and possible side effects. This is a prerequisite for the appropriate and safe use of these agents.

The classification of Vaughan-Williams,[1] which is based on microelectrode studies, used to characterize the effects of antiarrhythmic agents on the action potential of isolated cardiac cells. Class I antiarrhythmic agents depress fast response channels through their action on Na$^+$ current. These agents have been subdivided into three subgroups: class IA agents decrease the maximum rate of rise of phase 0 and prolong repolarization; a prototype of a class IA drug is quinidine. Class IB agents (*e.g.*, lidocaine) have slight effects on phase 0 and tend to shorten the action potential duration. Class IC agents exert their main effect by depressing the maximum rate of depolarization without marked repolarization alterations. A number of new antiarrhythmic agents belong to the class IC group and include encainide, flecainide, and cibenzoline. Class II agents cause sympathetic blockade and, therefore, include β-adrenergic blocking drugs. Class III agents are characterized by lengthening transmembrane action potential duration and are best represented by amiodarone. Class IV agents have slow calcium channel blocking properties and are often referred to as calcium antagonists. Verapamil and diltiazem belong to this group and are available in the United States. Bepridil is undergoing clinical evaluation and is available in Europe and the United States for treatment of coronary insufficiency. It also possesses sodium channel blocking properties.

MEXILETINE

Mexiletine (1-phenoxy-3-amino-isopropanol) is a local anesthetic antiarrhythmic agent that is similar to lidocaine both in chemical structure and pharmacologic characteristics. This drug has proven usefulness in the treatment of ventricular arrhythmias and is available for clinical use in Europe and the United States (Mexitil, Boeringher Ingelheim).

ELECTROPHYSIOLOGIC PROPERTIES. Mexiletine depresses the maximum rate of rise of phase 0 depolarization of cardiac cells without any significant change in resting membrane potential and in duration of action potential (class IB of Vaughan-Williams classification). Mexiletine decreases the effective refractory period of Purkinje fibers but to a lesser degree than the decrease in action potential duration.[2] It has no significant effect on the autonomic nervous system.

Given intravenously (125 mg to 250 mg over 5 to 10 minutes), mexiletine has little effect on heart rate and sinus node recovery time in patients with normal sinus node function. Similarly, no significant or consistent changes on cardiac conduction parameters are observed in patients with normal conduction. However, studies in patients with pre-existing abnormal sinus node automaticity or conduction disorders have been the subject of conflicting reports. Some advise caution in the use of mexiletine in this group of patients.[3,4] There are also conflicting results on the effect of mexiletine on accessory atrioventricular connections.

PHARMACOKINETICS. Given intravenously, the plasma half-life of mexiletine is about 12 hours. The drug is metabolized in the liver (80% to 90%), and its metabolites have no known antiarrhythmic activity. Drug elimination may be impaired in patients with renal insufficiency.

The oral form of mexiletine is virtually completely absorbed in normal subjects. Peak plasma concentrations occur 2 to 4 hours after administration, with a plasma half-life of 3 to 8 hours in patients with normal renal function, because 90% of excretion is urinary. The therapeutic range of serum concentrations is 0.7 μg to 1.5 μg/ml.

HEMODYNAMIC EFFECTS. Mexiletine exerts slight negative cardiac inotropic effects. Hemodynamic studies using intravenously administered mexiletine (1.5 mg to 3 mg/kg), or a single oral dose of 200 mg, have shown no significant effect on hemodynamic parameters. This may not be the case for rapid drug infusion or increased dose.

CLINICAL ANTIARRHYTHMIC SPECTRUM. Intravenous therapy with mexiletine has been proven to suppress ventricular arrhythmias related to acute myocardial infarction[5] and to digitalis toxicity. The success rate of mexiletine in suppressing more than 95% of ventricular extrasystoles ranged between 65% and 88%.[5-7] Controlled trials of mexiletine versus lidocaine[8] have shown that mexiletine is more effective than lidocaine. In 11 patients with sustained ventricular tachycardia, mexiletine given at an initial dose of 50 mg to 200 mg within 5 to 10 minutes, followed by 250 mg within the next 30 minutes, resulted in arrhythmia termination in 9 patients.[6]

Although in one report it has been suggested that intravenously administered mexiletine both terminated and prevented pacing-induced reciprocating supraventricular tachycardia using an accessory pathway in a significant percentage of patients, the usefulness of mexiletine for this indication remains to be determined.[9,10]

Mexiletine has been used to suppress both ventricular extrasystoles and ventricular tachycardias. It was able to suppress 90% or more of ventricular extrasystoles in 80% of patients.[6] I reviewed the results in 110 patients treated with a dosage of 600 mg to 800 mg/day, and a beneficial result occurred in 71 patients (64.5%). The beneficial results for a number of series varied from 55% to 86%. In one double-blind crossover study in patients with high-density premature ventricular complexes,[11] mexiletine (600 mg/day) suppressed 66% of the arrhythmia (versus 3% for placebo). A controlled study comparing mexiletine (600 mg/day) to disopyramide (600 mg/day) in patients with chronic ventricular arrhythmias showed that disopyramide was more effective. However, there was no difference when the dose of mexiletine was increased to 1000 mg/day.[12]

Given alone, mexiletine has been successful only in a minority of patients in preventing spontaneous recurrence of ventricular tachycardias or in suppressing pacing-induced sustained ventricular tachycardias. However, the efficacy of mexiletine is enhanced when combined with quinidine or another class I antiarrhythmic agent or amiodarone, which can be safely done in selected patients.[13-15] The usefulness of mexiletine in preventing supraventricular arrhythmias remains to be evaluated.

SIDE EFFECTS. Mexiletine is associated with side effects in 6.5% to 80% of patients. Because toxicity is dose dependent, the incidence decreases by lowering the dose. The drug had to be discontinued in up to 40% of patients.[16,17] Central nervous system disorders are similar to those of lidocaine and include dizziness, hallucinations, headaches, ataxia, confusion, and tremor, with the latter being the most common in my clinical experience. Gastrointestinal side effects are also common and include vomiting, nausea, gastric discomfort, and dyspepsia. Cardiac toxicity is rare. Mexiletine does not change PR, QRS, or QT intervals of the electrocardiogram. Conduction disturbances, bradycardia, and hypotension have been reported in rare instances. Proarrhythmic effect, including torsade de pointes, is a possible, although rare, complication of mexiletine.[18]

DOSAGE REGIMEN. An initial intravenous dose of 125 mg to 250 mg (1 mg to 3 mg/kg) over a minimum period of 10 minutes is recommended. The same dose may be repeated over a 1-hour period. If necessary, an infusion of 30 mg to 50 mg/hr may be undertaken. The oral dose is 200 mg every 6 to 8 hours (600 mg to 800 mg/day). Mexiletine may be usefully and safely combined with quinidine or amiodarone in selected patients.[19]

TOCAINIDE

Tocainide hydrochloride is an oral lidocaine analog with a primary amine structure available for clinical use in the United States and in some European countries (Tonocard, Merck, Sharp and Dohme).[20-28]

ELECTROPHYSIOLOGIC PROPERTIES. Tocainide is a class IB antiarrhythmic agent. Microelectrode studies have shown that tocainide decreases the duration of the action potential of the Purkinje fiber. Action potential upstroke velocity is depressed (concentration-related effect). There is a slight decrease in resting membrane potential, and the effective refractory period tends to decrease.

Clinical electrophysiologic studies[20] using intravenous tocainide have shown no change or a slight decrease in heart rate and no significant effect on QRS and conduction intervals. The atrial effective refractory period is increased, whereas the right ventricular effective refractory period is decreased. In four patients with accessory pathways, the effective refractory period increased in two and conduction was blocked in one and unchanged in the remaining patients.[21]

PHARMACOKINETICS. The bioavailability of tocainide is nearly 100%. The drug is metabolized in the liver, and 40% is excreted unchanged in the urine. The drug half-life is 13 hours.[22] The therapeutic range of plasma concentrations is 6 μg to 12 μg/ml. Peak plasma levels are reached 30 minutes to 4 hours after oral administration.

HEMODYNAMIC EFFECTS. Although tocainide does have a slight negative inotropic effect, it does not cause significant changes in hemodynamic parameters. In patients with left ventricular dysfunction, it may increase left ventricular end-diastolic pressure and peripheral vascular resistance.

CLINICAL ANTIARRHYTHMIC SPECTRUM. In the setting of acute myocardial infarction, intravenous tocainide has been successful in preventing ventricular arrhythmias (except for ventricular fibrillation) during the first 24 hours.[23] The main advantage of tocainide over lidocaine is that it allows for oral administration. The major indication is ventricular arrhythmias. Studies performed mainly in the United States have shown suppression of ventricular extrasystoles (greater than 70% reduction) in 66% to 73% of patients.[22-25] Tocainide was found to be effective in patients with ventricular tachycardias.[26] It was shown to prevent pacing-induced ventricular tachycardia in 35% of patients.[27]

SIDE EFFECTS. Intravenous therapy with tocainide may be occasionally associated with bradycardia, hypotension, and confusion. Oral therapy with tocainide may be responsible for three varieties of side-effects: neurologic disorder (tremor, headaches, diplopia, lightheadedness, dizziness, paresthesia, paranoid psychosis); gastrointestinal (anorexia, nausea, vomiting, abdominal pain); and cutaneous (rash). However, these side effects are often minor and seldom require drug discontinuation (less than 10%). Interstitial pneumonitis has also been reported.[27] The possible occurrence of agranulocytosis due to bone marrow depression, although rare (1 in 300 patients), requires regular complete blood cell counts during the first 12 weeks of therapy. Proarrhythmic effects such as aggravation of ventricular arrhythmia were noted in 14 of 288 patients.[26]

DOSE REGIMEN. Tocainide may be given as an infusion at a rate of 0.5 mg to 0.75 mg/kg/min over a 15-minute period. The recommended oral dose for tocainide is 400 mg to 800 mg every 8 hours.

ENCAINIDE

Encainide hydrochloride was developed in 1973. It was found to have potent antiarrhythmic activity in experimental animal models and in Europe and the United States is available for clinical use (Enkaid, Bristol-Myers).[29-41]

ELECTROPHYSIOLOGIC PROPERTIES. Encainide is the prototype of class IC antiarrhythmic agents. It slightly shortens the action potential duration in isolated cells and markedly depresses phase 0 upstroke of the action potential. It also lengthens the effective refractory period and slows phase 4 repolarization.

Clinical electrophysiologic studies using intravenous encainide (0.6 mg to 1 mg/kg) have shown significant dose-related increases in infranodal (HV) interval and QRS duration, corrected sinus node recovery time, and refractory periods of atrium, atrioventricular node, or right ventricle. Accessory pathway conduction is prolonged or abolished.

PHARMACOKINETICS. The bioavailability of encainide is roughly 50% with significant interindividual variations.[29] A high percentage of drug is bound to plasma proteins (80%). Hepatic metabolism results in several active metabolites, such as O-demethylencainide (ODE) or 3 methoxy-O-demethylencainide (MODE). The elimination half-life averages 3 to 4 hours for encainide and may be longer for metabolites. A therapeutic plasma concentration of encainide is 39 ng/ml for the intravenous form and 14 ng/ml for the oral form.

HEMODYNAMIC EFFECTS. Although intravenous therapy with encainide has been found to decrease cardiac output slightly, hemodynamic studies performed even in patients with impaired left ventricular function (ejection fraction 45% or less) showed no significant change.[30,31]

CLINICAL ANTIARRHYTHMIC SPECTRUM. Encainide has been found to be remarkably effective in ventricular arrhythmias.[31,32] Suppression of ventricular extrasystoles was achieved in 80% or more of patients treated with a daily dose of 75 mg to 225 mg in a French collaborative study, including 48 patients with stable ventricular extrasystoles. Suppression of more than 75% of ventricular extrasystoles was achieved in 75% of patients during the titration period. After a follow-up of 6 months, 62.5% of patients still showed a beneficial response.[33]

In sustained ventricular tachycardia refractory to conventional antiarrhythmic therapy, control of 50% or more of patients has been reported.[34-36] However, proarrhythmic effects have been noted in about 10% of the patients.[37] The proarrhythmic effect appears to be, in part, related to the rapidity of dose titration and occurs most frequently in patients with ventricular tachycardia or fibrillation or with altered left ventricular function.[30]

In supraventricular tachycardias, oral encainide has been reported to be successful in a variable percentage of patients. However, more data are needed to establish the role of encainide in this setting. The results appear better in patients with the Wolff-Parkinson-White syndrome, as opposed to patients with reentry confined to the atrioventricular node.[35,40,41]

SIDE EFFECTS. Intravenous therapy with encainide may be associated with central nervous system side effects such as tremor, blurred vision, or dizziness. Aside from proarrhythmic effects (*i.e.*, incessant ventricular tachycardia), these central nervous system side effects are common, although most often tolerable by dose adjustment. Long-term therapy is associated with an increase in PR, QRS, and QTc intervals. Caution should be observed in the use of encainide in patients with pre-existing conduction disturbances particularly at the His-Purkinje level. Other rare noncardiac side effects include elevated levels of serum liver enzymes, hepatitis, and gastrointestinal events (diarrhea, dyspepsia, abdominal pain, nausea).

DRUG INTERACTIONS. Encainide has no significant effect on digoxin blood levels. Combination therapy is feasible with β-blocking agents or calcium channel blockers, but electrocardiographic surveillance is recommended. Plasma concentrations of encainide are increased by the concomitant use of cimetidine.

DOSAGE REGIMEN. The intravenous dose is 0.5 mg to 1.5 mg/kg over 10 to 20 minutes. The oral dose is 25 mg to 50 mg every 8 hours (75 mg to 150 mg/day).

FLECAINIDE

Flecainide acetate is an interesting and highly effective antiarrhythmic agent that is available for clinical use in Europe and the United States (Tambocor, Flecaine, Riker Laboratories, 3M).[42-51]

ELECTROPHYSIOLOGIC PROPERTIES. Flecainide depresses the upstroke velocity of the action potential and lengthens action potential duration and refractory period of atrial and ventricular muscle. It is a class IC antiarrhythmic agent. No significant action was noted on slow channel currents.

Clinical electrophysiologic studies[47,50,51] have shown that flecainide lengthens PR, intra-atrial (PA), atrioventricular nodal (AH), and HV intervals and QRS complex duration. However, repolarization is not affected; the lengthening of the QT interval, when present, is due almost exclusively to an increase in QRS complex duration. The effective refractory periods of atria, atrioventricular node, and right ventricle are slightly increased. Spontaneous sinus cycle length is slightly increased by intravenous use of flecainide; the conduction over an accessory atrioventricular connection is either completely blocked or the antegrade and retrograde refractory periods are prolonged.[50]

PHARMACOKINETICS. Intravenous administration of flecainide (1 mg to 2 mg/kg over 10 minutes) results in peak concentration at 10 minutes. The half-life is about 14 hours. Forty percent of the drug is excreted unchanged in the urine.

The oral form of flecainide (200 mg to 400 mg/day) has a bioavailability of 90% or more, hepatic metabolism, and a long elimination half-life, ranging from 7 to 23 hours. Therapeutic plasma concentrations range from 200 ng to 1000 ng/ml. The excretion is predominantly renal; 27% of the drug is found unchanged, and known metabolites are inactive.

HEMODYNAMIC EFFECTS. Flecainide has a negative inotropic effect, as shown by depressed contractility in patients with coronary artery disease, and caution should be observed in patients with known congestive heart failure or altered left ventricular function.[42]

CLINICAL ANTIARRHYTHMIC SPECTRUM. Flecainide was found to be a potent antiarrhythmic agent for ventricular arrhythmias. Controlled studies in patients with ventricular extrasystoles have shown more than 80% reduction in premature ventricular contractions in 85% of patients and about 70% suppression of couplets and nonsustained ventricular tachycardia[45] and are consistent with previous reports in patients with resistant ventricular arrhythmias.[46] In a multicenter trial in patients with ventricular tachycardia (sustained or nonsustained), effective treatment was initially obtained in 72% of patients.[38] In patients with documented sustained ventricular tachycardia, prevention of pacing-induced ventricular tachycardia was achieved in 60% of patients.[47] Another study[39] showed that prevention of ventricular arrhythmia using programmed electrical stimulation predicted long-term efficacy. However, a proarrhythmic effect represents a potential complication[48,49] in about 5% of patients.

Flecainide may be useful in patients with reciprocating tachycardias, including accessory atrioventricular connection in the reentrant circuit. Intravenously administered[48,49] flecainide was able to block antegrade conduction in 75% of patients and retrograde conduction in about 50% of patients.[50,51] Intravenous flecainide was effective in converting atrial arrhythmias to sinus rhythm in a significant percentage of patients.[43,44] Reports suggest that oral flecainide may successfully prevent atrial and junctional tachycardias.

SIDE EFFECTS. Aside from an increase in PR interval and QRS complex duration, undesirable cardiac effects of flecainide include aggravation of pre-existing conduction disturbances or sinus node dysfunction. Caution should be observed in patients with congestive heart failure, cardiomegaly, and bundle branch block. Stimulation threshold is markedly increased by flecainide, suggesting that particular caution be used if the drug is administered to patients with permanent pacemakers. Extracardiac side effects are common (15% to 60%). Blurred vision, vertigo, tremor, headaches, paresthesias, ataxia, and metallic taste rarely require drug withdrawal. The most significant proarrhythmic effect is incessant ventricular tachycardia, which may be observed in 12% of patients with sustained ventricular tachycardia and/or left ventricular dysfunction (ejection fraction less than 30%). Treatment should be initiated in the hospital in this group of patients at risk.[52] Recent data (unpublished) from a prospective trial of IC agents show an excess mortality of treated post-infarction patients.

DOSAGE REGIMEN. The intravenous dose is 1 mg to 2 mg/kg in a slow 5- to 10-minute injection. Flecainide, 100 mg to 200 mg, can also be administered orally every 12 hours (200 mg to 400 mg/day).

PROPAFENONE

Propafenone chlorhydrate (Rythmonorm, Rythmol, Knoll Laboratories) was developed in West Germany and is effective in a wide range of cardiac arrhythmias. Its mode of action is not completely understood.

ELECTROPHYSIOLOGIC PROPERTIES. Propafenone depresses phase 0 of the action potential and belongs to class I of the Vaughan-Williams classification. It does not lengthen action potential duration; the amplitude of action potential is decreased without significant change of resting potential. The refractory periods of atria, myocardium, and His-Purkinje fibers are increased. Propafenone has a mild β-adrenergic antagonist action (class II) and, at high concentration, a slow channel blocking effect (class IV).

Intravenous therapy with propafenone in humans does not significantly affect the sinus cycle length and the sinus node recovery time. Conduction time intervals (PA, AH, HV) are significantly prolonged. Similarly, the effective refractory periods of atrial, atrioventricular node, and ventricle are lengthened. Oral propafenone prolongs the sinus cycle length, QRS, and QTc interval (due to QRS prolongation only). In patients with accessory atrioventricular connections, propafenone impairs conduction and prolongs the refractory period of the accessory pathway.

PHARMACOKINETICS. Taken orally, propafenone has an availability of 50%. A high percentage (90%) of the drug is bound to plasma proteins. Two metabolites have been identified: 5-hydroxypropafenone (an active metabolite) and methoxyhydroxypropafenone. The elimination half-life is short (3 to 4 hours) and longer for the active metabolite. The antiarrhythmic plasma concentrations range from 500 ng to 1000 ng/ml.

HEMODYNAMIC EFFECTS. Propafenone has a negative inotropic effect that is not detectable in patients with normal left ventricular function. However, in patients with left ventricular dysfunction, alteration of hemodynamic parameters has been established. Worsening of congestive heart failure has been reported in a limited number of patients.[53]

CLINICAL ANTIARRHYTHMIC SPECTRUM. The unique electrophysiologic properties of propafenone have prompted its use in various types of cardiac arrhythmias.

Controlled trials have shown that the oral form of propafenone was effective in suppressing more than 80% of ventricular extrasystoles, couplets, or nonsustained ventricular tachycardia in 60% to 75% of patients.[53]

In patients with recurrent ventricular tachycardia, propafenone prevented pacing-induced ventricular tachycardias in a limited number (25%) of patients.[54,55] Proarrhythmic effects, such as spontaneous recurrence of clinical ventricular tachycardia, or its transformation to the "incessant" form have been reported. This side effect occurs soon after drug administration (within hours) and subsides as the drug is discontinued.

Open trials suggest that propafenone may be useful in patients with paroxysmal atrial fibrillation or flutter. I have observed arrhythmia control in about 50% of such patients who are refractory to conventional therapy. Uncontrolled studies have suggested that propafenone may be more effective in patients with adrenergically dependent atrial arrhythmias.

In patients with the Wolff-Parkinson-White syndrome, oral therapy with propafenone prevented symptomatic tachycardia in about 40% of patients and improved an additional 40% in a long-term study. The combination of oral propafenone with β-blocking agents may improve the clinical results in selected patients.

SIDE EFFECTS. The use of propafenone is frequently associated with a slight (10% to 20%) prolongation of the PR interval and QRS complex duration. The oral form of the drug is well tolerated by the majority of patients. The reported side effects may be subdivided into three groups: gastrointestinal, central nervous system, and cardiac. Gastrointestinal side effects include metallic taste, dry mouth, nausea, and constipation; these side effects seldom require discontinuation of the drug. Occasional elevation of serum glutamic oxaloacetic or pyruvic transaminase levels has been reported. Central nervous system side effects, such as dizziness, lightheadedness, or disorientation are not uncommon. Aside from potential proarrhythmic effects, oral propafenone may expose or worsen pre-existing conduction disturbance or sinus node dysfunction. Caution should be observed in patients with impaired myocardial function. Torsade de pointes has been rarely observed. Polymorphous malignant ventricular tachycardias have been reported.

Intravenously administered propafenone is generally well tolerated (1 mg to 2 mg/kg). Metallic taste commonly follows the intravenous administration of this drug.

DOSAGE REGIMEN. The intravenous dose is 1 mg to 2 mg/kg over a 10-minute period followed when necessary by a 2-mg/min infusion. An oral dose of 300 mg, is administered every 8 hours; a lower dose of 150 mg three times a day or 300 mg twice daily may be sufficient in some patients.

CIBENZOLINE

Cibenzoline is a class I antiarrhythmic agent and is undergoing intensive clinical investigation.

ELECTROPHYSIOLOGIC PROPERTIES. Cibenzoline decreases the rate of rise of phase 0 and the amplitude of the action potential (class I effect). It also prolongs action potential duration (class III effect), except in Purkinje fibers, and reduces the slow current carried by calcium and sodium ions (class IV effect).

Clinical electrophysiologic studies have shown that cibenzoline does not significantly alter sinus cycle length, intra-atrial (PA), or atriohisian (AH) conduction time. Intraventricular conduction time (HV interval) and refractory periods of the right ventricle are significantly lengthened. Refractory periods of other structures are not significantly or consistently altered.[56] There is little information on the effect of cibenzoline on accessory atrioventricular connections.

PHARMACOKINETICS. The bioavailability of oral cibenzoline is more than 90%. The maximum plasma concentration is observed around 1½ hours after administration. Most of the drug (60%) is excreted unchanged in the urine. The elimination half-life of 4 hours in normal subjects,[57] may reach 7 to 10 hours in elderly patients. The only identified metabolite in humans (dehydrocibenzoline) has no antiarrhythmic effect.

HEMODYNAMIC EFFECTS. Cibenzoline has a negative inotropic effect, as shown by a study in patients with coronary artery disease; however, this effect seems to be mild.

CLINICAL ANTIARRHYTHMIC SPECTRUM. The intravenous dose of cibenzoline is 0.5 mg to 1.2 mg/kg. A review of its clinical use in 212 patients has shown that cibenzoline was effective in terminating various types of paroxysmal supraventricular tachyarrhythmias (15/24 patients), including those associated with the Wolff-Parkinson-White syndrome.[58] In patients with ventricular arrhythmias (ventricular extrasystoles or ventricular tachycardias), a good result, defined as a decrease of 75% or more of ventricular extrasystoles or termination of sustained ventricular tachycardia, was obtained in about 80% of patients (49/62 patients). A randomized study of the comparative effect of a bolus of cibenzoline (1.2 mg/kg) versus a bolus of lidocaine (1.4 mg/kg) in ventricular extrasystoles occurring in the setting of acute myocardial infarction showed that cibenzoline was as effective as lidocaine.

The oral form of cibenzoline has been used in treating a variety of cardiac arrhythmias. In patients with ventricular extrasystoles, a controlled study showed that 19 of 21 (90%) responded (more than 75% suppression) to a daily dose of 260 mg to 320 mg.[59] This is consistent with the results of uncontrolled trials.[60] Cibenzoline successfully suppressed spontaneous episodes of ventricular tachycardia in 8 of 16 patients unresponsive to conventional antiarrhythmic agents.[56] Further clinical investigation is needed to confirm these promising results and to determine the effect of cibenzoline on pacing-induced ventricular tachycardia.

The efficacy of cibenzoline (260 mg/day) in preventing paroxysmal atrial fibrillation in a double-blind study was compared with that of quinidine. The number of recurrences over a 6-month period was lower with cibenzoline (20%) than with quinidine (43%).[61]

There is little information regarding the effect of cibenzoline in preventing paroxysmal junctional tachycardias.

SIDE EFFECTS. Several studies have noted good tolerance to cibenzoline.[59-61] Intravenously administered cibenzoline (1 mg to 2 mg/kg) increases QRS and QT intervals. In one review, 18 of 212 patients (8.5%) developed side effects, including slight hypotension, conduction disturbances (bundle branch block, fascicular block, and atrioventricular block), and a proarrhythmic effect. Because most of the patients had an acute myocardial infarction, the actual incidence of side effects might have been overestimated. Gastrointestinal side effects (nausea and vomiting) have been reported in a few cases. I have observed conversion of atrial flutter with 2:1 block to 1:1 conduction due to slowing of the atrial flutter rate following intravenous therapy with cibenzoline.

Oral cibenzoline may be infrequently associated with side effects (nausea, vomiting, dyspepsia) and only rarely may require drug discontinuation. Anticholinergic effects (dry mouth and blurred vision) may occasionally occur. Cardiac side effects include proarrhythmic effects, which have been reported in 1 of 26 patients with ventricular arrhythmias in a recent report.[56] Elevated levels of serum glutamic oxaloacetic transaminase have been noted during long-term therapy.[61]

DOSAGE REGIMEN. The dose of intravenous cibenzoline is 1 mg/kg bolus over 2 to 5 minutes, if necessary, followed by an intravenous infusion of 8 mg/kg/day, or oral cibenzoline 1 hour after the bolus. The oral dose of cibenzoline is 130 mg three times a day (390 mg/day) or 4 mg to 6 mg/kg. This dose should be reduced by half in elderly patients. There is no known interaction of cibenzoline with digoxin.

AMIODARONE

Amiodarone, a benzofurane derivative, was discovered in 1961 and was initially used as an antianginal agent. This drug is structurally related to thyroxine (T_4) and has a high iodine content. The antiarrhythmic properties were recognized in 1970. Since then, amiodarone has become the most widely used antiarrhythmic agent in several European countries. Amiodarone is available for clinical use in the United States for the treatment of "documented, life-threatening recurrent ventricular arrhythmias, when these have not responded to documented adequate doses of other adequate available antiarrhythmics or when alternative agents could not be tolerated" (Cordarone, Wyeth Laboratories, Package insert)[52] Amiodarone has been the subject of an overwhelming number of reports concerning both its benefits and its side effects.

ELECTROPHYSIOLOGIC PROPERTIES. The main cellular electrophysiologic effect of amiodarone is to prolong the action potential duration of atrium and ventricle without altering the resting membrane potential. Amiodarone is the prototype of a class III antiarrhythmic drug. It prolongs the absolute refractory period by uniformly delaying repolarization in both atrium and ventricle. Amiodarone also exerts a minimal reduction in phase 0 of the action potential duration (class I effect) and exhibits "some antagonism to the action of catecholamines of a noncompetitive nature."

The clinical electrophysiologic properties of amiodarone have been studied by several investigators. Oral amiodarone decreases heart rate by an average of 15%. Atrioventricular nodal conduction (AH interval) is depressed. The effect on intra-atrial (PA interval) and infranodal (HV interval) conduction is variable. The effective refractory period of the atrium and atrioventricular node are increased. The antegrade refractory period of atrioventricular accessory pathways is generally prolonged, and the retrograde effective refractory period of about 50% of patients with the Wolff-Parkinson-White syndrome is increased.[62]

PHARMACOKINETICS. Little is known about the pharmacokinetics of amiodarone.

Given intravenously as an infusion of 600 mg over 24 hours, plasma concentrations of 0.5 μg/ml are obtained and the elimination half-life is around 20 hours after the drug has been discontinued.

Oral amiodarone has a slow gastrointestinal absorption (50% of the initial dose). The onset of action is delayed as amiodarone accumulates in tissues (fat and fat-ladened organs). The long elimination half-life (24 to 160 days; mean, 64 days) has been confirmed by the measurement of serum concentrations of amiodarone and desethylamiodarone. The maintenance serum amiodarone concentration ranged between 0.4 mg and 3.3 mg/liter.[63,64] A good correlation was found between serum levels and the daily dose. Control of arrhythmias was satisfactory at amiodarone levels of about 1.5 mg/liter. Reverse triiodothyronine (rT_3) was suggested as an alternative to monitoring amiodarone serum levels, since a good correlation was found between QTc measured on the electrocardiogram and rT_3. Tissue concentrations on postmortem studies were up to 300 times greater than plasma concentrations. The pharmacokinetics of amiodarone substantiates the necessity of a loading dose.

HEMODYNAMIC EFFECTS. Amiodarone may have a different hemodynamic effect if used intravenously, as opposed to orally. Hypotension may be observed as a side effect of the intravenous form, whereas the usual oral doses do not precipitate heart failure in patients with poor myocardial function. As a vasodilator, amiodarone increases coronary blood flow and reduces afterload, which counterbalances the negative inotropic effect.

CLINICAL ANTIARRHYTHMIC SPECTRUM. Amiodarone has been successfully used in a wide variety of cardiac arrhythmias.[65-69] Amiodarone (5 mg/kg infusion) has been reported in a large series[70] of patients with supraventricular tachyarrhythmias to restore sinus rhythm in 38% of cases with atrial fibrillation and in 21% with atrial flutter and to slow the ventricular response in 47% of cases. A beneficial effect was obtained in two thirds of patients, including patients with atrial tachycardia. Similar results were observed in the acute management of patients with ventricular arrhythmias. In a review of the reports from the French literature, I found that intravenous amiodarone (5 mg/kg over 2 to 5 minutes) restored sinus rhythm in 60% of cases of sustained ventricular tachycardia. This was consistent with a report in which acute control of the arrhythmia was obtained in 12 of 15 patients (80%) with ventricular tachycardia refractory to two or more antiarrhythmic agents.[65]

ORAL THERAPY. Successful results of oral therapy with amiodarone have been reported in a high proportion of patients with recurrent supraventricular tachyarrhythmias, both with or without the electrocardiographic features of the Wolff-Parkinson-White syndrome. In patients without the Wolff-Parkinson-White syndrome, effective symptomatic improvement was observed in more than 80% of the reported cases. In preexcitation, prevention of both atrial fibrillation and reciprocating tachycardia was achieved in 60% to 100% of patients. The figure of 60% parallels that of my personal experience.[66,67]

Amiodarone has a potent antiarrhythmic action at the ventricular level. Orally administered amiodarone was effective in suppressing persistent ventricular extrasystoles in about 90% of patients reported in the French literature. However, there have been no randomized, controlled trials, as the necessity of a loading dose makes performance of such trials difficult. The effect of amiodarone in the prophylaxis of recurrent ventricular tachycardia was seen as early as 1973 and confirmed by subsequent studies in 55% to 89% of patients. Controversy exists regarding the value of programmed electrical stimulation techniques in predicting drug efficacy of amiodarone.[68,69]

In summary, the oral form of amiodarone is a versatile antiarrhythmic agent with a wide antiarrhythmic spectrum that is efficient in preventing atrial, junctional, or ventricular tachyarrhythmias.

SIDE EFFECTS. The dramatic efficacy of amiodarone is, however, associated with a high incidence of side effects. Intravenous injection of amiodarone may be associated with flushing (5% of cases) or transient nausea and sweating (2%). Hypotension and cardiovascular collapse may occur in 5% of patients.[70] In order to prevent such complications, an intravenous bolus injection (5 mg/kg) should be slow (over 10 to 15 minutes), particularly in patients with altered myocardial function. Atrioventricular block (nodal) may occasionally occur. Venous inflammation with continuous infusion is possible and may be prevented by drug infusion through a central venous catheter.

The higher incidence of adverse effects reported in the United States may be due to higher maintenance doses (600 mg to 800 mg), as compared with the European experience, in which lower maintenance doses (200 mg to 400 mg) are used. Universal effects include QTc prolongation (marker of myocardial impregnation) and corneal microdeposits. In contrast, the dose-dependent side effects of oral amiodarone include cutaneous photosensitivity (3% to 7%), slate blue-gray discoloration, so-called visage mauve (1% to 2%), visual disturbances, gastrointestinal symptoms, and neurologic complications. In contrast, thyroid function disturbances do not seem to be dose related. Hypothyroidism and hyperthyroidism occur in less than 5% of patients. Because amiodarone blocks conversion of T_4 to T_3, an elevated T_4 level is a common laboratory finding. Hypothyroidism is more frequent than hyperthyroidism and subsides within a few months with drug discontinuation and thyroid replacement. Hyperthyroidism generally appears after several months of therapy. Atrioventricular block and sinus arrest may occur in predisposed patients. Worsening of cardiac arrhythmias and torsade de pointes have been reported, although the incidence seems to be less than that of conventional antiarrhythmic agents. Pulmonary fibrosis is rare with lower maintenance doses[71] and in most cases subsides spontaneously following drug discontinuation. Of concern are the reports of death related to this complication. Asymptomatic hepatic enzyme elevation also has been reported.

Despite these side effects, which can be lessened by careful surveillance, amiodarone is widely used in Europe and gaining popularity in the United States because of its extraordinary efficacy, although it is still restricted to refractory arrhythmia.

Amiodarone may be given as a slow intravenous injection (5 to 15 minutes) of 5 mg/kg. The onset of effect starts at the end of injection, and the duration of action ranges from 20 minutes to several hours. The dosage for an intravenous infusion is 600 mg to 1200 mg/day.

DOSAGE REGIMEN. A loading dose of 600 mg to 1000 mg for 7 to 14 days is required. The maintenance dosage of 200 mg to 400 mg/day, 5 days a week, is most commonly used in Europe. Higher maintenance doses of 600 mg to 1200 mg/day have been reported in the United States. Higher doses were used in order to obtain control of life-threatening arrhythmias refractory to conventional and investigational drugs.

Drug interaction has been reported in patients on digoxin. The serum levels of digoxin are increased. Caution should also be observed in patients taking warfarin, since potentiation of the anticoagulant effects may produce serious hemorrhage. Drug levels of class I antiarrhythmic agents may be increased when they are given in association with amiodarone.

In view of the possible side effects, amiodarone is mainly recommended for patients with refractory supraventricular arrhythmias, particularly those associated with the Wolff-Parkinson-White syndrome and a short refractory period of the accessory pathway, and for patients with life-threatening ventricular arrhythmias.

SOTALOL

Among β-blocking agents, sotalol chlorhydrate has unique electrophysiologic properties characterized by additional class III properties. Sotalol is a noncardioselective β-blocking agent with no membrane stabilizing activity or intrinsic sympathomimetic activity.

ELECTROPHYSIOLOGIC PROPERTIES. Sotalol prolongs repolarization, which results in QT interval prolongation and prolonged duration of the action potential (class III) and refractory periods. As a β-blocking agent, sotalol has a sympatholytic action (class II).

Clinical electrophysiologic properties of sotalol are common to β-blocking agents and additional effects, similar to those of amiodarone, are noted. The sinus cycle length, atrioventricular nodal conduction (AH interval), and effective refractory period are lengthened. The effective refractory period of the atrium and ventricle are increased, suggesting an antiarrhythmic action at the atrial and ventricular level.[72,73] In patients with the Wolff-Parkinson-White syndrome, sotalol lengthens the antegrade and retrograde accessory pathway effective refractory periods.[74]

PHARMACOKINETICS. The availability of sotalol is nearly 100%, because sotalol is completely absorbed and not metabolized. Excretion is renal. The maximum plasma concentration is rapidly reached (2 hours). The elimination half-life is about 11 hours.

HEMODYNAMIC EFFECTS. As a β-blocking agent, sotalol has a negative inotropic effect that is used in the treatment of hypertension and coronary insufficiency. However, in patients without heart failure, the hemodynamic status is generally not altered by sotalol.

CLINICAL ANTIARRHYTHMIC SPECTRUM. There is little information available on the use of the intravenous or oral form of the drug on supraventricular arrhythmias. When administered intravenously in ten patients with supraventricular tachyarrhythmias sotalol was able to restore sinus rhythm in five and to slow ventricular rate in four.[75]

In contrast, several studies have been performed in patients with ventricular arrhythmias. Sotalol was able to reduce the incidence of ventricular extrasystoles by 88% in a group of patients with coronary artery disease.[76] A lower incidence (about 50%) was stated in recent reports.

Intravenous therapy with sotalol prevented pacing-induced ventricular tachycardia in 12 of 18 patients (67%), and 9 of these put on oral therapy obtained effective prophylaxis against ventricular tachycardia.[77]

Although it is suggested that sotalol possesses more potent antiarrhythmic properties than other β-blocking agents, because of its unique electrophysiologic properties, more data are needed.

SIDE EFFECTS. Sotalol is generally well tolerated both in the intravenous and oral forms at usual doses. Cardiac side effects of oral sotalol include hypotension, aggravation of pre-existing conduction, or sinus node disturbances. Proarrhythmic effects were noted in a small percentage (<5%) of patients with ventricular extrasystoles. Noncardiac side effects are mild, provided the usual contraindications of β-blocking agents are observed. Dizziness and fatigue have occasionally been noted.

DOSAGE REGIMEN. Sotalol has been used intravenously at a dose of 0.6 mg to 1.2 mg/kg. The oral dose is 160 mg to 320 mg twice daily.

BEPRIDIL

Bepridil hydrochloride is a new calcium antagonist for the treatment of coronary insufficiency. It was found effective for control of ventricular arrhythmias, which gives this compound a unique position among the family of calcium antagonists.

ELECTROPHYSIOLOGIC PROPERTIES. Electrophysiologic studies at the cellular level have shown that bepridil is a slow and fast channel blocking agent and has properties in common with class I and class IV agents.

In humans, bepridil also has unique electrophysiologic properties.[78] As other calcium antagonists (except nifedipine), bepridil prolongs atrioventricular nodal conduction (AH interval) and refractoriness. In contrast to other class IV agents, bepridil prolongs atrial and ventricular refractoriness, which may explain its effectiveness for ventricular arrhythmias.

PHARMACOKINETICS. In humans, a single dose of bepridil has an availability of 60% and maximal serum concentration is reached 2 hours following administration. Bepridil may bind to a number of serum proteins and may be fixed to tissues, particularly to cardiac muscle. Bepridil is metabolized predominantly in the liver, and its elimination is both urinary and biliary. The elimination half-life is long (47 hours).

Using the recommended dose of 300 mg/day, the steady state is reached after 7 days. This delay may be shortened by using a loading dose (600 mg to 800 mg/day).

HEMODYNAMIC EFFECTS. Intravenously administered bepridil (2 mg and 4 mg/kg) used in patients with stable coronary insufficiency was found to reduce afterload and aortic pressure in a dose-dependent fashion, to slightly but significantly reduce contractility parameters (negative inotropic effect), and to increase coronary blood flow by 50%.[79] During exercise, intravenously administered bepridil improves ejection fraction and segmental contractility, as shown by isotope studies.[80] Hemodynamic parameters, including ejection fraction and cardiac index, are unchanged following oral administration of bepridil. The ejection fraction during exercise is significantly improved.[81]

CLINICAL ANTIARRHYTHMIC SPECTRUM. Intravenous therapy with bepridil (3 mg/kg over 5 minutes) was able to terminate paroxysmal, presumably junctional, tachycardia in 25 of 33 episodes (75.7%).[82] The success rate in ventricular tachycardia termination averaged 50%.[83-85] More information is needed on the usefulness of intravenously administered bepridil in tachycardia termination and prevention.

The oral form of the drug has been used mainly in ventricular arrhythmias. Suppression of 85% of ventricular extrasystoles was obtained in 70% of patients in uncontrolled trials,[86,87] using doses of 400 mg to 500 mg/day.

In patients with recurrent, sustained ventricular tachycardia, oral therapy with bepridil prevented pacing-induced ventricular tachycardia in about 60%.[83,88] However, data are lacking on the long-term results in a large group of patients.

SIDE EFFECTS. Intravenously administered bepridil (2 mg to 3 mg/kg) is well tolerated by the vast majority of patients. Transient flushing or nausea may occasionally occur.

The oral use of bepridil, aside from QT interval prolongation and changes of T wave morphology (flattening and biphasic changes), which are indicative of drug effect, may be associated in some patients with gastrointestinal side effects (nausea, dyspepsia, diarrhea, anorexia). One case of paralytic ileus has been observed.[83] The main concern has been the occurrence of torsade de pointes. An intensive search to collect cases of torsade de pointes in France, secondary to the use of bepridil, resulted in an incidence of about 1 in 1000 cases. Congestive heart failure in elderly patients and hypokalemia, most often related to a concomitant use of diuretics, are important precipitating factors.

DRUG INTERACTIONS. Digoxin may be used in association with bepridil, as there is no known clinically detectable pharmacokinetic interaction; however, this point deserves further investigation. Caution should be observed in the use of bepridil in association with diuretics and bradycardiac agents.

DOSAGE REGIMEN. The intravenous use of bepridil has exclusively been as a bolus of 2 mg to 3 mg/kg over a 5- to 10-minute period. Orally administered bepridil, in the treatment of cardiac arrhythmias, is effective in a dose of 400 mg to 600 mg/day. The long elimination half-life allows the dose to be administered once daily.

PIRMENOL

Pirmenol, a pyridine methanol derivative, is undergoing clinical investigation. Preliminary reports suggest that this agent may be effective in the treatment of a wide range of cardiac arrhythmias.

ELECTROPHYSIOLOGIC PROPERTIES. Pirmenol decreases the upstroke velocity of the action potential and action potential duration, properties similar to class IB drugs. However, it prolongs refractoriness and slows conduction in cardiac fibers as do class IA agents. Pirmenol depresses automaticity (both slow and fast responses) in Purkinje fibers.[89]

Electrophysiologic studies in patients with ventricular tachycardias showed a decrease in sinus cycle length (11-13%) and an increase in PR, QRS, QTc, and HV intervals.[90] Atrial and ventricular effective refractory periods were prolonged. AV nodal function is unchanged.

PHARMACOKINETICS. Pirmenol has a mean bioavailability of 80%. A high proportion (86%) of the plasma fraction is protein bound. Renal clearance is about 50%. Preliminary studies suggest the presence of active metabolites. The elimination half-life is long, averaging 8 to 12 hours. Clinical studies indicate a longer half-life of 12 to 48 hours. Therapeutic plasma concentrations range from 0.43 to 1.7 μg/ml.

HEMODYNAMIC EFFECTS. Experimental studies have suggested that myocardial contractility is decreased without significant change in stroke volume attributed to an increase in heart rate. Similar findings are suggested by available studies in humans, indicating no significant change following intravenous injection. Information on the hemodynamic effects of the oral form of pirmenol are needed.

CLINICAL ANTIARRHYTHMIC SPECTRUM. Intravenous therapy with pirmenol has been proven to suppress ventricular arrhythmias.[89-91] Reduction of stable ventricular extrasystoles was 76%[91] using a bolus dose of 150 mg over 30 minutes. Sustained pacing-induced ventricular tachycardia is also suppressed by intravenously administered pirmenol.[92] In 60% of patients with atrial fibrillation, conversion to sinus rhythm is obtained but pirmenol does not slow the rate of those patients whose rhythms where not converted.

Orally administered pirmenol was also found effective in suppressing ventricular extrasystoles. More information is needed on the efficacy of oral therapy with pirmenol in patients with supraventricular tachycardia.

A relative lack of potassium dependance suggests that pirmenol may be used if needed in patients with hypokalemia.

SIDE EFFECTS. Intravenously administered pirmenol is often associated with unusual taste. This is also reported in patients receiving the oral form. Constipation may occur in some patients.

DOSAGE REGIMEN. Pirmenol is given intravenously at an initial dose of 50 mg/min up to 1 to 2 g followed by a maintenance infusion of 2 mg/min.[92] The drug has been given orally in investigational use at doses of 150 to 250 mg in single or repeated doses in order to achieve plasma levels of 2 μg/ml.

LORCAINIDE

Lorcainide hydrochloride (Remivox) is a class I antiarrhythmic agent with local anesthetic activity.

ELECTROPHYSIOLOGIC PROPERTIES. Lorcainide decreases the rate of rise of transmembrane action-potential and conduction velocity in Purkinje fiber preparations. The refractory period of Purkinje of ventricular muscle fibers is prolonged, and phase 4 depolarization is slowed.[93]

Clinical electrophysiologic studies in humans have shown that the sinus cycle length is unchanged or slightly shortened, the AV nodal conduction time (AH) is unchanged or increased, the infranodal conduction (HV) is constantly prolonged. The atrial and ventricular effective refractory periods are prolonged. Lorcainide lengthens the refractory period of accessory AV pathways and may produce complete anterograde block.

PHARMACOKINETICS. Orally administered lorcainide has an initial availability of 50%, which reaches 100% at steady state. The drug is metabolized in the liver. An active metabolite (N-dealkylated or norlorcainide) with a slower plasma clearance is formed. The elimination half-life is slow (7 hours) and is significantly prolonged in heart failure and in hepatic dysfunction. The half-life of norlorcainide is longer, resulting in progressive increase in plasma levels during oral treatment up to and exceeding those of the mother compound. The excretion is urinary. Therapeutic plasma levels of lorcainide range from 100 to 500 ng/ml, and those of norlorcainide are from 100 to 1000 ng/ml. There is a good correlation between plasma levels and QRS complex widening.

HEMODYNAMIC EFFECTS. Experimental models and available studies in humans suggest that lorcainide has a negative inotropic effect. Intravenous injection of lorcainide is followed by a transient fall in blood pressure and a compensatory increase in heart rate.

CLINICAL ANTIARRHYTHMIC SPECTRUM. Intravenous therapy with lorcainide (2 mg/kg) was found to be as effective as lidocaine therapy in suppressing ventricular extrasystoles both in patients with and without acute myocardial infarction. Controlled trials have shown that the oral form of lorcainide is successful in reducing the number and severe forms of ventricular extrasystoles in about 60% of the patients.[94] In patients with sustained ventricular tachycardia or ventricular fibrillation, suppression of pacing induced arrhythmia is achieved in about 50% of patients.[94,95]

Except for patients with preexcitation syndrome in whom antegrade conduction is blocked or prolonged, the efficacy of lorcainide in the treatment of supraventricular arrhythmias remains to be demonstrated.

SIDE EFFECTS. Intravenous lorcainide injection may be associated with central nervous system side effects similar to those encountered with lidocaine such as paresthesia, dizziness, hot flashes, and headaches. Oral lorcainide may be associated in a significant percentage of patients with sleep disorders (insomnia, hallucinations, nightmare) or gastrointestinal disorders (nausea, vomiting).

DOSAGE REGIMEN. The intravenous dosage is 2 mg/kg in slow injection. The oral dosage is 200 to 400 mg/24 hr in divided doses.

MORICIZINE

Moricizine, or ethmozine, is structurally related to phenothiazine (ethyl ester hydrochloridine of 10 phenothiazine-2-carbonic acid). This class I antiarrhythmic agent was developed in the Soviet Union and is under clinical evaluation in the United States.[96-100]

ELECTROPHYSIOLOGIC PROPERTIES. Moricizine decreases the maximum upstroke of phase 0 and shortens the duration of the membrane action potential (class IC of Vaughan-Williams classification). An interesting property of moricizine is the observed suppression of automaticity in ischemic Purkinje fibers. In contrast, it does not affect the slope of phase 4 depolarization of spontaneous automatic Purkinje fibers. Clinical electrophysiologic studies have shown prolongation of AV nodal and infranodal (HV) intervals, resulting in significant PR interval lengthening. An important finding with oral moricizine is the prolongation of QRS complex duration at doses ranging from 750 to 1350 mg/day.[96] No significant effect is noted on sinus cycle length, on sinus node automaticity, or on QT interval. Atrial and ventricular effective refractory periods are not affected.

PHARMACOKINETICS. Orally administered moricizine is virtually totally absorbed. Peak plasma levels are reached rapidly (1 to 3 hours). The metabolism of moricizine is not clear. The drug half-life is 3 hours. In patients, the elimination half-life is longer (about 7 hours), suggesting the presence of an active metabolite. The therapeutic plasma level averages 0.42 µg/ml when the drug is given every 8 hours, for a total dose of 10 mg/kg.[97]

HEMODYNAMIC EFFECTS. No significant change of blood pressure is noted in patients on oral therapy with moricizine. Echocardiographic and radionuclide evaluation of left ventricular function shows no change.[97,100] No data are available on the effect of moricizine in patients with left ventricular dysfunction.

CLINICAL ANTIARRHYTHMIC SPECTRUM. Moricizine has been demonstrated to be effective in the treatment of ventricular arrhythmias. Suppression of ventricular extrasystoles is achieved in 50% to 80% of patients with a dose-dependent effect, as shown by placebo-controlled study.[97] Complex forms such as couplets and nonsustained ventricular tachycardias are abolished totally in 75% of patients.[96,100] Conflicting results are found in the literature regarding the preventive effect of moricizine on pacing-induced sustained ventricular tachycardias.[96-100] More studies are warranted in patients with life-threatening arrhythmias.

Little information is available on the effect of moricizine in patients with supraventricular tachycardias, but it suggests that moricizine may be effective in patients with accessory connections as it may block antegrade conduction.

SIDE EFFECTS. A proarrhythmic effect such as increase in arrhythmia frequency or facilitation of ventricular tachycardia induction has been reported.[96] Noncardiac side effects include dizziness, euphoria, perioral numbness, nausea, and diarrhea and occur in about 20% of patients. Rarely is discontinuation of the drug required. There is no known interaction with digoxin. The metabolism of moricizine is inhibited by cimetidine.

DOSAGE REGIMEN. The clinical trials have used an average of 7 mg/kg/day or 300 to 750 mg per 24 hours in three divided doses (every 8 hours).

REFERENCES

1. Vaughan-Williams EM: Classification of antiarrhythmic drugs. In Sandoe E, Flenstedt-Jensen E, Olesen KH (eds): Cardiac Arrhythmias. Sodertalje, Sweden, 1970
2. Woosley RL, Wang T, Stone W et al: Pharmacology, electrophysiology and pharmacokinetics of mexiletine. Am Heart J 107(part 2):1058, 1984
3. McComish M, Crook B, Kitson D et al: Clinical electrophysiologic effects of mexiletine, a new local anaesthetic type of antiarrhythmic drug. Circulation (Suppl II) 51/52:215, 1975
4. Roos JC, Paalman ACA, Dunning AJ: Electrophysiologic effects of mexiletine in man. Br Heart J 38:1262, 1976
5. Campbell RWF, Talbot RG, Dolder MA et al: Comparison of procainamide and mexiletine in the prevention of arrhythmias after acute myocardial infarction. Lancet 1:257, 1975
6. Talbot RA, Wilson J, Prescott LF: Treatment of ventricular arrhythmia with mexiletine (KO 1173). Lancet 2:399, 1973
7. Podrid PJ, Lown B: Mexiletine for ventricular arrhythmias. Am J Cardiol 47:895, 1981
8. Horowitz JD, Anavekar SN, Morris PM et al: Comparative trial of mexiletine and lignocaine in the treatment of early ventricular tachyarrhythmias after acute myocardial infarction. J Cardiovasc Pharmacol 3:409, 1981
9. Slatter SD, Simmons W, McCall JG: Mexiletine for supraventricular tachycardia. Br Med J 281:1072, 1980
10. Benditt DG, Pool-Schneider S, Dunnigan A et al: Suppression of paroxysmal supraventricular tachyarrhythmias with intravenous mexiletine. PACE 8:302, 1985
11. Mehta J, Conti CR: Mexiletine, a new antiarrhythmic agent, for treatment of premature ventricular complexes. Am J Cardiol 49:455, 1982
12. Breithart G, Seipel L, Lersmacher J et al: Comparative study of the antiarrhythmic efficacy of mexiletine and disopyramide in patients with chronic ventricular arrhythmias. J Cardiovasc Pharmacol 4:276, 1982
13. Duff HJ, Roden D, Primm RK: Mexiletine in the treatment of resistant ventricular arrhythmias: Enhancement of efficacy and reduction of dose-related side effects by combination with quinidine. Circulation 67:1124, 1983
14. DiMarco JP, Garan H, Ruskin JN: Mexiletine for refractory ventricular arrhythmias: Results using serial electrophysiologic testing. Am J Cardiol 47:131, 1981

15. Manz M, Steinbeck G, Nitsch J et al: Treatment of recurrent sustained ventricular tachycardia with mexiletine and disopyramide: Control by programmed ventricular stimulation. Br Heart J 49:222, 1983
16. Heger J, Nattel S, Rinkerburger RL: Mexiletine therapy in 15 patients with drug-resistant ventricular tachycardia. Am J Cardiol 45:627, 1980
17. Campbell NPS, Pantridge JF, Adgey AAJ: Long-term oral antiarrhythmic therapy with mexiletine. Br Heart J 40:796, 1978
18. Cocco G, Strozz C, Chu D: Torsade de pointes as a manifestation of mexiletine toxicity. Am Heart J 100:878, 1980
19. Waleffe A, Mary-Rabine L, Legrand V et al: Combined mexiletine and amiodarone treatment of refractory recurrent ventricular tachycardia. Am Heart J 100:788, 1980
20. Anderson JL, Mason JW, Winkle RA et al: Clinical electrophysiologic effect of tocainide. Circulation 57:685, 1978
21. Waleffe A, Brunnix P, Mary-Rabine L et al: Effects of tocainide studied with programmed electrical stimulation of the heart in patients with reentrant tachyarrhythmias. Am J Cardiol 43:292, 1979
22. Winkle RA, Meffin PJ, Fitzgerald JW et al: Clinical efficacy and pharmacokinetics of a new orally effective antiarrhythmic, tocainide. Circulation 54:885, 1976
23. Ryden L, Arnman K, Conradson TB et al: Prophylaxis of ventricular tachyarrhythmias with intravenous and oral tocainide in patients with and recovering from acute myocardial infarction. Am Heart J 100:1006, 1980
24. McDevitt DG, Nies AS, Wilkinson GR et al: Antiarrhythmic effects of a lidocaine congener, tocainide, 2-amino-2'6'-propion-oxylidide, in man. Clin Pharmacol Ther 19:396, 1976
25. Woosley RL, McDevitt DG, Nies AS et al: Suppression of ventricular ectopic depolarizations by tocainide. Circulation 56:980, 1977
26. Hohnloser SH, Lange HW, Raeder EA et al: Short and long-term therapy with tocainide for malignant ventricular tachyarrhythmias. Circulation 73:143, 1986
27. Braude AC, Downar I, Chamberlain DW et al. Tocainide-associated interstitial pneumonitis. Ann Intern Med 94:489, 1981
28. Winkle RA, Meffin PJ, Harrison DC: Long-term tocainide therapy for ventricular arrhythmias. Circulation 57:1008, 1978
29. Jaillon P: Antiarrhythmic Drugs I: Clinical pharmacology of quinidine, procainamide, disopyramide, encainide, propafenone and flecainide. In Lévy S, Scheinman MM (eds): Cardiac Arrhythmias: From Diagnosis to Therapy. Mount Kisco, NY, Futura Publishing, 1984
30. DiBianco R, Fletcher RD, Cohen AI: Treatment of frequent ventricular arrhythmia with encainide: Assessment using serial ambulatory electrocardiograms, intracardiac electrophysiologic studies, treadmill exercise tests, and radionuclide cineangiographic studies. Circulation 65:1134, 1982
31. Roden DM, Woosley RL: Clinical pharmacology of the new antiarrhythmic encainide. Clin Prog Pacing Electrophysiol 2:112, 1984
32. Chesnie B, Podrid P, Naccarelli GV et al: Encainide for refractory ventricular arrhythmia. Am J Cardiol 52:495, 1983
33. Dumoulin P, Jaillon P, Kher A et al: Etude de l'effet antiarythmique de l'encainide au long cours dans l'extrasystolie ventriculaire chronique. Arch Mal Coeur (Numero special) 78:105, 1985
34. Mason JW, Peters FA: Antiarrhythmic efficacy of encainide in patients with refractory recurrent ventricular tachycardia. Circulation 63:670, 1981
35. Brugada P, Abdollah H, Wellens HJJ: Suppression of incessant supraventricular tachycardia by intravenous and oral encainide. J Am Coll Cardiol 4:1255, 1984
36. Heger JJ, Nattel S, Rinkenberger R et al: Encainide therapy in patients with drug-resistant ventricular tachycardia (abstr). Circulation 60:SII-185, 1979
37. Winkle RA, Mason JW, Griffin JC et al: Malignant ventricular tachyarrhythmias associated with the use of encainide. Am Heart J 102:857, 1981
38. Flecainide Ventricular Tachycardial Study Group: Treatment of resistant ventricular tachycardia with flecainide acetate. Am J Cardiol 57:1299, 1986
39. Flowers D, O'Gallagher D, Torres W et al: Flecaine: Long-term treatment using a reduced dosing schedule. Am J Cardiol 55:79, 1985
40. Prystowsky EN, Klein GJ, Rinkenberger RL et al: Clinical efficacy and electrophysiologic effects of encainide in patients with Wolff-Parkinson-White syndrome. Circulation 69:278, 1984
41. Cassagneau B, Miquel JP, Puel JP et al: Effets électrophysiologiques et antiarythmiques de l'encainide dans les tachycardies supraventriculaires. Arch Mal Coeur (Numero special) 78:113, 1985
42. Legrand V, Vandormael M, Collignon P et al: Hemodynamic effects of a new antiarrhythmic agent, flecainide (R818), in coronary heart disease. Am J Cardiol 51:422, 1983
43. Goy JJ, Orbic M, Hurni M et al: Conversion of supraventricular arrhythmias to sinus rhythm using flecainide. Eur Heart J 6:518, 1985
44. Lacombe P, Cointe R, Metge M et al: Intravenous flecainidine in the management of acute supraventricular tachyarrhythmias. J Electrophysiol 1:19, 1988
45. Flecainide-Quinidine Research Group: Flecainide versus quinidine for treatment of chronic ventricular arrhythmias: A multicenter clinical trial. Circulation 67:1117, 1983
46. Duff HJ, Roden DM, Maffucci RJ et al: Suppression of resistant ventricular arrhythmias by twice daily dosing with flecainide. Am J Cardiol 48:1133, 1981
47. Anderson JL, Lutz JR, Allison SB: Electrophysiologic and antiarrhythmic effects of oral flecainide in patients with inducible ventricular tachycardia. J Am Coll Cardiol 2:105, 1983
48. Lui HK, Lee G, Dietrich P: Flecainide induced QT prolongation and ventricular tachycardia. Am J Heart 103:567, 1982
49. Oetgen WJ, Tibbits PA, Abt MEO et al: Clinical and electrophysiologic assessment of oral flecainide acetate for recurrent ventricular tachycardia: Evidence for exacerbation of electrical instability. Am J Cardiol 52:746, 1983
50. Fauchier JP, Cosnay P, Rouesnel PH et al: Effets de la flécainide injectable et orale chez les patients ayant une voie accessoire auriculoventriculaire (V.A—A.V). Arch Mal Coeur (Numero special) 78:81, 1985
51. Hellestrand K, Nathan A, Bexton R et al: Cardiac electrophysiologic effects of flecainide acetate for paroxysmal reentrant junctional tachycardias. Am J Cardiol 51:770, 1983
52. Horowitz LN, Morganroth J: Second-generation antiarrhythmic agents: Have we reached antiarrhythmic Nirvana? J Am Cardiol 9:459, 1987
53. Salerno DM, Granrud G, Sharkey P et al: A controlled trial of propafenone for treatment of frequent and repetitive ventricular premature complexes. Am J Cardiol 53:77, 1984
54. Connolly SJ, Kates RE, Lebsack CS et al: Clinical pharmacology of propafenone. Circulation 68:589, 1983
55. Cointe R, Lévy S, Metge M et al: Traitement des tachycardies ventriculaires recidivantes par la propafenone orale. Arch Mal Coeur (Numero special) 78:59, 1985
56. Browne KF, Prystowsky EN, Zipes DP et al: Clinical efficacy and electrophysiologic effects of cibenzoline therapy in patients with ventricular arrhythmias. J Am Coll Cardiol 3:857, 1983
57. Canal M, Flouvat B, Tremblay D et al: Pharmacokinetics in man of a new antiarrhythmic drug, cibenzoline. Eur J Clin Pharmacol 24:509, 1983
58. Haiat R, Aymard MF, Dufour A: La cibenzoline intra-veineuse dans le traitement des troubles du rhythme supraventriculaires et ventriculaires. Arch Mal Coeur (Numero special) 78:95, 1985
59. Kostis JB, Krieger S, Moreyra A et al: Cibenzoline for treatment of ventricular arrhythmias: A double-blind placebo-controlled study. J Am Coll Cardiol 4:372, 1984
60. Herpin D, Gaudeau B, Boutaud P et al: Clinical trial of a new antiarrhythmic drug: Cibenzoline (Cipralan). Curr Ther Res 30:742, 1981
61. Frances Y, Luccioni R, Delaage M et al: Prevention au long cours des récidives de fibrillation auriculaire par la cibenzoline (Etude multicentrique, à propos de 89 observations). Arch Mal Coeur (Numero special) 78:99, 1985
62. Wellens HJJ, Bar FW, Dassen WRM et al: Effects of drugs in the Wolff-Parkinson-White syndrome. Am J Cardiol 46:665, 1980
63. Haffajee CI, Love JC, Lesko LJ et al: Clinical pharmacokinetics and efficacy of amiodarone for refractory tachyarrhythmias. Circulation 67:1347, 1983
64. Staubli M, Bircher J, Galeazzi RL et al: Serum concentrations of amiodarone during long term therapy. Eur J Clin Pharmacol 24:485, 1983
65. Morady F, Scheinman MM, Shen E et al: Intravenous amiodarone in the acute treatment of recurrent symptomatic ventricular tachycardia. Am J Cardiol 51:156, 1983
66. Rosenbaum MB, Chiale PA, Halpern MS et al: Clinical efficacy of amiodarone as an antiarrhythmic agent. Am Heart J 38:934, 1976
67. Camm AJ, Ward DE, Al-Hamdi A et al: The use of amiodarone in the control of tachyarrhythmias associated with the Wolff-Parkinson-White syndrome. In Amiodarone in Cardiac Arrhythmias. Royal Society of Medicine 16:25, 1978
68. Waxman HL, Groh WC, Marchlinski FE et al: Amiodarone for control of sustained ventricular tachyarrhythmia: Clinical and electrophysiologic effects in 51 patients. Am J Cardiol 50:1066, 1982
69. McGovern B, Ruskin JN: The efficacy of amiodarone for ventricular arrhythmias can be predicted with clinical electrophysiological studies. Int J Cardiol 3:71, 1983
70. Benaim R, Denizeau JP, Melon J et al: Les effets antiarythmiques de l'amiodarone injectable: A propos de 100 cas. Arch Mal Coeur 59:513, 1976
71. Harris L, McKenna WJ, Rowland E et al: Side effects of long-term amiodarone therapy. Circulation 67:45, 1983
72. Touboul P, Atallah G, Kirkorian G et al: Clinical electrophysiology of intravenous sotalol, a beta-blocking drug with Class III antiarrhythmic properties. Am Heart J 107:888, 1984
73. Clementy J, Bricaud H: Variations in the electrophysiological properties of sotalol administered intravenously in relation to dose. In Lévy S, Gérard G (eds): Recent Advances in Cardiac Arrhythmias, Vol 1, p 323. London, John Libbey, 1983
74. Nathan AW, Hellestrand KJ, Bexton RS et al: Sotalol—more than just another beta-blocker? In Lévy S, Gérard R (eds): Recent Advances in Cardiac Arrhythmias, Vol 1, p 331. London, John Libbey, 1983
75. Prakash R, Parmley WW, Allen HN et al: Effects of sotalol on clinical arrhythmias. Am J Cardiol 29:397, 1972
76. Myburgh DP, Goldman AP, Cartoon J et al: The efficacy of sotalol in suppressing ventricular ectopic beats. Afr Med J 56:295, 1979
77. Senges J, Lengfelder W, Jauernig R et al: Sotalol for sustained ventricular tachycardia: Results using electrophysiological testing. In Lévy S, Gérard R (eds): Recent Advances in Cardiac Arrhythmias, Vol 1, p 224. London, John Libbey, 1983
78. Valere PE, Belin A, Chentir T et al: Effets électrophysiologiques du bépridil sur le coeur humain. Ann Cardiol Angeiol 31:409, 1982
79. Remme WJ, Kruijssen HACM, Krauss XH et al: Effets hémodynamiques aigus du bépridil administré en I.V. chez des patients porteurs d'une mala-

80. Amor M, Hocquard C, Karcher G et al: Amélioration sous bépridil intraveineux de la fonction ventriculaire gauche à l'effort chez le coronarien sévère. Rev Med 28:1293, 1983
81. Shapiro W, Narahara K, Park J: Evaluation du bépridil, un nouvel agent antiangineux: Etude en simple aveugle des modifications de la fraction d'éjection ventriculaire gauche appréciée par la scintigraphie, dans l'angor d'effort stable. Rev Med 28:1304, 1983
82. Medvedowsky JL, Barnay C, Arnaud C et al: Le bépridil dans le traitement des tachycardies paroxystiques supra-ventriculaires. Arch Mal Coeur (Numero special) 78:67, 1985
83. Lévy S, Cointe R, Metge M et al: Bepridil for recurrent sustained ventricular tachycardias: Assessment using electrophysiologic testing. Am J Cardiol 54:579, 1984
84. Fauchier JP, Cosnay P, Rouesnel PH et al: Traitement des tachycardies ventriculaires du coronarien par bépridil intraveineux et par voie orale. Rev Med 28:1341, 1983
85. Davy JM, Lainé JF, Sebag C et al: Bepridil: A new calcium antagonist for the treatment of ventricular tachycardia (abstr). Circulation (Suppl III) 68:III-310, 1983
86. Jullien JL, Baillon R, Benaim R et al: Etude de l'action du bépridil sur les extrasystoles ventriculaires. Rev Med 28:1327, 1983
87. Rio A, Pasco A, Dupont T et al: Efficacité du bépridil per os sur les troubles du rythme ventriculaires chez l'insuffisant coronarien stable. Arch Mal Coeur (Numero special) 78:75, 1985
88. Torres V, Flowers D, Butler B et al: Antiarrhythmic action of bepridil: A long-acting calcium blocker with antiarrhythmic properties (abstr). J Am Coll Cardiol 3:558, 1984
89. Kaplan HR, Mertz TE, Steffe TJ et al: Pirmenol. In Scriabine A (ed): New Drugs Annual, Cardiovascular Drugs, p 133. New York, Raven Press, 1983
90. Bring Liem L, Clay DA, Franz MR et al: Electrophysiology and antiarrhythmic efficacy of intravenous pirmenol in patients with sustained ventricular tachyarrhythmias (abstr). Circulation 74 (part 11):98, 1986
91. Hammil SC, Shand DG, Routledge PA et al: Pirmenol, a new antiarrhythmic agent: Initial study of efficacy, safety and pharmacokinetics. Circulation 65:369, 1982
92. Gold RL, Frumin H, Haffajee CI et al: The efficacy, electrophysiology and electrocardiographic effects of intravenous primenol, a new class I antiarrhythmic agent, in patients with ventricular tachycardia: Comparison with procainamide. PACE 11:308, 1988
93. Amery WK, Aerts T: Lorcainide. In Scriabine A (ed): New Drugs Annual, Cardiovascular Drugs, p 109. New York, Raven Press, 1983
94. Mead RH, Keffe DL, Kates RE et al: Chronic lorcainide therapy for symptomatic ventricular extrasystoles: Efficacy, pharmacokinetics and evidence for norlorcainide antiarrhythmic efficacy. Am J Cardiol 55:72, 1985
95. Sanberg JC, Butler B, Flowers D et al: Evaluation of lorcainide in patients with symptomatic ventricular tachycardia. Am J Cardiol 54:37B, 1984
96. Mann DE, Luck JC, Herre JM et al: Electrophysiologic effects of ethmozine in patients with ventricular tachycardia. Am Heart J 107:674, 1984
97. Pratt CM, Yepsen SC, Taylor AA et al: Ethmozine suppression of single and repetitive ventricular premature depolarizations during therapy and long-term safety. Am Heart J 106:85, 1983
98. Miura DS, Wynn J, Torres W et al: Antiarrhythmic efficacy of ethmozine in patients with ventricular tachycardias as determined by programmed electrical stimulation. Am Heart J 111:661, 1986
99. Podrid PJ, Lown B: Ethmozine therapy for malignant ventricular arrhythmia. Am J Cardiol 49:1015, 1982
100. Singh SS, Di Bianco R, Gottdiener JS et al: Effect of moricizine hydrochloride in reducing chronic high-frequency ventricular arrhythmia: Results of a prospective, controlled trial. Am J Cardiol 53:745, 1984

GENERAL REFERENCES

Chew CYC, Collett J, Singh BN: Mexiletine: A review of its pharmacological properties and therapeutic efficacy in arrhythmias. Drugs 17:161, 1979

Danilo P: Mexiletine. Am Heart J 97:399, 1979

Danilo P: Tocainide. Am Heart J 97:259, 1979

Ezri MD, Shima MA, Denes P: Amiodarone: A review of its clinical and electrophysiologic effects. Clin Prog Pacing Electrophysiol 1:20, 1983

Harrison DC, Winkle R, Sami M: Encainide: A new and potent antiarrhythmic agent. Am Heart J 100:1046, 1980

Jewitt DE: Hemodynamic effects of newer antiarrhythmic drugs. Am Heart J 100:984, 1980

Marcus F, Fontaine GH, Frank R et al: Clinical pharmacology and therapeutic applications of the antiarrhythmic agent amiodarone. Am Heart J 101:480, 1981

Mead H, Harrison DC: Therapy with investigational antiarrhythmic drugs. Med Clin North Am 68:1339, 1984

Nacarelli GV, Rinkenberger RL, Dougherty AH et al: Encainide, a review of its electrophysiology, pharmacology and clinical efficacy. Clin Prog Pacing Electrophysiol 3:268, 1985

Neuman M: Cibenzoline. Drugs of the Future 7:239, 1982

Prystowsky EN: Electrophysiologic and antiarrhythmic properties of bepridil. Am J Cardiol 55:59C, 1985

Ronfeld R: Comparative pharmacokinetics of new antiarrhythmic drugs. Am Heart J 100:978, 1980

Saksena S, Craelius W: The electropharmacology and therapeutic role of mexiletine. Clin Prog Pacing Electrophysiol 1:122, 1983

Salerno DM: Class IA and class IB antiarrhythmic drugs: A review of their pharmacokinetics, electrophysiology, efficacy and toxicity. J Electrophysiol 1:300, 1987

Salerno DM: Class IC drugs. A review of their pharmacokinetics, electrophysiology, efficacy and toxicity. J Electrophysiol 1:435, 1987

Singh BN, Ikeda N, Nademanee K et al: Cellular electrophysiology of the heart: Basis for elucidating the origin of cardiac arrhythmias and the action of antiarrhythmic agents. In Lévy S, Scheinman MM (eds): Cardiac Arrhythmias: From Diagnosis to Therapy. Mount Kisco, NY, Futura Publishing, 1984

Velebit V, Podrid P, Lown B et al: Aggravation and provocation of ventricular arrhythmias by antiarrhythmic drugs. Circulation 65:886, 1982

Winkle RA: Clinical pharmacology of new antiarrhythmic drugs. In Josephson ME, Wellens HJJ (eds): Tachycardias: Mechanisms, Diagnosis, Treatment. Philadelphia, Lea & Febiger, 1984

INVASIVE CARDIAC ELECTROPHYSIOLOGIC STUDIES: AN INTRODUCTION

CHAPTER 44 VOLUME 1

Masood Akhtar

The ability to record the electrical activity of the His bundle (HB) with an electrode catheter by Scherlag and associates more than 15 years ago has provided the impetus for the development of intracardiac electrophysiologic studies (EPS).[1] Although the HB recording provided an excellent marker of the atrioventricular (AV) junction, it was the introduction of programmed electrical stimulation (PES) that primarily contributed toward the rapid growth of EPS in the diagnosis and management of patients with cardiac arrhythmias.[2] Initially, the EPS were mainly used in the diagnosis of patients with sinus node dysfunction,[3,4] AV block,[5,6] and supraventricular tachycardia with or without associated Wolff-Parkinson-White syndrome.[7,8] Subsequently the technique found usefulness in the management of patients with ventricular tachyarrhythmias.[9,10] Currently, a variety of diagnostic and therapeutic uses exist for cardiac EPS. My purpose in this chapter is to provide an overview of the technique, major areas of utility, and limitations of this procedure. A detailed description of various tachycardias and conduction disturbances outlined here can be found elsewhere in these volumes.

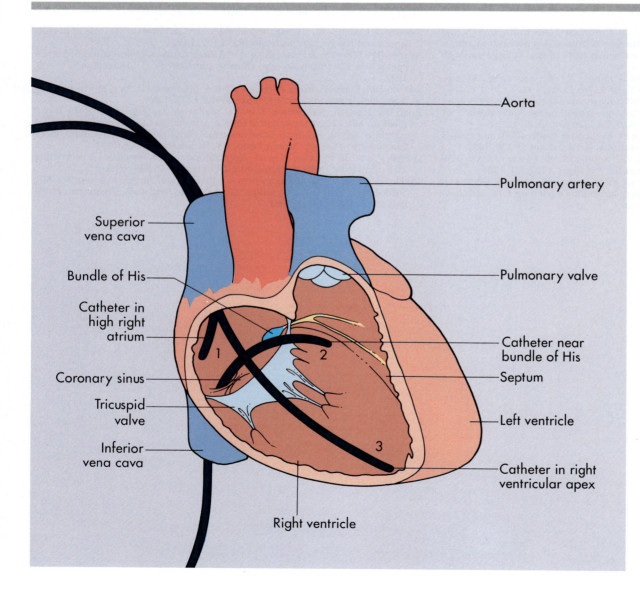

FIGURE 44.1 Usual location of intracardiac pacing and recording catheters during EPS. The position of the right atrial catheter is usually near the junction of the superior vena cava and right atrium (1) or right atrial appendage. The catheter across the AV junction is for recording from the His bundle from the right side of the interventricular septum (2). Advancement of this catheter will frequently permit recording from the right bundle branch. The third catheter is in the right ventricular apex.

INVASIVE ELECTROPHYSIOLOGIC EVALUATION

A thorough assessment of a patient with a problem arrhythmia being considered for electrophysiologic evaluation requires availability of both complex recording and pacing capability of the laboratory. In the current state of practice, both recording and pacing aspects are considered integral parts of a complete study. The studies are usually carried out in a nonsedated, postabsorptive state, although in apprehensive patients prior sedation is advisable. Any drugs that alter the behavior and responsiveness of the cardiac conduction system, atrial or ventricular myocardium, are discontinued to avoid misinterpretation of the data. Sufficient time is allowed for elimination of drugs. Roughly the duration of five half-lives is adequate for this purpose. Although the foregoing is a routine, the EPS should be designed to evaluate individual patients and modified as necessary to answer difficult medical questions. It may be important, for example, to carry out studies in the medicated state if an unexplained symptom (*e.g.,* as syncope, presyncope, palpitations) occurred while taking a given pharmacologic agent. We also do not discontinue other cardiovascular drugs that the patient must take for other cardiac problems (*e.g.,* diuretics, digitalis, vasodilators).

With the use of local anesthesia, electrode catheters (similar to temporary pacing catheters) are introduced into peripheral veins. We prefer percutaneous techniques rather than direct isolation of the vein for a variety of reasons, including (1) sutures are obviated; (2) there is less chance of venous spasm to hinder catheter progress (owing to the stiff sheath around the catheter); and (3) there are better chances of continued patency for subsequent use of the same vein. Several catheters can be accommodated in either of the femoral veins. For single catheters, either the medial or the lateral arm veins are adequate. Subclavian and jugular approaches are preferred by some, particularly when the catheters are to be left in place for an extended period of time. We generally insert two No. 6 F quadripolar catheters through the right or left femoral veins and one or two No. 6 F multipolar catheters via the arm veins. Immediately after insertion of the guide wires, intravenous administration of heparin (2000 to 3000 units) is desirable. The catheters are placed in appropriate areas with fluoroscopic guidance. As a matter of routine we position at least three catheters: (1) in right atrium or coronary sinus, (2) across the tricuspid valve for His bundle or right bundle (RB) recording, and (3) in the right ventricle (Fig. 44.1). The recording along the HB–RB axis can be obtained by gradual withdrawal of the catheter from the ventricular position (Fig. 44.2, position 1) initially to get the RB (position 2) and the HB (position 3) tracing. Further withdrawal of the catheter into the right atrium results in disappearance of the HB deflection and appearance of a large atrial deflection (position 5). The various electrodes are connected via isolated junction boxes and displayed on a multichannel oscilloscope and simultaneously recorded either on paper (ink, photographic, heat developed), via a tape recorder, or by both methods. It is more economical to record all data on tape and to use paper sparingly when necessary. All electrical equipment is carefully grounded, the power supply is isolated, and the cables are shielded.

As a matter of routine, at least three surface electrocardiographic (ECG) leads showing the three planes (*i.e.,* XYZ or leads I, II or aV$_F$, and V$_1$) are recorded in addition to the various intracardiac electrograms. Depending on the need, the intracardiac electrogram can be filtered at any frequency range. However, for most common clinical applications, the filter frequency settings between 30 Hz and 40 Hz on the low and 500 Hz at the higher range are satisfactory.[11] Well-placed

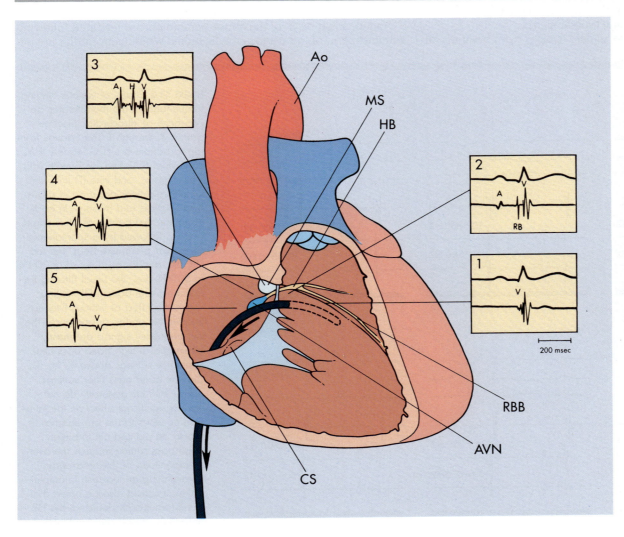

FIGURE 44.2 Intracardiac recordings from the specialized conduction system in the AV junction. The recording of various electrograms along the right side of the interventricular septum with gradual withdrawal of the catheter across the tricuspid valve is shown. (See text for further discussion.) Numericals 1 through 5 refer to intracardiac location of catheters along with corresponding electrogram. (CS, coronary sinus; SN, sinus node; Ao, aorta; MS, membranous septum; AVN, atrioventricular node; HB, His bundle; RBB, right bundle branch; A, atrial deflection; H and RB, His and right bundle potentials; V, ventricular deflection) (Reproduced and modified from Gallagher JJ, Damato AN: Technique of recording His bundle activity in man. In Grossman W (ed): Cardiac Catheterization and Angiography, pp 283–301. Philadelphia, Lea & Febiger, 1980)

catheters will record the appropriate signals at virtually all filtering frequencies (Fig. 44.3), but the low band pass filter settings would permit recording of undesirable low frequency signals, making interpretation of complex tracings more difficult. On the other hand, a high band pass filter setting (>100 Hz) for the low filter is helpful for elimination of undesirable low frequency atrial signals, such as in atrial fibrillation, and thus permits easier identification of the HB potential. It should also be pointed out that a minor alteration in the high band pass filter for surface ECG can markedly distort and diminish scalar ECG morphology. For accurate interpretation of electrophysiologic data it is important to obtain good recordings, which requires appropriate positioning of catheters, proper filtering, and amplification. Excessive amplification of intracardiac recordings (which may be necessary for HB deflection) often results in large atrial and ventricular electrograms, resulting in superimposition of these signals on several tracings. This problem can be controlled by applying a cut-off limit on the amplitude of the tracing. This limiting capability on the height and depth of the signal is available in some multichannel recorders.

The intracardiac electrograms are used primarily to detect the timing of local electrical activation. This can be accomplished by either recording from a pair of closely placed (preferably <1 cm) electrodes (bipolar recording) or by identifying the rapid intrinsic deflection from a unipolar electrogram. With the latter, the second electrode is remote and often extracardiac; therefore, the resultant tracing reflects more global depolarization and repolarization. The waveform analysis of the unipolar electrogram is useful in the study of a larger area, duration of Q wave, ST and T segment. The rapid local depolarization (intrinsic deflection) is sandwiched between the waveforms from more remote areas. Since many of these waveforms are of low frequency, a unipolar electrogram is best left unfiltered, which may, however, introduce baseline drift and undesirable signals. For routine intracardiac EPS there is only a limited advantage to recording of unipolar vs. bipolar electrograms, although the amplitude of unipolar electrograms is roughly twice that of a corresponding bipolar signal.

The introduction of undesirable signals (noise) from a variety of sources is a real problem and should be addressed in order to obtain interpretable recordings. Any signal that has a sufficient amplitude and is within the frequency range of those used during routine recordings may appear on the tracings. These include a variety of extraneous noises from sources both within and outside the electrophysiology laboratory. An example of an external source of noise is a radio frequency signal from a transmitter such as a paging system. More often, the causes of undesirable waveforms are within the laboratory, such as 60 Hz from power sources. Electrical noise can also be picked up from other monitoring and electrical equipment and parallel arrangement of power lines and monitoring cables. The overall noise level can be significantly reduced by proper grounding, isolation, and shielding of cables. A perpendicular arrangement between the noise sources and the recording cables is often helpful.

Once the catheters are in place and appropriate tracings are on line, programmed stimulation is initiated. The site and the specific protocol applied in a given patient depends on the particular clinical needs. However, a complete initial study generally takes several hours since it incorporates assessment of at least the following parameters:

1. Sinus node function
2. Intra-atrial, AV nodal, His-Purkinje system (HPS), and intramyocardial conduction and refractoriness during spontaneous and various paced rhythms
3. Initiation of supraventricular tachycardias
4. Initiation of ventricular tachycardias
5. Determination of the mechanism and site of tachycardia origin by pacing and mapping techniques
6. Determination of the presence, location, and electrophysiologic properties of accessory pathways when present

Often, some or all of the above parameters are repeated following administration of intravenous medications. When tachycardias are ini-

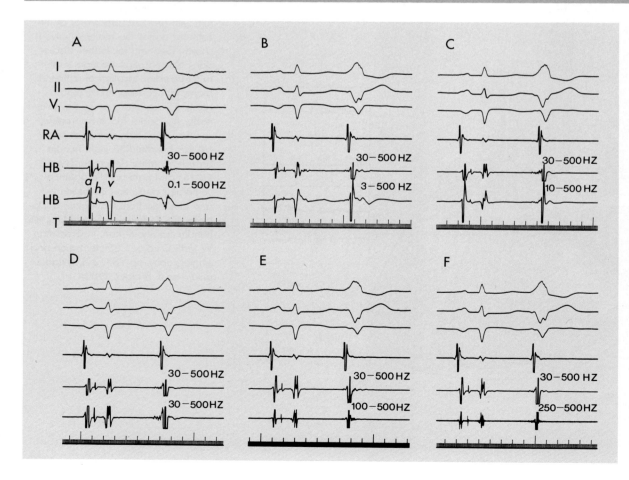

FIGURE 44.3 Effects of various filtering frequencies on the morphologic appearance of intracardiac electrograms. **A** through **F.** The tracings from top to bottom are ECG leads I, II, V_1, right atrial (RA), two His bundle (HB) electrograms, and time (T) line. Similar abbreviations are used in subsequent figures and tracings. In each panel the first beat is of sinus origin, which is followed by a spontaneous ventricular premature beat. The top HB, RA, and RV are filtered at 30 Hz to 500 Hz (i.e., the usual filtering frequencies). The bottom HB tracing shows the effect of various filtering frequencies on the appearance. The low frequency signals are mostly eliminated at high band pass filter frequency settings above 10 Hz (**C**). The low band pass filter settings above 500 Hz generally do not have a significant effect on the intracardiac electrogram appearance. It should be pointed out that high band pass setting reduces the overall magnitude of the electrogram, necessitating an increase in amplification. It should also be noted that at all frequencies depicted, the HB deflection can be clearly identified.

tiated during the EPS, most can also be terminated by overdrive pacing. However, a rapid ventricular tachycardia or a ventricular fibrillation frequently results in immediate hemodynamic deterioration and generally requires prompt external defibrillation. It should be emphasized that every electrophysiology laboratory should be equipped with at least one (preferably two) functioning direct-current cardioverter defibrillator.

At the completion of EPS the catheters are withdrawn and gentle pressure is applied at the area of catheter insertion. Unless arterial catheterization has been performed (*i.e.*, in the evaluation of ventricular tachycardia) patients are allowed to ambulate after approximately 6 hours of bed rest.

EPS FOR DIAGNOSTIC PURPOSES

Perhaps the key reason for the increasing acceptance of EPS for evaluation of patients with cardiac arrhythmias is the ability of these techniques to induce and replicate a patient's spontaneous abnormality in the controlled environment of the laboratory. The clinical settings in which EPS are found of diagnostic use have gradually expanded. A brief discussion of various entities that constitute diagnostic indications for EPS is presented below.

SINUS NODE DYSFUNCTION

Asymptomatic patients with ECG evidence of sinus node dysfunction (SND) are candidates neither for EPS nor for permanent pacemaker therapy. EPS are helpful in cases in which symptoms of SND, such as lightheadedness, dizziness, presyncope, or syncope, are present but SND cannot be documented because of the intermittent nature of the abnormality.[3,4,11] Demonstration of SND in the laboratory is often helpful in expediting the decision-making process. Other situations when EPS are useful are to define the potential aggravation of otherwise asymptomatic patients by drugs such as calcium channel blockers, β-blockers (Fig. 44.4), and Class I antiarrhythmic agents. These drugs may be necessary to control other conditions such as angina and tachyarrhythmias but may produce undesirable symptoms from bradycardia. This potential drug-induced bradycardia can be detected by the study of sinus node function before and after drug administration.

The most common test done for evaluation of sinus node function is overdrive suppression with atrial pacing, a test based on the observation that an abnormal sinus node takes longer to recover following overdrive as compared with normal. Following cessation of atrial pacing the interval between the last atrial paced beat and the sinus escape is measured. This interval is referred to as sinus node recovery time (SNRT). Mandel and associates found that the SNRT in patients with SND averaged 3087 msec, while the values for normals averaged 1073 msec.[3] Narula and co-workers introduced the concept of so-called corrected SNRT by subtracting the spontaneous sinus cycle length from the total SNRT. The corrected SNRT in their series for normals was less than or equal to 525 msec.[4]

There are a variety of other tests used in the evaluation of sinus node function, and these include direct and indirect assessment of sinoatrial conduction time and response to autonomic modulation. Evaluation of sinus node function is covered in detail elsewhere in this volume.

ATRIOVENTRICULAR CONDUCTION

HB electrocardiography has proven very useful in identifying the site of conduction delays and block.[5,6] Recording of the HB potential permits separation of AV conduction into intranodal, intra-His, and infra-His (bundle branches) components (see Figs. 44.2 and 44.3). Demonstration of intra-His or infra-His block is both of diagnostic and prognostic importance, frequently identifying candidates for permanent pacemaker therapy. Localization of block to the AV node (*i.e.*, proximal to HB) is associated with a generally benign outcome, and these cases seldom require permanent pacing. Although HB electrocardiography is used in a variety of AV conduction abnormalities, its greater usefulness is in patients with second-degree AV block where the site of block is not obvious from the surface ECG (Fig. 44.5).

The AV nodal conduction (atrio-His interval normal values, 60 msec to 140 msec) and HPS conduction times (His-ventricular interval normal values, 35 msec to 55 msec) are measured during sinus rhythm. If the block exists during spontaneous sinus rhythm, the location is identified. In patients with intermittent AV conduction abnormalities, the AV block can be provoked with atrial pacing at gradually increasing rates. Induction of AV block in the HPS (*i.e.*, within or below the HB) is abnormal with incremental pacing.[12] With abrupt onset of rapid atrial pacing, however, AV block in the HPS can be induced that is not necessarily indicative of an abnormality.[13] On the other hand, with increasing atrial rates, progressive AV nodal conduction delay and blocks are universal and this response is therefore considered physiologic. Although atrial pacing will produce an AV nodal Wenckebach phenomenon in virtually everyone at increasing rates, it is uncommon to see AV nodal block at rates less than or equal to 100 beats per minute. When atrial pacing does not result in HPS block in a suspect patient, intravenous procainamide (up to 10 mg/kg) can be used as a stress test.[14] In patients without spontaneous intermittent HPS block, procainamide rarely induces block in the HPS and it usually facilitates intranodal conduction.

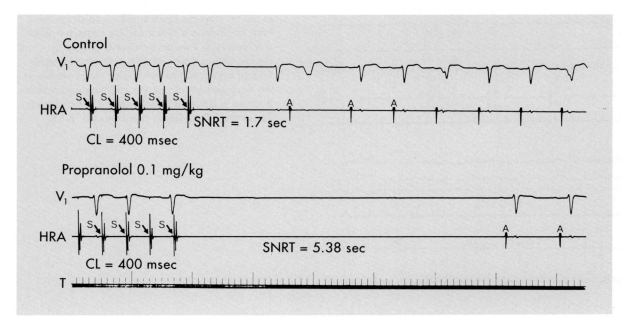

FIGURE 44.4 Aggravation of SND after propranolol. **Top.** Sinus node recovery time (*SNRT*) before drug therapy in an asymptomatic patient with SND. **Bottom.** After propanolol the patient experienced intermittent symptoms suggestive of aggravation in SND that could not be documented on ambulatory monitoring. A grossly abnormal SNRT of 5.38 seconds could be demonstrated during EPS. There was a marked increase in SNRT at the same cycle length of atrial pacing (400 msec). (Akhtar M: Clinical application of electrophysiologic studies in the management of patients requiring pacemaker therapy. In Barold S (ed): Modern Cardiac Pacing. Mount Kisco (NY), Futura Publishing Co, 1985)

With programmed electrical stimulation, the refractoriness of various components of the cardiac conduction system (*i.e.*, atria, AV node, HPS, ventricular myocardium) as well as the accessory pathways can be determined.[15] During the spontaneous or paced constant cycle length, programmed extrastimuli (*i.e.*, premature beats) are introduced, starting with a late coupled beat. The interval between the last beat of the constant cycle length drive and the premature beat is progressively decreased until there is no local response to stimulation. Either spontaneous sinus and/or paced atrial cycle length are used for determination of refractory periods during propagation of impulses in the antegrade direction. Similar assessment during retrograde impulse propagation can be accomplished by pacing the ventricle. The definitions of atrial, AV node, and HPS refractory periods are illustrated in Figure 44.6. The definition of ventricular refractory period is the same as depicted for atrial, except the word "atrium" can be replaced by "ventricle." Assessment of refractory periods is useful to determine the functional vs. abnormal behavior of a given component of the cardiac conduction system and is invaluable for evaluation of drug effects. For example, in patients with short refractory periods of the AV node or accessory pathway a rapid AV response via these routes can be predicted during an atrial arrhythmia. A prolongation in the refractory period after a drug will usually translate into slowing of the AV response during a similar arrhythmia.

DIFFERENTIAL DIAGNOSIS OF WIDE QRS TACHYCARDIA

The accurate diagnosis of the origin of a wide QRS tachycardia remains a significant clinical problem (Fig. 44.7). Even though careful analysis of a 12-lead ECG often provides good clues, the HB electrogram remains the gold standard for the distinction between ventricular tachycardia vs. supraventricular tachycardia with associated aberrant conduction.[16] In the latter cases all supraventricular impulses must travel over the HB and reach the ventricle; therefore, the His deflection precedes the QRS complex with a normal or prolonged HV interval (Fig. 44.8). In contrast, during ventricular tachycardia the activation of the His bundle occurs in the retrograde direction and the His potential is either obscured within the corresponding ventricular electrogram or its occurrence is noted following the onset of the QRS complex (Fig. 44.9). Wide QRS tachycardias can occur from mechanisms other than those mentioned above, particularly in patients with overt Wolff-Parkinson-White syndrome.[16] Anomalous conduction to the ventricle over the accessory pathway either during atrial tachyarrhythmias such as atrial fibrillation or the so-called antidromic tachycardia can result in wide QRS complexes (Fig. 44.10). The latter arrhythmia uses a reentry circuit in which the impulse reaches the ventricle via the accessory pathway and returns via the normal pathway or more commonly another accessory pathway, in which case the term *preexcited tachycardia* is used.[17] Wide QRS tachycardias in patients with the preexcitation syndrome are often quite complex, and EPS are very useful to define the nature of the problem, the origin of the arrhythmia, and the reentry circuits. Multiple recordings from both right and left atria (via the coronary sinus or patent foramen ovale) are needed in addition to the HB to get a thorough evaluation.

SUPRAVENTRICULAR TACHYCARDIA

Supraventricular tachycardia (SVT) is a relatively common arrhythmia in the absence of preexcitation syndromes. Excluding atrial fibrillation and flutter, the most common recurrent narrow QRS tachycardia is due to AV nodal reentry (commonly but incorrectly termed as paroxysmal atrial tachycardia [*PAT*]).[7,18,19] At the present time EPS are used for the differential diagnosis of SVT to define the mechanism that often leads to rational therapy (see Fig. 44.10). It should be pointed out that

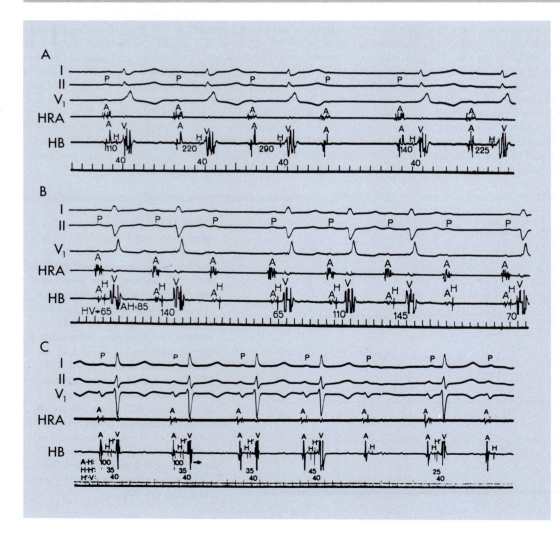

FIGURE 44.5 HB electrograms in AV block. The tracings are from three different patients with second-degree AV block. **A** and **B**. Conducted QRS complexes are wide and associated with bundle branch block (BBB). In **A** the block is in the AV node (*i.e.*, the A wave on HB is not followed by an HB deflection). In **B** it can be appreciated that the block is distal to the HB even though the surface ECG demonstrates a Wenckebach phenomenon. The latter can obviously occur in the His-Purkinje system as well, as depicted in this figure. **C**. Site of block is within the HB. This is suggested by split HB potentials (labeled H and H'), and the block is distal to the H but proximal to the H'. Intra-His block is difficult to diagnose from the surface ECG but can be suspected when a Mobitz type II occurs in association with a normal QRS complex and PR interval. (Akhtar M: Clinical application of electrophysiologic studies in the management of patients requiring pacemaker therapy. In Barold S (ed): Modern Cardiac Pacing. Mount Kisco (NY), Futura Publishing Co, 1985)

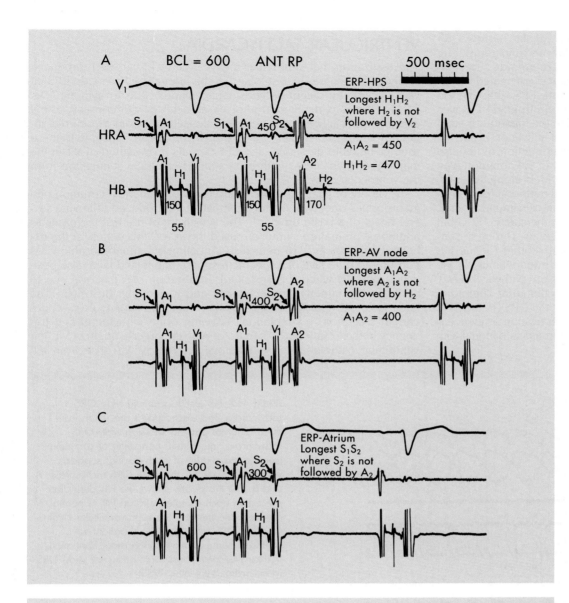

FIGURE 44.6 Determination of cardiac refractory periods during atrial pacing. **A** through **C**. During a basic cycle length pacing at 600 msec (S_1S_1 or A_1A_1), atrial premature stimulation (S_1 or A_2) at progressively shorter coupling intervals (S_1S_2 or A_1A_2) is depicted. The definition of the effective refractory period (*ERP*) of the HPS, AV node, and atrium are labeled. (*ANT RP*, antegrade refractory period)

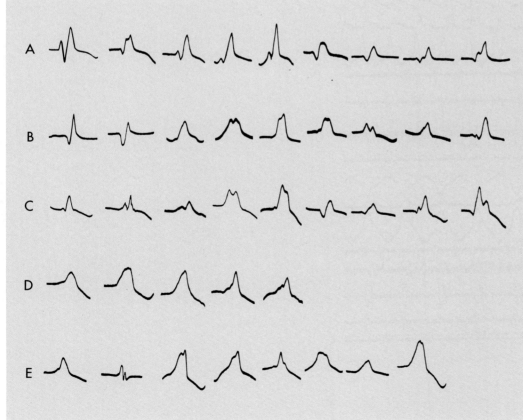

FIGURE 44.7 Origin of wide QRS complexes. The figures depict wide QRS complexes taken from 40 different patients showing a right bundle branch block pattern in V_1. **A** and **B**. Complexes are from aberrant conduction of supraventricular impulses. **C** and **D**. Complexes are of ventricular origin. **E**. Complexes are due to anomalous conduction in patients with Wolff-Parkinson-White syndrome. It can be clearly seen that there are several complexes in **C** and **D** that closely simulate complexes in **A**, **B**, and **E**. (Akhtar M: Electrophysiologic bases for wide QRS tachycardia. PACE 6:81, 1983)

roughly one third of patients presenting with a regular narrow QRS tachycardia who have no evidence of ventricular preexcitation during sinus rhythm use an accessory pathway in the retrograde direction during the SVT.[18-22] These cases with the so-called concealed Wolff-Parkinson-White syndrome are best identified with EPS, although the initial clue may be obtained from identification of retrograde P waves in the ST-T segment during SVT.[19-22] During EPS, the location of atrial activation relative to the QRS as well as the atrial activation sequence provide the all-important clues to the origin and direction of impulse propagation in a given type of SVT. For example, in the common type of AV nodal reentry the impulse proceeds antegradely along the slow, and retrogradely along the fast, pathway in such a temporal relation so that the atrial and ventricular activation occurs almost simultaneously. The P wave is therefore obscured by the QRS on the surface ECG but can be recognized on intracardiac atrial electrograms. During this arrhythmia the atrial activity on the low interatrial septum (in the HB tracing) or its immediate surroundings (OS or coronary sinus) is the earliest. On the other hand, the impulse in accessory pathway reentry must reach the ventricles before it can return to the atria. Therefore, the retrograde P wave almost always occurs after the QRS (in the ST-T segment).[21,22] Furthermore, the retrograde atrial activation sequence is clearly different than AV nodal reentry except perhaps in patients with septal accessory pathways.[23]

VENTRICULAR TACHYCARDIA

The realization that ventricular tachycardia (VT) can be reproduced safely and often easily terminated in the laboratory has made EPS invaluable for the diagnosis and management of this arrhythmia (Fig. 44.11). This is particularly true of VT associated with coronary artery disease, especially when it occurs in the setting of old myocardial infarction and/or aneurysm.[9,24,25] The arrhythmogenic substrate in these settings tends to be stable, and EPS permits provocation of VT in the majority of these cases with programmed electrical stimulation from the ventricular sites.

A variety of pacing protocols are used, but the most common one incorporates one, two, or three extrastimuli introduced following several beats of a basic drive.[25,26] The sensitivity of the test increases as additional premature stimuli are used; however, this occurs at the expense of specificity.[25] Nonetheless, induction of a monomorphic VT is considered reflective of a specific response and is seldom a false-positive, especially when it is sustained. Replication of VT allows one to establish the underlying mechanism and to identify the origin. The latter is of extreme importance since arrhythmia surgery (*e.g.*, endocardial resection, cryoablation) is being done with increasing frequency in these patients.[27,28] To determine the precise origin of VT, left ventricular catheterization is essential since most VT arise from left

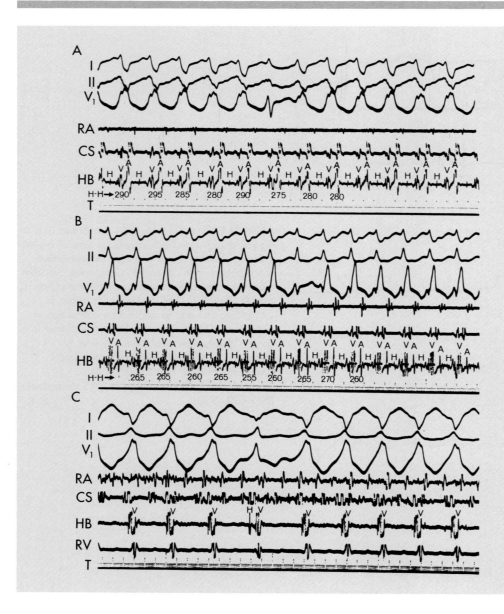

FIGURE 44.8 HB electrograms in wide QRS tachycardia. The electrograms are taken from three different patients showing wide QRS tachycardia. Intermittent narrowing of complexes (seen in the middle of each tracing) suggests ventricular origin for the wide QRS tachycardia. **A** and **B.** The HB clearly shows the His deflection preceding each complex with an HV of normal duration documenting the supraventricular origin. **C.** Wide QRS tachycardia in a patient with ventricular preexcitation during atrial fibrillation. (Akhtar M: Electrophysiologic bases for wide QRS tachycardia. PACE 6:81, 1983)

ventricular sites. The earliest point of activation during VT is considered closest to the endocardial breakthrough and, therefore, near the site of origin. If the origin of VT is properly determined, the earliest recorded intracardiac activity almost invariably precedes the surface QRS complex. When the induced VT is not well tolerated to permit endocardial mapping or if the VT is not induced or sustained, the technique of pace mapping can be safely applied instead.[29] During this technique, the 12-lead ECG morphology of the VT is reproduced during endocardial pacing (Fig. 44.12). The paced site producing QRS morphology identical to that of the previously recorded spontaneous VT is presumed to be near the endocardial breakthrough. With continued experience the pace mapping method may turn out to be as accurate as mapping to determine the VT origin. At the present time both should be applied for better localization of the origin of VT.

An understanding of the origin of VT with EPS is desirable prior to arrhythmia surgery since frequently VT cannot be initiated in the operating room. Similarly, localization of the VT circuit is important for application of electrical ablative procedures for VT control, a promising new and investigational technique for control of VT.

SURVIVORS OF SUDDEN CARDIAC COLLAPSE

A variety of cardiac arrhythmias and conduction disturbances can result in hemodynamic collapse. However, the literature indicates that VT–ventricular fibrillation (VF) is responsible for most sudden cardiac deaths.[10,31] EPS are very useful in identifying those cases in which the arrhythmia substrate persists, and in these patients the VT–VF can be induced in the laboratory. Noninducibility of VT–VF may also help to identify other dynamic causes (e.g., acute myocardial ischemia, changes in electrolyte balance) not readily replicated in the laboratory. Determination of the cause of initial collapse and its prevention by any means is of utmost importance since recurrence of VT–VF in this group without specific therapy is very high and unacceptable.

UNEXPLAINED SYNCOPE

Patients who have experienced a brief loss of consciousness are encountered often in clinical practice. In a good percentage of cases, the cause remains uncertain despite a thorough history and physical examination. Once the functional (e.g., vasovagal, hyperventilation) and metabolic causes are excluded, the workup focus shifts to the neurologic and cardiac etiologies. Without doubt, arrhythmias and conduction disturbances constitute common cardiac causes for syncope. Noninvasive tests for determining the cause of syncope such as Holter monitoring and exercise testing have a relatively poor yield. From the various studies available, EPS led to a presumptive cause of arrhythmic syncope in roughly one half of the cases, particularly those with structural heart disease.[32-35] Interestingly, the most common abnormality detected in most series is inducible VT, although some do have SND or diseased HPS. Since no documentation of rhythm is available from the episode of syncope in virtually all of these cases, there is always room for doubt whether laboratory-induced abnormalities indeed represent

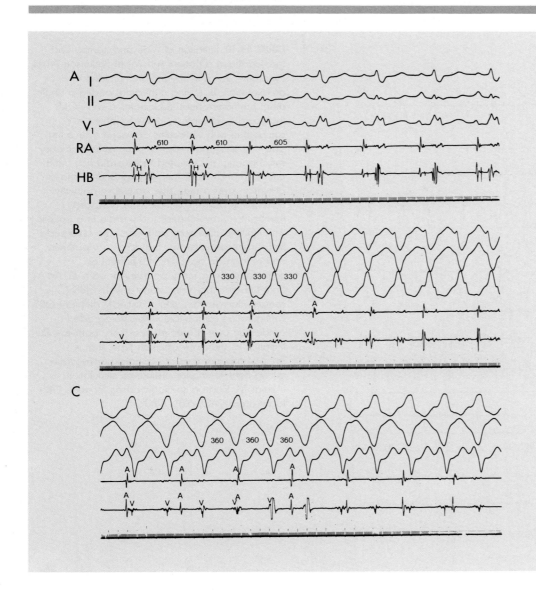

FIGURE 44.9 HB electrogram in ventricular tachycardia. **A.** Sinus rhythm and the HB deflection are clearly identifiable. **B** and **C.** During two different types of wide QRS tachycardia the HB deflection is obscured by the local ventricular electrogram and, therefore, follows the onset of ventricular activity and does not precede it (as seen in Figure 44.8). Also note AV dissociation during the tachycardia. These findings are usually diagnostic of ventricular tachycardia. (Akhtar M: Electrophysiologic bases for wide QRS tachycardia. PACE 6:81, 1983)

a true positive response. Nonetheless, some responses in the laboratory are quite specific, and these include demonstration of SND, second- or third-degree block in the HPS, and induction of sustained monomorphic VT. When these findings are encountered and specifically treated, symptoms of syncope are relieved in the majority of cases. The clinical significance of certain other abnormalities such as prolonged AV nodal conduction, induction of supraventricular tachycardia, and pleomorphic VT or VF in this patient population is not completely clear.

EPS FOR THERAPEUTIC PURPOSES

The use of EPS to gauge the effectiveness of pharmacologic control, as well as to explore other therapeutic options, has added to the popularity of these procedures for patient management.

PHARMACOLOGIC CONTROL OF TACHYCARDIA

Reproducible replication of either SVT or VT with PES forms the basis of this approach.[10,20,36-39] If tachycardia is inducible, then an intravenous therapeutic agent can be administered, reinduction is tried, and the response is judged. This information may help to decide in favor of or against a therapeutic agent. It is important to emphasize that the response to intravenous agents is not sufficient to decide on ultimate therapy but should be only used as a guide. Following the initial control study and the intravenous drug the patients are started on a comparable oral agent in the appropriate doses and frequencies. The choice of initial therapy is dependent on many factors, including prior history of specific drug intolerance, clinical failure to an agent, and the response to intravenous drug administration in the laboratory. The patients are treated with the oral agent until a steady state is achieved, which usually takes 48 to 72 hours for most conventional agents. During this time the patients are carefully observed for effect of drug on spontaneous rhythm, drug tolerance, absorption characteristics of the agent as detected by blood levels, and myocardial effects as manifested on the 12-lead ECG.

If a spontaneous arrhythmia occurs despite good levels or maximum tolerated doses or when significant side effects develop, a new drug regimen is initiated. The patients are brought back to the laboratory for follow-up drug testing when the spontaneous arrhythmia seems controlled, the drug regimen is well tolerated, and there is evidence of good drug absorption.

The purpose of the repeat study is to see drug effectiveness, failure, or possible aggravation as judged by the rate and stability of induced tachycardia. These so-called repeat or follow-up studies usually require use of a single multipolar catheter, which can be accomplished either by leaving the catheter at the completion of the first study or reinsertion of the catheter at the time of follow-up study. However, in patients with frequent episodes of tachycardia it is preferable to leave one of the catheters in the appropriate chamber for termination of the tachycardia until an effective drug regimen is established. This obviates the need of frequent direct-current countershocks before the tachycardia is controlled while the drug dosage is being titrated.

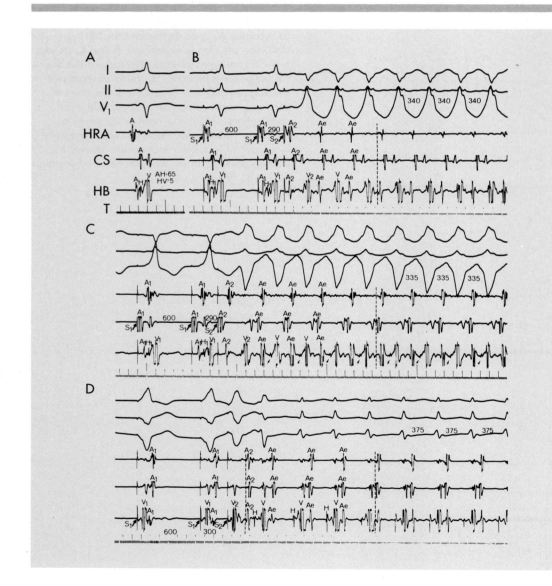

FIGURE 44.10 Initiation of wide and narrow QRS tachycardia in a patient with Wolff-Parkinson-White Syndrome. A. Sinus rhythm and ventricular preexcitation. B. During right atrial pacing a single atrial premature beat (S_2) initiates a wide QRS tachycardia showing a positive complex in V_1 compatible with ventricular activation over a left side accessory pathway. With left atrial (coronary sinus) pacing, the initiated tachycardia has a left bundle branch block morphology and ventricular activation over a right side accessory pathway. Both of the above examples are preexcited reentrant supraventricular tachycardia in a patient with multiple accessory pathways. The antegrade limb of the circuit is over the accessory pathway and retrograde via either the normal or contralateral accessory pathway or both. C. An A_2 from the coronary sinus starts a wide QRS complex tachycardia with a distinctly different QRS configuration compatible with anterograde conduction over a right AV accessory pathway. D. Initiation of the more common type, that is, orthodromic (narrow QRS complex) tachycardia during right ventricular premature stimulation. (Akhtar M: Electrophysiologic bases for wide QRS tachycardia. PACE 6:81, 1983)

During the conduct of follow-up studies, an effort is made to replicate the PES of the prior study, as well as the site of stimulation. As a matter of routine the entire pacing protocol for VT induction that is specific for the laboratory is tried from two right ventricular stimulation sites, including from the site where the VT was initiated during the first study. For induction of SVT arising in the AV junction (*i.e.*, reentry localized to the AV node or associated with preexcitation syndromes), both atrial, as well as ventricular stimulation sites must be tested. Complete suppression of inducibility on repeat study is the most desirable response and has an excellent correlation with clinical control of tachycardia both for SVT as well as for VT (Fig. 44.13).[38,40] The cardiac arrhythmias where this has been documented are AV nodal reentry, reentry using accessory pathways, and monomorphic sustained VT associated with coronary artery disease. Other favorable responses to programmed stimulation include conversion of a sustained to nonsustained form (Fig. 44.14), need for a more aggressive pacing protocol to initiate the arrhythmia, and significant slowing in the rate of tachycardia (Fig. 44.15). In contrast, unfavorable responses include no change or easier induction, conversion to a more sustained form, and acceleration in the rate of tachycardia. Any of the unfavorable responses generally dictate an unsatisfactory situation and need for one or more of the following: different drug, a higher dose, a combination of drugs, or nonpharmacologic therapy. In many patients serial follow-up EPS are carried out before an effective drug or combination is found. Overall, the conventional drugs are effective in controlling the arrhythmia in approximately one third of patients with tachycardia and new antiarrhythmic agents are needed in the remaining. In the process, however, a group of patients is identified (both among the SVT and VT groups) who do not respond to pharmacologic therapy, and the search for other therapeutic options becomes essential.

SELECTION OF PATIENTS FOR NONPHARMACOLOGIC CONTROL OF TACHYCARDIAS

A variety of procedures and devices are now used in the control of tachyarrhythmias. A complete electrophysiologic workup is important for selection of appropriate modality, some of which are discussed below.

PACING THERAPY

Tachycardias that are secondary to bradyarrhythmias such as AV block can be prevented with cardiac pacing. However, most of the regular tachycardias from reentrant mechanisms (both SVT and VT) can also be terminated with overdrive pacing.[41] The ease of termination depends on many factors, the most important being the rate of tachycardia and the proximity of reentry circuit to the site of stimulation. In general, the slower tachycardias are easier to terminate, particularly from a pacing site close to the origin of the arrhythmia. The latter provides easier access for the paced impulse to enter the reentry circuit. Since all tachycardias have the potential to accelerate during overdrive pacing, the safety of this technique has to be tested in each individual patient before final selection can be made. This is done by repeated induction and termination to define the safe but effective zone of tachycardia termination. Similarly, EPS are also desirable to determine the suitability of patients for implantable transvenous cardioverter and implantable automatic defibrillator.[42,43]

ABLATIVE THERAPY

Ablative therapy is gaining wider acceptance and has proven useful-

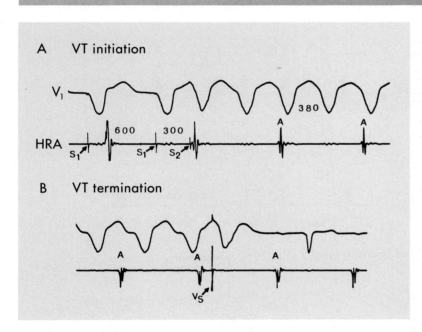

FIGURE 44.11 Initiation and termination of VT with a single programmed ventricular premature beat. **A.** VT is induced with a single extrastimulus (S_2) during basic pacing at 600-msec cycle length. **B.** VT is terminated with a single extrastimulus (V_S).

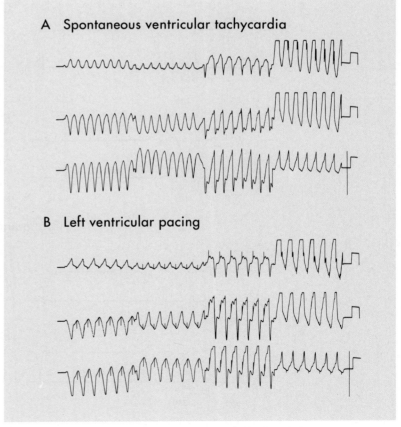

FIGURE 44.12 Pacemapping in VT. **A.** A 12-lead ECG of spontaneous VT. **B.** A similar 12-lead QRS complex morphology is reproduced during left ventricular stimulation.

ness in the control of SVT by producing AV block.[44] This is accomplished with catheters similar to those used for routine EPS. More recently, electrical ablation via the catheter has also been tried for VT with variable results.[45,46] Undoubtedly this technique will find greater use in the management of tachyarrhythmias as experience with electrical ablation is gathered. The details of the so-called ablative or fulguration methods are presented elsewhere in these volumes.

PROBLEMS ENCOUNTERED DURING EPS

Mechanical irritation from catheters during placement and even when not being manipulated can cause a variety of arrhythmias and conduction disturbance. These include induction of atrial, HB, and ventricular ectopic beats and right bundle branch block and therefore AV block in the HPS in patients with preexisting left bundle branch block during right ventricular catheterization (Fig. 44.16). Obviously, AV block in the HPS can occur in patients with preexisting right bundle branch block during left ventricular catheterization. Ventricular stimulation can also occur from physical movement of the ventricular catheter coincidental with atrial contraction, producing ECG patterns of ventricular preexcitation (Fig. 44.17). Recognition of all of these iatrogenic patterns is important to avoid misinterpretation of electrophysiologic phenomena and the significance of findings in the laboratory.[47]

Certain types of arrhythmias must be avoided at all costs such as atrial fibrillation and ventricular fibrillation. Atrial fibrillation will obviously not permit study of any other form of SVT, and ventricular fibrillation will require prompt cardioversion, making it difficult to continue the EPS. If atrial fibrillation must be initiated for diagnostic purposes (*i.e.*, to assess ventricular response over the accessory pathway in Wolff-Parkinson-White syndrome) it should be done at the end of the study (see Fig. 44.15). Patients with a prior history of atrial fibrillation are more prone to the occurrence of sustained atrial fibrillation in the laboratory. Frequently this will occur during initial placement of catheters, and excessive manipulation of catheters in the atria should therefore be avoided in such cases.

COMPLICATIONS

When only right-sided heart catheterization is done for EPS the complication rate is relatively low. Experience from the various laboratories indicates almost negligible mortality related to this procedure. In our own experience with more than 4000 EPS procedures, no mortality has been encountered either in the laboratory or remotely that could be ascribed to the EPS. Other complications include deep venous thrombosis, pulmonary embolism, infection at catheter sites, systemic infection, pneumothorax, and perforation of a cardiac chamber or coronary sinus.[48]

The occurrence of potentially lethal arrhythmias such as rapid VT or VF is common in the laboratory. However these are not necessarily counted as complications but are often expected and anticipated events. Nonetheless, the common occurrence of these events makes the electrophysiology laboratory a place for only highly trained personnel equipped to handle such problems on a daily basis.

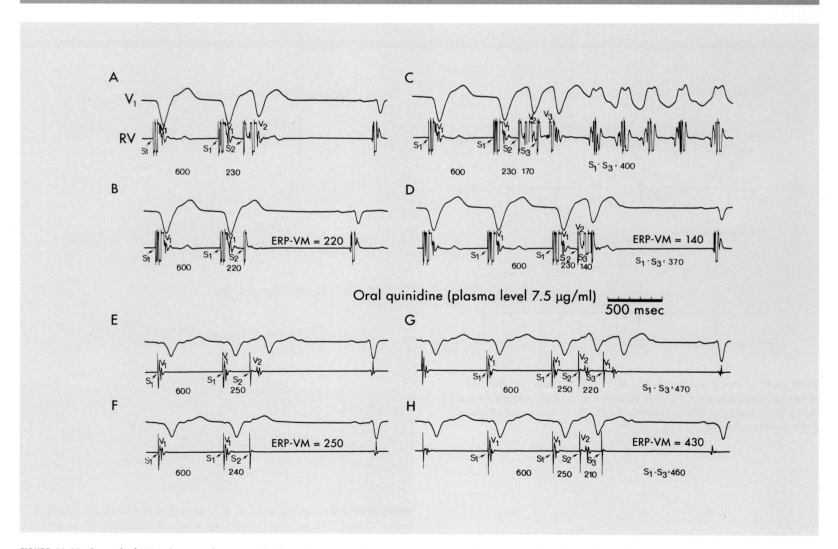

FIGURE 44.13 Control of VT induction after antiarrhythmic therapy. **A** through **D.** Attempted VT induction with single (S_2) and double (S_2S_3) premature beats; the VT is initiated with two extrastimuli. Panels **B** and **D** show the effective refractory period of ventricular myocardium in response to single and double extrastimuli, respectively. **E** through **H.** After quinidine the VT could not be initiated to the point of the ventricular effective refractory period, suggesting a favorable response.

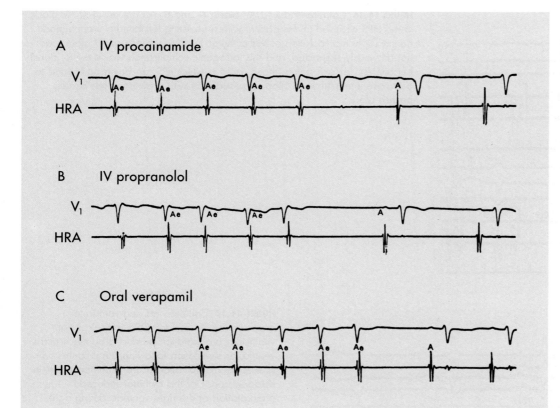

FIGURE 44.14 Control of inducible SVT with drugs. The effect of drugs on common AV nodal reentry is demonstrated on an induced tachycardia in the laboratory. Note the spontaneous termination of SVT with drugs and the site of drug action. **B** and **C.** Block in the reentry circuit occurs along the antegrade pathways; that is, there is an atrial echo beat (Ae), but there is block before the impulse reaches the ventricle. In **A** the tachycardia stops in the retrograde limb, that is, the ventricular response is not followed by an Ae beat.

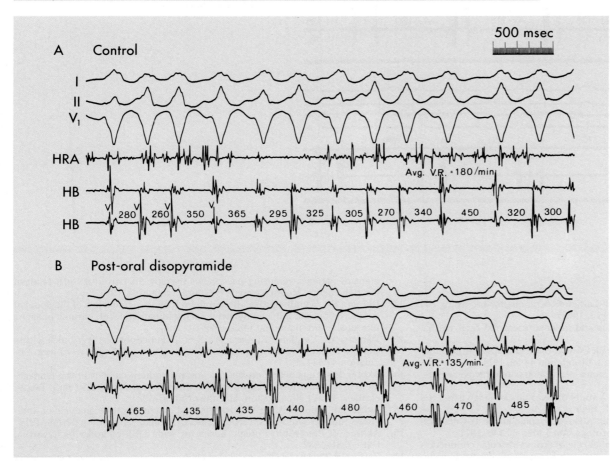

FIGURE 44.15 Effect of drug on accessory pathway conduction. **A.** Average ventricular response of 180 beats per minute over the accessory pathway during atrial fibrillation. **B.** The response slows to 135 beats per minute after oral disopyramide.

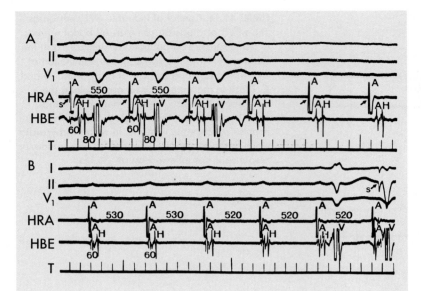

FIGURE 44.16 Catheter-induced AV block. **A** and **B.** Abrupt onset of AV block in the HPS occurred in this patient with preexisting left bundle branch block during slight manipulation of the catheter. Prior occurrence of AV block was not previously suspected, and this iatrogenic complication was easy to identify but can cause confusion in those cases in which EPS are being performed to diagnose intermittent AV block in association with preexisting left bundle branch block.

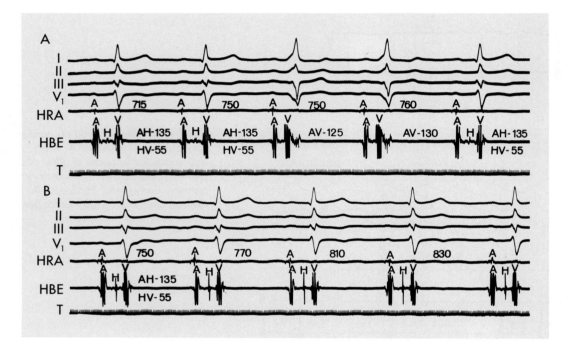

FIGURE 44.17 Catheter-induced ventricular preexcitation. **A.** Surface QRS typical of right ventricular preexcitation produced by mechanical ventricular stimulation following atrial contraction. **B.** A slight manipulation of the catheter results in disappearance of this catheter-induced preexcitation of the right ventricle during right-sided heart catheterization.

REFERENCES

1. Scherlag BJ, Lau SH, Helfant RH et al: Catheter technique for recording His bundle activity in man. Circulation 39:13, 1969
2. Goldreyer BN, Bigger JT: Spontaneous and induced reentrant tachycardia. Ann Intern Med 70:87, 1969
3. Mandel WJ, Hayakawa H, Danzig R et al: Evaluation of sino-atrial node function in many by overdrive suppression. Circulation 44:59, 1971
4. Narula OS, Samet P, Javier RP: Significance of the sinus node recovery time. Circulation 45:140, 1972
5. Damato AN, Lau SH, Helfant RH et al: A study of heart block in man using His bundle recordings. Circulation 39:297, 1969
6. Narula OS, Scherlag BJ, Samet P et al: Atrioventricular block: Localization and classification by His bundle recordings. Am J Med 50:146, 1971
7. Goldreyer BN, Damato AN: The essential role of atrioventricular conduction delay in the initiation of paroxysmal supraventricular tachycardia. Circulation 43:679, 1971
8. Wellens HJJ, Schuilenberg RM, Durrer D: Electrical stimulation of the heart in patients with the Wolff-Parkinson-White syndrome type A. Circulation 43:99, 1971
9. Mason JW, Winkel RA: Electrode catheter arrhythmia induction in the selection and assessment of antiarrhythmic drug therapy for recurrent ventricular tachycardia. Circulation 58:971, 1978
10. Ruskin JN, DiMarco JP, Garan H: Out of hospital cardiac arrest: Electrophysiologic observations in selection of long-term antiarrhythmic therapy. N Engl J Med 303:607, 1980
11. Akhtar M: Clinical application of electrophysiologic studies in the management of patients requiring pacemaker therapy. In Barold S (ed): Modern Cardiac Pacing. Mount Kisco, NY, Futura Publishing, 1985
12. Dhingra RC, Wyndham CRC, Bauernfiend R et al: Significance of block distal to the His bundle induced by atrial pacing in patients with chronic bifascicular block. Circulation 60:1455, 1979
13. Damato AN, Varghese PJ, Caracta AR et al: Functional 2:1 A-V block within the His-Purkinje system: Simulation of type II second-degree A-V block. Circulation 47:534, 1973
14. Akhtar M: Drugs acting on the fast inward sodium current in the management of tachycardias. In Surawicz B, Reddy CP, Prystowsky EN (eds): Tachycardias, pp 471–489. Boston, Martinus Nijhoff, 1984
15. Akhtar M, Damato AN, Batsford WP et al: A comparative analysis of antegrade and retrograde conduction patterns in man. Circulation 52:766, 1975
16. Akhtar M: Electrophysiologic bases for wide QRS complex tachycardia. PACE 6:81, 1983
17. Bardy GH, Packer DL, German LD et al: Preexcited reciprocating tachycardia in patients with Wolff-Parkinson-White syndrome: Incidence and mechanisms. Circulation 70:377, 1984
18. Wu D, Denes P, Amat-y-Leon F et al: Clinical electrocardiographic and electrophysiological observations in patients with paroxysmal supraventricular tachycardia. Am J Cardiol 41:1045, 1978
19. Akhtar M, Damato AN, Ruskin JN et al: Antegrade and retrograde conduction characteristics in three patterns of paroxysmal atrioventricular junctional reentrant tachycardia. Am Heart J 95:22, 1978
20. Akhtar M: Supraventricular tachycardias: Electrophysiologic mechanisms, diagnosis and pharmacologic therapy. In Josephson M, Wellens HJJ (eds): Tachycardias: Mechanisms, Diagnosis, and Treatment, pp 137–169. Philadel-

phia, Lea & Febiger, 1984
21. Akhtar M, Damato AN: Determination of site reentry from antegrade and retrograde conduction ratios in paroxysmal atrioventricular junctional reentrant tachycardia (abstr). Clin Res 24A, 1976
22. Josephson ME: Paroxysmal supraventricular tachycardia: An electrophysiologic approach. Am J Cardiol 41:1123, 1978
23. Gallagher JJ, Gilbert M, Svenson RH et al: Wolff-Parkinson-White syndrome: The problem, evaluation and surgical correction. Circulation 51:767, 1975
24. Wellens HJJ, Duren DR, Lie KI: Observations on mechanisms of ventricular tachycardia in man. Circulation 54:237, 1976
25. Brugada P, Green M, Abdollah H et al: Significance of ventricular arrhythmias initiated by programmed ventricular stimulation: The importance of the type of ventricular arrhythmia induced and the number of premature stimuli required. Circulation 69:87, 1984
26. Denker ST, Lehmann M, Mahmud R et al: Facilitation of ventricular tachycardia induction with abrupt changes in ventricular cycle length. Am J Cardiol 53:508, 1984
27. Josephson ME, Harken AH, Horowitz LN: Long-term results of endocardial resection from sustained ventricular tachycardia in coronary disease patients. Am Heart J: 104:51, 1982
28. Plumb VJ, McGiffin DC, Kirklin JK et al: Cryosurgery for ventricular tachycardia (abstr). J Am Coll Cardiol 5:409, 1985
29. Josephson ME, Waxman HL, Cain ME et al: Ventricular activation during ventricular endocardial pacing: II. Role of pace-mapping to localize origin of ventricular tachycardia. Am J Cardiol 50:11, 1982
30. Wellens HJJ, Farre J, Bar FW: Ventricular tachycardia: Value and limitation of stimulation studies. In Narula OS (ed): Cardiac arrhythmias: Electrophysiology, diagnosis and management, pp 436–456. Baltimore, Williams & Wilkins, 1979
31. Josephson ME, Horowitz LN, Spielman SR et al: Electrophysiologic and hemodynamic studies in patients resuscitated from cardiac arrest. Am J Cardiol 46:948, 1980
32. DiMarco JP, Garan H, Ruskin JN: Cardiac electrophysiologic techniques in recurrent syncope of unknown cause. Ann Intern Med 95:542, 1981
33. Akhtar M, Shenasa M, Denker S et al: Role of cardiac electrophysiologic studies in patients with unexplained recurrent syncope. PACE 6:192, 1983
34. Morady F, Scheinman MM: The role and limitations of electrophysiologic testing in patients with unexplained syncope. Int J Cardiol 4:229, 1983
35. Morady F, Shen E, Schwartz A et al: Long-term follow-up of patients with recurrent unexplained syncope evaluated by electrophysiologic testing. J Am Coll Cardiol 2:1053, 1983
36. Wu D, Wyndham CR, Denes P et al: Chronic electrophysiological study in patients with recurrent paroxysmal tachycardia: A new method for developing successful oral antiarrhythmic therapy. In Kulbertus HE (ed): Reentrant arrhythmias, p 294. Baltimore, University Park Press, 1976
37. Waxman HL, Buxton AE, Sadowski LM et al: The response to procainamide during electrophysiologic study for sustained ventricular tachyarrhythmias predicts the response to other medications. Circulation 67:30, 1983
38. Horowitz LN, Josephson ME, Farshidi A et al: Recurrent sustained ventricular tachycardia: Role of the electrophysiologic study in selection of antiarrhythmic regimens. Circulation 58:986, 1978
39. Mason JW, Winkle RA: Accuracy of ventricular tachycardia induction study for predicting long term efficacy and inefficacy of antiarrhythmic drugs. N Engl J Med 303:1073, 1980
40. Bauernfiend RA, Wyndham CR, Dhingra RC et al: Serial electrophysiologic testing of multiple drugs in patients with atrioventricular nodal reentrant paroxysmal tachycardia. Circulation 62:1341, 1980
41. Fisher JD, Kim SG, Furman S et al: Role of implantable pacemakers in control of recurrent ventricular tachycardia. Am J Cardiol 49:194, 1982
42. Zipes DP, Heger JJ, Mides WM et al: Early experience with an implantable cardioverter. N Engl J Med 311:485, 1984
43. Mirowski M, Reid PR, Winkle RA et al: Mortality in patients with implanted automatic defibrillators. Ann Intern Med 98:585, 1983
44. Scheinman MM, Morady F, Hess DS: Catheter-induced ablation of the atrioventricular junction to control refractory supraventricular arrhythmias. JAMA 248:851, 1982
45. Hartzler GO: Electrode catheter ablation of refractory focal ventricular tachycardia. J Amer Coll Cardiol 2:1107, 1983
46. Steinhaus D, Whitford E, Stavens C et al: Percutaneous transcatheter electrical ablation for recurrent sustained ventricular tachycardia. Circulation 70:II-100, 1984
47. Akhtar M, Damato AN, Gilbert-Leeds CJ et al: Induction of iatrogenic electrocardiographic patterns during electrophysiologic studies. Circulation 56:60, 1977
48. Di Marco JP, Garan H, Ruskin JN: Complications in patients undergoing cardiac electrophysiologic procedures. Ann Intern Med 97:490, 1982

MEASUREMENTS AND CLINICAL APPLICATION OF MONOPHASIC ACTION POTENTIALS

CHAPTER 45
VOLUME 1

Michael R. Franz

Monophasic action potentials (MAPs) are extracellular potentials that closely resemble transmembrane action potentials (TAPs) in shape and duration.[1,2] Unlike TAPs, which are recorded with an intracellular microelectrode, MAPs can be obtained in the intact beating heart and, most importantly, in patients. Basic studies in excised tissue preparations, although essential for defining cellular electrophysiologic properties, cannot faithfully reproduce the anatomical substrates and pathophysiology of human heart disease because the relevant cardiac arrhythmia often presents only in the context of the intact organ or organism. MAP recordings help bridge this gap between basic and clinical electrophysiology. In this chapter, the basic mechanisms, clinical applications, and limitations of MAP recordings are discussed.

ELECTROPHYSIOLOGIC PRINCIPLES AND DEVICES IN MAP RECORDING

EARLY TECHNIQUES

The first MAPs were recorded as early as 1883 by Burdon-Sanderson and Page[3] from frog myocardium by placing one electrode on an injured area of the heart and the other electrode on an uninjured area of the heart (Fig. 45.1). Since then, MAPs have been equated with "injury" potentials and methods to produce MAPs have employed various ways of tissue traumatization. In 1931, Schütz advocated the *Herzknoten* (heart knot), a tie around a circumscript piece of ventricular muscle, as a better means for producing the injury current.[4] This was followed by the introduction of the suction electrode,[5] which produced MAPs with greater simplicity and of better quality than the previous methods. The suction electrode remained the MAP recording method of choice for several decades and, in 1966, was introduced into the arena of clinical electrophysiologic research, when Korsgren and colleagues[6] recorded the first MAPs in patients. The method was adopted and refined by others,[7-9] most notably by Olsson and co-workers (Fig. 45.2).[10-12]

Certain restrictions, however, apply to the use of suction electrodes in humans and have hampered a more widespread clinical acceptance. Probably the most important is that suction causes myocardial injury at the site of the catheter tip, which has led to the recommendation not to exceed a 2-minute recording time at the same endocardial site.[10,12] Furthermore, suction electrode catheters require suction pumps, three-way stopcocks, air-bubble filters, and other precautions that make their clinical use cumbersome (see Fig. 45.2). Because of the risk of myocardial injury and arterial air emboli, suction electrode catheters have never been used in human left ventricles.

CONTACT ELECTRODE DEVICES FOR MAP RECORDING

A simpler and safer method for MAP recording was introduced in 1980 by Franz and co-workers,[13] who demonstrated that MAPs can be recorded from human endocardium without suction simply by bringing a special electrode in contact with the endocardium under gentle pressure. This observation contradicted the long-held contention that myocardial injury by suction or other means was a prerequisite for obtaining MAPs. The "contact electrode" technique not only is safer and simpler to use but also provides recordings that are more stable over time, making it possible to monitor MAPs over periods of several hours from the same endocardial site, both in the right and left human ventricle.[14]

ENDOCARDIAL MAP RECORDING CATHETERS

The basic design of the contact electrode catheter is illustrated in Figure 45.3, *A*. The tip of the catheter is formed by a rounded nonpolarizable electrode of 1 mm diameter, while another nonpolarizable electrode, the reference electrode, is located 5 mm proximal to the tip. The distal portion of the catheter shaft incorporates a flat spring wire that ensures that stable contact between the tip electrode and the endocardium is maintained throughout the cardiac contraction–relaxation cycle. The tip electrode lead is connected to the positive input and the proximal electrode lead to the negative input of the recording system. A high input-impedance differential preamplifier that is direct current (DC) coupled is recommended. The importance of DC amplification will be outlined later. The catheter size is usually 6F with a length of 100 to 130 cm. A modified version of the contact electrode catheter uses a retractable intraluminal spring wire. With the wire in the retracted position, the distal catheter portion flexes into a soft J configuration (Fig. 45.3, *B*). This facilitates maneuvering the catheter through tortuous vessels and allows easy passage of the catheter across the aortic valve. A special catheter for simultaneous pacing and MAP recording is described later.

EPICARDIAL MAP RECORDING PROBES

MAPs can also be recorded from the epicardium, using special spring-loaded contact electrode probes.[15] Figure 45.3, *C* shows a probe designed for use in the cardiac operating room.[16] Two nonpolarizable electrodes are mounted on a flat ribbon in such a configuration that only one electrode comes in direct contact with the epicardium; the other electrode is mounted at the base of the ribbon and gains electrical continuity with the epicardium through a small cap of saline-soaked foam rubber placed over the electrode assembly. The ribbon is made of a special alloy that makes it both malleable and elastic; this allows the surgeon to quickly adjust the ribbon's curvature and advance the probe through the epicardial-pericardial space to inferior or posterior ventricular sites. Another approach uses a small acrylic electrode housing that is held between the index and middle finger and placed directly over the desired epicardial location (Fig. 45.3, *D*).[17] These epicardial probes are useful for recording MAPs from many different epicardial sites of the human heart in the operating room, for instance for the purpose of mapping the ventricular repolarization sequence[16] or for localizing ischemic regions.[18]

ELECTRONIC RECORDING EQUIPMENT

The MAP signal contains low-frequency components, especially during the plateau phase (phase 2) and during the diastolic interval (phase 4). Accurate signal reproduction therefore requires the use of DC-coupled amplification without any high- or low-pass filtering. Electrocardiographic recording systems are alternating current (AC) coupled and tend to move the recorded potential toward the isoelectric line. Because the diastolic (resting) potential of the MAP has a negative value, AC coupling tends to move the diastolic MAP potential upward, thus artifactually mimicking spontaneous phase 4 depolarization. For optimal signal fidelity, MAPs should be recorded with high-bandwidth amplifiers and inertia-free paper recorders that can accurately reproduce a frequency range from 0 to 5000 Hz. Bandwidth settings used for conventional intracardiac electrophysiologic recordings (30 to 300 Hz) are not suitable for MAP recordings.

PROCEDURE OF CONTACT MAP RECORDING
ENDOCARDIAL MAP RECORDING

After gas sterilization, the MAP catheter is introduced into the femoral vein or artery by the Seldinger technique and advanced into the right or left ventricle, respectively. The electrode leads are then connected to the amplifier in order to monitor the intracardiac signal during further catheter manipulation. When the catheter tip is pressed gently against the endocardium, MAP signals develop and reach stable amplitudes usually within a few beats. MAP signals are negative during diastole and positive during early systole (Fig. 45.4, A and B). Once stable contact is established, MAPs can be recorded in continuous fashion, along with intracardiac and surface electrocardiograms normally obtained in electrophysiologic studies (Fig. 45.5). Catheter-tip dislodgement may occur, and repeated attempts may be necessary to bring the catheter into a stable position. Optimal recordings are obtained if the catheter is placed such that its distal, elastic portion is allowed to flex back and forth with each cardiac contraction–relaxation cycle. With such optimal conditions, MAPs can remain stable in amplitude and configuration for periods of up to 3 hours without further manipulation of the catheter or readjustment of the electrode position.[14]

MAP recordings from ventricular endocardium are characterized by a distinct plateau phase (phase 2) with a relatively steep phase of final repolarization (phase 3). In contrast, MAP recordings from atrial endocardium exhibit only a very short or absent plateau phase and a slower final repolarization time course, reproducing the triangular configuration typical of atrial muscle action potentials.

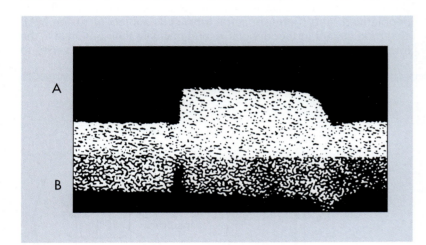

FIGURE 45.1 First monophasic action potential (MAP) recording obtained in 1883 by Burdon-Sanderson and Page from frog ventricle. **A.** MAP recording. **B.** Surface electrogram. (Burdon-Sanderson J, Page FJM: On the time-relations of the excitatory process in the ventricle of the heart of the frog. J Physiol 2:385, 1882).

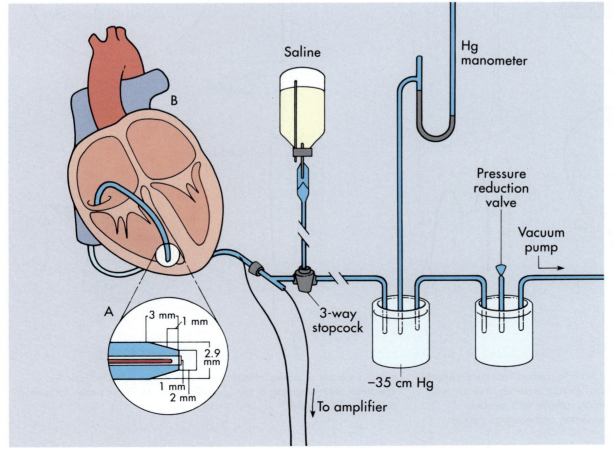

FIGURE 45.2 Suction electrode method by Olsson. **A.** Schematic view of catheter. **B.** Accessory equipment to suction electrode catheter. (Modified from Olsson B, Varnauskas E, Korsgren M: Further improved method for measuring monophasic action potentials of the intact human heart. J Electrocardiol 4:19, 1971).

EPICARDIAL MAP RECORDING

MAP recording from the epicardium by contact electrode technique is simple. The MAP tip electrode need only be held firmly against the epicardium, and stable recordings develop within seconds (see Fig. 45.4). It is possible to map the entire ventricular surface within a few minutes.[16,18] Epicardial MAP recordings from the human heart typically have amplitudes ranging from 15 to 60 mV, depending on the amount of pressure applied and on the surface area of the tip electrode. The tip electrode should be directed perpendicularly against the epicardium, avoiding placing probe parts other than the tip electrode against the epicardium. Such additional contact sites could produce depolarization of the myocardium adjacent to the exploring tip electrode and result in distortion of the electrical field that is measured by the MAP tip electrode (see below). Furthermore, as is apparent from the explanation of the genesis of the MAP given in the following section, MAP signals can only be obtained if the exploring electrode is in direct contact with heart muscle. Therefore, MAPs cannot be recorded in areas covered by fatty tissue. This provides a major obstacle for exploring epicardial repolarization properties in the human heart that is covered extensively by fatty tissue. MAPs also cannot be recorded from nonviable tissue such as a myocardial scar.

GENESIS OF THE MAP

Unlike intracellular microelectrode recordings, the MAP is measured with an extracellular catheter-tip electrode that has a diameter of 1 mm or more and therefore cannot enter a single cardiac cell. This has given rise to much discussion about how this technique can so reliably reproduce the voltage time course of the transmembrane action potential.[1,2,19-22] To date, a conclusive scientific explanation is still lacking but the following hypothesis, based on inference from available data,[1,2,19-23] seems plausible. Application of contact pressure against the myocardium depolarizes and inactivates the group of cells subjacent to the electrode while leaving the adjacent cells largely unaffected (Fig. 45.6). Because these adjacent normal cells retain their ability to depolarize and repolarize actively, there is an electrical gradient between the depolarized and inexcitable cells subjacent to the electrode and the adjacent normal cells. During electrical *diastole*, this gradient results in a source current emerging from the normal cells and a sink current descending into the depolarized cells subjacent to the MAP electrode. Under the volume conductor conditions provided by the surrounding tissue and blood pool, the sink current near the MAP electrode results in a negative electrical field that is proportional to the strength of current flow, which again is proportional to the potential gradient between the subjacent depolarized and the adjacent nonpolarized cells. During electrical *systole*, the normal cells adjacent to the MAP electrode undergo complete depolarization, which overshoots the zero potential in positive direction, whereas the already depolarized, and therefore refractory, cells subjacent to the MAP electrode cannot further depolarize and maintain their potential at the former reference level. As a result, the former current *sink* reverses to

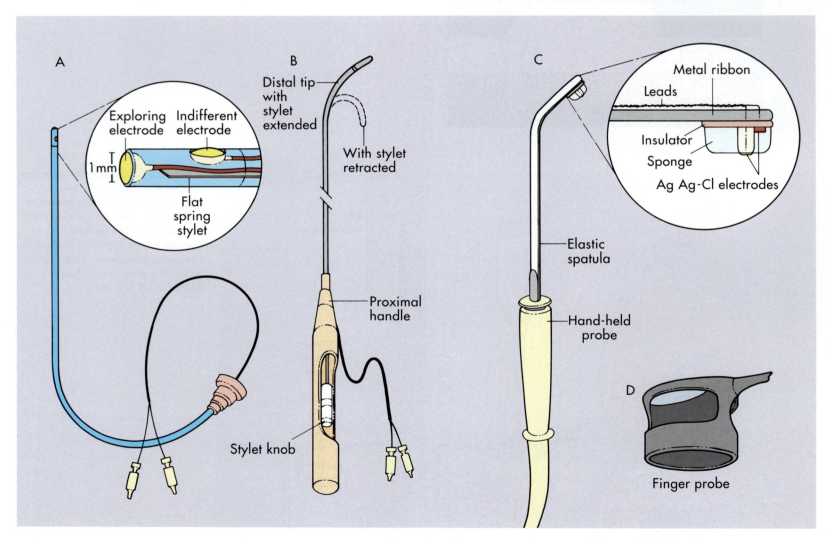

FIGURE 45.3 Design variations of contact electrode method with nonpolarizable silver–silver chloride electrodes. **A.** Standard contact electrode catheter with fixed intraluminal spring. **B.** Contact electrode catheter with movable intraluminal spring for easy catheter maneuvering and passage through tortuous vessels or across intracardiac valves. **C.** Spatula electrode for epicardial MAP recording in the operating room. **D.** Finger probe for manual placement by surgeon.

a current *source*, producing an electrical field of opposite polarity. The strength and polarity of the boundary current and the resulting electrical field reflect the potential gradient between the (depolarized and refractory) reference potential in the cells subjacent to the electrode and the voltage changes in the normal adjacent cells undergoing periodic depolarization and repolarization.

Because the amplitude of the MAP signal reflects the strength of extracellular current flow, which is proportional but not identical to the transmembrane voltage and which further may depend on the number of normal cells close enough to the contact electrode to contribute to the resting and action currents, both the degree of depolarization in individual cells as well as the number of cells depolarized by the contact pressure determine the amplitude of the MAP signal.[2] Accordingly, both greater contact pressure and greater muscle mass increase the amplitude of the MAP signal. Even using "maximal" pressure, the greatest MAP amplitude recorded from rabbit myocardium has been

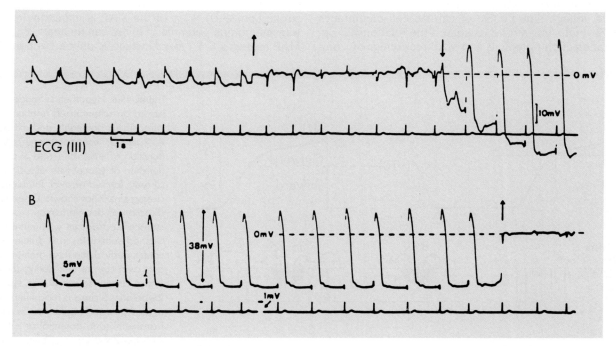

FIGURE 45.4 Procedure of MAP recording by contact electrode in right side of human heart. **A.** At the beginning of the upper tracing, the electrode contacts the atrial endocardium close to the tricuspid valve, giving rise to MAPs of triangular shape typical of atrial muscle (notches appearing in some potentials are due to unstable endocardial contact). Withdrawal of the catheter from the endocardium (arrow indicating upward) resulted in a sudden return to the intracavitary signal. During the subsequent seven heart beats the catheter was advanced through the tricuspid valve orifice into the apical region of the right ventricle, resulting in varying intracavitary electrograms. Firm contact of the tip electrode against the endocardium (downward arrow) produces successively increasing negative potentials during diastole and positive potentials during systole. **B.** Tracing shows stabilized MAP recordings. Withdrawal of the catheter from the endocardial surface is indicated by upward arrow. (Franz MR: Long-term recording of monophasic action potentials from human endocardium. Am J Cardiol 51:1629, 1983).

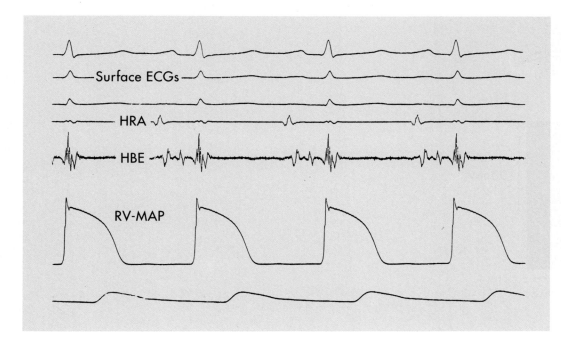

FIGURE 45.5 MAP recording from right ventricle (*RV*) during routine electrophysiologic study. (*HRA*, high right atrial electrogram; *HBE*, His-bundle electrogram).

reported to be 25 mV,[2] the greatest in dog left ventricular myocardium, 60 mV,[15] and the greatest in human left ventricular myocardium, 80 mV.[25] MAP recordings from human right ventricular free-wall myocardium seldom exceed 25 mV in amplitude, and from the human right atrial wall they usually range below 10 mV.[14,24,25]

ACCURACY OF MAP RECORDINGS

In contrast to intracellular microelectrode measurements, the MAP recorded by any of the extracellular techniques reported to date does not indicate the true magnitude of transmembrane potential changes. Despite this difference in absolute voltage magnitude, MAP recordings indicate the relative voltage time course of cardiac cell membranes with high fidelity. Several studies have examined the relationship between transmembrane action potentials and MAP recordings by comparing both signals from simultaneous recordings at closely adjacent myocardial sites.[1,2,23,26] These studies have confirmed that MAP recordings indicate the time of local activation and the duration and configuration of the entire cellular repolarization time course (phases 1 through 4) with high accuracy (Fig. 45.7). Figure 45.8 shows our preferred method of analyzing the MAP signal for duration at 90% repolarization.

UPSTROKE VELOCITY

The MAP recording technique cannot render information on the absolute rise velocity ($\dot{V}_{max}$) of the transmembrane action potential upstroke (phase 0). $\dot{V}_{max}$ of the MAP is markedly less than that of the transmembrane potential.[1,2] In the canine heart, $\dot{V}_{max}$ of the ventricular MAP averages 6.4 V/sec,[15] which is only a fraction of the transmem-

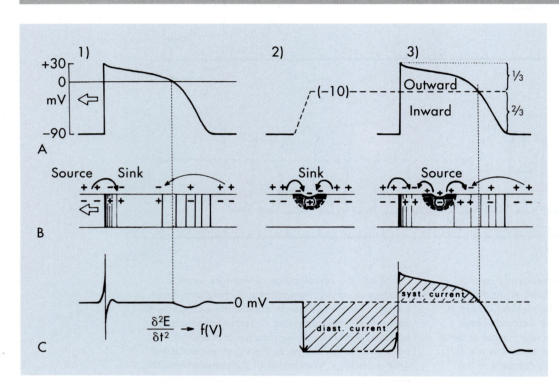

FIGURE 45.6 Hypothetical model of MAP genesis based on schematized relationship between intracellular potentials and extracellular recordings. **A.** 1 and 3: Transmembrane action potential (function of time). **B.** 1 and 3: Depolarization wave (function of space) with associated extracellular currents (curved arrows). Intracellular currents closing circuit not shown. Open arrows indicate direction of depolarization wave. **C.** 1: Myocardial surface electrogram with intrinsic deflection. Dashed semicircles in **B** delineate area of continuously diminished membrane potential, which acts as a current sink during diastole (column 2) and a current source during systole (column 3) (depolarized area is magnified with respect to excitation wavelength). An average transmembrane potential of −10 mV (dashed line in A) is assumed for the fibers under the electrode in an attempt to explain the ratio between diastolic and systolic current strengths proportionate to the measured ratio of negative and positive displacement of the MAP. For further discussion see text.

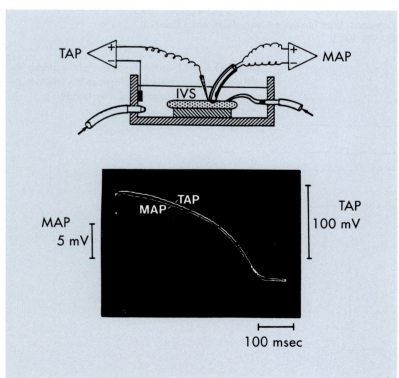

FIGURE 45.7 Comparison of monophasic action potential (MAP) and transmembrane action potential (TAP) recorded simultaneously from closely adjacent sites in an isolated perfused rabbit septum preparation.

brane $\dot{V}_{max}$ of ventricular cells (approximately 200 V/sec).[27] The smaller rise velocity of the MAP is in part due to its smaller amplitude and in part to the fact that the MAP electrode records from many cells whose depolarizations occur sequentially with time. Also in contrast to the transmembrane recording, small Q waves or notches may be seen just before or during the upstroke of the MAP, reflecting contamination of the local MAP recording with electrical activity from nearby tissue. The influence of remote electrical activity on the MAP can be minimized by an optimal placement of the MAP reference electrode and by using differential amplification.[14] When the catheter tip is directed axially (perpendicularly) against the endocardium, depolarization is confined to a small area subjacent to the tip electrode. With this orientation the reference electrode, located 5 mm proximal from the tip, is far enough away to serve as an indifferent electrode, yet close enough to cancel most of the remote electrical activity.[14] The influence of remote potentials on the MAP may increase with ectopic ventricular activation, which augments the magnitude of the intracavitary QRS vector. To minimize the interference from intracavitary potentials, it is recommended that MAP signals should be not less than 10 mV in amplitude.

EVALUATION OF RESTING POTENTIAL CHANGES

Using strict DC-coupled amplification, MAP recordings are capable of measuring transient changes in resting potential and action potential amplitude. For instance, acute ischemia mimicked by arresting perfusion in an isolated rabbit septum preparation not only causes marked changes in duration and configuration of the MAP but also a quantitatively similar decrease in resting potential magnitude, as confirmed by simultaneously recorded transmembrane action potentials.[24] Similarly, increases in extracellular potassium ion concentration from normal (4.5 mM) to 9 mM results in quantitatively parallel decreases in diastolic potential in both the transmembrane and MAP recordings.[2]

VENTRICULAR MUSCLE OR PURKINJE FIBER ACTIVITY: WHAT IS RECORDED?

An important question is whether endocardial MAP recordings reflect Purkinje fiber activity, ventricular muscle activity, or a mixture of both. Ino and co-workers[23] quantified the relative contributions of Purkinje fibers and ventricular fibers to the endocardial MAP signal and found that the MAP signal reflects predominantly "deeper" electrical activity, consisting of ventricular cells, with superficial Purkinje fibers contributing not more than 10%. Because Purkinje fiber action potentials are longer than those of ventricular muscle, the relative delayed repolarization of Purkinje fibers may mimic an "afterpotential" in the MAP recording.[23,28] However, this "artifact" has been reported only in isolated Purkinje/muscle preparations, which had a relative preponderance of conductive tissue, and does not seem to occur in endocardial recordings in humans.

EARLY AND DELAYED AFTERDEPOLARIZATIONS

Both early[29] and delayed[30] afterdepolarizations have been implicated in the genesis of so-called triggered arrhythmias, also known as automatic arrhythmias or polymorphous ventricular tachycardias. These afterdepolarizations cannot be detected by conventional intracardiac or surface electrocardiographic tracings but require a technique that faithfully reproduces the time course of cellular repolarization. (Afterdepolarizations are not to be confused with "late potentials." The latter can be detected with signal-averaged electrocardiograms and presumably reflect abnormal ventricular activation, not abnormal repolarization.[31]) MAP recording appears promising as a tool to identify and localize, in vivo, areas with afterdepolarizations. For instance, in isolated canine ventricular muscle, administration of cesium chloride produces afterdepolarizations not only in the intracellularly recorded transmembrane action potential but also in the adjacently recorded MAP.[26] In both excised tissue preparations and intact canine hearts, anthopleurin-A, a drug that greatly prolongs action potential duration, also produces afterdepolarizations, with similar appearance in the intracellular and MAP recording.[32] Clinical examples of the association of afterdepolarizations with polymorphous tachycardias are given below.

MAP RECORDINGS DURING CLINICAL ELECTROPHYSIOLOGIC STUDIES

Because MAP recordings represent both the time of local myocardial activation (depolarization) as well as the entire time course of local repolarization with high accuracy, they can not only supplant conventional electrode catheters during routine electrophysiologic studies but also offer additional information not available with other electrode catheters.

In MAP recordings, local activation time is reflected by the MAP upstroke, which is sharp and unambiguous in contrast to the often multiphasic deflections obtained with conventional catheters (see Fig. 45.5). This makes measurements of local activation time easier and more accurate. MAPs are obtained only when the catheter-tip electrode is in close contact with the endocardium, thus eliminating intracavitary potentials. With the use of conventional electrophysiologic catheters, fractionated, double, or late potentials have been observed and interpreted as markers of abnormal conduction in scarred myocardium, which is believed to be a substrate for reentry tachycardia[33,34]; however, concerns that some fractionated electrograms represent artifacts have been raised.[34,35] Comparisons between MAP signals and conventional electrograms may be helpful in further identifying the nature of these fractionated electrograms.

In contrast to conventional electrograms, MAP recordings provide accurate information on the entire repolarization time course.[1,2] The repolarization time course, or action potential duration and configura-

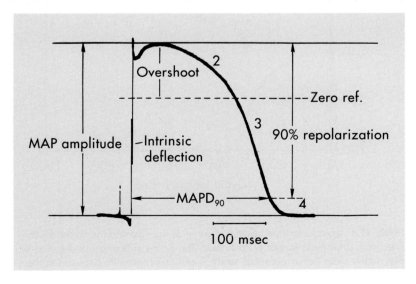

FIGURE 45.8 Method to analyze MAP amplitude and duration. This example shows evaluation of MAP duration at 90% repolarization. Note that the maximal amplitude is defined as the crest of the plateau, not as the peak of the upstroke. (Modified from Franz MR, Burkhoff D, Spurgeon H et al: In vitro validation of a new cardiac catheter technique for recording monophasic action potentials. Eur Heart J 7:34, 1986).

tion, is influenced by a variety of pathophysiologic and pharmacologic factors of clinical interest. The most notable among these are variations in the heart rate, myocardial ischemia, congenital or acquired long QT interval syndromes, other conditions causing triggered arrhythmias, and the effects of antiarrhythmic drugs with predominant effects on the APD (Table 45.1).

EFFECTS OF RATE AND RHYTHM ON THE HUMAN VENTRICULAR ACTION POTENTIAL DURATION

The cardiac APD decreases when the heart rate increases. This rate (or cycle length) dependence of the APD is a fundamental property of cardiac muscle that occurs independent of alterations in sympathetic tone.[36,37] In the body surface electrocardiogram, changes in APD are reflected by changes in the QT interval. However, precise measurement of the QT interval may be difficult, especially at high heart rates with superimposition of the P and T wave, or when prominent U waves make the definition of the terminal T wave doubtful. MAP recordings provide information on local myocardial depolarization and repolarization and, unlike the surface electrocardiogram, are not affected by superimposition of summated atrial and ventricular activity. MAP recordings therefore have become the method of choice to identify and accurately analyze changes in human APD, occurring as a result of changes in the heart rate or rhythm.[10,38,39]

Cycle-length dependent changes in APD must be distinguished between those that result from transient cycle length changes and those that develop over longer time. Transient APD changes are observed when the cycle length is abruptly decreased by premature atrial or ventricular beats or abruptly increased by a pause due to a blocked sinus discharge, blocked atrioventricular conduction, or postextrasystolic compensation. Long-term APD changes are seen if action potential recordings at different steady-state cycle length, such as during pacing or sustained ventricular tachycardia, are compared.[37,39]

EFFECT OF SINGLE CYCLE LENGTH ALTERATIONS: ELECTRICAL RESTITUTION CURVE

The cardiac APD is governed by a complex interplay of time- and voltage-dependent changes in membrane ion conductances. If insufficient time is available before a new stimulus, either no response (refractory state) or one with an abbreviated APD occurs. If a membrane response is preceded by a pause, a prolonged APD may result. The time course of this time-dependent recovery of APD, plotted as the function of the interval between a steady-state response and a subsequent premature or postmature extrastimulus, is described by the so-called *electrical restitution curve*.[40] (The electrical restitution curve thus describes all APDs that result from a *single* cycle length alteration of various length.) The earliest action potential that can be elicited by an extrastimulus is determined by the refractory period, which ends at approximately 70% repolarization of the preceding steady-state response. The duration of this most premature action potential is considerably less than the steady-state APD. With progressively increasing extrastimulus interval, APD increases to a maximum that is reached at coupling intervals above 1 second. In Purkinje fibers[41,42] this maximum is approached with a monophasic time course. In contrast, the electrical restitution curve of ventricular muscle of many mammalian species,[40,43–47] including humans,[38,39] is biphasic; APD first rises steeply to an early maximum at about 100 msec after the effective refractory period (or about 50 msec after 90% repolarization of the steady-state response), is followed by a transient decrease, and then gradually increases to a maximum value reached at a cycle length of approximately 1000 msec (Fig. 45.9). The premature action potentials responsible for the early peak of electrical restitution in ventricular muscle have a greater amplitude, plateau duration, and slope of phase 3 than those elicited at slightly shorter or longer extrastimulus intervals or the steady-state responses, and therefore have been termed *supernormal* premature action potentials.[37] Supernormal action potentials and a biphasic electrical restitution curve are not observed in ventricular muscle of guinea pig,[48] kitten,[49] and pig moderator band.[41]

The mechanism responsible for the early hump of electrical restitution is not yet fully understood but is believed to reflect the transient decrease in subsarcolemmal calcium concentration available during a premature depolarization.[47] This is supported by the observation that action potential plateau duration and contractile force are inversely related to each other.[38,50] The low activator calcium concentration available for the weaker premature beat results in an increased slow inward calcium current (a negative feedback to help restore intracellular calcium), which augments the action potential plateau duration and amplitude and, to a lesser degree, total APD. Consistent with this hypothesis, calcium channel blockers suppress supernormal action potentials and the early peak of electrical restitution.[47] Long pauses

TABLE 45.1 CLINICAL APPLICATIONS OF MONOPHASIC ACTION POTENTIAL RECORDINGS

Effects of rate and rhythm on action potential duration (APD)
Myocardial ischemia detection and infarct mapping
Afterdepolarizations and polymorphous ventricular tachycardias
  Congenital or acquired long QT syndromes
  Other forms of triggered arrhythmias (right ventricular outflow tract VT?)
Effects of antiarrhythmic drugs on APD
Effects of antiarrhythmic drugs on ERP/APD ratio
Evaluation of T wave changes
Automated signal analysis

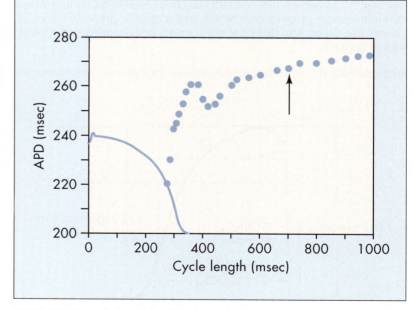

FIGURE 45.9 Typical electrical restitution curve of right ventricular myocardium. The basic drive cycle length is 700 msec. The arrow indicates the duration of the steady-state action potential, which is also schematically depicted in the graph.

result in increased contractility and action potentials that have a short plateau phase but a slowed final repolarization time course.[38,40,43,44,46] It follows that APD cannot be defined as a uniform variable but must take into consideration the repolarization level at which it is measured.

STEADY-STATE RELATIONSHIP

The cycle-length dependency of APD in the steady state (as during constant-rate pacing or during stable sinus rhythm) differs greatly from the APD relationship with single cycle length alterations. In the steady state, APD shows a completely linear relationship with cycle length, except for very long cycle lengths when APD attains a maximal, plateau value (Fig. 45.10). In general, over a range of steady-state cycle lengths from 350 to 800 msec, APD increases an average of 23 msec for each 100-msec increment in basic cycle length. In contrast to single cycle length–induced APD changes, steady-state APD changes are due to a change in phase 2 duration, with the slope of phase 3 remaining essentially unaltered (Fig. 45.10, inset). At any given cycle length, the steady-state APD may be larger or smaller than the non-steady-state APD, depending on whether the steady-state cycle length is less or greater than the premature or postmature cycle length; longer cycle lengths cause greater steady-state APD and shorter ones cause decreased steady-state APD as compared with effects of transient cycle length alterations (Fig. 45.11).[37,39]

The linearity of the steady-state relationship between cycle length and APD differs from Bazett's rate correction algorithm for the QT interval, which is based on a square root relationship.[51] Furthermore,

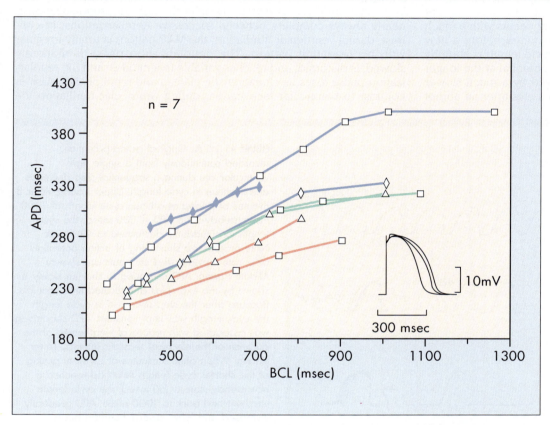

FIGURE 45.10 Relation between action potential duration (*APD*) and basic cycle length (*BCL*) in the steady state at a single right ventricular endocardial site (individual relations in seven patients). The inset exemplifies accompanying configurational changes of the MAP. (Modified from Franz MR: Long-term recording of monophasic action potentials from human endocardium. Am J Cardiol 51:1629, 1983).

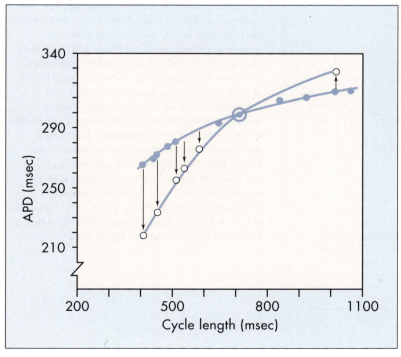

FIGURE 45.11 Comparison of APD following a single cycle-length alteration (*filled circles* = electrical restitution curve) with steady-state APD (*open circles*) at identical cycle lengths. The steady-state cycle length during which single cycle-length changes were introduced was 750 msec (the cycle length at which both curves intersect). The electrical restitution curve was truncated at 400 msec (the shortest steady-state cycle length in this patient) and therefore does not show the early supernormal phase. All recordings were from a single right ventricular site. (Franz MR, Swerdlow CD, Liem BL, Schaefer J: Cycle-length dependence of human action potential duration in vivo: Effects of single extrastimuli, sudden sustained rate acceleration and deceleration, and different steady-state frequencies. J Clin Invest 82:972, 1988).

Bazett's and other formulas[52,53] for rate correction of the QT interval assume a uniform relationship over the entire range of cycle lengths. In contrast, the correlation between APD and cycle length is linear for cycle lengths up to 800 msec and attains a plateau value at longer cycle lengths, suggesting that QT interval correction beyond steady-state cycle lengths of 1000 msec may not be necessary. The discrepancy between the steady-state and non-steady-state cycle length dependency further cautions against simple algebraic QT interval derivations that are not based on true steady-state conditions.

RATE ADAPTATION

The transition between the non-steady state and the steady state is described by the rate adaptation curve. Figure 45.12 shows the time course of action potential shortening and lengthening after a sequential step decrease and step increase in cycle length. The first action potential following the step *decrease* in cycle length shows abrupt shortening; thereafter, action potential shortening occurs with a much slower time course. Up to 3 minutes may be required before a new steady state is reached. Conversely, when the cycle length is abruptly *increased* to the baseline value, the first action potential at the longer cycle length shows abrupt prolongation, followed by a much slower time course of lengthening. During the first few beats after an abrupt cycle length decrease, APD may undergo regular or irregular oscillation (Fig. 45.13). These oscillations are due to the fact that, at a constant cycle length, each change in APD causes a reciprocal change in the diastolic interval that determines the subsequent APD according to the electrical restitution curve.[39] Corresponding changes following sudden rate acceleration have been reported for refractoriness of the human His-Purkinje system[54,55] and ventricular myocardium.[56]

VENTRICULAR TACHYCARDIA AND VENTRICULAR FIBRILLATION

MAP recordings reveal distinct differences between ventricular tachycardia and ventricular fibrillation, even under circumstances in which the surface ECG may be unreliable in differentiating these two types of arrhythmias (Fig. 45.14).[57] During ventricular tachycardia, the MAP shows a regular and repeating waveform with characteristics very similar to that during sinus rhythm. Despite the fast rate, repolarization is nearly always complete between successive depolarizations. In contrast, during ventricular fibrillation, the MAP pattern is totally irregular with no repeating pattern. The depolarization phase is markedly slowed, is distorted, and reaches variable magnitudes; and the repolarization phase loses its characteristic plateau and rapid phases. Also in contrast to ventricular tachycardia, during ventricular fibrillation the

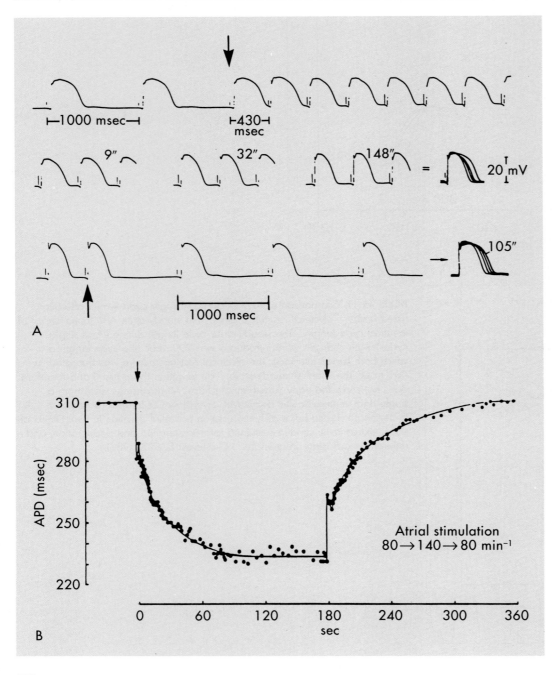

FIGURE 45.12 A. Original action potentials recorded continuously from a single right ventricular site during a sequential step decrease and increase in cycle length. *Upper tracing:* After 3 minutes of pacing at a basic cycle length of 1000 msec (steady-state APD = 330 msec), the cycle length was suddenly decreased to 430 msec. Note progressive shortening of action potentials after rate increase (first six beats are shown). *Middle tracing:* APD continued to shorten slowly as shown by the examples at indicated time intervals. Because after the step decrease in cycle length the cycle length was kept constant, APD shortening was associated with reciprocal lengthening of the duration of the electrical diastolic interval. *Lower tracing:* When after 3 minutes of constant pacing at the shorter cycle length APD had reached a new steady state (=210 msec), the cycle length was switched back to 1000 msec. APD gradually increased and, after several hundred beats, recovered to the initial steady-state duration. The superimposed recordings demonstrate that these slow changes in APD were mainly due to a change in plateau duration. (Franz MR, Swerdlow CD, Liem BL, Schaefer J: Cycle-length dependence of human action potential duration in vivo: Effects of single extrastimuli, sudden sustained rate acceleration and deceleration, and different steady-state frequencies. J Clin Invest 82:972, 1988). **B.** Time course of APD adaptation following a consecutive step decrease and increase in cycle length. Both the step increase and the decrease are followed by an initial rapid phase and a subsequent slow phase of action potential shortening and lengthening, respectively. The rapid phase of APD change showed "notching," which is explained in more detail in Figure 45.13.

potential never returns to its normal diastolic level but is interrupted by the subsequent depolarization at various degrees of incomplete repolarization, giving the MAP the appearance of "riding on" each other. These irregularities in the MAP pattern may, in part, reflect the irregular depolarization and repolarization of single cells during ventricular fibrillation[58,59] and, in part, the heterogeneity of depolarization and repolarization within the small group of cells from which the MAP is recorded. A somewhat less irregular MAP pattern has been recorded in atrial fibrillation.[60]

EFFECTS OF ANTIARRHYTHMIC DRUGS ON REPOLARIZATION AND REFRACTORINESS
EFFECT ON APD

Many antiarrhythmic drugs have distinct effects on APD, especially those in class IA and III, which, in addition to slowed impulse conduction, cause significant prolongation of the APD. The APD-prolonging effect of these agents has been implicated in their antiarrhythmic efficacy. For instance, a positive correlation has been found between

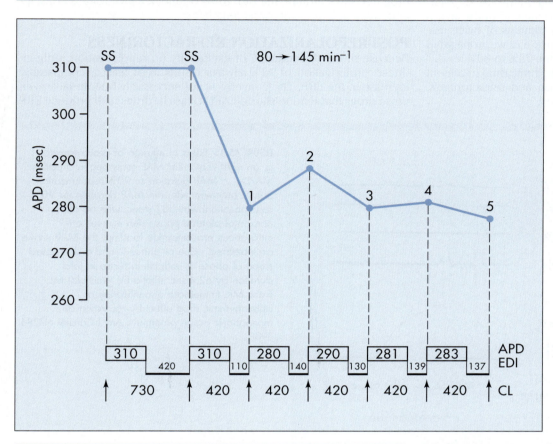

FIGURE 45.13 APD changes during the first five beats after a step decrease in cycle length (*CL*) from 730 to 420 msec are shown together with changes in electrical diastolic intervals (*EDI*). Because after the step change the new CL is kept constant, each APD change results in a reciprocal change in the EDI that precedes the subsequent action potential. A longer APD produces a shorter EDI, which in turn is followed by a shorter APD and a subsequently longer EDI. (Modified from Franz MR, Swerdlow CD, Liem BL, Schaefer J: Cycle-length dependence of human action potential duration *in vivo*: Effects of single extrastimuli, sudden sustained rate acceleration and deceleration, and different steady-state frequencies. J Clin Invest 82:972, 1988).

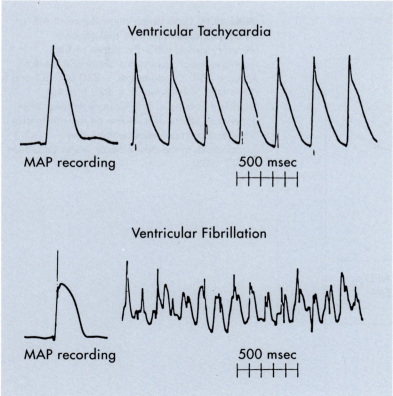

FIGURE 45.14 MAP recordings during ventricular tachycardia and ventricular fibrillation. (Liem BL, Swerdlow CD, Franz MR: Distinctive features of ventricular fibrillation and ventricular tachycardia detected by monophasic action potential recording in human subjects. J Electrophysiol 2:484, 1988).

atrial APD and susceptibility for atrial fibrillation; patients with longer atrial APD had a lesser chance for atrial fibrillation recurrence than those with shorter atrial APD.[61,62] Amiodarone produces QT interval and APD prolongation after chronic drug dosing, and this effect has been associated with the high efficacy of this drug for ventricular arrhythmias.[63] Using MAP recordings, an APD-prolonging effect has been demonstrated in patients for amiodarone,[64] quinidine[65,66] (Fig. 45.15), procainamide,[65] aprindine,[67] pirmenol,[68] and sotalol.[67,69]

RELATION BETWEEN APD AND REFRACTORINESS

Myocardial cells are refractory to a new stimulus during the depolarized state, with excitability recurring only toward the end of the action potential. In normal myocardium, an electrical stimulus of twice diastolic threshold strength is usually not able to elicit a new, propagated depolarization until repolarization has reached the 70% to 80% level.[70] Myocardial disease, such as ischemia, or antiarrhythmic drug treatment can alter this correlation between repolarization and refractoriness, leading to important implications for arrhythmias.

MAP studies have confirmed the relation between cellular repolarization and excitability for the *in vivo* heart.[71] In normal, drug-free myocardium, APD and the effective refractory period (ERP) both are linearly correlated to the cycle length of stimulation, with nearly identical linear regression slopes (Fig. 45.16). This means that in normal myocardium the relationship between APD and ERP is unaffected by the heart rate. When ERP is referenced to the repolarization level (at which excitability for twice diastolic threshold stimuli recurs), it falls between a rather narrow range of repolarization levels of 75% to 85%, regardless of the heart rate. It therefore can be stated that in normal, drug-free myocardium, the ERP to APD ratio at a given site is constant and independent of the cycle length.[62]

POST-REPOLARIZATION REFRACTORINESS

Because of the dependence of excitability on repolarization, drug-induced prolongation of APD always results in at least a comparable increase in the ERP. The converse is not necessarily true. In fact, even those drugs that tend to shorten APD (class IB drugs) still produce ERP

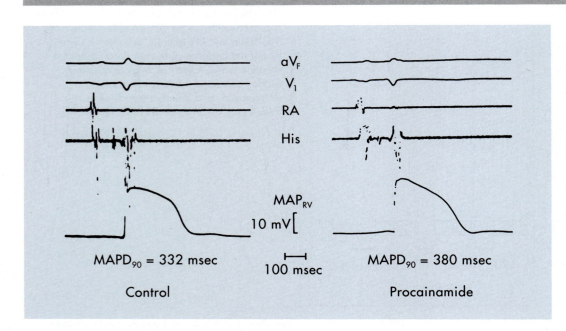

FIGURE 45.15 Effect of infusion of procainamide, 1 g, on right ventricular MAP recording in a patient. $MAPD_{90}$ = MAP duration at 90% repolarization. Before procainamide, the MAP duration (at 90% repolarization) was 332 msec, with an almost horizontal plateau phase. Ten minutes after intravenous procainamide loading, the MAP shows an increased slope of phase 2 and a decreased slope of phase 3, with an increase in total duration by 62 msec. (Platia EV, Weisfeldt ML, Franz MR: Immediate quantification of antiarrhythmic drug effect by recording of monophasic action potentials. Am J Cardiol 61:1284, 1988).

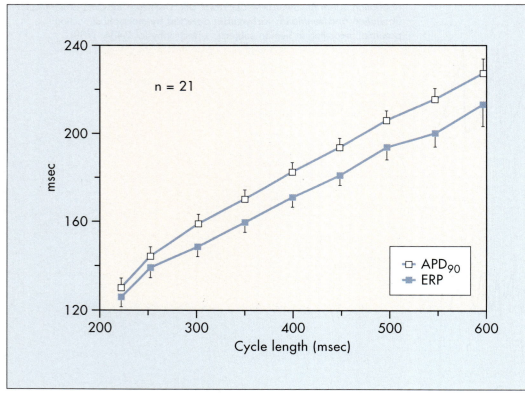

FIGURE 45.16 Cycle length dependence of APD at 90% repolarization (APD_{90}) and effective refractory period (*ERP*). The slopes of the respective linear regressions are nearly identical: $APD_{90} = 0.24 \times$ cycle length $+ 83.0$ (r = 1.0) and ERP $= 0.22 \times$ cycle length $+ 82.3$ (r = 1.0). (Modified from Franz MR, Costard A: Frequency-dependent effects of quinidine on the relationship between action potential duration and refractoriness in the canine heart *in situ*. Circulation 77:1177, 1988).

prolongation,[72] and APD prolonging drugs (class IA and III) cause relatively greater increases in ERP. This is exemplified in Figure 45.17, which shows the effect of an intravenous dose of pirmenol on the simultaneously recorded APD and ERP in a human subject.[68] Pirmenol produces a slight decrease in APD, most notable at the 50% repolarization level. Despite this decrease in APD, myocardial refractoriness, as assessed by the strength-interval method, increases. Similar, disproportionate increases on ERP relative to APD (resulting in an increased ERP/APD ratio) have been reported for lidocaine, quinidine, mexiletine, and other class I antiarrhythmic agents.[73–76] The increase in the ERP/APD ratio has been linked directly to the antiarrhythmic efficacy of the drugs, based on the rationale that ERP prolongation relative to APD provides a "window" of post-repolarization refractoriness that prevents the occurrence of early premature beats and rapid ventricular tachycardias.[77]

RATE DEPENDENCE OF ANTIARRHYTHMIC DRUG EFFECTS

In recent years, attention has focused on the rate dependence of the sodium channel blocking effect of antiarrhythmic drugs. Rate dependence (also called "use dependence") describes the property of antiarrhythmic drugs to increase their sodium channel blocking potential when the heart rate (or stimulation rate) is increased. With each successive depolarization, a certain amount of drug binds rapidly to the sodium channels while dissociating only slowly during the subsequent diastolic interval.[78,79] Therefore, as the rate of depolarization is increased, more drug is bound and less is dissociated, resulting in a rate-dependent accumulation of sodium channel block. Sodium channel block traditionally has been quantified by measuring the maximal depolarization velocity ($\dot{V}_{max}$) of the intracellular action potential, a method that cannot be duplicated in the beating heart. Using intracellular action potential[74,75] and MAP recordings,[72] it has been shown that an increase in the ERP/APD ratio also indicates rate dependence of sodium channel block in a quantitatively similar fashion as $\dot{V}_{max}$. As shown in Figure 45.18, quinidine produces only little change in the ERP/APD relationship at a moderate heart rate but with increasing heart rate the increase in ERP progressively exceeds the increase in APD. Thus, the size of the protective "window of post-repolarization refractoriness," which is offered by antiarrhythmic drugs, is heart rate dependent. In fact, such a rate-dependent mechanism of drug effect is expected to operate during ventricular tachycardias and may be an important factor in the "spontaneous" termination of otherwise sustained ventricular tachycardias.

MEASURING ANTIARRHYTHMIC DRUG EFFECTS IN THE CLINICAL LABORATORY

Platia and co-workers[67] performed serial MAP recordings during antiarrhythmic drug infusion in patients and found that an increase in APD during intravenous procainamide or quinidine administration correlates with the drug plasma concentration much better than either QT interval prolongation or increase in the ERP. Thus, MAP recordings can be used to quantitate the direct electrophysiologic effects of antiarrhythmic drugs and to ascertain that a sufficient antiarrhythmic drug dose is administered. This is particularly helpful in the setting of acute antiarrhythmic drug testing in the electrophysiology laboratory where it is important to know that an optimal dose is administered so that failure of arrhythmia suppression can be attributed to the drug's antiarrhythmic inefficacy rather than to an underdosage or overdosage. Besides being potentially more accurate in the assessment of drug-induced electrophysiologic and antiarrhythmic effects, MAP recordings can be obtained "on line" at the time of electrophysiologic study, in contrast to biochemical drug assays whose results usually are not available for several days after the study.

SIMULTANEOUS APD AND ERP DETERMINATIONS IN THE HUMAN HEART

Conventional electrode catheters used in electrophysiologic studies allow determination of the ERP at a given endocardial site but cannot elucidate the relationship between membrane repolarization and refractoriness. An extended, quadripolar version of the contact electrode catheter provides both pacing and MAP recording capabilities with a single catheter, thus allowing easy and accurate measurements of ERP and APD simultaneously and at the same site in the human heart.[80] Unlike conventional quadripolar electrode catheters, the pacing electrodes in this MAP recording/pacing combination catheter are oriented diametrically opposed halfway between the distal (tip) and proximal (reference) MAP electrode (Fig. 45.19). This electrode configuration provides for extremely low stimulus capture thresholds (0.02–0.25 mA, mean 0.09 mA),[80] resulting in minimal interference between the pacing artifact and the MAP signal and thus allowing precise, simultaneous determinations of both APD and ERP in vivo (Fig. 45.20).

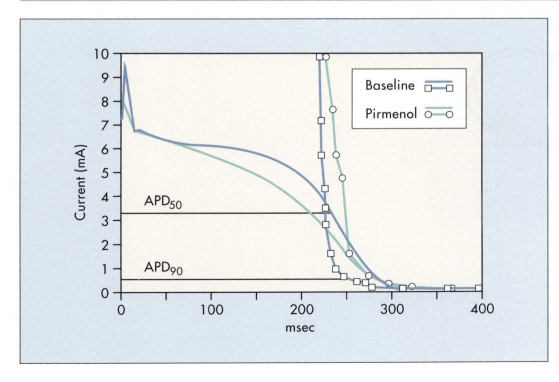

FIGURE 45.17 Effect of pirmenol on APD and strength interval curve, determined at the same right ventricular site in a patient. Refractoriness increases despite decreases in APD, particularly at the level of 50% repolarization. (Modified from Liem LB, Clay DA, Franz MR, Swerdlow CD: Electrophysiology and anti-arrhythmic efficacy of intravenous pirmenol in patients with sustained ventricular tachyarrhythmias. Am Heart J 113:1390, 1987).

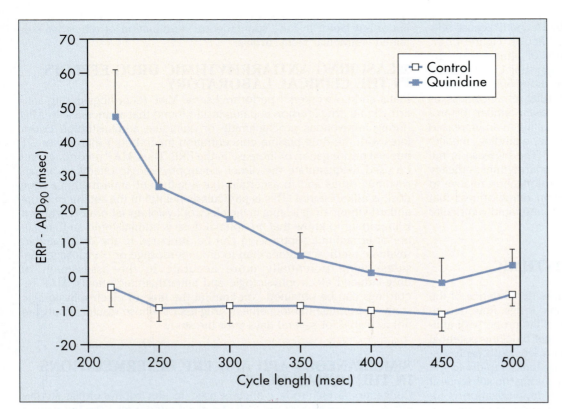

FIGURE 45.18 Difference between ERP and APD_{90} as a function of basic cycle length before and after quinidine administration. (Modified from Franz MR, Costard A: Frequency-dependent effects of quinidine on the relationship between action potential duration and refractoriness in the canine heart in situ. Circulation 77:1177, 1988).

FIGURE 45.19 Schematic of MAP recording/pacing combination catheter.

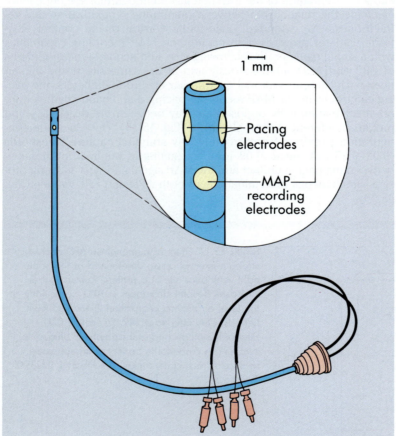

Simultaneous APD and ERP determinations can help characterize and quantitate antiarrhythmic drug effects in the clinical setting. By determining the ERP/APD relation at different pacing rates, information on the rate- (or use-) dependent effect of antiarrhythmic drugs can also be obtained.[81] Experimental studies have demonstrated that certain drug combination therapies that exhibit greater clinical efficacy and better tolerance than single drug treatment (such as quinidine–mexiletine combination),[82] produce rate-dependent post-repolarization refractoriness in an additive fashion.[72,82,83] The quantitative evaluation of antiarrhythmic drug effects on the ERP/APD relationship in the clinical laboratory, and its correlation with therapeutic efficacy, may increase our understanding of pharmacologic therapy and may aid in tailoring a specific antiarrhythmic drug regimen to an individual patient.

POLYMORPHOUS VENTRICULAR TACHYCARDIAS, THE LONG QT SYNDROME, AND AFTERDEPOLARIZATIONS

Polymorphous ventricular tachycardias may occur spontaneously or in response to antiarrhythmic drug treatment. In both settings they often, but not necessarily, are associated with a prolonged QT interval.[84] Often, such polymorphous ventricular tachycardia may have the appearance of "torsade de pointes," originally described in the setting of the long QT syndrome.[85] The classic long QT syndrome can be subdivided into two forms: idiopathic (congenital, familial)[86] and acquired. The familial form occurs in two main varieties: an autosomal dominant form associated with deafness[87] and an autosomal recessive form without deafness.[88,89] (Sporadic occurrences of the long QT syndrome also exist and are being increasingly acknowledged.[90]) The acquired form is seen in patients with electrolyte imbalances (such as hypomagnesemia) and in patients receiving antiarrhythmic drug treatment.[90] The drug-induced form is most commonly associated with class IA antiarrhythmic drugs that prolong the APD. Its occurrence does not seem to be related to the drug's plasma level, nor is it necessarily correlated with the degree of QT interval prolongation.[84] Drug-induced polymorphous ventricular tachycardia can occur even in the absence of QT interval prolongation and then is, strictly speaking, no longer part of the classic long QT syndrome.

Polymorphous ventricular tachycardia or torsade de pointes often requires a trigger. In the acquired form, torsade de pointes is usually precipitated by a premature beat and a subsequent pause. In the congenital form, it is induced by exercise, sudden emotions, or other factors provoking increased sympathetic stimulation, including isoproterenol infusion. Jackman and colleagues[90] therefore suggested classification of these two manifestations of "spontaneous" polymorphous ventricular tachycardia as either "pause dependent" or "adrenergic dependent." Both forms share the property of arrhythmia suppression by overdrive cardiac pacing. However, although in the acquired (pause dependent) form of long QT syndrome an increase in heart rate by β-agonists has been shown to be beneficial, arrhythmias in the congenital form (adrenergic dependent) are suppressed by β-blockers,[86] alone or in combination with pacing.

Despite this clinical divergence between the congenital and acquired long QT syndrome, there is growing consensus that the electrophysiologic mechanism underlying polymorphous ventricular tachycardias in both the congenital and acquired forms relates to abnormalities in cellular repolarization. Basic electrophysiologic stud-

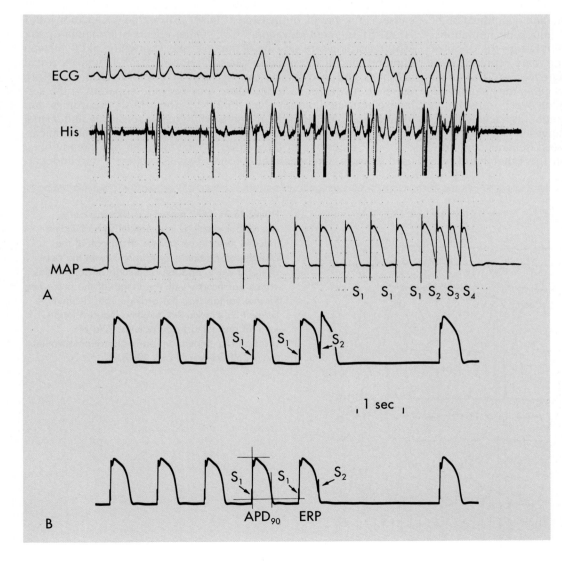

FIGURE 45.20 A. Simultaneous pacing and MAP recording during routine electrophysiologic study, using new combination catheter shown in Figure 45.19. **B.** Simultaneous in vivo measurement of APD and ERP with the combination catheter. S1 and S2 denote the basic and the extrastimulus artifacts. S1-stimulus artifacts are partially superimposed on the MAP upstroke but do not interfere with the ability to analyze the MAP duration. S2-stimulus artifacts are superimposed on the repolarization phase but do not affect its time course. (Franz MR, Chin MC, Sharkey HR, Scheinman MM: A new single-catheter technique for simultaneous measurement of action potential duration and refractory period in vivo. J Am Coll Cardiol (in press)).

ies have provided strong evidence that afterdepolarizations play a significant role in the genesis of torsade.[32,91-93] Unlike intracardiac or surface electrocardiographic tracings, MAP recordings can detect myocardial afterdepolarizations directly during electrophysiologic studies. Early afterdepolarizations (EADs) have been demonstrated in conditions mimicking both the congenital and acquired long QT syndrome. Priori and co-workers[93] reported that left stellate ganglion stimulation in dogs caused early afterdepolarizations in left ventricular MAP recordings accompanied by torsade de pointes–like ventricular arrhythmias, providing a possible explanation for polymorphic arrhythmias in the congenital long QT syndrome. El-Sherif and colleagues[94] reported clinical evidence that quinidine-induced polymorphic ventricular tachycardia of the torsade de pointes type was associated with prominent early afterdepolarizations and U waves (Fig. 45.21). Consistent with clinical observations on precipitating factors of torsade de pointes, these afterdepolarizations were enhanced by bradycardia and long pauses and suppressed by rapid pacing. These early afterdepolarizations coincided with a prominent U wave in the electrocardiogram, refueling the old debate on the genesis of the U wave.[95] These newer studies with the MAP recording technique support the view that the U wave reflects afterdepolarizations[96] rather than prolonged repolarization in Purkinje fibers, suggesting that what is often described as a prolonged QT interval may reflect fusion of the T wave with an enlarged U wave. On the other hand, prolonged QT intervals may result from abnormally long MAP durations without the presence of additional afterdepolarizations. Such excessively long MAP durations have been reported in a child with familial long QT syndrome and were shown to explain the associated 2:1 atrioventricular block.[97]

ASSESSING MYOCARDIAL ISCHEMIA BY MAP RECORDINGS

The electrocardiographic diagnosis, localization, and quantification of myocardial ischemia is hampered by several important limitations. Nonspecific ST segment changes may be present before the onset of ischemia, often mimicking ischemia (*e.g.*, secondary repolarization changes in left ventricular hypertrophy), and regression of ST segment changes following an ischemic event may reflect either the natural time course of infarct electrophysiology (due to healing over) or resolution of the ischemic process. This is because ST segment displacements do not directly reflect local electrophysiologic changes in ischemic myocardium but rather the electrical gradient between ischemic and nonischemic myocardium.[98] MAP recordings, on the other hand, are highly sensitive markers of myocardial ischemia that reflect electrophysiologic changes only at the recording site.[15]

Figure 45.22 shows electrocardiographic and MAP tracings from a 60-year-old woman with critical left anterior descending arterial stenosis who underwent an invasive pacing stress test. She began to experience typical anginal pain 3 minutes after the onset of right atrial pacing at a rate of 160 beats per minute. There were not yet any ischemic electrocardiographic changes in the body surface electrocardiogram. However, the MAP recording obtained from a right septal position showed marked changes in MAP recording and resting potential even before the onset of chest pain. The diastolic baseline rose and the MAP lost its plateau phase, assuming a more triangular shape. These changes are typical for myocardial ischemia, as previously shown in intracellular microelectrode studies.[99,100]

Several investigators have reported on the ability of endocardial and epicardial MAP recordings to detect myocardial ischemia in animal models[15,101] and human hearts during cardiac catheterization and cardiac surgery.[102] Kingaby and co-workers[103] examined the time course of changes in MAPs recorded from left ventricular epicardial sites following temporary coronary artery occlusion and reperfusion in porcine and canine hearts and found that MAP recordings provide a more sensitive and specific index of regional myocardial ischemia than electrocardiographic changes. They defined the level of myocardial underperfusion, and the time from its onset, required to detect electrophysiologic changes in ischemic myocardium by MAP recordings and found that a reduction in perfusion by 30% below normal caused noticeable changes in MAP recordings. Franz and associates[15] used the maximal upstroke velocity of epicardial MAP recordings as an index of myocardial viability and found that this index demarcates the infarct border with a precision of better than 5 mm. Ischemia-induced loss in MAP amplitude is due to both decreases in diastolic and systolic potential, allowing separation between electrophysiologic changes that cause TQ segment depression ("false" ST segment elevation) and "true" ST segment elevation.[15,103,104] Other effects of ischemia on the MAP recordings are slowing of the upstroke, shortening of the plateau duration, and a decrease in phase 3 slope.[15,102,105] Often, electrical alternans and arrhythmias can be seen in the MAP recording from ischemic myocardium long before they become apparent in the surface electrocardiogram (Fig. 45.23).[106] Thus, MAP recordings can identify and localize ischemic sites with greater sensitivity and spatial accuracy than ST segment changes in the electrocardiogram. Epicardial MAP recording in the cardiac operating room has already been used to assess the benefit of coronary bypass surgery,[102] and endocar-

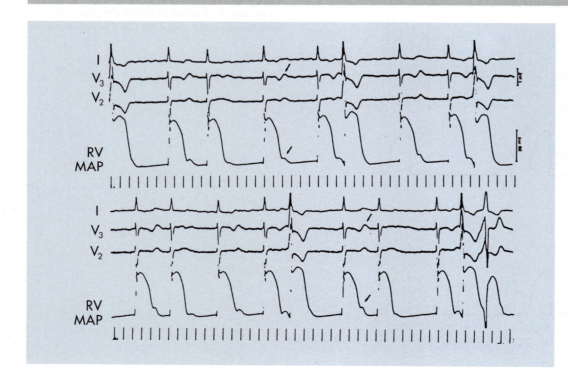

FIGURE 45.21 MAP recordings showing early afterdepolarizations in a patient with quinidine-induced torsade de pointes. The peak of the afterdepolarization is synchronous with the peak of the U wave, and the amplitude of both waves varies significantly with the length of the preceding RR interval (*arrows*). (Recordings from El-Sherif N, Bekheit SS, Henkin R: Quinidine-induced long QT interval and torsade de pointes: Role of bradycardia-dependent early afterdepolarizations. J Am Coll Cardiol 14:252, 1989).

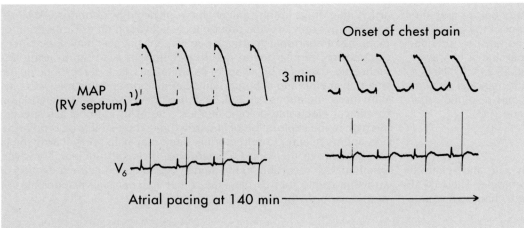

FIGURE 45.22 MAP recordings from right ventricular septum in a 60-year-old female patient with critical left anterior descending arterial stenosis undergoing pacing stress test. MAP changes characteristic of ischemia occurred during right atrial pacing before the onset of chest pain or ST segment changes.

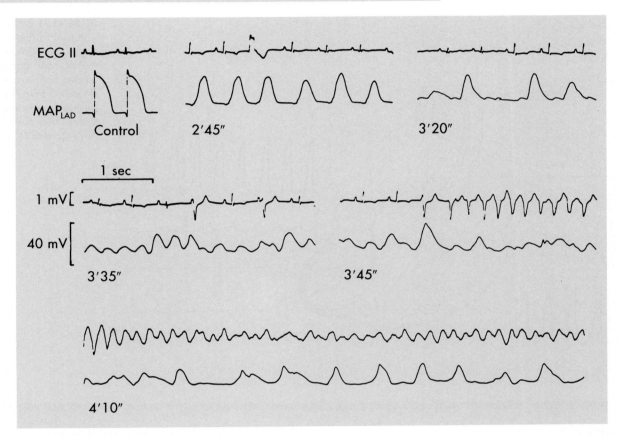

FIGURE 45.23 Development of electrical alternans and tachyarrhythmia in an ischemic region. Simultaneous surface electrocardiogram (*ECG*) and epicardial MAP recordings demonstrate superiority of MAP recording in the early detection of regional arrhythmias. MAP recordings were made from the ischemic region during a 5-minute period of left anterior descending artery (*LAD*) occlusion. Compared with control, at 2 minutes and 45 seconds after LAD occlusion, MAP recordings show decrease in resting potential, slurring of upstroke, loss of plateau, and decrease in systolic amplitude. A premature ventricular response (third complex) triggers electrical alternans in the MAP amplitude, not seen in the surface ECG. This alternans increases in magnitude until at 3 minutes, 20 seconds intermittent conduction block into the MAP recording site occurs. At 3 minutes, 35 seconds there is continuous electrical activity at the MAP recording site (local fibrillation), while in the surface ECG regular sinus rhythm still prevails, with only a few interruptions by premature ventricular beats. It took 10 seconds until "global" ventricular tachycardia, appreciable in the surface ECG, ensued (*panel 3'45"*). At 4 minutes, 10 seconds ventricular tachycardia degenerated into ventricular fibrillation. At the same time, depolarizations at the MAP recording site within the ischemic regions became more scarce, possibly indicating entrance block of ventricular fibrillation activity into the ischemic zone.

dial MAP recording in the catheterization laboratory before and after coronary angioplasty similarly may allow assessment of the efficacy of interventions designed to restore blood flow. In contrast to ischemic but viable myocardium, nonviable or scarred myocardium is characterized by the inability to record any MAPs at all (Fig. 45.24).[14,15] Hence, MAP recordings may be used to detect and localize regional myocardial ischemia with greater sensitivity, specificity, and resolution than are afforded by the body surface electrocardiogram.

CONCLUSIONS

The contact electrode technique allows clinically safe and relatively simple MAP recording even in the human left ventricle. These MAP recordings can reproduce the effects of cycle length changes and antiarrhythmic drugs in the clinical electrophysiology laboratory. MAP recordings not only provide precise local activation times (important for mapping of abnormal ventricular activation) but also may detect areas of abnormal repolarization due to ischemia or scarring. In using this technique, one must be aware of its limitations: lack of reproducing the true transmembrane action potential amplitude and upstroke velocity. With these limitations in mind, MAP recordings are a valuable addition to clinical electrophysiologic studies. The MAP method has specific strength in the exploration of antiarrhythmic drug effects on repolarization and its relation to refractoriness and may help unravel arrhythmia mechanisms in the long QT syndrome. It is still unclear, however, whether MAP recording in the human heart can aid in the detection of arrhythmogenic foci or elucidate other mechanisms responsible for ventricular arrhythmias.

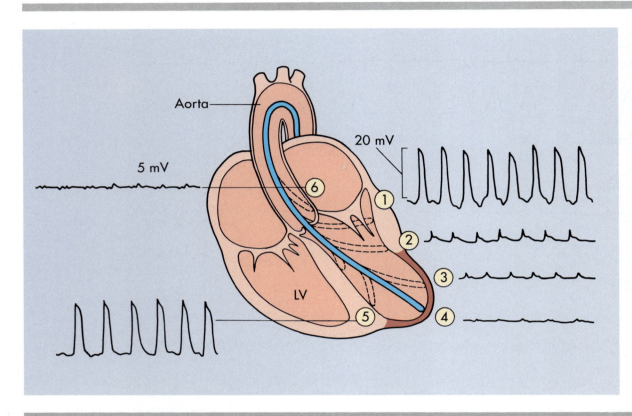

FIGURE 45.24 Left ventricular mapping with MAP catheter in a patient with large anteroapical aneurysm. Note that no MAP signals could be recorded from scarred myocardium. (Modified from Franz MR: Long-term recording of monophasic action potentials from human endocardium. Am J Cardiol 51:1629, 1983).

REFERENCES

1. Hoffman BF, Cranefield PF, Lepeschkin E et al: Comparison of cardiac monophasic action potentials recorded by intracellular and suction electrodes. Am J Physiol 196:1297, 1959
2. Franz MR, Burkhoff D, Spurgeon H et al: In vitro validation of a new cardiac catheter technique for recording monophasic action potentials. Eur Heart J 7:34, 1986
3. Burdon-Sanderson J, Page FJM: On the time-relations of the excitatory process in the ventricle of the heart of the frog. J Physiol 2:385, 1882
4. Schütz E: Einphasische Aktionsströme vom in situ durchbluteten Säugetierherzen. Z Biol 92:441, 1932
5. Schütz E: Elektrophysiologie des Herzens bei einphasischer Ableitung. Ergebn Physiol Exper Pharmakol 38:493, 1936
6. Korsgren M, Leskinen E, Sjostrand U, Varnauskas E: Intracardiac recording of monophasic action potentials in the human heart. Scand J Clin Lab Invest 18:561, 1966
7. Shabetai R, Surawicz B, Hamill W: Monophasic action potentials in man. Circulation 38:341, 1968
8. Gavrilescu S, Cotoi S, Pop T: The monophasic action potential of the right atrium. Cardiology 57:200, 1972
9. Puech P, Cabasson J, Latour H et al: Study of monophasic action potentials of the myocardium by endocavitary approach. Arch Mal Coeur 67:1117, 1974
10. Olsson B, Varnauskas E, Korsgren M: Further improved method for measuring monophasic action potentials of the intact human heart. J Electrocardiol 4:19, 1971
11. Olsson SB, Varnauskas E: Right ventricular monophasic action potentials in man: Effect of abrupt changes of cycle length and of atrial fibrillation. Acta Med Scand 191:159, 1972
12. Olsson SB: Right ventricular monophasic action potentials during regular rhythm: A heart catheterization study in man. Acta Med Scand 191:145, 1972
13. Franz M, Schöttler M, Schaefer J, Seed AW: Simultaneous recording of monophasic action potentials and contractile force from the human heart. Klin Wochenschr 58:1357, 1980
14. Franz MR: Long-term recording of monophasic action potentials from human endocardium. Am J Cardiol 51:1629, 1983
15. Franz MR, Flaherty JT, Platia EV et al: Localization of regional myocardial ischemia by recording of monophasic action potentials. Circulation 69:593, 1984
16. Franz MR, Bargheer K, Rafflenbeul W et al: Monophasic action potential mapping in human subjects with normal electrocardiograms: Direct evidence for the genesis of the T wave. Circulation 75:379, 1987
17. Runnalls ME, Sutton PM, Taggart P, Treasure T: Modifications of electrode design for recording monophasic action potentials in animals and humans. Am J Physiol 253:H1315, 1987
18. Taggart P, Sutton P, Runnalls M et al: Use of monophasic action potential recordings during routine coronary-artery bypass surgery as an index of localised myocardial ischaemia. Lancet 1:1462, 1986
19. Sugarman H, Katz LN, Sanders A, Jochim K: Observations on the genesis of the electrical currents established by injury to the heart. Am J Physiol 130:130, 1940
20. Cranefield PF, Eyster JAE, Gilson WE: Electrical characteristics of injury potentials. Am J Physiol 167:450, 1951
21. Eyster JAE, Gilson WE: The development and contour of cardiac injury po-

tential. Am J Physiol 145:507, 1946
22. Eyster JAE, Meek WJ, Goldberg H, Gilson WE: Potential changes in an injured region of cardiac muscle. Am J Physiol 124:717, 1938
23. Ino T, Karagueuzian HS, Hong K et al: Relation of monophasic action potential recorded with contact electrode to underlying transmembrane action potential properties in isolated cardiac tissues: A systematic microelectrode validation study. Cardiovasc Res 22:255, 1988
24. Franz MR, Burkhoff D, Lakatta EG, Weisfeldt ML: Monophasic action potential recording by contact electrode technique: In vitro validation and clinical applications. In Butrous GS, Schwartz PJ (eds): Clinical Aspects of Ventricular Repolarization, pp 81–92. London, Farrand Press, 1989
25. Franz MR: Eine neue Methode zur Ableitung kardialer monophasischer Aktionspotentiale: Experimentelle und klinische Ergebnisse, thesis. Hannover, Hannover Medical School, 1985
26. Levine JH, Spear JF, Guarnieri T et al: Cesium chloride–induced long QT syndrome: Demonstration of afterdepolarizations and triggered activity in vivo. Circulation 72:1092, 1985
27. Draper MH, Weidmann S: Cardiac resting and action potentials recorded with an intracellular electrode. J Physiol (Lond) 115:74, 1951
28. Gough WB, Raphael H: The early afterdepolarization as recorded by the monophasic action potential technique: Fact or artifact? Circulation 80 (suppl II):II-130, 1989
29. Cranefield PF: Action potentials, afterpotentials, and arrhythmias. Circ Res 41:415, 1977
30. Wit AL, Cranefield PF: Triggered and automatic activity in the canine coronary sinus. Circ Res 41:435, 1977
31. Hall PAX, Atwood JE, Myers J, Froelicher VF: The signal averaged surface electrocardiogram and the identification of late potentials. Prog Cardiovasc Dis 31:295, 1989
32. El-Sherif N, Zeiler RH, Craelius W et al: QTU prolongation and polymorphic ventricular tachyarrhythmias due to bradycardia-dependent early afterdepolarizations: Afterdepolarizations and ventricular arrhythmias. Circ Res 63:286, 1988
33. Wiener I, Mindich B, Pitchon R: Fragmented endocardial electrical activity in patients with ventricular tachycardia: A new guide to surgical therapy. Am Heart J 107:86, 1984
34. Josephson ME, Wit AL: Fractionated electrical activity and continuous electrical activity: Fact or artifact? Circulation 70:529, 1984
35. Ideker RE, Mirvis DM, Smith WM: Late, fractionated potentials. Am J Cardiol 55:1616, 1985
36. Carmeliet R: Repolarisation and frequency in cardiac cells. J Physiol (Paris) 73:903, 1977
37. Boyett MR, Jewell BR: Analysis of the effects of changes in rate and rhythm upon the electrical activity in the heart. Prog Biophys Mol Biol 36:1, 1980
38. Franz MR, Schaefer J, Schottler M et al: Electrical and mechanical restitution of the human heart at different rates of stimulation. Circ Res 53:815, 1983
39. Franz MR, Swerdlow CD, Liem BL, Schaefer J: Cycle-length dependence of human action potential duration in vivo: Effects of single extrastimuli, sudden sustained rate acceleration and deceleration, and different steady-state frequencies. J Clin Invest 82:972, 1988
40. Bass BG: Restitution of the action potential in cat papillary muscle. Am J Physiol 228:1717, 1975
41. Gettes LS, Morehouse N, Surawicz B: Effect of premature depolarization on the duration of action potentials in Purkinje and ventricular fibers of the moderator band of the pig heart: Role of proximity and the duration of the preceding action potential. Circ Res 30:55, 1972
42. Elharrar V, Atarashi H, Surawicz B: Cycle length-dependent action potential duration in canine cardiac Purkinje fibers. Am J Physiol 247:H936, 1984
43. Edmands RE, Greenspan K, Fisch C: Effect of cycle length alteration upon the configuration of the canine ventricular action potential. Circ Res 19:602, 1966
44. Greenspan K, Edmands RE, Fisch C: Effects of cycle-length alteration on canine cardiac action potentials. Am J Physiol 212:1416, 1967
45. Colatsky TJ, Hogan PM: Effects of external calcium, calcium channel-blocking agents, and stimulation frequency on cycle length-dependent changes in canine cardiac action potential duration. Circ Res 46:543, 1980
46. Gibbs CL, Johnson EA: Effect of changes in frequency of stimulation upon rabbit ventricular action potential. Circ Res 9:165, 1961
47. Iinuma H, Kato K: Mechanism of augmented premature responses in canine ventricular muscle. Circ Res 44:624, 1979
48. Gettes LS, Reuter H: Slow recovery from inactivation of inward currents in mammalian myocardial fibres. J Physiol (Lond) 240:703, 1974
49. Boyett MR, Jewell BR: A study of the factors responsible for rate-dependent shortening of the action potential in mammalian ventricular muscle. J Physiol (Lond) 285:359, 1978
50. Boyett MR, Jewell BR: Causes of shortening of the cardiac action potential during a tension staircase. J Physiol (Lond) 266:80P, 1977
51. Bazett HC: An analysis of the time relations of electrocardiograms. Heart 7:353, 1920
52. Adams W: Normal duration of electrocardiographic ventricular complex. J Clin Invest 15:335, 1936
53. Blair HA, Wedd AM, Young AC: The relation of the QT interval to the refractory period, the diastolic interval, the duration of contraction, and the rate of beating in the heart muscle. Am J Physiol 132:157, 1941
54. Tchou PJ, Lehmann MH, Dongas J et al: Effect of sudden rate acceleration on the human His-Purkinje system: Adaptation of refractoriness in a dampened oscillatory pattern. Circulation 73:920, 1986
55. Akhtar M, Denker ST, Lehmann MH, Mahmud R: Effects of sudden cycle length alteration on refractoriness of human His-Purkinje system and ventricular myocardium. In Butrous GS, Schwartz PJ (eds): Cardiac Electrophysiology and Arrhythmias, pp 399. London, Farrand Press, 1989
56. Marchlinski FE: Characterization of oscillations in ventricular refractoriness in man after an abrupt increment in heart rate. Circulation 75:550, 1987
57. Liem BL, Swerdlow CD, Franz MR: Distinctive features of ventricular fibrillation and ventricular tachycardia detected by monophasic action potential recording in human subjects. J Electrophysiol 2:484, 1988
58. Sano T, Tsuchiashi H, Shimamoto T: Ventricular fibrillation studied by the microelectrode method. Circ Res 6:41, 1958
59. Akiyama T: Intracellular recording of in situ ventricular cells during ventricular fibrillation. Am J Physiol 240:H465, 1981
60. Gavrilescu S, Cotoi S, Pop T: Monophasic action potential of the right atrium in paroxysmal atrial flutter and fibrillation. Br Heart J 35:585, 1973
61. Cotoi S, Gavrilescu S, Pop T, Vicas E: The prognostic value of right atrium monophasic action potential after conversion of atrial fibrillation. Eur J Clin Invest 2:472, 1972
62. Olsson SB, Cotoi S, Varnauskas E: Monophasic action potential and sinus rhythm stability after conversion of atrial fibrillation. Acta Med Scand 190:381, 1971
63. Singh BN, Venkatesh N, Nademanee K et al: The historical development, cellular electrophysiology and pharmacology of amiodarone. Prog Cardiovasc Dis 31:249, 1989
64. Olsson SB, Brorson L, Varnauskas E: Class 3 antiarrhythmic action in man: Observations from monophasic action potential recordings and amiodarone treatment. Br Heart J 35:1255, 1973
65. Platia EV, Weisfeldt ML, Franz MR: Immediate quantification of antiarrhythmic drug effect by recording of monophasic action potentials. Am J Cardiol 61:1284, 1988
66. Brugada J, Sassine A, Escande D et al: Effects of quinidine on ventricular repolarization. Eur Heart J 8:1340, 1987
67. Stroobandt R, Brachmann J, Kesteloot H et al: Effect of sotalol, aprindine and the combination aprindine-sotalol on monophasic action potential duration. Eur Heart J 7:47, 1986
68. Liem LB, Clay DA, Franz MR, Swerdlow CD: Electrophysiology and anti-arrhythmic efficacy of intravenous pirmenol in patients with sustained ventricular tachyarrhythmias. Am Heart J 113:1390, 1987
69. Way BP, Forfar JC, Cobbe SM: Comparison of the effects of chronic oral therapy with atenolol and sotalol on ventricular monophasic action potential duration and effective refractory period. Am Heart J 116:740, 1988
70. Hoffman BF, Cranefield PF: Electrophysiology of the Heart, pp 222–227. Mount Kisco, NY, Futura Press, 1960
71. Franz MR, Costard A: Frequency-dependent effects of quinidine on the relationship between action potential duration and refractoriness in the canine heart in situ. Circulation 77:1177, 1988
72. Costard A, Liem LB, Franz MR: Rate dependent effect of quinidine, mexiletine, and their combination on postrepolarization refractoriness in vivo. J Cardiovasc Pharmacol 14:810, 1989
73. Varro A, Elharrar V, Surawicz B: Frequency-dependent effects of several Class I antiarrhythmic drugs on V_{max} of action potential upstroke in canine cardiac Purkinje fibers. J Cardiovasc Pharmacol 7:482, 1985
74. Campbell TJ: Kinetics of onset of rate-dependent effects of Class I antiarrhythmic drugs are important in determining their effects on refractoriness in guinea-pig ventricle, and provide a theoretical basis for their subclassification. Cardiovasc Res 17:344, 1983
75. Nattel S, Zeng FD: Frequency-dependent effects of antiarrhythmic drugs on action potential duration and refractoriness of canine cardiac Purkinje fibres. J Pharmacol Exp Ther 229:283, 1984
76. Burke GH, Loukides JE, Berman ND: Comparative electropharmacology of mexilitine, lidocaine, and quinidine in a canine Purkinje fiber model. J Pharm Exp Ther 237:232, 1986
77. Rosen MR: Effects of pharmacological agents on mechanisms responsible for reentry. In Kulbertus HE (ed): Reentrant arrhythmias: Mechanisms and Treatment, pp 283–294. Baltimore, University Park Press, 1976
78. Hondeghem LM, Katzung BG: Time- and voltage-dependent interactions of antiarrhythmic drugs with sodium channels. Biochem Biophys Acta 472:373, 1977
79. Hondeghem LM: Antiarrhythmic agents: Modulated receptor applications. Circulation 75:514, 1987
80. Franz MR, Chin MC, Sharkey HR, Scheinman MM: A single-catheter technique for simultaneous measurement of action potential duration and refractory period in vivo. J Am Coll Cardiol (in press)
81. Lee RJ, Liem LB, Cohen TJ, Franz MR: Use dependent effect of class I antiarrhythmic drugs on the relationship between action potential duration and refractoriness in the human heart. Circulation 80(suppl II):II-327, 1989
82. Duff HJ, Roden D, Primm L et al: Mexiletine in the treatment of resistant ventricular arrhythmias: Enhancement of efficacy and reduction of dose-related side effects by combination with quinidine. Circulation 67:1124, 1983

83. Duff HJ, Kolodgie FD, Roden DM, Woosley RL: Electropharmacologic synergism with mexiletine and quinidine. J Cardiovasc Pharmacol 8:840, 1986
84. Nguyen PT, Scheinman MM, Seger J: Polymorphous ventricular tachycardia: Clinical characterization, therapy, and the QT interval. Circulation 74:340, 1986
85. Dessertenne F: La tachycardie ventriculaire à deux foyers opposés variables. Arch Mal Coeur 59:263, 1966
86. Schwartz PJ: The idiopathic long Q-T syndrome. Ann Intern Med 99:561, 1983
87. Jervell A, Lange-Nielsen F: Congenital deaf-mutism, functional heart disease, with prolongation of the QT interval and sudden death. Am Heart J 54:59, 1957
88. Romano C, Gemme G, Pongiglione R: Aritimie cardiache rare dell'et à pediatrica. Clin Pediatr 45:658, 1963
89. Ward OC: New familial cardiac syndrome in children. J Irish Med Assoc 54:103, 1964
90. Jackman WM, Friday KF, Anderson JL et al: The long QT syndromes: A critical review, new clinical observations and a unifying hypothesis. Prog Cardiovasc Dis 31:115, 1988
91. Ben-David J, Zipes DP: Differential response to right and left ansae subclaviae stimulation of early afterdepolarizations and ventricular tachycardia induced by cesium in dogs. Circulation 78:1241, 1988
92. Bailie DS, Inoue H, Kaseda S et al: Magnesium suppression of early afterdepolarizations and ventricular tachyarrhythmias induced by cesium in dogs. Circulation 77:1395, 1988
93. Priori SG, Mantica M, Schwartz PJ: Delayed afterdepolarizations elicited in vivo by left stellate ganglion stimulation. Circulation 78:178, 1988
94. El-Sherif N, Bekheit SS, Henkin R: Quinidine-induced long QT interval and torsade de pointes: Role of bradycardia-dependent early afterdepolarizations. J Am Coll Cardiol 14:252, 1989
95. Lepeschkin E: Physiologic basis of the U wave. In Schlant RC, Hurst JW (eds): Advances in Electrocardiography, pp 431–437. New York, Grune & Stratton, 1971
96. Bonatti V, Rolli A, Botti G: Recording of monophasic action potentials of the right ventricle in long QT syndromes complicated by severe ventricular arrhythmias. Eur Heart J 4:168, 1983
97. Van Hare GF, Franz MR, Scheinman MM, Roge C: Persistent functional atrioventricular block due to dramatic QT interval prolongation: Electrophysiologic study and monophasic action potential measurements. PACE (in press)
98. Holland RP, Brooks H: TQ-ST segment mapping: Critical review and analysis of current concepts. Am J Cardiol 40:110, 1977
99. Kleber AG, Janse MJ, van Capelle FJL, Durrer D: Mechanism and time course of S-T and T-Q segment changes during acute regional myocardial ischemia in the pig heart determined by extracellular and intracellular recordings. Circ Res 42:603, 1978
100. Downar E, Janse MJ, Durrer D: The effect of acute coronary artery exclusion on subepicardial transmembrane potentials in the intact porcine heart. Circulation 56:217, 1977
101. Platia EV, Franz MR, Rad PR et al: Endocardial monophasic action potentials: A sensitive index of subendocardial ischemia. Am J Cardiol 49:970, 1972
102. Taggart P, Sutton P, Runnalls M et al: Use of monophasic action potential recordings during routine coronary-artery bypass surgery as an index of localised myocardial ischaemia. Lancet 1:1462, 1986
103. Kingaby RO, Lab MJ, Cole AW, Palmer TN: Relation between monophasic action potential duration, ST segment elevation, and regional myocardial blood flow after coronary occlusion in the pig. Cardiovasc Res 20:740, 1986
104. Blake K, Clusin WT, Franz MR, Smith NA: Mechanism of depolarization in the ischaemic dog heart: Discrepancy between T-Q potentials and potassium accumulation. J Physiol (Lond) 397:307, 1988
105. Dilly SG, Lab MJ: Changes in monophasic action potential duration during the first hour of regional myocardial ischaemia in the anaesthetised pig. Cardiovasc Res 21:908, 1987
106. Franz MR: Unpublished observation

Ambulatory Holter Electrocardiography: Technology, Clinical Applications, and Limitations

Joel Morganroth • Harold L. Kennedy

The mechanism responsible for sudden death is a ventricular tachyarrhythmia in more than 80% of cases.[1] The presence of ventricular arrhythmias as detected by ambulatory electrocardiography (ECG) identifies patients at high risk from sudden cardiac death, and treatment is often given with the hope of decreasing morbidity and mortality.[2,3] As a result, in the past few years there has been a tremendous increase in the use and complexity of ambulatory or Holter ECG technology to detect and evaluate arrhythmias. The vast majority of ventricular arrhythmias are asymptomatic and do not correlate well with patient symptoms.[4] Furthermore, because of a high degree of spontaneous variability of ventricular arrhythmias,[5] their detection cannot be relied on by simple clinical means (*e.g.*, history or findings on physical examination) or even by a 12-lead resting ECG recording or exercise testing.[6,7]

Thus, Holter monitoring has emerged as the most sensitive and specific means of detecting and evaluating supraventricular and ventricular arrhythmias.

DEVELOPMENT

The first Holter monitoring device was an 85-pound backpack radio transmitter with limited range. It was then followed by a portable magnetic tape "electrocardiocorder" developed in the mid 1950s that weighed 4 pounds and could record the ECG for up to 10 hours.[8] In the 1960s, further technologic developments provided a system that allowed for the direct recording of the ECG from electrodes attached to a patient's chest over several hours during the day. The widespread adoption of Holter monitoring followed the early clinical[9] reports that identified a relationship between ventricular arrhythmias and mortality from heart disease. Further technologic advancements have increased the accuracy and reliability of analysis and recording methodology.[10,11] Furthermore, new recorders were able to be developed and capable of recording continuously for 8, 10, 12, and 24 hours. Additional technologic advancement consisted of printed circuit boards and small transistors that were able to allow recorders to be of smaller size, to be capable of longer periods of recording (24–48 hours), and to have playback systems that allowed for a variety of sophisticated and complex data analysis. In recent years, the introduction of solid-state microprocessors, microcomputers, and intergrated circuits have even further fostered a more flexible and versatile handling of data.

To date, there have been limited comparative studies evaluating the accuracy of Holter systems.[12-16] These studies call attention to the need for skilled, knowledgeable technicians to operate these systems[12-14] as well as to the inevitable variable degrees of human error.[13] Under the best conditions, accurate agreement in identifying various ventricular arrhythmias, based on the density and type of the ectopy, was achieved in 75% to 89% of instances.[13-15] Errors of underreading are almost six times more common than overreading when semiautomatic audiovisual methods are used.[12] Direct comparisons of different commercially available Holter systems are difficult to report without reflecting bias; nonetheless, one early study of two widely used Holter systems showed an absolute percent error to range from 13% to 16%.[15] Another study found the sensitivity of three commercial systems high (92%, 93%, and 95%) for detection of ventricular arrhythmia, with no differences in the absolute hand and system counts of total beats or ventricular ectopic beats.[16] These early studies regrettably did not address the repeatability of these instruments. Studies to define the relative cost and benefit of the various types of equipment are still unreported.

TYPES OF RECORDERS

The ambulatory ECG recorder includes bipolar skin electrodes that record the potential difference between two electrode sites. The conventional Holter recording obtains ECG data comparable to leads V_1 through V_5 positions of the standard 12-lead ECG. The skin electrodes are usually self-adhering electrodes in which a silver chloride sensing element is used. The electrodes are usually pre-gelled and disposable. The quality of the electrode adhesiveness and the degree of skin irritation are extremely important to ECG signal quality in regard to baseline wandering, degree of artifact, and duration of performance. The cable and the electrode leads are generally reusable. A source of artifacts and/or Holter recording malfunction might be due to these leads and the shielded cable that connects the leads to the Holter recorder. Therefore, the five-electrode lead system, which uses separate negative electrodes to complement each exploratory electrode, in addition to an external ground, is preferable. More recently, three-channel Holter recorders have been introduced, and they may use either a five- or seven-electrode lead system. Development of this expanded lead system was fueled predominantly by the need to detect ambulatory ST segment changes. As a result, there is renewed interest in bipolar lead systems and their capability to detect ST segment changes.[17] For anterior and inferior ischemia, current evidence favors the use of bipolar leads CM-V_3 and CM-V_5, which, for inferior ischemia, may be augmented by use of a modified aV_F.[17-19]

The recorder itself is powered by a battery using either a disposable alkaline or a rechargeable nickel cadmium system, and it is usually compact. From a single recording head a varying direct current is recorded onto magnetic tape in the recorder. A hysteresis-synchronous motor assembly transports the tape, and the electrical signal of 0.05 Hz to 100 Hz is recorded onto either a reel-to-reel or cassette magnetic tape. Reel-to-reel recorders are generally heavier than cassette recorders and thus less convenient for technicians to use and more cumbersome for the patients. Reel-to-reel recorders, however, offer better signal-to-noise ratio, better dynamic range, more consistent speed stability with less wow and flutter, and fewer recording failures than the cassette recorders. In addition, reel-to-reel recorders use ¼-inch tape, which is either chromium dioxide or ferric oxide. These recorders use wide two-track recording heads, and frequently three-phase motors are employed. This is in contrast to cassette recorders, which use ⅛-inch tape, usually of ferric oxide and typically of less thickness. Furthermore, narrow four-track recording heads and less stable motor transmission configurations have been used. Recorders are now available that can also simultaneously record ambulatory blood pressure, electroencephalographic findings, or respiratory rate. In the clinical setting, cassette recorders are predominantly used because of their smaller weight and size. More recently, the introduction of a microcassette recorder has decreased the size still further. However, reel-to-reel recorders are still the standard for Holter monitoring for research purposes, particularly in the evaluation of new antiarrhythmic agents. The features of some of the available Holter ECG recorders are compared in Table 46.1.

RECORDING MODES

In the past several years three types of recording modes have evolved: (1) continuous, (2) intermittent or patient-activated recording, and (3) real-time analytical or event recording. With a continuous Holter recording the ECG is recorded without alteration by the patient and/or a change in the ECG signal. Continuous recorders allow for a 24-hour recording of the ECG; if more than 24 hours of data are needed, the tape and battery must be changed. A millivolt calibration signal and time references are included in these recorders, and the patient can use these to mark an event on tape. In addition, the patient also notes such events in a diary.

The intermittent recording mode allows the patient to record the ECG by manual initiation of recording or an automatic time-activated initiation of ECG recording. Intermittent recording might be used transtelephonically by transmitting one channel of ECG data over the telephone to a receiving unit, which records a signal on a strip-chart recorder. Early devices had no internal storage and had to be used in real time; however, newer technology allows for storage of ECG data for later transmission over the telephone. This is a hybrid of a real-time event recorder with transtelephonic capability. The disadvantage of this system is that the ECG prior to the activation of the recorder is usually not obtained, and if the memory becomes filled before the patient can telephone to transmit the information, data can be lost.

Solid-state real-time analysis recorders are units consisting of a compact battery-operated microcomputer to analyze and record the Holter data, and a report generator that receives the data from the recorder, permits editing, generates analog and graphic hard copy, and permits data storage and retrieval. These devices are three to five times more expensive than the continuous recorders and usually weigh 50% to 100% more. Typically, this instrument also evaluates two or three continuous channels of electrocardiographic data from bipolar leads for 24 hours. Some instruments purport to examine continuous long-term electrocardiographic data (with battery changes) for extended periods up to 5 days. This continuous technology examines long-term electrocardiographic data as it occurs beat-by-beat (*i.e.,* during real time) to determine a variety of decision-analysis diagnoses within the capability of the algorithm of the specific microcomputer. Although this technique examines electrocardiographic data in a continuous manner, because of the constraints of data-storage technique in these microcomputers, they can usually only record and document selected electrocardiographic examples. Thus, most solid-state real-time analysis units store their decision analysis in a computational or summary data format, in either solid-state memory or on tape, and document that decision analysis with noncontinuous excerpted electrocardiographic examples. Recently, however, innovative data-compression techniques have resulted in some systems capable of storing

TABLE 46.1 COMPARISON OF TYPES OF HOLTER RECORDERS

Manufacturer, Model	Recording Media	Size (in)	Weight (oz)	Channels	Battery Type	Internal Calibration	Timing Track	Pacer Detection	Clock Display	Real-time System	Compatible Systems
ACS 8300	Reel-reel	1.75 × 6.5 × 3.25	11	2	9V	Yes	No	No	No	No	Most reel-reel
BioSensor Uni-day	Solid state	0.625 × 3 × 2	8	2	4 AA	Auto	N/A	No	Yes	Yes	None
CardioData DataCard	Solid state	7 × 2.8 × 1.6	24	2	5 AA	Auto	N/A	Yes	Yes	No	None
CardioData Superlite	Cassette	3.5 × 1 × 6	9	2	9V	Auto	Yes	No	Yes	No	All 1 mm/sec
Del Mar 457	Cassette	3.3 × 6.1 × 1.1	12.5	2	9V	Auto	Yes	Yes	Yes	No	3 ch., 1 mm/sec
Del Mar 463	Microcassette	3.77 × 2.36 × 0.98	6	3	9V	Auto	Yes	No	Yes	No	None
DMI Light Fantastic	Cassette	—	14	2	9V	Auto	Yes	No	Yes	No	All 1 mm/sec
Hewlett-Packard 43400B	Solid state	6.43 × 3.2 × 1.5	15.5	2	4 AA	Auto	N/A	Yes	Yes	Yes	None
Marquette 8500	Cassette	1.1 × 9.2 × 6.0	16	2/3	9V	Auto	Yes	Yes	Yes	No	Most 1 mm/sec
Marquette SEER	Solid state	3.6 × 5.3 × 1.7	15.5	2 ECG+ 2 paced	4 AA	Auto	N/A	Yes	Yes	Yes	Any Marquette charter
Oxford MR 35	Cassette	4.2 × 4.6 × 1.3	13	2	9V	Yes	Yes	No	Yes	No	Oxford (FM recorder)
Q-med Monitor One	Solid state	3.55 × 7.36 × 1.42	22	2	4 AA	Auto	N/A	No	Yes	Yes	None
Reynolds E-Ram	Solid state	—	16	2	Battery pack	Auto	N/A	Yes	Yes	No	None
Scole Omega IV	Cassette	4.3 × 3.1 × 1.2	8	2/3	6V	No	Yes	Yes	No	No	All 1 mm/sec
Zymed TriTrak	Cassette	1.4 × 3.3 × 5.6	16	3	9V	Auto	Yes	Yes	Yes	No	None

Adapted from Kennedy HL: Ambulatory electrocardiography, 2nd ed. Philadelphia, Lea & Febiger (in press).

all electrocardiographic complexes that occur during a continuous 24-hour examination. This is made possible by utilizing data-compression techniques that reduce the digital sampling rate of an electrocardiographic signal (usually from 256 or 128 Hz) by a factor of 2 to 4 (to 32 or 64 Hz) for storage. Later, when the data are recalled, playback computer techniques recreate these abbreviated waveforms (whose sampling is often "weighted" about the R wave) to reproduce stored "full disclosure" continuous electrocardiographic data. Whether important electrocardiographic data are lost with these techniques has not yet been determined. Whereas the major advantage of solid-state real-time analysis technology is cited to be the preprocessing of electrocardiographic data, making it available on completion of the examination, the major disadvantage of most systems is the lack of continuous storage of all electrocardiographic data for subsequent analysis and verification. Direct comparison of real-time analysis recorders to continuous recording techniques has been limited, but such studies are now being reported.[14,21,22]

ANALYSIS SYSTEMS

The analysis systems used to interpret the data obtained by Holter recordings differ greatly in hardware configuration, capabilities, and cost, despite their similarity in design and performance features. Sophisticated digital analysis systems arose from significant improvement in integrated computer processors, improvement in storage density with memory chips, and more powerful logic chips. These advances will translate into even faster, more accurate, and cost-effective equipment.

A modern analysis system includes a playback deck for either reel-to-reel or cassette tapes and an oscilloscope screen for operator interaction with the system. Recently, the playback scanners have incorporated analog-to-digital convertors and electronic memories. Therefore, the ECG can be memorized at high speed and portions can be played back through digital-to-analog converters to provide real-time ECG strip documentation. The oscilloscope screens can detail the superimposed sinus complexes in one location on the screen, ectopic ventricular complexes in a second sector, and ectopic supraventricular complexes in a third sector. The appearance of superimposed complexes is shown in Figure 46.1, A. Other systems used the oscilloscope to spread ECG data over time out on the screen for direct analyst interaction.[23] A freeze memory display of real time ranging from a few seconds to a few minutes can be shown. Incorporated into playback systems are an ECG chart printout that can provide real-time, trend, or graph presentations of data. The playback deck may read the oscilloscope display data at 30 to 480 times real time.

Currently available systems are so accurate that their microprocessor playback system can store QRS complex waveforms, creating "templates" that can be used for data correlations (Fig. 46.1, B). The normal QRS template is continuously updated and can be compared with new events that can be distinguished as artifacts or ectopic complexes. Thus separate templates can be counted for each patient. The operator might teach the computer to recognize and thus quantitate the various templates. When QRS complexes are grouped into templates and a cross-correlation algorithm is used to define the type of complex, a more accurate analysis results using data reduction. Cross-correlation techniques require a much more sophisticated computer system.

The high-speed data reduction processors that use semiautomated modes of processing are shown in Table 46.2. Representative examples have been chosen only for the three types of analysis systems.

The first group consist of those systems that use powerful 16-byte microcomputers as the central processing unit, which is buffered with a rigid-disk drive. The rigid-disk based analysis systems are the most advanced and filter original two-channel analog ECG tape for frequency and/or voltage artifacts localized in software. Analog-to-digital conversion occurs, and mass storage takes place on a hard disk. During a second pass of the ECG tape, digital QRS data are analyzed in core memory using an algorithm to detect ectopic complexes using both feature extraction and cross-correlation techniques. ECG strip documentation of "template" and special forms, such as salvos of ventricular tachycardia, are printed out as examples, and editing and formating of numerical data are generated (Figs. 46.2 and 46.3).

The algorithm driving the system is written in both low- and high-

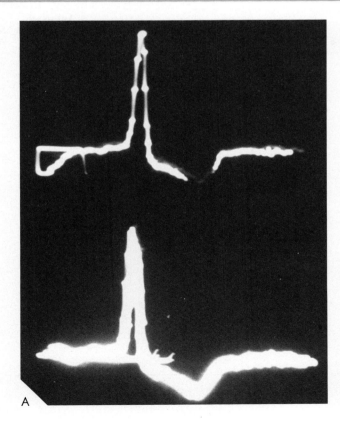

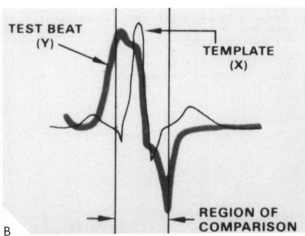

FIGURE 46.1 A. Audiovisual superimposed electrocardiographic presentation (AVSEP) in which ectopic beats are determined by change in the morphology or audio tone generated by superimposition of ongoing QRS complexes. **B.** Computerized template of the underlying normal QRS complex (X) and an ectopic complex termed a test beat (Y), which is matched to beat X by the computer during the region of comparison using cost correlation algorithms. (Morganroth J: Ambulatory Holter electrocardiography: Choice of technologies and clinical uses. Ann Intern Med 102:73, 1985)

level computer languages and is more adaptable for higher quality interpretation than the nonrigid disk-based system.

The second type of Holter analysis is one in which the entire ECG recording is displayed on a monitor or can be printed out in a miniaturized form of ECG data known as "full disclosure." Automatic ventricular arrhythmia detection is not usually performed (Fig. 46.4). This type of Holter analysis does not accurately quantitate the ECG data for manual analysis and is a tedious and fatiguing process. These systems are inexpensive and can be used in the office by physicians for arrhythmia screening; however, they are probably inaccurate for detection of infrequent but potentially important complex ECG forms such as ventricular triplets. In addition, they may not be able to provide an accurate quantitation of the frequency of ventricular arrhythmias.

The third type of analysis, detailed in Table 46.2, employs real-time analyzers. These systems are digitally based and automatic, using microprocessors to detect the arrhythmias on-line while being worn by the patient. These systems do not analyze the P wave and cannot be used, without risk of considerable error, in patients with atrial fibrillation or cardiac pacemakers.[24] Such systems by one specific manufacturer were recently reported to be accurate for detection of ST changes.[25,26] However, when significant ventricular arrhythmia density is present, caution must be exercised because of reported errors secondary to failure of accurate arrhythmia interpretation.[26] Advantages of the real-time analysis systems are thought to be overall lower cost, minimal technical and personnel time, and, depending on the sophistication of the arrhythmia analysis algorithms, presentation to the physician of presumably only significant electrocardiographic phenomena for analysis.[24] Disadvantages of the first generation of these devices include analysis of only a single channel and uneven ability to assess artifact. Their original inability to present all the data they examine has been overcome by "compression" storage of all beats for 24 hours. However, "full-disclosure" data must be viewed cautiously until it is clear what distortions may result from these techniques.[24] Moreover, accuracy and repeatability of such techniques have scarcely been reported.[14,21,22]

QUALITY CONTROL

To detail their accuracy, Holter analysis systems should be subjected to standard quality control programs. Each analysis system and Holter laboratory must be subjected to individual quality control standards using 24-hour tapes that have a high ECG abnormality and artifact frequency that has been quantitated by hand-counting in real time. Be cautious and wary of Holter monitor data that have not been subjected to rigid quality control programs to ensure accuracy and repeatability of the quantitated data.

DATA FORMATTING

The Holter system should detail precisely the types and frequency of supraventricular and ventricular arrhythmias detected as well as the changes in heart rate. These parameters should be displayed by detailing the low, high, and mean frequency of these events of the 24 hours as well as for each hour of the recording (see Fig. 46.2). In addition, important changes in the PR, QRS, and JT intervals should be noted.

Other parameters that should be monitored are the frequency and degree of ECG pauses, including second- and third-degree atrioventricular block, the presence of R-on-T phenomena, changes in the ST segment, and the presence of bradyarrhythmias and tachyarrhythmias. Since T waves are not recognized well by these systems, all R-on-T phenomena must be verified by the technician. ST segment changes are usually measured as the amount of negative deflection of the isoelectric level at 60 msec to 80 msec after the J point. The slope of the

TABLE 46.2 COMPARISON OF HOLTER MONITOR ANALYSIS SYSTEMS

Manufacturer, Model	User-accessible Microcomputer	Mass Storage	Analysis Method	Interactive Analysis	Full Disclosure	AVSEP	RR Display	Replay Speed	Channels Displayed	Strip Length	Automatic Arrhythmia Analysis	ST Analysis
BioSensor Uniday	Yes	Yes	Real-time	No	Yes	Yes	Yes	—	2	—	Yes	Yes
CardioData Prodigy Plus	Yes	Yes	Retrospective	Yes	Yes	Yes	No	×∼200	2	7.6 sec	Yes	Yes
Del Mar 750 Innovator	Yes	Yes	Interactive	Yes	Yes	Yes	Yes	×240	2/3	8 sec	Yes	Yes
DMI CardioView	No	No	Full disclosure	No	Yes	Yes	No	No	2	—	Yes	Yes
Hewlett-Packard 434200	Yes	Yes	Real-time	No	Yes	No	No	N/A	2	∼6 sec	Yes	Yes
Marquette LaserHolter XP	No	Yes	Retrospective	Yes	Yes	Yes	Yes	×500	2/3	8 sec	Yes	Yes
Marquette SEER	No	Yes	Real-time	No	Yes	No	No	N/A	2 ECG + 2 pacer	All 24 hours	Yes	Yes
Oxford Medilog Excel	Yes	Yes	Retrospective	Yes	Yes	Yes	Yes	×180	2	8 sec	Yes	Yes
Q-med Monitor-One	Yes	Yes	Real-time	Yes	Yes	No	No	N/A	2	—	Yes	Yes
Reynolds Pathfinder 3/ST	No	Yes	Full disclosure	Yes	Yes	Yes	Yes	×300	2	8 sec	Yes	Yes
Zymed QuickPage 1210	Yes	Yes	Interactive	Yes	Yes	Yes	No	×240	2	6 sec	Yes	Yes

Adapted from Kennedy HL: Ambulatory electrocardiography, 2nd ed. Philadelphia, Lea & Febiger (in press).

ST segment can be detailed or called flat, upward, or downward stroking.

Recently, automatic analysis of the ST segment has allowed simultaneous detection of the J point and ST segment point, permitting the automatic quantitation of ST segment episodes, duration, and integral area.[17] This methodology has undergone early clinical validation studies and, according to experienced workers, seems reasonably clinically acceptable.[17,25]

ADVERSE EFFECTS

Holter monitoring is a safe, noninvasive tool. However, several adverse effects are possible. Skin irritation or hypersensitivity from the electrode gel has been reported. The use of hydrocortisone cream can eliminate these allergic or irritative effects. Furthermore, electrical safety requirements for Holter recorders should be able to eliminate the potential for electrical charge leak.

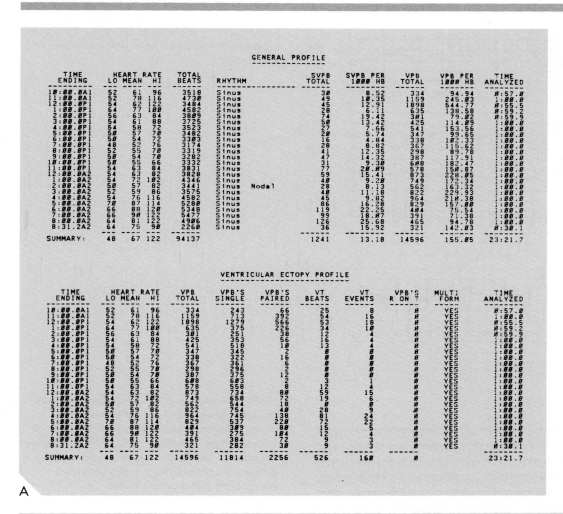

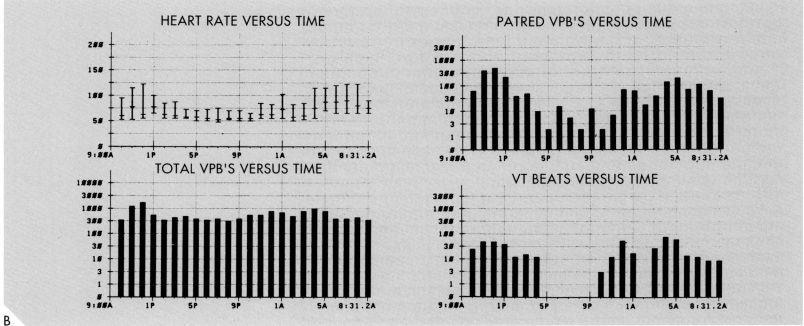

FIGURE 46.2 A. Suggested format for detailing data derived by quantitative analysis of Holter monitoring. The top represents a general profile, and the bottom provides a specific profile of ventricular ectopic beats. B. Data are displayed in graphic form. (SVPB, supraventricular premature beat; VPB, ventricular premature beat; VT, ventricular tachycardia) (Morganroth J: Ambulatory Holter electrocardiography: Choice of technologies and clinical uses. Ann Intern Med 102:73, 1985)

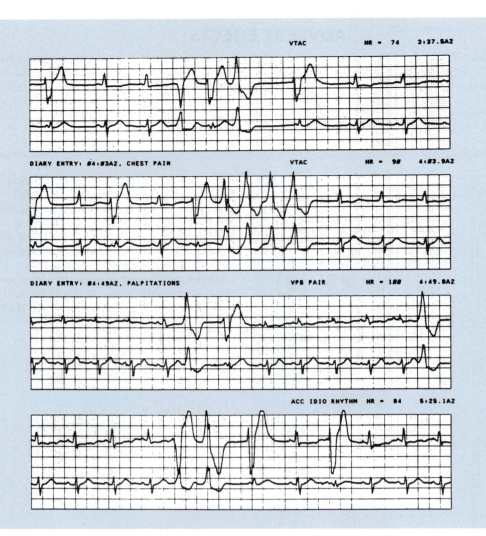

FIGURE 46.3 Four simultaneous pairs of ECG strips (representing ECG leads V₅ [top] and V₁ [bottom]) are displayed to document events that are reported in numerical and graphic displays of Holter data. The time of occurrence of the simultaneous ECG strips and the heart rate are noted as well as the type of arrhythmia defined by the technician-analysis system. In addition, the second and third set of ECG strips detail this patient's symptoms that can be correlated with the simultaneously recorded rhythm. (Morganroth J: Ambulatory Holter electrocardiography: Choice of technologies and clinical uses. Ann Intern Med 102:73, 1985)

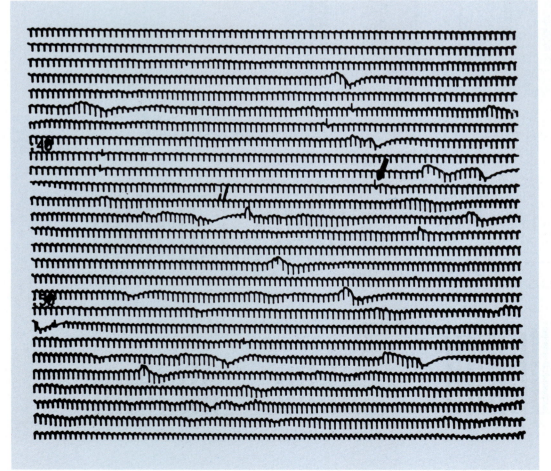

FIGURE 46.4 This mini-ECG format details the ECG recorded during a 24-hour Holter monitoring session. The single black arrow points out one of several ectopic complexes observed in this display. Deviations in the ECG's baseline due to motion artifact are frequently seen in this sample. (Morganroth J: Ambulatory Holter electrocardiography. Choice of technologies and clinical uses. Ann Intern Med 102:73, 1985)

It is important in applying a Holter monitor to sample the ECG output to be certain that the lead system chosen is one that will not provide too low a voltage. It is necessary that the ECG be recorded on the Holter monitor in sufficient magnitude to "trigger" the system. The demagnetization or extraneous magnetic induction of the recording tape can occur and must be safeguarded. Artifacts may occur on Holter monitoring, and if they are not properly detected, quantitative errors will result that may lead to erroneous clinical diagnosis. Equipment malfunction and/or the ambulatory nature of the patient are important reasons for artifacts. However, the use of two simultaneous ECG channels for analysis has been valuable in helping to identify artifacts and also to clarify ventricular from aberrant premature complexes. Pseudoectopic beats, pauses, and bradyarrhythmias and tachyarrhythmias can be produced by electrical, mechanical, and technician error. Finally, battery failure may cause pseudotachycardia or bradytachycardia, but usually all parts of the ECG complex become narrower or wider, depending on the problem (Fig. 46.5).

INDICATIONS

Holter monitoring is primarily indicated to detect ventricular and supraventricular arrhythmias, assess ST segment changes during daily activity in the known ischemic heart disease patient, and define the efficacy of various therapeutic interventions (antiarrhythmic, anti-ischemic, or pacemaker). This is best done by using a Holter analysis system that employs sophisticated software on hard disk microcomputers with accelerated analysis systems from continuous 24-hour ECG data recording. Using full quality control programs, accurate quantitation of the type and severity of arrhythmia must be ensured. It is becoming more popular to use commercial laboratories to provide Holter ECG analysis. Expensive quality control measures and availability of costly, constantly changing new technology are often more likely to be present in competitive commercial services than in the usual hospital-based laboratories. Nevertheless, a definite trend in decreasing cost of such instrumentation is evident with incorporation of personal microcomputers by several manufacturers.

For the patient who has an infrequent symptomatic arrhythmia, 24-hour Holter monitoring may be augmented with noncontinuously or continuously applied transtelephonic devices with or without memory.[27] These devices facilitate cost-effective examination of the patient over prolonged durations of time to record specific symptomatic events. Notwithstanding such adjunctive value, during the routine 24-hour Holter monitoring many patients disclose asymptomatic phenomena that permit diagnosis of the abnormality.

The clinical indications for Holter monitoring are (1) to correlate arrhythmias as the cause of specific patient complaints; (2) to detect the presence of supraventricular and/or ventricular arrhythmias in patients with conditions that place them at high risk for the occurrence of such arrhythmias; (3) to detect a change in the frequency or the severity of the arrhythmia after introduction of a therapeutic intervention, that is to determine the efficacy, inefficacy, or proarrhythmic effect of antiarrhythmic medications; (4) to evaluate ST segment morphology in patients with documented or suspected ischemic heart disease, including the important subgroups of silent ischemia and coronary spasm; and (5) to evaluate patients with potential pacemaker malfunction. Therefore, Holter monitoring has emerged as one of the most frequently used and important tools in the armamentarium of clinical medicine both for its diagnostic and therapeutic potentials.

SYMPTOM EVALUATIONS

Many ECG abnormalities occur without symptoms, and many symptoms of altered consciousness (dizziness, lightheadedness, palpitation, or syncope) are unrelated to ECG abnormalities. The correlation of arrhythmia with symptoms is critical in etiologic and therapeutic decisions.[28] For example, the symptom of palpitations might represent a variety of arrhythmias, sinus tachycardia, or even forceful normal heart beats; however, similar symptoms might be precipitated by ventricular or supraventricular arrhythmias. Ambulatory ECG recordings might help ascertain the precise diagnosis in a variety of clinical settings, particularly if the standard 12-lead ECG is of no diagnostic benefit.

Many patients reporting severe palpitations might have no evidence of underlying cardiovascular disease; however, the frequency of this complaint and the subsequent documentation of arrhythmia by ambulatory ECG recording is increased in patients with mitral valve prolapse,[29] idiopathic hypertrophic cardiomyopathy,[30] and valvular aortic stenosis.[31] We usually recommend no more than one or two 24-hour Holter monitors in patients with syncope. Often the patient may have no clear abnormality; yet at electrophysiologic testing a bradyarrhythmia or tachyarrhythmia will be induced that correlates with cerebral symptoms, thus leading to a definitive diagnosis and successful therapy. Occasionally, a similar outcome occurs with Holter monitoring in that "syncopal symptoms" are present in normal sinus rhythm leading to the etiology being correctly identified as noncardiovascular.

Palpitations are a subjective sensation and should be analyzed by ambulatory ECG monitoring for a correct diagnosis. The palpitations perceived in some patients may be due to the disturbance of the regular heart rhythm: some feel the premature beat, and some feel the compensatory pause after the extrasystole and are frightened. Many

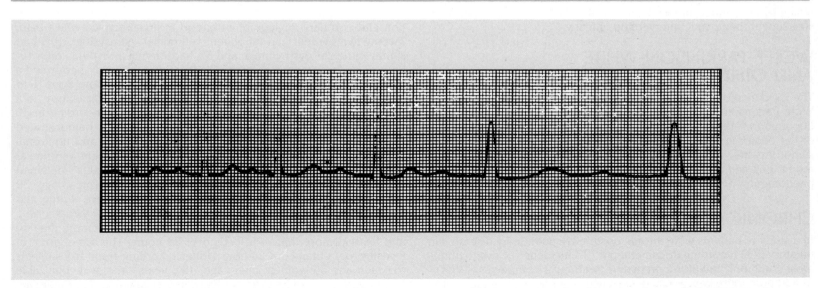

FIGURE 46.5 Example of pseudobradycardia in which the right side of the ECG strip details a marked bradycardia, which is caused by battery failure. This is recognized by a proportional prolongation of not only the RR interval but also the PR, QRS, and QT intervals.

experience at times a strong regular heart beat that they call palpitations, and a detailed history and ECG analysis in these individuals will reveal normal heart action. Palpitations are often a complaint in patients with paroxysmal supraventricular tachycardia. These patients have a characteristic history of feeling the sudden onset and offset of palpitations often preceded by extrasystoles.

Arrhythmias in ambulatory patients with a variety of systemic illness might predispose to sudden death. Long-term ambulatory ECG monitoring may help define this critical clinical problem and subsequently validate the efficacy of therapeutic intervention.[2,3]

CARDIOMYOPATHY

In patients with cardiomyopathy, both the frequency and complexity of ventricular ectopic beats appear related to sudden cardiac death. Ambulatory ECG monitoring might thus help guide therapeutic decisions in patients with congestive cardiomyopathy and high-grade ventricular ectopy.[32] Similarly, in patients with hypertrophic cardiomyopathy, ventricular arrhythmias are associated with an increased incidence of sudden death. It is still controversial whether better β-adrenergic blockade therapy alters the frequency of dysrhythmia and/or decreases the frequency of sudden death,[33,34] although the recent merit of amiodarone in improving survival of this subset of patients has been reported.[35]

MITRAL VALVE PROLAPSE AND AORTIC VALVE DISEASE

Patients with mitral valve prolapse commonly have ventricular ectopy that may be symptomatic or asymptomatic.[29] No correlation exists between the clinical features of mitral valve prolapse and the occurrence of arrhythmias. However, symptoms suggesting arrhythmia are often described concomitantly with a normal Holter recording.[36] Sudden death apparently related to repetitive ventricular arrhythmias has been reported.[37] However, there is no clear association per se of sudden death with the frequency or type of ventricular ectopic complexes in patients with mitral valve prolapse. Ambulatory Holter recording is diagnostically superior to exercise stress testing for arrhythmia identification in symptomatic patients with mitral valve prolapse.[36] Major ventricular ectopic activity, including ventricular tachycardia, is common in patients with aortic valvular disease.[28] Clinical correlations are necessary, since their significance has not been entirely established.

PROLONGED QT INTERVAL SYNDROME

Both congenital and acquired prolongation of the QT interval has been associated with sudden death, commonly in association with ventricular arrhythmias. However, the role of ambulatory ECG recording remains to be defined in documenting life-threatening arrhythmia and subsequent therapeutic intervention efficacy.

WOLFF-PARKINSON-WHITE AND OTHER PRE-EXCITATION SYNDROMES

The incidence of arrhythmia-related sudden death in patients with the Wolff-Parkinson-White syndrome remains to be defined but appears uncommon.[39] Patients with this syndrome require documentation both of the occurrence of asymptomatic arrhythmias and of whether their symptoms are, in fact, due to an arrhythmia. The ambulatory ECG monitoring can also confirm the diagnosis of preexcitation when this phenomenon occurs intermittently.

CHRONIC OBSTRUCTIVE PULMONARY DISEASE

In a study of patients with chronic obstructive pulmonary disease, ambulatory ECG recording documented a 72% incidence of dysrrhythmia, most commonly multiform premature ventricular complexes (PVCs).[40] In addition, there was a 52% occurrence of atrial dysrhythmia. Supraventricular arrhythmias are more common in hospitalized patients with acute respiratory failure than ventricular arrhythmias, which predominate in the chronic ambulatory state. The need for therapy in these patients is often defined more by the clinical setting than the prognostic significance of the arrhythmia.

CHRONIC HEMODIALYSIS

A 40% incidence of ventricular arrhythmias was identified during and after hemodialysis, with ventricular ectopy being more prominent in patients receiving digitalis and in those with left ventricular hypertrophy.[41] As the potassium level in the dialysate was increased the ventricular arrhythmias were reduced and decreased even further when quinidine was administered prior to dialysis. Therefore, in patients on dialysis who are receiving digitalis therapy or in those with left ventricular hypertrophy, ambulatory ECG monitoring might be of value. In another study by Malone and associates[42] it was reported that in patients on chronic hemodialysis, the increased incidence of arrhythmias was not related to electrolyte changes or to the dialysis per se.

DURING DIAGNOSTIC PROCEDURES

Arrhythmias occur in patients undergoing diagnostic procedures such as bronchoscopy, gastroscopy, and barium enema.[43] In one study, 40% of patients undergoing bronchoscopy had ventricular or supraventricular arrhythmias especially related to maximum oxygen desaturation but also during the passage of the bronchoscope through the vocal cords.[43] The arrhythmia occurred equally in patients with and without cardiovascular disease. There was no clinical impact of the arrhythmia.

Levy and Abinader[44] reported that ventricular and atrial ectopic complexes, tachyarrhythmias, and ST-T wave changes occurred in 38% of patients during gastroscopy. The incidence of the arrhythmias was equal among those with and without cardiovascular disease. The incidence of arrhythmia was diminished with premedication and spontaneously subsided after completion of the procedure.

Higgins and co-workers[45] reported that 40% of elderly patients developed new arrhythmias during a barium enema. The most common arrhythmias were frequent and multiform PVCs. A limitation to these studies was that no baseline Holter monitoring was performed.

DETECTION OF SUPRAVENTRICULAR AND VENTRICULAR TACHYARRHYTHMIAS
"NORMAL" POPULATION

The prevalence of arrhythmias in normal individuals is important to consider. DeMaria and colleagues[29] studied a group of 40 subjects who were free of cardiac disease as defined by normal cardiac catheterization and coronary angiography done to evaluate atypical chest pain. Twenty-five percent had infrequent ventricular extrasystole, 10% had supraventricular dysrhythmia, and 5% had varying arrhythmia on a 10-hour recording. In another study, Clarke and colleagues[46] performed a 48-hour ambulatory ECG recording in a normal population (aged 16 to 65 years) and showed that 12% had complex ventricular ectopy. In a study by Brodsky and co-workers,[47] a 24-hour ECG recording in 50 male medical students without apparent cardiac disease demonstrated that supraventricular arrhythmias, sinus bradycardia, and nocturnal atrioventricular block were common. However, frequent ventricular premature depolarizations were rare. Kostis and associates[48] obtained a 24-hour ECG recording from 100 men and women (mean age, 39 years) without cardiac disease after clinical noninvasive testing and cardiac catheterization with coronary angiography; 46% had at least 1 ventricular premature depolarization, but only 20% had more than 10 and 5% had more than 100 PVCs over 24 hours. The same group of investigators obtained a 24-hour Holter recording from 101 subjects (51 men and 50 women; mean age, 48.8 years) free of recognizable heart disease by noninvasive cardiac catheterization and coronary angiography.[49] They found fewer than 100 PVCs over 24 hours and no more than 5 PVCs in a given hour. No patient had repetitive PVCs (ventricular couplets or tachycardia).

Ventricular arrhythmias occur in normal populations in the absence of structural heart disease and with normal ventricular function; they are "benign" with regard to adverse outcome of morbidity or mortality. Even when such arrhythmias are frequent and complex, as they may be in 2% to 4% of the population, they are not associated with adverse clinical risk and should not be treated with antiarrhythmic agents.[50] This is particularly true when one appreciates that the proarrhythmic effects of antiarrhythmic drugs can lead to sudden cardiac death in such patients.[51]

SUPRAVENTRICULAR ARRHYTHMIAS

The value of Holter monitoring relative to standard ECG, exercise testing, and electrophysiologic testing in the diagnosis and management of supraventricular arrhythmias (Fig. 46.6) is still unclear. The frequency and severity of clinical symptoms may be sufficient for the management of these disorders. Guidelines are still to be defined for the clinician for the use of ambulatory ECG recording in the detection and management of symptomatic and asymptomatic supraventricular arrhythmias. The ability to detect paroxysmal bradyarrhythmias is an important use of Holter monitoring. A long sinus pause that may be seen in normal individuals requires clinical correlation (Fig. 46.7). Pauses of 2 to 3 seconds can be seen in normal healthy individuals and are probably due to excessive vagotonia.[47]

DETECTION OF HIGH-RISK PATIENTS WITH VENTRICULAR ARRHYTHMIAS

Sudden death can occur in patients with a variety of cardiac diseases (e.g., cardiomyopathy, congenital heart disease, valvular disease), but coronary artery disease is the underlying cause in more than 80%.[3] The incidence of sudden death is increased in patients with left ventricular dysfunction and ventricular arrhythmias.[2,3,52,53] The risk of sudden death is particularly high in survivors of acute myocardial infarction, particularly when the infarction is complicated by ventricular arrhythmias, left ventricular dysfunction, or both.[2] In this setting, Holter monitoring is helpful in the initial assessment of the risk of sudden death by detecting the frequency and complexity of ventricular arrhythmias, since the occurrence of PVCs, of only 240 per day and especially if complex (e.g., nonsustained ventricular tachycardia), indicates a severalfold increase in the risk of sudden death during the first year after infarction (Fig. 46.8).[2,52,53]

Studies of individuals who had sudden cardiac death while fortuitously wearing a Holter monitor have demonstrated that the mechanism of this condition (in approximately 80% of patients) was an acute ventricular tachyarrhythmia that led to ventricular fibrillation.[1]

Holter monitoring is the preferred diagnostic technique for detection of PVCs since it samples at least 100,000 QRS cycles in attempting to detect PVC frequency, compared with approximately 100 cycles detected by the routine 12-lead ECG.

It is not unreasonable to obtain a 24-hour Holter monitor recording to identify the high-risk subgroups for sudden death in patients with severe underlying structural heart disease. We often obtain this evaluation in patients with recent myocardial infarction, cardiomyopathy, or any cause of a reduced left ventricular ejection fraction of less than 40%. Recently, Kleiger et al showed that heart rate variability defined as the standard deviation of all normal RR intervals in a 24-hour Holter monitor obtained in 808 patients 11 ± 3 days after acute myocardial infarction had the strongest univariate correlation with mortality.[54] The relative risk of mortality was 5.3 times higher in the group with heart rate variability of less than 50 msec than in those with a variability of more than 100 msec.[54] Heart rate variability was a significant predictor of mortality after adjusting for clinical and demographic factors, ventricular arrhythmias, and ejection fraction.[54] Further studies by these workers indicate that parasympathetic nervous activity is substantially reduced in patients with low heart rate variability as compared with control patients. This suggests that low parasympathetic or high sympathetic activity decreases the electrical ventricular fibrillation threshold and increases the probability of ventricular fibrillation during myocardial ischemia.[55]

In other patient groups in which the risk for sudden death is less well defined (e.g., mitral valve prolapse), we usually only obtain a Holter monitor to evaluate symptoms, especially if they are as significant as syncope.

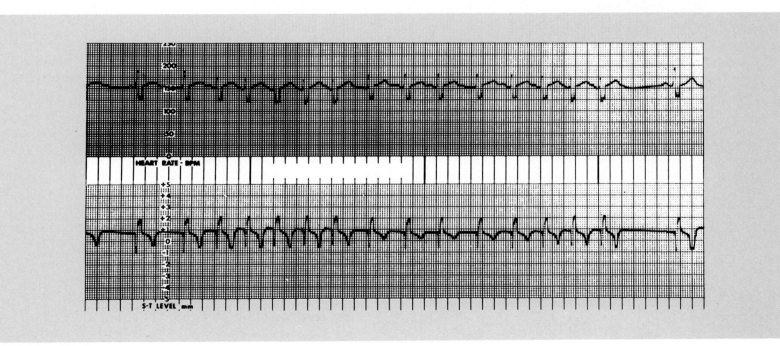

FIGURE 46.6 Episode of supraventricular tachycardia recorded on the simultaneous two leads of this Holter monitor recording. Its rate and regulatory onset and offset can be noted.

SPONTANEOUS VARIABILITY OF VENTRICULAR ECTOPY

Winkle and co-workers[56] studied 20 hospitalized patients undergoing evaluation of new antiarrhythmic drug therapy. Eleven 30-minute Holter monitoring segments were analyzed from a 5½-hour session for each patient. The initial 30 minutes were considered to be the control, and subsequent 30-minute periods were compared with that baseline. A large spontaneous variation in the frequency of ventricular ectopy was identified, with variations ranging from a 99% decline to a 1100% increase in frequency.

Morganroth and associates[5] reported on the degree of spontaneous variability present in ventricular ectopy in 15 hospitalized patients prior to evaluation with a new antiarrhythmic agent. These patients had to meet the requirements of having at least 30 PVCs per hour during placebo monitoring for 3 days and also had to demonstrate the presence of stable underlying cardiac conditions and medications. Before entry into the hospital, all patients had antiarrhythmic therapy discontinued for at least 7 days, and three consecutive 24-hour ambulatory recordings were used during controlled conditions on placebo therapy for this analysis. The analysis revealed quite clearly that the more frequent the control frequency the less the degree of spontaneous variability and the less the percent reduction required to define therapeutic efficacy. A sequential analysis of an additional 20 patients detailed the degree of spontaneous variability of beats of ventricular couplets and ventricular tachycardia.[57] These and other studies[58,59] have demonstrated that a reduction of at least 75% in PVC frequency on therapy compared with the pretreatment PVC level is required to define drug efficacy and to eliminate the likely chance that spontaneous variability is accounting for the observed change in PVC frequency. Although a higher degree of spontaneous variability will be present with lower baseline frequencies of ventricular arrhythmias (e.g., 10 PVCs per hour) one need only increase the percent reduction in PVCs required to show drug effect (e.g., ≥90%) when using such low frequencies. Because the spontaneous variability of ventricular arrhythmias is high, initial antiarrhythmic drug studies should be of short duration (e.g., 1 to 2 weeks). However, neither the use of repeated baseline Holter monitor measurements to establish initial ventricular arrhythmia variance nor the selection of an increased percentage suppression goal can prevent problems in the interpretation of apparent loss of efficacy during long-term antiarrhythmic drug therapy.[60] Kennedy and colleagues prospectively followed 28 patients with potentially lethal ventricular arrhythmias who had therapeutic suppression on moricizine therapy for 1 to 56 months, and found specific factors related to long-term antiarrhythmic drug therapy complicate the success of therapy.[60] These included (1) a transient loss of antiarrhythmic efficacy criteria, (2) a need for increased dose titration, (3) a loss of drug response to therapeutic doses, (4) the development of late proarrhythmic criteria, (5) the spontaneous resolution or diminution of ventricular arrhythmias during therapy, and (6) the development of delayed side effects necessitating drug withdrawal.[60] Long-term evaluation should employ short-term drug washout with placebo reintroduction every 6 to 12 months, with baseline reassessment of ventricular arrhythmia to demonstrate the continued presence of ventricular arrhythmias and the necessity for further treatment.[3,60]

DURATION OF RECORDING CYCLE AND ACTIVITY PROTOCOL

Bigger and co-workers[61] have examined the relationship between the probability of detecting PVCs and the duration of the Holter recording in two hundred 24-hour monitoring sessions in patients 2 weeks after

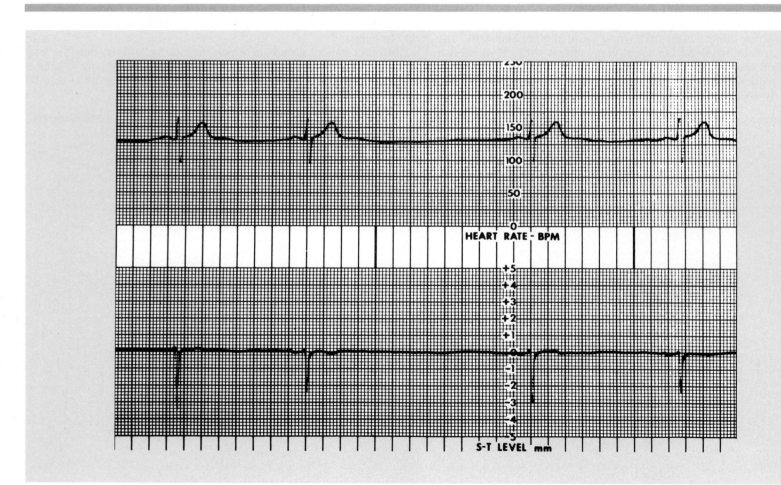

FIGURE 46.7 Pause of 2.6 seconds, a finding that requires clinical correlation since such pauses may be seen in normal individuals.

acute myocardial infarction. The percent of patients detected with PVCs related to duration of the recording and was for 1 minute, 11%; for 1 hour, 47%; 6 hours, 66%; and for 24 hours, 84%. Detection of repetitive forms of PVCs was also related to the duration of the recording. The incidence of ventricular tachycardia accumulated linearly over the 24-hour period, whereas other types of repetitive forms were not so related. The longer the Holter recording, the more was the likelihood of detecting patients with complex arrhythmias. This study also noted that only 10% of these patients with ventricular tachycardia would have been detected if only a 1-hour ECG recording (as the first hour) would have been chosen for the duration of monitoring. Examining the interaction of PVC frequency with PVC complexity showed a strong correlation if the frequency of PVCs was 10 or more in the first hour. This finding identified 12 of 18 (67%) of those patients who had ventricular tachycardia during the 24-hour recording period. Only 3 of these 18 patients had an episode of ventricular tachycardia in the first hour.

The spontaneous variability of lethal ventricular arrhythmias has not been specifically defined, but in such groups placebo periods are often impossible and the drug efficacy endpoint might be simply the lack of hemodynamic consequences from the manifested ventricular arrhythmias.

USE IN ST SEGMENT CHANGE EVALUATION

Early in the development of ambulatory ECG recording this technique was proposed as an alternate to the standard 12-lead ECG for identifying intermittent ischemic ST segment changes. However, the poor frequency response of the early recording instruments led to many false-positive ST segment changes. With recent technical improvements, many recorders now meet the requirements for diagnostic identification of ST segment changes. When ambulatory ECG recordings are used for the evaluation of ischemic ST segment changes, control recordings are needed in the supine, sitting, and standing positions with or without hyperventilation, just as one would obtain control recordings for an exercise stress test. Particular attention should be placed on lead placement. The recurrence of chest pain in association with ischemic ST changes on the ambulatory recording is clinically significant. In other patients in whom the ST segment changes occur without chest pain, the significance of these changes might be clarified by correlation with changes in heart rate, blood pressure, respiration, and food intake.[62] Although its clinical value had been reported previously, since the early 1980s Holter monitoring has been recognized as a valuable adjunctive diagnostic test to assess silent myocardial ischemia occurring during daily activities or spontaneously, with or without symptoms, during a diurnal 24-hour period.[63] Importantly, such observations should be confined to patients with documented coronary artery disease in order to avoid the false-positive changes associated with the confounding factors of myocardial hypertrophy, electrolyte imbalance, conduction abnormalities, pharmacologic agents, etc.[63] On a primary basis, Holter monitoring should not be used as the initial or solitary diagnostic test for coronary artery disease, perhaps with the only exception being suspected cases of Prinzmetal's variant angina associated with coronary spasm.[63,64] Numerous studies have failed to define specific characteristics unique to the ambulatory ECG detection of myocardial ischemia during daily activities.[63]

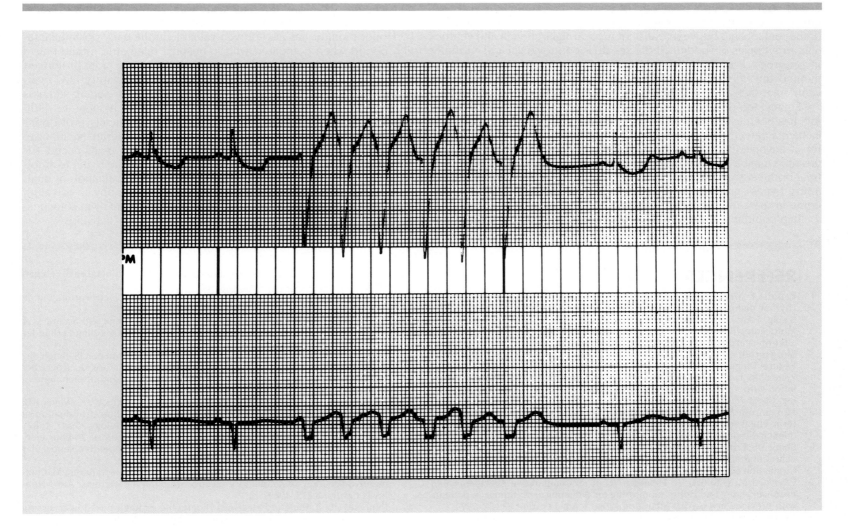

FIGURE 46.8 A six-beat episode of nonsustained, asymptomatic, ventricular tachycardia. This finding indicates an increased risk of sudden cardiac death when it occurs in the presence of underlying left ventricular dysfunction.

First, ambulatory ECG changes of ST segments in coronary artery disease patients may be detected during exercise as well as during rest periods, with a prevalence commonly varying from 75% to 90%, depending on the coronary artery disease population. Such stimuli as cold provocation, mental or emotional stress, or cigarette smoking have been substantiated to be the cause of ambulatory ECG ST segment changes and silent myocardial ischemia in patients with coronary artery disease. Second, dependent on the clinical state of the patient (e.g., unstable angina, nocturnal angina), an increased frequency, duration, and magnitude of silent myocardial ischemia are correlated with a severer degree of coronary artery disease. Third, examination of heart rates during the occurrence of ambulatory ECG ST segment changes discloses that myocardial ischemia throughout daily activities most frequently occurs at heart rates 10 to 20 beats per minute lower than the same ST segment changes exhibited during exercise testing. This indicates that spontaneously occurring myocardial ischemia throughout the day is mediated principally by mechanisms other than myocardial oxygen demand. The latter deductions have focused attention on the modulation of normal autonomic vascular tone as well as on coronary vasospasm. Fourth, examination of the most frequent time of occurrence of ambulatory ECG ST segment changes throughout the day has revealed a circadian distribution, with the greatest frequency of ST depression episodes occurring during the hours of 6 am to noon, while variant angina ST segment elevation episodes are most frequent from midnight to 6 am. This circadian variation parallels other neuroendocrine physiologic processes. Current perspective suggests that the increase in catecholamine and cortisol secretion seen in the early morning with the assumption of the upright posture is accompanied by an increase in heart rate and blood pressure, and is associated with the pathophysiology of myocardial ischemia and its sequelae—coronary thrombosis and myocardial infarction. Examination of the relationship between transient myocardial ischemia and ventricular arrhythmias or sudden cardiac death is controversial and currently in progress. Fortuitous ambulatory ECG examinations have documented the occurrence of transient ST segment changes preceding ventricular tachycardia, ventricular fibrillation, and cardiac arrest.[63]

Finally, the prognostic value of ambulatory ECG myocardial ischemia has been established in specific patient groups. Silent myocardial ischemia detected by ambulatory ECG has been shown to be a predictor of adverse cardiovascular morbidity and mortality in patients with unstable angina pectoris or stable angina, and after myocardial infarction, both early and late.[65–70] Although found in patients after coronary artery bypass grafting, its presence is not predictive of adverse outcome in the early years after surgery.[70]

In a comparison study of ST changes occurring during either exercise electrocardiography or ambulatory ECG recording in 70% of patients who subsequently underwent coronary angiography, the sensitivity of exercise testing was found to be 67% and that of ambulatory ECG recordings to be 62%. In addition, the specificity of the two tests was 75% and 61%, respectively.[71] In patients suspected of having variant angina, inferior lead sampling is valuable, since the ST-T wave elevation during coronary spasm is often recorded only from these leads. The ambulatory ECG recording can also be used to evaluate ST-T wave changes in patients who are unable to perform a treadmill or bicycle exercise test because of musculoskeletal or neurologic abnormalities.

USE IN PACEMAKER EVALUATION

Some patients after pacemaker implantation have a recurrence of symptoms such as dizziness, palpitations, or syncope. Transtelephonic ECG transmission and office monitoring may not indicate a malfunction. Ambulatory ECG recording might, however, identify those patients with intermittent pacemaker malfunction and provide a correlation with the symptoms. An ambulatory ECG recording for evaluation of pacemaker function should be carefully applied, and the technician should ensure adequate recording of the pacemaker artifact when the monitor is applied. It is important to realize that ambulatory ECG recording provides only a retrospective review of what has already happened and is not useful in signaling a potentially life-threatening malfunction of an implanted pacemaker. Because of the limited time of examination provided by the traditional pacemaker follow-up clinic visit and transtelephonic monitoring systems, the use of Holter monitoring for pacemaker evaluation over 24 hours or more during daily activities has increased the diagnostic yield in the detection of pacemaker dysfunction.[72] Enhanced detection of pacemaker dysfunction by Holter monitor has also proven valuable in the early postimplantation period when compared with in-hospital telemetric monitoring.[73] This increased diagnostic yield is not related simply to more prolonged time of examination. It has been facilitated by ambulatory ECG technology that permits detection and recognition of the pacing stimulus artifact through its amplification and recording on a separate dedicated channel.[74–76] Present technology can automatically provide information concerning failure to capture, sense, or generate an impulse, the number of pacing stimuli, and the percentage of beats paced. Although currently reliable for single chamber pacemakers, the technology needs additional refinement for the automatic evaluation of dual-chamber pacemakers. Ambulatory electrocardiography is of value, however, in the presence of dual-chamber pacemakers by making possible the visual interpretation of the ECG during daily activities.

REFERENCES

1. Panidis I, Morganroth J: Sudden death in hospitalized patients: Cardiac rhythm disturbances detected by ambulatory electrocardiographic monitoring. J Am Coll Cardiol 2:798, 1983
2. Multicenter Postinfarction Research Group: Risk stratification and survival after myocardial infarction. N Engl J Med 309:331, 1983
3. Morganroth J, Moore EN (eds): Sudden Cardiac Death and Congestive Heart Failure: Diagnosis and Treatment. Boston, Martinus Nijhoff, 1983
4. Zeldis SM, Levine BJ, Michelson EL et al: Cardiovascular complaints: Correlation with cardiac arrhythmias on 24-hour electrocardiographic monitoring. Chest 78:456, 1980
5. Morganroth J, Michelson EL, Horowitz LN et al: Limitations of routine long-term electrocardiographic monitoring to assess ventricular ectopic frequency. Circulation 58:408, 1978
6. Sheps DS, Ernst JC, Briese FR et al: Decreased frequency of exercise-induced ventricular ectopic activity in the second of two consecutive treadmill tests. Circulation 55:892, 1977
7. Crawford M, O'Rourke R, Henning NH et al: Comparative effectiveness of exercise testing and Holter monitoring for detecting arrhythmias in patients with previous myocardial infarction (abstr). Am J Cardiol 33:132, 1974
8. Gilson JS, Holter NJ, Glasscock WR: Clinical observations using the electrocardiorecorder: A VSEP continues electrocardiographic system: Tentative standards and typical patterns. Am J Cardiol 14:204, 1964
9. Hinkle LE Jr, Carver ST, Stevens M: The frequency of asymptomatic disturbances of cardiac rhythm and conduction in middle-aged men. Am J Cardiol 24:629, 1969
10. Kennedy HL: Ambulatory Electrocardiography. Philadelphia, Lea & Febiger, 1981
11. Wenger NK, Mock MB, Ringvist I (eds): Ambulatory Electrocardiographic Recordings. Chicago, Year Book Medical Publishers, 1981
12. Bjerregaard P: The quality of ambulatory ECG-recordings and accuracy of semiautomatic arrhythmia analysis: An evolution of the Medilog-Pathfinder system. Eur Heart J 1:417, 1980
13. DiBianco R, Katz RJ, Fletcher RD, Bortz Costello R, Gottdiener JS, Singh SN: Evaluation of technician audiovisual scanning of ambulatory electrocardiographic recordings utilizing the rapid oscillographic printout technique of validation. Clin Cardiol 5:39, 1982
14. Kennedy HL, Sprague MK, Shriver KK, Smith SC, Whitlock JA, Wiens RD: Real-time analysis ambulatory electrocardiography—clinical evaluation of cardiac arrhythmias by the Aegis system. J Electrocardiology 20:247, 1987
15. Salerno DM, Granrud G, Hodges M: Accuracy of commercial 24-hour electrocardiogram analyzers for quantitation of total and repetitive ventricular arrhythmias. Am J Cardiol 60:1299, 1987
16. Montague TJ, Rajaraman M, Montague PA, Spencer CA, Rautaharju PM: Comparative accuracy of ambulatory electrocardiographic systems. Am J Noninvas Cardiol 3:313, 1989
17. Kennedy HL: Ambulatory electrocardiographic strategies used in assessing silent myocardial ischemia. Eur Heart J Suppl V, 9:70, 1988
18. Tzivoni D, Benharin J, Gavish A, Stern S: Holter recording during treadmill testing in assessing myocardial ischemic changes. Am J Cardiol 55:1200, 1985
19. Quyyumi AA, Crake T, Mockus LJ et al: Value of the bipolar lead CM_5 in electrocardiography. Brit Med J 56:372, 1986

20. Bragg-Remschel DA, Winkle RA: Ambulatory monitoring of electrocardiograms: Current technology of recording and analysis. Physiologist 26:39, 1983
21. Silber S, Vogler AC, Spiegelsberger F, Vogel M, Theisen K: Validation of digital Holter ST segment analysis. J of Ambul Monitoring 1:145, 1988
22. Elfner R, Buss J, Heene DL: Beat-by-beat validation of the Oxford Medilog 4500: A 24-hour ambulatory ECG system with real-time analysis. J of Ambul Monitoring 1:17, 1988
23. Stein IM, Plunkett J, Troy M: Comparisons of techniques for examining long-term ECG recordings. Med Instrum 14:69, 1980
24. Kennedy HL, Wiens RD: Ambulatory (Holter) electrocardiography using real-time analysis. Am J Cardiol 59:1190, 1987
25. Barry J, Campbell S, Nabel EG, Mead K, Selwyn AP: Ambulatory monitoring of the digitized electrocardiogram for detection and early warning of transient myocardial ischemia in angina pectoris. Am J Cardiol 60:483, 1987
26. Jamal SM, Mitra-Duncan L, Kelly DT, Freedman SB: Validation of a real-time electrocardiographic monitor for detection of myocardial ischemia secondary to coronary artery disease. Am J Cardiol 60:525, 1987
27. Kennedy HL: Long-term electrocardiographic recordings. In Zipes DP, Rowlands DJ (eds): Progress in cardiology, p 238. Philadelphia, Lea & Febiger, 1988
28. Levine BJ, Zeldis SM, Morganroth J et al: Lack of correlation between symptoms and significant arrhythmias on long-term electrocardiographic analysis. Clin Res 26:247A, 1978
29. DeMaria AN, Amesterdam EA, Vismara LA et al: Arrhythmias in the mitral valve prolapse syndrome: Prevalence, nature and frequency. Ann Intern Med 84:656, 1976
30. Pratt CM, Vismara LA, DeMaria AN et al: Frequency and nature of ventricular arrhythmias in idiopathic hypertrophic subaortic stenosis: Importance of ambulatory electrocardiographic monitoring. Clin Res 25:245A, 1977
31. Amesterdam EA, Price JE, DeMaria AN et al: Ventricular ectopy in valvular heart disease: Evaluation by continuous ambulatory electrocardiographic monitoring and relation to coronary angioplasty. Clin Res 25:205A, 1977
32. Follansbee W, Michelson EL, Morganroth J: High risk of sudden death in clinically stable patients with nonsustained paroxysmal ventricular tachycardia. Clin Res 27:166A, 1979
33. McKenna WJ, Chetty S, Oakley CM et al: Exercise electrocardiographic and 48-hour ambulatory electrocardiographic monitor assessment of arrhythmia on and off beta-blocker therapy in hypertrophic cardiomyopathy. Am J Cardiol 43:420, 1979
34. Canedo MI, Frank MJ, Abdulla AM: Rhythm disturbances in hypertrophic cardiomyopathy: Prevalence, relation to symptoms and management. Am J Cardiol 45:848, 1980
35. McKenna WJ, Oakley CM, Krikler DM, Goodwin JF: Improved survival with amiodarone in patients with hypertrophic cardiomyopathy and ventricular tachycardia. Br Heart J 53:412, 1985
36. Winkle RA, Lopes MG, Fitzgerald JW et al: Arrhythmias in patients with mitral valve prolapse. Circulation 52:73, 1975
37. Jeresaty RM: Sudden death in the mitral valve prolapse-click syndrome. Am J Cardiol 37:317, 1976
38. Kennedy HL, Underhill SJ, Poblete PF et al: Ventricular ectopic beats in patients with aortic valve disease. Circulation 55:202, 1985
39. Hindman MC, Last JH, Rosen KM: Wolff-Parkinson-White syndrome observed by portable monitoring. Ann Intern Med 79:654, 1973
40. Kleiger RE, Senior RM: Long-term electrocardiographic monitoring of ambulatory patients with chronic airway obstruction. Chest 65:483, 1974
41. Morrison G, Brown ST, Michelson EL et al: Mechanism and prevention of cardiac arrhythmias during hemodialysis. Am J Cardiol 43:360, 1979
42. Malone D, deMello VR, Kleiger RE et al: Long-term electrocardiographic monitoring of patients with end-stage renal disease on chronic hemodialysis. Chest 72:405, 1977
43. Katz AS, Michelson EL, Stawicki J et al: Ear oximetry: A noninvasive method to identify patients at risk of arrhythmias during fiberoptic bronchoscopy. Am Rev Respir Dis 119:136, 1979
44. Levy N, Abinader E: Continuous electrocardiographic monitoring with Holter electrocardiocorder throughout all stages of gastroscopy. Dig Dis 22:1901, 1977
45. Higgins CB, Roeske WR, Karliner JS et al: Predictive factors and mechanism of arrhythmias and myocardial ischemic changes in elderly patients during barium enema. Br J Cardiol 49:1023, 1976
46. Clarke JM, Hamer J, Shelton JR et al: The rhythm of the normal human heart. Lancet 2:508, 1976
47. Brodsky M, Wu D, Denes P et al: Arrhythmias documented by 24 hour continuous electrocardiographic monitoring in 50 male medical students without apparent heart disease. Am J Cardiol 39:390, 1977
48. Kostis JB, Moreyra AE, Natarajan N et al: Ambulatory electrocardiography: What is normal (abstr)? Am J Cardiol 43:420, 1979
49. Kostis JB, McCrone K, Moreyra AE et al: Premature ventricular complexes in the absence of identifiable heart disease. Circulation 63:1351, 1981
50. Kennedy HL, Whitlock JA, Sprague MK et al: Long-term follow-up of asymptomatic healthy subjects with frequent and complex ventricular ectopy. N Engl J Med 312:193, 1985
51. Ruskin JN, McGovern B, Garan H, DiMarco JP, Kelly E: Antiarrhythmic drugs: A possible cause of out-of-hospital cardiac arrest. N Engl J Med 309:1302, 1983
52. Schultze RA, Strauss HW, Pi HB: Sudden death in the year following myocardial infarction: Relation to ventricular premature contractions in late hospital phase and left ventricular ejection fraction. Am J Med 62:192, 1977
53. Akhtar M: The clinical significance of the repetitive ventricular response. Circulation 63:773, 1981
54. Kleiger RE, Miller JP, Bigger JT et al: Decreased heart rate variability and its association with increased mortality after acute myocardial infarction. Am J Cardiol 59:256, 1987
55. Bigger JT, Kleiger RE, Fleiss JL et al: Components of heart rate variability measured during healing of acute myocardial infarction. Am J Cardiol 61:208, 1988
56. Winkle RA: Arrhythmia drug effect mimicked by spontaneous variability of ventricular ectopy. Circulation 57:1116, 1978
57. Michelson EL, Morganroth J: Spontaneous variability of complex ventricular arrhythmias detected by long-term electrocardiographic recordings. Circulation 61:690, 1980
58. Sami M, Kramemer H, Harrison DC et al: A new method of evaluating antiarrhythmic drug efficacy. Circulation 62:1172, 1980
59. Shapiro W, Canada WB, Lee G et al: Comparison of two methods of analyzing frequency of ventricular arrhythmias. Am Heart J 4:874, 1982
60. Kennedy HL, Sprague MK, Homan SM et al: Natural history of potentially lethal ventricular arrhythmias in patients treated with long-term antiarrhythmic drug therapy. Am J Cardiol 64:1289, 1989
61. Bigger JT, Rolnitzky LM, Leahey EB et al: Ambulatory ECG recording: Duration of recording and activity protocol. In Wenger NK, Mock MB, Ringvist I (eds): Ambulatory Electrocardiographic Recordings. Chicago, Year Book Medical Publishers, 1981
62. Crawford MH, Pesola A, Marzilli M et al: Coronary vasospasm in angina pectoris. Lancet 1:713, 1977
63. Kennedy HL, Wiens RD: Ambulatory (Holter) electrocardiography and myocardial ischemia. Am Heart J 117:164, 1989
64. Knoebel SB, Crawford MH, Dunn MI et al: Guidelines for ambulatory electrocardiography. A report of the American College of Cardiology/American Heart Association Task Force on assessment of diagnostic and therapeutic cardiovascular procedures (subcommittee on ambulatory electrocardiography). Circulation 79:206, 1989
65. Nademanee K, Intarachot V, Josephson MA, Rieders D, Mody FV, Singh BN: Prognostic significance of silent myocardial ischemia in patients with unstable angina. JACC 10:1, 1987
66. Gottlieb SO, Weisfeldt ML, Ouyang P, Mellits D, Gerstenblith KG: Silent ischemia predicts infarction and death during 2 year follow-up of unstable angina. JACC 10:756, 1987
67. Rocco MB, Nabel EG, Campbell S et al: Prognostic importance of myocardial ischemia detected by ambulatory monitoring in patients with stable coronary artery disease. Circulation 78:877, 1988
68. Tzivoni D, Gavish A, Zin D et al: Prognostic significance of ischemia episodes in patients with previous myocardial infarction. Am J Cardiol 62:661, 1988
69. Gottlieb SO, Gottlieb SH, Achuff SC et al: Silent ischemia on Holter monitoring predicts mortality in high-risk post-infarction patients. JAMA 259:1030, 1988
70. Kennedy HL, Seiler SM, Sprague MK et al: Relation of silent myocardial ischemia after coronary artery bypass grafting to angiographic completeness of revascularization and long-term prognosis. Am J Cardiol 65:14, 1990
71. Crawford M, O'Rourke RA, Ramakrishna N et al: Comparative effectiveness of exercise testing and continuous monitoring for detecting arrhythmias in patients with previous myocardial infarction. Circulation 50:301, 1974
72. Famularo MA, Kennedy HL: Ambulatory electrocardiography in the assessment of pacemaker function. Am Heart J 104:1086, 1982
73. Janosik DL, Redd RM, Buckingham TA, Blum RI, Wiens RD, Kennedy HL: The utility of ambulatory electrocardiography in detecting pacemaker dysfunction in the early post-implant period. Am J Cardiol 60:130, 1987
74. Kelen GJ, Bloomfield DA, Hardage M et al: A clinical evaluation of an improved Holter monitoring technique for artificial pacemaker function. PACE 3:192, 1980
75. Murray A, Jordan RS, Gold RG: Pacemaker assessment in the ambulant patient. Br Heart J 46:531, 1981
76. Tranesjo J, Fahraeus T, Nygards ME, Wigertz O: Automatic detection of pacemaker pulses in ambulatory ECG recording. PACE 5:120, 1982

THE SICK SINUS SYNDROME AND EVALUATION OF THE PATIENT WITH SINUS NODE DISORDERS

J. Anthony Gomes

The sinus node is the dominant pacemaker of the heart, whereby it has gained the distinction of being referred to as the "maestro" of the mammalian specialized conducting system.[1,2] Anatomically, the sinus node is a subepicardial structure and measures approximately 15 mm × 5 mm × 2 mm. It receives its blood supply from the sinus nodal artery, which arises from the proximal right coronary artery in 55% of subjects and from the circumflex artery in 45% of subjects.[3] In addition, it also receives blood via intracoronary and extracoronary anastomoses. The sinus node has a tripartite cellular population composed of "typical nodal cells," transitional cells, and working myocardial cells.[4,5] The typical nodal cells (also referred to as P cells) are thought to have the intrinsic property of automaticity and number in the thousands, accounting for the large reserve capacity of the sinus node and the gradual process of sinus pacemaker failure. Some of these pacemaker cells function as dominant pacemaker cells, whereas others function as latent or subsidiary pacemaker cells.[6,7] Both the dominant and subsidiary pacemaker cells have their own intrinsic rates, which are probably related to different ionic movements in diastole in the two groups of cells.[8] In addition, the intrinsic rates of these groups of cells are under the control of the autonomic nervous system. Boineau and co-workers[9] have suggested that the atrial depolarization wave has multicentric origins in the canine heart. Studies by Gomes and associates[10] have shown that the human sinus pacemaker can originate from different sites within the sinus node. Shifts in the sinus pacemaker complex from dominant to subsidiary pacemakers have been noted to occur spontaneously and particularly following carotid sinus massage and atrial stimulation. These findings are in disagreement with the observations made by Boineau and co-workers of the canine heart.

Abnormalities of sinus impulse generation and its transmission to the atrial myocardium can result in a variety of electrocardiographic (ECG) abnormalities. These abnormalities have been collectively referred to as the sick sinus syndrome (SSS).[11] However, this term should be restricted to only those patients who in addition to the ECG abnormalities have symptoms indicative of central nervous system dysfunction, such as episodes of lightheadedness, dizziness, and syncope. The ECG manifestations of SSS include varying degrees of sinus bradycardia (usually rates of ≤50 beats per minute), sinus arrest, sinoatrial block, and the tachy-brady syndrome. One or more of these ECG abnormalities may be seen in 38% to 100% of patients with SSS. In the tachy-brady syndrome the tachycardia component is usually atrial fibrillation (Fig. 47.1), but atrial flutter and paroxysmal atrial tachycardia may also be seen. The bradycardia component is a post-tachycardia pause as a result of sinus arrest and/or sinoatrial block. It is more likely that the post-tachycardia pause is a result of sinoatrial block rather than sinus arrest since studies in patients with SSS have demonstrated that the post-pacing pause is due to first-degree or high-degree sinoatrial block rather than to sinus arrest.[12,13] It is the bradycardia component that results in lightheadedness or syncope, whereas the tachycardia component may give rise to no symptoms or symptoms of palpitations or fluttering in the chest or angina pectoris in those patients who have coronary artery disease. The occurrence of syncopal episodes in the elderly should raise the suspicion of SSS. Of 49 male patients 65 years of age or older evaluated in our laboratory for syncope, 57% had electrophysiologic abnormalities suggestive of SSS. In contrast, 3 of 20 patients (15%) (≥65 years) without syncope had sinus node abnormalities in the laboratory. Other ECG abnormalities such as paroxysmal or sustained atrial fibrillation or flutter (Fig. 47.2) may be a manifestation of an underlying SSS.[14] It should also be suspected in those patients who do not promptly recover sinus rhythm following cardioversion. An association has been noted in some patients with the hypersensitive carotid sinus syndrome.[15,16] The SSS may coexist with other abnormalities of the conducting system such as atrioventricular conduction disturbance and bundle branch block. In addition, it has been suggested that patients with SSS have disease of distal pacemakers in the junction and the His-Purkinje system since these pacemakers do not readily escape during long sinus pauses.[17]

Over the past few years, the SSS has gained considerable importance. The latter is related to the fact that the SSS accounts for the majority of pacemakers implanted in the United States.[18] What also has become clear is that the ECG manifestations of the SSS may be seen in a substantial number of young subjects, athletes, and older individuals. Thus the proper recognition and management of the patient with symptomatic and asymptomatic sinus node disorders has gained considerable importance in cardiovascular medicine.

ETIOLOGY

The etiology of SSS is idiopathic in the majority of instances; however, it is likely related to a degenerative process of the sinus node and atrial myocardium. Nonetheless, SSS has been reported in a variety of disease entities (Table 47.1). It has been suggested that ischemic heart disease accounts for the majority of patients with SSS.[19] Except for a few instances, this contention is not based on solid pathologic or clinical grounds. On the basis of available data, coronary artery disease is unlikely to be playing a major role in the genesis of the SSS. The necropsy studies of Davies and Pomerance[20] have shown that muscle loss and increase in fibrosis in the sinus node and intranodal tracts is a slow but continuous process starting around the age of 60 years. Since the majority of patients with SSS are older than 60 years of age, this study supports the viewpoint that fibrosis is the likely underlying pathology in most patients with SSS. The familial and congenital nature of the syndrome seen in rare instances is suggested by the reports of the syndrome in young children and in families with and without the long QT interval syndrome.[21-23] One important entity is drug-induced abnormality of sinus node function. Cardioactive drugs such as digitalis glycosides, β-adrenergic blocking agents, calcium channel blockers (such as verapamil and diltiazem), quinidine, disopyramide, and procainamide may induce or unmask an underlying SSS.[24-29] Other drugs such as lithium, guanethidine, methyldopa, and clonidine have been reported to result in sinus node dysfunction. The importance of a good drug history in patients with suspected SSS cannot be overemphasized and will avoid unnecessary investigation.

PATHOPHYSIOLOGY AND NATURAL HISTORY

Sinus node function is dependent on a complex interaction between intrinsic sinus node automaticity, sinoatrial conduction, and autonomic regulatory mechanisms. The role of the autonomic nervous system in the pathophysiologic mechanism of the SSS has been clarified only recently. Studies in several independent laboratories have demonstrated that not all patients with SSS have an intrinsic abnormality of sinus node function.[30–33] Thus, mechanistically SSS can be classified into two types: (1) intrinsic SSS, in which there is an intrinsic abnormality in sinus node function, and (2) extrinsic SSS, in which the abnormality lies in autonomic regulation, with intrinsic sinus node function being normal. Studies in our laboratory in 22 patients with SSS demonstrated that approximately 60% of patients had intrinsic SSS whereas 40% had extrinsic SSS.[33] Jordan and colleagues[30] reported that 41% of 17 patients had intrinsic SSS whereas 59% of 17 patients had the extrinsic variety. Similarly Desai and co-workers[31] reported that 62% of 21 patients had extrinsic SSS whereas 38% of 21 patients had intrinsic SSS. They further classified their patients into three broad subgroups: (1)

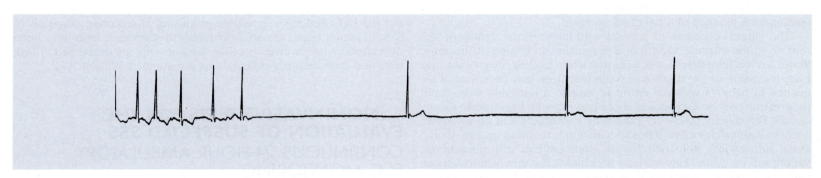

FIGURE 47.1 Monitor strip of a patient with the tachy-brady syndrome. The tachycardia component is atrial fibrillation, whereas the bradycardia component is a post-tachycardia pause that is followed by a junctional escape beat.

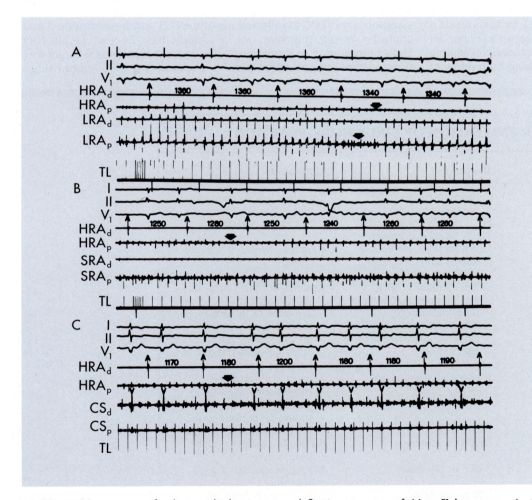

FIGURE 47.2 Coexistence of sick sinus rhythm in a patient with atrial flutter/fibrillation. From top to bottom are ECG leads I, II, and V₁ and the intracardiac recordings from the high right atrium (HRA) and low right atrium (LRA) in **A**; from the HRA and septal RA (SRA) in **B**; and from the HRA and coronary sinus (CS) in **C**. Note the distinct deflection at a rate of 44 to 51 beats per minute localized to the HRA whereas the remaining parts of the atrium are in either atrial flutter and/or fibrillation. (Gomes JAC, Kang PS, Gough W et al: Coexistence of sick sinus rhythm and atrial flutter-fibrillation. Circulation 63:80, 1981, by permission of the American Heart Association, Inc.)

TABLE 47.1 ETIOLOGY OF SSS

Idiopathic (degenerative)
Ischemic
Infiltrative
   Amyloid
   Hemochromatosis
   Scleroderma
   Tumor (metastatic)
Inflammatory
   Rheumatic fever
   Pericarditis
   Diphtheria
   Chagas' disease
Cardiomyopathy (dilated)
Collagen vascular disease
Surgical trauma
Familial
Congenital
Muscular dystrophies
Drug induced

those with extrinsic SSS but with relative hypervagotonia, (2) those with intrinsic SSS who are dependent on autonomic tone, and (3) those with intrinsic SSS unaffected by changes in autonomic tone. Our studies have in addition revealed that patients with the extrinsic variety in contrast to those with the intrinsic variety are younger and have a lower incidence of organic heart disease and the tachy-brady syndrome, whereas the incidence of sinus arrest or sinoatrial block is more or less equal in the two varieties. The extrinsic variety of SSS is probably related to vagal predominance. Although pathologic studies have not been performed in these patients, deficiency in atrial cholinesterase has been shown to result in a buildup of acetylcholine, which can result in episodes of sinus bradycardia and sinoatrial block. Rossi[34] has demonstrated histologic evidence for autonomic nerve damage leading to deficiency of atrial cholinesterase.

The clinical outcome of patients with the extrinsic variety of SSS relative to the intrinsic variety of SSS remains undefined at this time. However, it is tempting to speculate that whereas slow progression and even remission of the disease in some instances may be a natural sequence in patients with the extrinsic variety, a relatively more rapid progression may be expected in those patients with the intrinsic variety of SSS. Preliminary follow-up studies by Yamaguchi and co-workers[35] seem to support this view. If this speculation is found to be true, then it could substantially influence therapy since patients with the intrinsic variety will be more likely to need pacemaker therapy, whereas those with the extrinsic variety may be more amenable to initial medical therapy.

The natural history of the SSS is not well understood. A study by Lien and associates[36] of 52 patients with SSS found that in patients who presented with sinus bradycardia with sinoatrial block or sinus arrest it took 7 to 29 years (average, 13 years) for total sinus arrest to occur. Of additional interest was their observation that occasionally complete recovery of normal sinus mechanism was noted during the course of the disease. These observations are interesting and need further corroboration; nonetheless, they support the viewpoint that SSS is a disease of varying gradations, with a long natural history with occasional remission.

EVALUATION OF THE PATIENT WITH SUSPECTED SINUS NODE DISORDERS

The diagnosis of SSS can be suspected on the basis of a careful history and examination of the ECG. However, since a variety of medical and cardiovascular causes can result in syncope, dizzy spells, and palpitations and since sinus bradycardia and sinus pauses are not unusual in an otherwise ostensibly normal population, neither the history alone nor the ECG findings are reliable in making an accurate diagnosis of SSS. In recent years, several noninvasive and invasive tests have been described in the evaluation of the patient with suspected SSS. These tests and their merits and limitations are outlined in Table 47.2.

NONINVASIVE TESTS FOR THE EVALUATION OF SUSPECTED SSS
CONTINUOUS 24-HOUR AMBULATORY ECG MONITORING

A 24-hour ambulatory Holter monitor remains an important test in the diagnosis of suspected SSS since it affords correlation of symptoms with ECG abnormalities. Nonetheless, it is of importance to note that symptoms and ECG manifestations of the SSS may be intermittent and sporadic, events that may not be detected on 24-hour ambulatory Holter monitoring. It is not unusual to encounter patients who are free of symptoms for prolonged periods. Furthermore, ECG abnormalities

TABLE 47.2 TESTS FOR EVALUATION OF SINUS NODE FUNCTION

Test	Response	Comments
24-hour ECG monitoring	Sinus bradycardia (≤50 beats per minute) Sinus pauses ≥3 seconds Tachy-brady syndrome	Excellent test if correlation with symptoms; however, this rarely occurs
Atropine (1 mg to 2 mg or 0.4 mg/kg)	≤25% increase in sinus rate or sinus rate ≤90 beats per minute	Easy test, helpful if positive
Isoproterenol (2 μg to 3 μg/min)	≤25% increase in sinus rate or sinus rate ≤90 beats per minute	Same as atropine; may be dangerous in the presence of ischemic heart diease; sensitivity and specificity not known; results difficult to assess in elderly
Exercise test	≤90% of predicted maximal heart rate for age and sex	
Carotid sinus stimulation	≥3-second sinus pause	Seen in hypersensitive carotid sinus syndrome; may co-exist with SSS; should be performed in the evaluation of syncope
Sinus node recovery time	SNRTc > 450 msec	Moderate sensitivity; high specificity
Sinoatrial conduction	SACT ≥ 120 msec	Moderate specificity, high sensitivity
Intrinsic heart rate	IHR below 95% confidence limit of predicted IHR IHRP = 118.1 (0.53 × age)	Differentiation between extrinsic and intrinsic SSS
Sinus node refractoriness	≥500 msec	Value unclear; wide experience unavailable

alone that occur in patients with SSS may be seen in a substantial number of otherwise asymptomatic subjects. Southall and co-workers[37] reported Holter studies in 134 healthy full-term infants within the first 10 days of life. At their lowest rates, 81% of infants had sinus bradycardia and 19% had junctional escape rhythms. In a randomly selected subgroup of 71 infants, 72% had sinus pauses, 7% had sinus arrest, 11% had sinoatrial block, and 32% had Möbitz type I sinoatrial block. Scott and colleagues[38] reported their findings in 131 healthy boys 10 to 13 years of age. The heart rate ranged as low as 45 to 80 beats per minute during waking hours and as low as 30 to 70 beats per minute during sleeping hours. Complete sinoatrial block was seen in 8.4% of subjects, and slow junctional rhythm occurred in 13% during sleep. Brodsky and associates[39] studied 50 male medical students 23 to 27 years of age. During waking hours minimal heart rates ranged from 37 to 65 beats per minute and 33 to 55 beats per minute during sleeping hours. The longest pauses recorded during waking hours ranged from 1 to 1.68 seconds, whereas the longest pauses during sleeping hours were 1.2 to 2.06 seconds. In 12 subjects (24%), sinus bradycardia of less than 40 beats per minute was noted during the night. In long-distance runners, greater degrees of sinus bradycardia, sinoatrial block, and sinus arrest are seen. Talan and co-workers[40] reported minimum rates of 31 to 43 beats per minute during sleeping hours and 34 to 53 beats per minute during waking hours. The longest pauses ranged from 1.35 to 2.55 seconds during waking hours and from 1.6 to 2.81 seconds during sleep. Studies by Camm and colleagues[41] in 106 patients over 75 years of age from a general practice in Sussex, England, noted a lower incidence of sinus bradycardia in the elderly than in younger individuals reported in the studies discussed above. However, their subjects cannot be considered as normal since there was a high frequency of syncope, palpitations, dizziness, chest pain, and hypertension and a high intake of medications. Heart rates below 50 beats per minute were noted in 11 of 106 subjects (10%). In 7 of 11 subjects, sinus bradycardia occurred only during sleep. Atrial and junctional tachyarrhythmias were also noted in 14 patients. The studies discussed above suggest the following: (1) sinus rates in the 30s, particularly during sleep, occur rather frequently in young subjects and athletes and to a lesser extent in elderly subjects who are otherwise asymptomatic; (2) the presence of marked sinus bradycardia and sinus pauses during sleeping and awake hours cannot be considered as "abnormal" in the absence of symptoms; and (3) the diagnosis of SSS should be reserved for those patients in whom ECG Holter monitoring abnormalities are associated with and correlated with symptoms.

In patients with symptoms of syncope, palpitations, and dizziness, Lipski and associates[42] uncovered significant arrhythmias in 30 patients. Of these 30 patients, 21 had bradyarrhythmias that occurred during sleep. Five additional patients had severe sinus bradycardia. Reifel and co-workers[43] found evidence suggestive of SSS on 24-hour monitoring in 20 of 51 patients (39%) with suspected SSS. Gibson and Hertzman[44] reported on 24-hour Holter results in 1004 patients 60 years of age or older with possible SSS. All were referred for syncope. They found that 415 patients (41%) had one or more arrhythmias that may be associated with SSS depending on the definition of SSS. However, using stringent criteria of their own, which included (1) sinus bradycardia of a rate of less than 50 beats per minute (intermittent, persistent, and not during sleep); (2) sinus pause, sinus arrest, or sinoatrial block of 3.0 seconds or longer; (3) junctional rhythm (intermittent and persistent); (4) atrial fibrillation with intermittent slow ventricular response and RR intervals of 2.0 seconds or longer; and (5) tachy-brady syndrome, only 32 patients or 3% fell into the group with SSS. What is disturbing, however, is that symptom correlation occurred in only one patient who had syncope secondary to asystole of 7.8 seconds and in another who had chest pain secondary to supraventricular tachycardia. They concluded that an open referral 24-hour ambulatory monitoring service rarely results in identifying relevant symptom-related arrhythmias in patients with syncope and suspected SSS. Thus, the observations made in these studies can be summarized in the following manner:

1. ECG abnormalities suggestive of SSS may be observed frequently; however, correlation with symptoms is rare even in patients with syncope.
2. A 24-hour ambulatory Holter recording is associated with many asymptomatic arrhythmias that can compound the diagnostic problem in elderly patients and lead to unnecessary therapy.
3. The specificity of 24-hour Holter monitoring in patients with suspected SSS is low if ECG abnormalities are not associated with symptoms.
4. Holter criteria for the diagnosis of SSS should be stringent and pacemaker therapy should be initially reserved for those patients in whom a correlation has been noted between ECG abnormalities and symptoms.

PHARMACOLOGIC TESTING

The response of the sinus rate to atropine and isoproterenol has been used to assess sinus rate response in patients with SSS.[15,45,46] An increase in sinus rate of less than 25% or no more than 90 beats per minute is considered as abnormal. However, these pharmacologic tests have several limitations: (1) there is no standardization of dosages; (2) dose–response curves in normal patients are lacking for comparative purposes; (3) the sensitivity and specificity of the tests have not been determined; and (4) a normal response to pharmacologic agents does not preclude the diagnosis of SSS.

EXERCISE TESTING

The sinus rate response to exercise testing has been used in the evaluation of patients with SSS. Reduced heart rate response to exercise in patients with SSS was described by Mandel and colleagues,[15] Grant and Shaw,[47] and Abbott and co-workers.[48] Maximal upright, graded, bicycle stress testing was performed by Abbott and co-workers[48] in 16 patients with SSS. They observed that these patients were unable to achieve maximal heart rates comparable to age- and sex-matched controls. However, some SSS patients may respond normally to exercise. In addition to the fact that the sensitivity and specificity of exercise testing remains unknown in the diagnosis of the SSS, the value of the exercise test in patients with different gradations of the SSS has not been assessed. Furthermore, often maximal heart rates cannot be achieved in elderly patients owing to fatigue and poor conditioning.

CAROTID SINUS STIMULATION

Carotid sinus stimulation should be performed in the workup of patients who present with syncope and/or dizzy spells. The procedure is done by firmly massaging the right, then the left, carotid sinus for up to 10 seconds. This maneuver, however, should not be performed in patients who have audible carotid bruits. It is of importance to monitor the ECG and blood pressure continuously during carotid sinus massage. Carotid sinus hypersensitivity is indicated when a pause longer than 3 seconds occurs during carotid sinus massage. An association between carotid sinus hypersensitivity and the presence of SSS has been reported by Mandel and colleagues[15] and by Thorman and associates.[16] However, these two syndromes more often exist as separate entities.

ELECTROPHYSIOLOGIC EVALUATION OF SINUS NODE DYSFUNCTION

Over the past 14 years, a large body of investigative work has been done in an attempt to understand normal and abnormal physiology of the sinus node. These investigative endeavors have resulted in a variety of electrophysiologic tests for the evaluation of sinus node function in patients suspected of having SSS: These electrophysiologic tests include the following: sinus node recovery time, sinoatrial conduction time, determination of intrinsic heart rate and sinus node recovery time following pharmacologic autonomic blockade, direct recording of sinus node electrical activity, and sinus node refractoriness.

SINUS NODE RECOVERY TIME

Sinus node recovery time (SNRT) is assessed by overdrive stimulation of the atrium at rates above the spontaneous sinus rate for a period of 1 minute (range = 30 seconds to 2 minutes), after which atrial pacing is abruptly terminated.[15,49] Overdrive atrial pacing should be performed at multiple pacing rates in increments of 10 to 20 beats per minute up to a rate of approximately 200 beats per minute. SNRT is measured as the interval from the last paced atrial beat to the first spontaneous atrial deflection (A wave) or P wave of sinus origin (Fig. 47.3). The longest SNRT obtained at any pacing rate is taken as the representative SNRT. Because of the differences in spontaneous sinus rates between individuals, the SNRT has been expressed as the corrected SNRT (SNRTc),[49] which is obtained by subtracting the SNRT from the basic sinus cycle length or as a ratio of the sinus cycle length.[50] Overdrive suppression of the sinus node is seen in normal subjects as well as in patients with SSS; however, it is the degree of prolongation that defines an abnormal response. Unfortunately, a wide range of values for SNRT (1200 msec to 1740 msec) and SNRTc (375 msec to 525 msec) are reported using the mean value plus 2 standard deviations as the upper limit of normal for each study. When the SNRT is expressed as the ratio of sinus cycle length, the upper limit of normal for SNRT is defined as 1.61 times the pre-pacing sinus cycle length for subjects whose sinus cycle length is less than 800 msec and a value of 1.83 times the pre-pacing sinus cycle length for subjects with a pre-pacing sinus cycle length of greater than 800 msec. Most laboratories use the SNRTc to determine an abnormal recovery time. In our laboratory a value of more than 450 msec (SNRTc) is considered abnormal. An abnormal SNRT or SNRTc has been noted in 40% to 93% of patients with suspected SSS.[15,33,49,51] This wide variability in abnormal SNRT may be related to several of the following factors: (1) variability in patient selection: this may particularly be true when assessing the extrinsic variety of SSS due to autonomic dysfunction; (2) the severity of the SSS; (3) shift of the sinus pacemaker complex from a dominant to a subsidiary site; (4) induction of sinus node reentry; and (5) incomplete suppression of the sinus node due to entrance block. At times the administration of atropine may enhance atrio-sinus conduction or abolish entrance block, resulting in a longer recovery time,[52] whereas at other times analysis of secondary pauses may uncover an abnormal response.[50]

Until recently, the observation of an abnormally prolonged SNRT was taken to imply that sinus node automaticity was abnormal.[15,49] This hypothesis was based on the assumption that atrial electrical events in the region of the sinus node reflect sinus nodal events and that there is no significant change in sinoatrial conduction following overdrive atrial pacing. However, studies have shown that these assumptions are not necessarily true.[13] Studies using direct recordings of sinus nodal potentials in humans have demonstrated that the SNRT assessed by indirect methods described above is a reflection of sinus nodal automaticity as well as sinoatrial conduction.[13] What is of interest is that the prolonged SNRT seen in patients with SSS was not as much accounted for by depressed automaticity but rather by depressed sinoatrial conduction with the occurrence of marked first-degree or high-degree sinoatrial block.[12,13]

SINOATRIAL CONDUCTION TIME

Sinoatrial conduction time (SACT) defines the time it takes for the sinus impulse to depolarize the atrium. The SACT can be assessed by indirect and direct methods. The indirect methods used to assess SACT include the premature stimulation method[53] and the continuous pacing method.[54] The direct method involves recording a sinus node potential. Normal values for SACT have varied considerably between laboratories (50 msec to 120 msec). Usually a value of greater than or equal to 120 msec for unidirectional SACT is considered abnormal for most laboratories. Of the three methods currently used to assess SACT, the continuous pacing method is the simplest and least time consuming, whereas the premature stimulation method is more complex in its

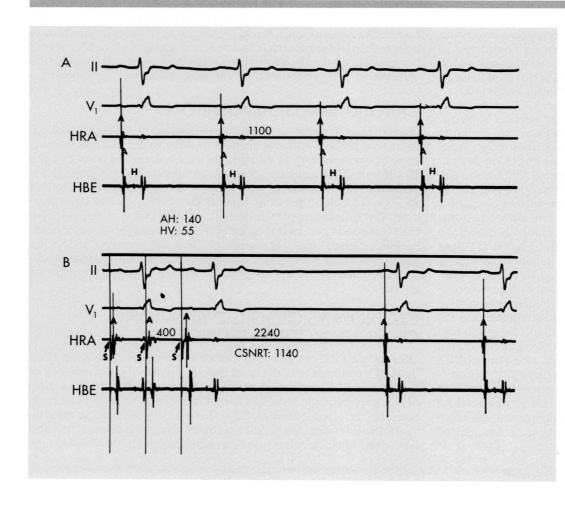

FIGURE 47.3 Assessment of SNRT in a patient with episodes of lightheadedness, syncope, and sinus bradycardia. From top to bottom are ECG leads II and V_1 and intracardiac recordings from the high right atrium (*HRA*) and His bundle (*HBE*). **A.** Sinus rhythm at a rate of 55 beats per minute. **B.** Last three beats of overdrive atrial pacing at a cycle length of 400 msec performed for 1 minute, following which pacing is abruptly terminated. The SNRT was 2240 msec, and the corrected SNRT, which is the SNRT-BCL, was grossly abnormal (1140 msec).

methodology and calculation. The direct method is dependent on obtaining close catheter contact with the atrial endocardium overlying the sinus node region and can be successfully obtained in 80% to 90% of patients. It is the most accurate and does not involve several assumptions that both the premature stimulation and continuous pacing methods take into account. However, any of the three methods may be used for estimation of SACT since generally there is a good correlation between the three methods, although appreciable differences can be observed in individual patients with SSS.[55] The direct method of measuring SACT is most useful in (1) confirming SACTs obtained by the indirect methods, particularly in patients with SSS since our studies and those of others have suggested that the direct method is superior in separating patients with SSS from those without; (2) assessing patients in whom the premature stimulation method is imprecise or in patients whom the absence of a zone of reset makes the measurement of SACT impossible; and (3) assessing patients with frequent premature atrial contractions that cannot be readily suppressed at rates less than or equal to 10 beats per minute above the sinus rate.

The incidence of abnormal prolongation of SACT in patients with and without SSS has varied considerably. Dhingra and co-workers[56] found a 2% incidence of abnormal SACT in 418 patients without sinus node dysfunction and in 29% of 52 patients with SSS. However, they used a value of 152 msec as abnormal, which may have decreased their false-positive as well as their true-positive results. Strauss and co-workers[57] reported abnormal values in 38% of patients with SSS, whereas Breithardt and associates[58] reported abnormal values in 45% of 41 patients with SSS. We also have reported abnormal values in 41% of 22 patients with SSS; however, we found that a greater proportion of patients (74%) with extrinsic SSS due to autonomic regulation had prolonged SACTs. In contrast, only 23% of patients with intrinsic SSS had abnormally prolonged SACTs.[33] It is of importance to note that the studies discussed above used indirect methods for measuring SACT.

Breithardt and co-workers[58] correlated prolongation of SNRT and SACT with specific ECG abnormalities in patients with SSS. They found that patients with symptomatic sinus bradycardia had significantly longer values of SACT and SNRT in contrast to asymptomatic subjects. Patients with spontaneous sinoatrial block demonstrated longer SACT values, whereas those with the tachy-brady syndrome had longer SNRT values. They observed that SNRT was a more sensitive parameter; however, the use of SNRT and SACT increased the diagnostic sensitivity of electrophysiologic testing. We studied sinus node function in 148 patients, who ranged in age from 19 to 94 years. Group I comprised 71 patients with symptomatic SSS, group II comprised 10 patients with paroxysmal atrial fibrillation or flutter without the bradycardia component, group III comprised 17 patients with sinus bradycardia alone, and group IV comprised 50 patients in whom there was no evidence of sinus node dysfunction. Abnormal sinus node function was defined as the presence of an abnormally prolonged SNRTc and/or SACT. Abnormal sinus node function was noted in 81.6% of group I, 50% of group II, 47% of group III, and 12% of group IV patients. On the basis of our findings in group I and group IV, assessment of sinus node function by determination of SNRTc and SACT had a sensitivity of 82% and a specificity of 88%. Of additional interest is the finding that abnormal sinus node function is dependent on the patient population being studied. Thus, whereas the majority of symptomatic SSS patients with two or more ECG manifestations of SSS have abnormal sinus node function, sinus node function is less often abnormal (47% to 50%) in patients with sinus bradycardia alone or in those with paroxysmal atrial fibrillation-flutter without the bradycardia component.

DETERMINATION OF INTRINSIC HEART RATE AND SINUS NODE RECOVERY TIME FOLLOWING PHARMACOLOGIC AUTONOMIC BLOCKADE

Intrinsic heart rate (IHR) is determined following pharmacologic autonomic blockade with propranolol (0.2 mg/kg) and atropine sulfate (0.04 mg/kg). The maximum spontaneous sinus rate observed 5 minutes after autonomic blockade is the IHR. Normal values for IHR can be determined by using the linear regression equation derived by Jose relating predicted IHR to age.[59,60] Thus, predicted IHR = 118.1 − (0.57 × age). For subjects under 45 years of age, the 95% confidence limit is predicted IHR ± 18%, and for subjects older than 45 years of age the 95% confidence limit is predicted IHR ± 14%. An IHR falling within 2 standard deviations of the predicted IHR is considered normal, whereas an IHR falling below and outside the 95% confidence limit of predicted IHR is considered abnormal. The determination of IHR and SNRT prior to and following pharmacologic autonomic blockade can provide an insight into the understanding of the pathophysiologic mechanism of the SSS[30-33] and increase the sensitivity of the SNRT.[33] Patients with an abnormal IHR have intrinsic SSS, whereas those with a normal IHR have the extrinsic variety of SSS. A minority of patients with extrinsic SSS have an abnormal SNRT prior to autonomic blockade. We found that in these patients the SNRT normalizes following autonomic blockade. An example of such a patient is shown in Figure 47.4. Prior to autonomic blockade, the sinus rate ranged from 38 to 43 beats per minute. The longest SNRTc was obtained following overdrive pacing at a cycle length of 800 msec and was grossly abnormal (1580 msec). Following autonomic blockade, the intrinsic heart rate was normal and the SNRTc normalized (405 msec). This subgroup of patients classically represents sinus node dysfunction due to abnormally exaggerated parasympathetic tone. The majority of patients with intrinsic SSS have an abnormal SNRT prior to autonomic blockade. However, in a minority of patients with intrinsic SSS who have a normal

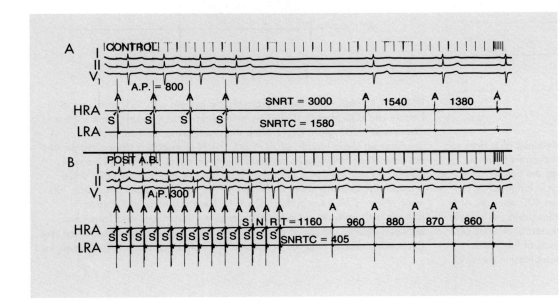

FIGURE 47.4 The measurement of SNRT in a patient with extrinsic SSS. From top to bottom are ECG leads I, II, and V₁ and intracardiac electrograms from the high right atrium (HRA) and low right atrium (LRA). **A.** During the control study the longest sinus nodal recovery time obtained after atrial pacing at a cycle length of 800 msec was 3000 msec. The calculated corrected SNRT was 1580 msec. **B.** After autonomic blockade the longest SNRT and corrected SNRT obtained after atrial pacing at a cycle length of 300 msec was 1160 msec and 405 msec, respectively. (Kang PS, Gomes JAC, El-Sherif N: Differential effects of functional autonomic blockade on the variables of sinus nodal automaticity in the sick sinus syndrome. Am J Cardiol 49:273, 1982)

SNRT prior to autonomic blockade the SNRT becomes abnormal only after autonomic blockade. An example of a tracing from such a patient is shown in Figure 47.5. The SNRTc was normal prior to autonomic blockade. Following autonomic blockade, the IHR was found to be abnormal. The longest SNRTc (602 msec) was also abnormal. Thus determination of SNRT following autonomic blockade increases the sensitivity of SNRT in patients with intrinsic SSS. Similar observations were also reported by Desai and co-workers.[31]

DIRECT RECORDINGS OF SINUS NODE POTENTIALS IN HUMANS

In 1978, Cramer and colleagues[61] reported successful recordings of sinus node potentials in a beating dog heart using hand-held probes and conventional catheters. In 1980, Hariman and associates[62] extended these methods to humans and described a catheter technique to record sinus node potentials. Later, Reifel and co-workers[63] and Gomes and associates[55] described modifications of the catheter technique that ensured either a higher success rate and/or stable sinus node electrograms free of baseline drifts. To record a sinus node electrogram, a No. 6 F quadripolar catheter with 10-mm interelectrode distance is inserted via the femoral vein and positioned at the junction of the superior vena cava and right atrial endocardium. The distal poles of the catheter are used for recording a sinus node electrogram using low-pass filter frequencies of 0.1 Hz to 50 Hz and high-gain amplification of 50 μV to 100 μV/cm. The proximal poles of the catheter are used for recording a high right atrial electrogram. We have found that close contact of the distal pole of the catheter with the atrial endocardium overlying the area of the sinus node ensures a higher success rate (86%) of recording a sinus node electrogram free of baseline drifts.[55] The sinus node electrogram is characterized by the presence of a diastolic slope and an upstroke slope that follows the T-U baseline and precedes the P wave and the high right atrial electrogram (Fig. 47.6).

Recordings of a sinus node electrogram have been used to measure the direct SACT, direct SNRT, and shifts in sinus pacemaker complex occurring spontaneously and following several interventions. Although at present it still remains unclear whether recording of sinus node electrograms will improve the diagnostic sensitivity of electrophysiologic tests, it has already had considerable impact in our understanding of the physiology and pathophysiology of the human sinus node.

On the sinus node electrogram, direct SACT is measured from the onset of the upstroke slope to the onset of the atrial activation on the sinus node electrogram or high right atrial electrogram, whichever comes first (see Fig. 47.6). Gomes and colleagues[55] have reported normal values of 50 msec to 112 msec, and Reifel and associates[63] reported normal values of 46 msec to 116 msec. In patients with SSS, Gomes and colleagues[55] found significantly longer direct SACT values when compared with subjects without SSS. Sinus node electrograms have also been used to assess direct SNRT (Fig. 47.7). These studies have found that (1) direct SNRT is significantly longer in patients with SSS (1263 ± 256 msec) when compared with patients without SSS (779 ± 89 msec)[12]; however further studies are needed to better quantify an abnormal direct SNRT in humans; (2) SACT is prolonged following overdrive atrial pacing both in patients with and without SSS, but the degree of prolongation is greater in patients with SSS; and (3) prolongation of indirect SNRT in patients with SSS is accounted for in the majority of instances by prolongation of SACT for the first post-pacing sinus beat (Fig. 47.8).

Asseman and associates[12] recorded sinus node electrograms in eight patients with SSS who had SNRTc of more than 1500 msec. They found persistent sinus nodal electrical activity during long atrial pauses following overdrive atrial pacing. They suggested that these pauses were the result of sinoatrial conduction block rather than depression of sinus nodal automaticity. Thus our studies[13] and those of Asseman and associates[12] suggest that although patients with SSS are likely to have

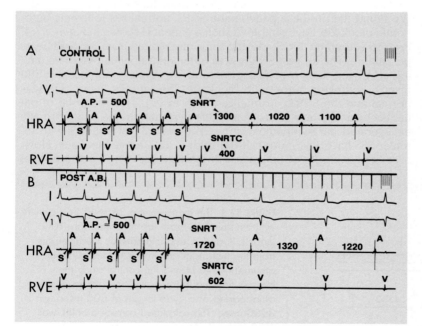

FIGURE 47.5 The measurement of SNRT in a patient with intrinsic SSS. From top to bottom are ECG leads I and V_1 and intracardiac electrograms from the high right atrium (HRA) and right ventricle (RVE). **A.** During the control study the longest SNRT obtained after atrial pacing (S) at a cycle length of 500 msec was 1300 msec. The calculated corrected SNRT was 400 msec. **B.** After autonomic blockade the longest SNRT obtained after atrial pacing at a cycle length of 500 msec was 1720 msec. The calculated corrected SNRT was 602 msec. (Kang PS, Gomes JAC, El-Sherif N: Differential effects of functional autonomic blockade on the variables of sinus nodal automaticity in the sick sinus syndrome. Am J Cardiol 49:273, 1982)

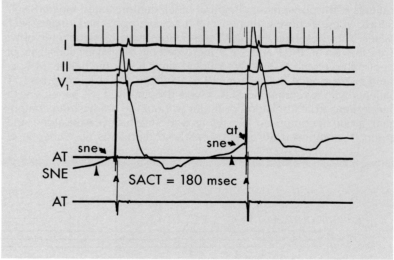

FIGURE 47.6 Sinus node electrogram from a patient with SSS. From top to bottom are ECG leads I, II, and V_1, intracardiac atrial electrograms (AT), and sinus node electrogram (SNE). Note the presence of marked sinus bradycardia (cycle length, 1800 msec). The SNE reveals a clear diastolic and upstroke slope followed by an atrial injury potential. The direct sinoatrial conduction time (SACT) is measured from the onset of the upstroke slope (straight arrow) to the atrial electrogram. The average direct SACT was 180 msec. (Gomes JAC, Kang PS, El-Sherif N: The sinus node electrogram in patients with and without sick sinus syndrome: Techniques and correlation between directly measured and indirectly estimated sinoatrial conduction time. Circulation 66:864, 1982, by permission of the American Heart Association, Inc.)

abnormalities of sinus nodal automaticity and sinoatrial conduction, abnormalities of conduction could be clinically more significant than those of automaticity. Studies in a large number of patients with different ECG manifestations of the SSS are needed before these questions can be conclusively answered.

SINUS NODE REFRACTORINESS

Kerr and Strauss[64] have assessed sinus nodal refractoriness in humans by defining the transition between the zone of reset and the zone of interpolation. They found a significant difference in sinus nodal refractoriness between normal subjects (250 msec to 350 msec) and patients with SSS (500 msec to 550 msec). However, the role of sinus node refractoriness relative to other well-established electrophysiologic tests in the diagnosis and treatment of patients with suspected SSS remains to be established.

INDICATIONS FOR ELECTROPHYSIOLOGIC TESTING OF SINUS NODE FUNCTION

The clinical approach to the patient with suspected SSS is shown in Figure 47.9. The SSS is a clinical diagnosis based on history, ECG findings, and 24-hour ambulatory Holter recordings. Thus in patients in whom a cause-and-effect relationship has been noted between ECG abnormalities and symptoms, pacemaker therapy is recommended. In these patients, electrophysiologic studies are confirmatory of the diagnosis if abnormal; however, they do not influence decision making regarding the need for pacemaker therapy if normal. If in the future it is

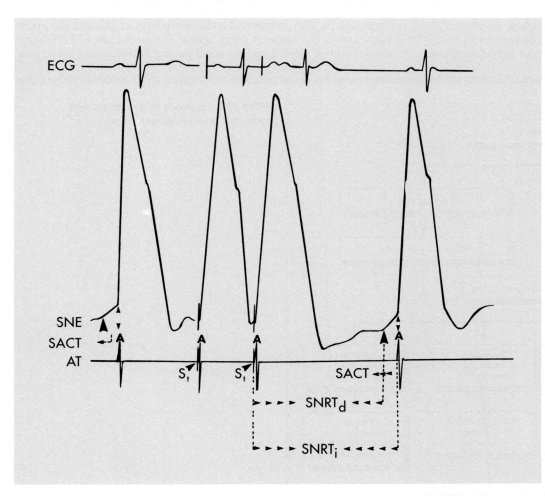

FIGURE 47.7 The measurement of SNRT and sinoatrial conduction time. From top to bottom are the electrocardiogram (*ECG*), sinus node electrogram (*SNE*), and atrial electrogram (*AT*). Sinoatrial conduction time (*SACT*) for sinus beats before and after pacing was measured from the onset of the upstroke slope to the onset of the atrial deflection (*A*). After overdrive pacing, the SNRTd was measured from the stimulus artifact (S_t) to the onset of the upstroke slope on the SNE. The SNRTi was measured from the onset of the stimulus artifact (S_t) to the atrial deflection (*A*). (Gomes JAC, Hariman RI, Chowdry IA: New application of direct sinus node recordings in man: Assessment of sinus node recovery time. Circulation 70:663, 1984, by permission of the American Heart Association, Inc.)

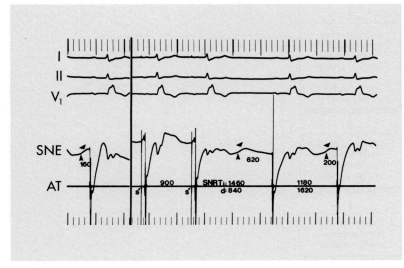

FIGURE 47.8 The measurement of SNRT in a patient with SSS. From top to bottom are ECG leads I, II, and V_1, sinus node electrogram (*SNE*), and atrial electrogram (*AT*). **Left.** A sinus beat before pacing. Note that the sinoatrial conduction time is abnormally prolonged (160 msec). **Right.** After overdrive pacing at a cycle length of 900 msec, the SNRT is 1460 msec and the SNRTd is 840 msec. Note the marked prolongation of conduction time (620 msec) for the first postpacing beat; for the second postpacing beat it shortens to 200 msec. (Gomes JAC, Hariman RI, Chowdry IA: New application of direct sinus node recordings in man: Assessment of sinus node recovery time. Circulation 70:663, 1984, by permission of the American Heart Association, Inc.)

shown that patients with extrinsic SSS, the majority of whom have a normal SNRTc, have a benign prognosis without pacemaker therapy, then the determination of IHR and SNRT may be of value in these patients. However, at this time this approach does not seem to be warranted.

Assessment of sinus node function may be helpful in the following groups of patients:

1. Patients with suspected SSS who have symptoms related to cerebral hypoperfusion such as syncope that are not documented on a 24-hour Holter recording. If an abnormally prolonged SNRT or SNRTc is found in such patients in the absence of any other cause for the symptoms, then permanent pacing is justified. A similar view was expressed by Gann and associates[65] in a long-term follow-up study of the value of SNRT in elderly patients with sinus bradycardia. However, it is important to note that the degree of SNRT prolongation as a guide to pacemaker therapy remains controversial. Gann and associates recommended pacing if the SNRTc was greater than or equal to 525 msec. The studies of Scheinman and co-workers[66] suggest that an SNRT of greater than or equal to 2 seconds is a probable indication for pacing. When only SACT is prolonged in such patients and SNRT is normal, the administration of atropine or pharmacologic autonomic blockade may uncover an abnormal SNRT.
2. Patients with suspected SSS who manifest normal sinus rhythm during asymptomatic periods. If sinus node function studies in these patients are normal, they should undergo pharmacologic autonomic blockade since occasionally abnormalities may be uncovered following the latter.
3. Patients who develop sinus node dysfunction on relatively small dosages of cardioactive drugs, such as digitalis glycosides, β-adrenergic blockers, verapamil, disopyramide, and quinidine.
4. Patients with asymptomatic sinus node dysfunction (*e.g.*, paroxysmal atrial fibrillation/flutter) who require drugs that may unmask or aggravate underlying SSS. An example of such a patient is shown in Figure 47.10. The patient had atrial flutter with a history of recurrent palpitations but without dizzy spells and/or syncope. Following conversion of atrial flutter by atrial pacing, the longest SNRTc was

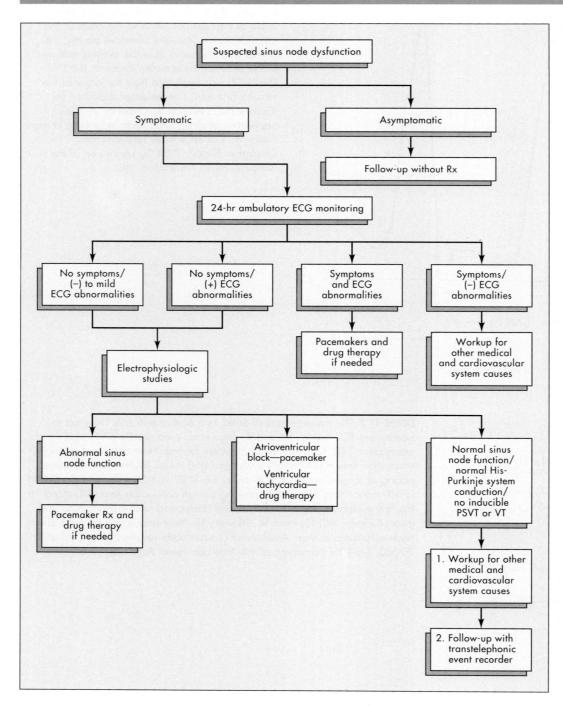

FIGURE 47.9 Approach to the patient with suspected sinus node dysfunction.

normal (300 msec). Following therapy with digoxin and quinidine the patient developed sinus bradycardia, sinus pauses, and dizzy spells. A repeat SNRT obtained after quinidine alone revealed a markedly abnormal SNRTc of 2000 msec.

5. Patients with suspected SSS with bundle branch block or bifascicular block. These patients should have evaluation of atrioventricular nodal and His-Purkinje system conduction since in such patients symptoms may be related to intermittent complete heart block. In addition, evaluation of atrioventricular nodal and His-Purkinje conduction should be performed in those patients in whom permanent atrial pacing is contemplated as the modality of therapy. Similarly, occasionally SSS may coexist with ventricular arrhythmias. In such patients, symptoms of syncope may be related to ventricular tachycardia rather than manifestation of SSS. If ventricular tachycardia is suspected, the patients should undergo programmed ventricular stimulation in addition to assessment of sinus node function.

THERAPY

No therapy is indicated for asymptomatic patients with ECG manifestations of sinus node dysfunction. Antiarrhythmic agents to suppress tachyarrhythmias such as paroxysmal atrial fibrillation and/or flutter in asymptomatic subjects should be used, with extreme caution since these agents have the propensity of compounding the bradyarrhythmia. The use of anticoagulants is justified in patients with tachy-brady syndrome if the tachycardia component is atrial fibrillation. Rubenstein and associates[67] noted a 24% incidence of peripheral emboli in patients with tachy-brady syndrome. Similarly, Fairfax and co-workers[68] found that embolic episodes occurred more frequently in patients with the tachy-brady syndrome who were over 50 years of age.

Medical management of bradyarrhythmias in SSS with atropine, belladonna alkaloids, and sympathomimetic agents has been tried, with dissappointing results.[67,69-71] However, Weiss and colleagues[72] reported amelioration of symptoms and a 20% or greater increase in heart rate with chronic hydralazine therapy in approximately 50% and 75% of normotensive and hypertensive patients, respectively, with symptomatic sinus bradycardia. Engel and associates[73] reported the effects of intravenous hydralazine, 0.15 mg/kg, in nine hypertensive patients with sinoatrial dysfunction. They found that although this dose of hydralazine caused no significant reduction in arterial blood pressure, it caused a significant increase in heart rate and a significant decrease in SNRT and junctional escape time. Thus the results of these studies would suggest that hydralazine may be useful in hypertensive as well as normotensive patients with sinus node dysfunction. However, long-term randomized studies are needed in a large number of patients before any conclusions can be drawn about the effectiveness of this agent. Benditt and co-workers[74] assessed the acute electrophysiologic effects of intravenous theophylline and clinical effects of chronic oral theophylline in ten young patients with symptoms of syncope and dizziness attributed to transient bradyarrhythmias, which included sinus pauses, marked sinus bradycardia, or atrioventricular block. Intravenous theophylline shortened sinus cycle length, sinoatrial conduction time, and SNRT. Chronic oral theophylline in a dose of 200 mg to 400 mg twice a day resulted in suppression of symptoms in six of eight patients over a 5- to 24-month follow-up. The authors suggested that theophylline treatment may be a useful therapeutic consideration in some patients with symptomatic bradycardia. Although it is unlikely that patients with intrinsic SSS with syncopal episodes will respond to agents such as hydralazine, atropine, theophylline, and sympathomimetic drugs, cautious use of these agents in mildly symptomatic patients, in those with dizzy spells alone, and in patients wth the extrinsic variety of SSS due to autonomic dysfunction seems justified. However,

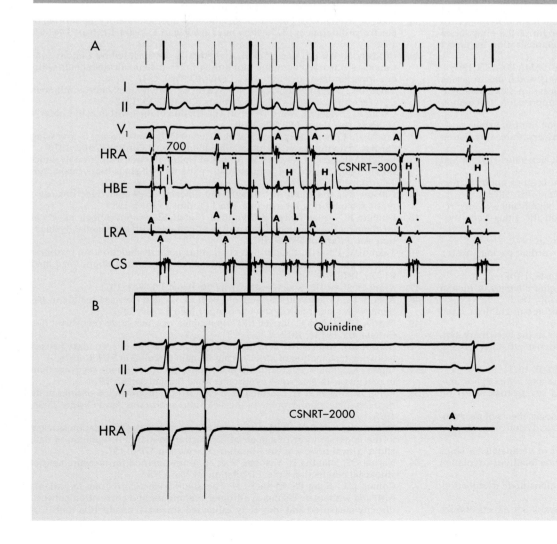

FIGURE 47.10 The measurement of SNRT during control (**A**) and following quinidine (**B**) in a patient with paroxysmal atrial flutter. From top to bottom are ECG leads I, II, and V_1 and intracardiac electrograms from the high right atrium (*HRA*), His bundle (*HBE*), low right atrium (*LRA*), and coronary sinus (*CS*). See text for further explanation.

it is important to note that only long-term prospective studies in a large number of patients can establish the role, if any, of these agents in the management of patients with sinus node dysfunction.

Permanent pacing remains the definitive treatment for symptomatic patients with SSS. Pacing can abolish the symptoms resulting from the bradycardia component and allow treatment of tachyarrhythmias with antiarrhythmic agents that otherwise have the propensity of aggravating the bradyarrhythmias. Ventricular demand (VVI), dual-chamber pacemakers, and atrial demand pacemakers (AAI) have been used in patients with SSS. The previous objections to atrial pacing such as perforation and dislodgement are no longer valid with the advent of new atrial leads and sophisticated atrial pulse generators. Therefore, AAI pacemakers are favored in the absence of atrioventricular conduction disease.[75,76] Furthermore, these pacemakers can increase cardiac output by preserving atrial contraction, which is of benefit to patients with left ventricular dysfunction. In addition, AAI pacing has the potential of decreasing the frequency of tachyarrhythmias, although results have not been promising. In patients with left ventricular dysfunction and atrioventricular conduction abnormalities, dual-chamber pacing is recommended. This form of pacing has also been shown to be superior to VVI pacing in patients with hypersensitive carotid sinus syndrome with a vasodepressor component.

REFERENCES

1. Keith A, Flack MW: The form and nature of the muscular connections between the primary divisions of the vertebrate heart. J Anat Physiol 41:172, 1907
2. Hudson REB: The human pacemaker and its pathology. Br Heart J 22:153, 1960
3. James TN: Anatomy of the human sinus node. Anat Rec 141:109, 1961
4. James TN, Sherf L, Fine G et al: Comparative ultrastructure of the sinus node in man and dog. Circulation 34:139, 1966
5. Becker AE: Relation between structure and function of the sinus node: General comments. In Bonke FIM (ed): The Sinus Node: Structure, Function and Clinical Relevance, p 212. The Hague, Martinus Nijhoff, 1978
6. Meck WJ, Eyster JAE: The effect of vagal stimulation and of cooling on the location of the pacemaker within the sinoauricular node. Am J Physiol 34:368, 1914
7. Bouman LN, Gerlings ED, Biersteker PA et al: Pacemaker shift in the sinoatrial node during vagal stimulation. Pflugers Arch 302:255, 1968
8. Lipsius SL, Vassalle M: Characterization of a two-component upstroke in the sinus node subsidiary pacemakers. In Bonke FIM (ed): The Sinus Node: Structure, Function and Clinical Relevance, p 233. The Hague, Martinus Nijhoff, 1978
9. Boineau JP, Schessler RB, Mooney CR et al: Multicentric origin of the atrial depolarization wave: The pacemaker complex: Relation to dynamics of atrial conduction, P wave changes and heart rate control. Circulation 58:1036, 1978
10. Gomes JA, Arora R, Novak H et al: Multicentric origin of the sinus node pacemaker complex in the intact human heart: Demonstration by direct sinus node recordings. J Am Coll Cardiol 5:496, 1985
11. Ferrer MI: The sick sinus syndrome in atrial disease. JAMA 206:645, 1968
12. Asseman P, Bergin B, Desry D et al: Persistent sinus nodal electrograms during abnormally prolonged post-pacing atrial pauses in sick sinus syndrome in humans: Sinoatrial block vs. overdrive suppression. Circulation 68:33, 1983
13. Gomes JAC, Hariman RI, Chowdry IA: New application of direct sinus node recordings in man: Assessment of sinus node recovery time. Circulation 70:663, 1984
14. Gomes JAC, Kang PS, Gough W et al: Coexistence of sick sinus rhythm and atrial flutter-fibrillation. Circulation 63:80, 1981
15. Mandel WJ, Hayakawa H, Allen HN et al: Assessment of sinus node function in patients with the sick sinus syndrome. Circulation 46:761, 1972
16. Thorman J, Schwarz F, Ensslen R et al: Vagal tone, significance of electrophysiological findings and clinical course in symptomatic sinus node dysfunction. Am Heart J 95:725, 1978
17. Ferrer MI: The sick sinus syndrome. Circulation 47:635, 1973
18. Parsonnet V, Crawford C: United States survey on cardiac pacing (abstr). PACE 6:A21, 1983
19. Scarpa W: The sick sinus syndrome. Am Heart J 92:648, 1976
20. Davies MJ, Pomerance A: Quantitative study of ageing changes in human sinoatrial node and internodal tracts. Br Heart J 34:150, 1972
21. Scott O, Macartney FJ, Deverall PB: Sick sinus syndrome in children. Arch Dis Child 51:100, 1976
22. Philips J, Tchinose H: Clinical and pathologic studies in the hereditary syndrome of a long QT interval, syncopal spells and sudden death. Chest 58:326, 1970
23. Spellberg RD: Familial sinus node disease. Chest 60:246, 1971
24. Margolis R, Strauss JC, Miller HC: Digitalis and the sick sinus syndrome: Clinical and electrophysiologic documentation of a severe toxic effect on sinus node function. Circulation 52:162, 1975
25. Strauss H, Gilbert M, Svenson R et al: Electrophysiologic effects of propranolol on sinus node function in patients with sinus node dysfunction. Circulation 54:452, 1976
26. Breithardt G, Seipel L, Wueburghaus E et al: Effect of verapamil on sinus node in patients with normal and abnormal sinus node function. Circulation 54:II-19, 1976
27. Colon AH, Ticzon AR, Akhtar M et al: Quinidine in sinus node dysfunction. Circulation 54:II-231, 1978
28. Le Barre A, Strauss H, Scheinman M et al: Electrophysiologic effects of disopyramide phosphate on sinus node function in patients with sinus node dysfunction. Circulation 59:226, 1979
29. Kim H, Friedman H: Procainamide-induced sinus node dysfunction in patients with chronic renal failure. Chest 76:699, 1979
30. Jordan JL, Yamaguchi I, Mandel WJ: Studies on the mechanism of sinus node dysfunction in the sick sinus syndrome. Circulation 57:217, 1977
31. Desai J, Scheinman MM, Strauss HC et al: Electrophysiologic effects of combined autonomic blockade in patients with sinus node disease. Circulation 63:953, 1981
32. Kang PS, Gomes JAC, Kelen G et al: Role of autonomic regulatory mechanisms in sinoatrial conduction and sinus node automaticity in the sick sinus syndrome. Circulation 64:832, 1981
33. Kang PS, Gomes JAC, El-Sherif N: Differential effects of functional autonomic blockade on the variables of sinus nodal automaticity in the sick sinus syndrome. Am J Cardiol 49:273, 1982
34. Rossi L: Histopathologic Features of Cardiac Arrhythmias. Milan, Casa Editrice Ambrosiana, 1969
35. Yamaguchi I, Kurusn T, Togo T et al: Follow-up study of patients with sinoatrial block by pharmacologic total autonomic blockade. Circulation 70:II-416, 1984
36. Lien WP, Lee YS, Cheng FZ et al: The sick sinus syndrome: Natural history of dysfunction of the sinoatrial node. Chest 72:628, 1977
37. Southall DP, Richards J, Mitchell P et al: Study of cardiac rhythm in healthy newborn infants. Br Heart J 43:74, 1980
38. Scott O, Williams GJ, Fiddler GI: Results of 24 hour ambulatory monitoring of electrocardiogram in 131 healthy boys aged 10 to 13 years. Br Heart J 44:304, 1980
39. Brodsky M, Wu D, Denes P et al: Arrhythmias documented by 24-hour continuous electrocardiographic monitoring in 50 male medical students without apparent heart disease. Am J Cardiol 39:390, 1977
40. Talan DA, Bauernfeind RA, Ashley WW et al: Twenty-four-hour continuous ECG recording in long-distance runners. Chest 82:19, 1982
41. Camm AJ, Evans KE, Ward DE et al: The rhythm of the heart in active elderly subjects. Am Heart J 99:598, 1980
42. Lipski JA, Cohen L, Espinoza J et al: Value of Holter monitoring in assessing cardiac arrhythmias in symptomatic patients. Am J Cardiol 37:102, 1976
43. Reifel JA, Bigger JT, Cramer M: Ability of Holter electrocardiogram dysfunction in symptomatic and asymptomatic patients with sinus bradycardia. Am J Cardiol 40:189, 1977
44. Gibson TC, Heitzman MR: Diagnostic efficacy of 24-hour electrocardiographic monitoring for syncope. Am J Cardiol 53:1013, 1984
45. Dhingra RC, Amat-Y-Leon F, Wyndham C et al: Electrophysiologic effects of atropine on the sinus node and atrium in patients with sinus nodal dysfunction. Am J Cardiol 38:848, 1976
46. Talano JV, Enler D, Randall WC et al: Sinus node dysfunction: An overview with emphasis on autonomic and pharmacologic consideration. Am J Med 64:773, 1978
47. Grant D, Shaw DB: Sinus bradycardia. Br Heart J 33:742, 1971
48. Abbott JA, Hirschheld DS, Kunkel FW et al: Graded exercise testing in patients with sinus node dysfunction. Am J Med 62:330, 1977
49. Narula OS, Samet P, Jarrier RP: Significance of sinus node recovery time. Circulation 45:140, 1972
50. Berditt DG, Strauss HC, Scheinman MM et al: Analysis of secondary pauses following termination of atrial pacing in man. Circulation 54:436, 1976
51. Gupta PK, Lichtein E, Chadda KD et al: Appraisal of sinus node recovery time in patients with sick sinus syndrome. Am J Cardiol 34:265, 1974
52. Reifel JA, Bigger JT Jr, Giardina EGV: Paradoxical prolongation of sinus node recovery time after atropine in the sick sinus syndrome. Am J Cardiol 36:98, 1975
53. Strauss HC, Saroff AL, Bigger JT Jr et al: Premature atrial stimulation as a key to the understanding of sinoatrial conduction in man: Presentation of data and a critical review of the literature. Circulation 47:86, 1973
54. Narula OS, Shantha N, Vasquez M et al: A new method for measurement of sinoatrial conduction time. Circulation 58:706, 1978
55. Gomes JAC, Kang PS, El-Sherif N: The sinus node electrogram in patients with and without sick sinus syndrome: Techniques and correlation between directly measured and indirectly estimated sinoatrial conduction time. Cir-

56. Dhingra RC, Amat-Y-Leon F, Wyndham C et al: Clinical significance of prolonged sinoatrial conduction time. Circulation 55:8, 1977
57. Strauss HC, Bigger JT Jr, Saroff AL et al: Electrophysiologic evaluation of sinus node function in patients with sinus node dysfunction. Circulation 53:763, 1976
58. Breithardt G, Seipel L, Loogen F: Sinus node recovery time and calculated sinoatrial conduction time in normal subjects and patients with sinus node dysfunction. Circulation 56:43, 1977
59. Jose AD: Effect of combined sympathetic and parasympathetic blockade on heart rate and cardiac function in man. Am J Cardiol 18:476, 1966
60. Jose AD, Collison D: The normal range and determinants of the intrinsic heart rate in man. Cardiovasc Res 4:160, 1970
61. Cramer M, Siegal M, Bigger JT Jr et al: Electrograms from the canine sinoatrial pacemaker recorded *in vitro* and *in situ*. Am J Cardiol 42:939, 1978
62. Hariman RJ, Krongrad E, Boxer RA et al: Method for recording electrical activity of the sinoatrial node and automatic atrial foci during cardiac catheterization in human subjects. Am J Cardiol 45:755, 1980
63. Reifel JA, Gang E, Glicklich J et al: The human sinus node electrogram: A transvenous catheter technique and a comparison of directly measured and indirectly estimated sinoatrial conduction time in adults. Circulation 62:1324, 1980
64. Kerr CR, Strauss HC: The measurement of sinus node refractoriness in man. Circulation 68:1231, 1983
65. Gann D, Tolentino A, Samet P: Electrophysiologic evaluation of elderly patients with sinus bradycardia: A long-term follow up study. Ann Intern Med 90:24, 1979
66. Scheinman MM, Strauss HC, Abbott JA: Electrophysiologic testing for patients with sinus node dysfunction. J Electrocardiol 12:211, 1979
67. Rubenstein JJ, Schulman CL, Yurchak PM et al: Clinical spectrum of sick sinus syndrome. Circulation 46:5, 1972
68. Fairfax AJ, Lambert CD, Leatham A: Systemic embolism in chronic sinoatrial disorder. N Engl J Med 295:190, 1976
69. Wan SH, Lee GS, Toh CCS: The sick sinus syndrome: A study of 15 cases. Br Heart J 34:942, 1972
70. Sigurd B, Jensen G, Meibom J et al: Adams-Stokes syndrome caused by sinoatrial block. Br Heart J 35:1002, 1973
71. Kulbertus HE, de Leval-Rutten F, Demoulin JC: Sinoatrial disease: A report on 13 cases. J Electrocardiol 6:303, 1973
72. Weiss AT, Rod JL, Gotsman MS et al: Hydralazine in the management of symptomatic sinus bradycardia. Eur J Cardiol 12:261, 1981
73. Engel TR, Leady C, Gonzalez AD et al: Electrophysiologic effects of hydralazine on sinoatrial function in patients with sick sinus syndrome. Am J Cardiol 41:763, 1978
74. Benditt DG, Benson DW Jr, Kreitt J et al: Electrophysiologic effects of theophylline in young patients with recurrent symptomatic bradyarrhythmias. Am J Cardiol 52:1223, 1983
75. Hayes DL, Furman S: Stability of AV conduction in sick sinus node syndrome patients with implanted atrial pacemakers. Am Heart J 107:644, 1985
76. Gilette PC, Wampler DG, Shannon C et al: Use of atrial pacing in a young population. PACE 8:94, 1985

BUNDLE BRANCH BLOCK AND ATRIOVENTRICULAR CONDUCTION DISORDERS

CHAPTER 48
VOLUME 1

Robert W. Peters ▪ *Melvin M. Scheinman*

The advent of implantable permanent pacemakers in the early 1960s provided, for the first time, effective therapy for patients with serious conduction system disorders. It is clear that permanent pacing is not required for all patients with transient neurologic symptoms and electrocardiographic (ECG) evidence of conduction system disease, since many have a benign course while in others symptoms are due to other causes. Newer techniques, such as intracardiac recording and stimulation, have allowed for more complete evaluation of disorders of atrioventricular (AV) conduction. In this chapter, we will review some of the fundamental concepts of the anatomy, histopathology, and physiology of the conduction system; the natural history of various types of conduction disorders; and the diagnostic and therapeutic modalities available to the clinician in dealing with patients with conduction system disease.

FUNCTIONAL ANATOMY OF THE LOWER CONDUCTION SYSTEM
AV NODE

In the human embryo, the AV node originates during the third and fourth weeks of gestation. It develops independently from the His bundle, from which it initially is separated by fibrous connective tissue coming from the primitive AV ring. In the normally developed heart, the atria and ventricles are connected by specialized structures, the AV node and bundle of His, which are located in the inferior border of the atrial septum (Fig. 48.1). As suggested by Puech and Wainwright, the phylogenetic separation of atria from ventricles can be considered a protective adaptation, preventing very rapid rates emanating from the atrium from being transmitted to the ventricles.[1] The atria are connected to the AV node by tracts that course through the atrial walls and septum. These tracts are composed in part of Purkinje tissue but are not insulated by fibrous tissue from surrounding atrial myocardium. The functional significance of these tracts remains controversial. Although their clinical significance is still open to question, stimulation or blockade of these fiber tracts can be shown to alter P wave morphology.

The AV node is a small ($7 \times 4 \times 1$ mm) ovoid structure located within the interatrial septum between the right atrial subendocardium and the central fibrous body of the heart. The central AV node is almost completely enclosed by the central fibrous body. The approaches to the node consist of two limbs extending toward the septal leaflet of the tricuspid valve and the mitral annulus, respectively. This relationship determines the electrical input into the AV nodal apparatus. The AV node is composed of a loose framework of collagen interspersed with small starlike P cells, Purkinje cells, ordinary "working" myocardial cells, and transitional cells extending from the atrium. The exact mechanism by which this grouping of diverse cells manages to conduct impulses has not been explained. The AV node has an abundant blood supply, mostly from the AV nodal artery, which originates from the distal right coronary artery in 90% of subjects and which also supplies part of the proximal His bundle. There is also extensive innervation of the area, with numerous autonomic ganglia found in the area between the AV node and coronary sinus. On the basis of both morphologic as well as functional differences, the node is divided into three regions: (1) the atrionodal portion, (2) the compact node, and (3) the nodohisian portion.

HIS BUNDLE

The common bundle consists of a parallel band of Purkinje fibers that converge from the AV node at a point that is morphologically ill defined to form a distinct bundle 1 mm to 2 mm wide. The His bundle penetrates the central fibrous body and descends through the membranous septum, usually along the left side, to the crest of the muscular septum, where it divides into the bundle branches. The division varies considerably, making it difficult to determine precisely where the His bundle ends and the bundle branches begin. Histologically, the His bundle consists of parallel strands of Purkinje fibers divided by a collagenous framework into separate compartments that are incompletely linked by relatively few fibrous septa. P cells are embedded in the collagen, particularly in the proximal portion of the His bundle. Although there is considerable variation in blood supply, there is usually a dual source to the area from branches of both the AV nodal and the left anterior descending coronary arteries.

BUNDLE BRANCHES

The right bundle branch (RBB) is a slender group of parallel Purkinje fibers that may appear as a direct continuation of the common bundle (when the His bundle is located in the right side of the septum) or, more commonly, may originate at an obtuse angle. In almost all cases, the RBB remains a slender unbranched structure until it reaches the base of the anterior papillary muscle, where it trifurcates into anterior, posterior, and lateral branches that terminate in the subendocardial Purkinje network of the free wall and lower septum. The left bundle branch (LBB) has a much more variable origin. Its initial portion may be either wide or narrow, but it eventually spreads out, fanlike, to all parts of the left ventricle with frequent anastomoses between its numerous branches. Since the classic description of Rosenbaum and others of the trifascicular nature of the specialized ventricular conduction system, there has been considerable debate about the configuration of the LBB and its divisions. Certainly the trifascicular or even quadrafascicular arrangement, as others have claimed, is a simplification of an immensely complex grouping of Purkinje fibers. However, at least in some hearts, there is a very broad anterior portion of the LBB that crosses the left ventricular outflow tract toward the anterior papillary muscle. A thicker, shorter tract of fibers, which may originate before the separation of the RBB, extends across the posterior aspect of the septum toward the posterior papillary muscle while a third discrete group of fibers is distributed to the septum itself. At autopsy, Demoulin and colleagues were able to identify separate and posterior divisions of the LBB in a large group of hearts and could also find a septal division in most of them.[2] In contrast, Massing and James were unable to identify separate fascicles in any of the hearts that they analyzed.[3]

There is considerable variation in the blood supply to the bundle branches, and anastomoses are abundant. In general, there is a dual supply to most of the septum from the AV nodal artery and septal branches of the left anterior descending coronary artery. Additional blood may be provided by Kugel's artery, septal branches of the posterior descending coronary artery, atrial arteries, and others. Only the anterior aspect of the LBB receives its predominant supply from septal branches of the left anterior descending coronary artery.

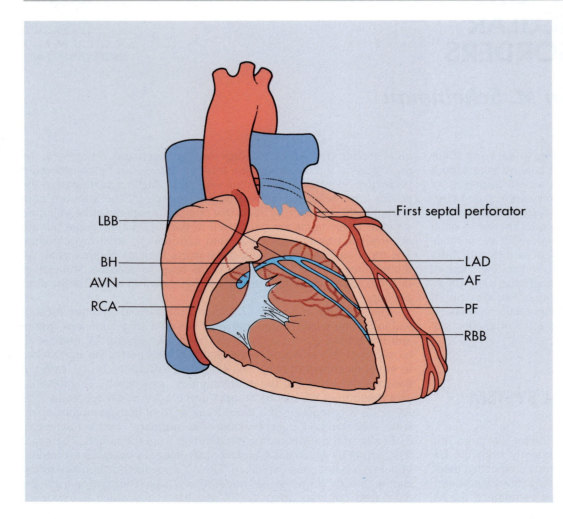

FIGURE 48.1 A schematic diagram of the anatomy and arterial blood supply of the lower conduction system. (AVN, atrioventricular node; BH, bundle of His; RBB, right bundle branch; LBB, left bundle branch; AF, anterior fascicle; PF, posterior fascicle; RCA, right coronary artery; LAD, left anterior descending coronary artery) (Modified from Peters RW et al: Bundle branch block: Anatomic, electrophysiologic and clinical correlates. Cardiology Update. New York: Elsevier Science Publishing Co., 1983.)

HISTOPATHOLOGY OF THE SPECIALIZED VENTRICULAR CONDUCTION SYSTEM

AV BLOCK

Because of the extensive network of fiber tracts entering the AV node from the atria and the ample blood supply of the area, high-grade AV nodal block is relatively uncommon. Congenital AV nodal block may be related to failure of fusion of the embryologically distinct primordia of the AV node and His bundle. Acquired AV nodal disease may be iatrogenic (surgical); traumatic; secondary to a variety of pathologic processes, including ischemic heart disease, neoplasms (i.e., mesotheliomas), infection, and infiltrative conditions such as amyloidosis; or due to a nonspecific sclerodegenerative process in individuals without demonstrable cardiac disease. Congenital AV block involving the His-Purkinje system (infranodal) is unusual and generally occurs in individuals with structural congenital heart disease (i.e., transposition of the great vessels). Acquired infranodal block is usually due to either degenerative or ischemic disease. Although the majority of patients with infranodal block have some clinical evidence of underlying organic heart disease, this may be an age-related, rather than a cause-and-effect, phenomenon.

PATHOLOGIC FINDINGS IN THE AV JUNCTION

The ECG provides only rough localization of the site of AV block. For example, Bharati and co-workers report two cases of chronic second-degree AV block in patients with LBB block, one of which had typical type I while the other had type II AV block.[4] In both cases, there was severe fibrosis of the AV node and both bundle branches. Ohkawa and associates describe an autopsy study of nine patients with complete AV block.[5] They found that while all five of the patients with wide QRS escape rhythms had severe bundle branch involvement, in three of the patients with narrow QRS escape rhythms the major histologic lesion was at or beyond the branching portion of the His bundle. Thus, AV block associated with narrow complex escape rhythm may actually be due to disease within the His bundle. In another report, Ohkawa and associates also found that lesions in the branching portion of the His bundle may produce complete heart block with either a wide or a narrow complex escape rhythm, depending primarily on the extent of disease in the adjacent bundle branches.[6] Rossi, in a review of the pathologic basis of cardiac arrhythmias, cites evidence that wide QRS complexes may arise from lesions in the junctional area.[7] These and other observations suggest segregation of fibers within the His bundle and with loss of transverse connections preferential ventricular conduction may be possible. Conceivably, lesions within the His bundle may result in an ECG pattern of bundle branch block. Hunt and co-workers reported on seven patients dying of acute myocardial infarction associated with AV block.[8] In the three patients with inferior wall myocardial infarction and narrow complex escape rhythms, there were ischemic changes in the AV node in two and in the distal conduction system in all three. The correlation between the histopathology and the ECG was better in the four patients dying of anteroseptal myocardial infarction where extensive infranodal disease was found in all.

PATHOLOGY OF BUNDLE BRANCH BLOCK

The pathologic processes associated with bundle branch block (BBB) are much the same as those associated with AV block, with ischemic heart disease and primary sclerodegenerative changes comprising the bulk of cases. As with AV block, diffuse disease is the rule, making it difficult to use the ECG pattern to predict the extent of the pathologic changes. Becker and associates described 22 patients developing BBB during acute myocardial infarction and found most of the pathologic changes to be located in the proximal bundle branches.[9] Necrosis was infrequent; hydropic swelling, probably indicative of ischemia, was the predominant histologic change. Lev and co-workers report pathologic findings in eight patients with LBBB, six of whom had marked left axis deviation.[10] In all cases, the major pathology was at the origin of the LBB but no differences were noted between those with normal frontal plane QRS axes and those with left axis deviation. Bharati and colleagues report three patients with chronic bifascicular block who had electrophysiologic studies shortly prior to death.[11] Severe degenerative changes were present in all three patients and were most severe in the anterior aspect of the LBB in the individual with left anterior fascicular block (LAFB). Takagi and Okada reviewed autopsy findings in 35 patients with chronic systemic hypertension whom they grouped according to mean QRS axis.[12] They found that 9 of 12 patients with marked left axis deviation had more severe pathologic lesions in the anterior portion of the LBB, while those with normal axes had more diffuse conduction disease. In contrast, Rossi describes a group of patients with RBBB and LAFB, whose conduction defects developed mostly during acute myocardial infarction.[13] The pathologic changes in the LBB were diffuse, rather than localized to the anterior portion, and the RBB was totally disrupted in almost all. Similarly, Demoulin and Kulbertus report 10 patients with LAFB who had diffuse disease of the LBB that was not perceptibly more severe in its anterior portion.[14] Myerburg and associates showed, in canine preparations, that destruction of the anterior aspect of the LBB had little effect on the ECG but that ligation of the many interconnections between the fascicles of the LBB caused an ECG pattern of LAFB.[15] Demoulin and Kulbertus report 13 patients with left posterior fascicular block (LPFB), nine of whom developed their conduction defect during acute MI.[16] Of these nine, four had major lesions in the posterior portion of the LBB, two had diffuse LBB disease, and three had no identifiable disease in the area of the posterior fascicle. Of the four with chronic conduction defects, all had major disease in the LBB that was maximal in its posterior portion. Rizzon and associates found that extensive damage to both the midseptal and posterior portions of the LBB was necessary for the ECG pattern of LPFB to occur.[17]

PHYSIOLOGY OF THE SPECIALIZED VENTRICULAR CONDUCTION SYSTEM

AV JUNCTIONAL AREA

The AV node can be considered to have several basic functions. It serves as the major pathway between atria and ventricles; it functions as an area of conduction delay allowing atrial contraction to prime the ventricular pump; it acts as a filter, preventing abnormally rapid atrial electrical activity from being transmitted to the ventricle; and tissue in the area of the AV node can spontaneously depolarize and serve as an escape rhythm if the sinoatrial node fails. In common with the sinoatrial node, AV nodal cells show characteristics of the calcium-dependent slow response. Transmembrane potentials recorded from this area are quite different from the remainder of the conduction system and reveal a slow upstroke velocity and reduced resting membrane potential, factors that decrease conduction velocity. In addition, recovery of excitability is both time and voltage dependent. These factors may help to account for differences between the AV node and the His-Purkinje system in the manner in which impulses are conducted. Atrial activation occurs through several different wavefronts, which have been described by some as fiber tracts. These wavefronts approach the AV node through a transitional zone. The large middle and anterior input appears to lead directly to the central AV node, while the posterior group leads to "dead end" areas whose impulses appear to have a minimal role in the normal activation of the His bundle and ventricles. The phylogenetic purpose of these dead-end pathways is unclear, but their potential for the generation of reentrant arrhythmias is obvious. Microelectrode recordings reported by Scherlag and co-workers suggest that the AV node can be divided into three different regions: the AN, the N (central), and the NH zones.[18] The AN zone displays a relatively high rate of spontaneous depolarization, the NH zone has a slower rate, and the central N region has no automaticity. The N zone appears to be responsible for the conduction delay that characterizes the classic Wenckebach cycle, typical of block at the AV node. In corresponding clinical studies, the same investigators were able to divide patients with "junctional" rhythms into two groups, one with an intrinsic rate of 45 to 60 beats per minute that increased with atropine administration and another, with a slower rate, that was unresponsive to atropine. Confirmation of these data comes from the experimental work in dogs of James and associates,[19] who found a mathematical relationship between two distinct junctional rhythms that may correspond to the rhythms described by Scherlag and co-workers.[18]

The lack of a clear separation between the AV node and the proximal His bundle exists both in the transmembrane potentials recorded as well as in the anatomical changes. Thus, there has been a longstanding controversy about the origin of the His bundle depolarization that is recorded on the intracardiac electrogram. As emphasized by James and Sherf, most data indicate that this potential arises in the very proximal His bundle, in an area of abundant P cells.[20] In individuals with intrahisian disease, the His bundle depolarization has been observed to fragment so that two potentials can be recorded. Bharati and colleagues describe a case of intrahisian AV block that was produced by a stab wound to the heart.[21] The origin of the split His potential is thought to be due to conduction delay within the His bundle, which may be due to either structural or functional changes in His bundle conduction. Rossi, for example, reported a patient with a split His potential who, at autopsy, had a morphologically normal His bundle.[22]

Surgical ablation of the His bundle as management of drug-resistant supraventricular tachycardia has provided a unique opportunity for study of His bundle automaticity in humans. Gonzalez and associates studied seven patients who had undergone surgical His bundle ablation and found an intrinsic His bundle rate of approximately 40 beats per minute that was unresponsive to atropine or mild exercise.[23] Similar findings were reported by Klein and co-workers.[24] Bexton and co-workers compared six who had undergone cryothermal His bundle ablation with 12 patients with congenital complete AV nodal block.[25] They found that the patients with congenital AV block could increase their heart rate in response to atropine while those with surgically induced block could not. These observations seem to provide further confirmation of the earlier work by Scherlag's group.

As alluded to in the section on anatomy, the division of the His bundle into a series of longitudinal compartments by means of collagenous septa provides the substrate for early separation of the various fascicles. Thus, a localized lesion in the pre-divisional part of the His bundle could produce the ECG pattern of bundle branch or fascicular block. Experimental and clinical evidence for such longitudinal separation of conduction has become available. El-Sherif and associates describe the production of BBB in association with intrahisian conduction delay in a group of dogs undergoing anterior septal artery ligation.[26] In the majority of dogs, distal His bundle pacing by means of plunge wire electrodes normalized the QRS complex duration. The authors report similar normalization of interventricular conduction in six patients with BBB, half of whom developed their conduction defect in the setting of acute myocardial infarction. Narula succeeded in normalizing the QRS complex duration by distal His pacing in 27 of 110 patients with BBB.[27] Castellanos and colleagues described four patients who developed RBBB associated with either LAFB or LPFB during insertion of a Swan-Ganz catheter in the right side of the heart, suggesting catheter-induced trauma to an area of the His bundle, since direct trauma to the left fascicles would appear to be unlikely during flow-directed right-sided heart catheterization.[28]

NORMAL VENTRICULAR ACTIVATION

Much of the information about normal ventricular activation stems from the work of Durrer and co-workers.[29] These investigators studied ventricular activation in seven isolated human hearts taken from individuals who died from noncardiac causes. In all cases, the heart was removed within 30 minutes of death and perfused in a physiologic solution while detailed mapping of the activation sequence was performed. Most of the hearts began beating spontaneously within 5 minutes of perfusion and continued beating for up to 6½ hours. Ventricular activation began simultaneously at three separate locations: high on the left anterior paraseptal wall, on the left central septal surface, and in the left posterior paraseptal area. Interestingly, these areas correspond to the three "fascicles" or portions of the LBB system described earlier. The right ventricle was activated earliest near the base of the anterior papillary muscle, shortly after earliest left ventricular activation. Control studies *in vivo* in dogs showed a similar activation pattern, suggesting that the findings in human hearts were not an artifact of the experimental preparation. Wyndham and associates report very similar findings after performing epicardial mapping in 11 patients undergoing open-heart surgery.[30]

Nakaya and co-workers provide further evidence of the importance of the septal portion of the LBB.[31] In a series of canine experiments they showed that selective septal block produced apical activation delay and anterior displacement of the vector loop. Selective block of the posterior portion of the LBB had little effect on activation until septal block was also produced, at which point there was marked delay to a large posterobasal area of the left ventricle. Thus, it appears that the numerous interconnections within the LBB network may serve as a type of safety valve should proximal fascicular damage occur.

EFFECT OF CONDUCTION DEFECTS ON VENTRICULAR ACTIVATION

Fascicular blocks are associated with alterations in ventricular activation, and these alterations tend to be more marked when the disease is located proximally. Much of the work that has been done recently has been aimed at determining the site of block, the specific ECG patterns caused by block at different sites, and the clinical significance of these differences.

RIGHT BUNDLE BRANCH BLOCK

In a canine preparation, Myerburg found that the action potential duration of Purkinje cells increases in a distal direction to a maximum at a point 2 mm prior to their termination in ventricular muscle and then progressively decreases.[32] Since refractoriness in the His-Purkinje system is voltage dependent and thus predominantly determined by the action potential duration, this sequence, termed the *gate* by some investigators, provides for block of premature impulses traveling in either direction. Myerburg also found that refractory periods within the RBB system are usually longer than those in the LBB, confirming the clinical impression that early premature impulses are more likely to conduct with a RBBB, rather than a LBBB, pattern. Glassman and Zipes, in a canine preparation on cardiopulmonary bypass, found that antegrade RBBB produced by this method was usually proximal whereas retrograde block tended to be distal, although multiple sites could occur in the same dog.[33] Similarly, Akhtar and associates induced RBBB by programmed stimulation in 14 patients with initially normal interventricular conduction.[34] They found that proximal block was the rule but that the site of block could vary within a given patient, sometimes with consecutive beats. Nagao and associates, in a canine preparation, found that ventricular activation during surgically induced RBBB occurred initially at the base of the anterior papillary muscle and shortly afterward in areas corresponding to the other two terminal branches of the right bundle.[35] Activation of the ventricular muscle in these areas was always preceded by Purkinje fiber activation and could be delayed by damage to any of the three branches. The authors conclude that the Purkinje system is essential to right ventricular activation and any interruption could cause the ECG pattern of incomplete RBBB.

Wyndham and co-workers performed epicardial mapping in three patients with RBBB undergoing open-heart surgery and found that right ventricular epicardial activation was abnormal and that the epicardial surface was activated slowly through the septum and then more rapidly through the right ventricular free wall.[36] Mayorga-Cortes and associates recorded His bundle and right ventricular apical electrograms in 13 patients with acute transmural myocardial infarction and RBBB and found that the conduction defect was proximal, either in the His bundle or in the proximal RBBB.[37] Using epicardial and endocardial electrodes to map the pattern of ventricular activation intraoperatively, Horowitz and co-workers determined the site of RBBB produced by surgical repair of ventricular septal defects.[38] They found that block could occur in three separate areas—proximal (near the septal defect), adjacent to the moderator band, and distal, in the terminal Purkinje network—and that these sites could be identified during electrophysiologic study by means of electrode catheters used for recording the His bundle and right ventricular apical electrograms. That this distinction has clinical relevance is suggested by the work of Wolff and colleagues, who found that the prognosis in post-repair tetralogy of Fallot patients is worse in those with RBBB due to proximal lesions.[39] Similarly, Alpert and co-workers, performing endocardial mapping in 10 apparently healthy subjects with RBBB, found a peripheral site of block in all cases and suggest that this type of lesion may be benign.[40] In contrast, Dancy and co-workers employed echocardiography to locate the site of block in 27 patients with chronic RBBB, 13 of whom had syncope.[41] Proximal lesions were characterized by late tricuspid valve closure, while in distal lesions tricuspid closure occurred normally but pulmonic valve opening was delayed. Of the 13 patients with distal delay, 12 had a history of syncope.

Body surface mapping was employed by Sohi and Flowers to study alterations in depolarization occurring in 14 patients with RBBB.[42] Their data suggested that the right ventricle is activated transseptally, after which the right-sided Purkinje network is engaged. The activation wave is inhomogeneous in speed and direction, perhaps reflecting additional disease within the peripheral conduction system.

LEFT BUNDLE BRANCH BLOCK

Left bundle branch block disrupts both activation of the left ventricle as well as the septum. Wyndham and associates evaluated left ventricular activation by means of epicardial mapping in five patients with LBBB and a normal QRS axis undergoing coronary artery bypass surgery.[43] They found that earliest ventricular activation occurred in the anterior right ventricle, with left ventricular activation occurring initially through the septum and then in an anteroinferior direction with probable terminal reengagement of the conduction system. Of interest is that part of the right ventricular septum was activated late, suggesting that it may normally be depolarized through the LBB system. This same group also performed intraoperative epicardial mapping in four patients with LAFB and found that all had terminal activation of the basal anterolateral left ventricle, as would be predicted from the ECG.[44] Barrett and associates studied 30 patients with chronic LBBB and found that despite the presence of "complete" LBBB electrocardiographically, left axis deviation could be elicited in some by atrial premature stimuli.[45] Their data suggest that the LBBB pattern represents an incomplete form of block, with premature beats producing further conduction delay. Rate-related LBBB offers a unique opportunity to study ventricular activation, with each individual serving as his own control. Cannon and co-workers recorded vectorcardiograms in nine patients with initially normal QRS complexes in whom LBBB was induced by atrial pacing.[46] They found that while septal activation was initially abnormal in four (who may have had partial forms of LBBB), all nine developed abnormal septal activation with the complete conduction defect, suggesting that abnormal septal activation is one of the hallmarks of LBBB. Swiryn and colleagues compared the frontal plane QRS axis during "normal" conduction to the axis during spontaneous rate-related LBBB.[47] They found that, in most, preexisting LAFB was not present prior to the development of LBBB. Abben and associates retrospectively analyzed ECGs of a large number of patients with LBBB.[48] They found preexisting "incomplete" conduction defects to be uncommon, suggesting that block is usually located within the His bundle or proximal LBB since simultaneous conduction failure in all fascicles would be unlikely.

FUNCTIONAL BUNDLE BRANCH BLOCK

Although the term *rate-related* aberrancy has been traditionally associated with a rapid rate, aberrancy due to slow heart rate has also been observed. The terms phase 3 and phase 4 block (referring to phase 3 and phase 4 of the membrane action potential) are used to describe tachycardia- and bradycardia-dependent block, respectively.[49,50] Phase 3 block (Fig. 48.2) can be explained by an impulse arriving relatively early in the cycle, when one of the bundle branches is refractory. In phase 4 block (Fig. 48.3), it is theorized that the interval between beats is sufficiently long that an area of the conduction system becomes depolarized and thus inexcitable. In support of this theory are two patients described by Fisch and Miles in whom varying degrees of LBBB-type aberrancy were directly related to the preceding cycle length.[51] Phase 4 block is usually associated with organic cardiac disease. Phase 3 and phase 4 blocks may be closely related, as illustrated by Goodfriend and Barold, who describe a patient with alcoholic intoxication who presented with high-degree AV block of the phase 3 variety that subsequently became phase 4 block before disappearing.[52] The presence of phase 4 block may predispose to a malignant form of block termed *paroxysmal AV block*.[53] In this situation, depolarization of an area of the conduction system associated with a pause (due, for example, to a nonconducted atrial premature beat) causes the area to become inexcitable until an escape beat from below manages to penetrate and restore the normal transmembrane potential.

ECG DIAGNOSIS OF AV BLOCK
FIRST-DEGREE AV BLOCK

First-degree AV block, characterized by a prolonged PR interval, may indicate delay anywhere within the conduction system (Table 48.1). In general, since most of the delay occurs at the AV node during normal conduction, the longer the PR interval, the greater the chances that the AV node is involved. However, since conduction disease is often diffuse, multiple areas may be affected. If the QRS complex is narrow, there is a 90% chance that the delay occurs at the AV node exclusively, whereas with a wide QRS there is greater than a 50% possibility that at least part of the delay is infranodal.[1]

SECOND-DEGREE AV BLOCK

The hallmark of second-degree AV block is a sinus P wave that is blocked prior to reaching the ventricles. Second-degree AV block has been traditionally divided into two varieties. Type I second-degree AV block is characterized by the Wenckebach phenomenon where the nonconducted beat is preceded by PR interval prolongation (Fig. 48.4). In typical cycles, every third or fourth P wave is blocked while in longer AV Wenckebach conduction cycles oscillation of the PR interval may be found prior to the blocked P wave. Long-cycle Wenckebach conduction may be confused with type II AV block. The change in PR interval between the last conducted beat in the sequence and the first beat after the pause is usually long (≥ 40 msec) in so-called atypical Wenckebach conduction. Type I block is usually located at the AV node and is accompanied by narrow QRS complexes, but both intrahisian and infrahisian Wenckebach conduction have been well documented, usually in association with a wide QRS complex. Type II second-degree AV block is characterized by a nonconducted sinus P wave without prior PR prolongation. It occurs within the His-Purkinje system and is usually associated with a wide QRS complex.

These traditional views have been challenged by El-Sherif and co-workers, who suggest that the two types of AV block may be different manifestations of the same process.[54-56] Using a canine preparation in which the anterior septal artery was ligated, they found that intrahisian block with a type II pattern gradually evolved into type I block. They were able to observe a similar progression in four patients with acute myocardial infarction and suggest that if high-speed recordings are carefully analyzed, some degree of PR interval prolongation at times in the order of only several milliseconds can be identified in all cases of second-degree AV block. Nevertheless, it would appear that the magnitude of change in AV conduction (large for AV nodal block) may still be useful in localizing the site of AV block.

HIGH DEGREES OF AV BLOCK

The anatomical site of block associated with the ECG pattern of fixed ratios of AV block (*i.e.*, 2:1, 3:1) may be difficult to predict (Fig. 48.5). However, data from Puech and Narula indicate that this type of block may be infranodal despite a narrow QRS complex.[1] The presence of a wide QRS complex strongly suggests infranodal block. The diagnosis of complete AV block can be made when atrial and ventricular rhythms are unrelated (none of the P waves are conducted) and the atrial rate is sufficiently slow that no atrial impulse falling outside the junctional refractory period is conducted (Fig. 48.6). The location of block can usually be deduced from the QRS complex width, but, as discussed above, the histopathology does not always correlate with the ECG findings. The diagnosis of AV block secondary to hypervagotonia is suggested by the presence of simultaneous slowing of the sinus rate (Fig. 48.7).[57] This distinction is of clinical importance because in patients with vagotonic AV block, the clinical course is often benign.

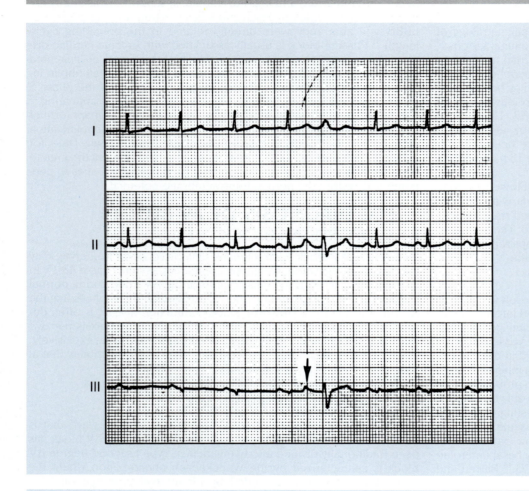

FIGURE 48.2 Simultaneous ECG leads I, II, and III showing an example of phase 3 block. A premature atrial beat (*arrow*) following the fourth QRS complex falls in the refractory period of part of the bundle branch system, producing a wide QRS complex characterized by a LBB block and superior axis.

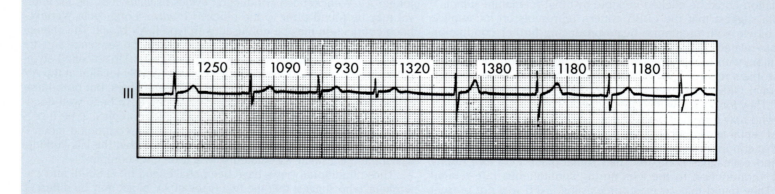

FIGURE 48.3 A rhythm strip (lead III) showing phase 4 block. The degree of aberrancy is related to the preceding cycle length so that the widest QRS complex follows the longest pause (1380 msec). An alternative explanation of this rhythm strip is an idioventricular escape rhythm with varying degrees of fusion.

TABLE 48.1 CLASSIFICATION OF AV BLOCK

Type	ECG Manifestation	Site of Block
First-degree	Prolongation (PR) ↑	AVN = HPS
Second degree		
Type I	PR ↑ precedes nonconducted P wave	AVN > HPS
Type II	No PR ↑ preceding nonconducted P wave	HPS
Vagotonic	PP ↑ precedes nonconducted P wave	AVN
2:1 or greater	Every other P wave not conducted	
Normal QRS		AVN = HPS
Wide QRS		HPS > AVN
Third-degree		
Normal QRS	All P waves not conducted	AVN > HPS
Wide QRS	All P waves not conducted	HPS > AVN

(AVN, AV node; HPS, His-Purkinje system)

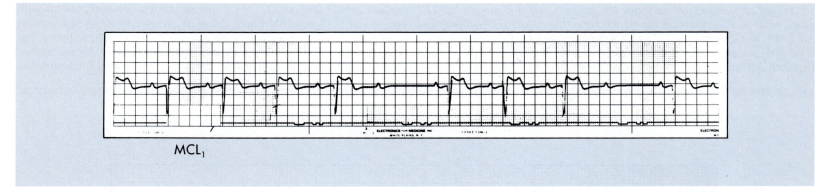

FIGURE 48.4 An example of type I second-degree block (Wenckebach phenomenon). Note the gradual PR prolongation followed by a "dropped" beat. (Morady F, Peters RW, Scheinman MM: Bradyarrhythmia and bundle branch block. In Scheinman MM (ed): Cardiac Emergencies. Philadelphia, WB Saunders, 1984)

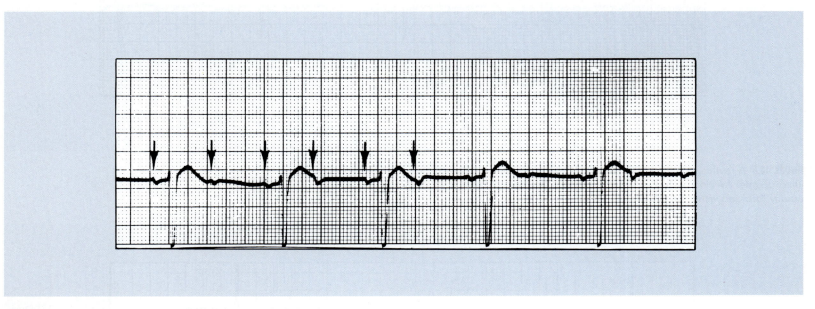

FIGURE 48.5 A rhythm strip from ECG lead MCL₁ showing fixed 2:1 AV block (*arrows* denote the P waves). A His bundle electrogram would be necessary to identify the site of block.

CLINICAL ASPECTS OF CHRONIC AV BLOCK

AV NODAL BLOCK

Chronic second-degree or third-degree AV nodal block is an uncommon condition of diverse etiologies. Although most often congenital, other causes include rheumatic disease, mitral annular calcification, ischemic heart disease, radiation, infiltrative diseases such as amyloidosis, tumors, and perhaps a variant of normal in young athletic people with hypervagotonia. Scott and co-workers reported a strong correlation between congenital complete heart block and maternal connective tissue disorders whereby a maternal antibody crosses the placenta and allows identification of individuals predisposed to heart block.[58] Whether this antibody is actually involved in the pathogenesis of heart block or is merely an innocent bystander is presently unclear. Approximately half of the cases of congenital complete heart block are associated with other cardiovascular abnormalities, especially transposition of the great vessels and ventricular septal defects. The traditional view that congenital AV block is a benign disorder not warranting permanent pacemaker insertion is now being challenged.

Young and associates describe 16 patients, aged 6 months to 17 years, who were asymptomatic at the time that type I second-degree AV block was discovered.[59] Over a follow-up period of up to 18 years, 7 have developed fixed third-degree AV block, including 2 who have required permanent pacing and several others whose lack of increase in rate with exercise suggest that they may become symptomatic later in life. Karpawich and associates, in a series of 24 children with congenital third-degree AV block followed for 1 to 19 years, found that a resting heart rate of 50 beats per minute or less was predictive of subsequent Stokes-Adams syncope and that other clinical and electrophysiologic factors had little prognostic value.[60] The site of block was located in the AV node in 19 of the 24 patients, in the bundle of His in 3, and in the distal conduction tissue in 1. Syncope occurred in 8 children, one of whom died following a bradycardic episode. Permanent pacemakers have been implanted in 10, all of whom have since become asymptomatic. Similarly, Besley and co-workers describe 13 patients, aged 15 to 37, who experienced marked symptomatic improvement following pacemaker implantation for congenital complete heart block.[61] Reid and co-workers found that bradycardia-related symptoms in infancy were the best predictors of subsequent pacemaker dependency in a group of 35 patients with congenital complete heart block.[62] Pacemakers were ultimately required in 21, including only 1 of 6 patients with associated congenital cardiac anomalies. In contrast, in two large series of patients with congenital heart block reported by Strasberg and associates and Pinsky and colleagues, prognosis was strongly related to the presence or severity of associated cardiovascular anomalies.[63,64] Of special interest are two patients with congenital complete AV block dying of congestive heart failure who displayed gradual slowing of their escape rhythms.[65] At autopsy, the expected destruction of the AV node was accompanied by severe disease in the His bundle and bundle branches, explaining the terminally

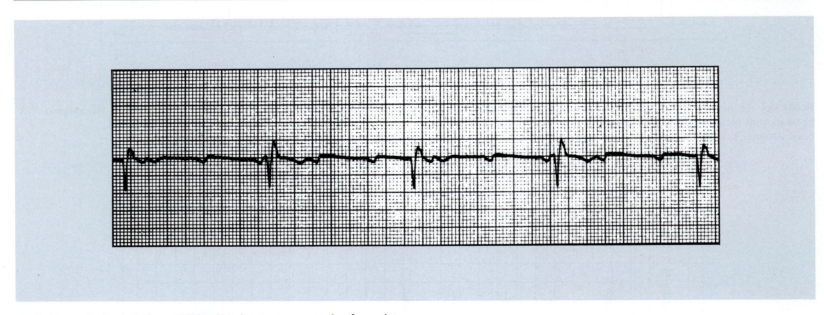

FIGURE 48.6 A rhythm strip from ECG lead V_1 showing an example of complete (third-degree) AV block with a wide QRS complex. This type of block is usually localized within the His-Purkinje system.

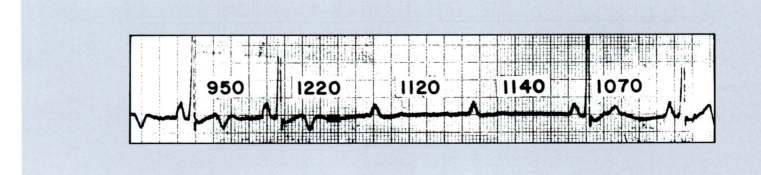

FIGURE 48.7 A rhythm strip from ECG lead II showing simultaneous sinus slowing and AV block. This combination is almost always due to hypervagotonia.

slow escape rhythm. The authors postulate that infranodal disease may have resulted from the long-term hemodynamic stress of bradycardia. Thus, it appears that although many children with congenital second-degree or third-degree AV nodal block are initially asymptomatic, some will eventually develop symptoms necessitating pacemaker insertion. Those individuals with slower rates and, perhaps, with significant underlying cardiovascular disease, seem most likely to develop problems, although the risk of sudden death is low.

INFRANODAL BLOCK

Chronic infranodal block is usually either ischemically mediated or secondary to nonspecific sclerodegenerative processes, although many other causes have been reported (Table 48.2). Most observers agree that chronic third-degree infranodal block is potentially malignant, because of the slow rate and unreliable nature of the escape rhythm, and warrants permanent pacemaker insertion at the time of diagnosis. Rosen and colleagues from the University of Illinois have reported a large series of patients with chronic high-grade AV block localized within or below the His bundle.[66] The vast majority were symptomatic and required permanent pacing.

CHRONIC BUNDLE BRANCH BLOCK

Patients with BBB and organic cardiac disease appear to have an increased incidence of progression to high-grade AV block and sudden death. In this section, we will review much of the available data and attempt to provide the clinician with a rational approach to the patient with BBB.

CLINICAL AND EPIDEMIOLOGIC STUDIES

A variety of retrospective studies have examined the prevalence of bifascicular block and the incidence of progression to high-grade AV block (Table 48.3). From these data it is apparent that the incidence of underlying cardiovascular disease in hospitalized patients with BBB is high and that prognosis is linked to the presence and severity of this disease.[67-73]

Several groups have examined the clinical significance of LBBB accompanied by marked ($-30°$ or greater) left axis deviation. Dhingra and colleagues found that patients with this conduction defect had worse left ventricular function, more advanced conduction system disease, and a higher cardiovascular mortality than those with LBBB and a normal frontal plane QRS axis.[74] In an autopsy study, Havelda and associates report that those with marked left axis deviation had larger myocardial infarcts.[75] In contrast, however, Barrett and coworkers could not correlate left axis deviation with any clinical or electrophysiologic descriptors.[45]

Several very large epidemiologic studies have contributed greatly to our knowledge of the long-term outlook of individuals with interventricular conduction defects (Table 48.4). Rotman and Triebwasser reviewed ECGs of 237,000 personnel at the United States School of Aerospace Medicine and found 394 with RBBB and 125 with LBBB, a combined incidence of 0.002%.[76] All were asymptomatic, and only 7% had any evidence of cardiovascular disease. In a 10-year follow-up period, only 2 subjects with conduction defects developed high-grade AV block and overall mortality was approximately 5%. Siegman-Igra and associates reviewed ECGs of 5204 working males aged 40 and over, representing a random sample of Israeli civil service employees, and found that 123 (2.4%) had interventricular conduction defects.[77] Ischemic heart disease was clinically apparent in 28% and was more common in those with LBBB. Approximately 147 of those with unifascicular block progressed to either bifascicular block (usually developing RBBB) or complete heart block. The Baltimore Longitudinal Study on Aging identified 24 otherwise healthy men (mean age, 64) with RBBB in an overall population of 1142 subjects.[78] Over an 8.4-year (mean) follow-up period, these individuals did not have a higher incidence of cardiovascular events than the remainder of the population.

The Manitoba study was begun in 1948 with 4000 male pilots (mean age, 31) who were initially free of cardiovascular disease by clinical and ECG criteria.[79,80] The investigators determined the prevalence of interventricular conduction defects that developed over the 28-year follow-up period. Right bundle branch block developed in 59 subjects, while 29 individuals developed LBBB. No progression to high-grade AV block was observed in either group. Prognosis in those with RBBB was especially benign; none died suddenly, and only 1 subject developed evidence of ischemic heart disease. In the LBBB group, however, 6 died suddenly; in 5 death occurred without prior clinical manifestations of ischemic heart disease.

Somewhat different results were obtained in the Framingham study, which began in 1949 and involved 5209 subjects initially free of clinically apparent cardiac disease.[81,82] Over an 18-year follow-up period, 70 people developed RBBB and 55 developed LBBB. Most of these 125 individuals had hypertension and cardiomegaly detected before they developed conduction defects. Although the onset of the conduction defects did not usually coincide with acute cardiac events, clinically manifest cardiac disease developed in the majority in the follow-up period and mortality and the incidence of sudden death was high. Conduction disease progressed slowly, however, and only four cases of high-grade AV block occurred, all in people with RBBB.

From these epidemiologic-type studies, it can be concluded that interventricular conduction defects are relatively uncommon and conduction system disease generally progresses slowly. The prognosis of people with BBB appears to depend on the population being studied. When the subjects are young and free of organic heart disease, the prognosis is generally excellent. If the population is older and has a high incidence of hypertension and other cardiac risk factors, clinical manifestation of heart disease including high-degree heart block and especially sudden death are found.

INVASIVE ELECTROPHYSIOLOGIC STUDIES

The standard 12-lead ECG has definite limitations in evaluating the functional status of the ventricular specialized conduction system. Disease of the fascicle may be inapparent until it is totally blocked while PR interval prolongation fails to differentiate between AV nodal and infranodal disease. Newer techniques involving intracardiac recording

TABLE 48.2 ETIOLOGY OF CHRONIC INFRANODAL BLOCK

Primary (sclerodegenerative)
Secondary
  Ischemic
  Trauma
  Valvular heart disease (calcific aortic stenosis)
  Solid tumors
  Malignant infiltrative
    Lymphoma
    Myeloma
  Other infiltrative
    Sarcoid
    Amyloid
    Rheumatoid arthritis
    Dermatomyositis
  Muscular dystrophy
  Diphtheria
  Luetic
  Iatrogenic (surgical closure of ventricular septal defect)
  Metabolic
    Myxedema
    Thyrotoxicosis
    Paget's disease
  Radiation

and pacing have been used in an attempt to identify a subset of individuals with BBB who are at greater risk for progression to high-grade AV block and/or sudden cardiac death (Fig. 48.8).

Early studies appeared to show that prolongation of the HV interval was associated with progression to higher grades of AV block. Narula and Samet recorded His bundle electrograms in 123 patients with interventricular conduction defects and found a high incidence of trifascicular involvement (prolonged HV) in those who had only bifascicular block patterns of ECG.[83] Levites and Haft found a poor correlation between PR interval and HV in 63 patients with bifascicular block and suggest that His bundle recordings are necessary to predict trifascicular disease.[84] The clinical importance of prolonged HV in patients with BBB was demonstrated by Vera and associates, who performed His bundle electrograms in 50 patients with chronic bifascicular block and episodic high-grade AV block.[85] HV was prolonged in 49 of the 50, and in 47 it was markedly prolonged.

TABLE 48.3 RETROSPECTIVE STUDIES OF PATIENTS WITH BBB

Study	Population	Incidence of Bifascicular Block	Incidence of High-Grade AV Block	Mortality	Length of Follow-up	Organic Heart Disease	Comments
Lasser et al[67]	5500 consecutive hospitalized patients	1% (55 patients)	9%				
Scanlon et al[68]	209 consecutive hospitalized patients	100%	7.2%/yr	9%/yr	2 yr	Approximately 80%	Prognosis related to underlying heart disease
DePasquale and Bruno[69]	83 hospitalized patients	100%	2%/yr	32%/yr	3.1 yr	94%	History of syncope in 11 patients
Kulbertus[70]	50 hospitalized patients	100%	8%/yr		4.8 yr		50% of patients with high-grade block had syncope and/or dizzy spells
Kulbertus[71]	20,000 subjects (routine ECG screening)	0.35% (70 subjects)	0	1 death	25 mo		
Pine et al[72]	108 patients	100%	2.5%/yr	6%/yr (17% of deaths were sudden)	12 yr	42%	Mortality, AV block more frequent than in age-matched controls
Wiberg et al[73]	34,160 hospitalized patients	0.9% (303 patients)	0.2%/yr	8%/yr	28 mo	54%	

TABLE 48.4 PROSPECTIVE LARGE EPIDEMIOLOGIC STUDIES OF BBB

Study	No. of Subjects	Initial Age (yr)	Initial Incidence of Cardiovascular Disease (%)	Follow-up (yr)	Subjects with BBB	No. Developing High-Grade Block	Mortality (%)	Sudden Death (%)
Rotman and Triebwasser[76]	237,000 healthy subjects	17–50	7	10	519 (0.002%)	2	5	0
Siegman-Igra et al[77]	5,204 Civil Service employees	54	48	10	123 (2.4%)	2	15	
Manitoba[77,80]	3,983 male pilots	31	0	28	88 (0.02%)	0		7
Framingham[81,82]	5,209 subjects without cardiovascular disease	50	70	18	125 (0.02%)	4	40	8
Baltimore Longitudinal Study on Aging[78]	1,142 healthy men	64 (mean)	0 (20% had hypertension)	8.4	24 (0.02%)	0	17	

Three similarly designed large prospective studies have contributed greatly to our knowledge of the natural history of BBB (Table 48.5). McAnulty and associates from the University of Oregon have reported their 3½-year (mean) follow-up of 554 patients with bifascicular and trifascicular disease.[86] High-grade AV block was documented in 19 patients and was not predicted by any clinical or electrophysiologic descriptor except syncope. Almost one third of their subjects died during the follow-up period, and more than half of the deaths were sudden. There was a high incidence of sinus node and atrial disease in their population, providing another possible explanation for syncope.[87]

Dhingra and co-workers from the University of Illinois followed 517 patients with chronic bifascicular block for a mean period of 3½ years.[88] They found that HV prolongation was a significant risk factor for progression to high-grade infranodal block. However, this finding was of limited predictive value in that only a very small percentage of those with prolonged HV intervals progressed to complete AV block. Their population had a higher incidence of organic heart disease and cardiomegaly than in the University of Oregon study, and mortality was correspondingly higher (over 42%). Both in their study and in that of McAnulty and associates, overall mortality was strongly related to presence and severity of underlying heart disease. They also found syncope to have little relation to prognosis and, in fact, to be nonrecurrent in the majority of patients.[89] Another finding of note from their data was the relatively high incidence of high-grade AV nodal block, emphasizing the diffuse nature of conduction system disease.

Scheinman and associates from the University of California, San Francisco, reported their findings in 401 patients with BBB followed for a mean interval of 2½ years.[90] In their data, the risk of high-degree block increased progressively with increasing HV. Of the 20 patients with markedly prolonged HV (≥ 100 msec), at least 5 (20%) had documented progression to high-degree block while another 10 received prophylactic permanent pacemakers so that the 20% figure may well underestimate the magnitude of progression for this subgroup. Their population was older than in the other two studies and had a considerably higher incidence of organic heart disease, syncope, and HV prolongation. The overall mortality (almost 50%) and the incidence of sudden death was correspondingly higher.

From these studies it seems apparent that the predictive value of HV prolongation for development of high-degree AV block varies according to the population being studied. In mass ECG screening trials, comprising less ill subjects, the value of the HV interval in predicting development of AV block appears to be limited. In contrast, studies of patients with organic heart disease and syncope show a higher incidence of HV prolongation as well as progressive conduction system disease.

PROPHYLACTIC PACEMAKERS

A major aim of the above studies has been to identify a subset of individuals with BBB who might benefit from the timely insertion of a permanent pacemaker. Scheinman and associates, having identified a high-risk group with markedly prolonged HV, have compared the clinical course of 77 patients undergoing prophylactic permanent pacemaker insertion (in the absence of documented second-degree or third-degree AV block) with that of the 302 unpaced patients.[90] Pacemakers were inserted at the discretion of the referring physician,

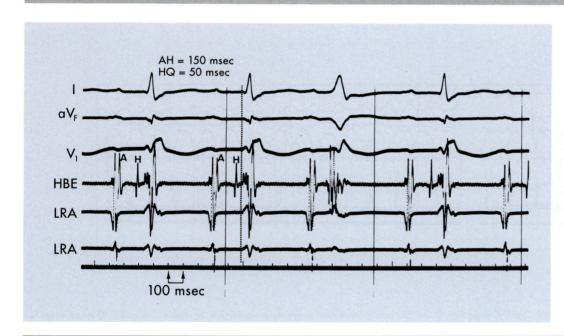

FIGURE 48.8 A His bundle electrogram (*HBE*) and simultaneous surface leads I, aV$_F$, and V$_1$ in a patient with right bundle branch block and a prolonged PR interval. Two intracardiac low right atrial leads (*LRA*) are also recorded. The dotted vertical line indicates the point of earliest ventricular activation from the three surface leads. The prolonged AH indicates that the cause of first-degree AV block is delay in the AV node, emphasizing the diagnostic limitations of the standard 12-lead ECG. (Peters RW, Scheinman MM: Anatomic and electrophysiologic aspects of fascicular block. In Scheinman MM, Levy S (eds): Cardiac Arrhythmias: From Diagnosis to Therapy. Mt. Kisco, NY, Futura Publishing, 1984)

TABLE 48.5 LARGE PROSPECTIVE STUDIES OF BBB USING INTRACARDIAC RECORDINGS

Study	No. of Patients	Follow-up (yr)	Mean Age (yr)	OHD (%)	CAD (%)	CHF (%)	↑HV (%)	Syncope (%)	HDB (No.) HQ < 55	HDB (No.) HQ > 55	Death (%)	Sudden Death (%)
McAnulty et al[86,87]	554	3½	64	74	25	25	54	25		19	29	12
Dhingra et al[88,89]	517	3½	61	80	13	14	38	14	2	9	42	17
Scheinman et al[90]	401	2½	65	86	30	39	65	39	4	15	47	17

(OHD, organic heart disease; CAD, coronary artery disease; CHF, congestive heart failure; HDB, high-degree AV block; HV, infranodal conduction time)

usually on the basis of unexplained transient neurologic symptoms, abnormal electrophysiology, or both. Over the 2½-year (mean) follow-up period, there was no significant difference between paced and unpaced patients in overall mortality, sudden death, or resolution of transient neurologic symptoms. Of the unpaced patients initially presenting with syncope, 73% had no recurrence, a finding similar to that reported by Dhingra and colleagues.

Somewhat different results were described by Altschuler and co-workers, who also compared the clinical course of paced and unpaced patients with BBB and transient neurologic symptoms.[91] They divided their population into three groups: One (15 patients) had prolonged HV and underwent permanent pacemaker insertion; a second group (18 patients) were not paced and had a normal HV; while the third group (17 patients) were not paced and had a prolonged HV. The decision to implant a permanent pacemaker was made by the private physicians. There were eight deaths and three progressions to high-grade block in the unpaced prolonged HV group, compared with no deaths in either of the other two groups. There were four progressions to high-grade block in the paced prolonged HV group and none in patients with normal HV. Altschuler's population differed from Scheinman's in that there was a much lower incidence of organic heart disease. In addition, in several of Altschuler's patients, pacemakers were not truly prophylactic in that high-degree block had previously been documented. Narula reports findings similar to those of Altschuler's group, again with a very similar population base.[92]

In an attempt to explain the lack of benefit from pacing in their symptomatic patients, Higgins and co-workers performed programmed premature ventricular stimulation in 25 patients with BBB and syncope.[93] Ventricular tachycardia was inducible in 14 (Fig. 48.9).

Similarly, Ezri and associates were able to induce ventricular tachycardia in 4 of 13 patients being evaluated for bifascicular block and syncope.[94]

Patients with BBB and syncope should undergo complete medical and neurologic evaluation including at least two 24-hour Holter recordings. Detailed electrophysiologic studies including programmed atrial and ventricular stimulation are necessary. If an HV interval of 100 msec or atrial pacing-induced infranodal block is found, permanent pacemaker insertion is indicated. Although the finding of an HV interval between 70 msec and 100 msec is associated with an increased risk of progression, this risk is quite small and no firm recommendation with regard to pacing is available. Sinus node dysfunction as well as induced sustained atrial and ventricular arrhythmias should be appropriately treated.

STRESSING THE CONDUCTION SYSTEM
PROVOCATIVE TESTING

Because of the low specificity of a prolonged HV interval in predicting subsequent high-degree block, some observers have recommended the use of provocative tests to "stress" the conduction system. Dhingra and colleagues studied the effects of atrial pacing in their population with bifascicular block.[95] Infranodal block during intact AV nodal conduction could only be induced in 15 patients, of whom, during follow-up, 7 developed spontaneous high-grade block, 1 developed exercise-induced AV block, and 2 died suddenly. Woelfel and associates described two patients with BBB and transient neurologic symptoms who developed exercise-induced infranodal block (Fig. 48.10).[96] In both cases, symptoms disappeared following permanent pacemaker

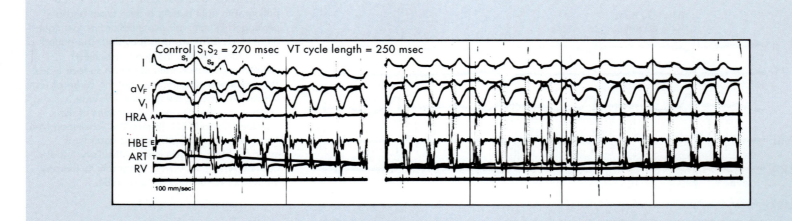

FIGURE 48.9 Simultaneous recording of surface leads I, aV$_F$, and V$_1$, together with His bundle (*HBE*) and right ventricular apical (*RV*) recordings. S$_1$ denotes the basic drive and premature ventricular complex induced 270 msec after S$_1$ produces stable sustained unimorphic ventricular tachycardia.

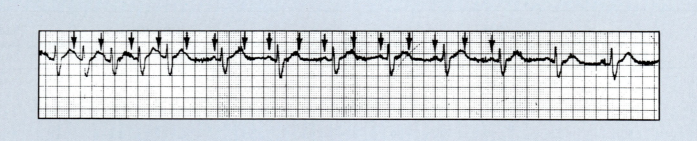

FIGURE 48.10 Standard ECG leads recorded during treadmill exercise showing the abrupt development of 2:1 AV block (*P waves denoted by arrows*). The patient is a 60-year-old man with right bundle branch block, left anterior fascicular block, and syncope.

insertion. Chiale and co-workers infused ajmaline, 1 mg/kg, intravenously into 12 patients with intermittent BBB and were able to elicit the conduction defect in 11.[97] The role of ajmaline as a means of inducing AV block has not been fully evaluated.

In summary, although further studies are needed, provocative testing holds promise as a means of improving the predictive power of electrophysiologic studies in discerning those patients with BBB at greater risk for development of AV block.

THERAPEUTIC USE OF ANTIARRHYTHMIC DRUGS

The use of potentially conduction-depressing antiarrhythmic drugs in patients with advanced conduction system disease has been a matter of very real concern to clinicians. Lidocaine, disopyramide, and other drugs have been reported to cause high-grade block in isolated instances.[98,99] Several series have shown that the risk of using these drugs is relatively low, especially in asymptomatic individuals.[100-102] However, until more complete information is available, it would seem prudent to administer antiarrhythmic medication with caution to patients with BBB, especially those with transient neurologic symptoms.

SURGERY

The risk of performing surgical procedures under general anesthesia in patients with interventricular conduction disturbances has been the subject of several investigations. Kunstadt and colleagues found no episodes of high-degree block during 38 procedures (most using general anesthesia) in 24 patients with chronic bifascicular block.[102]

Santini and co-workers found three episodes of high-grade block following administration of succinylcholine in 20 patients with BBB undergoing general anesthesia for surgical procedures.[103] Nineteen had a history of antecedent transient neurologic symptoms, including all three who developed AV block. Mikell and associates, reporting surgical procedures in 76 patients with bifascicular block (37 performed using general anesthesia), found no episodes of high-grade block.[104]

In conclusion, the risk of inducing AV block in patients with BBB undergoing surgical procedures appears to be quite low. Caution should be exercised, however, in patients with a history of prior unexplained neurologic symptoms. It might be advisable for these individuals to undergo either temporary pacemaker insertion or electrophysiologic evaluation prior to surgery.

CATHETER-INDUCED CONDUCTION DEFECTS

With the increase in cardiac catheterization procedures over the past decade, catheter-induced conduction defects have assumed greater clinical importance. Catheter-induced block has now been described at the level of the AV node, the His bundle, and the bundle branch–fascicular network.[105-107] These conduction defects seem to result from direct catheter trauma to the affected structure and are usually transient, lasting from seconds to, at most, a few days. However, the induction of RBBB in a patient with preexisting LBBB may have potentially disastrous consequences and has led some observers to recommend temporary pacemaker insertion for those with LBBB who undergo right-sided heart catheterization. However, with the advent of multipurpose electrode flotation catheters and R-V port flotation catheters, insertion of a separate temporary pacemaker catheter appears unnecessary during right-sided heart catheterization in patients with preexisting LBBB.

CLINICAL IMPLICATIONS

The structure and function of the AV node is designed to act as a weigh station modulating the atrial input into the ventricle. First- and second-degree block at the level of the node seldom require permanent pacemaker intervention. Third-degree AV block localized to the AV node is seldom associated with syncope but may require permanent pacing, owing to the slow rate. Congenital complete AV nodal block may run a benign clinical course, but about half of these patients will eventually require permanent pacemakers, especially those with underlying structural heart disease.

The ECG manifestations of bifascicular or trifascicular block may serve as a clue to the presence of infranodal disease. Infranodal block carries more serious clinical implications since the emerging ventricular rate is often slower and more erratic. Patients with second-degree or third-degree AV block localized to the His-Purkinje system should undergo permanent pacemaker insertion. Analysis of the surface ECG usually suffices for localization of the site of AV block. In difficult cases, intracardiac recordings may be helpful. In addition, they have allowed for a more detailed analysis of the functional status of the bundle branch system.

From an epidemiologic point of view, patients with the ECG pattern of BBB seldom show progression to complete AV block, but hypertension, coronary artery disease, and congestive heart failure are common associated findings.

In patients with BBB and syncope or dizziness, symptoms may be related to episodic high-grade AV block with ventricular asystole. If AV block is documented, then permanent cardiac pacing is indicated. If the cause of syncope is not found in spite of complete medical and neurologic evaluation, then invasive electrophysiologic studies are indicated for diagnosis of the arrhythmia.

AV CONDUCTION DISORDERS IN PATIENTS WITH ACUTE MYOCARDIAL INFARCTION

AV block occurring in the setting of acute myocardial infarction must be evaluated in terms of the coronary blood supply to the specialized conduction system. The right coronary artery provides the dominant blood supply to the AV node as well as to the inferior wall of the left ventricle. Thus, AV block in patients with inferior infarction is usually localized to the AV node. The AV block may be expressed as first-degree, Mobitz I (Wenckebach), or third-degree AV block. First-degree or AV Wenckebach conduction disorders generally require no specific therapy. Patients with third-degree AV block may require treatment owing to pronounced bradycardia, pump failure, or ventricular arrhythmias. Failing a trial of atropine therapy, insertion of a temporary transvenous pacemaker may be required for rate control. In survivors of inferior wall myocardial infarction complicated by AV block, the block is almost always transient and permanent pacing is rarely needed.

The dominant blood supply to the His bundle and proximal bundle branches is derived from the left anterior descending coronary artery. Thus, in patients with anterior wall myocardial infarction and AV block, the block is localized to the infranodal conducting system. Because infranodal pacemakers may prove unreliable, all patients with anterior wall myocardial infarction complicated by second-degree or third-degree AV block require emergent temporary pacemaker insertion. Since AV block in these patients is usually associated with severe heart failure, the ultimate prognosis (in spite of pacing) is still poor.

Bundle branch block in acute myocardial infarction is usually associated with anterior infarction. One exception is RBBB, which may occur in the setting of inferior wall infarction since the proximal RBB may be supplied from the AV nodal artery. Necrosis of the bundle branches reduces the safety margin for successful AV conduction.

BUNDLE BRANCH BLOCK

Numerous clinical studies have examined the prognosis of patients with BBB and acute myocardial infarction with the aim of determining whether temporary and/or permanent pacing will improve survival. Data involving 1279 patients with intraventricular conduction defects and acute myocardial infarction, most of whom had BBB in the setting of acute anteroseptal myocardial infarction, are summarized in Table 48.6.[108-120] It is clear from examining these data that the very high incidence of left ventricular power failure and ventricular tachyarrhyth-

TABLE 48.6 STUDIES OF BUNDLE BRANCH BLOCK AND ACUTE MYOCARDIAL INFARCTION

Study	No. Patients	Population	Acute HDB	Acute Mortality	Late HDB	Late Mortality	Comments/Conclusions
Godman et al[08]	68	BBB	21 (31%)	38 (56%)			CHF very frequent; PTP did not affect mortality
Scheinman and Brenman[109]	97	Any IVCD	13 (12%)	39 (40%)			Mortality related to CHF
Waters and Mizgala[110]	27	Bilateral BBB with PTP	15 (56%)	12 (44%)	0	1	PTP of little value; long-term prognosis good in survivors of acute episodes
Nimetz et al[111]	71	BBB	30 (42%)	22 (31%)	0	18 (14 SD)	Mortality correlates with CHF and unaffected by TP
Scanlon et al[112]	28	Bilateral BBB (3 admitted with HDB)	6 (21%)	8 (29%)	1	5 (not ↑ in 4 others)	PTP indicated in bilateral BBB and AMI
Atkins et al[113]	77	Any IVCD (30 with RBBB, LAFB)		7 (9%)		9 SD (7 in patients with RBBB, LAFD)	PTP indicated in RBBB, LAFB; PP indicated in all HDB, even if transient
Waugh et al[114]	116	Any IVCD	21 (18%)	34 (29%)			First-degree AVB plus LBB or bilateral BBB warrants PTP
Gann et al[115]	210	Any IVCD		111 (53%)	0		PP may be of value in patients with persisting RBBB
Ritter et al[116]	17	RBBB, LAFB & transient HDB				11 (65%)	All patients without PP died, 50% of those with PP survived; PP indicated in this population
Lie et al[117]	47	BBB & ASMI			0		17 (36%) had VF in 6 week period; prolonged monitoring recommended
Hauer et al[118]	42	ASMI & new BBB	3 (7%)*	24 (57%)	1	1	Patients surviving 6 weeks have good prognosis; SD usually second-degree to VF, not HDB
Hollander et al[119]	47	BBB	14 (30%)				Recommend PP in ASMI and either bifascicular block or LBBB
Hindman et al[120]	432	BBB without prior cardiogenic shock	95 (22%)	121 (28%)		87 (28%) of survivors	See text

(BBB, bundle branch block (R, right, L, left); IVCD, intraventricular conduction defect; LAFB, left anterior fascicular block; HDB, high-degree AV block; CHF, congestive heart failure; PTP, prophylactic temporary pacing; PP, permanent pacing; ASMI, anteroseptal myocardial infarction; *, 6 weeks of follow-up; VF, ventricular fibrillation; SD, sudden death; AMI, acute myocardial infarction)

TABLE 48.7 RISK FACTORS FOR ACUTE PROGRESSION TO HIGH-GRADE AV BLOCK DURING ACUTE MYOCARDIAL INFARCTION

Risk Factor	Risk of Progression to High-Grade AV Block (%)
1. First-degree AV Block	13
2. New or indeterminate onset of BBB	11
3. Bilateral BBB	10
1 and 2 combined	19
1 and 3 combined	20
2 and 3 combined	31
All 3 risk factors	38

(Data from Hindman MC, Wagner GS, Jaho M et al: The clinical significance of bundle-branch block complicating acute myocardial infarction: I. Clinical characteristics, hospital mortality and one-year follow-up. Circulation 58:679, 1978)

mias are a major cause of mortality in this population and that the role of both temporary and permanent pacing, accordingly, is limited. However, the large multicenter retrospective study of Hindman and co-workers has identified subgroups in which pacing may improve survival.[120] In their population, risk factors for acute progression to high-degree AV block were a new (or indeterminate) onset of the conduction defect, bilateral involvement of the bundle branches system, and first-degree AV block. The presence of any two of these risk factors was associated with a 19% or greater risk of acute progression, warranting prophylactic temporary pacing (Table 48.7). Patients who experienced high-degree AV block during the course of hospitalization had a 28% incidence of recurrent block or sudden death that was not substantially reduced if the conduction defect completely resolved prior to hospital discharge. In contrast, those without high-degree block acutely had a low incidence of block or sudden death in follow-up, even if they fulfilled the criteria for temporary pacing noted above.

The application of intracardiac recordings to patients with BBB and acute myocardial infarction promises to yield important prognostic information but most of the work so far is preliminary and involves relatively small numbers of patients. Information from six studies involving 202 patients is summarized in Table 48.8. In general, the data indicate that HV prolongation is common in these patients and predicts mortality but not necessarily progression to high-grade AV block.

Several studies have found an increased incidence of late sudden death among unpaced patients with transient AV block complicating anterior wall infarction.[116,121] The available data are not sufficiently persuasive to recommend permanent pacemaker insertion for these patients since a small number of patients have been reported and other associated risk factors for post-infarction late sudden death (*e.g.*, ventricular ectopy, ejection fraction, resting ST segmental abnormalities) were not controlled. In addition, prospective studies of patients with BBB complicating acute anterior infarction show a high incidence of sudden death due to ventricular arrhythmias.[117]

In summary, the following general points can be made:

1. AV block in the setting of inferior wall myocardial infarction is usually transient and responds readily to therapy. Permanent pacing is rarely required.
2. Patients who develop high-grade AV block during anteroseptal myocardial infarction have a very high mortality owing to left ventricular failure but temporary and permanent pacemakers are mandatory owing to the slow rate and unreliability of the escape rhythm.
3. BBB in the setting of acute myocardial infarction is also frequently accompanied by severe left ventricular dysfunction, but high-risk groups requiring temporary and permanent pacing have been tentatively identified.[120]
4. Intracardiac recordings can identify the site of AV block in acute myocardial infarction and may provide prognostic information in patients with BBB[122]; whether the finding of a prolonged infranodal conduction time predicts eventual development of complete AV block is not known.
5. Although several studies suggest a higher incidence of sudden death in unpaced patients with transient AV block complicating acute anterior myocardial infarction, the role of permanent pacing is still controversial.

TABLE 48.8 STUDIES OF BBB AND ACUTE MYOCARDIAL INFARCTION INVOLVING HIS BUNDLE ELECTROGRAMS

Study	No. Patients	Population	↑HV (Acute)	Acute HDB	Acute Mortality	↑HV (Late)	Late HDB	Late Mortality	Comments/Conclusions
Schoenfeld et al[122]	14	BBB	12 (86%)	6 (43%)	6 (43%)	5 (100%)		3	HV common and persists long-term
Lichstein et al[123]	15	Bilateral BBB	11 (73%)		7 (47%)			2	HV predicts mortality
Lie et al[124]	50	BBB in ASMI	16/35 (46%)	14 (28%)	37 (74%)				HV predicts HDB and mortality, but most die of CHF
Gould et al[125]	14	BBB	4 (29%)	0	7 (50%)		0	2	HV not predictive of mortality
Watson et al[126]	50	Persistent IVCD in survivors (2 wk) of AMI randomized to PP vs. unpaced	27 (59%)				0*	25 (50%)	HV not predictive of mortality; PP did not improve survival; ventricular arrhythmias are the major cause of death
Pagnoni et al[127]	59	IVCD discharged from hospital following AMI	14 (24%)			13 (23%)	1 (2%)	13 (23%)	HV predicts CHF and mortality; conduction disease not progressive in those with ↑HV

(BBB, bundle branch block; IVCD, intraventricular conduction defect; HV, infranodal conduction time; AMI, acute myocardial infarction; PP, permanent pacing; *, 2 year (mean) follow-up; ↑HV, abnormal infranodal conduction time)

REFERENCES

1. Puech P, Wainwright RJ: Clinical electrophysiology of atrioventricular block. Cardiol Clin 1:209, 1983
2. Demoulin JC, Simar LJ, Kulbertus HE: Quantitative study of left bundle branch fibrosis in left anterior hemiblock: A stereologic approach. Am J Cardiol 36:751, 1975
3. Massing GK, James TN: Anatomical configuration of the His bundle and bundle branches in the human heart. Circulation 53:609, 1976
4. Bharati S, Lev M, Dhingra RC et al: Electrophysiologic and pathologic correlation in two cases of chronic second-degree atrioventricular block with left bundle branch block. Circulation 52:221, 1975
5. Ohkawa S, Sugiura M, Itoh Y et al: Electrophysiologic and histologic correlations in chronic complete atrioventricular block. Circulation 64:215, 1981
6. Ohkawa S, Hackel DB, Ideker RE: Correlation of the width of the QRS complex with the pathologic anatomy of the cardiac conduction system in patients with chronic complete atrioventricular block. Circulation 63:938, 1981
7. Rossi L: The pathologic basis of cardiac arrhythmias. Cardiol Clin 1:13, 1983
8. Hunt D, Lie JT, Vohra J et al: Histopathology of heart block complicating acute myocardial infarction: Correlation with the His bundle electrogram. Circulation 43:1252, 1973
9. Becker AE, Lie KI, Anderson RH: Bundle-branch block: The setting of acute anteroseptal myocardial infarction: Clinicopathological correlation. Br

Heart J 40:773, 1978
10. Lev M, Unger PN, Rosen KM et al: The anatomic substrate of complete left bundle branch block. Circulation 50:479, 1974
11. Bharati S, Lev M, Dhingra R et al: Pathologic correlations in three cases of bilateral bundle branch disease with unusual electrophysiologic manifestations in two cases. Am J Cardiol 38:508, 1976
12. Takagi T, Okada R: An electrocardiographic-pathologic correlative study on left axis deviation in hypertensive hearts. Am Heart J 100:838, 1980
13. Rossi L: Histopathology of conducting system in left anterior hemiblock. Br Heart J 38:1304, 1976
14. Demoulin JC, Kulbertus HE: Histopathologic examination of concept of left hemiblock. Br Heart J 34:807, 1972
15. Myerburg RJ, Nilson K, Gelband H: Physiology of canine intraventricular conduction and endocardial excitation. Circ Res 30:217, 1972
16. Demoulin JC, Kulbertus HE: Histopathologic correlates of left posterior fascicular block. Am J Cardiol 44:1083, 1979
17. Rizzon P, Rossi L, Baissus C et al: Left posterior hemiblock in myocardial infarction. Br Heart J 37:711, 1975
18. Scherlag BJ, Lazzara R, Helfant RH: Differentiation of "AV junctional rhythyms." Circulation 48:304, 1973
19. James TN, Isobe JH, Urthaler F: Correlative electrophysiological and anatomical studies concerning the site of origin of escape rhythm during complete atrioventricular block in the dog. Circ Res 45:108, 1979
20. James TN, Sherf L: Fine structure of the His bundle. Circulation 44:9, 1971
21. Bharati S, Towne WD, Patel R et al: Pathologic correlations in a case of complete heart block with split His potentials resulting from a stab wound of the heart. Am J Cardiol 38:388, 1976
22. Rossi L: His bundle in electrocardiographic semantics of AV block: Anatomicoclinical considerations. PACE 3:275, 1980
23. Gonzalez R, Scheinman M, Thomas A et al: Electrophysiologic characterization of singly induced his bundle rhythm in man. PACE 4:152, 1981
24. Klein GJ, Sealy WC, Pritchett ELC et al: Cryosurgical ablation of the atrioventricular node–His bundle: Long-term follow-up and properties of the junctional pacemaker. Circulation 61:8, 1980
25. Bexton RS, Ward DE, Camm AJ: Electrophysiological characteristics of junctional pacemakers in congenital A-V block and following His bundle cryoablation. Clin Cardiol 5:577, 1982
26. El-Sherif N, Scherlag BJ, Lazzara R: Conduction disorders in the canine proximal His-Purkinje system following acute myocardial ischemia: I. The pathophysiology of intra-His bundle block. Circulation 49:837, 1974
27. Narula OS: Longitudinal dissociation in the His bundle: Bundle branch block due to asynchronous conduction within the His bundle in man. Circulation 56:996, 1977
28. Castellanos A, Ramirez AV, Mayorga-Cortes A et al: Left fascicular block during right-heart catheterization using Swan-Ganz catheter. Circulation 64:1271, 1981
29. Durrer D, Van Dam R, Freud GE et al: Total excitation of the isolated human heart. Circulation 41:899, 1970
30. Wyndham CRC, Meeran MK, Smith T et al: Epicardial activation of the intact human heart without conduction defects. Circulation 59:161, 1979
31. Nakaya Y, Inone H, Hiasa Y et al: Functional importance of the left septal Purkinje network in the left ventricular conduction system. Jpn Heart J 22:363, 1981
32. Myerburg RJ: The gating mechanism in the distal atrioventricular conducting system. Circulation 43:955, 1971
33. Glassman RD, Zipes DP: Site of antegrade and retrograde functional right bundle branch block in the intact canine heart. Circulation 64:1277, 1981
34. Akhtar M, Gilbert C, Al-Nourim M et al: Site of conduction delay during functional block in the His-Purkinje system in man. Circulation 61:1239, 1980
35. Nagao K, Toyama J, Kodama I et al: Role of the conduction system in the endocardial excitation spread in the right ventricle. Am J Cardiol 48:864, 1981
36. Wyndham C, Meeran M, Levitsky S et al: Epicardial mapping in three patients with right bundle branch block (abstr). Circulation 54:II-128, 1976
37. Mayorga-Cortes A, Rozanski JJ, Sung RJ et al: Right ventricular apical activation times in patients with conduction disturbances occurring during acute transmural myocardial infarction. Am J Cardiol 43:913, 1979
38. Horowitz LN, Alexander JA, Edmunds LH Jr: Postoperative right bundle branch block: Identification of three levels of block. Circulation 62:319, 1980
39. Wolff GS, Rowland TW, Ellison RC: Surgically induced right bundle branch block with left anterior hemiblock: An ominous sign in post-operative tetralogy of Fallot. Circulation 46:587, 1972
40. Alpert BL, Schnitzler RN, Treibwasser JH: Right ventricular conduction times in asymptomatic right bundle branch block (abstr). Am J Cardiol 41:385, 1978
41. Dancy M, Leech G, Leatham A: Significance of complete right bundle branch block when an isolated finding. Br Heart J 48:217, 1982
42. Sohi GS, Flowers NC: Body surface map patterns of altered depolarization and repolarization in right bundle branch block. Circulation 61:634, 1980
43. Wyndham CRC, Smith T, Meeran MK et al: Epicardial activation in patients with left bundle branch block. Circulation 61:696, 1980
44. Wyndham CR, Meeran MK, Smith T et al: Epicardial activation in human left anterior fascicular block. Am J Cardiol 44:636, 1979
45. Barrett PA, Yamaguchi I, Jordan JL et al: Electrophysiological factors of left bundle branch block. Br Heart J 45:594, 1981
46. Cannon DS, Wyman MG, Goldreyer DN: Initial ventricular activation in left-sided intraventricular conduction defects.
47. Swiryn S, Abben R, Denes P et al: Electrocardiographic determinants of axis during left bundle branch block: Study in patients with intermittent left bundle branch block. Am J Cardiol 46:53, 1980
48. Abben R, Rosen KM, Denes P: Intermittent left bundle branch block: Anatomic substrate as reflected in the electrocardiogram during normal conduction. Circulation 59:1040, 1979
49. Watanabe Y, Nishimura M: Terminology and electrophysiologic concepts in cardiac arrhythmias V, phase 3 block and phase 4 block: I. PACE 2:335, 1979
50. Watanabe Y, Nishimura M: Terminology and electrophysiologic concepts in cardiac arrhythmias VI, phase 3 block and phase 4 block: II. PACE 2:624, 1979
51. Fisch C, Miles WM: Deceleration-dependent left bundle branch block: A spectrum of bundle branch conduction delay. Circulation 65:1029, 1982
52. Goodfriend MA, Barold SS: Tachycardia-dependent and bradycardia-dependent mobitz type 2 atrioventricular block within the bundle of His. Am J Cardiol 33:908, 1974
53. Rosenbaum MD, Elizari MV, Levi RJ et al: Paroxysmal atrioventricular block related to hypopolarization and spontaneous diastolic depolarization. Chest 63:678, 1973
54. El-Sherif N, Scherlag BJ, Lazzara R: Conduction disorders in the canine proximal His-Purkinje system following acute myocardial ischemia: I. The pathophysiology of intra-His bundle block. Circulation 49:837, 1974
55. El-Sherif N, Scherlag BJ, Lazzara R: Conduction disorders in the canine proximal His-Purkinje system following acute myocardial ischemia: II. The pathophysiology of bilateral bundle branch block. Circulation 49:848, 1974
56. El-Sherif N, Scherlag BJ, Lazzara R: Pathophysiology of second-degree atrioventricular block: A unified hypothesis. Am J Cardiol 35:421, 1975
57. Massie B, Scheinman MM, Peters RW et al: Clinical and electrophysiologic findings in patients with paroxysmal slowing of the sinus rate and apparent Mobitz II atrioventricular block. Circulation 58:305, 1978
58. Scott JS, Maddison DJ, Taylor PV et al: Connective-tissue disease, antibodies to ribonucleoprotein, and congenital heart block. N Engl J Med 309:209, 1983
59. Young D, Eisenberg R, Fisch B et al: Wenckebach atrioventricular block (Mobitz type I) in children and adolescents. Am J Cardiol 40:393, 1977
60. Karpawich PP, Gilette PC, Garson A et al: Congenital complete atrioventricular block: Clinical and electrophysiologic predictors of need for pacemaker insertion. Am J Cardiol 48:1098, 1981
61. Besley DC, McWilliams GJ, Moodie DS et al: Long-term follow-up of young adults following permanent pacemaker placement for complete heart block. Am Heart J 103:332, 1982
62. Reid JM, Coleman EN, Doig W: Complete congenital heart block: Report of 35 cases. Br Heart J 48:236, 1982
63. Strasberg B, Amat-Y-Leon F, Dhingra RC et al: Natural history of chronic second-degree atrioventricular nodal block. Circulation 63:1043, 1981
64. Pinsky WW, Gilette PC, Garson A et al: Diagnosis, management, and long-term results of patients with congenital complete atrioventricular block. Pediatrics 69:728, 1982
65. Bharati S, Rosen KM, Strasberg B et al: Anatomic substrate for congenital atrioventricular block in middle-aged adults. PACE 5:860, 1982
66. Rosen KM, Dhingra RC, Loeb HS et al: Chronic heart block in adults: Clinical and electrophysiological observations. Arch Int Med 131:663, 1973
67. Lasser RP, Haft JI, Friedberg CK: Relationship of right bundle branch block and marked left axis deviation (with left parietal or peri-infarction block) to complete heart block and syncope. Circulation 37:429, 1968
68. Scanlon PJ, Pryor R, Blount SG Jr: Right bundle-branch block associated with left superior or inferior intraventricular block: Clinical setting, prognosis, and relation to complete heart block. Circulation 42:1123, 1970
69. DePasquale NP, Bruno MS: Natural history of combined right bundle branch block and left anterior hemiblock (bilateral bundle branch block). Am J Med 54:297, 1973
70. Kulbertus HE: The magnitude of risk of developing complete heart block in patients with LAD-RBBB. Am Heart J 86:278, 1973
71. Kulbertus HE: Reevaluation of the prognosis of patients with LAD-RBBB. Am Heart J 92:665, 1976
72. Pine MB, Uren M, Ciafone R et al: Excess mortality and morbidity associated with right bundle branch and left anterior fascicular block. J Am Coll Cardiol 1:1207, 1983
73. Wiberg TA, Richman HG, Gobel FL: The significance and prognosis of chronic bifascicular block. Chest 71:329, 1977
74. Dhingra RC, Amat-Y-Leon F, Wyndham C et al: Significance of left axis deviation in patients with chronic left bundle branch block. Am J Cardiol 42:551, 1978
75. Havelda CJ, Sohi GS, Flowers NC et al: The pathologic correlates of the electrocardiogram: Complete left bundle branch block. Circulation 68:445, 1982
76. Rotman M, Triebwasser JH: A clinical and follow-up study of right and left bundle branch block. Circulation 51:477, 1975
77. Siegman-Igra Y, Yahini JH, Goldbourt U et al: Intraventricular conduction disturbances: A review of prevalence, etiology, and progression for ten years within a stable population of Israeli adult males. Am Heart J 96:669, 1978

78. Fleg JL, Das DN, Lakatta EG: Right bundle branch block: Long-term prognosis in apparently healthy men. J Am Coll Cardiol 1:887, 1983
79. Rabkin SW, Mathewson FAL, Tate RB: Natural history of left bundle branch block. Br Heart J 43:164, 1980
80. Rabkin SW, Mathewson FAL, Tate RB: The natural history of right bundle branch block and frontal plane QRS axis in apparently healthy men. Chest 80:191, 1981
81. Schneider JF, Thomas HE, Kreger BE et al: Newly acquired left bundle-branch block: The Framingham study. Ann Intern Med 90:303, 1979
82. Schneider JF, Thomas HE Jr, Kreger DE et al: Newly acquired right bundle-branch block: The Framingham study. Ann Intern Med 92:37, 1980
83. Narula OS, Samet P: Right bundle branch block with normal, left or right axis deviation: Analysis by His bundle recordings. Am J Med 51:432, 1971
84. Levites R, Haft JI: Significance of first-degree heart block (prolonged P-R interval) in bifascicular block. Am J Cardiol 34:259, 1974
85. Vera Z, Mason DT, Fletcher RD et al: Prolonged His-Q interval in chronic bifascicular block: Relation to impending complete heart block. Circulation 53:46, 1976
86. McAnulty JH, Rahimtoola SH, Murphy E et al: Natural history of "high-risk" bundle-branch block: Final report of a prospective study. N Engl J Med 307:137, 1982
87. Wyse DG, McAnulty JH, Rahimtoola SH et al: Electrophysiologic abnormalities of the sinus node and atrium in patients with bundle branch block. Circulation 60:413, 1979
88. Dhingra RC, Palileo E, Strasberg D et al: Significance of the HV interval in 517 patients with chronic bifascicular block. Circulation 64:1265, 1981
89. Dhingra RC, Denes P, Wu D et al: Syncope in patients with chronic bifascicular block: Significance, causative mechanisms and clinical implications. Ann Intern Med 81:302, 1974
90. Scheinman MM, Peters RW, Sauvé MJ et al: The value of the HQ interval in patients with bundle branch block and the role of prophylactic pacing. Am J Cardiol 50:1316, 1982
91. Altschuler H, Fisher JD, Furman S: Significance of isolated H-V interval prolongation in symptomatic patients without documented heart block. Am Heart J 97:19, 1979
92. Narula OS: Intraventricular conduction defects: Current concepts and clinical significance. In Narula OS (ed): Cardiac Arrhythmias: Electrophysiology, Diagnosis, and Management, pp 114–132. Baltimore, Williams & Wilkins, 1979
93. Higgins J, Scheinman MM, Morady F et al: Electrophysiologic evaluation of patients with bundle branch block and syncope (abstr). Circulation 66(suppl II):147, 1982
94. Ezri M, Lerman DB, Marchlinski FE et al: Electrophysiologic evaluation of syncope in patients with bifascicular block. Am Heart J 106:693, 1983
95. Dhingra RC, Wyndham C, Bauernfeind R et al: Significance of block distal to the His bundle induced by atrial pacing in patients with chronic bifascicular block. Circulation 60:1455, 1979
96. Woelfel AK, Simpson RJ, Gettes LS, Foster JR: Exercise-induced distal atrioventricular block. J Am Coll Cardiol 2:578, 1983
97. Chiale PA, Przybylski J, Laino RA et al: Usefulness of the ajmaline test in patients with latent bundle branch block. Am J Cardiol 49:21, 1982
98. Gupta PK, Lichstein E, Chadda KD: Lidocaine-induced heart block in patients with bundle branch block. Am J Cardiol 33:487, 1974
99. Timins BI, Gutman JA, Haft JI: Disopyramide-induced heart block. Chest 79:477, 1981
100. Kunkel F, Rowland M, Scheinman MM: The electrophysiologic effects of lidocaine in patients with intraventricular conduction defects. Circulation 49:894, 1974
101. Desai JM, Scheinman M, Peters RW et al: Electrophysiological effects of disopyramide in patients with bundle branch block. Circulation 59:2151, 1979
102. Kunstadt D, Punja M, Cagin N et al: Bifascicular block: A clinical and electrophysiologic study. Am Heart J 86:173, 1973
103. Santini M, Carrara P, Benhar M et al: Possible risks of general anesthesia in patients with intraventricular conduction disturbances. PACE 3:130, 1980
104. Mikell FL, Weir EK, Chesler E: Perioperative risk of complete heart block in patients with bifascicular block and prolonged PR interval. Thorax 36:14, 1981
105. Peters RW, Nussbaum S, Mailhot J et al: Catheter-induced A-V nodal block occurring during electrophysiologic study. PACE 7:248, 1984
106. Jacobson LB, Scheinman M: Catheter-induced intra-hisian and intra-fascicular block during recording of His bundle electrogram. Circulation 49:579, 1974
107. Stein PD, Mathar VS, Herman MV et al: Complete heart block induced during cardiac catheterization of patients with pre-existent bundle branch block. Circulation 34:783, 1966
108. Godman MJ, Lassers BW, Julian DG: Complete bundle-branch block complicating acute myocardial infarction. N Engl J Med 282:237, 1970
109. Scheinman M, Brenman B: Clinical and anatomic implications of intraventricular conduction blocks in acute myocardial infarction. Circulation 46:753, 1972
110. Waters DD, Mizgala HF: Long-term prognosis of patients with incomplete bilateral bundle-branch block complicating acute myocardial infarction: Role of cardiac pacing. Am J Cardiol 34:1, 1974
111. Nimetz AA, Shubrooks SJ Jr, Hatter Am Jr et al: The significance of bundle-branch block during acute myocardial infarction. Am Heart J 4:439, 1975
112. Scanlon PJ, Pryor R, Blount SG Jr: Right bundle-branch block associated with left superior or inferior intraventricular block associated with acute myocardial infarction. Circulation 42:1135, 1970
113. Atkins JM, Leshin SJ, Blomquist G et al: Ventricular conduction blocks and sudden death in acute myocardial infarction: Potential indications for pacing. N Engl J Med 6:281, 1973
114. Waugh RA, Wagner GS, Haneg TL et al: Immediate and remote prognostic significance of fascicular block during acute myocardial infarction. Circulation 47:765, 1973
115. Gann D, Dalachandran PK, El-Sherif N et al: Prognostic significance of chronic versus acute bundle-branch block in acute myocardial infarction. Chest 67:298, 1975
116. Ritter WS, Atkins JM, Blomquist CG et al: Permanent pacing with patients with transient trifascicular block during acute myocardial infarction. Am J Cardiol 38:205, 1976
117. Lie KI, Liem KL, Schuilenberg RM et al: Early identification of patients developing late in-hospital ventricular fibrillation after discharge from the coronary care unit: A 5½ year retrospective and prospective study of 1897 patients. Am J Cardiol 41:674, 1978
118. Hauer RN, Lie KI, Liem KL et al: Long-term prognosis in patients with bundle branch block complicating acute anteroseptae infarction. Am J Cardiol 49:1581, 1982
119. Hollander G, Nadiminti V, Lichstein E et al: Bundle-branch block in acute myocardial infarction. Am Heart J 105:738, 1983
120. Hindman MC, Wagner GS, Jaho M et al: The clinical significance of bundle-branch block complicating acute myocardial infarction: I. Clinical characteristics, hospital mortality and one-year follow-up. Circulation 58:679, 1978
121. Hindman MC, Wagner GS, Jaho M et al: The clinical significance of bundle-branch block complicating acute myocardial infarction: II. Indications for temporary and permanent pacemaker insertion. Circulation 58:689, 1978
122. Schoenfeld CD, Mascarenhas E, Bhardwaj P et al: Clinical and electrophysiologic significance of bundle-branch block and acute myocardial infarction (abstr). Am J Cardiol 31:156, 1973
123. Lichstein E, Gupta PK, Chadda KD et al: Findings of prognostic value in patients with incomplete bilateral bundle branch block complicating acute myocardial infarction. Am J Cardiol 32:913, 1973
124. Lie KI, Wellers HJ, Schuilenburg RM: Factors influencing prognosis of bundle branch block complicating acute antero-septal infarction: The value of His bundle recordings. Circulation 50:935, 1974
125. Gould L, Reddy CVR, Kim SG et al: His bundle electrogram in patients with acute myocardial infarction. PACE 2:428, 1979
126. Watson RDS, Glover DR, Page AJF: The Birmingham Trial of permanent paving in patients with intraventricular conduction disorders after acute myocardial infarction. Am Heart J 108:496, 1984
127. Pagnori F, Finzi A, Valentini R: Long-term prognostic significance and electrophysiological evaluation of intraventricular conduction disturbances complicating acute myocardial infarction. PACE 9:91, 1986

SUPRAVENTRICULAR TACHYCARDIA

John M. Herre • Melvin M. Scheinman

A supraventricular tachycardia (SVT) is any tachycardia that requires the participation of tissues above the bifurcation of the bundle of His for propagation. In some reentrant SVTs, the ventricular muscle also participates as part of the reentrant loop. The basic mechanism of SVT appears to be related to abnormal automaticity, triggered rhythms, or reentry. These mechanisms are discussed in detail elsewhere in these volumes.

ELECTROCARDIOGRAPHIC DIAGNOSIS OF SUPRAVENTRICULAR TACHYCARDIA

A narrow QRS complex tachycardia with a rate greater than 100 beats per minute meets the criteria for SVT. However, some patients with SVT may have wide complex tachycardia owing to aberrant ventricular conduction or antecedent bundle branch block and thus may mimic ventricular tachycardia (VT). The presence of capture or fusion beats or atrioventricular (AV) dissociation is pathognomonic of VT. In addition, morphologic criteria suggestive of VT include QRS duration greater than 0.14 second, a markedly superior frontal plane QRS axis, and monophasic R or R/S pattern in V_1 for right bundle branch block morphology or a qR in V_6 for left bundle branch block morphology.[1] The morphology and axis of the P wave and the relationship between the P wave and the QRS complex may help to identify the mechanism of the tachycardia (Fig. 49.1).

HEMODYNAMIC EFFECTS OF SUPRAVENTRICULAR TACHYCARDIA

The hemodynamic response to SVT depends on a variety of factors related to heart rate, ventricular function, AV synchrony, coronary blood flow, volume status, and reflex autonomic adjustments.

While not identical to clinical tachycardia, the response to atrial pacing gives insight into hemodynamic response to systematic changes in rate during SVT. As atrial rate increases from 50 to 90 per minute, cardiac output increases. With further acceleration, cardiac output remains constant due to a progressive decline in left ventricular size, end-diastolic volume, and pressure.[2–4]

With the onset of SVT, there may be hypotension, decreased pulse pressure, and no detectable pulsatile flow for several beats. During the initial six tachycardia beats, Schleppes and co-workers[5] found that the left ventricular systolic pressure fell below arterial diastolic pressure. After six beats, left ventricular systolic pressure increased enough to open the aortic valve. By 9 minutes after the onset of tachycardia, arterial pressure and cardiac output were partially restored and contractility (dP/dt) was equal to pretachycardia levels although stroke volume remained depressed. Pulmonary venous pressures rise significantly during SVT, possibly accounting for the dyspnea that is so commonly observed.[5,6]

After the initial 5 to 15 tachycardia beats, there is a progressive tachycardia acceleration to peak rate after 20 to 30 seconds and then a gradual slowing of the tachycardia to a rate slightly faster than its initial rate. The initial rate increase seems related to increased sympathetic tone as manifested by shortened AV nodal refractoriness and conduction time. Later, there is compensatory restoration of blood pressure related to improved ventricular ejection. This is followed by increased vagal tone as manifested by prolonged AV nodal refractoriness and conduction time and slowing of the tachycardia rate.

Upright tilting accentuates the early hypotension and tachycardia acceleration. The magnitude of the early hemodynamic change is also accentuated when the change in rate is very rapid.[7] Thus, tolerance of SVT varies with time after onset, posture, and initial rate of the tachycardia.

In patients with cardiac disease, left ventricular end-diastolic pressure may rise acutely, decline, or remain unchanged with the onset of tachycardia.[8] Ventricular function may worsen with time depending on tachycardia rate and the severity of underlying disease.[9] Chronic SVT may cause a reversible cardiomyopathy.[10]

CORONARY BLOOD FLOW

Angina pectoris during tachycardia may occur in the absence of coronary artery disease,[6] probably resulting from a mismatch between myocardial oxygen demand and supply. At very rapid heart rates, reductions in ventricular filling and stroke volume limit coronary perfusion. In patients with cardiac disease, high subendocardial pressures and reduced coronary reserve may combine to increase risk for subendocardial ischemia during tachycardia.[11]

CLINICAL MANIFESTATIONS

With the onset of SVT, patients may be asymptomatic or complain of palpitations, pulsations in the neck, dyspnea, chest pain, or syncope. Polyuria may occur and is believed to be due to changes in antidiuretic hormone elaboration elicited by atrial stretch.[10] Structural cardiac lesions such as mitral stenosis, ventricular hypertrophy, or aortic stenosis influence clinical tolerance of supraventricular tachyarrhythmias by interfering with ventricular filling or emptying. Loss of the normal sequence of atrial contraction during atrial fibrillation may reduce ventricular diastolic filling with devastating functional effects on noncompliant, hypertrophied ventricles. Regional blood flow may be compromised during SVT in patients with pre-existing vascular disease leading to symptoms related to decreased cerebral, renal, or peripheral blood flow.

SINUS TACHYCARDIA

Sinus tachycardia is the normal physiologic response to increased sympathetic tone or reduced vagal tone. Sinus rate accelerates above 100 beats per minute and P wave morphology is identical to that during sinus rhythm, although P wave amplitude may increase and PR interval may shorten. Usually, sinus tachycardia develops and terminates gradually. Exercise, anxiety, fever, acute myocardial infarction, acute pulmonary embolism, hyperthyroidism, and pheochromocytoma cause increases in sinus rate through direct increases in sympathetic tone or increased cardiac sensitivity to adrenergic stimulation.

Occasionally, sinus tachycardia persists at rest. With resting sinus rates exceeding 100 beats per minute, patients may be annoyed by palpitations. Carotid sinus massage may slow tachycardia rate transiently but does not terminate sinus tachycardia. In seven patients with nonparoxysmal sinus tachycardia studied by Bauernfeind and associates, enhanced sinus node automaticity seemed related to increased sympathetic tone, reduced vagal tone, or both.[12] When palpitations are associated with symptoms and no underlying reversible illness can be found, a β-adrenergic agent may be required for symptomatic relief.

Sinoatrial reentry has been documented in as many as 3% of patients undergoing cardiac electrophysiologic evaluation for SVT.[13] In contrast to sinus tachycardia, sinoatrial reentry can be initiated and terminated by atrial pacing. Perinodal fibers that surround the sinus node are functionally similar to AV nodal fibers and provide the substrate for sinoatrial reentry.[14] Premature impulses conduct slowly through the sinoatrial and perinodal regions and exit to reexcite the surrounding atrial tissue. Sinoatrial reentrant tachycardia has a P wave morphology identical to that during sinus rhythm at comparable rates. P waves precede the QRS complex, and the PR interval is similar to that during sinus rhythm at comparable rates. Heart rates tend to be slower than rates common for AV node reentry, and the tachycardia tends to be nonsustained and minimally symptomatic.

Because of the generous vagal innervation in the region of the sinoatrial node, carotid sinus massage may terminate the arrhythmia. Digitalis, β-adrenergic blockers, or verapamil may be effective initial treatments but may adversely suppress sinus rate in patients with underlying sinus node dysfunction. In addition, class IA antiarrhythmic agents (procainamide, quinidine, and disopyramide) may prove effective in these patients.

ATRIAL ECTOPIC TACHYCARDIA

Ectopic tachycardias are believed to develop from enhanced automaticity in tissues lying above the bifurcation of the His bundle. In isolated human atrial tissue, spontaneous depolarizations recorded before or after full repolarization appear to be potential sources for pacemaker activity.[15] In patients, ectopic or automatic tachycardias are best distinguished from reentrant and triggered mechanisms by their response to pacing. After overdrive pacing there may be transient suppression or acceleration of tachycardia but never termination. The onset of atrial ectopic tachycardia may show a gradual increase in rate to a new steady-state rate.[16] The initiating P wave morphology is identical to all other tachycardia P waves. While a programmed premature atrial depolarization during tachycardia may reset the tachycardia, it seldom results in tachycardia termination. The P wave vector may help localize the atrial focus in the absence of atrial disease.[17-19]

Chronic ectopic tachycardia with one dominant P wave morphology has been described in children, but this form is rare in adults. Congestive heart failure commonly accompanies atrial ectopic tachycardia in the pediatric population.[20,21]

In adults, ectopic atrial tachycardia tends to be transient and may occur in the setting of acute myocardial infarction, exacerbation of chronic lung disease, ethanol excess, metabolic derangements, congestive heart failure, or digitalis excess. Underlying cardiac disease is almost always present.[13]

Treatment of the underlying illness is the cornerstone of treatment in adults with atrial ectopic tachycardia. If temporary or prolonged drug treatment is elected, the primary approach may be to suppress the atrial focus (class I agents) or to block impulse conduction at the level of the AV node (digitalis, β-adrenergic blockers, or calcium channel blockers). Drug selection is empiric and the response is variable.

In children with chronic or repetitive automatic atrial tachycardia, digoxin alone is not effective.[21] Class IA or IC agents or amiodarone may be effective in some cases. Gillette and associates have described the successful use of catheter ablation in 2 of 4 patients and mapping-guided surgical resection in 13 of 14 patients.[22]

MULTIFOCAL ATRIAL TACHYCARDIA

Multifocal atrial tachycardia (MAT) occurs in adult patients with underlying pulmonary or cardiac disease. Diagnostic electrocardiographic criteria include three or more P wave morphologies with variation in the PP and PR intervals. Isoelectric intervals are noted and the atrial rate is usually 100 to 250 beats per minute. When P wave amplitude is low, differentiation from atrial fibrillation may be difficult.

MAT occurs most often in elderly patients with acute worsening of a chronic obstructive pulmonary disease, coronary or hypertensive heart disease, or digitalis excess. Valvular heart disease, electrolyte imbalance, postanesthesia recovery, congenital heart disease, and pulmonary embolism are less common causes of MAT.

TREATMENT

MAT is often refractory to antiarrhythmic drug treatment but responds to control of the underlying illness. Digoxin is ineffective as a primary treatment but may help control symptoms of congestive heart failure owing to tachycardia. Phenytoin, quinidine, procainamide, lidocaine, and propranolol are often ineffective.

Verapamil has been shown to slow the atrial rate of multifocal atrial tachycardia and occasionally to restore sinus rhythm. Verapamil may be a useful adjunct for control of the arrhythmia before the precipitating illness can be effectively treated. However, it should be appreciated that hypoxia may worsen in those with chronic obstructive pulmonary disease because of pulmonary vasodilatation of unventilated lung segments by verapamil.[23]

ATRIAL FIBRILLATION

Atrial fibrillation is the most common sustained arrhythmia in clinical practice.[24] Atrial fibrillation may occur transiently during episodic illness, paroxysmally without obvious acute illness, or as a chronic sustained arrhythmia. In time, paroxysmal episodes of palpitations and rapid ventricular rates may evolve to chronic atrial fibrillation.

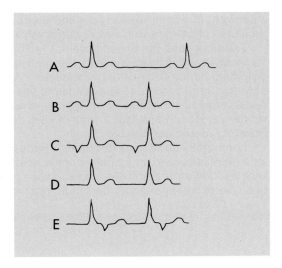

FIGURE 49.1 Electrocardiogram in supraventricular tachycardia, lead II. **A.** Normal sinus rhythm, rate < 100 beats per minute. Upright P wave precedes the QRS complex. **B.** Sinus tachycardia, sinoatrial reentrant tachycardia, intra-atrial tachycardia, or ectopic atrial tachycardia with the focus near the sinus node, rate > 100 beats per minute. Upright P wave precedes the QRS complex. **C.** Intra-atrial reentrant tachycardia or ectopic atrial tachycardia with a low atrial focus, unusual variety of AV nodal reentrant tachycardia, rate > 100 beats per minute. Inverted P wave precedes the QRS complex. **D.** AV nodal reentrant tachycardia (common variety), rate > 100 beats per minute. No P wave is visible. **E.** Atrioventricular reentrant tachycardia using an accessory pathway.

PREVALENCE

The prevalence of chronic atrial fibrillation depends on the population being observed. Twelve-lead electrocardiograms revealed atrial fibrillation in 8% to 14% of the hospitalized patients[24,25] but in only 5 of 122,043 healthy male Air Force flyers.[26] The Framingham population of 2325 men and 2866 women was followed for 22 years with biennial 13-lead electrocardiograms. Atrial fibrillation developed in 49 men and 49 women, for an incidence of 21.5 and 17.1 per thousand, respectively.[27]

Atrial fibrillation increases with age and with the presence of heart disease.[28] Atrial fibrillation is rare in infants and children, appearing almost exclusively in those with structural heart disease.[29,30] Even in hospitalized patients with atrial fibrillation, fewer than 1% of cases occur before age 9 and fewer than 5% before age 19.[31,32] In the Framingham study, the cumulative incidence of atrial fibrillation rose sharply after age 35[27] and began to plateau at 3% to 4% of the population at risk by the fifth and sixth decades.

MECHANISM

Atrial fibrillation is most likely due to intra-atrial reentry. Atrial fibrillation can be initiated by rapid pacing or by critically timed atrial premature stimuli and can be terminated by direct-current countershock.[33] Moe and associates[34] proposed that atrial fibrillation could develop from intra-atrial reentry of multiple wavelets moving over several pathways. Monitoring 192 unipolar electrograms during stable atrial fibrillation, Allessie and co-workers were able to detect three to four wavelets propagating simultaneously through each atrium.[35] Each wavelet existed for only a few hundred milliseconds before extinguishing by collision with other wavelets to produce functional conduction block. Merging of wavelets and septal breakthrough to excite the opposite atrium were also detected.

Both vagal and sympathetic tone influence the initiation and stability of atrial fibrillation.[35] Vagally induced fibrillation is seen typically in relatively young (age 30-40) athletic men. Attacks occur at rest or during sleep; may be aggravated by digitalis, verapamil, or β-adrenergic blocking drugs; and tend to respond to maneuvers that prevent relative bradycardia. Adrenergically induced atrial fibrillation is equally common in men and women, often occurs during daytime activity, may be reproduced by exercise or isoproterenol, and tends to respond to β-adrenergic blocker therapy.[36,37]

PATHOLOGIC FEATURES

The pathology of atrial fibrillation is diverse. Patients dying with acute pulmonary embolism and atrial fibrillation may have no atrial muscular abnormality, suggesting that sudden atrial stretch may cause atrial fibrillation. In others with atrial fibrillation and acute pericarditis, local atrial inflammation may be found. In chronic atrial fibrillation, sinus node cellular loss, and fibrotic replacement, disruption of atrial myocardium and atrial dilatation are common pathologic observations, but the relative roles of these changes are not defined. Thus, the pathologic substrate for atrial fibrillation may be acute stretch, acute inflammation, or replacement of atrial muscle by fibrous tissue or by an infiltrative process (such as amyloid or hemochromatosis). Structurally normal hearts have also supported sustained atrial fibrillation, although the mechanisms are not clear.[38]

CLINICAL PATTERNS AND PRECIPITATING ILLNESSES

Atrial fibrillation has paroxysmal or chronic patterns. Paroxysmal atrial fibrillation may occur with or without an acute clinical illness and is usually associated with normal atrial size. Pharmacologic therapy is often effective in the maintenance of sinus rhythm. In contrast, chronic atrial fibrillation tends to be sustained, develops in larger atria, and resists pharmacologic maintenance of sinus rhythm.[39]

The structural cardiac lesions associated with atrial fibrillation include rheumatic heart disease, hypertensive cardiomyopathy, dilated cardiomyopathy, alcoholic heart disease, and chronic pericarditis. Atrial fibrillation occurs in up to 75% of patients with hemodynamically significant mitral regurgitation[41] and in about 40% of patients needing surgery for mitral stenosis.[40] In these patients, the risk for atrial fibrillation appears to increase with the magnitude of left atrial enlargement, but the risk does not correlate with hemodynamic severity of mitral stenosis or pulmonary vascular resistance. Sinus rhythm and paroxysmal atrial fibrillation become less common in those with gross atrial enlargement, but there is considerable overlap between the groups.[39]

With the decline of acute rheumatic fever in developed countries, hypertensive heart disease has supplanted rheumatic mitral disease as the most common precursor of atrial fibrillation. Hypertension was present in half of the Framingham population with atrial fibrillation, and risk was primarily reserved for those with ventricular hypertrophy.[27] McIntosh and co-workers suggested that atrial fibrillation may be present in up to one fourth of patients dying with hypertensive cardiovascular disease.[8]

In hypertrophic cardiomyopathy, atrial fibrillation occurs only in well-advanced disease. Significant hemodynamic deterioration is common, and risk for systemic embolization is high. As in rheumatic disease, risk for atrial fibrillation increases with left atrial enlargement. In one study of patients with hypertrophic cardiomyopathy,[41] atrial fibrillation occurred in 16 of 167 patients (10%). The risk was unrelated to the severity of atrial or ventricular end-diastolic pressure elevation, but 13 of the 16 patients had left atrial enlargement. The average duration of illness was 16 years, suggesting a relationship between risk and the extent of atrial muscular disease. Similarly, atrial fibrillation occurs late in patients dying of severe obesity and its associated cardiomyopathy.[42,43]

Risk for atrial fibrillation is high in primary cardiac muscle disorders including dilated, restrictive, and infiltrative cardiomyopathies. Dilated cardiomyopathy is complicated by atrial fibrillation in up to 25% of patients.[44] Occult alcoholic cardiomyopathy with superimposed binge drinking can induce atrial fibrillation in up to 60% of patients.[45] Similarly, chronic obstructive pulmonary disease with superimposed bronchitis may lead to atrial fibrillation, which improves with control of the infection. Transient atrial fibrillation may complicate reversible cardiomyopathy in the peripartum period,[46] acute lupus myocarditis,[47] and idiopathic or uremic pericardial disease with inflammation. Thyrotoxicosis is complicated by atrial fibrillation in 12% to 18% of patients, especially in the elderly where it may be the only clue of thyroid excess. Hoffman and Lowrey found no atrial fibrillation in thyrotoxic patients under age 30 but a 20% incidence in those over age 50.[48,49]

Atrial fibrillation is uncommon in ischemic heart disease unless complicated by cardiopulmonary congestion or acute myocardial infarction.[27,50] Autopsy data reveal isolated coronary artery disease in fewer than 5% of patients dying of atrial fibrillation and in fewer than 0.8% with demonstrable high-grade coronary artery disease at angiography.[50] Similarly, atrial fibrillation is uncommon in aortic valvular disease without mitral involvement and its development reflects poor prognosis in patients with severe aortic valvular obstruction.

Transient atrial fibrillation develops in 10% to 18% of patients with acute myocardial infarction either related to atrial ischemia[51] or to distention during congestive heart failure.[52] As a group, these patients have poorer prognosis because of larger infarctions and greater functional ventricular impairment or because of advanced age.[53] Control of ventricular rate is important to limit oxygen demand and curtail further ischemic ventricular damage.

Lone atrial fibrillation describes a group of patients with stable atrial fibrillation and structurally normal hearts. Evans and Swann described lone atrial fibrillation in otherwise healthy males. These patients were asymptomatic, had moderate ventricular rates, resisted cardioversion to sinus mechanism, and had an excellent long-term prognosis.[54,55] Structural heart disease was not identified in 31% of patients with atrial fibrillation followed in the Framingham study.[27]

ELECTROCARDIOGRAPHIC FINDINGS

The hallmarks of atrial fibrillation are irregular baseline oscillations or atrial F waves and an irregularly irregular ventricular rate. When F waves are discernible, the atrial fibrillation rate varies from 400 to 700 per minute but fine F waves or no observable atrial activity may be present. In such cases, random irregularity in the ventricular response is present in the absence of drug treatment. Concealed conduction occurs primarily at the AV node but decremental conduction could develop in the atrium, His-Purkinje system, or Purkinje-myocardial junction. Partial penetration leaves tissue refractory so that subsequent early impulses are slowed or blocked at various levels within the AV junction. Random impulse arrival, penetration, and slowing appear to account for the irregular ventricular response during atrial fibrillation.[56,57] The irregularity may be less obvious at very fast ventricular rates, and careful scrutiny with calipers may be needed to confirm atrial fibrillation. Extremely regular ventricular rates during atrial fibrillation suggest the presence of complete AV block as a result of drug therapy or because of intrinsic disease of the AV conduction system[58] or ventricular tachycardia. Ventricular bigeminy during atrial fibrillation may slow the ventricular rate further due to retrograde concealed conduction in the AV node.

PHYSICAL FINDINGS

Physical findings during atrial fibrillation include variation in the intensity of the first heart sound, absence of a waves in the jugular venous pulse, and variance between the apical and radial pulses due to feeble ventricular ejection with short diastolic filling times. Hypotension, diaphoresis, or loss of consciousness with the onset of atrial fibrillation is unusual and suggests poor left ventricular compliance. Regularization of the radial pulse usually means conversion to another rhythm.

COMPLICATIONS

Systemic embolization is a dreaded complication for patients with either paroxysmal or chronic atrial fibrillation. Embolic risk is highest soon after the onset of atrial fibrillation[59] or with rhythm change. Elective direct-current cardioversion is complicated by a 1% to 4% incidence of clinical embolic events[60] usually within 2 weeks of the procedure.[59] Similarly, in 59 patients in the Framingham study with atrial fibrillation and cerebrovascular accidents, 14 patients (24%) were already hospitalized for a cerebrovascular accident when atrial fibrillation was first detected and an additional 8 patients (14%) developed strokes over the subsequent year. The incidence of embolization remained at 5% per year over the next 30 years.[59] However, 30% to 40% or more of patients with chronic atrial fibrillation will have peripheral emboli at autopsy.[60-63]

Risk for embolization is highest in those with atrial fibrillation complicating rheumatic mitral disease,[64,65] large myocardial infarctions,[63] hypertrophic cardiomyopathy,[40,66] and dilated cardiomyopathy.[67] In patients with prior myocardial infarction, mural thrombi have been found in the left atrium or near a left ventricular aneurysm.[63] Of autopsied patients with atrial fibrillation, 40% to 70% show cerebral involvement.[60,63] Coronary, renal, mesenteric, and splenic emboli are less common.[63]

Prior embolization is a strong indication for chronic anticoagulation. Once systemic embolization has occurred, the recurrence rate is 25% to 42%. Recurrences tend to cluster near the initial event with nearly half occurring within 2 weeks of the first event and an additional one fourth within 4 months.[59] Early anticoagulation is safe and effective in these patients. Bleeding and poor patient compliance are contraindications to long-term therapy. Anticoagulation should be delayed until hemorrhage has been excluded by computed tomography or magnetic resonance imaging and examination of the cerebrospinal fluid for red blood cells.[63] In the absence of bleeding, anticoagulation may be instituted 24 to 48 hours after a cerebral embolic event. Anticoagulant therapy is clearly indicated for those patients with mitral stenosis and atrial fibrillation given the high (30%–75%) incidence of cerebral and peripheral emboli.[64]

In patients without rheumatic heart disease or previous emboli, few firm guidelines for anticoagulation exist. Anticoagulation may reduce the risk for embolization during cardioversion from 5% to less than 1%,[68] but some argue for anticoagulating only high-risk patients in this setting given the low incidence and significant potential risk of bleeding.[69,70] In those at high risk, anticoagulation should be instituted at least 2 weeks before and continued for 1 week after elective cardioversion.[71] If atrial fibrillation recurs, chronic anticoagulation should be considered strongly for those in high-risk groups.[72]

In patients with hemodynamically unstable arrhythmias, emergency direct-current cardioversion is necessary. In more stable patients drug therapy should be directed at slowing the ventricular rate. In those with recent-onset atrial fibrillation and nearly normal atrial size, conversion to sinus rhythm should be attempted.

Patients with a single episode of hemodynamically stable atrial fibrillation and normal left atrial dimensions may not require long-term therapy. In patients with hemodynamically unstable arrhythmias, emergency direct-current cardioversion is necessary. In more stable patients, initial drug therapy should be directed at slowing the ventricular rate. Pharmacologic conversion may be accomplished with intravenous therapy with procainamide in doses up to 1 g[73] or with oral therapy with procainamide or quinidine. Pharmacologic conversion is more likely when the atrial fibrillation is of recent onset and left atrial size is normal or near normal.

Long-term treatment with class IA or IC antiarrhythmic agents may reduce the recurrence of atrial fibrillation. Amiodarone may be partially or completely effective in 50% to 75% of patients with paroxysmal atrial fibrillation who failed to respond to quinidine.[74]

ATRIAL FLUTTER

Experimental and clinical evidence favors a reentrant mechanism for classic atrial flutter. The arrhythmia can be initiated and terminated by extrastimulation or rapid atrial pacing[75-77] and is terminated by direct-current cardioversion. Unlike atrial rhythms related to enhanced automaticity, circulating intracardiac impulses can be recorded throughout most of the atrial cycle in atrial flutter.[78,79]

ELECTROCARDIOGRAPHIC FINDINGS

The electrocardiographic criteria for atrial flutter are based primarily on rate. In the absence of drug treatment, the atrial rate is 280 to 320 beats per minute with sawtooth undulations of the baseline best seen in inferior frontal leads II, III, and aV_F and in precordial lead V_1. The QRS complex is usually narrow and 2:1 AV conduction yields a ventricular rate of 150 beats per minute. Carotid sinus massage may increase the degree of AV block and unmask the flutter waves. Four-to-one penetration may result from block of the first and third impulse in the upper AV node (AN region) and the second impulse block in a lower (NH) area. Watanabe[80] has observed deeper penetration of first and third impulses to the mid AV node (N region). Occasionally, variation in the PR interval and ventricular irregularity occur during atrial flutter, reflecting a more random pattern of decremental conduction. Ventricular rate may be slowed in patients with intrinsic AV node or His-Purkinje disease or quite rapid in those with short AV node refractory periods or accessory pathways.[81] One-to-one AV conduction and extremely rapid ventricular rates can lead to syncope or sudden death. Using bipolar atrial electrogram recordings in postsurgical patients,

Waldo[76] has described typical or type I flutter demonstrating regular, uniform atrial deflections, rates averaging 240 to 340 beats per minute, and entrainment or termination of the tachycardia with atrial pacing. Atypical or type II flutter also occurs with constant beat-to-beat morphology, amplitude, and cycle length but has faster rates (340–433 beats per minute) and fails to terminate with atrial overdrive pacing.

The atria contract in atrial flutter and the arrhythmia tends to be transient, factors probably accounting for the low incidence of systemic emboli. Flutter waves in the jugular venous pulse or alternating cannon waves may allow bedside diagnosis. Atrial flutter is rare in patients with structurally normal hearts but may occur after an acute pulmonary embolus,[82] with hyperthyroidism,[83] after cardiac surgery,[76] or with other reversible illnesses.

Atrial flutter is seen in three groups in the pediatric population: (1) otherwise normal infants, either prenatally or in the early postpartum period; (2) children with atrial abnormalities; and (3) children and young adults after repair of congenital heart disease, particularly with Mustard, Senning and Fontan procedures, and of atrial septal defects. In the newborn population, flutter rates as high as 400 beats per minute are seen. One-to-one AV conduction is possible, leading to congestive heart failure or hemodynamic collapse. Following cardioversion, the arrhythmia may not recur and treatment beyond 6 months of age is rarely necessary.[84] Atrial flutter may present at any age in children with atrial abnormalities, particularly sinus venosus atrial septal defect.

In the postoperative patient, atrial flutter is common and, with 1:1 AV conduction, has been implicated in the pathogenesis of sudden cardiac death. Often, coexistent sinus node dysfunction requires permanent pacing in order to allow adequate medical treatment.[85]

TREATMENT

When atrial flutter is tolerated poorly, prompt direct-current cardioversion is required. Transthoracic energy as low as 10 to 25 joules may be effective. When atrial flutter is tolerated, initial treatment strategy is often aimed at slowing the ventricular rate. Pharmacologic block of the atrioventricular node is usually attempted with β-adrenergic blockers, verapamil, or digitalis. In contrast to atrial fibrillation, atrial flutter tends to resist ventricular rate control by digitalis, even after large intravenous doses. Patients ill with acute pulmonary embolus, unstable angina, pneumonitis with fever and tachypnea, or thyrotoxicosis appear to have increased sympathetic tone. Digitalis acts through baroreceptor reflexes to increase vagal tone and reduce sympathetic tone in experimental settings[86] but heightened sympathetic tone may overwhelm the reflex digitalis effects. Low-dose β-adrenergic blockers may slow ventricular rates impressively in this setting. Verapamil may also assist in slowing ventricular rates in digitalized patients.[58] Combined verapamil and propranolol should be used cautiously when ventricular function is severely compromised or when atrial flutter is due to the sick sinus syndrome.

In an alternative strategy, conversion to sinus rhythm may be attempted. Class IA antiarrhythmic agents may encourage conversion to sinus rhythm. The class IC agents (encainide, flecainide and propafenone) may also be effective. However, these agents have not been approved for supraventricular arrhythmias and recent preliminary data from the CAST suggests an unacceptable incidence of arrhythmia aggravation, particularly in patients with ischemic heart disease and recent myocardial infarction. Quinidine and disopyramide have indirect autonomic effects that shorten AV refractoriness while slowing atrial flutter rates and may result in 1:1 AV conduction. Pretreatment with propranolol, verapamil, diltiazem, or digoxin prevents this potential risk.

Type I atrial flutter may be terminated by transvenous right atrial pacing and obviates the need for general anesthesia, which is required for direct-current cardioversion. Prolonged pacing for 30 seconds or more with increased current may be required for arrhythmia termination.

After conversion to sinus rhythm, clinical assessment of risk for recurrent atrial flutter should be made. Predisposing factors include congestive heart failure, acute myocardial infarction or ischemia, recurrent pulmonary emboli, thyrotoxicosis, acid–base or electrolyte imbalance, intracardiac or extracardiac infection, and severe anemia. In those with identifiable risk for recurrent atrial flutter or resultant fibrillation, quinidine may reduce atrial ectopy and prevent atrial flutter. Verapamil or propranolol may help control ventricular rate during recurrences.

ATRIOVENTRICULAR JUNCTIONAL TACHYCARDIAS

Atrioventricular junctional tachycardias represent those arrhythmias requiring the AV junction for their maintenance. Tachycardias requiring the AV junction but also incorporating an accessory pathway will be discussed separately.

ATRIOVENTRICULAR NODAL TACHYCARDIAS
MECHANISM

In 1956, Moe and co-workers[87] described the relationship between the coupling interval of a premature cardiac extrastimulus and the conduction of that impulse. Abrupt lengthening of conduction time was often associated with an echo complex (*i.e.*, a complex that returned to the chamber of origin). On the basis of these observations, they postulated the existence of dual AV nodal conduction pathways with different properties of conduction and refractoriness. The slow pathway showed slower impulse propagation but was associated with a shorter refractory period. In contrast, the fast pathway showed more rapid conduction but a longer refractory period. A critically timed premature impulse could block in the fast pathway and conduct over the slow pathway. If conduction velocity was sufficiently slow, the retrograde impulse could then engage the fast pathway when it was no longer refractory and initiate a circus movement tachycardia confined to the AV node. The above sequence of events is believed to explain the common type of AV nodal reentrant tachycardia.

In the so-called atypical form of AV nodal reentry,[88] the tachycardia circuit is reversed so that antegrade conduction occurs over the fast and retrograde conduction over the slow pathway (Fig. 49.2). It is often very difficult to distinguish retrograde conduction over a slow AV nodal pathway from that due to retrograde conduction over an accessory pathway with nodelike properties.[89] Present evidence suggests that most patients with the permanent form of junctional reentrant tachycardia (PJRT) use an atypical accessory pathway for retrograde conduction.

CLINICAL AND ELECTROCARDIOGRAPHIC FINDINGS

The common form of AV nodal reentrant tachycardia is generally paroxysmal (abrupt onset and termination). The heart rate varies from 115 to 230 beats per minute and is usually regular and narrow unless coexistent bundle branch block is present.[90] While functional right bundle branch block may be present during tachycardia, functional left bundle branch block is seldom present. During tachycardia, the P wave either just precedes or falls within the QRS in two thirds of the patients. In a minority of patients, the P wave falls at the terminal portion of the QRS. Because the P wave originates from the region of the AV junction, its vector is oriented superiorly and anteriorly. When visible, the P wave will, therefore, inscribe a negative deflection in leads II, III, aV$_F$ (pseudoinfarction pattern) or a late positive deflection in V$_1$ (pseudo RR' pattern).[90] In contrast, patients with the atypical form of AV junctional reentrant tachycardia will show a P wave clearly preceding the QRS (short PR) and a long interval between QRS and the subsequent retrograde P wave. The P wave vector will be oriented anteriorly and superiorly. The tachycardia in these patients tends to be slower (<150 beats per minute) and virtually incessant.

CLINICAL ELECTROPHYSIOLOGIC FINDINGS

Rosen and associates were the first to describe discontinuous AV nodal conduction in humans.[91] Progressively, premature atrial extrastimuli resulted in an abrupt increase in AV nodal conduction. These findings were interpreted as showing conduction over the fast pathway by relatively late atrial extrastimuli. Critically timed earlier atrial depolarizations blocked in the fast pathway and conducted over the slow pathway. Although approximately 10% of adults[92] and 35% to 46% of children[93,94] show discontinuous AV nodal conduction properties, approximately 80% of patients with AV nodal reentrant tachycardia show this finding.[13] Typically, block in the fast pathway and conduction over the slow pathway are attended by atrial echoes or sustained tachycardia (Fig. 49.3). Evidence for dual AV nodal conduction may also be found in response to rapid atrial or ventricular pacing by an abrupt increase in propagation of the paced impulse at a critical paced cycle length. Most authors accept a 40-msec to 50-msec increase in conduction time in response to a 10-msec decrement in delivered stimuli. In addition, retrograde dual pathway conduction may be elicited by abrupt increases in retrograde conduction by critically timed ventricular premature impulses. The characteristic electrophysiologic features of AV nodal reentrant tachycardia include (1) finding of a critical atrium-to-His (AH) interval for tachycardia initiation, (2) presence of the atrial depolarization within the QRS complex during tachycardia, (3) His-to-ventricle (HV) interval greater than or equal to conducted impulses, and (4) presence of dual AV nodal conduction curves. It should be emphasized that the incidence of the latter finding will be dependent on both the number of drive cycle lengths tested as well as the site of stimulation (*i.e.*, right atrium, coronary sinus, or right ventricle).

Direct proof of intranodal reentry is not possible and hence this diagnosis is made by excluding participation of both the atrium and ventricle. Exclusion of the atrium is suggested by inability to affect the tachycardia by inducing progressively premature atrial depolarizations throughout the tachycardia cycle.[95] In addition, termination of the tachycardia by critically timed ventricular impulses that fail to reach the atrium excludes an atrial tachycardia. Continuation of the tachycardia in the face of AV block serves to exclude participation of the ventricles.[96] The inability to provide direct proof of sole intranodal reentry as well as the finding of a constant short retrograde His-to-atrial interval both during tachycardia as well as during ventricular pacing has suggested incorporation of specialized atriojunctional fibers in the tachycardia circuit.[97] This hypothesis is strengthened by three additional findings: (1) different described exit points for fast and slow pathways,[98] (2) different electropharmacologic effects of drugs on the two pathways (see below), and (3) results of surgical perinodal dissection that controls tachycardia without affecting AV conduction.[99]

TREATMENT

Drugs that tend to prolong refractoriness and delay AV nodal conduction (*i.e.*, digitalis, β-adrenergic blockers, or calcium channel blockers)[100] exert their predominant effects on the slow pathway.[100] The calcium channel blockers may also affect retrograde pathway conduction and refractoriness.[101] In contrast, class IA antiarrhythmic agents have relatively minor effects on the slow pathway but show predominant effect on retrograde fast pathway conduction.[102] Similarly, class IC drugs (encainide, flecainide)[103] appear to act predominantly on retrograde fast pathway conduction. Some drugs appear to exert blocking effects on both AV nodal pathways and include aprindine, propafenone, amiodarone, and sotalol.[104] In contrast, atropine appears to improve conduction and shorten refractoriness over both pathways.[105]

The common form of AV reentrant tachycardia is usually paroxysmal. If the paroxysms are infrequent and well tolerated, the patient is instructed in the use of vagal maneuvers and chronic antiarrhythmic therapy is not used. If the paroxysms are frequent but well tolerated, then empiric therapy guided by understanding of pharmacologic effects of antiarrhythmic drugs may be used. For example, the clinician may decide to initiate therapy with an AV nodal blocking agent (*i.e.*, digitalis, β-adrenergic blocker, or calcium channel blocker) and if the patient remains refractory to this approach, then use of class IA or IC drugs may be tried. The same considerations regarding arrhythmia aggravation with the I-C agents may be applicable to patients with AV

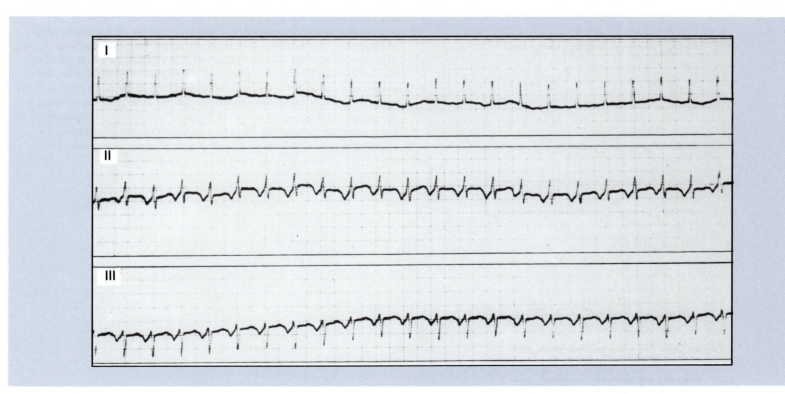

FIGURE 49.2 Rhythm strips from leads I, II, and III showing supraventricular tachycardia with short PR interval. Note that the P waves are inverted in the inferior leads. The electrocardiogram was taken from a patient with "atypical" AV nodal reentry. The tachycardia circuit involves antegrade conduction over the fast pathway (short PR) and retrograde conduction over a slow pathway (long RP).

nodal re-entry. Therapy guided by invasive studies is indicated if the arrhythmia proves refractory to conventional drugs or if tachycardia is associated with alarming symptoms (*i.e.*, syncope, heart failure, angina pectoris, or transient ischemic episodes). In the latter situation, invasive studies are indicated in order to devise an effective drug regimen as quickly as possible. The purpose of these studies is to determine the weak link in the tachycardia circuit and test the efficacy of drug therapy. Intermittent drug therapy applied only during episodes of tachycardia has been described. Such therapy involves use of high doses of antiarrhythmic drugs, and it is prudent to test any projected regimen under controlled conditions with a temporary cardiac pacemaker in place as tachycardia termination may result in prolonged and symptomatic pauses. In addition, invasive studies are required if nonpharmacologic treatment modalities are contemplated (see below).

NONPHARMACOLOGIC TREATMENT

A variety of effective nonpharmacologic modalities are currently available for patients with AV nodal reentrant tachycardia. These patients may prove responsive to antitachycardia pacing. The rationale, efficacy, and potential problems with antitachycardia pacing are described elsewhere in these volumes. Another therapeutic option includes catheter or surgical ablation of the AV junction. The chief undesirable effects of the latter approach include induction of complete AV block and the necessity of permanent cardiac pacing. A newer surgical technique that involves atrial dissection in the area of earliest atrial activation during tachycardia has been described recently.[99] Patients undergoing this procedure have experienced tachycardia control without impairment of AV conduction. The technique of catheter ablation of posteroseptal accessory pathways for patients with the permanent form of junctional reentrant tachycardia is discussed elsewhere in these volumes.

NONPAROXYSMAL JUNCTIONAL TACHYCARDIA

Nonparoxysmal junctional tachycardia was originally described by Pick and Dominguez.[106] The tachycardia is usually relatively slow, 80 to 120 beats per minute, nonparoxysmal in onset, and often associated with AV dissociation. The available data suggest that this arrhythmia is due to delayed afterdepolarizations[107] and has none of the features of a reciprocating tachycardia. It is usually manifest in the course of digitalis toxicity, acute myocardial infarction, chronic pulmonary disease, or after cardiac surgery.

Treatment is directed at the underlying condition but atrial overdrive pacing may be required for those who manifest hemodynamic instability owing to AV dissociation.

JUNCTIONAL ECTOPIC TACHYCARDIA

Junctional ectopic tachycardia has been described as a rare arrhythmia occurring predominately in infancy. The tachycardia is often rapid and is usually repetitive or incessant. This tachycardia cannot be initiated or terminated by pacing and is believed to be due to abnormal automaticity. One histologic study of a patient with this disorder showed focal degenerative changes within the His bundle.[108] In infancy, the tachycardia is often resistant to conventional drugs but some patients may respond to amiodarone.[109] Garson and Gillette[110] have stressed the poor prognosis of these children in terms of development of a tachycardia myopathy as well as sudden death.

Our own studies in adults suggest that this arrhythmia may be more common than originally appreciated.[111] In a period of 2 years, we found five young adults with this arrhythmia. The arrhythmia in adults tends to be less incessant and is associated with an irregular ventricular

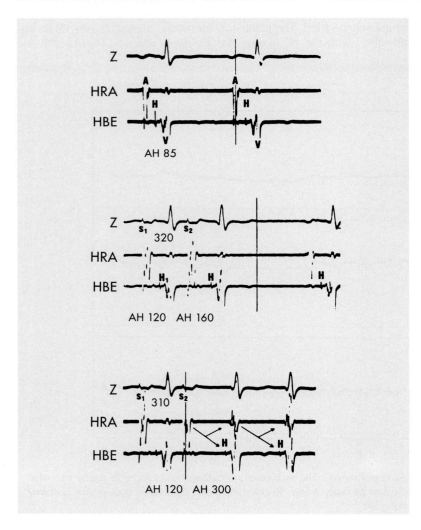

FIGURE 49.3 The top panel shows simultaneous tracings from surface lead Z (Frank lead system), the high right atrial electrogram (*HRA*), and the His bundle electrogram (*HBE*). The control AV nodal conduction time (*AH*) is 85 msec. The middle panel illustrates the effects of an atrial extrastimulus (S_2) induced 320 msec after the basic drive cycle (S_1). The atrial depolarization falls in the relative refractory period of the AV node and results in prolongation of the AH interval. The bottom panel shows the effects of an atrial extrastimulus inserted 10 msec earlier. Note the marked increase in AH (300 msec) compared with that observed in the middle panel. In addition, this extrastimulus initiates an episode of supraventricular tachycardia. The sudden increase in AH is taken to represent block of the atrial impulse in the fast pathway with antegrade conduction over the slow pathway allowing for retrograde atrial activation with dual AV nodal conduction and initiation of AV nodal reentrant tachycardia. Note that during tachycardia the atrial electrogram occurs simultaneously with the ventricular electrogram.

response. It is commonly misdiagnosed as paroxysmal atrial fibrillation or multifocal atrial tachycardia (Figs. 49.4 and 49.5). The treatment of choice in adults appears to be β-adrenergic blockers, but more aggressive treatment including His bundle ablation is required for some.

WOLFF-PARKINSON-WHITE SYNDROME

A syndrome consisting of "bundle branch block with short P-R interval in healthy young people prone to paroxysmal tachycardia" was described first by Wolff, Parkinson, and White in 1930.[112] However, Kent and others had noted multiple bands of muscular tissue connecting the atria and ventricles outside the normal conducting system as early as 1893.[113] The relationships between the AV connection or accessory pathway and the observations of Wolff, Parkinson, and White were suggested in 1933 by Wolferth and Wood,[114] who noted that (1) the interval from the beginning of the P wave to the end of the QRS complex was normal; (2) the QRS complex duration shortened as the PR interval lengthened; and (3) the slurring of the QRS complex always involved the initial deflection. Finally, Wood[115] in 1943 and Ohnell[116] in 1944 demonstrated AV bypass tracts in autopsy specimens from patients known to have had the Wolff-Parkinson-White (WPW) syndrome during life.

PATHOLOGIC FINDINGS

The anatomical basis for the WPW syndrome was summarized by Lev and Bharati[117] in 1979. Of 31 cases reported, AV (Kent) connections were found in 24 and fasciculoventricular or nodoventricular (Mahaim) fibers in four. In the remaining three cases, no anatomical basis for pre-excitation was found. Mean width of the AV pathways was 1.3 mm (range, 0.1 mm–7 mm). Multiple strands were identified in nearly half of the specimens studied. Multiple pathways are found in approximately 5% of patients.[118] Accessory pathways may be located anywhere along the AV ring except in the region of the aortic-mitral valve continuity (Fig. 49.6).

Pre-excitation is found in one to two per thousand individuals in

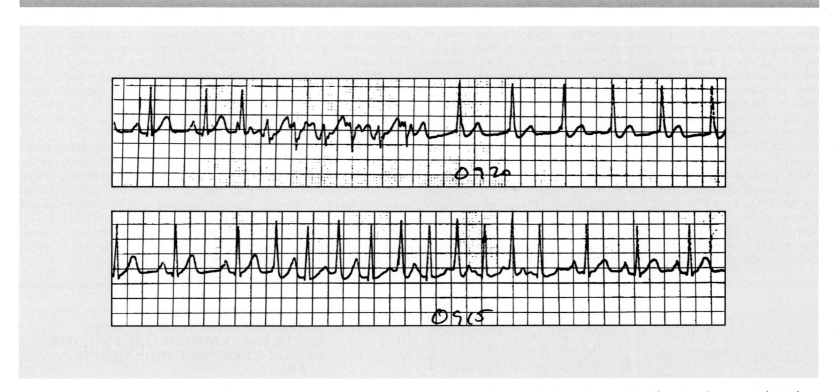

FIGURE 49.4 Simultaneously recorded rhythm strips from a patient with recurrent episodes of supraventricular tachycardia. During tachycardia, the P waves are dissociated from the QRS complex and the ventricular cycle length is irregular. These features are characteristic of junctional ectopic tachycardia. The intracardiac recordings for this patient are shown in Figure 49.5.

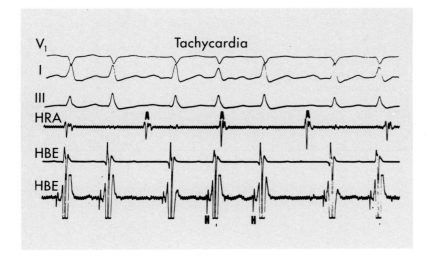

FIGURE 49.5 Simultaneous recordings of surface leads V_1, I, and III together with recordings from the high right atrium (*HRA*) and His bundle electrogram (*HBE*). Each QRS is preceded by a His bundle deflection (*H*) and the sinus P waves (*A*) are dissociated from the QRS.

whom an electrocardiogram is obtained.[119] The incidence of accessory pathways capable of only retrograde conduction is unknown, but these pathways may account for up to 30% of cases of paroxysmal supraventricular tachycardia. Ebstein's anomaly may be associated with one or more right-sided pathways[120,121] and mitral valve prolapse with left-sided pathways.[122]

ELECTROCARDIOGRAPHIC FINDINGS

The electrocardiographic diagnosis of the WPW syndrome is based on (1) a PR interval less than 0.12 second, (2) a QRS complex duration greater than or equal to 0.12 second, and (3) initial slurring of the QRS complex (delta wave). The morphology of the delta wave on the electrocardiogram may indicate roughly the location of the accessory pathway (Table 49.1). QRS forces are positive when a wave of depolarization approaches the lead and negative when it proceeds away from the lead. Thus, the delta wave will be negative in those leads adjacent to the ventricular insertion site of the accessory pathway and positive in those leads opposite or at a distance from the accessory pathway. The older terminology of type A (delta wave positive in V_1) and type B (delta wave negative in V_1) is no longer used because comparisons between surface electrocardiograms and the results of intraoperative mapping have allowed more accurate localization of accessory pathways from the 12-lead surface electrocardiogram. Figure 49.6 shows the arrangement of surface electrocardiograph leads around the AV ring, and Table 49.1 lists the electrocardiographic expressions of accessory pathways located around the AV ring. This scheme is limited by (1) multiple accessory pathways, (2) fusion with impulses conducted over the AV mode, and (3) other congenital or acquired cardiac disease.[121] Accessory pathways capable only of retrograde conduction cannot be identified or localized on a routine electrocardiogram.

Accessory pathways have widely varying refractory periods, ranging from less than 200 msec to greater than 1 second. Conduction velocity generally is rapid, accounting for the short PR intervals observed. The relationships between antegrade and retrograde conduction and refractoriness of the accessory pathway and the AV node determine the mechanism and rate of tachycardia.

ASSOCIATED ARRHYTHMIAS

Orthodromic AV reentry is the most common arrhythmia associated with the WPW syndrome. The tachycardia is regular, with narrow QRS complex, reflecting antegrade conduction over the AV node and specialized conduction system. The P wave has a superior axis and follows the QRS, reflecting retrograde activation of the atria via the accessory pathway. The tachycardia generally begins with an atrial premature depolarization that blocks in the accessory pathway and conducts solely over the AV node and specialized conducting system (Fig. 49.7). Thus, the first beat of tachycardia has a normal QRS complex and a normal or long PR interval (Fig. 49.8, A). In order for tachycardia to begin in this manner, the accessory pathway refractory period must be longer than the AV node refractory period. While this condition may not be met at rest, vagal withdrawal and increased sympathetic outflow as seen during exercise or emotion may allow the AV node refractory period to shorten sufficiently to allow an atrial premature depolarization to block first in the accessory pathway. The wave of depolarization then proceeds retrogradely over the accessory pathway to activate the atria (see Fig. 49.7). The cycle repeats itself indefinitely. Alternatively, the tachycardia may be initiated by a ventricular premature beat that blocks retrogradely in the AV node and conducts over the accessory pathway (Fig. 49.8, B). The rate of the tachycardia depends on conduction velocities of the AV node, accessory pathway, atrial muscle, and ventricular muscle, but it is generally between 140 and 250 beats per minute. The tachycardia terminates when block occurs in either the AV node (antegrade, Fig. 49.8, C) or accessory pathway (retrograde, Fig. 49.8, D). Vagal maneuvers may be effective for termination of tachycardia by prolonging AV node refractoriness or may slow tachycardia by slowing AV conduction.

The only reliable electrocardiographic criterion that distinguishes AV reentry using an accessory pathway from AV nodal reentry is the presence of the P wave after the QRS complex in patients with accessory pathways. QRS complex alternation, a characteristic that has been associated with AV reentry, is seen frequently with both AV nodal and AV reentry at rates greater than 200 beats per minute.[123] It should be appreciated, however, that atrial tachycardia (either ectopic or reentrant) may mimic the patterns of either AV nodal reentry or AV reentrant tachycardia depending on the length of the PR interval.

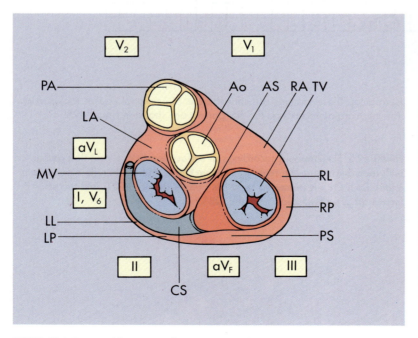

FIGURE 49.6 Potential locations of accessory pathways and their relationships to the surface ECG leads. (PA, pulmonary artery; RA, right anterior; Ao, aorta; TV, tricuspid valve; RL, right lateral; CS, coronary sinus; RP, right posterior; PS, posterior septal; LP, left posterior; LL, left lateral; MV, mitral valve; LA, left anterior; AS, anterior septal.)

TABLE 49.1 ORIENTATION OF INITIAL FORCES (DELTA WAVE) DURING SINUS RHYTHM (SURFACE ELECTROCARDIOGRAPHIC LEAD)

Accessory Pathway Location	I	II	III	aV_L	aV_F	V_1	V_2	V_6
Right anterior	+	+	+	+	+	−	−	+
Right lateral	+	+ or ±	−	+	±	±	±	+
Right posterior	+	−	−	+	−	±	±	+
Posterior septal	+	−	−	+	−	±	+	+
Left posterior	+	−	−	+	−	+	+	+
Left lateral	−	±	+	−	±	+	+	−
Left anterior	−	+	+	−	+	+	+	±

(+, upright delta wave; −, inverted delta wave; ±, variable delta wave)

When bundle branch block occurs during AV reentrant tachycardia, the VA interval increases and the rate of tachycardia generally decreases if the bundle branch block is present in the bundle ipsilateral to the accessory pathway. This occurs because the reentrant circuit is lengthened as the impulse must travel down the contralateral bundle and across the septum before reaching the accessory pathway for retrograde conduction. This phenomenon may be useful in the localization of accessory pathways, particularly if pre-excitation is not manifest on the electrocardiogram during normal sinus rhythm.

Atrial fibrillation or atrial flutter is observed in up to 40% of patients with the WPW syndrome. In patients with otherwise normal hearts, atrial fibrillation often develops during AV reentrant tachycardia. Patients with anatomically abnormal hearts and WPW may develop atrial fibrillation without antecedent AV reentry.[124] The ventricular response to atrial fibrillation depends on the refractory periods of the accessory pathway and AV node. Patients with long accessory pathway refractory periods may conduct solely over the AV node during atrial fibrillation. However, patients with very short accessory pathway refractory periods may conduct very rapidly over the accessory pathway. Rates in excess of 300 beats per minute have been observed during atrial fibrillation in patients with the WPW syndrome. Sudden cardiac death due to ventricular fibrillation occurs more frequently in patients with the WPW syndrome than in normal persons of similar age. Patients with the WPW syndrome who had been resuscitated from ventricular fibrillation have a higher incidence of AV reentrant tachycardia, atrial fibrillation, and multiple accessory pathways than those patients with the WPW syndrome but without ventricular fibrillation. Both the mean RR interval and the shortest RR interval during atrial fibrillation are shorter in these patients.[125]

Antidromic reentrant tachycardia is present when an accessory pathway is responsible for antegrade conduction, and the AV node and specialized conducting system or a second accessory pathway are responsible for retrograde conduction. The QRS complex is fully pre-excited on the electrocardiogram. Wide complex, regular tachycardia also occurs in patients with the WPW syndrome when bundle branch block is present during orthodromic AV reentrant tachycardia, when nodoventricular or fasciculoventricular fibers pre-excite the ventricle during tachycardia, when atrial tachycardia or flutter results in 1:1 or 2:1 conduction over the accessory pathway, or when ventricular tachycardia occurs.[126]

NONINVASIVE EVALUATION

Asymptomatic patients with the incidental electrocardiographic finding of pre-excitation do not require further evaluation or treatment unless the patient is involved in vigorous athletics. Noninvasive data suggesting a long refractory period of the accessory pathway include intermittent pre-excitation and loss of pre-excitation with exercise or after administration of drugs. Exercise testing has been used in patients with the WPW syndrome in order to identify those with long accessory pathway refractory periods and who, therefore, are at low risk for sudden cardiac death. The abrupt normalization of the QRS during exercise suggests rate-related block in the accessory pathway. However, the usefulness of exercise testing as an indicator of accessory pathway refractory period is limited by the enhancement of AV node conduction that occurs normally with exercise. Thus, the QRS complex may narrow despite continued conduction over the accessory pathway.[127]

ELECTROPHYSIOLOGIC STUDIES

Patients with symptomatic arrhythmias associated with the WPW syndrome should undergo electrophysiologic studies in order to (1) determine the mechanism of tachycardia, (2) localize the accessory pathway or pathways, (3) assess the risk for sudden cardiac death, and

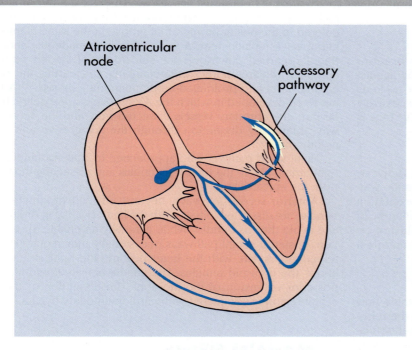

FIGURE 49.7 Propagation of orthodromic AV reentrant tachycardia using an accessory pathway. Antegrade conduction is over the AV node. Retrograde conduction is over the accessory pathway.

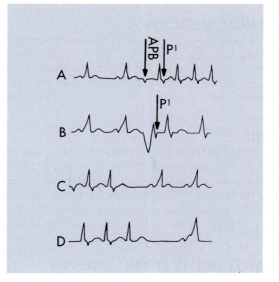

FIGURE 49.8 Patterns of spontaneous initiation and termination of orthodromic AV reentrant tachycardia. **A.** Initiation of orthodromic AV reentry by an atrial premature beat (APB). Note the absence of a delta wave following the APB, signifying antegrade block in the accessory pathway. **B.** Initiation of orthodromic AV reentry by a ventricular premature beat. Note the retrograde P wave following the ventricular premature beat. **C.** Termination of orthodromic AV reentry by antegrade block in the AV node. The last event is a blocked P wave. **D.** Termination of orthodromic AV reentry by retrograde block in the accessory pathway. The last event is a QRS complex.

(4) delineate therapy. At the time of electrophysiologic study, antegrade and retrograde refractoriness of the accessory pathway are determined before and after administration of drugs. Tachycardia is induced by atrial or ventricular overdrive, or both, or by programmed pacing. If orthodromic AV reentry is induced, then the atria are mapped by exploring the tricuspid annulus and coronary sinus in order to identify the earliest site or sites of atrial activation that correspond to the atrial insertion of the accessory pathway(s). If orthodromic tachycardia cannot be induced, then mapping may be performed during ventricular pacing. Mapping during ventricular pacing may be limited by retrograde conduction over the AV node, which leads to an area of early atrial activation at the low septal right atrium. Atrial fibrillation is induced with rapid atrial pacing or atrial extrastimuli in order to determine the shortest pre-excited RR interval achievable. The effect of the drug on inducibility of tachycardia and atrial fibrillation and on the ventricular response to atrial fibrillation is assessed. A drug that prevents the induction of AV reentry and atrial fibrillation is likely to be successful. A drug that slows AV reentry or makes it nonsustained or slows the ventricular response to atrial fibrillation is likely to be partially successful. The tachycardia response to isoproterenol is often assessed because the electrophysiology laboratory may be an inadequate milieu for assessing increased sympathetic tone. Patients who have AV reentry as their only arrhythmia may respond well to overdrive pacing by an implanted antitachycardia pacemaker.

TREATMENT
DIGITALIS GLYCOSIDES
Digitalis preparations may be effective treatment for atrioventricular reentrant tachycardia as they slow AV node conduction and prolong AV node refractory period. However, because digitalis may increase the likelihood of ventricular fibrillation in a subset of adult patients with the WPW syndrome and atrial fibrillation, its use should be avoided in patients with manifest pre-excitation unless its safety is confirmed by electrophysiologic studies.[128,129]

β-ADRENERGIC BLOCKERS
β-Adrenergic blockers have little effect on either antegrade or retrograde accessory pathway conduction. As AV node blocking agents, they may prevent or terminate AV reentry involving the AV node as the antegrade limb. In addition, β-blockers may prevent excessively rapid rates during atrial fibrillation when increased sympathetic tone is present.

VERAPAMIL
Verapamil is highly effective for termination of AV reentrant tachycardia by means of AV node block. However, it may accelerate the ventricular response to atrial fibrillation in patients with pre-excitation during atrial fibrillation. Thus, it is useful for acute termination of orthodromic AV reentry in a monitored patient but should not be used acutely during atrial fibrillation in patients with manifest pre-excitation.[130]

CLASS I ANTIARRHYTHMIC AGENTS
The class IA agents procainamide, quinidine, and disopyramide may be effective both in AV reentrant tachycardia by increasing the retrograde refractory period of the accessory pathway and in atrial fibrillation by increasing the antegrade refractory period of the accessory pathway. Responses are variable among patients, particularly with respect to the ventricular response during atrial fibrillation. Thus, it is important to establish the effect of the drug in each patient during induced atrial fibrillation.[131] In general, refractoriness is significantly increased only in those with relatively long baseline refractory periods (>270 msec).

The class IC agents flecainide[132] and encainide[133,134] prolong antegrade and retrograde refractory periods, may prevent SVT, and slow the ventricular response to atrial fibrillation. These agents have proven to be remarkably effective in patients with the WPW syndrome. Unfortunately, there is no long-term safety data and these agents have not yet been approved for use in SVT by the Food and Drug Administration.

AMIODARONE
Amiodarone lengthens both accessory pathway and AV nodal refractory periods and may abolish AV reentrant tachycardia because of its effects on either pathway. In addition, amiodarone may slow the ventricular response to atrial fibrillation.[135] Even when low doses are used, its use in patients with the WPW syndrome is limited primarily by side effects.

NONPHARMACOLOGIC TREATMENT
When drug therapy has proved ineffective or intolerable or when arrhythmias are potentially life threatening, operative resection or catheter ablation of the accessory pathway is indicated. Patients should be considered for accessory pathway ablation or resection if ventricular fibrillation has occurred in association with atrial fibrillation or when the shortest RR interval during atrial fibrillation is less than 250 msec.[125] When the accessory pathway is localized to the region of the posterior septum (earliest atrial activation during AV reentry or ventricular pacing at or near the os of the coronary sinus), the discharge of the 200 to 300 joules through an electrode catheter just outside the coronary sinus os may be curative.[136] Preliminary studies suggest that pathways at other locations around the AV ring might be approached by catheter ablation.[137]

Accessory pathways at any location in the septum or AV ring may be divided surgically. At the time of operation, the ventricular insertion of the accessory pathway is localized by determining the site of earliest activation of the ventricle during sinus rhythm or atrial pacing with pre-excitation. The atrial insertion is confirmed by determining the earliest site of atrial activation during ventricular pacing or AV reentrant tachycardia. Two approaches are available for left free wall accessory pathways. In the most commonly used approach, the left atrium is entered in the posterior interatrial groove in the same manner as for a mitral valve replacement. A wide incision is made just above the AV ring and carried down over the epicardium of the left ventricle. This approach requires aortic cross-clamping and carries the risks of air embolization and prolonged cardiopulmonary bypass.[138] A technique has been developed in which the AV groove is approached in a closed fashion, the coronary vessels dissected free, and the accessory pathway ablated by dissection through the AV groove and the use of cryothermia.[139]

Right-sided pathways are approached by making an incision in the right atrium above the tricuspid annulus and dissecting the fat pad free from the epicardium.

Anterior septal pathways, because of their proximity to the His bundle, are dissected initially with the heart beating in order to localize and avoid the His bundle. While generally amenable to catheter ablation, posterior septal pathways occasionally may require operative intervention. Again, with the heart beating, the right atrium is opened above the tricuspid annulus. His bundle activity is monitored during posterior extension of the incision. The dissection of the posterior septal region is completed with cardiopulmonary bypass.[138]

MAHAIM FIBERS
Two additional accessory pathways have been described. Presumed nodoventricular fibers may yield normal or short PR intervals on the electrocardiogram depending on the location of the proximal insertion and the characteristics of the pathway. The initial portion of the QRS complex may or may not demonstrate a delta wave, depending on the site of the distal insertion. Fasciculoventricular fibers result in a normal PR interval and variable slurring of the initial portion of the QRS complex. Together, these pathways have been called Mahaim fibers.[140]

Reentrant arrhythmias are associated with nodoventricular fibers. The QRS complex is wide and has a left bundle branch block morphology because the Mahaim fibers insert into the right ventricle. Retrograde conduction may occur over the normal conducting system. In addition, the tachycardia mechanism may be due to AV nodal reentry with the nodoventricular tract acting as bystander. Ventriculoatrial conduction may or may not be intact. During electrophysiologic study, SVT (atrial tachycardia, AV nodal reentrant tachycardia, or orthodromic AV reentrant tachycardia) may be excluded by the absence of a His bundle deflection before the QRS complex. The reproduction of the QRS morphology of the tachycardia by atrial pacing excludes VT. The long AV interval excludes antidromic AV reentrant tachycardia.

Arrhythmias in patients with fasciculoventricular fibers appear to be coincidental, and the Mahaim fibers act as bystander.[141] In addition, fasciculoventricular fibers may be distinguished from nodoventricular fibers by atrial and His bundle pacing in the electrophysiology laboratory. When the fasciculoventricular fibers take off below the site of His bundle pacing, neither atrial nor His bundle pacing will alter the pre-excited QRS complex. With nodoventricular fibers, atrial pacing enhances pre-excitation while His bundle pacing causes normalization of the QRS complex.

The anatomical presence of nodoventricular fibers has not been proved. Evidence suggests that these fibers may be AV fibers with AV node–like properties. Tchou and associates[142] have demonstrated that atrial tissue is a necessary component of the tachycardia circuit, suggesting that the antegrade limb is an AV or atriofascicular pathway and that the retrograde limb is the AV node and His bundle. Klein and associates,[143] using selective cooling intraoperatively, showed insertion of the accessory pathway at a distance from the AV node.

PERMANENT FORM OF JUNCTIONAL RECIPROCATING TACHYCARDIA

The permanent form of junctional reciprocating tachycardia is an unusual form of SVT in which antegrade conduction is over the AV node and retrograde conduction occurs over an atypical posterior septal pathway with decremental retrograde conduction.[144] Coumel and associates[145] described the tachycardia in 1967 as follows: (1) it occurs primarily in infants and children, (2) it is nearly incessant, (3) it begins with a short PP interval, (4) the RP interval exceeds the PR interval, and (5) the P wave is inverted in the inferior leads. The tachycardia may be poorly responsive to conventional treatment. Catheter or surgical ablation of the AV node or accessory pathway may be curative.[144,146]

REFERENCES

1. Wellens HJJ, Bar FWHM, Vanagt EJDM et al: Medical treatment of ventricular tachycardia: Considerations in the selection of patients for surgical treatment. Am J Cardiol 49:186, 1982
2. Segal N, Samet P: Physiologic aspects of cardiac pacing. In Samet P, El-Sherif N (eds): Cardiac Pacing, pp 111–147. New York, Grune & Stratton, 1980
3. Samet P, Castillo C, Bernstein WJ: Hemodynamic results of right atrial pacing in 33 normal subjects. Chest 52:652, 1967
4. Samet P, Castillo C, Bernstein WH: Hemodynamic results of right atrial pacing in cardiac subjects. Chest 52:133, 1968
5. Schleppes M, Weppner HG, Merle H: Haemodynamic effects of supraventricular tachycardias and their alterations by electrically and verapamil induced termination. Cardiovasc Res 12:28, 1978
6. Goldreyer BN, Kastor JA, Kershbaum KL: The hemodynamic effects of induced supraventricular tachycardia in man. Circulation 54:783, 1976
7. Waxman MB, Wald RW: Effects of autonomic tone on tachycardias. In Surawicz B, Reddy CP, Prystowsky EN (eds): Tachycardias, pp 67–102. Boston, Martinus Nijhoff, 1984
8. McIntosh HD, Kong Y, Moms JJ Jr: Hemodynamic effects of supraventricular arrhythmia. Am J Med 37:712, 1964
9. Swiryn S, Pavel D, Byrom E et al: Assessment of left ventricular function by radionuclide angiography during induced supraventricular tachycardia. Am J Cardiol 47:555, 1981
10. Bellet S: In: Hemodynamics. Clinical Disorders of the Heart Beat, 3rd ed, pp 105–114. Philadelphia, Lea & Febiger, 1971
11. Hoffman JIE, Grattan MT, Hanley FL et al: Total and transmural perfusion of the hypertrophied heart. In ter Keurs HEDJ, Schipperheyn JJ (eds): Cardiac Left Ventricular Hypertrophy. Boston, Martinus Nijhoff, 1983
12. Bauernfeind RA, Amat-Y-Leon F, Dhingra RC et al: Chronic nonparoxysmal sinus tachycardia in otherwise healthy persons. Ann Intern Med 91:702, 1979
13. Wu D, Denes P, Amat-Y-Leon F et al: Clinical, electrocardiographic and electrophysiologic observations in patients with paroxysmal supraventricular tachycardia. Am J Cardiol 41:1045, 1978
14. Josephson ME, Seides SF: Clinical Cardiac Electrophysiology: Techniques and Interpretations, pp 147–190. Philadelphia, Lea & Febiger, 1979
15. Mary-Rabin L, Hordof AJ, Danilo P Jr et al: Mechanisms for impulse initiation in isolated human atrial fibers. Circ Res 47:267, 1980
16. Goldreyer BN, Gallagher JJ, Damato AN: The electrophysiologic demonstration of atrial ectopic tachycardia in man. Am Heart J 85:205, 1973
17. Leon DF, Lancaster JF, Shaver JA et al: Right atrial ectopic rhythms: Experimental production in man. Am J Cardiol 25:6, 1970
18. Lau SH, Cohen SI, Stein E et al: P waves and P loops in coronary sinus and left atrial rhythms. Am Heart J 79:201, 1971
19. Massumi R, Tawkkol AA: Direct study of left atrial P waves. Am J Cardiol 20:331, 1967
20. Scheinman MM, Basu D, Hollenberg M: Electrophysiologic studies in patients with persistent atrial tachycardia. Circulation 50:266, 1974
21. Garson A, Gillette PC: Electrophysiologic studies of supraventricular tachycardia in children: I. Clinical electrophysiologic correlations. Am Heart J 102:233, 1981
22. Gillette PC, Wampler DG, Garson A Jr et al: Treatment of atrial automatic tachycardia by ablation procedures. J Am Coll Cardiol 6:405, 1985
23. Levine JH, Michael JR, Guarnieri T: Treatment of multifocal atrial tachycardia with verapamil. N Engl J Med 312:21, 1985
24. Katz LN, Pick A: Clinical Electrocardiography, Part I, The Arrhythmias. Philadelphia, Lea & Febiger, 1956
25. Campbell M: Etiology of cardiac arrhythmias. Guy's Hosp Rev 85:471, 1935
26. Hess RG, Lamb LE: Electrocardiographic findings in 122,043 individuals. Circulation 25:947, 1962
27. Kannel WB, Abbott RD, Savage DD et al: Epidemiologic features of chronic atrial fibrillation. N Engl J Med 306:1018, 1982
28. Morris DC, Hurst JW: Atrial fibrillation. Curr Probl Cardiol 5:1, 1980
29. Radford DJ, Izukawa T: Atrial fibrillation in children. Pediatrics 59:250, 1977
30. Mehta AV, Casta A, Wolff GS: Supraventricular tachycardia. In Roberts NK, Gelband H (eds): Cardiac Arrhythmias in the Neonate, Infant, and Child. Norwalk, CT, Appleton-Century-Crofts, 1983
31. Cookson H: Auricular fibrillation in children. Lancet 2:1139, 1929
32. McEachern D, Caer BM Jr: Auricular fibrillation: Its etiology, age, incidence and production by digitalis therapy. Am J Med Sci 183:35, 1932
33. Hoffman BF, Dangmen KH: Demonstration of the mechanisms for arrhythmias in experimental animals. Ann NY Acad Sci 432:17, 1984
34. Moe GK, Rheinboldt WC, Abildskov JA: A computer model of atrial fibrillation. Am Heart J 67:200, 1964
35. Allessie MA, Camers WJEP, Bonke FIM et al: Experimental evaluation of Moe's multiple wavelet hypothesis of atrial fibrillation. In Zipes DP, Jalife J (eds): Cardiac Electrophysiology and Arrhythmias, pp 265–275. Orlando, FL, Grune & Stratton, 1985
36. Coumel P, Leclercq JF, Attuel P et al: Autonomic influences in the genesis of atrial arrhythmias: Atrial flutter and fibrillation of vagal origin. In Narula OS (ed): Cardiac Arrhythmias: Electrophysiology, Diagnosis and Management, pp 243–255. Baltimore, Williams & Wilkins, 1979
37. Coumel P, Leclercq JF: Cardiac arrhythmias and autonomic nervous system. In Levy S, Scheinman MM (eds): Cardiac Arrhythmias from Diagnosis to Therapy, pp 37–55. Mt. Kisco, NY, Futura Publishing, 1984
38. Davies MJ, Pomerance A: Pathology of atrial fibrillation in man. Br Heart J 34:520, 1972
39. Probst P, Goldschlager N, Selzer A: Left atrial size and atrial fibrillation in mitral stenosis: Factors influencing their relationship. Circulation 18:572, 1973
40. Bentivoglo LC, Uriccho JF, Waldo A et al: An electrocardiographic analysis of sixty-five cases of mitral regurgitation. Circulation 18:572, 1958
41. Glancy DL, O'Brien KP, Gold HK et al: Atrial fibrillation in patients with idiopathic hypertrophic subaortic stenosis. Br Heart J 32:652, 1970
42. Alexander JK: The cardiomyopathy of obesity. Prog Cardiovasc Dis 27:325, 1985
43. Balsaver AM, Morales AR, Whitehouse FN: Fat infiltration of myocardium as a cause of cardiac conduction defect. Am J Cardiol 19:261, 1967
44. Reyes MP, Lerner M: Coxsackie virus myocarditis—with special reference to acute and chronic effects. Prog Cardiovasc Dis 27:373, 1985
45. Ettinger PO, Wu CF, Dela Cruz C et al: Arrhythmias and the "Holiday Heart": Alcohol associated cardiac rhythm disorders. Am Heart J 95:555, 1978
46. Walsh JJ, Burch GE, Black WC et al: Idiopathic cardiomyopathy of the puerperium (post partum heart disease). Circulation 32:19, 1965
47. Ansari A, Larson PH, Bates HD: Cardiovascular manifestations of systemic lupus erythematosus: Current perspective. Prog Cardiovasc Dis 27:421,

48. Hoffman I, Lowrey RD: The electrocardiogram in thyrotoxicosis. Am J Cardiol 6:893, 1960
49. Sandler G, Wilson GM: The nature and prognosis of heart disease in thyrotoxicosis. Q J Med 52:347, 1958
50. Kramer RJ, Zeldis SM, Hamby RI: Atrial fibrillation—a marker for abnormal left ventricular function in coronary heart disease. Br Heart J 47:606, 1982
51. James TN: Myocardial infarction and atrial arrhythmias. Circulation 24:761, 1961
52. Lown B, Vassaux C, Hood WB et al: Unresolved problems in coronary care. Am J Cardiol 20:494, 1967
53. Sugiura T, Iwasaka T, Ogawa A et al: Atrial fibrillation in acute myocardial infarction. Am J Cardiol 56:27, 1985
54. Evans W, Swann P: Lone auricular fibrillation. Br Heart J 16:189, 1954
55. Peter RH, Gracey JG, Beach TB: A clinical profile of idiopathic atrial fibrillation: A functional disorder of atrial rhythm. Ann Intern Med 68:1288, 1968
56. Moore EN: Microelectrode studies on concealment of multiple premature atrial responses. Circ Res 18:660, 1966
57. Sung RJ, Myerberg RJ, Castellanos A: Electrophysiological demonstration of concealed conduction in the human atrium. Circulation 58:940, 1978
58. Singh BN: New perspectives in the pharmacologic therapy of cardiac arrhythmias. Prog Cardiovasc Dis 22:243, 1980
59. Wolf PA, Kannel WB, McGee DL et al: Duration of atrial fibrillation and imminence of stroke: The Framingham study. Stroke 14:664, 1983
60. Mancini GBJ, Goldberger AL: Cardioversion of atrial fibrillation: Consideration of embolization, anticoagulation, prophylactic pacemaker, and long-term success. Am Heart J 104:617, 1982
61. Vost A, Wolochow DA, Howell DA: Incidence of infarcts of the brain in heart disease. J Pathol Bacteriol 88:463, 1964
62. Wolf PA, Dawber TR, Thomas HE, Kannel WB: Epidemiologic assessment of chronic atrial fibrillation and risk of stroke: The Framingham study. Neurology 28:973, 1978
63. Hinton RC, Kistler JP, Fallon JT et al: Influence of etiology of atrial fibrillation on incidence of systemic embolism. Am J Cardiol 40:509, 1977
64. Easton JD, Sherman DG: Management of cerebral embolism of cardiac origin. Stroke 11:433, 1980
65. Sherman DG, Goldman L, Whiting RB et al: Thromboembolism in patients with atrial fibrillation. Arch Neurol 41:708, 1984
66. Henry WL, Morganroth J, Pearlman AS et al: Relation between echocardiographically determined left atrial size and atrial fibrillation. Circulation 53:273, 1976
67. McDonald CD, Burch GE, Walsh JJ: Prolonged bedrest in the treatment of idiopathic cardiomyopathy. Am J Med 52:41, 1972
68. Bjerkelund CJ, Orning OM: The efficacy of anticoagulant therapy in preventing embolism related to D.C. electrical conversion of atrial fibrillation. Am J Cardiol 23:208, 1969
69. Lown B: Electrical reversion of cardiac arrhythmias. Br Heart J 29:469, 1967
70. Forfar JC: Prediction of hemorrhage during long-term oral coumarin anticoagulation by excessive prothrombin ratio. Am Heart J 103:445, 1982
71. Goldman MJ: The management of chronic atrial fibrillation: Indications for and method of conversion to sinus rhythm. Prog Cardiovasc Dis 2:465, 1960
72. Rogers PL, Sherry S: Current status of antithrombotic therapy in cardiovascular disease. Prog Cardiovasc Dis 19:235, 1976
73. Fenster PE, Comess KA, Marsh R et al: Conversion of atrial fibrillation to sinus rhythm by acute intravenous procainamide infusion. Am Heart J 106:501, 1983
74. Horowitz LN, Spielman SR, Greenspan AM et al: Use of amiodarone in the treatment of persistent and paroxysmal atrial fibrillation resistant to quinidine therapy. J Am Coll Cardiol 6:1402, 1985
75. Rytand DA: Editorial: Atrial flutter and the circus movement hypothesis. Circulation 34:713, 1966
76. Waldo AL, Wells JL Jr, Plumb VJ et al: Studies of atrial flutter following open heart surgery. Annu Rev Med 30:259, 1979
77. Rytand DA: The circus movement (entrapped circuit wave) hypothesis and atrial flutter. Ann Intern Med 65:125, 1966
78. Frame LH, Page RL, Hoffman BF: Atrial reentry around an anatomic barrier with a partially refractory excitable gap: A canine model of atrial flutter. Circ Res 58:495, 1986
79. Schuessler RB, Boineau JP, Wylds AC et al: Dynamics of atrial activation. In Little RC (ed): Physiology of Atrial Pacemakers and Conductive Tissues, pp 187–206. Mt. Kisco, NY, Futura Publishing, 1980
80. Watanabe Y, Dreifus LS: Cardiac Arrhythmias: Electrophysiologic Basis for Clinical Interpretation. New York, Grune & Stratton, 1977
81. Moleiro F, Mendoza IJ, Medina-Ravell V et al: One to one atrioventricular conduction during atrial pacing at rates of 300/minute in absence of Wolff-Parkinson-White syndrome. Am J Cardiol 48:789, 1981
82. Johnson JC, Flowers NC, Horan LG: Unexplained atrial flutter: A frequent herald of pulmonary embolism. Chest 60:29, 1971
83. Deutsch PG, Koronzon I, Weiss EC: Unusually rapid atrial rate in a patient with thyrotoxicosis and atrial flutter. Chest 67:350, 1975
84. Dunnigan A, Benson W Jr, Benditt DG: Atrial flutter in infancy: Diagnosis, clinical features and treatment. Pediatrics 75:725, 1985
85. Vetter VL, Tanner CS, Horowitz LN: Electrophysiologic consequences of the Mustard repair of d-transposition of the great arteries. J Am Coll Cardiol 10:1265, 1987
86. Gillis RA, Pearle DL, Levit B: Digitalis: A neuroexcitatory drug. Circulation 52:739, 1975
87. Moe GK, Preston JB, Burlington H: Physiologic evidence for dual AV transmission system. Circ Res 4:357, 1956
88. Wu D, Denes P, Amat-Y-Leon F et al: An unusual variety of atrioventricular nodal reentry due to retrograde dual atrioventricular nodal pathways. Circulation 56:50, 1977
89. Gallagher JJ, Sealy WC: The permanent form of junctional reciprocating tachycardia: Further elucidation of the underlying mechanism. Eur J Cardiol 8:415, 1978
90. Farre J, Wellens HJJ: The value of the electrocardiogram in diagnosis of the site of origin and mechanism of supraventricular tachycardia. In Wellens HJJ, Kulbertus HE (eds): What Is New in Electrocardiography, p 120. Boston, Martinus Nijhoff, 1981
91. Rosen KM, Metha A, Miller RA: Demonstration of dual atrioventricular pathways in man. Am J Cardiol 33:291, 1974
92. Denes P, Wu D, Dhingra R et al: Dual atrioventricular nodal pathways: A common electrophysiological response. Br Heart J 37:1069, 1975
93. Thapar MK, Gillette PC: Dual atrioventricular nodal pathways: A common electrophysiologic response in children. Circulation 60:1369, 1979
94. Casta A, Wolf GS, Mehta AV: Dual atrioventricular nodal pathways: A benign finding in arrhythmia-free children with heart disease. Am J Cardiol 46:1013, 1980
95. Josephson ME, Kastor JA: Paroxysmal supraventricular tachycardia: Is the atrium a necessary link? Circulation 54:430, 1976
96. Wellens HJJ, Wesdorp JC, Duren DR et al: Second-degree block during reciprocal atrioventricular nodal tachycardia. Circulation 53:595, 1976
97. Gomes JAC, Dhatt MS, Rubenson DS et al: Electrophysiologic evidence for selective retrograde utilization of a specialized conducting system in atrioventricular nodal reentrant tachycardia. Am J Cardiol 43:687, 1979
98. Sung RJ, Waxman HL, Saksena S et al: Sequence of retrograde atrial activation in patients with dual atrioventricular nodal pathways. Circulation 64:1059, 1981
99. Ross DL, Johnson DC, Denniss AR et al: Curative surgery for atrioventricular junctional ("AV nodal") reentrant tachycardia. J Am Coll Cardiol 6:1381, 1985
100. Wu D, Denes P, Dhingra R et al: The effects of propranolol on induction of A-V nodal reentrant paroxysmal tachycardia. Circulation 50:665, 1974
101. Wellens HJJ, Tan SL, Bar FWH et al: Effect of verapamil studied by programmed electrical stimulation of the heart in patients with paroxysmal reentrant supraventricular tachycardia. Br Heart J 39:1058, 1977
102. Wu D, Hung JS, Juo CT et al: Effects of quinidine on atrioventricular nodal reentrant paroxysmal tachycardia. Circulation 64:823, 1981
103. Hellestrand KJ, Nathan AW, Bexton RS et al: Cardiac electrophysiologic effects of flecainide acetate for paroxysmal reentrant junctional tachycardia. Am J Cardiol 51:770, 1983
104. Garcia-Civera R, Sanjuan R, Morell S et al: Effects of propafenone on induction and maintenance of atrioventricular nodal reentrant tachycardia. PACE 7:649, 1984
105. Nuess H, Schlepper M, Spies HF: Effects of heart rate and atropine on dual AV nodal conduction. Br Heart J 37:1216, 1975
106. Pick A, Dominguez P: Nonparoxysmal AV nodal tachycardia. Circulation 16:1022, 1957
107. Rosen MR, Fisch C, Hoffman BF et al: Can accelerated atrioventricular junctional escape rhythms be explained by delayed afterdepolarizations? Am J Cardiol 45:1272, 1980
108. Brechenmacher C, Coumel P, James TN: Intractable tachycardia in infancy. Circulation 53:377, 1976
109. Coumel P, Fidelle JE, Attuel P et al: Tachycardies focales hissiennes congenitales. Arch Mal Coeur 69:899, 1976
110. Garson A, Gillette PC: Junctional ectopic tachycardia in children: Electrocardiography, electrophysiology and pharmacologic response. Am J Cardiol 44:298, 1979
111. Ruder MA, Davis JC, Eldar M et al: Clinical and electrophysiological characterization of automatic junctional ectopic tachycardia in adults. Circulation 73:930, 1986
112. Wolff L, Parkinson J, White PD: Bundle branch block with short P-R interval in healthy young people prone to paroxysmal tachycardia. Am Heart J 5:685, 1930
113. Kent A: Researches on the structure and function of the mammalian heart. J Physiol 14:233, 1893
114. Wolferth CC, Wood FC: The mechanism of production of short P-R intervals and prolonged QRS complexes in patients with presumably undamaged hearts: Hypothesis of an accessory pathway of auriculoventricular conduction (bundle of Kent). Am Heart J 8:297, 1933
115. Wood FC, Wolferth CC, Geckeler GD: Histologic demonstration of accessory muscular connections between auricle and ventricle in a case of short P-R interval and prolonged QRS complex. Am Heart J 25:454, 1943
116. Ohnell R: Preexcitation, a cardiac abnormality. Acta Med Scand (Suppl) 152:1, 1944
117. Lev M, Bharati S: Anatomic basis for preexcitation. In Narula O (ed): Cardiac Arrhythmias: Electrophysiology, Diagnosis and Management, p 556. Baltimore, Williams & Wilkins, 1979
118. Gallagher JJ, Sealy WC, Kasell J et al: Multiple accessory pathways in patients with the preexcitation syndrome. Circulation 54:571, 1976

119. Ferrer M: Preexcitation. Mt. Kisco, NY, Futura Publishing, 1976
120. Lev M, Gibson S, Miller RA: Ebstein's disease with Wolff-Parkinson-White syndrome. Am Heart J 49:724, 1955
121. Gallagher JJ, Pritchett ELC, Sealy WC et al: The preexcitation syndromes. Prog Cardiovasc Dis 20:285, 1978
122. Josephson ME, Horowitz LN, Kastor JA: Paroxysmal supraventricular tachycardia in patients with mitral valve prolapse. Circulation 57:111, 1978
123. Kay NG, Pressley JC, Packer DL et al: Value of the 12-lead electrocardiogram in discriminating atrioventricular nodal reciprocating tachycardia from circus movement atrioventricular tachycardia utilizing a retrograde accessory pathway. Am J Cardiol 59:296, 1987
124. Bauernfeind RA, Wyndham CR, Swiryn SP et al: Paroxysmal atrial fibrillation in the Wolff-Parkinson-White syndrome. Am J Cardiol 47:562, 1981
125. Klein G, Bashore T, Sellers T et al: Ventricular fibrillation in the Wolff-Parkinson-White syndrome. N Engl J Med 301:1080, 1979
126. Benditt DC, Pritchett ELC, Gallagher JJ: Spectrum of regular tachycardia with wide QRS complexes in patients with accessory atrioventricular pathways. Am J Cardiol 42:828, 1980
127. Strasberg B, Ashley WW, Wyndham CRC et al: Treadmill exercise testing in the Wolff-Parkinson-White syndrome. Am J Cardiol 45:742, 1980
128. Dhingra RC, Palileo EV, Strasberg B et al: Electrophysiologic effects of ouabain in patients with preexcitation and circus movement tachycardia. Am J Cardiol 47:139, 1981
129. Sellers TD, Bashore TM, Gallagher JJ: Digitalis in the preexcitation syndrome: Analysis during atrial fibrillation. Circulation 56:260, 1977
130. Gulamhusein S, Ko P, Carruthers G et al: Acceleration of the ventricular response during atrial fibrillation in the Wolff-Parkinson-White syndrome after verapamil. Circulation 65:348, 1982
131. Sellers TD Jr, Campbell RWF, Bashore TM et al: Effects of procainamide and quinidine sulfate in the Wolff-Parkinson-White syndrome. Circulation 55:15, 1977
132. Kim SS, Lal R, Ruffy R: Treatment of paroxysmal reentrant supraventricular tachycardia with flecainide acetate. Am J Cardiol 58:80, 1986
133. Prystowsky EN, Klein GJ, Rinkenberger RL et al: Clinical efficacy and electrophysiologic effects of encainide in patients with Wolff-Parkinson-White syndrome. Circulation 69:278, 1984
134. Abdollah H, Brugada P, Green M et al: Clinical efficacy and electrophysiologic effects of intravenous and oral encainide in patients with accessory atrioventricular pathways and supraventricular arrhythmias. Am J Cardiol 54:544, 1984
135. Wellens HJJ, Lie KI, Bar FW et al: Effect of amiodarone in the Wolff-Parkinson-White syndrome. Am J Cardiol 38:189, 1976
136. Morady F, Scheinman MM, Winston SA et al: Efficacy and safety of transcatheter ablation of posteroseptal accessory pathways. Circulation 72:170, 1985
137. Warin JF, Haissaguerre M: Catheter ablation of accessory pathway in all locations: Report of 50 patients (abstr). PACE 11:908, 1988
138. Gallagher JJ, Sealy WC, Cox JL et al: Results of surgery for preexcitation caused by accessory atrioventricular pathways in 267 consecutive cases. In Josephson ME, Wellens HJJ (eds): Tachycardias: Mechanisms, Diagnosis, and Treatment. Philadelphia, Lea & Febiger, 1984
139. Guiraudon GM, Klein GJ, Sharma AD et al: Surgical treatment of Wolff-Parkinson-White syndrome: The epicardial approach. In Benditt DG, Benson DW (eds): Cardiac Preexcitation Syndromes, pp 535–541. Boston, Martinus Nijhoff, 1986
140. Mahaim I, Winston MR: Recherches d'anatomie comparée et du pathologie experimentale sur les connexions hautes de faisceau de His-Tawara. Cardiologia 5:189, 1941
141. Gallagher JJ, Smith WM, Kasell JH et al: Role of Mahaim fibers in cardiac arrhythmias in man. Circulation 64:176, 1981
142. Tchou P, Lehmann MH, Jazayeri M et al: Atriofascicular connection or a nodoventricular Mahaim fiber? Electrophysiologic elucidation of the pathway and associated reentrant circuit. Circulation 77:837, 1988
143. Klein GJ, Guiraudon GM, Kerr CR et al: "Nodoventricular" accessory pathway: Evidence for a distinct accessory atrioventricular pathway with atrioventricular node-like properties. J Am Coll Cardiol 11:1035, 1988
144. Critelli G, Gallagher JJ, Monda V et al: Anatomic and electrophysiologic substrate of the permanent form of junctional reciprocating tachycardia. J Am Coll Cardiol 4:601, 1984
145. Coumel P, Cabrol C, Fabiato A et al: Tachycardie permanente par rhythme reciproque. Arch Mal Coeur 60:1830, 1967
146. Gallagher JJ, German LD, Broughton A et al: Variants of the preexcitation syndromes. In Rosenbaum MB, Elizari MV (eds): Frontiers of Cardiac Electrophysiology. The Hague, Martinus Nijhoff, 1983

VENTRICULAR ARRHYTHMIAS

John M. Miller • Mark E. Josephson

Ventricular arrhythmias continue to be a major cause of cardiovascular morbidity and mortality in the United States, as well as a major cause of confusion and concern among physicians who treat them. The causes, clinical presentations, and prognosis vary widely depending in large part on the type and extent of heart disease. In this chapter, we will attempt to draw distinctions between various subsets of patients as well as outline a general approach to the management of patients with ventricular arrhythmias.

DEFINITIONS

PREMATURE VENTRICULAR COMPLEXES. Premature ventricular complexes (PVCs) are premature impulses originating in the ventricles. These may be single or multiform and simple (single, isolated PVCs of varying frequency) or complex (two or more PVCs occurring in sequence or multiform configuration). Additional significance has been attached by some investigators to PVCs occurring on the T wave of the preceding QRS complex (so-called R on T phenomenon).

VENTRICULAR TACHYCARDIA. Ventricular tachycardia (VT) is generally defined as three or more successive beats of ventricular origin at a rate in excess of 100 beats per minute. VT may be nonsustained (3 beats to an arbitrary length, usually less than 30 seconds and self-terminating) or sustained (lasting longer than 30 seconds or requiring cardioversion because of hemodynamic compromise). VT is generally of uniform morphology, that is, each successive beat is morphologically identical to all previous beats (Fig. 50.1). A special subset of VT is *polymorphic VT*, in which each beat is slightly different in electrocardiographic (ECG) configuration, especially when multiple ECG leads are evaluated (see Fig. 50.1). The rate of polymorphic VT is usually in excess of 200 beats per minute and is usually slightly irregular. Polymorphic VT may be nonsustained or sustained, just as can VT of uniform morphology. A final, somewhat arbitrary subclassification of VT is *ventricular flutter*, which is usually defined as a sinusoidal QRS complex without a clear isoelectric point between beats, at a rate of 250 beats per minute or greater. This is usually associated with rapid hemodynamic collapse and requires immediate cardioversion.

VENTRICULAR FIBRILLATION. Ventricular fibrillation (VF) is defined as extremely rapid, disorganized ventricular depolarization characterized by an undulating baseline on the ECG. VF may on rare occasion be self-terminating but generally is sustained, and if it is not quickly terminated by electrical shock it results in death.

PVCs may be a source of symptoms such as palpitations, skipped beats, or dyspnea. They are not in themselves life threatening, but may be markers for serious underlying heart disease and are often associated with more significant arrhythmias, such as VT and VF. PVCs will be discussed in the remainder of this chapter only insofar as they relate to the pathogenesis, diagnosis, and treatment of VT and VF.

UNIFORM SUSTAINED VENTRICULAR TACHYCARDIA

Sudden cardiac death is a major cause of mortality in the United States, accounting for several hundred thousand deaths a year. Studies have shown that the majority of cases of sudden death are caused by VT or VF rather than by bradyarrhythmia.[1] Prevention of recurrences of VT or VF is a major concern, in that patients with sustained VT have up to 20% mortality rates in the first year after the initial episode, and that survivors of cardiac arrest may have up to a 30% to 50% annual recurrence rate.[2] As more cases are reported in which Holter monitors were in place at the time of onset of sudden death, it becomes evident that uniform VT is a frequent inciting event, occurring in up to 50% of cases. Much of this chapter will be concerned with the evaluation and management of the patient with uniform sustained VT.

DIFFERENTIATION OF VT FROM SUPRAVENTRICULAR TACHYCARDIA WITH ABERRANT INTRAVENTRICULAR CONDUCTION

It is important to make sure one is dealing with VT rather than supraventricular tachycardia (SVT) with aberration, since the pathogenesis, significance, and treatment differ significantly between these two arrhythmias. Careful application of the following criteria can separate most cases of VT from SVT with aberration; the majority of these criteria were developed by Wellens and co-workers,[3] in a study of 100 consecutive patients with VT and 100 with SVT:

1. The presence of atrioventricular (AV) dissociation during tachycardia. AV dissociation is present in 50% of cases of VT but is extremely rare, although not impossible, in supraventricular tachycardia with aberrant conduction.
2. Left axis deviation (more negative than $-30°$). This occurred in 68% of cases of VT, but only 7% of cases of SVT in Wellens and co-workers' series.[3]
3. QRS complex duration in excess of 0.14 second. The QRS complex was wider than 0.14 second in 59% of cases of VT, but in no cases of SVT with aberration.
4. QRS morphology in leads V_1 and V_6
   a. Right bundle branch block (RBBB) tachycardias (defined as a terminal R wave in V_1). A monophasic R wave in V_1 or a QR complex in V_1 is very suggestive of VT and extremely uncommon in SVT with aberration. Likewise an rS or QS complex in lead V_6 (or, R/S ratio <1) is very suggestive of VT.
   b. Left bundle branch block (LBBB) tachycardias (defined as terminal S wave in V_1). An R wave greater than 30 msec in duration in lead V_1 or an interval between the onset of the QRS complex and the nadir of the S wave in V_1 greater than 70 msec suggests VT. Additionally, the presence of a Q wave in V_6 also suggests VT, since this is very unusual in LBBB aberration.[4]
5. In patients with preexisting bundle branch block in sinus rhythm, a significant difference in QRS morphology during tachycardia (not just axis shift) suggests VT.[5]
6. Fusion beats. Intermittent narrowing or normalization of the QRS complex during tachycardia is strongly suggestive of VT and implies that supraventricular capture of all or part of the ventricle is occurring; this tends to correlate with AV dissociation. It is important to recall that PVCs occurring during either VT or SVT with aberration may cause fusion beats without implying a tachycardia mechanism. Fusion beats are uncommon overall and are generally observed in slower tachycardias.
7. Some researchers have suggested that the presence of Q waves during a wide QRS tachycardia suggests VT, but one should recall

that Q waves during tachycardia can be seen as well in patients with cardiomyopathy and patients with SVT and a history of prior myocardial infarction; additionally, pseudo Q waves due to inverted P waves at the onset of the QRS complex may be evident in some cases of SVT.

8. Concordance. A concordant precordial R wave pattern is defined as all positive (R waves) or all negative (QS or Qr waves) complexes from V_1 to V_6 during tachycardia. Although uncommon during VT (only 10% of cases showing precordial concordance),[6] this does not occur at all in SVT with aberration. Patients with preexcited tachycardias in the Wolff-Parkinson-White syndrome can occasionally have precordial R wave concordance, but this constitutes a small percentage of the total number of tachycardias exhibiting this pattern.

It is very important to recall that most of the above criteria were derived from groups of patients with a normal QRS complex in sinus rhythm. The sensitivity and specificity of criteria 2, 3, 4, and 7 are diminished in the presence of preexisting bundle branch block in sinus rhythm. Additionally, patients on antiarrhythmic drugs may have nonspecific prolongation of QRS duration that can lessen the discriminating capacity of the third criterion.

Another source of confusion between VT and SVT are cases of the Wolff-Parkinson-White syndrome with antegrade conduction (atrium to ventricle) over the bypass tract simulating VT. This is fortunately not a common clinical problem, occurring in less than 10% of patients with Wolff-Parkinson-White syndrome.[7] Supraventricular arrhythmias that can mimic VT in this setting are atrial tachycardias or atrial flutter with conduction over the bypass tract. Differentiation of SVT from VT in these instances often requires invasive electrophysiologic study. In other cases in which the differentiation between SVT and VT is unclear, the simple recording of a His bundle electrogram during tachycardia may make the diagnosis. It was once believed that observing a dissociated His-potential was a helpful means of distinguishing VT from SVT with aberration, since all cases of SVT should have a 1:1 H:QRS relationship; unfortunately, only 2% of VT have truly dissociated His-potentials, making this criterion less helpful than had once been believed. Similarly, cases of SVT with aberration should have a His-ventricle (HV) interval the same or greater than that during sinus rhythm, but this also occurs in up to 40% of cases of VT where a 1:1 H:QRS relationship also frequently exists.[8]

MECHANISMS

Several different mechanisms of arrhythmia are potentially operative during uniform sustained VT, as described below.

Automaticity is defined as spontaneous phase IV depolarization until threshold is reached. This does not ordinarily occur in ventricular muscle at rates sufficient for VT, although "abnormal" automaticity has been observed in diseased human ventricular tissue.[9] A special case of presumed automaticity arising in the ventricles is accelerated idioventricular rhythm (AIVR), which can occur in the early hours following acute myocardial infarction. Experimental studies have shown that automaticity appears to be responsible for some ventricular arrhythmias within the first 48 hours after coronary occlusion,[10] but it is generally agreed that true "automatic VT" is uncommon clinically.

Triggered activity as a cause of clinical arrhythmias is a relatively new concept.[11] It is characterized by the observation in cellular preparations that small depolarizations following the repolarization downstroke of an action potential (so-called afterdepolarizations) can, under certain circumstances, achieve amplitude sufficient to reach threshold potential and result in a second, triggered depolarization. As the name implies, arrhythmias caused by triggered activity are not spontaneously arising but must have a "trigger." The afterdepolarizations responsible for triggered activity have been divided into early and late, according to timing on the repolarization downslope of the action potential. Early afterdepolarizations may be responsible for certain cases of the long QT interval syndrome, especially when associated with bradycardias, drug toxicity, or electrolyte imbalance. Late afterdepolarizations have been observed in cellular preparations that have been made digitalis toxic or when large amounts of catecholamines have been added to the bath. The role of either early or late afterdepolarizations and triggered activity in the genesis of clinical ventricular arrhythmias is speculative, but this mechanism does not appear to account for a significant proportion of cases of ventricular arrhythmia.

Reentry, as originally defined by Mines, is characterized by heterogeneous refractoriness and conduction in muscle such that unidirec-

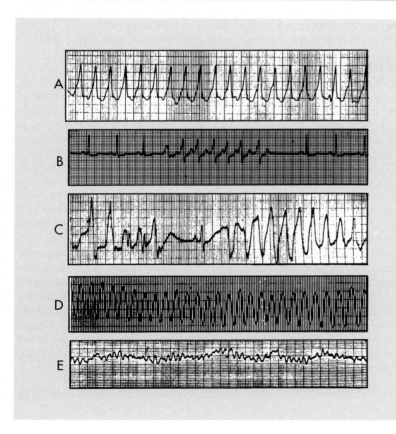

FIGURE 50.1 Differentiating forms of ventricular arrhythmia. **A.** Uniform, sustained VT. **B.** Uniform, nonsustained VT. **C.** Polymorphic VT (torsades de pointes). Note constantly changing QRS. **D.** Ventricular flutter (very rapid VT with sine wave configuration). **E.** Ventricular fibrillation.

tional block of an impulse in one portion of the muscle can occur, with slow conduction through other areas of muscle, circumventing the area of initial block. If conduction is slow enough to provide sufficient time for recovery of excitability of the area where block initially occurred, reentry of the impulse retrogradely through the area initially blocked can take place. Because of the electrophysiologic heterogeneity required, reentry within the ventricle generally requires significant underlying heart disease. This mechanism is believed to account for the majority of VT in humans. Reentry as classically described can be very difficult to differentiate from triggered activity, in that both rhythms can be initiated and terminated by rapid pacing or premature extrastimuli, techniques commonly used in evaluating clinical VT. Although this differentiation can be difficult, VT in humans exhibits several other phenomena that suggest that reentry, and not triggered activity, is the mechanism (such as reset of tachycardia by premature extrastimuli, entrainment of the tachycardia by rapid overdrive pacing, with resumption of the tachycardia after pacing, and certain responses to antiarrhythmic drugs). These characteristics have been well set forth elsewhere.[12]

The clinical features of uniform sustained VT may be palpitations, syncope or presyncope, cardiac arrest, or a more stable sustained VT. Other symptoms, such as dyspnea or angina, may be present, especially when coronary artery disease is responsible, but ordinarily no new myocardial event (such as infarction) has occurred with the VT episode. The frequency of episodes in a given person varies widely; single episodes of VT occur in a minority of patients if followed long enough, while other patients have multiple episodes or even incessant VT (with only rare interludes of sinus rhythm even after termination by pacing or cardioversion).

ETIOLOGIES OF VENTRICULAR ARRHYTHMIAS BY UNDERLYING HEART DISEASE

CORONARY ARTERY DISEASE

The major underlying cause of sustained VT in Western countries is coronary artery disease (CAD). The most frequent clinical setting for VT in CAD is in the chronic phase of myocardial infarction, often with left ventricular aneurysm formation and decreased left ventricular function.[13] Uniform sustained VT can occur in other settings in CAD, such as during treadmill exercise test, with or without concurrent ischemia,[14] or in the very early hours of an acute myocardial infarction, but these instances account for a small minority of cases of VT in patients with CAD. The incidence of sustained VT after myocardial infarction is difficult to assess, but is probably in the 5% to 7% range. The first episode can occur at any time after infarction (from 1 week to over 10 years), but is generally 1 to 2 years after infarction. As mentioned earlier, most patients have recurrent episodes of tachycardia and high mortality if untreated.

Because of its prevalence, more is understood about sustained VT after myocardial infarction than other forms of VT. VT in this setting is believed to be due to reentry in the majority of cases. The so-called substrate for reentry (the fixed anatomical and electrophysiologic milieu that allows reentry to occur) is generally believed to reside in the surviving layers of subendocardial myocardium arranged in isolated longitudinal bundles that reach the borders of the infarction.[15] Conduction through these bundles of surviving muscle appears to occur very slowly, presumably owing to poor cell-to-cell coupling, and thus could serve as one of the necessary elements of a reentrant circuit. Evidence for reentry involving subendocardial tissues includes the following:

1. Mapping studies (done by sampling endocardial electrical activity during VT either in the catheterization laboratory or intraoperatively and comparing the timing of the local electrograms to the surface QRS[16]) have demonstrated that the earliest electrical activity during VT in cases of chronic infarction occurs on the left ventricular endocardium, as opposed to epicardial or intramural tissues.

2. Surgical alteration or ablation of small circumscribed areas having early electrical activity during VT results in cessation of tachycardia and cure from further episodes of VT postoperatively.[17]
3. Cellular electrophysiologic studies of human subendocardium removed at surgery have demonstrated a wide range of electrophysiologic derangements,[9] including abnormal resting membrane potential, delayed upstroke of the action potential, and prolonged refractoriness, all of which could play a role ("substrate") in the genesis and perpetuation of ventricular arrhythmias.

CARDIOMYOPATHY

The second major etiologic group for sustained VT is dilated cardiomyopathy.[18] Approximately 20% of patients with New York Heart Association Class III or IV congestive heart failure have cardiac arrest or sustained VT. As in CAD, episodes of VT in these patients are generally recurrent and, in some, occur in clusters with relatively long arrhythmia-free intervals. The most common mechanism of VT in this group of patients is also believed to be reentry, in that many of these tachycardias can be induced, terminated, and entrained or reset by extrastimuli or rapid pacing in the electrophysiologic laboratory. Less is known about the nature of the substrate for VT in cardiomyopathy than in CAD. It is likely that several diverse disease states lead to the final expression of "idiopathic" dilated cardiomyopathy and that the pathophysiologic substrate thus may not be the same in all instances. In diseases in which the pathologic process is more clearly defined (*e.g.*, hypertrophic obstructive cardiomyopathy, Chagas' disease, sarcoidosis), too few cases have been carefully studied to allow insight into the mechanisms or substrate for reentry.

TETRALOGY OF FALLOT

Survivors of corrective surgery for tetralogy of Fallot are known to be at increased risk of sudden death. Many studies have shown a significant incidence of spontaneous nonsustained VT and a lesser incidence (5% to 10%) of inducible sustained VT at electrophysiologic study. These patients generally have persistent elevations of right ventricular pressures as well as clinical right ventricular failure, as compared with patients without arrhythmias. Some students have shown that sustained VT in these patients results from a wavefront of electrical activity circulating around the healed incision in the right ventricular infundibulum (through which the repair was accomplished). Incising this scar tissue at a second operation has resulted in cessation of VT and prevention of postoperative recurrences in several reported cases.[19] Other workers have reported mapping studies that suggest that VT in these patients may originate near the region of the ventricular septal defect.[20]

ARRHYTHMOGENIC RIGHT VENTRICULAR DYSPLASIA

Marcus and colleagues[21] reported a series of patients with right ventricular contractile abnormalities on ventriculography, abnormal surface QRS complexes, tachycardias, and distinctive late electrical activity on the epicardium of the right ventricle corresponding to abnormal waves in the ST segment on the surface ECG. The characteristic sinus rhythm ECG shows inverted right precordial T waves, occasionally complete or incomplete right bundle branch block, and abnormal low-amplitude ripples in the ST segment. They termed this disorder *arrhythmogenic right ventricular disorder* (ARVD). It has since been shown that sustained VT arises in areas of very delayed epicardial activation in these patients, suggesting a reentrant mechanism. Furthermore, programmed stimulation can almost always induce VT in these patients. Histologically, abnormal areas are characterized by isolated bundles of surviving muscle cells separated by fat. There are three general areas in the right ventricle in which dysplastic changes most commonly occur: near the apex; the right ventricular outflow tract/infundibulum; and the lateral basal right ventricle (all on the free wall). An individual patient may have one or more of these areas involved. The reasons for development of dysplasia are not clear. Similar findings are occasionally observed in the left ventricular free wall.

MITRAL VALVE PROLAPSE

Many patients with the mitral valve prolapse syndrome have palpitations; on rare occasions, these are shown to be due to sustained uniform VT. The mechanism of arrhythmia in these instances is unclear, but it has been hypothesized that tension on the posteroinferior papillary muscle is arrhythmogenic, either due to automaticity or perhaps reentry. The results of programmed electrical stimulation in these patients are variable, although if spontaneous uniform sustained VT is present, it can usually be induced.[22]

LOCALIZED LEFT VENTRICULAR ABNORMALITIES

Occasional cases of left ventricular aneurysm not associated with coronary disease have been associated with VT. Some cases have shown the same pathologic findings as in ARVD, but occurring in the left ventricle. The mechanism of VT in cases of so-called idiopathic left ventricular aneurysm is not clear, but has been presumed to be reentry, based on the response of these arrhythmias to programmed stimulation, as noted above. Sustained uniform VT has been reported in a variety of diseases, including sarcoidosis, myotonic dystrophy, and cardiac tumors.[23]

NORMAL HEART

Two distinct patterns of VT exist in patients without discernible heart disease. The first of these is that of VT with a left bundle branch block, inferior axis, which generally occurs in salvos of uniform nonsustained VT, but which can occasionally be sustained (so-called repetitive monomorphic VT).[24] This VT can more often be brought out by exercise or rapid pacing than by extrastimuli introduced using programmed electrical stimulation and responds well to β-blockers and often other agents as well. These findings suggest that reentry is not responsible for this form of VT, but few cases have been studied extensively. Mapping studies in some have revealed an earliest site of activation during VT in the right ventricular outflow tract.

A second clinical setting of VT arising in a normal heart is that of VT with a right bundle branch block, left axis morphology, which is often induced by atrial or ventricular pacing as well as extrastimuli.[25] This would imply reentry as the mechanism of tachycardia, although some have suggested triggered activity. A retrograde His deflection is often seen at or near the onset of the QRS complex in VT, suggesting participation of the specialized conducting system. Mapping studies in some patients have shown earliest activation in the mid-inferior septum on the left ventricular endocardium, and these VTs respond well to β-blockade or calcium channel blockade. Both syndromes of VT in normal hearts tend to occur in younger patients and are usually associated with palpitations or presyncope. The tachycardias are generally well tolerated hemodynamically and almost never result in death.

UNIFORM NONSUSTAINED VENTRICULAR TACHYCARDIA

Uniform nonsustained ventricular tachycardia is a more frequent finding than sustained VT in patients with all types of heart disease.[26-29] This arrhythmia usually signifies the presence of serious underlying heart disease in most, but not all, patients,[30] a significant exception being those with the repetitive monomorphic tachycardia. Less is known about the underlying mechanisms of this arrhythmia, since it has not been as thoroughly studied as sustained VT. Several studies have shown that programmed electrical stimulation can induce nonsustained VT in 20% to 65% of patients and sustained VT (similar in morphology to nonsustained VT) in 15% to 20% of patients with nonsustained VT, thus suggesting reentry as the underlying mechanism in at least these patients. These observations are more frequent in patients with CAD. The underlying mechanism responsible for the remainder of nonsustained VT cases is far from clear. The overall prognosis in nonsustained VT generally depends on the severity and type of underlying heart disease; in one study, all patients with CAD who had sudden death over a nearly 3-year follow-up had ejection fractions less than 40%. Patients with cardiomyopathy had twice the incidence of sudden death compared with patients with nonsustained VT in the presence of underlying coronary artery disease.[31]

POLYMORPHIC VENTRICULAR TACHYCARDIA

Polymorphic VTs can be generally divided into those associated with a long QT interval in sinus rhythm,[32] in which case the term *torsades de pointes* is applied, and those cases with a normal QT interval in sinus rhythm. The long QT interval syndromes will be discussed extensively elsewhere in this volume.

NORMAL QT INTERVALS: POLYMORPHIC VT

Polymorphic VT may occur in patients with normal QT intervals, most commonly in the setting of acute ischemia.[33] The arrhythmia is most usually nonsustained in these persons, being a cause of syncope in some, but uncommonly causing death. It is of note that in these instances, type I antiarrhythmic drugs (which aggravate long QT interval syndrome–associated polymorphic VT) may be reasonable therapeutic agents in preventing further episodes. The mechanism is unclear, but the prognosis appears good overall. Finally, polymorphic VT in patients with normal QT intervals is commonly induced with programmed stimulation at electrophysiologic study, in which cases it is most usually nonsustained. This appears to represent a nonspecific response of the myocardium to intensive stimulation, with no prognostic significance. If the induction of uniform sustained VT is facilitated by type I drugs, however, the resultant arrhythmia may be clinically significant.

VENTRICULAR FIBRILLATION

Any of the previously noted underlying heart diseases can be associated with ventricular fibrillation, although certain categories are of special note. These include acute ischemia or infarction, coronary reperfusion (with streptokinase, or spontaneously after an acute infarction), hypothermia, hypocalcemia, and rarely in persons with normal hearts. The mechanism is presumed to be extremely rapid reentry of multiple small wavefronts throughout the heart. Ideker and co-workers[34] have shown in experimental models that the surface ECG manifestations of the early stages of VF can be produced by electrical activity moving in organized wavefronts across the epicardium, each one starting at one heart border before the others have finished their transit across the heart. This in essence may represent accelerating ventricular tachycardia that breaks down into fibrillation. We have observed similar organized activity at the outset of catheter-induced VF.

MANAGEMENT

The approach to the management of the patient with ventricular arrhythmias consists of delineation of the relevant rhythm disturbance, whether uniform sustained VT, nonsustained VT, polymorphic VT, or VF, as well as the setting in which it occurs, and of determination of the type and severity of underlying heart disease. Several methods are available for treatment and assessing the efficacy of these therapeutic modalities. The outlook for these patients is considerably less bleak than even a decade ago and likely will continue to improve as new techniques and antiarrhythmic drugs become available in the future.

DIAGNOSTIC STUDIES (TABLE 50.1)

PASSIVE METHODS

Several "passive" methods for detection of ventricular arrhythmias are available. These include incidental detection on routine ECG. This is unusual except in instances of nonsustained VT, which may occur frequently enough to be recorded on a routine ECG. Generally, however, patients present to their physician complaining of a history of palpitations, syncope, or presyncope or have had a cardiac arrest or documented sustained VT. In these cases it is necessary to document the arrhythmia and relationship to symptoms, if it is not already apparent. Studies useful in this regard include in-hospital telemetry monitoring, which may give an indication of the frequency of arrhythmia as well as providing a means of rapidly treating an arrhythmia should this be required. Long-term ambulatory ECG monitoring (Holter, from 24 to 48 hours) is useful for detection of arrhythmias as well as correlation with symptoms. It is most beneficial in instances in which the arrhythmia occurs frequently enough to have a reasonable chance of being recorded in a 24- to 48-hour period of monitoring. For less frequent arrhythmia episodes, a patient-activated transient arrhythmia monitoring system, of which several are available, may be more useful. Using this system, the patient carries a portable recording device the size of a transistor radio with him for a month or longer. When an episode of palpitations or presyncope occurs, the patient applies the unit (which has several metal electrodes on its back for skin contact) to his chest and activates the unit by pressing a button. The unit then records a rhythm strip for 30 seconds or longer, stores the information, and is able to replay the rhythm strip transtelephonically at the patient's convenience. This type of recording device is obviously of limited usefulness in cases of syncope or severe presyncope, in that the patient would not be able to apply the device before losing consciousness. Another limitation is the fact that some of these devices use only single-channel recordings, which can make distinction of uniform from polymorphic VT difficult. Two-channel recorders circumvent this limitation to a large degree.

PROVOCATIVE METHODS

When the above methods, such as Holter monitoring or transtelephonic telemetry devices, are successful in documenting the clinical arrhythmia, it is possible that no further testing is necessary to elucidate the nature of the rhythm disturbance. However, these methods are unrevealing in the majority of patients. In patients eventually found to have serious ventricular arrhythmias, several provocative methods of arrhythmia detection are available, which may be used both for confirmation of the diagnosis and as a therapeutic guide. If the arrhythmia can be reproducibly initiated with some method, and a therapeutic intervention made that prevents the same method of initiation, the therapy would be predicted to be effective in preventing further episodes of arrhythmia. Two general methods of provoking arrhythmias are exercise testing and electrophysiologic studies.

EXERCISE TESTING. Exercise testing is especially useful in instances of repetitive monomorphic tachycardia,[35] which generally occurs in persons with no underlying heart disease. Occasionally, patients with ischemic disease will have reproducible initiation of either uniform VT (sustained or nonsustained) or ventricular fibrillation. In all such instances in which symptomatic ventricular arrhythmias are reproducibly provoked by exercise testing, the efficacy of therapy (e.g., drugs, coronary bypass surgery) may be reasonably evaluated by repeat exercise testing. This method will be dealt with in further detail in a later section.

ELECTROPHYSIOLOGIC STUDIES. Electrophysiologic studies use rapid ventricular pacing or programmed ventricular extrastimuli (premature beats delivered at precise intervals after the preceding beat) to induce arrhythmias.[36] This is based on the hypothesis that a pathophysiologic "substrate" for VT exists that, when appropriately "stressed" can lead to the development of VT. The effect of premature extrastimuli is generally to impinge on refractoriness of some tissues (block of impulse transmission) at the same time causing slow conduction of the impulse in other areas. If conduction is slow enough that the initially blocked area can recover excitability, reentry may occur. Electrophysiologic studies would be expected to have their greatest uses in diagnosis and management of patients with paroxysmal reentrant arrhythmias, such as the majority of instances of uniform sustained VT appear to be, and likewise relatively little efficacy inducing automatic rhythms, since they require spontaneous phase IV depolarization and not heterogeneous conduction and refractoriness within the ventricles. Triggered activity may be induced with rapid pacing or programmed extrastimuli (although less reproducibly),[11] but, as mentioned earlier, current evidence is that triggered activity has little role in the genesis of clinical ventricular arrhythmias.

The electrophysiologic study is performed with the patient in a postabsorptive state with little or no sedation. Several multipolar electrode catheters (usually No. 6 or 7 F in diameter) are introduced percutaneously from femoral or antecubital veins and are positioned in the heart using fluoroscopic guidance. Catheter positions include the high right atrium, atrioventricular junction (for recording the His bundle electrogram), right ventricular apex, and right ventricular outflow tract or left ventricle (via a femoral arterial approach) as needed. Programmed ventricular extrastimuli are introduced during sinus rhythm and following a train of 8 to 10 paced ventricular beats (usually at 600- and 400-msec paced cycle lengths). The extrastimulus is introduced at progressively decreasing coupling intervals (increasing prematurity) until it no longer propagates (the effective refractory period). Approximately 25% of the time, a single ventricular extrastimulus will result in the initiation of sustained VT. If no ventricular arrhythmia is induced with a single extrastimulus, a second extrastimulus is introduced after the first. This protocol will be successful at initiating uniform sustained VT in 60% to 80% of patients who presented with the same arrhythmia.[37,38] Addition of a third extrastimulus or occasionally burst pacing will increase the yield of the study to approximately 95% among patients with a history of spontaneous sustained VT.[39] The reproducible induction of VT allows the assessment of drug therapy and, where indicated, mapping procedures can be performed. VT thus initiated is

---

TABLE 50.1 DIAGNOSTIC STUDIES IN PATIENTS WITH VENTRICULAR ARRHYTHMIAS

Passive (useful for arrhythmia determination, but generally inadequate for guiding therapy)
   Routine ECG (nonsustained VT)
   In-hospital telemetry
   Ambulatory ECG (Holter) monitoring
   Patient-activated transient arrhythmia detection device

Provocative
   Exercise testing
      Patients with arrhythmia, but no discernible heart disease
      Patients with coronary artery disease
   Electrophysiologic study
      Rapid atrial or ventricular pacing
      Programmed extrastimuli
      Isoproterenol infusion

occasionally hemodynamically unstable, in which case rapid overdrive ventricular pacing will usually terminate VT. Occasionally, cardioversion is required to return the patient to sinus rhythm. Overall, electrophysiologic studies are quite safe, with a 2% complication rate per procedure (generally minor bleeding at the site of catheter insertion in the skin, deep venous thrombosis, local wound infections).[40] Death as a result of electrophysiologic studies is an extremely rare occurrence.

The role of electrophysiologic studies in the evaluation of nonsustained VT is less clear. Buxton and associates[41] studied 83 patients with a variety of underlying cardiac disorders who had a history of nonsustained VT. Fifty patients (60%) had nonsustained VT induced by electrophysiologic studies in whom 15 had sustained VT (18%) initiated; 40% (31 patients) had no inducible arrhythmia at electrophysiologic studies. Thus, the yield of inducible arrhythmia is substantially less in cases of nonsustained VT than in sustained VT. The prognostic implications of inducible VT in this subset of patients is less clear as well.

Among survivors of cardiac arrest, sustained ventricular arrhythmias (mainly VT) can be initiated in from 60% to 80% of patients,[42-44] with relatively more patients having inducible arrhythmia (80%) when CAD is present, rather than other heart disease.

Electrophysiologic studies have limited use in the diagnosis and management of patients with polymorphic VT (especially in the long QT interval syndrome) in which only rare patients have the reproducible initiation of polymorphic or uniform VT. In patients with a normal QT (such as in a coronary disease population), polymorphic VT can often be initiated, but frequently this requires the delivery of multiple ventricular extrastimuli. This is important in that the specificity of electrophysiologic studies decreases with the addition of increasing numbers of extrastimuli, generally resulting in the induction of polymorphic VT (usually nonsustained, 10 to 15 beats maximum). This nonspecific response can be observed in 6% of normal persons given two extrastimuli, 15% to 30% of normal persons given three extrastimuli and up to 25% after four extrastimuli.[45] Thus, the documentation of the nature of the clinical arrhythmia (uniform VT, polymorphic VT, VF) assumes an even greater importance. The response of polymorphic VT to type I drugs may enhance the specificity of electrophysiologic studies. If this results in inducible uniform sustained VT, we believe this arrhythmia to be clinically significant. Higher doses of type I drugs frequently abolish inducible VT in these patients.

Findings of electrophysiologic studies are highly reproducible over time in patients with CAD. In a small study[46] of 17 patients with ventricular arrhythmias who had two separate electrophysiologic studies without any antiarrhythmic drugs separated by a mean of 18 months, 11 patients with underlying CAD had inducible VT, but only 1 of 6 patients without coronary disease had inducible VT on the follow-up study. These results suggest that, at least in coronary disease, the substrate for arrhythmia is stable over time and that electrophysiologic studies are effective in studying the arrhythmia and its response to therapeutic intervention.

DELINEATION OF TYPE AND SEVERITY OF UNDERLYING HEART DISEASE (TABLE 50.2)

Determination of the type and severity of underlying heart disease is important in the management of patients with ventricular arrhythmias, in that the selection of the most appropriate therapeutic modality (e.g., drugs, pacemakers, surgery) often hinges more on the status of the underlying heart disease than on which particular ventricular arrhythmia is present. For instance, two patients with uniform sustained VT, one with no underlying heart disease and exercise-provoked VT and the other with prior extensive myocardial infarction and depressed left ventricular function, would be treated quite differently based more on their underlying heart disease rather than on the arrhythmia itself. The first patient would be expected to respond to β-blockers or calcium channel antagonists. The same therapy used in the second patient would produce further depression of already marginal left ventricular function and no beneficial effect on the arrhythmia. Studies that may aid in the elucidation of the type and severity of underlying heart disease include the following:

1. History (including family history, for family members with early or sudden death, history of coronary artery disease, cardiomyopathy, prior heart surgery, and congenital heart disease)
2. Physical examination (presence of congestive heart failure, valvular disease, a dyskinetic impulse suggesting an aneurysm, or evidence of hypertrophic obstructive cardiomyopathy)
3. Electrocardiography (evidence of old myocardial infarction or ischemia, arrhythmogenic right ventricular dysplasia, a long QT interval, drug effects)
4. Some assessment of global and segmental left ventricular function, such as gated blood pool scan or echocardiography. Echocardiography is especially useful for evaluation of valvular heart disease (mitral valve prolapse, aortic valve disease), as well as hypertrophic obstructive cardiomyopathy and dilated cardiomyopathy. These studies may also reveal discrete wall motion abnormalities or aneurysm.
5. Exercise testing. This test may be used to provoke arrhythmias in instances of exercise-induced VT in the absence of ischemia or ischemic-associated arrhythmias (VT, either uniform or polymorphic, or VF). The test can also be used to uncover underlying ischemia, which again may alter the therapeutic approach.
6. Cardiac catheterization. This procedure, especially with left ventriculography, is used for evaluation of discrete wall motion abnormalities/aneurysm as well as global left ventricular function; coronary arteriography is also useful in patients with CAD, especially when cardiac surgery for control of ventricular arrhythmias is contemplated.
7. Right ventriculography. This study may be indicated in some instances in which arrhythmogenic right ventricular dysplasia is a possibility.
8. Right ventricular endomyocardial biopsy has been advocated by some in elucidating underlying cardiac disease in patients with no discernible cardiac abnormalities on other testing or suspicion of acute myocarditis. Some studies have shown clinically unsuspected lymphocytic myocarditis, as well as other histologic abnormalities,

TABLE 50.2 DELINEATION OF TYPE/SEVERITY OF UNDERLYING HEART DISEASE

All Patients
1. History
    a. Personal: duration of history of symptoms, syncope, cardiac arrest, hypertension, prior myocardial infarction, surgery for congenital heart disease
    b. Family: coronary artery disease, early sudden death, hypertrophic obstructive cardiomyopathy
2. Physical examination (congestive heart failure, dyskinetic impulse, valvular disease, congenital heart disease)
3. ECG (Q waves/persistent ST segment elevation, left ventricular hypertrophy, long QT interval, drug effects, right ventricular dysplasia)
4. Assessment of global/regional left ventricular function (left ventriculography; gated blood pool scan; 2D echocardiogram)
5. Exercise testing (functional capacity, detection of ischemia, provocation of arrhythmia)

Selected Patients
6. Coronary arteriography (especially operative candidates)
7. Right ventriculography (in suspected right ventricular dysplasia)
8. Endomyocardial biopsy

which may be responsible for arrhythmias in certain select groups of patients.[47] The therapeutic implications of this finding are not clear.

TREATMENT
ACUTE SETTING

The acute management of a patient with serious ventricular arrhythmias at the time of evaluation is an important part of clinical practice. The proper course of therapy depends on a rapid recognition of the type of arrhythmia present and specific action. The most important element of therapy is the condition of the patient. Obviously, if loss of consciousness, severe hypotension, or uncontrollable angina is present, even a relatively slow tachycardia should be immediately cardioverted. Ventricular fibrillation and sustained polymorphic VT require immediate countershock as soon as they are recognized.

ACUTE THERAPY FOR SUSTAINED UNIFORM VT. As noted previously, if the patient is severely compromised by the arrhythmia, sedation and cardioversion are in order. If the arrhythmia is hemodynamically and symptomatically tolerated, our practice is to obtain 12-lead ECGs whenever possible. The reasons for this are twofold: (1) to confirm the diagnosis of VT as opposed to SVT with aberrant conduction and (2) to compare the 12-lead ECG morphology of tachycardia with subsequent VT episodes, either spontaneous or induced in the laboratory. At least 20% of patients with VT in the presence of prior myocardial infarction have spontaneously occurring multiple morphologically distinct VTs, and up to 80% have multiple VTs induced in the laboratory.[48]

After obtaining a 12-lead ECG, attempts can be made to terminate the arrhythmia. The first line of therapy is pharmacologic. Lidocaine is the most commonly employed initial drug, administered as a rapid (over 5 to 15 minutes) intravenous infusion of 3 to 5 mg/kg of the drug. This regimen will be effective in terminating VT in less than 10% of cases and has little effect on VT rate, which may in some cases paradoxically increase. However, because the drug is rapidly administered, well tolerated, has few side effects, and does not impair the ability to give other agents subsequently, it has been the first-line drug in many institutions. If lidocaine is unsuccessful in terminating the tachycardia, the next agent of choice is procainamide, given as a 10 mg to 15 mg/kg intravenous infusion at roughly 50 mg/min, depending on the response of the systemic pressure. This will be effective in 20% to 30% of cases; even if the tachycardia does not cease, it very often slows in rate such that patient tolerance of VT is improved. As a result, we favor procainamide as the first pharmacologic option. If both lidocaine and procainamide are unsuccessful in converting VT to sinus rhythm, other drugs have a low likelihood of success but an increased likelihood of side effects. In some institutions, amiodarone, given as a 5-mg/kg intravenous loading dose followed by an infusion of 1 g/day for 2 to 3 days, has been effective; the drug is associated with significant hypotension in many cases and has variable efficacy rates. Few institutions are currently approved to use this investigational agent. Other drugs, such as bretylium or quinidine, have rather low success rates and are associated with significant side effects (mainly hypotension). Of note, verapamil (an agent with marked efficacy in supraventricular tachyarrhythmias) is very unlikely to convert sustained VT to sinus rhythm in cases with underlying coronary disease, and if given intravenously, often results in severe hypotension and occasional conversion of VT to VF. Because of this, verapamil should not be given in the acute setting of sustained VT unless there are compelling reasons to do so (such as a high degree of confidence that the VT is one of the unusual types associated with no underlying heart disease).

If antiarrhythmic drugs are unsuccessful in terminating VT, the arrhythmia can either be terminated with synchronized DC cardioversion or, in some cases, by temporary transcutaneous pacing.[49] If cardioversion is chosen to terminate VT, the patient can be mildly sedated with medazolam, diazepam, or a short-acting barbiturate, after which a synchronized shock of 150 to 200 joules can be delivered (as little as 2 joules may be effective); this usually results in reversion to sinus rhythm. The applicability of transcutaneous overdrive pacing to terminate VT is limited by the maximum rate of the pacing device (180 beats per minute) as well as factors related to the ability to capture the heart with this pacing mode (e.g., body habitus, skin condition). Either underdrive or overdrive pacing modes may be successful with this method, analogous to transvenous pacing (see below). At least in the acute setting, patients tolerate transcutaneous stimulation fairly well, and VT can frequently be terminated with this form of pacing. Although experience is limited, it appears that this method may be useful in certain cases.[5] Depending on the clinical setting, it may be necessary to maintain the patient on antiarrhythmic drugs that seemed to have some beneficial effect either during the current episode or previously or are given simply empirically to prevent further episodes.

If VT recurs after drug or electrical conversion, such that multiple cardioversions will be necessary, a temporary pacemaker can be placed in the right ventricle and, using a variety of pacing modalities, VT can generally be terminated.[50] (Alternatively, transcutaneous pacing may be attempted, but this method is less suitable if pacing will be needed repeatedly for more than a few hours due primarily to patient discomfort). Underdrive pacing (regular pacing at a rate slower than the VT rate) may result in random capture of the ventricles with cessation of VT; however, programmed single or double ventricular extrastimuli result in termination in a significant number of cases in a shorter period of time. Rapid overdrive pacing (at rates 115% to 130% of the VT rate) for 8 to 10 beats is the most successful pacing modality but also is more likely to cause acceleration of the tachycardia or VF, requiring cardioversion.

An experimental modality that has received attention is transvenous, low-energy cardioversion.[51] This device consists of a catheter that is inserted through a peripheral or central vein, with a wide bipole through which the shock is delivered. The tip of the catheter is positioned in the RV apex, and the proximal electrode is in the right atrium or superior vena cava. When VT occurs, the operator charges the device, which then delivers a synchronous, low-energy (usually less than 1 to 2 joules) shock between the two poles. This device has obvious advantages in patients with very frequent episodes of VT, who would ordinarily require repeated transthoracic cardioversion. The device is currently being used only on an experimental basis, and although promising, it has several important drawbacks. Unacceptable pain is often associated with the shock (even with less then 0.1 joule), and acceleration of VT to VF is unfortunately frequent. The device can, however, serve as a useful interim form of therapy until antiarrhythmic drugs have had time to take effect (e.g., amiodarone), or surgical procedures can be arranged.

ACUTE TREATMENT OF NONSUSTAINED VT. In general, no specific therapy is needed for nonsustained VT unless it causes significant symptoms or develops into sustained VT or VF. This is certainly true for patients with otherwise normal hearts and short runs of repetitive monomorphic VT.

POLYMORPHIC VT ASSOCIATED WITH LONG QT INTERVAL SYNDROME. The treatment of polymorphic VT[32,50,52,53] associated with the long QT syndrome is discussed elsewhere in these volumes.

NORMAL QT INTERVAL. Since a major cause of polymorphic VT in the setting of a normal QT interval is myocardial ischemia, relief of ischemia (for example, with nitrates or calcium channel blocking agents) is a necessary first step in many instances. Other instances of polymorphic VT in the setting of a normal QT interval respond to type I antiarrhythmic agents (e.g., procainamide, quinidine).[52]

VF IN THE SETTING OF ACUTE MYOCARDIAL INFARCTION. There is good evidence that VF is prevented by lidocaine (bolus followed by infusion) in the first 24 hours after acute myocardial infarction.[54] Several investigators have argued, however, that since defibrillation for VF can be performed effectively and rapidly in a coronary care unit setting, the potential toxicity of lidocaine can be avoided. (This toxicity is especially likely to occur in low cardiac output states or in the elderly—a substantial proportion of the population with myocardial infarction.) Our belief is that the benefits of a short-term infusion of lidocaine outweigh the risks, in that the trauma of cardioversion and potential for aspiration pneumonitis may be avoided.

VF IN OTHER SETTINGS. Evidence is that the earlier sinus rhythm is restored in cases of VF, the better is the long-term prognosis. This translates into immediate defibrillatory shocks of 300 to 400 joules as soon as the rhythm is recognized, with repeated shocks delivered as soon as possible if VF persists. These may be more efficacious than the initial shock in that subsequent shocks reduce chest wall impedance, resulting in delivery of more energy to the heart. Valuable time in restoring sinus rhythm should not be wasted by starting drug infusions while VF continues. In the event of recurrent episodes, lidocaine in a 3-mg to 5-mg/kg rapid intravenous infusion followed by a 2-mg to 4-mg/min constant infusion may prevent further episodes. If this is unsuccessful, bretylium (5 mg/kg intravenous loading dose with 1 mg to 2 mg/min infusion) may be successful. Finally, procainamide, 10 mg to 15 mg/kg over 20 minutes intravenously, followed by a 4-mg/min drip is occasionally a useful alternative. The recurrence of multiple episodes of VF usually points to an ongoing underlying cause, such as severe ischemia or severe congestive heart failure. Attempts should be made to reverse these conditions while continuing to try to maintain the patient in sinus rhythm.

LONG-TERM MANAGEMENT (TABLE 50.3)

Ideally, a particular drug or other therapy could be prescribed for a specific arrhythmia based on some distinguishing features in the clinical setting with 100% predictive accuracy, obviating the need for prolonged monitoring or provocative testing. In certain cases, such as repetitive monomorphic tachycardia or right bundle branch block/left axis deviation VT in persons with otherwise normal hearts, verapamil or β-blocking agents very often accomplish this end. In these rare instances, once the diagnosis is confirmed and serious organic heart disease excluded, these drugs may be started. No further evaluation may be needed in these circumstances. Unfortunately, for the majority of serious ventricular arrhythmias, there are no distinguishing features that would allow selection of specific therapeutic modalities with any degree of confidence. Thus, the efficacy of any particular therapeutic regimen must be evaluated by its effect on the spontaneous occurrence of arrhythmia or, when rare and sporadic episodes occur, provocative testing is required.

PHARMACOLOGIC THERAPY. The mechanisms of actions of antiarrhythmic drugs have been dealt with in an earlier chapter and will not be discussed in detail here.

EMPIRIC THERAPY. Initial studies in pharmacologic therapy for sustained ventricular arrhythmias were done using "therapeutic blood levels" of type I antiarrhythmic agents (e.g., procainamide, quinidine).[55] In one study, six of six patients with a history of VT or VF had no recurrences when "therapeutic" antiarrhythmic drug levels were maintained, but eight of ten patients with nontherapeutic (low) blood levels had recurrences of VT or VF. This was a small study, and since therapeutic blood levels in one patient may not be therapeutic in another instance,[56] this principle has not gained widespread acceptance.

HOLTER MONITORING. Some investigators have found that the elimination of nonsustained VT in patients with a history of sustained VT or VF accurately predicts the outcome of therapy at 2 years' follow-up. In one such study, 52 patients were treated with investigational antiarrhythmic agents (after conventional agents had failed to prevent spontaneous VT) until "symptomatic" VT was controlled.[57] In patients in whom nonsustained VT was eliminated during Holter monitoring, no deaths occurred in long-term follow-up. In contrast, if nonsustained VT persisted despite the use of investigational antiarrhythmic agents, one third of patients had sudden death or recurrent syncope during the follow-up period. Of note, however, only two thirds of patients had elimination of nonsustained VT on 24-hour Holter monitoring, even with the use of investigational antiarrhythmic drugs (which are not widely available). One of the most important limitations of Holter monitoring is that approximately one fourth of patients with sustained VT or VF have too few PVCs, either simple or complex, on Holter monitoring to be able to use this method to guide therapy. In addition, there is a substantial degree of variability from day to day in Holter monitoring findings, and these variations may simulate a salutary response to an antiarrhythmic drug.[58] Finally, there is often no constant relationship between clinical success of a therapeutic modality in preventing recurrence of VT or VF and the elimination of PVCs or nonsustained VT on Holter monitoring.[59]

EXERCISE TESTING. Due to the limitations of the above methods, Lown and co-workers[60] devised a method of treatment of ventricular arrhythmias by suppressing both ambient PVCs as well as exercise-provoked nonsustained VT. In this method, the elimination of nonsustained VT on exercise, as well as ambient frequent or complex ventricular ectopic activity, is the major therapeutic endpoint, and, in contrast to electrophysiologic studies, the induction of sustained arrhythmias is an undesirable outcome. After baseline exercise testing, patients treated with this method are given a relatively large oral dose of an

TABLE 50.3 LONG-TERM MANAGEMENT OF VENTRICULAR ARRHYTHMIAS

Modality	Uniform Sustained VT	Polymorphic VT		Ventricular Fibrillation
		Long QT	*Normal QT*	
Pharmacologic	EPS Exercise testing (Holter monitoring, empiric)	Empiric	EPS	EPS Exercise testing
Electrotherapy	Pacemakers AID (catheter ablation, cardioverter/defibrillator)	Pacemaker (rate support)	AID	AID
Surgery	Subendocardial resection Encirclement Cryoablation Disarticulation—ARVD	Stellectomy/cardiac sympathectomy		Subendocardial resection (coronary artery bypass)

(VT, ventricular tachycardia; EPS, electrophysiologic study; AID, automatic internal defibrillator; ARVD, arrhythmogenic right ventricular dysplasia; modalities in parentheses denote alternative managements for selected cases)

antiarrhythmic drug that is predicted to result in therapeutic blood levels. Exercise testing is repeated, and arrhythmia frequency is assessed. This process is repeated after washout of successive antiarrhythmic drugs until one or more effective regimens are identified (as characterized by no further nonsustained VT on exercise testing, no R on T PVCs, and a decrease in ambient PVCs by 50%). Once an effective regimen has been identified, exercise testing is repeated after 48 to 96 hours on maintenance antiarrhythmic dosing designed to replicate more closely the conditions the patient will be experiencing after hospital discharge. These investigators usually employ two antiarrhythmic drugs in the final regimen, as a safety factor. Of 123 patients with sustained ventricular arrhythmias,[61] a successful antiarrhythmic regimen was identified using this method in 80%; among these patients, there was a 2.3% annual mortality rate during a 2-year follow-up. This is contrasted to the patients for whom no effective regimen was found, among whom 17 of 25 died during the follow-up. Unfortunately, most patients with sustained VT or cardiac arrest either are unable to exercise adequately or have no exercise-induced arrhythmia. Exercise-induced nonsustained VT is not a good predictor of sudden death. It correlates with severity of underlying disease, but offers little independent predictive value once coronary anatomy and left ventricular ejection fraction are known.[26] Because of these factors, this method of assessing drug therapy for ventricular arrhythmias is not widely used.

ELECTROPHYSIOLOGIC STUDIES. Some centers use electrophysiologic studies as the sole method of evaluating antiarrhythmic drug efficacy (electropharmacologic studies). In instances in which nonsustained VT can neither be provoked by exercise nor detected by Holter monitoring (such that its suppression by drugs could be followed as a therapeutic endpoint), electrophysiologic studies are a useful method for assessing success of treatment regimens. Once a sustained ventricular arrhythmia (VT or VF) has been induced by electrophysiologic studies according to the previously detailed protocol, serial drug testing to prevent the arrhythmia induction can be undertaken. At least one antiarrhythmic agent can be tested at the initial study. This is usually procainamide, owing to its ease of administration and low incidence of side effects. Once an agent has been found that is successful in preventing induction of the previously identified arrhythmia when given intravenously, a blood sample is drawn and the drug concentration is determined. The oral antiarrhythmic drug is then initiated, and when the same plasma levels have been obtained, repeat electrophysiologic studies are undertaken. Several conventional and investigational agents may have to be tested before a successful agent or combination of agents can be identified. This is possible in 60% to 70% of unselected cases of sustained ventricular arrhythmia in most studies[62,63]; among individual antiarrhythmic drugs, type I agents (*e.g.*, procainamide, quinidine, disopyramide) have a 25% to 30% success rate in preventing initiation of VT or VF; lidocaine, 10%; mexiletine (an oral lidocaine analog), 20%; propranolol, 10%; and phenytoin, 3%. Combinations of agents may be used that slightly increase the success rate. If a regimen has been identified by electrophysiologic studies as successful, the likelihood of its preventing spontaneous arrhythmia recurrence on long-term follow-up is approximately 90%; on the other hand, if a regimen is predicted to be unsuccessful by electrophysiologic studies, there is a 50% to 90% arrhythmia recurrence rate on follow-up.

Since identification of the successful therapeutic regimen usually requires testing of multiple drugs, several groups have attempted to identify specific characteristics of patients to streamline the process. These studies have shown that women, patients with less severe coronary disease, and patients with fewer arrhythmia episodes prior to treatment are more likely to have a successful regimen identified by electrophysiologic studies.[64] Other variables predictive of successful response to drugs include ejection fraction greater than 50%, age under 45 years, absence of organic heart disease, and hypokinesia as the worst wall motion abnormality.[65] Unfortunately, most patients presenting with sustained ventricular arrhythmias are men, older than age 45, with depressed left ventricular function, associated coronary disease, and large areas of myocardial akinesia or aneurysm. Another variable that has been shown by some to predict the success of conventional antiarrhythmic drugs is the response to high-dose (1 g to 2.5 g) procainamide on acute testing.[66] If arrhythmia is still inducible on procainamide, there is less than a 15% chance that other conventional antiarrhythmic agents will be successful in suppressing the arrhythmia. Our current practice is to test procainamide intravenously in the laboratory, and if unsuccessful (in at least 70% of cases), discontinue testing other conventional agents and move on to investigational agents (usually amiodarone) or other treatments (particularly surgery).

Amiodarone, an investigational antiarrhythmic drug, has had good success rates in preventing VT or VF recurrence.[67,68] Unfortunately, in the experience of most investigators, the use of electrophysiologic studies in predicting amiodarone success or failure is quite limited. Only 5% to 10% of patients have no inducible arrhythmia on amiodarone therapy, although 50% to 70% have no arrhythmia on long-term follow-up. The reason for this discrepancy is unclear. As a consequence, electrophysiologic studies are not repeated once amiodarone has been initiated in many centers. Other investigational agents, such as sotalol (a type III agent with β-blocking effects), appear to behave similarly to amiodarone in that electrophysiologic studies are poor predictors of long-term outcome.

In many cases, no drug regimen can be found that is effective at completely suppressing VT induction at electrophysiologic study. Other endpoints of stimulation on drug regimens have been evaluated as potential indicators of successful clinical outcomes on the same medications, despite persistent VT inducibility, and include the following:

1. Induction of only relatively slow, well-tolerated VT. In one series of 258 patients undergoing electropharmacologic therapy for VT, those who still had inducible VT, but with a cycle length at least 100 msec slower than baseline arrhythmia and not accompanied by untoward symptoms, had the same low incidence of sudden death on follow-up as patients who had no inducible arrhythmia on medications (despite having the same frequency of tachycardia recurrences, although nonfatal, as patients who had persistently inducible/poorly tolerated VT.)[69]
2. Rendering VT more difficult to initiate. Among 88 patients with sustained VT tested on drug therapy in one series, 34 had no inducible VT, 18 had inducible VT, but required more vigorous stimulation to induce the arrhythmia, and 36 had inducible VT but without change in the ease of VT inducibility. On follow-up, 10 patients in the latter group had arrhythmia recurrence, whereas only 1 in the noninducible group and 2 in the harder-to-induce group had tachycardia recurrences.[70]
3. Conversion of sustained to nonsustained VT on drug therapy. One group of investigators found no difference in the frequency of arrhythmia recurrences between 66 patients who had no inducible VT on drug therapy and 44 patients with only nonsustained VT on therapy, all of whom had sustained VT inducible baseline.[71]

Experience using these alternative endpoints of stimulation on drug therapy is limited, but the above studies suggest that complete suppression of VT inducibility on drugs may not be the only acceptable outcome in electropharmacologic testing.

Electrophysiologic studies have not been shown to be very useful in guiding therapy for patients with polymorphic VT, *unless* associated with a normal QT interval and coronary disease. In this subset, type I antiarrhythmic drugs (which aggravate polymorphic VT in the long QT interval syndrome) have been shown to be of reasonable efficacy. There is less information available on the use of electrophysiologic studies in patients with nonsustained VT; in patients with nonsustained VT in whom sustained VT or VF is initiated on electrophysiologic studies, the response to drugs as guided by electrophysiologic studies appears to be the same as for patients with spontaneous sustained VT or

VF. There is not enough information to make firm conclusions about this population of patients at present.

As previously mentioned, VT occurring in patients without underlying heart disease commonly responds to either calcium channel blockers or β-blockers. In patients with the so-called repetitive monomorphic tachycardia (left bundle branch block, inferior axis), electrophysiologic studies are not as useful either in inducing VT or in predicting drug responders, compared with those with coronary disease. In patients with normal hearts and right bundle branch block, left axis deviation VT, electrophysiologic studies can reliably induce the arrhythmia. In this latter instance the clinical use of electrophysiologic studies for drug testing is as good or better than that for VT associated with coronary disease.

Immunosuppressive agents have been used in an uncontrolled fashion in small numbers of patients with no evidence of heart disease or cardiomyopathy, in whom endomyocardial biopsy shows lymphocytic myocarditis.[72] In small numbers of patients, control of arrhythmias has been reported over the short term, in some cases without addition of specific antiarrhythmic drugs. This form of therapy is highly investigational at this point and appears to apply to a very small subset of patients.

The true efficacy of these methods of assessing therapy for VT (*i.e.*, capacity to predict arrhythmia recurrence) has been difficult to determine owing to several factors, such as changing natural history of the underlying diseases and interindividual variability in frequency of arrhythmic episodes.[73] There are some data to suggest that electrophysiologic studies are superior to either the empiric method[74] or Holter monitoring[75,76] to guide antiarrhythmic therapy for VT. There has been no direct comparison of the use of exercise testing ("Lown method") with other methods.

There are several caveats in the use of antiarrhythmic drugs for ventricular arrhythmias. First, drug levels are subject to change as a function of patient compliance and gastrointestinal absorption. If blood levels of antiarrhythmic drugs fall below what is "therapeutic" for the individual patient, effective arrhythmia prophylaxis may be lacking. Second, allergic reactions or unacceptable side effects may develop over time, necessitating discontinuation of an effective antiarrhythmic drug. Finally, there is a significant incidence of proarrhythmic effects of "antiarrhythmic" drugs,[77,78] either making the "clinical" tachycardia more likely to occur or causing other forms of tachycardia (especially type I agent-associated torsades de pointes). Thus, antiarrhythmic drugs, while frequently effective and usually well tolerated, must be used with due respect for their possible ill consequences.

ELECTROTHERAPY. Several types of implantable electrical devices have been developed for clinical use in patients with ventricular arrhythmias. These include various forms of pacemakers, implantable low-energy cardioverters, implantable defibrillators (high-energy), and the special case of catheter ablation of VT foci using electrical discharges. These devices will be discussed in detail elsewhere in these volumes.

SURGERY. Surgical therapy can be undertaken in patients with drug-refractory sustained VT, those with unacceptable side effects from effective antiarrhythmic drugs, and those in whom electrotherapy is not feasible or is declined. Several different procedures are available for differing indications.[23,79]

PREOPERATIVE ASSESSMENT. Patients considered for surgical treatment of VT should undergo cardiac catheterization with coronary arteriography and left ventriculography to define surgical anatomy and need for coronary artery bypass grafting. Patients considered for surgical therapy usually have readily inducible sustained VT, which has been refractory to all antiarrhythmic drugs tested.[80]

Endocardial catheter mapping can be performed during VT in the majority of patients (Fig. 50.2).[81] This study is analogous to intraoperative studies and consists of sampling of multiple endocardial sites during VT to pinpoint areas requiring surgical attention (having presystolic or "early" sites of activation during VT). Although the sampling density is considerably less than that available at surgery, catheter mapping has several advantages. First, time is not as pressing a consideration as during intraoperative study (which is usually limited to 1 hour). Second, not all morphologically distinct VT can be initiated intraoperatively in all cases, and thus the information derived from catheter VT mapping can be used to guide surgery. In cases in which the tachycardia is poorly tolerated, such that prolonged mapping is not possible, procainamide infusion will often slow the VT sufficiently to allow hemodynamic tolerance. Additionally, VT can in some cases be repeatedly started and stopped while the catheter is being moved from site to site. Endocardial catheter mapping is obviously also essential before attempts at catheter ablation can be considered.

In cases in which VT rapidly degenerates to ventricular fibrillation or quickly results in hemodynamic collapse, other methods have been used in an attempt to locate arrhythmogenic areas within the left ventricle. One of these, pace mapping, attempts to replicate the surface 12-lead ECG of VT by endocardial pacing in the left ventricle at various sites.[82] The assumption is that, when pacing from the exact area where earliest endocardial activity during VT would be mapped, the 12-lead ECG should be identical to that of the native VT. There are several limitations to this procedure, however. First, the accuracy is limited, in that pacing from widely separated areas in the ventricle can occasionally yield very similar 12-lead ECGs, and conversely, markedly different ECGs can result from pacing as little as 1 cm away from the area proven to be the earliest site during VT. Second, the procedure is time consuming, and thus appears to offer no advantage over activation mapping during VT when the latter procedure can be safely performed. Sinus rhythm endocardial catheter mapping has been performed in the hope that certain characteristics of endocardial electrograms (*e.g.*, markedly abnormal or fractionated, double potentials, extremely long electrograms) would be of sufficient specificity to obviate the need for mapping during VT.[83] This has unfortunately not proven true, either in the catheterization laboratory or during intraoperative studies.[84] No characteristics of sinus rhythm endocardial electrograms have been found that can help specify areas in the ventricle requiring surgical attention. Finally, the 12-lead ECG of VT has been shown to contain valuable localizing information in about half of patients with infarct-related VT. Several distinct combinations of bundle branch block type, axis, and precordial R wave pattern during VT exist that, using endocardial mapping, have been shown reliably to arise from relatively specific endocardial regions.[6] Although not by any means a substitute for endocardial catheter mapping during VT, one can apply the criteria developed in these studies to place the catheter at sites likely to display presystolic activity during VT, and thus facilitate and shorten the duration of mapping. Predicting regions of tachycardia origin using the 12-lead ECG during VT should be used only to aid in mapping studies.

INDIRECT METHODS. *Coronary artery bypass grafting (CABG)* has been used in the past for sustained uniform VT, with poor results.[85] The major use of this procedure thus has not been in sustained VT in the presence of prior myocardial infarction, but rather in exercise-induced VF or VT associated with ischemia. No large series of patients exists, but isolated reports and small series have yielded encouraging results in these subsets of patients.

Aneurysmectomy has resulted in cures in a minority of patients with uniform sustained VT due to underlying CAD. This is presumably because the areas responsible for arrhythmogenesis appear to lie in the border zone between an aneurysm and more normal myocardium. Standard aneurysmectomy involves removal of only a portion of the infarcted area, leaving a fibrous cuff of tissue suitable for holding sutures. It is in this fibrous cuff, or just beyond it, that most VT reentrant zones appear to reside.

DIRECT METHODS. In the past decade, several other procedures have been introduced as surgical therapy for VT, largely due to the advent of endocardial mapping of VT.[16] Mapping has become a valuable tool in the understanding and surgical therapy of sustained VT. This procedure consists of a comparison of the timing of local electrical activity sampled at multiple points (usually greater than 50) in the heart to detect areas where the earliest electrical activity during VT is located with the onset of the surface QRS complex. Initial studies were done using intraoperative epicardial and endocardial mapping during VT, but the best correlate of cure of tachycardia was found with endocardial mapping.[86] Many groups currently use only endocardial intraoperative mapping. Techniques are being developed that employ large multielectrode arrays and computerized analysis, which may allow more rapid acquisition and interpretation of mapping data.

The most common surgical procedure for VT currently in use is *subendocardial resection*, in which a 1-mm to 3-mm thick layer of endocardium and underlying tissues is dissected from the heart. The most common application of this method is with endocardial mapping to direct the surgeon to areas that require resection (map-directed subendocardial resection). With the use of this procedure, the chest is opened through a median sternotomy and the heart is cannulated in routine manner for cardiopulmonary bypass. Reference electrodes are placed in the right and left ventricle, and the aneurysm or infarct is opened after the patient has been placed on normothermic cardiopulmonary bypass. VT is initiated with programmed electrical stimulation, and endocardial mapping is performed, usually with a roving bipolar probe electrode with a 1-mm to 2-mm interelectrode distance. Most patients with CAD have multiple morphologically distinct tachycardias,

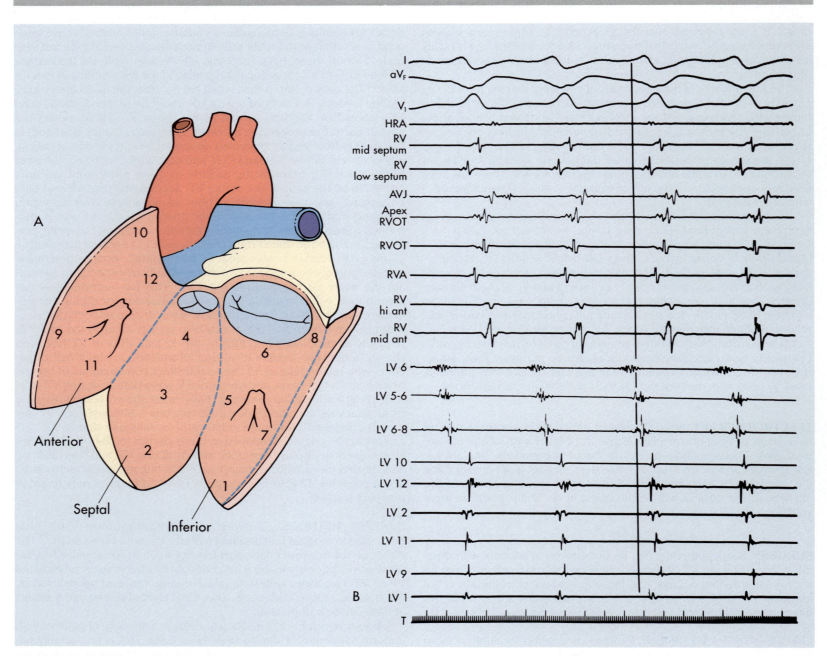

FIGURE 50.2 A. Typical catheter mapping schema. The heart has been opened along the lateral border, and 12 areas or sites for endocardial mapping are displayed. Each site is approximately 6 to 8 sq cm in area. **B.** Catheter map analog data. Individual endocardial electrograms during VT from sites corresponding to the schema in **A** are time aligned and compared with the onset of the surface QRS. The earliest site is LV_6, an inferobasal site. (*HRA*, high right atrium; *RV*, right ventricle; *LV*, left ventricle; *sep*, septum; *RVOT*, RV outflow tract; *RVA*, RV apex; *T*, time lines [10-msec intervals]) (**A**, Modified from Cassidy DM, Vassallo JA, Buxton AE et al: The value of catheter mapping during sinus rhythm to localize site of origin of ventricular tachycardia. Circulation 69:1103, 1984; **B**, from Josephson ME, Horowitz LN, Spielman SR et al: Role of catheter mapping in the preoperative evaluation of ventricular tachycardia. Am J Cardiol 49:207, 1982)

which may arise in the same or nearby areas (within 2 cm), but in 15% of these patients, tachycardias arise at "disparate sites," more than 5 cm distant from one another.[48] Most centers try to map each VT as thoroughly as possible, attempting to localize the earliest endocardial activation (usually 40 msec to 100 msec prior to the onset of the surface QRS complex). Once all VT mapping is completed, endocardial resection can be performed on the areas identified by mapping, including a 1-cm to 2-cm margin of surrounding subendocardium. Additional procedures can then be performed, such as cryotherapy of areas not amenable to subendocardial resection (such as papillary muscle), aneurysmectomy and repair, and coronary artery bypass grafting as indicated.

This procedure has a 10% to 15% operative mortality, regardless of preexisting left ventricular dysfunction, and approximately 70% efficacy in preventing inducibility of VT postoperatively. In patients with persistent VT postoperatively, antiarrhythmic drugs that had been ineffective preoperatively control the majority of VT postoperatively. This gives an overall efficacy rate of 85% to 90% for subendocardial resection with occasional adjunctive antiarrhythmias among operative survivors. Five-year survival is in excess of 60%.[87]

Several modifications of the basic subendocardial resection procedure have been developed in recent years:

1. Use of adjunctive cryoablation in inferior-infarct–related VT, applying the cryoprobe to the isthmus of surviving endocardium between the posterior basal edge of the infarct/aneurysm and mitral valve annulus. This procedure was developed because of evidence that in at least some cases of inferior-infarct–related VT, the reentrant wavefront travels around the perimeter of the infarct/aneurysm with a critical narrow portion of the circuit traveling in the isthmus of muscle between the edge of the infarct and the mitral annulus. Destruction of this tissue has been associated with dramatic improvement in surgical success (over 90% are free of inducible VT postoperatively versus 50% having inducible VT prior to using this procedure).[88]
2. Sequential subendocardial resection, in which attempts are made to reinitiate VT in the operating room after subendocardial resection has been performed (either on the normothermic heart or immediately after rewarming, if cold cardioplegia is used). Approximately 20% of patients in whom intraoperative stimulation is repeated after subendocardial resection have inducible uniform sustained VT; in these cases, mapping is repeated as before and additional resection of cryoablation performed of the arrhythmogenic tissue. The process of stimulation, mapping, and resection/cryoablation is repeated until VT is no longer inducible in the operating room. This procedure has yielded good success rates with no significant increment in operative mortality despite attendant small increases in total bypass time, as well as aortic cross clamp time.[89]
3. Regional subendocardial resection, in which all endocardium displaying any presystolic activity during VT is resected (whether scarred or not). Although the theoretical basis for this procedure is less clear than other modifications of subendocardial resection, it has resulted in improvement in the antiarrhythmic success rate of the operation without increasing operative mortality.[90]
4. Extended subendocardial resection, or visually directed surgery.[91] Mapping is not necessary with this procedure in that all visible scar tissue is resected. Although attractive in concept, this procedure has several limitations, among which is the necessity of removing papillary muscles in 20% to 25% patients because of involvement in the endocardial scar, with attendant mitral valve replacement. Also, in VT occurring very early after infarct there is no clear border between scar tissue and more normal myocardium, such that visual inspection could identify the areas requiring resection. Finally 10% to 15% of VT sites may be found in areas with relatively normal appearing endocardium.
5. Implantation of automatic internal cardioverter-defibrillator (AICD) patches at the time of surgery. Some centers have advocated implantation of patches as well as the AICD generators in patients undergoing directed surgical treatment of VT, citing published spontaneous VT recurrence rates in patients with and without inducible VT at the postoperative electrophysiologic study.[92] This procedure has not been adopted generally however because of an unfavorable balance between the relatively low risk of VT recurrence (5% to 10% per year at worst) compared with the expense and risk of initial AICD implantation and generator/battery replacement (currently every 1½ to 2 years). Many centers have begun implanting AICD patches in all or only select cases at the time of surgery for VT and implanting AICDs in only those patients in whom VT is inducible and poorly tolerated postoperatively.[93]

Cryoablation or cryosurgery (freezing of local areas with a cryoprobe at $-60°C$ to $-70°C$) has been used alone or in conjunction with other procedures, such as subendocardial resection in some cases of VT. The object is to kill the cells responsible for the arrhythmia without disrupting the structural integrity of the remaining myocardial wall, as well as leaving nearby areas unaffected. There are no controlled studies on the efficacy or long-term effects of this procedure, but several reports attest to its efficacy in certain cases.

Several forms of *laser photoablation* have seen limited use in the surgical treatment of VT. Some groups have used neodymium:YAG photocoagulation to ablate either endocardial or epicardial tissue with promising results.[94] Potential advantages are (as with cryoablation) effective killing of the tissue responsible for VT without destruction of the fibrous stroma of the myocardial wall as well as slightly less time required per lesion than cryoablation. Other forms of laser energy, such as argon and CO_2 lasers are less attractive because of their tendency to vaporize or carbonize target tissues.

There are reports on the use of another technique for both intraoperative mapping and VT ablation termed *balloon shock ablation*. This involves insertion of an electrode-studded latex balloon into the left ventricle via ventriculotomy or, in some cases, left atriotomy with passage of the balloon to the left ventricular cavity via the mitral valve. The balloon is then inflated to appose the electrodes to the endocardium, VT is induced and mapped using computer techniques, and the electrode having the earliest diastolic activity in VT can be used as a conduit to deliver direct-current or radiofrequency energy to ablate the underlying endocardium. Experience with this technique is thus far limited but promising.[95]

Among *encirclement procedures*, encircling endocardial ventriculotomy (EEV) was developed in the past decade to treat VT from a different viewpoint, that is, transecting presumed reentrant circuits or preventing VT from spreading to the rest of the ventricle.[96] Using this procedure, the area of endocardial scar or areas to which VT has been mapped are excluded from the remaining ventricle by a nearly transmural incision, from endocardium to just beneath the epicardial surface. The entire area can thus be encircled, which either incises existing reentrant circuits or prevents spread of impulses to the remaining portions of the ventricle. As initially devised, mapping during VT is not essential since the border of scar in normal tissue can usually be readily identified. This procedure has been used less commonly than subendocardial resection and has a slightly higher operative mortality (owing largely to intractable congestive heart failure), as well as lower overall efficacy rate (VT cure). Two modifications of this procedure have been developed. First, partial EEV consists of an incision to only one third to one half of the wall thickness, and occasionally the incision does not entirely circumscribe the arrhythmogenic area, especially if papillary muscles would be damaged. Mapping is generally performed with this procedure, and good results have been obtained (5% to 10% operative mortality, with 65% to 70% of survivors free of inducible VT postoperatively).[97] A second modification, encircling endocardial cryoablation, consists of placing adjacent cryolesions along the endocardial rim of scar tissue to complete the encirclement. Although experience with this technique is limited, and a significant disadvantage is the time required for placement of sequential freezes lasting 3 or more minutes each, encircling endocardial cryoablation appears to have a role in certain cases in which endocardial resection would jeopardize papillary muscles.

Right ventricular disarticulation, a novel surgical procedure, is occasionally used in patients with ARVD when large and sometimes multiple areas of the right ventricle are involved in the dysplastic process. This procedure, right ventricular disarticulation,[98] involves incision of the right ventricle along the septal margins anteriorly and posteriorly and freezing at the right ventricular infundibulum. The incision lines are then reopposed and sutured. In some cases, VT persists in the disarticulated right ventricle but does not spread to the left ventricle. The hemodynamic consequences of this procedure have been variable, and it has been attempted in only a small number of patients.

REFERENCES

1. Josephson ME, Horowitz LN, Spielman SR et al: Electrophysiologic and hemodynamic studies in patients resuscitated from cardiac arrest. Am J Cardiol 46:948, 1980
2. Schaffer WA, Cobb LA: Recurrent ventricular fibrillation and modes of death in survivors of out-of-hospital ventricular fibrillation. N Engl J Med 293:259, 1975
3. Wellens HJJ, Bar FW, Vanagt EJ et al: The differentiation between ventricular tachycardia and supraventricular tachycardia with aberrant conduction: The value of the 12-lead electrocardiogram. In Wellens HJJ, Kulbertus KE (eds): What's New in Electrocardiography?, pp 184–199. The Hague, Martinus Nijhoff, 1981
4. Kindwall KE, Brown J, Josephson ME: Electrocardiographic criteria for ventricular tachycardia in wide complex left bundle branch block morphology tachycardias. Am J Cardiol 61:1279, 1988
5. Dongas J, Lehmann MH, Mahmud R et al: Value of preexisting bundle branch block in the electrocardiographic differentiation of supraventricular from ventricular origin of wide QRS tachycardia. Am J Cardiol 55:717, 1985
6. Miller JM, Marchlinski FE, Buxton AE, Josephson ME: Relationship between the 12-lead electrocardiogram during ventricular tachycardia and endocardial site of origin in patients with coronary artery disease. Circulation 77:759, 1988
7. Benditt DG, Pritchett ELC, Gallagher JJ: Spectrum of regular tachycardias with wide complex QRS complexes in patients with accessory atrioventricular pathways. Am J Cardiol 42:828, 1978
8. Miller JM, Gottlieb GD, Lesh MD et al: His-Purkinje activation during ventricular tachycardia: A determinant of QRS duration. J Am Coll Cardiol 13:21A, 1989
9. Spear JF, Horowitz LN, Hoden AB et al: Cellular electrophysiology of human myocardial infarction: I. Abnormalities of cellular activation. Circulation 59:247, 1979
10. Lazarra R, El-Sheriff N, Scherlag BJ: Electrophysiological properties of canine Purkinje cells in one-day old myocardial infarction. Circ Res 33:722, 1973
11. Brugada P, Wellens JHH: The role of triggered activity in clinical ventricular arrhythmias. PACE 7:260, 1984
12. Josephson ME, Buxton AE, Marchlinski FE et al: Sustained ventricular tachycardia in coronary artery disease: Evidence for a reentrant mechanism. In Zipes DP, Jalife J (eds): Cardiac Electrophysiology and Arrhythmias, pp 409–418. Orlando, FL, Grune & Stratton, 1985
13. Josephson ME, Horowitz LN, Farshidi A et al: Recurrent sustained ventricular tachycardia: I. Mechanisms. Circulation 57:431, 1976
14. Woelfel A, Foster JR, Simpson RJ et al: Reproducibility and treatment of exercise-induced ventricular tachycardia. Am J Cardiol 53:751, 1984
15. Fenoglio JL, Pham TD, Harken AH et al: Recurrent sustained ventricular tachycardia: Structure and ultrastructure of subendocardial regions in which tachycardia originates. Circulation 68:518, 1983
16. Gallagher JJ, Kasell JH, Cox JL et al: Techniques of intraoperative electrophysiologic mapping. Am J Cardiol 49:221, 1982
17. Mason JW, Stinson EB, Winkle RA et al: Relative efficacy of blind left ventricular aneurysm resection for the treatment of recurrent ventricular tachycardia. Am J Cardiol 49:241, 1982
18. Poll DS, Marchlinski FE, Buxton AE et al: Sustained ventricular tachycardia in patients with idiopathic dilated cardiomyopathy: Electrophysiologic testing and lack of response to antiarrhythmic drug therapy. Circulation 70:451, 1984
19. Horowitz LN, Vetter VL, Harken AH et al: Electrophysiologic characteristics of sustained ventricular tachycardia occurring after repair of tetralogy of Fallot. Am J Cardiol 46:446, 1980
20. Kugler JD, Pinsky WW, Cheatham JP et al: Sustained ventricular tachycardia after repair of tetralogy of Fallot: New electrophysiologic findings. Am J Cardiol 51:1137, 1983
21. Marcus FI, Fontaine GH, Guiradon G et al: Right ventricular dysplasia: A report of 24 adult cases. Circulation 65:384, 1982
22. Morady F, Shen E, Bhandari A et al: Programmed ventricular stimulation in mitral valve prolapse: Analysis of 36 patients. Am J Cardiol 53:135, 1984
23. Fontaine G, Guiradon G, Frank R et al: Surgical management of ventricular tachycardia unrelated to myocardial ischemia or infarction. Am J Cardiol 49:397, 1982
24. Rahilly GT, Prystowsky EN, Zipes PP et al: Clinical and electrophysiologic findings in patients with repetitive monomorphic ventricular tachycardia and otherwise normal electrocardiogram. Am J Cardiol 50:459, 1982
25. Lin FC, Finley CS, Rahimtoola SH et al: Idiopathic paroxysmal ventricular tachycardia with a QRS pattern of right bundle branch block and left axis deviation: A unique clinical entity with specific properties. Am J Cardiol 52:95, 1983
26. Califf RM, McKinnis RA, McNeer JF et al: Prognostic value of ventricular arrhythmias associated with treadmill exercise testing in patients studied with cardiac catheterization for suspected ischemic heart disease. J Am Coll Cardiol 2:1060, 1983
27. Bigger JT, Weld FM, Rolnitzky LM: Prevalence, characteristics, and significance of ventricular tachycardia (3 or more complexes) detected with ambulatory electrocardiographic recording in the late hospital phase of acute myocardial infarction. Am J Cardiol 48:815, 1981
28. Huang SK, Messer JV, Denes P: Significance of ventricular tachycardia in idiopathic dilated cardiomyopathy: Observations in 35 patients. Am J Cardiol 51:507, 1983
29. Maron BJ, Savage DD, Wolfson JK et al: Prognostic significance of 24-hour ambulatory electrocardiographic monitoring in patients with hypertrophic cardiomyopathy: A prospective study. Am J Cardiol 48:252, 1981
30. Buxton AE, Waxman HL, Marchlinski FE, Josephson ME: Electrophysiologic studies in nonsustained ventricular tachycardia: Relation to underlying heart disease. Am J Cardiol 52:985, 1983
31. Buxton AE, Marchlinski FE, Waxman HL et al: Prognostic factors in nonsustained ventricular tachycardia. Am J Cardiol 53:127, 1984
32. Jackman WM, Clark M, Friday KJ et al: Ventricular tachyarrhythmias in the long QT syndrome. Med Clin North Am 68:1079, 1984
33. Coumel P, LeClercq J, Dessertenne F: Torsades de Pointes. In Josephson ME, Wellens HJJ (eds): Tachycardias: Mechanisms, Diagnosis, Treatment, pp 325–352. Philadelphia, Lea & Febiger, 1984
34. Ideker RE, Bardy GH, Worley SJ et al: Patterns of activation during ventricular fibrillation. In Josephson ME, Wellens HJJ (eds): Tachycardias: Mechanisms, Diagnosis, Treatment, pp 519–536. Philadelphia, Lea & Febiger, 1984
35. Palileo EV, Ashley WW, Swiryn S et al: Exercise-provokable right ventricular outflow tract tachycardia. Am Heart J 104:185, 1982
36. Fisher JD: Role of electrophysiologic testing in the diagnosis and treatment of patients with known and suspected bradycardias and tachycardias. Prog Cardiovasc Dis 24:25, 1981
37. Livelli FD, Bigger JT, Reifell JA et al: Response to programmed ventricular stimulation: Sensibility, specificity, and relation to heart disease. Am J Cardiol 50:452, 1982
38. Robertson JF, Cain ME, Horowitz LN et al: Anatomic and electrophysiologic correlates of ventricular tachycardia requiring left ventricular stimulation. Am J Cardiol 48:263, 1981
39. Buxton AE, Waxman HL, Marchlinski FE et al: Role of triple extrastimuli during electrophysiologic study of patients with documented sustained ventricular tachyarrhythmias. Circulation 69:532, 1984
40. DiMarco JP, Garan H, Ruskin JN: Complications in patients undergoing cardiac electrophysiologic procedures. Ann Intern Med 97:490, 1982
41. Buxton AE, Waxman HL, Marchlinski FE et al: Electropharmacology of nonsustained ventricular tachycardia: Effects of Class I antiarrhythmic agents, verapamil and propranolol. Am J Cardiol 53:738, 1984
42. Ruskin JN, Dimarco JP, Garan H: Out-of-hospital cardiac arrest: Electrophysiologic observations and selection of long-term antiarrhythmic therapy. N Engl J Med 303:607, 1980
43. Morady F, Scheinmann MM, Hess D: Electrophysiologic testing in the management of survivors of out-of-hospital cardiac arrest. Am J Cardiol 51:85, 1982
44. Roy D, Waxman HL, Kienzle MG et al: Clinical characteristics and long-term follow-up in 119 survivors of cardiac arrest: Relation to inducibility at electrophysiologic testing. Am J Cardiol 52:969, 1983
45. Brugada P, Abdollah H, Heddle B et al: Results of a ventricular stimulation protocol using a maximum of 4 premature stimuli in patients without documented or suspected ventricular arrhythmias. Am J Cardiol 52:1214, 1983
46. Schoenfeld M, McGovern B, Garan H et al: Long-term reproducibility of responses to programmed cardiac stimulation in spontaneous ventricular tachyarrhythmias. Am J Cardiol 54:564, 1984
47. Sugrue DD, Holmes DR, Gersh BJ et al: Cardiac histologic findings in patients with life threatening ventricular arrhythmias of unknown origin. J Am Coll Cardiol 4:952, 1984
48. Miller JM, Kienzle MG, Harken AH et al: Morphologically distinct sustained ventricular tachycardias in coronary artery disease: Significance and surgical results. J Am Coll Cardiol 4:1073, 1984
49. Rosenthal ME, Stamato NJ, Marchlinski FE, Josephson ME: Noninvasive cardiac pacing for termination of sustained uniform ventricular tachycardia. Am

50. Weiner I: Pacing techniques in the treatment of tachycardias. Ann Intern Med 93:326, 1980
51. Zipes DP, Jackman WJ, Heger JJ et al: Clinical transvenous cardioversion of recurrent life-threatening ventricular tachyarrhythmias: Low energy synchronized cardioversion of ventricular tachycardia and termination of ventricular fibrillation in patients using a catheter electrode. Am Heart J 103:789, 1982
52. Horowitz LN, Greenspan AM, Spielman SR et al: Torsades de pointes: Electrophysiologic studies in patients without transient pharmacologic or metabolic abnormalities. Circulation 63:1120, 1981
53. Tzivoni D, Karen A, Cohen AM et al: Magnesium therapy for torsades de pointes. Am J Cardiol 53:528, 1984
54. Lie KI, Wellens HJJ, van Cappelle FJ et al: Lidocaine in the prevention of primary ventricular fibrillation: A double-blind, randomized study of 212 consecutive patients. N Engl J Med 291:1324, 1974
55. Myerburg RJ, Conde C, Sheps DS et al: Antiarrhythmic drug therapy in survivors of prehospital cardiac arrest. Circulation 59:855, 1979
56. Greenspan AM, Horowitz LN, Spielman SR et al: Large dose procainamide therapy for ventricular tachyarrhythmia. Am J Cardiol 46:453, 1980
57. Vlay SC, Kallman CH, Reid PR: Prognostic assessment of survivors of ventricular tachycardia and ventricular fibrillation with ambulatory monitoring. Am J Cardiol 54:87, 1984
58. Michelson EL, Morganroth J: Spontaneous variability of complex arrhythmias detected by long-term electrocardiographic recording. Circulation 61:690, 1980
59. Herling IM, Horowitz LN, Josephson ME: Ventricular ectopic activity after medical and surgical treatment for recurrent sustained ventricular tachycardia. Am J Cardiol 45:633, 1980
60. Lown B, Podrid PJ, DeSilva RA et al: Sudden cardiac death: Management of the patient at risk. Curr Prob Cardiol 4:1, 1980
61. Graboys TB, Lown B, Podrid PJ et al: Long-term survival of patients with malignant ventricular arrhythmia treated with antiarrhythmic drugs. Am J Cardiol 50:437, 1982
62. Mason JW, Winkle RA: Accuracy of ventricular tachycardia induction study for predicting long-term efficacy and inefficacy of antiarrhythmic drugs. N Engl J Med 303:1073, 1980
63. Horowitz LN, Josephson ME, Kastor JA: Intracardiac electrophysiologic studies as a method for the optimization of drug therapy in chronic ventricular arrhythmia. Prog Cardiovasc Dis 23:18, 1980
64. Swerdlow CD, Gong G, Echt DS et al: Clinical factors predicting successful electrophysiologic-pharmacologic study in patients with ventricular tachycardia. J Am Coll Cardiol 1:409, 1983
65. Spielman SR, Schwartz JS, McCarthy DM et al: Predictors of the success or failure of medical therapy in patients with chronic recurrent sustained ventricular tachycardia: A discriminant analysis. J Am Coll Cardiol 1:401, 1983
66. Waxman HL, Buxton AE, Sadowski LM et al: The response to procainamide during electrophysiologic study for sustained ventricular tachyarrhythmias predicts the response to other medications. Circulation 67:30, 1983
67. Saksena S, Rothbart ST, Shah Y et al: Clinical efficacy and electropharmacology of continuous intravenous amiodarone infusion and chronic oral amiodarone in refractory ventricular tachycardia. Am J Cardiol 54:347, 1984
68. Heger JJ, Prystowsky EN, Jackman WJ et al: Amiodarone: Clinical efficacy and electrophysiology during long-term therapy for recurrent ventricular tachycardia or ventricular fibrillation. N Engl J Med 305:539, 1981
69. Waller TJ, Kay HR, Speilman SR et al: Reduction in sudden death and total mortality by antiarrhythmic therapy evaluated by electrophysiologic drug testing: Criteria of efficacy in patients with sustained ventricular tachyarrhythmia. J Am Coll Cardiol 10:83, 1987
70. Borggrefe M, Trampisch H-J, Breithardt G: Reappraisal of criteria for assessing drug efficacy in patients with ventricular tachyarrhythmias: Complete versus partial suppression of inducible arrhythmias. J Am Coll Cardiol 12:140, 1988
71. Schoels W, Brachmann J, Schmitt C et al: Conversion of sustained into non-sustained ventricular tachycardia during therapy assessment by programmed ventricular stimulation: Criterion for a positive drug effect? Am J Cardiol 64:329, 1989
72. Vignola PA, Aonuma K, Swaye PS et al: Lymphocytic myocarditis presenting as unexplained ventricular arrhythmias: Diagnosis with endomyocardial biopsy and response to immunosuppression. J Am Coll Cardiol 4:812, 1984
73. McGovern B, Garan H, Ruskin JN: Treatment of ventricular arrhythmias: Suppression, survival, and the problem of bias. Ann Intern Med 101:123, 1984
74. Ferguson D, Saksena S, Greenberg E et al: Management of recurrent ventricular tachycardia: Economic impact of therapeutic alternatives. Am J Cardiol 53:531, 1984
75. Platia EV, Reid PR: Comparison of programmed electrical stimulation and ambulatory electrocardiographic (Holter) monitoring in the management of ventricular tachycardia and ventricular fibrillation. J Am Coll Cardiol 4:493, 1984
76. Mitchell LB, Duff HJ, Manyari DE, Wyse DG: A randomized clinical trial of the noninvasive and invasive approaches to drug therapy of ventricular tachycardia. N Engl J Med 317:1681, 1987
77. Velebit V, Podrid PJ, Lown B et al: Aggravation and provocation of ventricular arrhythmias by antiarrhythmic drugs. Circulation 65:886, 1982
78. Stanton MS, Prystowsky EN, Fineberg NS et al: Arrhythmogenic effects of antiarrhythmic drugs: A study of 506 patients treated for ventricular tachycardia or fibrillation. J Am Coll Cardiol 14:209, 1989
79. Horowitz LN, Harken AH, Josephson ME et al: Surgical treatment of ventricular arrhythmias in coronary artery disease. Ann Intern Med 95:88, 1981
80. Wellens HJJ, Bar FW, Vanagt EJ et al: Medical treatment of ventricular tachycardia: Considerations in the selection of patients for surgical treatment. Am J Cardiol 49:186, 1982
81. Josephson ME, Horowitz LN, Spielman SR et al: Role of catheter mapping in the preoperative evaluation of ventricular tachycardia. Am J Cardiol 49:207, 1982
82. Josephson ME, Waxman HL, Cain ME et al: Ventricular activation during ventricular endocardial pacing: II. Role of pace-mapping to localize origin of ventricular tachycardia. Am J Cardiol 50:11, 1982
83. Cassidy DM, Vassallo JA, Buxton AE et al: The value of catheter mapping during sinus rhythm to localize site of origin of ventricular tachycardia. Circulation 69:1103, 1984
84. Kienzle MG, Miller JM, Falcone RA et al: Intraoperative endocardial mapping during sinus rhythm: Relationship to site of origin of ventricular tachycardia. Circulation 70:957, 1984
85. Garan H, Ruskin JN, DiMarco JP et al: Electrophysiologic studies before and after myocardial revascularization in patients with life-threatening ventricular arrhythmias. Am J Cardiol 50:519, 1982
86. Horowitz LN, Harken AH, Kastor JA et al: Ventricular resection guided by epicardial and endocardial mapping for treatment of recurrent ventricular tachycardia. N Engl J Med 302:589, 1980
87. Miller JM, Kienzle MG, Harken AH et al: Subendocardial resection for ventricular tachycardia: Predictors of surgical success. Circulation 70:624, 1984
88. Hargrove WC, Miller JM, Vassallo JA, Josephson ME: Improved results in the operative management of ventricular tachycardia related to inferior wall infarction: Importance of annular isthmus. J Thorac Cardiovasc Surg 92:726, 1986
89. Kron IL, Lerman BB, Nolan SP et al: Sequential endocardial resection for the surgical treatment of refractory ventricular tachycardia. J Thorac Cardiovasc Surg 94:843, 1987
90. Krafchek J, Lawrie GM, Roberts R et al: Surgical ablation of ventricular tachycardia: Improved results with a map-directed regional approach. Circulation 73:1239, 1986
91. Moran JM, Kehoe RF, Loeb JM: The role of papillary muscle resection and mitral valve replacement in the control of refractory ventricular arrhythmia. Circulation 68(II):154, 1983
92. Platia EV, Lawrence SCG, Watkins L et al: Treatment of malignant ventricular arrhythmias with endocardial resection and implantation of the automatic cardioverter-defibrillator. N Engl J Med 314:213, 1986
93. Manolis AS, Rastegar H, Estes NAM: Prophylactic automatic implantable cardioverter-defibrillator patches in patients at high risk for postoperative ventricular tachyarrhythmias. J Am Coll Cardiol 13:1367, 1989
94. Svenson RH, Gallagher JJ, Selle JG et al: Neodymium:YAG laser photocoagulation: A successful new map-guided technique for the intraoperative ablation of ventricular tachycardia. Circulation 76:1319, 1987
95. Downar E, Mickleborough L, Harris L, Parson I: Intraoperative electrical ablation of ventricular arrhythmias: A "closed heart" procedure. J Am Coll Cardiol 10:1048, 1987
96. Guiradon G, Fontaine G, Frank R et al: Encircling endocardial ventriculotomy: A new surgical treatment for life-threatening ventricular tachycardias resistant to medical treatment following myocardial infarction. Ann Thorac Surg 26:438, 1978
97. Ostermeyer J, Borggrefe M, Breithardt G et al: Direct operations for the management of life-threatening ischemic ventricular tachycardia. J Thorac Cardiovasc Surg 94:848, 1987
98. Guiradon G, Klein GJ, Gulambusein SS et al: Total disconnection of the right ventricular free wall: Surgical treatment of right ventricular tachycardia associated with right ventricular dysplasia. Circulation 67:463, 1983

GENERAL REFERENCES

Buxton AE, Josephson ME: Ventricular tachycardias—1983. PACE 7:90, 1984
Singh BN, Weiss JN, Nademanee K et al: Recent trends in the management of life-threatening ventricular arrhythmias. West J Med 141:649, 1984
Waldo AL, Arciniegas JG, Klein H: Surgical treatment of life-threatening ventricular arrhythmias: The role of intraoperative mapping and consideration of the presently available surgical techniques. Prog Cardiovasc Dis 23:247, 1981

RIGHT VENTRICULAR TACHYCARDIAS

*Guy Fontaine • Robert Frank
Fabrice Fontaliran • Gilles Lascault
Joelice Tonet*

Ventricular tachycardia has long been recognized as a dangerous cardiac arrhythmia.[1,2] In some cases it is the harbinger of ventricular fibrillation, which can result in sudden death.[3] In other cases, especially in the chronic form, episodes of ventricular tachycardia can be well tolerated over long periods of time, provided the heart rate is not inordinately rapid.[4]

RIGHT VT AFTER MYOCARDIAL INFARCTION

In patients suffering from coronary artery disease, ventricular tachycardia is frequently observed during the acute or chronic phase after myocardial infarction.[1,2,5] Programmed pacing techniques have provided evidence of the reentrant nature of this arrhythmia.[6-9] It generally shows a right bundle branch block pattern, and originates in the left ventricle at the border zone between normal and abnormal tissue.[10]

However, in some cases VT can have a left bundle branch block pattern, and can originate either in the left ventricular septum or in the right ventricle, as demonstrated by endocardial mapping.[11] This localization allows for surgical or catheter ablative procedures (Fig. 51.1).[12]

RIGHT VT IN THE NONCORONARY PATIENT

Ventricular tachycardia can also be observed in noncoronary patients. It is frequently associated with idiopathic dilated cardiomyopathy, and may be the first presenting symptom of this disease.[13] The QRS morphology generally suggests that the tachycardia originates in the left ventricle. With the exception of sudden death, which can occur at any time during the evolution of the disease, the prognosis is related to the involvement of the left ventricle.[14]

ARRHYTHMOGENIC RIGHT VENTRICULAR DYSPLASIA

Ventricular tachycardia showing a left bundle branch block pattern may be observed in young patients with no evidence of heart disease on physical examination.[15,16] The good left ventricular function explains why these patients can tolerate multiple episodes of ventricular tachycardia relatively well. However, there is a risk of ventricular fibrillation, which is generally manifested during strenuous exercise.[17-19]

Ventricular tachycardia of right ventricular origin with a clinically normal heart has been identified in our institution as a particular subgroup termed *arrhythmogenic right ventricular dysplasia* (ARVD).[20,21] Our study of 24 cases of presumed right ventricular dysplasia was reported in a paper by Marcus and colleagues.[22] This syndrome was originally identified by analyzing electrophysiologic as well as anatomic data obtained at surgery, with particular attention to right-sided abnormalities.[20] ARVD has been also observed in the pediatric age group.[23,24]

With time, this syndrome has come to be more and more frequently recognized, and exhibits a wide spectrum of clinical manifestations.[25]

In typical forms, the diagnosis is suggested by recurrent ventricular tachycardia, or by extrasystoles with a left bundle branch block pattern. These arrhythmias are frequently exacerbated by exercise. The patient is generally a young adult, more frequently male. A recent review of our series of 52 patients[26] showed a 80% predominance of males. The age of first symptoms was 33 ± 14 years and ranged from 13 to 73 years. Features of spontaneous arrhythmias in our series are reported in Table 51.1. Generally, the patient has no complaint other than palpitations, but some experience syncopal episodes. Other cases may have ventricular arrhythmias but remain asymptomatic. Routine clinical examination may be completely normal.[22]

FAMILIAL OCCURRENCE OF ARVD

Familial forms of right ventricular dysplasia (RVD) as well as ARVD have been reported.[22,27-33] In our series of 52 cases, a familial history of ARVD was proven in 2 and likely in 4 more.[26] It was concluded in a study made by a group in Padua that the genetic pattern of RVD is characterized by an autosomal dominant inheritance with incomplete penetrance and variable expression.

ELECTROCARDIOGRAPHY AND OTHER DIAGNOSTIC MODALITIES

ECG testing in patients with VT shows a left bundle branch block pattern suggesting delayed activation of the left ventricular chamber (Fig. 51.2). The QRS axis is normal or shifted to the right when the tachycardia originates in the pulmonary infundibulum, or it may show extreme left axis deviation when arising from the diaphragmatic wall or near the apex of the right ventricle.[22] These two areas of origin for ventricular tachycardia may alternate in the same patient. Precordial leads help localize posterior or anterior origin of VT. However, peripheral conduction disturbances may lead to inaccurate predictions as compared with the results of endocardial mapping. ECG data during documented VT in our series of 52 cases are presented in Table 51.1.

Sinus rhythm may also show ECG changes suggesting a right-sided abnormality.[34] An increase in the size of P waves to over 2.5 mm is observed in 13% of cases, and ECG signs of right ventricular hypertrophy appear in 15%. T wave inversion from V_1 to V_4–V_5 is found in 54%. Varying degrees of delayed right ventricular activation may also be observed, going from complete (15% of cases) to, more frequently, incomplete right bundle branch block pattern (18%) with low voltage of the rapid phase potentials (Fig. 51.3). Recent data derived from correlation of surface ECGs and epicardial mapping have suggested that these patterns are due to a parietal block without definite alteration of the bundle branches.[35] However, involvement of the conducting system has been also described.[36] Table 51.1 indicates the standard ECG findings observed in our updated series of 52 cases.

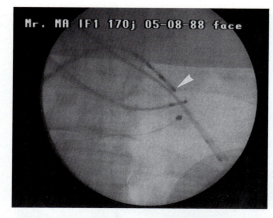
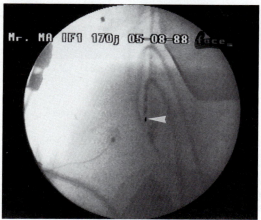
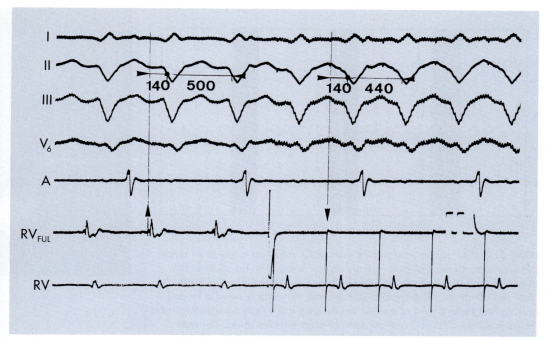

FIGURE 51.1 Fulguration in the upper part of the right ventricle in a patient with an anteroseptal myocardial infarction referred for incessant resistant monomorphic VT. Endocardial recording and pacing with the same coupling interval of 140 msec in addition to a perfect pacemapping indicates the appropriate site for VT ablation. Two sessions of fulguration performed in the same place in the right ventricle led to control of the arrhythmia with a follow-up period of 1 month.

TABLE 51.1 CHARACTERISTICS OF 52 PATIENTS WITH RIGHT VENTRICULAR TACHYCARDIA

Surface ECG Abnormalities	Types of Ventricular Arrhythmias	Morphology of Sustained VT
Atrial fibrillation (2%)	Ventricular fibrillation (12%)	LBBB (98%)
QRS axis (19 ± 42°)	SVT (81%)	RBBB (2%)
Right atrial hypertrophy (13%)	NSVT (6%)	QRS axis (13 ± 66°)
Right ventricular hypertrophy (15%)	PVCs (2%)	QRS duration (135 ± 20 msec)
Incomplete RBBB (18%)		Rate (198 ± 50 bpm)
Complete RBBB (15%)		
Inverted T waves (V_1–V_3) (54%)		

ECG, electrocardiographic; VT, ventricular tachycardia; LBBB, left bundle branch block; SVT, sustained ventricular tachycardia; RBBB, right bundle branch block; NSVT, nonsustained ventricular tachycardia (≥5 ventricular premature beats); PVCs, premature ventricular contractions.

FIGURE 51.2 Typical pattern of ventricular tachycardia originating in the right ventricle in a patient with ARVD. The left axis deviation suggests that the site of origin is localized on the diaphragmatic aspect of the right ventricle.

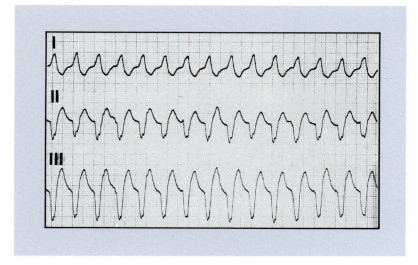

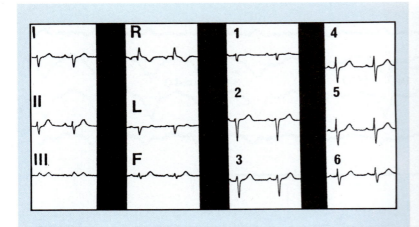

FIGURE 51.3 ECG pattern in a patient with ARVD, recorded a few days before the operation. (Epicardial map in sinus rhythm is shown in Fig. 51.8.) In this particular case, the T wave was not inverted in the right precordial leads. Note the abnormal left precordial pattern and the deep S wave in leads I and V_6. This patient died of cardiac insufficiency more than 5 years later, and the postmortem disclosed a major form of adipomatosis cordis. The right ventricle is covered by fatty tissue (R) and there is a large layer of fatty tissue penetrating from the epicardium toward the endocardium (L) on the left ventricle.

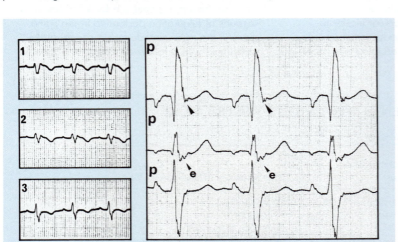

FIGURE 51.4 Recording of post-excitation epsilon waves (e) in a patient with ARVD. On the left, the recording is made from leads V_1–V_3 with thermosensitive recording paper at standard speed and amplification. On the right, bipolar precordial leads are recorded by an ink-jet recorder, after increasing the amplification to its maximum and recording at a speed of 50 mm/sec. The three bipolar precordial lead system consists of electrodes located at the two extremities of the sternum and one lead on the left precordium in the position of ECG lead V_4. Note the widening of the QRS complexes in the right precordial leads V_1 and V_2. The epsilon waves are clearly seen in the right part of the figure.

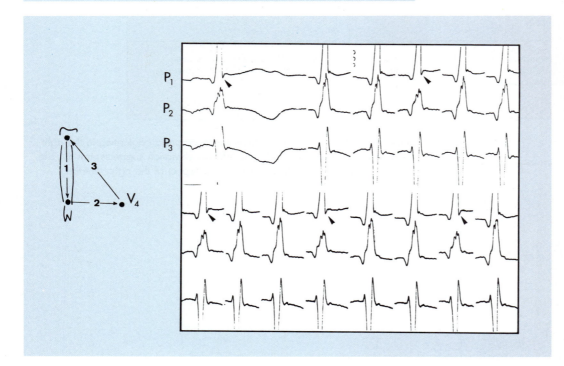

FIGURE 51.5 Beat-to-beat analysis of spontaneous modification of QRS complex morphology (arrow) showing cyclic abrupt changes of an S wave seen at the end of the QRS complexes. These modifications were independent of respiration. The beats were recorded at 50 mm/sec and high amplification. The left part of the panel shows the position of recording electrodes (described in Fig. 51.3).

In 30% of cases, more specific changes may be recorded, such as ventricular post-excitation waves.[37] These are potentials of small amplitude which have been called "epsilon waves." They occur after the QRS complex at the beginning of the ST segment.[20] These waves are better demonstrated by recording the precordial ECG from three bipolar suction electrodes applied at the superior and inferior poles of the sternum, in addition to another electrode placed over a rib close to the precordial lead V_4, and by increasing the sensitivity of the ECG machine two or three times (Fig. 51.4). Abnormalities of myocardial conduction in these patients can sometimes be observed even in sinus rhythm, using beat-to-beat analysis of amplified QRS complexes. These changes should be independent of respiration-related artifacts (Fig. 51.5). Another approach is to use the summation and averaging method to process the signal, in order to increase the gain without distortion induced by the exceedingly large noise produced by muscle potentials (Fig. 51.6).[20] We believe that these post-excitation waves are the surface counterpart of "delayed" or "late" potentials detected during endocardial or epicardial mapping.

M-MODE AND 2D ECHOCARDIOGRAPHY

Echocardiographic studies show isolated dilatation of right heart cavities, especially the right ventricle, with an increased RV/LV ratio or localized abnormalities.[38,39] However, in minor forms only an experienced echocardiographer will be able to detect the abnormality.[40] The study of 16 patients with ARVD suggested that this examination was of value only in cases where more relevant clinical data suggested ARVD. The specificity of this investigation was poor, however, since there are many other disorders which mimic this condition.[41]

CHEST RADIOGRAPHY

X-ray studies generally show a moderate cardiac enlargement with a convexity between the aortic knob and the left ventricle, without pulmonary vascular redistribution. The cardiothoracic index is less than 0.6 in most cases. However, a wide spectrum from a completely normal cardiac silhouette to a definitely enlarged heart may be found.[42,43]

RIGHT VENTRICULAR ANGIOGRAPHY

Angiography shows a global dilatation of the right ventricular cavity, with marked reduction in its contractility and complete wash-out of dye from the ventricle at the end of the injection.[44] The contrast medium may stagnate for up to 20 beats in the abnormal regions. These signs are not specific, however, and may be observed in other cases of poor ventricular function. Localized dilatations like small aneurysms may also be observed at the infundibulum, the apex, or the postero-diaphragmatic right ventricular wall below the tricuspid valve.[23,45] These abnormalities can be isolated or associated in the same patient, constituting a triangle of dysplasia.[22] Right ventricular abnormalities recently seen at our center are presented in Table 51.2. Their appearance contrasts with the normal size and contractility of the left chamber.

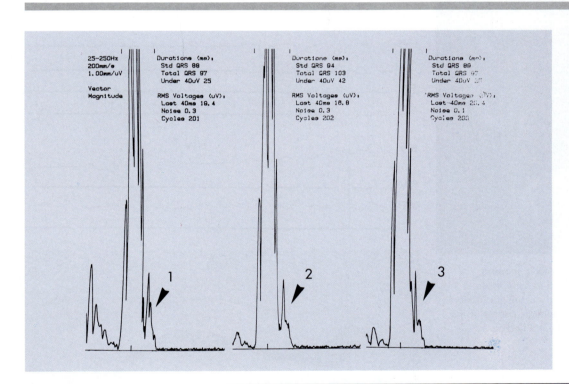

FIGURE 51.6 Recording of late potentials by the summation-averaging technique in a young patient with ARVD. Delayed potentials are recorded at the end of the QRS complexes (1). Changes in delayed potentials are observed after the first (2) and second (3) fulguration procedures. These changes suggest that the substrate has been modified. This sign is not in itself a marker of success. However, no change after fulguration could be a marker of failure.

TABLE 51.2 ANGIOGRAPHIC DATA IN PATIENTS WITH ARVD

Left ventricular angiographic and/or echocardiographic segmental abnormalities	15%
Mean ejection fraction (n = 20)	60 ± 9%
Right ventricular angiographic abnormalities:	
Apex	9.8%
Infundibulum	15.7%
Inferior wall	5.9%
Anterolateral wall	3.9%
Multiple segments	9.8%
RV dilatation	23.5%
"Abnormal RV"	31.4%

However, abnormalities of contraction at the inferior part of the septum are frequently found.[46] Abnormalities of the coronary arteries are independent of the syndrome.

Clinical cardiac catheterization sometimes shows an increase in the presystolic A wave, but there are no hemodynamic changes in the left ventricle at rest.[47]

NUCLEAR ANGIOSCINTIGRAPHY

This examination provides data concerning the size of the ventricles, their contraction pattern, and the originating site of VT. It is also an excellent way of studying both left and right ejection fractions.[48]

Moderate dysfunction of the left ventricle has been reported during exercise, suggesting that dysplasia may not be solely localized in the right ventricle but may represent a generalized form of cardiomyopathy with major involvement of the right ventricle.[49]

MAGNETIC RESONANCE IMAGING (MRI)

This new and promising technique can be used to analyze the dimensions as well as the dynamic behavior of the cardiac chambers, and is also used to identify adipose tissue within ventricular myocardium (Fig. 51.7).[50–52] MRI may be the most effective noninvasive examination for detecting fatty infiltration of the myocardium.

ELECTROPHYSIOLOGIC INVESTIGATIONS

These studies should be carried out after localization of the dysplasia zones by 2D echo and angiography, in order to facilitate positioning of the exploratory catheter in the abnormal zones where delayed potentials are most likely to be recorded (Fig. 51.8). These potentials are tiny waves occurring after the QRS complex in addition to the normal synchronous potential. Their dynamic behavior exhibits time-dependent properties which can be of significance for intramyocardial reentrant phenomena.[53] In addition, it is sometimes possible to observe a delay of more than 80 msec between stimulus and ventricular activation—this phenomenon also showing time-dependent properties.[53]

An increase in pacing threshold is frequently seen in the abnormal areas.[54,55] Nevertheless, programmed stimulation or bursts of rapid ventricular stimulation usually induce and terminate VT.[20–22,55] In some cases it may be difficult to induce VT, and many attempts may be necessary to bring on the first attack. Pacing should be carried out at

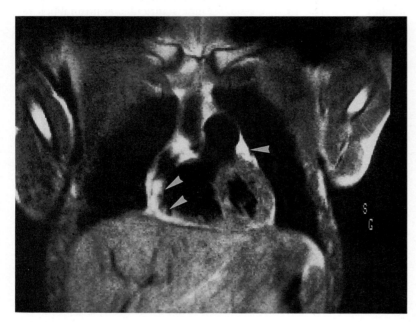

FIGURE 51.7 Magnetic resonance imaging in a case of ARVD, showing increased signals in the right ventricle, which are related to fatty tissue. Horizontal arrow points to the left AV groove, where fatty tissue is a normal finding. Oblique arrows point to the lateral or diaphragmatic aspect of the right ventricular free wall, where fatty tissue is an abnormal finding suggesting dysplasia.

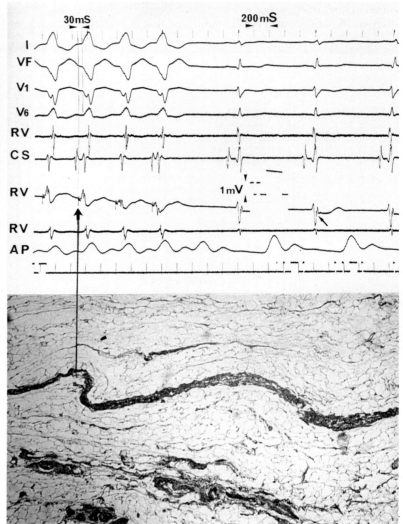

FIGURE 51.8 *Upper panel:* Endocardial recording of an episode of ventricular tachycardia, and spontaneous resumption of sinus rhythm. A presystolic potential is recorded in the right ventricle (*RV*) 30 msec before the QRS onset in ventricular tachycardia and just after the QRS complex in sinus rhythm. This thin deflection could be related to a histologic structure (discovered in a different case, *lower panel*) showing isolated strands of myocardial fibers inside the fatty tissue. (*CS*, coronary sinus; *AP*, atrial blood pressure)

several places in the right ventricle, using different basic cycle lengths, introducing several extrastimuli and even burst pacing, or a more premature stimulus at the end of the burst. In contrast, when the initial episode of VT has been induced, reinitiation is easier. These maneuvers may induce spontaneous or undocumented episodes of VT, the axis of which is generally consistent with the area involved.

Programmed pacing may be used to evaluate induction of repetitive VT in asymptomatic cases, but its sensitivity is poor.[56] Some groups are now using isoproterenol infusion during electrophysiologic study to increase its sensitivity. We use the same method to induce VT under general anesthesia during the fulguration procedure.

In some cases programmed pacing can induce ventricular fibrillation.[57] Table 51.3 shows the arrhythmias induced in the electrophysiologic laboratory in our updated series.[26]

EPICARDIAL MAPPING

This procedure used in sinus rhythm demonstrates delayed activation of the right ventricular free wall globally consistent with ECG data. However, bunching of the isochrones are always observed over the dysplastic areas (Fig. 51.9). The amplitude of right ventricular epicardial potentials is generally reduced markedly.

These potentials are probably the result of delayed conduction in the abnormal myocardium, and especially in the strands of surviving fibers. These delayed potentials could be part of the substrate for the development of reentry phenomena, provided that delayed activity could reactivate adjacent normal myocardium. Epicardial maps show delayed activation of the right ventricle, even if the activation of the free wall is within the normal range, suggesting a preserved conduction system in these cases.[35]

When the map is drawn from the most delayed potentials instead of from the initial QRS-synchronous activation, a post-excitation map is obtained that clearly demonstrates the most abnormal zones of activation (see Fig. 51.8). In some cases, a good correlation is observed between the zones of most delayed activation in sinus rhythm and the originating site of VT.[37,53,58,59] However, this concept may not be valid when the arrhythmia originates from the right side of the interventricular septum. This area seems to be the originating site of VT in some cases of ARVD.[59]

Epicardial mapping during VT localizes the emergence of the abnormal activation and determines the area where surgery should be performed.[60]

ANATOMIC APPEARANCE

Gross pathology confirms that the right ventricle is dilated and covered with fatty tissue (Fig. 51.10). Inside this fat, vessels are more visible than in areas of the heart where normal fat is found. After the right ventricular free wall is opened, the thinness of the myocardial wall is readily apparent, and there is major fatty infiltration of subepicardial areas. Therefore, if the thickness of the right ventricular free wall is globally increased, remaining apparently normal myocardium has in fact undergone a major reduction in thickness. Endocardium seen from the inside of the heart looks normal. However, in one of our cases plaques of thick fibrosis not related to dysplastic areas were observed (see Fig. 51.13). In another case right ventricular endocardium looked chamois-colored. Histology demonstrated fibrous tissue infiltration.

When the macroscopic appearance suggests thinning of the ventricular wall and an exaggerated amount of epicardial fat, the histologic study demonstrates strands of surviving or partially degenerated fibers in restricted areas. These strands of partially degenerated myofibrillar fascicles, having in some places a plexiform structure exchanging fibers with normal myocardium, may provide a comprehensive basis for slow conduction (delayed potentials) and reentry[61] (Fig. 51.11). Finally, although the pathological substrate seems specific, this structure is mainly observed in the subepicardial layers, and therefore endocardial biopsies may exhibit a lack of specificity.[62-65]

HISTOLOGIC BASIS OF VENTRICULAR ARRHYTHMIAS

Strands of surviving fibers observed inside the fatty tissue are bordered by a thin rim of fibrosis (see Fig. 51.11). This suggests that the fatty tissue is in fact the result of degeneration of myocytes, and also explains why the coronary arteries, although normal in number, are clearly seen inside the yellow fatty tissue. The thin rim of fibrosis indicates that what was originally considered to be the mechanism of dysplasia is the result of a different kind of degeneration, not transforma-

TABLE 51.3 ELECTROPHYSIOLOGIC TESTING BY PROGRAMMED RV STIMULATION IN 50 PATIENTS WITH ARVD

	Induced Arrhythmias	
	SVT, VF	NSVT, VPBs
Spontaneous Arrhythmia		
SVT	37	0
NSVT	6	0
None	5	2
Rate: 194 ± 43 bpm		

	Clinical	Nonclinical	Both	Unknown
Induced Arrhythmia				
Sustained	20	9	7	1
Nonsustained	2	3	0	1

SVT, sustained ventricular tachycardia; VF, ventricular fibrillation; NSVT, nonsustained ventricular tachycardia (≥5 VPBs); VPBs, ventricular premature beats.

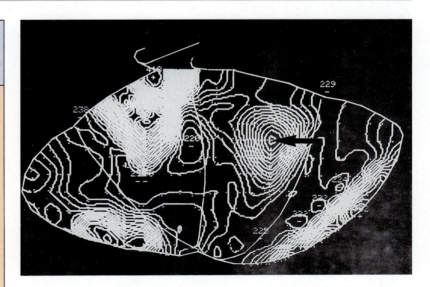

FIGURE 51.9 Epicardial map in a patient with right ventricular dysplasia. This map, drawn from the latest delayed potentials recorded in the epicardium (post-excitation mapping), indicates a major delay of activation in the anterior aspect of the right ventricle as well as the right paraseptal areas. In addition, there is a major delay of activation in the middle of the anterior aspect of the left ventricle, which is not artifactual (single point with high aberrant delay). Note also a delayed activation of the left septal area adjacent to the right septal area.

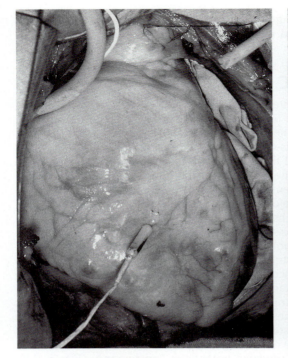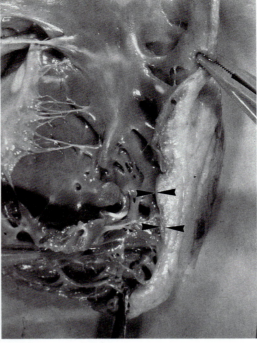

FIGURE 51.10 Operative exposure of the right ventricle in a patient with ARVD. There is no normal muscle in this dilated right ventricle. When the ventricle was opened (postmortem performed seven years later), there was a major thinning of ventricular myocardium bracketed by arrows.

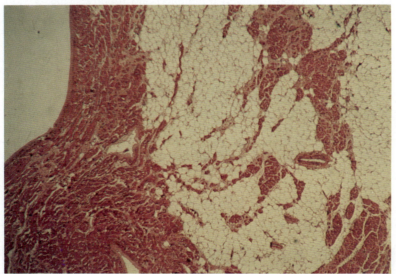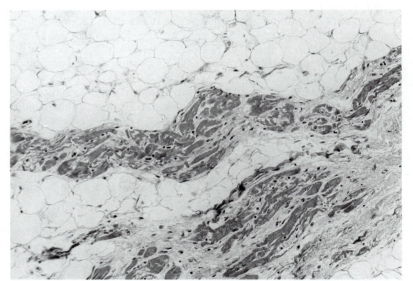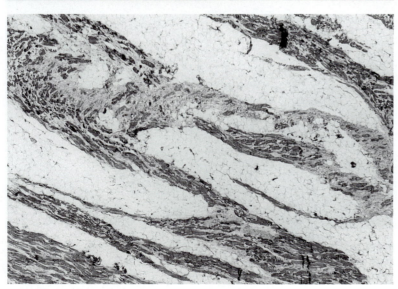

FIGURE 51.11 Some examples of myofat. **A.** Note the large amount of fatty tissue. Surviving fibers can be observed in the medial layers, embedded in a thin rim of fibrosis. (*EPI*, epicardium) (×40). **B.** Longitudinal section of fibers in the same clinical setting (×120). **C.** Interconnections of surviving fibers can explain how a reentry pathway can exist in such a structure (×120).

tion into fatty tissue. Leiomyocytes constituting the coronary arteries are not involved in this fatty degeneration, except that these vessels, which may in some areas be completely normal, can in other places display increased thickness of the media, leading in some instances to the almost-complete obstruction of their lumen. Direction of the leiomyocytes can also be altered (Fig. 51.12). Major thicknesses of fibrotic plaque may be observed over the endocardium (Fig. 51.13).

MYOFAT

This structure should be considered from a topographic point of view to include endocardial, medial, and subepicardial layers (see Fig. 51.11). This term has been chosen instead of fibro-myofat because fibrosis is not the typical form of the disease and is only observed around the surviving myocytes. Endocardial biopsy from the right ventricle (which can be dangerous for these patients) has confirmed descriptions made from surgical samples. However, in some patients fibrous tissue, which may be observed in endocardial plaques (as shown in Fig. 51.13) or in the interstitium, could be the result of a more advanced form of the disease or could suggest a different mechanism (Fig. 51.14).

ELECTRON MICROSCOPY

Ultrastructural changes have been observed in patients with ARVD. They mainly concern the structure of the intercalated disks, where the convolutions of sarcolemma are flattened, with abnormalities in the desmosomes.[66,67] These features can, at least in part, explain the abnormal conduction observed in these fibers.

DELAYED POTENTIALS

Delayed, doubled, and fragmented potentials have been recorded from the dysplastic areas. During rapid pacing, their coupling interval increases. This may provide the basis for reentry, if activity is delayed long enough to overcome the refractory period of adjacent healthy fibers. However, prolonged intervals between the onset of QRS and delayed potentials were recorded without any visible propagated activity on the surface ECG. This suggests that a certain proportion of arrhythmogenic areas may remain isolated in a region unable to transmit the activation to adjacent fibers. The significance of delayed potentials should therefore be interpreted with caution. Although they appear to accompany intraventricular reentry, they may not be sufficient in

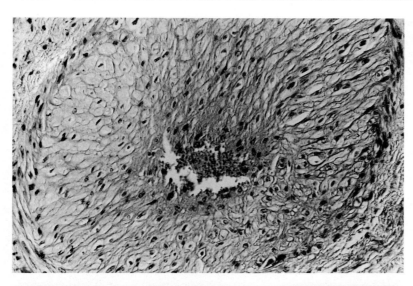

FIGURE 51.12 Major thickening of the media of one vessel in a dysplastic zone, with a longitudinal deposition of the leiomyocytes. Proliferation of the media led to a near-complete obstruction of this vessel. There were no atheromatous signs of coronary artery disease.

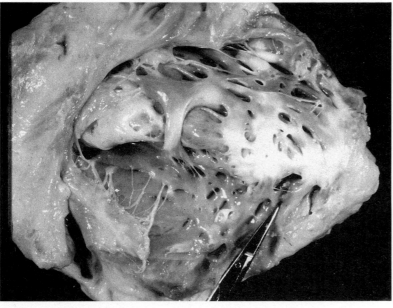

FIGURE 51.13 Endocardial view toward the right septum of the same heart shown in Fig. 51.9. Note the hypertrophy of trabeculations, and especially the moderator band. This is partially covered by areas of fibrosis which are

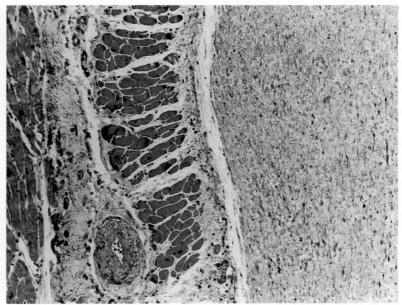

better documented on the histologic preparation. Note also the thickening of the media of the vessel presented in the lower left part of this figure.

themselves for the initiation of VT. The finding of abnormal conduction properties within the myocardium does not imply that any delayed potential is capable of reactivating adjacent tissues.[68] Delayed conduction may and probably does result from attenuation in the adipose and fibrous tissue which surrounds these zones. It is well known that propagation can take place only when the safety factor of propagation of the activation front is adequate.[69] When it is reduced, conduction may be blocked.

This idea was well illustrated in a recent experimental study explaining unidirectional conduction in a Wolff–Parkinson–White-type accessory pathway. A portion of myocardium was modeled so that a narrow strip communicated with a wider portion.[70] Conduction was normal in one direction (from the wider to the narrower portion) but not in the other. It is easy to conceive a similar situation in several abnormal zones of ventricular myocardium. The transmission of activation from the narrower to the wider zone appears, therefore, to be a critical determinant of further propagation. Recent data concerning the electrophysiologic and pathologic basis of paroxysmal junctional reciprocating tachycardia provide the concept of decremental conduction in a long Kent bundle-like accessory pathway.[71] It is not difficult to conceive that a similar structure may be operating in the isolated strands of fiber connecting two areas of normal myocardium. Our findings indicate that stimulation in an abnormal zone is unquestionably capable of activating the rest of the myocardium, and this appears to be of paramount importance in the understanding of arrhythmic mechanisms.[53]

PATHOGENESIS

This is still unclear. According to one mechanism, we hypothesized that ARVD was the result of an abnormality in the structure of myocardial fibers that was already present in the embryo. This reasoning was based on the fact that ARVD was observed in other members of the same family as the patient (siblings or father), suggesting some genetic factor.[22,30] The abnormality was presumed to become apparent with time, as myocardial fibers were replaced by fatty tissue. This occurs mainly in the medial and subepicardial layers. When this process is advanced, only the subendocardial layers consist of normal myocardial tissue, the remaining part of the wall being fatty tissue.[42] Thinning of endocardium and the plexiform structure of surviving fibers could explain slow conduction and the setup for reentry.

A second mechanism has recently been suggested which may be even more plausible. Dysplasia may be the result of acquired myocardial damage produced by a remote inflammatory or infectious process, manifest or occult during its acute phase, and disappearing with few or even no indications of residual disease (see Fig. 51.14). This theory has

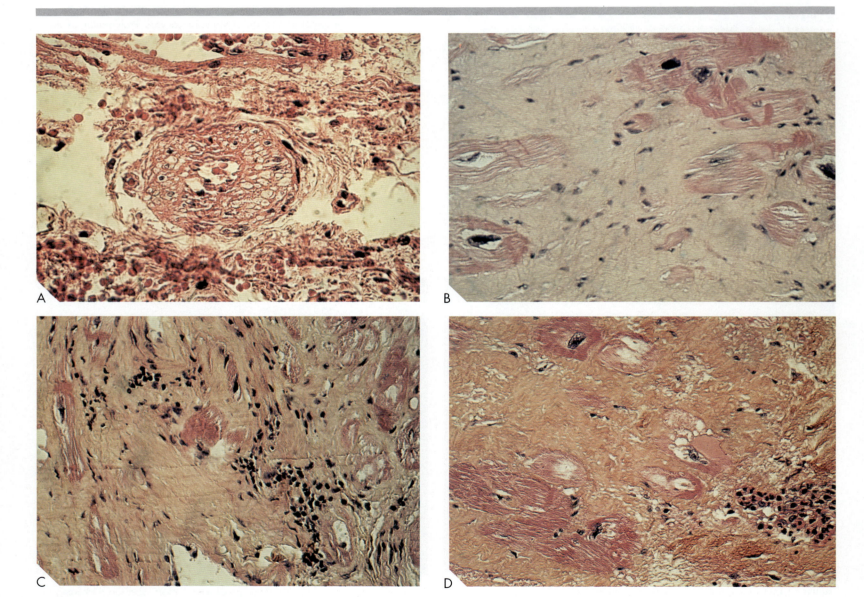

FIGURE 51.14 One of the cases of ARVD, in a patient who died shortly after the fulguration procedure. Pathologic studies show many zones of major fibrosis containing lymphocytes. **A.** Vessel with proliferation of the media (×320). **C.** Strands of fibers isolated in a zone of sclerosis (×320). **B–D.** Fibrous tissue with lymphocytes (×120).

ARRHYTHMOGENIC RIGHT VENTRICULAR TACHYCARDIA, AN UNAPPRECIATED CAUSE OF SUDDEN DEATH IN YOUNG ADULTS

Sudden death in young adults without cardiac abnormality is generally considered extremely rare. However, a number of cardiac pathologists have recently focused on this phenomenon. They reported fatty and fibrous infiltration of myocardium in which they demonstrated right ventricular cardiomyopathy and which appeared similar to what we have termed ARVD.[31] In any case, the available data show that sudden death may occur as the first presenting symptom in a patient with an apparently normal heart. Intense physical effort appears to be an important risk factor.[76]

In a study of 29 cases, Maron found myocardial abnormalities in 22 athletes below 35 years of age who died suddenly during competitive sports.[77] The most common finding was hypertrophic cardiomyopathy, followed by abnormal anatomy of coronary arteries, idiopathic concentric hypertrophy, and coronary heart disease.

In a series of 12 cases studied by Thiene,[31] 4 young athletes had a localized abnormality in the right ventricle compatible with chronic myocarditis, or dilated cardiomyopathy of the right ventricle. One patient who had fatty infiltration of the right ventricle died suddenly while playing tennis. It is possible that a form of dysplasia was present in some of these patients.

In our own series, we have data on 4 patients who died suddenly. In 2, death occurred during sports or major exercise. In 2, syncope or near-syncope was reported.

Olsson and colleagues were the first to report histologic proof of dysplasia found in a patient who had syncopal episodes due to ventricular fibrillation.[78]

An interesting paper by Virmani and others[79] from the Armed Forces Institute of Pathology described sudden death occurring during exercise in 3 cases, two involving black American basketball players. The authors observed an almost complete disappearance of myocardium in the free wall of the right ventricle, but the histologic study showed this not to be the typical pattern of Uhl's anomaly. The study was published before the classical paper by Marcus and colleagues, and it is now clear that their patients had arrhythmogenic right ventricular dysplasia. (Robinowitz M, personal communication, ACC Heart House Conference, Washington, D.C., 1984).

Sugrue and colleagues have reported the case of a 20-year-old patient who had syncopal episodes during a basketball game.[80] The electrocardiogram displayed ventricular tachycardia degenerating into ventricular fibrillation and necessitating an external DC shock.

Virmani and others, as well as Olsson and colleagues confirmed that sudden death can appear as the first manifestation of the disease. In one of two cases reported by Waller and co-workers,[81] the patient died suddenly with no previous sign of cardiac dysfunction, although he suffered from cardiac failure and his cardiac disease was complicated by atrial as well as ventricular arrhythmia.

A possible case of dysplasia mixed with adipomatosis cordis is suggested in a report by Voigt and colleagues in a patient who died suddenly during a ball game. This man had no cardiac symptoms before his death. Autopsy showed a fatty infiltration of the right ventricular wall, and the myocardial picture suggested dysplasia. Further, the patient had a brother who died suddenly at the age of 17 during exercise.[82]

One case, classified as a localized form of Uhl's anomaly diagnosed by echocardiography, has been reported by Laurenceau and others. The patient died suddenly a short time after a game of hockey.[83] Other suggestive reports can be found in the literature.[33,50]

Based on our previous experience and our reading of the literature, we think that the cause of death in these cases was arrhythmic. It is possible to imagine several mechanisms. Increased venous return to the right ventricle could increase distension of the myocardial wall, resulting in conduction slowing in the dysplastic area, in turn causing reentrant ventricular tachycardia, and finally ventricular fibrillation. The circulating catecholamines mediated through the autonomous nervous system could also play an adjuvant role in this mechanism. In addition, increased heart rate could also produce conduction block by "use-dependent" effects.

SUBGROUPS OF ARVD

Data provided by surgical samples as well as by careful pathology of patients who died suddenly lead us to believe that the histologic patterns are not constant. The population includes cases referred by other centers as well as those from our own extensive experience.[72-74,84] These patients appear to fall into several subgroups, which are tentatively listed below.

UHL'S ANOMALY

Uhl's anomaly is to our mind a syndrome different from arrhythmogenic right ventricular dysplasia, from both the histologic and the clinical standpoint. This syndrome is very rare, and appears in two groups. In the newborn, Uhl's anomaly generally leads to fatal heart failure within days or weeks.[43] A second group consists of adults who suffer from cardiac failure associated with or independent of ventricular tachycardia.[81] These patients present with an enormous cardiac silhouette in which trabeculations of the right ventricle have disappeared. The wall is extremely thin, accounting for the terms "parchment heart" or "paper-thin right ventricle."[84] Because of the extreme thinning of the wall, all the distal coronary vessels are displayed on the same surface, giving the impression of a surprising increase in the number of vessels. This pattern in the right ventricle contrasts with a left ventricle that is completely normal in size and thickness.

We do not know at the present time if Uhl's anomaly involves the same pathogenetic mechanism as dysplasia.[22] Up to now, no case of dysplasia has been reported in the newborn, and patients with dysplasia may lead a normal life well into the sixties without cardiac failure or dilatation of the right ventricle. Familial cases of Uhl's anomaly have been reported.[85]

LOCALIZED FORM OF UHL'S ANOMALY

In a small number of cases reported in the literature, localized Uhl's anomaly has been observed. Because of the localization, the cardiac silhouette may be completely normal on routine examination, and therefore this anomaly may be first discovered at postmortem.[86-89] In some forms it may be limited to a few centimeters in size; in others it can involve the entire anterior aspect of the right ventricle. A schematic representation of these different aspects is presented in Fig. 51.15.

ADIPOMATOSIS CORDIS

This is also a rare anomaly; we are now aware of 2 cases in our series, one referred from abroad. In this disease, the fatty infiltration involves the left ventricle, and fatty tissue seems to extend very deeply into the left myocardium toward the endocardium. This situation can lead to cardiac failure and/or cardiac arrhythmia. One of our patients who had undergone surgery for ventricular tachycardia with left ventricular conduction delay, and had initially been considered to have arrhythmogenic right ventricular dysplasia, died several years later of a noncardiac cause. Postmortem examination revealed major fatty infiltration of both ventricles. This pattern was consistent with the diagnosis of essential adipomatosis cordis. The interesting point in this case was that the patient had delayed potentials on the left side of the heart (see Fig. 51.9).[20] He also had ventricular tachycardia originating near the septum in the anterior aspect of the left ventricle.[90]

SEQUELAE OF MYOCARDITIS

This differential diagnosis is difficult to establish clinically when there is no definite proof of the original infection. In a group of 4 cases of ventricular tachycardia originating in the right ventricle, Thiene and Coll have reported 2 in which this diagnosis was suspected.[76] We have one well-documented case in a 27-year-old patient. She experienced episodes of sustained ventricular tachycardia, for which the diagnosis of ARVD was made on a clinical basis. She had had a previous myocarditis at the age of 7, and the ejection fraction of the left ventricle was abnormal.

Sequelae of myocarditis can produce generalized or localized fatty and fibrotic degeneration of myocardial muscle. It usually heals in a period of a few weeks, leaving no sequelae. However, we believe that in some patients modification of myocardium can produce an arrhythmogenic substrate which could be operative decades later.

The combination of dysplasia and myocarditis has also been discussed by Bharati and Lev.[36] Conceivably a patient with the classical form of dysplasia could also develop myocarditis. It is not known if this is a coincidental association, or a particular sensitivity of already-abnormal myocardium to an infectious problem.

CARDIOMYOPATHIES

Since in some patients arrhythmogenic right ventricular dysplasia is the result of sequelae of myocarditis, it is understandable that some forms of healed myocarditis, can be difficult to distinguish from dilated cardiomyopathy.[20,91]

However, when the pathologic substrate exhibits a large amount of fibrosis with depressed cardiac function, it may represent some form of idiopathic dilated cardiomyopathy complicated by ventricular tachycardia originating in the right ventricle.[92] In these patients, there is generally a decrease in cardiac function at rest, or at least during exercise.

Left ventricular involvement can be better explained if dysplasia is the result of myocarditis or cardiomyopathy resulting from myocarditis. The infection may have disappeared completely. The involvement of the left ventricle reported by many authors is therefore more easily understood.[49,81,93–95]

OCCULT ARVD

An occult form of ARVD is also suspected. We have seen previously that patients with ventricular arrhythmias can be asymptomatic. It is possible to go one step further and to suggest that an individual without arrhythmia could already have a silent arrhythmogenic substrate. Such an individual could under certain circumstances develop a possibly dangerous arrhythmia.

As the arrhythmogenic substrate is in fact the most basic prerequisite for these arrhythmias, and its detection is feasible by a noninvasive method such as the high amplification technique, it seems logical to perform this examination on anyone entering a profession at risk.

ANTIARRHYTHMIC THERAPIES
DRUG TREATMENT

This is the first and most frequently used therapy. If, as is generally the case, left ventricular function is preserved, class I antiarrhythmic drugs can be safely used. If the left ventricular function is depressed, we believe that amiodarone therapy is the treatment of choice. Combination therapies including amiodarone plus class I agents or amiodarone plus β-blocking agents have been used.[96] Table 51.4 shows the selection of treatments used in our patients at hospital discharge. Table 51.5 indicates the drug selection at discharge and during the last clinic visit.

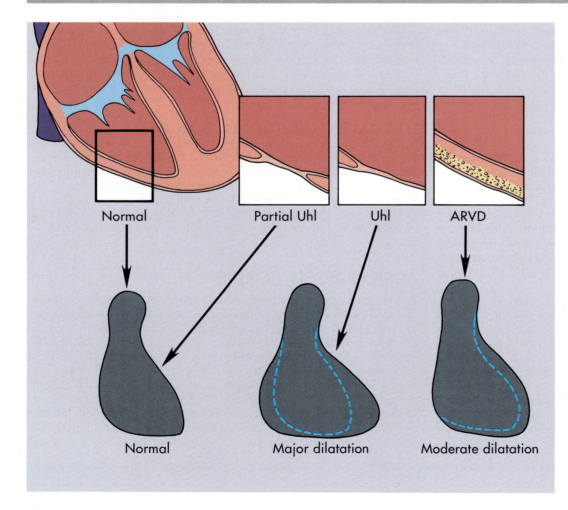

FIGURE 51.15 Schematic representation of different forms of dysplasia as compared with normal. The upper part of the diagram shows myocardial structure, and the lower part the cardiac silhouette. *Left to right*: normal, typical Uhl's anomaly as well as localized (partial) form of Uhl's anomaly, and ARVD.

SURGERY

Our group has used surgical techniques to treat chronic VT in patients without coronary artery disease.[97] A simple ventriculotomy or transmural incision of the ventricular wall at the originating site of the ventricular tachycardia can prevent recurrence of ventricular arrhythmias for long periods. Because of the reduced ventricular wall thickness in ARVD, the point of epicardial breakthrough is immediately proximal to the originating site of VT, at the point where it exits from the zone of delayed conduction and enters the healthy myocardium.[98] If other clinically recognized originating sites of VT are found at the time of surgery, they too should undergo a simple ventriculotomy.

DISARTICULATION OF THE RIGHT VENTRICLE

This procedure has been proposed for the treatment of ARVD associated with VT of several different forms for which simple ventriculotomy may be inadequate.[99] The aim of the operation is to isolate completely the right ventricular free wall by performing an incision along the right border of the interventricular septum, up around the pulmonary artery, and then sectioning the right atrioventricular groove as far as the crux of the heart. This operation is based on the principle that the right ventricle makes only a small contribution to cardiac hemodynamics, and that the isolation of its free wall will prevent the transmission of abnormal rhythms to the left ventricle. Epicardial recordings have shown electrical activity at a rate of 300/min arising from the right ventricle while the left ventricle continued to beat at its usual rate. The efficacy of this operation in the prevention of VT is unquestioned. Nevertheless, because of hemodynamic alterations, this extensive surgical approach should be used with caution.[100]

FULGURATION

Catheter fulguration or ablation for the treatment of ventricular tachycardia was introduced by P. Puech in 1983,[101] and was investigated by our center in a series of 15 patients with a mean follow-up period of 45 months.[102] Seven were treated after a first session, and 8 after a second. Two patients died during the second session, one due to an inappropriate protocol at the beginning of the study. The second was in the terminal stages of cardiac failure with recurrent VTs which proved to be due to a form of dilated idiopathic cardiomyopathy as a probable result of myocarditis. The pathology of this patient is presented in detail in Fig. 51.9. No death was directly related to the fulguration procedure.

The initial fears of perforation of the right ventricle due to DC ablation were not justified by our study, or by other reports.[103] However, in our second case of death, an unusual amount of blood was observed in the pericardium. It was later found that this was related to the me-

TABLE 51.4 SELECTION OF TREATMENT IN 52 PATIENTS WITH ARVD

Procedure	No. of Patients
Treatment at hospital discharge (n = 52)	
Antiarrhythmic drugs*	36 (70%)
Surgery	8 (15%)
Fulguration	7 (13%)
None	1 (2%)
Second approach in case of drug inadequacy (n = 9)	
Surgery + drugs	1 (11%)
Fulguration + drugs	8 (89%)

* Amiodarone was the most frequently used drug (47% of the cases, alone or in combination).

TABLE 51.5 DRUG THERAPIES FOR ARVD

	Treatment at Hospital Discharge (n = 47)	Treatment at Last Clinic Visit (n = 43)
Monotherapy		
Amiodarone	9	15
β-blockers	7	3
Class I-a	6	1
Class I-b	0	0
Class I-c	3	3
Combination		
Amiodarone + β-blockers	0	3
Amiodarone + Class I-a	7	5
Amiodarone + Class I-b	4	1
Amiodarone + Class I-c	2	9
Class I + β-blockers	4	2
Unknown	5	1
Amiodarone alone or in combination	47%	77%
Untreated: 5 patients		

TABLE 51.6 FOLLOW-UP RESULTS IN 52 PATIENTS WITH ARVD

Mean duration of follow-up (mo): 41.3 ± 30.7 (0–150)	
Follow-up > 3 mo: 44.7 ± 29.5 (6–150)	
Outcome	
Alive	42
Died	
During fulguration procedure	2
Cardiac failure	1 (21 mo)
Suicide (cardiac failure)	1 (7 mo)
Total	4
Uncertain	
Lost to follow-up since hospital discharge	2
No news for more than 2 yr	4
Total	6

chanical manipulation of the catheter inside the cavities and was not the result of barotrauma. In addition, an investigational catheter with stylet was used, and the stiffness of this device could explain a small mechanical perforation observed in the infundibular area.

A previous report[104] cited a smaller series which demonstrated ($P < 0.01$) a direct relation between the isoenzyme CK MB release and the successful outcome of catheter fulguration, which suggests that ventricular tachycardia can only be controlled when sufficient myocardial damage has been produced.

Therefore, at present we think that the fulguration procedure is an acceptable alternative treatment for patients with ARVD. In our center it has essentially replaced surgery in drug-resistant cases.[105]

LONG-TERM EVOLUTION

Few studies have followed the long-term evolution of the disease.[93] Blomstrom-Lundqvist reported the outcome of a series of 15 cases.[106] In a large series from France including some of our own cases the death rate was 5% over a mean follow-up period of more than 5 years.[107] In a survey of the literature Marcus reported 11 deaths out of 90 cases followed, and observed an increased risk of death in patients who experienced syncopal episodes.[108] This symptom should therefore prompt a properly controlled form of treatment. In our own series (included in the Marcus report) no case of arrhythmic death was observed.[26] However, we have documented two recent cases of syncopal episodes experienced 4 and 6 years previously, one of them resulting in documented arrhythmogenic death. This occurred after inadequate modification of drug treatment performed outside of our institution, and not reevaluated by programmed pacing methods. This emphasizes the fact that management of these cases should only be undertaken at centers experienced in clinical electrophysiology. Table 51.6 reports the follow-up results in our series.

CONCLUSION

Patients with right ventricular tachycardia appear to have a spectrum of right ventricular abnormalities, and this condition seems to be more frequent than is reported in the medical literature. Further study is clearly needed, for this disease is emerging as an important cause of sudden death in young and otherwise healthy individuals.

REFERENCES

1. Armbrust CA, Levine SA: Paroxysmal ventricular tachycardia: A study of one hundred and seven cases. Circulation 1:28–40, 1950
2. Bouvrain Y, Slama R, Motte G et al: Les tachycardies ventriculaires: Etiologie et evolution: A propos de 161 malades. Arch Mal Coeur 61:909–920, 1968
3. Greene HL, Reid PR, Schaeffer AH: The repetitive ventricular response in man: A predictor of sudden death. N Engl J Med 299:729, 1978
4. Gallavardin L: Extrasystole ventriculaire a paroxysmes tachycardiques prolonges. Arch Mal Coeur 15:298, 1922
5. Ruberman W, Weinblatt E, Goldberg JD et al: Ventricular premature beats and mortality after myocardial infarction. N Engl J Med 297:750, 1977
6. Wellens HJJ, Schuilenburg RM, Durrer D: Electrical stimulation of the heart in patients with ventricular tachycardia. Circulation 46:216, 1972
7. Wellens HJJ, Lie KI, Durrer D: Further observations on ventricular tachycardias as studied by electrical stimulation of the heart. Circulation 49:647, 1974
8. Wellens HJJ, Duren DR, Lie KI: Observations on mechanisms of ventricular tachycardia in man. Circulation 54:237, 1976
9. Sung RJ, Shen EN, Morady F et al: Electrophysiologic mechanism of exercise-induced sustained ventricular tachycardia. Am J Cardiol 51:525–530, 1983
10. Josephson ME, Horowitz LN, Farshidi A et al: Recurrent sustained ventricular tachycardia: IV-Pleomorphism. Circulation 59:459, 1979
11. Josephson ME, Horowitz LN, Farshidi A et al: Recurrent sustained ventricular tachycardia: II-Endocardial mapping. Circulation 57:440, 1978
12. Fontaine G, Tonet JL, Frank R et al: Electrode catheter ablation of ventricular tachycardia by fulguration and antiarrhythmic therapy: Experience of 43 patients with a mean follow-up of 29 months. Chest 95:785–797, 1989
13. Huang SK, Jones J, Denes P: Significance of ventricular tachycardia in primary congestive cardiomyopathy. Am J Cardiol 49:1006, 1982
14. Giles TD: Cardiomyopathy. PSG Pub Co, Littleton, 1988
15. Deal BJ, Miller SM, Scagliotti D et al: Ventricular tachycardia in a young population without overt heart disease. Circulation 6:1111–1118, 1986
16. Rossi P: Arrhythmogenic right ventricular dysplasia: Clinical features. Eur Heart J 10:supp-D, 7–9, 1989
17. Berg KJ: Multifocal ventricular extrasystoles with Adams-Stokes syndrome in siblings. Am Heart J 60:965, 1960
18. Lesch M, Lewis E, Humphries JO et al: Paroxysmal ventricular tachycardia in the absence of organic heart disease. Ann Intern Med 66:950–960, 1967
19. Furlanello F, Bettini R, Bertoldi A et al: Arrhythmia patterns in athletes with arrhythmogenic right ventricular dysplasia. Eur Heart J 10:supp-D, 16–19, 1989
20. Fontaine G, Guiraudon G, Frank R et al: Stimulation studies and epicardial mapping in ventricular tachycardia: Study of mechanisms and selection for surgery. In Kulbertus HE (ed): Reentrant Arrhythmias, pp 343–350. Lancaster, MTP Pub, 1977
21. Frank R, Fontaine G, Vedel J et al: Electrocardiologie de quatre cas de dysplasie ventriculaire droite arythmogene. Arch Mal Coeur 71:963–972, 1978
22. Marcus FI, Fontaine G, Guiraudon G et al: Right ventricular dysplasia: A report of 24 cases. Circulation 65:384–399, 1982
23. Tomisawa M, Onouchi Z, Masakutsu G et al: Right ventricular aneurysm with ventricular premature beats. Br Heart J 36:1182–1185, 1974
24. Dungan WT, Garson A, Gillette PC: Arrhythmogenic right ventricular dysplasia: A cause of ventricular tachycardia in children with apparently normal hearts. Am Heart J 102:745–750, 1981
25. Rizzon P: Polymorphism of the clinical picture. Eur Heart J 10:supp-D, 10–12, 1989
26. Lascault G, Laplaud O, Frank R et al: Ventricular tachycardia features in right ventricular dysplasia (abstract). Circulation 78:Supp-II, 300, 1988
27. Diggelmann U, Baur HR: Familial Uhl's anomaly in the adult. Am J Cardiol 53:1402–1403, 1984
28. Nava A, Scognamiglio R, Thiene G et al: A polymorphic form of familial arrhythmogenic right ventricular dysplasia. Am J Cardiol 59:1405–1409, 1987
29. Waynberger M, Courtadon M, Peltier JM et al: Tachycardie ventriculaire familiale: A propos de 7 cas. Nouv Presse Med 3:1857–1860, 1974
30. Blomstrom-Lundqvist C, Enestrom S, Edvardsson N et al: Arrhythmogenic right ventricular dysplasia presenting with ventricular tachycardia in a father and a son. Clin Cardiol 10:277–283, 1987
31. Thiene G, Nava A, Corrado D et al: Right ventricular cardiomyopathy and sudden death in young people. N Engl J Med 318:129–133, 1988
32. Ruder MA, Winston SA, Davis JC et al: Arrhythmogenic right ventricular dysplasia in a family. Am J Cardiol 56:799–800, 1985
33. Rakovec P, Rossi L, Fontaine G et al: Familial arrhythmogenic right ventricular disease. Am J Cardiol 58:377–378, 1986
34. Gaita F, Mangiardi LM, Uslenghi E et al: Electrocardiography in patients with arrhythmogenic right ventricle displasia. In Mariani M (ed): Cardiology Up to Date: Diagnosis and Therapy, pp 383–386. Bologna, Monduzzi editore Pub, 1989
35. Fontaine G, Frank R, Guiraudon G et al: Signification des troubles de conduction intraventriculaires observes dans la dysplasie ventriculaire droite arythmogene. Arch Mal Coeur 77:872–879, 1984
36. Bharati S, Feld AW, Bauernfeind RA et al: Hypoplasia of the right ventricular myocardium with ventricular tachycardia. Arch Pathol Lab Med 107:249–253, 1983
37. Fontaine G, Guiraudon G, Frank R: Intramyocardial conduction defects in patients prone to ventricular tachycardia: I-The postexcitation syndrome in sinus rhythm. In Sandoe E, Julian DG, Bell JW (eds): Management of Ventricular Tachycardia: Role of Mexiletine, pp 39–55. Amsterdam, Excerpta Medica Pub, 1978
38. Laurenceau JL, Dumesnil JG: Right and left ventricular dimensions as determinants of ventricular septal motion. Chest 69:388–393, 1976
39. Scognamiglio R, Fasoli G, Nava A et al: Relevance of subtle echocardiographic findings in early diagnosis of the concealed form of right ventricular dysplasia. Eur Heart J 10:supp-D, 27–28, 1989
40. Baran A, Nanda NC, Falkoff MD et al: Two-dimensional echocardiographic detection of arrhythmogenic right ventricular dysplasia. Am Heart J 103:1066–1067, 1982
41. Kisslo JA: Two-dimensional echocardiography in arrhythmogenic right ventricular dysplasia. Eur Heart J 10:supp-D, 22–26, 1989
42. Fontaine G, Tereau Y, Frank R et al: Dysplasie ventriculaire droite arythmogene et maladie de Uhl. Arch Mal Coeur 75:361, 1982
43. Uhl HS: A previously undescribed congenital malformation of the heart: Almost total absence of the myocardium of the right ventricle. Bull John Hopkins Hosp 91:197–205, 1952
44. Drobinski G, Verdiere C, Fontaine G et al: Diagnostic angiocardiographique des dysplasies ventriculaires droites. Arch Mal Coeur 78:544–551, 1985
45. Daubert C, Descaves C, Foulgoc JL et al: Critical analysis of cineangiographic criteria for diagnosis of arrhythmogenic right ventricular dysplasia. Am Heart J 115:448–459, 1988
46. Blomstrom-Lundqvist C: The syndrome of arrythmogenic right ventricular

47. Chiddo A, Locuratolo N, Gaglione A et al: Right ventricular dysplasia: Angiographic data. Eur Heart J 10:supp-D, 42–45, 1989
48. Le Guludec D, Slama M, Frank R et al: Fourier analysis of gated blood pool studies in the detection of arrhythmogenic right ventricular dysplasia (abstract). Circulation 80:4, SUPP-II, 155, 1989
49. Manyari DE, Klein GJ, Gulamhusein SS et al: Arrhythmogenic right ventricular dysplasia: A generalized cardiomyopathy. Circulation 68:251–257, 1983
50. Fontaine G, Fontaliran F, Frank R et al: La dysplasie ventriculaire: Nosologie et mort subite. Ann Cardiol Angeiol 37:347–355, 1988
51. Klersy C, Raisaro A, Salerno JA et al: Arrhythmogenic right and left ventricular disease: Evaluation by computed tomography and nuclear magnetic resonance imaging. Eur Heart J 10:supp-D, 33–36, 1989
52. Wolf JE, Rose-Pittet L, Page E et al: Mise en evidence par l'IRM des lesions parietales au cours de dysplasies arythmogenes du ventricule droit. Arch Mal Coeur 82:1711–1717, 1989
53. Fontaine G, Guiraudon G, Frank R: Intramyocardial conduction defects in patients prone to ventricular tachycardia: II-A dynamic study of the post-excitation syndrome. In Sandoe E, Julian DG, Bell JW (eds): Management of Ventricular Tachycardia: Role of Mexiletine, pp 56–66. Amsterdam, Excerpta Medica Pub, 1978
54. Bharati S, Ciraulo DA, Bilitch M et al: Inexcitable right ventricle and bilateral bundle branch block in Uhl's disease. Circulation 57:636–644, 1978
55. Belhassen B, Webb CR, Shapira I et al: Unusual features of ventricular tachycardia during respiration and exercises in arrhythmogenic right ventricular dysplasia. Am J Cardiol 54:1280, 1984
56. DiBiase M, Favale S, Assari VM et al: Programmed stimulation in patients with minor forms of right ventricular dysplasia. Eur Heart J 10:supp-D, 49–53, 1989
57. Panidis IP, Greenspan AM, Mintz GS et al: Inducible ventricular fibrillation in arrhythmogenic right ventricular dysplasia. Am Heart J 110:1067–1069, 1985
58. Fontaine G, Guiraudon G, Frank R: Intramyocardial conduction defects in patients prone to ventricular tachycardia: III-The post-excitation syndrome during ventricular tachycardia. In Sandoe E, Julian DG, Bell JW (eds): Management of Ventricular Tachycardia: Role of Mexiletine, pp 67–79. Amsterdam, Excerpta Medica Pub, 1978
59. Fontaine G, Guiraudon G, Frank R et al: Correlations between latest delayed potentials in sinus rhythm and earliest activation during chronic ventricular tachycardia. In Bircks E, Loogen F, Schulte HD et al (eds): Medical and Surgical Management of Tachyarrhythmias, pp 138–154. Berlin, Springer-Verlag Pub, 1980
60. Guiraudon G, Fontaine G, Frank R et al: Is the reentry concept a guide to the surgical treatment of chronic ventricular tachycardia? In Bircks E, Loogen F, Schulte HD et al (eds): Medical and Surgical Management of Tachyarrhythmias, pp 155–172. Berlin, Springer-Verlag Pub, 1980
61. Fontaine G, Guiraudon G, Frank R et al: The pathophysiology of chronic disturbances of ventricular rhythm. In Masoni A, Alboni P (eds): Cardiac Electrophysiology Today, pp 251–271. London, Academic Press Pub, 1982
62. Fitchett DH, Mac Arthur CG, Oakley CM et al: Right ventricular cardiomyopathy presenting with recurrent ventricular tachycardia. Am J Cardiol 47:402, 1981
63. Morgera T, Salvi A, Alberti E et al: Morphological findings in apparently idiopathic ventricular tachycardia: An echocardiographic haemodynamic and histologic study. Eur Heart J 6:323–334, 1985
64. Strain JE, Grose RM, Factor SM et al: Clinically normal patients with spontaneous ventricular tachycardia: Endomyocardial biopsy results. Circulation 66:SUP.II, 1371, 1982
65. Billingham ME, Tazelaar HD: Cardiac biopsy. In Parmley WW, Chatterjee K (eds): Cardiology, Vol 1, Ch 54. Philadelphia, JB Lippincott Pub, 1987
66. Guiraudon CM: Histological diagnosis of right ventricular dysplasia: A role for electron microscopy? Eur Heart J 10:Supp-D, 95–96, 1989
67. Roncali L, Nico B, Locuratolo N et al: Right ventricular dysplasia: An ultrastructural study. Eur Heart J 10:Supp-D, 97–99, 1989
68. Janse MJ, van Capelle FJL, Morsink H et al: Flow of injury current and patterns of excitation during early ventricular arrhythmias in acute regional myocardial ischemia in isolated porcine and canine hearts: Evidence for two different arrhythmogenic mechanisms. Circ Res 47:151, 1980
69. Spach MS, Miller WT, Geselowitz DB: The discontinuous nature of propagation in normal canine cardiac muscle: Evidence for recurrent discontinuities of intracellular resistance that affect the membrane currents. Circ Res 48:39–54, 1981
70. de la Fuente D, Sasyniuk BJ, Moe GK: Conduction through a narrow isthmus in isolated canine atrial tissue: A model of the WPW syndrome. Circulation 44:803, 1971
71. Critelli G, Perticone F, Coltorti F et al: Antegrade slow bypass conduction after closed-chest ablation of the his bundle in permanent junctional reciprocating tachycardia. Circulation 67:687–692, 1983
72. Fontaine G, Fontaliran F, Linares-Cruz E et al: The arrhythmogenic right ventricle. In Iwa G, Fontaine G (eds): Cardiac Arryhthmias: Recent Progress in Investigation and Management, pp 189–202. The Hague, Elsevier Science Pub, 1988
73. Fontaine G, Fontaliran F, Mesnildrey P et al: Acquired and transmitted dysplasia. In Cardiomyopathy Update, Vol 3, pp 173–181. Tokyo, Univ of Tokyo Press, 1990
74. Fontaine G, Fontaliran F, Martin de la Salle E et al: Right ventricular dysplasias. In Aliot E, Lazzara R (eds): Ventricular Tachycardias: From Mechanism to Therapy, pp 113–133. Dordrecht, Martinus Nijhoff Pub, 1987
75. Dallavolta S: Arrhythmogenic cardiomyopathy of the right ventricle: Thoughts on aetiology. Eur Heart J 10:supp-D, 2–6, 1989
76. Thiene G, Gambino A, Corrado D et al: The pathological spectrum underlying sudden death in athletes. New Trends in Arrhythmias 3:323–331, 1985
77. Maron BJ, Roberts WC, McAllister HA: Sudden death in young athletes. Circulation 62:218, 1980
78. Olsson SB, Edvardsson N, Emanuelsson H et al: A case of arrhythmogenic right ventricular dysplasia with ventricular fibrillation. Clin Cardiol 5:591–596, 1982
79. Virmani R, Robinowitz M, Clark MA et al: Sudden death and partial absence of the right ventricular myocardium. Arch Pathol Lab Med 106:163–167, 1982
80. Sugrue DD, Edwards WD, Olney BA: Histologic abnormalities of the left ventricle in a patient with arrhythmogenic right ventricular dysplasia. Heart and Vessels 1:179–181, 1985
81. Waller BF, Smith ER, Blackbourne BD et al: Congenital hypoplasia of portions of both right and left ventricular myocardial walls: Clinical and necropsy observations in two patients with parchment heart syndrome. Am J Cardiol 46:885, 1980
82. Voigt J, Agdal N: Lipomatous infiltration of the heart: An uncommon cause of sudden, unexpected death in a young man. Arch Pathol Lab Med 106:497–498, 1982
83. Laurenceau JL, Liehnart JF, Malergue MC et al: Donnees echocardiographiques dans le syndrome du ventricule droit papyrace. Arch Mal Coeur 72:258, 1979
84. Vedel J, Frank R, Fontaine G et al: Tachycardies ventriculaires recidivantes et ventricule droit papyrace de l'adulte: A propos de deux observations anatomo-cliniques. Arch Mal Coeur 71:973–981, 1978
85. Hoback J, Adicoff A et al: A report of Uhl's disease in identical adult twins: Evaluation of right ventricular dysfunction with echocardiography and nuclear angiography. Chest 79:306–310, 1981
86. Gould L, Gutman B, Carrasco J et al: Partial absence of the right ventricular musculature: A congenital lesion. Am J Med Sci 42:636–641, 1967
87. Reeve R, Mac Donald CD: Partial absence of the right ventricular musculature: Partial parchment heart. Am J Cardiol 14:415–419, 1964
88. Slama R, Leclercq JF, Coumel P: Paroxysmal ventricular tachycardia in patients with apparently normal hearts. In Zipes DP, Jalife J (eds): Cardiac Electrophysiology and Arrhythmias, pp 545–552. Orlando, Grune & Stratton Pub, 1985
89. Sugiura M, Hayashi T, Ueno K: Partial absence of the right ventricular muscle in an aged patient. Jpn Heart J 11:582–585, 1970
90. Chomette G, Koulibali M, Linares-Cruz E et al: Dysplasie arythmogene: Parentes nosologiques avec le syndrome de Uhl et la lipomatose: A propos de trois observations anatomo-cliniques. Arch Anat Cytol Path 34:46–50, 1986
91. Nishikawa T, Sekiguchi M, Kunimine Y et al: An infant with dilated cardiomyopathy confirmed as myocarditis by endomyocardial biopsy. Heart and Vessels 3:108–110, 1987
92. Ibsen HHW, Baandrup U, Simonsen EE: Familial right ventricular dilated cardiomyopathy. Br Heart J 54:156–159, 1985
93. Higuchi S, Caglar NM, Shimada R et al: 16-Year follow-up of arrhythmogenic right ventricular dysplasia. Am Heart J 108:1363–1365, 1984
94. Robertson JH, Bardy GH, German LD et al: Comparison of 2-dimensional echocardiographic and angiographic findings in arrhythmogenic right ventricular dysplasia. Am J Cardiol 55:1506–1508, 1985
95. Webb JG, Kerr CR, Huckell VF et al: Left ventricular abnormalities in arrhythmogenic right ventricular dysplasia. Am J Cardiol 58:568–570, 1986
96. Fontaine G: Amiodarone drug interactions: Potential beneficial and adverse effects. Clin Cardiol 10:I-17–I-20, 1987
97. Fontaine G, Guiraudon G, Frank R et al: La cartographie epicardique et le traitement chirurgical par simple ventriculotomie de certaines tachycardies ventriculaires rebelles par reentree. Arch Mal Coeur 68:113–124, 1975
98. Fontaine G, Guiraudon G, Frank R: Mechanism of ventricular tachycardia with and without associated chronic myocardial ischaemia: Surgical management based on epicardial mapping. In Narula OS (ed): Cardiac Arrhythmias: Electrophysiology, Diagnosis and Management, pp 516–545. Philadelphia, Williams and Wilkins Pub, 1979
99. Guiraudon G, Klein GJ, Gulamhusein SS et al: Total disconnection of the right ventricular free wall: Surgical treatment of right ventricular tachycardia associated with right ventricular dysplasia. Circulation 67:463–470, 1983
100. Cox JL, Bardy GH, Damiano RJ et al: Right ventricular isolation procedures for nonischemic ventricular tachycardia. J Thorac Cardiovasc Surg 90:212–224, 1985
101. Puech P, Gallay P, Grolleau R et al: Traitement par électrofulguration endocavitaire d'une tachycardie ventriculaire récidivante par dysplasie ventriculaire droite. Arch Mal Coeur 77:826–835, 1984
102. Fontaine G, Frank R, Rougier I et al: Electrode catheter ablation of resistant ventricular tachycardia in arrhythmogenic right ventricular dysplasia: Experience of 15 patients with a mean follow-up of 45 months. Heart and Vessels (in press)

103. Leclercq JF, Chouty F, Cauchemez B et al: Results of electrical fulguration in arrhythmogenic right ventricular disease. Am J Cardiol 62:220–224, 1988
104. Fontaine G, Frank R, Rougier I et al: Electrode catheter ablation of resistant ventricular tachycardia in arrhythmogenic right ventricular dysplasia: Experience of 13 patients with a mean follow-up of 45 months. Eur Heart J 10:Supp-D, 74–81, 1989
105. Fontaine G, Frank R, Tonet JL et al: Arrhythmogenic right ventricular dysplasia: A clinical model for the study of chronic ventricular tachycardia. Jpn Circ J 1984:48, 515–538
106. Blomstrom-Lundqvist C, Sabel KG, Olsson SB: A long-term follow-up of 15 patients with arrhythmogenic right ventricular dysplasia. Br Heart J 58:477–488, 1987
107. Leclercq JF, Coumel P: Characteristics, prognosis and treatment of the ventricular arrhythmias of right ventricular dysplasia. Eur Heart J 10:supp-D, 61–67, 1989
108. Marcus FI, Fontaine G, Frank R et al: Long term follow-up in patients with arrhythmogenic right ventricular disease. Eur Heart J 10:supp-D, 68–73, 1989

DEVICES FOR THE MANAGEMENT OF RHYTHM DISORDERS: PACEMAKERS AND DEFIBRILLATORS

CHAPTER 52
VOLUME 1

Jerry C. Griffin

Implantable devices have been used for the management of disorders of cardiac rhythm since 1958 when Elmquist and Senning[1] implanted the first battery-powered pulse generator in a patient with atrioventricular (AV) block. The first device with a permanent battery was constructed by Greatbatch and implanted in a patient in the United States by Chardack in the following year.[2] Over the next 5 years, implantable pacemakers became an accepted way of managing patients with symptomatic AV block. Since that time, improvements in pacemaker and electrode design have occurred, many as a result of the enormous advances occurring in integrated electronics. Progressively larger scale integration and the development of the microprocessor have allowed the incorporation of sufficient memory and computing capability within an implantable pacemaker to handle multiple and complex interactions between sensed and paced events. Parallel advances in battery construction and design have allowed these sophisticated electronics to be long lived and protected from the hostile environment of the human body. With appropriate patient selection and programming, present-day devices can restore the cardiac rhythm to normal or near-normal despite severe and permanent disorders of the cardiac rhythm.[3]

BRADYCARDIA
INDICATIONS

Because of recent concerns regarding the appropriate use of cardiac pacemakers, a joint committee of the American College of Cardiology and the American Heart Association drafted a summary of recommendations for appropriate indications for cardiac pacing.[4] The reader is referred to these recommendations as well as to the guidelines of the Department of Health and Human Services for Medicare use.[5] Both documents recognize the fact that indications for permanent pacing in an individual patient may not always be clear-cut.

PACING SYSTEM DESIGN AND MODES OF PACING
PULSE GENERATOR DESIGN

During the evolution of cardiac pacing systems, some of the most striking changes have been in the design of the electronic circuits. Early devices consisted of only a few hand-soldered transistors, resistors, and capacitors. Presently, highly advanced techniques of microcircuit fabrication are employed (Fig. 52.1). Many devices now contain a microprocessor similar in capability to that found in most personal computers. These highly integrated circuits may contain tens of thousands of transistors and other elements, all on a silicon chip less than half an inch square. The microprocessor performs the logical chores of the pacemaker, such as the storage and location of various programmable settings, the interaction between various sensed and paced events, and the control of communications with external programmers. It depends on a highly precise timer circuit based on a crystal oscillator. The most advanced of these devices also contain both of the types of memory found in computers. The first is "read only memory" (ROM), which usually contains the pacing algorithm. There is also a small quantity of volatile "read and write memory" or "random access memory" (RAM), in which temporary values are stored. These may consist of the present programmed settings, entered data such as model number, serial number, data of implant, and so on, or accumulated data such as the ratio of sensed vs. paced beats or the frequency of various modes of pacing within a multimodal system such as DDD. All of these circuit elements may be described as digital since they deal in numeric quantities such as time and numbers. Also necessary are certain analog elements such as filters and amplifiers for detecting intrinsic cardiac activity and output circuits for collecting a quantity of energy from the battery and delivering that energy to the myocardium in appropriate amounts at appropriate intervals as instructed by the microprocessor. All of these elements are mounted on a circuit board with a minimum of hand soldering. This board is then placed in a hermetically sealed metal box for protection against body fluids. Pacemaker circuits may be single or dual channel depending on whether they are capable of single- or dual-chamber performance. A DDD pacemaker, for example, contains analog elements for both atrial and ventricular channels as well as the digital logic elements necessary to integrate the functions of both.[3]

The ability of an implanted pulse generator to communicate with an external device or programmer has become standard. Generally this communication is bidirectional, allowing both the input of new programmed values that define the pulse generator's function as well as the output of measured or accumulated data. This is usually performed using a serial, binary, data stream that is alternately broadcast and detected by coils within both the pulse generator and the programmer head.[6]

At the present time, the lithium battery, specifically the lithium iodide cell, is the industry standard. It has proved to be a striking improvement over its predecessor, the mercury zinc battery, for three reasons: (1) it has a higher energy density, thus a longer functioning life; (2) it has a longer end-of-life decay; and (3) it may be hermetically sealed, preventing the influx of body fluids. These characteristics have contributed both to the longevity of the battery and to the likelihood that the pulse generator will function successfully until the end of battery life.[7-11]

ELECTRODE SYSTEM DESIGN

Electrodes may be broadly classified into two categories depending on whether the positive pole, or anode, is in contact with active myocardium. If so, the pacing system is termed *bipolar;* if not, it is termed *unipolar.* The case of the pulse generator generally serves as the anode in the unipolar design and is the site for returning current. In both systems, the cathode is in contact with the myocardium. Although popular for many years because of smaller lead size, the unipolar configuration has recently become less popular. New materials and lead designs have largely eliminated the advantages of size and handling characteristics, and long-term follow-up studies have demonstrated the absence of any superiority of unipolar pacing or sensing.[12] Therefore, in the face of a significant incidence of either symptomatic false inhibition due to skeletal muscle myopotentials or pacing of extracardiac muscle, the choice of a unipolar pacing system seems unwarranted.[13]

Like pulse generators, significant progress has also been made in electrode design. Polyurethane has largely replaced silicon rubber as an insulating material because of its greater structural strength (which allows a thinner coating and smaller lead) and its superior surface wetting properties (which allow two leads to slide against each other easily when wet). Problems with certain models of polyurethane leads have attracted a great deal of attention and concern, but these problems appear to be isolated and not a result of inherent defects in polyurethane in general.[14] The development of both passive and active fixation mechanisms such as tines and small endocardial screws have essentially eliminated electrode displacement.[15] New electrode materials featuring porous surfaces of platinum, carbon, and others are being evaluated. Early data from these trials suggest that chronic pacing with these leads at an output of 2.5 V to 3 V may provide as much safety margin as present leads offer with a standard 5-V pacemaker.[16]

ELECTROPHYSIOLOGY OF PACING AND SENSING

The passage of an electrical current through viable myocardium results in hyperpolarization of the cell membrane near the anode and the lowering of membrane potential in the vicinity of the cathode. If enough current is applied, depolarization of a portion of myocardium will occur. If a critical mass is brought to threshold, a propagated action potential will spread throughout the myocardium as a result of its syncytial nature. The magnitude of the stimulus necessary to produce a propagated depolarization is termed the *excitation threshold*. This is a reasonably stable factor that may be modified by certain metabolic and pharmacologic conditions. These include alterations of acid–base balance and changes in intracellular and extracellular content of electrolytes (principally sodium and potassium). Drugs generally have only very modest effects. In general, physiologic and pharmacologic factors probably cause the threshold to vary no more than 40% to 50% at most.

The measured excitation threshold is a function of the intensity of the electrical field generated by the stimulating pulse, which is in turn a result of the current density or the amount of current passed across the electrode per unit of its surface area. Thus, a larger electrode will require more total current in order to achieve the required current density for excitation. In a similar fashion, the development of an inexcitable fibrous capsule around the electrode results in a larger virtual electrode surface area, causing the current necessary to reach threshold to rise. This is likely to be the underlying mechanism for the development of electrode "exit block" in most patients. The other important factor in the determination of the excitation threshold is impulse duration. As impulse duration increases, the stimulus amplitude required for excitation decreases in an exponential fashion. However, beyond a pulse duration of approximately 2 msec, this curve becomes essentially flat (rheobase).[17,18]

Most implantable pulse generators are designed to supply a fixed output voltage, allowing the resistance of the electrode system to determine the current flow to the myocardium according to Ohm's law (Fig. 52.2). Pulse duration is usually programmable within a range of 0.1 msec to 2.5 msec. The standard pulse generator output is 5 V to 6 V but may be programmable within a range from 1.5 V to 10 V. A pulse generator should usually be programmed to provide approximately a 100% voltage safety margin. This allows the maintenance of pacing in the face of short-term fluctuations resulting from changes in physiology such as those described above (Fig. 52.3).

Pacemakers also have the capacity to detect intrinsic cardiac activity. Electrograms generated by the electrical activity of the heart are

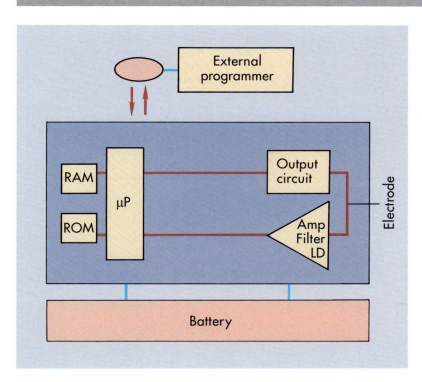

FIGURE 52.1 A modern cardiac pacemaker consists of analog and digital components, both of which are powered by a lithium battery and hermetically sealed within a metallic container (usually titanium). The microprocessor (μP) of the pacemaker can communicate with the external programmer and receive instructions that are held in volatile memory (RAM). The basic format of the pacing scheme is contained in nonvolatile memory (ROM). These elements constitute the digital portion, while the R wave detector system and output circuit are the analog elements. The R wave detection system generally consists of amplifier(s), band-pass filter(s), and level detector(s).

detected on the electrode system and amplified by the sensing circuits of the pacemaker. Amplification increases the low biologic voltages (millivolts) to a level commonly employed in electronic circuits (volts). This signal is then filtered to remove extraneous content such as environmental "noise," skeletal muscle activity, and T waves. Thus, the object of filtering is to produce a waveform that represents only local activation. The bandpass of the filter is selected to "pass" those frequencies and progressively attenuate all others. The portion of the waveform that represents local activation is the intrinsic deflection. Its slew rate or dV/dt can be measured clinically and is an index of frequency content. Slew rates of 0.5 V to 3 V/sec are optimal for most pulse generators. Complexes with slew rates lower than 0.5 V/sec may be substantially attenuated by the filters. Finally, the amplified, filtered complex is "sensed" if it is of a predetermined amplitude. The amplitude level for sensing may also be varied by programming.[19,20]

MODES OF CARDIAC PACING

The mode of pacing refers to the way in which the pacemaker interacts with the underlying cardiac rhythm. The various modes may be described by a shorthand code suggested by the Intersociety Commission for Heart Disease Resources (ICHD) report of 1983.[21] The basic code consists of three letters, the first of which refers to the chamber paced; the second, the chamber sensed; and the third, the response to a sensed event. The various modes are outlined in Table 52.1. They may be functionally divided according to whether the pacing is at a fixed rate simply becoming inhibited by faster intrinsic rates or whether they are rate responsive and thus have the capability to provide ventricular pacing in synchrony with an intrinsic atrial rhythm.

FIXED-RATE PACEMAKERS. The ventricular-inhibited pulse generator is the most commonly used of this group. It provides a single channel of operation, thus performing all pacing and sensing activity in one chamber using a single electrode. The ICHD designation is VVI, indicating a ventricular implantation with an inhibited response to a sensed ventricular event. The same pulse generator, if implanted in the atrium, would offer AAI pacing in a similar manner. The function of a pulse generator can be understood in more detail by examining its timing cycle (Fig. 52.4). The timing cycle of a single-chamber–inhibited pulse generator begins with either a sensed or a paced event. The initial portion of the cycle is the refractory period, during which the sensing

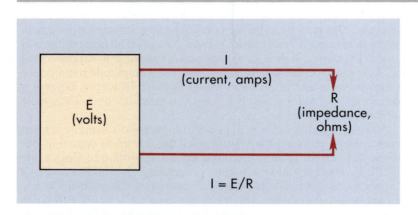

FIGURE 52.2 Ohm's law relates the current (in amperes) to the electromotive force (in volts) propelling that current and the resistance (in ohms) that tends to impede it. The battery of the pulse generator serves as the source of electromotive force, typically 5 V (programmable from 1.5 V to 10 V in some devices). Electrode system impedance may vary from 300 to 1000 ohms, resulting in stimulus currents of 5 mA to 15 mA.

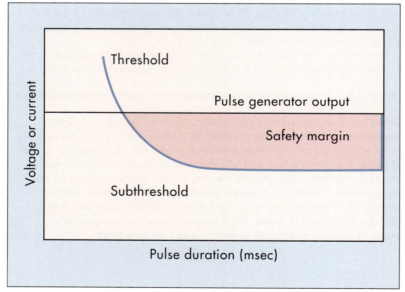

TABLE 52.1 ATTRIBUTES OF CURRENT MODES OF ARTIFICIAL CARDIAC PACING

Mode*	Paces Atrium	Paces Ventricle	Senses Atrium	Senses Ventricle	Tracks Atrium
AAI	Yes	No	Yes	No	
VVI	No	Yes	No	Yes	
DVI	Yes	Yes	No	Yes	No
DDI	Yes	Yes	Yes	Yes	No
VDD	No	Yes	Yes	Yes	Yes
DDD	Yes	Yes	Yes	Yes	Yes

* Chamber paced (*first letter*)—A, atrial; V, ventricular; D, both. Chamber sensed (*second letter*)—same as chamber paced. Response to a sensed event (*third letter*)—I, inhibited; T, triggered; D, both.

FIGURE 52.3 The bold line labeled "threshold" indicates the relationship between stimulus intensity (voltage and current) and stimulus duration. Capture may be obtained by applying a stimulus of any combination indicated by the threshold curve. The thin horizontal line is placed at the level of the output of the pulse generator, nominally 5 V. The shaded area, therefore, represents the margin of safety between pulse generator output and that stimulus intensity/duration required for capture. It should be noted that beyond a certain point, rheobase (generally 2 to 3 msec), no further extension of stimulus duration improves safety margin. Stimulus intensity/duration combinations falling below the bold line are subthreshold and will not result in capture of the myocardium.

amplifier is blinded to any electrical signals occurring on the electrode. This effectively prevents the sensing of any leftover current from the stimulus pulse (afterpotential) or ventricular repolarization. At the end of the pulse generator refractory period (usually 250 msec to 350 msec in duration), the amplifier is reactivated and the sensing period begins. If during this period an electrical event meets the amplitude and frequency criteria described above, it is sensed, the timing cycle is ended, and a new cycle is initiated. If no event is sensed before the pacemaker reaches the end of its escape interval (*i.e.*, the refractory period plus the sense interval), a pacing stimulus will be provided. The response to a sensed event determines whether the device operates in the inhibited or triggered mode. In the inhibited mode (VVI, AAI), the output stimulus is inhibited and the timing cycle is reinitiated. In the triggered mode (VVT, AAT), the occurrence of a sensed event causes the immediate release of a pacing stimulus and the reinitiation of the timing cycle.

AV sequential pacing may also be done in a fixed rate mode. The most common form is DVI in which the capacity for pacing both chambers is present but sensing occurs only on the ventricular channel. When sensing occurs on the ventricular channel, both atrial and ventricular channels are inhibited. DVI pacing may be in one of two forms, committed or noncommitted. The fundamental difference between these two is that in the committed mode the ventricular pulse is obligatory once the atrial pulse is delivered, thus sensing does not occur during the AV interval.[22] The DDI mode of pacing is similar to DVI in that tracking of atrial events at rates above the programmed rate does not occur, but unlike in DVI, sensing is present on the atrial channel, preventing atrial competition.[23]

RATE-RESPONSIVE PACING. Rate-responsive pacemakers (VDD, DDD) differ from fixed-rate devices in that sensing an event in the atrial channel causes or "triggers" an event on the ventricular channel after a period of delay. Such a pacemaker may (DDD) or may not (VDD) provide for pacing in both chambers as well. Timing cycles for such devices are much more complex, consisting of two channels of activity, the atrial and ventricular, linked by a third, the AV delay (see Fig. 52.3). In its simplest form, there are refractory and sensing periods in

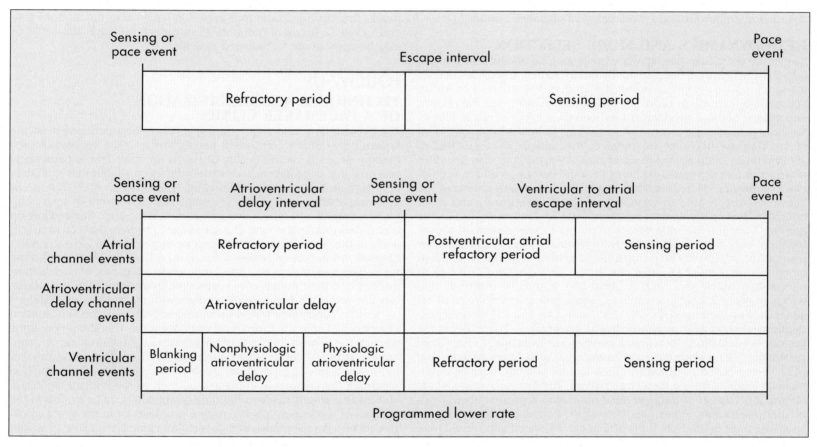

FIGURE 52.4 The upper bar is a very simple timing diagram representative of that of a single chamber pulse generator. The cycle is initiated by a stimulus or pace event that is immediately followed by a period of refractoriness. Following refractoriness, the device initiates a sensing period that ends at the conclusion of the escape interval with a pace event. The sense event may be interrupted at any time by an intrinsic depolarization reinitiating the cycle. The more complex timing diagram is that of a dual-chamber pacemaker. Either a pace or sense event occurring in the atrium initiates an AV delay. This period is concluded by a ventricular stimulus or may be interrupted by sensing an intrinsic ventricular event. Refractory periods are initiated in both channels following either. These are in turn followed by sense periods in both chambers. As with a single chamber device, the sense period is concluded by a stimulus event, in this case, in the atrium. The escape interval, however, consists not of the total atrial-atrial interval but the ventricular to atrial interval (atrial to atrial interval or lower rate cycle length minus the AV delay), which is the fundamental interval for timing for most dual-chamber pacing systems. The timing system illustrated also incorporates "nonphysiologic AV delay" or "ventricular safety" pacing. The ventricular channel AV delay period is divided into three phases. First is the blanking period, which is a time of absolute refractoriness. The next block of time, ending 100 msec to 110 msec after the atrial recycling event, is termed the *nonphysiologic AV delay period*. Events sensed during this time will initiate a stimulus event at the conclusion of the nonphysiologic AV delay phase and recycle the atrial and ventricular channels. The final portion of the AV delay is the physiologic period.

The rationale is that events sensed during this period are not the result of normal conduction of the preceding atrial event (sensed or initiated) to the ventricles. Therefore, it may represent ectopic ventricular activity or cross-talk. Since it may be cross-talk, stimulation must occur. Since it may also be true ventricular depolarization, stimulation should occur earlier (at the end of the nonphysiologic AV delay period) rather than later (at the programmed AV delay time) to minimize pacing during the vulnerable period. Events sensed during this time will result in inhibition of the ventricular stimulus and recycling of the pacemaker. An absence of a sensed event will result in a ventricular stimulus at the appropriate programmed AV delay.

both channels, with the atrial channel being refractory throughout the AV delay while the ventricular channel generally is not. The ventricular channel does undergo a brief period of refractoriness coincident with and for a short period after (15 msec to 50 msec) the atrial stimulus. The DDD pacemaker functions as an AV sequential device, pacing both the atria and ventricles when no intrinsic activity is detected on either lead. If spontaneous atrial activity exceeds the basic rate of the pacemaker, it is sensed and will, after an AV delay period, trigger a ventricular pace event. In such a way the pacemaker will "track" the spontaneous atrial rhythm until its cycle length is just shorter than the pacemaker's total atrial channel refractory period. At that point, only every other atrial event will be sensed and in effect a 2:1 ventricular response will occur. Some devices, in order to prevent this rapid deceleration during sinus tachycardia, provide a more complex upper rate structure, allowing a Wenckebach type of behavior.[24]

Certain new pacemakers also feature rate responsiveness based not on atrial activity but rather on some independent indicator of exercise.[25] These devices may use physiologic markers such as shortening of the QT interval, increases in respiratory rate, increases in central blood temperature, or skeletal muscle activity. Although largely investigational at present, they may, in the future, offer a simple, single chamber alternative to more complex dual chamber systems.

HEMODYNAMICS AND MODE SELECTION

Single-rate ventricular pacing, while preventing significant bradycardia, falls short of restoring the cardiac rhythm to normal. It provides neither for synchronous activity between the atria and ventricles nor for an appropriate increase in heart rate with exercise. Although the relative importance of these two factors has been the subject of much debate, for most patients, rate responsiveness seems to be the more important factor. They are, of course, interrelated. For example, as rate increases, AV synchrony becomes more significant. AV synchrony also becomes more important as ventricular filling pressure decreases and as ventricular compliance decreases. Rate responsiveness is less critical in the individual who is able to vary stroke volume significantly and more critical in those patients who function with very limited stroke volume reserve.[26] Despite the wide variety of pacing modes described above, basically only three exist in hardware form: (1) the single-chamber pacemaker, which may be programmed to either triggered or inhibited mode and implanted in either the atrium or ventricle; (2) the DDD pacemaker, which uses both an atrial and ventricular electrode and which, in general, contains within its programming repertoire all of the lesser modes such as VDD, DVI, VVI, and AAI; and (3) the independently rate responsive, or sensor-based, pacemaker. Therefore, at the time of implantation, four broad choices are available: (1) an atrial pacemaker, (2) a ventricular pacemaker, (3) a DDD pacemaker, and (4) a sensor-based pacemaker. Three factors in large measure determine the optimal device for a given patient. The first is the status of the atrium. If persistent or frequent atrial fibrillation is present, then a ventricular pacemaker, either fixed-rate (VVI) or independently rate responsive, must be chosen. If the atrium can be paced and sensed, one must next consider the need for concomitant ventricular pacing. If AV block is persistently or intermittently present, then pacing in the ventricle is required. However, if it is absent, then atrial pacing (AAI) may be quite effective, particularly in patients having sinus node dysfunction, with primarily sinus pauses and sinus bradycardia. Atrial pacing in this group provides an inexpensive, simple, noncompetitive form of pacing that prevents symptoms and provides AV synchrony as well. If the atrium can be paced and sensed and AV block is present, then a DDD pacemaker can be used. This device will be most effective if the sinus rate (and thereby atrial) increases normally with exercise. In patients lacking a normal sinus response, a sensor-based rate-responsive pacemaker can be considered as an alternative approach. The factors listed above only determine the optimal pacing system. Other factors must also be considered before deciding whether an optimal system is warranted. These include the status of ventricular function and filling pressures; the nature, frequency, and duration of both bradyarrhythmias and concomitant tachyarrhythmias; and any intercurrent medical problems. At present, there are no simple or objective tests that allow us to make these decisions. They must be based on medical judgments formed after consideration of the factors outlined above.[26]

PACEMAKER IMPLANTATION

Specific and comprehensive details of pacemaker implantation are beyond the scope of this chapter, and the reader is referred elsewhere.[27] However, it is important to know that pacemaker implantation is a highly specialized procedure involving the implantation of foreign bodies in both the subcutaneous tissues and in the vascular system. Much attention should be given to operative technique and sterility. One should strive for the same level of sterile environment used for other cardiovascular operative procedures. Of course, this must be balanced against the requirements for good fluoroscopic imaging and electrophysiologic testing, which are usually absent in the operating room. Pacemaker implantation involves multiple skills, both surgical and electrophysiologic. It may be performed by a cardiologist and a surgeon or by either alone if he is willing to learn the extra skills that are required. Postimplant care dictates a period of continuous ECG monitoring by individuals well versed in pacemaker function. In general, 36 to 72 hours of monitoring is prudent, although shorter stays may be appropriate for selected patients.[21]

FOLLOW-UP
TECHNIQUES AND ORGANIZATION OF A PACEMAKER CLINIC

The prescription, selection, and implantation of a permanent pacing system only initiates permanent pacing therapy. The success of such therapy depends on the quality of follow-up care. This is particularly true now that pacemakers have extraordinary capabilities for modification of their function by programming.[28] In order to make full use of these capabilities and avoid the complications inherent in such complexity, careful and interactive follow-up is necessary. Such follow-up is best delivered in the form of a specialized program that caters specifically to the pacemaker patient. Such a program would have a number of goals, among them patient education, record keeping, monitoring for pacing system abnormalities, differential diagnosis of such abnormalities and their noninvasive correction, detection of the end of battery life, and a general periodic contact with the health care system.[29]

Ideally, pacemaker follow-up should begin before the implantation of a pacemaker in the form of patient education. This should continue through the in-hospital phase of pacemaker implantation and throughout the patient's subsequent course. Much in the way of pacemaker follow-up depends on accurate record keeping. Specific information regarding the equipment implanted, as well as the implant technique and measurements made at the time of implant, may be critical in the analysis of subsequent pacing system problems or in the event of device recalls. A major value of a pacemaker clinic is its ability to assimilate and maintain such a record system. Obviously, the principal purpose of a pacemaker clinic is to monitor the patient periodically for evidence of pacing system malfunctions, the annual risk of which is 4% to 8%. Preferably, problems will be detected prior to having caused clinical events. Once problems are detected, the pacemaker clinic may play a critical role in determining the exact nature of a malfunction and, in the majority of patients, in correcting it using programmability. A traditional and important role of pacemaker follow-up is the extension of pulse generator life by periodically monitoring it for evidence of battery depletion. In this way, elective replacement is avoided and the maximum safe use of the battery is obtained. Although an important function of pacemaker follow-up, battery depletion is now a less frequent event than other causes of pacing system malfunction.[30]

In general, two techniques are used in pacemaker follow-up, clinical evaluation and telephone surveillance. Clinical evaluation allows a much more detailed examination. The patient can be questioned regarding symptoms and the physical site of the pacemaker can be examined. Interval measurements, complete telemetry information, pacing thresholds, and sensing thresholds can be obtained, and various provocative maneuvers can be performed. These allow a much more detailed and sensitive evaluation for underlying pacing system problems, which might not be detected during a brief electrocardiographic recording.

Telephone surveillance is particularly useful for the detection of battery depletion and clinical problems of the pacemaker system that are sufficient to be manifest in the electrocardiogram. In addition, with newer pulse generators, measured and telemetry values may also be transmitted via the telephone, allowing more extensive pacing system evaluation. The obvious advantages of transtelephonic surveillance are that it is efficient and inexpensive both for the patient and for the health care system. It is especially useful in those elderly patients for whom it is not easy to travel long distances to a pacemaker clinic facility. Unfortunately, it as yet does not allow the sort of interactive evaluation of programmable devices that can be performed in person. Likewise, if problems are detected, they cannot be corrected by programming. An effective pacemaker follow-up program should therefore offer both periodic clinic evaluation and interim telephone surveillance.

It is necessary that the clinic have certain specialized equipment for pacemaker evaluation. A three-channel electrocardiograph is preferable, and some form of precise digital interval counter is mandatory. A storage oscilloscope may be extremely useful for recording the pacemaker stimulus artifact. This may indicate electrode fractures, insulation defects, and other problems. Programmers and telemetry receivers are necessary for all of the types of pacemakers in the clinic. For nonprogrammable pacemakers and other specialized circumstances, it may be useful to have a temporary pulse generator for pacemaker inhibition by chest wall stimulation. Equipment must be available and personnel trained in techniques for cardiopulmonary resuscitation. No pacemaker evaluation, especially one involving pacemaker reprogramming, should be performed in locations where these are unavailable. In addition to the equipment described above, the clinic should have access to other diagnostic modalities, such as fluoroscopy, echocardiography, Holter monitoring, and exercise electrocardiography. The latter studies may be particularly useful in the delineation of problems with rate-responsive pacing systems.

It is difficult to make specific recommendations with regard to the frequency of pacemaker follow-up. Many factors affect not only the frequency of follow-up but also the partition of follow-up between clinic and telephone surveillance (Table 52.2). In general, problems are more frequent early in the life of a pacemaker system and as it nears its end of life.[30] Follow-up should be arranged accordingly. It is our practice to follow patients more closely in the first year and after the third year of implantation. Because of a greater likelihood of pacing system dysfunction and the greater need for programming adjustment, dual-chamber pacemakers generally require more frequent follow-up than single-chamber systems, particularly in the first several months when the basic pacing parameters are being determined. Thus, it is clear that frequency of follow-up should not be predicted solely on the expectations of battery or pulse generator performance but rather on that of the entire pacing system.

THE PACEMAKER PRESCRIPTION

The pacemaker prescription is that set of programmed values chosen for a particular patient at a particular time. In general, certain programming changes should be made in the pacing system at the time of implant, in order to better assess the pacing system during postimplant telemetry monitoring. Patients are seen prior to discharge, and the pulse generator is reprogrammed to compensate for expected physiologic changes that occur early in the postimplant period. At 1 month after implantation, it can be assumed that stable functioning has been reached in most patients, and this is confirmed by threshold and sensitivity testing. If these values are acceptable, then final programming for long-term functioning is performed. The patient is rechecked 3 to 6 months later to confirm that long-term values are stable, and any necessary, final programming changes are made. Obviously, changes in the pacemaker prescription may also occur at any time a problem is detected with the pacing system. The reader is referred to recent reviews regarding the diagnosis and management of specific pacing system problems.[29,31,32]

THE IMPLANT PRESCRIPTION. At the time of implantation, changes are made in the pulse generator to allow observation of pacing function. When possible, a pacing rate is chosen to allow evidence of both pacing and sensing. Output is adjusted to maintain a wider than usual safety margin to allow for any changes in threshold that may occur early after lead implantation. Sensitivity is adjusted to allow an extra safety margin as well. For dual-chamber pacemakers, the AV delay is sometimes intentionally shortened to result in more ventricular pacing. The patient is brought to the clinic prior to discharge where thresholds for pacing and sensing are determined.

If the system is to be used in the DDD mode (or some DVI, DDI, or VDD modes), susceptibility to cross-talk and pacemaker-mediated tachycardia are sought. Cross-talk is the sensing of the atrial stimulus on the ventricular channel, resulting in false inhibition of ventricular output. This is potentially the most hazardous complication of DDD pacing, since it can be manifest as a paced atrial rhythm with the absence of ventricular pacing stimuli despite ventricular asystole (Fig. 52.5). Cross-talk may be provoked by increasing both the atrial output and the ventricular sensitivity. It may be prevented by decreasing one or both of these parameters or by increasing the duration of the blanking period if this is programmable.

Pacemaker-mediated tachycardia (PMT) results from retrograde conduction to the atrium of a stimulated ventricular complex. This atrial activity is then sensed on the atrial channel and a subsequent stimulus triggered to the ventricle, repeating the cycle (Fig. 52.6). This may be initiated in one of several ways (Table 52.3). For testing in the clinic, one method is to decrease the atrial output during AV sequential pacing sufficient to result in transient atrial noncapture. This sets up the conditions for retrograde conduction to the atrium, if capability for such conduction is present. It may also be prevented in several ways, depending on the method of initiation (Table 52.4). In general, extension of the post-ventricular portion of the atrial refractory period (PVARP) is effective in all cases, but at the expense of the maximum tracking rate. If PMT results from ventricular premature beats, it may be prevented by automatic refractory period extension following ventricular premature complexes (available in some models). On the other hand, this technique will not prevent PMT resulting from events such as pectoral muscle oversensing on the atrial channel since the events in

TABLE 52.2 FACTORS AFFECTING THE TYPE AND FREQUENCY OF FOLLOW-UP

Pulse generator performance
   Complexity
   Programmed settings and configuration
   Years since implant
   Performance record:
      Individual pacemaker
      Total model group (longevity, recall)
Electrode performance
   Years since implant
   Performance record
Patient characteristics
   Degree of pacemaker dependence
   Age
   Mobility
   Economics

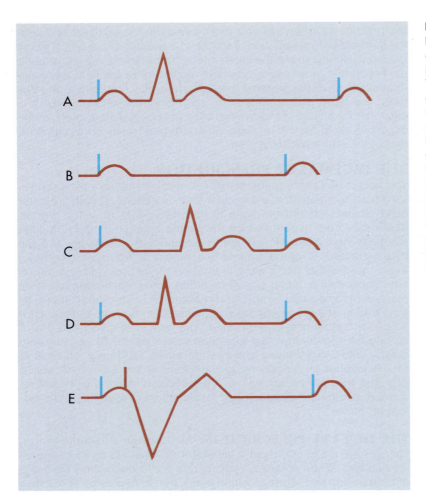

FIGURE 52.5 Various manifestations of cross-talk. **A.** A normally functioning DDD pacing system, illustrating atrial pacing with a normally conducted QRS complex occurring slightly prior to the end of the AV delay. A normal VA time is illustrated between the QRS complex and the subsequent atrial stimulus. **B.** The most devastating manifestation of cross-talk: atrial stimulation with a complete absence of either normally initiated or paced ventricular activity. Cross-talk is suggested by the shortening of the interval between atrial stimuli. Measurement of this interval will demonstrate that it is only slightly longer than the programmed VA time. **C.** Cross-talk is also present in this example; however, AV conduction is present although impaired, resulting in a longer atrial stimulus to the R interval than the programmed AV delay allows (indicating the absence of the ventricular stimulus). Cross-talk is further manifest by the abnormal VA time for the values programmed. **D.** Here is illustrated the most subtle form of cross-talk. AV conduction is normal with a PR interval that would inhibit ventricular pacing. The only clue to the presence of cross-talk is the shortened VA time. **E.** Cross-talk in a pacing system featuring a nonphysiologic AV delay or ventricular safety pacing. Cross-talk is suggested by dual-chamber pacing with a shortened AV delay.

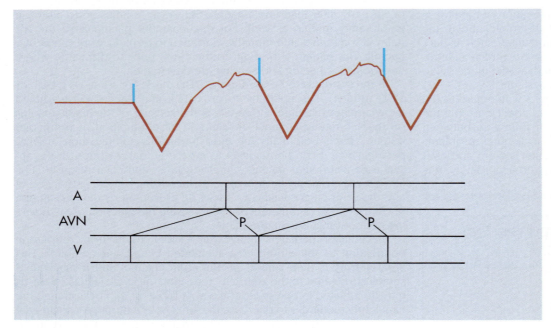

FIGURE 52.6 Pacemaker-mediated tachycardia. Following a ventricular (V) paced beat there is retrograde conduction through the AV conduction system (AVN), resulting in retrograde capture of the atria (A). This atrial activity is sensed, triggering a stimulus (P) to the ventricle. Once established, this system is self-perpetuating and will result in sustained tachycardia as long as retrograde atrial activation persists.

TABLE 52.3 COMMON METHODS OF INITIATION OF PACEMAKER-MEDIATED TACHYCARDIA

Retrograde atrial activation
    Ventricular premature beat
    Junctional premature beat
    Transient ventricular pacing without atrial pacing
    Low rate pacing in VDD mode
    VOO pacing in magnet mode
    Echo beats associated with abnormal AV pathway
Atrial sensing of electromagnetic interference
Pectoral muscle oversensing
External electromagnetic interference

question will not be perceived by the pacemaker as ventricular premature beats. Some devices contain algorithms for the recognition and termination of PMTs after a brief period by intermittently failing to trigger a ventricular stimulus after an atrial sensed event. Owing to the nature of PMT, a single such cycle (or placing a magnet over the pacemaker briefly) is sufficient for its termination.

THE PREDISCHARGE PRESCRIPTION. Output on both channels should be adjusted to a wide safety margin to allow for physiologic changes that can occur in the first 1 to 2 weeks after electrode implantation. A similar approach is taken with sensitivity programming. The pacemaker should be programmed to facilitate control by the patient's underlying rhythm—encouraging sinus rhythm in VVI mode, for example, by programming to rates less than typical and to adequate sinus rates, or in DDD mode by providing sufficient AV delay to allow normal AV conduction, or lower rate limits that allow VDD mode pacing. Patients should be questioned regarding exercise tolerance and symptoms during exercise. If there is evidence that the patient is likely to exceed the upper rate limit and develop pacemaker block, then additional upper rate capability should be programmed if possible. In some patients this may not be possible since it would require shortening the post-ventricular atrial refractory period, thus increasing the vulnerability to PMT. It is important to remember that it is only the post-ventricular portion of the atrial refractory period that protects against PMT. However, since the total atrial refractory period or upper tracking cycle length is the sum of the AV delay and post-ventricular atrial refractory period, it may also be reduced by shortening the AV delay.

This will allow higher upper rate limits, without sacrificing the post-ventricular portion of the refractory period and increasing the susceptibility to PMT. This may be a critical improvement if it increases the upper rate limit from 125 to 150 beats per minute in a patient whose maximum sinus rate is typically 130 to 140 beats per minute.

THE PACEMAKER PRESCRIPTION DURING STABLE FUNCTION. At each clinic evaluation, the patient must be assessed for evidence of problems. Changes in threshold may be compensated for by programming of either pulse duration or amplitude. As discussed above, the most efficient pulse durations are in the range of 1 msec; therefore amplitude should be adjusted accordingly (Fig. 52.7). When available, bipolar/unipolar or configuration programmability may also be useful in seeking an acceptable threshold.[12] Oversensing in unipolar systems most commonly results from skeletal muscle sensing. This may be dealt with in one of several ways: by configuration programming if present, by mode programming (VVT or AAT rather than VVI), or by sensitivity programming. Frequently, sensitivity programming alone is inadequate to deal with symptomatic pectoral muscle inhibition since the inhibiting skeletal muscle electromyograms may be larger than the R waves.[13] Although rare, oversensing may occur with bipolar electrodes. It is less frequently correctable by programmability since it is usually the result of an electrode fracture or other structural problem. Undersensing may be improved by increasing sensitivity levels or by configuration programming if available. Extracardiac muscle stimulation occurring at the case of the pulse generator of a unipolar system may be corrected by configuration programming. Output programming

TABLE 52.4 PROGRAMMMING AND THE CORRECTION OF PACEMAKER-MEDIATED TACHYCARDIA

Method	Corrects	Problems
Longer PVARP	All causes of PMT	Limits upper tracking rate
Automatic lengthening of PVARP	PMT due to premature beats	Does not correct other causes
Automatic detection and termination of PMT	All causes of PMT	Will not detect if less than URL. Allows short periods of PMT.
Atrial synchronous activity in DDD	PMT due to atrial oversensing	Does not correct other causes

(PMT, pacemaker-mediated tachycardia; PVARP, post-ventricular atrial refractory period; URL, upper rate limit)

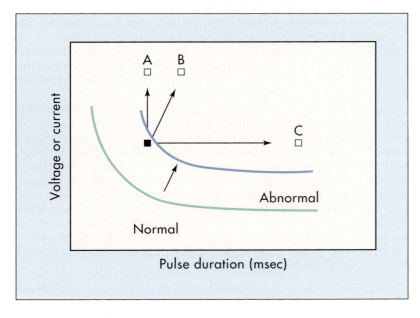

FIGURE 52.7 Several approaches to a patient with rising thresholds. The initial curve (*normal*) has shifted to one (*abnormal*) requiring more energy for ventricular capture. One might restore a safety margin by programming amplitude (A); however, this would leave the patient on the very steep portion of the strength duration curve and be relatively inefficient with regard to energy conservation. Programming only pulse duration (C) would not achieve an adequate safety margin owing to reaching rheobase. The best approach (B) would result from increasing both amplitude and pulse duration, resulting in an adequate safety margin at an efficient range of pulse duration.

may be effective if the threshold for stimulating skeletal muscle is significantly greater than that for cardiac muscle. In general, amplitude programming is more effective than pulse duration programming in this regard.

Pacemaker syndrome is a loose symptom-complex manifest by varying degrees of awareness of pacing.[33] It commonly occurs in patients with normal or near-normal ventricular function, in those with intermittent pacing and frequent transitions from paced to nonpaced rhythm, and in those with retrograde conduction. The exact mechanism is not clearly defined but appears to be more complex than the simple hydraulic problems of the loss of atrial synchrony. Symptoms with ventricular pacing can range from mild awareness to complete syncope. The syndrome is most effectively dealt with by replacement of the ventricular pacemaker by a dual-chamber system, preferably DDD. In some cases, lowering the ventricular escape rate may be helpful by reducing the frequency of transitions between paced and nonpaced rhythms, preserving pacing only for those periods of severe asystole. Alternatively, some patients may be helped by pacing at a faster rate to achieve persistent pacing.

Elevations of measured threshold may result from exit block, electrode/connector discontinuities, or insulation defects. Accompanying oversensing suggests an electrode problem while undersensing is more often seen with peri-electrode fibrosis. Telemetry information such as lead impedance and current drain may also be helpful in reaching a diagnosis. In general, with high thresholds due to peri-electrode fibrosis, lead impedance is normal and the voltage and current at threshold are both high. With disruption of the electrode conductor, impedance is high, as is the voltage at threshold. However, because the defect is one of an impedance to current flow, the current at threshold is normal. With an insulation defect, the opposite is true; impedance is low due to short circuiting through the defect, allowing a normal threshold voltage to result in an increased current flow.

TACHYCARDIAS
INDICATIONS
EVOLUTION OF PACING FOR TACHYCARDIAS

Pacing for the control of tachycardia is intertwined with the earliest uses of cardiac pacing. Ventricular tachycardia and fibrillation occurring in the setting of bradycardia secondary to complete AV block was noted by Zoll and co-workers[34] as a cause of Stokes-Adams syncope. These arrhythmias could be prevented by restoring the cardiac rate to normal levels. Sowton and colleagues[35] noted that in patients with normal heart rates, ventricular ectopy could be suppressed by pacing at more rapid rates. McCallister and co-workers[36] implanted a permanent pacemaker to achieve this end. The current role for pacing in tachycardias stems from reports in 1967 by Massumi[37] and Durrer[38] and their associates regarding the role of premature extrastimuli in the initiation and termination of reentrant tachyarrhythmias. This not only indicated the potential efficacy in spontaneous arrhythmias but provided the tools for more detailed electrophysiologic testing. In the same year, Haft and co-workers[39] reported the first successful termination of atrial flutter by cardiac pacing. Atrial rather than ventricular overdrive was used by Kastor[40] and Cohen[41] and their associates for the suppression of ventricular arrhythmias. Lister and colleagues[42] expanded on the report of Haft describing the termination of a variety of supraventricular tachycardias. Bennett and Pentecost[43] reported the first successful terminations of clinically occurring ventricular tachycardia. Slow asynchronous pacing at rates well below that of the tachycardia were used by Hunt and associates[44] in a method of arrhythmia termination that they termed *underdrive*. This method was attractive since it could easily be implemented using standard implantable pacemakers activated by a magnet. Ryan and colleagues[45] took advantage of this capability using implanted pacemakers for the long-term treatment of a patient with supraventricular tachycardia and the Wolff-Parkinson-White syndrome. In 1971, the externally controlled radiofrequency pacemaker, designed specifically for arrhythmia therapy, was used by Urbaszek and co-workers[46] for ventricular tachycardia and by Dreifus and associates[47] for supraventricular tachycardia. Moss and Rivers[48] modified this technique for use in patients with ventricular tachycardia. The next increase in complexity was reported by Fisher and colleagues,[49] who used a permanently implanted pacemaker that could be activated by the application of a magnet to control ventricular tachycardia using brief bursts of rapid pacing. This type of device was shortly replaced by multiprogrammable pacemakers capable of automatically detecting and terminating tachycardias with bursts of pacing. Early experience with these devices was reported by Fisher and colleagues[50] and by Griffin and Mason.[51] Krikler and co-workers[52] used a pacemaker that automatically employed the underdrive technique responding to both bradyarrhythmias and tachyarrhythmias with asynchronous normal rate pacing, the dual-demand pacemaker. Limited flexibility for adaptation of the termination pattern was incorporated in a device that allowed scanning of a portion of diastole by single or double extrastimuli.[53] Further flexibility has recently been provided by pacemakers capable of automatically adapting the termination cycle length to the underlying tachycardia cycle length (adaptive behavior).

The problem of sudden cardiac death has been the focus of a decade of basic and clinical device research. A new tool to aid in the management of such patients is the automatically activated, implanted defibrillator (AICD). This device is capable of detecting the occurrence of ventricular tachycardia or fibrillation (VT/VF) and restoring normal rhythm by means of single or repetitive DC shocks. Clinical use began in 1980,[54] and preliminary results indicate that it may be an important adjunct in the therapy of life-threatening ventricular tachyarrhythmias.[55-57] Using a level of energy intermediate between pacing and defibrillation, Zipes and associates[58] demonstrated the successful termination of ventricular tachycardia using synchronous cardioversion.

INDICATIONS FOR PACING IN SUPRAVENTRICULAR TACHYCARDIAS

A number of the more common paroxysmal supraventricular tachycardias are amenable to pacing termination including AV nodal reentry, AV reentry incorporating either manifest or concealed accessory pathways, atrial flutter, and intra-atrial reentry.[59] The principal question in pacing for supraventricular tachycardia is usually at what point should such an expensive and aggressive therapy be applied. Certainly those patients who are effectively treated with drugs that are safe and well tolerated are not generally considered candidates. Pacing is indicated in those patients with recurrent sustained tachycardia in whom symptomatic episodes are not prevented by drug therapy or in whom drug therapy is attendant with unacceptable side effects. In general, it is our practice to use pacing in such patients, when it is effective, rather than AV conduction system ablation, since both would require a pacemaker and a tachycardia-terminating device does not require destruction of the conduction system. Other patients who may be considered for pacing therapy are those with problematic tachycardia that can be controlled with drug therapy but who prefer freedom from drug side effects, a regimen of daily medication, and periodic sustained tachycardias, since even successful drug therapy is occasionally attendant with a recurrence of arrhythmia.[60]

Pacing may be contraindicated in some patients with supraventricular tachycardia. Patients with any form of AV conduction having excessively short effective refractory periods are at risk from very rapid conduction during atrial fibrillation.[61] Pacing for arrhythmia termination may be associated with the induction of atrial fibrillation,[59] thereby, in such patients, converting a benign though bothersome rhythm to one that is potentially life-threatening. These patients may also be placed at risk by 1:1 AV conduction of rapid atrial pacing during termination attempts. Thus, it is imperative that all candidates for pacing therapy of supraventricular tachycardia have invasive electrophysiologic study to define the arrhythmia mechanism and characterize its electrophysiology.

INDICATIONS FOR PACING IN VENTRICULAR TACHYCARDIA

Indications for device therapy in patients with ventricular arrhythmias are less well established. At the present time, pacing as a sole modality cannot be recommended on any wide scale because of the problems of arrhythmia acceleration. Pacing, particularly with externally activated devices, has been used as an effective therapy in drug-resistant patients who have infrequent and well-tolerated arrhythmias.[62] It has also been used as an adjunct to primary drug or surgical therapy as a means of serial assessment, and in control of intercurrent arrhythmia.[63]

INDICATIONS FOR THE AUTOMATIC IMPLANTED DEFIBRILLATOR

The automatic implantable defibrillator plays a significant and expanding role in the therapy of recurrent ventricular arrhythmias. In devising therapy for patients with life-threatening VT/VF, the AICD is most often chosen to play a supporting role. Rather than being the sole or primary treatment, it is most often employed as a "safety net" for those patients in whom VT/VF recurrence is likely despite our best efforts at drug, ablation, and/or surgical therapy (Table 52.5). The likelihood of success of the AICD as a sole therapy of VT/VF is inversely proportional to the frequency of arrhythmia episodes. Shocks are delivered either with the patient awake (most often with VT) or unconscious (very fast VT or VF). Neither condition is acceptable if episodes are frequent. Awake shocks are very uncomfortable, while frequent episodes of unconsciousness pose even greater problems such as falling, injury, and so on. Finally, device longevity may be seriously impacted if frequent shocks are required. Thus, another modality, most often drugs, is usually provided as a primary therapy to reduce as much as possible the frequency of arrhythmia. In selected cases, one may consider the use of both an implanted pacemaker and defibrillator. The combination of pacing or cardioversion and defibrillation in a single unit will allow much more flexibility and wider application of devices for ventricular tachycardia. The majority of episodes can then be terminated using low-energy techniques, reserving defibrillation only for acceleration or primary ventricular fibrillation.

New indications will continue to be defined and old indications redefined as we gain more experience with the device and its implantation, as refinements occur in the devices themselves, and as other therapies gain or lose favor in the treatment of life-threatening arrhythmias.

Certain other clinical findings may also complicate use of the AICD. Nonsustained ventricular tachycardia episodes of greater than 5 to 10 seconds can meet detection criteria and cause the unit to charge. Once "charge-up" begins, the unit is committed to shock, even if the arrhythmia terminates spontaneously. This can result in frequent, unnecessary shocks, prematurely depleting the battery and causing patient discomfort. Uncontrolled atrial arrhythmias, paroxysmal supraventricular tachycardia, and atrial fibrillation/flutter may also be a cause of unnecessary shocks. In patients with good functional capacity, sinus tachycardia with exercise can also provoke the device to shock unnecessarily. Slow ventricular tachycardia, of rates less than the tachycardia detect rate, will not be terminated and will remain a clinical problem. These considerations do not constitute contraindications to the device necessarily, since many of them can be manipulated through appropriate drug therapy or the use of other than standard rate units. It is important to anticipate them, however, in order to secure a unit with the proper characteristics prior to implantation. When the cardiac drug regimen is changed, it is important to determine the effects, if any, on sinus rate or ventricular response (if in atrial fibrillation) and on defibrillation threshold.

PACING SYSTEM DESIGN AND MODES OF PACING

GENERAL CONCEPTS

The effectiveness of pacing therapy depends on the presence of a reentrant arrhythmia. Since these arrhythmias result from an advancing wavefront circling a functional or anatomical obstacle, they may be terminated by depolarizing a portion of the loop ahead of the advancing wavefront. For a stimulus to be successful, it must be able to enter the reentrant loop (Fig. 52.8). The factors that determine this are the refractoriness, conduction characteristics, and distance between the site of pacing and the reentrant loop, as well as characteristics of the reentrant loop itself.[64] Thus the period in the cycle between the moment of refractoriness and the subsequent depolarization is termed the *window of termination*. In general the duration of the window is directly proportional to the cycle length of the tachycardia. If a single stimulus is unable to penetrate this window, the application of successive stimuli may be able to do so. Successively closer stimuli allow for peeling back of refractoriness of intervening tissue, thus enhancing penetration of a critically timed stimulus into the termination zone. Trains of stimuli may gradually push the site of collision toward the reentrant circuit, eventually allowing entry into it. Thus, depending on the nature of the arrhythmia, single stimuli, serial extrastimuli of decreasing cycle length, and/or longer series of extrastimuli of fixed cycle length may be effective. In general, the slower the tachycardia, the more likely that it can be terminated and by fewer pacing stimuli at longer cycle lengths. The closer the electrode to the reentrant circuit, the more likely fewer stimuli will be successful. The comparative effectiveness of single and multiple stimuli have been studied for both ventricular and supraventricular tachycardias.[59,65] Clearly, "trains" or "bursts" of rapid pacing are the most effective. Unfortunately, they are also attendant with a significant complication, a tendency to accelerate the tachycardia or cause fibrillation. For most supraventricular tachycardias (except for some previously mentioned patients with the Wolff-Parkinson-White syndrome), this is usually clinically inconsequential, is of brief duration, and quickly converts spontaneously to sinus rhythm. In ventricular tachycardia it occurs in perhaps 10% to 20% of episodes and has, of course, catastrophic consequences.

Defibrillation converts arrhythmias by the simultaneous depolarization of all nonrefractory tissue, allowing a nonsynchronous repolariza-

TABLE 52.5 POTENTIAL APPLICATIONS FOR THE AICD

Failure of Diagnosis	Failure of Therapy	Demonstration of Risk Despite Best Efforts at Therapy
Arrhythmia not induced with programmed stimulation or observed during monitoring following an episode of documented life-threatening ventricular arrhythmia	Clinical recurrence of VT/VF on a drug predicted to be effective by electrophysiology testing Clinical recurrence of VT/VF on amiodarone Clinical recurrence of VT/VF following catheter or surgical ablation	Inducible VT despite adequate drug levels of the most effective Type I drug available (amiodarone excluded) Recurrent nonsustained VT in the presence of amiodarone in a patient with LV dysfunction and history of sudden death or syncope Inducible VT/VF following catheter or surgical ablation

tion, which in turn allows the dominant pacemaker to achieve control of the rhythm.[66] As such, it differs from pacing in that it is a "final common pathway" form of therapy effective against all types of arrhythmia. Obviously, if the source of tachycardia is an automatic focus, termination may be very short-lived, perhaps only a cycle or so. Cardioversion is less well understood, uses less energy than defibrillation, and probably has a mechanism of termination intermediate between pacing and defibrillation. It is effective only against ventricular tachycardia and like pacing tends to become less effective as tachycardia cycle length decreases. It also shares with pacing a significant incidence of acceleration of arrhythmia or fibrillation.[58]

Many implanted devices are designed to detect the occurrence of tachycardia automatically and respond with an attempt at termination. Early devices use rate as the sole criterion for this, and as a result, confusion between supraventricular tachycardia and sinus tachycardia and among ventricular tachycardia and the entire spectrum of supraventricular tachycardias can be seen. More recently, additional algorithms have been incorporated using other timing features such as the rapidity of tachycardia onset, taking advantage of the abrupt onset of most paroxysmal reentrant rhythms. Other features such as the stability of cycle length in reentrant tachycardia as opposed to sinus tachycardia or atrial fibrillation may offer additional specificity.[67] Recent reports suggest that morphology of the endocardial electrogram may also contain significant information with respect to normal versus abnormal rhythm.[68]

SYSTEM DESIGN

The general design and construction of pacemakers for tachycardia are similar to those described for pacemakers for bradycardia. Many use the same microprocessor, which is simply reprogrammed to provide antitachycardia function. Initially, devices tended to be mode specific, providing either programmed extrastimuli or bursts of pacing but not both. Presently, all of these functions and many others can be found as programmable options of the same unit. An effective device should provide for one up to large numbers of sequential pacing stimuli. Fewer stimuli may be used to decrease the risk of acceleration, more stimuli for greater effectiveness. Some form of adaptation to changes in termination window and underlying cycle length should be provided. This may be done either by scanning, by adaptive behavior, or preferably both. Stimulus patterns may be of three varieties: (1) fixed, in which the time between successive stimuli is constant both within a train of stimuli and among successive trains; (2) scanning, in which the cycle length of stimuli vary among successive trains; or (3) autodecremental/incremental, in which cycle lengths vary within a train but are constant among successive trains (Fig. 52.9). Each of these forms may be either preset (in which all cycle lengths and successive changes in cycle length are programmed in fixed values of rate or millisecond) or adaptive (in which cycle lengths and changes are programmed as a fraction of the observed tachycardia cycle length). Multiple modes of tachycardia identification should be available to increase the specificity of the automated diagnosis. Bipolar configura-

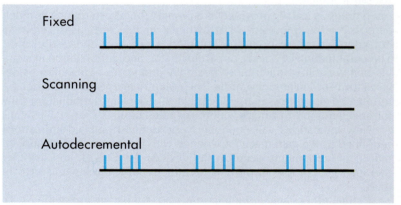

FIGURE 52.9 Fixed stimulus patterns are characterized by having constant intervals between stimuli of a train and a constant pattern from train to train. In other words, the same stimulus pattern is applied repetitively. Scanning is characterized by gradually changing cycle lengths within the stimulus pattern on successive applications of the pattern. Autodecremental pacing provides for progressively changing cycle lengths within a train of stimuli but repetitively applies this decremental pattern. Newer devices may allow each of these to be in either a preset or an adaptive mode and may even allow combinations of some of these basic patterns.

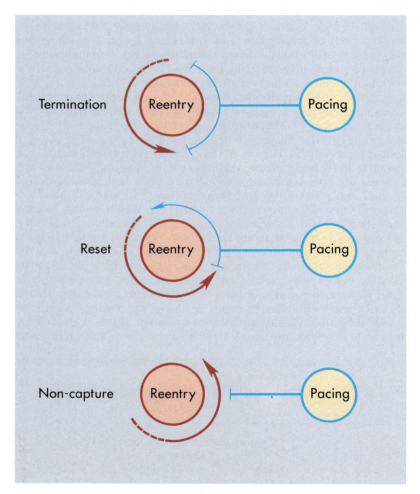

FIGURE 52.8 A pacing stimulus may interact with a reentrant circuit in one of several ways, depending on their relative timing. The stimulus may not be able to enter the circuit because of refractoriness at the entry site (lower panel); it may enter and block in only one limb (middle panel), thus resetting but not terminating the tachycardia since the advancing limb simply reinitiates the tachycardia; or the stimulus may enter the block in both limbs, resulting in termination (upper panel).

tion is mandatory for its increased resistance to intrinsic and extrinsic electromagnetic interference. The ability to provide externally controlled noninvasive electrophysiologic testing is important. The effective use of pacing devices depends on the ability to repeatedly induce the arrhythmia and observe the effectiveness of the recognition and termination capability of the device. Finally, the device should offer some amount of record-keeping capability to assist in developing the most effective pacemaker prescription. The characteristics of a representative cross-section of available devices are outlined in Table 52.6.

At present, cardioverting and particularly defibrillating devices are substantially larger than their pacing counterparts. This results not only from a greater battery capacity but also from the presence of large capacitors necessary to achieve the extremely high voltages necessary for defibrillation. The initial AICD weighed nearly 300 grams and was capable of detecting only ventricular fibrillation by calculation of the probability-density function (PDF), which is a measure of randomness of the electrogram baseline, recorded from the defibrillating electrodes. In order to better detect ventricular tachycardia, this unit was superceded by models AICD-B and AICD-BR, which featured a heart-rate criterion for the definition of an abnormal rhythm in addition to calculation of PDF (rate is the sole criterion for the model BR unit). Currently available devices are the Ventak* models 1500, 1510, 1520, and 1530. They are distinguished by the presence of only a rate criterion (1520 and 1530) and/or higher output for the initial shock (1510, 1520). They weigh 250 grams and measure 10.8 cm × 7.6 cm × 2.0 cm. They require 10 to 20 seconds for tachycardia identification and 5 to 15 seconds to charge the unit's capacitors before a shock can be delivered. The wave shape is that of a truncated exponential pulse, 5 msec to 8 msec in duration, with an intensity of 23 to 28 joules, at 645 V to 710 V. Subsequent shocks in a continuous series are 28 to 37 joules. Up to four shocks can be delivered in a single series, after which the device becomes quiescent until at least 35 seconds of rhythm is detected that does not meet the definition of tachycardia or fibrillation. In the case of models 1500 and 1510, both PDF and rate criteria must be met before a discharge will occur. The device is not programmable but can be ordered with a variety of rate criteria (126–209 beats per minute).[69]

---

* Ventak, Cardiac Pacemakers, Inc., St. Paul, MN.

IMPLANTATION TECHNIQUES
PACEMAKERS

The implantation of a device for tachyarrhythmia management must be preceded by complete electrophysiologic testing in order to establish the mechanism and characteristics of the tachycardia. The rhythm must be demonstrated to be both inducible and terminable by pacing stimuli. The characteristics of the tachycardia must be well understood, since its effects on hemodynamic and overall cardiovascular function must be considered when choosing the mode of tachycardia recognition and termination. The presence of an accessory pathway and its capability for antegrade conduction is of particular concern. Pacing in such patients may precipitate dangerous arrhythmias. Once the mechanism has been established, its susceptibility to pacing termination must be documented. At the conclusion of the initial study, an electrode catheter can be left in place for subsequent testing during the next 12 to 24 hours. In this way, the effects of changes in autonomic tone, induced by changes in posture, exercise, and so on, may be evaluated along with the success of the termination method selected, during any spontaneous arrhythmias that might occur. The techniques of pacemaker implantation are in general the same as those used for pacemakers for bradyarrhythmias. One exception is that thresholds and electrograms should be obtained both in sinus rhythm and during the induced tachycardia. There may be substantial changes in electrogram morphology between the two, owing to changes in activation pattern or the superimposition of atrial and ventricular components of the electrogram in tachycardias such as AV nodal reentry. Thus pacing and particularly sensing may be acceptable during one rhythm and not the other.

THE AUTOMATIC IMPLANTABLE DEFIBRILLATOR

At the present time, implanting an automatic defibrillator is a much more substantial undertaking than implanting a cardiac pacemaker. This is because of the large size of the device and the necessity for placing at least one electrode on the epicardial surface. The subxiphoid operation was used initially but has largely been replaced by the subcostal approach, midline sternotomy, or the left lateral thoracotomy.[70] In a similar fashion transvenous leads used in early implants have largely been abandoned by implanters in favor of an all-epicardial lead configuration.

TABLE 52.6 CHARACTERISTICS OF VARIOUS PACEMAKERS

Manufacturer/ Device	Termination Method	Termination Algorithm	Tachycardia Recognition
Cordis			
Orthocor II	Pacing	Scanning and/or adaptive	Heart rate
Intermedics			
Cybertach-60	Pacing	Programmed	Heart rate
Intertach 262-12	Pacing	Scanning and/or adaptive	Heart rate, RC, RS, SR
Medtronic			
RF 5998	Pacing	Programmed	External
SPO 502	Pacing	Programmed	External
Symbios 7008	Pacing	Programmed	Heart rate
Cardioverter	2J	N/A	Heart rate, RC
Siemens			
Tachylog	Pacing	Scanning	Heart rate, RC
Telectronics			
PASAR	Pacing	Scanning	Heart rate
CPI			
AICD-B	25-30J	N/A	Heart rate, PDF

(PDF, probability density function; RC, rate of change of rate; RS, rate stability; SR, sustained high rate; N/A, not applicable)

At the time of surgery, both the clinical arrhythmia and ventricular fibrillation (if it is not the clinical arrhythmia) should be induced so that thresholds can be tested. Conversion thresholds obtained during ventricular tachycardia may be excellent, while those for fibrillation may be unacceptable. Since with device therapy every patient is susceptible to ventricular fibrillation (either clinically or by acceleration of a ventricular tachycardia by a shock), a lead position with acceptable defibrillation thresholds is mandatory. In general, defibrillation energies of 15 joules or less are preferred. The impact of the healing process on the threshold for defibrillation is not yet well documented. In rare patients, adequate defibrillation thresholds cannot be achieved in the operating room with any lead position/configuration or use of a high-energy device.[56,57] In addition, in some patients the device will not successfully defibrillate postoperatively despite acceptable defibrillation thresholds at the time of implantation.[56,57] Our current practice is to retest the implanted system in the electrophysiologic laboratory prior to hospital discharge.[71]

FOLLOW-UP
GENERAL TECHNIQUES
Many techniques for the follow-up of patients with pacemakers for supraventricular tachycardia are the same as for those with pacemakers for bradyarrhythmias, although certain significant differences exist. Telephone monitoring plays only a minor role and is used only during periods of symptoms. End-of-life monitoring may be much less rigorous since few of these patients are pacemaker-dependent. Clinic evaluation should include the induction and termination of episodes of tachycardia for the assessment of the selected termination pattern and measurement of pacing and sensing thresholds during both supraventricular tachycardia and sinus rhythm. Our current practice is to see patients quarterly for 1 year and every 6 months thereafter for routine evaluation.

Telephone transmission is of no benefit for functional or battery assessment of the AICD though it may be useful for rhythm assessment during periods of symptoms or repeated shocks. Because of the end-of-life characteristics of the device, routine evaluation every other month is necessary. When charge time begins to rise, or after 1 year, monthly follow-up is needed.[71]

The automatic response of the implanted device can be either temporarily or permanently inhibited by the presence of a magnet. Magnet application in the active state is evidenced by the presence of a tone, synchronous with each sensed ventricular contraction. Continued application of the magnet for 30 to 40 seconds causes the unit to switch to the permanently inhibited state, signaled by the emission of a continuous tone. Removal and reapplication of the magnet for a similar time will convert the device back to the active state. Brief application and removal of the magnet during the active state causes the unit to charge the capacitors and then discharge the energy across an internal test resistor. As an indicator of battery status, the capacitor charging time can be determined using the AIDCHECK-B unit. A signal is also emitted indicating the total number of pulses the device has delivered to the lead terminals, that is, the patient. The lack of an accurate elective replacement indicator (ERI) has been a clinical problem. Current recommendations are to replace the unit when the second of two charge times (done 10 minutes apart) is greater than or equal to 20% more than that recorded eight months after implantation, or 12 seconds if earlier data are not available.[69]

THE DEVICE PRESCRIPTION
DEVICES FOR SUPRAVENTRICULAR TACHYCARDIA. Programming for the assessment and selection of basic pacing variables such as output and sensitivity are performed as described for bradycardia pacing. It is important to realize, however, that these choices must satisfy two rhythms, sinus and the pathologic tachycardia. In addition, there are several variables unique to tachycardia pacing that are found in most devices.

TACHYCARDIA RECOGNITION CRITERIA. Tachycardia recognition criteria are those rules by which an implanted device accepts a given rhythm as a pathologic tachycardia (as opposed to a sinus tachycardia). These may be as simple as rate only (rate > criteria = pathologic tachycardia) or complex, using additional criteria for the rapidity of tachycardia development, the regularity of the tachycardia, and the duration of tachycardia, among others. The principal use of these algorithms is to prevent attempts to "terminate" sinus tachycardia or both sinus and supraventricular tachycardia in the case of devices for ventricular arrhythmias. Maximum exercise sinus rate can best be determined by treadmill exercise testing. If there is a significant gap between the sinus and tachycardia rates, the heart rate criterion is simply set between them. If the gap is narrow or the two rates overlap, other criteria can be used, if available, to minimize false triggering. One must be careful in doing so, however, in order not to lessen sensitivity of the device to actual tachycardias. For example, use of the rapid-onset algorithm may cause the device to miss an abnormal tachycardia if it begins in the midst of a sinus tachycardia such as during exercise.

Care must also be taken to adjust tachycardia criteria downward if drugs that might slow the tachycardia rate are to be initiated. If secondary recognition algorithms are unavailable, other approaches may be used. An exercise program can improve fitness, reducing the sinus rate for a given workload without affecting tachycardia rate. β-Blocking drugs may also be tried but frequently decrease both sinus and tachycardia rates proportionally.

Sensing problems should be searched for carefully since even occasional undersensing or oversensing may result in the induction of tachycardia, which in return requires termination. With undersensing, unnecessary stimuli may be delivered at the bradycardia escape cycle length, thus falling in the relative refractory period of the unsensed

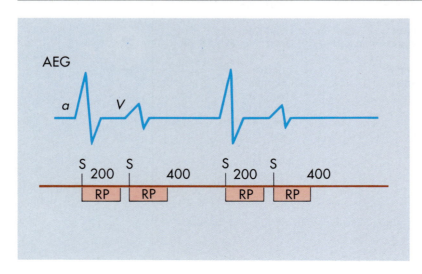

FIGURE 52.10 Tachycardia sensing devices, triggered by rates exceeding a preset criteria, may exhibit "double counting." The mechanism for this may vary but in most cases probably results from sensing both the atrial (a) and ventricular (V) depolarizations on the atrial electrogram (AEG). These pacemakers require that cycle lengths be shorter than the programmed criterion. They do not require constancy of cycle length. Thus, as in this example, alternating 200-msec (A to V) and 400-msec (V to A) sense intervals will trigger a pulse generator with a 175-msec refractory period (RP) and a 425-msec tachycardia criterion, even though the actual heart rate is only 100 beats per minute. (600 msec).

sinus beat, a point at which tachycardia may be induced. If this cannot be corrected by adjustment of sensing level, some devices offer a mode in which bradycardia pacing is eliminated but pacing for tachycardia is preserved. The atrial electrogram has both near-field (atrial depolarization) and far-field (ventricular depolarization) components usually separated by 120 msec to 280 msec.[72] Excessive sensitivity may allow both of these to be detected (since the refractory period for these pacemakers is necessarily short) resulting in an effective doubling of the "perceived" rate and identification of a tachycardia (Fig. 52.10).

TACHYCARDIA TERMINATION ALGORITHMS. The effectiveness of termination of supraventricular tachycardia should be assessed at each visit by serial tachycardia induction and termination. In general, approaches documented during inpatient testing remain valid long-term, though an increase in tachycardia rate is sometimes seen when patients are fully ambulatory and are no longer treated with antiarrhythmic drugs. Thus, fixed-format devices may need to be programmed to shorter termination cycle lengths and/or to greater numbers of stimuli. If fibrillation becomes a clinical problem, it can sometimes be resolved either with a change in termination pattern toward fewer stimuli and longer cycle lengths if these remain effective. If not, the concomitant use of tachycardia-slowing drugs, such as β-blockers or calcium antagonists, may allow such algorithms to be effective.

DEVICES FOR VENTRICULAR TACHYCARDIA. The automatic defibrillator is not programmable; thus, the device prescription must be determined before implantation. Careful attention should be given to the selection of detection rate. Minimum tachycardia rate and maximum sinus tachycardia rate must be determined and a device chosen to take advantage of any gap between the two. If a pacemaker for ventricular tachycardia termination is also to be used, the detection rate of the AICD should be high (probably > 200 beats per minute) so that the AICD is not activated by pacing but only by ventricular flutter/fibrillation.

REFERENCES

1. Elmquist R, Senning A: Implantable pacemaker for the heart. In Smyth CN (ed): Medical Electronics, Proceedings of the Second International Conference on Medical Electronics, Parish, June 1959. London, Iliffe & Sons, 1960
2. Chardack WM, Gage AD, Greatbatch W: A transistorized self-contained, implantable pacemaker for the long-term correction of heart block. Surgery 48:643, 1960
3. Parsonnet V, Bernstein AD: Cardiac pacing in the 1980s: Treatment and techniques in transition. J Am Coll Cardiol 1:339, 1983
4. Frye RL, Collins JJ, DeSanctis RW et al: Guidelines for permanent cardiac pacemaker implantation, May 1984: A report of the Joint American College of Cardiology/American Heart Association Task Force on Assessment of Cardiovascular Procedures (Subcommittee on Pacemaker Implantation). J Am Coll Cardiol 4:434, 1984
5. Medicare Hospital Manual. CIA 65-6, Cardiac Pacemakers Rev 439. HFCA publication No. 10. US Department of Health and Human Services, May 1985
6. Hardage ML, Barold SS: Pacemaker programming techniques. In Barold SS, Mujica J (eds): The Third Decade of Cardiac Pacing: Advances in Technology and Clinical Application. Mt. Kisco, NY, Futura Publishing, 1982
7. Greatbatch W, Lee JH, Mathis W et al: The solid-state lithium battery: A new improved chemical power source for implantable cardiac pacemakers. Trans Bio-Med Eng 18:317, 1971
8. Parsonnet V: Cardiac pacing and pacemakers VII: Power sources for implantable pacemakers: I. Am Heart J 94:517, 1977
9. Parsonnet V: Cardiac pacing and pacemakers VII: Power sources for implantable pacemakers: II. Am Heart J 94:658, 1977
10. Hurzeler P, Morse D, Leach C et al: Longevity comparisons among lithium anode power cells for cardiac pacemakers. PACE 3:555, 1980
11. Bilitch M, Hauser RG, Goldman BS et al: Performance of cardiac pacemaker pulse generators. PACE 7:311, 1984
12. Nielsen AP, Cashion WR, Spencer WH et al: Long-term assessment of unipolar and bipolar stimulation and sensing thresholds using a lead configuration programmable pacemaker. J Am Coll Cardiol 5:1198, 1985
13. Secemsky SI, Hauser RG, Denes P et al: Unipolar sensing abnormalities: Incidence and clinical significance of skeletal muscle interference and undersensing in 228 patients. PACE 5:10, 1982
14. Raymond RD, Nanian KB: Insulation failure with bipolar polyurethane pacing leads. PACE 7:378, 1984
15. Robicsek F, Tarjan P, Harold NB Jr et al: Self-anchoring endocardial pacemaker leads: Current spectrum of types, advances in design and clinical results. Am Heart J 102:775, 1981
16. Weidlich E, Richter GJ, Mund K et al: Threshold measurements using stimulating electrodes of different materials in the skeletal muscles of cats. Med Progr Technol 7:11, 1980
17. Furman S, Hurzeler P, Mehra R: Cardiac pacing and pacemakers IV: Threshold of cardiac stimulation. Am Heart J 94:115, 1977
18. Irnich W: The electrode myocardial interface. Clin Prog Electrophysiol Pacing 3:338, 1985
19. Furman S, Hurzeler P, DeCaprio V: Cardiac pacing and pacemakers III: Sensing the cardiac electrogram. Am Heart J 93:794, 1977
20. Irnich W: Intracardiac electrograms and sensing test signals: Electrophysiological, physical, and technical considerations. PACE 8:870, 1985
21. Parsonnet V, Furman S, Smyth N et al: Optimal resources for implantable cardiac pacemakers. Circulation 68:227A, 1983
22. Calfee RV: Dual-chamber committed mode pacing. PACE 6:387, 1983
23. Floro J, Castellanet M, Florio J et al: DDI: A new mode for cardiac pacing. Clin Prog Pacing Electrophysiol 2:255, 1984
24. Hauser RG: The electrocardiography of AV universal DDD pacemakers. PACE 6:399, 1983
25. Rickards AF, Donaldson RM: Rate responsive pacing. Clin Prog Pacing Electrophysiol 1:12, 1983
26. Griffin JC: Pacemaker selection for the individual patient. In Barold SS (ed): Modern Cardiac Pacing, p 411. Mt. Kisco, NY, Futura Publishing, 1985
27. Parsonnet V: Pacemaker implantation. In Blades' Surgical Diseases of the Chest, 4th ed, p 699. St. Louis, CV Mosby, 1978
28. Hayes DL, Maloney JD, Merideth J et al: Initial and early follow-up assessment of the clinical efficacy of a multiparameter-programmable pulse generator. PACE 4:417, 1981
29. Griffin JC, Schuenemeyer TD: Pacemaker follow-up: An introduction and overview. Clin Prog Pacing Electrophysiol 1:30, 1983
30. Griffin JC, Shuenemeyer TD, Hess KR et al: Pacemaker follow-up: Its role in the detection and correction of pacemaker system malfunction. PACE 9:387, 1986
31. Mond HG, Sloman JG: The malfunction pacemaker system: I. PACE 4:49, 1981
32. Mond HG, Sloman JG: The malfunctioning pacemaker system: II. PACE 4:168, 1981
33. Alicandri C, Fouad FM, Tarazi RC et al: Three cases of hypotension and syncope with ventricular pacing: Possible role of atrial reflexes. Am J Cardiol 42:137, 1978
34. Zoll PM, Linenthal AJ, Zarsky LRN: Ventricular fibrillation: Treatment and prevention by external electric currents. N Engl J Med 262:105, 1960
35. Sowton E, Leatham A, Carson P: The suppression of arrhythmias by artificial pacemaking. Lancet 2:1098, 1964
36. McCallister BD, McGoon DC, Connolly DC: Paroxysmal ventricular tachycardia and fibrillation without complete heart block. Am J Cardiol 18:898, 1966
37. Massumi RA, Kistin AD, Tawakkol AA: Termination of reciprocating tachycardia by atrial stimulation. Circulation 36:637, 1967
38. Durrer D, Schoo L, Schuilenburg RM et al: Role of premature beats in the initiation and termination of supraventricular tachycardia in the Wolff-Parkinson-White syndrome. Circulation 36:644, 1967
39. Haft JI, Kosowsky BD, Lau SH et al: Termination of atrial flutter by rapid electrical pacing of the atrium. Am J Cardiol 20:239, 1967
40. Kastor JA, DeSanctis RW, Harthorne JW et al: Transvenous atrial pacing in the treatment of refractory ventricular irritability. Ann Intern Med 66:939, 1967
41. Cohen HE, Meltzer LE, Lattimer G et al: Treatment of refractory supraventricular arrhythmias with induced permanent atrial fibrillation. Am J Cardiol 28:472, 1971
42. Lister JW, Cohn LS, Bernstein WH et al: Treatment of supraventricular tachycardias by rapid atrial stimulation. Circulation 38:1044, 1968
43. Bennett MA, Pentecost BL: Reversion of ventricular tachycardia by pacemaker stimulation. Br Heart J 33:922, 1971
44. Hunt NC, Cobb FR, Waxman MB et al: Conversion of supraventricular tachycardias with atrial stimulation: Evidence for reentry mechanism. Circulation 38:1060, 1968
45. Ryan GF, Easley RM, Zaroff LI et al: Paradoxical use of a demand pacemaker in treatment of supraventricular tachycardia due to the Wolff-Parkinson-White syndrome. Circulation 38:1037, 1968
46. Urbaszek W, Gunther K, Trenckmann H: Zur Therapie tachycarder rhythmusstorungen mit der intermittierenden Electrostimulation des Herzens nach dem Sender-empfanger-prinzip. Z Gesamte Inn Med 26:475, 1971
47. Dreifus LS, Arriaga J, Watanabe Y et al: Recurrent Wolff-Parkinson-White tachycardia in an infant: Successful treatment by a radio-frequency pacemaker. Am J Cardiol 28:586, 1971
48. Moss AJ, Rivers RJ: Termination and inhibition of recurrent tachycardias by implanted pervenous pacemakers. Circulation 50:942, 1974
49. Fisher JD, Furman S, Mehra R: Ectopic ventricular tachycardia treated with

bursts of pacing at 300 per minute from an implanted ventricular pacer. Circulation 52(suppl II):II-182, 1975
50. Fisher JD, Furman S, Kim SG: Implanted automatic burst pacemakers for termination of ventricular tachycardia (abstr). Am J Cardiol 45:458, 1980
51. Griffin JC, Mason JW: Clinical use of an implantable automatic tachycardia terminating pacemaker (abstr). Clin Res 28:177A, 1980
52. Krikler D, Curry P, Buffet J: Dual-demand pacing for reciprocating atrioventricular tachycardia. Br Med J 1:1114, 1976
53. Spurrell RAJ, Nathan AW, Bexton RS et al: Implantable automatic scanning pacemaker for terminating of supraventricular tachycardia. Am J Cardiol 49:753, 1982
54. Mirowski M, Reid PR, Mower MM et al: Termination of malignant ventricular arrhythmias with an implanted automatic defibrillator in human beings. N Engl J Med 303:322, 1980
55. Mirowski M: The automatic implantable cardioverter-defibrillator: An overview. J Am Coll Cardiol 6:461, 1985
56. Echt DS, Armstrong K, Schmidt P et al: Clinical experience, complications and survival in 70 patients with the automatic implantable cardioverter/defibrillator. Circulation 71:289, 1985
57. Marchlinski FE, Flores BT, Buxton AE et al: The automatic implantable cardioverter-defibrillator: Efficacy, complications, and device failures. Ann Intern Med 104:481, 1986
58. Zipes DP, Heger JJ, Miles WM et al: Early experience with an implantable cardioverter. N Engl J Med 311:485, 1984
59. Ward DE, Camm AJ, Spurrell RAJ: The response of regular reentrant supraventricular tachycardia to right heart stimulation. PACE 2:586, 1979
60. Pritchett ELC, Hammill SC, Reiter MJ et al: Life-table methods for evaluating antiarrhythmic drug efficacy in patients with paroxysmal atrial tachycardia. Am J Cardiol 52:1007, 1983
61. Wellens HJJ, Durrer D: Wolff-Parkinson-White syndrome and atrial fibrillation. Am J Cardiol 34:777, 1974
62. Ruskin JN, Garan H, Poulin F et al: Permanent radiofrequency ventricular pacing for management of drug-resistant ventricular tachycardia. Am J Cardiol 46:317, 1980
63. Herre JM, Griffin JC, Nielsen AP et al: Permanent triggered antitachycardia pacemakers in the management of recurrent sustained ventricular tachycardia. J Am Coll Cardiol 6:206, 1985
64. Wellens HJJ: Value and limitations of programmed electrical stimulation of the heart in the study and treatment of tachycardias. Circulation 57:845, 1978
65. Naccarelli GV, Zipes DP, Rahilly GT et al: Influence of tachycardia cycle length and antiarrhythmic drugs on pacing termination and acceleration of ventricular tachycardia. Am Heart J 105:1, 1983
66. Zipes DP: Electrophysiological mechanisms involved in ventricular fibrillation. Circulation (suppl III)51/52:III-120, 1975
67. Tomaselli G, Scheinman M, Griffin J: The utility of timing algorithm from supraventricular tachycardias (abstr). PACE 10:415, 1987
68. Langberg JJ, Gibb WJ, Griffin JC, Auslander DM: Identification of ventricular tachycardia with use of morphology of the endocardial electrogram. Circulation 77:1363, 1988
69. Physicians Manual for the Automatic Implantable Cardioverter Defibrillator. Document #16J0155, Rev A. St. Paul, Cardiac Pacemakers, Inc, August 1986
70. Mirowski M: The automatic implantable cardioverter-defibrillator: An overview. J Am Coll Cardiol 6:461, 1985
71. Winkle RA, Stinson EB, Echt DS et al: Practical aspects of automatic cardioverter/defibrillator implantation. Am Heart J 108:1335, 1984
72. Griffin JC: Sensing characteristics of the right atrial appendage electrode. PACE 6:22, 1983

SURGICAL TREATMENT OF CARDIAC ARRHYTHMIAS

CHAPTER 53 · VOLUME 1

T. Bruce Ferguson, Jr · James L. Cox

The first successful surgical procedure for the Wolff-Parkinson-White syndrome was performed in 1968.[1] Since that initial clinical experiment, surgical intervention has come to be recognized as an integral part of the armamentarium used to treat virtually all types of cardiac arrhythmias. The development of specific surgical techniques based on an increase in understanding of the anatomical basis of arrhythmias has occurred, as well as technologic advances that have facilitated electrophysiologic evaluation. During this same time interval, newer and more effective pharmacologic agents have been developed for the treatment of cardiac arrhythmias, as well as other therapeutic techniques not requiring full cardiac surgical intervention. This virtual explosion of therapeutic alternatives has proved most of all to be of benefit to those patients afflicted by these disabling and sometimes life-threatening arrhythmias. The surgical methods available for the treatment of these relatively common disorders of the heart are discussed in this chapter.

ANATOMY OF THE CARDIAC CONDUCTION SYSTEM AND RELATED STRUCTURES

The sinoatrial (SA) node is a small subepicardial group of highly specialized cells in the sulcus terminalis just lateral to the junction of the superior vena cava and the right atrium.[2] Experimental studies suggest that the SA node consists of three distinct regions, each responsive to a separate group of neural and circulatory stimuli.[3] Under normal conditions, these cells are the only ones in the heart capable of spontaneous phase 4 depolarization, thus establishing the SA node as the site of origin of the normal cardiac impulse. This impulse traverses the atrial septum preferentially via the crista terminalis and the limbus of the fossa ovalis, although these muscle bundles do not represent specialized, insulated conduction tracts comparable to ventricular bundle branches.

The atrioventricular (AV) junctional area, where functionally a normal delay in AV conduction occurs, corresponds to a group of cells histologically distinct from working myocardium.[4] A "transition zone" of specialized cells located anteriorly in the base of the atrial septum surrounds the atrial aspect of the "compact AV node" where the major conduction delay occurs. The lower, longitudinal portion of the compact AV node penetrates the central fibrous body of the heart to become the bundle of His. The AV node, its transition zone, and its penetrating bundle are all contained within the triangle of Koch, an anatomically discrete region bounded by the tendon of Todaro, tricuspid valve annulus, and thebesian valve of the coronary sinus (Fig. 53.1).

As seen in Figure 53.2, the attachment of the tricuspid valve is lower down (more apical) on the interventricular septum than in the mitral valve; sitting on top of the interventricular septum at this point is the compact AV node and, more anteriorly, the His bundle. The triangle of Koch contains these important structures, which lie at a variable depth between the endocardium of the right and left atria.

The His bundle travels along the posteroinferior rim of the membranous portion of the intraventricular septum and divides into the right bundle branch and a broad band of fasciculi, forming the left bundle branch that extends down the left side of the septum. The distal branches of the conduction system terminate in an intermediate zone,

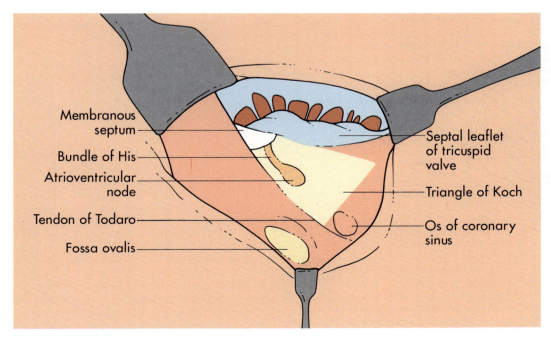

FIGURE 53.1 The right atrial septum viewed through a longitudinal right atriotomy. The patient's head is to the left and the feet are to the right. The boundaries of the triangle of Koch are the tendon of Tadaro, the tricuspid valve annulus, and a line connecting the two at the level of the os of the coronary sinus. Within the triangle of Koch resides the AV node and proximal portion of the His bundle, which enters the ventricular septum immediately posterior to the membranous portion of the interatrial septum. (Modified from Cox JL, Holman SL, Cain ME: Cryosurgical treatment of atrioventricular node reentry tachycardia. Circulation 76:1329, 1987)

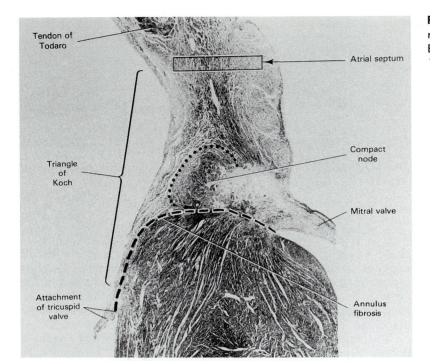

FIGURE 53.2 The boundaries of the triangle of Koch in cross-section and the relation of the compact node to the triangle. (In Davies MJ, Anderson RH, Becker AE (eds): The Conduction System of the Heart. London, Butterworth, 1983. With permission.)

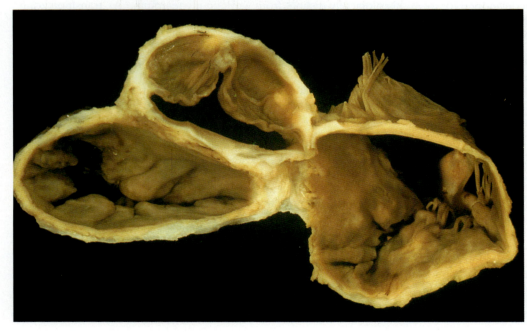

FIGURE 53.3 Dissection showing the fibrous cardiac skeleton after it has been removed from the ventricles. (Anderson RH, Becker AE: Cardiac Anatomy. London, Gower Medical Publishing, 1980.)

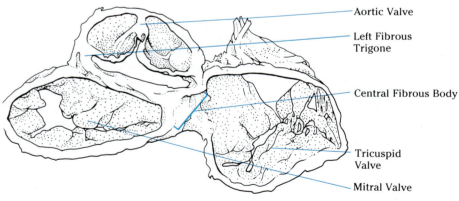

6.186

SURGICAL TREATMENT OF CARDIAC ARRHYTHMIAS ▪ CHAPTER 53

where the cells gradually lose their Purkinje characteristics and take on the characteristics of myocardial cells.

The cardiac skeleton is strongest at the central fibrous body, where the annuli of the mitral, tricuspid, and aortic valves meet (Fig. 53.3). The mitral and aortic valve annuli contribute significantly to the structural integrity of the fibrous skeleton and are further strengthened at their left junction to form the left fibrous trigone. The left anterior portion of the central fibrous body is designated as the right fibrous trigone, and the fibrous continuity between these two trigones is the only area in the AV groove where atrial muscle is not in juxtaposition to ventricular muscle. For this reason, accessory AV pathways are not found between the left and right fibrous trigones.

INTRAOPERATIVE COMPUTERIZED MAPPING SYSTEMS

The first data acquisition systems for intraoperative mapping were single-point mapping systems, employing one fixed and one roving electrode recording epicardial data related to the surface of the heart by using an arbitrary grid.[5] Local activation was determined on a point-by-point basis with the hand-held electrode, and the difference in activation times recorded by this electrode and the fixed reference electrode was determined using an activation timer. This basic system has been used for intraoperative mapping of both supraventricular and ventricular tachyarrhythmias for more than a decade.

A number of limitations with this single-point system were encountered, however, when it was used to map both types of arrhythmias. In patients with Wolff-Parkinson-White syndrome and only intermittent anterograde conduction across the accessory pathway, it was frequently impossible to identify the site of ventricular pre-excitation. The problem was further compounded if the patient had atrial fibrillation with only intermittent anterograde pre-excitation, because the retrograde map could not be performed. With the single-point system excessive cardiac manipulation was necessary in order to map the posterior aspect of the heart, frequently resulting in conduction block across the accessory pathway and precluding further mapping until conduction returned. Cardiopulmonary bypass was also required for adequate mapping in most instances. Identification of multiple pathways was difficult with the single-point system, particularly if one of the pathways was concealed.

The short duration and multifocality of ventricular arrhythmias in the operating room further demonstrated the shortcomings of single-point mapping systems for ventricular tachycardia surgery. Multipoint analog systems were developed for generating epicardial maps, but endocardial mapping was done with a single-point electrode, plunge needle electrodes, or an intracavitary egg electrode array.[6] With these multipoint analog systems, intraoperative data analysis often could not be performed in time to base an operative approach on the results.

An automated computerized mapping system that could record a virtually unlimited number of electrograms simultaneously was developed in 1984 by Witkowski and Corr.[7] The original 48-channel clinical system has been upgraded and is now capable of recording 160 bipolar electrograms simultaneously, analyzing the data, and displaying it in various forms within 2 minutes after data acquisition. Analog data recorded from the heart enter the front-end system located in the operating theater, where each electrogram is individually filtered and digitized. The digitized data are transferred over a fiberoptic cable to a remote computer facility approximately 1500 meters away. The personnel in the operating room and computer facility are connected by both audio and video display systems. Only 16 channels of the system are used for mapping patients undergoing surgery for Wolff-Parkinson-White surgery, but all 160 channels are used to map other atrial and ventricular arrhythmias (Fig. 53.4).[8]

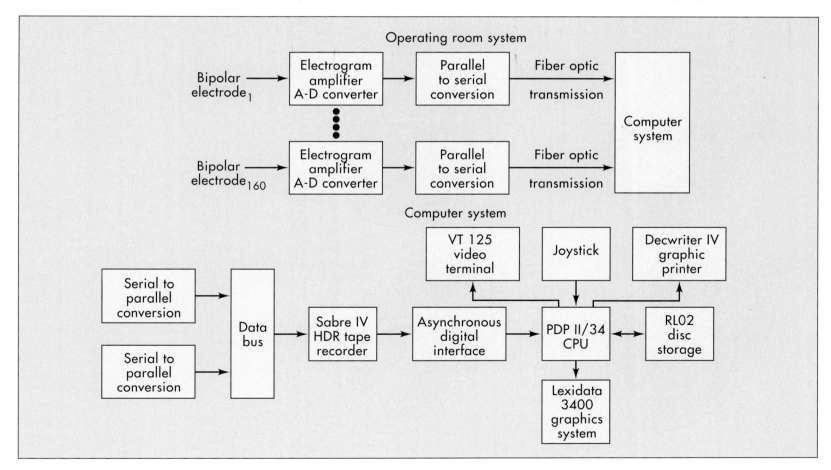

FIGURE 53.4 Schematic diagram of computerized mapping system illustrating separate data acquisition and analysis components. See text for discussion. (Modified from Cain ME, Cox JL: Surgical treatment of supraventricular tachyarrhythmias. In Platia EV [ed]: Management of Cardiac Arrhythmias—The Nonpharmacologic Approach. Philadelphia, JB Lippincott, 1987)

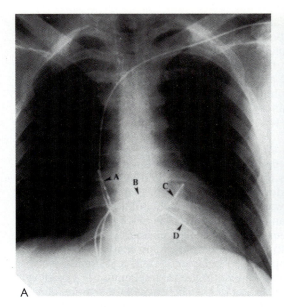

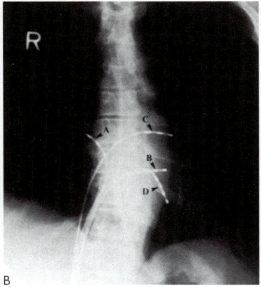

FIGURE 53.5 Catheter positioning for patients undergoing electrophysiologic study for supraventricular tachycardia. **A.** Coronary sinus catheter (C) is inserted via the left subclavian vein. Other catheters are inserted via the femoral approach. **B.** Left atrial catheter (C), advanced across a patent foramen ovale, is used in place of a coronary sinus catheter. (A, high right atrial catheter; B, His bundle catheter; D, right ventricular catheter). (Platia EV: The electrophysiologic study. In Platia EV [ed]: Management of Cardiac Arrhythmias—The Nonpharmacologic Approach. Philadelphia, JB Lippincott, 1987)

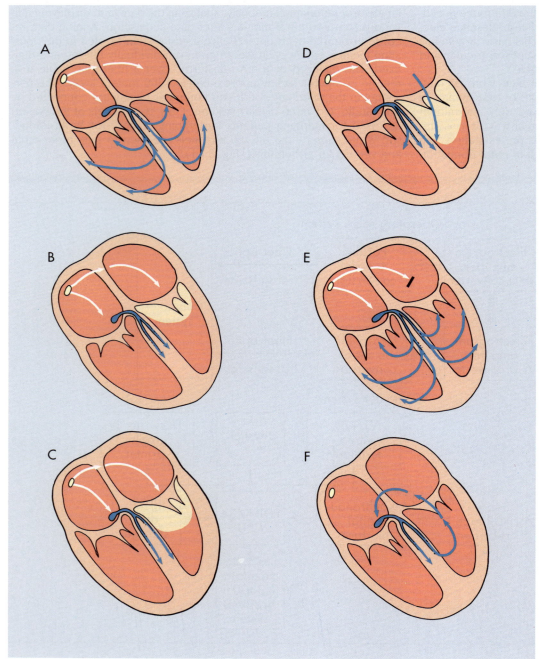

FIGURE 53.6 A. Normal spread of electrical activation in the heart during sinus rhythm. The electrical impulse is delayed approximately 100 msec in the AV node. **B** through **F.** Spread of electrical activation during sinus rhythm in the Wolff-Parkinson-White syndrome with an accessory pathway in the left free-wall position. See text for discussion. (Modified from Cox JL: The surgical management of cardiac arrhythmias. In Sabiston DC, Spencer FC [eds]: Gibbon's Surgery of the Chest, 5th ed. Philadelphia, WB Saunders, 1988)

SURGICAL TREATMENT OF SUPRAVENTRICULAR TACHYARRHYTHMIAS
PREOPERATIVE ELECTROPHYSIOLOGIC EVALUATION

All patients who are to be subjected to surgery for supraventricular arrhythmias should first undergo an endocardial catheter electrophysiologic study (Fig. 53.5). This preoperative electrophysiologic study should (1) document that the arrhythmia is supraventricular in origin, (2) evaluate the response of the supraventricular tachycardia to programmed electrical stimulation to determine if it is reentrant or automatic, (3) establish the conduction properties of the normal specialized conduction tissue, (4) document the etiology of the arrhythmia, and (5) define the location of the accessory pathway and/or arrhythmogenic focus.

WOLFF-PARKINSON-WHITE SYNDROME

In 1930 Dr. Louis Wolff combined a series of patients followed by Dr. Paul Dudley White with a similar series followed by the English physician Dr. John Parkinson and published the reported observations.[9] Both groups of patients were young and apparently healthy, had pre-excitation on their electrocardiograms, and had frequent bouts of supraventricular tachycardia. The anatomical substrate for these lesions was hypothesized in 1933 by Wolferth and Wood as being due to the accessory pathway connection described in mammals by Kent in 1893, and these physicians demonstrated an accessory pathway histologically at autopsy 10 years later.[10] Another 25 years passed, however, before surgical interruption of the Kent bundle was successfully performed.

The Wolff-Parkinson-White syndrome is characterized by the presence of an abnormal muscular connection between the atrium and ventricle, and this connection is believed to be a congenital abnormality. Electrophysiologically, the patients have two routes by which an electrical impulse can travel from the atrium to the ventricle during sinus rhythm: via the normal AV node–His bundle pathway (Fig. 53.6, A) and by the accessory pathway (Fig. 53.6, B through D). However, normal anterograde (atrium-to-ventricle) conduction is delayed because of the conduction delay that occurs in the AV node, and the electrical activity reaches the ventricle first at the site of insertion of the accessory pathway onto the ventricle. This initial activation of the ventricle at a site remote from the His bundle causes slurring of the initial portion of the QRS complex and is known as a delta wave. Normal conduction through the His bundle–Purkinje system continues during this pre-excitation, and the wavefronts eventually fuse, resulting in a wide QRS complex. Thus the three electrocardiographic abnormalities found during sinus rhythm in patients with the Wolff-Parkinson-White syndrome are a short PR interval, a delta wave, and a wide QRS complex (Fig. 53.7).

Three types of supraventricular arrhythmias complicate the Wolff-Parkinson-White syndrome, including orthodromic (the most common) or antidromic reciprocating tachycardias and atrial fibrillation/flutter.[11] In order for orthodromic reciprocating tachycardia to occur, anterograde conduction across the accessory pathway must be blocked. Under these circumstances, propagation down the AV node–His bundle pathway occurs and ventricular activation proceeds normally. When the activation front reaches the nondepolarized accessory pathway, however, retrograde (ventricle-to-atrium) conduction occurs, quickly reactivating the atria and establishing the macroreentrant circuit characteristic of the Wolff-Parkinson-White syndrome. Antegrade block in the accessory pathway may result from a number of causes, including premature atrial or ventricular beats and sudden changes in autonomic tone. During antidromic reciprocating tachycardia, anterograde conduction to the ventricle occurs through the accessory pathway and retrograde conduction to the atria occurs through

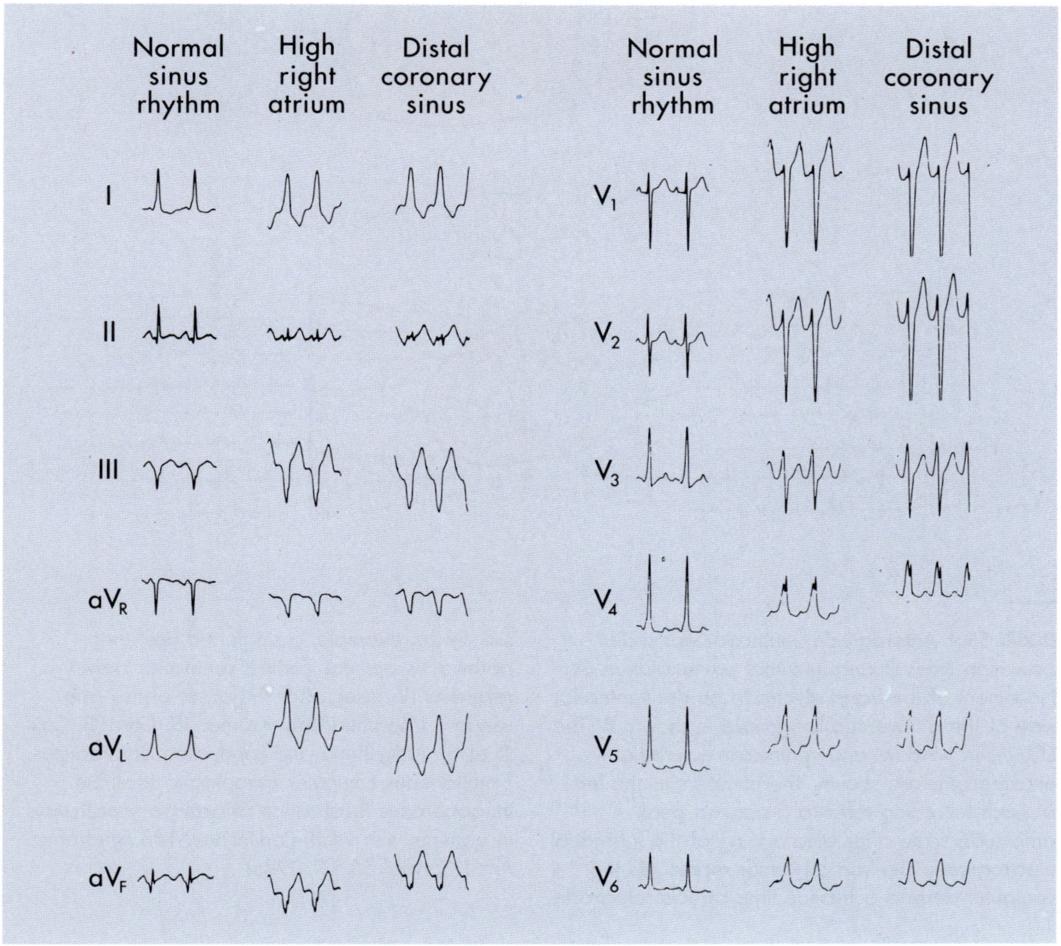

FIGURE 53.7 Comparison of 12-lead ECGs from a patient having a single left free-wall accessory pathway during normal sinus rhythm, during pacing from the high right atrium at a cycle length of 400 msec, and during pacing from the distal coronary sinus at a cycle length of 400 msec. Pacing from either atrium results in a similar pattern of ventricular pre-excitation. (Cain ME, Cox JL: Surgical treatment of supraventricular tachyarrhythmias. In Platia EV [ed]: Management of Cardiac Arrhythmias—The Nonpharmacologic Approach. Philadelphia, JB Lippincott, 1987)

the normal AV conduction system. Atrial fibrillation/flutter occurring in a patient with an accessory pathway may be associated with a rapid and potentially life-threatening ventricular rate because there is no AV node proximal to the accessory pathway to filter the number of impulses that can reach the ventricle.

INDICATIONS FOR SURGERY

Candidates for surgical ablation of accessory pathways include (1) patients with recurrent reciprocating tachycardia who are poorly controlled on medical therapy or have developed significant toxicity to an otherwise successful medical regimen; (2) patients with Wolff-Parkinson-White syndrome having symptomatic supraventricular arrhythmias who are undergoing cardiac surgery for other indications; and (3) patients with atrial fibrillation/flutter having an excessive ventricular rate even if it can be attenuated with antiarrhythmic agents.[12] Among these, the major indication for surgical intervention is medical refractoriness. In addition, surgery for younger, healthy patients is now recommended due to its safety and curative nature as the conservative alternative to a life time of dependence on antiarrhythmic drugs.

Patients with symptomatic arrhythmias due to atrio-His (AH), nodoventricular, and fasciculoventricular fibers should undergo surgery only if they are resistant or intolerant to medical therapy, as operative procedures for these patients are still under development.

INTRAOPERATIVE ELECTROPHYSIOLOGIC MAPPING

Epicardial pacing and sensing electrodes are sutured onto the atrium and ventricle near the suspected site of the accessory pathway. An epicardial band electrode[13] (Fig. 53.8) containing 16 bipolar button electrodes is used for epicardial mapping. The band is placed on the ventricular side of the AV groove, and electrograms are recorded simultaneously from the 16 bipolar electrodes during normal sinus rhythm and during atrial pacing to assess anterograde ventricular activation during maximal pre-excitation. Two minutes later, three digitized tracings from the standard ECG are displayed on the color graphics terminals in the operating theater and in the computer facility. A pre-excited QRS complex is selected, and the activation sequence of

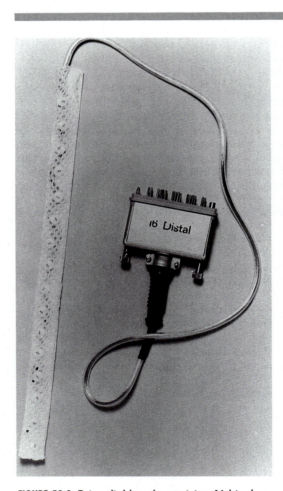

FIGURE 53.8 Epicardial band containing 16 bipolar button electrodes used for mapping multiple sites simultaneously around the AV groove. (Kramer JB, Corr PB, Cox JL et al: Arrhythmia and conduction disturbances: Simultaneous computer mapping to facilitate intraoperative localization of accessory pathways in patients with Wolff-Parkinson-White syndrome. Am J Cardiol 56:571, 1985)

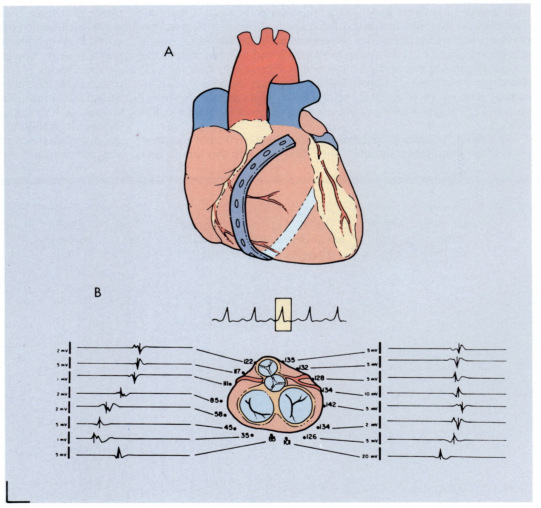

FIGURE 53.9 Anterograde ventricular epicardial activation times during maximal pre-excitation. **A.** Placement of the band electrode on the ventricular side of the atrioventricular groove is shown. **B.** The ECG, time window, and ventricular epicardial electrograms are shown. The numbers to the left of each recording refer to a peak-to-peak amplitude scale after autoranging of the individual electrograms. The vertical cursor represents the computer-derived activation time at each electrode site. In this example, a single left posterior pathway is present. Earliest ventricular activity is recorded 35 msec after the onset of the time window. (Modified from Kramer JB, Corr PB, Cox JL et al: Arrhythmia and conduction disturbances: Simultaneous computer mapping to facilitate intraoperative localization of accessory pathways in patients with Wolff-Parkinson-White syndrome. Am J Cardiol 56:571, 1985)

the 16 electrodes is determined by the computer. The local activation time (point of maximal deflection) for each of the 16 digitized electrograms is displayed by a vertical cursor on each electrogram. The electrogram recorded from the electrode located nearest the site of the ventricular insertion of the accessory pathway shows the earliest activation (Fig. 53.9).

The band electrode is then moved to the atrial side of the AV groove, and retrograde atrial activation is assessed during orthodromic reciprocating tachycardia induced with programmed electrical stimulation or with ventricular pacing. Only a few cycles of tachycardia are allowed to occur as hemodynamic compromise is common and the patients are not on cardiopulmonary bypass. Because only retrograde atrial data are of interest, the portion of the electrocardiographic tracing that contains the retrograde p wave is analyzed. This display of atrial data is especially important because it demonstrates unsuspected concealed accessory pathways that would have gone undetected until this point in the mapping procedure (Fig. 53.10). In addition, rapid identification of multiple pathways (Fig. 53.11) and pathways manifesting intermittent conduction (Fig. 53.12) is greatly facilitated. In most circumstances, complete atrial and ventricular mapping and data analysis can be completed in approximately 10 minutes, and only a single beat is required for analysis of ventricular or atrial activation times.

The anterograde and retrograde mapping techniques described above are capable of detecting not only free-wall accessory pathways but also anterior septal and posterior septal accessory pathways. However, if either is detected during the computerized mapping procedure, the patient is placed on cardiopulmonary bypass; a right atriotomy and endocardial mapping are performed using the hand-held single-point mapping system prior to proceeding with surgical dissection. In addition, endocardial mapping is also routinely performed for right free-wall accessory pathways.

SURGICAL TECHNIQUES

The anatomical location of accessory AV connections may be classified into (1) left free-wall, (2) right free-wall, (3) anterior septal, and (4) posterior septal regions (Fig. 53.13). In decreasing order of frequency, accessory pathways are located in the left free-wall, posterior septal, right free-wall, and anterior septal locations.[14] Approximately 20% of patients in the Duke–Washington University series have had multiple (two–four) pathways.[15]

The accessory pathway(s) responsible for the Wolff-Parkinson-White syndrome must by definition connect atrial and ventricular muscle, and both the atrial and ventricular connections must be located between the annulus of one of the AV valves and the epicardial reflection that covers the AV groove fat pad. As such, all accessory pathways must course through the AV groove fat pad unless they are located immediately adjacent to the valve annulus or immediately underneath the epicardium. The surgical objective is to divide the accessory connection, either at the atrial or the ventricular end of the pathway.

The techniques for dividing accessory pathways have evolved considerably in recent years.[16] The first surgical procedures used relatively limited incisions that bracketed the presumed location of the pathway, and the dissection was largely directed at the endocardial layers. A more detailed understanding of the variability of accessory pathway location along with increased experience led to the practice of more extensive dissection of the entire anatomical space in each patient.[17]

Two surgical approaches are now commonly employed to divide accessory AV connections. The endocardial technique is designed to

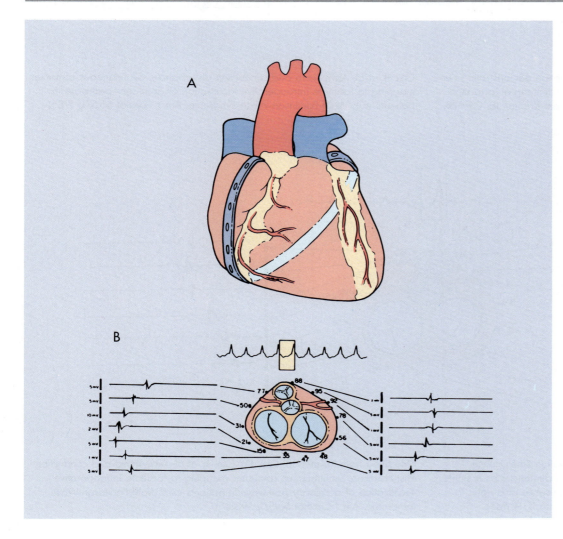

FIGURE 53.10 Retrograde atrial epicardial activation times during sustained orthodromic supraventricular tachycardia. **A.** Placement of the band electrode on the atrial side of the atrioventricular groove is shown. **B.** The atrial activation map indicates the presence of a single left posterior accessory pathway, where the activation time is 15 msec. (Modified from Kramer JB, Corr PB, Cox JL et al: Arrhythmia and conduction disturbances: Simultaneous computer mapping to facilitate intraoperative localization of accessory pathways in patients with Wolff-Parkinson-White syndrome. Am J Cardiol 56:571, 1985)

divide the ventricular end of the accessory pathway, and the epicardial technique is directed toward division of the atrial end of the pathway (Fig. 53.14).[18] Excellent results may be obtained with both techniques;[14,19,20] at Washington University, however, the endocardial technique is performed exclusively.

A median sternotomy is employed in all patients regardless of the suspected pathway location. The patients are cannulated for cardiopulmonary bypass using single aortic and superior and inferior vena caval cannulae, and the pacing/sensing electrodes are placed as described previously. Once the atrial and ventricular insertions of the accessory pathways have been identified by intraoperative epicardial mapping, cardiopulmonary bypass is begun and endocardial mapping via a right atriotomy is performed if necessary.

LEFT FREE-WALL ACCESSORY PATHWAYS. A left atriotomy in the posterior interatrial groove is performed after the aorta is cross-clamped and the heart is arrested with cold potassium cardioplegic solution. Currently, all patients with left free-wall pathways undergo the same surgical dissection regardless of the precise location of the pathway within the left free-wall space. A supra-annular incision is made 2 mm above the mitral valve annulus extending from the left fibrous trigone anteriorly to the junction of the free wall and septum posteri-

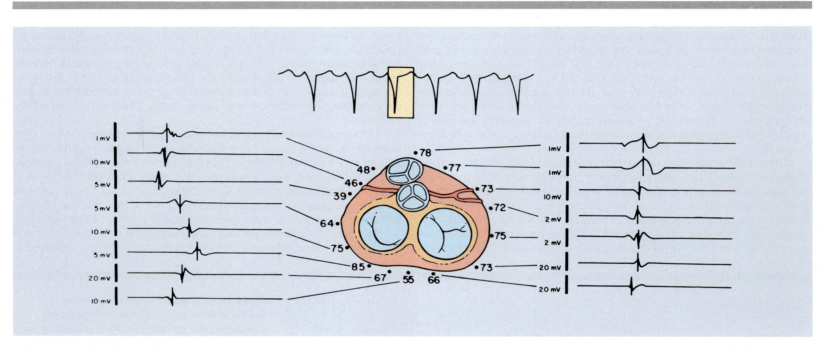

FIGURE 53.11 Anterograde ventricular epicardial activation demonstrating two distinct accessory pathways: left anterolateral and posteroseptal (activation times are 39 and 55 msec, respectively). (Modified from Kramer JB, Corr PB, Cox JL et al: Arrhythmia and conduction disturbances: Simultaneous computer mapping to facilitate intraoperative localization of accessory pathways in patients with Wolff-Parkinson-White syndrome. Am J Cardiol 56:571, 1985)

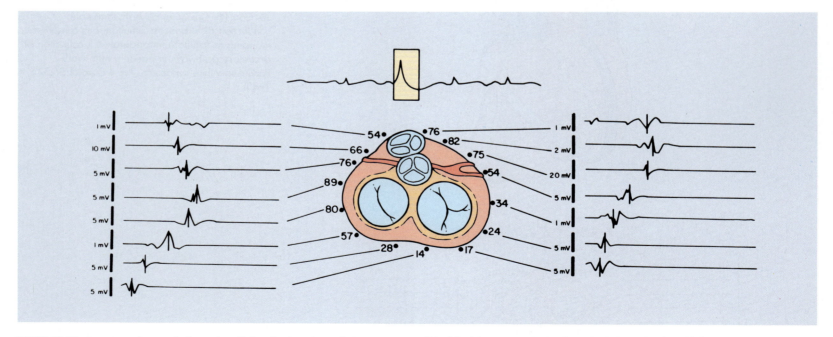

FIGURE 53.12 Anterograde ventricular epicardial activation times during intermittent ventricular pre-excitation. The electrogram demonstrates a single pre-excited beat. The activation map indicated the presence of a right paraseptal accessory pathway, where the activation time is 14 msec. (Modified from Kramer JB, Corr PB, Cox JL et al: Arrhythmia and conduction disturbances: Simultaneous computer mapping to facilitate intraoperative localization of accessory pathways in patients with Wolff-Parkinson-White syndrome. Am J Cardiol 56:571, 1985)

orly (Fig. 53.15). A plane of dissection is established between the underlying AV groove fat pad and the top of the posterior left ventricle throughout the length of the supra-annular incision. This plane of dissection is carried to the epicardium as it reflects off the posterior left ventricle onto the AV groove fat pad. The ends of the supra-annular incision are then "squared off" to the level of the mitral annulus to isolate the rim of atrial tissue above the mitral annulus (Fig. 53.16). This maneuver precludes any problem with accessory pathways that might lie immediately adjacent to the mitral annulus. When this technique of dissecting the entire anatomical space was used in every patient, not a single reoperation has been required and no patient has had an early or late recurrence. Following the dissection, the supra-annular incision is closed with a nonabsorbable suture. The epicardial technique for left free-wall pathways has been described elsewhere.[17,18,20]

POSTERIOR SEPTAL ACCESSORY PATHWAYS. Historically, posterior septal pathways have been considered the most difficult to interrupt successfully, and because the His bundle is located in this space the dissection was frequently complicated by AV block.[21] These pathways may be located anywhere in the pyramidal space that lies above the interventricular septum posteriorly.[22] This space is bounded anteriorly by the central fibrous body and posteriorly by the epicardium overlying the crux of the heart. The floor of this space comprises the interventricular septum and the posterosuperior process of the left ventricle (Fig. 53.17). The lateral walls of the pyramidal space are formed by diverging walls of the right and left atria. A greater appreciation of the complex anatomy of this pyramidal space has made posterior septal pathways perhaps the easiest to treat surgically and has made the problem of postoperative heart block a matter of historical interest only.[14]

Epicardial mapping with the band electrode is first performed. After institution of cardiopulmonary bypass at normothermia, endocardial atrial mapping with a hand-held electrode is then performed around the tricuspid annulus during induced orthodromic reciprocating tachycardia and/or ventricular pacing to identify the atrial insertion of the pathway. In addition, the His bundle is identified. A supra-annular incision is placed well posterior to the site of the His bundle and continued in a counterclockwise direction onto the posterior right atrial free wall (Fig. 53.18). A plane of dissection is established between the fat pad and the top of the posterior interventricular septum. This plane is developed in the anterior portion of the posterior septal space closest to the His bundle, approaching the central fibrous body

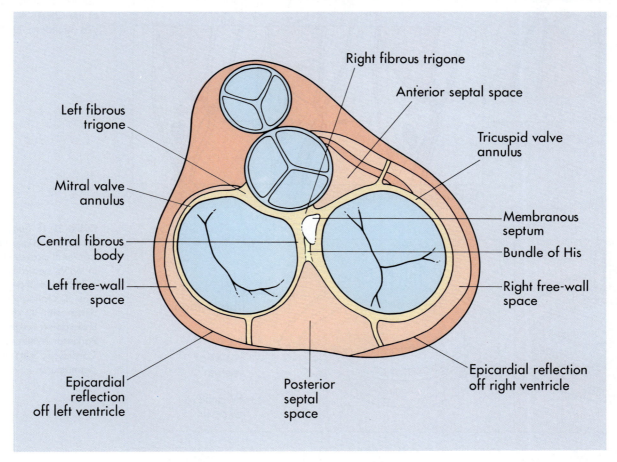

FIGURE 53.13 Diagram of the superior view of the heart with the atria cut away demonstrating the boundaries of each of the four anatomical areas where accessory pathways can occur in the Wolff-Parkinson-White syndrome. The boundaries of the left free-wall space are the mitral valve annulus and the ventricular epicardial reflection extending from the left fibrous trigone to the posterior septum. The boundaries of the posterior septal space are the tricuspid valve annulus, the mitral valve annulus, the posterior superior process of the left ventricle, and the ventricular epicardial reflection. The boundaries of the right free-wall space are the tricuspid valve annulus and the epicardial reflection extending from the posterior septum to the anterior septum. The boundaries of the anterior septal space are the tricuspid valve annulus, the membranous portion of the interatrial septum, and the ventricular reflection. All accessory atrioventricular connections must insert into the ventricle somewhere within these anatomical boundaries. (Modified from Cox JL: The surgical management of cardiac arrhythmias. In Sabiston DC, Spencer FC [eds]: Gibbon's Surgery of the Chest, 5th ed. Philadelphia, WB Saunders, 1988)

from the posterior direction. While this portion of the dissection may be performed prior to the institution of cardioplegic arrest, a better understanding of the anatomy of this region has made this unnecessary. If performed prior to arresting the heart, then atrial pacing or inducing orthodromic tachycardia with careful monitoring of the AV interval will prevent injury to the AV node-His bundle complex. The dissection is carried medially to the mitral valve annulus and posteriorly to the epicardial reflection off the posterior ventricular surface. The left corner of the pyramidal space overlying the posterosuperior process of the left ventricle at the site where the posterior interventricular septum is juxtaposed to the posterior left ventricular free wall is carefully dissected to complete the procedure. It is absolutely essential to divide all structures penetrating the posterior ventricular septum in the posterior septal space, including the AV nodal artery, which leaves the fat pad to enter the posterior ventricular septum within the posterior septal space in approximately 50% of patients with posterior septal

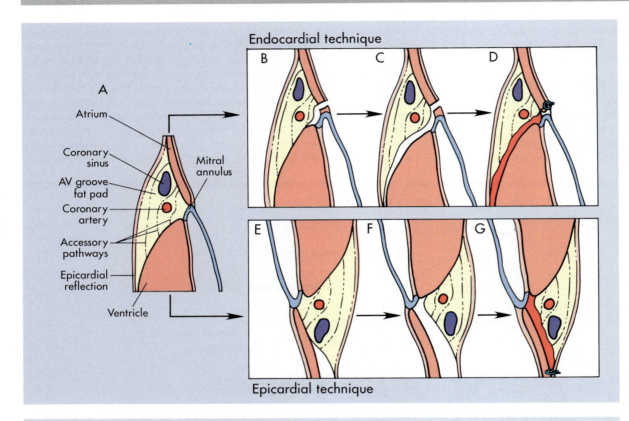

FIGURE 53.14 **A.** Diagrammatic representation of a cross-section of the posterior left heart showing the different depths that left free-wall pathways can be located in relation to the mitral annulus and epicardial reflection. **B** through **D.** Endocardial surgical technique. **E** through **G.** Epicardial surgical technique. See text for further discussion. (Modified from Cox JL: The surgical management of cardiac arrhythmias. In Sabiston DC, Spencer FC [eds]: Gibbon's Surgery of the Chest, 5th ed. Philadelphia, WB Saunders, 1988)

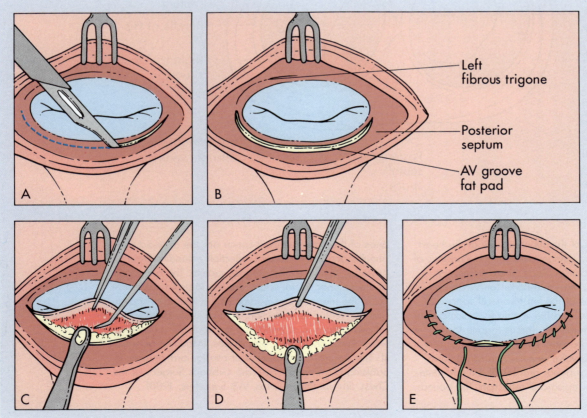

FIGURE 53.15 Surgeon's view of endocardial technique for dividing left free-wall accessory pathways (**A–E**) in WPW syndrome. See text for detailed description. (Adapted from Cox JL, Gallagher JJ, Cain ME: Experience with 118 consecutive patients undergoing surgery for the Wolff-Parkinson-White syndrome. J Thorac Cardiovasc Surg 90:490, 1985. With permission.)

pathways. Ligation of the AV nodal artery does not produce early or late AV node dysfunction. The supra-annular incision is closed with a nonabsorbable suture.

RIGHT FREE-WALL ACCESSORY PATHWAYS. The surgical approach to right free-wall accessory pathways may be performed from the epicardial or endocardial approach, but we prefer the latter. After institution of cardioplegic arrest, a supra-annular incision is placed 2 mm above the tricuspid annulus around the entire right free wall. A plane of dissection is established between the underlying AV groove fat pad and the top of the right ventricle throughout the length of the incision. The plane is developed all the way to the epicardial reflection off the ventricle. Again, each end of the supra-annular incision is connected to the annulus ("squared off") to isolate the supra-annular rim of the right atrial tissue so that juxta-annular accessory pathways will be rendered inoperative. In general, the plane of dissection between the AV groove fat pad and the heart (atrium or ventricle) is not as well defined on the right side as on the left side of the heart. This is especially true in patients with Ebstein's anomaly, whether the patient has the classic anomaly or only the forme fruste of the disease. This is due to the "folding over" of the atrial and ventricular tissues on the right side of the heart (Fig. 53.19) and to the fact that the tricuspid annulus is less well-developed than the mitral annulus (see Fig. 53.3). The incision is closed with a nonabsorbable suture.

ANTERIOR SEPTAL ACCESSORY PATHWAYS. Accessory pathways in this location are frequently adjacent to the right fibrous trigone and are typically situated just anterior to the recorded His deflection. Thus, endocardial mapping around the tricuspid annulus during orthodromic reciprocating tachycardia is particularly useful for defining the precise location of the accessory pathway relative to the His bundle. Anterior septal pathways appear to be more frequently located adjacent to the His bundle (anteriorly) than are posterior septal pathways (posteriorly). On the ventricular aspect, these accessory pathways are directly related to the crista supraventricularis. A supra-annular incision is placed just anterior to the His bundle 2 mm above the tricuspid annulus and extended in a clockwise direction well onto the right anterior free wall. A plane of dissection is established between the fat pad occupying the anterior septal space and the top of the right ventricle and developed medially to the aorta and anteriorly to the epicardial reflection off the ventricle. The initial portion of the dissection is usually performed with the heart beating and during continual recording of the His bundle potential. Cardioplegic arrest may be used for the remainder of the dissection of the anterior septal space, which is just anterior to the membranous portion of the interatrial septum between the pericardial reflection of the ascending aorta and the medial wall of the right atrium. The fat pad in this space contains the right coronary artery before it inserts into the AV groove and must be retracted very gently during the dissection. The incision is closed with a nonabsorbable suture.

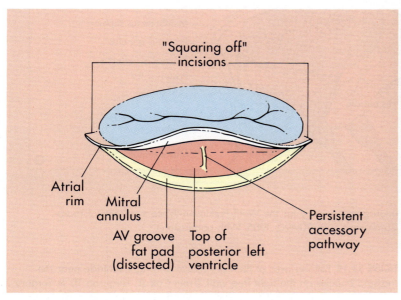

FIGURE 53.16 Diagrammatic representation of the adjunctive procedure necessary to ensure complete interruption of a "juxta-annular" pathway. The 2-mm rim of atrial tissue is "squared off" at either end down to the valve annulus to isolate the rim from surrounding atrial tissue. (From Cox JL, Ferguson TB Jr: Surgery for the Wolff-Parkinson-White syndrome: The endocardial approach. Semin Thorac Cardiovasc Surg 1:34, 1989. With permission.)

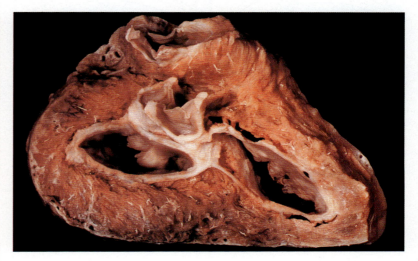

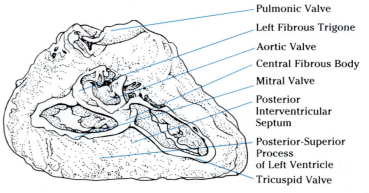

FIGURE 53.17 The atrioventricular junction viewed from the surgical orientation following removal of the atria and great arteries. (Modified from Anderson RH, Becker AE: Cardiac Anatomy. London, Gower Medical Publishing, 1980.)

CONCEALED ACCESSORY ATRIOVENTRICULAR CONNECTIONS

In addition to the accessory pathways responsible for the classic Wolff-Parkinson-White syndrome, accessory pathways connecting the atrium and ventricle may be present in which conduction across the pathway can occur in the retrograde direction only. Such pathways are said to be "concealed," because the ventricles are activated only through the normal AV node–His bundle complex and thus the QRS complex is normal during sinus rhythm. Because these pathways are capable of conducting in the retrograde direction, however, a macroreentrant reciprocating tachycardia can occur just as it does in the classic Wolff-Parkinson-White syndrome. This condition results in the clinical arrhythmia termed *paroxysmal supraventricular tachycardia* (PSVT), characterized by the sudden onset of the arrhythmia in a patient with an otherwise normal electrocardiogram. The intraoperative approach involves only retrograde atrial mapping during ventricular pacing or induced reciprocating tachycardia, because the absence of

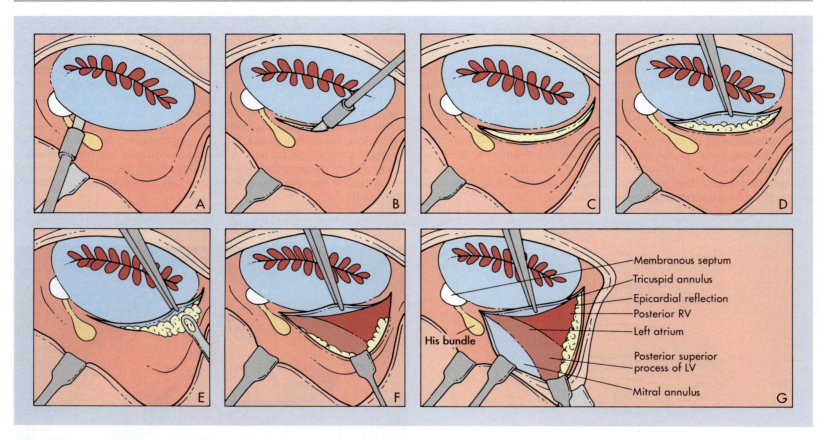

FIGURE 53.18 Endocardial technique for surgical division of posterior septal accessory pathways in WPW syndrome. (*RV,* right ventricle; *LV,* left ventricle) (From Cox JL, Gallagher JJ, Cain ME: Experience with 118 consecutive patients undergoing surgery for the Wolff-Parkinson-White syndrome. J Thorac Cardiovasc Surg 90:490, 1985. With permission.)

FIGURE 53.19 Folding over of the right atrium and right ventricle near the tricuspid annulus on the right free wall. (From Cox JL, Ferguson TB Jr: Surgery for the Wolff-Parkinson-White syndrome: The endocardial approach. Semin Thorac Cardiovasc Surg 1:34, 1989. With permission).

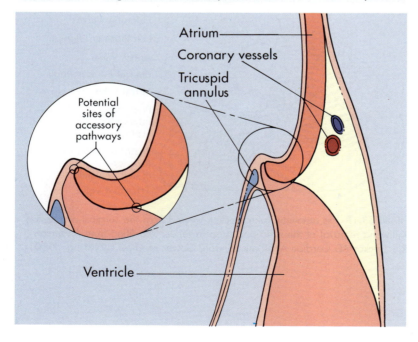

antegrade conduction across the pathway precludes any benefit from antegrade ventricular mapping. The surgical technique employed to divide concealed accessory pathways is the same as for patients with the classic Wolff-Parkinson-White syndrome.

ATRIOVENTRICULAR NODAL REENTRY

Reentry within the AV node is the most common form of PSVT.[23] The tachycardia is caused by a reentrant circuit that is confined to the AV node or to the perinodal tissues of the lower atrial septum. The anatomical-electrophysiologic substrate for this reentrant circuit is the presence of dual AV node conduction pathways, one fast and one slow, through the AV nodal tissue.[24]

While this condition is frequently successfully treated with antiarrhythmic agents, interruption or alteration of AV conduction is occasionally required in patients who are refractory to or intolerant of medical therapy. Prior to 1982, the only surgical therapy available for patients with medically refractory AV node reentrant tachycardia was elective cryoablation of the bundle of His and insertion of a ventricular pacemaker.[25] This did not ablate the AV node reentry but did confine the tachycardia to the atria, thus relieving the patient's symptoms. In 1982, Scheinman and co-workers[26] developed a closed-chest technique for permanent His bundle ablation in which 200 to 500 joules were delivered through a His bundle catheter, and this procedure has effectively replaced surgical cryoablation for the treatment of this arrhythmia.[27] Because of the disadvantages associated with permanent AV block and a ventricular pacemaker, we developed a surgical technique capable of interrupting the actual reentrant circuit responsible for AV node reentrant tachycardia without blocking normal AV conduction. Results of studies in experimental animals using multiple discrete (3 mm) cryolesions around the AV node delineated by the triangle of Koch demonstrated that AV node conduction could be attenuated.[28] In studies performed on animals with dual AV node conduction pathways, this discrete cryosurgical procedure was capable of selectively ablating only one of the pathways, while leaving normal AV conduction intact.[29,30] Discrete cryosurgical modification of AV node conduction has now been performed in patients with AV node reentrant tachycardia, accessory nodoventricular connections (Mahaim fibers), and accessory atrio-His connections (James fibers) with excellent results.[31]

The preoperative electrophysiologic study should provide an accurate diagnosis of AV nodal reentry as the mechanism responsible for the clinical arrhythmia as well as excluding other conditions associated with PSVT, principally a concealed accessory pathway.[32] After preparation for cardiopulmonary bypass through a median sternotomy or right anterior thoracotomy, incremental atrial pacing and induction and termination of AV node reentrant tachycardia are performed. After institution of normothermic cardiopulmonary bypass, a right atriotomy is performed and a hand-held electrode is used to confirm the location of the His bundle at the apex of the triangle of Koch. Throughout the cryothermia portion of the procedure, the AV interval is monitored on a beat-to-beat basis during atrial pacing. A nitrous oxide cryoprobe with a 3-mm diameter tip is used to apply a series of discrete cryolesions encompassing the triangle of Koch (Fig. 53.20). When the cryolesions approximate the AV nodal tissue, the cryothermia application prolongs the AV interval in a linear fashion, and prolongation of the AV interval to 200 msec to 300 msec indicates impending complete AV block (Fig. 53.21). The cryothermia is terminated immediately on development of complete heart block, and the freeze point is irrigated with warm saline. Resumption of normal AV conduction occurs within two or three beats, and the AV interval usually returns to near its control value during the ensuing 10 to 15 beats. In this manner, the cryoprobe acts as a "reversible knife," allowing cryoablation to be applied to as much of the perinodal tissue as possible without causing permanent AV conduction block.

In patients with AV node reentry tachycardia and concomitant Wolff-Parkinson-White syndrome, the latter problem must be surgically corrected first. In the presence of a functioning accessory pathway, exclusive monitoring of conduction through the AV node–His bundle complex on a beat-to-beat basis (required for the cryosurgical procedure) is not possible due to preferential conduction anterograde down the accessory pathway.

AUTOMATIC (ECTOPIC) ATRIAL TACHYCARDIAS

Automatic (ectopic) atrial tachycardias are often incessant.[33] Clinical data suggest that derangements in automaticity and not reentry underlie the genesis of these arrhythmias. These tachycardias appear to have a focal origin and usually originate from the body of the right atrium or left atrium, but they may occasionally arise from the interatrial septum (Fig. 53.22). During atrial tachycardia, the ventricular rate depends on conduction through the AV node. Reversible abnormalities that may precipitate atrial tachycardias (e.g., hyperthyroidism, electrolyte imbal-

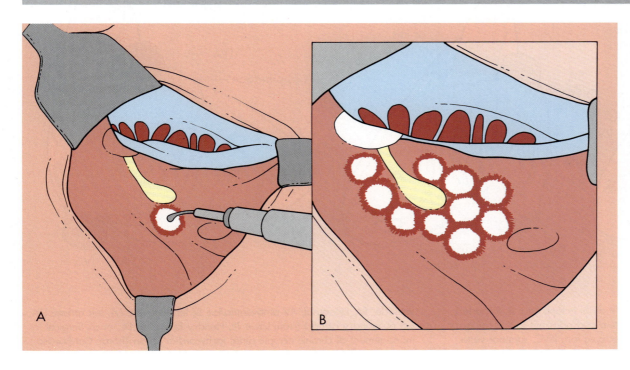

FIGURE 53.20 Discrete cryosurgical procedure for the treatment of AV node reentry tachycardia. A 3-mm cryoprobe is employed to place nine cryolesions around the periphery of the AV node (**B**), beginning at the upper edge of the os of the coronary sinus (**A**). See text for detailed description. (Modified from Cox JL et al: Cryosurgical treatment of atrioventricular node reentry tachycardia. Circulation 76:1329, 1987)

ance, digitalis toxicity) should be excluded before considering surgical treatment.

Preoperative electrophysiologic evaluation is necessary to discern the mechanism of the arrhythmia, regionalize the origin of the tachycardia, and exclude concomitant electrophysiologic derangements that may contribute to the rapid ventricular rate. Accurate preoperative localization is particularly important in patients with automatic atrial tachycardias if surgical ablation of the ectopic focus is contemplated. These tachycardias are frequently suppressed by general anesthesia and, as a result, intraoperative mapping to localize their site of origin may not be possible. In addition, automatic tachycardias are not inducible by standard programmed stimulation techniques. If the arrhythmia does happen to persist intraoperatively so that it can be precisely localized, or if a multipoint intraoperative mapping system is available so that the atria can be mapped from only a few beats of tachycardia (Fig. 53.23), treatment by surgical excision or cryoablation is performed.[34]

Without accurate intraoperative localization, however, elective His bundle ablation has been the only surgical alternative in the past. For the same reasons that this treatment was unsatisfactory for AV node reentrant tachycardias, alternative surgical techniques that leave the normal atrioventricular conduction intact while isolating the arrhythmogenic atrial myocardium from the remainder of the heart have been developed.

As illustrated in Figure 53.22, left atrial tachycardias usually originate in the body of the left atrium. A technique to isolate the entire left atrium from the remainder of the heart, which then persists in normal sinus rhythm, has been developed (Fig. 53.24).[35] Following the left atrial isolation procedure patients remain in normal sinus rhythm despite the presence of an incessant tachycardia confined to the left atrium (Fig. 53.25). No adverse sequelae have been noted over a 5-year follow-up period with this procedure.

Right atrial tachycardias may occur on the basis of automaticity or

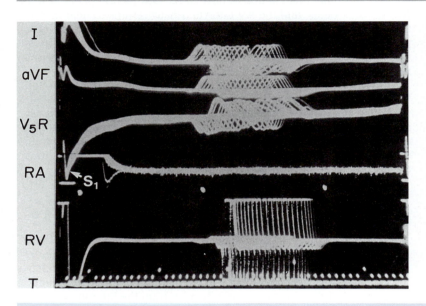

FIGURE 53.21 This photograph was taken directly from the screen of the oscilloscope used intraoperatively to monitor AV node conduction during application of the discrete cryolesions. Leads I, aV_F, and V_5R are displayed along with the electrograms recorded from the right atrium and right ventricle and time lines. The sweep of the oscilloscope is timed to the S_1 stimulus, so that the right ventricular bipolar electrogram appears at the same spot on the oscilloscope on each beat as long as the AV interval is stable. During application of the cryothermia along the tricuspid annulus prolongation of the AV interval occurs on each succeeding beat. This prolongation is seen on the oscilloscope as a progressively later occurrence of the QRS complex and of the right ventricular electrogram with each succeeding beat. If complete AV block develops during the application of the cryolesions, the cryothermia is immediately stopped and the area is irrigated with copious amounts of warm saline. Within 3 to 5 beats, AV conduction invariably returns, and within 15 to 30 seconds the AV interval gradually decreases to the range of its preoperative value. (From Cox JL, Holman WL, Cain ME: Cryosurgical treatment of atrioventricular node reentrant tachycardia. Circulation 76:1329, 1987)

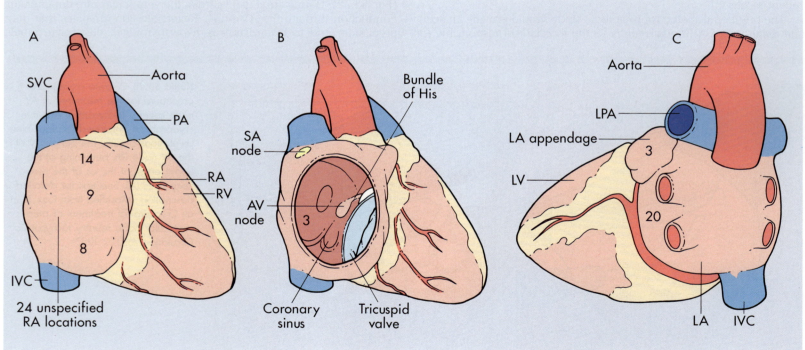

FIGURE 53.22 A. Reported locations of right atrial ectopic foci. B. Reported locations of ecotopic foci in the atrial septum and adjacent to the coronary sinus. C. Reported locations of left atrial ectopic foci. (SVC, superior vena cava; RA, right atrium; IVC, inferior vena cava; PA, pulmonary artery; RV, right ventricle; SA, sinoatrial; AV, atrioventricular; LV, left ventricle; LA, left atrium; LPA, left pulmonary artery.) (From Lowe JE, Hendry PJ, Packer DL, et al: Surgical management of chronic ectopic atrial tachycardia. Semin Thorac Cardiovasc Surg 1:58, 1989. With permission.)

reentry and are usually confined to the body of the right atrium. Although these right atrial arrhythmias are less suppressed by general anesthesia than are left atrial automatic tachycardias, and reentrant right atrial tachycardias can usually be induced by programmed stimulation, failure to localize the site of origin of the arrhythmia and their multifocal nature have previously required AV node ablation and pacemaker insertion. A right atrial isolation procedure that isolates the body of the right atrium while leaving the atrial pacemaker complex in continuity with the atrial septum and the ventricles has been developed (Fig. 53.26).[36] Early clinical results with this technique have demonstrated successful isolation of the tachycardias with no adverse sequelae during a 2-year follow-up period (Fig. 53.27).

ATRIAL FLUTTER AND ATRIAL FIBRILLATION

Atrial fibrillation is the second most lethal of all cardiac arrhythmias, second only to ventricular fibrillation. Available statistics indicate that approximately 0.4% of the United States population, one million people, suffer from atrial fibrillation.[37] The diagnosis of atrial flutter or atrial fibrillation can usually be made from the surface electrocardiogram. A preoperative electrophysiologic study should be performed in operative candidates in order to confirm that conduction occurs exclusively via the normal AV conduction system and that an accessory pathway does not exist. Until recently, surgery for atrial fibrillation/flutter has been directed toward alleviating the hemodynamic effects of these arrhythmias rather than toward ablation of the arrhythmia itself and has consisted of elective surgical interruption of AV conduction using cryothermia.[38] This therapy has been effective in controlling the ventricular rate during these arrhythmias in patients resistant to medical control, thus taking care of the problem of irregular heartbeat that these patients experience. However, this cryoablative procedure does not address the other two problems associated with atrial fibrillation: 1) the loss of atrioventricular synchrony, resulting in loss of atrial transport function; and 2) thromboembolism. Any truly effective therapy for atrial fibrillation must alleviate all three of these problems.

Studies by Boineau and colleagues[39,40] and Allessie and associates[41] have documented that both atrial flutter and fibrillation most likely occur on the basis of macroreentrant circuits. These authors have demonstrated that atrial geometry, local refractory distribution, and the resultant local conduction velocity of atrial tissues determine whether reentry will occur, how many wavefronts will form, and whether the process will be sustained.

Multipoint, computerized intraoperative mapping of patients in sinus rhythm, atrial flutter, and atrial fibrillation have confirmed these experimental findings (Fig. 53.28), with the observation that human atrial fibrillation is even more complex in terms of the number of reentrant pathways and the rapidity with which they change position in the atria. It became clear that even if all the reentrant circuits could be recorded and computer-analyzed, this information would be of limited benefit as a guide for surgical interruption of the multiple, transient reentrant circuits. The only way that atrial fibrillation could be ablated surgically would be to create a specific pathway from SA node to the

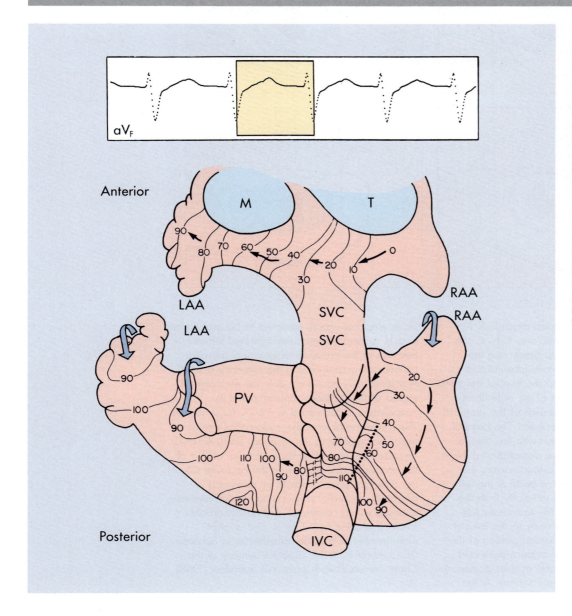

FIGURE 53.23 Focal right atrial tachycardia. The top panel shows the standard ECG lead aV_F recording during tachycardia. The boxed area is the time window analyzed to produce the activation sequence map shown beneath. The dotted line on the posterior atrium is the site of the previous atriotomy. The activation starts in the anterior right atrium and proceeds across the anterior intraatrial band (Bachmann's bundle) and through the atrial septum (exiting posteriorly) to activate the left atrium. The activation also proceeds inferiorly to activate the posterior right atrium, but is blocked at the junction between the right atrium and left atrium. (M, mitral valve; T, tricuspid valve; LAA, left atrial appendage; SVC, superior vena cava; RAA, right atrial appendage; PV, pulmonary veins; IVC, inferior vena cava.) (From Canavan TE, Schuessler RB, Cain ME et al: Computerized global electrophysiological mapping of the atrium in a patient with multiple supraventricular tachyarrhythmias. Ann Thorac Surg 46:232, 1988. With permission.)

AV node through which all electrical activity originating in the former would have to pass to reach the latter. All functional atrial myocardium would have to be activated by this sinus impulse in order for the atrium to maintain its normal transport function and to eliminate the problem of thromboembolism. A surgical procedure satisfying these criteria has been developed, appropriately named the maze procedure (Fig. 53.29). Early clinical results have been excellent.

POSTOPERATIVE ELECTROPHYSIOLOGIC ASSESSMENT

The initial postoperative assessment of the efficacy of surgery should be performed immediately after completion of the surgical procedure, with the patient on normothermic cardiopulmonary bypass. This initial study is designed to test the results of the operative intervention. A later study should be performed prior to hospital discharge to assess definitively the efficacy and sequelae of the operative intervention.

In patients operated on for the WPW syndrome, incremental atrial and ventricular pacing should be performed. During atrial pacing, the QRS complex should be normal, there should be no evidence of ventricular pre-excitation, and the AV interval should increase as the atrial pacing rate increases (decremental AV conduction). During ventricular pacing, patients should develop VA block or decremental VA conduction, a pattern of response typical of retrograde conduction through the normal conduction system.[42]

In the predischarge study, temporary atrial and ventricular epicardial pacing wires placed at the time of surgery are used to confirm the findings of the postoperative study. In rare cases the accessory pathway may only be traumatized and not actually divided during the operative procedure; in these instances, abnormal conduction usually returns within 72 hours and can be demonstrated on the predischarge study.

In patients undergoing operation for attenuation of AV node conduction for AV node reentrant tachycardia, intraoperative evaluation

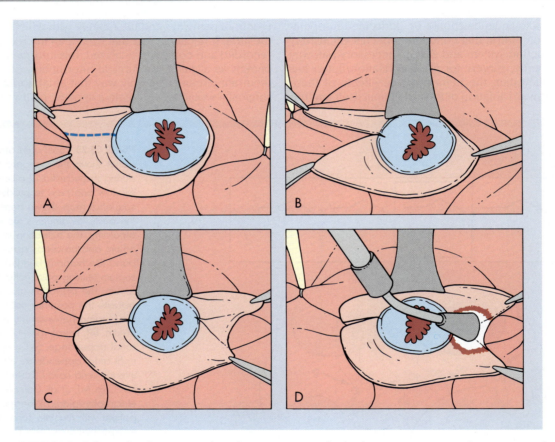

FIGURE 53.24 Left atrial isolation procedure. **A.** Following a standard left atriotomy incision, the interatrial septum is retracted gently and the atriotomy is extended anteriorly (*dashed line*) across Bachmann's bundle to the level of the mitral valve annulus just to the left of the right fibrous trigone. **B.** The anterior extension of the standard left atriotomy has been completed. The base of the aorta and its juxtaposition with the anterior leaflet of the mitral valve are demonstrated. Note that the anterior atriotomy extends across the mitral valve annulus. The main body of the left atrium has been separated anteriorly from the remainder of the heart. **C.** The transmural left atriotomy is extended posteriorly to the level of the coronary sinus. The remaining portion of the incision is made through the endocardium and extends across the mitral valve annulus posteriorly just to the left of the interatrial septum. At this point, electrical activity continues to be propagated in a 1:1 fashion between the right and left atria because of the presence of interatrial muscular connections accompanying the coronary sinus. **D.** A cryoprobe is positioned over the endocardial aspect of the posterior atriotomy, and its temperature is decreased to −60°C for 2 minutes. This cryolesion ablates the endocardial interatrial fibers accompanying the coronary sinus. A similar cryolesion is created on the epicardial aspect of the atrioventricular groove on the opposite side of the coronary sinus to ablate all remaining interatrial epicardial connections. The left atriotomy is closed with a continuous 4-0 nonabsorbable suture. (Modified from Cox JL: The surgical management of cardiac arrhythmias. In Sabiston DC, Spencer FC [eds]: Gibbon's Surgery of the Chest, 5th ed. Philadelphia, WB Saunders, 1988)

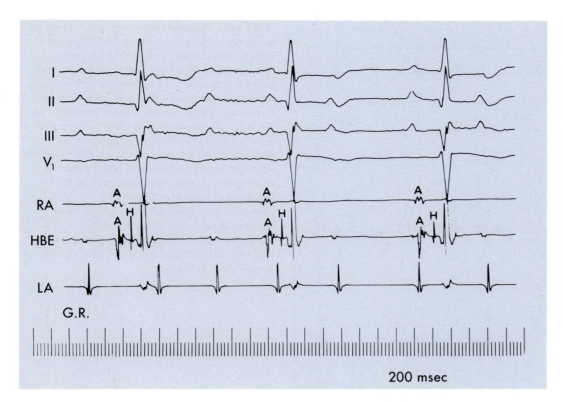

FIGURE 53.25 Postoperative recordings following surgical exclusion of the left atrium.

Recordings from the top down are surface ECG leads I to III, V$_1$, bipolar catheter recordings of the right atrium and the His bundle, and a bipolar recording obtained by permanent electrodes sutured to the left atrial appendage.

The right and left atria are dissociated. Right atrial activity proceeds from the catheter positioned in the high-right atrium to the atrial septum as recorded on the His bundle catheter, followed by conduction to the ventricle. An irregular left atrial tachycardia is present, which fails to propogate to either the right atrium or to the ventricles. Note that the surface P wave correlates with left atrial activity although the ventricles are responding to activity initiated in the right atrium. (Gallagher JJ et al: Non-pharmacologic treatment of supraventricular tachycardia. In Josephson ME, Wellens HJJ [eds]: Tachycardias: Mechanisms, Diagnosis, Treatment. Philadelphia, Lea & Febiger, 1984)

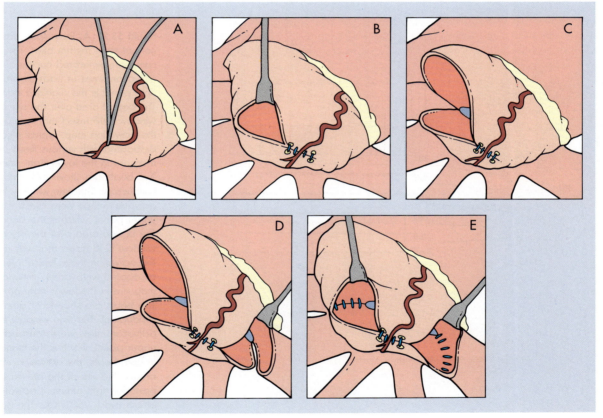

FIGURE 53.26 Right atrial isolation. **A.** Initially, the sinoatrial node artery is dissected free from the atrial tissue 5 mm anterior to the crista terminalis. A 2-cm incision parallel to the crista terminalis is placed beneath the artery. **B.** The incision beneath the sinoatrial node artery is closed with a continuous nonabsorbable 5-0 suture, taking care not to damage the artery. The small pledgets are used above and below the artery to reinforce the incision. The right atriotomy is then extended to a point anterior to the junction of the superior vena cava and the base of the right atrial appendage. **C.** The atriotomy is extended along the anterior limbus of the fossa ovalis to the anteromedial tricuspid valve annulus, just anterior to the membranous interatrial septum. **D.** Caudad extension of the right atriotomy around the posterior right atrial–inferior vena cava junction to the posterorlateral tricuspid valve annulus. A cryolesion (–60°C for 2 minutes) is placed at the end of the incision to ensure complete interruption of connecting atrial muscle fibers between the body of the right atrium and the remainder of the heart. **E.** The atriotomy is closed with a continuous 4-0 nonabsorbable suture. (Modified from Harada A et al: Right atrial isolation: A new surgical treatment for supraventricular tachycardia. I. Surgical technique and electrophysiologic effects. J Thorac Cardiovasc Surg 95:643, 1988)

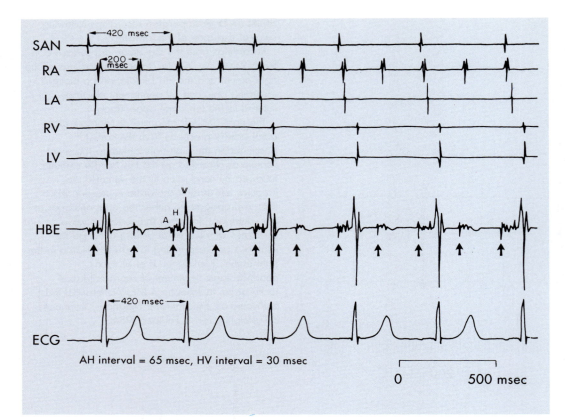

FIGURE 53.27 Postoperative electrograms recorded simulated tachycardia in the isolated right atrium. Tachycardia is simulated by rapid RA pacing at a cycle length of 200 msec and is confined to the isolated right atrium. The simulated right atrial tachycardia does not affect sinus rhythm or the normal conduction sequence in the remainder of the heart. Arrows mark right atrial pacing spikes reflected in the His bundle electrogram. (*SAN*, sinoatrial node; *RA*, right atrium; *LA*, left atrium; *RV*, right ventricle; *LV*, left ventricle; *HBE*, His bundle electrogram; *A*, atrial depolarization; *H*, His bundle depolarization; *V*, ventricular depolarization). (Harada A et al: Right atrial isolation: A new surgical treatment for supraventricular tachycardia. I. Surgical technique and electrophysiologic effects. J Thorac Cardiovasc Surg 95:643, 1988)

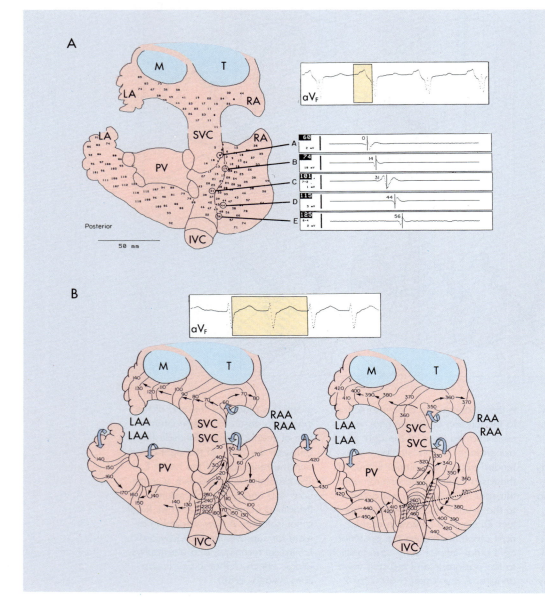

FIGURE 53.28 A. Raw data recorded from a single normal sinus rhythm beat. The left panel shows the computer-generated outline of the atrium with activation times at each electrode site. The upper right panel is the digitized standard ECG lead aV_F. The boxed area over the signal is the time window (248 msec) that was analyzed to produce the activation map. Typical electrograms associated with various times on the activation map are in the lower right panel. **B.** Atrial flutter. Two beats are shown (2:1 atrioventricular conduction). The time window from which the activation maps were constructed is shown on the upper panel, which is the standard ECG lead aV_F. The boxed area over the signal is the time window (248 msec) that was analyzed to produce the activation map. Typical electrograms associated with various times on the activation map are in the lower right panel. **B.** Atrial flutter. Two beats are shown (2:1 atrioventricular conduction). The time window from which the activation maps were constructed is shown on the upper panel, which is the standard ECG lead aV_F. In both beats, the activation wave is seen to rotate around the site of the previous atriotomy on the posterior right atrium; it activates the rest of the atrium every 260 msec. The dotted line in the activation map of the second beat is the site of the surgical incision used to interrupt the reentrant wave. (*M*, mitral valve; *T*, tricuspid valve; *SVC*, superior vena cava; *PV*, pulmonary vein; *IVC*, inferior vena cava; *LAA*, left atrial appendage; *RAA*, right atrial appendage.) (Modified from Canavan TE, Schuessler RB, Cain ME et al: Computerized global electrophysiological mapping of the atrium in a patient with multiple supraventricular tachyarrhythmias. Ann Thorac Surg 46:232, 1988. With permission.)

following cryosurgery should include assessment of AV node refractory curves in response to programmed atrial extrastimuli. It is important to use the same paced cycle lengths and coupling intervals that were found during the preoperative study to result in disparate AV node refractory curves. Postoperatively, the AV conduction interval should increase smoothly in response to progressively premature atrial extrastimuli until AV node refractoriness is reached. In addition, in our experience, VA block has been present in all patients at the completion of the operative procedure, although it returned to normal in all but one patient by the time of the predischarge study. In these patients a formal predischarge study should measure AV node refractory curves more definitively and it should demonstrate the inability of AV nodal reentrant tachycardia to be induced.

In patients operated on to isolate either the left or right atrial free wall, incremental pacing from the isolated side should not influence normal ventricular activation and pacing from the nonisolated side should result in normal conduction to both ventricles. Isolation of the dissociated electrical activity should be demonstrated in the formal predischarge study.

CLINICAL SURGICAL RESULTS
WOLFF-PARKINSON-WHITE SYNDROME
In the first 200 patients undergoing surgery for the Wolff-Parkinson-White syndrome at Duke University Medical Center there was an overall 86% success rate for division of the accessory pathway.[43] However, approximately 20% of those patients required more than one operation to accomplish this success rate. In other words, the success rate with the initial operation was only approximately 66%. In the combined Duke-Washington University series since 1981 the incidence of successful surgical correction of the Wolff-Parkinson-White syndrome using the techniques described is 100% with the initial operation, with an operative mortality for elective, uncomplicated cases of 0.5%.[14] In our series, 20% of patients have had multiple pathways, 12% Ebstein's anomaly, 34% other arrhythmias, 6% cardiomyopathy, 6% coronary artery disease, and 22% congenital heart disease other than Ebstein's anomaly.[12] There have been no early or late recurrences following surgery using the endocardial technique and thus no reoperations have been required. The epicardial closed-heart technique developed by Guiraudon has also been performed successfully in patients having free-wall as well as posterior septal accessory pathways.[44] The recurrence rate following the epicardial technique is also small.[20]

Patients with the permanent form of junctional reciprocating tachycardia (PJRT) are handled surgically exactly as patients with the classic type of Wolff-Parkinson-White syndrome, and the results are the same.[45]

AUTOMATIC ATRIAL TACHYCARDIAS
Results of direct surgical procedures for automatic atrial tachycardia have been reported in only small numbers of patients.[46] If preoperative or intraoperative localization was possible, the procedures have been uniformly successful. Several partial atrial isolation procedures have been attempted.[47] As mentioned above, the total left atrial isolation procedure has now been performed on five patients and the right atrial isolation procedures has been performed on three patients in our series, without adverse sequelae.

ATRIOVENTRICULAR NODAL REENTRY
Attenuation of input to the AV node using the discrete cryothermia technique has been performed in 32 patients in our institution with AV nodal reentrant tachycardia. In all cases postoperative electrophysiologic study has demonstrated the persistence of only a single AV conduction pathway, and the reentrant tachycardia could not be induced postoperatively. No recurrences have occurred during a 5-year follow-up period.

Johnson and co-workers have described their experience with an alternative surgical technique for this lesion, with favorable results in short-term follow-up.[48,49]

ATRIAL FIBRILLATION/FLUTTER
Direct surgical cryoablation of the normal AV conduction system is nearly always successful (89%) if the His bundle has been identified properly.[25] The maze procedure has been performed in seven patients over the past two years. All patients have remained in sinus rhythm, have objectively-demonstrated evidence of atrial transport function,

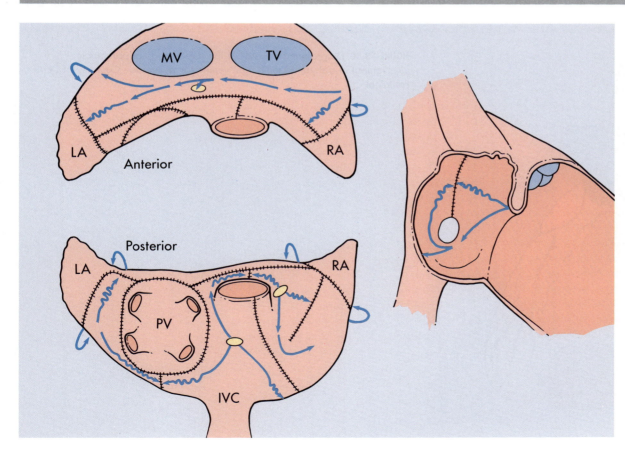

FIGURE 53.29 The maze procedure. See text for discussion. (LA, left atrium; MV, mitral valve; TV, tricuspid valve; RA, right atrium; PV, pulmonary vein; IVC, inferior vena cava.) (From Cox JL, Schuessler RB, Cain ME et al: Surgery for atrial fibrillation. Semin Thorac Cardiovasc Surg 1:67, 1989. With permission.)

and are free from thromboembolic complications. These early results warrant further application of this still-experimental form of therapy.

The surgical treatment for the Wolff-Parkinson-White syndrome is a well-established procedure, and the excellent surgical results warrant liberalization of the previously limited surgical indications for this curable congenital cardiac abnormality. At this point in time, however, surgical intervention for other types of supraventricular arrhythmias should be considered experimental.

SURGERY FOR VENTRICULAR TACHYARRHYTHMIAS

Surgical management of life-threatening ventricular tachyarrhythmias has progressed considerably in recent years.[6] Advances in pharmacologic and pacemaker therapies for these common arrhythmias have likewise occurred, but a substantial number of patients do not respond to medical treatment alone. The encouraging results with surgical intervention, discussed below, suggest that surgery should play an increasing role in the management of these most common and lethal of arrhythmias.

Differences in the clinical presentations and anatomical substrates of these arrhythmias allow them to be separated into two groups. Ischemic ventricular tachycardia, by far the most common form, results from chronic myocardial ischemia secondary to coronary artery disease. Nonischemic ventricular tachycardias occur in the absence of coronary artery disease.

NONISCHEMIC VENTRICULAR TACHYCARDIAS

Nonischemic forms of ventricular tachyarrhythmias usually arise in the right ventricle and in general are extremely resistant to medical therapy. They have been classified into five categories based on their pathologic and/or clinical characteristics.

Idiopathic ventricular tachycardia refers to patients in whom the only clinical manifestation of cardiac disease is the arrhythmia. Both the macroscopic appearance of the heart at operation and the pathologic data acquired at the time of autopsy in such patients fail to show any evidence of primary cardiac disease. The repetitive episodes of tachycardia may produce heart failure and global dilatation of the heart. A majority of these arrhythmias have been shown to arise in the septum, making initial surgical approaches difficult.[50] More recently, surgical procedures have been reported in which the arrhythmogenic area of myocardium is locally isolated if the site of origin is in the right ventricular free wall.[51] Multipoint map-guided cryoablation techniques have been used if the site of origin is in the septum.[52]

Patients with diffuse *cardiomyopathy* may present with sustained monomorphic ventricular tachycardia that is tolerated hemodynamically. These patients have angiographic and catheter data indicating some type of abnormal myocardial contractility associated with recurrent ventricular tachycardia. Pathologically, there is diffuse dilatation of both ventricles with widespread patchy myocardial fibrosis. In general, these patients are often refractory to medical therapy.[53] Unlike arrhythmias associated with coronary artery disease in which the anatomical substrate (endocardial fibrosis) is easy to identify visually at the time of surgery, the substrate for arrhythmogenesis in nonischemic cardiomyopathy can be much more difficult to identify. More extensive mapping techniques, including computerized multipoint data acquisition systems, may be required for accurate localization. Because these tachyarrhythmias frequently arise in the right ventricle, a combination of surgical isolation and cryoablation has provided treatment in this setting.[17] Following surgery, however, the potential exists for other areas of myocardium involved with the diffuse myopathic process to act as future arrhythmogenic foci.[54]

Fontaine and associates have described a previously unrecognized form of cardiomyopathy localized to the right ventricle, termed *arrhythmogenic right ventricular dysplasia*.[55] This congenital myopathy is remarkable pathologically for transmural infiltration of adipose tissue resulting in weakness and aneurysmal bulging of three pathologic areas of the right ventricle: the infundibulum, apex, and/or posterior basilar region (Fig. 53.30). Ventriculography demonstrates diffuse dilatation of the right ventricle with a significant reduction in contractility and marked delay in right ventricular emptying. Ventricular bulges or frank aneurysms are seen in one or all of the three pathologic areas noted above, and hypertrophic muscular bands in the infundibulum and anterior right ventricular wall result in apparent pseudodiverticula, the so-called feathering appearance of the right ventricular outflow tract.[56] Because the origin of the tachycardia is the right ventricle, the 12-lead ECG shows a pattern consistent with a left bundle branch block pattern during the tachycardia, and right ventriculography should be per-

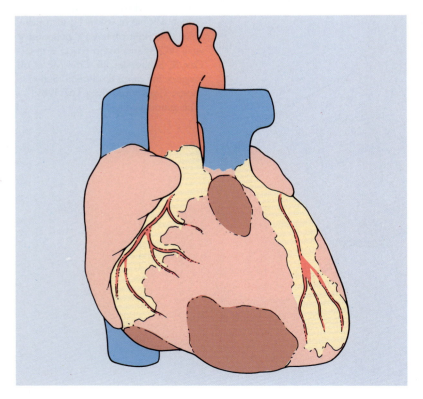

FIGURE 53.30 Diagrammatic sketch of the three areas of pathologic involvement in arrhythmogenic right ventricular dysplasia. (Courtesy of Dr. G. Fontaine)

formed in any patient with ventricular tachycardia and this QRS complex configuration.

The objective of surgical intervention in these cases is to isolate the arrhythmogenic myocardium from the remainder of the heart. During the intraoperative mapping, it is important to recognize the possibility that the three pathologically abnormal regions of the right ventricle in arrhythmogenic right ventricular dysplasia may exhibit electrical silence on epicardial mapping. The actual site of origin of the ventricular tachycardia may be in the electrically silent region and only appear to arise from the border of the silent region because a certain critical mass of synchronously depolarized myocardium is necessary to produce an electrogram large enough to be detected by the exploring electrode.

The operation consists of a transmural encircling ventriculotomy that effectively isolates the arrhythmogenic myocardium from the remainder of the heart.[51] The surgically isolated pedicle is based on a vascular supply originating from the right coronary artery (Fig. 53.31).

Two cryolesions are placed at the proximal and distal aspect of the incision at the level of the tricuspid valve annulus to ensure complete separation of all ventricular muscle fibers on either side of the incision (Fig. 53.32). In certain instances, intraoperative mapping has suggested that the entire right ventricular free wall may be arrhythmogenic, giving rise to multiple morphologic types of tachycardia. In such cases, surgical isolation of the entire right ventricular free wall has been undertaken to relieve the life-threatening sequelae of this arrhythmia, but only in the most dire of circumstances (Fig. 53.33).[6] Postoperatively, the right ventricle may undergo progressive dilatation, and cardiac transplantation in a suitable patient with this arrhythmia would be the most likely surgical approach today.

An adult form of the congenital lesion of *Uhl's syndrome* occurs in which the associated ventricular tachycardia is the dominant feature.[57] Uhl's syndrome is a rare congenital anomaly that may be considered from the anatomical standpoint to be a more complete form of arrhythmogenic right ventricular dysplasia.[56] There is complete absence

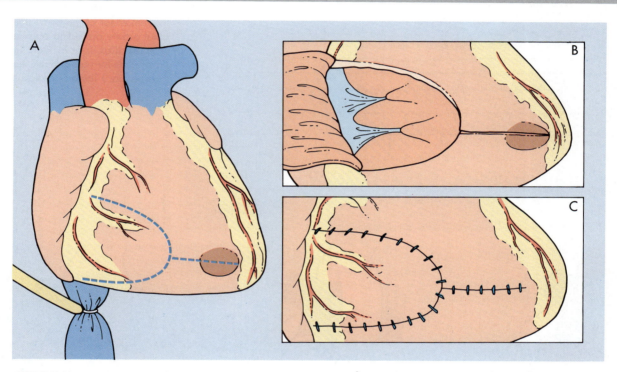

FIGURE 53.31 A. Appearance of the right ventricle in a patient with arrhythmogenic right ventricular dysplasia. Note the three coronary arteries coursing from the atrioventricular groove across the surface of the right ventricle. The acute margin of the right ventricle corresponded to the location of the middle coronary artery depicted in this drawing. An area approximately 2 × 3 cm near the upper coronary artery was electrically silent. Epicardial mapping during ventricular tachycardia demonstrated the earliest site of activation to be located near the lower edge of the electrically silent region just below the midsegment of the middle coronary artery on the posterobasilar region of the right ventricle. A transmural ventriculotomy was placed around the electrically silent area and included the apparent site of origin of the ventricular tachycardia on the posterobasilar region of the heart (*dashed line*). The two ends of this incision were based at the AV groove, where cryolesions were applied to ensure isolation of the arrhythmogenic region of myocardium from the remainder of the heart. In addition, a second transmural incision was made from the apex of the semicircular incision to the apex of the right ventricle to include the small saccular aneurysm in that region.

B. The isolated pedicle of the right ventricular myocardium containing the electrically silent area and the apparent site of origin of the ventricular tachycardia has been reflected to demonstrate the internal anatomy of the right ventricle. Note the extension of the incision to the right ventricular apex to open the small aneurysm located in that region.

C. The transmural encircling ventriculotomy around the arrhythmogenic region of the right ventricle and the simple ventriculotomy through the right ventricular apical aneurysm have been closed with a continuous 3-0 nonabsorbable suture. Following completion of this procedure for arrhythmogenic right ventricular dysplasia, the isolated pedicle was paced at a rapid rate, but the paced impulses were not conducted to the remainder of the heart. In addition, the remainder of the right ventricle was then paced rapidly, but those paced impulses were not conducted into the isolated pedicle, confirming total isolation of the arrhythmogenic right ventricular myocardium from the remainder of the heart. (Modified from Cox JL: The surgical management of cardiac arrhythmias. In Sabiston DC, Spencer FC [eds]: Gibbon's Surgery of the Chest, 5th ed. Philadelphia, WB Saunders, 1988)

of myocardium in the right ventricular free wall, resulting in the endocardial and epicardial layers being in direct contact without interposition of myocardial fibers. The right ventricle is dilated in this lesion, but the tricuspid valve remains in normal position, differentiating it from Ebstein's anomaly.

Patients with familial or idiopathic prolonged QT interval syndrome and recurrent ventricular arrhythmias have been managed with a variety of medical and surgical therapies. The electrocardiographic abnormality has been associated with several congenital syndromes and noted as a sequelae of acute myocardial infarction.[58]

Ventricular tachycardia occurring in association with the long QT interval syndrome is frequently of a distinct type called torsade de pointes, characterized by changes in QRS complex polarity during tachycardia. Accumulated data suggest that torsade de pointes represents an abnormality of myocardial repolarization, in contradistinction to other types of ventricular tachycardias, which are believed to be abnormalities of myocardial depolarization. As such, this arrhythmia should be susceptible to alterations in autonomic tone, and medical therapy with β-adrenergic blockade has been successful.[59] Surgically, left cervicothoracic sympathectomy with removal of the left stellate ganglion and the first three to four left thoracic sympathetic ganglia has been advocated.[60] Some authors have reported abolition of symptoms

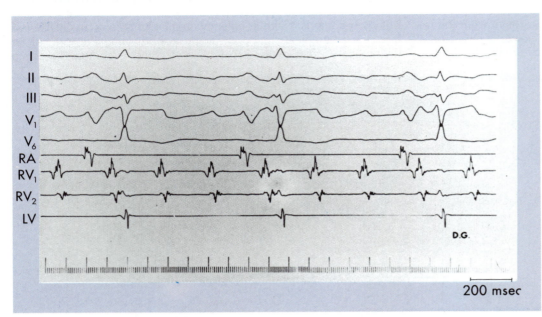

FIGURE 53.32 Surface recordings and intracardiac electrograms in a 16-year-old boy during an episode of right ventricular tachycardia following the right ventricular isolation procedure. The limb lead (I–III) and precordial lead (V_1 and V_6) electrograms demonstrated normal sinus rhythm in the remainder of the heart documented by right atrial activity preceding each left ventricular complex. (Cox JL et al: Right ventricular isolation procedures for non-ischemic ventricular tachycardia. J Thorac Cardiovasc Surg 90:212, 1985)

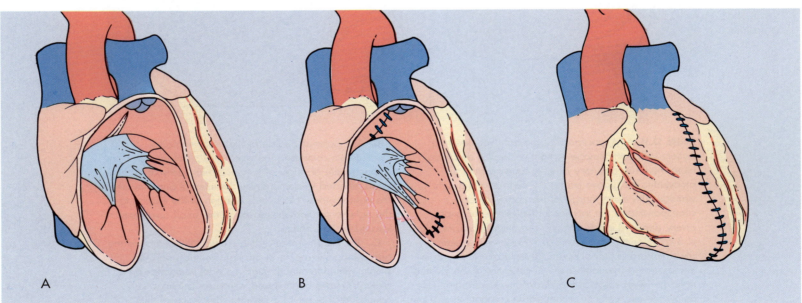

FIGURE 53.33 Right ventricular disconnection procedure. **A.** A transmural right ventriculotomy is placed parallel to and 5 mm from the interventricular septum extending from just across the pulmonic valve annulus anteriorly to the tricuspid valve posteriorly. It is necessary to divide several large infundibular muscular bundles and to divide the moderator band of the right ventricle. Although the entire incision is transmural, special care must be taken to avoid injury to the right coronary artery lying in the AV groove at the posterior extent of this incision. After identification of the location of the His bundle and right bundle branch, a second transmural incision is placed from the posterior pulmonic valve annulus to the anterior medial tricuspid valve annulus, exposing the underlying aortic root. If the tricuspid portion of this incision is placed too far anteriorly, the bundle of His may be inadvertently divided. **B.** After completion of the two transmural incisions, the papillary muscle attached to the anterior leaflet of the tricuspid valve is divided at its base and reimplanted on the lower ventricular septum using interrupted 3-0 pledgeted Prolene suture. Cryolesions are placed at each end of the anteroposterior ventriculotomy and at each end of the ventriculotomy between the posterior pulmonic valve annulus and the anterior medial suture, followed by closure of the long free-wall ventriculotomy with continuous 3-0 nonabsorbable suture (**C**). (Modified from Cox JL: Surgery for cardiac arrhythmias. Curr Probl Cardiol 8(4), 1983)

following the procedure in a number of patients with the long QT interval syndrome,[61] but others have found the results to be characterized by early success and late failure.[62,63] Because of these equivocal surgical results, implantation of an automatic defibrillator has been advocated as an adjunct to sympathectomy, to serve as backup therapy in those with a history of life-threatening arrhythmias.[64] Recently, permanent atrial or ventricular pacing in combination with β-blocker therapy has been tried in a subset of patients with promising early results.[65]

ISCHEMIC VENTRICULAR TACHYCARDIA

The most common ventricular tachyarrhythmias are those that occur in association with ischemic heart disease. Serious ventricular arrhythmias of this type are harbingers of sudden cardiac death within the first year after an acute myocardial infarction[66] and are frequently unresponsive to medical management.

Surgical treatment for ventricular tachycardias in the setting of ischemic heart disease dates to 1959, when Couch and associates performed a simple aneurysmectomy in an attempt to ablate the tachycardia.[67] Since then, much progress has been made through the development of a number of surgical procedures designed to cure the patient of the tachycardia. Nevertheless, the role of surgery as primary therapy for ventricular arrhythmias in the setting of ischemic heart disease is still in the process of evolution.

Experimental studies performed 20 years ago documented the heterogeneity of tissue injury in acute myocardial infarction.[68] The process of acute infarction results in the juxtaposition of normal and injured myocardium, and ventricular irritability, tachycardia, and fibrillation frequently occur during the initial and early phases of the infarct. These manifestations of acute ischemic injury are usually transient and tend to be responsive to medical management. On occasion, patients will develop life-threatening tachyarrhythmias during the setting of an acute infarction, during exercise-induced ischemia, or during episodes of angina pectoris. In this subset of patients coronary revascularization as primary therapy has been quite successful.[69,70]

In the majority of patients, however, there is subsequent progression of the acutely ischemic tissue to cell death, leaving a fibrous scar in place of the injured myocardium. The interlacing anisotropic pattern of the remaining scar and normal myocardium may harbor local areas of slow conduction, unidirectional block, uneven refractoriness, and nonuniform repolarization, which are the electrophysiologic substrates for the development of reentrant circuits.[71-73] These regions are located primarily in the endocardium and subendocardium, especially at the periphery of myocardial infarcts or ventricular aneurysms. Electrical activity is believed to be identifiable as part of the reentrant tachycardia circuit if it precedes the onset of ventricular depolarization evident on the surface electrocardiogram and is required for the initiation and perpetuation of the tachycardia. The site of origin of the tachycardia is believed to be the area exhibiting the earliest presystolic electrical activity in the latter half of diastole and represents the region of myocardium that must be identified and removed at the time of surgery in order to prevent the arrhythmias.[74]

PREOPERATIVE ELECTROPHYSIOLOGIC AND HEMODYNAMIC EVALUATION

All patients who are surgical candidates should undergo complete electrophysiologic, angiographic, and ventriculographic evaluation. The catheter electrophysiologic study should confirm that the arrhythmia is ventricular and not supraventricular in origin and should demonstrate that the arrhythmia is reentrant by induction and termination with programmed electrical stimulation techniques.[75] In addition, identification of the earliest site of origin on the endocardium of all morphologically distinct tachycardias using "catheter mapping" techniques is performed. Monomorphic ventricular tachycardias originate from a single region of the left or right ventricle and are usually stable enough to permit catheter localization on the preoperative study. Nonsustained monomorphic tachycardias, however, may not be stable enough to permit localization. *Multiple monomorphic ventricular tachycardia* is a term applied to ventricular tachycardias arising from several different regions of the left ventricle, giving rise to different morphologic types of tachycardia. In contrast, polymorphic ventricular tachycardia is characterized by a beat-to-beat variation in the QRS complex during the tachycardia. These polymorphic ventricular tachycardias originate from one region of the ventricle but are associated electrophysiologically with excessive fragmentation such that the individual depolarization complexes may be difficult to identify. This fragmentation may be due to afterdepolarizations or in fact may indicate a multifocal origin. From a surgical point of view, however, it is convenient to distinguish between simple monomorphic ventricular tachycardia and other more complex types, including the multiple monomorphic and polymorphic forms.

Polymorphic tachycardias may be sustained or nonsustained and commonly deteriorate into ventricular fibrillation. Polymorphic nonsustained ventricular tachycardia that quickly deteriorates into ventricular fibrillation must be distinguished from primary ventricular fibrillation. This latter arrhythmia is characterized by the absence of any type of induced ventricular tachycardia prior to the onset of ventricular fibrillation following programmed electrical stimulation and is not yet amenable to surgical therapy.

SURGICAL INDICATIONS AND CONTRAINDICATIONS

The final decision regarding surgical therapy for ischemic ventricular tachycardia is based on a variety of preoperative clinical factors. The primary indication for surgery is refractoriness to medical therapy. Controversy exists, however, as to whether patients who have failed amiodarone therapy should be included in this group. Amiodarone has been shown to depress left ventricular function, and this depressant effect is aggravated by ischemic cardioplegic arrest in the majority of patients on the drug.[76,77] Because therapy with amiodarone can complicate surgical intervention in patients requiring a procedure for ventricular tachycardia and coronary revascularization, and because it fails to control the arrhythmia in a significant number of patients,[77,78] it would appear logical to make the decision regarding surgical intervention prior to the institution of amiodarone therapy, after the patient has been shown to be refractory to all other medications.

In a review of the available literature, virtually all demographic, clinical, catheterization, and electrophysiologic factors that might predispose to an increased operative risk have been evaluated.[79] Only three preoperative variables clearly increase the operative mortality rate: (1) in a patient with a ventricular aneurysm, the nonaneurysmal portion of the left ventricle is so dysfunctional that class III or IV heart failure exists preoperatively; (2) in a patient without a ventricular aneurysm, global dysfunction is so severe that class III or IV heart failure exists preoperatively; and (3) if emergency surgical intervention is required. Thus the only absolute contraindication to surgery for ischemic ventricular tachycardia is left ventricular dysfunction so severe that the operative risk is prohibitive. Because most patients with ischemic heart disease and ventricular tachycardia have a left ventricular aneurysm, accurate determination of the ejection fraction is often difficult in these patients, and the absolute number is not an accurate predictor of operative mortality.[79] Poor systolic function in the nonaneurysmal portion of the ventricle would, as indicated, appear to increase operative risk.[80]

The availability of computerized mapping systems that permit localization of the majority of the areas of arrhythmogenic myocardium have made the presence of nonsustained polymorphic ventricular tachycardia no longer a contraindication to surgery.

INTRAOPERATIVE ELECTROPHYSIOLOGIC MAPPING

The role of intraoperative mapping is closely related to the type of procedure that is performed. With the advent of intraoperative mapping techniques,[81,82] the concept existed that intraoperative localization of the region of origin of the tachycardia would permit a relatively limited procedure to be performed. These types of procedures have been termed *localized* and include the subendocardial resection originally described by the Pennsylvania group,[83] endocardial cryoablation, laser protoablation, and the partial encircling endocardial ventriculotomy popularized by Ostermeyer and co-workers.[84] The other category of procedures is termed *generalized* and includes the original encircling endocardial ventriculotomy,[85] the extended endocardial resection procedure,[86] and procedures that completely encircle the visible scar with contiguous cryolesions or laser photoablation. These generalized procedures do not depend on intraoperative mapping, because they are directed toward the entire visible anatomical substrate (endocardial fibrosis) associated with the ventricular tachycardia. If any of these procedures are performed without intraoperative mapping, they are referred to as "blind" or "visually guided" procedures, while if they are performed with intraoperative mapping they are referred to as "guided" procedures.

A number of authors have argued that performance of a procedure that resects more potentially arrhythmogenic tissue (*i.e.*, a generalized procedure) would minimize the assumed benefit associated with intraoperative mapping. A review of the literature provides data that are inconclusive;[79] however, in the one intrainstitutional study where map-guided and blind procedures performed by the same surgical group were compared, the reinducibility rate was significantly lower in the map-guided group.[87] Furthermore, the operative mortality for map-guided procedures reported in the literature is 11.6% and for "blind" procedures it is 11.4%, indicating that performance of extensive intraoperative mapping in these patients did not increase their operative risk.[79] This same analysis demonstrated that the reinducibility rate of tachycardia was slightly lower with generalized as opposed to localized procedures, although this difference was not significant. A logical conclusion from these findings is to employ intraoperative mapping as a guide and that wide excision or exclusion of the suspected arrhythmogenic tissue should be performed. The development of more sophisticated multipoint computerized mapping systems will undoubtedly produce an overall beneficial effect on the results of ventricular tachycardia surgery.

The detailed intraoperative mapping procedure is performed as follows in our institution. All 160 channels of the computerized system are used to map the heart in patients with ventricular tachycardia. An epicardial map employing a 96-electrode sock array (Fig. 53.34) is recorded, and this information is used to guide the subsequent placement of plunge needle electrodes to delineate further the specific site of arrhythmogenesis (Fig. 53.35). The epicardial map is also most useful in characterizing nonclinical arrhythmias that may be induced during programmed electrical stimulation.

Subsequently, multiple plunge needle electrodes containing four bipolar pairs of electrodes are inserted into the ventricle in the region of earliest epicardial activation (Fig. 53.36). If the tachycardia appears to be arising from the intraventricular septum, a right atriotomy is performed and up to 15 plunge needle electrodes are inserted into the septum from the right side. A total of up to 160 endocardial, intramural, and epicardial data points can be simultaneously recorded from the septum and free wall. A ventriculotomy, which can prevent further inducibility of the ventricular tachycardia and necessitate performance of a "blind" procedure, does not have to be performed in order to obtain an endocardial map. The results of the 160-point plunge needle map are automatically analyzed for activation times by the computer, edited, and displayed on the CRT in the operating room. The earliest epicardial site of activation is displayed on the screen (Fig. 53.37) and then the entire activation sequence is displayed cinematically.

GUIDED SURGICAL TREATMENT OF ISCHEMIC VENTRICULAR TACHYCARDIA

The encircling endocardial ventriculotomy (EEV) was introduced in 1978 by Guiraudon and colleagues and was the first technique specifically designed to control refractory ischemic ventricular tachycardia.[82] The objective of the encircling endocardial incision just outside the junction of endocardial fibrosis and normal myocardium was either to interrupt the reentrant circuit or to encompass it entirely and isolate it from the remainder of the ventricle. Laboratory studies demonstrated, however, that the encompassed myocardium was made more ischemic, thus suppressing the reentrant circuit responsible for the tachy-

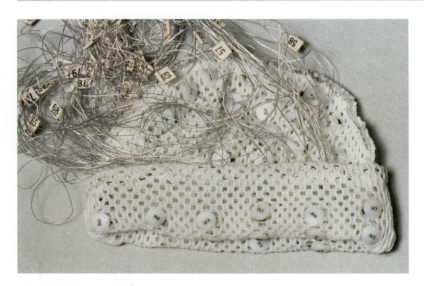

FIGURE 53.34 Ninety-six-electrode sock that fits over both ventricles to record epicardial activation data during sinus rhythm and during different morphologic types of ventricular tachycardia.

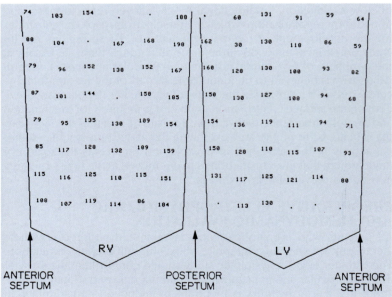

FIGURE 53.35 Hard copy of the color graphics terminal display of data recorded from the 96 epicardial electrodes in the sock electrode array during induced ventricular tachycardia. The epicardial data show that the earliest area of epicardial breakthrough is over the upper anterior ventricular septum. (Cox JL: Intraoperative computerized mapping techniques. In Brugada P, Wellens HJJ [eds]: Cardiac Arrhythmias: Where to Go From Here? Mount Kisco, NY, Futura Publishing Company, 1987)

cardia. This increased ischemia caused by the EEV resulted in poorer left ventricular function following the procedure in these studies, and clinically the EEV was associated with an unacceptable incidence of postoperative low output syndrome and operative mortality.[88-91]

In 1979, the group in Philadelphia introduced the concept of a directed procedure based on intraoperative mapping and then resection of the endocardial fibrosis in the arrhythmogenic region, thus either interrupting or removing the reentrant circuit (Fig. 53.38).[85] This local endocardial resection procedure (ERP) was later modified by Moran and co-workers so that all of the endocardial fibrosis was removed regardless of the location of the arrhythmogenic tissue, an extended endocardial resection procedure (EERP) (Fig. 53.39).[86] The addition of cryothermic techniques was combined with the EERP to ablate arrhythmogenic tissue that was located near the aortic or mitral valve annuli or on the base of the papillary muscles.[91] It has been demonstrated that the base of the papillary muscles can be cryoablated without causing mitral regurgitation.[92]

More recently, Ostermeyer and associates have used a partial EEV technique in which an endocardial incision is placed only in the region of arrhythmogenesis with excellent results,[84,92] and Krafchek and associates have reported superior results with a technique that combines wide endocardial resection with endocardial cryosurgery.[93]

The current technique employed at our institution involves the initial intraoperative mapping sequence described above, usually on cardiopulmonary bypass. Then with the heart in the normothermic beating state and preferably in ventricular tachycardia, the ventricle is opened through the infarct or aneurysm and all of the associated endocardial fibrosis is resected except that which extends onto the base of the papillary muscles. Approximately 10% of patients will still have inducible tachycardia following resection of the fibrosis, indicating that the actual site of origin of the tachycardia in these patients is deeper in the myocardium than the visible border of the fibrosis. Endocardial cryolesions are applied to the site(s) of origin of the tachycardia(s) as determined from the intraoperative mapping data, thus destroying the myocardium underneath the visible fibrosis responsible for the tachycardia (Fig. 53.40). Resection of endocardial fibrosis extending onto the base of the papillary muscles is not performed; instead, as mentioned above, one or more cryolesions are placed directly on the base of the involved papillary muscle. The clinical and laboratory experience with this method of dealing with fibrosis extending onto the base of the papillary muscle argues strongly against the practice of resecting papillary muscles for ventricular tachycardia as has been reported in the past.[86]

Following completion of the extended endocardial resection and endocardial cryoablation, programmed electrical stimulation is applied in an attempt to reinduce the arrhythmia. If ventricular tachycardia is still inducible, mapping is again performed and the remaining arrhythmogenic myocardium is cryoablated. If the arrhythmia is no longer inducible in this setting intraoperatively there is a 98% chance that it has been ablated.[79] If coronary bypass grafting or other procedures are to be performed, then they are carried out after completion of the antiarrhythmic portion of the operation and confirmation of the result. The reason for the strict insistence that cardioplegic solution not be administered until the antiarrhythmic portion of the operative procedure is successfully completed is that the cardioplegia itself may temporarily alter the delicate reentry circuits causing the tachycardia. If the antitachycardia procedure is performed under cardioplegic arrest, it is impossible to determine intraoperatively whether the surgical procedure has ablated the arrhythmia.

Promising results using endocardial mapping followed by ablation of the arrhythmogenic myocardium using the ND-YAG laser has been reported.[94,95] This technique is easy and quick to perform and can be applied to the normothermic beating heart, which is a major advantage as described above. Immediate reapplication of programmed stimulation to determine the efficacy of the procedure has facilitated excellent surgical results.

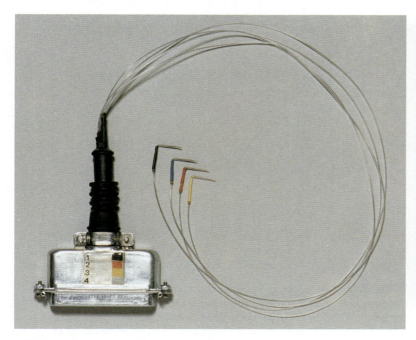

FIGURE 53.36 One bay of four needle electrodes. Each needle shaft contains four bipolar electrodes to record data from four different layers of the ventricular free wall and/or septum; thus, this one bay carries signals recorded from 16 individual sites in the heart. By inserting multiple needle electrodes, endocardial maps of the left and/or right ventricles (in addition to intramural and epicardial maps) can be constructed without a ventriculotomy. (Cox JL: Intraoperative computerized mapping techniques. In Brugada P, Wellens HJJ [eds]: Cardiac Arrhythmias: Where to Go From Here? Mount Kisco, NY, Futura Publishing Company, 1987)

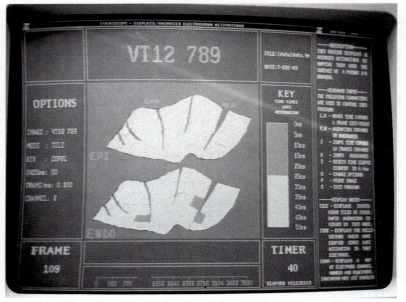

FIGURE 53.37 Photograph taken directly from the CRT in the operating room, illustrating the earliest endocardial activation on either side of the interventricular septum for this morphologic type of tachycardia in a patient undergoing surgical ablation. Subsequent frame displays would illustrate the remaining activation sequence.

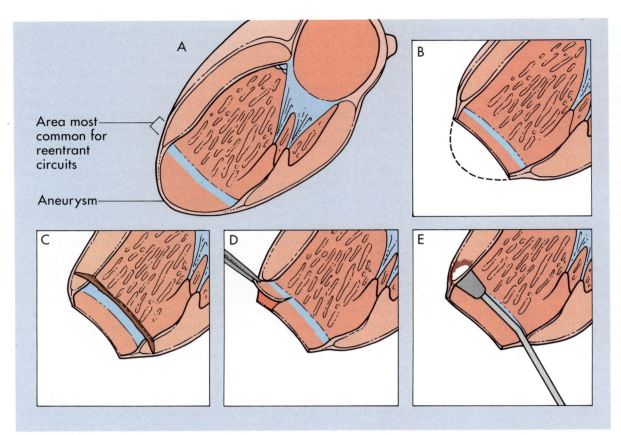

FIGURE 53.38 Diagrammatic cross-section of an anterior left ventricular aneurysm showing more proximal extension of the associated fibrosis at the endocardial level than at the epicardial level (**A**). Since the reentrant circuits responsible for ischemic ventricular tachycardia occur most commonly at the junction of this endocardial fibrosis and normal myocardium, a standard left ventricular aneurysm resection (**B**) does not ablate or remove them. The encircling endocardial ventriculotomy (**C**), localized endocardial (or "subendocardial") resection (**D**), and endocardial cryoablation (**E**) were all introduced specifically to ablate ventricular tachycardia associated with left ventricular aneurysms or infarcts. (Modified from Cox JL: Anatomic-electrophysiologic basis for the surgical treatment of refractory ischemic ventricular tachycardia. Ann Surg 198:119, 1983)

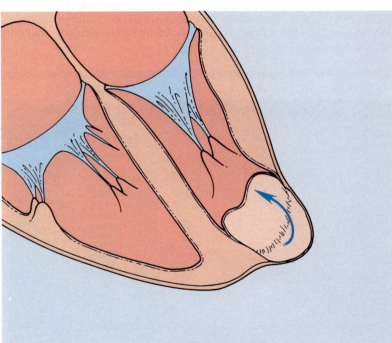

FIGURE 53.39 Diagrammatic sketch of an extended endocardial resection procedure (EERP) in an anterior left ventricular aneurysm. The principle involved in this procedure is the same as that for localized ERP, but in this procedure all of the endocardial fibrosis associated with the aneurysm is resected except that involving the papillary muscle. (Modified from Cox JL: Surgical treatment of ischemic and non-ischemic ventricular tachyarrhythmias. In Cohn LH [ed]: Modern Technics in Surgery. Mount Kisco, NY, Futura Publishing Company, 1985)

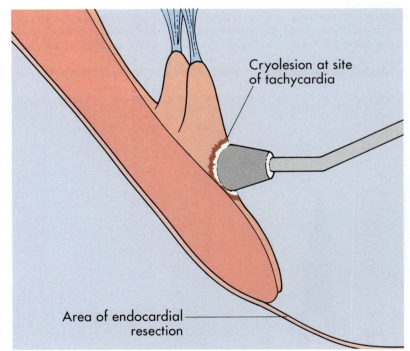

FIGURE 53.40 After resecting all of the endocardial scar as a preliminary measure, endocardial cryolesions are placed at the site or sites of origin of the ventricular tachycardia as determined by intraoperative mapping. In addition, any remaining scar on the papillary muscle is cryoablated as shown. (Modified from Cox JL: Surgical treatment of ischemic and nonischemic ventricular tachyarrhythmias. In Cohn LH [ed]: Modern Technics in Surgery. Mount Kisco, NY, Futura Publishing Company, 1985)

SURGICAL RESULTS AND CURRENT PROBLEMS

The lack of consensus regarding the optimal surgical technique for ventricular tachycardia surgery would suggest that problems regarding this type of surgery exist; these relate to operative mortality and surgical failure, that is, persistence of the preoperative tachycardia(s) postoperatively. A complete review of the cumulative experience during the past decade demonstrates an average operative mortality rate of 12.4% (range 0–21%) and an average postoperative reinducibility rate of 23.8% (range 0–38%).[79] Nevertheless, these data must be weighed against the fact that currently the medical therapy has failed in the majority of patients coming to surgery for ventricular tachycardia.

The preoperative and intraoperative variables that impact on operative mortality have been alluded to in the previous discussion. Amiodarone therapy, evidence of severe left ventricular dysfunction, and the requirement for emergent surgical intervention appear to be associated with an increased operative risk. Intraoperatively, the only variables known to represent an incremental risk factor for operative death in ventricular tachycardia surgery are the use of the EEV and the inability to perform an aneurysmectomy.[84,91] The probable reason for the paucity of intraoperative variables correlating with operative mortality is that preoperative left ventricular dysfunction is such a powerful predictor of operative mortality that the majority of other intraoperative factors are rendered insignificant. Importantly, aortic cross-clamp time, cardiopulmonary bypass time, intraoperative mapping, and the avoidance of cardioplegic arrest cannot be correlated with the operative mortality in surgery for ventricular tachycardia.[79]

Thus a significant lowering of operative mortality for ventricular tachycardia surgery can only be achieved by more optimal selection of patients for surgery and development of methodologies to manage patients considered to be too high a surgical risk.

Regarding the reinducibility rate of tachycardia, the only two preoperative variables that have been demonstrated to be a predictor of surgical failure are the presence of complex (polymorphic or multiple monomorphic) ventricular tachycardia, and the anatomical-electrophysiologic character of the arrhythmia.[79] Ventricular tachycardia associated with a posteroinferior infarct or aneurysm is more difficult to eradicate than that arising in the anterior portion of the left ventricle.[74,79,80] Several authors have suggested, however, that intraoperative measures such as more extensive mapping and/or the use of adjunctive procedures such as cryosurgery may be capable of overcoming the increased risk of surgical failure in this group (Fig. 53.41).

The intraoperative factors that affect the reinducibility rate of ventricular tachycardia are the operative procedure performed (generalized or localized), whether intraoperative mapping is used ("guided" or "blind"), and whether the surgical procedure for ventricular tachycardia is performed under cardioplegic arrest or in the normothermic, beating heart. The results of this analysis suggest that generalized procedures are probably more effective in curing ventricular tachycardia than are localized procedures, the use of intraoperative mapping to guide surgical procedures for ventricular tachycardia results in a higher cure rate than can be attained with "blind" surgical procedures, and ventricular tachycardia surgery performed in the normothermic, beating heart probably results in a higher cure rate than surgery performed under cardioplegic arrest.[79] This last point is not yet conclusive, but we feel strongly that the practice of performing ventricular tachycardia surgery under cardioplegic arrest is the major reason for the high reinducibility rates at the time of the postoperative electrophysiologic study reported in most series.[79] The ability to induce ventricular tachycardias during the postoperative electrophysiologic study has a profound effect on subsequent prognosis, increasing the incidence of spontaneous ventricular tachycardia and/or sudden death sixfold in this postoperative population.[74,80,84,86,93,95,96]

The final aspect in evaluating the results of surgical intervention for ventricular tachycardia is assessment of the long-term follow-up results of surgery. A review of the five series with over 50 patients and greater than 5-year follow-up in the literature[74,79,84,87,97] demonstrates a 64% overall 5-year survival rate for these patients, most of whom are critically ill at the time of surgical intervention.[79] More importantly, of those patients who survive surgery, 96% were either cured by surgery alone or were able to have their arrhythmia controlled postoperatively by medical therapy, a remarkable success rate in these patients with a life-threatening problem.

ALGORITHM FOR THE OPTIMAL SURGICAL MANAGEMENT OF REFRACTORY ISCHEMIC VENTRICULAR TACHYCARDIA

Using the previous discussion as a basis, an algorithm for the optimal surgical treatment of refractory ventricular tachycardia can be constructed. As indicated in Figure 53.42, this scheme proposes a therapeutic and preventative role for the automatic internal cardioverter-

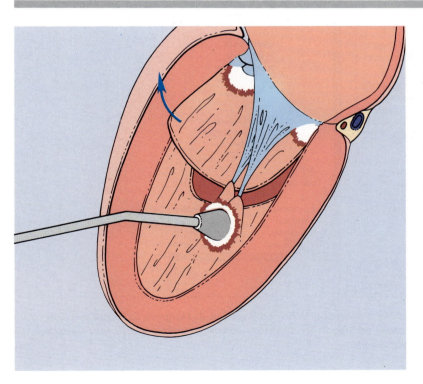

FIGURE 53.41 Extended endocardial resection of the fibrosis associated with a posterior myocardial infarction or aneurysm and cryoablation of the lower two thirds of the posterior papillary muscle. The endocardial fibrosis is resected to within 5 mm of the aortic and mitral valve annuli. Because the site of origin of ventricular tachycardia is frequently adjacent to the junction of the aortic and mitral valve annuli, endocardial cryolesions (*white circles*) are applied at the base of the aortic and mitral valve annuli to ablate any reentrant circuits that might reside in the remaining endocardial fibrosis immediately beneath the valve annuli. In addition, endocardial cryolesions are applied to the site or sites of origin of ventricular tachycardia as determined by intraoperative mapping, but only after removal of all endocardial scar. (Modified from Cox JL: Surgical treatment of ischemic and nonischemic ventricular tachyarrhythmias. In Cohn LH [ed]: Modern Technics in Surgery. Mount Kisco, NY, Futura Publishing Company, 1985)

defibrillator (AICD) in ventricular tachycardia surgery. With this algorithm as a guide, the following points can be emphasized:

1. The evaluation regarding surgical intervention for medically refractory ischemic ventricular tachycardia should be made prior to institution of amiodarone therapy.
2. This evaluation should be based primarily on the determination that the patient has a sufficient degree of normal left ventricular function to survive operative intervention.
3. If the patient has a prohibitive degree of left ventricular dysfunction, amiodarone therapy should be begun. If this therapy is unsuccessful, then implantation of an AICD should be undertaken, provided that the episodic rate of the patient's tachycardia is low enough so as to not exhaust the battery supply of the device or make the patient's life prohibitively uncomfortable due to an excessive number of device discharges.
4. If the patient's tachycardia is uncontrolled on amiodarone with an AICD, then cardiac transplantation should be considered. If the patient is not a transplant candidate, then ventricular tachycardia surgery is the only therapeutic option available.
5. If the patient's left ventricular function is acceptable for surgery, then the surgical approach outlined above is recommended.
6. If the institution does not have the capability of performing computerized intraoperative mapping or cryosurgery, if a "blind" proce-

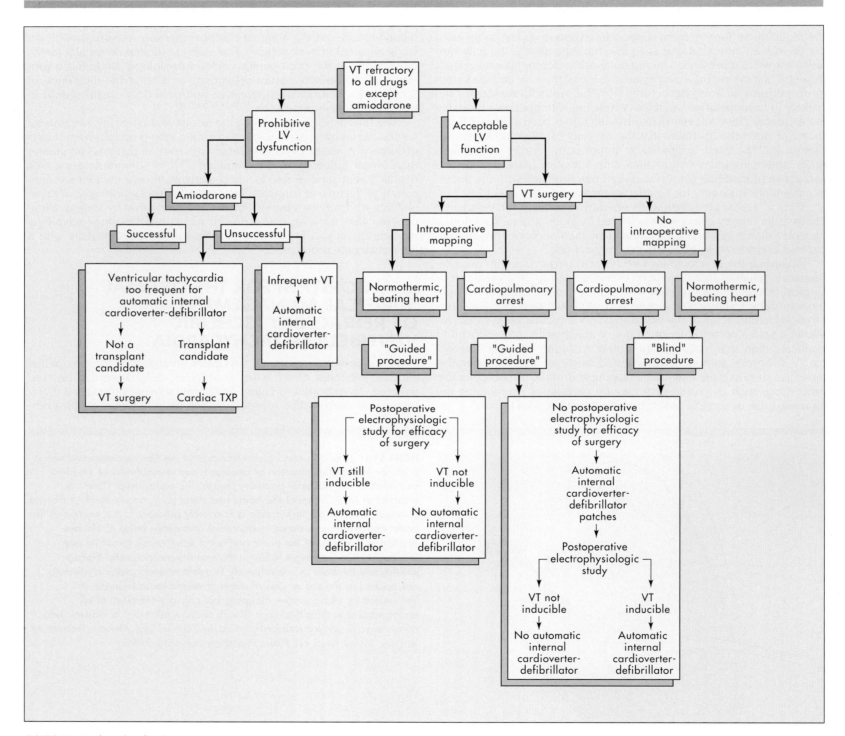

FIGURE 53.42 Algorithm for the selection and treatment of patients with ischemic ventricular tachycardia that is refractory to all antitachycardia drugs except amiodarone. The decision regarding surgery or amiodarone is made at this point because of the increased risk of surgery in patients who are taking amiodarone. (Modified from Cox JL, Hargrove C: Patient selection criteria and results for refractory ischemic ventricular tachycardia. Circulation, [in press])

dure is performed, or if the surgical procedure is performed under cardioplegic arrest then it seems prudent to place AICD patches in these patients at the time of their ventricular tachycardia surgery. The rationale for this recommendation is that approximately 25% of these patients will have inducible tachycardia following the surgical procedure. If the tachycardia is inducible at the time of the postoperative electrophysiologic study then the device should be implanted. On the other hand, if the rationale recommended here for surgical intervention is employed, implantation of the AICD device and patches would then only be necessary in the few patients in whom tachycardia was inducible on the postoperative electrophysiologic study.

7. Careful scrutiny of the operative and long-term follow-up results for ventricular tachycardia surgery would appear to argue strongly against routine implantation of the AICD device and performance of coronary bypass surgery as a therapeutic modality for ventricular tachycardia, as has been advocated by some.[98] Furthermore, it should be recognized that the AICD device actually provides an extremely viable therapeutic option for those patients in whom performance of ventricular tachycardia surgery has been fraught with an excessive mortality, namely, patients with extreme degrees of left ventricular dysfunction. Judicious selection of these patients for the much-simplified operative procedure of AICD implantation should reduce the operative mortality rate in this subset of ventricular tachycardia patients and thus reduce the overall operative mortality rate for ventricular tachycardia procedures as well.

The long-term success rate for ventricular tachycardia surgery should provide an extremely strong impetus in the future to optimize the preoperative evaluation, operative selection, and intraoperative management of this critically ill but potentially curable group of cardiac surgical patients.

REFERENCES

1. Cobb FR, Blumenschein SD, Sealy WC et al: Successful surgical interruption of the bundle of Kent in a patient with Wolff-Parkinson-White syndrome. Circulation 38:1018, 1968
2. Anderson RH, Becker AE: Cardiac anatomy for the surgeon. In Danielson GK (ed): Lewis' Practice of Surgery, Chap 16. Hagerstown, MD, Harper & Row, 1979
3. Boineau JP, Mooney C, Hudson R et al: Observations on re-entrant excitation pathways and refractory period distribution in spontaneous and experimental atrial flutter in the dog. In Kulbertus HE (ed): Re-entrant Arrhythmias, pp 79–98. Baltimore, MD, University Park Press, 1977
4. Anderson RH, Becker AE: Morphology of the human atrioventricular junction area. In Wellens HJJ, Lie KI, Janse MJ et al (eds): The Conduction System of the Heart: Structure, Function and Clinical Implications, p 264. Philadelphia, Lea & Febiger, 1976
5. Gallagher JJ, Kasell JH, Sealy WC et al: Epicardial mapping in the Wolff-Parkinson-White syndrome. Circulation 57:854, 1978
6. Cox JL: Surgery for cardiac arrhythmias. Curr Probl Cardiol 8(4):46, 1983
7. Witkowski FX, Corr PB: An automated simultaneous transmural cardiac mapping system. Am J Physiol 247:H661, 1984
8. Cox JL: Intraoperative computerized mapping techniques. In Brugada P, Wellens HJJ (ed): Cardiac Arrhythmias: Where to Go From Here? Mount Kisco, NY, Futura Publishing Company, 1987
9. Wolff L, Parkinson J, White PD: Bundle branch block with short PR interval in healthy young people prone to paroxysmal tachycardia. Am Heart J 5:685, 1930
10. Wolferth CC, Wood FC: The mechanism of production of short P-R intervals and prolonged QRS complexes in patients with presumably undamaged hearts: Hypothesis of an accessory pathway of auriculo-ventricular conduction (bundle of Kent). Am Heart J 8:297, 1933
11. Bardy GH, Packer DL, German LD et al: Pre-excited reciprocating tachycardia in patients with Wolff-Parkinson-White syndrome: Incidence and mechanisms. Circulation 70:377, 1984
12. Cain ME, Cox JL: Surgical treatment of supraventricular tachyarrhythmias. In Platia EV (ed): Management of Cardiac Arrhythmias—The Nonpharmacologic Approach. Philadelphia, JB Lippincott, 1987
13. Kramer JB, Corr PB, Cox JL et al: Arrhythmia and conduction disturbances: Simultaneous computer mapping to facilitate intraoperative localization of accessory pathways in patients with Wolff-Parkinson-White syndrome. Am J Cardiol 56:571, 1985
14. Cox JL, Gallagher JJ, Cain ME: Experience with 118 consecutive patients undergoing surgery for the Wolff-Parkinson-White syndrome. J Thorac Cardiovasc Surg 90:490, 1985
15. Cox JL, Cain ME: Surgery for pre-excitation syndromes. In Benditt DG, Benson DW Jr (eds): Pre-excitation Syndromes: Origins, Evaluation, and Treatment. Hingham, MA, Martinus Nijhoff, 1986
16. Cox JL: A clarification of the techniques most commonly employed for the surgical treatment of the Wolff-Parkinson-White syndrome. Ann Thorac Surg (in press)
17. Cox JL: The surgical management of cardiac arrhythmias. In Sabiston DC, Spencer FC (eds): Gibbon's Surgery of the Chest, 5th ed. Philadelphia, WB Saunders, 1988
18. Guiraudon GM, Klein GJ, Sharma AD et al: Surgical ablation of posterior septal accessory pathways in the Wolff-Parkinson-White syndrome by a closed heart technique. J Thorac Cardiovasc Surg 92:406, 1986
19. Klein GJ, Guiraudon GM, Perkins DG et al: Surgical correction of the Wolff-Parkinson-White syndrome in the closed heart using cryosurgery: A simplified approach. J Am Coll Cardiol 3:405, 1984
20. Guiraudon GM, Klein GJ, Sharma AD et al: Closed-heart technique for Wolff-Parkinson-White syndrome: Further experience and potential limitations. Ann Thorac Surg 42:651, 1986
21. Gallagher JJ, Sealy WC, Cox JL et al: Results of surgery for pre-excitation caused by accessory atrioventricular pathways in 267 consecutive cases. In Josephson ME, Wellens HJJ (eds): Tachycardias: Mechanisms, Diagnosis, and Treatment, pp 259–269. Philadelphia, Lea & Febiger, 1984
22. Sealy WC: Arrhythmia surgery: An overview. In Iwa T, Fontaine G (eds): Cardiac Arrhythmias: Recent Progress in Investigation and Management. Amsterdam, Elsevier, 1988
23. Josephson ME, Kastor JA: Supraventricular tachycardia: Mechanisms and management. Ann Intern Med 87:346, 1977
24. Wu D: Reentrant tachycardia within normal conduction system: Atrioventricular nodal tachycardia, junctional reciprocating tachycardia, and His-Purkinje system tachycardia. In Iwa T, Fontaine G (eds): Cardiac Arrhythmias: Recent Progress in Investigation and Management. Amsterdam, Elsevier, 1988
25. Sealy WC, Gallagher JJ, Kasell JH: His bundle interruption for control of inappropriate ventricular responses to atrial arrhythmias. Ann Thorac Surg 32:429, 1981
26. Scheinman MM, Morady F, Hess DS et al: Catheter-induced ablation of the atrioventricular junction to control refractory supraventricular arrhythmias. JAMA 248:851, 1982
27. Morady F: Interventional electrophysiology: Catheter ablation techniques. In Platia EV (ed): Management of Cardiac Arrhythmias—The Nonpharmacologic Approach. Philadelphia, JB Lippincott, 1987
28. Holman W, Ikeshita M, Lease J et al: Elective prolongation of atrioventricular conduction by multiple discrete cryolesions: A new technique for the treatment of paroxysmal supraventricular tachycardia. J Thorac Cardiovasc Surg 84:554, 1982
29. Holman WL, Ikeshita M, Lease JG et al: Alteration of antegrade atrioventricular conduction by cryoablation of periatrioventricular nodal tissue. J Thorac Cardiovasc Surg 88:67, 1984
30. Holman WL, Ikeshita M, Lease JG et al: Cryosurgical modification of retrograde atrioventricular conduction: Implications for the surgical treatment of atrioventricular node reentry tachycardia. J Thorac Cardiovasc Surg 91:826, 1986
31. Cox JL, Holman WL, Cain ME: Cryosurgical treatment of atrioventricular node reentry tachycardia. Circulation 76:1329, 1987
32. Denes P, Wu D, Dhingra R et al: Dual atrioventricular nodal pathways: A common electrophysiological response. Br Heart J 37:1069, 1975
33. Gillette PC, Garson A Jr: Electrophysiologic and pharmacologic characteristics of automatic ectopic atrial tachycardia. Circulation 56:571, 1977
34. Gallagher JJ, Cox JL, German LD et al: Nonpharmacologic treatment of supraventricular tachycardia. In Josephson ME, Wellens HJJ (eds): Tachycardias: Mechanisms, Diagnosis, and Treatment, pp 271–285. Philadelphia, Lea & Febiger, 1984
35. Williams JM, Ungerleider RM, Lofland GK et al: Left atrial isolation: New technique for the treatment of supraventricular arrhythmias. J Thorac Cardiovasc Surg 80:373, 1980
36. Harada A, D'Agostino HJ Jr, Schuessler RB et al: Right atrial isolation: A new surgical treatment for supraventricular tachycardia. I. Surgical technique and electrophysiologic effects. J Thorac Cardiovasc Surg 95:643, 1988
37. Cox JL, Schuessler RB, Cain ME et al: Surgery for atrial fibrillation. Semin Thorac Cardiovasc Surg 1:67, 1989
38.. Klein GJ, Sealy WC, Pritchett ELC et al: Cryosurgical ablation of the atrioventricular node-His-bundle: Long-term follow-up and properties of the junctional pacemaker. Circulation 61:8, 1980
39. Boineau JP, Schuessler RB, Mooney CR et al: Natural and evoked atrial flutter due to circus movement in dogs. Am J Cardiol 45:1167, 1980
40. Boineau JP, Wylds AC, Autry LJ et al: Mechanisms of atrial flutter as determined from spontaneous and experimental models. In Josephson ME, Wellens HJJ (eds): Tachycardias: Mechanisms, Diagnosis and Treatment, pp 91–111. Philadelphia, Lea & Febiger, 1984
41. Allessie MA, Lammers WJEP, Bonke IM et al: Intra-atrial reentry as a mecha-

42. Akhtar M, Damato AN, Batsford WP et al: A comparative analysis of antegrade and retrograde conduction patterns in man. Circulation 52:766, 1975
43. Gallagher JJ, Sealy WC, Cox JL et al: Results of surgery for pre-excitation in 200 cases (abstr). Circulation 64:IV-164, 1981
44. Guiraudon GM, Klein GJ, Gulamhusein S et al: Surgical repair of Wolff-Parkinson-White syndrome: A new closed-heart technique. Ann Thorac Surg 37:67, 1984
45. Guarnieri T, Sealy WC, Kasell JH et al: The nonpharmacologic management of the permanent form of junctional reciprocating tachycardia. Circulation 69:269, 1984
46. Josephson ME, Spear JF, Harken AH et al: Surgical excision of automatic atrial tachycardia: Anatomic and electrophysiologic correlates. Am Heart J 104:1076, 1982
47. Yee R, Guiraudon GM, Gardner MJ et al: Refractory paroxysmal sinus tachycardia: Management by subtotal right atrial exclusion. J Am Coll Cardiol 3:400, 1984
48. Ross DL, Johnson DC, Denniss AR et al: Curative surgery for atrioventricular junctional ("AV nodal") reentrant tachycardia. J Am Coll Cardiol 6:1383, 1985
49. Johnson DC: Results of surgical cure for atrioventricular junctional reentrant tachycardia. In Iwa T, Fontaine G (eds): Cardiac Arrhythmias: Recent Progress in Investigation and Management. Amsterdam, Elsevier, 1988
50. Fontaine G, Guiraudon G, Frank R et al: Surgical management of ventricular tachycardia not related to myocardial ischemia. In Josephson ME, Wellens HJJ (eds): Tachycardias: Mechanisms, Diagnosis, Treatment, p 451. Philadelphia, Lea & Febiger, 1984
51. Cox JL, Bardy GH, Damiano RJ et al: Right ventricular isolation procedures for nonischemic ventricular tachycardia. J Thorac Cardiovasc Surg 90:212, 1985
52. Iwa T, Mikai K, Misaki T et al: Surgical management of the Wolff-Parkinson-White syndrome. In Iwa T, Fontaine G (eds): Cardiac Arrhythmias: Recent Progress in Investigation and Management. Amsterdam, Elsevier, 1988
53. Poll DM, Marchlinski FE, Buxton AE et al: Sustained ventricular tachycardia in patients with idiopathic dilated cardiomyopathy: Electrophysiologic testing and lack of response to antiarrhythmic drug therapy. Circulation 70:451, 1984
54. Marchlinski FE, Josephson ME: Surgical treatment of ventricular tachyarrhythmias. In Platia EV (ed): Management of Cardiac Arrhythmias—the nonpharmacologic approach. Philadelphia, JB Lippincott, 1987
55. Fontaine G, Guiraudon G, Frank R: Management of chronic ventricular tachycardia. In Narula OS (ed): Innovations in Diagnosis and Management of Cardiac Arrhythmias. Baltimore, Williams & Wilkins, 1979
56. Fontaine G, Fontaliran F, Linares-Cruz E et al: The arrhythmogenic right ventricle. In Iwa T, Fontaine G (eds): Cardiac Arrhythmias: Recent Progress in Investigation and Management. Amsterdam, Elsevier, 1988
57. Bharati S, Ciraulo DA, Bilitch M et al: Inexplicable right ventricle and bilateral bundle branch block in Uhl's disease. Circulation 57:636, 1978
58. Schwartz PJ, Periti M, Malliani A: The long Q-T syndrome. Fund Clin Cardiol 89:378, 1975
59. Moss AJ, Schwartz PJ, Crampton RS et al: The long QT syndrome: A prospective international study. Circulation 71:17, 1985
60. Schwartz PJ: The idiopathic long QT syndrome. Ann Intern Med 99:561, 1983
61. Malliani A, Schwartz PJ, Zanchetti A: Neural mechanisms and life-threatening arrhythmias. Am Heart J 100:705, 1980
62. Benson DW Jr, Cox JL: Surgical treatment of cardiac arrhythmias. In Roberts NK, Gelband H (eds): Cardiac Arrhythmias in the Neonate, Infant and Child, 2nd ed, pp 341–366. New York, Appleton-Century-Crofts, 1982
63. Bhandari AK, Scheinman MM, Morady F et al: Efficacy of left cardiac sympathectomy in the treatment of patients with the long QT syndrome. Circulation 70(6):1018, 1984
64. Platia EV, Griffith LSC, Watkins L et al: Management of the prolonged QT syndrome and recurrent ventricular fibrillation with an implantable automatic cardioverter-defibrillator. Clin Cardiol 8:490, 1985
65. Eldar M, Griffin JC, Abbott JA et al: Permanent cardiac pacing in patients with the long QT syndrome. J Am Coll Cardiol 10:600, 1987
66. Breithardt G, Broggrefe M, Podczeck A et al: Prognostic significance of programmed ventricular stimulation for identification of patients at risk of ventricular tachyarrhythmias. In Iwa T, Fontaine G (eds): Cardiac Arrhythmias: Recent Progress in Investigation and Management. Amsterdam, Elsevier, 1988
67. Couch OA Jr: Cardiac aneurysm with ventricular tachycardia and subsequent excision of aneurysm. Circulation 20:251, 1959
68. Cox JL, McLaughlin VW, Flowers NC et al: The ischemic zone surrounding acute myocardial infarction: Its morphology as detected by dehydrogenase staining. Am Heart J 76:650, 1968
69. Zheutlin T, Steinman R, Summers C et al: Long-term outcome in survivors of cardiac arrest with non-inducible ventricular tachycardia during programmed stimulation. Circulation 70:II-399, 1984
70. Bryson AL, Parisi AF, Schechter E et al: Life-threatening ventricular arrhythmias induced by exercise. Am J Cardiol 32:995, 1973
71. Boineau JP, Cox JL: Slow ventricular activation in acute myocardial infarction: A source of re-entrant premature ventricular contractions. Circulation 48:702, 1973
72. Boineau JP, Cox JL: Rationale for a direct surgical approach to control ventricular arrhythmias. Am J Cardiol 49:381, 1982
73. Cox JL: Anatomic-electrophysiologic basis for the surgical treatment of refractory ischemic ventricular tachycardia. Ann Surg 198:119, 1983
74. Miller JM, Kienzle MG, Harken AH et al: Subendocardial resection for ventricular tachycardia: Predictors of surgical success. Circulation 70:624, 1984
75. Miller JE, Josephson ME: Intracardiac electrophysiologic studies in sustained ventricular tachycardia. In Iwa T, Fontaine G (eds): Cardiac Arrhythmias: Recent Progress in Investigation and Management. Amsterdam, Elsevier, 1988
76. Landymore R, Marble A, MacKinnon G et al: Effects of oral amiodarone on left ventricular function in dogs: Clinical implications for patients with life-threatening ventricular tachycardia. Ann Thorac Surg 37:141, 1984
77. Klein RC, Machell C, Rushforth N et al: Efficacy of intravenous amiodarone as short-term treatment for refractory ventricular tachycardia. Am Heart J 115:96, 1988
78. Hockings BE, George T, Mahrous F et al: Effectiveness of amiodarone on ventricular arrhythmias during and after acute myocardial infarction. Am J Cardiol 60:967, 1987
79. Cox JL: Patient selection criteria and results of surgery for refractory ischemic ventricular tachycardia. Circulation (in press)
80. Garan H, Nguyen K, McGovern B et al: Perioperative and long-term results after electrophysiologically directed ventricular surgery for recurrent ventricular tachycardia. J Am Coll Cardiol 8:201, 1986
81. Wittig JH, Boineau JP: Surgical treatment of ventricular arrhythmias using epicardial transmural and endocardial mapping. Ann Thorac Surg 20:117, 1975
82. Gallagher JJ, Oldham HN Jr, Wallace AG et al: Ventricular aneurysm with ventricular tachycardia: Report of a case with epicardial mapping and successful resection. Am J Cardiol 35:696, 1975
83. Guiraudon G, Fontaine G, Frank R et al: Encircling endocardial ventriculotomy: A new surgical treatment of life-threatening ventricular tachycardias resistant to medical treatment following myocardial infarction. Ann Thorac Surg 26:438, 1978
84. Ostermeyer J, Borggrefe M, Breithardt G et al: Direct operations for the management of life-threatening ischemic ventricular tachycardia. J Thorac Cardiovasc Surg 94:848, 1987
85. Josephson ME, Harken AH, Horowitz LN: Endocardial excision—a new surgical technique for the treatment of recurrent ventricular tachycardia. Circulation 60:1430, 1979
86. Moran JM, Kehoe RF, Loeb JM et al: Extended endocardial resection for the treatment of ventricular tachycardia and ventricular fibrillation. Ann Thorac Surg 34:538, 1982
87. Swerdlow CD, Mason JW, Stinson EB et al: Results of operations for ventricular tachycardia in 105 patients. J Thorac Cardiovasc Surg 92:105, 1986
88. Ungerleider RM, Holman WL, Stanley TE III et al: Encircling endocardial ventriculotomy (EEV) for refractory ischemic ventricular tachycardia. I. Electrophysiologic effects. J Thorac Cardiovasc Surg 83:840, 1982
89. Ungerleider RM, Holman WL, Stanley TE III et al: Encircling endocardial ventriculotomy (EEV) for refractory ischemic ventricular tachycardia. II. Effects on regional myocardial blood flow. J Thorac Cardiovasc Surg 83:850, 1982
90. Ungerleider RM, Holman WL, Calcagno D et al: Encircling endocardial ventriculotomy (EEV) for refractory ischemic ventricular tachycardia. III. Effects on regional left ventricular function. J Thorac Cardiovasc Surg 83:857, 1982
91. Cox JL, Gallagher JJ, Ungerleider RM: Encircling endocardial ventriculotomy (EEV) for refractory ischemic ventricular tachycardia. IV. Clinical indications, surgical technique, mechanism of action, and results. J Thorac Cardiovasc Surg 83:865, 1982
92. Ostermeyer J, Breithardt G, Borggrefe M et al: Surgical treatment of ventricular tachycardias: Complete versus partial encircling endocardial ventriculotomy. J Thorac Cardiovasc Surg 87:517, 1984
93. Krafchek J, Lawrei GM, Roberts R et al: Surgical ablation of ventricular tachycardia: Improved results with a map-directed regional approach. Circulation 73:1239, 1986
94. Selle JG, Svenson RH, Sealy WC et al: Successful clinical laser ablation of ventricular tachycardia: A promising new therapeutic method. Ann Thorac Surg 42:380, 1986
95. Svenson RH, Gallagher JJ, Selle JG et al: Neodymium:YAG laser photocoagulation: A successful new map-guided technique for the intraoperative ablation of ventricular tachycardia. Circulation 76:1319, 1987
96. Kron IL, Lerman BB, Nolar SP et al: Sequential endocardial resection for the surgical treatment of refractory ventricular tachycardia. J Thorac Cardiovasc Surg 94:843, 1987
97. McGiffin DC, Kirklin JK, Plumb VJ et al: Relief of life-threatening ventricular tachycardia and survival after direct operation. Circulation 76:V-93, 1987
98. Fonger JD, Guarnieri T, Griffith LSC et al: Impending sudden cardiac death: Treatment with myocardial revascularization and automatic implantable cardioverter defibrillator. Presented at the Twenty-third Annual Meeting of The Society of Thoracic Surgeons, Toronto, Ontario, Canada, September 22, 1987

CATHETER ABLATION FOR CARDIAC ARRHYTHMIAS

CHAPTER 54 — VOLUME 1

Melvin M. Scheinman

In recent years, techniques have been developed using standard electrode catheters for ablation of the atrioventricular (AV) junction, accessory AV pathways, and arrhythmic foci. These techniques have proven to be of value for selected patients with drug-refractory cardiac arrhythmias.

HISTORICAL PERSPECTIVE

A number of closed-chest animal models for disruption of AV conduction have been described.[1-3] These techniques generally involve injection of caustic substances into the region of the AV junction. In 1976, Beazell and associates[4] described a technique of closed-chest ablation of the AV junction in dogs using direct-current shocks delivered via a catheter positioned by fluoroscopy in the region of the AV junction. This technique was later modified by Gonzalez and co-workers[5] to allow for ready and reproducible production of complete AV block in dogs. Careful anatomical evaluation of these dogs showed no evidence of atrial septal perforation or disruption of the cardiac valvular apparatus.[6] My colleagues and I performed the first catheter ablative procedure in humans in March 1981.

Brodman and colleagues[7] described pathologic changes in the left annulus resulting from direct-current discharges delivered to the coronary sinus. This technique was first used by the same group for attempted ablation of left free wall accessory pathways in patients with the Wolff-Parkinson-White syndrome.[8] Hartzler[9] was first to describe use of a catheter technique for attempted ablation of ventricular tachycardia foci in humans.

CATHETER ABLATION OF THE AV JUNCTION

TECHNIQUE

The procedure involves insertion of an electrode catheter by vein against the apex of the right ventricle, which is used for cardiac pacing after ablation. A second multipolar electrode catheter is introduced by vein and manipulated in order to record a unipolar His bundle of greatest amplitude (Figs. 54.1 and 54.2). The patient is anesthetized with a short-acting anesthetic agent, and one or more direct-current shocks are delivered from the catheter electrode in close proximity to the His bundle to a patch positioned over the left scapula (Fig. 54.3). Temporary pacing is instituted via the catheter inserted into the right ventricle, and the patient is carefully monitored in a coronary care unit. A permanent cardiac pacemaker is inserted after stable complete AV block has been established for at least 24 hours.

CLINICAL USE

Prior to the introduction of catheter ablative procedures, patients with supraventricular tachycardia refractory to drug or anti-tachycardia pacemaker devices were treated by direct surgical ablation of the His bundle. The surgical technique involves open-heart surgery with direct severance of the His bundle. Most of the reported cases to date involve use of this technique for patients with atrial fibrillation or flutter that is resistant to drug therapy. It should be noted that catheter disruption of

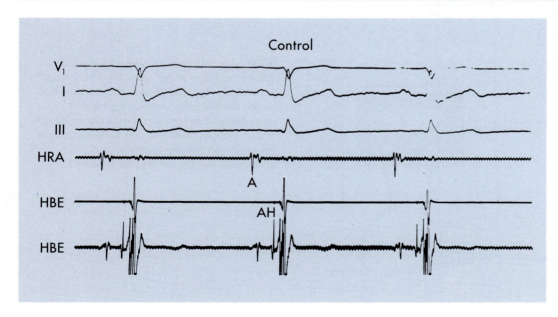

FIGURE 54.1 Surface leads V_1, I, and III are recorded simultaneously with intracardiac electrograms from the high right atrium (*HRA*) and His bundle electrograms (*HBE*). The catheter electrode with the largest unipolar His deflection is chosen as the cathode.

the AV junction may be applied for any supraventricular arrhythmia using the AV junction as a conduit to the ventricles. Thus, patients with drug-refractory atrial tachycardia, AV junctional reentry tachycardia, or AV tachycardia involving a bypass tract may potentially benefit from catheter ablative procedures. In patients with the Wolff-Parkinson-White syndrome, the usual tachycardia circuit involves antegrade conduction over the AV node–His axis and retrograde conduction over the bypass tract. Successful ablation of the AV junction completely suppresses this tachycardia (Fig. 54.4). Catheter ablation has been used successfully for such patients who have failed medical therapy as well as anti-tachycardia pacing or attempts at direct surgical incision of the bypass tract. It should be emphasized that patients with the Wolff-Parkinson-White syndrome must be carefully evaluated prior to attempted AV junctional ablation. First, it must be demonstrated that the AV junction is an obligatory participant of the tachycardia circuit. Second, the accessory pathway refractory period should not allow for rapid transmission of impulses to the ventricle should atrial fibrillation supervene. Furthermore, it is recommended that these patients undergo insertion of a permanent "backup" ventricular pacemaker since the natural history of successful long-term conduction over the bypass tract is not known (Fig. 54.5). Another subset of patients who may benefit from catheter ablation of the AV junction involves those with AV reentrant tachycardia incorporating a nodoventricular Mahaim tract. In these patients, careful evaluation is required to define the mechanisms of the tachycardia.[10,11] His bundle ablation would be expected to be universally successful in those whose tachycardia circuit involves antegrade conduction over the Mahaim pathway and retrograde conduction via the His bundle. In contrast, if the tachycardia mechanism is related to AV node reentry (with the Mahaim tract as passive bystander) then AV junctional ablation distal to the takeoff of the Mahaim tract may not prevent tachycardia (Fig. 54.6). In addition, preliminary experience with a small number of patients with nodoventricular pathways who have undergone AV junctional ablation suggests that permanent pacemaker insertion may not be required.[12,13]

CLINICAL EXPERIENCE

A number of reports from throughout the world have documented the efficacy of catheter-induced AV junctional ablation.[14-17] The widest experience to date has been summarized by the Percutaneous Map-

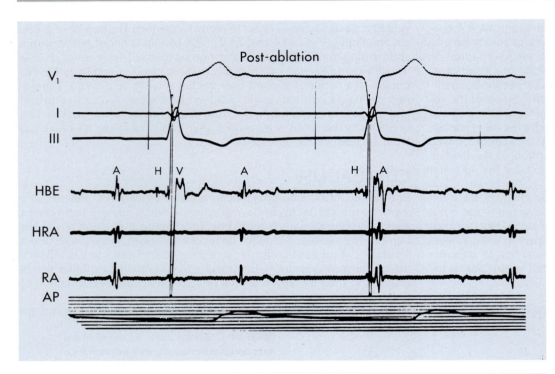

FIGURE 54.2 After delivery of one shock of 200 joules, simultaneous V_1, I and III surface leads are recorded with His bundle electrogram (*HBE*), high right atrial (*HRA*) and mid-right atrial electrograms (*RA*). The arterial pressure (top scale = 200 mm Hg) is recorded at the bottom. Post ablation complete atrioventricular block is present with emergence of a junctional pacemaker. Atrial deflection (*A*) and His bundle deflection (*H*) are noted.

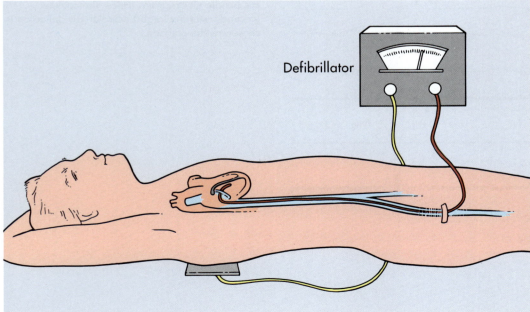

FIGURE 54.3 Schematic showing technique of catheter ablation of the atrioventricular junction. A catheter is inserted by vein and positioned to record the maximum unipolar His bundle electrogram. One or more shocks are delivered from a standard direct-current defibrillator from the electrode catheter (cathode) to a patch positioned over the left scapula (anode).

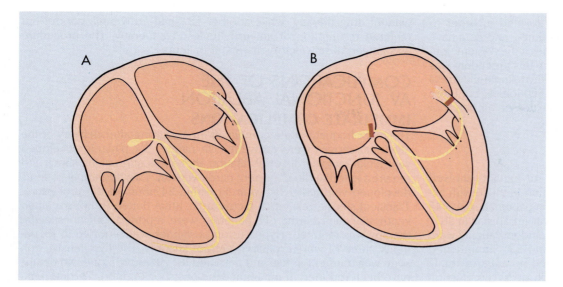

FIGURE 54.4 A. Schema showing typical reentrant circuit for patients with the Wolff–Parkinson–White syndrome. Conduction occurs antegradely over the atrioventricular node–His axis and retrogradely via the accessory pathway. **B.** Since both the atrioventricular junction and accessory pathway are necessary components of the tachycardia circuits, successful ablation of either structure should eliminate reentrant tachyarrhythmias.

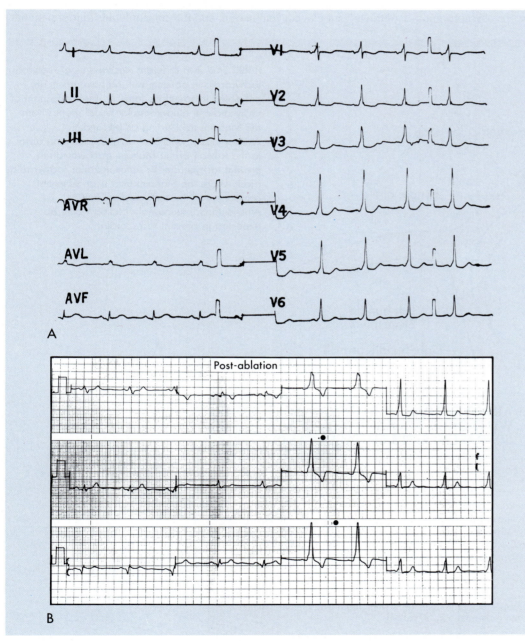

FIGURE 54.5 A. Twelve-lead ECG from a patient with the Wolff–Parkinson–White syndrome and frequent drug-resistant episodes of paroxysmal orthodromic atrioventricular tachycardia. The ECG shows fusion complexes resulting from simultaneous activation of the ventricles from both normal and accessory pathways. **B.** Twelve-lead ECG following atrioventricular junctional ablation in the same patient with the Wolff–Parkinson–White syndrome. Post ablation, the ECG shows maximal preexcitation since the ventricles are totally activated from the accessory pathway.

ping and Ablation Registry.[18] This registry was formed in order to monitor the safety and efficacy of ablative procedures, and data have been provided for 367 patients undergoing ablation of the AV junction. The types of supraventricular arrhythmias for which this procedure was instituted are listed in Table 54.1. The magnitude of single electrical shocks used for ablation varied between 80 and 500 joules, but more recent reports confirm successful ablation with lesser amounts of energy.[19]

CLINICAL RESPONSE

Immediately after delivery of the shock(s), 90% of patients showed either complete AV block (or maximal preexcitation in those with accessory pathways). The average rate of the escape pacemaker was 45 (±15) beats per minute. The escape pacemaker was infrahisian in 58%, suprahisian in 32%, and indeterminate in the remainder. Patients were followed over a mean of 11 (±10) months, and 63% maintained chronic stable third degree AV block and required no antiarrhythmic drugs. The remaining patients showed resumption of AV conduction within a mean of 6 (±18) days after the procedure. Ten percent of patients who had resumption of AV conduction were asymptomatic without drug therapy, while another 12% had arrhythmia control but required resumption of antiarrhythmic drug therapy. The procedure was judged unsatisfactory in 15% of patients.

COMPLICATIONS OF THE AV JUNCTIONAL ABLATION
IMMEDIATE COMPLICATIONS

The most frequent acute complications occurring after delivery of the electrical shocks were arrhythmic in nature. Six patients developed ventricular tachycardia or fibrillation after application of the shock and required external direct-current cardioversion. Two additional patients developed ventricular tachycardia within 24 hours of the procedure. Transient sinus arrest, atrial tachycardia, atrial flutter, or nonsustained ventricular tachycardia (17 patients) were reported, but no specific therapy was required. Hypotension postshock was reported in six patients, three of whom required pressor support. The hypotensive episode was transient in five and persisted for 72 hours in one. No deaths have been reported in the immediate postshock period. Thromboembolic complications included a pulmonary embolus in one, thrombosis of the left subclavian vein in one, and thrombophlebitis in four patients.

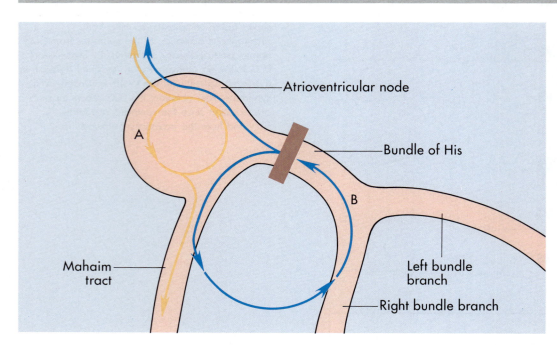

FIGURE 54.6 Two different mechanisms of reentrant tachycardia in patients with Mahaim tracts are presented in schematic form. **A.** The mechanism of tachycardia is atrioventricular nodal reentry with the Mahaim tract acting as bystander. Atrioventricular junctional ablation occurring distal to the takeoff of the Mahaim tract would not prevent tachycardia. **B.** Atrioventricular tachycardia circuit where the Mahaim tract is an essential component of the tachycardia circuit. Atrioventricular junctional ablation would be expected to prevent tachycardia.

TABLE 54.1 ARRHYTHMIAS IN PATIENTS WITH DRUG-REFRACTORY SUPRAVENTRICULAR TACHYCARDIA

Diagnosis	Percent*
Atrial fibrillation/flutter	61
Atrioventricular node reentry	17
Accessory pathway	14
Atrial tachycardia	9
Permanent junctional reciprocating tachycardia	2
Other	2

* The percentages total more than 100% since more than one arrhythmia may have been present in a given patient.

(Scheinman MM, Evans-Bell T, and the Executive Committee of the Percutaneous Mapping and Ablation Registry: Catheter ablation of the atrioventricular junction: A report of the Percutaneous Mapping and Ablation Registry. Circulation 70:1024, 1984, by permission of the American Heart Association)

One patient developed a large right atrial thrombus despite prior anticoagulant therapy. In addition, infectious complications, all related to pacemaker insertion, were recorded in four patients. One patient in a presumed immunodeficient state died of overwhelming sepsis. One patient had diaphragmatic pacing and ventricular tachycardia, which resolved on repositioning of the temporary pacing electrode.

LATE COMPLICATIONS

Late complications included a cerebrovascular accident 17 months after ablation in a patient with atrial fibrillation; another had a probable arterial embolus after the procedure. Long-term pacemaker complications included a pacemaker-mediated tachycardia in three, pacemaker tracking of supraventricular tachycardia in two, pacemaker inhibition resulting from myopotential sensing in one, and symptoms owing to acute pacemaker failure in two. A slow, underlying pacemaker emerged in the latter two patients.

FOLLOW-UP MORTALITY STATISTICS

A total of 19 patients died in the follow-up period. The death was sudden and of natural causes in eight and occurred in the period from 3 days to 13 months after ablation. Seven of these patients had underlying organic cardiac disease, and one was free of known heart disease. Four patients died of severe congestive heart failure, which was present prior to the ablative procedure, one died two years after the procedure from infective endocarditis, and one following surgical attempts at accessory pathway division. Noncardiac deaths were recorded as a result of sepsis (after pacemaker revision in one), severe chronic lung disease (one patient), and cerebral hemorrhage (one patient). The cause of death was unknown in one.

CHOICE OF PACEMAKER

Serious consideration must be given to the type of cardiac pacing required after ablation of the AV junction. In my experience, most of the elderly patients with drug-resistant atrial fibrillation or flutter have done well with simple VVI pacing. In contrast, physically active patients with intact sinus node function benefit from atrial tracking and AV synchronous pacing. In some of the younger patients, actual generator replacement was required in order to achieve heart rates necessary for their level of exertion. A special problem of pacemaker choice pertains to those patients with the Wolff-Parkinson-White syndrome who undergo AV junctional ablation. It must be remembered that these patients have intact retrograde conduction via a bypass tract and are thus liable to develop pacemaker-mediated tachycardias following insertion of DDD units. These patients require careful pre-pacer implant studies of retrograde ventriculoatrial conduction in order to eliminate the possibility of pacemaker-mediated tachycardia. In more active patients, often a balance has to be struck between providing adequate heart rate for that individual and avoiding pacemaker-mediated tachycardia syndrome.

CLINICAL ROLE

The catheter technique has largely supplanted the direct surgical method as the preferred mode of therapy for patients with drug- and/or anti-tachycardia-resistant supraventricular tachyarrhythmias. The catheter technique is associated with lower morbidity, mortality, and cost compared with the surgical approach.[20] Direct surgical ablation of the AV junction appears to be reserved for those patients who fail attempted catheter ablation or those patients with resistant tachycardia who require surgical correction of other cardiac lesions.

Although the technical aspects of AV junctional ablation are relatively simple to master, the decision to perform this procedure is often a difficult one. Ideally, the clinician would prefer a procedure that sufficiently modifies AV conduction resulting in tachycardia control without sacrificing the normal AV conduction system. Even application of relatively small energy discharges (50 joules) to the AV junction may produce chronic complete AV block.[19] At this point, catheter ablation of the AV junction must still be considered a technique of last resort since chronic cardiac pacing is obligatory and because of postablative ventricular arrhythmias as well as risk of sudden death.

CATHETER ABLATION OF ACCESSORY BYPASS TRACTS

Accessory extranodal bypass tracts are located either in the region of the cardiac annulus (free wall) or the septum. Approximately 70% of these pathways occur either in the septum or the left free wall. Surgical ablation of these pathways has proved to be both effective and safe.[21] Recently, techniques have been introduced allowing for attempted catheter ablation of these pathways.[8,22-25] The technique involves insertion of a multipolar electrode catheter in close proximity to the bypass tract as guided by endocardial retrograde atrial activation sequences. One or more shocks are delivered from an electrode catheter in close proximity to the tract to an indifferent patch placed on the chest wall.

CATHETER ABLATION OF FREE WALL ACCESSORY PATHWAYS

The coronary sinus lies in the left AV groove and hence in close proximity to left free wall accessory pathways. Fisher and associates[8] have described a technique for attempted catheter ablation of left free wall pathways by delivery of direct-current shocks from electrode catheters in the coronary sinus placed in close proximity to the bypass tract. Prior animal experiments showed that shocks delivered in the coronary sinus produced fibrosis of surrounding atrial and ventricular myocardium.[7] This technique was used in eight patients, and chronic modification of accessory pathway conduction occurred in two. One patient developed acute tamponade owing to disruption of the coronary sinus. Preliminary results from the Percutaneous Mapping and Ablation Registry suggest a similar low rate of efficacy and a 25% incidence of tamponade due to disruption of the coronary sinus.[26] At this time direct surgical ablation of left free wall pathways would appear to be far preferable to attempted catheter ablation. Data are insufficient to assess the safety and efficacy of catheter ablation of right free wall pathways.

CATHETER ABLATION OF POSTEROSEPTAL ACCESSORY PATHWAYS

Posteroseptal pathways are defined as those pathways occurring in the region between the ostium of the coronary sinus and the AV junction. Morady and Scheinman[27] described a catheter technique for ablation of posteroseptal accessory pathways whose earliest retrograde activation occurs at the ostium of the coronary sinus. The technique involves insertion of a quadripolar electrode catheter into the coronary sinus. The distal electrodes are anchored into the coronary sinus, while the proximal electrodes are positioned just outside the coronary sinus ostium in close apposition to the atrial insertion of the bypass tract. One or more direct-current shocks are delivered from the catheter to an external chest wall patch (Fig. 54.7). An ongoing combined series with Morady (University of Michigan) is following 25 patients who underwent attempted catheter ablation of a posteroseptal accessory pathway. In 19 patients, the arrhythmia is controlled without need for drugs. Four of the remaining six patients underwent cardiac electrosurgery, and two were controlled with drug therapy. To date in our series, two major complications have occurred: One patient developed rupture of the coronary sinus and required emergency pericardiocentesis, and one developed complete AV block. It is important to emphasize that the shocks are delivered just outside the coronary sinus os. Special care is used to avoid giving the shocks in the coronary sinus. Other smaller series with similar results have been reported.[23-25]

The initial reports detailing results of catheter ablation of posteroseptal accessory pathways appear to be especially promising. If this early experience is confirmed, then this technique should supplant cardiac electrosurgery for these patients. My experience thus far suggests a high efficacy rate and no significant morbidity. Catheter ablation of these pathways should be considered for patients with symptomatic arrhythmias refractory to medical therapy or in younger patients with a desire to avoid lifelong drug therapy for arrhythmia control.

CATHETER ABLATION OF VENTRICULAR TACHYCARDIA FOCI

Patients with drug-refractory recurrent sustained symptomatic ventricular tachycardia may be candidates for map-directed surgical extirpation of the arrhythmia focus. This technique involves induction of ventricular tachycardia during cardiac surgery together with cardiac mapping procedures in order to detect the earliest cardiac potential relative to reference surface leads.[26] In prior studies, the earliest electrical breakthrough always occurred over the endocardium at the border between scar and normal muscle.[28] Various surgical techniques including ventriculotomy,[29] encircling procedures,[30] or endocardial resection[31] have been described. The surgical techniques are associated with high mortality (10% to 15%) since the patient population often consists of those with associated severe coronary artery disease, prior myocardial infarction, and poor left ventricular function. Seventy-five to 80% of survivors achieve benefit in that arrhythmia control is achieved either without drugs or with drugs that previously failed in arrhythmia control.

New techniques for catheter ablation of ventricular foci have been introduced in recent years.[9,32-36] These techniques depend on careful localization of the arrhythmia focus. The latter is achieved by insertion of electrode catheters into both the right and left ventricles. The tachycardia is induced using standard methods, and both ventricles are explored by catheter during tachycardia in order to detect the earliest endocardial potential relative to three orthogonal surface electrocardiographic leads (Fig. 54.8). In addition, pacemapping is used to confirm the exit point of the tachycardia focus. The latter technique involves cardiac pacing in close proximity to the assumed focus and comparison of the QRS complex morphology during pacing with that of the spontaneous tachycardia. The electrode catheter is then positioned against the ventricular area showing earliest endocardial activation, and one or more direct-current shocks are applied from the catheter to an indifferent conductive patch placed over the chest wall (Fig. 54.9). An additional procedure has been described for patients

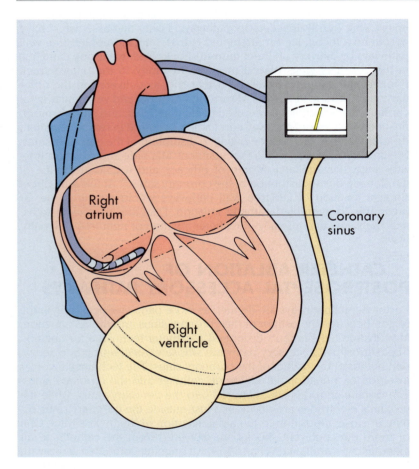

FIGURE 54.7 Catheter ablation of posteroseptal accessory pathway. Schematic showing placement of quadripolar electrode catheter into the coronary sinus for attempted ablation of a posteroseptal accessory pathway. The distal electrodes are anchored into the root of the coronary sinus while the proximal electrode pair are positioned just outside the os of the coronary sinus. The proximal electrode pair are tied together as the cathode and a patch placed on the chest wall serves as the anode. Shocks are delivered from a direct-current defibrillator.

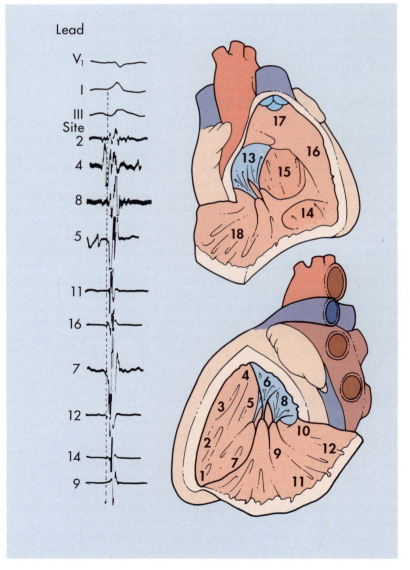

FIGURE 54.8 Schema showing endocardial mapping procedure during ventricular tachycardia. The column on the left shows simultaneous surface leads V_1, I, and III and endocardial electrograms from various ventricular sites. The numerical schema follows that proposed by Dr. Mark Josephson.

with septal foci.[34] In these patients, electrode catheters are used to explore both sides of the ventricular septum. The right and left heart catheters are positioned so that the earliest endocardial potentials from both right and left septal surfaces are found. One or more shocks are then delivered from one electrode to another. After delivery of shocks, the patient is retested to determine whether the tachycardia is still inducible. The patient must be monitored in a coronary care unit, and treatment is similar to that of a patient with acute myocardial infarction. Complications resulting from this technique include myocardial perforation, deterioration of myocardial performance, and induction of more serious cardiac arrhythmias.

Tachycardia arising from the right ventricle has been described in patients with cardiomyopathy,[27] with arrhythmogenic right ventricular dysplasia,[37] following correction of congenital cardiac abnormalities (*i.e.*, repair of tetralogy of Fallot),[38] with right ventricular outflow tract tachycardia without apparent cardiac disease,[39] and rarely with ischemic heart disease. Various centers have reported the use of this technique in patients with right ventricular foci,[32,33] and although the experience is limited, those with ventricular tachycardia associated with post–tetralogy of Fallot repair appear to respond best in terms of arrhythmic control without need for antiarrhythmic drugs.[33] Other patients with right ventricular foci may, after ablation, respond to drugs that were previously ineffective.

Catheter ablation of tachycardia foci arising from the left ventricle is usually related to coronary artery disease with prior infarction or idiopathic cardiomyopathy.[40] A few reports of tachycardia arising from the posterior septum in otherwise normal hearts[41] or bundle branch reentry[42] have been reported. In preliminary reports, good to excellent responses have been reported in 60% to 90% of patients undergoing ablative procedure.[9,32–36]

CLINICAL STUDIES

As of December 1986, a total of 141 patients who underwent attempted electrical ablation of ventricular tachycardia foci have been reported to the Registry. The clinical data are summarized in Table 54.2. The mean age was 53 (±15) years, and there was a large predominance of males (86% of the group). The most frequent cardiac diagnoses included coronary artery disease (63%), cardiomyopathy (17%), and arrhythmogenic right ventricular dysplasia (12%). The most frequent symptoms included palpitations (68%), syncope or presyncope (66%), and one or more episodes of cardiac arrest (26%). Patients proved unresponsive or intolerant to a variety of treatments including type I antiarrhythmic drugs (94%), amiodarone (80%), cardiac electrosurgery (5%), automatic internal defibrillation (2%), or antitachycardia pacing (2%). A total of 85 patients required one or more external direct-current shocks for arrhythmia control.

CLINICAL RESPONSE

The patients were followed for a mean of 12 (±10) months, and their response to catheter ablation was varied. Thirty-four patients (24%) are currently asymptomatic without antiarrhythmic drugs, while 59 pa-

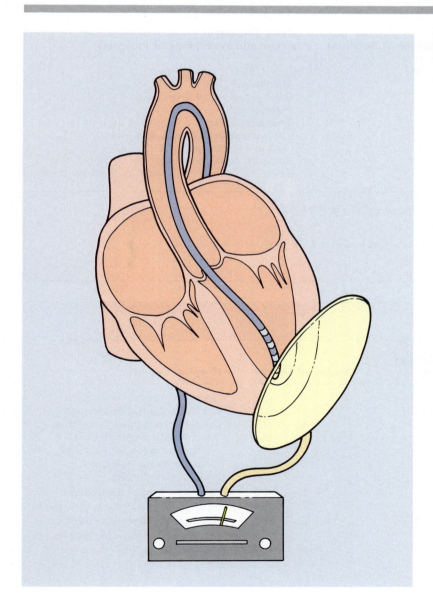

FIGURE 54.9 Schema for ablation of ventricular tachycardia originating from the left ventricle. The multipolar electrode catheter is inserted in close proximity to the earliest endocardial potential registered during ventricular tachycardia (see Fig. 54.8). One or more shocks are delivered from the electrode catheter to a patch placed on the chest wall from a direct-current defibrillator.

tients (42%) have arrhythmia control but require antiarrhythmic agents and 48 patients (34%) failed to respond.

COMPLICATIONS

A procedure-related death was defined as any death occurring within 24 hours of the ablative shocks. Seven procedure-related deaths were reported (Table 54.3) and consisted of electromechanical dissociation in four, intractable ventricular fibrillation in one, and severe low-output state leading to death in two. New sustained ventricular arrhythmias occurred in eight patients after shock. One patient had ventricular fibrillation five days after the ablative procedure. Other in-hospital complications included hypotension in 12 patients, pericarditis in 4, systemic embolization in 3, myocardial infarction in 2, ventricular perforation in 1, and sepsis in 2.

MORTALITY

Over a mean follow-up of 12 months, 31 patients died. Seven patients had procedure-related deaths and 14 died suddenly. (Documented ventricular tachycardia was found in 9 of these 14.) The sudden deaths occurred in the period from 2 weeks to 23 months after ablation. Seven patients died of congestive heart failure, and three were noncardiac deaths (gastrointestinal hemorrhage in one, cerebrovascular accident in one, suicide in one).

It is premature to define the precise role of catheter ablation for those with ventricular tachycardia. Although some of the reported catheter ablation series show results that are quite favorable compared with the surgical series, no long-term follow-up comparisons are available. At this time it would appear to be reasonable to use the catheter technique in patients in whom all available drug therapy has failed and in those considered at high risk for surgical intervention.

FUTURE OF CATHETER TECHNIQUES

The introduction of catheter ablative procedures for patients with cardiac arrhythmias introduces an exciting chapter in interventional electrophysiology. Although the experience is still limited, certain observations are appropriate: The technique of catheter ablation of the AV junction is preferable to direct surgical intervention since it is associated with a lower morbidity, mortality, and cost. The use of this technique will remain limited until procedures are introduced that modify AV junction function and allow for tachycardia control without com-

---

TABLE 54.2 CLINICAL FINDINGS IN 141 PATIENTS WITH DRUG- AND/OR PACEMAKER-RESISTANT VENTRICULAR TACHYCARDIA

Heart Disease (Type and Percentage of Patients)	Symptoms (Type and Percentage of Patients)	Prior Treatment (Type and Percentage of Patients)
Coronary artery disease, 63%	Palpitations, 74%	Type I, 95%
Cardiomyopathy, 16%	Dizziness, 41%	Amiodarone, 78%
Arrhythmogenic right ventricular dysplasia, 10%	Syncope, 36%	Other experimental drugs, 55%
Valvular heart disease, 6%	Dyspnea, 34%	Digitalis, 36%
Others, 6%	Cardiac arrest, 25%	β-blockers, 33%
Hypertensive cardiovascular disease, 2%	Fatigue, 18%	Calcium channel blockers, 29%
No organic disease, 6%	Angina, 18%	Cardiac electrosurgery, 6%
	Chest pain, 10%	Antitachycardia pacemaker, 4%
	Other, 7%	Automatic internal cardioverter defibrillator, 2%

The percentages total more than 100% since more than one parameter may have been present in a given patient.

(Type I, Type I antiarrhythmic drug)

(Scheinman MM, Evans-Bell T: Percutaneous mapping and ablation registry [Personal Communication] January, 1986)

TABLE 54.3 PROCEDURE-RELATED DEATHS

Diagnosis	Number of Deaths	Total Energy (Joules)	Number of Shocks	Hospital Course
Coronary artery disease	3	300	1	Electromechanical dissociation
		480	2	Electromechanical dissociation
		900	3	Four hours postshock, ventricular tachycardia recurred. Died following pump failure during anesthesia for ventricular tachycardia surgery
Arrhythmogenic right ventricular dysplasia	2	1140	5	Electromechanical dissociation
		340	2	
Cardiomyopathy	1	240	1	Electromechanical dissociation
Coronary artery disease/cardiomyopathy	1	300	1	Hypotension, intra-aortic balloon assist

plete disruption of AV conduction. Catheter ablation of posteroseptal pathways appears to be especially promising, since, if successful, it offers the patient the prospect of a complete cure of the arrhythmia. Catheter ablation of ventricular tachycardia foci remains highly experimental, but its use is worthy of consideration for those patients with drug-refractory symptomatic ventricular tachycardia who are considered to be high-risk candidates for direct surgical intervention.

Much more work is required in refining the catheter ablation procedures to make them even more effective. First, better endocardial mapping systems are needed. These systems should include both more steerable catheters as well as multiple flange electrodes to allow for simultaneous multiple electrode recordings. In addition, the present techniques of applying high energy shocks results in substantial damage to surrounding normal tissues. Other more focused energy such as laser or radiofrequency waves may prove more effective with less damage to surrounding muscle.

REFERENCES

1. Randall OS, Westerhof N, Van de Boss G et al: Production of chronic heart block in closed-chest dogs: An improved technique. Am J Physiol H279, 1981
2. Steiner C, Kovalik ATW: A simple technique for production of chronic complete heart block in dogs. J Appl Physiol 25:631, 1968
3. Turina MI, Babotai I, Wegmann W: Production of chronic atrioventricular block in dogs without thoracotomy. Cardiovasc Res 2:389, 1968
4. Beazell J, Tan K, Criley J et al: The electrosurgical production of heart block without thoracotomy (abstr). Clin Res 24:137, 1976
5. Gonzalez R, Scheinman MM, Margaretten W et al: Closed chest electrode catheter technique for His bundle ablation in dog. Am J Physiol 241:283, 1981
6. Gonzalez R, Scheinman MM, Bharati S et al: Closed chest permanent atrioventricular block in dogs. Am Heart J 105:461, 1983
7. Brodman R, Fisher JD: Evaluation of a catheter technique for ablation of accessory pathways near the coronary sinus using a canine model. Circulation 67:923, 1983
8. Fisher JD, Brodman R, Kim SG et al: Attempted nonsurgical electrical ablation of accessory pathways via the coronary sinus in the Wolff-Parkinson-White syndrome. J Am Coll Cardiol 4:685, 1984
9. Hartzler GO: Electrode catheter ablation of refractory focal ventricular tachycardia. J Am Coll Cardiol 2:1107, 1983
10. Ward DE, Camm AJ, Spurrell RAJ: Ventricular preexcitation due to anomalous nodo-ventricular pathways. Eur J Cardiol 49:995, 1982
11. Gallagher JJ, Smith WM, Benson DW: Role of Mahaim fibers in cardiac arrhythmias in man. Circulation 64:176, 1981
12. Bhandari A, Morady F, Shen EN et al: Catheter-induced His bundle ablation in a patient with reentrant tachycardia associated with a nodoventricular tract. J Am Coll Cardiol 4:611, 1984
13. Ellenbogen K, O'Callaghan WG, Colavita PG et al: Catheter atrioventricular junction ablation for recurrent supraventricular tachycardia with nodoventricular fibers. Am J Cardiol 55:1227, 1985
14. Nathan AW, Bennett DH, Ward DE et al: Catheter ablation of atrioventricular conduction. Lancet 1:1280, 1984
15. Wood D, Hammill S, Holmes DR et al: Catheter ablation of the atrioventricular system in patients with supraventricular tachycardia. Mayo Clin Proc 58:793, 1983
16. Gillette PC, Garson A, Porter CJ et al: Junctional automatic ectopic tachycardia: New proposed treatment by transcatheter His bundle ablation. Am Heart J 106:619, 1983
17. Manz M, Steinbeck G, Luderitz B: His-Bundel-Ablation: Eine neue Methode zur Behandlung bedrohlicher supraventrikulärer Herzrhythmusstorungen. Der Internist 24:95, 1983
18. Scheinman MM, Evans-Bell T, and the Executive Committee of the Percutaneous Mapping and Ablation Registry: Catheter ablation of the atrioventricular junction: A report of the Percutaneous Mapping and Ablation Registry. Circulation 70:1024, 1984
19. McComb JM, McGovern BA, Garan H et al: Modification of atrioventricular conduction using low energy transcatheter shocks (abstr). J Am Coll Cardiol 5:454, 1985
20. German LD, Pressley J, Smith MS et al: Comparison of cryoablation of the atrioventricular node versus catheter ablation of the His bundle (abstr). Circulation 70:II-412, 1984
21. Gallagher JJ, Svenson RH, Sealy WC et al: The Wolff-Parkinson-White syndrome and the preexcitation dysrhythmias: Medical and surgical management. Med Clin North Am 60:101, 1976
22. Weber H, Schmitz L, Wesselhoeft H: A new technique of mapping for localization and closed-chest ablation of reentry pathways. Circulation 68:III-175, 1983
23. Bardy GH, Poole JE, Coltorti F et al: Catheter ablation of a concealed accessory pathway. Am J Cardiol 54:1366, 1984
24. Kunz KP, Kuck KH: Transvenous ablation of accessory pathways in patients with incessant atrioventricular tachycardia (abstr). Circulation 70:II-412, 1984
25. Nathan AW, Davies DW, Creamer JE et al: Successful catheter ablation of abnormal atrioventricular pathways in man. Circulation 70:II-99, 1984
26. Scheinman MM, Evans-Bell T: Percutaneous mapping and ablation registry (Personal communication), January 1986
27. Morady F, Scheinman MM: Transvenous catheter ablation of a posteroseptal accessory pathway in a patient with the Wolff-Parkinson-White syndrome. N Engl J Med 310:705, 1984
28. Josephson ME, Horowitz LN, Spielman SR et al: Comparison of endocardial catheter mapping with intraoperative mapping of ventricular tachycardia. Circulation 61:395, 1980
29. Fontaine G, Guiraudon G, Frank R et al: Epicardial mapping and surgical treatment in six cases of resistant ventricular tachycardia not related to coronary artery disease. In Wellens HJ, Lie KI, Janse MJ (eds): The Conduction System of the Heart, pp 545–566. Philadelphia, Lea & Febiger, 1976
30. Guiraudon G, Fontaine G, Frank R et al: Apports de la ventriculotomie circulaire d'exclusion dans le traitement de la tachycardie ventriculaire recidivante après infarctus du myocarde. Arch Mal Couer 75:1013, 1982
31. Miller JM, Kienzle MG, Harken AH et al: Morphologically distinct sustained ventricular tachycardias in coronary artery disease: Significance and surgical results. J Am Coll Cardiol 4:1073, 1984
32. Fontaine G, Tonet JL, Frank R et al: La fulguration endocavitaire: Une nouvelle methode de traitement des troubles du rhythme? Ann Cardiol Angeiol 33:543, 1984
33. Winston SA, Morady F, Davis JC et al: Catheter ablation of ventricular tachycardia (abstr). Circulation 70:II-412, 1984
34. Winston SA, Davis JC, Morady F et al: A new approach to electrode catheter ablation for ventricular tachycardia arising from the ventricular septum (abstr). Circulation 70:II-412, 1984
35. Downar E, Parson I, Cameron D et al: Unipolar and bipolar catheter ablation techniques for management of ventricular tachycardia: Initial experience (abstr). J Am Coll Cardiol 5:472, 1985
36. Huang SK, Marcus FI, Ewy GA: Clinical experience with endocardial catheter ablation for refractory ventricular tachycardia (abstr). J Am Coll Cardiol 5:473, 1985
37. Marcus FL, Fontaine GH, Giraudon G et al: Right ventricular dysplasia: A report of 24 adult cases. Circulation 65:384, 1982
38. Horowitz LN, Vetter VL, Harken AH et al: Electrophysiologic characteristics of sustained ventricular tachycardia occurring after repair of tetralogy of Fallot. Am J Cardiol 46:446, 1980
39. Buxton AE, Waxman HL, Marchlinski MD et al: Right ventricular tachycardia: Clinical and electrophysiologic characteristics. Circulation 68:917, 1983
40. Kastor JA, Horowitz LN, Harken AH et al: Clinical electrophysiology of ventricular tachycardia. N Engl J Med 304:1004, 1981
41. German LD, Packer DL, Bardy GH et al: Ventricular tachycardia induced by atrial stimulation in patients with symptomatic cardiac disease. Am J Cardiol 52:1202, 1983
42. Camons JP, Varenne A, Banza R et al: Tachycardia bidirectionalle d'origine infra-hisienne: Arguments en faveur d'un rhythm reciproque. Arch Mal Coeur 69:533, 1976

GENERAL REFERENCES

Fontaine G: Les methodes ablatives. Arch Mal Coeur 77:1299, 1984
Scheinman MM: Editorial: Interventional electrophysiology. Mayo Clin Proc 58:832, 1983

Syncope

Fred Morady

Determination of the cause of syncope, which is defined as transient loss of consciousness with spontaneous recovery, often presents a significant diagnostic challenge. A thorough history, physical examination, and laboratory evaluation often is helpful in identifying a potential cause of syncope. However, because syncope is usually a sporadic and infrequent event, it is rarely possible to examine a patient or obtain an electrocardiographic (ECG) recording during an actual episode. Therefore, the diagnosis arrived at based on the results of clinical evaluation is usually a presumptive one. Unfortunately, abnormalities uncovered that might potentially cause syncope may simple be incidental findings unrelated to the syncope. Furthermore, when the patient with syncope is treated based on a presumptive diagnosis, if syncope recurs it is often unclear whether the recurrence was due to failure to correctly identify the cause of syncope or to ineffective treatment of a correctly identified cause.

In some patients syncope is a benign condition with no prognostic implications (*e.g.*, in the patient who has vasodepressor syncope triggered by emotional distress). On the other hand, syncope may be a harbinger of cardiac arrest or sudden cardiac death (*e.g.*, in the patient with syncope caused by short bursts of ventricular tachycardia). It is therefore always important to attempt to establish the cause of syncope.

ETIOLOGY

METABOLIC CAUSES

Metabolic causes of syncope include hypoxemia, hypocapnia, and hypoglycemia (Table 55.1). The most common circumstance in which syncope is caused by hypoxemia is when there is a rapid ascent to high altitude. Oxygen saturation is approximately 90% at 10,000 feet and 60% at 20,000 feet. At altitudes greater than 20,000 feet there is the insidious onset of mental deterioration associated with headache, breathlessness, and eventually loss of consciousness. In patients with heart disease and a diminished cardiac output or anemia, symptoms caused by hypoxia may occur at lower altitudes.

Hypocapnia occurs in the hyperventilation syndrome, which is usually precipitated by anxiety. Hypocapnia results in a decrease in cerebral blood flow due to vasoconstriction of the vascular supply to the brain. As hypocapnia becomes progressively more severe, symptoms may include dyspnea, chest tightness, numbness or a tingling sensation in the fingers and toes and around the mouth, palpitations, lightheadedness, confusion, and, rarely, complete loss of consciousness.

Because glucose is the major energy source for the brain and there are limited glycogen stores in the brain, hypoglycemia can cause cerebral dysfunction and loss of consciousness. Although there is no fixed relationship between symptoms and the plasma glucose level, symptoms usually do not occur until the plasma glucose level falls below 55 mg/dl. Symptoms depend on the magnitude and rate of fall in the plasma glucose level and on the duration of hypoglycemia. A rapid and severe fall in the plasma glucose level can cause loss of consciousness, which is transient because of compensatory mechanisms that act to increase the plasma glucose level. Syncope caused by hypoglycemia is preceded by weakness, tremulousness, diaphoresis, hunger, and palpitations, which are caused by sympathetic overactivity. Profound and persistent hypoglycemia results in coma instead of syncope. Causes of hypoglycemia include exogenous insulin administration, insulinoma, glycogen storage diseases, severe liver disease, extrapancreatic neoplasms, and alcohol abuse.

CEREBROVASCULAR AND NEUROLOGIC CAUSES

Brain stem ischemia, due to basilar artery insufficiency or posterior circulation transient ischemic attacks, can result in transient loss of consciousness but rarely in the absence of other symptoms of brain stem ischemia (*e.g.*, diplopia, vertigo, dysphasia, dysarthria, or sensory or motor symptoms). In the syndrome of basilar artery migraine there is vasoconstriction of the basilar artery that produces symptoms similar to basilar artery transient ischemic attacks. Symptoms of cerebral isch-

TABLE 55.1 CAUSES OF SYNCOPE

I. Metabolic
  A. Hypoxemia
  B. Hypocapnia
  C. Hypoglycemia
II. Cerebrovascular and Neurologic
  A. Posterior circulation transient ischemic attack
  B. Migraine
  C. Partial complex seizure*
  D. Akinetic temporal lobe seizure*
III. Cardiovascular
  A. Vagally mediated (cardioinhibitory or vasodepressor)
    1. Common faint
    2. Carotid sinus hypersensitivity syndrome
    3. Glossopharyngeal syncope
    4. Swallow syncope
    5. Micturition syncope
  B. Orthostatic hypotension
    1. Drug-induced
    2. Hypovolemia
    3. Autonomic insufficiency
    4. Idiopathic
  C. Obstructive diseases
    1. Aortic stenosis
    2. Hypertrophic obstructive cardiomyopathy
    3. Atrial myxoma
    4. Pulmonary vascular disease
  D. Arrhythmias
    1. Sinus node dysfunction
    2. Atrioventricular block
    3. Supraventricular tachycardia
    4. Ventricular tachycardia
IV. Miscellaneous
  A. Myocardial infarction/ischemia
  B. Post-tussive syncope
  C. Hysterical syncope

* Included because this type of seizure may mimic syncope.

emia may also occur in the subclavian steal syndrome, in which there is occlusive disease in a subclavian artery, with shunting of blood away from the vertebral artery through the circle of Willis to the distal subclavian artery; cerebral ischemia typically occurs during arm exercise, because of a decrease in vascular resistance in the affected limb during exercise.

Episodic loss of consciousness due to classic grand mal seizures is usually readily differentiated from other causes of syncope. Although syncope caused by cerebral hypoperfusion is often accompanied by seizure-like motor activity, the clonic or repetitive movements are generally irregular and short-lived, whereas in true seizures the clonic movements are more pronounced and regular.[1] In addition, the confusional state that may follow an episode of syncope usually lasts less than 30 seconds, whereas true seizures are followed by a longer postictal confusional state. However, partial complex or akinetic temporal lobe seizures are not associated with many of the features typical of epilepsy, such as tonic-clonic jerking, tongue biting, or urinary incontinence. These types of seizures may be associated with olfactory, gustatory, or déjà-vu auras and auditory or somatosensory symptoms. The seizures are followed by a postictal state that is usually limited to a few minutes of disorientation.

CARDIOVASCULAR CAUSES

Cardiovascular causes of syncope include those that are vagally mediated and those due to orthostatic hypotension, obstructive cardiac lesions, severe pulmonary hypertension, and bradyarrhythmias or tachyarrhythmias.

VAGALLY MEDIATED SYNCOPE

Vagally mediated syncope is the most common cause of syncope in the general population.[2,3] There is vagal overactivity and sympathetic withdrawal, which results in a cardioinhibitory response (bradycardia), a vasodepressor response (vasodilatation and hypotension), or both. The common "fainting spell" falls into the category of vagally mediated syncope. Episodes are usually triggered by emotional distress, pain, the sight of blood, phlebotomy, or instrumentation. Contributing factors may be fatigue and a hot or crowded environment. There is typically a prodrome of weakness, lightheadedness, nausea, epigastric discomfort, pallor, and diaphoresis. As consciousness is lost, the patient falls to the ground. There may at times be some tonic, opisthotonic, or tonic-clonic seizure-like movements. The individual usually regains consciousness shortly after assuming a horizontal position. Symptoms of weakness, lightheadedness, and nausea commonly persist for at least several minutes. The patient may experience the urge to have a bowel movement. Syncope may recur if the individual attempts to stand shortly after regaining consciousness.

In the carotid sinus hypersensitivity syndrome, episodes of syncope may be triggered by pressure on the carotid sinus by a tight collar, turning the neck, manual compression, or a neck mass. Carotid sinus hypersensitivity is manifested by a long pause (>3 seconds) or hypotension in response to extrinsic pressure on the carotid sinus. Patients with syncope and carotid sinus hypersensitivity may not have any identifiable mechanical stimulus during spontaneous episodes of syncope.[4] As is the case in all other types of vagally mediated syncope, the cardiovascular response that results in cerebral ischemia and syncope may be cardioinhibitory, vasodepressor, or both.[4,5]

Glossopharyngeal syncope is due to excitation of the dorsal motor nucleus of the vagus by afferent impulses from the glossopharyngeal nerve. Episodes of syncope are preceded by severe pain at the base of the tongue, pharynx, larynx, tonsillar area, or external auditory meatus and may be triggered by pressure at these sites.[6]

Closely related to glossopharyngeal syncope is swallow syncope, in which syncope is provoked by swallowing.[7] Vagal hyperactivity triggered by swallowing and resulting in syncope is usually associated with an abnormality of the esophagus such as diverticula, stricture, or tumor.[7,8]

Micturition syncope is limited almost completely to males, presumably because of the standing position during urination. Syncope may occur during or after urination and is secondary to vagal discharge associated with emptying of a distended bladder. Orthostatic hypotension occurring after arising from sleep may be a contributing factor.[9]

ORTHOSTATIC HYPOTENSION

Syncope due to orthostatic hypotension typically occurs shortly after the patient arises rapidly from a recumbent or sitting position.[10,11] Prolonged motionless standing or standing after prolonged bed rest may also precipitate syncope. Orthostatic hypotension may occur after a meal in elderly patients, owing to splanchnic pooling.

There are many types of pharmacologic agents that may cause orthostatic hypotension. These drugs include diuretics, ganglionic blocking agents, vasodilators, tricyclic antidepressants, and phenothiazines.

Hypovolemia due to dehydration or hemorrhage may result in orthostatic hypotension and syncope when the patient attempts to stand.

Orthostatic hypotension and syncope may also result from surgical sympathectomy or autonomic insufficiency associated with peripheral or central nervous system diseases. Peripheral neuropathies that may cause orthostatic hypotension include diabetes mellitus, alcoholic neuropathy, amyloidosis, and Guillain-Barré syndrome. Central nervous system lesions that may cause orthostatic hypotension include Wernicke's encephalopathy, the myelopathy of multiple sclerosis, and tabes dorsalis.

Idiopathic orthostatic hypotension may occur as an isolated abnormality in blood pressure control or in association with other symptoms of sympathetic and parasympathetic dysfunction, including anhydrosis, sphincter abnormalities, impotence, lack of tears, and extrapyramidal disorders (Shy-Drager syndrome). There is usually little or no compensatory sinus tachycardia accompanying the postural drop in blood pressure.

OBSTRUCTIVE CARDIOVASCULAR LESIONS

Syncope may be due to a markedly reduced cardiac output and cerebral ischemia caused by severe aortic valve (or pulmonic valve) stenosis. Syncope may be particularly prone to occur during exercise, when an increase in blood flow to large muscle groups diverts blood flow away from the cerebral circulation. However, syncope in aortic stenosis may also be caused by a burst of ventricular tachycardia that spontaneously terminates.

Syncope may also be a symptom of hypertrophic obstructive (or nonobstructive) cardiomyopathy. Because left ventricular outflow tract obstruction is aggravated by an increase in inotropic state, a reduced cardiac output and syncope may be precipitated by exercise. Patients with hypertrophic cardiomyopathies are at risk of having ventricular tachycardia, which is a second potential cause of syncope in these patients. A third potential cause of syncope is related to reduced ventricular compliance; ventricular filling during systole may be dependent on a vigorous and synchronous atrial contraction. A precipitous fall in blood pressure causing syncope may occur with the onset of atrial fibrillation or other types of supraventricular tachycardia (Fig. 55.1).

Myxomas occur most commonly in the left atrium and may cause syncope either by intermittent obstruction of the mitral valve or by embolization to the brain stem. Less commonly, myxomas may cause intermittent or persistent obstruction of the tricuspid valve or may simulate aortic or pulmonary stenosis.

Pulmonary vascular disease causes syncope because of cerebral ischemia related to a markedly diminished cardiac output. Syncope may occur in association with a massive pulmonary embolus, primary pulmonary obstruction, Eisenmenger's syndrome, or other types of obstructive pulmonary vascular diseases.

ARRHYTHMIAS

Syncope can be caused by either a bradyarrhythmia or a tachyarrhythmia. With either type of arrhythmia, syncope is caused by a reduction in cardiac output and cerebral ischemia. This is more likely to occur when the patient is upright; however, if there is a severe drop in cerebral blood flow, syncope may of course occur even in the supine position. Although the rate of a bradyarrhythmia or tachyarrhythmia is one of the factors that determines the severity of cerebral symptoms, there is not an absolute relationship between the rate of the arrhythmia and syncope.[12] Other factors that influence the magnitude of fall in blood pressure and the extent of cerebral symptoms include the presence and severity of structural heart disease, the presence of obstructive lesions in the cerebrovascular bed, and the ability of compensatory mechanisms such as peripheral vasoconstriction to prevent a drastic fall in blood pressure. At times, syncope occurs at the outset of a bradyarrhythmia or tachyarrhythmia and the patient regains consciousness, despite the continuation of the arrhythmia at the same rate; this may be attributed to assumption of a supine position and the action of homeostatic mechanisms (such as the baroreceptor reflex) that result in an increase in blood pressure and cerebral blood flow despite persistence of the arrhythmia.

Syncope due to a bradyarrhythmia can be caused by either sinus node dysfunction or atrioventricular (AV) block. Manifestations of sinus node dysfunction include marked sinus bradycardia or pauses caused by either sinus arrest or sinoatrial exit block. In the sick sinus syndrome, bradyarrhythmias may alternate with episodes of supraventricular tachycardia. Long pauses and syncope may occur on termination of the supraventricular tachycardia, owing to overdrive suppression of the sinus node (Fig. 55.2).

When syncope is caused by AV block, the level of the block in the

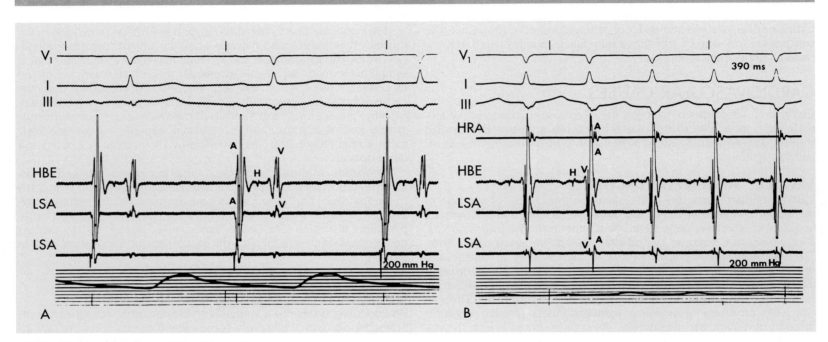

FIGURE 55.1 Electrograms of a patient with nonobstructive cardiomyopathy in whom syncope was caused by supraventricular tachycardia. **A.** During sinus rhythm, the patient's blood pressure was 180/90 mm Hg. From top to bottom are ECG leads V₁, I, and III, the His bundle electrogram (*HBE*), the low septal right atrial electrogram (*LSA*), and an arterial blood pressure recording. **B.** Supraventricular tachycardia (AV nodal reentry) was induced during an electrophysiologic study. Although the rate of the tachycardia was not excessively rapid (154 beats per minute, cycle length 390 msec), the patient's blood pressure fell rapidly to 60/40 mm Hg and the patient experienced near-syncope, in the supine position. If upright, the patient almost certainly would have experienced syncope. In this patient with hypertrophic cardiomyopathy, the syncope was caused by the deleterious hemodynamic effects of tachycardia and a loss of AV synchrony. Time lines represent 1-second intervals. (*A*, atrial electrogram; *H*, His bundle depolarization; *V*, ventricular electrogram; *HRA*, high right atrial electrogram)

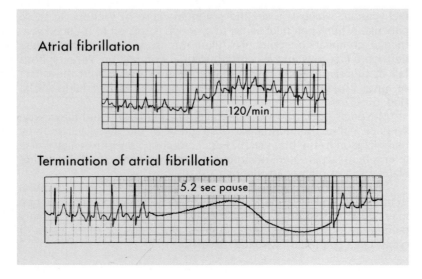

FIGURE 55.2 A 5.2-second sinus pause occurring on spontaneous termination of atrial fibrillation in a patient with the sick sinus syndrome. The patient had a history of syncope occurring immediately after the abrupt cessation of palpitations. The long pause was caused by overdrive suppression of the sinus node by the atrial fibrillation. (Morady F, Peters RW, Scheinman MM: Bradyarrhythmias and bundle branch block. In Scheinman MM [ed]: Cardiac Emergencies, pp 135–149. Philadelphia, WB Saunders, 1984)

conduction system is usually below the AV node. Block in the AV node is usually associated with a stable junctional escape rhythm at a rate of 50 to 60 beats per minute, which is sufficient to maintain hemodynamic stability. In contrast, high-degree infranodal block is associated with a slow idioventricular escape rhythm, which may be as slow as 15 to 20 beats per minute and which is prone to suddenly fail.[13] Syncope may occur in association with intermittent second- or third-degree infranodal block or at the outset of persistent high-degree infranodal block. In the latter situation, loss of consciousness may be only transient because of gradual warm-up of an escape rhythm in addition to the assumption of the supine position and to homeostatic cardiovascular reflexes.

Syncope may at times be caused by vagotonic AV block. This type of AV block occurs at the level of the AV node and is related to the depressant effects of vagal discharge on conduction through the AV node. The hallmark of this type of AV block is slowing of the sinus rate in association with the AV block (Fig. 55.3).[14] This is due to the concomitant effects of vagal discharge on the sinus node and AV node. In classic Mobitz II second-degree AV block, the sinus rate remains constant or accelerates in association with the AV block. Vagotonic AV block may occur during sleep in healthy individuals or during episodes of vagal discharge in patients, as might occur during instrumentation or pain. Although often not associated with cerebral symptoms, vagotonic AV block may at times result in long pauses and syncope.

Supraventricular tachycardia usually does not cause syncope unless the rate is extremely rapid (>250 beats per minute) or the patient has underlying heart disease. Although any type of supraventricular tachycardia can potentially be rapid enough to cause syncope, this is most likely to occur in patients who have an accessory AV connection and episodes of atrial fibrillation (the Wolff-Parkinson-White syndrome). In the Wolff-Parkinson-White syndrome, the ventricular rate during atrial fibrillation may exceed 300 beats per minute. This may result not only in syncope but also in degeneration into ventricular fibrillation and a cardiac arrest.[15]

Loss of consciousness is more commonly associated with ventricular than with supraventricular tachycardia. The patient who has syncope due to ventricular tachycardia typically has coronary artery disease or some other form of structural heart disease. Ventricular tachycardia may rarely cause syncope in otherwise healthy individuals who do not have identifiable structural heart disease.

In a group of 113 patients presenting to the hospital with sustained ventricular tachycardia not associated with cardiac arrest, 15% of patients had experienced syncope before arriving at the hospital.[16] The rate of ventricular tachycardia in these patients was 224 ± 29 beats per minute (mean ± one standard deviation) and was significantly higher than the mean ventricular tachycardia rate in patients without syncope. Patients who had underlying congestive heart failure had a higher incidence of syncope during ventricular tachycardia than patients without congestive heart failure (24% vs. 7%, P < .05). When the rate of ventricular tachycardia exceeded 200 beats per minute, the incidence of syncope was 37%, whereas only 5% of patients with a ventricular tachycardia rate of less than 200 beats per minute experienced syncope (P < 0.005). Therefore, the rate of ventricular tachycardia and the status of underlying cardiac function are factors that clearly influence whether a patient with ventricular tachycardia has syncope. However, it is also clear that other factors must also play a role; these factors may include the presence of atherosclerotic disease in the cerebrovascular circulation, the status of homeostatic circulatory reflexes, and the presence of ventriculoatrial conduction during ventricular tachycardia. At a given rate of ventricular tachycardia, blood pressure may fall to a greater degree when there is one-to-one ventriculoatrial conduction than when there is AV dissociation, possibly because of more atrial distention and activation of atrial stretch receptors when the atria and ventricles contract simultaneously.

MISCELLANEOUS CAUSES

Syncope may at times be the major presenting symptom in patients with myocardial infarction or ischemia.[17,18] There are several potential mechanisms by which syncope may occur in the setting of a myocardial infarction or severe ischemia: (1) a marked drop in cardiac output due to pump dysfunction; (2) marked sinus bradycardia, usually occurring in the early stages of myocardial infarction; (3) high-degree AV block, usually associated with anterior myocardial infarction; (4) ventricular tachycardia; and (5) a vagally mediated vasodepressor or cardioinhibitory response to pain.

Post-tussive syncope is an unusual form of syncope in which a prolonged bout of severe coughing results in a fall in cardiac output and cerebral ischemia. Cardiac output falls because the increase in intrathoracic pressure impedes venous return to the heart, as would a prolonged Valsalva maneuver. Cerebral blood flow may also be impeded by an increase in intracranial pressure, which occurs during a cough paroxysm. In some patients, a vagally mediated cardioinhibitory or vasodepressor response may be triggered by a coughing fit.

Hysterical syncope generally occurs in patients who are young or who have a prior history of hysterical reactions to stress. There may be circumstances that suggest secondary gain. This type of syncope typically is associated with a lack of prodromal symptoms, a lack of pallor, bizarre postures or movements, and prolonged unconsciousness.

RELATIVE INCIDENCE OF THE VARIOUS CAUSES OF SYNCOPE

The relative frequency of the various causes of syncope will depend on the age and clinical characteristics of the patient population. In an unselected population of patients presenting with syncope to an emergency department, the most common cause of syncope is typical vasovagal syncope (the common faint) or some other form of vagally mediated syncope. If patients with a clear-cut seizure disorder are excluded, vagally mediated syncope accounts for 13% to 43% of episodes of syncope.[2,3] The presumed cause of syncope in an unselected population of patients with syncope is a cardiac arrhythmia (most commonly ventricular tachycardia) in 7% to 20%, orthostatic hypotension in 5% to 7%, a miscellaneous cardiovascular cause (e.g., aortic stenosis, pulmonary embolus, myocardial infarction) in 5% to 6%, a neurologic abnormality or cerebrovascular insufficiency in 4% to 5%, and hysteria in 1% to 5%.[2,3] The other causes of syncope listed in Table 55.1 are uncommon in patients presenting for evaluation of syncope, proba-

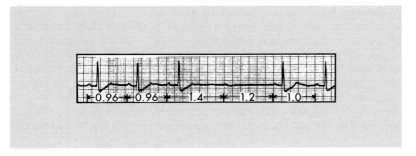

FIGURE 55.3 Vagotonic AV block. The sinus cycle length increases from 0.96 to 1.4 seconds in association with AV block. The concomitant sinus slowing and AV block is caused by the effects of hypervagotonia on the sinus and AV nodes. In contrast, there is an increase or no change in the sinus rate during classic second-degree AV block. Vagotonic AV block is rarely the cause of recurrent syncope and usually does not require treatment with a permanent pacemaker.

bly accounting for less than 1% of episodes of syncope. In a significant proportion of unselected patients with syncope (17% to 50%), a likely cause for the syncope cannot be identified.[2,3]

DIAGNOSTIC EVALUATION

The cornerstone of the diagnostic evaluation of syncope is a thorough history and physical examination. Among patients in whom a likely cause of syncope can be identified, the history and physical examination yield the presumed diagnosis in 50% to 75% of patients.[2,3] Routine blood tests, a chest roentgenogram, and an ECG are virtually always indicated, except perhaps in otherwise healthy individuals who experience a typical vagally mediated fainting spell. The need for further evaluation with neurologic testing, continuous ECG monitoring, echocardiography, exercise treadmill testing, tilt-table testing, cardiac catheterization, and invasive electrophysiologic studies must be determined on an individual basis and will depend on the results of the initial clinical evaluation.

HISTORY AND PHYSICAL EXAMINATION

In regard to metabolic causes of syncope, the occurrence of syncope at high altitude, with prodromal symptoms of headache, dyspnea, and confusion, suggests that hypoxemia was the cause. A history of dyspnea, chest tightness, tingling in the extremities and circumorally, and prolonged syncope (>5 to 10 minutes) would be clues that syncope may have been due to the hyperventilation syndrome. There may not always be an identifiable emotional or environmental trigger for the hyperventilation. If hyperventilation syndrome is suspected, it is often helpful to have the patient voluntarily hyperventilate for 1 to 2 minutes to see if the symptoms associated with syncope can be reproduced. Hypoglycemia should be suspected whenever there is a history of exogenous insulin use or if typical symptoms of hypoglycemia precede loss of consciousness.

A posterior circulation transient ischemic attack should be considered the likely cause of syncope if syncope occurs in association with other symptoms of brain stem ischemia (e.g., diplopia, tinnitus, focal weakness or sensory loss, vertigo, or dysarthria). Syncope in association with a throbbing unilateral headache, scintillating scotomata, and nausea suggests the possibility of migraine syncope. Basilar insufficiency due to the subclavian steal syndrome should be suspected if syncope occurs during arm exercise. Physical examination will demonstrate a bruit emanating from the subclavian artery, and an attempt should be made to at least partially reproduce the patient's symptoms by arm exercise.

It is always important to attempt to distinguish loss of consciousness due to a seizure from true syncope. Clues suggestive of a seizure disorder include a history of an aura preceding the sudden loss of consciousness; depending on the location of the seizure focus, the aura may be olfactory, gustatory, or déjà-vu or it may consist of visual scotomata or focal sensory or motor symptoms. Generalized tonic-clonic movements are common in grand mal seizures; however, they may be absent in temporal lobe seizures or partial complex seizures. When syncope is caused by cerebral ischemia, there may be decorticate rigidity with flexion of the arms but pronounced tonic-clonic movements are uncommon. A history of a few jerking movements is of little value in the differential diagnosis because this may occur either with a seizure or with syncope due to cerebral ischemia. Urinary incontinence may also occur in either situation but is more commonly associated with seizures, as is tongue biting.

If the episode of syncope was witnessed, an attempt should be made to elicit information on the patient's color and breathing pattern during the loss of consciousness. Cyanosis and a stertorous breathing pattern are often observed during a seizure. In contrast, pallor is common in vagally mediated syncope and may also occur during any type of syncope associated with a diminished cardiac output. Syncope due to an arrhythmia may be associated with a marked redness or blush.[19] Pallor is distinctly uncommon during seizures. Respirations may be shallow or not apparent during syncope due to cardiovascular causes.

Another distinguishing feature of seizures is a postictal state following the seizure, usually consisting of disorientation for several minutes and a headache. In contrast, consciousness and orientation are usually regained simultaneously in vagally mediated syncope. However, syncope associated with several minutes of cerebral ischemia may also be associated with a period of altered consciousness following the episode.

In the evaluation of patients with syncope, information on the environmental circumstances at the time of syncope should be sought. Syncope occurring in a warm and/or crowded environment should raise the suspicion of a vagally mediated fainting spell, as should a history of syncope preceded by emotional distress, pain, the sight of blood, or instrumentation. In vagally mediated fainting spells there is a prodrome of weakness, lightheadedness, nausea, diaphoresis, and sometimes visual blurring or diminished hearing. On recovering consciousness, the patient often has a persisting sensation of weakness, lightheadedness, and/or nausea and may have the urge to defecate. A history of a recurrence of syncope on attempting to stand shortly after recovering consciousness is compatible with a vagally mediated fainting spell. Historical clues suggesting that a vagally mediated fainting spell is an unlikely possibility are the complete absence of prodromal or residual symptoms and the occurrence of syncope when the individual is in the horizontal position.

Patients with syncope should be questioned about possible external pressure on the neck just prior to loss of consciousness. A history of syncope while wearing a tight collar or during rotation or extension of the neck is suggestive of the carotid sinus hypersensitivity syndrome. However, in a significant proportion of patients with the carotid hypersensitivity syndrome, no mechanical trigger for spontaneous episodes of syncope can be identified. In the course of the physical examination, left and right carotid sinus massage should be performed during an ECG recording, if the patient does not have carotid bruits. A pause of 3 seconds or more indicates that the patient has a hypersensitive carotid sinus reflex but is not necessarily diagnostic of the hypersensitive carotid sinus syndrome. Pauses of 3 seconds or more may be elicited in response to carotid sinus massage in elderly patients with no history of syncope.[20] If the patient's symptoms are reproduced by carotid sinus massage, this would suggest that the patient did indeed have the hypersensitive carotid sinus syndrome (Fig. 55.4).

As in other types of vagally mediated syncope, cerebral ischemia and loss of consciousness may occur in the hypersensitive carotid sinus syndrome due to a peripheral vasodepressor response, without significant slowing of the heart rate. Therefore, blood pressure should be measured when carotid sinus massage is performed as a diagnostic maneuver in the course of the clinical evaluation. If a long pause or cerebral symptoms are not elicited when the patient is supine, carotid sinus massage should be repeated with the patient upright, because this may accentuate a vasodepressor response and reproduce the patient's symptoms.

The diagnosis of other types of vagally mediated syncope relies heavily on historical information. Syncope associated with severe pain in the tongue, throat, or ear, with swallowing, or with urination suggests the diagnosis of glossopharyngeal, swallow, and micturition syncope, respectively.

A history of syncope occurring shortly after rising from a lying or sitting position suggests that the cause may have been orthostatic hypotension. A complete drug history should be obtained to determine whether the patient was being treated with one or more drugs that could cause hypotension. Syncope occurring while standing in a warm environment or after a meal are other clues that orthostatic hypotension may have been responsible. During the physical examination, blood pressure and heart rate should be measured both in the supine and standing positions. A postural drop in blood pressure of more than 15 to 20 mm Hg without an accompanying increase in heart rate would suggest that the patient may have autonomic insufficiency and should prompt further questioning in regard to other symptoms of autonomic insufficiency (*e.g.*, impotence, incontinence, anhydrosis). Because the onset of orthostatic hypotension may be delayed in elderly patients, it is important to measure the blood pressure after several minutes of standing in place.

Syncope occurring during or immediately after exertion may be a clue that the patient has an obstructive cardiac lesion (or an exercise-induced arrhythmia). The physical examination should be directed specifically toward the identification of signs of aortic stenosis, hypertrophic cardiomyopathy, atrial myxoma, and pulmonary hypertension.

A history of palpitations or sensation of rapid heart beat preceding loss of consciousness suggests that a tachyarrhythmia may have caused the syncope. However, other causes of syncope that are associated with sinus tachycardia may also be preceded by a sensation of palpitations (*e.g.*, hypoglycemia, hyperventilation syndrome, and orthostatic hypotension related to intravascular volume depletion). A history of syncope immediately after the abrupt termination of palpitations is strongly suggestive of the sick sinus syndrome, in which a long sinus pause may occur on cessation of a supraventricular tachycardia. The absence of a history of palpitations preceding syncope would make paroxysmal supraventricular tachycardia an unlikely possibility. However, it is important to note that many patients with ventricular tachycardia do not experience a sensation of rapid or abnormal heart beating, and therefore the absence of a history of palpitations preceding syncope by no means rules out the possibility that syncope was caused by ventricular tachycardia.[16]

A history of syncope occurring in the first few days or weeks after initiation of treatment with a type I antiarrhythmic drug (quinidine, procainamide, or disopyramide) suggests the possibility of drug-induced ventricular tachycardia (torsade de pointes).[21]

There are no aspects of the history that are specific for syncope due to AV block. When syncope is due to either AV block or ventricular tachycardia, loss of consciousness may be abrupt, with no prodrome whatsoever, or it may be preceded by a few seconds of progressive lightheadedness.

Syncope occurring in association with chest pressure or pain may occur due to the hyperventilation syndrome, vagally mediated syncope, aortic stenosis, hypertrophic cardiomyopathy, severe pulmonary hypertension, tachyarrhythmias, or myocardial infarction or ischemia.

The patient with syncope should be questioned regarding family history. A positive family history for syncope or sudden death suggests that the patient with syncope may have a hypertrophic cardiomyopathy or the congenital long QT interval syndrome.

Historical clues suggestive of hysterical syncope include a history of multiple episodes of syncope without any resultant injuries and a history of bizarre symptoms in association with syncope. It should be kept in mind that a several-year history of recurrent syncope, at times with bizarre or unusual associated symptoms, may also occur in the carotid hypersensitivity syndrome.

ELECTROCARDIOGRAPHY

ECG findings that are helpful in identifying a likely cause of syncope include the findings typical of an acute myocardial infarction, prolongation of the QT interval, a short PR interval and delta waves indicative of the Wolff-Parkinson-White syndrome, and high-degree AV block. Many other abnormal findings on the 12-lead ECG either may be related to the cause of syncope or may be incidental findings (*e.g.*, left or right ventricular hypertrophy, bundle branch block, first-degree AV block, and premature ventricular or atrial complexes).

AMBULATORY ELECTROCARDIOGRAPHIC MONITORING

If the history, physical examination, and 12-lead ECG have not yielded a likely cause of syncope, continuous ambulatory ECG monitoring should be performed for at least 24 hours in an attempt to uncover an arrhythmic etiology for the syncope (Fig. 55.5). Because syncope is often sporadic and infrequent, ambulatory ECG monitoring is unfortunately only rarely diagnostic. A survey of over 1500 patients who underwent ambulatory monitoring for the evaluation of syncope indicated that only 1% of patients had syncope during the monitoring period.[22] It should be emphasized that unless syncope (or at least near-syncope) occurs in association with an arrhythmia, it should not be assumed that the arrhythmia is the cause of syncope. Abnormalities such as a sinus pause, AV Wenckebach block, or bursts of ventricular tachycardia that are not associated with cerebral symptoms may be incidental findings unrelated to syncope (Fig. 55.6).

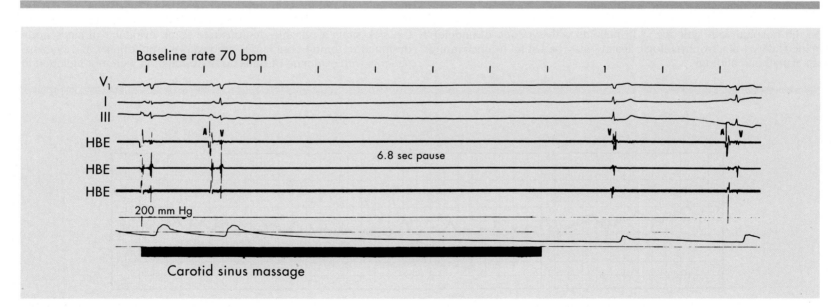

FIGURE 55.4 Demonstration of carotid sinus hypersensitivity in a patient with recurrent syncope preceded by several seconds of lightheadedness. Left carotid sinus massage resulted in a 6.8-second period of asystole, associated with lightheadedness. No other potential cause of syncope was found in this patient. Syncope did not recur after a permanent pacemaker was implanted. Although carotid sinus hypersensitivity may sometimes be an incidental finding, the partial reproduction of the patient's symptoms during carotid massage and the favorable response to pacing suggest that this patient did have the carotid hypersensitivity syndrome. As may be the case in the carotid hypersensitivity syndrome, there was no identifiable trigger for the patient's spontaneous syncopal episodes. (*A*, atrial electrogram; *H*, His bundle depolarization; *V*, ventricular electrogram)

TREADMILL TESTING

An exercise treadmill test should be performed as part of the diagnostic evaluation of the patient who has had syncope during or after exercise or in association with chest pain, unless the patient has clear-cut evidence of severe aortic stenosis. The treadmill test may be helpful by demonstrating an exercise-induced arrhythmia or evidence of myocardial ischemia.

ECHOCARDIOGRAPHY

M-mode and/or two-dimensional echocardiography may at times be helpful in the evaluation of the patient with syncope by demonstrating a cardiac abnormality that could be related to syncope (e.g., hypertrophic cardiomyopathy, aortic valve disease, or a myxoma). In most cases, these cardiac abnormalities can be identified (or at least suspected) based on the physical examination. The echocardiogram has an extremely low diagnostic yield in the evaluation of patients with syncope who have no abnormal cardiac findings on physical examination.

TILT-TABLE TESTING

Evaluation on a tilt table is an effective means of provoking vagally mediated syncope. Although the sensitivity and specificity of tilt-table testing in detecting vagally mediated syncope remain to be determined, helpful diagnostic information may be obtained if a patient's typical symptom-complex is reproduced on the tilt table. In addition, based on the hemodynamic response to tilting, the efficacy of therapies aimed at preventing vagally mediated syncope can be assessed.

CARDIAC CATHETERIZATION

Cardiac catheterization may be indicated if, based on history, physical examination, or noninvasive cardiac evaluation, there is the suspicion of an obstructive cardiac lesion or myocardial ischemia as the cause of syncope.

ELECTROPHYSIOLOGIC TESTING

Despite a thorough history, physical examination, neurologic evaluation, and noninvasive cardiac evaluation, a likely cause of syncope cannot be identified in at least 10% of unselected patients who present to the hospital with syncope.[2,3] In patients with syncope of undetermined cause, electrophysiologic testing may be useful in uncovering an arrhythmic etiology.

INDICATIONS

Because many patients who experience an episode of syncope may never have a recurrence, evaluation with an invasive electrophysiologic study generally should be considered only in patients who have had recurrent syncope. However, there are two situations in which an electrophysiologic study may be appropriate even after only one episode of syncope. In the patient who has been severely injured as a result of syncope and in whom a likely cause of syncope cannot be identified by standard methods, electrophysiologic testing may be indicated in order to maximize the diagnostic yield of the evaluation, thus minimizing the risk of additional injury. In addition, an electrophysiologic study is indicated in the patient with unexplained syncope who has a form of heart disease associated with an increased risk of sudden death (e.g., coronary artery disease and a history of myocardial infarction, hypertrophic cardiomyopathy, or dilated cardiomyopathy). In these patients it is possible that the syncope was caused by ventricular tachycardia and is a harbinger of sudden death or cardiac arrest.

An electrophysiologic study for the evaluation of syncope should be preceded by a thorough clinical evaluation and at least 24 hours of continuous ECG monitoring. As stated earlier, an arrhythmia noted during monitoring may be a clue to the cause of syncope but should not be assumed to be the cause of syncope unless the patient's symptoms are reproduced. For example, in a patient who has had syncope and who is found to have bursts of asymptomatic nonsustained ventricular tachycardia during continuous monitoring, an electrophysiologic study should be performed to assess whether symptomatic ventricular tachycardia or other potential arrhythmic causes of syncope can be elicited.

It should be noted that 15% to 20% of patients with recurrent ventricular tachycardia or ventricular fibrillation have either infrequent or absent ventricular premature depolarizations during continuous monitoring between the episodes of tachycardia.[23] Therefore, in the patient at risk of sudden death who has had an episode of unexplained syncope, an electrophysiologic study should be performed even when continuous ECG monitoring demonstrates no ventricular ectopic activity.

EVALUATION OF SINUS NODE FUNCTION

Sinus node function is evaluated during electrophysiologic testing by determination of the sinus node recovery time,[23] sinoatrial conduction time,[24] and sinus node refractory period.[25] Because most patients with the sick sinus syndrome demonstrate some evidence of sinus node dysfunction during continuous ambulatory monitoring[26] and because patients with evidence of sinus node dysfunction were not included in

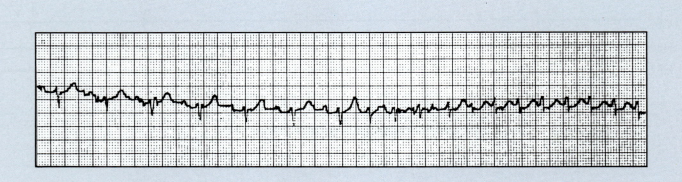

FIGURE 55.5 Ambulatory ECG recording obtained during an episode of syncope in a patient with a prosthetic aortic valve and a history of several episodes of syncope preceded by a brief period of lightheadedness and palpitations. Syncope was caused by supraventricular tachycardia (rate, 187 beats per minute). Shortly after falling to the ground, he regained consciousness even though the supraventricular tachycardia continued. Cerebral blood flow presumably increased because of assumption of a supine position and homeostatic cardiovascular mechanisms.

studies of the yield of electrophysiologic testing in patients with unexplained syncope, abnormal sinus node function has been reported to be an infrequent cause of syncope in patients undergoing electrophysiologic testing. In three studies, among a total of 108 patients with recurrent, unexplained syncope who did not have any evidence of sinus node dysfunction during ambulatory monitoring and who underwent electrophysiologic testing, only 6% of patients were found to have a sinus node abnormality as the presumed cause of syncope.[27-29]

Demonstration of abnormal sinus node function by electrophysiologic testing does not necessarily imply that the cause of syncope has been correctly identified. In some patients, especially the elderly, sinus node dysfunction may be an incidental finding, unrelated to syncope. An abnormal sinus node recovery time is more likely to be a clinically significant finding if the post-pacing pause is longer than 2 seconds and if the patient's symptoms are at least partially reproduced during the pause (Fig. 55.7). On the other hand, a mildly prolonged sinus node recovery time or an isolated abnormality of the sinoatrial conduction time may often have no clinical significance in the patient with unexplained syncope. Patients who have these types of abnormalities and who undergo implantation of a permanent pacemaker may have recurrent syncope despite normal pacemaker function.[29]

Electrophysiologic testing is not necessary if continuous monitoring has demonstrated a sinus pause or marked sinus bradycardia in association with syncope. In elderly patients with syncope, a more common finding during ECG monitoring is an asymptomatic sinus pause or sinus bradycardia. In these patients, it cannot be assumed that syncope is secondary to the sick sinus syndrome. An abnormal sinus node recovery time may be useful in identifying patients with syncope and chronic sinus bradycardia who benefit from implantation of a permanent pacemaker. In a group of 16 patients with sinus bradycardia and a history of syncope, the sinus node recovery time was abnormal and symptoms did not recur after pacemaker implantation.[30] In contrast, among 18 patients with sinus bradycardia, a history of syncope, and a normal sinus node recovery time, 9 of 10 unpaced patients be-

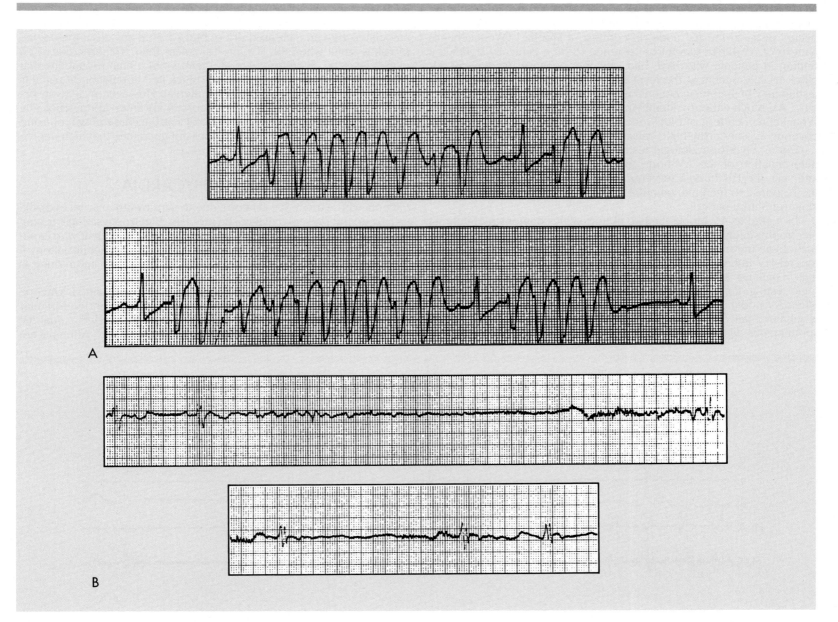

FIGURE 55.6 Continuous ECG monitoring in a patient with a history of two syncopal episodes. **A.** Initial recordings demonstrated several episodes of nonsustained ventricular tachycardia up to 11 beats in duration. The ventricular tachycardia was associated with palpitations but not lightheadedness or syncope. Ventricular tachycardia was presumed to be the cause of syncope in this patient. **B.** On the seventh day of continuous ECG monitoring, the patient experienced a typical syncopal episode and was found to have a severe bradyarrhythmia, with an 8.4-second period of asystole. In this patient, ventricular tachycardia was an incidental finding, unrelated to syncope. This case demonstrates a potential pitfall of continuous ECG monitoring as a diagnostic aid in patients with syncope. An arrhythmia that does not reproduce the patient's symptoms should not be presumed to be the cause of syncope.

came asymptomatic and 2 of 8 patients who underwent pacemaker implantation continued to have syncope. Therefore, a prolonged sinus node recovery time may predict a beneficial response to pacing in patients with syncope and sinus bradycardia. However, as stated previously, the clinical significance of a mildly prolonged sinus node recovery time should be interpreted with caution.

ATRIOVENTRICULAR BLOCK

Syncope may be caused by intermittent high-degree AV block that cannot be documented despite repeated ambulatory ECG recordings because the AV block is an infrequent occurrence. Electrophysiologic testing may be helpful in identifying patients with unexplained syncope and no documented AV block in whom intermittent high-degree AV block is the likely cause of syncope.

In addition, electrophysiologic testing may be helpful in patients with syncope who have had documented but asymptomatic episodes of AV block. If a patient with syncope is found to have an asymptomatic episode of classic Mobitz II second-degree AV block, implantation of a permanent pacemaker is indicated, because this type of AV block occurs distal to the AV node. In contrast, a Mobitz I (Wenckebach) pattern of AV block cannot be assumed to be a clinically significant finding in patients who have had syncope, because this type of AV block usually occurs at the level of the AV node. Electrophysiologic testing may be helpful in patients with syncope and asymptomatic Mobitz I AV block either by identifying the occasional patient in whom a Wenckebach pattern of block occurs distal to the AV node or by uncovering another arrhythmic cause of syncope.

During electrophysiologic testing, AV conduction is evaluated by determination of the AV node to His bundle conduction time (AH interval), the His bundle to ventricular activation time (HV interval), the response to incremental atrial pacing, and AV nodal and His-Purkinje refractory periods.

In regard to AV block, the two abnormalities demonstrable during electrophysiologic testing that have the highest diagnostic value are pathologic infranodal block during atrial pacing and a markedly prolonged HV interval (≥100 msec). Both are relatively infrequent findings in patients with unexplained syncope who undergo electrophysiologic testing. Pathologic infranodal block during atrial pacing occurs when AV nodal conduction is intact and the atrial pacing cycle length is greater than 300 msec (Fig. 55.8).[31] This finding is predictive of spontaneous high-degree AV block. Pathologic infranodal block must be distinguished from "functional" infranodal block, which occurs when there is AV nodal Wenckebach block; AV nodal block results in a pause that lengthens His-Purkinje refractoriness, causing infranodal block in the second beat of the next Wenckebach cycle (Fig. 55.9). Functional infranodal block has a benign prognosis and is not of diagnostic value in patients with unexplained syncope.[31]

Although the clinical significance of an abnormal HV interval (>55 msec) in the patient with unexplained syncope may be unclear, it appears that a markedly prolonged HV interval (≥100 msec) is associated with approximately a 25% risk of high-degree AV block over a 3-year follow-up period.[32] Therefore, in a patient with unexplained syncope who has no other abnormalities, an HV interval greater than or equal to 100 msec suggests that AV block may be the cause of syncope.

There is controversy regarding the prognostic implications of an HV interval of 55 msec to 100 msec. Some studies in patients with bundle branch block have suggested that the HV interval cannot be used to determine which patients with bundle branch block are at increased risk of developing high-degree AV block,[33] whereas other studies have indicated that an HV interval of 55 msec to 70 msec is associated with an increased risk of block.[32,34] In any case, the degree of risk is small when the HV interval is less than 100 msec (i.e., 12% over 3 years).[32] Therefore, overall there is not a high probability that syncope is related to intermittent AV block in a population of patients with syncope and an abnormal HV interval. However, in a given patient, a mildly prolonged or even a normal HV interval does not rule out the possibility of intermittent AV block as the cause of syncope and a markedly prolonged HV interval does not guarantee that high-degree block is the cause of syncope.[35]

SUPRAVENTRICULAR TACHYCARDIA

Patients who experience syncope due to supraventricular tachycardia usually do not present a diagnostic problem. Electrophysiologic testing may be helpful as a diagnostic tool in the occasional patient who experiences sporadic episodes of syncope as the major manifestation of supraventricular tachycardia and in whom ambulatory monitoring is unrevealing.

Electrophysiologic testing in patients with unexplained syncope should include incremental and programmed atrial and ventricular pacing to uncover the presence of an accessory pathway,[36,37] dual AV nodal pathways,[38] and enhanced AV nodal conduction.[39] Attempts are

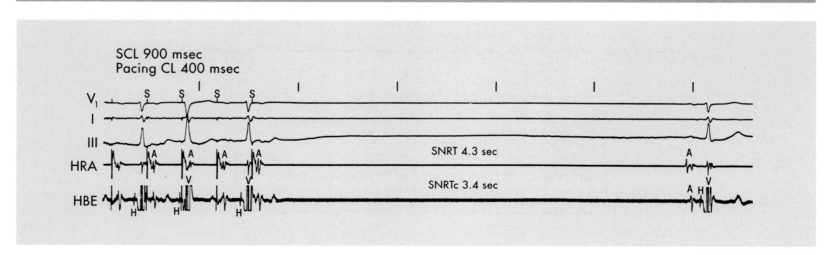

FIGURE 55.7 Markedly prolonged sinus node recovery time. The patient had a history of several episodes of syncope and near-syncope. Ambulatory ECG recordings demonstrated sinus pauses up to 2 seconds in duration, but without associated symptoms. It was therefore unclear whether this patient's symptoms were due to the sick sinus syndrome. On cessation of right atrial pacing at a cycle length (CL) of 400 msec, the sinus node recovery time (SNRT) was 4.3 seconds. The patient's spontaneous cycle length (SCL) was 900 msec, and the corrected SNRT (SNRTc) was 3.4 seconds. During the pause, the patient experienced near-syncope. Based on this abnormality, a permanent pacemaker was implanted. The patient had no recurrence of syncope or near-syncope, suggesting that this patient did have the sick sinus syndrome. (S, pacing stimulus; A, atrial electrogram; H, His bundle electrogram; V, ventricular electrogram) (Morady F, Peters RW, Scheinman MM: Bradyarrhythmias and bundle branch block. In Scheinman MM [ed]: Cardiac Emergencies, pp 135–149. Philadelphia, WB Saunders, 1984)

made to induce AV nodal reentrant tachycardia, reciprocating tachycardia using an overt or concealed accessory pathway, atrial tachycardia, and atrial fibrillation/flutter. If the patient describes a prodrome of rapid palpitations in association with syncope, or if ambulatory ECG monitoring demonstrates short runs of supraventricular tachycardia, this increases the likelihood that supraventricular tachycardia is the cause of syncope, and attempts at inducing supraventricular tachycardia during electrophysiologic testing should be vigorous.

Supraventricular tachycardia induced during electrophysiologic testing is unlikely to be the cause of syncope unless it is rapid and/or associated with hypotension. Although a patient with syncope caused by supraventricular tachycardia may not lose consciousness when supraventricular tachycardia is induced in the supine position in the electrophysiology laboratory, the patient will usually experience lightheadedness or near-syncope. Supraventricular tachycardia may be an incidental finding unrelated to syncope if it is not associated with a fall in blood pressure or cerebral symptoms when it is induced in the electrophysiology laboratory.

VENTRICULAR TACHYCARDIA

The most common abnormality that is found by electrophysiologic testing in patients with unexplained syncope is inducible ventricular tachycardia.[27-29] In some cases, there is good reason to presume that ventricular tachycardia is in fact the cause of syncope, but in others there is not. The type of ventricular tachycardia induced and the

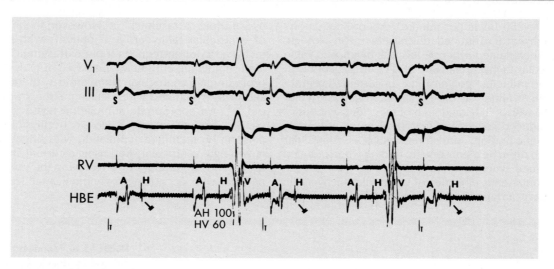

FIGURE 55.8 Pathologic infranodal AV block during atrial pacing at a cycle length of 500 msec. The AH interval remains constant at 100 msec. Alternate His bundle depolarizations (H) are not followed by a ventricular depolarization (V), indicating 2:1 infranodal AV block. The AV block is "pathologic" because it occurs at a relatively slow atrial pacing rate, when AV nodal conduction is intact. In patients with unexplained syncope who undergo electrophysiologic testing, the finding of pathologic infranodal AV block suggests that syncope may be due to intermittent high-degree AV block. (RV, right ventricular apex electrogram; S, pacing stimulus; A, atrial electrogram; H, His bundle electrogram; V, ventricular electrogram) (Morady F: Electrophysiologic testing in the management of patients with unexplained syncope. In Mandel WJ [ed]: Cardiac Arrhythmias, 2nd ed. Philadelphia, JB Lippincott, 1985)

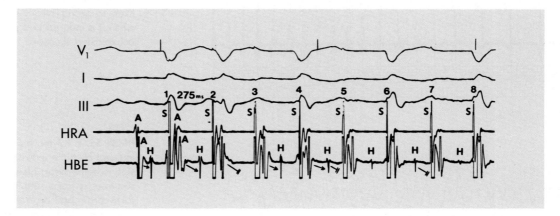

FIGURE 55.9 Functional infranodal AV block during atrial pacing at a cycle length of 275 msec. There is AV nodal Wenckebach block, and stimulus No. 2 is followed by AV nodal block. Because of the long HH interval that results from the AV nodal block, His-Purkinje refractoriness is lengthened and stimulus No. 4 is followed by infranodal block. In this case, infranodal AV block is "functional" because it occurs during a relatively rapid atrial pacing rate, in the setting of AV nodal Wenckebach block. Functional infranodal AV block is not a clinically significant finding in patients with unexplained syncope who undergo electrophysiologic testing. (S, pacing stimulus; A, atrial electrogram; H, His bundle electrogram) (Morady F: Electrophysiologic testing in the management of patients with unexplained syncope. In Mandel WJ [ed]: Cardiac Arrhythmias, 2nd ed. Philadelphia, JB Lippincott, 1985)

method of its induction must be taken into account when assessing its clinical significance.

Sustained, unimorphic ventricular tachycardia is rarely inducible in patients who have not had spontaneous ventricular tachycardia, but it can be induced in approximately 20% of patients with unexplained syncope.[40-44] If sustained, unimorphic ventricular tachycardia is induced during electrophysiologic testing in a patient with unexplained syncope, it is likely that the ventricular tachycardia is a clinically significant abnormality (Fig. 55.10). Treatment aimed at suppression of the unimorphic ventricular tachycardia usually is associated with no recurrence of syncope, suggesting that the cause of syncope was correctly identified and treated.[29]

Depending on the stimulation protocol used, ventricular tachycardia can be induced in up to 37% to 45% of patients who have no documented or suspected history of ventricular tachycardia.[42-44] The nonclinical ventricular tachycardia induced in these patients is usually polymorphic and rapid (>250 beats per minute). Accordingly, polymorphic ventricular tachycardia induced during electrophysiologic testing in patients with unexplained syncope has less diagnostic value than unimorphic ventricular tachycardia (Fig. 55.11). In patients with unexplained syncope and inducible polymorphic, unsustained ventricular tachycardia, treatment aimed at the suppression of ventricular tachycardia is associated with a 40% incidence of recurrent syncope.[29] This suggests that the induced arrhythmia may have been, at least in some patients, a nonspecific finding, unrelated to syncope. Ventricular fibrillation appears to also often be a nonspecific finding when induced in patients with unexplained syncope.[45]

In some patients, spontaneous episodes of ventricular tachycardia are polymorphic and have an appearance similar to the nonclinical polymorphic ventricular tachycardia that may be a nonspecific response to an aggressive stimulation protocol. Therefore, when polymorphic ventricular tachycardia is induced in a patient with unexplained syncope, it cannot be assumed that this is always a laboratory artifact. The yield of nonclinical forms of polymorphic ventricular tachycardia is directly related to the number of extra-stimuli used during programmed stimulation.[42-44] Therefore, the probability that polymorphic ventricular tachycardia is a clinically significant abnormality is highest when it is induced by a single estrastimulus and lowest when it is induced by triple extrastimuli. If the induced episode of ventricular tachycardia reproduces the patient's symptom-complex, this may increase the likelihood that the ventricular tachycardia is not an artifact.

Because the clinical significance of ventricular tachycardia induced during electrophysiologic testing may be unclear, it is important to use a stimulation protocol that has maximum sensitivity and specificity. The yield of nonclinical arrhythmias is increased significantly by the use of triple extrastimuli.[42-44] However, the induction of clinical forms of ventricular tachycardia in patients with documented ventricular tachycardia often requires triple extrastimuli.[46] In contrast, the use of high stimulating current strength (>5 mA) decreases the specificity of programmed ventricular stimulation without significantly improving sensitivity compared with a current strength of twice-diastolic threshold.[47,48] An appropriate stimulation protocol in patients with unexplained syncope who undergo electrophysiologic testing would be to perform programmed stimulation with single and double extrastimuli at two right ventricular sites, using a current strength between twice-diastolic threshold and 5 mA, reserving the use of triple extrastimuli for patients who do not have ventricular tachycardia induced by fewer extrastimuli.

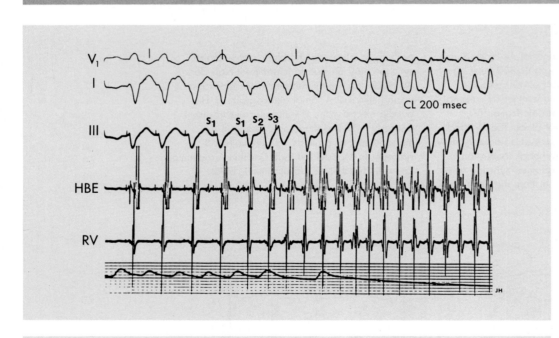

FIGURE 55.10 Monomorphic ventricular tachycardia, induced by double extrastimuli ($S_2 S_3$) in a patient who had a dilated cardiomyopathy and a history of two syncopal episodes. Ambulatory ECG monitoring demonstrated occasional ventricular premature depolarizations but not symptomatic ventricular tachycardia. The induced ventricular tachycardia had a cycle length (CL) of 200 msec (rate 300 beats per minute) and was associated with loss of consciousness. Induction of ventricular tachycardia was suppressed by procainamide, and syncope did not recur with chronic procainamide therapy. Monomorphic ventricular tachycardia is likely to be a clinically significant abnormality when it is induced in a patient with otherwise unexplained syncope.

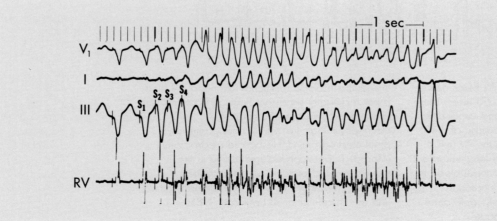

FIGURE 55.11 Polymorphic ventricular tachycardia induced by triple extrastimuli ($S_2 S_3 S_4$) in a patient with ischemic heart disease and a history of recurrent syncope. The induced ventricular tachycardia had an average cycle length of 180 msec (rate, 330 beats per minute) and was nonsustained, lasting 3.5 seconds. This type of polymorphic ventricular tachycardia is less likely than monomorphic ventricular tachycardia to be a clinically significant abnormality in patients with unexplained syncope, especially when it is induced by triple extrastimuli.

Left ventricular stimulation may be considered if right ventricular stimulation does not induce ventricular tachycardia. However, the yield of left ventricular stimulation will be small (<5%) when preceded by right ventricular stimulation at two sites.[46] Because of its low yield and potential morbidity, left ventricular stimulation may not be appropriate unless there is a high clinical suspicion that ventricular tachycardia is the cause of syncope.

Isoproterenol may facilitate the induction of ventricular tachycardia by programmed stimulation in some patients and can be used as an additional provocative maneuver if ventricular tachycardia is not induced during baseline ventricular stimulation.[49,50] The use of isoproterenol as a provocative maneuver is particularly appropriate in patients who have had syncope during or shortly after exercise.

PROBABILITY OF A POSITIVE STUDY

On the basis of clinical variables, many patients with unexplained syncope can be stratified into subgroups with high and low probability of having an electrophysiologic abnormality that is likely to be related to syncope. In patients who have had unexplained syncope, the most powerful predictor of a positive electrophysiologic study is a left ventricular ejection fraction of less than 0.40, followed by the presence of bundle branch block, coronary artery disease, remote myocardial infarction, use of type I antiarrhythmic drugs, injury related to loss of consciousness, and male sex.[51] A negative electrophysiologic study is associated with an ejection fraction greater than 0.40, the absence of structural heart disease, a normal ECG, and normal results of ambulatory monitoring.[51] The probability of a negative study increases as the number and duration of syncopal episodes increases.

Another noninvasive method for identifying patients with unexplained syncope who are likely to have a positive electrophysiologic study is the signal-averaged ECG. The signal-averaged ECG detects late potentials that reflect the myocardial substrate for reentrant ventricular tachycardia. The sensitivity and specificity of the signal-averaged ECG in detecting the subgroup of patients with unexplained syncope who have inducible ventricular tachycardia during electrophysiologic testing are approximately 80% and 90%, respectively.[52-54] The signal-averaged ECG has the greatest predictive value in patients with coronary artery disease who do not have a bundle branch block.

LIMITATIONS

Diagnosis of the cause of syncope based on the results of electrophysiologic testing is inferential and often is based on probability analysis. At times it is unclear whether an abnormality demonstrated during electrophysiologic testing is a clinically significant finding or a laboratory artifact or incidental finding unrelated to syncope. In some patients, electrophysiologic testing demonstrates two or more abnormalities that could potentially cause syncope, creating confusion as to which abnormality is the cause of syncope.[55] Programmed ventricular stimulation generally induces tachycardias that are caused by reentry. Because some patients may experience syncope caused by an automatic tachycardia, a negative electrophysiology study does not rule out an arrhythmic etiology of syncope.[55,56]

TREATMENT

In most cases, once the cause (or likely cause) of syncope is established, the most appropriate form of therapy to prevent a recurrence of syncope is obvious. Treatment may vary from aortic valve replacement in patients with severe aortic stenosis, to elimination of the offending agent in drug-induced orthostatic hypotension, to psychotherapy or counseling in patients with hysterical syncope or the hyperventilation syndrome. The specific treatment of metabolic and obstructive cardiovascular causes of syncope and orthostatic hypotension will not be discussed in detail here.

VAGALLY MEDIATED SYNCOPE

Vagally mediated syncope may occur in some individuals as an isolated event and therefore may not require specific therapy. When vagally mediated syncope is a recurrent problem and a precipitating factor that is avoidable can be identified, appropriate management may consist of simply avoiding the precipitating factor. However, in many patients with vagally mediated syncope there is no identifiable trigger. In such patients, loss of consciousness may be prevented if prodromal symptoms are of sufficient duration to allow the patient to assume a supine position with legs raised. Pharmacologic therapy with an anticholinergic agent or xanthine derivative may at times be helpful in decreasing the severity of symptoms.[57,58] An occasional patient with recurrent simple fainting spells that are vagally mediated may require a permanent pacemaker.[59]

Appropriate treatment for patients with recurrent syncope due to the carotid sinus hypersensitivity syndrome or with recurrent swallow or micturition syncope usually consists of implantation of a permanent pacemaker[60] or carotid sinus denervation.[61]

In all types of vagally mediated syncope, an important consideration before pacemaker implantation is whether the syncope is caused by a cardioinhibitory response or vasodepressor response. It is extremely useful to be able to identify a trigger that can reproduce the patient's symptoms (e.g., phlebotomy, carotid sinus massage, or the sight of blood). If episodes can be triggered, this should be performed while blood pressure is monitored and during ventricular and AV synchronous pacing. In patients who have a pure or predominantly cardioinhibitory response, a ventricular demand pacemaker is appropriate. If a mixed cardioinhibitory and peripheral vasodepressor response is found, an AV synchronous pacemaker may be more effective in preventing hypotension than a ventricular pacemaker. However, in patients with a pure vasodepressor response, a permanent pacemaker is not helpful. The vasodepressor type of vagally mediated syncope may be difficult to prevent. Therapies that may be successful include administration of fludrocortisone, wearing of tight stockings, or use of a phosphodiesterase inhibitor (e.g., aminophylline).

Carbamazepine is the drug of choice for treatment of glossopharyngeal syncope.[62]

SYNCOPE CAUSED BY ARRHYTHMIAS

Implantation of a permanent pacemaker is generally the treatment of choice when syncope is caused by sinus node dysfunction or high-degree AV block. However, before a permanent pacemaker is implanted, correctable causes of the bradyarrhythmia should be ruled out (e.g., drug toxicity or a metabolic abnormality).

When syncope is caused by a supraventricular or ventricular tachycardia that is inducible by programmed stimulation, long-term drug therapy to prevent a recurrence should be guided by the results of electropharmacologic testing.[63] However, electropharmacologic testing is not useful in some patients (e.g., patients with the congenital long QT interval syndrome[64] or with automatic tachycardias). If ventricular tachycardia was drug induced, appropriate therapy consists of discontinuing the use of the offending agents.

In patients with syncope caused by a tachyarrhythmia that is refractory to pharmacologic therapy, other therapeutic options include an antitachycardia pacemaker, an automatic implanted defibrillator,[64] cardiac electrosurgery,[65] or percutaneous transcatheter ablation.[66-68]

RECURRENT SYNCOPE IN A PATIENT WITH A NEGATIVE ELECTROPHYSIOLOGIC STUDY

There is a high spontaneous remission rate (70% to 85%) in patients with unexplained syncope who undergo an electrophysiologic study that does not demonstrate any abnormalities.[29] It may be that some of these patients have a psychiatric basis for syncope and benefit from a placebo effect associated with undergoing electrophysiologic testing.

There appears to be little or no role for empiric implantation of a permanent pacemaker in patients with unexplained syncope who have no documented bradyarrhythmia and a negative electrophysiologic study.[29]

Empiric antiarrhythmic drug treatment is generally of little value in patients with recurrent unexplained syncope who have no documented symptomatic tachyarrhythmia and a normal electrophysiologic study.

In patients who have a negative electrophysiologic study but continue to have syncope and have an asymptomatic bradyarrhythmia during ECG monitoring, a trial of pacemaker therapy may at times be appropriate, especially if the syncope causes injuries.

If the patient with recurrent syncope who has a negative electrophysiologic study has asymptomatic bursts of nonsustained ventricular tachycardia during ECG monitoring, a clinical trial of antiarrhythmic therapy should be considered, especially if the patient has underlying heart disease associated with a risk of sudden death.

REFERENCES

1. Aminoff MJ, Scheinman MM, Griffin JC et al: Electrocerebral accompaniments of syncope associated with malignant ventricular arrhythmias. Ann Intern Med 108:791, 1988
2. Day SC, Cook EF, Funkenstein H et al: Evaluation and outcome of emergency room patients with transient loss of consciousness. Am J Med 73:15, 1982
3. Kapoor WN, Karpf M, Wieand S et al: A prospective evaluation and follow-up of patients with syncope. N Engl J Med 309:197, 1983
4. Thomas JE: Hyperactive carotid sinus reflex and carotid sinus syncope. Mayo Clin Proc 44:127, 1969
5. Walter PF, Crawley IS, Dorney ER: Carotid sinus hypersensitivity and syncope. Am J Cardiol 42:396, 1978
6. Kong Y, Heyman A, Entman ML et al: Glossopharyngeal neuralgia associated with bradycardia, syncope, and seizures. Circulation 30:109, 1964
7. Levin B, Posner JR: Swallow syncope: Report of a case and review of the literature. Neurology 22:1086, 1972
8. Wik B, Hillestad L: Deglutition syncope. Br Med J 3:747, 1975
9. Schoenberg BS, Kuglitsch JF, Karnes WE: Micturition syncope—not a single entity. JAMA 229:1631, 1974
10. Ziegler MG: Postural hypotension. Annu Rev Med 31:239, 1980
11. Thomas JE, Schirger A, Fealey RD et al: Orthostatic hypotension. Mayo Clin Proc 56:117, 1981
12. Hamer AWF, Rubin SA, Peter T et al: Factors that predict syncope during ventricular tachycardia in patients. Am Heart J 107:997, 1984
13. Morady F, Peters RW, Scheinman MM: Bradyarrhythmias and bundle branch block. In Scheinman MM (ed): Cardiac Emergencies, pp 135–149. Philadelphia, WB Saunders, 1984
14. Massie B, Scheinman MM, Peters R: Clinical and electrophysiologic findings in patients with paroxysmal slowing of the sinus rate and apparent Mobitz type II atrioventricular block. Circulation 58:305, 1978
15. Klein GJ, Bashore TM, Sellers TD et al: Ventricular fibrillation in the Wolff-Parkinson-White syndrome. N Engl J Med 301:1080, 1979
16. Morady F, Shen EN, Bhandari A et al: Clinical symptoms in patients with sustained ventricular tachycardia. West J Med 142:341, 1985
17. Pathy MS: Clinical presentation of myocardial infarction in the elderly. Br Heart J 29:190, 1967
18. Librach G, Schadel M, Seltzer M et al: The initial manifestations of acute myocardial infarction. Geriatrics 31:41, 1976
19. Burch GE: A sign of cardiac arrest. Am Heart J 86:138, 1973
20. Brown KA, Maloney JD, Smith HC et al: Carotid sinus reflex in patients undergoing coronary angiography: Relationship of degree and location of coronary artery disease to response to carotid sinus massage. Circulation 62:697, 1980
21. Smith WM, Gallagher JJ: "Les torsade de pointes": An unusual ventricular arrhythmia. Ann Intern Med 93:578, 1980
22. Gibson TC, Heitzman MR: Diagnostic efficacy of 24-hour electrocardiographic monitoring for syncope. Am J Cardiol 53:1013, 1984
23. Podrid PJ, Schoeneberger A, Lown B et al: Use of nonsustained ventricular tachycardia as a guide to antiarrhythmic drug therapy in patients with malignant ventricular arrhythmia. Am Heart J 105:181, 1983
24. Strauss HC, Saroff AL, Bigger JT Jr: Premature atrial stimulation as a key to the understanding of sinoatrial conduction in man: Presentation of data and critical review of the literature. Circulation 47:86, 1973
25. Kerr CR, Strauss HC: The measurement of sinus node refractoriness in man. Circulation 68:1231, 1983
26. Moss AJ, Davis RJ: Brady-tachy syndrome. Prog Cardiovasc Dis 16:439, 1974
27. DiMarco JP, Garan H, Harthorne JW et al: Intracardiac electrophysiologic techniques in recurrent syncope of unknown cause. Ann Intern Med 95:542, 1981
28. Akhtar M, Shenasa M, Denker S et al: Role of cardiac electrophysiologic studies in patients with unexplained recurrent syncope. PACE 6:192, 1983
29. Morady F, Shen E, Schwartz A et al: Long-term follow-up of patients with recurrent unexplained syncope evaluated by electrophysiologic testing. J Am Coll Cardiol 2:1053, 1983
30. Gann D, Tolentino A, Samet P: Electrophysiologic evaluation of elderly patients with sinus bradycardia: A long-term follow-up study. Ann Intern Med 90:24, 1979
31. Dhingra RC, Wyndham C, Bauernfeind R et al: Significance of block distal to the His bundle induced by atrial pacing in patients with chronic bifascicular block. Circulation 60:1455, 1979
32. Scheinman MM, Peters RW, Sauve MJ et al: Value of the H-Q interval in patients with bundle branch block and the role of prophylactic permanent pacing. Am J Cardiol 50:1316, 1982
33. McAnulty JH, Rahimtoola SH, Murphy E et al: Natural history of "high-risk" bundle-branch block: Final report of a prospective study. N Engl J Med 307:137, 1982
34. Dhingra RC, Palileo E, Strasberg B et al: Significance of the HV interval in 517 patients with chronic bifascicular block. Circulation 64:1265, 1981
35. Kereiakes DJ, Morady F, Ports TA: High-degree atrioventricular block after radiation therapy. Am J Cardiol 53:1403, 1984
36. Sung RJ, Castellanos A, Mallon SM et al: Mode of initiation of reciprocating tachycardia during programmed ventricular stimulation in the Wolff-Parkinson-White syndrome: With reference to various patterns of ventriculoatrial conduction. Am J Cardiol 40:24, 1977
37. Farshidi A, Josephson ME, Horowitz LN: Electrophysiologic characteristics of concealed bypass tracts: Clinical and electrocardiographic correlates. Am J Cardiol 41:1052, 1978
38. Rosen KM, Mehta A, Miller RA: Demonstration of dual atrioventricular nodal pathways in man. Am J Cardiol 33:291, 1974
39. Benditt DG, Pritchett EL, Smith WM et al: Characteristics of atrioventricular conduction and the spectrum of arrhythmias in Lown-Ganong-Levine syndrome. Circulation 57:454, 1978
40. Vandepol CJ, Farshidi A, Spielman SR et al: Incidence and clinical significance of induced ventricular tachycardia. Am J Cardiol 45:725, 1980
41. Livelli FD Jr, Bigger JT Jr, Reiffel JA et al: Response to programmed ventricular stimulation: Sensitivity, specificity and relation to heart disease. Am J Cardiol 50:452, 1982
42. Mann DE, Luck JC, Griffin JC et al: Induction of clinical ventricular tachycardia using programmed stimulation: Value of third and fourth extrastimuli. Am J Cardiol 52:501, 1983
43. Brugada P, Abdollah H, Heddle B et al: Results of a ventricular stimulation protocol using a maximum of 4 premature stimuli in patients without documented or suspected ventricular arrhythmias. Am J Cardiol 52:1214, 1983
44. Morady F, Shapiro W, Shen E et al: Programmed ventricular stimulation in patients without spontaneous ventricular tachycardia. Am Heart J 107:85, 1984
45. DiCarlo LA Jr, Morady F, Schwartz AB et al: Clinical significance of ventricular fibrillation-flutter induced by ventricular programmed stimulation. Am Heart J 109:959, 1985
46. Morady F, DiCarlo L, Winston S et al: A prospective comparison of triple extrastimuli and left ventricular stimulation in studies of ventricular tachycardia induction. Circulation 70:52, 1984
47. Brugada P, Abdollah H, Wellens HJJ: Sensitivity of a ventricular stimulation protocol using two ventricular extrastimuli at twice diastolic threshold and 20 mA (abstr). J Am Coll Cardiol 3:609, 1984
48. Herre JM, Mann DE, Luck JC et al: Effect of third and fourth extrastimuli and increased current on programmed ventricular stimulation—a prospective study. Circulation (Suppl III) 68:III-243, 1983
49. Reddy CP, Gettes LS: Use of isoproterenol as an aid to electric induction of chronic recurrent ventricular tachycardia. Am J Cardiol 44:705, 1979
50. Freedman RA, Swerdlow CD, Echt DS et al: Facilitation of ventricular tachyarrhythmia induction by isoproterenol. Am J Cardiol 54:765, 1984
51. Krol RB, Morady F, Flaker GC et al: Electrophysiologic testing in patients with unexplained syncope: Clinical and noninvasive predictors of outcome. J Am Coll Cardiol 10:358, 1987
52. Kuchar DL, Thorburn CW, Sammel NL: Signal-averaged electrocardiogram for evaluation of recurrent syncope. Am J Cardiol 58:949, 1986
53. Gang ES, Peter T, Rosenthal ME et al: Detection of late potentials on the surface electrocardiogram in unexplained syncope. Am J Cardiol 58:1014, 1986
54. Winters SL, Stewart D, Gomes J: Signal averaging of the surface QRS complex predicts inducibility of ventricular tachycardia in patients with syncope of unknown origin: A prospective study. J Am Coll Cardiol 10:775, 1987
55. Morady F, Higgins J, Peters RW et al: Electrophysiologic testing in bundle branch block and unexplained syncope. Am J Cardiol 54:587, 1984
56. Morady F, Scheinman MM: The role and limitations of electrophysiologic testing in patients with unexplained syncope. Int J Cardiol 4:229, 1983
57. Sugrue DD, Wood DL, McGoon MD: Carotid sinus hypersensitivity and syncope. Mayo Clin Proc 59:637, 1984
58. Benditt DG, Kriett JM, Haugland JM et al: Effects of aminophylline on sinus and atrioventricular node function in young adults with vasovagal syncope

59. Sapire DW, Casta A, Safley W et al: Vasovagal syncope in children requiring pacemaker implantation. Am Heart J 106:1406, 1983
60. Davies AB, Stephens MR, Davies AG: Carotid sinus hypersensitivity in patients presenting with syncope. Br Heart J 42:583, 1979
61. Cheng LH, Norris CW: Surgical management of the carotid sinus syndrome. Arch Otolaryngol 97:395, 1973
62. Crill WE: Carbamazepine. Ann Intern Med 79:844, 1973
63. Horowitz LN, Josephson ME, Kastor JA: Intracardiac electrophysiologic studies as a method for the optimization of drug therapy in chronic ventricular arrhythmia. Prog Cardiovasc Dis 23:81, 1980
64. Mirowski M, Reid PR, Winkle RA et al: Mortality in patients with implanted automatic defibrillators. Ann Intern Med 98(part I):585, 1983
65. Josephson ME, Harken AD, Horowitz LN: Long-term results of endocardial resection for sustained ventricular tachycardia in coronary disease patients. Am Heart J 104:51, 1982
66. Scheinman MM, Morady F, Hess DS et al: Catheter-induced ablation of the atrioventricular junction to control refractory supraventricular arrhythmias. JAMA 248:851, 1982
67. Morady F, Scheinman MM: Transvenous catheter ablation of a posteroseptal accessory pathway in a patient with the Wolff-Parkinson-White syndrome. N Engl J Med 310:705, 1984
68. Morady F, Scheinman MM, DiCarlo LA et al: Catheter ablation of ventricular tachycardia with intracardiac shocks: Results in 33 patients. Circulation 75:1037, 1987

EVALUATION AND TREATMENT OF PATIENTS WITH ABORTED SUDDEN DEATH

David J. Wilber • Hasan Garan • Jeremy N. Ruskin

The successful resuscitative combination of artificial ventilation, sternal compression, and external electrical defibrillation was first introduced by Jude and co-workers in 1960.[1] Subsequent modification and widespread application of these techniques by effective prehospital emergency care systems made possible the resuscitation of an increasing number of victims of unexpected out-of-hospital cardiac arrest.[2,3] However, early investigators reported an alarmingly high rate of late mortality in patients with aborted sudden death—approximately 30% of patients died within the first year following hospital discharge.[4,5] The majority of deaths were secondary to recurrent cardiac arrest,[6] and empirical therapy with antiarrhythmic agents available at the time did not alter the high risk of late sudden death. In the last decade, the care of these patients has undergone continued evolution as new insights into the pathophysiology of sudden death and new therapeutic techniques have emerged.

OBSERVATIONS AT THE TIME OF CARDIAC ARREST

Sudden death is defined as sudden and unexpected collapse occurring within seconds to minutes of symptom onset during normal activity in either a previously healthy person, or in a patient with previously stable heart disease. The initial rhythm documented by emergency personnel several minutes after collapse is ventricular fibrillation (VF) in 65% to 80% of patients.[7-10] In an additional 5% of patients, ventricular tachycardia (VT) is observed. Profound sinus bradycardia, slow idioventricular rhythms, or asystole are found in the remaining patients. However, relatively few patients with brady–asystolic arrest are successfully resuscitated;[8,9] the overwhelming majority of survivors admitted to the hospital have been resuscitated from a ventricular tachyarrhythmia.

While VF is the rhythm most commonly documented several minutes after collapse, when the onset of cardiac arrest is recorded fortuitously during ambulatory monitoring, VF is generally preceded by a brief period of monomorphic or polymorphic VT.[11-15] These tachycardias are characterized by short cycle lengths (<300 msec) and rapid degeneration into VF within seconds to minutes (Fig. 56.1). Sustained monomorphic VT lasting more than a few minutes is uncommon. When VF recurs within several hours after the initial resuscitation, nonsustained VT precedes VF in 75% of episodes.[16]

Chest discomfort or dyspnea immediately precedes collapse in a minority of sudden death survivors,[4,5] and is often associated with subsequent objective evidence of myocardial necrosis.[5,10] However, the frequent occurrence of retrograde amnesia in survivors,[17] and the unreliability of bystander reporting, may result in underestimation of prodromal symptoms. Approximately 25% of patients are engaged in moderate or strenuous physical activity at the time of collapse.[18,19] In relation to the amount of time spent in such activities, this frequency represents a disproportionately high risk of sudden death during exercise.

Out-of-hospital cardiac arrest is uncommon in the absence of structural heart disease, though the structural abnormality may have been previously unrecognized in up to 35% of patients.[5] Most survivors (72%–85%) have evidence of significant obstructive coronary artery disease.[10,20-30] In autopsy series of patients in whom attempted resuscitation was unsuccessful, the prevalence of coronary artery disease is even greater (at least 90%).[7,31] Most other patients have either primary myocardial disease, valvular heart disease, or congenital abnormalities. In a few, no cardiac abnormalities are found despite extensive investigation.

CHARACTERISTICS OF SURVIVORS WITH ISCHEMIC HEART DISEASE
CLINICAL PRESENTATION

Fifty percent of sudden-death survivors with ischemic heart disease have electrocardiographic evidence of remote myocardial infarction and a similar number have a history of previous angina pectoris.[20,22,23] Coronary arteriography usually discloses extensive multivessel obstructive lesions, although single vessel disease is found in 12% to 35% of patients.[20-23] At least two thirds of the patients have one or more occluded vessels and single or multiple regional wall motion abnormalities.[20,22,23] Global ventricular function is commonly impaired, but up to 30% of survivors have a left ventricular ejection fraction of greater than 50%.[20-23,32] Thus, while the typical sudden-death survivor with ischemic heart disease has multivessel coronary obstructions and remote myocardial infarction, the extent of structural abnormalities varies over a wide spectrum.

ROLE OF ACUTE MYOCARDIAL INFARCTION

The frequency of acute myocardial infarction in survivors of out-of-hospital cardiac arrest has not been settled. In a widely cited study by Baum and coworkers, only 19% of 305 sudden-death survivors with ischemic heart disease had evolution of new Q waves in the days following resuscitation.[5] However, in 10% of patients, Q waves of uncertain age were noted. Thirty-eight percent of patients had isoenzyme evidence (LDH1 > LDH2) evidence of myocardial injury. More recently, Goldstein and co-workers reported a 44% incidence of new Q waves in 142 sudden-death survivors with ischemic heart disease.[10] An additional 27% of patients had new ST-T wave changes associated with isoenzyme evidence (elevated CK–MB or LDH1) of myocardial injury. Myerburg and coworkers reported a 36% incidence of myocardial infarction (new Q waves, or persistent ST segment or T wave abnormalities), although no enzyme data were specified.[21] Thus, evidence for new myocardial infarction or ischemic injury is present in a substantial number of sudden-death survivors with coronary artery disease, although a majority will not evolve new Q waves (a specific but insensitive marker of myocardial necrosis). In this latter group of patients, it may be difficult to determine whether injury was the result of events preceding (and precipitating) cardiac arrest, or, alternatively, resulted from hypoperfusion, defibrillation,[33] or mechanical trauma[34] during resuscitation.

Longterm prognosis following hospital discharge is more favorable for patients with definite evidence of new myocardial infarction. Cumulative mortality (all causes) at one year and two years after discharge is two to three times greater in patients without new Q waves.[5,10] Cobb and co-workers also found a much higher risk of recurrent cardiac arrest within one year of hospital discharge in patients without new Q waves after the initial arrest (22% versus 2%).[35] Previous reports of patients with acute myocardial infarction suggest that the occurrence of cardiac arrest within the early hours of infarction, *in the absence of pump failure*, has no independent effect on longterm prognosis.[36,37]

SPONTANEOUS ARRHYTHMIAS

Frequent and complex ventricular ectopy is common in sudden-death survivors with ischemic heart disease, both in the initial days following resuscitation[21] and at later intervals.[30,38] During 24-hour ambulatory monitoring, performed within several months of the initial cardiac arrest, Weaver and co-workers found complex ectopy (> Lown class II) in 70% of patients and repetitive beats in 53% of patients.[38] Complex ectopy was more common in patients with recurrent cardiac arrest (84% versus 60%). In a later analysis from this group, following adjustment for the degree of left ventricular dysfunction, no arrhythmia variable had additional predictive value for subsequent sudden or non-sudden death.[32] Myerburg and coworkers found a similar incidence of complex ectopy and repetitive forms during 24-hour recordings at multiple intervals following hospital discharge.[30] Nonsustained VT was observed in 20% of patients. The findings on ambulatory monitoring were poor predictors of recurrent cardiac arrest.

In contrast to these observations, large-scale longitudinal studies of patients following myocardial infarction have documented that frequent (>10 complexes/hr) and repetitive ventricular ectopy each have independent predictive power for subsequent cardiac mortality and sudden death in that population.[39-41] Failure to identify this relationship during followup of sudden-death survivors may be related to the smaller sample sizes of these studies, and to differences in definition of high-risk arrhythmia variables.

OTHER PROGNOSTIC FACTORS

In a Seattle study, determinants of late mortality and recurrent cardiac arrest after hospital discharge have been examined in a large group of sudden-death survivors with ischemic heart disease. Recurrent cardiac arrest was more common in patients with previous myocardial infarction, congestive heart failure, three-vessel coronary disease, and depressed left ventricular function.[20,38] More recently, the same group reported a multivariate survival analysis that included clinical and hemodynamic variables as well as the results of exercise testing and am-

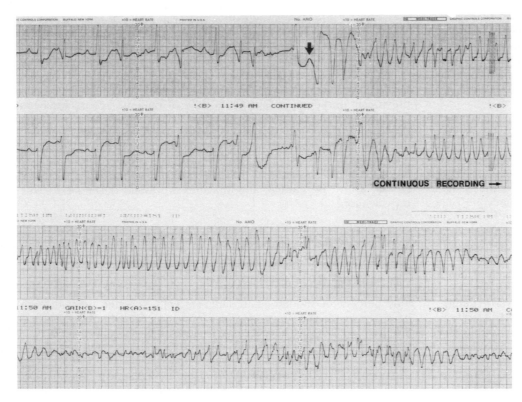

FIGURE 56.1 Ambulatory recording during the onset of cardiac arrest in a patient with chronic left bundle branch block and a remote anterior myocardial infarction. The arrow indicates the onset of polymorphic ventricular tachycardia (preceded by a fusion complex) that rapidly degenerates to ventricular fibrillation.

bulatory monitoring. Left ventricular ejection fraction was the single most powerful predictor of recurrent cardiac arrest and cardiac death. Inclusion of the remaining variables provided little additional prognostic information. Of 154 sudden-death survivors followed for a minimum of two years, 96% of patients with a left ventricular ejection fraction of greater than 50% survived (Fig. 56.2). Therapy was not standardized and 60% of patients received antiarrhythmic drugs.[32]

PATHOPHYSIOLOGY OF CARDIAC ARREST IN ISCHEMIC HEART DISEASE
CHRONIC ELECTRICAL INSTABILITY

From the preceding discussion, it is evident that survivors of cardiac arrest with a history of remote myocardial infarction and depressed ventricular function are at particularly high risk of recurrent cardiac arrest. Ventricular arrhythmias, predominantly due to re-entry,[42] can be reproducibly provoked during intracardiac electrophysiologic studies in most of these patients.[24-29] The propensity for both spontaneous ectopy and inducible ventricular arrhythmias may be related to the abnormal electrophysiologic properties of surviving cells within and around an area of remote myocardial infarction.[43,44] In addition, disrupted intercellular connections produced by patchy fibrosis and necrosis of individual muscle fibers[45,46] may also predispose to disordered impulse propagation and re-entrant arrhythmias. The presence of this chronic electrically unstable substrate appears to greatly enhance the risk of recurrent cardiac arrest.

TRIGGERING MECHANISMS

Left ventricular dysfunction and repetitive ventricular ectopy are common in survivors of cardiac arrest. While both may be independent markers of an electrically unstable substrate, the events that trigger a cardiac arrest at a particular point in time are less certain. The initial complex of a lethal ventricular tachyarrhythmia is often viewed as an independent event, which by virtue of its appropriate timing triggers the sustained arrhythmia. The concept of a critically timed premature complex introduced during the vulnerable period of cardiac repolarization (R on T phenomenon) has been useful in understanding the artificial induction of ventricular arrhythmias in the laboratory. However, in over 100 reported cases of cardiac arrest recorded by ambulatory monitoring,[11-15] the R on T phenomenon was observed in only one third, and the initial complexes frequently occurred in late diastole. For many patients, the features and timing of the initial complexes may not play a critical role in the genesis of spontaneous cardiac arrest. The precipitating event is more likely an additional, often transient, alteration in the electrophysiologic environment of the heart that permits spontaneous ectopy to become sustained and, more importantly, to become rapidly disorganized.

ISCHEMIA

The incidence of VF is 19% in patients with definite evidence of acute myocardial infarction observed within one hour of the onset of chest pain.[47] The lower incidence reported in most other series relates to a relative delay in observation, since 75% of episodes occur within two hours of symptom onset. The initially high risk of VF is related to marked regional alterations in conduction and the temporal dispersion of refractoriness,[48] which promote the progressive fractionation of successive activation fronts as they pass through ischemic myocardium. The severity of these abnormalities subsides rapidly as muscle necrosis evolves.

Definite evidence of myocardial infarction at the time of collapse is not present in the majority of sudden-death survivors with ischemic heart disease. However, there is accumulating experimental evidence from animal models of multivessel coronary disease that suggests that even brief periods of myocardial ischemia may be highly arrhythmogenic in the setting of previous myocardial infarction.[49,50] The risk of VF during acute ischemia appears to be greatest in the setting of remote myocardial infarction *and* chronic electrical instability, as demonstrated by inducible ventricular tachyarrhythmias during baseline (nonischemic) conditions.[51]

The importance of transient ischemia as a mechanism of sudden death following myocardial infarction is also suggested by recent clinical studies. Schuster and Bulkley found a 27% incidence of sudden death over an average followup of three months in patients who manifested postinfarction angina during their early convalescence.[52] Theroux and coworkers studied 210 patients without angina or clinical heart failure by submaximal exercise testing two weeks after myocardial infarction.[53] Patients with 1 mm or more of ST segment depression during exercise had a 15% incidence of sudden death at one year compared to a less than 1% incidence in patients without ST segment depression. Exertional angina associated with fixed coronary stenoses is only one potential cause of ischemia-related sudden death. Post-

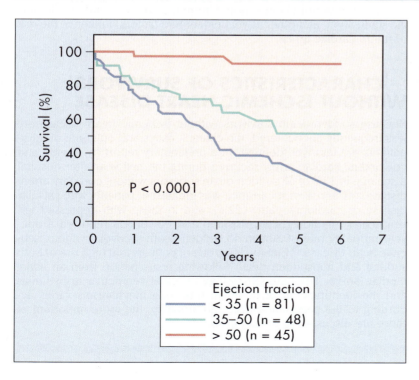

FIGURE 56.2 Longterm survival following resuscitation from cardiac arrest stratified according to left ventricular function. Eighty percent of deaths were sudden. (Modified from Ritchie JL, Hallstrom AP, Troubaugh GB et al: Out-of-hospital sudden coronary death: Rest and exercise radionuclide left ventricular function in survivors. Am J Cardiol 55:645, 1985)

mortem examination of sudden-death victims frequently discloses acute nonocclusive intracoronary lesions (plaque rupture, endothelial platelet, and fibrin thrombi) that may have contributed to transient ischemia preceding fatal cardiac arrest.[54]

Coronary vasospasm is a potential cause of out-of-hospital cardiac arrest and sudden death. In patients with a clinical history of variant angina, many of whom have significant coronary artery disease, the occurrence of serious ventricular arrhythmias accompanying the episode of spasm is well documented.[55-57] While experimental investigations have emphasized the significance of reperfusion arrhythmias,[58] clinical studies indicate that arrhythmias occur with equal or greater frequency soon after the onset of ischemia, and prior to reperfusion.[58] Sudden death occurred in 17% of 114 patients with known variant angina during a mean followup of 26 months,[59] and occurred with equal frequency in patients with and without significant concomitant coronary disease. Over half of the sudden deaths occurred in patients already taking calcium channel blockers or nitrates. It may be inappropriate to extend these findings to all sudden-death survivors, since a large majority of these patients manifest no previous or subsequent clinical evidence of classical variant angina.[26,27] The contribution of less dramatic changes in vasomotor tone to the production of transient ischemia, particularly in patients with severe obstructive coronary disease, may be important but requires further investigation.

HYPOKALEMIA

Despite abundant experimental and circumstantial evidence attesting to the arrhythmogenic potential of hypokalemia,[60] its relative importance as a primary cause of lethal ventricular arrhythmias in humans remains controversial.[61] Hypokalemia is associated with an increased risk of early VF in patients with acute myocardial infarction.[62] Not uncommonly, depression of serum K^+ is noted during initial laboratory studies following successful resuscitation. A serum K^+ < 3.6 millimolar (mM) was noted in 50% of 115 patients resuscitated from out-of-hospital VF, and in 17%, the value was less than 3 mM.[63] Surprisingly, hypokalemia could not be related to previous diuretic use. This finding suggests that in many patients, the observed hypokalemia does not reflect cellular potassium depletion; rather, potassium may have been shifted intracellularly as a result of administered and endogenous epinephrine, excessive bicarbonate administration, and mechanical hyperventilation during resuscitation.

Potassium depletion alone may give rise to dispersion of ventricular repolarization associated with prolongation of the QT interval and polymorphic VT.[64] More often, hypokalemia is a contributing factor when this syndrome complicates antiarrhythmic drug therapy. Hypokalemia also potentiates the ventricular arrhythmias associated with digitalis therapy.[60] In the absence of these factors, and without knowledge of previous potassium balance, caution should be exercised in attributing cardiac arrest to hypokalemia alone on the basis of mildly depressed postresuscitation serum potassium levels.

DRUGS

Aggravation of ventricular arrhythmias by antiarrhythmic drug therapy is observed in 5% to 15% of all drug trials.[65,66] While the adverse effect is often an increase in the frequency and complexity of ventricular ectopy beyond that expected by statistical variability, the precipitation of sustained arrhythmias and cardiac arrest may also occur. In two large series of sudden-death survivors referred for electrophysiologic testing, antiarrhythmic therapy was identified as the primary cause of cardiac arrest in 5% of patients.[26,27] This complication of antiarrhythmic therapy is not always related to toxic serum drug levels, and may not emerge for several months after the initiation of therapy.[67] Programmed ventricular stimulation may facilitate identification of such potential complications, particularly in patients who have no previous history of spontaneous or inducible sustained arrhythmias in the absence of drug therapy.[66,67]

Virtually all antiarrhythmic drugs are potentially arrhythmogenic.[65,66] Other drugs, notably the phenothiazines and tricyclic antidepressants, have also been implicated in the precipitation of lethal ventricular arrhythmias. The most well-described syndrome—prolongation of the QT-interval-associated paroxysms of polymorphous VT or VF—is a common mechanism of arrhythmogenesis involving Type IA drugs such as quinidine and procainamide.[64] However, these same agents may precipitate cardiac arrest in the absence of QT prolongation.[67] Type IC drugs such as flecainide have little influence on cardiac repolarization, and their arrhythmogenic potential may be related to marked slowing of intraventricular conduction, particularly in patients with pre-existing cardiac diseases.[68] It is likely that a variety of mechanisms lead to arrhythmia exacerbation during antiarrhythmic therapy.[69]

OTHER TRIGGERING MECHANISMS

The autonomic nervous system plays an important role in the regulation of cardiac repolarization. *Nonuniform* adrenergic stimulation, resulting in heterogeneous ventricular repolarization,[70] has an arrhythmogenic effect in a variety of animal models.[71] While this condition is produced experimentally by selective stimulation or interruption of cardiac nerve fibers, Barber and coworkers reported that destruction of sympathetic nerve fibers by transmural myocardial infarction may result in selective denervation of adjacent normal myocardium.[72] During periods of heightened adrenergic stimulation, the resultant inhomogeneities in repolarization may precipitate lethal arrhythmias. The role of abnormal autonomic regulation in the genesis of sudden death in patients with ischemic heart disease is suggested by the frequent finding of abnormally prolonged QT intervals in survivors of sudden death.[73] In addition, patients with prolonged QT intervals following myocardial infarction have a higher mortality[74] and incidence of subsequent sudden death.[75] Mechanical and hemodynamic events (changes in loading conditions) may independently alter the electrophysiologic properties of ventricular myocardium.[76] The clinical relevance of this mechanism is suggested by the extremely high recurrence rate of sudden death among patients with depressed left ventricular function, severe wall motion abnormalities, and clinical heart failure.

The occurrence of sudden death in patients with ischemic heart disease, therefore, is best viewed as a variable interaction between an electrically unstable substrate and transient triggering events. In the case of acute myocardial infarction, the presence of pre-existing structural and electrophysiologic abnormalities play a minor role, and the risk of recurrence is low. In other patients, both the severity of pre-existing abnormalities, and the likelihood of recurring trigger events (such as transient ischemia, nonuniform increases in cardiac adrenergic stimulation, and other as yet unidentified factors) influence the risk of future cardiac arrest.

CHARACTERISTICS OF SURVIVORS WITHOUT ISCHEMIC HEART DISEASE

Because sudden-death survivors without ischemic heart disease are less frequently encountered, the characteristics and outcome of these patients are less well defined. In a preliminary report by Oseran and coworkers, cardiac arrest recurred during the first year after hospital discharge in 13% of 53 sudden-death survivors without coronary artery disease.[77] The risk of recurrence was greatest in patients with valvular disease or cardiomyopathy (22%), and in those with depressed left ventricular function (32%). Rosman and coworkers reported a one-year mortality rate of 30% in 43 sudden-death survivors without ischemic heart disease.[78] Clearly this group of patients is at high risk of both sudden and nonsudden death following resuscitation from an initial cardiac arrest. The pathophysiology of lethal ventricular arrhythmias and the identification of potential triggering mechanisms varies according to the particular cardiac abnormality; the more important of these are discussed in detail below.

HYPERTROPHIC CARDIOMYOPATHY

Sudden death is the most common cause of death in patients with hypertrophic cardiomyopathy (HCM), with an annual incidence of 2% to 4%.[79-81] Ventricular tachyarrhythmias are the usual cause, though in a minority of cases; conduction system disease and bradyarrhythmias may play a role. In a series of 78 patients with sudden death (including 17 survivors of cardiac arrest) reported from the NIH, a disproportionate number of episodes (39%) occurred during moderate or strenuous exercise.[82] The median age of death was 19 years and 71% of patients were less than 30 years old. In patients over the age of 40, significant coronary artery disease was usually found. In 42% of patients, sudden death was the first manifestation of cardiac disease. No symptomatic, hemodynamic, electrocardiographic, or echocardiographic variables differentiated those who would later suffer sudden death from other HCM patients. One quarter of sudden-death victims were taking propranolol in doses of at least 120 mg/d, suggesting that beta blockade alone may not provide adequate protection from lethal arrhythmias; higher doses of propranolol (>320 mg/d) may provide more effective protection from sudden death.[83] Septal myotomy does not prevent sudden death.[79,84]

Only a family history of sudden death[79] and the presence of nonsustained VT (usually asymptomatic) on prolonged ambulatory monitoring have been identified as predictors of fatal outcome.[80] Such high-risk patients frequently have inducible ventricular arrhythmias during programmed stimulation;[85] the substrate for these arrhythmias is myocardial hypertrophy and disordered fiber architecture. Pre-excitation syndromes may coexist with HCM, and contribute to the genesis of cardiac arrest.

DILATED CARDIOMYOPATHY

Sudden death accounts for up to half of all deaths in patients with dilated cardiomyopathy (DCM). In series that included mildly symptomatic patients, sudden death occurred in 7% to 19% after more than five years of followup.[86,87] In severely symptomatic patients with DCM, a higher incidence of sudden death has been reported (up to 20% within one year).[88-90] Nonsustained VT is detected on ambulatory monitoring in as many as 50% of patients with symptomatic DCM.[88-93] The prognostic significance of this finding is uncertain. Some investigators have found that patients with frequent ventricular ectopy[91] or frequent episodes of nonsustained VT[89] are more likely to die suddenly. However, other researchers could not identify a relationship between the presence of either complex ectopy or nonsustained VT and the subsequent risk of sudden or nonsudden death.[90,92,93] The prognosis of sudden-death survivors with DCM is most strongly related to the degree of left ventricular dysfunction.[77] Interstitial fibrosis, myocardial hypertrophy, and subendocardial scarring, the potential substrate of lethal arrhythmias, are universal findings.[94] Patients with a history of sustained ventricular arrhythmias have inducible VT during electrophysiologic study.[95]

MITRAL VALVE PROLAPSE

The precise incidence of sudden death in this extremely common and usually asymptomatic valvular disorder is uncertain, but it is probably less than 1%.[96] A ventricular tachyarrhythmia is the most common mechanism, although autopsy studies of sudden-death victims have implicated ruptured chordae[97] or extensive fibrosis of the conduction system[98] as causal factors in several patients. Most, but not all, reported sudden deaths occurred in symptomatic women who had systolic murmurs. The majority had evidence of at least moderately severe prolapse during echocardiography, angiography, or at autopsy.[97,99-101] Ventricular ectopy and abnormal electrocardiograms (ST-T wave changes) were frequently noted prior to death;[99-101] complex ventricular arrhythmias appear to be related to the severity of mitral regurgitation.[102] Excessive adrenergic stimulation may be an arrhythmogenic influence in this population,[96] and may trigger some episodes of cardiac arrest. Ventricular tachyarrhythmias can be induced in many patients with mitral valve prolapse, particularly those with a prior history of sustained VT or VF.[103]

PRE-EXCITATION SYNDROMES

A small number of patients with accessory atrioventricular connections will develop cardiac arrest. The predominant mechanism of cardiac arrest is the degeneration of rapidly conducting, pre-excited atrial fibrillation to VF.[104] Therapeutic attempts to terminate atrial fibrillation with drugs such as digoxin[104] or verapamil[105] may precipitate VF in some patients. However, in 30% of patients reported from Duke, cardiac arrest occurred during strenuous exercise.[106] The majority of these patients had no, or only minimal, previous symptoms, and the diagnosis of pre-excitation had not been previously established.

In patients who develop VF, age, symptom duration, and associated cardiac conditions are similar to patients with pre-excitation and no history of VF.[104] Pre-excitation is nearly always present on the surface electrocardiogram, and a history of previous atrial fibrillation is present in 75% of cases. No particular location of the accessory pathway occurs with greater frequency in patients with VF, but multiple pathways are more common. During induced atrial fibrillation, all patients with a previous cardiac arrest had a shortest RR interval between pre-excited beats that was less than or equal to 250 msec. Rapid conduction over the accessory pathway, in association with sympathetic stimulation[107] secondary to hypotension, increases the vulnerability to VF in these patients.

CONGENITAL HEART DISEASE

Nine percent of all deaths in a large pediatric cardiology clinic were reported to be sudden;[108] one half of the sudden deaths were observed late after the surgical repair of congenital cardiac defects. Sudden death is reported in 3% to 6% of patients following intracardiac repair of the tetralogy of Fallot.[109-111] Frequent ventricular ectopy and postoperative right ventricular hypertension are common findings in patients who subsequently die suddenly. Extensive fibrosis associated with right ventricular dysfunction, and scarring secondary to the previous ventriculotomy have been implicated as the anatomical substrates of lethal arrhythmias.[111] Late sudden death has also been reported following closure of ventricular septal defects[112] and the Mustard procedure.[113]

IDIOPATHIC LONG QT SYNDROME

Since its initial description in 1957, the syndrome of idiopathic QT interval prolongation—associated with a structurally normal heart, stress-related syncope, and with or without congenital deafness—has been recognized with increasing frequency. This syndrome has been reviewed extensively,[114,115] but a few points merit emphasis. Family studies have documented that exertion-related sudden death without overt QT prolongation may occur in the siblings of patients with the typical syndrome. While the traditional guideline for determining abnormally prolonged repolarization (QTc > 440 msec) remains useful, repolarization abnormalities may be subtle and intermittent. The primary abnormality appears to be asymmetric adrenergic neural input to the ventricular myocardium that gives rise to heterogeneous repolarization. During generalized increases in adrenergic tone (exertion, excitement), this heterogeneity is accentuated and lethal arrhythmias may be triggered. In keeping with the apparent absence of structural *myocardial* disease, sustained ventricular arrhythmias are rarely induced in patients with the idiopathic long QT syndrome.[116] Patients with congenital deafness and a previous history of syncope are at greatest risk of cardiac arrest.

NO STRUCTURAL HEART DISEASE

In a small number of sudden-death survivors, no obvious structural abnormalities can be detected by invasive and noninvasive testing. In some of these patients, cardiac arrest is precipitated by drug therapy or electrolyte imbalance. More commonly, these factors precipitate cardiac arrest in patients with pre-existing structural abnormalities. A small number of patients (usually children or young adults) have a history of exertional syncope and cardiac arrest, but no evidence of repolarization abnormalities on multiple electrocardiograms.[117,118] Such patients may represent a variant of the long QT syndrome. Myocardial biopsy has been reported to disclose evidence of structural abnormalities in a large number of patients with "unexplained" life-threatening arrhythmias after a normal routine diagnostic evaluation.[119-121] In most instances, the pathologic findings are nonspecific interstitial fibrosis or cellular hypertrophy. Occasionally, clinically inapparent myocarditis is detected.

MANAGEMENT OF SUDDEN-DEATH SURVIVORS

INITIAL HOSPITAL COURSE

Of patients initially resuscitated and admitted to the hospital, 40% to 60% die prior to discharge.[3,10,30] Recurrent arrhythmias and cardiac arrest are common within the first 24 hours.[4,21] However the vast majority of early deaths are due to shock or the complications of persistent anoxic coma.[3,21] These complications are less frequent when early aggressive resuscitation is initiated at the time of cardiac arrest.[3] Of patients who are unconscious at the time of hospital admission, slightly more than half will ultimately regain consciousness (90% within three days).[122] Unresponsive patients with intact pupillary reflexes and localized motor responses to noxious stimuli at the time of admission are more likely to regain consciousness.[17,122]

Parenteral antiarrhythmic therapy is recommended during the initial several days of stabilization and diagnostic assessment. Administration of lidocaine should be carefully monitored, particularly in patients with severe left ventricular dysfunction, as toxic manifestations may be easily confused with the sequelae of cerebral anoxic injury. In most patients, parenteral therapy can be discontinued after several days to allow baseline assessment of spontaneous and inducible ventricular arrhythmias.

Serial cardiac isoenzymes and electrocardiograms should be obtained in all patients. The diagnosis of acute myocardial infarction remains difficult in the absence of newly evolved Q waves. However, myocardial infarction as the precipitant of cardiac arrest should also be considered in patients with significant elevations of cardiac isoenzymes associated with new and persistent ST segment or ST-T wave abnormalities. Myocardial imaging with technetium pyrophosphate 24 hours to 72 hours after cardiac arrest may be useful in equivocal circumstances,[123] though the technique appears to be less sensitive for the detection of non-Q-wave infarctions.[124] In sudden-death survivors with definite evidence of new myocardial necrosis, subsequent management and prognostic stratification is similar to other patients with myocardial infarction.[125]

Other immediate, precipitating factors should be identified and corrected, including the withdrawal of arrhythmogenic drugs, and the correction of metabolic abnormalities. Medical therapy to relieve symptoms of congestive heart failure and to improve ventricular performance is recommended, although the impact of these measures on longterm survival is unknown. The psychological burden of resuscitation, complex diagnostic and therapeutic interventions, and uncertainty with regard to future functional status is considerable. The recognition and treatment of anxiety, depression, and denial are an integral part of management.[126] The goals of education are to enhance compliance with treatment and to ensure that patients have reasonable expectations with regard to subsequent treatment alternatives and future lifestyle.

DIAGNOSTIC EVALUATION

In sudden-death survivors without definite evidence of new myocardial infarction, cardiac anatomy and the physiologic consequences of structural abnormalities should be defined as completely as possible. The clinical history, physical examination, and electrocardiogram will provide important diagnostic information in many patients. In view of the overwhelming prevalence of coronary artery disease, and the common occurrence of sudden death as the initial clinical presentation, the authors perform cardiac catheterization and coronary arteriography in all patients unless strong contraindications exist. Because of its powerful prognostic utility, an objective measure of left ventricular function should be obtained in all patients; evaluation of symptoms alone frequently underestimates the severity of left ventricular dysfunction. The physiologic significance of fixed angiographic lesions can be evaluated by exercise testing in association with perfusion scintigraphy or radionuclide ventriculography. Symptom-limited maximal exercise testing may be safely undertaken in patients with previous cardiac arrest, and the provocation of sustained arrhythmias is rare.[127] In selected patients, myocardial biopsy may be useful in disclosing myocarditis, particularly in those with unexplained global ventricular dysfunction of recent onset.

ANTIARRHYTHMIC DRUG THERAPY

The major objectives of antiarrhythmic therapy are to reduce symptoms from intermittent arrhythmias and to prevent recurrent cardiac arrest. Antiarrhythmic therapy can modify the chronic electrophysiologic environment of the heart so that rapid repetitive ventricular ectopy and sustained arrhythmias can no longer be maintained. Most commonly used antiarrhythmic agents have multiple effects, reviewed in detail in an earlier chapter. In addition to influencing spontaneous depolarization, conduction, and refractoriness in cardiac tissue, many drugs alter systemic hemodynamics, autonomic function, and myocardial perfusion. These latter effects may also be beneficial in reducing the likelihood of recurrent cardiac arrest.

Empirical antiarrhythmic therapy, administered in variable dosage and without specific therapeutic endpoints, has not altered mortality nor the risk of recurrent cardiac arrest in sudden-death survivors.[32] Attempts to maintain chronic plasma concentrations of quinidine, procainamide, or disopyramide at adequate levels may reduce the risk of recurrent cardiac arrest. Using this method, Myerburg and coworkers reported recurrent cardiac arrest in 15% of 61 sudden-death survivors within two years of hospital discharge; mean plasma drug concentrations tended to be lower at the time of last followup in patients who had recurrent cardiac arrest.[30] However, there is accumulating evidence that the suppression of VT (either spontaneous or induced) as a specific therapeutic endpoint for antiarrhythmic drug trials may be a more effective means of guiding therapy and predicting freedom from recurrent cardiac arrest.

SUPPRESSION OF SPONTANEOUS ARRHYTHMIAS

Complex and frequent ventricular ectopy is ubiquitous in sudden-death survivors. There is no evidence that the suppression of either frequent ectopy or most complex forms is a necessary or sufficient condition for successful antiarrhythmic therapy.[30,128] However, the suppression of spontaneous repetitive complexes and particularly of nonsustained VT may alter the risk of recurrent cardiac arrest. In a series of 123 patients (50% survivors of cardiac arrest), short-term serial drug testing (4 months–5 months after arrhythmia onset) was performed, using suppression of frequent and complex ectopy during ambulatory monitoring and exercise testing as an endpoint for selecting effective therapy.[129] Ninety percent of patients had spontaneous VT (three or more complexes) in the absence of antiarrhythmic therapy. When patients were divided into those in whom runs of VT were completely suppressed and those without suppression, a striking difference in the actuarial incidence of sudden death within one year of discharge was noted (2.3% in suppressed versus 43.6% in nonsuppressed).

In contrast to these findings, Platia and Reid examined the predictive accuracy of predischarge ambulatory monitoring in 44 patients with recurrent VT or VF who were undergoing antiarrhythmic drug testing.[130] Nonsustained VT was suppressed in 34 patients and was not suppressed in 10 patients. Over 12 months to 32 months of followup, 50% of suppressed and 70% of nonsuppressed patients had sustained VT or sudden death. While failure to suppress nonsustained VT on ambulatory monitoring in these high-risk patients is clearly associated with a poor outcome, the predictive value of VT suppression on ambulatory monitoring is less certain. The current practice of the authors is to use ambulatory monitoring as a guide for antiarrhythmic therapy only in patients with frequent episodes of nonsustained VT, or when programmed stimulation cannot be performed. A drug regimen is judged to be effective if nonsustained VT is completely suppressed during at least 48 hours of ambulatory monitoring.

THE ROLE OF PROGRAMMED ELECTRICAL STIMULATION

Programmed electrical stimulation has assumed an increasingly important role in the management of patients with a variety of cardiac arrhythmias and has been discussed in detail in a previous chapter. In this section, attention will be focused on those aspects specifically related to the management of sudden-death survivors.

Ventricular tachyarrhythmias are induced in 60% to 90% of patients with previous out-of-hospital cardiac arrest (Table 56.1).[25-29,131] The determinants of inducible ventricular arrhythmias were examined in 146 sudden-death survivors without acute myocardial infarction who were studied by programmed stimulation at the Massachusetts General Hospital. The stimulation protocol was limited to one or two ventricular extrastimuli and burst ventricular pacing introduced at the right ventricular apex in 92 patients. In 54 patients, more aggressive stimulation was employed, including up to three ventricular extrastimuli introduced from the right ventricular apex, the right ventricular outflow tract, and the left ventricular apex. With limited stimulation, 28% of patients had sustained monomorphic VT, 9% had polymorphic VT degenerating to VF, 36% had nonsustained VT, and 27% had no inducible arrhythmias. With more aggressive stimulation, 45% of patients had sustained monomorphic VT, 20% had polymorphic VT–VF, 26% had nonsustained VT, and only 9% had no inducible arrhythmias. The most powerful independent determinants of the ability to induce sustained arrhythmias were the use of an aggressive stimulation protocol and the degree of ventricular dysfunction (as reflected by left ventricular ejection fraction). The initial cycle length of induced sustained arrhythmias is short (260 ± 31 msec) and cardioversion is required for termination of the sustained arrhythmia in two thirds of patients. Similar characteristics have been reported in other series.[27]

The clinical significance of ventricular arrhythmias induced in survivors of sudden death, particularly nonsustained VT and polymorphic VT degenerating to VF, has been controversial. These arrhythmias (as well as sustained monomorphic VT) may be induced in patients with structural heart disease but without a previous history of cardiac arrest or sustained arrhythmias.[132] Each of these rhythms may also be observed at the onset of cardiac arrest, although in most patients, the morphology of the initiating rhythm will be unknown. The ability to induce ventricular arrhythmias is, in part, related to the chronic structural and electrophysiologic abnormalities commonly observed in sudden-death survivors. These abnormalities (and inducible ventricular arrhythmias) are not specific to survivors of cardiac arrest, nor are they the sole determinants of future sudden death. As reviewed above, the spontaneous initiation of cardiac arrest involves a variety of additional triggers (ischemia, nonhomogeneous adrenergic stimulation, mechanical factors) which may not be reproduced at the time of electrophysiologic study. Despite these considerations, there is evidence that modification of the chronic electrically unstable substrate by pharmacologic therapy or surgery (as reflected by the subsequent inability to induce ventricular arrhythmias) is associated with a reduction in the likelihood of recurrent cardiac arrest.

Of 97 sudden-death survivors who underwent programmed stimulation at the Massachusetts General Hospital, 73 patients had inducible ventricular arrhythmias at baseline study.[29] In 75% of these patients, a drug regimen was identified that completely suppressed the induction of ventricular arrhythmias. Patients discharged on antiarrhythmic agents that completely suppressed inducible ventricular arrhythmias (including nonsustained VT and polymorphic VT degenerating to VF) had a 9% incidence of sudden death over an average followup of 22 months. In contrast, patients discharged on a drug regimen that failed to suppress inducible ventricular arrhythmias had a 36% incidence of recurrent sudden death over a similar followup period.

The value of programmed ventricular stimulation as a method of identifying effective longterm antiarrhythmic therapy in sudden-death survivors has been confirmed by several other investigators (Table

TABLE 56.1 ELECTROPHYSIOLOGIC TESTING IN SUDDEN-DEATH SURVIVORS: OUTCOME OF MEDICAL THERAPY

	Northwestern†	UCSF‡	Indiana§	MGH‖	Penn#	Minnesota**
Patients (n)	44	45	63	97	119	31
IVA (%)	64	76	75	75	61	87
IVA suppressed (%)	18	26	34	75	33	78
Mean followup (mo)	14	20	18	22	17	17
Recurrent SD (IVA suppressed) (%)	0	22	0	9	17	6
Recurrent SD (IVA not suppressed) (%)	78	*	41	36	22	40
Reference	25	27	131	29	26	28

(*IVA*, inducible ventricular arrhythmias; *SD*, sudden death)

* Patients with persistently inducible arrhythmias were treated empirically with amiodarone, and did not undergo repeat electrophysiologic testing.

† Northwestern Memorial Hospital, Northwestern University

‡ Moffit Hospital, University of California at San Francisco

§ Indiana University

‖ Massachusetts General Hospital

University of Pennsylvania

** University of Minnesota

56.1). At Stanford, a series of 239 patients with recurrent VT or cardiac arrest was studied by programmed stimulation. The suppression of inducible ventricular arrhythmias predicted greater longterm survival and freedom from subsequent sudden death.[133] The predictive value of electrophysiologic testing was independent of all other clinical variables, including the type of structural heart disease, and the degree of left ventricular dysfunction.

Failure to induce ventricular arrhythmias in survivors of cardiac arrest has been associated with a variable prognosis (Table 56.2).[26,29,131,134,135] Interpretation of these studies is hampered by nonuniform stimulation protocols (even within the same series), exclusion of patients with nonsustained VT in some but not all series, and variable longterm therapy. In the reports of Morady[134] and Tomaso,[135,136] a large subgroup of patients had normal ventricular function, no remote myocardial infarction, exertion-related cardiac arrest, and provocable ischemia during exercise. These patients were treated with revascularization and/or beta adrenergic blockade. Other patients had cardiac arrest in association with drug therapy or hypokalemia. Thus, in selected patients without inducible ventricular arrhythmias, particularly those with normal ventricular function and a readily identified precipitating cause of cardiac arrest, longterm prognosis appears to be good without specific antiarrhythmic therapy.

The current protocol for programmed ventricular stimulation in survivors of sudden death at the Massachusetts General Hospital involves the introduction of up to three extrastimuli initially from the right ventricular apex. If no sustained ventricular arrhythmias are induced, stimulation is performed at the right ventricular outflow tract, and subsequently at the left ventricular apex. All studies are initially performed in the absence of antiarrhythmic therapy. Sequential drug testing (usually one traditional Type IA drug, one combination of Type IA and IB drugs, and one or more investigational drugs) is performed on subsequent days following oral or intravenous loading. Drug therapy is considered effective if sustained ventricular arrhythmias can no longer be induced from the right ventricular apex and, if initially required to provoke the arrhythmia, from additional ventricular sites. For patients in whom only nonsustained VT can be induced at baseline study, therapeutic endpoints are less certain. In those who are at high risk of recurrent cardiac arrest (depressed ejection fraction, prior infarction), attempts to eliminate inducible nonsustained VT by serial drug testing are undertaken. The purpose of aggressive stimulation is to maximize the exposure of sustained ventricular arrhythmias, so that subsequent drug trials may be undertaken. In patients without previous cardiac arrest, and with a lower risk of subsequent sudden death, such aggressive stimulation may not be appropriate.

While the formal electrophysiologic study of patients with aborted sudden death emphasizes the exposure of ventricular tachyarrhythmias, patients should undergo evaluation of atrial and conduction system function as well. Two subgroups of patients deserve special comment. Intraventricular conduction defects and so-called bifascicular block are common among survivors of cardiac arrest, and are associated with higher subsequent mortality.[4,21] A prolonged HV interval is frequently observed, but unless markedly prolonged (>100 msec), this finding is a poor predictor of future AV block or bradyarrhythmic sudden death.[137,138] An additional predictor of spontaneous AV block in such patients is the development of infranodal block during rapid atrial pacing in the presence of intact AV nodal conduction.[139] The emergence of spontaneous or pacing-induced infranodal block following initiation of antiarrhythmic drug therapy should be managed by permanent pacing if alternative effective antiarrhythmic therapy cannot be found. However, most sudden deaths in patients with bifascicular block are a result of ventricular tachyarrhythmias.[140,141] Incremental atrial pacing is also of value in exposing ventricular pre-excitation in an occasional patient in whom the resting electrocardiogram is nondiagnostic. In patients with ventricular pre-excitation, the antegrade effective refractory period of the accessory pathway should be evaluated using extrastimulus techniques, and the maximum pre-excited ventricular response during induced atrial fibrillation should be determined.

AMIODARONE

Empirical therapy with amiodarone has been widely advocated in the treatment of sudden-death survivors. In four small series of patients resuscitated from cardiac arrest treated with amiodarone, recurrent sudden death occurred in 7% to 12% over followup periods averaging 12 months to 18 months.[142-145] Recently, the efficacy and toxicity of amiodarone was examined in 1307 patients (72% with previous sustained VT or VF).[146] The actuarial incidence of arrhythmia recurrence and death after one year of therapy was 29% and 23%, respectively. After three years of therapy, ventricular arrhythmias recurred in 49% of patients and death in 40% of patients. Adverse drug reactions were common, and required dose reduction or drug discontinuation in 49% of patients. While amiodarone may be effective therapy for many sudden death survivors, significant problems of arrhythmia recurrence and undesirable side effects remain.

Several variables have been examined in an attempt to predict the risk of arrhythmia recurrence in patients treated with amiodarone for recurrent VT or VF. Recurrent sudden death or symptomatic sustained VT is more common in patients with persisting frequent ectopy (>10 complexes/hr) or nonsustained VT on 24-hour ambulatory monitoring after one week to two weeks of therapy,[147,148] although the predictive

TABLE 56.2 ELECTROPHYSIOLOGIC TESTING IN SUDDEN-DEATH SURVIVORS: OUTCOME IN PATIENTS WITHOUT INDUCIBLE ARRHYTHMIAS

	Northwestern*	Moffitt†	Indiana‡	MGH§	Penn‖
Patients (n)	32	19	15	24	47
Diagnosis (% IHD)	50	74	70	76	72
Mean followup (mo)	24	26	18	28	20
Recurrent SD (%)	3	5	14	7	32
Reference	135	134	131	29	26

(*IHD*, ischemic heart disease; *SD*, sudden death)

* Northwestern Memorial Hospital, Northwestern University

† University of California at San Francisco

‡ Indiana University

§ Massachusetts General Hospital

‖ University of Pennsylvania

value of these findings is limited for the individual patient. Left ventricular dysfunction is an independent predictor of arrhythmia recurrence, regardless of the findings during ambulatory monitoring.[148] Finally, recent data suggest that information obtained during electrophysiologic study after one week to two weeks of high dose amiodarone therapy has prognostic significance despite the persistence of inducible arrhythmias in a majority of patients.[149,150] Recurrence of symptomatic VT or sudden death was observed almost exclusively in patients with persistently inducible ventricular arrhythmias. In those in whom the induced tachycardia during therapy was slow and well-tolerated, fatal recurrence was rare; patients with rapid, poorly tolerated induced tachycardias during amiodarone therapy had a high incidence of subsequent sudden death.[149]

NONPHARMACOLOGIC TREATMENT ALTERNATIVES

Map-guided resection or cryoablation of endocardial tissue overlying and adjacent to scarred myocardium is an effective method of reducing arrhythmia recurrences in patients with drug refractory sustained VT.[151] This approach requires extensive multisite recordings of endocardial activation during well-organized and well-tolerated tachycardias. In a majority of sudden-death survivors, the extremely rapid and poorly tolerated tachycardias induced during programmed stimulation preclude this systematic approach. However, nondirected excision of all visible endocardial scar tissue has been successful in the prevention of recurrent sudden death in a series of 22 survivors of out-of-hospital VF, all with rapid, poorly tolerated inducible arrhythmias during programmed stimulation.[152]

The development of the automatic implantable cardioverter/defibrillator (AICD), designed not to prevent arrhythmias but rather to terminate potentially lethal episodes, represents a major advance in the treatment of sudden-death survivors.[153] A detailed discussion of this device is presented in another chapter. Current models require at least one epicardial patch electrode for reliable defibrillation and, thus, cannot be placed transvenously. Many patients require concomitant antiarrhythmic drug therapy to suppress frequent episodes of nonsustained VT or rapid supraventricular rhythms that could lead to inappropriate defibrillator discharge. Experience with the most recent device (AICD–B) suggests an extremely low incidence of death due to recurrent cardiac arrest (2% at one year) in a series of patients with drug refractory ventricular tachyarrhythmias (80% with previous cardiac arrest).[154] With the development of better arrhythmia detection algorithms and endocardial electrodes capable of effective cardioversion and defibrillation, such devices may find an even wider application in the management of sudden-death survivors.

TREATMENT OF ISCHEMIA AND OTHER TRIGGER MECHANISMS

The relative importance of ischemia as a precipitant of cardiac arrest in the absence of definite myocardial infarction is often difficult to determine for an individual patient. The presence of viable but jeopardized myocardium (as indicated by exercise testing or scintigraphic imaging) is helpful in identifying patients in whom intensive efforts to treat ischemia should be made. In those without significant myocardial scar tissue (the usual substrate of recurrent arrhythmias), and particularly in the absence of inducible arrhythmias during programmed stimulation, a primary ischemic event is the likely cause of cardiac arrest. Medical or surgical therapy directed against recurrent ischemia alone may be sufficient to prevent future sudden death. However, in the majority of patients with significant coronary disease, anti-ischemic therapy should be combined with specific antiarrhythmic therapy, even in the absence of a prior history of angina.

The role of coronary revascularization in the prevention of recurrent cardiac arrest merits additional comment. In selected survivors with inducible VT or VF, severe coronary artery disease, and adequate left ventricular function, coronary revascularization alone may render as many as 50% noninducible during postoperative electrophysiologic study; such patients do well without additional antiarrhythmic therapy.[155] In a study of primary prevention in a high-risk group (patients with surgically approachable coronary anatomy enrolled in the Coronary Artery Surgery Study [CASS] registry), medically treated patients had a three-fold higher incidence of sudden death at five years relative to patients who had surgical revascularization.[156] This difference was independent of left ventricular function, the extent of CAD, or the amount of jeopardized myocardium. In a selected group of sudden death survivors undergoing coronary revascularization, recurrent sudden death occurred in 3% at two years, compared with 17% in medically treated survivors matched for age, sex, ejection fraction, complex ectopy on ambulatory monitoring, and histories of remote infarction or angina.[157] Whether surgical revascularization or angioplasty should be undertaken in an individual patient depends upon the presence of appropriate anatomy and ventricular function, prior symptoms, and the amount of residual jeopardized myocardium. It should be noted that survivors of sudden death, even in the absence of previous angina or episodic dyspnea, are not asymptomatic, and thus revascularization should not be excluded on this basis alone.

Beta adrenergic blockade has been established as moderately effective in the primary prevention of sudden death in the initial year or two following myocardial infarction (approximately 30% risk reduction).[158,159] Several mechanisms—direct electrophysiologic effects, reduction of adrenergic stimulation and heart rate, prevention of ischemia, prevention or amelioration of recurrent infarction—may be responsible. Whether anti-adrenergic therapy is equally effective in the secondary prevention of recurrent cardiac arrest remains speculative. It is the authors' practice to administer beta adrenergic antagonists to most sudden-death survivors, provided that at least moderate doses can be tolerated.

GENERAL GUIDELINES FOR THERAPY

The authors' approach to the treatment of sudden-death survivors is outlined below. All patients undergo coronary angiography and left ventriculography. Antiarrhythmic therapy is then discontinued. If frequent, spontaneous, nonsustained VT is subsequently observed, patients undergo serial antiarrhythmic drug trials guided by ambulatory monitoring. In the majority of patients, frequent nonsustained VT is not observed, and programmed ventricular stimulation with serial drug testing is performed. If spontaneous or inducible VT cannot be suppressed by pharmacologic therapy, or if intolerable side effects emerge, patients are considered candidates for an AICD, or in selected cases, endocardial resection. Patients without inducible or spontaneous arrhythmias, but at high risk for recurrent cardiac arrest (depressed ventricular function, absence of treatable precipitating factors) are also considered candidates for an AICD.

In patients with ischemic heart disease, the potential for recurring myocardial ischemia is treated aggressively. Patients with active inflammatory myocarditis are treated with immunosuppressive drugs in addition to antiarrhythmic therapy. When cardiac arrest complicates medically refractory heart failure, cardiac transplantation is considered. In sudden-death survivors with ventricular pre-excitation and atrial fibrillation, serial testing may identify drugs which prevent tachyarrhythmia induction or significantly lengthen the effective refractory period of the accessory pathway. However, pharmacologic therapy is frequently ineffective in this group, and surgical section or cryoablation of the pathway is safe and essentially curative treatment.[160] Finally, in patients with the long QT syndrome, serial drug testing guided by electrophysiologic study is not helpful,[116] and therapy with beta blockers alone or in combination with chronic pacing is recommended.[114]

☐ CONCLUSION

The etiology of out-of-hospital cardiac arrest is multifactorial; the approach to the management of each patient requires a precise knowledge of underlying structural heart disease and an accurate assessment of risk for future recurrence. Ideal therapy would possess minimal toxicity and a high degree of efficacy. Unfortunately, current pharmacologic therapy is frequently ineffective and is often accompanied by significant adverse effects (20% to 30% for most drugs). At the present time, alternative nonpharmacologic treatment is available only at specialized referral centers. Considerable gains have been made in the identification and treatment of high-risk patients; however, methods for determining therapeutic efficacy remain imprecise, costly, and time consuming. While new insights into the mechanism of cardiac arrest and new therapeutic options will undoubtedly modify the future care of patients with aborted sudden death, the present approach remains complex, and must be individualized for each patient.

REFERENCES

1. Jude JR, Kouwenhoven WB, Knickerbocker GG: A new approach to cardiac resuscitation. Ann Surg 154:311, 1961
2. Eisenberg MS, Copass MK, Hallstrom AP et al: Treatment of out-of-hospital cardiac arrest with rapid defibrillation by emergency medical technicians. N Engl J Med 302:1379, 1980
3. Thompson RG, Hallstrom AP, Cobb LA: Bystander-initiated cardiopulmonary resuscitation in the management of ventricular fibrillation. Ann Intern Med 90:737, 1979
4. Liberthson RR, Nagel EL, Hirschman JC, Nussenfeld SR: Prehospital ventricular defibrillation: Prognosis and followup course. N Engl J Med 291:317, 1974
5. Baum RS, Alvarez H, Cobb LA: Survival after resuscitation from out-of-hospital ventricular fibrillation. Circulation 50:1231, 1974
6. Schaffer WA, Cobb LA: Recurrent ventricular fibrillation and modes of death in survivors of out-of-hospital ventricular fibrillation. N Engl J Med 293:259, 1975
7. Liberthson RR, Nagel EL, Hirschman JC et al: Pathophysiologic observations in prehospital ventricular fibrillation and sudden cardiac death. Circulation 49:790, 1974
8. Iseri LT, Humphrey SB, Siner EL: Prehospital brady-asystolic cardiac arrest. Ann Intern Med 88:741, 1978
9. Myerburg RJ, Estes D, Zaman L et al: Outcome of resuscitation from bradyarrhythmic or asystolic prehospital cardiac arrest. J Am Coll Cardiol 4:1118, 1984
10. Goldstein S, Landis JR, Leighton R et al: Characteristics of the resuscitated out-of-hospital cardiac arrest victims with coronary heart disease. Circulation 64:977, 1981
11. Pratt CM, Francis MJ, Luck JC et al: Analysis of ambulatory electrocardiograms in patients during spontaneous ventricular fibrillation. J Am Coll Cardiol 2:789, 1983
12. Panidis IP, Morganroth J: Sudden death in hospitalized patients: Cardiac rhythm disturbances detected by ambulatory electrocardiographic monitoring. J Am Coll Cardiol 2:798, 1983
13. Kempf FG, Josephson ME: Cardiac arrest recorded on ambulatory electrocardiograms. Am J Cardiol 53:1577, 1984
14. Lewis BH, Antman EM, Graboys TB: Detailed analysis of 24 hour ambulatory electrocardiographic recordings during ventricular fibrillation. J Am Coll Cardiol 2:426, 1983
15. Nikolic G, Bishop RL, Singh JB: Sudden death recorded during Holter monitoring. Circulation 66:218, 1982
16. Fellows CL, Weaver WD, Dennis D: Mechanism of refibrillation following successful resuscitation in pre-hospital cardiac arrest (abstr). J Am Coll Cardiol 5:463, 1985
17. Caronna JJ, Finklestein S: Neurologic syndromes after cardiac arrest. Stroke 9:517, 1978
18. McManus BM, Waller BF, Graboys TB et al: Exercise and sudden death. Curr Probl Cardiol 6:10, 1981
19. Weaver WD, Cobb LA, Hallstrom AP: Characteristics of survivors of exertion- and nonexertion-related cardiac arrest: Value of subsequent exercise testing. Am J Cardiol 50:671, 1982
20. Weaver D, Lorch GS, Alvarez HA, Cobb LA: Angiographic findings and prognostic indicators in patients resuscitated from sudden cardiac death. Circulation 54:895, 1976
21. Myerburg RJ, Cone CA, Sung RJ et al: Clinical, electrophysiologic and hemodynamic profile of patients resuscitated from prehospital cardiac arrest. Am J Med 68:568, 1980
22. Tresch DD, Grove R, Siegal R et al: Survivors of prehospitalization sudden death: Characteristic clinical and angiographic features. Arch Intern Med 141:1154, 1981
23. Josephson ME, Horowitz LN, Spielman SR et al: Electrophysiologic and hemodynamic studies in patients resuscitated from cardiac arrest. Am J Cardiol 46:948, 1980
24. Ruskin JN, DiMarco JP, Garan H: Out-of-hospital cardiac arrest: Electrophysiologic observations and selection of long term antiarrhythmic therapy. N Engl J Med 303:607, 1980
25. Kehoe RF, Moran JM, Zheutlin T et al: Electrophysiologic study to direct therapy in survivors of pre-hospital ventricular fibrillation (abstr). Am J Cardiol 49:928, 1982
26. Roy D, Waxman HL, Kienzle MG et al: Clinical characteristic and long-term follow-up in 119 survivors of cardiac arrest: Relation to inducibility at electrophysiologic testing. Am J Cardiol 52:969, 1983
27. Morady F, Scheinman MM, Hess DS et al: Electrophysiologic testing in the management of survivors of out-of-hospital cardiac arrest. Am J Cardiol 51:85, 1983
28. Benditt DG, Benson DW, Klein GJ et al: Prevention of recurrent sudden cardiac arrest: Role of provocative electropharmacologic testing. J Am Coll Cardiol 2:418, 1983
29. Ruskin JN, Garan H: Electrophysiologic observations in survivors of out-of-hospital cardiac arrest. In Lucchesi BR (ed): Clinical Pharmacology of Antiarrhythmic Therapy, p 241. New York, Raven Press, 1984
30. Myerburg RJ, Kessler KM, Estes D et al: Long-term survival after prehospital cardiac arrest: Analysis of outcome during an 8 year study. Circulation 70:538, 1984
31. Reichenbach DD, Moss NS, Meyer E: Pathology of the heart in sudden cardiac death. Am J Cardiol 39:865, 1977
32. Ritchie JL, Hallstrom AP, Troubaugh GB et al: Out-of-hospital sudden coronary death: Rest and exercise radionuclide left ventricular function in survivors. Am J Cardiol 55:645, 1985
33. Eshani A, Ewy GA, Sobel BE: Effects of electrical countershock on serum creatine phosphokinase (CPK) isoenzyme activity. Am J Cardiol 37:12, 1976
34. Bynum WR, Connell RM, Hawk WA: Causes of death after external cardiac massage: Analysis of observations on fifty consecutive autopsies. Cleve Clin Q 30:147, 1963
35. Cobb LA, Werner JA, Trobaugh GB: Sudden cardiac death, II. Outcome or resuscitation, management and future directions. Modern Concepts of Cardiovascular Disease 49:37, 1980
36. Goldberg R, Szklo M, Tonascia J, Kennedy HL: Acute myocardial infarction: prognosis complicated by ventricular fibrillation or cardiac arrest. JAMA 241:2024, 1979
37. Lawrie DM: Long-term survival after ventricular fibrillation complicating acute myocardial infarction. Lancet 2:1085, 1969
38. Weaver WG, Cobb LA, Hallstrom AP: Ambulatory arrhythmias in resuscitated victims of cardiac arrest. Circulation 66:21, 1982
39. Moss AJ, Davis HT, DeCamilla J, Bayer LW: Ventricular ectopic beats and their relation to sudden and nonsudden cardiac death after myocardial infarction. Circulation 60:998, 1979
40. Multicenter Postinfarction Research Group: Risk stratification and survival after myocardial infarction. N Engl J Med 309:331, 1983
41. Bigger JT, Fleiss JL, Kleiger R et al: The relationships among arrhythmias, left ventricular dysfunction and mortality in the 2 years after myocardial infarction. Circulation 69:250, 1984
42. Josephson ME, Buxton AE, Marchlinski FE et al: Sustained ventricular tachycardia in coronary artery disease—evidence for reentrant mechanism. In Zipes DP, Jalife J (ed): Cardiac electrophysiology and arrhythmias, p 409. Orlando, Grune and Stratton, 1985
43. Spear JF, Horowitz LN, Hodess AB et al: Cellular electrophysiology of human myocardial infarction. Circulation 59:247, 1979
44. Gilmour RF, Heger JJ, Prystowsky EN, Zipes DP: Cellular electrophysiologic abnormalities of diseased human ventricular myocardium. Am J Cardiol 51:137, 1983
45. Fenoglio JJ, Pham TD, Harken A et al: Recurrent sustained ventricular tachycardia: Structure and ultrastructure of subendocardial regions in which tachycardia originates. Circulation 68:518, 1983
46. Spach MS, Kootsey JM: The nature of electrical propagation in cardiac muscle. Am J Physiol 244:H3, 1983
47. Pantridge JF, Adgey AJ: Arrhythmias in the first hours of myocardial infarction. Prog Cardiovas Dis 23:265, 1981
48. Wit AL: Electrophysiological mechanisms of ventricular tachycardia caused by myocardial ischemia and infarction in experimental animals. In Josephson ME (ed): Ventricular tachycardia, p 33. Mount Kisco, Futura, 1982
49. Kabell G, Brachmann J, Scherlag BJ et al: Mechanisms of ventricular arrhythmias in multivessel coronary disease: The effects of collateral zone ischemia. Am Heart J 108:447, 1984
50. Schwartz PJ, Billman GE, Stone HL: Autonomic mechanisms in ventricular fibrillation induced by myocardial ischemia during exercise in dogs with healed myocardial infarction. Circulation 69:790, 1984
51. Wilber DJ, Lynch JJ, Montgomery D et al: Postinfarction sudden death: Significance of inducible ventricular tachycardia and infarct size in a conscious canine model. Am Heart J 109:8, 1985
52. Schuster EH, Bulkley BH: Early post-infarction angina. N Engl J Med 305:1101, 1981
53. Theroux P, Waters DD, Halphen C et al: Prognostic value of exercise testing soon after myocardial infarction. N Engl J Med 301:341, 1979
54. Davies MJ, Thomas A: Thrombosis and acute coronary-artery lesions in sudden cardiac ischemic death. N Engl J Med 310:1137, 1984
55. Szlachcic J, Waters DD, Miller D, Theroux P: Ventricular arrhythmias during

56. ergonovine-induced episodes of variant angina. Am Heart J 107:20, 1984
57. Previtali M, Klersy C, Salerno JA et al: Ventricular tachyarrhythmias in Prinzmetal's variant angina: Clinical significance and relation to the degree and time course of ST segment elevation. Am J Cardiol 52:19, 1983
58. Plotnick GD, Fisher ML, Becker LC: Ventricular arrhythmias in patients with rest angina. Am Heart J 105:32, 1985
59. Balke CW, Kaplinsky E, Michelson EL et al: Reperfusion ventricular tachyarrhythmias. Am Heart J 101:449, 1981
60. Miller DD, Waters DD, Szlachcic J, Theroux P: Clinical characteristics associated with sudden death in patients with variant angina. Circulation 66:588, 1982
61. Lloyd EA, Surawicz B: Tachycardia related to electrolyte imbalance. In Surawicz B (ed): Tachycardias, p 407. Boston, Martinus Nijhoff, 1984
62. Hulting J: In-hospital ventricular fibrillation and its relation to serum potassium. Acta Med Scand 206:177, 1979
63. Harrington JT, Isner JM, Kassirer JP: Our national obsession with potassium. Am J Med 73:155, 1982
64. Thompson RG, Cobb LA: Hypokalemia after resuscitation from out-of-hospital ventricular fibrillation. JAMA 248:2860, 1982
65. Smith WM, Gallagher JJ: "Les torsades de pointes": An unusual ventricular arrhythmia. Ann Intern Med 93:578, 1980
66. Velebit V, Podrid P, Lown B et al: Aggravation and provocation of ventricular arrhythmias by antiarrhythmic drugs. Circulation 65:886, 1982
67. Torres V, Flowers D, Somberg JC: The arrhythmogenicity of antiarrhythmic agents. Am Heart J 109:1090, 1985
68. Ruskin JN, McGovern B, Garan H et al: Anitarrhythmic drugs: A possible cause of out-of-hospital cardiac arrest. N Engl J Med 309:1302, 1983
69. Estes NM, Garan H, Ruskin J: Electrophysiologic properties of flecainide acetate. Am J Cardiol (suppl)53:26B, 1984
70. Goldstein RE, Tibbits PA, Oetgen WJ: Proarrhythmic effects of antiarrhythmic drugs. Ann NY Acad Sci 427:94, 1984
71. Kralios FA, Martin L, Burgess MJ, Millar K: Local ventricular repolarization changes due to sympathetic nerve-branch stimulation. Am J Physiol 228:1621, 1975
72. Malliani A, Schwartz PJ, Zanchetti A: Neural mechanisms in life-threatening arrhythmias. Am Heart J 100:705, 1980
73. Barber MJ, Mueller TM, Henry DP et al: Transmural myocardial infarction in the dog produces sympathectomy in noninfarcted myocardium. Circulation 67:787, 1983
74. Haynes RE, Hallstrom AP, Cobb LA: Repolarization abnormalities in survivors of out-of-hospital ventricular fibrillation. Circulation 57:654, 1978
75. Ahnve S, Gilpin E, Madsen EB et al: Prognostic importance of QTc interval at discharge after acute myocardial infarction: A multicenter study of 865 patients. Am Heart J 108:395, 1984
76. Schwartz JF, Wolf S: QT interval prolongation as predictor of sudden death in patients with myocardial infarction. Circulation 57:1074, 1978
77. Lab MJ: Contraction-excitation feedback in myocardium: Physiological basis and clinical relevance. Circ Res 50:757, 1982
78. Oseran DS, Speck SM, Weaver WD et al: Ventricular fibrillation in patients with normal coronary arteries (abstr). Circulation 68(suppl III):107, 1983
79. Rosman H, Golstein S, Acheson A et al: Sudden death in patients without coronary atherosclerosis (abstr). J Am Coll Cardiol 5:443, 1985
80. McKenna W, Deanfield J, Faruqui A et al: Prognosis in hypertrophic cardiomyopathy. Am J Cardiol 47:532, 1981
81. Maron BJ, Savage DD, Wolfson JK, Epstein SE: Prognostic significance of 24-hour ambulatory electrocardiographic monitoring in patients with hypertrophic cardiomyopathy. Am J Cardiol 48:252, 1981
82. Frank S, Braunwald E: Idiopathic hypertrophic subaortic stenosis. Circulation 37:759, 1968
83. Maron BJ, Roberts WC, Epstein SE: Sudden death in hypertrophic cardiomyopathy. Circulation 65:1388, 1982
84. Frank MJ, Abdulla AM, Caneido MI, Saylors RE: Long-term medical management of hypertrophic obstructive cardiomyopathy. Am J Cardiol 42:993, 1978
85. Morrow AG, Koch JP, Maron BJ et al: Left ventricular myotomy and myectomy in patients with obstructive hypertrophic cardiomyopathy and previous cardiac arrest. Am J Cardiol 46:313, 1980
86. Watson RM, Liberati JM, Tucher E et al: Inducible ventricular fibrillation in patients with hypertrophic cardiomyopathy. J Am Coll Cardiol 5:395, 1985
87. Segal JP, Stapleton JF, McClellan JR et al: Idiopathic cardiomyopathy: Clinical features, prognosis and therapy. Curr Probl Cardiol 3:9, 1978
88. Hatle L, Orjavik O, Storstein O: Chronic myocardial disease. Acta Med Scand 199:399, 1976
89. Franciosa JA, Wilen M, Ziesche S, Cohn JN: Survival in men with severe chronic left ventricular failure due to either coronary heart disease or idiopathic dilated cardiomyopathy. Am J Cardiol 51:831, 1983
90. Meinertz T, Hoffman T, Wolfgang K: Significance of ventricular arrhythmias in idiopathic dilated cardiomyopathy. Am J Cardiol 53:902, 1984
91. Wilson JR, Schwarts S, Sutton MS, Ferraro N, Horowitz LN, Josephson ME: Prognosis in severe heart failure: Relations to hemodynamic measurements and ventricular ectopic activity. J Am Coll Cardiol 2:403, 1983
92. Homes J, Spencer HK, Cody RJ, Kligfield P: Arrhythmias in ischemic and nonischemic dilated cardiomyopathy. Am J Cardiol 55:146, 1985
93. Huang SK, Messer JV, Denes P: Significance of ventricular tachycardia in idiopathic dilated cardiomyopathy. Am J Cardiol 51:507, 1983
94. Von Olshausen K, Schafer A, Mehmel HC et al: Ventricular arrhythmias in idiopathic dilated cardiomyopathy. Br Heart J 51:195, 1984
95. Johnson RA, Palacios I: Dilated cardiomyopathies of the adult. N Engl J Med 307:1051, 1982
96. Poll DS, Marchlinski FE, Buxton AE et al: Sustained ventricular tachycardia in patients with idiopathic dilated cardiomyopathy. Circulation 70:451, 1984
97. Cheitlin MD, Byrd RC: Prolapsed mitral valve. Curr Probl Cardiol 8:7, 1984
98. Davies MJ, Moore BP, Baimbridge MV: The floppy mitral valve: Study of incidence, pathology and complications in surgical, necropsy and forensic material. Br Heart J 40:468, 1978
99. Bharati S, Bauernfeind R, Miller LB: Sudden death in three teenagers. J Am Coll Cardiol 1:879, 1983
100. Chesler E, King RA, Edwards JE: The myxomatous mitral valve and sudden death. Circulation 67:632, 1983
101. Jeresaty RM: Sudden death in the mitral valve prolapse-click syndrome. Am J Cardiol 37:317, 1976
102. Pocock WA, Bosman CK, Chesler E et al: Sudden death in primary mitral valve prolapse. Am Heart J 107:378, 1984
103. Hochreiter C, Kramer HM, Kligfield P: Arrhythmias in mitral valve prolapse: Effect of additional mitral regurgitation. J Am Coll Cardiol 1:6, 1983
104. Morady F, Shen E, Bhandari A et al: Programmed ventricular stimulation in mitral valve prolapse. Am J Cardiol 53:135, 1985
105. Klein GJ, Bashore TM, Sellers TD et al: Ventricular fibrillation in the Wolff–Parkinson–White syndrome. N Engl J Med 301:1080, 1979
106. Gulamhusein S, Ko P, Carruthers SG, Klein GJ: Acceleration of the ventricular response during atrial fibrillation in the Wolff–Parkinson–White syndrome after verapamil. Circulation 65:348, 1982
107. Bardy GH, Packer DL, German LD, Gallagher JJ: Utility of electrophysiologic studies in the management of tachycardia, sudden death and syncope. Ann NY Acad Sci 427:16, 1984
108. Wellens HJ, Brugada P, Roy D et al: Effect of isoproterenol on the anterograde refractory period of the accessory pathway in patients with the Wolff–Parkinson–White syndrome. Am J Cardiol 50:180, 1982
109. Garson A, McNamara DG: Sudden death in a pediatric cardiology population: J Am Coll Cardiol 5:134B, 1985
110. Garson A, Nihill MR, McNamara DG: Status of the adult and adolescent after repair of the tetralogy of Fallot. Circulation 59:1232, 1979
111. Fuster V, McGoon DC, Kennedy MA: Long-term evaluation of open heart surgery for tetralogy of Fallot. Am J Cardiol 46:635, 1980
112. Kobayashi J, Hirose H, Nakano S et al: Ambulatory electrocardiographic study of the frequency and cause of ventricular arrhythmias after correction of tetralogy of Fallot. Am J Cardiol 54:1310, 1984
113. Blake RS, Chung EE, Wesley H, Hallidies–Smith KA: Conduction defects, ventricular arrhythmias, and late death after surgical closure of ventricular septal defect. Br Heart J 47:305, 1982
114. Flinn CJ, Wolff GS, Dick M et al: Cardiac rhythm after the Mustard operation for complete transposition of the great arteries. N Engl J Med 310:1635, 1984
115. Schwartz PJ: Idiopathic long QT syndrome: Progress and questions. Am Heart J 109:399, 1985
116. Moss AJ, Schwartz PJ, Cramptom RS et al: The long QT syndrome: A prospective international study. Circulation 71:17, 1985
117. Bhandari AK, Shapiro WA, Morady F et al: Electrophysiologic testing in patients with the long QT syndrome. Circulation 71:63, 1985
118. Shaw TR: Recurrent ventricular fibrillation associated with normal QT intervals. Q J Med 200:451, 1981
119. Von Bernuth G, Bernsau U, Gutheil H et al: Tachyarrhythmic syncopes in children with structurally normal hearts with and without QT prolongation in the electrocardiogram. Eur J Pediatr 138:206, 1982
120. Strain JE, Grose RM, Factor SM, Fisher JD: Results of endomyocardial biopsy in patients with spontaneous ventricular tachycardia but without apparent structural heart disease. Circulation 68:1171, 1983
121. Vignola PA, Kazutaka A, Swayne PS et al: Lymphocytic myocarditis presenting as unexplained ventricular arrhythmias. J Am Coll Cardiol 4:812, 1984
122. Sugrue DD, Holmes DR, Gersh BJ et al: Cardiac histologic findings in patients with life-threatening ventricular arrhythmias of unknown origin. J Am Coll Cardiol 4:952, 1984
123. Longstreth W, Diehr P, Inui T: Prediction of awakening after out-of-hospital cardiac arrest. N Engl J Med 308:1378, 1983
124. Davison R, Spies S, Przybylek J, Hai H, Lesch M: Technetium-99m stannous pyrophosphate myocardial scintigraphy after cardiopulmonary resuscitation with cardioversion. Circulation 60:292, 1979
125. Massie BM, Botvinick EH, Werner JA et al: Myocardial scintigraphy with technetium-99m stannous pyrophosphate: An insensitive test for nontransmural myocardial infarction. Am J Cardiol 43:186, 1979
126. Sniderman A (ed): Symposium on the patient postinfarction: New knowledge and new therapeutic strategies. Am J Cardiol 52:657, 1983
127. Vlay SC, Fricchione GL: Psychosocial aspects of surviving sudden cardiac death. Clin Cardiol 8:237, 1985
128. Young DZ, Lampert S, Graboys TB: Safety of maximal exercise testing in patients at high risk for ventricular arrhythmia. Circulation 70:184, 1984
129. Herling IM, Horowitz LN, Josephson ME: Ventricular ectopic activity after medical and surgical treatment for recurrent sustained ventricular tachy-

129. Graboys TB, Lown B, Podrid PJ, DeSilva R: Long-term survival of patients with malignant ventricular arrhythmia treated with antiarrhythmic drugs. Am J Cardiol 50:437, 1982
130. Platia EV, Reid PR: Comparison of programmed electrical stimulation and ambulatory electrocardiographic monitoring in the management of ventricular tachycardia and ventricular fibrillation. J Am Coll Cardiol 4:493, 1984
131. Skale BT, Miles WM, Heger JJ et al: Survivors of cardiac arrest: Results of management guided by electrophysiologic testing or electrocardiographic monitoring (abstr). Circulation 68(suppl III):244, 1983
132. Brugada P, Waldecker B, Wellens HJ: Characteristics of induced ventricular arrhythmias in four subgroups of patients with myocardial infarction (abstr). Circulation 70(suppl II):29, 1984
133. Swerdlow CD, Winkle RA, Mason JW: Determinants of survival in patients with ventricular tachyarrhythmias. N Engl J Med 308:1436, 1983
134. Morady F, DiCarlo L, Winston S et al: Clinical features and prognosis of patients with out of hospital cardiac arrest and a normal electrophysiologic study. J Am Coll Cardiol 4:39, 1984
135. Zheutlin TE, Steinman R, Summers C et al: Long-term outcome in survivors of cardiac arrest with noninducible ventricular tachycardia during programmed stimulation (abstr). Circulation 70(suppl II):399, 1984
136. Tomaso C, Kehoe R, Koransky A, Meyers S: Clinical, angiographic and electrophysiologic features of sudden death survivors: Differing mechanism of ventricular fibrillation in ischemic heart disease (abstr). Circulation 64(suppl IV):241, 1981
137. Dhingra RC, Palileo E, Straberg B et al: Significance of the HV interval in 517 patients with chronic bifascicular block. Circulation 64:1265, 1981
138. McAnulty JH, Rahimtoola SH, Murphy E et al: Natural history of "high-risk" bundle branch block. N Engl J Med 307:137, 1982
139. Dhingra RC, Wyndham C, Bauerfeind R et al: Significance of block distal to the His bundle induced by atrial pacing in patients with chronic bifascicular block. Circulation 60:1455, 1979
140. Denes P, Dhingra RC, Wu D et al: Sudden death in patients with chronic bifascicular block. Arch Intern Med 137:1005, 1977
141. McAnulty JH, Rahimtoola SH, Murphy ES et al: A prospective study of sudden death in "high-risk" bundle-branch-block. N Engl J Med 299:209, 1978
142. Peter T, Hamer A, Weiss D, Mandel WJ: Prognosis after sudden cardiac death without associated myocardial infarction: One year followup of empiric amiodarone therapy. Am Heart J 107:209, 1984
143. Nadamanee K, Singh BN, Cannon DS et al: Control of sudden recurrent arrhythmic deaths: Role of amiodarone. Am Heart J 106:895, 1983
144. Haffajee CI, Love JC, Alpert JS et al: Efficacy and safety of long-term amiodarone in treatment of cardiac arrhythmias: Dosage experience. Am Heart J 106:935, 1983
145. Morady F, Sauve MJ, Malone P et al: Long-term efficacy and toxicity of high-dose amiodarone therapy for ventricular tachycardia or ventricular fibrillation. Am J Cardiol 52:975, 1983
146. Mason JW: Toxicity of amiodarone (abstr). Circulation (in press)
147. Marchlinski FE, Buxton AE, Flores BT et al: Value of holter monitoring in identifying risk for sustained ventricular arrhythmia recurrence on amiodarone. Am J Cardiol 55:709, 1985
148. DiCarlo LA, Morady F, Sauve MJ et al: Cardiac arrest and sudden death in patients treated with amiodarone for sustained ventricular tachycardia or ventricular fibrillation: Risk stratification based on clinical variables. Am J Cardiol 55:372, 1985
149. Horowitz LN, Greenspan AM, Spielman SR et al: Usefulness of electrophysiologic testing in evaluation of amiodarone therapy for sustained tachyarrhythmias associated with coronary heart disease. Am J Cardiol 55:367, 1985
150. McGovern B, Garan H, Malacoff RF et al: Long-term clinical outcome of ventricular tachycardia or fibrillation treated with amiodarone. Am J Cardiol 53:1558, 1984
151. Josephson ME, Harken AH, Horowitz LN: Long-term results of endocardial resection for sustained ventricular tachycardia. Circulation 64:203, 1981
152. Moran JM, Kehoe RF, Loeb JM et al: Extended endocardial resection for the treatment of ventricular tachycardia and ventricular fibrillation. Ann Thorac Surg 34:538, 1982
153. Mirowski M, Reid PR, Winkle RA et al: Mortality in patients with implanted automatic defibrillators. Ann Intern Med 98:585, 1983
154. Echt DS, Armstrong K, Schmidt P et al: Clinical experience, complications, and survival in 70 patients with the automatic implantable cardioverter/defibrillator. Circulation 71:289, 1985
155. Garan H, Ruskin JN, DiMarco JP et al: Electrophysiologic studies before and after myocardial revascularization in patients with life-threatening ventricular arrhythmias. Am J Cardiol 51:519, 1983
156. Holmes DR, Davis KB, Mock MB et al: The effect of coronary artery surgery on sudden cardiac death: A report from the coronary artery surgery (CASS) registry (abstr). Circulation 70(suppl II):22, 1984
157. Cobb LA, Hallstrom AP, Zia M, Trobaugh GB et al: Influence of coronary revascularization on recurrent sudden cardiac death syndrome (abstr). J Am Coll Cardiol 1:688, 1983
158. Frishman WH, Furberg CD, Friedewald: β-adrenergic blockade for survivors of acute myocardial infarction. N Engl J Med 310:830, 1984
159. Prevention of myocardial reinfarction and of sudden death in survivors of acute myocardial infarction: Role of prophylactic β-adrenoceptor blockade. Am Heart J 107:189, 1984
160. Cox JL: The status of surgery for cardiac arrhythmias. Circulation 71:413, 1985

CARDIOPULMONARY RESUSCITATION

James T. Niemann ▪ J. Michael Criley

Coronary heart disease is the leading cause of death in the industrially developed world[1]; nearly two thirds of patients who die from coronary heart disease do so before they can reach a hospital and benefit from advances in emergency and coronary care.[2,3] In the United States, sudden cardiac death claims about 1200 lives daily, or about one victim every minute of every day. Nearly 25% of sudden death victims are ostensibly healthy and without prior symptoms of heart disease before what is usually an abrupt and terminal event.[1]

There has been a decline in coronary deaths. This decline is due in part to prevention, through risk factor interventions or aggressive treatment of patients considered to be at high risk for sudden cardiac death, and through intervention in the setting of acute myocardial infarction, for example, antiarrhythmia drug therapy and myocardial salvage by pharmacologic therapy or recanalization. A third area has been largely ignored, but could have a substantial impact on the outcome of cardiac arrest due to coronary heart disease, namely, improved basic and advanced life support of the victim of cardiac arrest.

SUDDEN CARDIAC DEATH: PATHOPHYSIOLOGIC CONSIDERATIONS

Sudden cardiac death is most commonly defined as unexpected, nontraumatic death occurring within 1 hour of the onset of symptoms. Among epidemiologic investigators, this definition may vary from instantaneous death to death within 24 hours of the onset of symptoms. Semantic problems notwithstanding, the vast majority of victims of sudden cardiac death have significant coronary atherosclerosis. In autopsy studies of victims of sudden cardiac death, more than 60% of victims have more than 75% stenosis in all three of the major coronary vessels. More than 70% of victims will have at least one artery with 90% obstruction.[4] Fewer than 10% have no significant coronary lesions.[5] A similar distribution of coronary arterial obstructions has been demonstrated in patients successfully resuscitated from prehospital cardiac arrest.[6] In only about 15% of victims of sudden cardiac death is atherosclerotic coronary artery disease not presumed to be the basis of cardiac arrest. In these patients, other etiologies have been established (Table 57.1).

Despite the extent and severity of atherosclerotic coronary artery disease in survivors and nonsurvivors, few victims have demonstrable evidence of acute occlusion or fresh myocardial infarction.[2] Such studies make it clear that sudden cardiac death is not frequently associated with, or the result of, acute myocardial infarction.

THE ARRHYTHMIAS OF SUDDEN CARDIAC DEATH/CARDIAC ARREST

The key element in the majority of victims of sudden cardiac death appears to be an electrophysiologic derangement leading to life-threatening cardiac arrhythmias, the result of underlying coronary artery disease and ischemia. It has been suggested that widespread, significant atherosclerotic stenoses may render the chronically ischemic myocardium susceptible to repetitive ventricular electrical activity.[1] This suggestion has been supported by observations made by advanced prehospital rescuers using electrocardiographic monitoring and telemetric capabilities, and by several cases of sudden death recorded during outpatient ambulatory (Holter) monitoring.[7]

In the vast majority of instances, ventricular fibrillation or ventricular tachycardia is the first arrhythmia observed by paramedical personnel. In selected instances, these rhythm disturbances are usually preceded by high-grade ventricular ectopy as confirmed by ambulatory monitoring of patients who experience cardiac arrest. Most studies of prehospital cardiac arrest have been limited to patients in whom ventricular fibrillation was the initial rhythm disturbance as documented by prehospital rescue personnel. Because of this, the exact prevalence of rhythm disturbances associated with sudden cardiac death cannot be accurately determined. Based upon information from unselected populations, ventricular fibrillation or tachycardia is the mechanism of arrest in 50% to 70% of prehospital sudden cardiac deaths. A bradyarrhythmia or asystole is the first encountered rhythm in 30% to 50% of patients. This wide variation in first encountered rhythms cannot be exclusively explained by differences in advanced medical response times but is an important consideration.

Bradyarrhythmia or asystole may occur as a terminal or agonal event after prolonged ventricular fibrillation or following ventricular tachycardia, or may occur as a primary event. The importance of these slow rhythm disturbances in several settings has received recent attention[8]: (1) based on natural history studies of chronic bifascicular block, complete heart block is seldom the cause of sudden cardiac death; (2) vagotonic bradycardia and hypotension (Bezold-Jarisch reflex) occurs in the setting of inferior wall ischemia and may follow interventional coronary reperfusion; (3) asystole and bradyarrhythmias may precede or lead to cardiac arrest in critically ill patients.

Bradycardia/asystole at the onset of sudden death may be more common than previously expected, based on findings in witnessed and monitored prehospital and hospital cardiac arrests, but is almost universally unresponsive to recommended drug therapy. The clinical settings in which cardiac arrest due to potentially lethal bradyarrhythmias

TABLE 57.1 ETIOLOGIES OF SUDDEN DEATH/CARDIAC ARREST IN ADULTS

Atherosclerotic coronary artery disease
Valvular heart disease
Hypertrophic cardiomyopathy
Drug toxicity
Prolonged QT syndrome
Preexcitation syndromes
Coronary artery spasm
Coronary or pulmonary embolism
Dissecting aortic aneurysm
Complete heart block

or asystole may be encountered are listed in Table 57.2. Bradyarrhythmias and asystole are usually fatal (hospital discharge rate no greater than 3%), due to limited knowledge of their mechanisms and therefore their appropriate treatment. Ventricular fibrillation and ventricular tachycardia are more favorably responsive to emergency management, with a 10% to 30% hospital discharge rate.

CARDIAC ARREST: THE EFFECTIVENESS OF CARDIOPULMONARY RESUSCITATION (CPR)

The introduction of closed-chest "cardiac massage" rapidly followed observations by Kouwenhoven and coworkers.[9] In their pioneering studies on transthoracic electrical countershock of the fibrillating heart, these investigators noted that restoration of spontaneous and effective myocardial contractions was unlikely to follow countershock if ventricular fibrillation lasted for more than a few minutes, limiting the use of the then-promising technique of transthoracic defibrillation. These investigators also noted that arterial pressure rose when firm pressure was applied to the transthoracic defibrillation paddles, and later that rhythmic manual compression of the chest produced arterial pressure pulses and flow. It was believed that thoracic compressions "massaged" or compressed the heart; they found that if this form of artificial circulation during ventricular fibrillation was provided, successful defibrillation and restoration of spontaneous circulation could follow 30-minute periods of ventricular fibrillation.[9] These investigators recognized that combining early artificial circulation and early defibrillation yielded more successful outcomes in arrest due to ventricular fibrillation, now recognized as the most common rhythm disturbance underlying sudden cardiac death.

Although the physiology of blood flow during arrest and rhythmic thoracic compressions had not been well substantiated, this simple technique offered obvious advantages over open-chest cardiac massage. The technique was readily accepted by the medical community worldwide. When later combined with artificial ventilation, basic CPR was developed and was later endorsed by the American Heart Association and the American Red Cross. Lay instruction through community programs soon followed.

A number of recent laboratory studies have demonstrated that CPR, as currently practiced, produces limited systemic perfusion and that blood flow to vital organs may be below that necessary to meet metabolic requirements to sustain life or normal postresuscitation function.[10,11] At the same time, a number of clinical studies have indicated that early application of CPR is life-saving, especially if cardiac arrest is due to ventricular fibrillation.[12] Early CPR may not improve the prehospital resuscitation rate but may lower subsequent hospital mortality, suggesting that a viable level of vital organ perfusion occurs during CPR.

TABLE 57.2 CARDIAC ARREST DUE TO BRADYCARDIA/ASYSTOLE

Inferior MI and bradycardia
Anterior MI and high-degree heart block
MI and asystole
Drug-induced bradycardia or asystole
Cardiac rupture after acute MI
Bradycardia/hypotension-induced VF
Sudden death due to primary asystole/bradycardia

PHYSIOLOGY OF BLOOD FLOW DURING CLOSED-CHEST CPR

When closed-chest "cardiac massage" was introduced in the early 1960s, it was assumed that rhythmic depression of the sternum during cardiac arrest selectively compressed the ventricles against the vertebral column and that perfusion resulted from the simulation of open-chest cardiac massage.[9] This hypothesis had not been tested and was at variance with both the anatomical relationships within the thorax and the observation that sternal depression resulted in pulsations of equal magnitude in arteries and veins. However, these conflicting observations were overlooked because of pragmatic considerations—the clinical effectiveness and avoidance of thoracotomy afforded by external compression. Early hospital experience indicated that closed-chest CPR combined with prompt application of electrical countershock produced at least as good survival statistics (25%) as open-chest massage performed outside of the operating room (17%).[13]

The observation that rhythmic coughing generated pulsatile arterial pressure and systemic perfusion in a group of patients who developed cardiac arrest or bradyarrhythmias during coronary arteriography provided an alternative closed-chest resuscitation method that was not dependent on sternal depression or selective ventricular compression.[14] This observation also led to a reassessment of closed-chest CPR, in which there were many similarities to "cough CPR." When CPR was performed in experimental animals, intrathoracic pressure was found to rise in parallel with intravascular pressure, and improved carotid flow could be achieved when the lungs were inflated (as in coughing) during pressurization of the thorax to increase the magnitude of the pressure. Although equal pressure rises were again observed in the systemic arteries and major veins, the brachiocephalic veins had pressure rises of significantly less magnitude which in turn resulted in a positive arteriovenous gradient across this vascular bed.[15] Cineangiographic studies demonstrated a lack of significant cardiac compression as well as simultaneous opening of both left heart valves during chest compression, with flow through the left heart chambers from the lungs. The pulmonic valve was closed during chest compression. The tricuspid valve was incompetent during compression, as were the mitral and aortic valves between compressions. The site of the pressure drop within the venous system was found to be at the thoracic inlets, where closure of competent venous valves protected the brachiocephalic veins from retrograde surges of blood and high pressure from the thorax during chest compression, and maintained the low pressure necessary for forward flow from arteries to veins in this vascular compartment.[16]

The functional anatomy of the heart during CPR has also been studied by two-dimensional echocardiography in human subjects undergoing CPR, with findings similar to those of the animal studies.[17] These studies confirmed the lack of significant ventricular compression and the simultaneous opening of mitral and aortic valves and closure of the pulmonic valve during chest compression, as well as the incompetence of the cardiac valves that was noted in the animal work.

From these observations has emerged a new concept of blood flow during CPR which is in concert with most of the hemodynamic observations that have been made in animals and in human subjects undergoing CPR. The application of phasic pressure to the thorax, through either sternal depression, cough, or combinations of airway inflation and chest splinting and/or abdominal compression, extends equally to all of the thoracic and abdominal contents. These phasic pressure rises cause blood to move along lines of least resistance. Blood flows through the left heart chambers toward the brachiocephalic vascular bed because of the low-pressure veins therein (a result of the thoracic inlet valves closing). Thus the left heart is a passive conduit during "CPR systole." Closure of the pulmonic valve ensures forward flow from the lungs to the periphery, but incompetence of the tricuspid valve permits reflux from the right heart into the inferior vena cava. The superior vena cava receives little or no reflux because the closure of valves at the thoracic inlets creates a closed compartment.

Between applications of intrathoracic pressure, or during "CPR diastole," there is passive filling of the pulmonary vascular bed through the right heart from the systemic veins—the right heart is also a passive conduit. The mitral valve fails to close during diastole, and the aortic valve is also incompetent, so that some aortic blood refluxes into the left atrium during diastole. Coronary blood flow occurs during diastole, and is dependent on the magnitude of the aortic-right atrial pressure gradient.

There is an ebb and flow phenomenon in the inferior vena cava, with systolic reflux and minimal forward flow during diastole, yielding very little net forward flow from this vascular bed, while perfusion of the brachiocephalic vascular bed is more substantial.[18]

The traditional concept of the mechanism of blood flow during CPR, that is, closure of the atrioventricular valves and opening of the semilunar valves with ventricular stroke volume resulting from cardiac compression, is not supported by hemodynamic, cineangiographic, or echocardiographic observations in animals or man. It is possible that in some instances direct application of pressure or compression of cardiac chambers does occur, and that the intracardiac pressure could exceed the intrathoracic pressure as a result. However, in experimental studies in which cardiac compression is purposely achieved by exaggerated sternal depression, cineangiograms reveal that the left heart "conduit" is distorted and narrowed, and forward flow decreases.[16]

An understanding of the mechanisms responsible for blood flow during artificial support is of critical importance, since there is considerable room for improvement in vital organ flow. This advanced understanding of the mechanism of blood flow during CPR has led to the investigation of a number of experimental modifications of CPR as well as to alternative means of providing circulatory support, but at this time no clinically applicable changes in CPR technique have emerged. It must be appreciated that perturbations of CPR which may appear to be advantageous may be technically cumbersome to perform or may have undesirable side effects. For example, simultaneous ventilation and chest compression will increase aortic pressure and carotid blood flow, but requires endotracheal intubation, modification of resuscitator valves to withstand high airways pressures (60 mm Hg to 100 mm Hg), and the need for synchronization of two different modalities. Abdominal binding during CPR will also increase the aortic pressure and carotid blood flow, but will decrease the coronary perfusion gradient by increasing right atrial pressure. Alternative devices that have shown promise in the experimental laboratory have yet to be extensively tested in man.[19]

PREDICTORS OF CPR SUCCESS IN CARDIAC ARREST

In the setting of prehospital cardiac arrest, the following variables are considered to be important determinants of successful cardiac resuscitation and survival to hospital discharge: (1) witnessed or unwitnessed arrest; (2) initial rhythm encountered; (3) initiation of basic CPR by lay bystanders; (4) level of advanced rescuer response (defibrillation capability); and (5) response time of advanced rescuer care.[20] These predictors have led to the concept of an advanced cardiac life-support score that is largely representative of outcome.

Other important variables have been defined in studies of survival rates in the setting of hospital cardiac arrest.[21] In the hospital setting, the degree of metabolic acidemia during CPR and the duration of arrest have been shown to be inversely related to the likelihood of successful defibrillation. In addition, the outcome of cardiac arrest and CPR in hospitalized patients has identified patient subsets who are unlikely to respond to resuscitative efforts.

In the basic research laboratory, an aortic diastolic pressure (aortic pressure during the CPR relaxation phase) greater than 40 mm Hg, a peak CPR diastolic coronary perfusion gradient (aortic minus right atrial pressure difference) of greater than 16 mm Hg to 20 mm Hg, and a myocardial flow of greater than 20 ml/min/100 g myocardial tissue have been shown to facilitate restoration of spontaneous circulation despite prolonged ventricular fibrillation and artificial circulation (CPR). Peak systolic pressures recorded during CPR chest compression are not predictive of outcome, nor are arterial blood gas values (PaO_2 or pH).[22]

VENTRICULAR DEFIBRILLATION

The history of the clinical use of electrical countershock spans several decades, and a comprehensive review of its contribution to resuscitation is beyond the scope of this chapter. The reader is referred to a recent work by Ewy for a thorough review of defibrillators and defibrillation.[23]

A renewed and growing interest in resuscitation, coupled with bioengineering and biophysical considerations, has resulted in a greater understanding of the use and effect of electrical countershock/defibrillation. The following observations have been well substantiated and are accepted clinical considerations about countershock in treating ventricular fibrillation:

1. Countershock in ventricular fibrillation is most successful when used early after circulatory arrest.
2. Interim CPR applied early may facilitate a favorable outcome when a defibrillator is not immediately available.
3. Ventricular fibrillation is most probably due to multiple reentrant circuits, is self-sustaining, and is dependent upon a critical myocardial mass for perpetuation. Reducing the excitable mass to a value less than the critical mass by countershock should terminate ventricular fibrillation.
4. During transthoracic (closed-chest) countershock, the delivered transmyocardial current is the major determinant of the success of defibrillation.
5. Transthoracic impedance is a major determinant of delivered transmyocardial current, is highly variable (50 ohms to 100 ohms), may decrease after repeated countershocks, and can be decreased with application of electrode pastes, proper electrode position, and proper manual pressure applied to the defibrillation paddles.
6. Body weight in adults is not a major determinant of energy dose required for defibrillation.
7. Electrical countershock may produce myocardial damage, especially if used repeatedly and at high energies (electrical overdose).
8. Drug use, metabolic status, and duration of arrest may affect defibrillation energy threshold and outcome.

At present, the initial use of low-energy countershocks (200 J to 300 J) is recommended. Anteroposterior electrode placement offers no advantage over the conventional sternal-apical placement. Recent work by Kerber and associates suggests that transthoracic impedance can be calculated/predicted and more effective current levels delivered.[24]

DRUG USE DURING ADVANCED CARDIAC LIFE SUPPORT (TABLE 57.3)
EPINEPHRINE

Epinephrine is an endogenous catecholamine with α- and β-adrenergic agonist effects. When epinephrine is administered, β-agonist effects (increase in heart rate, myocardial contractility, and cardiac output) predominate at doses of ≤ 0.1 μg/kg. α-Agonist effects (increase in peripheral arterial vascular resistance and decrease in venous capacitance) are seen in the higher dose range.[25] During cardiac arrest and advanced cardiac life support, both adrenergic agonist effects are expected when epinephrine is administered as an intravenous bolus in the recommended dose (0.5 mg to 1 mg).

On the basis of experimental observations made during cardiac arrest caused by ventricular fibrillation or pulseless bradyarrhythmias (induced by asphyxia), it appears that the α-adrenergic agonist effects of epinephrine are responsible for improved survival.[26] When epinephrine is administered as a bolus during cardiac arrest and CPR, a gradual rise in arterial systolic and diastolic pressures can be seen within 2 to 5 minutes. CPR coronary perfusion pressure (the mean or diastolic aortic minus right atrial pressure difference) also increases and is associated with an increase in myocardial blood flow.[27] Although epinephrine increases right atrial pressure during CPR systole (chest compression), it has little effect on right atrial diastolic pressure (chest relaxation phase). An increase in myocardial perfusion pressure and flow therefore results. Several experimental studies suggest that there is a critical coronary perfusion gradient and level of myocardial blood flow which must be reached to ensure successful resuscitation from prolonged cardiac arrest.[27,28] Prearrest β-adrenergic blockade with propranolol does not significantly alter the hemodynamic effects of epinephrine or resuscitation outcome. Prearrest α-blockade with phenoxybenzamine attenuates the hemodynamic effects of administered epinephrine during CPR and significantly decreases the likelihood of successful resuscitation, that is, restoration of spontaneous circulation.[26]

Whether the β-agonist effects of epinephrine are of particular value in the setting of cardiac arrest and resuscitation has not been established. During ventricular fibrillation, epinephrine may increase the contractile force of the fibrillating myocardium and "convert" electrocardiographic fine ventricular fibrillation to coarse ventricular fibrillation. Although experimentally untested and unproven, anecdotal experience suggests that countershock of coarse ventricular fibrillation is more often successful than countershock of fine ventricular fibrillation. A clinical study indicates that both fine and coarse ventricular fibrillation are equally reponsive to countershock, that is, fibrillation is terminated. However, countershock of fine ventricular fibrillation is more likely to be followed by a nonperfusing rhythm and a high mortality.[29] After prolonged ventricular fibrillation and CPR, epinephrine does not significantly affect defibrillation threshold energy. In the experimental setting of asphyxia-induced cardiac arrest due to bradyarrhythmias, β-agonist effects appear to be of limited importance. In asystole or pulseless bradyarrhythmias following countershock of ventricular fibrillation, epinephrine and methoxamine, a pure α-agonist, appear equally effective in restoring spontaneous circulation.

It has been suggested that the β-agonist actions of epinephrine may, in fact, be detrimental during cardiac arrest and CPR.[30] Administration of epinephrine may increase the oxygen demand of the fibrillating heart beyond the oxygen supply afforded by the observed increase in coronary perfusion pressure. The significance of this observation with respect to resuscitation outcome has not been studied, but in our opinion is not likely to be of independent consequence in an assessment of long-term survival. Epinephrine remains the vasopressor of choice in cardiac arrest due to ventricular fibrillation, a pulseless bradyarrhythmia, or asystole. Although other "pure" α-agonist vasopressors, that is, methoxamine and phenylephrine, may be of equal value in restoration of a spontaneous circulation, they have not been shown to improve long-term survival from prehospital or hospital cardiac arrest in patients or in experimental animals.

ISOPROTERENOL

Isoproterenol hydrochloride is a synthetic, pure β-adrenergic agonist. Any potential value in the setting of cardiac arrest can therefore be ascribed only to its β_1- and β_2-adrenergic effects. Intravenous administration of isoproterenol in the noncardiac arrest setting usually produces an increase in heart rate (chronotropy) and an increase in myocardial contractility (inotropy). If improved cardiac output follows the administration of isoproterenol in the setting of a spontaneous cardiac rhythm, it is usually accompanied by an increase in myocardial oxygen

TABLE 57.3 DRUGS COMMONLY USED IN RESUSCITATION

Drug	How Supplied	Adult Dose	Infusion Rate	Comments
Atropine sulfate	10 ml prefilled syringe; 0.1 mg/ml	0.5 mg–1 mg (5 ml–10 ml); may repeat Q 5 min up to total dose of 2 mg	—	Drug of choice for symptomatic bradycardia
Calcium chloride	10 ml prefilled syringe; 100 mg/ml (10% solution—1.36 mEq Ca^{+2}/100 mg of salt)	500 mg (5 ml); may repeat Q 5 min	—	Do not mix with sodium bicarbonate solutions
Epinephrine hydrochloride	10 ml prefilled syringe (1:10,000 dilution) (0.1 mg/ml)	0.5 mg–1 mg (5 ml–20 ml) may repeat Q 5 min	Mix 1 mg in 250 ml 5% dextrose (4 μg/ml). Titrate rate to BP response	Do not mix with sodium bicarbonate solutions. Endotracheal administration may not be effective during arrest and CPR
Isoproterenol hydrochloride	5 ml prefilled syringe (0.2 mg/ml)	IV bolus not recommended	Mix 1 mg in 250 ml 5% dextrose (4 μg/ml). Titrate rate (2 mg–20 mg/min) to response	Do not mix with sodium bicarbonate solutions
Sodium bicarbonate	50 ml prefilled syringe (7.5% solution) 44.5 mEq/50 ml	0.5 mEq–1 mEq/kg; dose should be guided by pH	—	Complications: hyperosmolality, alkalemia, sodium overload
Bretylium tosylate	10 ml ampule; 50 mg/ml	500 mg (5 ml) as first dose; 1 g (10 ml) as second dose	Mix 500 mg in 500 ml 5% dextrose (1 mg/ml); infuse at 1 mg–2 mg/min	Hypotension may complicate therapy. May be useful in refractory VF
Lidocaine hydrochloride	10 ml prefilled syringe (10 mg/ml)	75 mg–100 mg (7.5 ml–10 ml); may give 50 mg Q 5 min to total dose of 225 mg	Mix 2 g in 500 ml 5% dextrose (4 mg/ml); infuse at 1 mg–4 mg/min	Use lower doses in hypotensive patients; kinetics during arrest and CPR not established

demand. This demand may not be met by improved cardiac output, as coronary perfusion pressure may decrease due to arterial β-adrenergic stimulation and a decrease in diastolic arterial pressure.

Administration of isoproterenol during cardiac arrest and CPR may decrease myocardial perfusion pressure (mean or CPR diastolic aortic minus right atrial pressure difference) and myocardial blood flow due to its peripheral β-mediated adrenergic effects.[31] Isoproterenol has not been shown to be an effective pharmacologic agent in the management of the arrhythmias of sudden cardiac death/cardiac arrest. Widespread use of this pharmacologic agent in the management of cardiac rhythm disturbances following acute myocardial ischemia/infarction and/or cardiac arrest is no longer supported, considering its known effects on the myocardial demand/supply relationship and its demonstrated effects on myocardial and cerebral blood flow during cardiac arrest and CPR.

ATROPINE

Atropine sulfate is a parasympatholytic drug; in animal models and human subjects, its effects are dose dependent. After an effective parasympatholytic dose, atropine enhances sinus node discharge rate and increases atrioventricular conduction velocity. When administered in low, nonparasympatholytic doses, atropine may slow the rate of sinus discharge by a poorly understood mechanism.

Atropine has been shown to be an effective agent in prehospital and hospital management of life-threatening rhythm disturbances that frequently accompany inferior or inferoposterior myocardial ischemia/infarction, that is, sinus bradycardia or second-degree atrioventricular blocks with hypotension/hypoperfusion. Cardiac rhythm and perfusion abnormalities in this setting have been ascribed to cardiac reflex vagotonia (Bezold-Jarisch reflex) or to atrioventricular nodal ischemia, and have also been observed following thrombolytic therapy and reperfusion of the right coronary artery. Bradyarrhythmias or prolonged ventricular asystole may also be encountered during coronary arteriography, and have been ascribed to the calcium-binding properties of radiographic contrast agents.[8] In the clinical settings of inferior or inferoposterior myocardial ischemia/infarction, a vasovagal physiologic response, or bradyarrhythmias/asystole following the intracoronary injection of contrast media, atropine is an effective pharmacologic agent. In the clinical setting of cardiac arrest due to bradycardia/asystole, its utility remains unproven.[8] In prehospital advanced rescuer (paramedic) observations of sudden cardiac death due to bradycardia/asystole, atropine has been shown to be of limited value in restoring circulation. In the hospital and experimental setting, atropine has been shown to be of limited value in cardiac arrest due to bradycardias/asystole or in the management of postcountershock bradycardia/asystole.

CALCIUM CHLORIDE

Transcellular fluxes of calcium ions play a major role in myocardial electrical excitation-contraction and the regulation of vascular smooth muscle tone. These effects make it a logical pharmacologic agent to be used in cardiac arrest, which is characterized by a nonbeating or ineffectively beating heart.

The beneficial effects of physiologic concentrations of calcium on ventricular function have been known since 1882. In experimental animal preparations and *in vitro* studies of the heart, lowering the plasma ionized calcium or decreasing the calcium concentration of the myocardial perfusate has been shown to depress left ventricular function. Restoring calcium concentration to normal increases ventricular pump function. However, increasing calcium concentration from a normal to a supranormal value produces only a small and statistically insignificant improvement in ventricular pump performance.[32]

Calcium chloride had been recommended for the management of several cardiac rhythm disturbances that may be encountered during cardiac arrest and attempted resuscitation. These recommendations are largely based upon a single human study (four pediatric patients who arrested during cardiac surgery and who received multiple drugs) and limited observations in the experimental laboratory without an appropriate control group. Studies now suggest that administered calcium is of limited therapeutic value in the setting of cardiac arrest and advanced cardiac life support. In addition, the role of calcium accumulation in the process of irreversible cellular injury (cell death) has received renewed attention.

In retrospective and prospective studies of prehospital cardiac arrest and advanced cardiac life support by trained advanced rescuers, calcium chloride has not been shown to be of value in the management of patients with asystole or pulseless bradyarrhythmias.[33,34] Calcium administration does not improve the rate of immediate resuscitation or survival to hospital discharge of patients with these rhythm disturbances.

In the laboratory setting, with appropriate controls, calcium chloride has not been shown to be of value in the treatment of pulseless bradyarrhythmias following asphyxia or the management of asystole or bradyarrhythmias following countershock of ventricular fibrillation.[35]

In the population of sudden cardiac death victims, electrolyte abnormalities are an uncommon cause of cardiac arrest. Although plasma total or ionized calcium levels have not been studied in a large representative population of cardiac arrest victims, in our opinion it is unlikely that such values would be low. Limited data in the clinical population suggest that total plasma calcium is normal in cardiac arrest patients and that administration of 500 mg calcium chloride results in hypercalcemia without improved outcome.[36] Such a result could be predicted from laboratory observations. Intracellular calcium accumulation plays a major role in the process of irreversible cellular injury, and it has been suggested that administered calcium and resulting hypercalcemia may accelerate or worsen this potential outcome. This concern is theoretical and not supported by laboratory or clinical investigations.

Calcium administration is now recommended only in patients with cardiac arrest due to hyperkalemia or hypocalcemia. In addition, it may be of value in the management of cardiac arrest patients who are taking calcium channel-blocking agents, since the hemodynamic complications of calcium blockade often respond to calcium administration. The latter instance has not been studied, but is of obvious clinical interest, as patients with atherosclerotic coronary artery disease (those most likely to experience sudden cardiac death) are often treated with calcium-blocking agents.

MANAGEMENT OF COMMON CARDIAC ARREST RHYTHMS IN ADULTS
VENTRICULAR FIBRILLATION (FIG. 57.1)

Ventricular fibrillation (VF) is the first rhythm encountered by rescue personnel in 50% to 70% of victims of prehospital sudden cardiac death and in 30% to 40% of patients who suffer cardiac arrest in hospital.

If cardiac arrest due to VF is witnessed in an adult and a defibrillator is readily available, immediate countershock should be attempted at an energy level of 200 J delivered. If VF persists, a second shock at 200 J to 300 J should be given immediately. If VF persists after the second countershock, a third countershock at 360 J should be given. Chest compressions should be initiated and artificial ventilation with supplemental oxygen begun if VF persists. Epinephrine, 0.5 mg to 1 mg, should be administered intravenously as a bolus. Administration into the central venous circulation may be the preferred route, but the drug will produce its hemodynamic effect if delivered peripherally.[37] Sodium bicarbonate administration is not necessary if the duration of arrest and artificial circulatory support is less than 10 minutes. A sodium bicarbonate dose of 0.5 mEq/kg is recommended at ten-minute intervals during CPR.

Two to three minutes after epinephrine administration, a third countershock of 360 J should be delivered. If VF persists, lidocaine

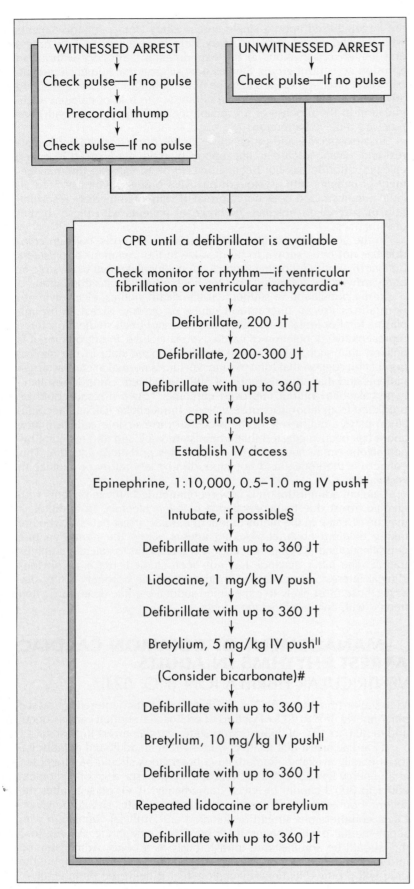

FIGURE 57.1 Ventricular fibrillation (and pulseless ventricular tachycardia). This sequence was developed to assist in teaching how to treat a broad range of patients with ventricular fibrillation (VF) or pulseless ventricular tachycardia (VT). Some patients may require care not specified herein. This algorithm should not be construed as prohibiting such flexibility. Flow of algorithm presumes that VF is continuing.

* Pulseless VT should be treated identically to VF.

† Check pulse and rhythm after each shock. If VF recurs after transiently converting (rather than persists without ever converting), use whatever energy level has previously been successful for defibrillation.

‡ Epinephrine should be repeated every 5 minutes.

§ Intubation is preferable. If it can be accomplished simultaneously with other techniques, then the earlier the better. However, defibrillation and epinephrine are more important initially if the patient can be ventilated without intubation.

∥ Some may prefer repeated doses of lidocaine, which may be given in 0.5-mg/kg boluses every 8 minutes to a total dose of 3 mg/kg.

Value of sodium bicarbonate is questionable during cardiac arrest, and it is not recommended for routine cardiac arrest sequence. Consideration of its use in a dose of 1 mEq/kg is appropriate at this point. Half of original dose may be repeated every 10 minutes if it is used. (Modified from Standards for CPR and ECC. JAMA 255:2947, 1986)

hydrochloride (100 mg) should be given, CPR continued, and repeated countershock with 360 J attempted. Large clinical studies comparing lidocaine and bretylium have failed to demonstrate a clear benefit of one drug over the other in the setting of refractory VF.[38] Between countershocks, arterial blood gases (if available) should be analyzed to assess adequacy of ventilation and oxygenation. Repeated doses of epinephrine (0.5 mg to 1 mg) can be administered at 5-minute intervals in an attempt to maintain an adequate coronary perfusion pressure during CPR.

Mortality increases as the number of required countershocks increases. In many instances, repeated countershocks will often be followed by asystole or pulseless bradyarrhythmia, usually an accelerated ventricular rhythm.

If a perfusing spontaneous supraventricular rhythm follows the first or a subsequent countershock, a lidocaine infusion should be started (2 mg to 4 mg/min), preceded by a lidocaine bolus of 100 mg, if lidocaine was not used between defibrillation attempts. Ventilation, oxygenation, and acid-base status should be assessed with frequent blood gas determinations. Vasopressors may be required following restoration of spontaneous circulation. Dopamine hydrochloride, 5 μg to 15 μg/kg/min, is the drug of choice. Postresuscitative care will frequently necessitate invasive hemodynamic monitoring (flow-directed pulmonary artery catheter) to assess ventricular filling pressure and systemic perfusion.

If cardiac arrest due to VF is unwitnessed or is witnessed but a defibrillator is not immediately available, artificial circulatory and ventilatory support should immediately be initiated and continued until countershock can be applied. After three sequential countershocks at 200 J, 200 J–300 J, and 360 J, epinephrine can be administered as described above, and repeated countershocks should be given. Antiarrhythmia agents (lidocaine then bretylium) should be given if VF is refractory to countershock.

POSTCOUNTERSHOCK ASYSTOLE/BRADYCARDIA

Asystole or a pulseless bradyarrhythmia may follow countershock of VF in 30% to 40% of first or second attempts. This is more likely to occur when countershock of low-amplitude VF (<0.2 mV) is attempted. Such an outcome is usually fatal. Low-amplitude VF is most likely to be encountered in prolonged VF in the absence of early CPR.[29]

The appropriate treatment of postcountershock or "secondary" asystole/bradycardia has not been established. α-Adrenergic agonist therapy combined with continued effective CPR may result in a perfusing spontaneous cardiac rhythm.[31] Immediate artificial cardiac pacing using transvenous endocardial stimulation, or the technique of transcutaneous cardiac pacing, has not been shown to be of value in this setting. In addition, calcium chloride has been shown to be of no value.[35]

PRIMARY BRADY/ASYSTOLIC ARREST (FIG. 57.2)

Asystole or a pulseless bradyarrhythmia is the first encountered rhythm disturbance in 30% to 40% of victims of prehospital cardiac arrest and is noted in a similar proportion of patients who suffer hospital cardiac arrest. In the prehospital setting, the frequency with which asystole is encountered may be related to the response time of advanced rescuers with electrocardiographic monitoring and whether or not early CPR was performed. Primary brady/asystolic cardiac arrest is a true clinical entity; it has been noted during ambulatory electrocardiographic monitoring and is often the arrest rhythm of hospitalized, critically ill patients.[8] Even when primary brady/asystolic arrest is witnessed by paramedics or intensive care unit personnel, current therapy appears ineffective and the mortality rate exceeds 98%. The mechanism(s) for primary brady/asystolic arrest is poorly understood.

CPR should be started immediately. After an intravenous line has been established, epinephrine, 0.5 mg to 1 mg should be given. If a rhythm is not restored or a pulseless bradycardia persists, atropine sulfate, 0.5 mg to 2 mg can be given, or a dopamine or epinephrine infusion may be started. Epinephrine can be infused at a rate of 8 μg/kg/min.

Although isoproterenol is recommended and frequently used in this clinical setting, its benefits are unproven and its selective β-adrenergic agonist effects may, in fact, be detrimental. Peripheral β stimulation will produce a decrease in arterial vascular resistance and tone. In our laboratory experience, isoproterenol decreases CPR diastolic aortic pressure, the coronary perfusion gradient (aortic-right atrial pressure), and myocardial blood flow during resuscitation from postcountershock brady/asystole.[31] In an early study by Redding and Pearson, isoproterenol had no effect on brady/asystole induced by asphyxia.[39] In a later study by Holmes and associates,[40] isoproterenol had no significant effect on regional perfusion during VF and CPR, whereas epinephrine increased myocardial and cerebral perfusion. Although myo-

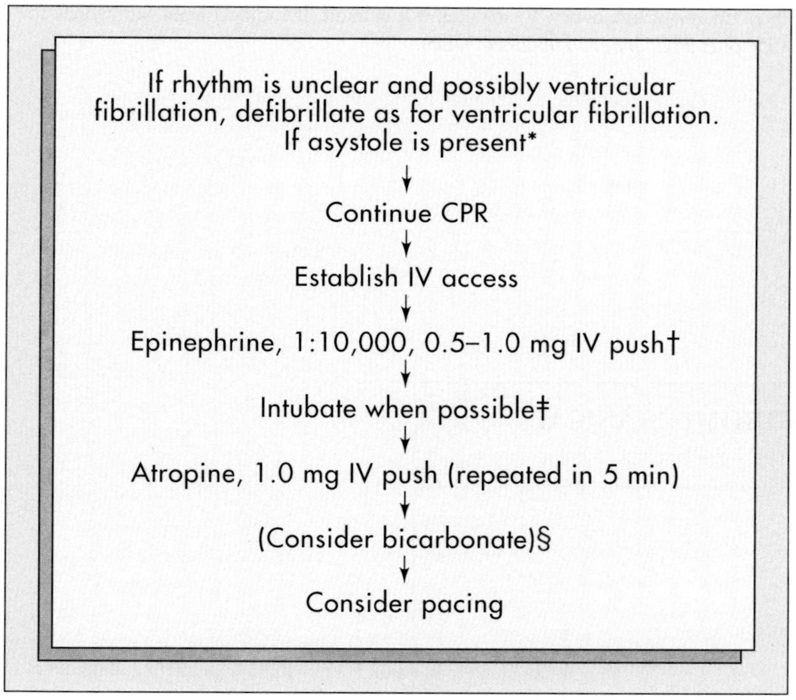

If rhythm is unclear and possibly ventricular fibrillation, defibrillate as for ventricular fibrillation. If asystole is present*
↓
Continue CPR
↓
Establish IV access
↓
Epinephrine, 1:10,000, 0.5–1.0 mg IV push†
↓
Intubate when possible‡
↓
Atropine, 1.0 mg IV push (repeated in 5 min)
↓
(Consider bicarbonate)§
↓
Consider pacing

FIGURE 57.2 Asystole (cardiac standstill). This sequence was developed to assist in teaching how to treat a broad range of patients with asystole. Some patients may require care not specified herein. This algorithm should not be construed to prohibit such flexibility. Flow of algorithm presumes asystole is continuing. VF indicates ventricular fibrillation.

* Asystole should be confirmed in two leads.

† Epinephrine should be repeated every 5 minutes.

‡ Intubation is preferable; if it can be accomplished simultaneously with other techniques, then the earlier the better. However, CPR and use of epinephrine are more important initially if patient can be ventilated without intubation. (Endotracheal epinephrine may be used.)

§ Value of sodium bicarbonate is questionable during cardiac arrest, and it is not recommended for the routine cardiac arrest sequence. Consideration of its use in a dose of 1 mEq/kg is appropriate at this point. Half of original dose may be repeated every 10 minutes if it is used. (Modified from Standards for CPR and ECC. JAMA 255:2947, 1986)

cardial β-adrenergic agonist effects are theoretically beneficial in this setting, peripheral effects may offset such benefits by reducing vital organ perfusion.

Temporary artificial cardiac pacing in the setting of primary or postcountershock brady asystole is of limited value. Use of endocardial, percutaneous transthoracic, or cutaneous electrodes for pacing has resulted in few long-term survivals.[41] Percutaneous transthoracic pacing, in which a needle is used to insert an electrode into the cavity of the right ventricle, can result in myocardial or coronary artery lacerations with tamponade.

ELECTROMECHANICAL DISSOCIATION (EMD) (FIG. 57.3)

By definition, EMD is characterized by electrocardiographic evidence of organized cardiac electrical activity not associated with arterial pressure fluctuations, that is, absence of effective ventricular contractile function. Such a definition most appropriately applies to a supraventricular rhythm with narrow QRS complexes; the most common etiologies are listed in Table 57.4. Pulseless, wide complex bradyarrhythmias encountered during cardiac arrest may be mechanistically different and are unlikely to respond to conventional pharmacologic treatment.

When a supraventricular rhythm with narrow QRS complexes not associated with arterial pressure fluctuations is encountered, CPR should be initiated, and a volume challenge with an intravenous crystalloid or colloid solution should be given. If EMD is due to relative or absolute intravascular volume depletion, such a fluid challenge may have beneficial results. If a fluid challenge fails to produce arterial pressure fluctuations, infusion of epinephrine or dopamine should then be considered. Although pericardial tamponade is a well-recognized cause of EMD and is treatable by pericardiocentesis, it is an infrequent cause of prehospital sudden cardiac death. It is more likely to occur in patients at risk, that is, patients with recent myocardial infarction in the intensive care unit, patients with known malignancy, patients on chronic hemodialysis, or patients subjected to a recent invasive hemodynamic insult (such as pacemaker wire insertion, or left or right heart catheterization). In such clinical settings, pericardiocentesis should be attempted early during resuscitative efforts and preferably under electrocardiographic guidance.

THE POSTRESUSCITATION SYNDROME

About 50% of patients who suffer a prehospital or hospital cardiac arrest will be resuscitated, that is, spontaneous circulation will be restored. Many of these patients will die hours to days later due to anoxic encephalopathy, cardiogenic shock, or intractable cardiac rhythm disturbances. These complications may be related to postreperfusion tissue injury.

Postreperfusion neuronal injury after restoration of circulation has been demonstrated in animal models.[42] After return of spontaneous circulation, there is a brief period of hyperemic cerebral flow, followed soon after by a gradual decrease in perfusion to nearly zero within 3 to 4 hours. This no-reflow phenomenon has been ascribed to calcium influx and increased cerebrovascular resistance. Experimentally, early use of calcium-blocking agents has been shown to alleviate postreperfusion neuronal injury. Decompartmentalization of cellular iron stores may also play a role in postreperfusion neuronal injury, and iron-chelating agents (desferroxamine) have also been shown to attenuate neuronal injury after restoration of circulation.[43]

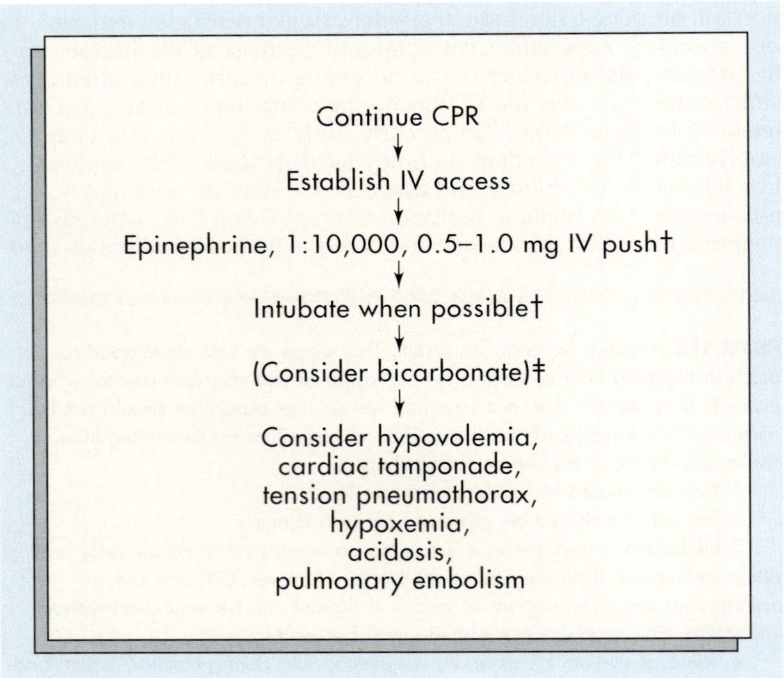

Continue CPR
↓
Establish IV access
↓
Epinephrine, 1:10,000, 0.5–1.0 mg IV push†
↓
Intubate when possible†
↓
(Consider bicarbonate)‡
↓
Consider hypovolemia,
cardiac tamponade,
tension pneumothorax,
hypoxemia,
acidosis,
pulmonary embolism

FIGURE 57.3 Electromechanical dissociation. This sequence was developed to assist in teaching how to treat a broad range of patients with electromechanical dissociation. Some patients may require care not specified herein. This algorithm should not be construed to prohibit such flexibility. Flow of algorithm presumes that electromechanical dissociation is continuing.

* Epinephrine should be repeated every 5 minutes.

† Intubation is preferable. If it can be accomplished simultaneously with other techniques, then the earlier the better. However, epinephrine is more important initially if the patient can be ventilated without intubation.

‡ Value of sodium bicarbonate is questionable during cardiac arrest, and it is not recommended for routine cardiac arrest sequence. Consideration of its use in a dose of 1 mEq/kg is appropriate at this point. Half of original dose may be repeated every 10 minutes if it is used. (Modified from Standards for CPR and ECC. JAMA 255:2947, 1986)

TABLE 57.4 CAUSES OF ELECTROMECHANICAL DISSOCIATION

Hypovolemia
Cardiac tamponade
Massive pulmonary embolism
Tension pneumothorax
Severe myocardial contractile dysfunction

A no-reflow phenomenon has also been demonstrated following regional myocardial ischemia, and has been ascribed to microvascular injury or white cell capillary occlusion.[44] A similar phenomenon may follow resuscitation from global myocardial ischemia and may account for worsening cardiac function and cardiogenic shock. Postreperfusion injury of the heart subjected to normothermic global ischemia and subsequently "resuscitated" has not been well studied, but is very likely, based on regional myocardial ischemia models.

Similar postreperfusion injury might also be encountered in other vascular beds and lead to multiorgan failure following resuscitation. A "postresuscitation syndrome" may limit successful CPR outcome and is being actively investigated.

OPEN-CHEST CPR

Available data in the clinical population suggest that early use of open-chest CPR and defibrillation in the hospital setting of cardiac arrest due to ventricular fibrillation result in a resuscitation rate equal to that of early closed-chest CPR and defibrillation in the prehospital setting.[12,13] Early use of either technique may result in a favorable outcome.

There are no data to support the use of open-chest CPR after an unfavorable outcome using closed-chest CPR in a clinically relevant model. Although open-chest CPR may produce better regional perfusion during prolonged cardiac arrest due to ventricular fibrillation, there are no data to support its use after failure of closed-chest CPR and transthoracic defibrillation.

Open-chest CPR is recommended in the following clinical situations:[45] (1) cardiac arrest during thoracotomy, (2) suspected intrathoracic trauma, (3) suspected massive pulmonary embolism, (4) cardiac arrest due to hypothermia, and (5) absence of large artery pressure fluctuation during closed-chest CPR. In the latter three instances, open-chest CPR has not been shown to be effective in large clinical series.

REFERENCES

1. Lown B: Sudden cardiac death: The major challenge confronting contemporary cardiology. Am J Cardiol 43:313, 1979
2. Guerci A: Sudden death. West J Med 133:313, 1980
3. Kuller L, Lilienfeld A, Fisher R: Epidemiological study of sudden and unexpected deaths due to arteriosclerotic heart disease. Circulation 34:1056, 1966
4. Perper JA, Kuller LH, Cooper M: Arteriosclerosis of coronary arteries in sudden, unexpected deaths. Circulation (Suppl III) 52:27, 1975
5. Reichenbach D, Moss N, Meyer E: Pathology of the heart in sudden cardiac death. Am J Cardiol 39:865, 1977
6. Weaver WD, Lorch GS, Alarez HA et al: Angiographic findings and prognostic indicators in patients resuscitated from sudden cardiac death. Circulation 54:895, 1976
7. Nikolic G, Bishop RL, Singh JB: Sudden death recorded during Holter monitoring. Circulation 66:218, 1982
8. Greenberg HM: Bradycardia at onset of sudden death: Potential mechanisms. Ann N Y Acad Sci 427:241, 1984
9. Kouwenhoven WB, Jude JR, Knickerbocker GG: Closed-chest cardiac massage. JAMA 173:1064, 1960
10. Criley JM, Niemann JT, Rosborough JP: Cardiopulmonary resuscitation research 1960-1984: Discoveries and advances. Ann Emerg Med 13:756, 1984
11. Niemann JT: Differences in cerebral and myocardial perfusion during closed-chest resuscitation. Ann Emerg Med 13:849, 1984
12. Cummins RO, Eisenberg MS: Prehospital cardiopulmonary resuscitation: Is it effective? JAMA 253:2408, 1985
13. Stephenson HE, Reid LC, Hinton JW: Some common denominators in 1200 cases of cardiac arrest. Ann Surg 137:731, 1953
14. Criley JM, Blausfuss AH, Kissel GL: Cough-induced cardiac compression. JAMA 236:1246, 1976
15. Rudikoff MT, Maughan WL, Effron M et al: Mechanisms of blood flow during cardiopulmonary resuscitation. Circulation 61:345, 1980
16. Niemann JT, Rosborough JP, Hausknecht M et al: Pressure-synchronized cineangiography during experimental cardiopulmonary resuscitation. Circulation 64:985, 1981
17. Werner JA, Greene HL, Janko CL et al: Visualization of cardiac valve motion in man during external chest compression using two-dimensional echocardiography. Implications regarding the mechanism of flow. Circulation 63:1417, 1981
18. Niemann JT, Rosborough JP, Ung S et al: Hemodynamic effects of continuous abdominal binding during cardiac arrest and resuscitation. Am J Cardiol 53:269, 1984
19. Niemann JT, Rosborough JP, Niskanen RA et al: Mechanical "cough" cardiopulmonary resuscitation during cardiac arrest in dogs. Am J Cardiol 55:199, 1985
20. Eisenberg MS, Bergner L, Hearne T: Out-of-hospital cardiac arrest: A review of major studies and a proposed uniform reporting system. Am J Public Health 70:236, 1980
21. Bedell SE, Delbanco TL, Cook F et al: Survival after cardiopulmonary resuscitation in the hospital. N Engl J Med 309:569, 1983
22. Niemann JT, Criley JM, Niskanen RA et al: Predictive indices of successful resuscitation after prolonged arrest and experimental cardiopulmonary resuscitation. Ann Emerg Med 14:521, 1985
23. Ewy GA: Cardiac arrest and resuscitation: Defibrillators and defibrillation. Curr Prob Cardiol 11:8, 1978
24. Kerber RE, Kouba C, Martins J et al: Advance prediction of transthoracic impedance in human defibrillation and cardioversion: Importance of impedance in determining the success of low-energy shocks. Circulation 70:303, 1984
25. Weiner N: Norepinephrine, epinephrine, and the sympathomimetic amines. In Gilman A, Goodman LS, Gilman A (eds): The Pharmacologic Basis of Therapeutics, pp 144–151. New York, Macmillan, 1980
26. Yakaitas RW, Otto CW, Blitt CD: Relative importance of alpha and beta adrenergic receptors during resuscitation. Crit Care Med 7:293, 1979
27. Michael JR, Guerci AD, Koehler RC et al: Mechanisms by which epinephrine augments cerebral and myocardial perfusion during cardiopulmonary resuscitation in dogs. Circulation 69:822, 1984
28. Ralston SH, Voorhees WD, Babbs CF: Intrapulmonary epinephrine during prolonged cardiopulmonary resuscitation: Improved regional blood flow and resuscitation in dogs. Ann Emerg Med 13:79, 1984
29. Weaver WD, Cobb LA, Dennis D et al: Amplitude of ventricular fibrillation waveform and outcome after cardiac arrest. Ann Int Med 102:53, 1985
30. Otto CW, Yakaitas RW: The role of epinephrine in CPR: A reappraisal. Ann Emerg Med 13:840, 1984
31. Haynes K, Niemann JT, Garner D et al: Postcountershock asystole and pulseless bradyarrhythmias: Response to CPR, adrenergic agonists, and glucagon, a non-adrenergic stimulator of adenyl cyclase. Ann Emerg Med 14:496, 1985
32. Drop LJ, Geffin GA, O'Keefe DD et al: Relation between ionized calcium concentration and ventricular pump performance in the dog under hemodynamically controlled conditions. Am J Cardiol 47:1041, 1981
33. Stueven HA, Thompson BM, Aprahamian C et al: Calcium chloride: Reassessment of use in asystole. Ann Emerg Med 13:820, 1984
34. Harrison EE, Amey BD: Use of calcium in electromechanical dissociation. Ann Emerg Med 13:844, 1984
35. Niemann JT, Adomian GE, Garner D et al: Endocardial and transcutaneous cardiac pacing, calcium chloride, and epinephrine in postcountershock asystole and pulseless bradyarrhythmias. Crit Care Med 13:699, 1985
36. Dembo DH: Calcium in advanced life support. Crit Care Med 9:358, 1981
37. Doan LA: Peripheral versus central venous delivery of medications during CPR. Ann Emerg Med 13:784, 1984
38. Haynes RE, Chin T, Copass M et al: Comparison of bretylium tosylate and lidocaine in the management of out of hospital ventricular fibrillation: A randomized clinical trial. Am J Cardiol 48:353, 1981
39. Redding JS, Pearson JW: Evaluation of drugs for cardiac resuscitation. Anesthesiology 24:203, 1963
40. Holmes HR, Babbs CF, Voorhees WD et al: Influence of adrenergic drugs upon vital organ perfusion during CPR. Crit Care Med 8:137, 1980
41. Hedges JR, Syverud SA, Dalsey WC: Developments in transcutaneous and transthoracic pacing during bradyasystolic arrest. Ann Emerg Med 13:822, 1984
42. White BC, Wiegenstein JG, Winegar CD: Brain ischemic anoxia. Mechanisms of injury. JAMA 251:1586, 1984
43. White BC, Aust SD, Arfors KE et al: Brain injury by ischemic anoxia: Hypothesis extension—a tale of two ions? Ann Emerg Med 13:862, 1984
44. Kloner RA, Ganote CE, Jennings RB: The "no-reflow" phenomenon after temporary coronary occlusion in the dog. J Clin Invest 54:1496, 1974
45. Safar P: Cardiopulmonary cerebral resuscitation: A manual for physicians and paramedical instructors, p. 172. World Federation of Societies of Anesthesiologists. Philadelphia, WB Saunders, 1981

Supported in part by AHA Investigative Group Award #421G11 and a grant from Physio-Control Corporation, Redmond, Washington

CONGENITAL AND ACQUIRED LONG QT SYNDROMES

Anil K. Bhandari • Phuc Tito Nguyen
Melvin M. Scheinman

The association of prolongation of the QT interval with recurrent attacks of syncope, sudden death, and malignant ventricular arrhythmias is known as the *long QT syndrome* (LQTS).[1-8] The syndrome may be congenital with or without heritable features, or acquired secondary to drug use, electrolyte imbalance, metabolic disorders, or central nervous system lesions. In patients with either form of the syndrome, there is an increased vulnerability of the myocardium to ventricular tachyarrhythmias, often of a peculiar variety known as *torsade de pointes*. This tachycardia is characterized by cyclic changes in the amplitude and polarity of QRS complexes such that their peaks appear to be twisting around an imaginary isoelectric baseline (Fig. 58.1). Most paroxysms of torsade de pointes resolve spontaneously, but some may degenerate to ventricular fibrillation. At times, episodes of monomorphic ventricular tachycardia (VT) may also alternate with torsade de pointes.

During the past two decades the syndrome has received considerable attention from the medical community, and significant new information has been accumulated regarding the natural history, clinical presentation, and prognostic features of the syndrome. The object of this chapter is to summarize and update current knowledge of the syndrome, and to critically examine some of the recent experimental and clinical observation on the syndrome.

NORMAL QT INTERVAL

The QT interval is an electrocardiographic measurement of the period between the earliest ventricular activation and the completion of ventricular recovery.[5,9] At the cellular level, it parallels the duration of the ventricular action potential. Although the QT interval is generally considered a reflection of the ventricular repolarization, the measurement of the interval also includes the ventricular depolarization phase (the QRS duration) and, therefore, is altered by conditions affecting the ventricular depolarization. A better index of ventricular repolarization may be the JT interval obtained by subtracting QRS duration from the QT interval. However, this index has only rarely been used and its superiority over the QT interval remains to be determined.

The QT interval is measured from the earliest onset of ventricular activation inscribed on the surface electrocardiogram (ECG) leads to the terminal inscription of the T wave. Accurate measurement of the QT interval requires several simultaneously recorded limb and precordial leads. There are potential sources of error in the measurement of the QT interval. Determination of the end of the T wave may be difficult to accomplish because of a gradual slope of the terminal portion of the T wave, or when a prominent or a bizarrely shaped U wave appears to fuse with the preceding T wave. At times, conditions causing prominent U waves are also associated with a prolongation of the QT interval, and the interval is then best referred to as the QT-U interval.

Heart rate is a major determinant of the duration of the QT interval; it shortens with increasing heart rate and lengthens with decreasing heart rate.[10-12] However, adjustment to a change in heart rate is not instantaneous, and a steady-state QT measurement is obtained only after the rhythm remains regular for several cycles. Many formulas have been proposed to correct the QT interval for heart rate such as square root, cube root, logarithmic, exponential, or linear formulas.[9] However, none is completely satisfactory for a wide range of heart rates. Of these, the most widely used is Bazett's formula, in which the corrected QT (QT_c) is obtained by dividing the measured QT interval by the square root of the preceding R-R interval in seconds. The upper limit of normal for QT_c in both sexes has been arbitrarily considered as 440 msec. The measured QT interval may also be compared against Simonson's age- and rate-adjusted normal range of values of the QT interval.[9]

The QT interval is also significantly influenced by variations in autonomic tone. Augmentation of adrenergic activity with exercise or inhibition of cholinergic tone by atropine shortens the QT interval independent of changes in the heart rate.[12,13]

ETIOLOGY OF LQTS

The syndrome can be broadly categorized into a congenital or an acquired form (Table 58.1). The congenital syndrome may be genetically determined or may occur sporadically. The acquired syndrome is far more common than the congenital syndrome. The distinction between the congenital and the acquired syndrome is of clinical and therapeutic significance. In the congenital syndrome, ventricular arrhythmias are often precipitated by sudden changes in sympathetic activity and are generally suppressed by β-adrenergic blockers. On the other hand, in patients with acquired LQTS, isoproterenol infusion generally suppresses the malignant ventricular arrhythmia, and the β-adrenergic blockers may potentially exacerbate arrhythmias. However, it must be appreciated that exceptions to each of the above generalizations have been reported and the separation of the two forms may not always be clearcut.

CONGENITAL SYNDROME

The congenital syndrome was first described in 1957 by Jervell and Lange-Nielsen in a Norwegian family in which four of six siblings had congenital deafness, marked prolongation of the QT interval, and multiple syncopal attacks induced by exercise or emotion.[14] Three of the four affected siblings died suddenly at ages 4, 5, and 9 years. A similar syndrome but without deafness was reported by Romano and coworkers in 1963[15] and by Ward in 1964.[16] Both investigators documented transient ventricular arrhythmias as the mechanism of syncope. Since then, numerous case reports have appeared in the literature,[17-23] but much has been learned about this syndrome by the experience (in over 300 patients) provided by the worldwide prospective registry started in 1979 by Moss, Schwartz, and Crampton.[4,7,8]

The congenital syndrome is an uncommon syndrome, which may occur with or without deafness. The syndrome with deafness (Jervell and Lange-Nielsen syndrome) is inherited through an autosomal recessive mechanism; the auditory and cardiac defects are probably pleiotropic manifestations of the same abnormal gene in its homozygous form.[20,21] Patients heterozygous for this gene may be completely normal or may have only borderline QT prolongation. A high incidence of consanguinity has been reported in patients with Jervell and Lange-

Nielsen syndrome. The mode of transmission in the inherited syndrome without deafness (Romano-Ward syndrome) is autosomal dominant with good penetrance of the gene. A recent report by Itoh and co-workers has suggested a close linkage of this dominant gene with HLA locus.[22] They performed HLA typing in 16 members of a family with Romano-Ward syndrome; all 10 affected persons with Romano-Ward syndrome had the same haplotype (A9-BW54), whereas none of the six unaffected ones had this haplotype. At times, significant overlap may exist in the mode of inheritance, and patients in the same family may have this syndrome with or without congenital deafness.[23]

CLINICAL PRESENTATION

The natural history of the syndrome is extremely variable.[1] Patients may be entirely asymptomatic with the only abnormality being prolongation of the QT interval. Typically, the patient presents in early childhood or adulthood with recurrent attacks of presyncope and syncope due to torsade de pointes (Fig. 58.2). Symptoms may appear as early as the first month of life or well into adulthood. The late development of syncope appears to be more common in sporadic forms of the syndrome. The symptoms are stated to be provoked during periods of sudden surges in sympathetic activity induced by emotional or physical stress. In the prospective worldwide study, 58% of the patients had at least one of their syncopal episodes with acute emotional or physical stress.[24] Most of the patients experience multiple syncopal attacks, and sudden death is common. In one retrospective analysis, the mortality was reported to be as high as 78% (73 of 94 patients) in untreated symptomatic patients with congenital LQTS.[4] The risk for sudden death appears to be increased in patients who have congenital deafness, history of syncope, family history of sudden death, and documented malignant ventricular arrhythmias. The degree of QT prolongation was not associated with increased mortality risk in the prospective worldwide study.[24]

Some patients with congenital LQTS may have a low resting heart rate, sinus pauses, and impaired chronotropic response to exercise.[4,8] Isolated case reports have also described atrioventricular (AV) dissociation and high-grade AV block.[25,26] We recently had the opportunity of observing 2:1 AV block during treadmill exercise in a 9-year-old boy with congenital LQTS (Fig. 58.3). The level of block was shown to be infrahisian during subsequent electrophysiologic testing. The significance of these unusual conduction abnormalities in congenital LQTS is not known.

DIAGNOSIS

Most of the patients with congenital LQTS demonstrate obvious QT prolongation unrelated to any secondary abnormality, and establishment of a correct diagnosis is relatively simple. Most patients also have abnormal T waves (bifid, notched, or biphasic) and may have T wave alternans prior to episodes of torsade de pointes. The degree of QT prolongation can vary from day to day, and it must be appreciated that approximately one third of these patients will have ECGs showing a normal QT interval but may demonstrate marked QT prolongation just prior to syncopal attacks or during emotional stress (Fig. 58.4).[8,27] These cases are more difficult to diagnose. On occasion, the diagnosis may be made with provocative tests; for example, valsalva maneuver, treadmill testing, sudden startling noise, or infusion of catecholamines.[8,28,29,30] These tests increase sympathetic activity, reflexly or directly, thereby resulting in abnormal QT prolongation with or without T wave changes. In our experience such tests have seldom proved of value in documenting the diagnosis.

PATHOGENESIS

The fundamental pathogenetic mechanism of the syndrome remains undefined. In a detailed autopsy study of eight deaths associated with this syndrome, James and co-workers[31] failed to find any significant anatomical evidence of organic heart disease; the single consistent abnormality was focal neuritis and neural degeneration within the sinus node, A-V node, His bundle, and ventricular myocardium. Djonlagic and co-workers[32] reported two patients with LQTS in whom round cell ganglionitis was found in both stellate ganglia. The exact prevalence and significance of these neuropathologic lesions are not known.

Yanowitz and co-workers[33] in 1966 demonstrated that right stellate

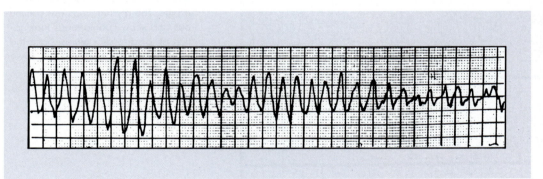

FIGURE 58.1 Rhythm strip showing torsade de pointes in a patient receiving quinidine. Phasic variation in the peaks of the QRS complexes around the baseline is evident.

TABLE 58.1 ETIOLOGY OF LONG QT SYNDROMES

Congenital Syndrome	Acquired Syndrome	
Inherited forms	Drugs	Metabolic abnormalities
Jervell and Lange-Nielsen syndrome	Antiarrhythmic agents	Hypothyroidism
Autosomal recessive	Psychotropic agents	Liquid-protein-modified-fast diet
Romano-Ward syndrome	Phenothiazines	Bradyarrhythmias
Autosomal dominant	Tricyclic compounds	High-grade AV blocks
Sporadic form	Tetracyclic compounds	Sick sinus syndrome
	Miscellaneous	Central nervous system diseases
	Organophosphorous insecticides	Intracranial hemorrhage
	Prenylamine	Acute cerebral thrombosis
	Electrolyte imbalance	Structural heart disease
	Hypokalemia	Ischemic heart disease
	Hypomagnesemia	Mitral valve prolapse
	Hypocalcemia	

ganglionectomy or left stellate stimulation in the open-chest dog produced QT prolongation and T wave changes accompanied by heterogeneous changes in the ventricular refractory periods. Right ganglionectomy produced marked prolongation of the refractory period over the anterior surface, and left ganglionectomy produced the greatest prolongation over the posterior surface of the heart. The clinical significance of this finding for LQTS first became apparent in 1971 when Moss and McDonald demonstrated shortening of the QT interval with left stellate ganglion block in a patient with congenital LQTS.[34] This patient underwent left cervicothoracic sympathectomy and became symptom free. The hypothesis of sympathetic imbalance with relative dominance of left-sided adrenergic activity was first proposed in 1975 by Schwartz and Malliani as the basic defect of the syndrome.[35] In experimental animals, both anesthetized and unanesthetized, stimulation of the left stellate ganglion and/or ablation of the right stellate ganglion have been shown to produce: (1) prolongation of the QT interval,[35,36] (2) episodes of T wave alternans,[35] (3) increased incidence of ventricular arrhythmias during acute myocardial ischemia or intense psychological stress,[37] and (4) decreased threshold for ventricular fibrillation.[38] In some patients with congenital LQTS the effects of right stellate ganglion block or left stellate stimulation have been reported to be similar to those observed in animal preparations.[39] This hypothesis was further supported by an apparent success of left cervicothoracic sympathectomy in the suppression of symptoms in patients with this syndrome.[3,4,8,40] However, none of the above observations prove a direct cause-and-effect relationship between sympathetic imbalance and congenital LQTS. In fact, several patients have been reported in whom left cervicothoracic sympathectomy failed to provide sustained remission of symptoms.[41–43] Furthermore, sympathectomy almost never restores the abnormally prolonged QT interval to the normal range despite providing relief of symptoms in some patients.[43] It is possible that the basic defect may be at the myocardial level involving some complex electrophysiologic mechanisms (see below) as yet undefined, and the sudden surges in left-sided adrenergic activity merely provide the trigger for malignant ventricular arrhythmias.

ACQUIRED LQTS

Acquired LQTS is a heterogeneous syndrome related to diverse etiologies[44,45] (see Table 58.1). With few exceptions, torsade de pointes has been reported to occur in association with almost all known causes of QT prolongation. However, the precise relationship of QT prolongation with torsade de pointes still remains unclear for several reasons. First, torsade de pointes occurs in only a small minority of patients with QT prolongation, and no clinical or electrocardiographic variable is known that can identify all patients developing torsade de pointes from those who do not develop this arrhythmia. Second, in some clinical situations, for example, hypocalcemia or organophosphorous insecticide poisoning, torsade de pointes is very rare although the QT interval is markedly prolonged. Finally, prolongation of the QT interval is the predominant mechanism by which some antiarrhythmic drugs (amiodarone) exert their antiarrhythmic effect. What determines whether QT prolongation will provide antiarrhythmic effect in one patient and make another patient vulnerable to torsade de pointes remains enigmatic.

ANTIARRHYTHMIC DRUG-INDUCED LQTS

Antiarrhythmic drugs are the most common cause of torsade de pointes. All drugs that cause prolongation of the QT interval have also been associated with torsade de pointes (Table 58.2). Although quinidine was the drug mainly implicated in earlier reports,[46,47] procainamide and disopyramide[48–53] (Class Ia agents of Vaughan Williams classification[54]) cause this arrhythmia probably with equal frequency. Less commonly, torsade de pointes has been reported to occur with flecainide,[55] encainide and indecainide (Class Ic agents), and with amiodarone[56–58] and sotalol[59] (Class III agents). The occurrence of

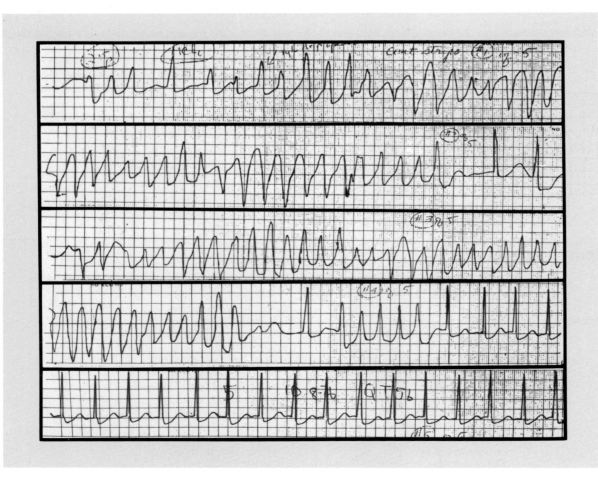

FIGURE 58.2 Typical episodes of torsade de pointes in a patient with sporadic form of the long QT syndrome. The rhythm strips are continuous and show spontaneous termination of torsade de pointes. Note the marked QT prolongation in the lowermost rhythm strip.

torsade de pointes has not been reported with drugs that shorten the QT interval such as mexiletine, tocainide, and lidocaine (Class Ib agents). Pure β-adrenergic blockers or calcium-channel antagonists do not cause torsade de pointes, but drugs with mixed effects (*i.e.*, sotalol[59] and bepridil[60]) may produce torsade. Torsade de pointes has also been reported to complicate therapy with prenylamine (coronary vasodilator).[61]

CLINICAL PRESENTATION AND DIAGNOSIS

In about one half of patients, drug-induced torsade de pointes occurs within the first 3 to 4 days of initiation of drug therapy.[6,44,45] However, others may develop this arrhythmia after many months or even years of therapy. The late onset of torsade de pointes has been associated with a change in drug dose, electrolyte imbalance, or onset of bradyarrhythmias. Typically, the onset of torsade de pointes is almost always preceded by the appearance of pauses. The pauses may be caused by sinus arrest, irregular ventricular rates during atrial fibrillation, sinus bradycardia, or high-grade AV blocks. More often, the pauses occur in association with new onset late-cycle premature ventricular complexes (PVCs) often in a bigeminal fashion. The PVCs are generally of the same morphology with a coupling interval ranging from 400 msec to 800 msec. The T wave of the beat terminating the pause (postpause T wave) frequently exhibits bizarre changes in its shape and amplitude. Preliminary data suggest that the degree of postpause T wave changes may bear a direct relationship with the duration of the preceding pause.[6] Torsade de pointes is generally initiated by a late-cycle PVC occurring on the summit of a markedly abnormal postpause T wave (Fig. 58.5).

In most patients, short repetitive runs of polymorphic ventricular tachycardia (VT) may occur along with episodes of classic torsade de pointes. The episodes may not always self-terminate and can deteriorate into ventricular fibrillation. The typical morphology of torsade de pointes may not always be evident in the monitored lead and, at times, even multiple electrocardiographic leads may not show the typical undulating pattern of QRS complexes. Therefore, an accurate early diagnosis of drug-induced torsade de pointes requires a high degree of clinical suspicion, and sole reliance should not be placed on the classical pattern of torsade de pointes.

Several warning signs of impending drug-induced torsade de pointes have been proposed. Keren and co-workers[62] suggested that prolongation of the uncorrected QT interval above 0.60 second may be an important warning sign for development of torsade de pointes. However, review of the literature indicates a very low sensitivity of this finding because the majority of reported cases of drug-induced torsade de pointes had had an uncorrected QT interval of less than 0.60 seconds. In fact, there is no known critical value of QT or QT_c that would distinguish patients developing torsade de pointes from those who receive such drugs without developing this arrhythmia. Other warning signs that have been proposed include a widening of the QRS complex of more than 25% and a new appearance of bradyarrhythmia[62]; both findings are relatively infrequent and of low specificity. More reliable warning signs of an impending drug-induced torsade de pointes may be the new appearance of a peculiar ventricular bigeminy with late-cycle PVCs and bizarre postpause T wave changes in association with a moderate QT prolongation.[6,50,63]

No definite information exists on how frequently torsade de pointes occurs during therapy with antiarrhythmic agents. In one prospective study, 6 of the 71 patients (8.4%) developed torsade de pointes or ventricular fibrillation within the first 4 days of starting quinidine.[64] The actual incidence is probably much lower (1% to 2%).[65] Torsade de pointes appears to be an idiosyncratic reaction to the antiarrhythmic agent. Serum levels of the drug are often in the therapeutic range or may be even subtherapeutic, and there is usually no other clinical evidence of drug toxicity.[44,45,63]

PSYCHOTROPIC DRUG-INDUCED LQTS

Phenothiazines and tricyclic antidepressant drugs have electrophysiologic properties similar to those of quinidine.[66] In therapeutic doses,

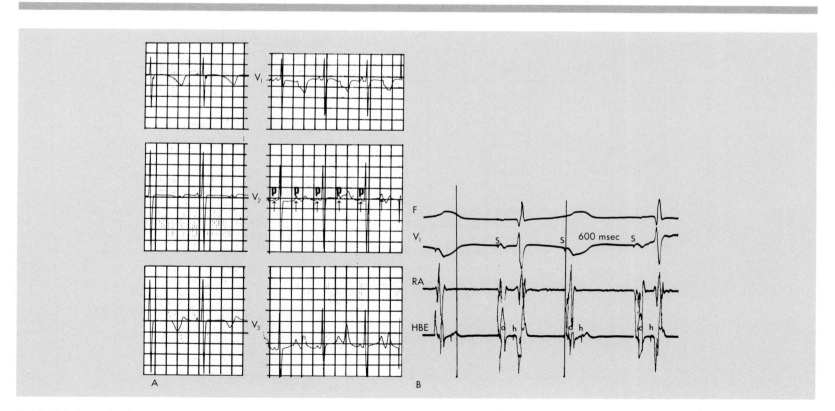

FIGURE 58.3 Example of exercise-induced 2:1 AV block in a 9-year-old boy with congenital LQTS. **A.** Simultaneous ECG leads V_1, V_2, and V_3 show sinus rhythm at a rate of 60 beats/min with marked prolongation of the QT interval (0.68 sec) with patient at rest (*left panel*). With exercise, atrial rate increases to 150 beats/min with 2:1 AV conduction (*right panel*). **B.** Right atrial pacing study in the same patient. Recordings show surface leads F and V_1 and bipolar intracardiac electrograms from the lower right atrium (*RA*) and the region of the His bundle (*HBE*). With atrial pacing at a cycle length of 600 msec (S-S interval) patient developed 2:1 AV block below the His bundle. The paper speed is 100 mm/sec. (*a*, atrial electrogram; *h*, His bundle potential; *v*, ventricular electrogram)

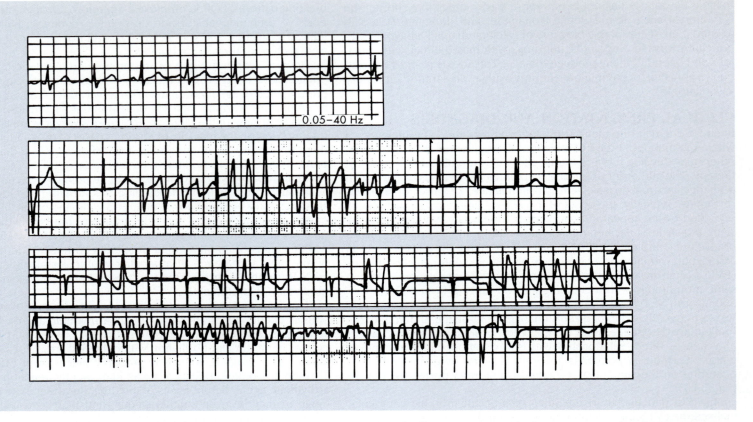

FIGURE 58.4 Spontaneous variability of the QT interval in a patient with congenital LQTS. In the top tracing, sinus rhythm is present at a rate of 78/min and QT interval is 400 msec. The three lower rhythm strips show spontaneous episodes of self-terminating torsade de pointes. Note that QT interval is markedly prolonged at 560 msec–600 msec prior to episodes of torsade de pointes.

TABLE 58.2 ANTIARRHYTHMIC DRUGS AND LQTS

Class*	Drugs	QT	Occurrence of Torsade de Pointes
1a	Quinidine Procainamide Disopyramide	↑↑	Common
1b	Lidocaine Tocainide Phenytoin Mexiletene	↓	Not reported
1c	Flecainide Encainide Indecainide	↑	Uncommon
2	β-Adrenergic antagonists	↔	Not reported†
3	Amiodarone	↑↑	Less common
4	Calcium channel antagonists	↔	Not reported‡

* Vaughan Williams Classification of antiarrhythmic agents[54]

† Except for sotalol

‡ Except for bepridil

(↑, Mild increase; ↓, mild decrease; ↑↑, modest increase; ↔, no effect)

phenothiazines increase the duration of the QRS complex, prolong the QT interval, and cause flattening of the T wave with prominence of the U wave. These electrocardiographic changes occur in approximately 50% of treated patients and are more marked with thioridazine than with chlorpromazine or trifluoperazine.[5,66] Tricyclic antidepressants produce similar changes in about 20% of treated patients.[67]

In toxic doses, both phenothiazines and tricyclic antidepressants frequently lead to increased ventricular irritability.[68] However, there are reports of fatal ventricular arrhythmias in patients receiving these drugs even in therapeutic doses.[69,70] Well-documented cases of torsade de pointes have been reported in association with almost all psychotropic drugs, but thioridazine (Mellaril) appears to be the major culprit.[66,69] Although no available prospective study has assessed the incidence of torsade de pointes in patients receiving psychotropic drugs, the risk appears to be relatively low. In the Boston Collaborative Drug Surveillance Program of 11,526 hospitalized patients, no significant increase in the frequency of sudden death or ventricular arrhythmias was noted in 260 patients who received psychotropic medications.[71]

ELECTROLYTE IMBALANCE AND LQTS

The electrocardiographic effects of hypokalemia include QT prolongation, T wave abnormalities, and prominent U waves. Hypokalemia, when severe, can cause torsade de pointes by itself.[72] More often hypokalemia precipitates torsade de pointes in association with other antiarrhythmic or psychotropic drugs.[50,63] Torsade de pointes has also been reported with hypomagnesemia alone or in combination with hypokalemia.[73] Although hypocalcemia is a known cause of QT prolongation, it has only rarely been associated with the development of torsade de pointes.[74]

METABOLIC ABNORMALITIES AND LQTS

Although QT prolongation is a frequent finding in hypothyroidism, the development of torsade de pointes in association with hypothyroidism has never been well documented. Malignant ventricular arrhythmias have been described in six patients with hypothyroidism and prolonged QT interval.[75,76] However, the morphology of the tachycardia was never documented to be of the torsade de pointes type, and in all cases additional contributing factors were present that might have contributed to the development of ventricular arrhythmias.

Torsade de pointes is a known but rare complication of liquid-protein-modified-fast dieting.[77,78] Prior to onset of ventricular arrhythmias, all reported patients had lost a massive amount of weight over a relatively short span of time. QT prolongation was present in all and was unrelated to any electrolyte abnormality or other recognizable cause of QT prolongation. In one series of 17 autopsies of patients who died suddenly during use of a liquid-protein diet,[78] histopathologic studies of the heart were unremarkable except for the nonspecific finding of an attenuation and pigmentation of the myocardial fibers.

BRADYARRHYTHMIA-INDUCED LQTS

For many years bradyarrhythmias have been known to be a cause of torsade de pointes. Ventricular tachyarrhythmias have been implicated as a cause of syncope in 10% to 60% of patients with high-grade AV block and syncope, and in 4% to 7% with sick sinus syndrome and syncope.[79,80] In some instances, the tachycardia has been documented to be torsade de pointes in morphology (Fig. 58.6).

CENTRAL NERVOUS SYSTEM DISEASES AND ACQUIRED LQTS

The typical electrocardiographic pattern associated with central nervous system diseases is characterized by deeply inverted or tall T waves, prolongation of the QT interval, and prominent U waves.[5] This pattern is seen most commonly in patients with subarachnoid hemorrhage, but may occur infrequently in patients with intracranial aneurysms, acute cerebral thrombosis, and brain metastases. The mechanism of QT prolongation is probably related to an altered central sympathetic discharge from the hypothalamus. Serious ventricular arrhythmias, as a rule, are uncommon and most reported cases have provided no information either on the morphology of the arrhythmia or the QT prolongation. Nevertheless, well-documented cases of torsade de pointes have been described, albeit rarely, in association with subarachnoid hemorrhages.[81–83]

ISCHEMIC HEART DISEASE AND QT PROLONGATION

QT_c prolongation has been observed in 30% to 40% of the survivors of acute myocardial infarction and has been claimed to be predictive of poor prognosis in such patients. Schwartz and Wolf[84] observed 55 postmyocardial infarction patients for 7 years and reported a significantly higher QT_c in 28 patients who died suddenly (443 ± 27 msec) than in 27 survivors (429 ± 20 msec). However, the diseased patients were often on antiarrhythmic drugs and had an increased duration of the QRS complexes as compared to the survivors, and it is unclear if

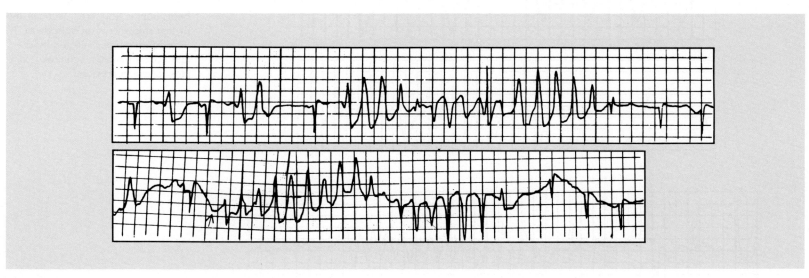

FIGURE 58.5 Procainamide-induced torsade de pointes. (*Top*) Rhythm strip shows late cycle premature ventricular complexes in bigeminal pattern and a nonsustained run of torsade de pointes. (*Bottom*) Arrow marks a large deformed postpause T wave associated with the emergence of another episode of torsade de pointes.

QT_c had any independent prognostic significance. Furthermore, an absolute prolongation of the QT_c interval (>440 msec) was seen in only a minority of the patients and the magnitude of prolongation was usually mild. Haynes and co-workers[85] reported a significantly higher QT_c in 125 survivors of out-of-hospital cardiac arrest with coronary artery disease as compared to 98 matched ambulatory postmyocardial infarction patients without ventricular arrhythmias (426 ± 4 msec versus 412 ± 3 msec). However, two other large studies by Ahnve and co-workers[86] and Vedin and co-workers[87] failed to find any predictive value of the QT_c prolongation for subsequent occurrence of ventricular arrhythmias. Therefore, QT_c prolongation in patients with ischemic heart disease appears to be of no independent prognostic significance, and there is no evidence to suggest that it plays any role in the genesis of ventricular arrhythmias in these patients.

Attention has been drawn to the occurrence of polymorphic ventricular tachycardia (often with characteristic morphology of torsade de pointes) in patients with coronary artery disease and normal or borderline prolonged QT_c interval.[88] The recognition of this arrhythmia is important because it often responds favorably to treatment with conventional type I antiarrhythmic agents. Torsade de pointes without QT prolongation has also been reported to occur, albeit rarely, in the setting of acute myocardial infarction and portends a very poor prognosis. In one reported study of 1771 consecutive patients with acute myocardial infarction, 22 (1.2%) developed torsade de pointes with no other predisposing factor and only a mildly prolonged QT_c interval.[89] These arrhythmias were resistant to treatment with bretylium, overdrive pacing, and direct current countershock, but some responded to intravenous verapamil. Six of the nine patients died during hospitalization (67% mortality) and the remaining three patients died within 6 months after discharge.

MITRAL VALVE PROLAPSE AND QT INTERVAL

QT_c prolongation has been reported to occur in 7% to 64% of patients with idiopathic mitral valve prolapse and has been associated with a higher prevalence of ventricular arrhythmias.[90] However, the QT_c is rarely if ever markedly prolonged, and the significance of this finding is unclear.[91]

TORSADE DE POINTES: ELECTROPHYSIOLOGIC MECHANISM

Controversy exists as to whether torsade de pointes is reentrant or automatic in origin. Reentry has been cited as the favored mechanism.[92-94] In his classic description of this arrhythmia in a patient with complete heart block, Dessertenne favored the theory of two competitive automatic ventricular foci that were discharging slightly out of phase, and alternately controlling the heart.[92] Bardy and co-workers studied the epicardial activation sequence during electrically induced episodes of torsade de pointes and demonstrated that each change in the QRS morphology was associated with a change in the site of epicardial breakthrough of the activation wavefront.[93] They could also produce a morphologic pattern of torsade de pointes by simultaneously pacing both ventricles at slightly different heart rates. Nhon and co-workers hypothesized that rapid ventricular tachycardia from a single focus could produce a pattern of torsade de pointes if the tachycardia wavefronts had varying exit sites in the myocardium.[94] For example, if the cycle length of the tachycardia was shorter than the refractory period of certain portions of the myocardium, this would produce successive wavefronts with different sites of epicardial breakthrough.

Controversy also exists relative to the importance of dispersion of ventricular refractoriness in the genesis of torsade de pointes. Gavrilescu and Luca studied three patients with LQTS (two cases acquired, one case congenital) and demonstrated that the right ventricular monophasic action potentials not only were prolonged, but also differed significantly in duration when recorded at different sites in the right ventricle.[95] Bonatti and co-workers also reported large differences in the duration of monophasic action potentials recorded from areas of the right ventricle in ten patients with LQTS (eight cases acquired, two cases congenital).[96] This dispersion of refractoriness has been shown to favor induction of reentrant ventricular arrhythmias.[97] However, programmed ventricular stimulation studies have been uniformly ineffective in inducing sustained ventricular tachycardia or ventricular fibrillation in patients with congenital LQTS.[27,97] In one study of 15 patients with this syndrome, sustained ventricular tachyarrhythmias were not induced in any of the patients.[27] Furthermore, no significant

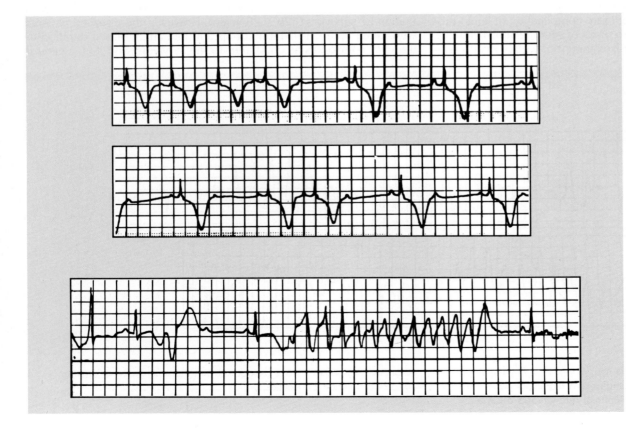

FIGURE 58.6 Torsade de pointes associated with high-grade AV block in a patient with repeated syncopal attacks. (Upper two panels) Mobitz II AV block and deep inverted T waves. QT interval in the first four sinus beats (top) is 460 msec. (Bottom) The rhythm strip shows an episode of torsade de pointes initiated by a late-cycle premature ventricular complex following a pause.

differences were found in the effective refractory periods measured at different sites in the ventricles. These findings make reentry an unlikely mechanism of torsade de pointes in the congenital form of the syndrome. Recently, attention has been drawn to the presence of a low-frequency, late-diastolic wave (following the T wave) on the intracavitary electrograms of some patients with congenital LQTS.[98,99] It has been hypothesized that this late-diastolic wave may represent an abnormally prominent delayed afterdepolarization which may be enhanced in size by catecholamines so as to achieve the threshold potential and initiate tachycardia (triggered activity). Afterdepolarization and triggered activity may also be the mechanism of torsade de pointes in patients with acquired LQTS. Brachmann and co-workers have pointed out the similarities in the ventricular arrhythmias produced by cesium chloride *in vivo* in dogs to the clinical syndrome of torsade de pointes induced by antiarrhythmic drugs: prolongation of the QT or QT-U interval, bizarre changes in T and U waves, and the undulating morphology of the polymorphic ventricular tachycardia and its bradycardia dependence.[100] They also demonstrated that *in vitro* superfusion of the isolated Purkinje fibers with cesium led to prolongation of repolarization and induction of early afterdepolarizations that generated triggered firing, especially at slower heart rates.[100] This interesting hypothesis needs further clinical investigation.

THERAPY
CONGENITAL LQTS

Since the symptoms of LQTS occur in the setting of excess sympathetic activity, the therapy is directed toward blunting of sympathetic activity.[1–8] β-Adrenergic antagonists are the primary mode of therapy and in full doses completely suppress or significantly reduce the frequency of symptoms, although the QT interval remains unaffected. In one large retrospective analysis, the mortality in 133 patients treated with β-adrenergic antagonists was 6% as compared to 78% in 107 untreated patients.[4] Although the largest experience has been with propranolol, other β-adrenergic antagonists (in equivalent doses) are likely to be equally effective. In patients who report only partial relief of symptoms on full-dose β blockers, addition of phenytoin and/or phenobarbital is thought to decrease the frequency of the symptoms. Therapy with digoxin or atropine is of no proven benefit and should not be used.

Left cervicothoracic sympathectomy has been recommended for patients who have symptoms refractory to β-adrenergic antagonists or who develop disabling side effects to them.[3,4,7,9,40] Surgery is performed extrapleurally by a supraclavicular or transaxillary approach and includes resection of the lower half of the left stellate ganglion and the first three to five left thoracic sympathetic ganglia. The upper half of the left stellate ganglion need not be removed as it provides no sympathetic innervation to the heart, and its removal leads to an unnecessary and cosmetically disfiguring complication of Horner's syndrome. The surgery is technically simple and has no significant complications. Although the initial results with sympathectomy were described as very encouraging, patients have been reported who had had recurrent syncope or cardiac arrest after a brief initial symptom-free interval.[41–43] In our experience of ten patients with LQTS who underwent sympathectomy, three developed cardiac arrest and five had recurrence of presyncope or syncope over a mean follow-up of 3 years.[43] The recurrent symptoms in these patients did not always respond to the addition of β-adrenergic antagonists. For such patients, chronic overdrive cardiac pacing with or without β-adrenergic antagonists appears to be promising. Cardiac pacing (atrial or ventricular) is also useful in patients who develop significant bradyarrhythmias on β-adrenergic antagonists.[42,43] For patients with severe manifestations of the syndrome (*e.g.*, recurrent cardiac arrest) or symptoms refractory to all of the above modalities, implantation of an automatic implantable cardioverter defibrillator (AICD) should be strongly considered.

The importance of therapy in symptomatic patients with congenital LQTS cannot be too strongly emphasized. Patients with congenital deafness, syncope, and family history of sudden death are in a very high-risk subgroup and treatment is mandatory. Drugs that prolong the QT interval are absolutely contraindicated in patients with congenital LQTS. However, the natural history of asymptomatic patients is unknown and the issue of prophylactic therapy is not clear. Although there is a general consensus not to treat them, therapy is probably indicated for a subgroup of asymptomatic patients who have marked QT prolongation and a family history of sudden death and/or congenital deafness. Another problem lies in our inability to evaluate reliably the efficacy of a given treatment modality. The symptoms, being sporadic in nature, are unreliable end-points for therapy. The QT prolongation shows a marked variability from day to day, and therefore the degree of QT shortening is a poor guide to successful therapy. Furthermore, the protective effects of β blockers or left cervicothoracic sympathectomy bear no relationship to the extent of QT shortening. Prolonged ambulatory monitoring often fails to reveal significant ventricular arrhythmias. Programmed ventricular stimulation almost never induces sustained VT or ventricular fibrillation in these patients. In one study of programmed ventricular stimulation in 15 symptomatic patients with congenital LQTS, only nonsustained polymorphic VT was induced in six patients (40%); neither the inducibility of tachycardia nor the results of electropharmacologic therapy with the β blockers proved to be of any prognostic value during the mean follow-up of 28 ± 17 months.[27]

ACQUIRED LQTS

The most important aspect of therapy is early identification of torsade de pointes and correction of its etiologic factor(s).[6,44,45,63] Failure of diagnosis leads not only to the continual use of the offending agent, but also to the use of antiarrhythmic agents that may prolong the QT interval. Both may lead to more frequent episodes of torsade de pointes resulting in fatal arrhythmias.

Immediate therapy should be instituted in all patients once the diagnosis of torsade de pointes is made and etiologic factors are identified. This includes withdrawal of the offending agent(s) and correction of any electrolyte abnormality. Electrical defibrillation is acutely successful in terminating sustained episodes of torsade de pointes, but subsequent recurrences can be prevented only by accelerating heart rate with isoproterenol infusion or temporary cardiac pacing. The beneficial effects of acceleration of the heart rate have been attributed to a rate-dependent shortening of the QT interval leading to decreased temporal dispersion of the ventricular refractoriness. Isoproterenol infusion (1 μcg to 4 μcg/minute) can be instituted rapidly and is effective within a few minutes. However, isoproterenol is not uniformly effective and carries some risks in patients with acute myocardial infarction, angina pectoris, or uncontrolled systemic hypertension.[6,44,50] Therefore, temporary cardiac pacing is the preferred mode of therapy, since it proves successful in rapidly abolishing torsade de pointes.[44,45] Pacing can also be safely instituted in all patients including those in whom isoproterenol is contraindicated. In the absence of AV block, atrial pacing may be advantageous since it maintains AV synchrony as well as a normal depolarization sequence of the ventricles. Others have preferred ventricular pacing since consistent atrial pacing may be less reliable; however, insertion of the ventricular electrode may cause PVCs that can initiate episodes of torsade de pointes.

Other drugs that have been used in the acute treatment of torsade de pointes have included lidocaine,[44,59,63] atropine,[6] phenytoin,[44] magnesium sulfate,[101] and bretylium tosylate.[102] Lidocaine infusion is inconsistently effective, but rarely if ever results in arrhythmia aggravation. Atropine has been reported to be effective in some patients when it raised the heart rate; however, the available experience is limited. Preliminary data suggest that magnesium sulfate (1 g to 2 g intravenously administered) may be effective in suppressing torsade de pointes even in normomagnesemic patients.[101] There are reports of occasional efficacy of bretylium tosylate in abolishing drug-induced torsade de pointes.[102]

After torsade de pointes has subsided, the need for continuing antiarrhythmic treatment should be reassessed. The risk of redevelopment of torsade de pointes is very high when these patients are retreated with the same or related antiarrhythmic/psychotropic agents.[103,104] In patients requiring antiarrhythmic therapy, drugs that shorten the QT interval (tocainamide, mexiletene, or phenytoin) may be safer to use. There are some recent preliminary data to suggest that amiodarone may be successfully used on a long-term basis in some of these patients.[104]

CLINICAL OVERVIEW

It should be emphasized that rapid ventricular arrhythmias showing near beat-to-beat variation in QRS morphology (so-called polymorphous ventricular tachycardia) may be drug-induced arrhythmias and their treatment identical to that outlined for torsade. In our experience,[104] failure to recognize this association often leads to delay in appropriate therapy or administration of inappropriate drugs. It is impossible to distinguish pathologic QT prolongation subjecting the patient to the risk of torsade de pointes from benign prolongation of the QT interval owing to drug effect. The decision to treat is made independently of the degree of QT prolongation. In addition, it should be remembered that short-term drug safety presents no guarantee of long-term protection against development of torsade de pointes. For example, patients successfully treated with type I antiarrhythmic agents should be carefully monitored when agents or conditions causing hypokalemia or bradycardia are instituted. Available data strongly suggest that patients with transient neurologic symptoms associated with the congenital LQTS should be treated with adequate β blockade. More aggressive therapy (as outlined) is required for those who remain symptomatic in spite of β-blocker therapy.

REFERENCES

1. Vincent GM, Abildskov JA, Burges MJ: QT interval syndromes. Prog Cardiovasc Dis 16:523, 1974
2. Schwartz PJ, Periti M, Malliani A: The long QT syndrome. Am Heart J 89:378, 1975
3. Moss AJ, Schwartz PJ: Sudden death and the idiopathic long QT syndrome. Am J Med 66:6, 1979
4. Schwartz PJ: The long QT syndrome. In Kulbertus HE, Wellens HJJ (eds): Sudden Death, p. 358. The Hague, M. Nijhoff, 1980
5. Surawicz B, Knoebel SB: Long QT: Good, bad or indifferent? J Am Coll Cardiol 4:398, 1984
6. Jackman WM, Clark M, Friday KJ et al: Ventricular tachyarrhythmias in the long QT syndromes. Med Clin NA 68:1079, 1984
7. Moss AJ, Schwartz PJ: Delayed repolarization (QT or QTU prolongation) and malignant ventricular arrhythmias. Mod Concept Cardiovasc Dis 51:85, 1982
8. Schwartz PJ: Idiopathic long QT syndrome: Progress and questions. Am Heart J 109:399, 1985
9. Simonson E, Cady LD, Woodbury M: The normal QT interval. Am Heart J 63:747, 1962
10. Milne JR, Ward DE, Spurell RAJ et al: The ventricular paced QT interval—the effects of rate and exercise. Pace 5:352, 1982
11. Akhras F, Rickards A: The relationship between QT interval and heart rate during physiologic exercise and pacing. Jpn Heart J 22:345, 1980
12. Ahnve S, Vallin H: Influence of heart rate and inhibition of autonomic tone on the QT interval. Circulation 65:435, 1982
13. Browne K, Prystowsky E, Heger J et al: Modulation of the QT interval by autonomic nervous system. PACE 6:1050, 1983
14. Jervell A, Lange-Nielsen F: Congenital deaf-mutism, functional heart disease with prolongation of the QT interval and sudden death. Am Heart J 54:59, 1957
15. Romano C, Gemme G, Pongiglione R: Aritme cardiache rare dell'eta pediatrica. Clin Pediatr (Bologna) 45:656, 1963
16. Ward OC: New familial cardiac syndrome in children. J Irish Med Assoc 54:103, 1964
17. Fraser GR, Frogatt P, James TN: Congenital deafness associated with electrocardiographic abnormalities. Q J Med 33:361, 1964
18. Garza LA, Vick RL, Nora J et al: Heritable QT prolongation without deafness. Circulation 41:39, 1970
19. Ratshin R, Hunt D, Russell R et al: QT interval prolongation, paroxysmal ventricular arrhythmias and convulsive syncope. Ann Int Med 75:919, 1971
20. Roy P, Emanuel R, Ismail S et al: Hereditary prolongation of the QT interval. Genetic observations and management in three families with twelve affected members. Am J Cardiol 37:237, 1976
21. Chaudron JM, Heller F, Vanden Berghe HB et al: Attacks of ventricular fibrillation and unconsciousness in a patient with prolonged QT interval. A family study. Am Heart J 91:783, 1976
22. Itoh S, Munemura S, Satoh H: A study of the inheritance pattern of Romano-Ward syndrome. Clin Pediatr 21:20, 1982
23. Mathews EC, Blount AN, Townsend JI: QT prolongation and ventricular arrhythmias with and without deafness in the same family. Am J Cardiol 29:702, 1972
24. Moss AJ, Schwartz PJ, Crampton RS et al: The long QT syndrome: A prospective international study. Circulation 71:17, 1985
25. Southall DP, Oakley JR, Anderson RH et al: Prolonged QT and cardiac arrhythmias in two neonates: Sudden infant death syndrome in one case. Arch Dis Child 54:776, 1979
26. Ramon JR, Espinosa AG, Reverte F et al: QT alargado, conduccion A-V 2:1 y crisis syncopales. Rev Esp Cardiol 25:557, 1973
27. Bhandari AK, Shapiro WA, Morady F et al: Electrophysiologic testing in patients with the long QT syndrome. Circulation 71:63, 1985
28. Ruben SA, Brundage B, Mayer W et al: Usefulness of Valsalva maneuver and cold pressor test for evaluation of arrhythmias in long QT syndrome. Br Heart J 42:490, 1979
29. Mitsutake A, Takeshita A, Kuroiwa A et al: Usefulness of the Valsalva maneuver in management of the long QT syndrome. Circulation 63:1029, 1981
30. Curtiss E, Heibel R, Shaver J: Autonomic maneuvers in hereditary QT interval prolongation. Am Heart J 95:420, 1978
31. James TN, Frogatt P, Alkinson WJ Jr et al: De subitaneis mortibus: Observations on the pathophysiology of the long QT syndrome with special reference to the neuropathology of the heart. Circulation 57:1221, 1978
32. Djonlagic H, Bos I, Diederich HW: Grenzstrang-Ganglionitis bei erblichem syndrom der QT-verlängerung (Romano-Ward syndrom). Dtsch Med Wochenschr 107:655, 1982
33. Yanowitz R, Preston JB, Abildskov JA: Functional distribution of right and left stellate innervation to the ventricles: Production of neurogenic electrocardiographic changes by unilateral alternation of sympathetic tone. Circ Res 18:416, 1966
34. Moss AJ, McDonald J: Unilateral cervicothoracic sympathetic ganglionectomy for the treatment of long QT interval syndrome. N Engl J Med 285:903, 1970
35. Schwartz PJ, Malliani A: Electrical alternation of the T-wave: Clinical and experimental evidence of its relationship with the sympathetic nervous system and with the long QT syndrome. Am Heart J 89:45, 1975
36. Schwartz PJ: Experimental reproduction of the long QT syndrome. Am J Cardiol 41:374, 1978
37. Schwartz PJ, Stone HL, Brown AM: Effects of unilateral stellate ganglion blockade on the arrhythmias associated with coronary occlusion. Am Heart J 89:45, 1975
38. Schwartz PJ, Smebold HG, Brown AM: Effects of unilateral cardiac sympathetic denervation on the ventricular fibrillation threshold. Am J Cardiol 37:1034, 1976
39. Crampton RS: Preeminence of left stellate ganglion in the long QT syndrome. Circulation 59:769, 1979
40. Coyer BH, Pryor R, Kirsh WM et al: Left stellectomy in the long QT syndrome. Chest 74:584, 1978
41. Baudouy PH, Andreassian B, Attuel P et al: Syndrome de Romano-Ward et stellectomie gauche: Revue générale á propos d'un nouveau cas. Arch Mal Coeur 70:645, 1977
42. Chaudron J, Lebacq E: Romano-Ward syndrome treated by left stellectomy and intracavitary stimulation. Am Heart J 100:131, 1980
43. Bhandari AK, Scheinman M, Morady F et al: Efficacy of left cardiac sympathectomy in the treatment of patients with the long QT syndrome. Circulation 70:1018, 1984
44. Smith WM, Gallagher JJ: "Les torsades de pointes": An unusual ventricular arrhythmia. Ann Int Med 93:578, 1980
45. Fontaine G, Frank R, Grosgogeat Y: Torsade de pointes: Definition and management. Mod Concepts Cardiovasc Dis 51:103, 1982
46. Selzer A, Wray HW: Quinidine syncope. Paroxysmal ventricular fibrillation occurring during treatment of chronic atrial arrhythmias. Circulation 30:17, 1964
47. Oravetz J, Sloaki SJ: Recurrent ventricular fibrillation precipitated by quinidine. Arch Int Med 122:63, 1968
48. Strasberg B, Sclarovsky S, Erdberg A et al: Procainamide-induced polymorphous ventricular tachycardia. Am J Cardiol 47:1309, 1981
49. Olshansky B, Martins J, Hunt S: N-acetyl-procainamide causing torsade de pointes. Am J Cardiol 50:1439, 1982
50. Kay GN, Plumb VJ, Arciniegas JG et al: Torsade de pointes: The long short initiating sequence and other clinical features. J Am Coll Cardiol 2:806, 1983
51. Nicholson WJ, Martin LE, Gracey J et al: Disopyramide-induced ventricular fibrillation. Am J Cardiol 43:1053, 1979
52. Wald RW, Waxman M, Coman J: Torsade de pointes ventricular tachycardia: A complication of disopyramide shared with quinidine. J Electrocardiol 14:301, 1981
53. Tzivoni D, Keren A, Stern S et al: Disopyramide-induced torsade de pointes.

Arch Int Med 141:946, 1981
54. Vaughan Williams E: A classification of antiarrhythmic actions reassessed after a decade of new drugs. J Clin Pharmacol 24:129, 1984
55. Lui H, Lee G, Dietrich P et al: Flecainide induced QT prolongation and ventricular tachycardia. Am Heart J 103:567, 1982
56. Keren A, Tzivoni D, Gottlieb S et al: Atypical ventricular tachycardia (torsade de pointes) induced by amiodarone: Arrhythmia previously induced by quinidine and disopyramide. Chest 81:384, 1982
57. Sclarovsky S, Lewin RB, Kracoff O et al: Amiodarone-induced polymorphous ventricular tachycardia. Am Heart J 105:6, 1983
58. Bhandari AK, Quock C, Sung RJ: Polymorphous ventricular tachycardia associated with a marked prolongation of the QT interval induced by amiodarone. PACE 7:341, 1984
59. Neuvoven PJ, Elonen E, Vuorenmaa J et al: Prolonged QT interval and severe tachyarrhythmias. Common features of sotalol intoxication. Eur J Clin Pharmacol 20:85, 1981
60. Leclercq J, Kural S, Valere P: Bepridil el-torsades de point. Arch Mal Coeur 76:341, 1983
61. Abinader E, Shahar J: Possible female preponderance in prenylamine induced torsade de pointes tachycardia. Cardiology 70:37, 1983
62. Keren A, Tzivani D, Gavish D et al: Etiology, warning signs and therapy of torsade de pointes. A study of 10 patients. Circulation 64:1167, 1981
63. Sclarovsky S, Strasberg B, Lewin R et al: Polymorphous ventricular tachycardia: Clinical features and treatment. Am J Cardiol 44:339, 1979
64. Ejvinsson G, Prinius E: Prodromal ventricular premature beats preceded by a diastolic wave. Acta Med Scand 208:445, 1980
65. Roden D, Woosley R, Bostick D et al: Quinidine induced long QT syndrome: Incidence and presenting features (abstr). Circulation 68(suppl III):276, 1983
66. Fowler N, McCall D, Chou T et al: Electrocardiographic changes and cardiac arrhythmias in patients receiving psychotropic drugs. Am J Cardiol 37:223, 1976
67. Giardina E, Bigger J, Glassman A et al: The electrocardiographic and antiarrhythmic effects of imipramine hydrochloride at therapeutic plasma concentrations. Circulation 60:1045, 1979
68. Fasoli R, Glauser F: Cardiac arrhythmias and ECG abnormalities in tricyclic antidepressant overdose. Clin Toxicol 18:155, 1981
69. Kemper A, Dunlap R, Pietro D: Thioridazine-induced torsade de pointes: Successful therapy with isoproterenol. JAMA 249:2931, 1983
70. Herrmann H, Kaplan L, Bierer B: QT prolongation and torsade de pointes ventricular tachycardia produced by the tetracyclic antidepressant agent Maprotiline. Am J Cardiol 51:904, 1983
71. Collaborative Drug Surveillance Program: Report from Boston: Adverse reaction to the tricyclic-antidepressant drugs. Lancet 1:529, 1971
72. Tamura K, Tamura T, Yoshida S et al: Transient recurrent fibrillation due to hypopotassemia with special note on the U wave. Jap Heart J 8:652, 1967
73. Topol E, Lerman B: Hypomagnesemic torsade de pointes. Am J Cardiol 52:1367, 1983
74. Giustiniani S, Roustelli D, Sardeo C et al: Torsade de pointes induced by hypocalcemia. G Ital Cardiol 12:889, 1982
75. Fredlung B, Olsson S: Long QT interval and ventricular tachycardia of "torsade de pointe" type in hypothyroidism. Acta Med Scand 213:231, 1983
76. Hansen JE: Paroxysmal ventricular tachycardia associated with myxedema. A case report. Am Heart J 61:692, 1961
77. Singh B, Gaarder T, Kanegae T et al: Liquid protein diets and torsade de pointes. JAMA 240:115, 1978
78. Isner J, Sours H, Paris A et al: Sudden unexpected death in avid dieters using the liquid-protein-modified-fast diet. Observations in 17 patients and the role of the prolonged QT interval. Circulation 60:1401, 1979
79. Jensen G, Sigurd B, Sandoe E: Adams-Stokes seizures due to ventricular tachyarrhythmias in patients with heart block: Prevalence and problems of management. Chest 67:43, 1975
80. Gascho JA, Schierken R: Congenital complete heart block and long QT syndrome requiring ventricular pacing for control of refractory ventricular tachycardia and fibrillation. J Electrocardiol 12:331, 1979
81. Carruth JE, Silverman ME: Torsade de pointe: Atypical ventricular tachycardia complicating subarachnoid hemorrhage. Chest 78:886, 1980
82. Hust M, Nitsche K, Holnloser S et al: QT prolongation and torsade de pointes in a patient with subarachnoid hemorrhage. Clin Cardiol 7:44, 1984
83. Ranquin R, Parziel G: Ventricular fibrilloflutter (torsade de pointes): An established electrocardiographic and clinical entity—report of 8 cases. Angiology 28:115, 1977
84. Schwartz PJ, Wolf S: QT interval prolongation as predictor of sudden death in patients with myocardial infarction. Circulation 57:1074, 1978
85. Haynes RE, Hallstrom AP, Cobb LA: Repolarization abnormalities in survivors of out-of-hospital ventricular fibrillation. Circulation 57:654, 1978
86. Ahnve S, Helmers C, Lundman T: QTc intervals at discharge after acute myocardial infarction and long term prognosis. Acta Med Scand 208:55, 1980
87. Vedin A, Wilhelmsen L, Wedel H et al: Predictor of cardiovascular deaths and nonfatal reinfarctions after myocardial infarction. Acta Med Scand 201:309, 1977
88. Horowitz L, Greenspan A, Spielman S et al: Torsade de pointes: Electrophysiologic studies in patients without transient pharmacologic or metabolic abnormalities. Circulation 63:1120, 1981
89. Newsletter Communication: Torsade points to poor prognosis. Cardiology Observer 1(6):1, 1984
90. Bekheit SG, Ali A, Deglin A: Analysis of QT interval in patients with idiopathic mitral valve prolapse. Chest 61:820, 1982
91. Savage D, Devereux R, Garison RJ et al: Mitral valve prolapse in the general population. 2. Clinical features: The Framingham Study. Am Heart J 106:577, 1983
92. Dessertenne F: La tachycardie ventriculaire a deux foyers opposes variables. Arch Mal Coeur 59:263, 1966
93. Bardy G, Ungerleider R, Smith et al: A mechanism of torsade de pointes in a canine model. Circulation 67:52, 1983
94. Nhon N, Hope RR, Kabell G: Torsade de pointes: Electrophysiology of atypical ventricular tachycardia. Am J Cardiol 45:494, 1980
95. Gavrilescu W, Luca S: Right ventricular monophasic action potential in patients with long QT syndrome. Br Heart J 40:1014, 1978
96. Bonatti V, Rolli A, Botti G: Recording of monophasic action potentials of the right ventricle in long QT syndromes complicated by severe ventricular arrhythmias. Eur Heart J 4:168, 1983
97. Kuo C, Munakata K, Reddy C et al: Characteristics and possible mechanisms of ventricular arrhythmia dependent on the dispersion of action potential durations. Circulation 67:1356, 1983
98. Hartzler GO, Osborn MJ: Invasive electrophysiologic study in the Jervell and Lange-Nielsen syndrome. Br Heart J 45:225, 1981
99. Schechter E, Freeman C, Lazzara R: After-depolarizations as a mechanism for the long QT syndrome: Electrophysiologic studies of a case. J Am Coll Cardiol 3:1556, 1984
100. Brachmann J, Scherlag B, Rosenshtraukh L et al: Bradycardia-dependent triggered activity: Relevance to drug-induced multiform ventricular tachycardia. Circulation 68:846, 1983
101. Tzivani D, Keren A, Cohen A et al: Magnesium therapy for torsade de pointes. Am J Cardiol 53:528, 1984
102. Vander Ark C, Reynolds E, Kahn D: Quinidine syncope: A report of successful treatment with bretylium tosylate. J Thorac Cardiovasc Surg 72:464, 1976
103. Clark M, Friday K, Anderson J et al: Drug induced torsade de pointes: High concordance rate among antiarrhythmic drugs and amiodarone (abstr). J Am Coll Cardiol 5:450, 1985
104. Nguyen PT, Scheinman M, Seger J: Polymorphous ventricular tachycardia: Clinical characterization, therapy and the QT interval. Circulation 74:340, 1986